SURGERY OF THE FOOT AND ANKLE

SURGERY OF THE FOOT AND ANKLE

EIGHTH EDITION

VOLUME I

Michael J. Coughlin, MD
Private Practice of Orthopaedic Surgery
St. Alphonsus Regional Medical Center
Director, Idaho Foot and Ankle Fellowship
Boise, Idaho
Clinical Professor, Department of Orthopaedic Surgery and Rehabilitation
Oregon Health Sciences University
Portland, Oregon
Past President, American Orthopaedic Foot and Ankle Society

Roger A. Mann, MD
Private Practice of Orthopaedic Surgery
Director of Foot Fellowship Program
Oakland, California
Associate Clinical Professor
Department of Orthopaedic Surgery
University of California at San Francisco School of Medicine
San Francisco, California
Past President, American Orthopaedic Foot and Ankle Society

Charles L. Saltzman, MD
Professor and Chair
Department of Orthopaedics
University of Utah School of Medicine
Salt Lake City, Utah

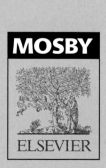

MOSBY

ELSEVIER

1600 John F. Kennedy Blvd.
Ste 1800
Philadelphia, PA 19103-2899

SURGERY OF THE FOOT AND ANKLE

ISBN-13: 978-0-323-03305-3
ISBN-10: 0-323-03305-9

Previous editions copyrighted 1999, 1993, 1986, 1978.

Library of Congress Cataloging-in-Publication Data
Surgery of the foot and ankle.—8th ed. / editors, Michael J. Coughlin, Roger A. Mann, Charles Saltzman.
   p. ; cm.
   Includes bibliographical references and index.
   ISBN-13: 978-0-323-03305-3   ISBN-10: 0-323-03305-9
   1. Foot—Surgery. 2. Ankle—Surgery. I. Coughlin, Michael J. II. Mann, Roger A., 1936–
III. Saltzman, Charles, MD.
   [DNLM: 1. Ankle—surgery. 2. Foot—surgery. 3. Foot Diseases—surgery. WE 880 S9602 2007]
RD563.S87 2007
617.5'85059—dc22   2006044407

Publishing Director: Kim Murphy
Developmental Editor: Pamela Hetherington
Publishing Services Manager: Linda Van Pelt
Design Direction: Ellen Zanolle
Cover Direction: Ellen Zanolle

ISBN-13: 978-0-323-03305-3
ISBN-10: 0-323-03305-9
Printed in China

Last digit is the print number: 9 8 7 6 5 4 3 2

Contributors

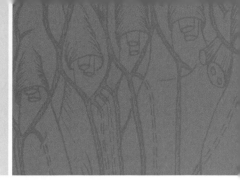

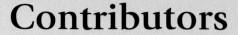

Robert B. Anderson, MD
Chief, Foot and Ankle Service
Assistant Chief
Department of Orthopedic Surgery
Carolinas Medical Center
Co-Director, Foot and Ankle Fellowship
OrthoCarolina
Charlotte, North Carolina

David P. Barei, MD, FRCS
Assistant Professor
Harborview Medical Center
University of Washington
Seattle, Washington

Philip A. Bauman, MD
Assistant Clinical Professor of Orthopaedic Surgery
Columbia University College of Physicians and
  Surgeons
Senior Attending of Orthopaedic Surgery
St. Luke's-Roosevelt Hospital Center
New York, New York

Douglas N. Beaman, MD
Portland Orthopaedic Specialists
Portland, Oregon

James H. Beaty, MD
Professor of Orthopaedics
Department of Orthopaedic Surgery
University of Tennessee
Chief of Staff
Campbell Clinic
Memphis, Tennessee

Carlo Bellabarba, MD
Associate Professor
Orthopaedics and Sports Medicine
Harborview Medical Center
University of Washington Medical Center
Seattle, Washington

Gary Berke, MS, CP
Adjunct Clinical Instructor
Department of Orthopaedic Surgery
Stanford University
Palo Alto, California

James W. Brodsky, MD
Clinical Professor
Department of Orthopedic Surgery
University of Texas Southwestern Medical School
Fellowship Director
Fellowship in Surgery of the Foot and Ankle
Baylor University Medical Center
University of Texas Southwestern Medical School
Chief, Foot and Ankle Surgery
Department of Orthopaedic Surgery
Dallas Veterans Administration Medical Center
Dallas, Texas

Thomas O. Clanton, MD
Professor and Chairman
Department of Orthopaedic Surgery
The University of Texas Medical Center at Houston
Houston, Texas
Team Physician, Rice University
Lead Team Physician, Houston Rockets
Team Orthopaedist, Houston Texans

Michael P. Clare, MD
Attending Physician
Foot and Ankle Fellowship
Florida Orthopaedic Institute
Tampa, Florida

Bruce E. Cohen, MD
Fellowship Director
Foot and Ankle Fellowship
OL Miller Foot and Ankle Institute
OrthoCarolina
Clinical Faculty
Carolinas Medical Center
Charlotte, North Carolina

Michael J. Coughlin, MD

Private Practice of Orthopaedic Surgery
St. Alphonsus Medical Center
Boise, Idaho
Clinical Professor
Department of Orthopaedics and Rehabilitation
Oregon Health Sciences University
Portland, Oregon

W. Hodges Davis, MD

Medical Director
OL Miller Foot and Ankle Institute
OrthoCarolina
Clinical Faculty
Carolinas Medical Center
Charlotte, North Carolina
Clinical Professor
Department of Orthopaedics
Tulane University
New Orleans, Louisiana

Robert Dehne, MD

Central Texas Pediatric Orthopedics
Austin, Texas

James K. DeOrio, MD

Associate Professor
Mayo Clinic College of Medicine
Rochester, Minnesota
Director of Foot and Ankle Fellowship Program
Department of Orthopedic Surgery
Mayo Clinic Jacksonville
Jacksonville, Florida

Richard D. Ferkel, MD

Associate Clinical Professor
UCLA School of Medicine
Los Angeles, California
Attending Surgeon and Director of Sports Medicine
    Fellowship Program
Southern California Orthopedic Institute
Van Nuys, California

Richard E. Gellman, MD

Portland Orthopaedic Specialists
Portland, Oregon

Brett R. Grebing, MD

Assistant Professor
Foot and Ankle Service
Department of Orthopaedic Surgery
Washington University
St. Louis, Missouri

J. Speight Grimes, MD

Assistant Professor
Texas Tech University Health Sciences Center
Lubbock, Texas

Gregory P. Guyton, MD

Attending Physician
Orthopaedics
Union Memorial Hospital
Baltimore, Maryland

Steven L. Haddad, MD

Associate Professor of Clinical Orthopaedic Surgery
Northwestern University School of Medicine
Chicago, Illinois
Section Head
Foot and Ankle Surgery
Evanston Northwestern Healthcare
Evanston, Illinois

William G. Hamilton, MD, BSE

St. Luke's-Roosevelt Hospital
The Hospital for Special Surgery
New York, New York
The Keller Army Hospital
West Point, New York
Clinical Professor of Orthopaedic Surgery
The College of Physicians and Surgeons
Columbia University
New York, New York

Andrew Haskell, MD

Assistant Clinical Professor
University of California, San Francisco
San Francisco, California

Jan Pieter Hommen, MD

Director of Sports Medicine
Orthopaedic Institute at Mercy Hospital
Miami, Florida

Greg A. Horton, MD

Associate Professor
Department of Orthopaedic Surgery
Kansas University Medical Center
Kansas City, Kansas

Carroll P. Jones, MD

Clinical Faculty
Carolinas Medical Center
OL Miller Foot and Ankle Institute
OrthoCarolina
Charlotte, North Carolina

Douglas W. Kress, MD

Clinical Associate Professor
Department of Dermatology
University of Pittsburgh
Pittsburgh, Pennsylvania

Thomas H. Lee, MD

Ohio Foot and Ankle Center
Grant Medical Center
Columbus, Ohio

L. Scott Levin, MD, FACS

Division Chief
Plastic and Reconstructive Surgery
Duke University Medical Center
Professor
Orthopaedic and Plastic Surgery
Duke University School of Medicine
Durham, North Carolina

Eric Lindvall, MD

Private Practice
Fresno, California

Jeffrey A. Mann, MD

Private Practice
Oakland, California

Roger A. Mann, MD

Private Practice of Orthopaedic Surgery
Director of Foot Fellowship Program
Oakland, California
Associate Clinical Professor
Department of Orthopaedic Surgery
University of California at San Francisco School of
    Medicine
San Francisco, California

Peter B. Maurus, MD

Foot and Ankle Surgeon
Steindler Orthopedic Clinic
Mercy Hospital
Iowa City, Iowa

William M. McGarvey, MD

Associate Professor
Department of Orthopaedic Surgery
University of Texas Health Science Center at Houston
    Medical School
Houston, Texas

James A. Nunley, MD

J. Leonard Goldner Professor of Orthopaedics
Chief, Division of Orthopaedic Surgery
Duke University Medical Center
Durham, North Carolina

Steven Papp, MD, FRCSC, MSc

Assistant Professor
University of Ottawa
Ottawa, Ontario, Canada

David I. Pedowitz, MD, MS

Chief Resident
Department of Orthopedic Surgery
University of Pennsylvania Hospital
Philadelphia, Pennsylvania

Walter J. Pedowitz, MD

Clinical Professor of Orthopedic Surgery
Department of Orthopedic Surgery
Columbia University
New York, New York
Union County Orthopedic Group
Linden, New Jersey

Charles L. Saltzman, MD

Professor and Chair
Department of Orthopaedics
University of Utah School of Medicine
Salt Lake City, Utah

Roy W. Sanders, MD

Chief, Department of Orthopaedics
Tampa General Hospital
Director, Orthopedic Trauma Services
Florida Orthopedic Institute
Tampa, Florida

Lew C. Schon, MD

Assistant Professor
Johns Hopkins School of Medicine
Baltimore, Maryland
Associate Professor
Georgetown School of Medicine
Washington, District of Columbia
Director of Foot and Ankle Fellowship
Director of Orthobiologic Lab
Union Memorial Hospital
Baltimore, Maryland

Paul S. Shurnas, MD

Foot and Ankle Service
The Columbia Orthopaedic Group
Columbia, Missouri

Elly Trepman, MD

Associate Professor
Department of Surgery
Professional Associate
Department of Medical Microbiology
University of Manitoba
Winnipeg, Manitoba, Canada

Arthur K. Walling, MD

Clinical Professor of Orthopaedics
University of South Florida
Foot and Ankle Fellowship Director
Florida Orthopaedic Institute
Tampa, Florida

Keith L. Wapner, MD

Clinical Professor
University of Pennsylvania
Adjunct Professor
Drexel College of Medicine
Director
Foot and Ankle Fellowship
Pennsylvania Hospital
Philadelphia, Pennsylvania

Alastair S. E. Younger, MB, ChB, MSc, ChM, FRCSC

Clinical Associate Professor
Division of Lower Extremity Reconstruction and
    Oncology
Department of Orthopaedics
The University of British Columbia
Director
British Columbia's Foot and Ankle Clinic
St. Paul's Hospital
Vancouver, British Columbia, Canada

Preface

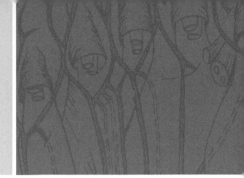

Fifty years ago, Henri L. DuVries, MD, of Chicago, Illinois, commenced work on the first edition of *Surgery of the Foot*, which was eventually published in 1959. This text contained his personal views regarding the diagnosis and treatment of foot and ankle disorders. The book was significant because it was written by a physician who had obtained his initial training as a podiatrist and then subsequently became a doctor of medicine. His 30 years of experience in treating disorders, deformities, and injuries of the foot were presented in this work, which became a classic reference text in the treatment of common foot disorders. In 1965, Dr. DuVries expanded the book to include several contributors, including Verne T. Inman, MD (Chairman of the Department of Orthopaedic Surgery at the University of California, San Francisco), and Roger A. Mann, MD, a senior resident in orthopaedics. Eight years later, in 1973, Dr. Inman succeeded Dr. DuVries as the editor of the third edition of *Surgery of the Foot*. Again the text was expanded, this time to include the ankle joint as well as an in-depth analysis of the biomechanics of the foot and ankle. Five years later, in 1978, Dr. Mann edited the fourth edition. Having been a resident under Dr. Inman and having served a fellowship under Dr. DuVries, Dr. Mann provided a means of blending the special interests of these two unique individuals—the basic biomechanical interests of Dr. Inman and the wealth of clinical knowledge of Dr. DuVries. In 1986, Dr. Mann updated and published an expanded fifth edition.

As Dr. Mann's first foot and ankle fellow in 1978, I had the opportunity to be exposed to both his philosophy of patient care and the creativity with which he addressed the evaluation and treatment of his patients. His meticulous surgical technique and comprehensive postoperative program were coupled with an introspective method of assessing the results of specific procedures in order to delineate the preferred treatment regimen. Dr. Mann's 40 years in private practice, stimulated by more than 50 foot and ankle fellows, have complemented my interaction with him. In 1999, I initiated my own fellowship program and have learned a great deal from the 10 fellows that I have trained. I have frequently reviewed the surgical procedures used in my everyday practice, with the common goal of defining the strengths of individual procedures as well as their weaknesses. For the 28 years that I have been in private practice in Boise, Idaho, I believe that the principles initially espoused by Drs. Inman and DuVries and expanded on by Dr. Mann have given me a unique perspective. In 1993, Dr. Mann and I collaborated on the sixth edition, which was expanded to a comprehensive two-volume text. In 1999, this was revised by us as the seventh edition.

This is a living text and has continued to evolve from the initial work of Henri L. DuVries. Much of our orthopaedic careers have been involved with this text—Dr. Mann has contributed to or edited all but one of the editions, and I have contributed to or edited half of the editions. However, change and growth are important! So in this current edition of *Surgery of the Foot and Ankle*, 17 authors continue to contribute, but 29 new authors have been added. Most important, Charles L. Saltzman, MD, a fellow of Kenneth A. Johnson, MD, joins Dr. Mann and me as an editor of this text. Dr.

Saltzman brings a wealth of basic science and clinical knowledge to this association. Just as Dr. DuVries complimented his text by adding Dr. Inman, we feel strongly that Dr. Saltzman's addition will make this a stronger and more well-rounded work. The eighth edition is also enhanced by the work of many of our excellent fellows and colleagues from around the nation who have made substantial sacrifices to contribute to this textbook. These contributing authors are at the forefront of their specific area of foot and ankle surgery. Each contributing author has covered a specific topic in a comprehensive fashion, which we believe will leave the reader with a clear, concise appreciation of that subject. While this book is not meant to be encyclopedic in nature, our goal has always been to provide the reader with a method of evaluating and treating a particular problem.

A dramatic change occurs with this edition with the addition of color photographs and illustrations which, we believe, will markedly improve the didactic experience of reading this text. This new edition has been divided into 10 sections that have been subdivided into individual chapters. Specific surgical techniques within the chapters are described and illustrated in detail to afford the reader an understanding of the indications for each procedure as well as insight into the performance of a specific surgical technique. Although many different treatment regimens are presented, our goal is to recommend a specific treatment plan for each pathologic entity. Furthermore, some topics are presented in more than one section, enabling the reader to appreciate the varying points of view presented by individual contributors. In specific chapters dealing with clinical problems written by either Dr. Mann or myself, the treatment protocol we present is a result of our continued collaboration and evaluation of specific techniques. Assisted by both our former fellows and our colleagues, we continue to carefully reassess the clinical results of major surgical procedures about the foot and ankle. These results have been included in this updated eighth edition. Our patients are frequently recalled and carefully evaluated, and new radiographs are obtained as we continue to assess specific procedures and make necessary technical changes when appropriate. Likewise, new procedures have been developed since our last edition, and we have assessed them as well to determine whether they warrant inclusion in this text. Thus, it is our goal to provide the reader with an accurate assessment of both the attributes and the deficiencies of specific orthopaedic foot and ankle procedures, new and old. In this current edition, we present our most current, up-to-date thinking regarding the diagnosis, treatment, and specific surgical care of foot and ankle problems.

In Part I, *General Considerations*, the biomechanics, examination, and conservative treatment of foot and ankle problems are addressed. In large part, the initial principles advocated by both Dr. DuVries and Dr. Inman and presented in their initial work are included in this portion of the text. Anesthetic techniques are covered in detail and have been updated to include sciatic and femoral blocks. Imaging of the foot and ankle, an integral part of the evaluation process for foot and ankle disorders, has been updated and includes in-depth coverage of magnetic resonance imaging, computed tomography, and bone scanning. It also includes algorithms to assist the clinician in choosing appropriate imaging techniques.

In Part II, *Forefoot*, an extensive analysis of deformities of the great toe along with complications associated with individual hallux valgus procedures has been completely revised to make the reader aware of primary surgical techniques as well as salvage techniques following postsurgical complications. The chapter on juvenile hallux valgus has been incorporated into the hallux valgus chapter to provide a comprehensive section on the treatment of this complex problem. The chapter on lesser toes has been completely rewritten and updated because of the vast number of advances made in this area during the past decade. In particular, the treatment of complex forefoot deformities, including subluxation and dislocation of the lesser metatarsophalangeal joints, has been revised because of rapidly evolving techniques. The chapter on sesamoids and accessory bones has been updated as well. The chapter on keratotic disorders and intractable plantar keratosis has been separated from the bunionette section in order to provide a more clear understanding of the differential diagnosis and the appropriate conservative and surgical treatments for these difficult problems.

Part III, *Nerve Disorders,* has been completely rewritten and covers both acquired and static neurologic disorders, including entrapment and impingement syndromes of both the young and the skeletally mature patient. In Part IV, *Miscellaneous,* the chapters on heel pain, soft tissue and bone tumors, and toenail abnormalities have been rewritten and updated. A new chapter on workers' compensation and liability issues has been added to complement the surgical treatment of the working patient contained in other sections of this textbook.

Part V, *Arthritis, Postural Disorders, and Tendon Disorders,* has been completely revamped, updating our current knowledge and treatment of systemic inflammatory arthritis, traumatic arthritis, and osteoarthritis. A separate chapter on arthritis of the ankle has been added by Dr. Saltzman, and another chapter on deformity correction and distraction arthroplasty compliments this section. Extensive revisions of the chapters on pes planus and pes cavus are included. The chapter on arthrodesis of the foot has been updated, reflecting the results of surgical techniques and our personal in-depth review of these procedures. The chapter on tendon abnormalities has been extensively rewritten to reflect significant technical advances in this area. A separate section on diabetes (Part VI, *Diabetes)* is now included. The three chapters on diabetes, amputations, and prostheses of the foot and ankle have been completely updated.

Part VII, *Sports Medicine,* includes a comprehensive chapter on athletic soft tissue injuries as well as specific chapters regarding stress fractures of the foot and ankle and foot and ankle injuries in dancers. The chapter on foot and ankle arthroscopy has been revised and updated in color to familiarize the reader with this exciting and evolving area of orthopaedic technology.

Pediatrics is covered in Part VIII, and *Soft Tissue Disorders of the Foot and Ankle* are discussed in Part IX. A new chapter on soft tissue trauma to the foot and ankle has been added.

Part X, *Trauma,* has been expanded and extensively rewritten under the direction of Roy Sanders, with new chapters on fracture-dislocations of the ankle and updates of the remaining chapters.

In 1990, Dr. Mann and I published the *Video Textbook of Foot and Ankle Surgery,* the second volume of which appeared in 1995. This enabled foot and ankle surgeons to view a surgical procedure while simultaneously reading about the operative technique. Encouraged by the success of this endeavor, we proposed that we incorporate a markedly edited version of the original videos into an accompanying DVD. This eighth edition thus incorporates for the very first time both written and video versions of surgical procedures. We believe that this will be a valuable addition.

As Roger Mann stated in the preface of the fifth edition, "As medicine continues to progress, the information of this textbook will again need to be upgraded. The principles presented, however, are basic in their approach and will not change significantly over the years." We believe that the eighth edition of *Surgery of the Foot and Ankle* will strongly enhance this dynamic and exciting field of orthopaedics and will complement the learning experience of both the resident and fellow-in-training as well as the practicing surgeon.

Michael J. Coughlin, MD

Acknowledgments

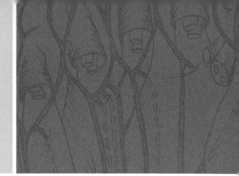

We would like to acknowledge those who have assisted us in the preparation of this text: Joe Kania (video support), Steadman Hawkins Clinic, Vail, Colorado; Tom Hadzor, Wide-Eye Productions, Boise, Idaho (video support), Penny Dunlap, RN (word processing and editing), Barbara Kirk (color illustrations), and Sandra Hight and Therese Borgerding (librarians, Kissler Family Health Sciences Library), St. Alphonsus Regional Medical Center, Boise, Idaho.

Michael J. Coughlin, MD
Roger A. Mann, MD
Charles L. Saltzman, MD

Contents

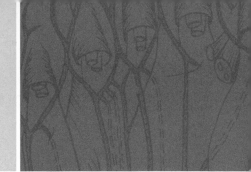

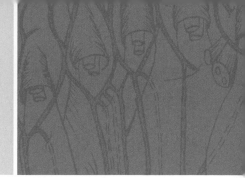

List of Video Clips

GENERAL CONSIDERATIONS

Biomechanics of the Foot and Ankle

Roger A. Mann • Andrew Haskell

The initial chapters of this text on surgery are not concerned with anatomy, as is customary, but rather with discussion of the biomechanics of the foot and ankle. The specific relationships are emphasized, and some methods for functional evaluation of the foot are presented. These alterations were initiated for several reasons.

First, it has been assumed that the orthopaedic surgeon possesses an accurate knowledge of the anatomic aspects of the foot and ankle. If this knowledge is lacking, textbooks of anatomy are available that depict in detail the precise anatomic structures constituting this part of the human body.[70]

Second, any textbook on surgery of the foot should begin with a discussion of the biomechanics of the foot and ankle as an integral part of the locomotor system. The human foot is an intricate mechanism that functions interdependently with other components of the locomotor system. No text is readily available to the surgeon that clearly enunciates the functional interrelationships of the various parts of the foot. Interference with the functioning of a single part may be reflected in altered functions of the remaining parts. Yet the surgeon is called on constantly to change the anatomic and structural components of the foot. When making these changes, the surgeon should be fully aware of the possible consequences of his or her actions.

Third, wide variations occur in the component parts of the foot and ankle, and these variations are reflected in the degree of contribution of each part to the function of the entire foot. Depending on the contributions of an individual component, the loss or functional modification of that component by surgical intervention can result in either minor or major alterations in the function of adjacent components. An understanding of basic interrelationships can assist the surgeon in explaining why the same procedure performed on the foot of one person produced a satisfactory result, whereas in another person the result was unsatisfactory.

Fourth, by being alert to the mechanical behavior of the foot, the physician may find that some foot disabilities caused by malfunction of a component part can be successfully treated by nonsurgical procedures rather than approached surgically, as has been customary. Furthermore, if some operative procedure fails to completely achieve the desired result, the result can be improved by minor alterations in the behavior of adjacent components through modification of the shoe or the use of inserts. An understanding of the biomechanics of the foot and ankle therefore should be an essential aid in surgical decision making and contributes to the success of postoperative treatment.

LOCOMOTOR SYSTEM

The human foot too often is viewed as a semirigid base whose principal function is to provide a stable support for the superincumbent body. In reality the foot is poorly designed for this purpose. Standing for prolonged periods can result in a feeling of fatigue or can produce actual discomfort in the feet. One commonly prefers to sit rather than stand. Furthermore, it is far less tiring to walk, run, jump, or dance on normally functioning feet, either barefoot or in comfortable shoes, than it is to stand. The foot therefore appears to have evolved as a dynamic mechanism functioning as an integral part of the locomotor system, and it should be studied as such rather than as a static structure designed exclusively for support.

Inasmuch as human locomotion involves all major segments of the body, certain suprapedal movements demand specific functions from the foot, and alterations in these movements from above may be reflected below by changes in the behavior of the foot. Likewise, the manner in which the foot functions may be reflected in patterns of movement in the other segments of the body. Therefore the basic functional interrelationships between the foot and the remainder of the locomotor apparatus must be understood clearly.

To begin a review of the locomotor system, one must recognize that the ambulating human is both a physical machine and a biologic organism. The human as physical machine is subject to the physical laws of motion; the human as biologic organism is subject to the laws of muscular action. All characteristics of muscular behavior are exploited in locomotion; for example, when called on to perform such external work as initiating or accelerating angular motion around joints, muscles rarely contract at lengths below their resting lengths.[16,20,69] When motion in the skeletal segments is decelerated or when external forces work on the body, activated muscles become efficient. Activated muscles, in fact, are approximately six times as efficient when resisting elongation as when shortening to perform external work.[1,6,7] In addition, noncontractile elements in muscles and specific connective tissue structures assist muscular action. Thus human locomotion is a blending of physical and biologic forces that compromise to achieve maximum efficiency at minimum cost.

Humans use a unique and characteristic orthograde bipedal mode of locomotion. This method of locomotion imposes gross similarities in the way all of us walk. However, each of us exhibits minor individual differences that allow us to be recognized, even from a distance. The causes of these individual characteristics of locomotion are many. Each of us differs somewhat in the length and distribution of mass of the various segments of the body, segments that must be moved by muscles of varying fiber length. Furthermore, individual differences occur in the position of axes of movement of the joints, with concomitant variations in effective lever arms. These and many more such factors combine to establish in each of us a final idiosyncratic manner of locomotion.

A smoothly performing locomotor system results from the harmonious integration of many components. This final integration does not require that the specific contribution of a single isolated component be identical in every person, nor must it be identical even within the same person. The contribution of a single component varies under different circumstances. Type of shoe, amount of fatigue, weight of load carried, and other such variables can cause diminished functioning of some components, with compensatory increased functioning of others. An enormous number of variations in the behavior of individual components are possible; however, the diversely functioning components, when integrated, are complementary and produce smooth bodily progression.

Average values of single anthropometric observations in themselves have little value. The surgeon should be alert to the anthropometric variations that occur within the population, but it is more important to understand the functional interrelationships among the various components. This is particularly true in the case of the foot, where anatomic variations are extensive. If average values are the only bases of comparison, it becomes difficult to explain why some feet function adequately and asymptomatically, although their measurements deviate from the average, whereas others function symptomatically, even though their measurements approximate the average. It appears reasonable therefore to use average values only to provide a mathematical reference for demonstrating the extent of possible deviations from these averages. Therefore emphasis is placed on functional interrelationships and not on descriptive anatomy.

Human locomotion is a learned process; it does not develop as the result of an inborn reflex. This statement is supported by Popova,[64] who studied the changing gait in growing children. The first few steps of an infant holding onto his or her mother's hand exemplify the learning process necessary to achieve orthograde progression. Scott,[72] of the Canadian National Institute for the Blind, noted that congenitally blind children never attempt to stand and walk spontaneously but must be carefully taught. The result of this learning process is the integration of the neuromusculoskeletal mechanisms, with their gross similarities and individual variations, into an adequately functioning system of locomotion. Once a person has learned to walk and has attained maximum growth, a built-in regulatory mechanism is a part of his or her physiologic makeup and works whether the person is an amputee learning to use a new prosthesis, a long-distance runner, or a woman wearing high-heeled shoes.

Ralston[65] has noted that the locomotor system is one that will take us from one spot to another with the least expenditure of energy.

Walking Cycle

Human gait is a rhythmic, cyclical forward progression involving motion of all body segments. A single cycle is often defined as the motion between the heel strike of one step and the heel strike of the same foot on the subsequent step. Gait parameters such as stride length, velocity, and cadence can be measured based on this definition. A single cycle can be divided further.

The walking cycle consists of the stance phase and the swing phase of the same leg. The stance phase usually consumes about 62% of the cycle and the swing phase 38%. The stance phase is further divided into a period of double limb support (0% to 12%) in which both feet are on the ground followed by a period of single limb support (12% to 50%) and a second period of double limb support (50% to 62%), after which the swing phase begins (Fig. 1–1).

During the walking cycle, foot flat is observed by 7% of the cycle, opposite toe-off at 12%, heel rise beginning at 34% as the swing leg passes the stance foot, and opposite heel strike at 50% (Fig. 1–2).

In a patient with spasticity, the initial foot strike may be toe contact, and foot flat might not occur by 7% of the cycle. Heel rise may be premature if spasticity or a contracture is present, or it can be delayed in the case of weakness of the gastrocnemius–soleus muscle group.

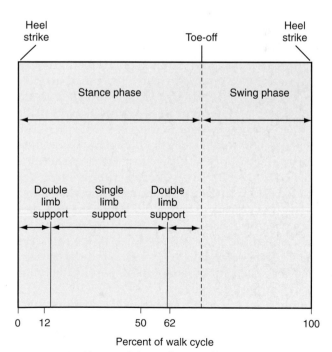

Figure 1–1 Phases of the walking cycle. Stance phase constitutes approximately 62% and swing phase 38% of the cycle. Stance phase is further divided into two periods of double limb support and one period of single limb support.

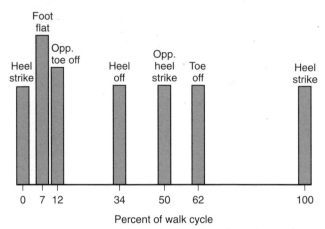

Figure 1–2 Events of the walking cycle. While observing the patient walk, the clinician should note events to help identify gait abnormality. Opp, opposite.

The pronation that occurs at initial ground contact is a passive mechanism, and the amount of motion appears to depend entirely on the configuration of the articulating surfaces, their capsular attachments, and the ligamentous support. No significant muscle function appears to play a role in restricting this motion at initial ground contact.

Because of the specific linkage of the leg to the foot, which occurs through the subtalar joint, the eversion of the calcaneus is translated proximally by the subtalar joint into inward rotation that is transmitted across the ankle joint into the lower extremity. Distally this eversion unlocks the transverse tarsal joint (Fig. 1–3E).

The walking cycle, being one of continuous motion, is difficult to describe in its entirety because so many events occur simultaneously. However, a reasonably accurate summary of the events can be presented if the stance phase is divided into three intervals: the first interval, extending from heel strike to foot flat; the second interval, occurring from the period of foot flat as the body passes over the foot; and the third interval, extending from the beginning of ankle joint plantar flexion to toe-off.

First Interval

The first interval occurs during approximately the first 15% of the walking cycle. The center of gravity of the body is decelerated by ground contact then immediately accelerated upward to carry it over the extending lower extremity. The body's impact and shift of the center of gravity account for a vertical floor reaction that exceeds body weight by 15% to 25% (Fig. 1–3A). The ankle joint undergoes rapid plantar flexion until foot flat, at 7% of the cycle, after which dorsiflexion begins (Fig. 1–3B). The plantar flexion is under the control of the anterior compartment muscles, which undergo an eccentric contraction to prevent foot slap. The posterior calf muscles all are electrically quiet, as are the intrinsic muscles in the sole of the foot (Fig. 1–3C). There is no muscle response in those muscles usually considered important in supporting the longitudinal arch of the foot.

At this time, the foot is being loaded with the weight of the body, and the longitudinal arch flattens. Gait analysis during walking reveals rapid eversion of the calcaneus and flattening of the longitudinal arch as a result of the impact of the body weight. This flattening of the arch originates in the subtalar joint and reaches a maximum during this interval (Fig. 1–3D).

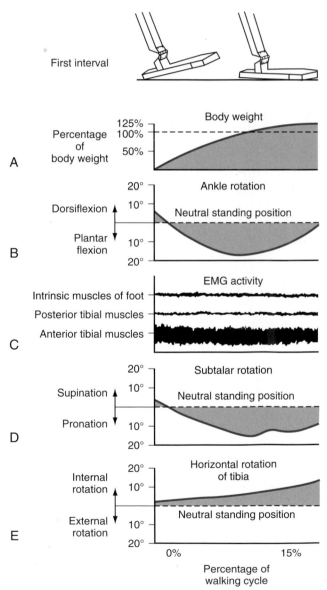

Figure 1–3 Composite of events of the first interval of walking, or the period that extends from heel strike to foot flat.

The main thrust of what occurs during the first interval is that of absorption and dissipation of the forces generated by the foot's striking the ground.

Second Interval

The second interval extends from 15% to 40% of the walking cycle. During this interval the body's center of gravity passes over the weight-bearing leg at about 35% of the cycle, after which it commences to fall. Force plate recordings show that the foot is supporting less than actual body weight. The load on the foot may be as low as 70% to 80% of actual body weight (Fig. 1–4A).

The ankle joint is undergoing progressive dorsiflexion, reaching its peak at 40% of the walking cycle. This is when the force across the ankle joint has reached a maximum of four and one half times body weight. Heel rise begins at 34% of the cycle and precedes the

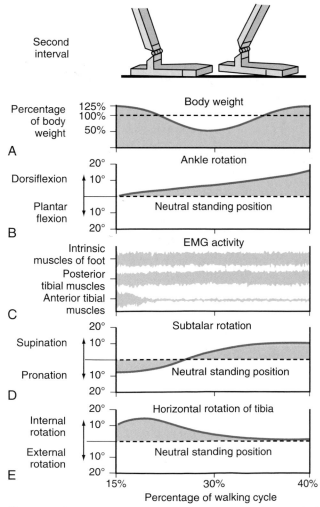

Figure 1–4 Composite of events of the second interval of walking, or the period of foot flat.

onset of plantar flexion, which begins at 40% (Fig. 1–4B).

During the second interval, important functional changes occur in both the foot and leg as the result of muscle action. The triceps surae, peroneals, tibialis posterior, long toe flexors, and intrinsic muscles in the sole demonstrate electrical activity (Fig. 1–4C). The activity in the intrinsic muscles of the normal foot begin at 30% of the cycle, whereas in flatfoot the activity begins at 15% of the cycle. The posterior calf musculature is functioning to control the forward movement of the tibia over the fixed foot, which permits the contralateral limb to increase its step length.

Subtalar joint motion demonstrates progressive inversion at about 30% of the cycle in a normal foot and at about 15% of the cycle in a flatfoot (Fig. 1–4D). The inversion is brought about by several factors, and precisely which plays the greatest role is unclear. The factors occurring above the subtalar joint consist of the external rotation of the lower extremity brought about by the swinging contralateral limb, its transmittal to the stance limb as an external rotation torque, its transmittal across the ankle joint, and its translation by the subtalar joint into inversion. The oblique nature of the ankle joint axis, the oblique setting of the metatarsal break, and the function of the plantar aponeurosis all act in concert to bring about this inversion. Because the forefoot is fixed to the floor, inversion of the subtalar joint is passed distally into the foot, increasing the stability of the transverse tarsal articulation. The progressive inversion rearranges the skeletal components of the foot, which helps transform the flexible midfoot into a rigid structure. During this interval, full body weight is not borne on the foot, which might make this transition somewhat easier.

Third Interval

The third interval constitutes the last of the stance phase and extends from 40% to 62% of the walking cycle.

Force plate recordings demonstrate an increase in the percentage of body weight as a result of the fall of the center of gravity at the beginning of this interval; the load on the foot again exceeds body weight by approximately 20%. The vertical floor reaction promptly falls to zero during this period as the body weight is being transferred to the opposite foot (Fig. 1–5A).

The ankle joint demonstrates rapid plantar flexion during this interval. The flexion is caused primarily by the concentric contraction of the posterior calf musculature, in particular the triceps surae (Fig. 1–5B). The plantar flexion leads to relative elongation of the

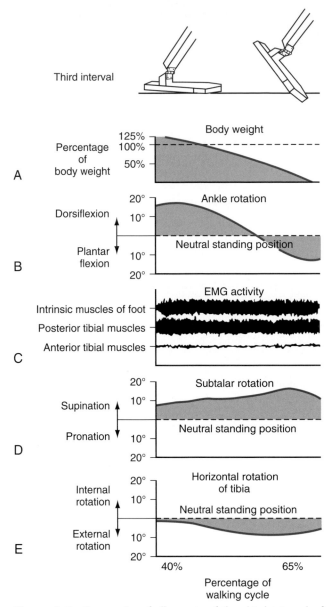

Figure 1–5 Composite of all events of the third interval of walking, or the period extending from foot flat to toe-off.

extremity. Although full plantar flexion at the ankle joint occurs during this interval, electrical activity is observed only until 50% of the cycle, after which there is no longer electrical activity in the extrinsic muscles (Fig. 1–5C). The remainder of ankle joint plantar flexion occurs because of the transfer of weight from the stance leg to the contralateral limb.

The intrinsic muscles of the foot are active until toe-off. Although the intrinsic muscles help to stabilize the longitudinal arch, the main stabilizer is the plantar aponeurosis, which is functioning maximally during this period as the toes are brought into dorsiflexion and the plantar aponeurosis is wrapped around the

metatarsal heads, forcing them into plantar flexion and elevating the longitudinal arch. The anterior compartment muscles become active in the last 5% of this interval, probably to initiate dorsiflexion of the ankle joint immediately after toe-off. The subtalar joint continues to invert during this interval, reaching its maximum at toe-off (Fig. 1–5D). As mentioned, the inversion probably is the result of the limb above the foot externally rotating and the passage of this movement across the ankle and subtalar joints to help bring about inversion. The inversion, however, is enhanced by the obliquity of the ankle joint, the function of the plantar aponeurosis, and oblique metatarsal break.

Distally, the transverse tarsal joint is converted from a flexible structure into a rigid one by the progressive inversion of the calcaneus. This then completes the conversion of the forefoot from the flexible structure observed in the first interval at the time of weight acceptance to a rigid structure at the end of the third interval in preparation for toe-off.

The talonavicular joint also is stabilized during this period by the pressure brought to bear across this joint by both body weight and the intrinsic force created by the plantar aponeurosis.

KINEMATICS OF HUMAN LOCOMOTION

Walking is more than merely placing one foot before the other. During walking, all major segments of the body are in motion and displacements of the body occur that can be accurately described.

Vertical Body Displacements

The rhythmic upward and downward displacement of the body during walking is familiar to everyone and is particularly noticeable when someone is out of step in a parade. These displacements in the vertical plane are a necessary concomitant of bipedal locomotion. When the legs are separated, as during transmission of the body weight from one leg to the other (double weight bearing), the distance between the trunk and the floor must be less than when it passes over a relatively extended leg, as during midstance. Because the nature of bipedal locomotion demands such vertical oscillations of the body, they should occur in a smooth manner for conservation of energy. Figure 1–6 shows that the body's center of gravity does displace in a smooth sinusoidal path; the amplitude of displacement is approximately 4 to 5 cm.[69,71]

Although movements of the pelvis and hip modify the amplitude of the sinusoidal pathway, the knee, ankle, and foot are particularly involved in converting

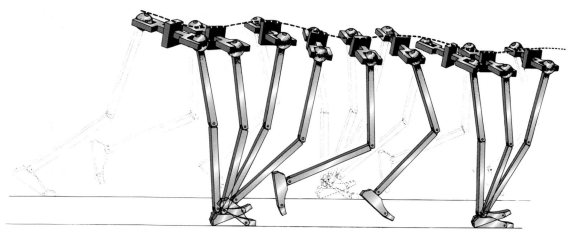

Figure 1–6 Displacement of center of gravity of body in smooth sinusoidal path. (From Saunders JB, Inman VT, Eberhart HD: *J Bone Joint Surg Am* 35:552, 1953.)

what would be a series of intersecting arcs into a smooth sinusoidal curve.[71] This conversion requires both simultaneous and precise sequential motions in the knee, ankle, and foot.

The body's center of gravity reaches its maximum elevation immediately after passage over the weight-bearing leg, then begins to fall. This fall must be stopped at the termination of the swing phase of the other leg as the heel strikes the ground. If one were forced to walk stiff-kneed and without the foot and ankle, the downward deceleration of the center of gravity at this point would be instantaneous. The body would be subjected to a severe jar and the locomotor system would lose kinetic energy. In fact, the falling center of gravity of the body is smoothly decelerated, because relative shortening of the leg occurs at the time of impact against a gradually increasing resistance. The knee flexes against a graded contraction of the quadriceps muscle; the ankle plantar flexes against the resisting anterior tibial muscles. After foot-flat position is reached, further shortening is achieved by pronation of the foot to a degree permitted by the ligamentous structures within.

Although the occurrence of this pronatory movement is more important in regard to other functions of the foot, it must be mentioned here because it constitutes an additional factor to that of knee flexion and ankle plantar flexion needed to smoothly decelerate and finally to stop the downward path of the body.

After decelerating to zero, the center of gravity must now evenly accelerate upward to propel it over the opposite leg. The kinetics of this phenomenon are complex, but the kinematics are simple. The leg is relatively elongated by transitory extension of the knee; further plantar flexion of the ankle elevates the heel, and the foot supinates. Elevation of the heel is the major component contributing to upward acceleration of the center of gravity at this time.

Horizontal Body Displacements

In addition to vertical displacements of the body, a series of axial rotatory movements occurs that can be measured in a horizontal plane. Rotations of the pelvis and the shoulder girdle are familiar to any observant person. Similar horizontal rotations occur in the femoral and tibial segments of the extremities. The tibias rotate about their long axes, internally during swing phase and into the first part of stance phase and externally during the latter part of stance. This motion continues until the toes leave the ground; the degree of these rotations is subject to marked individual variations. Levens et al,[53] in a study of a series of 12 male subjects, recorded the minimum amount of horizontal rotation of the tibia in space at 13 degrees and the maximum at 25 degrees (average, 19 degrees). A great portion of this rotation occurs when the foot is firmly placed on the floor; the shoe normally does not slip but remains fixed. The rotations, however, generate a torque of 7 to 8 newton-meters, which is of considerable magnitude.[23]

For these movements to occur, the foot must have a mechanism that permits the rotations but offers resistance to them of such magnitude that they are transmitted through the foot to the floor and are recorded on the force plate as torques. The ankle and subtalar joints are such mechanisms and will be described.

Lateral Body Displacements

When a person is walking, the body does not remain precisely in the plane of progression but oscillates slightly from side to side to keep the center of gravity approximately over the weight-bearing foot. Everyone has experienced this lateral shift of the body with each step but may not have consciously appreciated its cause. Everyone has at some time walked side by side with a companion. If one gets out of step with the other, their bodies are likely to bump.

The body is shifted slightly over the weight-bearing leg with each step; therefore a total lateral displacement of the body of approximately 4 to 5 cm occurs from side to side with each complete stride. This lateral displacement can be increased by walking with the feet more widely separated and can be decreased by keeping the feet close to the plane of progression (Fig. 1–7). Normally the presence of the tibiofemoral angle (slight genu valgum) permits the tibia to remain essentially vertical and the feet close together while the femurs diverge to articulate with the pelvis. Again, the lateral displacement of the body is through a smooth sinusoidal pathway.

KINETICS OF HUMAN LOCOMOTION

The forces resulting from displacement of the body's center of gravity have been measured using a force plate. The force plate measurements are based on Newton's third law, which states that for every action there is an equal and opposite reaction. It is used to accurately record the gravitational effects on the whole body while walking.[23] The principle of the force plate can be demonstrated by the bathroom scale. When one stands on the scale quietly and then flexes and extends the knees to raise and lower the body, the indi-

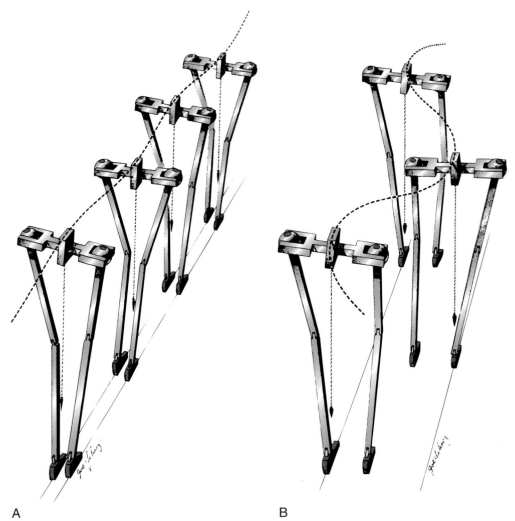

A   B

Figure 1–7 **A,** Slight lateral displacement of the body occurring during walking with feet close together. **B,** Increased lateral displacement of the body occurring during walking with feet wide apart. (From Saunders JB, Inman VT, Eberhart HD: *J Bone Joint Surg Am* 35:552, 1953.)

cator on the dial moves abruptly as vertical floor reaction is registered.

The only forces that can produce motion in the human body are those created by gravity, by muscle activity, and in a few instances by the elasticity of specific connective tissue structures. The force plate instantaneously records the forces imposed by the body on the foot, which are transmitted through the interface between the sole of the shoe and the walking surface. These measurements include vertical floor reactions, fore and aft shears, medial and lateral shears, and horizontal torques. During the stance phase of walking, the floor reactions in all four categories are continuously changing. The changes indicate that the foot is being subjected to varying forces imposed on it by movements of the superincumbent body.

Using the force plate, the ground reaction can be identified and graphed. Figure 1–8 demonstrates the force plate data obtained during normal walking. These include the vertical force, the fore and aft shears,

the medial and lateral shears, and the torque. The slower a person walks, the less movement of the center of gravity and the less the recorded force. Conversely, the faster the gait, the greater the movement of the center of gravity and hence a larger force. To demonstrate this, the vertical force recorded during jogging is shown in Figure 1–9.

The vertical force curve demonstrates an initial spike against the ground, after which the force declines. This initial spike is the reaction of the heel against the ground. The magnitude of the spike can be altered by the shoe material: A softer heel results in a smaller initial spike and a harder heel in a larger spike. Then the first peak occurs that is 10% to 15% greater than body weight and is caused by the upward acceleration of the body's center of gravity. This is followed by a dip in which the weight against the ground is approximately 20% less than body weight. This dip occurs because after the initial force has been exerted to raise the center of gravity, the stance foot is unloaded as the

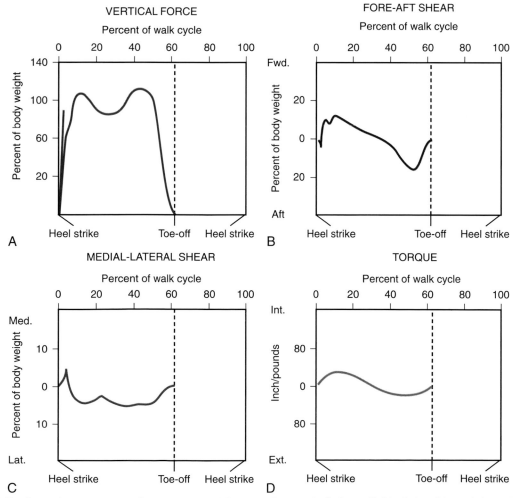

Figure 1–8 Ground reaction to walking. **A,** Vertical force. **B,** Fore and aft shear. **C,** Medial and lateral shear. **D,** Torque.

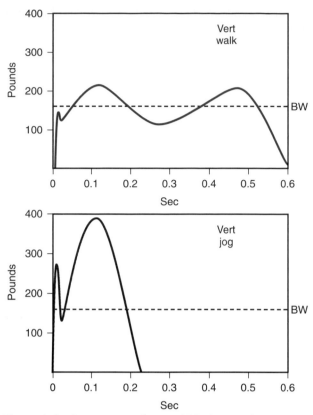

Figure 1–9 Comparison of vertical (Vert) ground reaction to walking versus jogging. Note that this is expressed in pounds rather than percentage of body weight. Time scale is in tenths of seconds rather than percentage of gait cycle. Vertical force during jogging for a 150-pound person reaches a maximum of almost 400 pounds, compared with the same person walking, which reaches a maximum of approximately 215 pounds.

center of gravity reaches the top of its trajectory before starting to fall. A second peak, again 10% to 15% greater than body weight, is caused by the falling of the center of gravity, after which the force rapidly declines to zero at toe-off and subsequent weight transfer to the opposite limb (see Fig. 1–8A).

Fore shear represents the initial braking of the body at the time of heel strike and occurs because the center of gravity is behind the foot at the time of heel strike. After the center of gravity has passed in front of the weight-bearing foot, an aft shear is noted. The aft shear reaches a maximum as the opposite limb strikes the ground at 50% of the walking cycle, at which time a fore shear is noted. The magnitude of the fore–aft shear, however, is only about 10% to 15% of body weight (see Fig. 1–8B).

Medial shear is the force exerted toward the midline at the time of heel strike, after which there is a persistent lateral shear until opposite heel strike at 50% of the cycle, when the medial shear occurs again. A medial shear is always observed except in persons with

an above-the-knee amputation, in whom a lateral shear mode is always present because of lack of abductor control of the prosthesis. The magnitude of the medial–lateral shear is about 5% of body weight (see Fig. 1–8C).

Torque measurement against the ground is in response to the rotation occurring in the lower extremity during the stance phase. Following heel strike there is an internal torque that reaches maximum at the time of foot flat, after which there is a progressive external torque that reaches a maximum just prior to toe-off. This torque corresponds to the inward and outward rotation of the lower extremity (see Fig. 1–8D).

Another way of visualizing the force against the ground is to observe the movement of the center of pressure. The movement of the center of pressure along the bottom of the foot in a normal person follows a consistent pattern (Fig. 1–10).[46] Following heel strike, the center of pressure moves rapidly along the bottom of the foot until it reaches the metatarsal area, where it dwells for about half of the stance phase and then passes distally to the great toe. A greater appreciation of the movement of the center of pressure is observed in a patient with rheumatoid arthritis who has a hallux valgus deformity and significant metatarsalgia (Fig. 1–11).[28] In this circumstance the center of pressure remains in the posterior aspect of the foot, avoiding the painful metatarsal area, then rapidly passes over the metatarsal heads along the middle of the foot, compared with weight bearing under the great toe in the normal foot. In a study carried out in patients with amputation of the great toe, the center of pressure passed in a more lateral direction (Fig. 1–12).[55]

COMPONENT BIOMECHANICS

Although floor reactions are important in demonstrating the totality of the forces transmitted through the foot, they give little information concerning the movements of the various articulations of the foot and ankle or about the activity of the muscles controlling these movements. Continuous geometric recordings and electromyographic studies are required to indicate joint motion and phasic activity of the intrinsic and extrinsic muscles. From the moment of heel strike to the instant of toe-off, floor reactions, joint motions, and muscle activity are changing constantly. Thus we cannot summarize this information for the entire period of stance or even hope to approximate what in reality is occurring in the foot and ankle. To make it easier to understand the various events that occur during a step, a discussion of the biomechanics of the various articulations and muscles that control their function is presented.

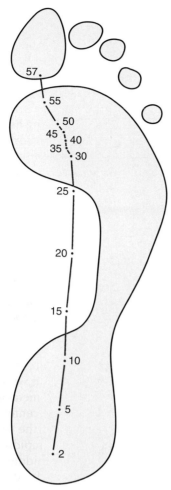

Figure 1–10 Progression of the center of pressure during the walking cycle. Center of load or pressure represents points of summation of forces through which load on the foot can be considered to act during the stance phase of walking. Note that the center of pressure moves distally rapidly after heel strike, as demonstrated by wide spacing between the data points. Pressure then dwells beneath the metatarsal head area from approximately 30% to 55% of the cycle, after which it moves rapidly out toward the great toe. (From Hutton WC, Stott JRR, Stokes JAF. In Klenerman L [ed]: *The Foot and Its Disorders*. Oxford, Blackwell Scientific, 1982, p 42.)

Ankle Joint

The direction of the ankle axis in the transverse plane of the leg dictates the vertical plane in which the foot will flex and extend. In the clinical literature this plane of ankle motion in relation to the sagittal plane of the leg is referred to as the *degree of tibial torsion*. Although it is common knowledge that the ankle axis is directed laterally and posteriorly as projected on the transverse plane of the leg, it is not widely appreciated that the ankle axis is also directed laterally and downward as seen in the coronal plane. Inman,[48] in anthropometric studies, found that in the coronal plane the axis of

the ankle can deviate 88 to 100 degrees from the vertical axis of the leg (Fig. 1–13A). Because the axis of the ankle passes just distal to the tip of each malleolus, the examiner should be able to obtain a reasonably accurate estimate of the position of the empirical axis by placing the ends of the index fingers at the most distal bony tips of the malleoli (Figs. 1–13B and 1–14).

A horizontal axis that remains normal to the vertical axis of the leg can affect only the amount of toeing out or toeing in of the foot; no rotatory influence can be imposed in a transverse plane on either the foot or the leg during flexion and extension of the ankle. However, because the ankle joint axis is obliquely oriented, it allows horizontal rotations to occur in the foot or the leg with movements of the ankle.

These rotations are clearly depicted in Figures 1–15 and 1–16. With the foot free and the leg fixed, the oblique ankle joint axis causes the foot to deviate outward on dorsiflexion and inward on plantar flexion. The projection of the foot onto the transverse plane, as shown by the shadows in the sketches, reveals the extent of this external and internal rotation of the foot (see Fig. 1–15). The amount of this rotation varies with the obliquity of the ankle axis and the amount of dorsiflexion and plantar flexion.

With the foot fixed on the ground during midstance, the body passing over the foot produces dorsiflexion of the foot relative to the leg (see Fig. 1–16). The oblique ankle axis then imposes an internal rotation on the leg.[53] Again, the degree of internal rotation of the leg on the foot depends on the amount of dorsiflexion and the obliquity of the ankle axis. As the heel rises in preparation for lift-off, the ankle is plantar flexed. This flexion in turn reverses the horizontal rotation, causing the leg to rotate externally.

When the horizontal rotations of the leg are studied independently, the foregoing sequence of events can be seen to be precisely what occurs in human locomotion. The lower part of the leg rotates internally during the first third and externally during the last two thirds of stance. The average amount of this rotation is 19 degrees, within a range of 13 to 25 degrees.[53] The recording of torques imposed on a force plate substantiates these rotations. Magnitudes vary from person to person but range from 7 to 8 newton-meters.[23]

In summary, the oblique ankle axis produces the following series of events: From the instant of heel contact to the time the foot is flat, plantar flexion occurs and the foot appears to toe in. The more oblique the axis, the more apparent the toeing in. During midstance the foot is fixed on the ground; relative dorsiflexion, with resulting internal rotation of the leg, occurs as the leg passes over the foot. As the

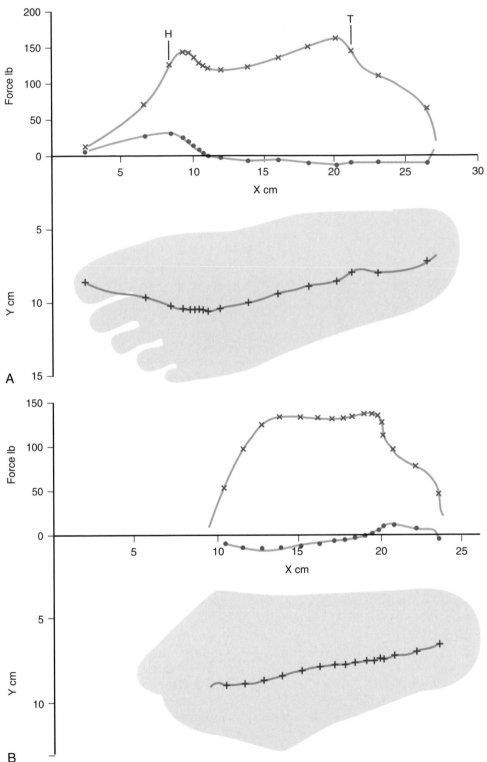

Figure 1–11 Progression of the center of pressure in a normal and an abnormal foot. **A,** Note progression of the center of pressure from the heel toward the toes during the normal walking cycle. As in Figure 1–10, the center of pressure moves rapidly from the heel, dwells in the metatarsal head region, then passes rapidly to the great toe at toe-off. **B,** Progression of the center of pressure in a patient with rheumatoid arthritis with severe hallux valgus deformity and significant metatarsalgia. Note that center-of-pressure points remain toward the heel, then rapidly progress across the metatarsal head area with little or no participation by the great toe in weight bearing. A patient with rheumatoid arthritis or significant metatarsalgia keeps weight in the posterior aspect of the foot to avoid pressure over the painful portion of foot. This leads to a shuffling type of gait. (From Grundy M, Tosh PA, McLeish RD, et al: *J Bone Joint Surg Br* 57:98-103, 1975.)

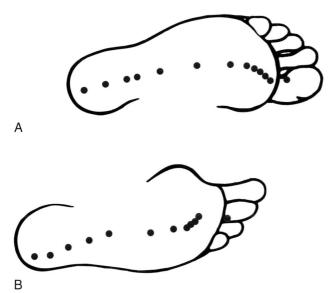

A

B

Figure 1–12 Movement of the center of pressure after amputation of the great toe. **A,** Normal progression of the center of pressure. **B,** Abnormal movement of the center of pressure after amputation of the great toe. Note that pressure tends to dwell more laterally in the metatarsal area, then passes out toward the third toe rather than the great toe. (From Mann RA, Poppen NK, O'Konski M: *Clin Orthop* 226:192-205, 1988.)

heel rises, plantar flexion takes place and causes external rotation of the leg.

Rotations of the leg and movements of the foot caused by an oblique ankle axis, when observed independently, are seen to be qualitatively and temporarily in agreement. However, when the magnitudes of the various displacements are studied, irreconcilable disparities are evident. In normal locomotion, ankle motion ranges from 20 degrees to 36 degrees, with an average of 24 degrees.[10,69] The obliquity of the ankle axis ranges from 88 to 100 degrees, with an average of 93 degrees from the vertical.[48] Even in the most oblique axis and movement of the ankle through the maximum range of 36 degrees, only 11 degrees of rotation of the leg around a vertical axis will occur. This is less than the average amount of horizontal rotation of the leg as measured independently in normal walking. The average obliquity of the ankle, together with the average amount of dorsiflexion and plantar flexion, would yield values for the horizontal rotation of the leg much smaller than the degree of horizontal rotation of the leg that actually occurs while the foot remains stationary on the floor and is carrying the superincumbent body weight.

The range of motion of the ankle demonstrates that at heel strike, rapid plantar flexion occurs at the ankle joint, reaching a maximum at about 7% of the cycle when foot flat has occurred. Following this, progressive dorsiflexion occurs until approximately 40% of

the gait cycle, at which time plantar flexion once again begins, reaching a maximum at the time of toe-off. During swing phase, dorsiflexion occurs at the ankle joint (Fig. 1–17). The muscle function about the ankle joint demonstrates that the anterior compartment muscles function as a group. Following heel strike, anterior compartment muscle activity continues until plantar flexion is complete, at about 7% of the cycle. During this time the muscle undergoes an eccentric (lengthening) contraction. Clinically, if the anterior tibial muscle group is not functioning, there is a foot-drop gait during swing phase that is characterized by increased flexion of the hip and knee to accommodate for the lack of dorsiflexion of the ankle joint. If this muscle group fails to function following heel strike, a foot slap results from lack of control of initial plantar flexion. Beginning at about 55% of the cycle and throughout swing phase, the anterior compartment muscles bring about dorsiflexion of the ankle. The dorsiflexion is achieved by a concentric (shortening) contraction.

The posterior calf muscles basically function as a group, although the tibialis posterior and peroneus longus muscles usually begin functioning by about 10% of the stance phase, whereas the other posterior calf muscles tend to become functional at about 20% of the stance phase. During the initial period of activity, the ankle joint undergoes progressive dorsiflexion until 40% of the cycle, and these muscles are undergoing eccentric contraction until plantar flexion begins, when they undergo concentric contraction. It is interesting to note, however, that by 50% of the cycle the electrical activity in these muscles ceases and the remainder of the plantar flexion of the ankle joint is rather passive. High-speed motion pictures have demonstrated that at the time of toe-off the foot literally is lifted from the ground and the toes do not demonstrate any plantar flexion, which leads us to believe that active push-off does not occur during steady-state walking. During running and changing direction, as well as acceleration and deceleration, the toes play an active role in push-off, but it is minimal during steady-state walking.

The function of the posterior calf group during stance phase is to control the forward movement of the tibia on the fixed foot.[74,79] During this portion of the gait cycle the body is moving forward over the fixed foot, and the control of the forward movement of the tibia is essential. This control of the forward movement of the stance leg tibia permits the contralateral leg to take a longer step. In pathologic states in which the calf muscle is weak, dorsiflexion occurs at the ankle joint after heel strike because it is a position of stability.

Observation of the forces across the ankle joint demonstrate that they reach a peak at approximately

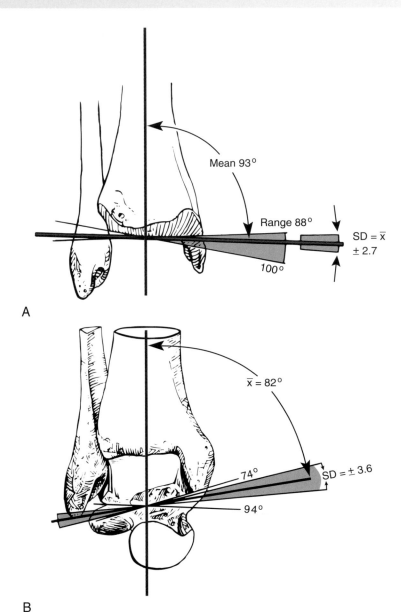

A

B

Figure 1–13 A, Variations in angle between midline of the tibia and plafond of the mortise. **B,** Variations in angle between midline of the tibia and empirical axis of the ankle. SD, standard deviation; x̄, arithmetic mean. (From Inman VT: *The Joints of the Ankle*. Baltimore, Williams & Wilkins, 1976.)

40% of the cycle, which is when the transition from dorsiflexion to plantar flexion occurs (Fig. 1–18). The force across the ankle joint reaches approximately four and one half times body weight. This much force confined to a small surface area probably is the reason the components of total ankle joints loosen.

Subtalar Joint

It is necessary to examine other articulations in the foot that could, in cooperation with the ankle, allow the leg to undergo the additional amount of internal and external rotation. The mechanism that appears to be admirably designed for this function is the subtalar joint.

The subtalar joint is a single axis joint that acts like a mitered hinge connecting the talus and the calcaneus. The axis of the subtalar joint passes from medial to lateral at an angle of approximately 16 degrees and from the horizontal plane approximately 42 degrees (Fig. 1–19).[20,57] Individual variations are extensive and imply variations in the behavior of this joint during locomotion. Furthermore, the subtalar joint appears to be a determinative joint of the foot, influencing the performance of the more distal articulations and modifying the forces imposed on the skeletal and soft tissues. Therefore we must understand the anatomic and functional aspects of this joint.

Based on the anatomic fact that the subtalar joint moves around a single inclined axis and functions

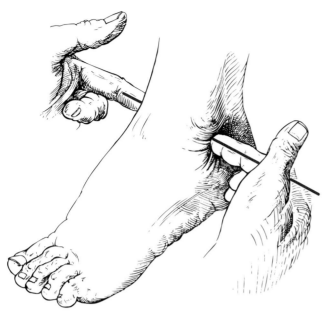

Figure 1–14 Estimation of obliquity of the empirical ankle axis by palpating the tips of the malleoli.

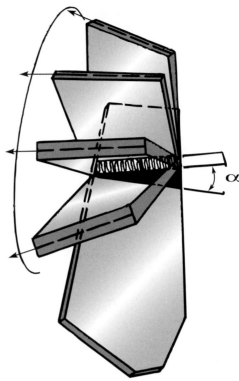

Figure 1–16 Foot fixed to the floor. Plantar flexion and dorsiflexion of the ankle produce horizontal rotation of the leg because of obliquity of the ankle axis. α, angle of flexion.

essentially like a hinge connecting the talus and the calcaneus, the functional relationships that result from such a mechanical arrangement are easily illustrated. Figure 1–20A shows two boards jointed by a hinge. If the axis of the hinge is at 45 degrees, a simple torque converter has been created. Rotation of the vertical member causes equal rotation of the horizontal member. Changing the angle of the hinge alters this one-on-one relationship. A more horizontally placed hinge causes a greater rotation of the horizontal

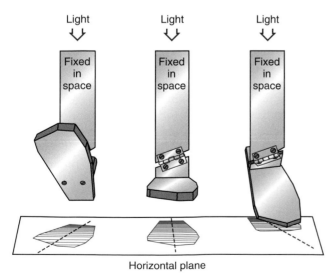

Horizontal plane

Figure 1–15 Effect of obliquely placed ankle axis on rotation of the foot in the horizontal plane during plantar flexion and dorsiflexion, with the foot free. Displacement is reflected in shadows of the foot.

member for each degree of rotation of the vertical member; the reverse holds true if the hinge is placed more vertically. In Figure 1–20B, to prevent the entire horizontal segment from participating in the rotatory displacement, the horizontal member has been divided into a short proximal and a long distal segment, with a pivot between the two segments. This pivot represents the transverse tarsal joint, which consists of the talonavicular and calcaneocuboid joint. The specific mechanics of this joint are discussed in the following section. Thus the distal segment remains stationary, and only the short segment adjacent to the hinge rotates.

To approach more closely the true anatomic situation of the human foot, in Figures 1–21A and B the distal portion of the horizontal member has been replaced by two structures. The medial represents the three medial rays of the foot that articulate through the cuneiform bones to the talus; the lateral represents the two lateral rays that articulate through the cuboid to the calcaneus. In Figure 1–21C and D, the entire mechanism has been placed into the leg and foot to demonstrate the mechanical linkages resulting in specific movements in the leg and foot. External rotation of the leg causes inversion of the heel, elevation of the medial side of the foot, and depression of the lateral side.

Internal rotation of the leg produces the opposite effect on the foot.

In persons with flatfeet the axis of the subtalar joint is more horizontal than in persons with normal feet; therefore the same amount of rotation of the leg imposes greater supinator and pronatory effects on the foot. This phenomenon can partially explain why some persons with asymptomatic and flexible pes planus break down their shoes and often prefer to go without shoes, which they find restrictive. Further-

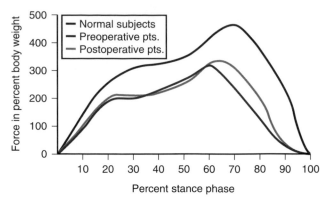

Figure 1–18 Compressive forces across the ankle joint during the stance phase of walking. Note that for normal subjects, force across the ankle joint is approximately four and one half times body weight at 60% to 70% of stance phase. This corresponds to 40% of the walking cycle when ankle plantar flexion is beginning. pts, patients. (From Stauffer RN, Chao EYS, Brewster RC: *Clin Orthop* 127:189, 1977.)

more, people with asymptomatic flatfeet usually show a greater range of subtalar motion than do persons with normal feet. The reverse holds true for people with pes cavus; in them, the generalized rigidity of the foot and the limited motion in the subtalar joint often are surprising.

Motion of the subtalar joint during walking was described by Wright and colleagues.[88] At the time of heel strike there is eversion in the subtalar joint, which reaches a maximum at foot flat, after which progressive inversion occurs until the time of toe-off, when eversion resumes. Approximately 6 degrees of rotation occurs in the normal foot, and in flatfoot rotation is approximately 12 degrees. Although the quantitation of the subtalar joint motion remains elusive because of the complexity of the movement, subsequent studies have qualitatively demonstrated the direction of movement to be in agreement, namely, eversion after heel strike until foot flat, after which inversion until toe-off (Fig. 1–22). Also, the phasic activity of the intrinsic muscles of the foot seems to correlate fairly closely with the degree of subtalar joint rotation. In the normal foot the intrinsic muscles become active at about 30% of the walking cycle, whereas in flatfoot they become active during the first 15% of the walking cycle (Fig. 1–22B).[54]

Transverse Tarsal Articulation

The calcaneocuboid and talonavicular articulations together often are considered to make up the transverse tarsal articulation. Each possesses some independent motion and has been subjected to intensive study.[26] However, from a functional standpoint they perform together.

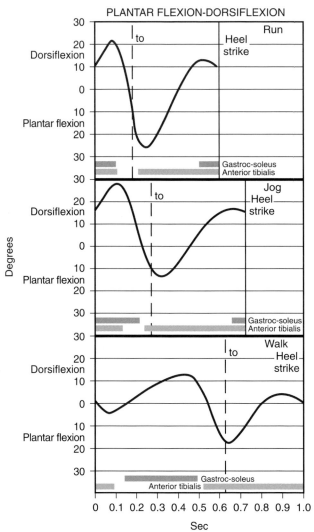

Figure 1–17 Ankle joint dorsiflexion–plantar flexion during running, jogging, and walking. Note that time of the walking cycle decreases from 1 second for walking to approximately 0.6 second for running. Stance phase time decreases significantly, as well. Muscle function is characterized by the gastrocnemius–soleus muscle group and the anterior tibial muscle. Note that the gastrocnemius–soleus muscle group becomes active in the late swing phase for jogging and running, compared with stance phase muscle for walking. Gastroc, gastrocnemius. (From Mann RA: In Nicholas JA, Hershmann EB [eds]: *The Lower Extremity and Spine in Sports Medicine*, ed 2. St Louis, Mosby, 1995.)

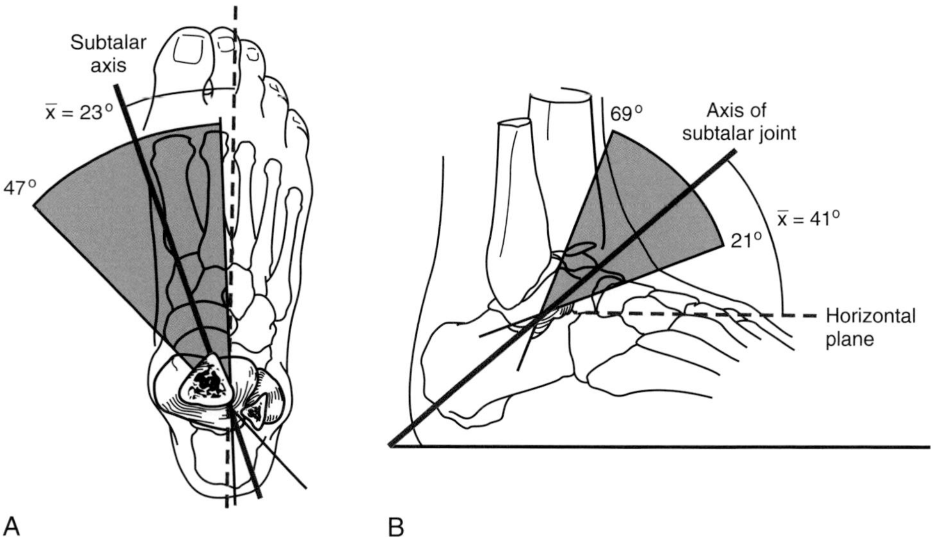

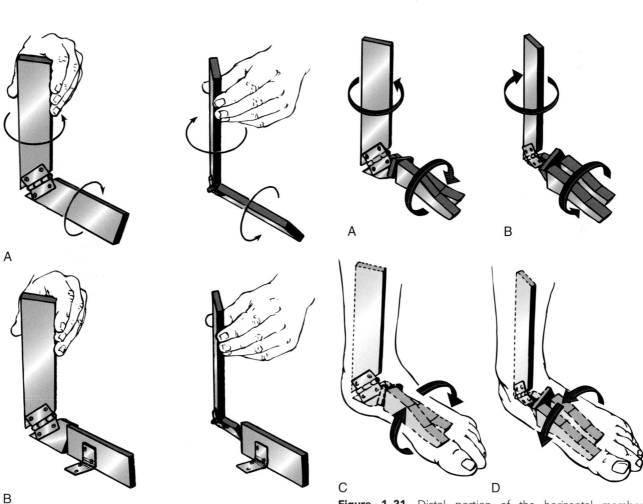

Figure 1–19 Variations in subtalar joint axes. **A,** In the transverse plane, the subtalar axis deviates approximately 23 degrees medial to the long axis of the foot, with a range of 4 to 47 degrees. **B,** In the horizontal plane, the axis approximates 41 degrees, with a range of 21 to 69 degrees. x̄, arithmetic mean. (Adapted from Isman RE, Inman VT: *Bull Prosthet Res* 10:97, 1969.)

Figure 1–20 Simple mechanism demonstrating functional relationships. **A,** Action of mitered hinge. **B,** Addition of pivot between two segments of the mechanism.

Figure 1–21 Distal portion of the horizontal member replaced by two structures. **A** and **B,** Mechanical analog of principal components of the foot. **C** and **D,** Mechanical components inserted into the foot and leg.

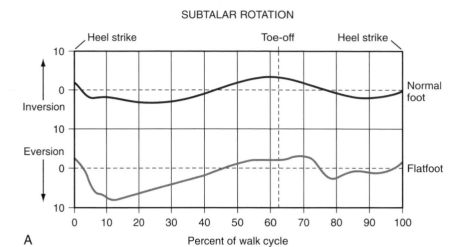

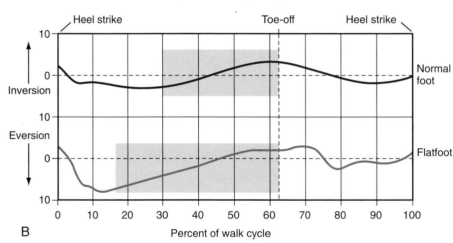

Figure 1–22 Subtalar joint motion. **A,** Motion in normal foot and flatfoot. **B,** Shaded areas indicate the period of activity of intrinsic muscles in the normal foot and flatfoot.

Elftman[26] demonstrated that the axes of these two joints are parallel when the calcaneus is in an everted position and are nonparallel when the calcaneus is in an inverted position. This relative position is important because when the axes are parallel there is flexibility within the transverse tarsal joint, whereas when the axes are nonparallel there is rigidity at the transverse tarsal joint (Fig. 1–23). As indicated in Figure 1–21, the transverse tarsal joint transmits the motion that occurs in the calcaneus distally into the forefoot, which is fixed to the ground. At the time of heel strike, as the calcaneus moves into eversion there is flexibility in the transverse tarsal joint, and at the time of toe-off the calcaneus is in an inverted position, resulting in stability of the transverse tarsal joint and hence the longitudinal arch of the foot. Motion in this joint has not been quantitated, but Figure 1–24 visually demonstrates the degree of motion that occurs in the transverse tarsal joint.

From a clinical standpoint, the importance of this joint is observed if a subtalar arthrodesis is placed into too much inversion, resulting in stiffness of the midfoot region and causing excessive weight on the lateral border of the foot and a tendency to vault over the rather rigid midfoot region.

The importance of the transverse tarsal articulation lies not in its axes of motion while non–weight bearing but in how it behaves during the stance phase of motion when the foot is required to support the body weight. Some specific changes occur in the amount of motion sustained by the transverse tarsal articulation with the forefoot fixed and the heel everted or inverted. Everting the heel produces relative pronation of the foot; varying amounts of flexion and extension in the sagittal plane, adduction and abduction in the transverse plane, and rotation between the forefoot and the heel then occur. The examiner gets the impression that the midfoot has become unlocked and that maximum motion is possible in the transverse tarsal articulation. However, if the forefoot is held firmly in one hand, something happens in the transverse tarsal articulation to make it appear locked. The previously elicited motions all become suppressed and the midfoot becomes rigid (Fig. 1–25).

Metatarsophalangeal Break

After wearing a new pair of shoes for awhile, one notices the appearance of an oblique crease in the area overlying the metatarsophalangeal articulation (Fig.

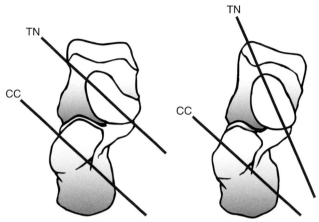

Figure 1–23 Function of the transverse tarsal joint, as described by Elftman, demonstrates that when the calcaneus is in eversion, resultant axes of the talonavicular (TN) and the calcaneocuboid (CC) joints are parallel. When the subtalar joint is in an inverted position, the axes are nonparallel, giving increased stability to the midfoot.

1–26). Its obliquity is a result of the unequal forward extension of the metatarsals. The head of the second metatarsal is the most distal head; that of the fifth metatarsal is the most proximal. Although the first metatarsal usually is shorter than the second (because the first metatarsal head is slightly elevated and is supported by the two sesamoid bones), it often functionally approximates the length of the second.

When the heel is elevated during standing or at the time of lift-off, the weight of the body normally is shared by all the metatarsal heads. To achieve this fair division of the body weight among the metatarsals, the foot must supinate slightly and deviate laterally. The oblique crease in the shoe gives evidence that these motions occur with every step. It has been demonstrated that the angle between the metatarsophalangeal break and the long axis of the foot can vary from 50 to 70 degrees.[49] The more oblique the metatarsophalangeal break, the more the foot must supinate and deviate laterally.

If the leg and foot acted as a single rigid member without ankle, subtalar, or transverse tarsal articulations, the metatarsophalangeal break would cause lateral inclination and external rotation of the leg (Fig. 1–27A). However, to permit the leg to remain in a vertical plane during walking, an articulation must be provided between leg and foot (Fig. 1–27B). Such an articulation is supplied by the subtalar joint (Fig. 1–27C). Because of its anatomic arrangement, it is

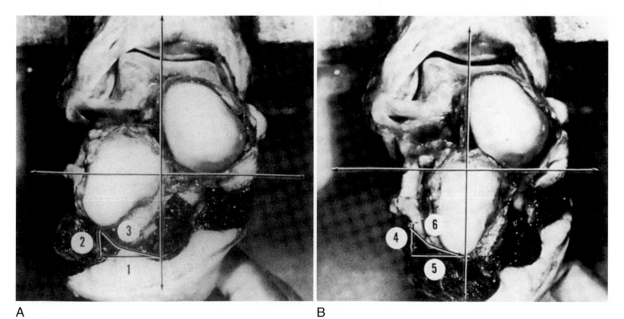

A   B

Figure 1–24 Anatomic model of the hindfoot demonstrating the relationship between the talus and calcaneus. **A,** Valgus position of the os calcis involving abduction (1), extension (2), and pronation (3). **B,** Varus position of the calcaneus involving flexion (4), adduction (5), and supination (6). When the calcaneus is in valgus position, the transverse tarsal joint is mobile. When the calcaneus is in varus position, the transverse tarsal joint is locked. (From Sarrafian SK: *Anatomy of the Foot and Ankle.* Philadelphia, JB Lippincott, 1983, p 391.)

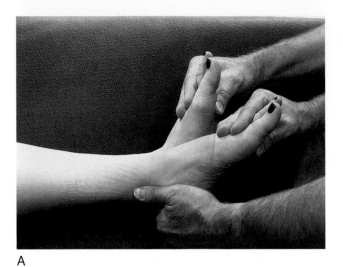

A

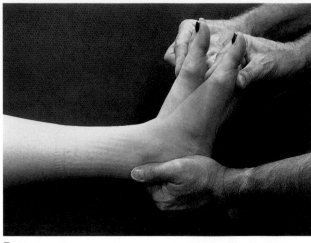

B

Figure 1–25   Rearrangement of skeletal components of the foot. **A,** Supination of the forefoot and eversion of the heel, permitting maximal motion in all components of the foot. **B,** Pronation of the forefoot and inversion of the heel, resulting in locking of all components of the foot and producing a rigid structure.

ideally suited to permit the foot to respond to the supinatory forces exerted by the oblique metatarsophalangeal break and still allow the leg to remain in a vertical plane.

All of the essential mechanisms discussed in this chapter are pictorially summarized in Figure 1–28. The two lower photographs, taken with the subject standing on a barograph, reveal the distribution of pressure between the foot and the weight-bearing surface. (A barograph records reflected light through a transparent plastic platform; the intensity of the light is roughly proportionate to the pressure the foot imposes on the plate.)

In Figure 1–28A, the subject was asked to stand with muscles relaxed. Note that the leg is moderately rotated internally and the heel is slightly everted (in valgus position). The body weight is placed on the heel, the outer side of the foot, and the metatarsal heads.

In Figure 1–28B, the subject was asked to rise on his toes. Note that the leg is now externally rotated, the heel is inverted (in varus position), and the longitudinal arch is elevated. The weight is concentrated on the metatarsal heads and is shared equally by the metatarsal heads and the toes.

Even though such movements cannot be illustrated pictorially, it is easy to imagine the contraction of the intrinsic and extrinsic muscles that is necessary to stabilize the foot and ankle as the body weight is transferred to the forefoot and the heel is raised. It should also be recalled that dorsiflexion of the toes tightens the plantar aponeurosis and assists in inversion of the heel. The supinatory twist activates the "locking"

mechanism in the foot, thus converting a flexible foot (see Fig. 1–28A) into a rigid lever (see Fig. 1–28B), an action that is necessary at lift-off.

Transverse Plane Rotation

During walking, transverse rotation occurs within the lower extremity. This rotation has been fairly well documented and quantitated. It demonstrates that at heel strike, progressive inward rotation occurs in the lower extremity, which consists of the pelvis, femur, and tibia, and this inward rotation reaches a maximum at the time of foot flat. Following contralateral toe-off, at about 12% of the cycle, progressive outward rotation occurs, which reaches a maximum at the time of toe-off, when inward rotation resumes (Fig. 1–29). The internal rotation at heel strike is initiated by the collapse of the subtalar joint into valgus, and its magnitude is determined by the flexibility of the foot and its ligamentous support. As a result of the loading of the subtalar joint and its collapse into eversion, two other events occur: Proximally the lower extremity internally rotates, and distally the transverse tarsal joint unlocks, resulting in flexibility of the longitudinal arch. This is a passive energy-absorbing mechanism.

Once the foot is on the ground, progressive external rotation occurs, probably initiated by the contralateral swinging limb, which rotates the pelvis forward, imparting a certain degree of external rotation to the stance limb. This external rotation subsequently is passed from the pelvis distally to the femur and tibia and across the ankle joint and is translated by the subtalar joint into inversion, which reaches its maximum

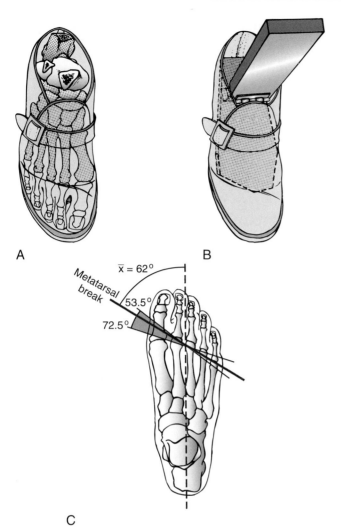

Figure 1–26 Diagram of location of oblique metatarsophalangeal crease. **A,** Skeletal foot in shoe. **B,** Wooden mechanism in shoe. **C,** Variations in the metatarsal break in relation to the longitudinal axis of the foot. x̄, arithmetic mean. (From Isman RE, Inman VT: *Bull Prosthet Res* 10:97, 1969.)

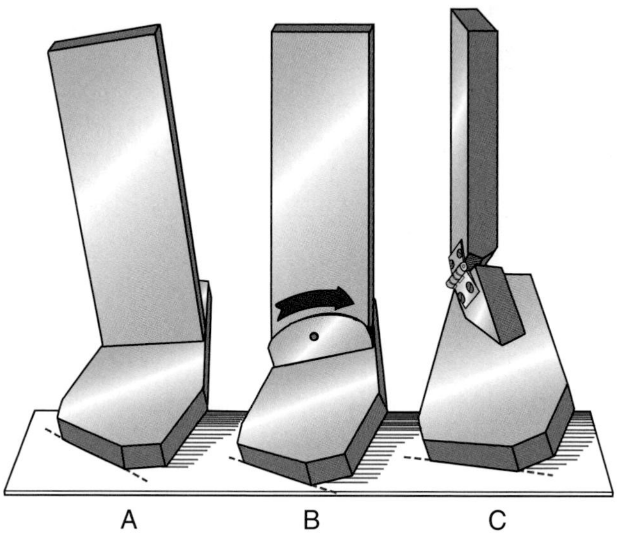

Figure 1–27 Supination and lateral deviation of the foot during raising of the heel caused by an oblique metatarsophalangeal break. **A,** Wooden mechanism without articulation. If no articulation is present, the leg deviates laterally. **B,** Wooden mechanism with articulation. The leg remains vertical; hence some type of articulation must exist between the foot and leg. **C,** Articulation similar to that of the subtalar joint. In addition to its other complex functions, the subtalar joint also functions to permit the leg to remain vertical.

at toe-off. The external rotation is enhanced by the external rotation of the ankle joint axis, the oblique metatarsal break, and the plantar aponeurosis after heel rise begins.

Plantar Aponeurosis

The plantar aponeurosis arises from the tubercle of the calcaneus and passes distally to insert into the base of the proximal phalanx. As the plantar aponeurosis passes the plantar aspect of the metatarsophalangeal joint it combines with the joint capsule to form the plantar plate. The function of the plantar aponeurosis has been described by Hicks,[34] who demonstrated that mechanically it is a windlass mechanism (Fig. 1–30). As the proximal phalanges are dorsiflexed as the body

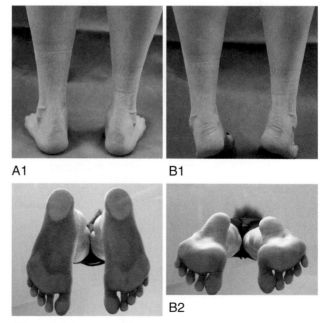

Figure 1–28 Feet and legs of person standing on barograph. **A,** Weight bearing with muscles relaxed. **B,** Rising on toes.

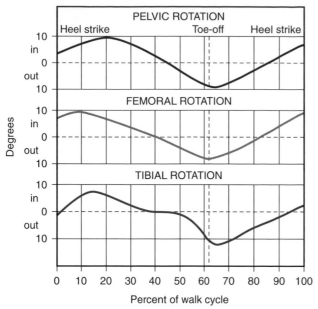

Figure 1–29 Transverse rotation occurring in the lower extremity during walking. Internal rotation occurs until approximately 15% of the cycle, at which time progressive external rotation occurs until toe-off, when internal rotation begins again.

moves across the fixed foot, they pull the plantar aponeurosis over the metatarsal heads, which results in a depression of the metatarsal heads and hence an elevation of the longitudinal arch (Fig. 1–31). This is a somewhat passive mechanism in that no muscle

function per se brings about this stabilizing mechanism, which is the most significant stabilizer of the longitudinal arch. The plantar aponeurosis is most functional on the medial side of the foot, and it becomes less functional as one moves laterally toward the fifth metatarsophalangeal articulation.

In addition to causing elevation of the longitudinal arch, the plantar aponeurosis brings about inversion of the calcaneus, which in turn results in some external rotation of the tibia. This mechanism can be demonstrated clinically by having a person stand and forcing the great toe into dorsiflexion. As this occurs, one observes elevation of the longitudinal arch by the depression of the first metatarsal by the proximal phalanx, and at the same time inversion of the calcaneus. Careful observation of the tibia demonstrates that it externally rotates in response to this calcaneal inversion.

Talonavicular Joint

The talonavicular joint adds stability to the longitudinal arch when force is applied across it during the last half of the stance phase. In the anteroposterior and lateral projections, a circle of differing diameters is noted (Fig. 1–32). When force is applied across a joint of this shape, stability is enhanced. This occurs at toe-off, when the plantar aponeurosis has stabilized the longitudinal arch and most of the body weight is being borne by the forefoot and medial longitudinal arch.

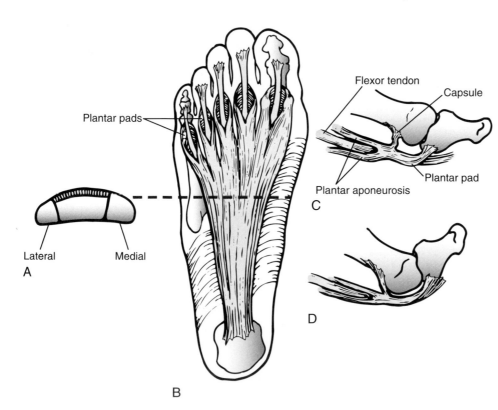

Figure 1–30 Plantar aponeurosis. **A,** Cross section. **B,** Division of the plantar aponeurosis around the flexor tendons. **C,** Components of the plantar pad and its insertion into the base of the proximal phalanx. **D,** Extension of toes draws the plantar pad over the metatarsal head, pushing it into plantar flexion.

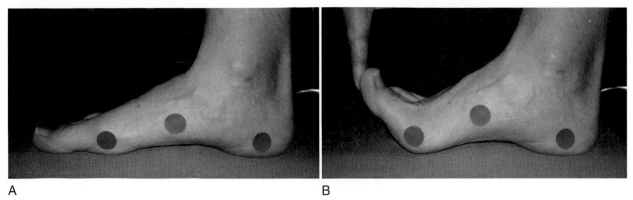

A   **B**

Figure 1–31   Dynamic function of plantar aponeurosis. **A,** Foot at rest. **B,** Dorsiflexion of metatarsophalangeal joints, which activates windlass mechanisms, brings about elevation of the longitudinal arch, plantar flexion of the metatarsal heads, and inversion of the heel.

The talonavicular joint enhances the stability of the longitudinal arch.

Ligaments of the Ankle Joint

The configuration and alignment of the ligamentous structures of the ankle are such that they permit free movement of the ankle and subtalar joints to occur simultaneously. Because the configuration of the trochlear surface of the talus is curved in such a manner as to produce a cone-shaped articulation whose apex is directed medially, the single fan-shaped deltoid ligament is adequate to provide stability to the medial side of the ankle joint (Fig. 1–33). On the

lateral aspect of the ankle joint, however, where there is a larger area to be covered by a ligamentous structure, the ligament is divided into three bands: the anterior and posterior talofibular ligaments and the calcaneofibular ligament. The relationship of these ligaments to each other and to the axes of the subtalar and ankle joints must always be considered carefully when these joints are examined or ligament surgery is contemplated.

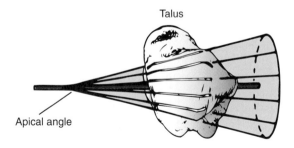

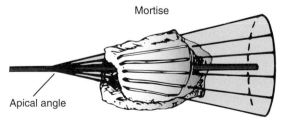

Figure 1–33   Curvature of the trochlear surface of the talus creates a cone whose apex is based medially. From this configuration one can observe that the deltoid ligament is well suited to function along the medial side of the ankle joint, whereas laterally, where more rotation occurs, three separate ligaments are necessary. (From Inman VT: *The Joints of the Ankle.* Baltimore, Williams & Wilkins, 1976.)

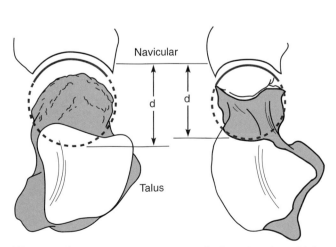

Figure 1–32   Talonavicular joint. *Left,* Anterior view. *Right,* Lateral view. Relationship of the head of the talus to the navicular bone shows differing diameters (d) of the head of the talus. (From Mann RA: In Nicholas JA, Hershman EB [eds]: *The Lower Extremity and Spine in Sports Medicine,* ed 2. St Louis, Mosby, 1995.)

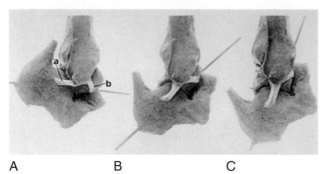

A   B   C

Figure 1–34 The calcaneal fibular ligament (a) and anterior talofibular ligament (b). **A,** In plantar flexion, the anterior talofibular ligament is in line with the fibula and is providing most of the support to the lateral aspect of the ankle joint. **B,** In neutral position of the ankle joint, both the anterior talofibular and calcaneofibular ligaments provide support to the joint. The relationship of the calcaneofibular ligament to the subtalar joint axis, depicted in the background, is noted. Note that this ligament and the axis are parallel to each other. **C,** In dorsiflexion, the calcaneofibular ligament is in line with the fibula and provides support to the lateral aspect of the ankle joint. (From Inman VT: *The Joints of the Ankle.* Baltimore, Williams & Wilkins, 1976.)

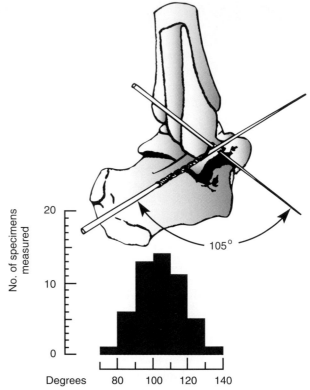

Figure 1–35 Average angle between the calcaneofibular and talofibular ligaments in the sagittal plane. Although the average angle is 105 degrees, there is considerable variation, from 70 to 140 degrees. (From Inman VT: *The Joints of the Ankle.* Baltimore, Williams & Wilkins, 1976.)

Figure 1–34 demonstrates the anterior talofibular and calcaneofibular ligaments in relation to the subtalar joint axis. The calcaneofibular ligament is parallel to the subtalar joint axis in the sagittal plane. As the ankle joint is dorsiflexed and plantar flexed, this relationship between the calcaneofibular ligament and the subtalar joint axis does not change. Furthermore, the calcaneofibular ligament crosses both the ankle and the subtalar joint. Construction of this ligament permits motion to occur in both of these joints simultaneously.

It is important to appreciate that when the ankle joint is in neutral position the calcaneofibular ligament is angulated posteriorly, but as the ankle joint is brought into more dorsiflexion the calcaneofibular ligament is brought into line with the fibula, thereby becoming a true collateral ligament. Conversely, as the ankle joint is brought into plantar flexion the calcaneofibular ligament becomes horizontal (parallel) to the ground. In this position it provides little or no stability insofar as resisting inversion stress. The anterior talofibular ligament, on the other hand, is brought into line with the fibula when the ankle joint is plantar flexed, thereby acting as a collateral ligament. When the ankle joint is brought up into dorsiflexion, the anterior talofibular ligament becomes sufficiently horizontal that it does not function as a collateral ligament. Therefore, depending on the position of the ankle joint, either the calcaneofibular or the anterior talofibular ligament will be a true collateral ligament

with regard to providing stability to the lateral side of the ankle joint.

The relationship between these two ligaments has been quantified and is presented in Figure 1–35. This demonstrates the relationship of the angle produced by the calcaneofibular and the anterior talofibular ligaments to one another. The average angle in the sagittal plane is approximately 105 degrees, although there is considerable variation, from 70 to 140 degrees. This is important because from a clinical standpoint it probably explains why some persons have lax collateral ligaments. If we assume that when the ankle is in full dorsiflexion the calcaneofibular ligament provides most of the stability and that in full plantar flexion the anterior talofibular ligament provides stability, then as we pass from dorsiflexion to plantar flexion and back there will be a certain period in which neither ligament is functioning as a true collateral ligament. If we assume there is an average angle of approximately 105 degrees between these ligaments, then generally speaking, an area in which an insufficient lateral collateral ligament is present is unusual; however, if we have angulation of 130 to 140 degrees between these two ligaments, there is a significant interval while the ankle is passing from dorsiflexion to plantar flexion and back in which neither ligament is functioning as a collateral ligament. This may explain why some persons are susceptible to chronic ankle sprains. Some patients who are thought to have ligamentous laxity may in reality possess this anatomic configuration of lateral collateral ligaments.

The other factor that needs to be considered is the relationship of the calcaneofibular ligament to subtalar joint motion. Motion in the subtalar joint occurs about an axis that deviates from medial to lateral as it passes from dorsal to plantarward direction. Figure 1–36 demonstrates the position of the subtalar joint axis in relation to a cadaver specimen. If a probe is placed along the calcaneofibular ligament, it is noted that a V-shaped or cone-shaped arc has been created. This cone-shaped arc of motion permits the calcaneofibular ligament to move in such a way as to prevent restriction of subtalar joint or ankle joint motion (Fig. 1–37). This relationship of the calcaneofibular ligament to the ankle and subtalar joint axes is critical when contemplating ligamentous reconstruction, because any ligament reconstruction that fails to take this normal anatomic configuration into consideration results in a situation in which motion in one or both of these joints is restricted.

From a clinical standpoint, when one is evaluating the stability of the lateral collateral ligament structure,

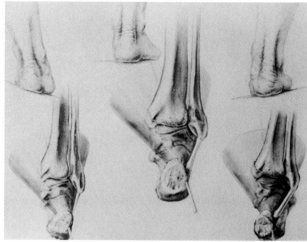

Figure 1–37 Functional arrangement of the calcaneofibular ligament. The drawing represents the concept that explains the mechanism in which free motion is permitted in the subtalar joint without restriction by the calcaneofibular ligament. An imaginary cone has been drawn around the axis of the subtalar joint. The calcaneofibular ligament is shown converging from its fibular attachment to the calcaneus. Because the ligament lies on the surface of the cone, whose apex is the point of intersection of the functional extensions of the ligament and the axis of the subtalar joint, motion of the calcaneus under the talus is allowed without undue restriction from the ligament, which is merely displaced over the surface of the cone. (From Inman VT: *The Joints of the Ankle.* Baltimore, Williams & Wilkins, 1976.)

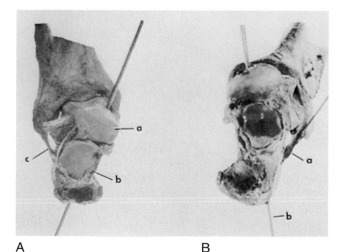

A   B

Figure 1–36 A, Anterior view of the transverse tarsal joint. Head of talus (a); head of calcaneus (b); calcaneofibular ligament (c). Rod passing through the head of the talus and exiting on the lateral aspect of the calcaneus demonstrates the axis of the subtalar joint. **B,** The same specimen viewed from below. A Kirschner wire has now been placed through the fibers of the calcaneofibular ligament (a). Note the direction of the ligament extending from the malleolus to the lateral side of the calcaneus. (From Inman VT: *The Joints of the Ankle.* Baltimore, Williams & Wilkins, 1976.)

the ankle joint should be tested in dorsiflexion to demonstrate the competency of the calcaneofibular ligament and in plantar flexion to test the competency of the anterior talofibular ligament. If both ligaments are completely disrupted, there will be no stability in either position. Furthermore, to test for stability of the anterior talofibular ligament, the anterior drawer sign should be elicited, with the ankle joint in neutral position, when the anterior talofibular ligament is in a position to resist anterior displacement of the talus from the ankle mortise (Fig. 1–38).

MECHANICS OF RUNNING

With increased attention being given to athletics in general and to running in particular, it is essential that the physician have a basic knowledge of the mechanics that occur during running. The same basic mechanisms that have been described for the biomechanics of the foot and ankle are not significantly altered during running. The same stabilization mechanism within the foot occurs during running as during walking.

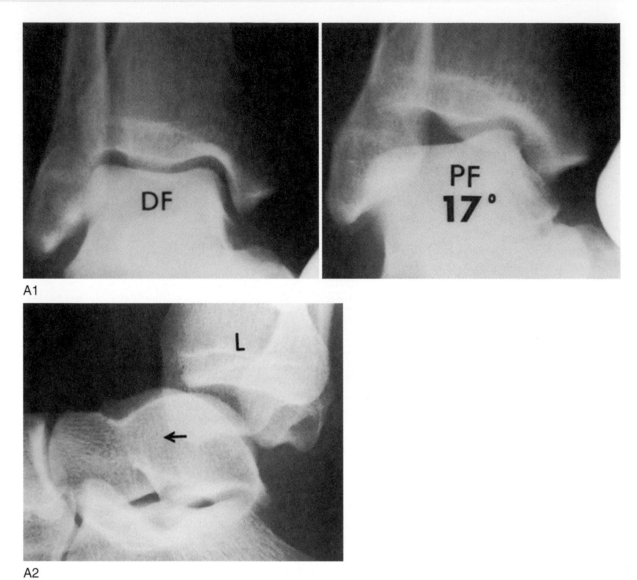

Figure 1–38 **A1,** *Left,* Stress x-ray film of ankle in dorsiflexion (DF) demonstrates no instability in the calcaneofibular ligament. *Right,* The same ankle stressed in plantar flexion (PF) demonstrates loss of stability caused by disruption of the anterior talofibular ligament. **A2,** Note the anterior subluxation present when this ligament (L) is torn *(arrow)* (anterior drawer sign).

The major differences observed during running are that the gait cycle is altered considerably; the amount of force generated, as measured by force plate data, is markedly increased; the range of motion of the joints of the lower extremities is increased; and the phasic activity of the muscles of the lower extremities is altered. The changes that occur in the gait cycle are illustrated in Figure 1–39. During walking, one foot is always in contact with the ground; as the speed of gait increases, a float phase is incorporated into the gait cycle, during which both feet are off the ground. There also is no longer a period of double limb support. As the speed of gait continues to increase, the time the foot spends on the ground, both in real time and in percentage of cycle, decreases considerably.

The forces involved during running are considerable (see Fig. 1–9). Displacement of the center of gravity increases as the speed of gait increases, and the forces generated are in large part related to this. The main function of the body at initial ground contact is absorption of these forces. This is carried out by increasing the range of motion at the ankle, knee, and hip joints. As the speed of gait further increases, the degree of motion in these joints also increases to help absorb the added impact.

Along with this increase in the range of motion and in the forces generated during running, the muscle function in the lower extremity also is altered. In general, in real time the phasic activity of most muscles is decreased; however, when considered as a percent-

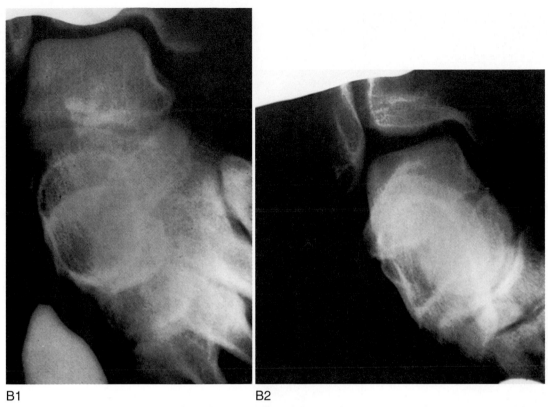

B1   B2

Figure 1–38—cont'd   B, *Left,* Stress x-ray film of ankle in plantar flexion demonstrates no ligamentous instability. *Right,* The same ankle stressed in dorsiflexion demonstrates laxity of calcaneofibular ligament.   *Continued*

age of the gait cycle, the period of activity of these muscles is increased considerably. Generally speaking, at initial ground contact the majority of the muscles about the hip, knee, and ankle joints are active, and their period of activity, which begins during the late float phase, increases as the speed of gait increases. This is probably related to the rapid motion required by these joints in preparation for the impact of ground contact. During walking there is adequate time for most of the preparation for ground contact to be carried out rather passively, but with the markedly increased range and speed of motion of these joints during running, muscle function plays a more active role.

Looking briefly at the events that occur at the ankle joint when comparing walking with jogging or running, one notes the progressive decrease in the cycle time from 1 second to 0.6 second (see Fig. 1–17). The magnitude of total range of motion increases from 30 degrees during walking to 45 degrees during running. This motion occurs during 0.6 second for walking and 0.2 second for running. The direction of motion also changes: During walking, plantar flexion occurs at heel strike, whereas during jogging and running there is progressive dorsiflexion. Rapid plantar

flexion occurs at toe-off during all speeds of gait. As the speed of gait increases, the muscle function in the posterior calf group changes significantly. During walking the posterior calf group functions in stance phase, and during jogging and running it performs in late swing phase; its activity is ongoing from the time of initial ground contact through most of the stance phase. The muscle group controls the ankle dorsiflexion that occurs after initial ground contact, the forward movement of the tibia, and brings about plantar flexion of the ankle joint. Similar changes in both the magnitude of motion and muscle function occur about the hip and knee joint as well.

Briefly stated, what occurs biomechanically during running is that the stance phase is diminished from approximately 0.6 second while walking to 0.2 second while sprinting. During this brief period of stance phase the forces involved in the vertical plane are increased to two and one half to three times body weight. The range of motion of the joints is increased approximately 50%, and the muscles in the lower extremity are called on to bring about and control these motions over a short time when measured in real time but over a considerable period when expressed as percentage of the gait cycle. It is probably because of

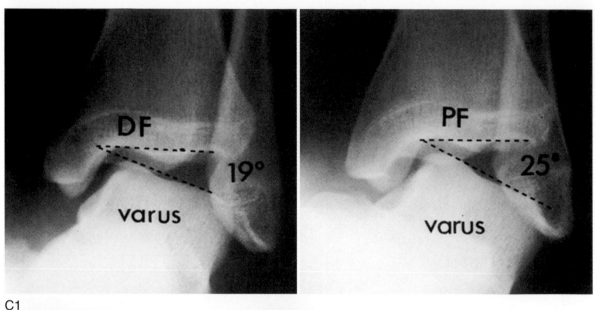

C1

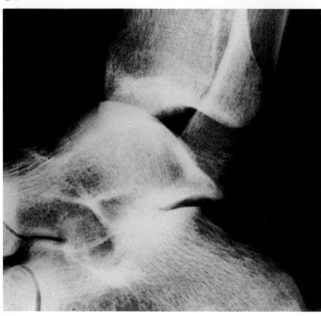

C2

Figure 1–38—cont'd   C1, Stress x-ray films of ankle joint in dorsiflexion *(left)*, plantar flexion *(right)*, and anteriorly **(C2)** all demonstrate evidence of ligamentous disruption. This indicates a complete tear of the lateral collateral ligament structure.

the previously mentioned factors and the repetitive nature of the sport that injuries occur during running.

PLANTAR PRESSURE AND FORCE MEASUREMENTS

Studying the foot's interaction with the ground has a long history ranging from examining footprints in soil to real-time mapping of plantar pressure under natural conditions. Investigation of the pressures experienced by the various regions of the plantar foot has provided insight into the pathogenesis and treatment of many foot and ankle disorders. Assessment of the forces and torques imparted by the ground on the lower extremity has illuminated the biomechanical processes at work during gait.

Plantar pressure and ground reaction force measurements are well established in the research realm and have been instrumental in refining our understanding of foot and ankle biomechanics. In conjunction with other technology, including high-speed

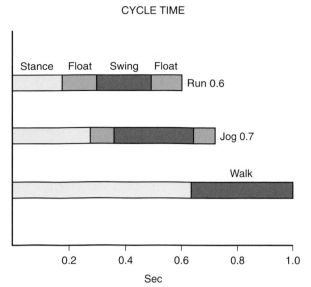

CYCLE TIME

Figure 1–39 Variations in the gait cycle for running, jogging, and walking. Note that as the speed of the gait increases, the stance phase decreases. In this illustration, the subject is walking 1 mile per 16 minutes, jogging about 1 mile per 9 minutes, and running about 1 mile per 5 minutes.

cameras, video motion-sensing equipment, electrogoniometers, and electromyography (EMG) devices, the study of the ground–foot interface has aided the understanding of gait kinetics and kinematics. Unfortunately, a large number of measurement systems and an equally large number of data-analysis techniques have clouded the useful data that have been obtained.

Despite improvements in available measurement methods, practical collection of clinically novel information remains difficult. While confirmation of areas of excess pressure and monitoring the effects of treatment may prove useful, there is little specificity between plantar pressure patterns and clinical syndromes. The wide variability of normal measures makes clinical comparisons difficult.

Types of Studies

A variety of measurement techniques have been used to study the interaction of the foot with the ground. Direct measurement techniques rely on physical properties or electronic transducers to translate the interaction between the foot and the ground into a measurable quantity. Over time, their precision, spatial resolution, responsiveness, flexibility, and ease of use have all improved. A number of temporal and spatial parameters can be measured and analyzed in tabular or graphic formats. The cost of these systems varies considerably based on factors such as the type of measurement made; size of the measurement platform;

density, precision, and speed of measurement cells; and the computational power of associated equipment. Indirect techniques rely on correlating other measurable gait parameters to plantar characteristics and offer the advantage of not relying on expensive and often bulky equipment. For example, an estimation of ground reaction force can be made based on a simple-to-measure temporal variable, foot–ground contact time.[15]

Several direct measurement systems are available that use a variety of strategies to record plantar pressure or ground reaction force. Two factors to consider are the ability of a system to temporally record over a gait cycle versus statically summarize a gait cycle into one measurement, and the ability to spatially distinguish regions of the foot versus average the forces distributed across the whole foot. Unfortunately, results obtained with different systems under similar conditions are not always similar, and even qualitative comparisons might not be appropriate.[42] Different measurement resolutions and sample rates affect the ability of a system to record true peak plantar pressures and to isolate particular areas under the foot. Understanding of the strengths of different measurement strategies is critical when assessing a study's validity.

Physical Transduction

The earliest methods relied on physical properties of various materials to capture the interaction of the foot with the ground. Casts of the foot in clay, plaster, or soil were used with the assumption that areas of deeper penetration represented areas of highest pressure.[11,25] Rubber mats incorporating longitudinal ridges[59] or pyramidal projections[25] used the elastic property of rubber to improve on these techniques (Fig. 1–40). When stood on or walked on, the rubber ridges or projections distort in proportion to the applied pressure.

This technique gained widespread use when Harris and Beath, in 1947, described a modification of the technique that is still used for a variety of clinical and research applications. The modification uses a mat composed of a three-level grid, with the deeper levels more finely gradated. The grid is coated with a thin layer of ink and covered with paper. When the subject stands or takes a step onto the mat, areas of higher pressure transfer ink from the more finely gradated grids, and light pressure only prints on the widely spaced ridges. The resulting footprint shows the distribution of plantar pressure exerted by the foot. Advantages of this system include its ease of use, speed, low cost, and portability. Disadvantages include low measurement resolution (0.27 to 4.8 kg/cm^2 in seven steps)[73] and lack of a temporal component of the measurement. Despite these limitations, numerous

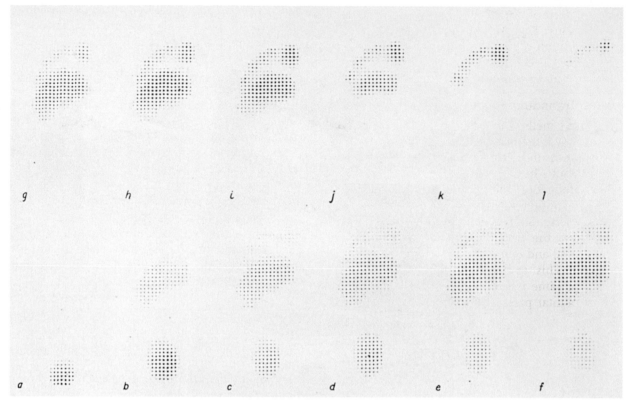

Figure 1–40 Pressure distribution on plantar aspect of foot during walking as demonstrated by use of a barograph. As dots get larger and denser, pressure distribution is greater. (From Elftman H: *Anat Rev* 59:481, 1934.)

clinical studies have been based on the Harris–Beath mat for a variety of clinical conditions including metatarsalgia,[73,87] posterior tibial tendon dysfunction,[58,90] hallus rigidus,[21] pes planus,[80] hallux valgus correction,[17] and changing plantar pressure patterns in youth[85] and the elderly.[44]

Optically Based Systems

Optically based systems rely on visualizing the plantar aspect of the foot during stance or gait. The simplest allows observation or photographic recording of the plantar foot during stance or gait through a clear platform (see Fig. 1–28). This provides an accurate, dynamic, qualitative representation of foot morphology. Addition of a rubber mat device between the foot and glass plate allows some quantification of the regionalized plantar pressures experienced by the foot and adds the temporal component missed using an ink-and-paper–based mat system.[25]

A further refinement is the pedobarograph, which relies on the pressure-sensitive diffraction properties of a thin plastic sheet placed over the clear plate.[4] The sheet is illuminated at the edges, allowing the light to reflect within the plastic. Pressure on the plastic distorts the light in proportion to the pressure applied and allows it to come through the glass plate beneath.

The images are recorded and digitized to quantify the data. The system is calibrated with reference force transducers placed at the edges of the platform. This provides a spatial resolution and temporal responsiveness not found with the Harris–Beath mat. However, slow responsiveness at high forces can bias results.[40]

Force Plate

The force transducers used to calibrate the pedobarograph can be configured in orthogonal planes at the corners of a section of floor, creating a force plate. A force plate measures the ground reaction force, that is, the force exerted by the ground on the foot in three degrees of freedom (vertical force, forward shear, side shear) and allows calculation of the torques around the foot and ankle (axial torque, sagittal torque, coronal torque). The resulting data are measured over the gait cycle and provide a representation of the average forces experienced by the foot. (see Fig. 1–8)

This type of measurement has been useful in describing whole body kinematics with pedal forces such as the torques about the ankle, knee, and hip throughout the gait cycle. One advantage of this type of system is that shear forces and torques can be measured in addition to vertical force. The limitations include the lack of ability to map specific regions of plantar pressure. This limitation can be circumvented with the addition of an optical diffraction system to the force plate, as described above, or with a series of smaller force plates placed in tandem.[78]

Pressure Transducer Array

A more direct method of measuring plantar pressure has evolved over the last 40 years that relies on transducers that measure electronic parameters based on an applied pressure. Initially, they were placed on strategic points of the foot. The size of these transducers has shrunk to the point that an array can be created to map the pressures exerted by the foot during stance or gait. The data from the array are sampled over time, providing a spatial and temporal map of plantar pressure (Fig. 1–41). This technologic improvement allows study of the same issues that prompted the earliest studies of plantar pressure with more refined, objective data.[59,66]

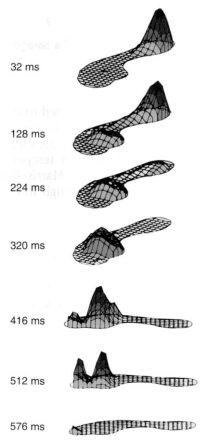

32 ms

128 ms

224 ms

320 ms

416 ms

512 ms

576 ms

Figure 1–41 Pressure distribution under bare foot during walking. Height of display above ground is proportional to pressure. ms, milliseconds. (From Clarke TE: *The Pressure Distribution under the Foot during Barefoot Walking* [doctoral dissertation]. University Park, Penn, Pennsylvania State University, 1980.)

Many of these systems use a floor mat or platform built into the floor with a grid of pressure-sensitive transducers that can measure the pressure applied during gait. Subjects typically walk barefoot down a short runway timed such that one foot strikes the mat in stride. In this way, natural gait is recorded. An alternative is to place a thin film containing a pressure transduction array into a shoe. In this way, the plantar pressures experienced by the foot can be measured in a wider variety of settings and under multiple impacts and can account for the effect of shoe wear as well.[47,86] For example, feet experience 10% to 50% higher plantar pressures in a flat flexible shoe compared to a soft shoe with a firm rubber sole.[67] The floor mat and in-shoe methods correlate well when the patient wears a shoe with a firm sole or goes barefoot.[8]

A number of system-specific and analysis-dependent factors affect the results of pressure transducer array measurements. Pressure transducer density, responsiveness, linearity, and resolution and the range of the transducers all affect the measurements. Methods of analyzing the data also differ, including reporting results as force or pressure, reporting results as peak values or sum of values over time, and strategies of regionalizing the foot's plantar surface.

The density of pressure transducers is important when defining areas of study on the foot. Relatively higher density allows for better spatial representation of plantar pressure, whereas systems with relatively lower transducer density can underestimate measurements such as peak pressure because the true peak can be missed. The transducer resolution affects the precision of the measurement, that is, how well the system is able to differentiate between small changes in pressure. Some transducers have a nonlinear response at the extremes of their measurable range or have a low-level cutoff. These can affect results during extreme measurement conditions or measurements that summate the pressure experienced by a region of the foot. The sample rate affects contact time measurements. Low sample rates can underestimate peak pressure measurements because the true peak pressure might be missed.

Data Representations

Output from the different measurement systems reflects the nature of their measurement mechanisms. The force plate reports a true ground reaction force. The Harris mat reports pedal pressure but does not vary with time. The optical systems and the transduction arrays each report pedal pressure that varies with time. The data measured by these systems are subject to the sensor density, resolution, and sample rate limitations discussed above. In order to simplify the abundant amount of information the data provide and to allow comparisons between subjects or after treatments, parameters have been defined based on these data. Not all systems or measurement methods are able to derive all of these measurements.

The ground reaction force is a vector quantity that varies temporally and spatially over the gait cycle and that represents the average reciprocal force exerted by the floor in response to the foot. It has a magnitude and direction, and the starting point can be projected onto a representation of the plantar foot at the point of average maximum vertical force (see Figs. 1–10 to 1–12). The ground reaction force can be deconstructed into many components. The vertical ground reaction force represents the force of the ground pushing upward on the foot. It typically has two peaks separated by a valley. The first peak occurs as the body weight is transferred from dual to single leg stance, and the second occurs as the body weight moves forward over the metatarsal heads. Other components include anterior–posterior shear and medial–lateral shear. The fore–aft torque, side–side torque, and axial torque around a joint can be calculated from these measurements and knowledge of the joint's position relative to the force plate. Studies of ground reaction forces may focus on the magnitude of one or the other peak or the timing of the peaks and valleys. The vertical component of ground reaction force can be calculated from systems that measure plantar pressure for the whole foot or for defined regions of the foot.[84]

Another frequently reported measurement is the maximum pressure recorded, or peak pressure. It is usually reported over a spatially subdivided map of the plantar foot. Peak pressure for areas such as the heel, individual or grouped metatarsal heads, and toes are common. Alternatively, peak pressure can be reported as a temporally varying measure by displaying its location and magnitude on a diagram of the foot. Peak force can be calculated from peak pressure because the size of the pressure transducers is known.

Timing measurements can also be made. The intervals from heel strike to metatarsal strike, toe strike, heel-off, metatarsal-off, and toe-off can be calculated. The pressure•time integral, or impulse, for the whole foot or defined regions can be calculated. This may be standardized for each region as a percentage of the total impulse for a given foot. The impulse might characterize plantar loading better than peak pressure by taking both pressure and time into consideration.

Finally, the pattern of plantar loading can be categorized based on the pressure measurements. Patients can tend to load the medial ray, the medial and central rays, the central rays, or the central and lateral rays.[39] Put another way, there is an inverse relationship between peak pressure under the first metatarsal head

and toe relative to peak pressure under the lesser metatarsal heads.[29] As walking speed increases, forefoot pressure is medialized such that peak pressure increases under the first metatarsal head and decreases under the lesser metatarsal heads.[68]

Measurement Variability

Many sources of variability affect the results of these measurements. Separating important clinical or research findings from differences based on testing apparatus, measurement methodology, patient demographic factors, or analysis methodology requires an understanding of how these factors affect the measured results. Differences between the different testing apparatus have been described above. Other sources of variability can be divided into methodology, analysis, and patient-specific factors.

Methodology Factors

Walking speed affects the magnitude of plantar pressures during gait. Velocity is linearly related to peak vertical and fore–aft ground reaction forces[3,62] and inversely related to the pressure•time integral.[91] As velocity increases, peak pressures in the heel, medial metatarsal heads, and the first toe increase while peak pressure in the fifth metatarsal head decreases.[43,68] This medialization may be related to increased magnitude and velocity of hindfoot eversion and medial shear force at heel strike with increased walking speed. Timing measurements also change with increasing speed. The normalized time to peak pressure is decreased in the heel but unchanged in the midfoot and forefoot, suggesting the rollover process is mainly accelerated by reducing the time from heelstrike to foot flat.[68]

To minimize variability introduced due to walking speed, some researchers have subjects walk at a fixed rate and others have subjects walk at their natural pace. Subjects can be trained to walk at a given speed using a metronome.[91] However, this might not be a reliable method of regulating speed.[43] Alternatively, measurements made when subjects are asked to walk at their most comfortable rate are reproducible but make comparisons between subjects difficult.[42]

Deviations from a normal gait pattern can occur if the subject has to take a long or short stride in an effort to place the foot in the appropriate measurement area of floor-based systems. To minimize this effect, the measurement platform is placed flush with the floor and hidden from the subject with a thin, uniform floor covering. The traditional midgait method is then to have subjects walk a predetermined distance taking numerous steps before having a foot step on the platform. This results in a reproducible gait but requires a large space to allow adequate lead-up to the platform. Shorter lead-ups have been studied to try to limit the distance a subject has to walk before measurements are made. A three-step or two-step lead-up is as reproducible as the midgait methods, but a one-step lead-up is not adequate.[18,61]

Variability of the measurements also depends on the reproducibility of a normal gait. Even when using one system of measurement, the methods by which these measurements are made affect the results. For example, plantar pressures measured when standing differ from pressures measured during gait.[11] Both have clinical or research interest depending on the questions being asked. Variations in walking patterns, such as a shuffling gait, alter the peak forces on the foot.[92] Gait pattern alteration can be seen in certain conditions such as after ankle fracture fixation or with concurrent knee disorder.[3,9]

Drift and calibration of the measurement systems affect the variability of measurements. Plantar pressure measurement systems need to be calibrated to known standards to allow comparisons between different studies using different systems. Transducer output varies between different transducers, with temperature, when an in-shoe system is removed and reinserted, and with the number of trials performed. Pressure can vary by as much as 20% with repeated measurements on the same insert.[67] When compared to ground-based force plate systems, thin film transducers systems were found to be linearly related but have an offset that drifts with time.[61] The measurements may be adequate for relative ranking purposes but need repeated calibration with a fixed system if accurate values are required, such as for threshold measurements of plantar pressure.

Analysis Factors

Variability is also introduced in the methods by which the acquired data are analyzed. A number of frequently used measurements have been described earlier, including peak pressure. Peak pressure can be reported for the whole surface of the foot during a gait cycle, but its clinical utility is limited because different regions of the foot experience different plantar pressures during the gait cycle. Whole-foot measurements can be used as a method of calculating ground reaction force.

Subdividing the regions of the plantar foot and recording peak pressures in each of these areas over the gait cycle provides more meaningful data. The heel is often represented as a single region but may be subdivided into medial, central, and lateral regions.[68] Midfoot peak pressures are less informative in normal gait as the weight transfers rapidly from the hindfoot to the forefoot, but it can be useful in pathologic

conditions such as rocker-bottom deformity. Study of the distribution of pressure through the midfoot can classify foot morphology into planus, normal, and cavus categories.[68] The base of the fifth metatarsal can be included as part of the midfoot or can be identified as a separate pressure zone. Measurement of forefoot pressures is helpful for defining normal biomechanics and studying abnormal conditions.[29,41] Improvements in sensor technology have allowed isolation of individual metatarsal heads and toes for plantar pressure measurement. Older studies often grouped the metatarsal heads, a practice that might have led to erroneous conclusions.

How these regions are defined affects the results. The definition of these regions (masks) is still a manual process and is repeated for each trial. Having a single person define the regions can decrease variability.[41] Older systems did not have adequate resolution to pick out each metatarsal head. With improvements in transducer density and software strategies to improve repeatability of definition of regions, multiple distinct regions can be mapped and studied.

Subject-Specific Factors

Subject-specific characteristics can also introduce variability. Factors such as the patient's age, ethnicity, side dominance, and body weight can affect plantar pressure characteristics. Children's feet have a dramatically different loading pattern and lower peak pressure due to high relative foot area (Fig. 1–42).[31] Differences in joint mobility and forefoot pressure based on a subject's ethnicity have been shown in patients with diabetic neuropathy.[81] The patient's dominant side can experience greater static and dynamic vertical force,[47] although others have found no side dominance.[33] Similarly, there is an inverse correlation between sides such that if one side has higher overall forces, the other will have lower forces.

Foot morphology also affects plantar pressure. Cavus feet have different midfoot loading characteristics and hindfoot eversion extent and velocity than flatfeet.[68] During running, fatigued subjects tend to have decreased step time, decreased peak and integral force and pressure under the heel, and medialization of forces.[86] After a hindfoot fusion, greater contact force at heel strike has been observed.[50,76] This could be due to the inability of the calcaneus to move into a valgus position after heel strike.[2]

The effect of body weight on plantar pressure is less direct than might be expected. Whereas some studies have correlated maximum vertical force during gait and body weight,[47] many other studies found little correlation.[30,31,39] In children, the correlation of body weight to peak plantar pressures is clear and plays a greater role in determining peak pressure than in

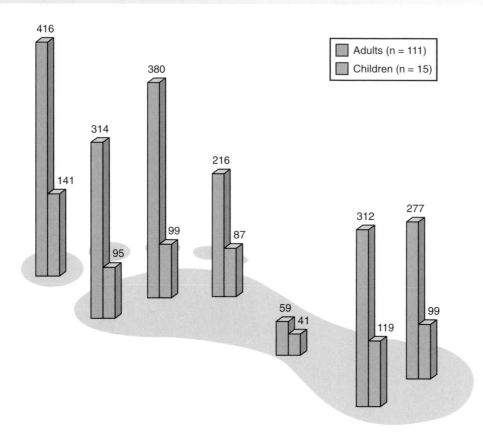

416
380
314
141
216
99
95
87
59
41
312
277
119
99

Adults (n = 111)
Children (n = 15)

Figure 1–42 Peak pressure values (in KPA) under selected foot regions demonstrate impact in the heel region, minimal weight bearing in the midfoot, buildup of pressure beneath the metatarsal heads, and most important, transfer of weight to the great toe region. (From Hennig EM, Rosenbaum D: *Foot Ankle* 11:306-311, 1991.)

adults.[31,39] The area of peak pressure most highly correlated with body weight in children and adults is the fourth metatarsal head[39] and in adults is the midfoot.[31]

Individual persons load the foot in different spatial patterns during gait. After heel strike, the forefoot can be loaded more medially or laterally across the metatarsal heads and can load the metatarsals and toes simultaneously or in turn. Various classification systems have been proposed to group these types of loading, and biomechanical theories have been proposed to explain the different loading patterns.[39,41,84]

Finally, there is an inherent variability in a person's gait from step to step that ranges from less than 1% for vertical ground reaction force to much higher for timing dependent variables and values calculated as a product of measures.[33] Measured values can vary by more than 10% under identical testing conditions. A strategy of taking an average of multiple trials has been used to reduce the variability.[42] Averaging data from as few as three trials improves the reliability of the measurement.[43]

Clinical Correlations

Research studies based on plantar pressure measurements have added to our understanding of gait

biomechanics. Unfortunately, clinical application of this technology has lagged behind. A number of clinically relevant areas of study have emerged that provide useful information for practitioners.

Hallux Valgus

Patients with hallux valgus often have pain under the lesser metatarsal heads as part of their clinical presentation. A variety of theories have been proposed to explain this finding. Plantar pressure measurements have helped to demonstrate the disorder associated with hallux valgus as well as the resolution of this disorder after surgical correction.

A number of studies in patients with hallux valgus have shown a relation between metatarsalgia under the second metatarsal head and increased plantar pressure in this region. Compared to normal feet, patients with hallux valgus have increased plantar pressure under the lesser metatarsal heads and decreased plantar pressure under the first toe.[13,45] In a large group of subjects with hallux valgus, those with lesser toe metatarsalgia have greater peak pressure and peak pressure•time integral under the second through fifth metatarsal heads than those without metatarsalgia.[82] A pressure cutoff was established such that no patients with less than 20 N/cm² peak pressure had metatarsalgia and all patients with more than 70 N/cm² peak pressure had metatarsalgia. A transfer of peak pressure from the medial to lateral forefoot could be shown from the nonmetatarsalgia to metatarsalgia groups. There is a correlation between the first to second intermetatarsal angle and the plantar pressure under the second and third metatarsal heads such that the greater the intermetatarsal angle, the higher the peak pressures under the lesser metatarsal heads.[89]

Studies of plantar pressure after hallux valgus correction have also shown clinical utility. Comparisons of Keller resection arthroplasty and first metatarsophalangeal joint fusion showed decreased weight-bearing ability of the first toe after Keller resection and correlated the degree of postoperative metatarsalgia under the lesser metatarsal heads with the ability to bear weight on the first toe after fusion.[24,32,45,77] One study of a distal chevron osteotomy for mild to moderate hallux valgus found increased pressure under the second and third metatarsal heads.[51] However, this result can be explained by another study that correlated the degree of plantar displacement of the distal first metatarsal osteotomy to the degree of increased pressure under the first metatarsal head and to a decrease in clinical metatarsalgia.[83] Finally, proximal first metatarsal osteotomy and distal soft tissue procedure for hallux valgus has been shown to decrease peak pressure under the second and third metatarsal head.[89] A study by Beverly et al[12] of patients who had undergone silicone (Silastic) arthroplasty of the hallux demonstrated a decrease of 46% in the peak load transmitted by the hallux and an increase of 65% in the peak load beneath the second and third metatarsal heads. The peak pressure beneath the first metatarsal head fell by 23% (Fig. 1–43). Careful observation of these data demonstrates the importance of maintaining the function of the first metatarsophalangeal joint when planning surgical procedures about the hallux. Procedures that destabilize the first metatarsophalangeal joint result in significant alteration of the weight-bearing pattern.

Forefoot Pressure

Forefoot pressures without hallux valgus have also been studied in the context of metatarsalgia. A soft pad placed proximal to the metatarsal heads decreases metatarsal head pressure between 12% and 60%.[38] The effect of a heel wedge on forefoot pressure can affect clinical metatarsalgia. Placement of a half-inch lateral heel wedge decreased pressure under the third through fifth metatarsal heads by 24% and increased pressure under the first and second metatarsal heads by 21%.[67] A half-inch medial heel wedge decreased the pressure under the first and second metatarsal heads by 28% and under the first toe by 31%. Ground contact time was unchanged.

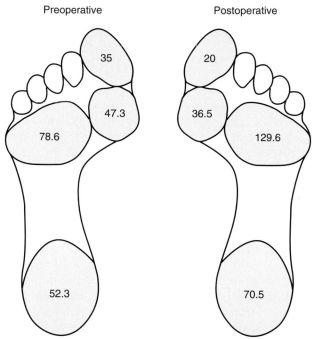

Preoperative | Postoperative

Figure 1–43 Peak forces (in newtons) measured in four areas of the foot. Preoperatively there is significant weight bearing by the first metatarsal and the great toe relative to lateral metatarsals. Postoperatively (silicone arthroplasty of first metatarsophalangeal joint) there is decreased weight bearing by the first metatarsal and the great toe and increased weight bearing beneath the lesser metatarsal head region. This demonstrates the effect of loss of the windlass mechanism, by which pressure is transferred to the great toe, which in turn depresses the first metatarsal head. (From Beverly MC, Horan FT, Hutton WC: *Int Orthop* 9:101-104, 1985.)

Forefoot pressure is also important in development of neuropathic forefoot ulcers. Plantar forefoot pressure is increased in patients with neuropathic ulcers and Charcot joint changes relative to normal and neuropathic nonulcerated feet.[5] In the diabetic and neuropathic foot, areas of ulceration correlate well with the areas demonstrating maximum vertical and shear forces.[63] The weight-bearing pattern in these patients tends to shift from the medial to the lateral border of the forefoot,[75] and the load taken by the toes is reduced.[22] The rheumatoid foot demonstrates findings similar to those of the neuropathic foot.[2] Side-to-side differences in these patients were notable for increased plantar forefoot pressure on the side of ulceration, but there were no side-to-side differences if no ulcers were present.

Achilles Tendon

The relationship of the Achilles tendon, plantar fascia, and metatarsophalangeal joints influences plantar pressure and gait biomechanics. The windlass mechanism describes the effect of metatarsophalangeal joint dorsiflexion on the plantar fascia. During the foot-flat phase of the gait cycle, the tibia moves forward and the ankle dorsiflexes, increasing tension in the Achilles tendon, leading to heel rise and metatarsophalangeal joint dorsiflexion. The plantar fascia tightens, the hindfoot inverts, and the transverse tarsal joint locks.[19] These changes stabilize the midfoot and allow the foot to act as a rigid lever during the toe-off phase of gait. The Achilles tendon contributes to heel rise, leading to a reduction in the vertical displacement of the center of gravity and minimizing energy expenditure during gait.[52] Gastrocnemius–soleus work increases with step length, effectively lengthening the limb by plantarflexing the ankle.[36]

Force plate analysis has been used to study the function of the gastrocnemius–soleus complex during walking, running, and jumping, highlighting the importance of the elastic component of the musculotendinous unit.[37] During the stance phase of gait, energy is stored in the gastroc–soleus complex as the ankle dorsiflexes and the tendon is elastically stretched. This energy is returned after heel rise as the ankle plantarflexes. This elastic recoil allows shortening of the gastroc–soleus complex at rates well above those possible by maximal muscle contraction. This also allows the muscles to act relatively isometrically at a rate and length of maximum efficiency over the gait cycle. This mechanism allows preservation of energy in the gastroc–soleus complex during the transition from eccentric to concentric contraction.[35,36] The gastroc–soleus contribution to forward propulsion is minimal during normal walking but plays a larger role as walking speed increases.[27]

Force plate analysis has also been used to study the effects of failed Achilles repair. Achilles insufficiency can lead to a paradoxical ankle rigidity that results from overactivity of toe dorsiflexors. Gait characteristics with an elongated or ruptured tendon demonstrate a paradoxically rigid ankle and excess toe dorsiflexor activity.[14] Midstance dorsiflexion is decreased and time to initial peak vertical force is shortened, resulting in a loss of shock absorption. The second peak vertical force, representing metatarsal head pressure, is not diminished in contrast to what might be expected. However, when the toe flexors and the gastroc–soleus complex are made nonfunctional by blocking the tibial nerve, the secondary peak vertical force is increased.[79] This suggests that excess toe dorsiflexion to compensate for loss of gastroc–soleus function causes the paradoxical ankle rigidity.

This relationship among the Achilles tendon, plantar fascia, and metatarsophalangeal joint motion has been studied in diabetic patients with plantar ulceration. Adding Achilles tendon lengthening to total contact casting in these patients leads to increased rate of healing and decreased recurrence of neuropathic ulcers.[60] Ankle dorsiflexion is increased and both plantarflexion torque and peak plantar pressure are reduced after Achilles tendon lengthening.[60] The increase in ankle dorsiflexion remains at 7 months, but plantar flexor peak torque and peak plantar pressures return to baseline. This return to baseline suggests that the decrease in peak plantar pressure might be related to a weakening of ankle plantar flexors rather than to an increase in ankle dorsiflexion.

SURGICAL IMPLICATIONS OF BIOMECHANICS OF THE FOOT AND ANKLE

The purpose of this section is to correlate the biomechanical principles discussed thus far with some of the surgical procedures carried out about the foot and ankle. The decisions made by the orthopaedic surgeon when planning and undertaking a surgical procedure depend on a thorough understanding of biomechanical principles.

Rotation occurs in the transverse plane during normal walking. This transverse rotation increases as we proceed from the pelvis to the ankle. Internal rotation occurs at initial ground contact, followed by external rotation until toe-off, when internal rotation begins again (see Fig. 1–29). This transverse rotation passes across the ankle joint and is translated by the subtalar joint to the calcaneus and hence into the foot. If this transverse rotation cannot be dissipated, increased stress is placed on the ankle joint. The loss of subtalar joint motion can result from trauma, arthritis, surgery, or congenital abnormality. This loss of rotation causes increased stress on the joint above (ankle) and below (transverse tarsal) the immobile joint. This increased stress can cause secondary changes to occur in some patients, which may take the form of a ball-and-socket ankle joint (Fig. 1–44). At other times, beaking can occur in the talonavicular joint in a patient with a subtalar coalition (Fig. 1–45). In adults, the increased stress placed on the ankle and transverse tarsal joint by lack of subtalar joint function can lead to chronic pain.

Biomechanical Considerations in Ankle Arthrodesis

An arthrodesis of the ankle joint places increased stress on the subtalar joint below and the knee joint above. Because the subtalar and ankle joints work together during gait, it is important that certain anatomic facts

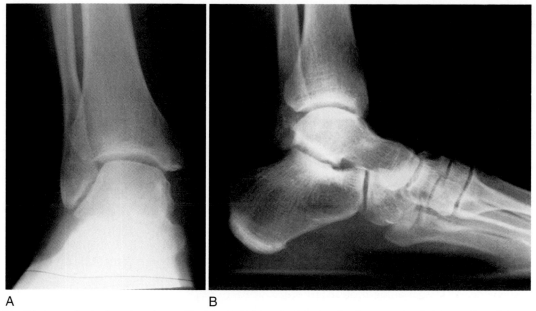

A   B

Figure 1–44   Etiology of a ball-and-socket ankle joint in adults. **A,** As a result of a congenital abnormality of the subtalar joint that eliminated subtalar motion, the ankle joint absorbed transverse rotation that normally occurs in the subtalar joint. **B,** A congenital talonavicular fusion, which results in loss of subtalar joint motion and causes the ankle to absorb transverse rotation, resulting in a ball-and-socket ankle joint.

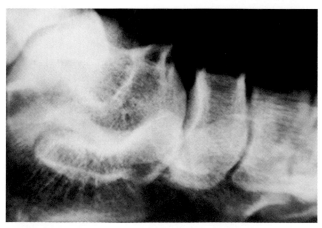

Figure 1–45   Talar breaking following increased stress as a result of subtalar coalition.

be kept in mind when carrying out an ankle arthrodesis. The degree of internal or external tibial torsion, genu varum or genu valgum, proximal muscle weakness, and configuration of the longitudinal arch should be considered. When an ankle arthrodesis is carried out, the degree of transverse rotation placed in the ankle mortise must be carefully considered so that increased stress is not caused within the foot.

If the ankle is placed into excessive internal rotation, the patient experiences difficulty when the center of gravity passes over the foot. The position of internal rotation places increased stress on the subtalar and midtarsal joint region, which may become painful as a result of increased stress. Knee pain and possibly hip pain also can develop secondarily as a result of attempts to externally rotate the lower limb to help compensate for the abnormal position of the foot.

If the ankle is placed into too much external rotation, the patient tends to roll over the medial border of the foot. This position permits the patient to easily roll over the foot, but it in turn places increased stress on the medial side of the first metatarsophalangeal joint, which can lead to a hallux valgus deformity. It may also cause increased stress along the medial side of the knee joint.

The degree of varus or valgus tilt of the ankle joint must be carefully considered and should be related to the degree of subtalar joint motion and the overall alignment of the knee and tibia. If the subtalar joint is stiff and unable to compensate for any malalignment, it is imperative to place the ankle joint into sufficient valgus position to obtain a plantigrade foot. If the ankle joint is placed into varus position, the patient will walk on the lateral border of the foot. Not only does this cause the patient discomfort because of localized weight bearing in a relatively small area, but also the persistent varus position of the subtalar joint keeps the transverse tarsal joint in a semirigid state, resulting in a rather immobile forefoot that is difficult for the body to pass over during the stance phase.

The degree of dorsiflexion and plantar flexion of the ankle joint must also be carefully considered when carrying out an ankle arthrodesis. If there is a short lower extremity or an unstable knee joint as a result of weakness or loss of quadriceps function, the ankle joint should be placed into plantar flexion (10 to 15 degrees) to help give stability to the knee joint. If the pathologic process involves only the ankle joint, 0 degrees (neutral position) for men and 0 to 5 degrees of plantar flexion for women are considered the positions of choice. If the ankle joint is placed into excessive plantar flexion, the involved limb is lengthened, which in turn causes a back-knee thrust on the knee joint, uneven gait pattern, and stress across the midfoot. If the ankle is placed into too much dorsiflexion, the impact of ground contact is concentrated in one small area of the heel, which can result in chronic pain.

Following an ankle arthrodesis, patients usually develop increased motion in the sagittal plane, which helps to compensate for loss of ankle motion. In our study of 81 ankle fusions, the sagittal arc of motion of the talar first metatarsal averaged 24 degrees (9 to 43 degrees), at the talonavicular joint it averaged 14 ± 5 degrees, and at the talocalcaneal joint it averaged 8 ± 6 degrees (Fig. 1–46).[56]

Hindfoot Alignment

When a subtalar joint is fused, the transverse rotation that occurs in the lower extremity is partially absorbed in the ankle joint because it no longer can pass through the subtalar joint into the foot. The varus or valgus alignment of the subtalar joint affects the position of the forefoot, so accurate alignment is essential. If the subtalar joint is placed into too much varus, the forefoot is rotated into supination and the weight-bearing line of the extremity then passes laterally to

the calcaneus and fifth metatarsal. This results in increased stress on the lateral collateral ligament structure and abnormal weight bearing along the lateral aspect of the foot. This position also holds the forefoot in a semirigid position, so the patient must either vault over it or place the foot in external rotation to roll over the medial aspect.

The position of choice is a valgus tilt of about 5 degrees in the subtalar joint, because this permits satisfactory stability of the ankle joint, and the weight-bearing line of the body will pass medial to the calcaneus; therefore, no stress will be placed on the lateral collateral ligament structure. This position results in slight pronation of the forefoot, which permits even distribution of weight on the plantar aspect of the foot. The slight valgus position also allows the forefoot to remain flexible so that the body can easily pass over it.

Midfoot Alignment

When the talonavicular or transverse tarsal joint is surgically stabilized, motion in the subtalar joint is eliminated. For motion to occur in the subtalar joint, the navicular must rotate over the head of the talus. If it cannot, there is essentially no subtalar joint motion. An isolated fusion of the calcaneal cuboid joint results in about a 30% loss of subtalar joint motion. Motion of the subtalar joint directly affects the stability of the foot through its control of the transverse tarsal joint. When the subtalar joint is in valgus position, the transverse tarsal joint is unlocked and the forefoot is flexible. Conversely, when the subtalar joint is inverted, the transverse tarsal joint is locked and the forefoot is fairly rigid. Because of the role the transverse tarsal joint plays in controlling the forefoot, it is essential

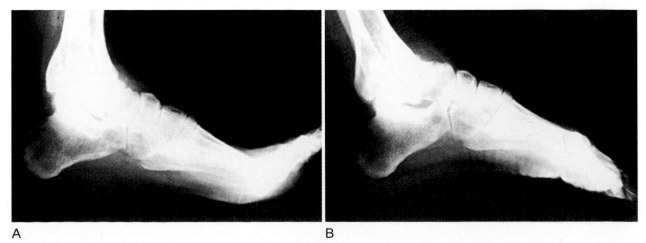

A   B

Figure 1–46 Increased motion in transverse tarsal and subtalar joints to compensate for ankle arthrodesis. **A,** Dorsiflexion. **B,** Plantar flexion.

that the foot be placed in a plantigrade position when the joints are stabilized. If the foot is placed into too much supination, the medial border of the foot is elevated and undue stress is placed on the lateral aspect of the foot. It also creates a rigid forefoot. The position of choice is neutral rotation or slight pronation, which ensures a flexible plantigrade foot.

When a triple arthrodesis is carried out, the position of choice is 5 degrees of valgus for the subtalar joint and neutral rotation of the transverse tarsal joint. It should be emphasized, however, that it is better to err on the side of too much valgus and pronation to keep the weight-bearing line medial to the calcaneus, because that produces a more flexible plantigrade foot. When carrying out a plantar arthrodesis, the same basic principles apply.

The intertarsal and tarsometatarsal joints can be surgically stabilized with minimal loss of function or increased stress on the other joints in the foot. The intertarsal joints, which are distal to the transverse tarsal joint and proximal to the metatarsophalangeal joints, have little or no motion between them.

Forefoot Principles

Removal of the base of the proximal phalanx of the great toe causes instability of the medial longitudinal arch as a result of disruption of the plantar aponeurosis and the windlass mechanism. This leads to decreased weight bearing of the first metatarsal head, which results in weight being transferred to the lesser metatarsal heads. If the base of the proximal phalanx

of one of the lesser toes is removed, a similar problem of instability occurs, but to a much lesser degree, particularly moving laterally across the foot. Conversely, resection of the metatarsal head, except in severe disease states such as rheumatoid arthritis or diabetes, results in a similar problem because the windlass mechanism is destroyed as a result of the relative shortening of the ray. This also causes increased stress and callus formation beneath the adjacent metatarsal head, which is subjected to increased weight bearing.

When carrying out an arthrodesis of the first metatarsophalangeal joint for such conditions as hallux rigidus, recurrent hallux valgus, or degenerative arthritis, the alignment of the arthrodesis site is critical. The metatarsophalangeal joint should be placed into approximately 10 to 15 degrees of valgus and 15 to 25 degrees of dorsiflexion in relation to the first metatarsal shaft. The degree of dorsiflexion depends to a certain extent on the heel height of the shoe that the patient desires to wear. An arthrodesis of the first metatarsophalangeal joint has a minimum effect on gait. The arthrodesis places increased stress on the interphalangeal joint of the hallux. This increased stress can result in degenerative changes over time, but these rarely become symptomatic. In theory, increased stress is placed on the first metatarsocuneiform joint following arthrodesis of the metatarsophalangeal joint, but it is unusual to see any form of degenerative change.

An isolated arthrodesis of the interphalangeal joint of the great toe does not seem to have any significant effect on the biomechanics of gait, nor does an

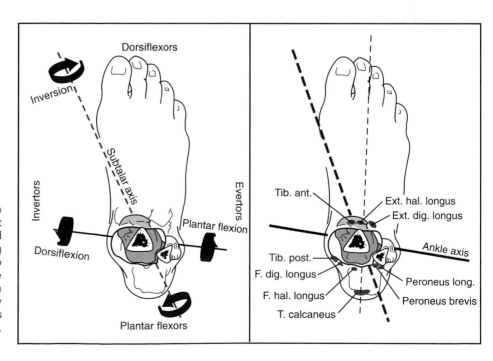

Figure 1–47 *Left,* Diagram demonstrates rotation that occurs about the subtalar and ankle axes. *Right,* Drawing demonstrates the relationship of various muscles about the subtalar and ankle axes. (From Mann RA. In American Academy of Orthopaedic Surgeons: *Atlas of Orthotics,* ed 3. St Louis, Mosby, 1997.)

arthrodesis of the proximal and distal interphalangeal joints of the lesser toes.

Resection of a single sesamoid bone because of a pathologic condition such as a fracture, avascular necrosis, or intractable plantar keratosis may be done with relative impunity. If, however, one sesamoid already has been removed, the second sesamoid probably should not be removed because of risk of a cock-up deformity of the metatarsophalangeal joint. This occurs because the intrinsic muscle insertion into the proximal phalanx of the great toe encompasses the sesamoids, and when the sesamoid is removed this insertion is impaired to a varying degree. If adequate intrinsic function is not present, flexion of the proximal phalanx cannot be brought about, and a cock-up deformity results.

Tendon Transfers

When evaluating muscle weakness or loss about the foot and ankle, the diagram in Figure 1–47 can be useful. It demonstrates the motion that occurs around each joint axis and the location of the muscles in relation to the axes. By considering the muscles in relation to the axes it is possible to carefully note which muscles are functioning and thereby determine which muscles might be transferred to rebalance the foot and ankle. Generally speaking, if inadequate strength is present to balance the foot adequately, it is important to establish adequate plantar flexion function over that of dorsiflexion; an equinus gait is not as disabling as a calcaneal-type gait. Also keep in mind that it is much more difficult to retrain a muscle that has been a stance-phase muscle to become a swing-phase muscle than to retrain a swing-phase muscle to become a stance-phase muscle. Therefore, if possible, an in-phase muscle transfer will produce a more satisfactory result, because no phase conversion is necessary.

REFERENCES

1. Abbott BC, Bigland B, Ritchie JM: The physiological cost of negative work. *J Physiol* 117:380-390, 1952.
2. Alexander IJ, Chao EY, Johnson KA: The assessment of dynamic foot-to-ground contact forces and plantar pressure distribution: A review of the evolution of current techniques and clinical applications. *Foot Ankle* 11:152-167, 1990.
3. Andriacchi TP, Ogle JA, Galante JO: Walking speed as a basis for normal and abnormal gait measurements. *J Biomech* 10:261-268, 1977.
4. Arcan M, Brull MA: A fundamental characteristic of the human body and foot, the foot–ground pressure pattern. *J Biomech* 9:453-457, 1976.
5. Armstrong DG, Lavery LA: Elevated peak plantar pressures in patients who have Charcot arthropathy. *J Bone Joint Surg Am* 80:365-369, 1998.
6. Asmussen E: Positive and negative muscular work. *Acta Physiol Scand* 28:364-382, 1953.
7. Banister E, Brown S: The relative energy requirements of physical activity. In Falls H (ed): *Exercise Physiology.* New York, Academic Press, 1968.
8. Barnett S, Cunningham JL, West S: A comparison of vertical force and temporal parameters produced by an in-shoe pressure measuring system and a force platform. *Clin Biomech* 15:781-785, 2000.
9. Becker HP, Rosenbaum D, Kriese T, et al: Gait asymmetry following successful surgical treatment of ankle fractures in young adults. *Clin Orthop Relat Res* 311:262-269, 1995.
10. Berry FR: *Angle Variation Patterns of Normal Hip, Knee, and Ankle in Different Operations.* Berkeley, Prosthetic Devices Research Project, 1952.
11. Betts RP, Franks CI, Duckworth T, Burke J: Static and dynamic foot-pressure measurements in clinical orthopaedics. *Med Biol Eng Comput* 18:674-684, 1980.
12. Beverly MC, Horan FT, Hutton WC: Load cell analysis following Silastic arthroplasty of the hallux. *Int Orthop* 9:101-104, 1985.
13. Blomgren M, Turan I, Agadir M: Gait analysis in hallux valgus. *J Foot Surg* 30:70-71, 1991.
14. Boyden EM, Kitaoka HB, Cahalan TD, An KN: Late versus early repair of Achilles tendon rupture: Clinical and biomechanical evaluation. *Clin Orthop Relat Res* 317:150-158, 1995.
15. Breit GA, Whalen RT: Prediction of human gait parameters from temporal measures of foot–ground contact. *Med Sci Sports Exerc* 29:540-547, 1997.
16. Bresler B, Berry F: *Energy and Power in the Leg during Normal Level Walking.* Berkeley, Prosthetic Devices Research Project, 1951.
17. Broughton NS, Winson IG: Keller's arthroplasty and Mitchell osteotomy: A comparison with first metatarsal osteotomy of the long-term results for hallux valgus deformity in the younger female. *Foot Ankle* 10:201-205, 1990.
18. Bryant A, Singer K, Tinley P: Comparison of the reliability of plantar pressure measurements using the two-step and midgait methods of data collection. *Foot Ankle Int* 20:646-650, 1999.
19. Carlson RE, Fleming LL, Hutton WC: The biomechanical relationship between the tendoachilles, plantar fascia and metatarsophalangeal joint dorsiflexion angle. *Foot Ankle Int* 21:18-25, 2000.
20. Close J, Inman V: *The Action of the Subtalar Joint.* Berkeley, Prosthetic Devices Research Project, 1953.
21. Coughlin MJ, Shurnas PS: Hallux rigidus: Demographics, etiology, and radiographic assessment. *Foot Ankle Int* 24:731-743, 2003.
22. Ctercteko GC, Dhanendran M, Hutton WC, Le Quesne LP: Vertical forces acting on the feet of diabetic patients with neuropathic ulceration. *Br J Surg* 68:608-614, 1981.
23. Cunningham D: *Components of Floor Reaction During Walking.* Berkeley, Prosthetic Devices Research Project, 1950.
24. Duckworth T, Betts RP, Franks CI, Burke J: The measurement of pressures under the foot. *Foot Ankle* 3:130-141, 1982.
25. Elftman H: A cinematic study of the distribution of pressure in the human foot. *Anat Rev* 59:481-491, 1934.
26. Elftman H: The transverse tarsal joint and its control. *Clin Orthop Relat Res* 16:41-46, 1960.
27. Fujita M, Matsusaka N, Norimatsu T, Suzuki R: The role of the ankle plantar flexors in level walking. In Winter DA, Norman RW, Wells RP, et al (eds). *Biomechanics IX-A.* International Series on Biomechanics. Champaign, Ill, Human Kinetics Publishers, 1985, pp 484-488.
28. Grundy M, Tosh PA, McLeish RD, Smidt L: An investigation of the centres of pressure under the foot while walking. *J Bone Joint Surg Br* 57:98-103, 1975.

29. Hayafune N, Hayafune Y, Jacob HAC: Pressure and force distribution characteristics under the normal foot during push-off phase in gait. *The Foot* 9:88-92, 1999.
30. Hennig EM, Rosenbaum D: Pressure distribution patterns under the feet of children in comparison with adults. *Foot Ankle* 11:306-311, 1991.
31. Hennig EM, Staats A, Rosenbaum D: Plantar pressure distribution patterns of young school children in comparison to adults. *Foot Ankle Int* 15:35-40, 1994.
32. Henry AP, Waugh W, Wood H: The use of footprints in assessing the results of operations for hallux valgus. A comparison of Keller's operation and arthrodesis. *J Bone Joint Surg Br* 57:478-481, 1975.
33. Herzog W, Nigg BM, Read LJ, Olsson E: Asymmetries in ground reaction force patterns in normal human gait. *Med Sci Sports Exerc* 21:110-114, 1989.
34. Hicks JH: The mechanics of the foot. II. The plantar aponeurosis and the arch. *J Anat* 88:25-30, 1954.
35. Hof AL: In vivo measurement of the series elasticity release curve of human triceps surae muscle. *J Biomech* 31:793-800, 1998.
36. Hof AL, Geelen BA, Van den Berg J: Calf muscle moment, work and efficiency in level walking; role of series elasticity. *J Biomech* 16:523-537, 1983.
37. Hof AL, Van Zandwijk JP, Bobbert MF: Mechanics of human triceps surae muscle in walking, running and jumping. *Acta Physiol Scand* 174:17-30, 2002.
38. Holmes GB, Jr., Timmerman L: A quantitative assessment of the effect of metatarsal pads on plantar pressures. *Foot Ankle* 11:141-145, 1990.
39. Hughes J, Clark P, Jagoe JR, et al: The pattern of pressure distribution under the weightbearing forefoot. *Foot* 1:117-124, 1991.
40. Hughes J, Clark P, Klenerman L: The importance of the toes in walking. *J Bone Joint Surg Br* 72:245-251, 1990.
41. Hughes J, Clark P, Linge K, Klenerman L: A comparison of two studies of the pressure distribution under the feet of normal subjects using different equipment. *Foot Ankle* 14:514-519, 1993.
42. Hughes J, Kriss S, Klenerman L: A clinician's view of foot pressure: A comparison of three different methods of measurement. *Foot Ankle* 7:277-284, 1987.
43. Hughes J, Pratt L, Linge K, et al: Reliability of pressure measurements: The EMED F system. *Clin Biomech* 6:14-18, 1991.
44. Hung LK, Ho YF, Leung PC: Survey of foot deformities among 166 geriatric inpatients. *Foot Ankle* 5:156-164, 1985.
45. Hutton WC, Dhanendran M: The mechanics of normal and hallux valgus feet—a quantitative study. *Clin Orthop Relat Res* 157:7-13, 1981.
46. Hutton WC, Stott JRR, Stokes JAF: The mechanics of the foot. In Klenerman L (ed). *The Foot and Its Disorders.* Oxford, Blackwell Scientific Publications, 1982, p 42.
47. Imamura M, Imamura ST, Salomao O, et al: Pedobarometric evaluation of the normal adult male foot. *Foot Ankle Int* 23:804-810, 2002.
48. Inman VT: *The Joints of the Ankle.* Baltimore, Williams & Wilkins, 1976.
49. Isman R, Inman V: Anthropometric studies of the human foot and ankle. *Bull Prosthet Res* 10/11:97-129, 1969.
50. Katoh Y, Chao EY, Laughman RK, et al: Biomechanical analysis of foot function during gait and clinical applications. *Clin Orthop Relat Res* 177:23-33, 1983.
51. Kernozek TW, Sterriker SA: Chevron (Austin) distal metatarsal osteotomy for hallux valgus: Comparison of pre- and post-surgical characteristics. *Foot Ankle Int* 23:503-508, 2002.
52. Kerrigan DC, Della Croce U, Marciello M, Riley PO: A refined view of the determinants of gait: Significance of heel rise. *Arch Phys Med Rehabil* 81:1077-1080, 2000.
53. Levens A, Inman V, Blosser J: Transverse rotation of the segments of the lower extremity in locomotion. *J Bone Joint Surg Am* 30:859, 1948.
54. Mann R, Inman VT: Phasic activity of intrinsic muscles of the foot. *J Bone Joint Surg Am* 46:469-481, 1964.
55. Mann RA, Poppen NK, O'Konski M: Amputation of the great toe. A clinical and biomechanical study. *Clin Orthop Relat Res* 226:192-205, 1988.
56. Mann RA, Rongstad KM: Arthrodesis of the ankle: A critical analysis. *Foot Ankle Int* 19:3-9, 1998.
57. Manter J: Movements of the subtalar and transverse tarsal joints. *Anat Rec* 80:397, 1941.
58. Mizel MS, Temple HT, Scranton PE Jr, et al: Role of the peroneal tendons in the production of the deformed foot with posterior tibial tendon deficiency. *Foot Ankle Int* 20:285-289, 1999.
59. Morton DJ: Structural factors in static disorders of the foot. *Am J Surg* 9:315-328, 1930.
60. Mueller MJ, Sinacore DR, Hastings MK, et al: Effect of Achilles tendon lengthening on neuropathic plantar ulcers. A randomized clinical trial. *J Bone Joint Surg Am* 85:1436-1445, 2003.
61. Mueller MJ, Strube MJ: Generalizability of in-shoe peak pressure measures using the F-scan system. *Clin Biomech* 11:159-164, 1996.
62. Nilsson J, Thorstensson A: Ground reaction forces at different speeds of human walking and running. *Acta Physiol Scand* 136:217-227, 1989.
63. Pollard JP, Le Quesne LP, Tappin JW: Forces under the foot. *J Biomed Eng* 5:37-40, 1983.
64. Popova T: Quoted in issledovaniia po biodinamike lokomotsii. In Bernstein N (ed). *Biodinamika khod'by normal'nogo vzroslogo muzhchiny,* vol. 1. Moscow, Idat Vsesoiuz Instit Eksper Med, 1935.
65. Ralston HJ: Energy–speed relation and optimal speed during level walking. *Int Z Angew Physiol* 17:277-283, 1958.
66. Rodgers MM, Cavanagh PR: Pressure distribution in Morton's foot structure. *Med Sci Sports Exerc* 21:23-28, 1989.
67. Rose NE, Feiwell LA, Cracchiolo A 3rd: A method for measuring foot pressures using a high resolution, computerized insole sensor: The effect of heel wedges on plantar pressure distribution and center of force. *Foot Ankle* 13:263-270, 1992.
68. Rosenbaum D, Hautmann S, Gold M, Claes L: Effects of walking speed on plantar pressure patterns and hindfoot angular motion. *Gait Posture* 2:191-197, 1994.
69. Ryker NJ: *Glass Walkway Studies of Normal Subjects during Normal Walking.* Berkeley, Prosthetic Devices Research Project, 1952.
70. Sarrafian SK: *Anatomy of the Foot and Ankle.* Philadelphia, JB Lippincott, 1993.
71. Saunders JB, Inman VT, Eberhart HD: The major determinants in normal and pathological gait. *J Bone Joint Surg Am* 35A:543-558, 1953.
72. Scott E: Personal communication, 1975.
73. Silvino N, Evanski PM, Waugh TR: The Harris and Beath footprinting mat: Diagnostic validity and clinical use. *Clin Orthop* 151:265-269, 1980.
74. Simon SR, Mann RA, Hagy JL, Larsen LJ: Role of the posterior calf muscles in normal gait. *J Bone Joint Surg Am* 60:465-472, 1978.
75. Soames RW: Foot pressure patterns during gait. *J Biomed Eng* 7:120-126, 1983.
76. Stein H, Simkin A, Joseph K: The foot–ground pressure distribution following triple arthrodesis. *Arch Orthop Trauma Surg* 98:263-269, 1981.
77. Stokes IA, Hutton WC, Stott JR, Lowe LW: Forces under the hallux valgus foot before and after surgery. *Clin Orthop Relat Res* 142:64-72, 1979.

78. Stott JR, Hutton WC, Stokes IA: Forces under the foot. *J Bone Joint Surg Br* 55:335-344, 1973.

79. Sutherland DH, Cooper L, Daniel D: The role of the ankle plantar flexors in normal walking. *J Bone Joint Surg Am* 62:354-363, 1980.

80. Tareco JM, Miller NH, MacWilliams BA, Michelson JD: Defining flatfoot. *Foot Ankle Int* 20:456-460, 1999.

81. Veves A, Sarnow MR, Giurini JM, et al: Differences in joint mobility and foot pressures between black and white diabetic patients. *Diabet Med* 12:585-589, 1995.

82. Waldecker U: Metatarsalgia in hallux valgus deformity: A pedographic analysis. *J Foot Ankle Surg* 41:300-308, 2002.

83. Wanivenhaus A, Brettschneider W: Influence of metatarsal head displacement on metatarsal pressure distribution after hallux valgus surgery. *Foot Ankle* 14:85-89, 1993.

84. Wearing SC, Urry SR, Smeathers JE: Ground reaction forces at discrete sites of the foot derived from pressure plate measurements. *Foot Ankle Int* 22:653-661, 2001.

85. Welton EA: The Harris and Beath footprint: Interpretation and clinical value. *Foot Ankle* 13:462-468, 1992.

86. Willson JD, Kernozek TW: Plantar loading and cadence alterations with fatigue. *Med Sci Sports Exerc* 31:1828-1833, 1999.

87. Winson IG, Rawlinson J, Broughton NS: Treatment of metatarsalgia by sliding distal metatarsal osteotomy. *Foot Ankle* 9:2-6, 1988.

88. Wright DG, Desai SM, Henderson WH: Action of the subtalar and ankle-joint complex during the stance phase of walking. *J Bone Joint Surg Am* 46:361-382, 1964.

89. Yamamoto H, Muneta T, Asahina S, Furuya K: Forefoot pressures during walking in feet afflicted with hallux valgus. *Clin Orthop* 000:247-253, 1996.

90. Yeap JS, Singh D, Birch R: Tibialis posterior tendon dysfunction: A primary or secondary problem? *Foot Ankle Int* 22:51-55, 2001.

91. Zhu H, Wertsch JJ, Harris GF, Alba HM: Walking cadence effect on plantar pressures. *Arch Phys Med Rehabil* 76:1000-1005, 1995.

92. Zhu HS, Wertsch JJ, Harris GF, et al: Foot pressure distribution during walking and shuffling. *Arch Phys Med Rehabil* 72:390-397, 1991.

Principles of the Physical Examination of the Foot and Ankle

W. Hodges Davis • *Roger A. Mann*

You may not see it, but it sees you.

JACK HUGHSTON, MD,
discussing the physical examination

The foot, ankle, and leg are parts of the body that are readily accessible to careful physical examination. In the vast majority of cases, a definitive diagnosis can be reached by obtaining a careful history, conducting a proper physical examination, and using the indicated ancillary laboratory procedures. Examination techniques available to the practitioner to gather information concerning the foot and to make a proper diagnosis vary with the patient's age and receptiveness to examination.

In this chapter, the focus is on examination of the mature foot and ankle. The reader will receive a framework for a systematic approach to the normal examination. This will give a background for understanding the pathology described in subsequent chapters. In addition, a detailed description of the topographic anatomy of the foot and ankle is provided. It is with this knowledge that the practitioner can best evaluate the abnormalities in this easily palpable body part. It must be stressed that one sees only what one is looking for, or, in the words of a wise Southern gentleman physician "you may not see it [foot pathology], but it sees you." Keep your eyes wide open.

OVERVIEW

To prevent overlooking pertinent findings, the examiner should follow a rigorous routine. The particular routine adopted will vary depending on personal preference and arrangement of office facilities. The suggestion is to consciously formulate this routine and school oneself to deviate rarely from it. This will best assure nothing is missed. However, no matter what procedure is used, the examiner must consider the foot and ankle from three different points of view.

First, the foot and ankle should be seen systemically or as part of the greater body. In the detailed examination, the effects of systemic problems cannot be underestimated. The foot examination can reveal the presence of systemic disease as well as give evidence of circulatory, neuropathic, metabolic, and cutaneous abnormalities. One should not be so focused on the foot as to miss a much more illustrative and often treatable global disease.

Second, the foot and ankle should be considered an important component of the locomotor system. They play reciprocal roles with the suprapedal segments, and abnormal function of any part of the locomotor apparatus is reflected in adaptive changes in the normal parts. Therefore it is helpful for the examiner to observe the patient walking over an appreciable distance.

Third, the human foot and ankle should be viewed as relatively recent evolutionary acquisitions; thus they are subject to considerable individual anatomic and functional variation. It is regrettable that in most of the anatomic and orthopaedic literature, only average values for the positions of axes of the major articulations and for ranges of motion about these axes are given (see Chapter 1). It so happens that an average person is difficult to find, particularly among patients seeking help in our offices. The examiner should be aware of these variations and should also be cognizant of their functional implications. Only with such knowledge and insight can the examiner determine the proper therapeutic course and realistically evaluate the chances of success or failure of that choice.

SEQUENCE OF EXAMINATION

When examining the foot and ankle, the examiner should follow as closely as possible the procedural sequence taught in courses in introductory physical diagnosis. After taking an adequate history, the examiner first inspects, then palpates, and finally (in an orthopaedic examination) manipulates. This sequence must be modified and repeated several times as the patient performs tasks in various positions and under various stresses.

The following outline for the examination of the foot and ankle has proved useful. In subsequent sections we detail specific portions of the particular examination that should be stressed.

It is helpful for the patients to be in shorts, skirts, or loose-fitting trousers to allow for easy observation of the legs and knees. Generally all socks or hose are removed. The examination area should allow for gait and stance observation from front and rear.

The usual sequence of examination begins with the examiner first observing the patient walking because this often can be done even prior to taking the history. Second is the standing examination, which is done from front and rear. Third, the bulk of the examination is done with the patient sitting on a table slightly above the examiner. This allows for easy inspection, palpation, and manipulation of both extremities. Examination with the patient prone or supine is optional and is done as the first three portions of the examination dictate. The amount of time spent on each portion of this examination sequence depends on the patient's presentation.

TOPOGRAPHIC ANATOMY

The importance of topographic anatomy to the examination of the foot and ankle cannot be overstated. The experienced examiner can palpate the vast majority of the pathologic structures and use radiographic tests for confirmation only. We divide this discussion into anatomic regions, with the palpable bones, joints, nerves and vascular structures, and ligaments and tendons highlighted.

Ankle and Hindfoot

The examination of the osteology of the lateral ankle begins with the easily palpable tip of the fibula (Fig. 2–1). From the tip, the distal fibula *(A)* and the shaft *(B)* can be felt in its entirety by running one's fingers

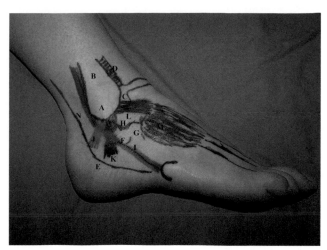

Figure 2-1 Lateral ankle and hindfoot topography, anterior lateral view. *A,* Distal fibula; *B,* fibular shaft; *C,* lateral gutter of the ankle; *D,* distal syndesmosis; *E,* lateral wall of the calcaneus; *F,* the peroneal tubercle; *G,* sinus tarsi; *H,* lateral talar process; *I,* peroneal tendons; *J,* insertion point of the superior peroneal retinaculum; *K,* calcaneofibular ligament; *L,* anterior talofibular ligament; *M,* extensor digitorum brevis muscle; *N,* sural nerve.

proximally. The lateral gutter of the ankle joint *(C)* can be found by running one's thumb medially over the anterior and medial edge of the fibula. The lateral shoulder of the talus can be felt at the joint line by dorsiflexing and plantar flexing the ankle. The distal syndesmosis *(D)* is felt by following the medial edge of the fibula superior to the joint line. The lateral wall of the calcaneus *(E)* can be palpated with little difficulty inferior and posterior to the tip of the fibula. If this lateral wall is palpated distal and inferior to the tip of the fibula, the peroneal tubercle *(F)* can be felt as the calcaneal neck nears the calcaneocuboid joint. The sinus tarsi *(G)* (the space in front of the posterior facet of the subtalar joint) is a palpable soft spot approximately 1 cm distal and 1 cm inferior to the tip of the fibula. The anterior portion of the posterior facet of the subtalar joint can be located with deep thumb palpation into the sinus tarsi. The lateral talar process *(H)* is palpated on the posterior wall of the sinus tarsi. The anterior process of the calcaneus is the anterior wall of the sinus tarsi.

The palpable tendons, muscles, and ligaments in the lateral ankle and hindfoot can best be referenced from the tip of the fibula. Superior and posterior to the tip of the fibula are the peroneal tendons *(I).* The peroneus brevis is deep to the peroneus longus. The tendons can be felt in the groove, and the anterior edge of the fibular groove is sharp and is the insertion point of the superior peroneal retinaculum *(J).* Inferior and extending posterior and inferior is the calcaneofibular

ligament *(K).* It passes deep to the peroneal tendons as the tendons clear the fibula. From the tip of the fibula, if one runs a finger 1 to 1.5 cm along the anterior edge, the anterior talofibular ligament *(L)* can be felt. In the uninjured patient it can be felt as a soft tissue thickening that can be rolled against the anterior lateral talar shoulder.

If one continues to run a finger superior on the anterior fibula up to the junction with the distal tibiofibular connection, the most inferior fibers of the syndesmotic ligament *(D)* can be felt (anterior distal tibiofibular ligament). The remainder of the anterior syndesmotic ligament can be felt by palpating directly superior to the tibia and fibula junction. To truly assess this portion of the syndesmosis requires deep palpation. The extensor digitorum brevis muscle *(M)* can be located by palpating the sinus tarsi *(G)* because this muscle covers this space. The peroneal tendons can be felt on the lateral calcaneal wall extending from the distal end of the fibular groove, which runs inferior then distal. The brevis is dorsal as the tendons turn distal. The peroneus brevis is also dorsal at the peroneal tubercle, and the peroneus longus is plantar. In this area the tendons can be felt in their separate sheaths created by the inferior peroneal retinaculum and the tubercle.

The nervous topography in this region is fairly straightforward. The sural nerve can be felt in the fatty soft spot directly posterior to the peroneal tendons in the fibular groove (Fig. 2-2). In a thin patient this nerve can be rolled under one's finger just posterior to the course of the peroneal tendons as they enter the midfoot. The superficial peroneal nerve can first be

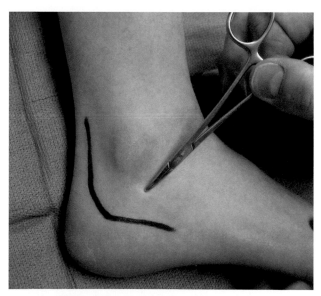

Figure 2-2 Sural nerve, surface anatomy.

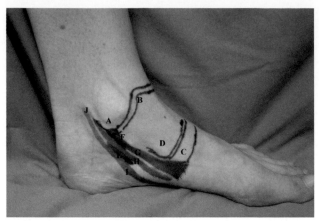

Figure 2–3 Medial ankle and hindfoot topography, direct medial view. *A,* Tip of the medial malleolus; *B,* anterior medial tibiotalar joint line; *C,* navicular bone; *D,* the talar head; *E,* sustentaculum tali; *F,* superficial deltoid ligament; *G,* posterior tibial tendon; *H,* flexor digitorum longus; *I,* flexor hallucis longus; *J,* pulse of the posterior tibial artery.

palpated as a number of branches just superior to the distal ankle syndesmosis. Again, it is best felt by rolling the branch under a finger as the ankle is plantar flexed.

Medial

The topography of the medial ankle and hindfoot (Fig. 2–3) is as accessible as the lateral. The reference point here is the tip of the medial malleolus *(A),* which also allows for a reference for medial ankle osteology. The tip of the malleolus is the most distal bony prominence palpated on the medial tibia. From this point the anterior medial tibiotalar joint line *(B)* can be located by sliding a thumb 2 cm superior and then lateral until one's thumb feels a soft spot. This is the medial gutter, the articular space between the medial malleolus and the medial talar body. Following the gutter proximally allows palpation of the anterior distal tibial plafond. This can be followed laterally across the joint. Following the malleolus posteriorly and proximally allows one to palpate the entire posterior medial edge of the malleolus and tibia.

From the tip of the medial malleolus, with the ankle at neutral, a line drawn distal and slightly plantar will run through the navicular bone *(C).* The navicular is best felt with the hindfoot slightly supinated. With the hindfoot pronated and the midfoot abducted, the talar head *(D)* can be felt on the medial foot just proximal to the navicular. The medial talonavicular joint can be delineated by adducting and abducting the trans-

verse tarsal joint. If one divides the line between the navicular and the medial malleolus in half and drops plantarward 1 to 1.5 cm, the sustentaculum tali *(E),* a medial ossicle of the calcaneus, can be palpated.

The palpable tendons and ligaments of the medial hindfoot can also be referenced from the tip of the medial malleolus. The superficial deltoid ligament *(F)* fans out from the malleolus but can best be palpated anterior and distal to it. The anterior fascicles of the deltoid can be felt by following the anterior edge of the malleolus only 1 cm. If one feels the medial gutter, the origin of the superficial deltoid has been passed. The most anterior fascicles of the superficial deltoid (anterior tibionavicular and anterior tibioligamentous) can be palpated as they originate from the anterior ridge of the malleolus. The portion of the superficial deltoid originating from the tip of the malleolus can be located as it courses deep to the tendons of the medial ankle. The deep deltoid ligament cannot be isolated by palpation. The more posterior aspects of the superficial deltoid cannot be palpated directly.

The posterior tibial tendon *(G)* can be felt along its entire course. It begins at the musculotendinous junction, 5 to 7 cm from the tip of the medial malleolus, just off the posterior bony margin of the distal tibia and travels distally, almost adherent to the posterior aspect of the medial malleolus. The tendon curves around the medial malleolus and heads distally to the plantar medial insertion on the navicular.

The flexor digitorum longus (FDL) *(H)* is easily palpated posterior and medial to the posterior tibialis tendon at a level 1 to 2 cm from the tip of the malleolus. It can be felt again in the midfoot as it crosses deep to the flexor hallucis longus (FHL) tendon. The FHL tendon *(I)* is best palpated in the ankle slightly posterior and deep to the posterior tibial artery and nerve at the level 1 to 2 cm proximal to the medial malleolus. The FHL also can be felt as it passes plantar to the sustentaculum tali. The superomedial aspect of the spring ligament (superomedial calcaneonavicular ligament) is palpated plantar and deep to the posterior tibial tendon just proximal to the tendon's insertion on the plantar–medial navicular (Fig. 2–4).

The neurovascular structures of the medial ankle are important to locate. The pulse of the posterior tibial artery (see Fig. 2–3, *J*) can be felt 1 to 2 cm posterior and medial to the medial edge of the medial malleolus. The pulse is strongest approximately 2 cm from the malleolar tip (Fig. 2–5). The posterior tibial nerve runs with the artery in the tarsal tunnel. The nerve bifurcates into the medial and lateral plantar nerves at

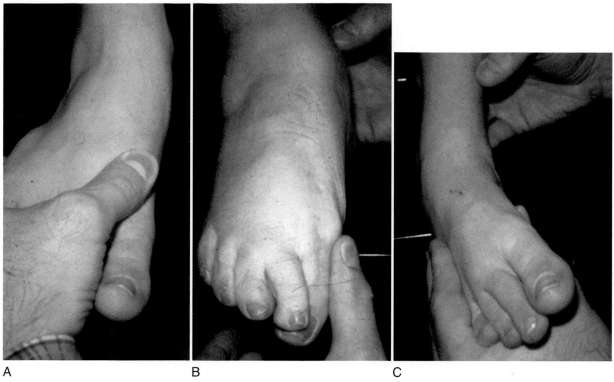

A   B   C

Figure 2–4 Examination of the posterior tibial tendon. **A,** The foot is plantar flexed and abducted to neutralize the pull of the anterior tibial tendon. **B,** The posterior tibial tendon is palpated. **C,** The patient attempts to adduct the foot, and the strength of the posterior tibial tendon is assessed.

the level of the tip of the malleolus. The medial branch courses distally and plantarly and can be palpated as it runs under the abductor hallucis muscle at the level of the medial gutter of the ankle joint (Fig. 2–6). The

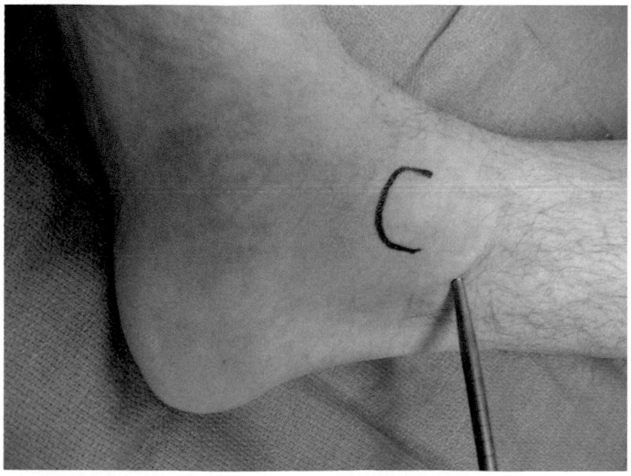

Figure 2–5 The posterior tibial artery pulse is best felt 2 cm from the malleolar tip.

lateral plantar nerve travels straight inferior from the tarsal tunnel and can be palpated as it runs deep to the abductor hallucis. The saphenous nerve can sometimes be palpated on the medial malleolus by rolling it gently under one's fingers.

Posterior

The Achilles tendon (Fig. 2–7, *A*) defines the posterior ankle and hindfoot. This large tendon can best be examined with the patient prone. The tendon transects the posterior ankle and can be easily palpated because of the tendon's subcutaneous course. The tendon inserts into the calcaneus broadly, and the Achilles insertional ridge of the calcaneus *(B)* is palpated at the distal insertion of the tendon. The posterior calcaneus is palpated medially, laterally, and posteriorly. The retrocalcaneal space *(C)*, which is deep to the Achilles at its insertion, can be easily pinched by pressure from either medial or lateral. The space or its bursa (or both) is an area that is easily delineated from the Achilles proper. The posterior lateral ankle is another access point for the peroneal tendons *(D)* as they pass posterior to the fibula and can be an easier way to feel both tendons in the fibular groove. The same can be

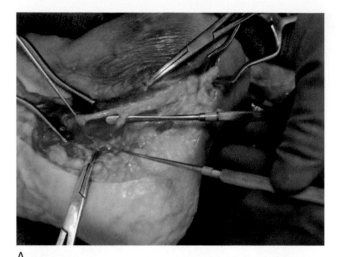

A

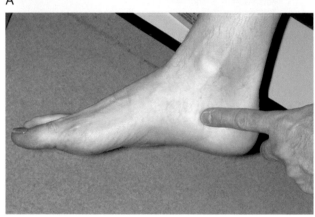

B

Figure 2–6 A, Anatomic specimen demonstrating the posterior tibial nerve. **B,** The posterior tibial nerve may be palpated just inferior to the medial malleolus.

said for the FHL tendon *(E)*, which is a posteromedial ankle tendon at this point (Fig. 2–8).

Anterior

The anterior ankle (Fig. 2–9) is defined by the easily palpable anterior tibialis tendon *(A)*. The tendon is found by asking the patient to actively dorsiflex the ankle. The anterior tibialis, first felt at or near the midanterior ankle just above the malleoli, is the largest tendon structure that passes more medially as it travels distally. Its insertion on the plantar medial cuneiform and first metatarsal is defined with the same dorsiflexion maneuver (Fig. 2–10).

On either side of the anterior tibialis tendon, the anterior ankle joint *(B)* can be felt by deep palpation. The distinction between the tibia and the talus is more easily felt with gentle dorsiflexion and plantar flexion of the ankle joint. The transition from anterior tibia to anterior fibula is quite superficial and can help to

guide the estimation of the location of the less superficial midanterior tibia and talus. The branches of the superficial peroneal nerve (see Fig. 2–9, *C*) are palpated by gently rolling one's fingers over the superficial portions of the anterior ankle (Fig. 2–11). All of these branches are found lateral to the anterior tibialis. The pulse of the dorsalis pedis artery is usually felt not at the ankle but in the dorsal midfoot.

The remaining tendons of the anterior ankle (refer again to Fig. 2–9) are all found lateral to the anterior tibialis. From medial to lateral these easily palpable tendons are the extensor hallucis longus (EHL) *(D)*, the extensor digitorum longus (EDL) *(E)*, and the peroneus tertius *(F)* (found in most people). The examination of these tendons can be made easier by active dorsiflexion or passive plantar flexion of the toes and ankle. Medial to the anterior tibialis, no tendons are normally present.

Plantar

Examination of the plantar–lateral aspect of the hindfoot is all about defining the anatomy of the

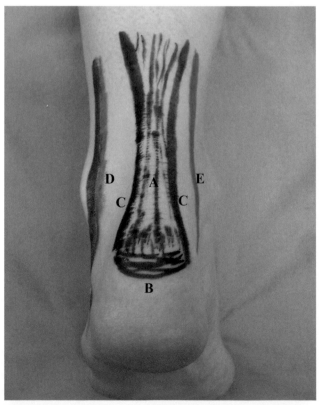

Figure 2–7 Posterior ankle and hindfoot. *A,* Achilles tendon; *B,* the Achilles insertional ridge of the calcaneus; *C,* retrocalcaneal space; *D,* the peroneal tendons; *E,* flexor hallucis longus tendon.

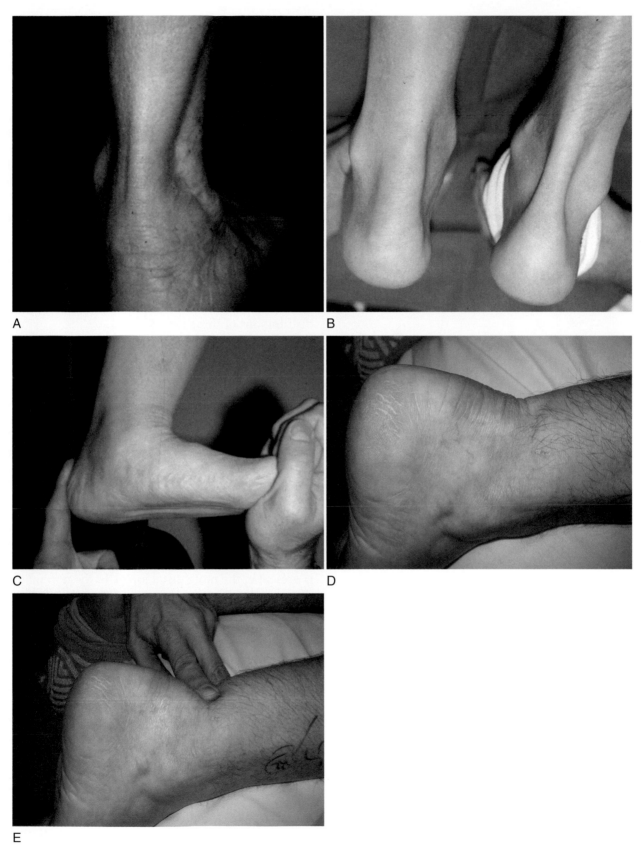

Figure 2–8 Achilles tendon. **A,** The normal tendon is examined from behind. **B,** Tendinosis is seen in the Achilles tendon on the left. **C,** Excursion of the ankle joint is noted. A defect in the Achilles tendon following a rupture is observed **(D)** and palpated **(E)** on examination.

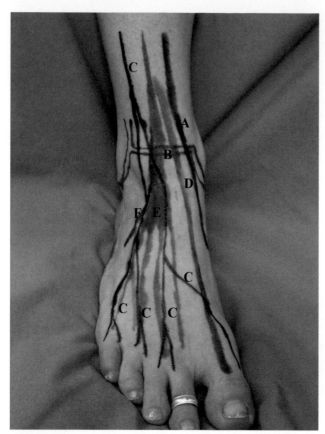

Figure 2–9 Anterior ankle. *A,* Anterior tibialis tendon; *B,* anterior ankle joint; *C,* branches of the superficial peroneal nerve; *D,* extensor hallucis longus; *E,* extensor digitorum longus; *F,* peroneus tertius.

plantar–medial calcaneus and extends distally to insert on the plantar–medial first metatarsophalangeal (MTP) joint. The medial cord of the plantar fascia *(C)* is palpated just plantar and lateral to the abductor hallucis. It is felt most readily by passively dorsiflexing the toes.

The origin of the medial cord of the plantar fascia is best felt by passively dorsiflexing the toes and then running a thumb posterior until it is felt on the proximal plantar calcaneus. Deep palpation is required, as one feels posterior, because the thick plantar fat pad *(D)* dominates this area by covering the posterior–plantar calcaneus. The heel pad is thinner as the plantar hindfoot transitions to the non–weight-bearing arch. There are no palpable neural or vascular structures in the plantar hindfoot, but the medial and lateral plantar nerves are just deep to the abductor hallucis muscle as they cross into the plantar hindfoot. Deep palpation can elicit tenderness in the respective distributions of these nerves.

Midfoot

Osteology

The structures of the dorsal midfoot, in most cases, can be appreciated with a careful examination (Fig. 2–14A and B). In addition, the bones of the midfoot can all be palpated nicely on the dorsum. The osteology of the dorsal midfoot is best felt by starting proximal at the talonavicular joint *(A)*. The bones can be defined by the palpable joints. The talonavicular joint can be felt as the most mobile joint on the medial side. By moving the foot into abduction and supination, the mobility of the joint can be felt. Whereas some motion is present in the more distal joints, in the normal foot the talonavicular joint is more mobile.

Once the talonavicular joint is found medially, the dorsal joint can be felt by running a finger along the navicular. Palpating distally while staying dorsal, one will feel a subtle ridge or thickening at the navicular cuneiform joint and the first tarsometatarsal joint *(B)*. The edges of the joints can be followed to define the bony architecture of the corresponding bones. The bases of the lesser tarsometatarsal joints are best isolated by following the lesser metatarsal shafts proximally. The second base is proximal to the first base, inset between the first and the third *(C)*.

The lateral aspect of the midfoot is more mobile than the medial and is best referenced from the prominent base of the fifth metatarsal *(D)*. This is the most lateral bony area on the lateral midfoot. It is both prominent and mobile. The calcaneocuboid joint *(E)* is isolated by holding the hindfoot stable and then dorsiflexing and plantar flexing the midfoot. The calcaneocuboid

lateral calcaneal area (Fig. 2–12). If one begins at the posterior-most aspect of the calcaneus and runs a finger distal to it, the lateral edge of the calcaneus can be felt as separate from the lateral aspect of the plantar fat pad (Fig. 2–13). The fat pad begins to be prominent as the skin texture changes from thin to thick as the weight-bearing surface of the heel becomes apparent. On the plantar surface (refer again to Fig 2–12), the lateral band of the plantar fascia and the abductor digiti minimi *(A)* are most often indistinguishable as a pinchable band originating from the palpable lateral calcaneus and extending distal to the fifth metatarsal head. The sural nerve can be felt as a cord just plantar to the peroneal tendons as they run along the calcaneal wall.

The plantar–medial hindfoot is best located from the posterior calcaneus by running a finger along the plantar–medial border of the bone. Quickly the bone becomes less subcuticular as the soft tissues of the arch are more prominent. The abductor hallucis muscle *(B)* can be palpated as it originates from the

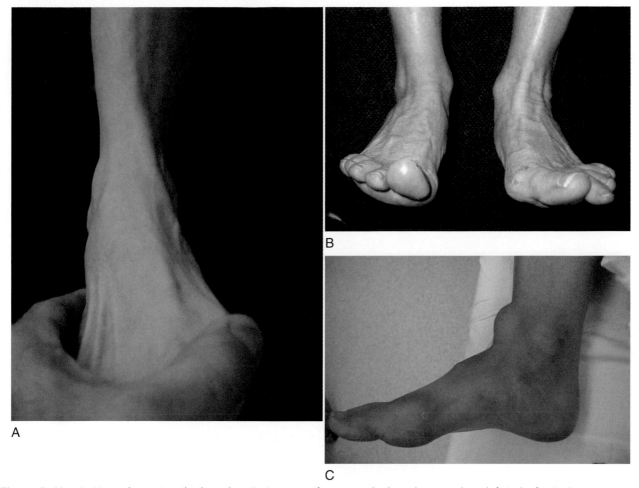

Figure 2–10 **A,** Normal anterior tibial tendon. **B,** Rupture of anterior tibial tendon noted on *left* (right foot). **C,** Rupture and contraction leaves a mass on the anterior ankle. (**B** and **C** courtesy of L. Schoen, MD.)

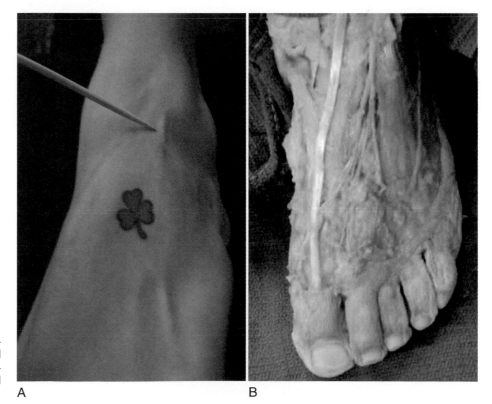

Figure 2–11 Superficial peroneal nerves. **A,** Superficial anatomy. **B,** Anatomic dissection demonstrating superficial peroneal nerve branches.

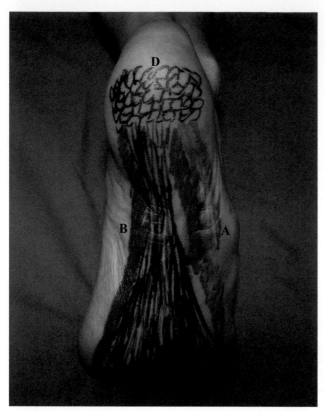

Figure 2–12 Plantar hindfoot. *A,* Lateral band of the plantar fascia and the abductor digiti minimi; *B,* abductor hallucis muscle; *C,* medial cord of the plantar fascia; *D,* plantar fat pad.

an area that can be mobile with peroneus longus activity. Asking the patient to actively plantar flex the first metatarsal can isolate the peroneus longus tendon (see Fig. 2–14C and D).

The medial midfoot is an area where the examiner can palpate extrinsic tendons that insert distal in the forefoot. Directly plantar to the medial cuneiform (Fig. 2–15), the point where the FHL and FDL cross (refer again to Fig. 2–14), the master knot of Henry *(I)*, can be located by deep palpation. This is made easier by active plantar flexion of the five toes. The medial cord of the plantar fascia covers the knot, but the moving tendons can be felt deep and medial to the medial cord of the static fascia. The EHL and EDL cross the dorsal medial midfoot and also are best palpated after active dorsiflexion of the toes.

On the lateral side, the peroneus brevis insertion *(J)* on the base of the fifth metatarsal is best appreciated with active eversion. The peroneus longus can be

joint is the mobile segment just proximal to the base of the fifth metatarsal as one feels along the lateral calcaneal wall. The anterior process of the calcaneus *(F)* is found by running a finger dorsally on the calcaneocuboid joint. The most dorsal palpable bony structure on the line is the anterior process of the calcaneus. The fourth and fifth tarsometatarsal joint can be located by the same dorsiflexion and plantar flexion used for the calcaneocuboid joint, but the fifth joint is at the base of the fifth metatarsal and the fourth joint is slightly medial and dorsal to the fifth metatarsal.

The midfoot represents the insertion area of many of the ankle tendons. The medial midfoot is the insertion area for the posterior tibialis, the anterior tibialis, and the peroneus longus tendons. The insertion of the posterior tibialis *(G)* is best felt at the navicular. When a patient actively supinates and inverts the foot, the tendon can be isolated proximally at the medial malleolus and followed to its insertion. The same can be done for the anterior tibialis *(H)* as it inserts on the plantar-medial aspect of the cuneiform and proximal first metatarsal.

The insertion of the peroneus longus cannot be palpated specifically except in very thin patients, but its insertion on the plantar base of the first metatarsal is

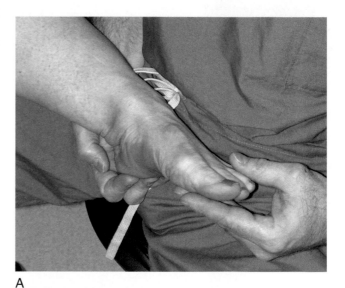

A

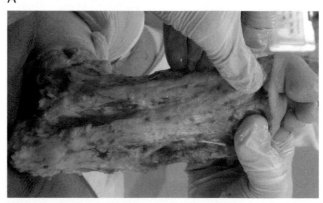

B

Figure 2–13 Plantar fascia. **A,** Clinical examination of plantar fascia. **B,** Anatomic dissection demonstrating the plantar fascia.

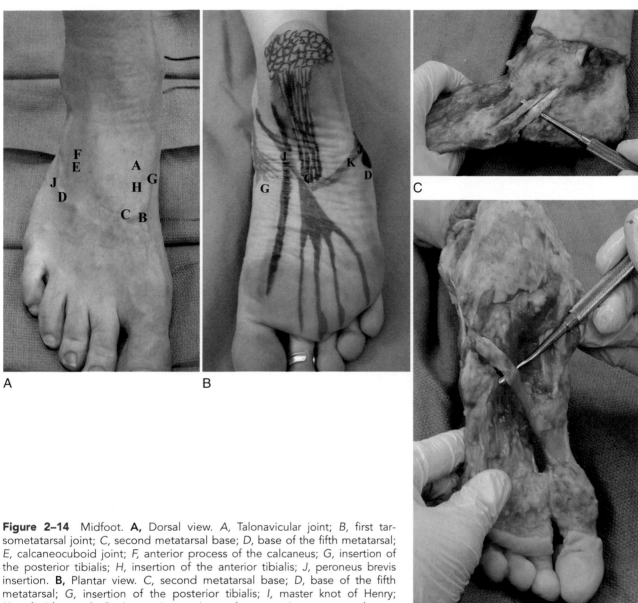

Figure 2–14 Midfoot. **A,** Dorsal view. *A,* Talonavicular joint; *B,* first tarsometatarsal joint; *C,* second metatarsal base; *D,* base of the fifth metatarsal; *E,* calcaneocuboid joint; *F,* anterior process of the calcaneus; *G,* insertion of the posterior tibialis; *H,* insertion of the anterior tibialis; *J,* peroneus brevis insertion. **B,** Plantar view. *C,* second metatarsal base; *D,* base of the fifth metatarsal; *G,* insertion of the posterior tibialis; *I,* master knot of Henry; *K,* cuboid tunnel. **C,** Anatomic specimen demonstrating peroneus longus and brevis. **D,** Plantar view of peroneus longus insertion.

palpated as it exits the inferior peroneal retinaculum plantar to the peroneus brevis. As the peroneus longus crosses superficial to the calcaneocuboid joint, it is felt as it dives plantar to head into the cuboid tunnel *(K)* and then across the bottom of the foot to the base of the first metatarsal. The cuboid tunnel and the peroneus longus in it can be palpated by deep pressure at the plantar–lateral cuboid.

The plantar fascia (PF) can be appreciated on the plantar foot with passive dorsiflexion of the toes. At the midfoot, the PF is wider than and not as thick as it is in the hindfoot. At this point one also can see the PF heading to the five toes. The intrinsic foot muscles can be palpated, but other than the abductor hallucis

(medial) and abductor digiti minimi (lateral), the specific muscles cannot be isolated.

Forefoot

Hallux Complex

The forefoot examination must begin with the hallux and its surrounding complex (Fig. 2–16). The first metatarsal can be palpated along its entire course. Beginning with the base of the proximal metatarsal, the first metatarsal can be followed distally to the head of the metatarsal *(A)*. At the first metatarsal's distal plantar extent, the tibial (medial) *(B)* and fibular (lateral) sesamoids *(C)* can be appreciated. They can

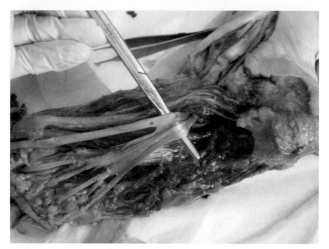

Figure 2–15 Anatomic specimen demonstrating the knot of Henry.

best be felt by passive dorsiflexion of the hallux MTP joint and deep palpation of the fat pad plantar to the joint. The proximal phalanx is very superficial and can be felt almost circumferentially. The hallux interphalangeal joint and the distal phalanx of the hallux can also be palpated circumferentially.

The sensory nerves of the hallux are very superficial and can often be palpated in a thin patient. The clinically significant nerves are the dorsal hallucal nerve and the plantar medial hallucal nerve. The dorsal hallucal nerve *(D)* is felt as a rounded cord on the dorsomedial edge of the medial eminence of the first metatarsal. The plantar–medial hallucal nerve *(E)* is found on the plantar–medial first metatarsal, just medial and dorsal to the tibial sesamoid bone and the dorsal lateral hallucal nerve *(F)* on the lateral aspect of the hallux. The dorsalis pedis artery pulse is appre-

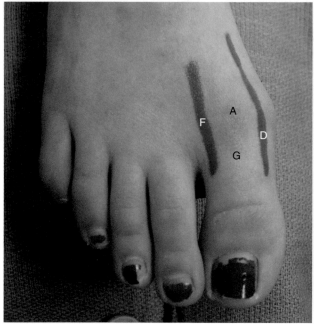

A

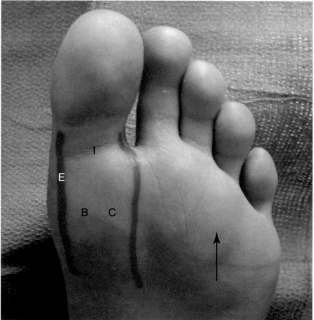

B

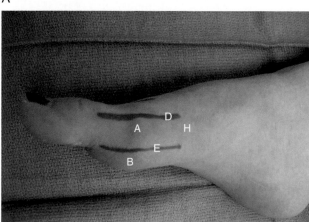

C

Figure 2–16 Hallux complex. **A,** Dorsal view. *A,* Head of the first metatarsal; *D,* dorsal medial hallucal nerve; *F,* dorsal lateral hallucal nerve; *G,* extensor hallucis longus. **B,** Plantar view. *B,* Tibial (medial) sesamoid; *C,* fibular (lateral) sesamoid; *E,* plantar medial hallucal nerve; *I,* flexor hallucis longus. **C,** Medial view. *A,* Head of the first metatarsal; *B,* tibial (medial) sesamoid; *D,* dorsal medial hallucal nerve; *E,* plantar medial hallucal nerve; *H,* abductor hallucis tendon.

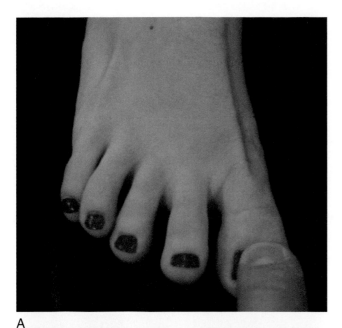

A

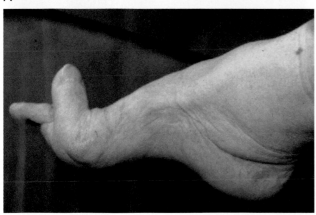

B

Figure 2–17 **A,** Normal appearance of the extensor hallucis longus (EHL). **B,** Following a cerebrovascular accident, an overactive EHL causes excess dorsiflexion of the hallux.

ciated proximal to the bases of the first and second metatarsals as the artery goes to the plantar foot.

The tendons of the hallux are palpated circumferentially. Dorsally the EHL *(G)* (larger) and EHB (smaller and lateral) can best be seen with active dorsiflexion of the hallux (Fig. 2–17). The abductor hallucis tendon (refer again to Fig. 2–16) *(H)* is appreciated dorsal to the tibial sesamoid at the joint line of the hallux MTP joint. The FHL *(I)* is appreciated between the sesamoids plantarly. It can be found lying on the proximal phalanx by rolling a finger across the plantar proximal phalanx all the way to the FHL insertion on the plantar base of the distal phalanx. The flexor hallucis brevis cannot be felt directly, but its location can be estimated by allowing a finger to slide proximally and distally on the sesamoids.

Lesser Metatarsals and Toes

The lesser metatarsals and the corresponding toes can be discussed as a group (Fig. 2–18A and B). As in the hallux, the bony anatomy is quite superficial. The metatarsal shafts can be palpated their entire length dorsally. The shafts are best located at the mid metatarsal and a finger run distally or proximally as needed. The plantar metatarsals cannot be directly palpated until the distal end or head. The metatarsal heads are always felt, but the detail is variable depending on the thickness of the plantar fat pad. The dorsal toe bones are easier to palpate than the plantar bones. Regardless, the MTP joints can be appreciated by passive plantar and dorsiflexion of the toes. The proximal interphalangeal (PIP) and distal interphalangeal (DIP) joints can be appreciated by passive or active plantar flexion of the joints (Fig. 2–18C and D). As the toes get smaller, the joints become less active and more passive. The fifth toe has little active control.

The tendons of the lesser toes move as a unit and are best examined together. The EDL can be seen best with active dorsiflexion of the toes. The EDB can usually be seen with the same maneuver in the second and third toes, but it is less accessible in the fourth. The FDL can be best palpated plantar at the base of the toes with a finger sweep in the transverse direction. Active flexion of the toes can help with this. The plantar plate of the MTP joint is in the space between the plantar metatarsal head and the base of the proximal phalanges.

EXAMINATION IN SEQUENCE

As mentioned earlier, the systematic sequence of the foot and ankle examination allows the examiner to be thorough and complete. Observation of gait and stance is followed by a sitting examination, which depends on mastering topographic anatomy, and the supine and prone examinations for special situations. At the same time, it is helpful to examine the patient's shoe and shoe wear patterns.

Gait

It is usually convenient at the beginning of the examination to observe the patient walking at various speeds and with shoes on and off. The hands should be empty and arms hanging freely at the sides. The following observations should be made.

1. *Detect obvious abnormalities of locomotion.* This is best observed, for examination purposes, by trying to examine each leg through a number of strides individually. This allows the examiner to

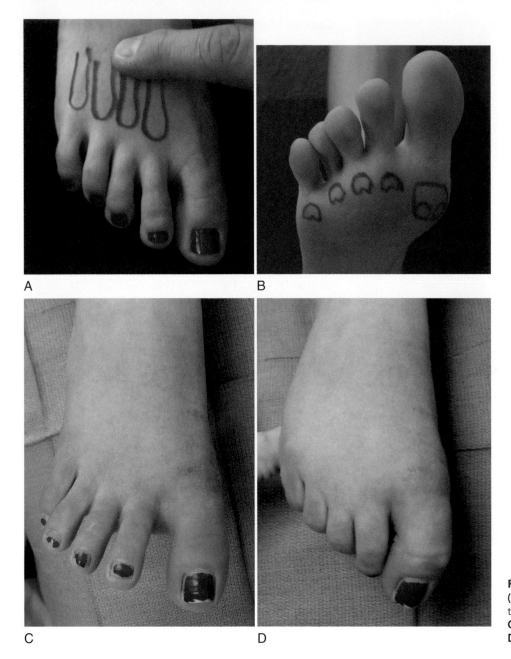

A

B

C

D

Figure 2–18 Forefoot. Dorsal **(A)** and plantar **(B)** views of the lesser metatarsals and toes. **C,** Extension of lesser toes. **D,** Flexion of lesser toes.

separate out sidedness on loss of stride length and gait phase of a limp.

2. *Perceive asymmetric behavior of the two sides of the body.* This asymmetry can be in torso rotation, upper extremity swing, or lower extremity unilateral gait disturbances. As a rule, the shoulders rotate 180 degrees out of phase with the pelvis; this is a passive response to pelvic rotation. If there are no abnormalities in the spine or upper extremities, rotation of the shoulders is reflected in equal and symmetric arm swing. If the arm swing is asymmetric, horizontal rotation of the pelvis also is asymmetric. Because such asymmetric pelvic rotation can be the result of abnor-

mality in any of the components of the lower extremity, it is mandatory that the practitioner take extra care in examining not only the foot and ankle but also the knees and hips.

3. *Observe the position of the patellas and tibial tubercles in standing and walking.* They are indicators of the degree of horizontal rotation of the leg in the horizontal plane and can guide the examiner to look more proximal for the primary pathologic process.

4. *Observe the degree of toeing in or out* (Fig. 2–19). The phase of gait when this deformity occurs is the key to understanding the cause. At toe-off, the leg has achieved its maximal external rotation and

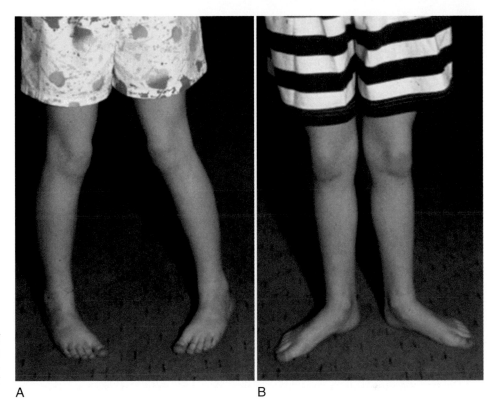

Figure 2–19 Examination of patella and tibial tubercle position. **A,** Intoeing in a child. **B,** External rotation of lower extremities.

A   B

the foot toes out slightly. During swing phase, the entire leg and foot rotate internally. The average amount of rotation is about 15 degrees, but this varies greatly from person to person. It may be almost imperceptible (3 degrees) or considerable (30 degrees).[2] At the time of heel strike, the long axis of the foot has approached, to a varying degree, the plane of progression. The degree of parallelism between the long axis of the foot and the plane of progression at this point is subject to considerable individual variation. However, the transition from heel strike to foot flat, which occurs rapidly, should be carefully observed. Some persons show an increase in toe-in during the very short period of plantar flexion of the ankle, indicating a greater degree of obliquity of the ankle axis (see Chapter 1).

5. *Observe the longitudinal arch during the first half of stance phase walking* (Fig. 2–20). Look for dynamic pronation or supination at the stance phase to assess for midstance stability. Normally the foot pronates as it is loaded with the body weight during the first half of stance phase. The amount of pronation is subject to extreme individual variation. The important factor, however, is whether the foot remains pronated during the period of heel rise and lift-off. In the normally functioning foot, as the heel rises there is almost instantaneous inversion of the heel. If the heel fails to invert at this time, the examiner should

check the strength of the intrinsic and extrinsic muscles of the foot and the range of motion in the articulations of the hindfoot and midfoot.

6. *Note the amount of heel inversion and supination of the foot* during lift-off and the presence or absence of rotatory slippage of the forefoot on the floor. Except on slippery surfaces, the shoe does not visibly rotate externally or slip on the floor at the time of lift-off. Failure of the ankle and subtalar joints to permit adequate external rotation of the leg during this phase of walking can result in direct transmission of the rotatory forces to the interface between the sole of the shoe and the walking surface, with resultant rotatory slippage of the shoe on the floor. On noting slippage, the examiner should look for possible muscle imbalance and should check the obliquity of the ankle axis and the range of motion in the subtalar joint (Fig. 2–21).

7. *Observe the position of the foot in relation to the floor at the time of heel strike.* Normally the heel strikes the ground first, followed by rapid plantar flexion. If this sequence does not occur, further investigation is indicated. In pathologic conditions, the patient might contact the ground with the foot flat or possibly on the toes. The time of heel rise also should be carefully noted; it occurs normally at 34% of the walking cycle just after the swinging leg has passed the stance foot. Early heel rise can indicate tightness of the

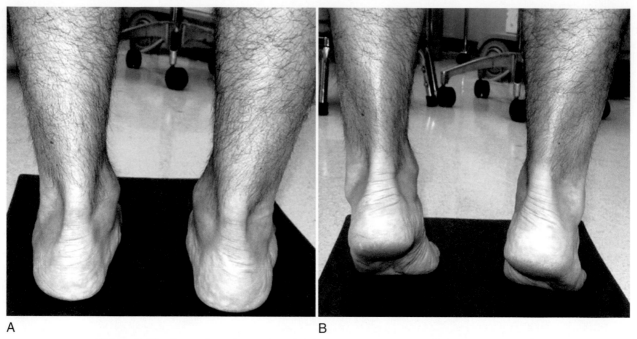

A   B

Figure 2–20 Dynamic arch creation. **A,** Flatfoot at stance. **B,** Arch creation at toe-off.

gastrocnemius–soleus muscle complex. A delay in heel rise can indicate weakness in the same muscle group.

If the implications of the preceding statements are not readily apparent, it is suggested that the reader review Chapter 1

Shoe Examination

Because the type of shoe and the heel height affect the way a person walks, they must be noted in the history and in the examination sequence. When wearing high heels, for example, women show less ankle-joint motion than when wearing flat heels, and in tennis shoes they show little difference from men in gait.

It is most convenient for the examiner to inspect the shoes after the gait analysis. This often is done during the history taking. The examination should include:

1. Path of wear from heel to toe. Early lateral hind-shoe and midshoe wear indicates a supination deformity. Loss of the medial sole and counter indicates a pronation deformity.

2. Presence of supportive devices or corrections in the shoes. Arch supports, heel pads, heel wedges, leather manipulation to accommodate deformity, or forefoot pads indicate previous difficulties.

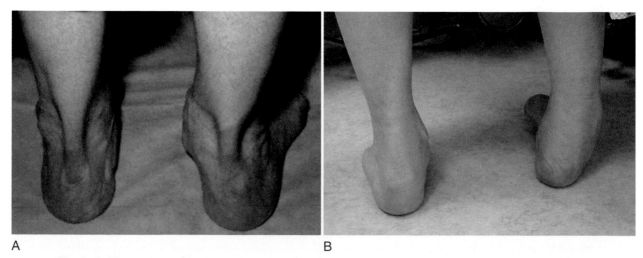

A   B

Figure 2–21 Position of heel in stance phase. **A,** Excess heel valgus *(right).* **B,** Excess heel varus *(right).*

3. Obliquity of the angle of the crease in the toe of the shoe. The angle varies from person to person; the greater the obliquity of the crease in the shoe to its long axis, the greater the amount of subtalar motion required to distribute the body weight evenly over the metatarsal heads.

4. Impression the forefoot has made on the insole of the shoe. This can often give important information about the patient's force distribution on the plantar foot.

5. Presence or absence of circular wear on the sole of the shoe. Such wear indicates rotatory slippage of the foot on the floor during lift-off from lack of subtalar motion.

6. The shape of the shoe compared to the shape of the foot. This gives the examiner clues as to the proper sizing of the patient's shoes. The shape of the shoe (e.g., narrow pointed shoe or broad toe box) and the overall shape of the foot when the patient is weight bearing should be carefully observed.

Standing Examination

The standing examination, in the normal setting (patient is able to stand), can give the examiner a tremendous amount of information. The whole issue of asymmetry can best be addressed on standing examination because the direct visual comparison can be accomplished with a hard, careful look.

First, the patient is asked to stand facing the examiner on a raised stool (Fig. 2–22). This allows visualization of the anterior pelvis, the patellas, and the tibial tubercle. Using these anatomic landmarks, the rotation of the foot in relation to the tibia, hip, and pelvis

can be established. To estimate pelvic tilt from the front, the examiner places an index finger on either the anterior superior iliac spines or the iliac crests. An anatomic or functional shortening of one leg can be seen readily if the shortening is greater than 1/4 inch. Inspection of the popliteal creases reveals whether major shortening is in the thigh or in the lower leg. Gross abnormalities of components of the lower extremity best located standing include differences in circumference of the thighs and calves and excessive deviation in skeletal alignment in all planes (varus, valgus, flexion, extension, and rotation).

This front-facing standing examination gives the best view of the medial longitudinal arch. The presence of pes planus or pes cavus can be determined. There are least two general categories of pes planus for the purposes of the physical examination. In one category, the longitudinal arch is depressed, without the complicating factors of everted heel, abducted forefoot, or longitudinal rotation of the metatarsals and phalanges (Fig. 2–23A and B). In the other category, the foot appears to have fallen inward, like the tilting of a half-hemisphere (Fig 2–23C and D). The heel is everted, the outer border of the foot shows angulation at the midfoot, and the forefoot is abducted, creating a more impressive deformity. In the first category, the Achilles tendon remains relatively straight; in the second, the Achilles tendon deviates laterally when the patient bears weight on the relaxed foot. The pathologic implications of these two types of flatfoot are different.

The pes cavus or high arch also has two main types. In the first, the heel is in neutral to slight valgus but the forefoot flexibility allows the forefoot good ground accommodation. This prevents forefoot adduction on standing examination. In the second, the heel is

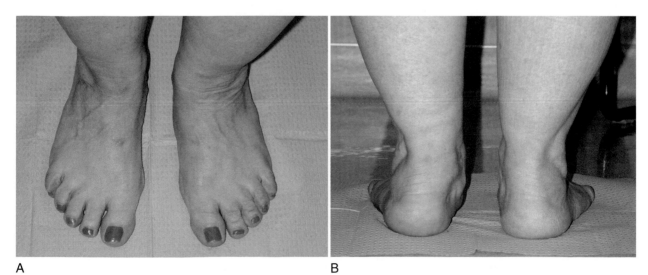

A   B

Figure 2–22 Standing examination. **A,** Patient facing the examiner. **B,** Patient facing away from the examiner.

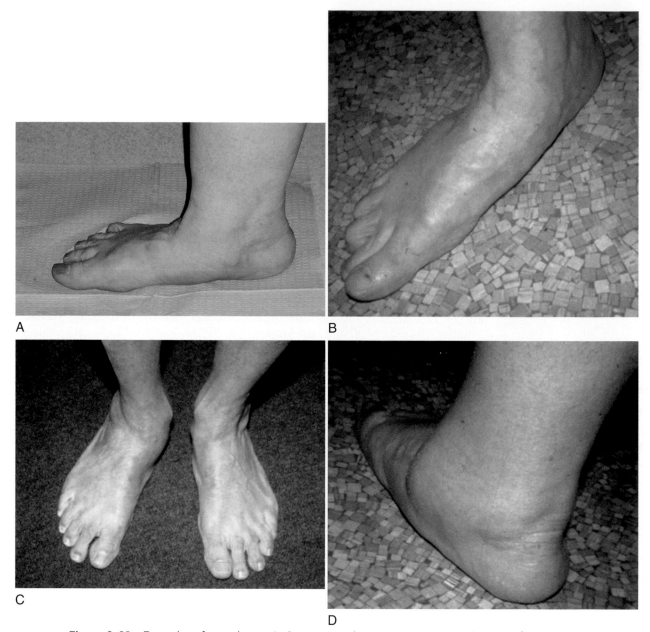

Figure 2–23   Examples of pes planus. **A,** Severe pes planus. **B** to **D,** Varying degrees of pes planus.

fixed in varus and the midfoot and forefoot have compensated by forefoot adduction and lateral overload. Again, the pathologic process associated with the two types is different. A consistent definition of "normal" when speaking of flatfoot and cavus foot is unclear.

Finally, the front-facing standing examination gives a good view of the toes and how they contact the ground. The valgus or varus position of the hallux is highlighted with weight bearing. The pronation of the hallux in relation to the rest of the foot is seen best in this posture. The lesser toes can also be appreciated in this way. Cross-over deformities, cock-up deformities, joint contractures, floating toes, and dynamic location of callus (terminal or dorsal) are most efficiently exam-

ined with the patient standing on a stool. The examiner also should note whether the toes touch the ground.

At this point the patient can step off the stool and face away from the seated examiner (see Fig. 2–22A). The pelvis, femur, thigh, knee, tibia, and calf symmetry is re-examined from this view. In particular, the relationship of the heel axis to the ankle joint and the rest of the foot are appreciated. The lateral metatarsal and toes are seen normally from this view. Asymmetry in this examination goes a long way in illustrating the cause and solution in hindfoot, midfoot, and ankle disorder.

It is helpful to have the patient elevate to balance on the toes. If the foot is functioning normally, the heel promptly inverts, the longitudinal arch rises, and the

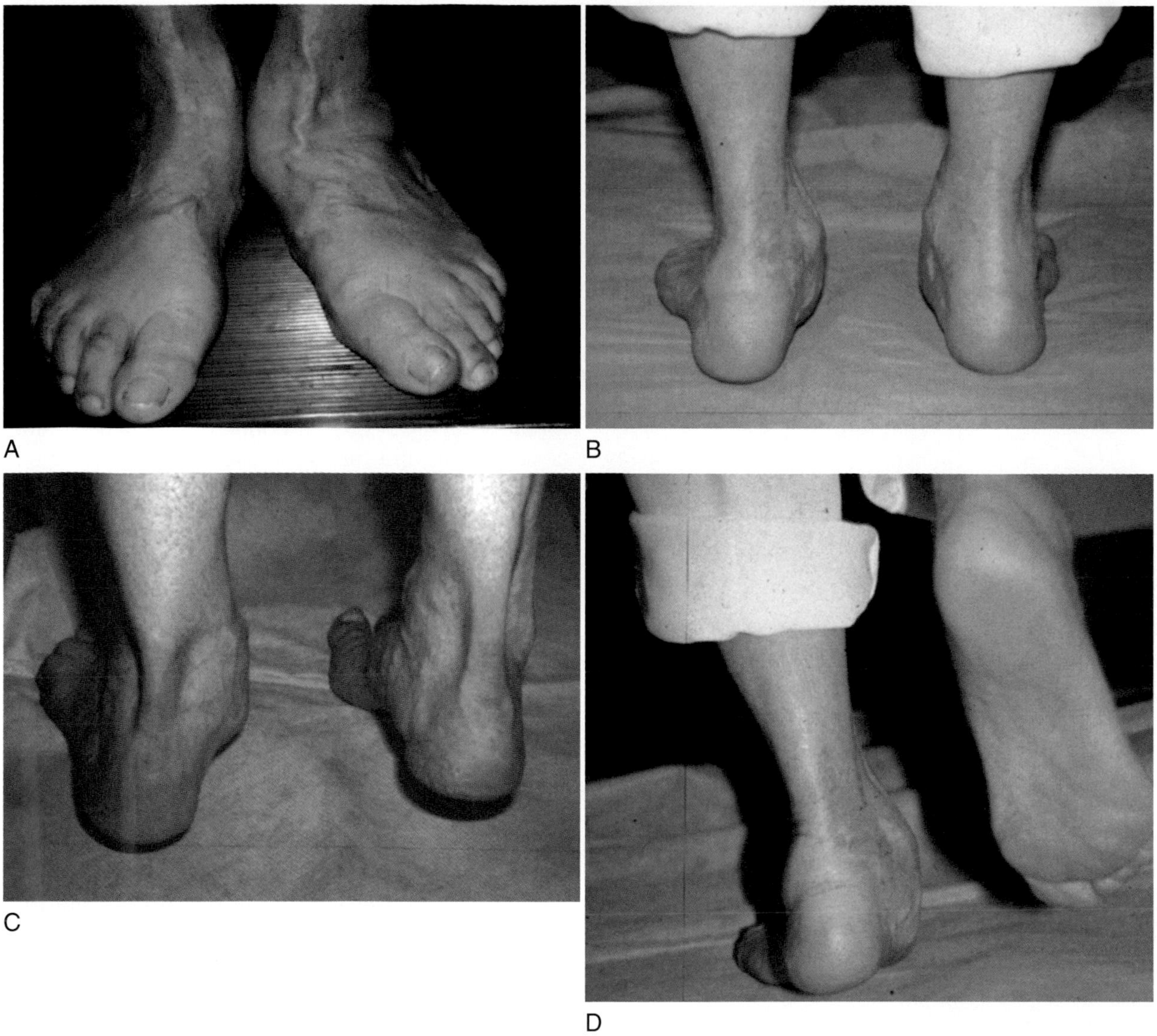

Figure 2–24 Single-limb toe-raise examination. **A,** Anterior view. **B,** Posterior view prior to examination (patient's left foot has a ruptured posterior tibial tendon). **C,** Patient is able to stand on tip toe on the right foot without difficulty. **D,** On the left foot, the arch sags; the patient is not able to perform a repetitive toe rise.

leg rotates externally (see Fig. 2–20). Failure of these movements to occur can indicate a weak foot or a specific pathologic process.

Inversion of the heel is achieved through proper performance of the subtalar and transverse tarsal articulations and the tendons that act across these joints. Failure of the heel to invert should immediately focus the examiner's attention on possible malfunction of these structures. Some conditions that can limit activity in these joints are muscle weakness, dysfunction of the tibialis posterior, arthritic changes in the hindfoot, and such skeletal abnormalities as vertical talus and tarsal coalition. The patient should also be asked to single-limb toe raise on each foot (Fig. 2–24). This can demonstrate early weakness, especially when the patient is asked to do it multiple times, or marked weakness if the patient is unable to single-limb toe

raise at all. Do not put too much stock in the single-limb toe raise in elderly patients, because many elderly patients cannot do this maneuver even when all joints and tendons are normal.

Sitting Examination

The patient is asked to sit on the edge of the table with the legs dangling over the edge (Fig. 2–25). The examiner should sit lower on a stool. This allows for easy inspection, palpation, and manipulation of both extremities. It is at this point that the lessons learned in the topographic anatomy section are best used.

General Visual Overview

Any visible abnormalities should be noted at this time. Varicosities, areas of telangiectasia, erythema, and

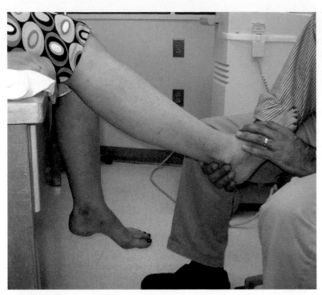

Figure 2–25 Sitting examination. Note the position of the examiner.

ecchymosis, and generalized edema should be noted. The dorsalis pedis and posterior tibial pulses should be palpated. The speed of capillary filling after compression of the nail bed should be checked. The skin is examined for local areas of swelling, and the structures in these areas are palpated. The skin over joints normally is cooler than the skin over muscular areas of the extremity. One should observe the various muscle groups, looking for atrophy in the anterior, lateral, and posterior calf region, as well as the medial side of the foot.

The distribution of hair on the foot should be carefully noted. Loss of distal foot or toe hair can suggest a systemic disorder such as peripheral vascular disease or lupus.

The skin on the plantar aspect of the foot and about the toes is inspected carefully for callus formation, which often indicates abnormal pressure on the foot. All scars, wounds, and ulcerations should be noted, surgical or otherwise, because this can give the examiner insight into the history of that particular foot.

General Skeletal Overview

Gross skeletal deformities are readily discernible and can hardly be overlooked even by the most inexperienced examiner. Deviation in the hallux MTP joints, lesser toe deformities, and asymmetric midfoot deformity can be observed grossly at this point. The bony prominences about the foot are carefully noted. A prominence over the region of the tarsometatarsal joints may be the first sign of arthrosis of these joints, and a prominence over the fifth metatarsal head can indicate a bunionette deformity. Difficulties in making a diagnosis are more likely to arise in

patients whose feet, on casual inspection, appear relatively normal.

Range of Motion of the Joints

While the patient remains on the table, the joints of the foot and ankle should be assessed for motion. The passive and active range of motion of all major articulations of the foot should be checked for limitation of motion, painful movement, and crepitus. These findings can occur separately or in any combination or sequence.

ANKLE JOINT

The ankle joint should be moved through its full range of motion (Fig. 2–26). Although the ankle is essentially a single-axis joint, its axis is skewed to both the transverse and the coronal planes of the body, passing downward and backward from the medial to the lateral side. A reasonably accurate estimate of the location of the ankle axis is obtained by placing the tips of the index fingers just below the most distal projections of the two malleoli (Fig. 2–27). Depending on the degree of obliquity of the axis, dorsiflexion and plantar flexion produce medial and lateral deviation of the foot. Because an oblique axis of the ankle assists in absorbing the horizontal rotation of the leg, its range of motion on gross examination is related to the range of motion in the subtalar joint. Normally there is no lateral play of the talus in the mortise even when the foot is in full plantar flexion. Often the talus can be displaced forward and backward a millimeter or so in the mortise, but this is a normal finding. Any lateral or medial displacement of the talus in the mortise that is seen on examination indicates an abnormality of the mortise.

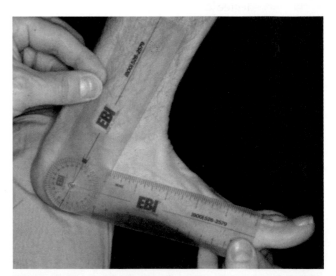

Figure 2–26 Ankle range of motion documented on the lateral aspect with a goniometer.

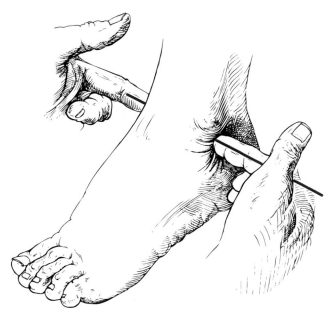

Figure 2–27 Estimating the location of the ankle axis.

SUBTALAR JOINT

The amount of motion in the subtalar joint varies. Isman and Inman[1] found a minimum of 20 degrees and a maximum of 60 degrees of motion in a series of feet in cadaver specimens. A gross method of determining the degree of subtalar motion is to apply rotatory force on the calcaneus while permitting the rest of the foot to move passively. When rotatory force is applied to the forefoot, abnormally large displacements can be obtained through movements of the articulations in the midfoot that are additive to subtalar motion. This method allows gross analysis but is not specific enough for making treatment decisions.

The most accurate, but not practical, method of determining the degree of subtalar motion is to place the patient prone and flex the knee to approximately 135 degrees. The axis of the subtalar joint now lies close to the horizontal plane. The examiner then passively inverts and everts the heel while measuring the extent of motion with a gravity goniometer or level (Fig. 2–28). This method is used primarily for research purposes.

A more practical method, for the office setting, of determining the degree of subtalar motion is accomplished while the patient is sitting on the examining table. The calcaneus is placed in line with the long axis of the tibia. With the calcaneus held in one hand and the forefoot, including the transverse tarsal joint, in the other, the subtalar joint is brought into inversion and eversion. While carrying out this motion, it is important to note not only the total range of motion but also the amount of inversion and eversion. There usually is twice as much inversion as eversion. Occasionally in a patient with flatfoot, although there is full total range of motion, the plane of motion is such that little or no inversion occurs. It also is important to observe any asymmetry of subtalar motion in a percentage fashion. This is often the most reproducible measurement for this joint. Lack of subtalar motion should alert the examiner to the possibility of arthrosis of the subtalar joint, peroneal spastic flatfoot, or an anatomic abnormality such as tarsal coalition.

TRANSVERSE TARSAL JOINT

The motion of the transverse tarsal joint is observed by holding the calcaneus in line with the long axis of the tibia (the subtalar neutral position) and the forefoot parallel to the floor. Adduction and abduction of this joint can be isolated (Fig. 2–29). Although these measurements are somewhat variable, a general rule is that there is twice as much adduction as abduction at the transverse tarsal joint. As with the subtalar joint, it is imperative that the total range of motion is noted as well as the degree of adduction and abduction. In some pathologic states such as posterior tibial tendon dysfunction or arthrosis of the midtarsal joints, the foot is maintained in a chronically abducted position, and a neutral position cannot be achieved. This fixed abduction should be noted to highlight the joints with the primary disorder.

METATARSOPHALANGEAL JOINTS

Motion at the MTP joints is measured by placing the ankle at a right angle and having the patient actively dorsiflex and plantar flex the MTP joints and the interphalangeal joints. Then passive motion can be determined at the same time. Again, there is a great deal of individual variability, with dorsiflexion ranging from 45 to 90 degrees and plantar flexion from 10 to 40 degrees, depending on the mobility of the individual joints. The critical factor is, again, to compare the sides for asymmetry. Motion of the interphalangeal joints is likewise observed (Fig. 2–30).

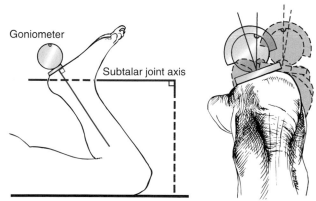

Figure 2–28 Spherical goniometer attached to the calcaneus to measure the degree of subtalar motion.

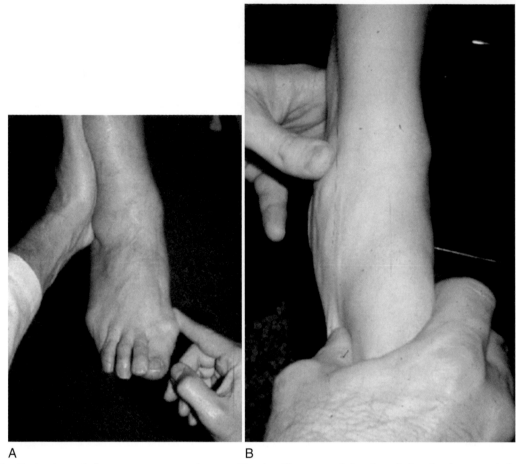

A   B

Figure 2–29 Evaluation of the transverse tarsal joint. The hindfoot is stabilized and the forefoot is abducted **(A)** and adducted **(B)**.

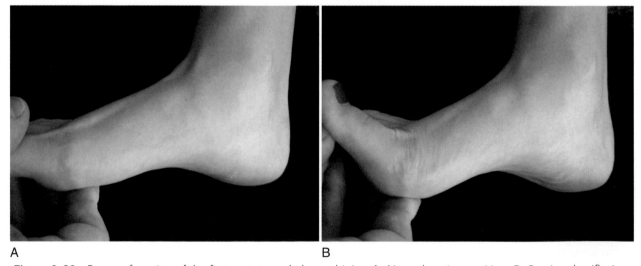

A   B

Figure 2–30 Range of motion of the first metatarsophalangeal joint. **A,** Normal resting position. **B,** Passive dorsiflexion.

Relationship of Forefoot to Hindfoot

After the range of motion of the foot has been determined, the relationship of the hindfoot to the forefoot should be ascertained. This relationship is important because it can be the underlying cause of the patient's clinical problem. Determination of this relationship is best carried out with the patient sitting on the examining table with the knees flexed at 90 degrees.

The hindfoot is grasped and placed into its neutral position (the calcaneus in line with the long axis of the leg or the Achilles). When examining the right foot, the heel is grasped with the examiner's right hand and the area of the fifth metatarsal head is grasped with the left hand. The examiner's right thumb is placed over the talonavicular joint, and this joint is manipulated until the examiner feels that the head of the talus is covered by the navicular. This movement is brought about by the examiner's left hand moving the forefoot in relation to the hindfoot. Once neutral hindfoot position has been achieved, the relationship of the forefoot as projected by a plane parallel to the metatarsals is related to a plane perpendicular to the long axis of the calcaneus.

Based on this measurement, the forefoot will be in one of three positions in relation to the hindfoot:

- *Neutral*: The plane of the metatarsals and the plane of the calcaneus are perpendicular to each other.

- *Forefoot varus*: The lateral aspect of the foot is more plantar flexed than the medial aspect, placing the forefoot in a supinated position (Fig. 2–31).

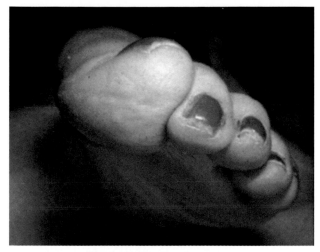

Figure 2–31 Forefoot varus.

- *Forefoot valgus*: The medial border of the foot is more plantar flexed in relation to the lateral border of the foot, placing the foot in a pronated position.

This measurement should be carried out two or three times to be sure an error is not made (Fig. 2–32).

The importance of this measurement is that by relating the position of the forefoot to the hindfoot, various types of clinical problems can be identified. In the normal foot, the forefoot and hindfoot planes are almost perpendicular to each other, although a moderate degree of variability in the measurement is of no clinical significance. The relation of the forefoot to the

Figure 2–32 Relationship of hindfoot to forefoot. **A,** Normal alignment; forefoot perpendicular to calcaneus. **B,** Forefoot varus (uncompensated); lateral aspect of the forefoot is plantar flexed in relation to the medial aspect. **C,** Forefoot varus (compensated); with the forefoot flat on the floor, the heel assumes a valgus position, which can result in impingement of the calcaneus against the fibula. **D,** Forefoot valgus (uncompensated); the medial aspect of the forefoot is plantar flexed in relation to the lateral aspect. **E,** Forefoot valgus (compensated); with the forefoot flat on the floor, the heel assumes a varus position.

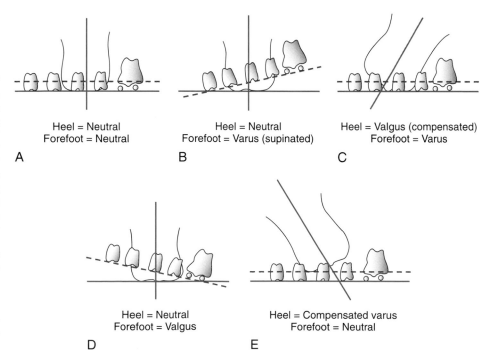

A   Heel = Neutral / Forefoot = Neutral

B   Heel = Neutral / Forefoot = Varus (supinated)

C   Heel = Valgus (compensated) / Forefoot = Varus

D   Heel = Neutral / Forefoot = Valgus

E   Heel = Compensated varus / Forefoot = Neutral

hindfoot may be supple or rigid. This determination is important when considering surgery to create a plantigrade foot. A fixed varus or valgus forefoot deformity does not permit the foot to become plantigrade once the hindfoot is placed into neutral position, and thus the extent of the fusion mass needs to include the transverse tarsal joint in order to realign the forefoot. Conversely, when the forefoot is supple or neutral, realignment of the hindfoot alone permits the forefoot to be plantigrade.

Direct Palpation

The importance of direct palpation cannot be emphasized enough in the examination of the foot and ankle. The ready access to the bony, tendinous, and ligamentous structures in combination with a focused history is essential to finally determining the exact structure that is pathologic. The distance between the tender area in the two medial tendons, FHL and posterior tibialis, is only a few millimeters but makes a world of difference in treatment and prognosis. Careful study of the topographic anatomy (see earlier) allows for a mastery of this portion of the seated examination. The systematic palpation must be done carefully and directly. The tools used most often are the tip of the examiner's dominant index finger or, for deeper structures, the tip of the thumb. It is not unusual to arrive at a diagnosis after a careful history and a single palpation with a question: Does it hurt here?

Muscle Function

Muscle function about the foot and ankle should be carefully tested. Most of the testing is done while the patient is seated. It is important to observe the strength of each muscle, particularly in a patient who has demonstrated some evidence of muscle weakness. It is also helpful to palpate each tendon to be sure that compensation by another muscle is not masking loss of function. The anatomically adept examiner can readily perform this, although several specific muscles sometimes lead to confusion.

The tibialis posterior function may be difficult to differentiate from the tibialis anterior insofar as inversion function is concerned. In addition to having the patient actively invert the foot and palpating the tibialis posterior tendon, the foot should be placed into an everted position and the patient then asked to invert against some resistance. This maneuver can isolate weakness of the tibialis posterior. In some patients this can be done easiest with the patient's leg crossed (Fig. 2–33).

The extrinsic muscles of the lateral foot can lead to similar difficulties. The peroneus brevis muscle functions mainly to evert the foot, and the peroneus longus functions mainly to bring about plantar flexion of the medial border of the foot. The eversion function of the peroneus longus is quite weak, and to isolate the longus the patient should be asked to plantar flex the medial side of the foot. The examiner should resist beneath the first metatarsal head.

Not only should the strength of this muscle group be tested, but also it is important to determine whether a contracture is present. In the hindfoot, the most common contracture is the calf muscle complex. To check the gastrocnemius–soleus complex for contracture, with the knee flexed, the hindfoot is first placed into neutral position and the navicular is centered over the head of the talus. With the foot in neutral position, passive dorsiflexion of the ankle to approximately 10 to 15 degrees should be possible. If not, there is an

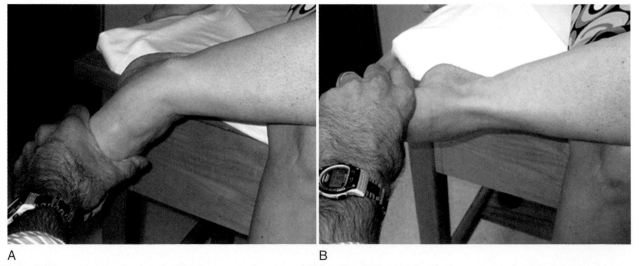

A   B

Figure 2–33 Isolation of posterior tibialis muscle function. **A,** The muscle is tested with the patient's foot dependent to gravity with the legs crossed. **B,** The strength is tested from full eversion to full inversion.

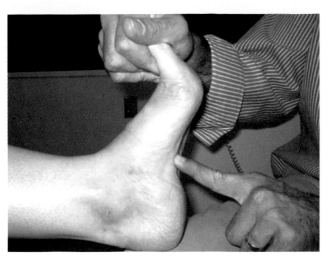

Figure 2–34 Palpation of the plantar aponeurosis facilitated by dorsiflexion of the toes.

element of contracture of the muscle group. The knee is then fully extended and the same maneuver carried out. If dorsiflexion past neutral cannot be achieved, then the gastrocnemius portion of the gastrocnemius–soleus complex is contracted. If the subtalar joint is permitted to pass into valgus while the examiner is attempting to measure dorsiflexion at the ankle joint, the presence of a contracture can easily be masked.

Plantar Fascia

The plantar aponeurosis or plantar fascia should be palpated along its entire surface. Dorsiflexion of the toes makes the fascia more prominent and facilitates palpation (Fig. 2–34).

Peripheral Nerves

The detailed peripheral nerve evaluation is best directed by the history. When the patient complains of a burning type of pain, often accompanied by a feeling of numbness, a careful sensory examination should be conducted because this is most often nerve pain. Such complaints often indicate peripheral nerve disorders and may be early symptoms of a generalized neuritis or neuropathy. Systemic disorders such as diabetes and sensory axonal neuropathy are commonly first suspected after a careful foot examination. Simple office tools such as the Semmes–Weinstein monofilament test (Fig. 2–35) can be used to assess the degree of sensory deficit in the patient. The examiner should check not only for deficits in cutaneous sensation and reflexes but also for diminished positional and vibratory sensation.

There are several areas in the foot in which the peripheral nerves may be locally entrapped and irri-

tated. The most common site is the posterior tibial nerve as it passes through the tarsal tunnel, which is located behind the medial malleolus. Percussion along the course of the nerve as it passes through the tunnel to elicit tingling over the nerve can indicate compression or irritation of the nerve.

The deep peroneal nerve can be entrapped beneath the extensor retinaculum on the dorsum of the foot and ankle; this is known as *anterior tarsal tunnel syndrome*. When the diagnosis is suspected, the examiner should carefully percuss over the extensor retinaculum and along the course of the deep peroneal nerve to look for evidence of tingling, which indicates irritability of the nerve. Besides being compressed at the level of the extensor retinaculum, the nerve may be involved as it passes over a dorsal exostosis at the talonavicular joint or more distally at the tarsometatarsal articulation.

Burning pain that radiates to the web space between the second and third toes should make one suspicious of interdigital neuroma. Firm palpation in the plantar web space usually reproduces the neuritic symptoms. Mediolateral compression of the foot, particularly when examining the third web space, can result in a click and pain radiating toward the toes.

On rare occasions a tight band of transverse crural fascia entraps the superficial peroneal nerves. This is detected by carefully percussing along the inferior margin of the crural fascia when examining a patient who complains of discomfort over the dorsum of the foot. Nerve entrapment also can occur around a surgical scar or in an area that has been crushed, and these areas should be carefully noted.

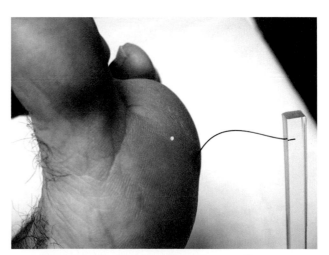

Figure 2–35 Semmes–Weinstein monofilament.

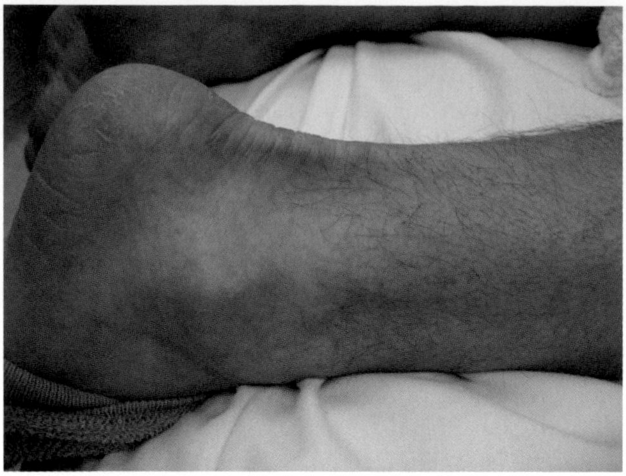

Figure 2–36 Prone examination.

Supine Examination

The supine examination is mentioned for completeness. The most common use of the supine examination is for a detailed inspection of the plantar foot. In particular, in an obese patient, body habitus prevents adequate inspection of the bottom of the foot while sitting.

Prone Examination

The prone examination is a specialty examination that can make certain areas of the foot and ankle more readily accessible (Fig. 2–36). In particular, the posterior calcaneus, Achilles tendon, and calf are best examined prone. The tendon can be palpated along its entirety under direct vision. This allows for access to defects and masses. The skin over the tendon can be manipulated in this position to differentiate between a number of Achilles pathologies. The posterior calcaneus can best be viewed from this approach. The ability to palpate this subcutaneous bone can give valued insights into its problems.

REFERENCES

1. Isman RE, Inman VT: Anthropometric studies of the human foot and ankle. *Bull Prosthet Res* 10-11:97-129, 1969.
2. Levens AS, Inman VT, Blosser JA: Transverse rotation of the segments of the lower extremity in locomotion. *J Bone Joint Surg Am* 30:859-872, 1948.

Imaging of the Foot and Ankle

Carroll P. Jones • Alastair S. E. Younger

Imaging of the foot and ankle is essential to the surgeon for the diagnosis and treatment of multiple lower extremity conditions including fractures, neoplasms, arthritides, deformities, and infections. Radiologic modalities are evolving rapidly, and the surgeon must have a firm understanding of the ideal imaging technique for specific conditions. Understanding the advantages and limitations of different types of imaging will facilitate an accurate, cost-efficient diagnostic evaluation.

The purpose of this chapter is to review the most commonly used radiologic techniques for foot and ankle problems. The major options are presented to provide a basic understanding of the procedures and a general overview of their role in patient evaluation. Pertinent normal anatomy and important congenital variation are included when possible, although a full review is beyond the scope of this chapter.

The chapter ends with a discussion of several common foot and ankle problems, offering simple algorithms to guide the clinician's choice of imaging. A thorough review of the initial material should allow one to substitute imaging options in the decision-making process, depending on institutional strengths and individual patient needs.

ROUTINE RADIOGRAPHY

Plain-film radiography is the mainstay of foot and ankle imaging and is usually employed at the initial patient evaluation. Standard weight-bearing projections are recommended if clinically practical, with supplemental special views obtained to evaluate a specific problem or condition. Inherent limitations exist and should be kept in mind, including technical variations in beam angulations, strength, and distance; inter- and intraobserver variability in radiographic assessments; and inconsistencies in patient positioning and weight-bearing efforts.

Radiographic Evaluation of the Foot

The foot is anatomically divided into the forefoot, midfoot, and hindfoot. The forefoot consists of the phalanges and metatarsals and is separated from the midfoot by Lisfranc's joint, or the tarsometatarsal articulation. The midfoot includes the navicular, cuboid, and three cuneiform bones and is separated from the hindfoot by Chopart's joint. The hindfoot contains the talus and calcaneus.

Standard projections of the foot include anteroposterior (AP), lateral, internal oblique, and external oblique views (Fig. 3–1). Non–weight-bearing views are adequate for assessing structural anatomy, including common normal variants (Fig. 3–2), but do not view the foot in a physiologic position.

The AP projection provides excellent imaging of the forefoot and midfoot, including the tarsometatarsal and transverse tarsal articulations. The x-ray beam is centered on the third metatarsal and angled 15 degrees cephalad from the vertical (Fig 3–3 and see Fig 3–1). The lateral view demonstrates the anatomy of the talus and calcaneus, as well as their relationship to the midfoot and ankle joint (Fig. 3–4). Lateral radiographs are obtained with the beam directed perpendicular to a point just above the base of the fifth metatarsal.

A medial (internal) oblique image is part of the routine three-view foot series (see Fig. 3–1). This view complements both the AP and lateral views in evaluating the forefoot and hindfoot, respectively. One of its primary roles is in assessing the lateral tarsometatarsal articulations, which is particularly impor-

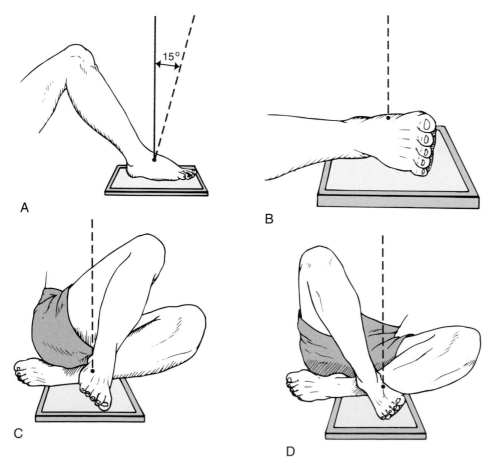

Figure 3–1 Standard positioning of foot for non–weight-bearing views. **A,** Anteroposterior. **B,** Lateral. **C,** Medial (internal) oblique with lateral border of foot elevated 30 degrees. **D,** Lateral (external) oblique with medial border of foot elevated 30 degrees.

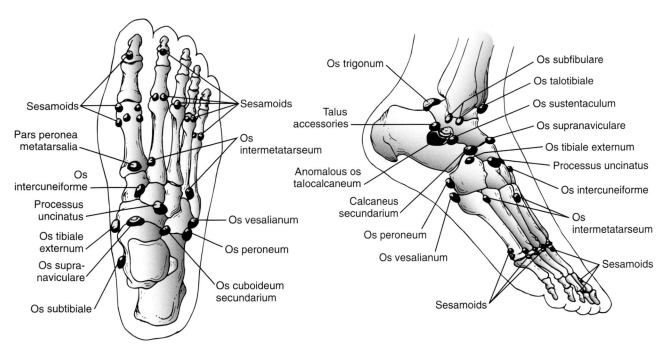

Figure 3–2 Accessory ossicles and sesamoid bones of foot and ankle. Sesamoid bones occasionally are bipartite, whereas accessory ossicles may be multicentric or even fused to adjacent bone.

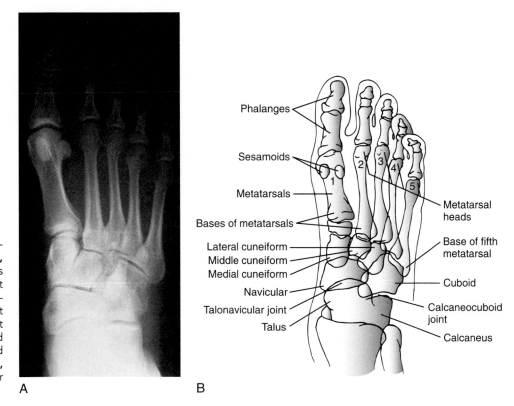

Figure 3–3 Anteroposterior projections of foot. **A,** Angled x-ray beam provides improved detail of midfoot anatomy, particularly illustrating normal alignment of lateral border of first tarsometatarsal joint and medial border of second tarsometatarsal joint. **B,** Anatomic drawing for correlation.

A

B

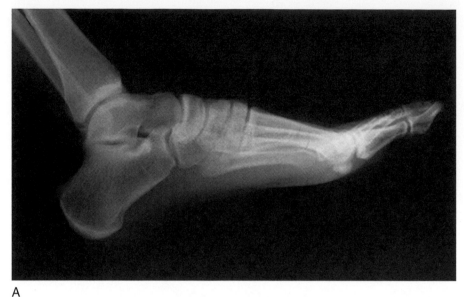

A

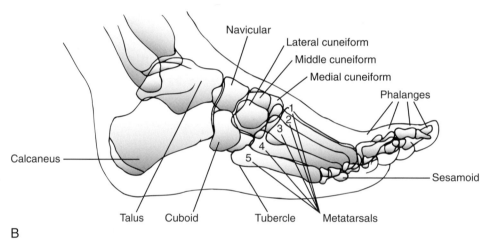

B

Navicular
Lateral cuneiform
Middle cuneiform
Medial cuneiform
Phalanges
1
2
3
4
5
Calcaneus
Sesamoid
Talus   Cuboid   Tubercle   Metatarsals

Figure 3–4 Lateral projection of foot. **A,** Radiograph illustrates anatomic relationships of midfoot and hindfoot. **B,** Anatomic drawing for correlation.

tant if a Lisfranc injury is suspected (Fig. 3–5). A calcaneonavicular tarsal coalition can also be visualized with the internal oblique projection. The lateral oblique view offers additional information about the tarsals and Chopart's joint (Fig. 3–6) and can aid in identifying an accessory navicular bone. Occasionally it demonstrates lateral capsular or ligamentous avulsions not seen on other views.

Weight-bearing views of the foot offer insight with regard to function in response to the physiologic stress of standing and are recommended for all evaluations unless clinically contraindicated. Shereff et al[21] have demonstrated significant measurement differences between weight-bearing and non–weight-bearing views when assessing conditions such as arch align-

ment and foot splaying. Bilateral AP views can be obtained simultaneously, if desired, but the lateral views are taken individually (Figs. 3–7 and 3–8). Special techniques are required to obtain adequate views in young children and infants. These involve active immobilization and compression by a gloved assistant or a static immobilization system (Fig. 3–9). Radiographs of the contralateral foot may be helpful for comparison views.

Phalanges

When clinical concerns about the phalanges are not addressed on routine foot projections, additional views are obtained, usually a lateral oblique view (Fig. 3–10) and a lateral view (Fig. 3–11).

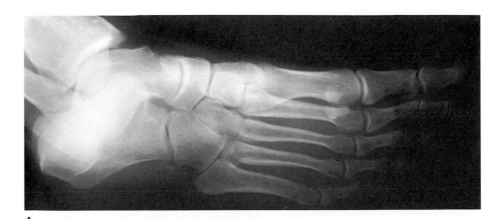

A

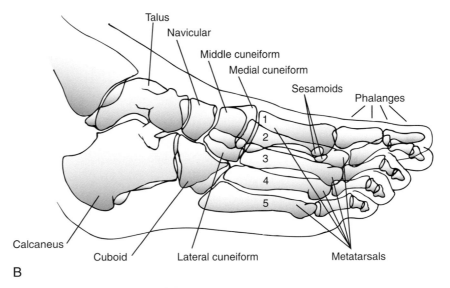

Talus
Navicular
Middle cuneiform
Medial cuneiform
Sesamoids
Phalanges
1
2
3
4
5
Calcaneus
Cuboid
Lateral cuneiform
Metatarsals

B

Figure 3–5 Medial oblique projection of foot. **A,** Radiograph demonstrates normal medial border alignment of third and fourth tarsometatarsal joints. It also allows evaluation of talonavicular and calcaneocuboid relationships. **B,** Anatomic drawing for correlation.

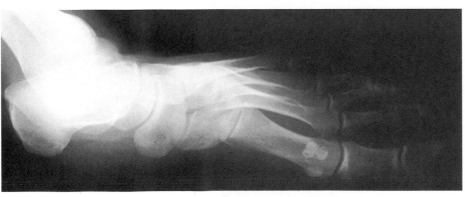

A

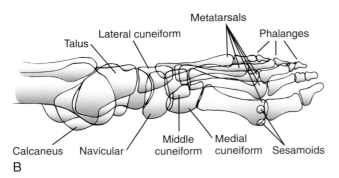

Metatarsals
Phalanges
Talus
Lateral cuneiform
Calcaneus   Navicular   Middle cuneiform   Medial cuneiform   Sesamoids

B

Figure 3–6 Lateral oblique projection of foot. **A,** Radiograph profiles lateral and dorsal surfaces of tarsal bones. **B,** Anatomic drawing for correlation.

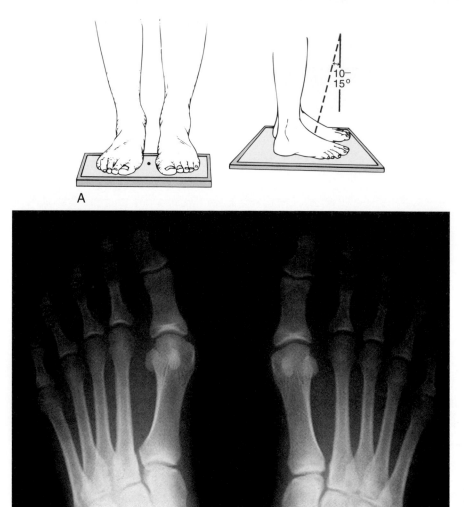

Figure 3–7 Anteroposterior (AP) weight-bearing feet. **A,** Frontal and side views show patient positioning for simultaneous AP views with centering between feet at first metatarsophalangeal joint. **B,** Weight-bearing AP radiograph.

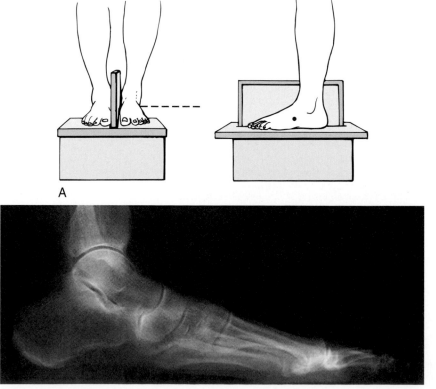

Figure 3–8 Lateral weight-bearing feet. **A,** Frontal and side views show patient positioning for lateral views. **B,** Weight-bearing lateral radiograph.

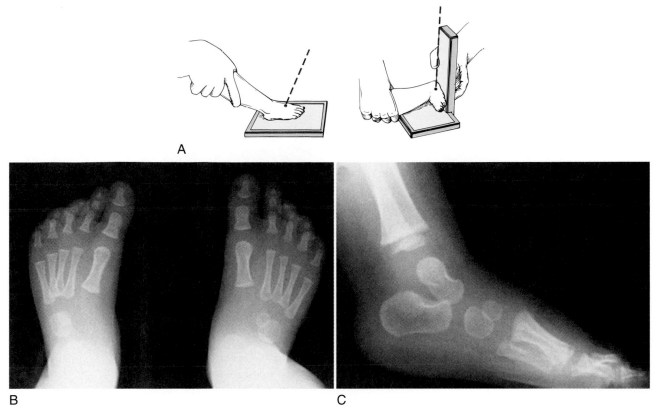

Figure 3–9 Infant weight-bearing projections. **A,** Positioning for anteroposterior (AP) and lateral views with immobilization technique. **B,** AP radiograph shows anatomic relationships. **C,** Lateral radiograph shows anatomic relationships.

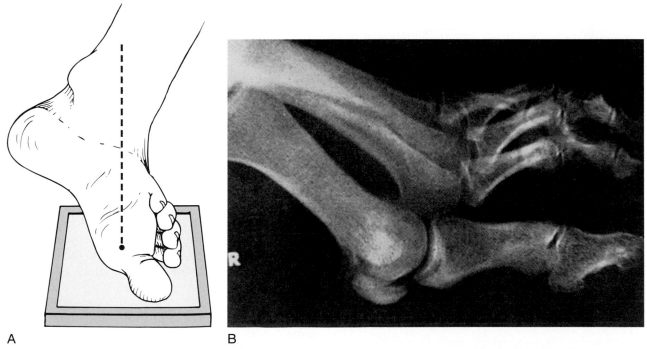

Figure 3–10 Lateral oblique phalanges. **A,** Patient positioning shows oblique orientation of plantar surface of foot. **B,** Radiograph illustrates improved visualization of phalanges, particularly great toe. (**B** from Clarke KC: *Positioning in Radiography,* ed 9. London, Ilford, 1973.)

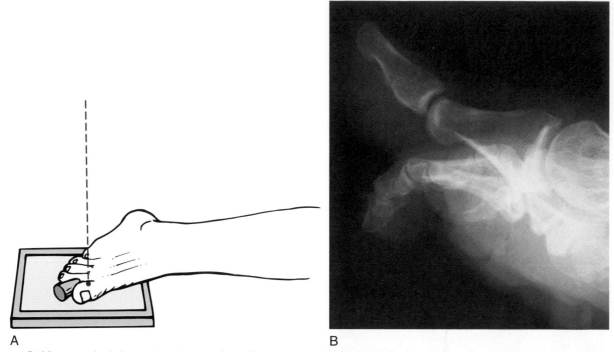

Figure 3–11 Lateral phalanges. **A,** Foot is laterally positioned with uninvolved toes flexed and, if possible, involved toe extended by padding or other means. **B,** Lateral radiograph of great toe illustrates fracture.

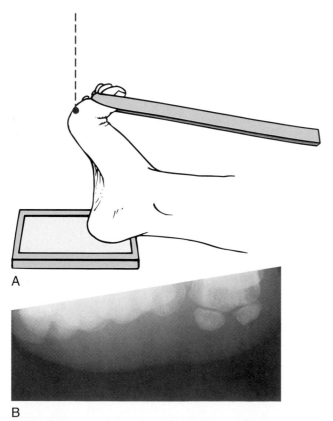

Figure 3–12 Sesamoid axial projection. **A,** Patient positioning with toes dorsiflexed and plantar foot surface at 75-degree angle with respect to cassette. **B,** Radiograph shows congruent fit of sesamoids with respect to sulci of first metatarsal head. No arthritic changes or displacement is noted.

Sesamoid Bones

The hallux sesamoids are the sesamoid bones most commonly involved by pathologic conditions, including arthritis, trauma (stress fracture), osteomyelitis, and osteonecrosis. The relationship of the sesamoid bones to the first metatarsal head is illustrated on the AP view of the foot. Osseous detail, however, is best seen on the axial view (Fig. 3–12) and lateromedial tangential projections (Fig. 3–13). Anderson[1] has recommended a dorsiflexion lateral stress view of the sesamoids if a plantar complex injury is suspected (Fig. 3–14).

Hindfoot

The complex anatomy of the hindfoot presents a diagnostic challenge that can require special views and advanced imaging for full evaluation. The os calcis may be involved by both acquired and congenital conditions. The calcaneus has important anatomic landmarks that are useful in evaluating the structural integrity of the foot. The axial and lateral projections represent the initial means for evaluating the calcaneus (Figs. 3–15 and 3–16). Oblique views are often added to complete the plain-film evaluation. One of the more commonly used oblique hindfoot projections is the Brodén view.[4] This technique provides a reliable image of the posterior facet and is often used to evaluate intraarticular calcaneus fractures and subtalar

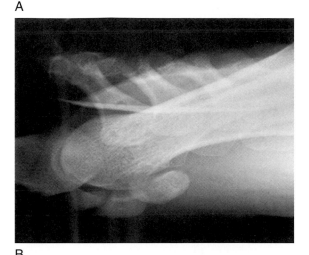

A

B

Figure 3–13 Sesamoid lateromedial projection. **A,** Patient positioning with foot lateral and transverse axis of first metatarsal joint approximately perpendicular to cassette. X-ray beam is angled 40 degrees toward heel. **B,** Radiograph illustrates separation of sesamoids and improved anatomic detail.

fusions. A Brodén view is obtained with the ankle placed in neutral dorsiflexion, the leg internally rotated 30 degrees, and the x-ray beam centered over the lateral malleolus with different angles (Fig 3–17).

The talus is a unique structure that has a functional relationship to the ankle joint and hindfoot as well as the midfoot. It is less commonly fractured than the calcaneus, and fractures occur most often in adults. When fractured it is at risk for avascular necrosis, particularly if the fracture is in the talar neck.[6] Routine evaluation of the talus usually is completed with an ankle series including AP, lateral, and mortise views. Routine foot series can provide additional information, particularly in trauma if talar neck or subtle avulsion fractures are suspected.[3] Canale and Kelly[6] have described a talar neck view for fracture evaluation that may be obtained

by placing the ankle in maximal equinus with the foot pronated 15 degrees. The x-ray beam is centered on the talar neck and angled 15 degrees cephalad (Fig. 3–18).

The subtalar or talocalcaneal joint may be affected by trauma, arthritis, or congenital coalition. Axial and lateral views are combined with oblique views for initial evaluation. The axial view is usually a weight-bearing or Harris–Beath view, which allows analysis of the medial and posterior facets of the talocalcaneal joint, as well as the alignment of the heel. The oblique view usually is a 45-degree medial oblique view of the foot. The medial oblique view assesses the sinus tarsi and the subtalar joint. It should be obtained if a tarsal coalition is suspected. Numerous special positions have been described to further evaluate the three artic-

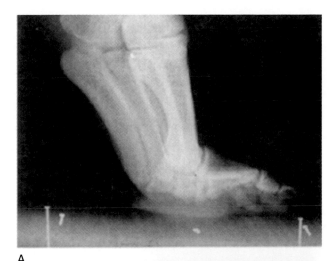

A

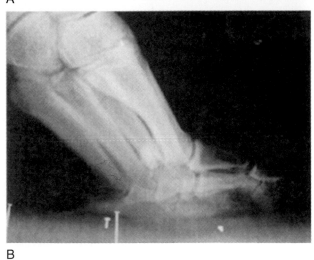

B

Figure 3–14 A lateral radiograph with the hallux metatarsophalangeal joint in forced dorsiflexion can demonstrate proximal migration of the sesamoids if the plantar complex is disrupted. (From Anderson RB: *Techniques in Foot and Ankle Surgery* 1[2]:102-111, 2002.)

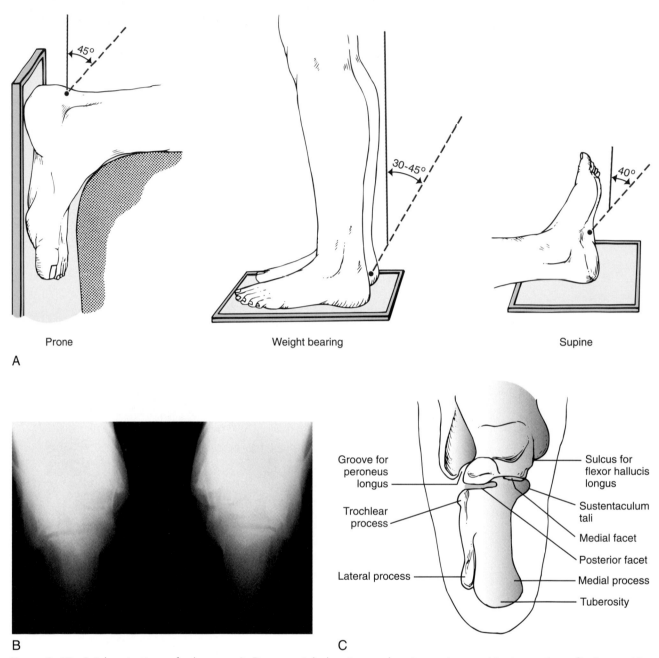

Prone   Weight bearing   Supine

A

B   C

Groove for
peroneus
longus

Trochlear
process

Lateral process

Sulcus for
flexor hallucis
longus

Sustentaculum
tali

Medial facet

Posterior facet

Medial process

Tuberosity

Figure 3–15   Axial projections of calcaneus. **A,** Prone, weight-bearing, and supine patient positioning options. Supine position often is used in trauma, but it does not optimally visualize articulations. **B,** Axial weight-bearing radiograph of calcaneus. **C,** Anatomic drawing for correlation details medial and posterior facets.

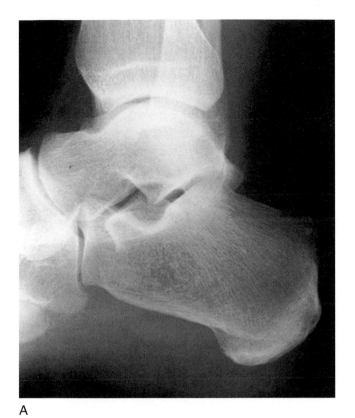

A

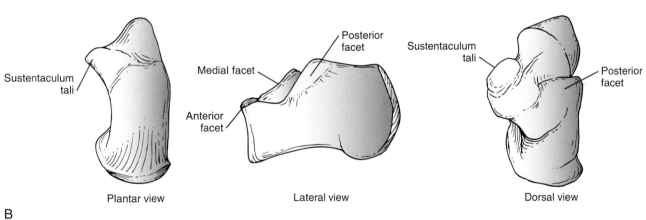

Sustentaculum tali

Plantar view

Posterior facet

Medial facet

Anterior facet

Lateral view

Sustentaculum tali

Posterior facet

Dorsal view

B

Figure 3–16   Os calcis anatomy. **A,** Lateral radiograph. **B,** Disarticulated calcaneus demonstrates anatomy.

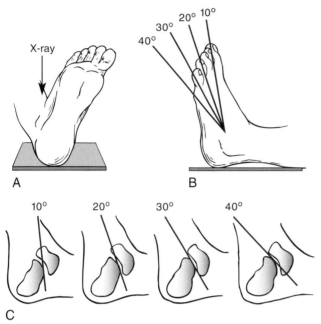

C

Figure 3–17 Brodén's view. **A,** Positioning of foot. **B** and **C,** Views of 10 to 40 degrees are obtained by moving the x-ray beam tangential to the facet. (Redrawn from Burdeaux BD Jr: *Clin Orthop Relat Res* 290:96-107, 1993.)

ulations. Oblique medial projections with varying tube angulation toward the head have been used (Fig. 3-19). Feist et al,[11] Isherwood,[13] and Pinsky[18] have detailed discussions of these views and other views including lateral oblique projections.

Radiographic Evaluation of the Ankle

Anatomically the ankle, or talocrural joint, is formed by the talus, distal tibia, and lateral malleolus.

A routine ankle series includes AP, lateral, and internal oblique (mortise) views (Fig. 3–20). Additional special views can be added to evaluate areas of concern. A number of accessory ossification centers that can confuse interpretation occur around the ankle and deserve recognition (see Fig. 3–2).

The AP view allows evaluation of the tibiotalar joint, distal tibia and fibula, peripheral borders of the tarsals, and talar dome (Fig. 3–21). The lateral view assesses the ankle for effusion, talocalcaneal relationships, tibiofibular integrity, and tibiotalar joint congruity. It is critical that the proximal metatarsals be included on the film. One of the most common inversion injuries is fracture of the fifth metatarsal base (Fig. 3–22).[10]

Oblique views provide additional information, particularly about the ankle mortise, talar dome, and malleoli. The mortise view is commonly used because it provides the best assessment of mortise congruity and the talar dome (Fig. 3–23). The internal oblique view assesses those areas less optimally, but it does provide additional information regarding the lateral malleolus and talocalcaneal relationships (Fig. 3–24A and B). The external oblique view primarily adds information about the medial malleolus (Fig. 3–24C and D).

Stress Views

Stress views may be obtained to assess ligamentous stability in patients with suspected soft tissue injuries.

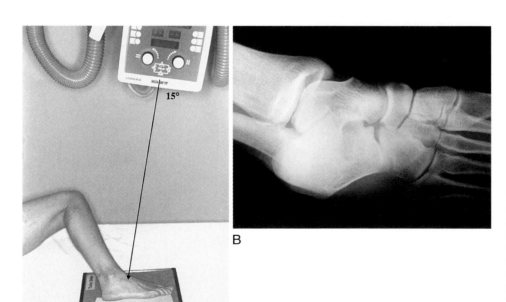

Figure 3–18 Talar neck view. **A,** The ankle is in maximum equinus and the foot is pronated 15 degrees on a wedge. The beam is angled 15 degrees cephalad and centered on the talar neck. **B,** The talar neck is viewed in the frontal plane. (From Myerson M [ed]: *Foot and Ankle Disorders,* vol 1. Philadelphia, WB Saunders, 1999, p 115.)

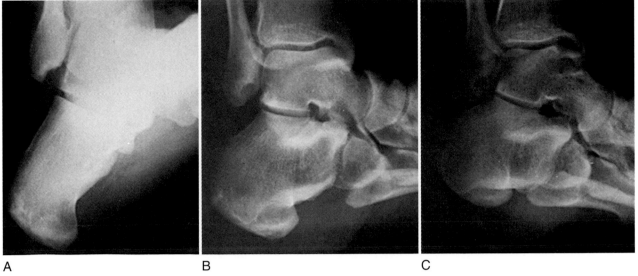

A   B   C

Figure 3–19   Talocalcaneal, subtalar, and medial oblique special projections. **A,** 40-degree angulation toward head demonstrates anterior portion of posterior facet. **B,** Angulation of 20 to 30 degrees demonstrates the medial facet. **C,** Angulation of 10 degrees demonstrates posterior portion of posterior facet.

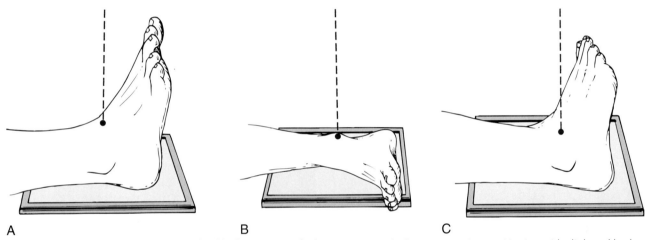

A   B   C

Figure 3–20   Standard positioning of ankle for non–weight-bearing views. **A,** Anteroposterior positioning with slight ankle dorsiflexion. **B,** Lateral (medial lateral) with slight ankle dorsiflexion and centering just proximal to medial malleolus. **C,** Mortise view with ankle dorsiflexion in 15 to 20 degrees of internal rotation.

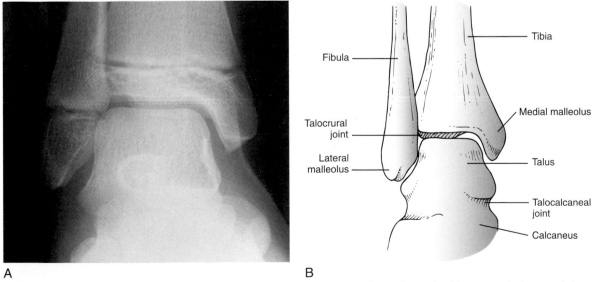

A   B

Figure 3–21   Anteroposterior views of the ankle. **A,** Radiograph illustrates relationships of ankle joint including medial mortise. **B,** Anatomic drawing for correlation.

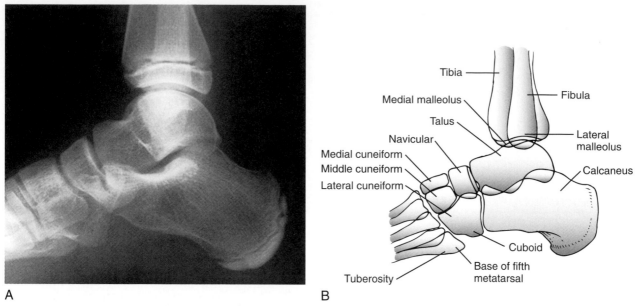

A   B

Figure 3–22   Lateral views of the ankle. **A,** Radiograph demonstrates osseous anatomy of lateral ankle including proximal fifth metatarsal. **B,** Anatomic drawing for correlation.

Stress can be applied manually or with a mechanical device. Local analgesia probably increases accuracy.[15] Multiple stress views including varus, valgus, anterior drawer, flexion, extension, and subtalar inversion have been described.[16] Varus, valgus, and anterior drawer views are most commonly used clinically (Figs. 3–25 and 3–26).

Varus stress views are used to assess the lateral stability of the ankle. Comparison with the contralateral ankle is recommended because absolute measure-

ments are less reliable.[16] The most common measurements are lateral ankle joint opening distance and the angle of talar tilt. Lateral ankle joint opening distance is measured from the most lateral aspect of the talar dome to the adjacent tibial articular surface. A 3-mm or greater discrepancy between the injured and normal side is abnormal.[14] The angle of talar tilt is obtained by drawing a line along the talar dome and another along the tibial plafond (Fig. 3–27). The resultant angle is compared with the contralateral stressed

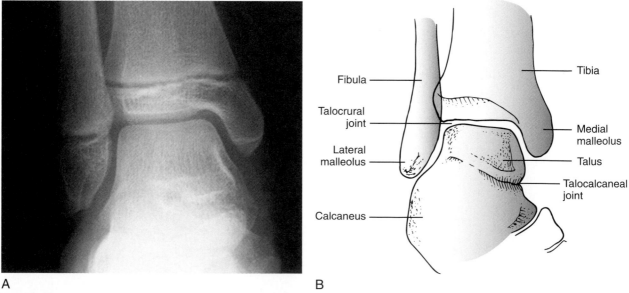

A   B

Figure 3–23   Mortise view of the ankle. **A,** Radiograph demonstrates uniform joint space of mortise. **B,** Anatomic drawing for correlation.

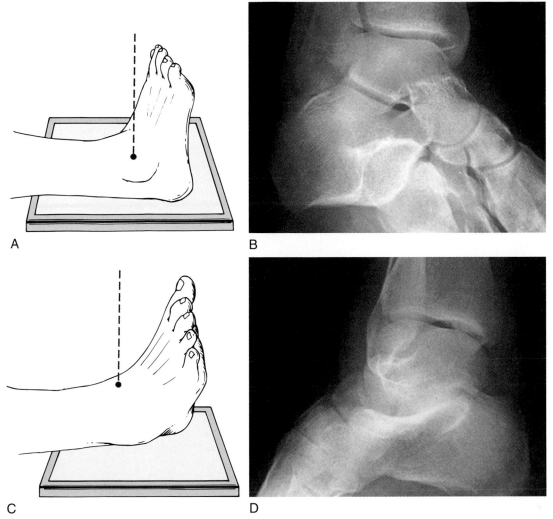

Figure 3–24 Patient positioning for special oblique ankle projections. **A,** Internal oblique view is obtained similarly to mortise view but with more plantar flexion and 45 degrees of internal rotation. **B,** Radiograph demonstrates improved visualization of talus and calcaneus compared with mortise view. **C,** External oblique view is obtained with 45 degrees of external rotation. **D,** Radiograph demonstrates improved detail over medial malleolus.

ankle. A difference of 10 degrees or greater is considered significant.[5,7,14,28]

Anterior drawer stress evaluation also usually compares one side with the other. A static radiograph is taken, followed by a stress view (Fig. 3–28). A change of 4-mm or greater anterior displacement of the talus with respect to the tibia on the stress view compared with the static view is considered significant.[7] A difference between the two stressed ankles of 2 mm or greater also is abnormal.[2]

Weight-Bearing Views

AP and lateral weight-bearing views are used to assess structural changes that occur with physiologic loading. Lateral views are obtained using the same basic technique used for the foot (see Fig. 3–8). The AP view of

the two ankles is obtained simultaneously (Fig. 3–29). These radiographs are used to evaluate the symmetry of the tibiotalar joints, which normally have similar width and tilt.

Deformity Evaluation

Plain-film evaluation of the lower extremity is used to evaluate malalignments ranging from complex tibial shaft malunions to simple hallux valgus deformities. Numerous linear and angular relationships have been described in the literature, but this section focuses on the measurements most commonly applied clinically.

If a limb-length discrepancy or deformity above the ankle is suspected, radiographic evaluation begins with standing bilateral hip-to-knee AP and lateral films

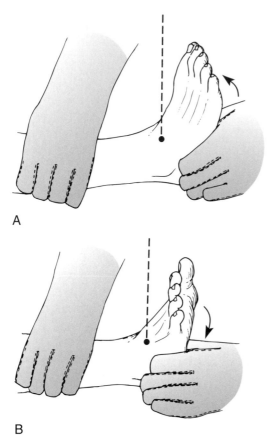

A

B

Figure 3–25   Patient positioning for varus and valgus stress views. **A,** Varus stress with foot plantar flexed particularly evaluates anterior talofibular ligament and calcaneofibular ligament for lateral stability. **B,** Valgus stress evaluates for medial stability, particularly deltoid ligament injury.

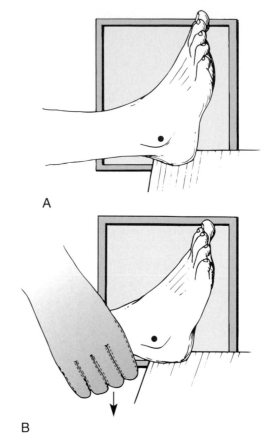

A

B

Figure 3–26   Patient positioning for anterior drawer stress. **A,** Cross-table lateral with heel at rest on 2 to 3 inches of support. **B,** Cross-table lateral with vertical stress applied to assess for anterior talofibular ligament instability.

on long cassettes. The mechanical axis is determined by drawing a line from the center of the femoral head to the center of the ankle. A deviation of the mechanical axis by more than one centimeter from the center of the knee joint suggests a deformity in the more proximal tibia or femur.[12] Normal values of joint angles have been reported and can be used to define the deformity (Fig. 3–30).[17]

Even in the setting of an isolated foot or ankle deformity, it is important to determine alignment relative to the tibia using radiographs. In the frontal plane, the average angle between the anatomic, or mid-diaphyseal axis of the tibia and the talar dome is 89 degrees (range, 86 to 92 degrees) (Fig. 3–30).[17] The axis of the tibia in the frontal plane is typically slightly medial to the center of the talus (Fig. 3–31). On a standing lateral radiograph, the mid axis of the tibia passes through the lateral talar process and normally forms an angle of 80 degrees with the anterior-to-posterior distal tibial line (Fig. 3–32). Comparison films of the contralateral extremity are recommended.

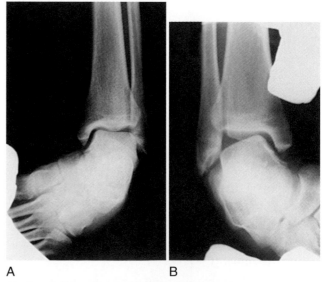

A   B

Figure 3–27   Abnormal varus stress examination. Radiographs of normal **(A)** and abnormal **(B)** ankles with varus stress. Note that the degree of talar tilt on the abnormal side is more than 10 degrees greater than on the normal side.

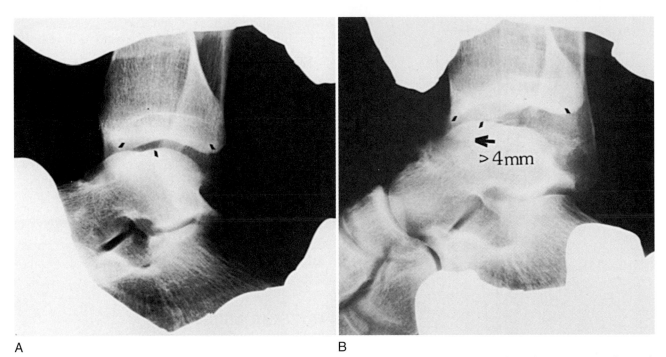

A   B

Figure 3–28 Abnormal anterior drawer stress examination. **A,** Cross-table lateral radiograph with ankle at rest. **B,** Radiograph of cross-table lateral with vertical stress demonstrates abnormal anterior displacement of talus with respect to tibia that exceeds 4 mm.

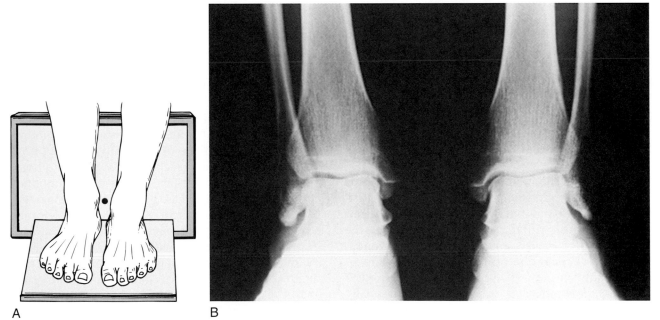

A   B

Figure 3–29 Patient positioning for anteroposterior weight-bearing ankle views. **A,** Frontal view of patient positioned on 2-inch block with film cassette in holder behind heels. Horizontal x-ray beam is centered between ankle joints. **B,** Radiograph illustrates symmetric joints with slight tilt of talar articular surface. The angle of the talar articular surface can normally be a few degrees off horizontal in either a medial or lateral direction.

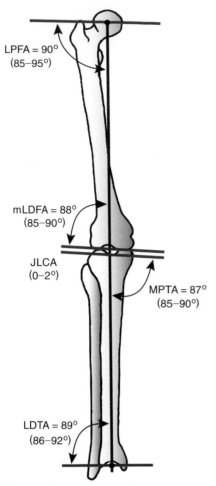

LPFA = 90°
(85–95°)

mLDFA = 88°
(85–90°)

JLCA
(0–2°)

MPTA = 87°
(85–90°)

LDTA = 89°
(86–92°)

Figure 3–30 Mechanical axis in frontal plane and normal values. JLCA, joint line congruency angle; LDTA, lateral distal tibial angle; LPFA, lateral patellofemoral angle; mLDFA, mechanical lateral distal femoral angle; MPTA, medial proximal tibial angle. (Redrawn from Paley D: *Principles of Deformity Correction.* Berlin, Springer-Verlag, 2002.)

Alignment of the hindfoot relative to the tibia was first described by Cobey in 1976.[8] The hindfoot alignment view is obtained with the patient standing on an elevated platform with the x-ray beam posterior to the heel, angled 20 degrees caudal from the horizontal. The cassette is placed in front of the patient, perpendicular to the beam, angles 20 degrees off the vertical (Fig. 3–33). The midline of the calcaneus normally lies lateral to the mid-diaphyseal axis of the tibia (Fig. 3–34).

Commonly used angular and linear measurements to evaluate foot deformities are depicted in Figure 3–35.[2,20,22] Sangeorzan et al[19] first described the talonavicular coverage angle, which may be particularly helpful in evaluating pes planus deformities and planning the appropriate surgical reconstruction (Fig 3–36). It should be emphasized that there can be a

wide variation of normal and that any apparent radiographic abnormality should be viewed in the clinical context.

Hallux valgus is one of the most common conditions seen by foot and ankle specialists, and weight-bearing radiographs are an integral part of the diagnostic evaluation. These deformities are typically defined based on the hallux valgus and one or two intermetatarsal angles. Unfortunately, the methods of measuring and reporting these values are often inconsistent. To standardize these angular measurements, Coughlin et al[9] published radiographic guidelines endorsed by the American Orthopaedic Foot and Ankle Society. Mid-diaphyseal reference points are used to define the axes of the first metatarsal, hallux proximal phalanx, and second metatarsal (Fig. 3–37).

NUCLEAR MEDICINE

Nuclear medicine diagnostic imaging has the dual advantage of providing both anatomic and physiologic information when evaluating the foot and ankle.[29,30] Nuclear medicine diagnostic imaging is based on the development of radiopharmaceutical agents, which are radionuclides that have been adapted for medical use.[29] These short-lived radiopharmaceuticals emit radiation that can be detected clinically. A large number of these agents have been developed to address a wide variety of medical concerns.

After administration of a radiopharmaceutical agent, the Anger gamma camera is used to record the pattern of radiopharmaceutical distribution in the patient. The radioactivity emitted passes through a lead collimator and interacts with sodium iodide crystals in the camera. A resultant reaction gives off photons of light, which are recorded by photomultiplier tubes, which in turn release an amplified number of electrons that are proportional to the intensity of the incident light. The electrons emitted produce an image recorded on film or by computer for later processing. The collimator is a major factor determining image resolution.[30] Pinhole, parallel hole, converging, and diverging collimators are commonly used. The type of collimator used depends on imaging needs, for example, magnification of small body parts.[29,30]

Single-photon emission computed tomography (SPECT) is an imaging alternative to routine planar images.[29,30] It can obtain images with improved contrast and spatial resolution. A series of planar images are obtained by means of a gamma camera traveling in an arc around the patient. Information from these acquisitions is processed by a computer, and axial

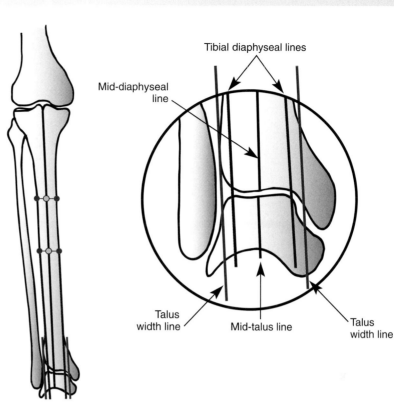

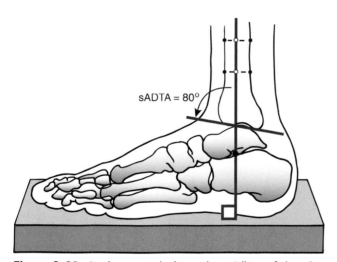

Figure 3–31 In the frontal plane, the midline of the tibia passes through the lateral process of the talus. (Redrawn from Paley D: *Principles of Deformity Correction.* Berlin, Springer-Verlag, 2002.)

Figure 3–32 In the sagittal plane, the midline of the tibia passes through the lateral process of the talus when the foot is plantigrade. The anterior distal tibial angle is normally 80 degrees. sADTA, sagittal anterior distal tibial angle. (Redrawn from Paley D: *Principles of Deformity Correction.* Berlin, Springer-Verlag, 2002.)

images are reconstructed. Sagittal and coronal images can be reformatted from those images.

Indications for nuclear medicine imaging include evaluation of tumors or tumor-like conditions, metabolic disorders, trauma, avascular necrosis, arthritis, infection, reflex sympathetic dystrophy, or pain of unknown cause.[29,30] The radionuclides most commonly used for evaluation of the musculoskeletal system include ^{99m}Tc-diphosphonates, ^{67}Ga-citrates, ^{111}In-labeled white blood cells (leukocyte scan), and ^{99m}Tc-leukocyte scans. Indications for the specific agent and the imaging technique depend on the clinical problem.

^{99m}Tc methylene diphosphonate (MDP) is a commonly used bone scanning agent. The primary bone scan imaging options include three-phase bone scans for focal areas of interest, complete body scan, or a combination of the two options. The three-phase bone scan includes a vascular flow acquisition, blood pool image, and delayed planar images over a specific body part (Fig. 3–38). A complete body scan has delayed imaging of the whole skeleton (Fig. 3–39). Imaging usually can be completed 3 to 4 hours after injection of radionuclides. Bone scans take advantage of the fact that there is normally a continuous balance between bone breakdown and new bone formation in the skeleton. Increased or decreased uptake of the bone scan agent, particularly if focal, can be recognized as abnormal. It is critical that one recognize that abnormal increased metabolic activity represents a final common pathway for many diseases that alter normal osteoblast activity.[29]

^{67}Ga is an agent that accumulates in infections or other areas of inflammation and in tumors.[30] It is a weak bone scanning agent. Its lack of specificity,

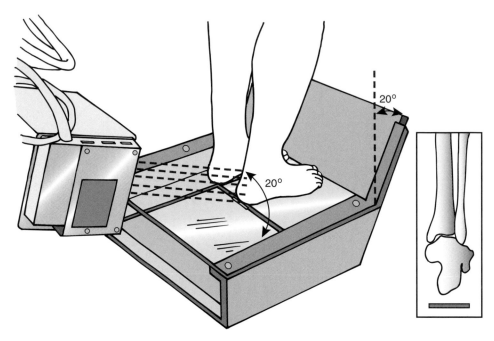

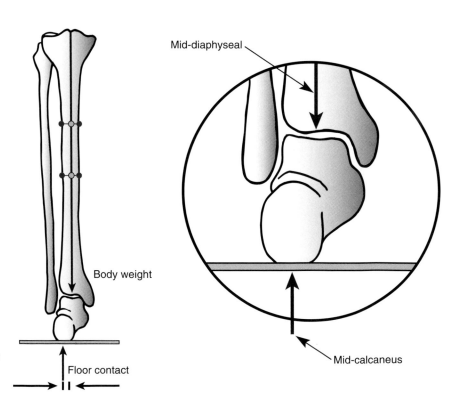

Figure 3–33 The hindfoot alignment view with the beam angled 20 degrees from the horizontal. (Redrawn from Paley D: *Principles of Deformity Correction*. Berlin, Springer-Verlag, 2002.)

Figure 3–34 The center of the calcaneus is lateral to the midline tibia. (Redrawn from Paley D: *Principles of Deformity Correction*. Berlin, Springer-Verlag, 2002.)

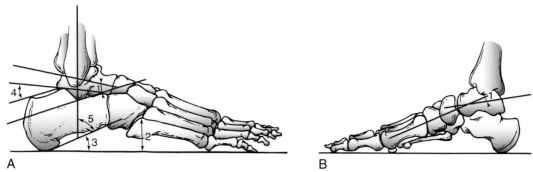

A   **B**

Figure 3–35 Linear and angular relationships of the foot. **A,** Lateral illustration of lateral aspect of the foot. *1,* Lateral talocalcaneal angle; normal is 25 to 30 degrees. *2,* Fifth metatarsal base height; normal is 2.3 to 3.8 cm. *3,* Calcaneal pitch angle; normal is 10 to 30 degrees. *4,* Bohler's angle; normal is 22 to 48 degrees. *5,* Tibiocalcaneal angle; normal is 60 to 90 degrees. **B,** Lateral illustration of medial aspect of foot. *1,* Talar–first metatarsal angle; normal is –4 degrees to +4 degrees.

delayed imaging times, and bone scan activity somewhat limit its clinical utility. After administration of ^{67}Ga, imaging usually is performed at 24, 48, and 72 hours. Whole-body imaging usually is performed, but scanning can be limited to the area of interest.

Leukocyte imaging for detection of infection or inflammation depends on labeling of leukocytes with a radionuclide in vitro, then injecting them intravenously into the patient.[27] The leukocytes usually are harvested from the patient for labeling, although alternatively white blood cells from an appropriate donor

can be labeled and used in the leukopenic patient.[30] Imaging of the body can be performed at 4 hours and again at 24 hours (Fig. 3–40).[33,38]

Bone scanning remains the primary means of evaluating the entire skeleton for a potentially polyostotic

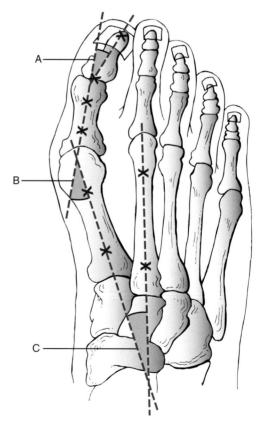

Figure 3–37 Mid-diaphyseal lines are determined using midpoints at the metadiaphyseal region. These are drawn and used to measure the hallux valgus interphalangeal angle (*A*), hallux valgus angles (*B*), and the angle between the first and second metatarsals (*C*).

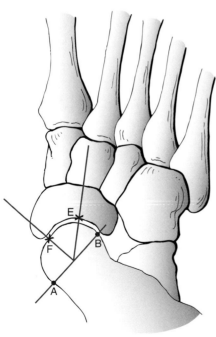

Figure 3–36 The midlines of the talus and navicular bones are identified and marked by points *F* and *E* at their intersection with the articular surfaces. The angle subtended by these lines is the talonavicular coverage angle.

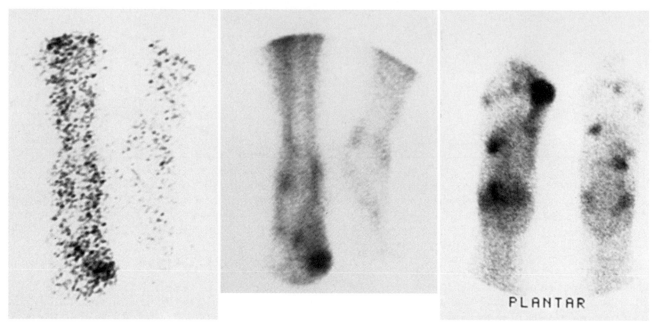

Figure 3–38   Three-phase bone scan. Note increased vascular flow, blood pool, and delayed planar activity focally over the first metatarsal in the involved foot compared fully with the contralateral foot in a patient with osteomyelitis. Radiograph was normal except for arthritis, explaining other areas of activity seen on delayed planar images.

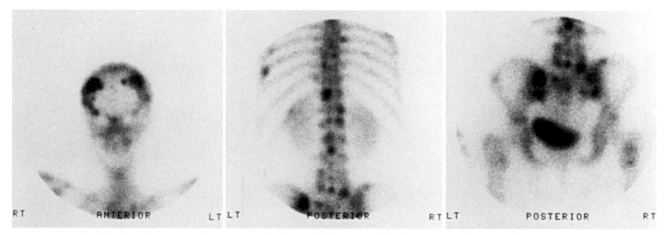

Figure 3–39   Whole body bone scan (representative images). Note multiple focal areas of abnormal increased metabolic activity in skeleton, consistent with metastatic disease in patient with breast cancer.

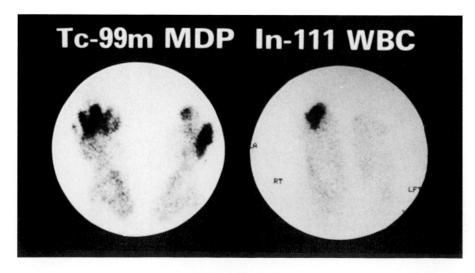

Figure 3–40   Leukocyte scan shows focal leukocyte uptake in right third and fourth metatarsals, consistent with osteomyelitis. (Courtesy of Kathryn Morton, MD, Department of Nuclear Medicine, Veterans Administration Medical Center, Salt Lake City, Utah.)

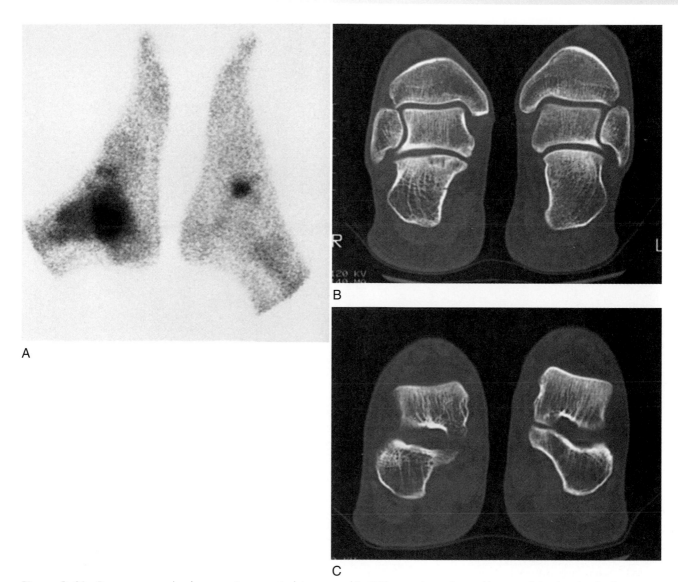

Figure 3–41 Bone scan and subsequent computed tomographic (CT) scan in patient with unexplained pain. **A,** Bone scan demonstrates intensely abnormal right subtalar joint with increased metabolic activity. **B,** Coronal CT image confirms right subtalar posterior facet osteoarthritis as cause of abnormal activity on nuclear medicine bone scan. **C,** Coronal CT image illustrates congenitally deficient right medial facet as cause of posterior facet arthritis.

process such as metastatic neoplasm or diffuse arthritis.[28,29] If there is a high degree of concern over a focal area of abnormality, MRI is more sensitive in tumor detection.[28] When a focal bone lesion suspected of being a tumor or tumor-like lesion—for example, eosinophilic granuloma or fibrous dysplasia—is being evaluated, it is recommended that a three-phase bone scan be performed in conjunction with a complete body scan at the same setting, to exclude a polyostotic process.

Infection is another common indication for radionuclide scanning, although some reports indicate that MRI may be more accurate and provide more

detailed information regarding the extent of involvement.[35,40,44] ^{111}In-leukocyte imaging is considered more sensitive and specific than ^{67}Ga for diagnosis of infection.[33,34] ^{111}In-labeled leukocyte scan combined with three-phase bone scan is a common method used to diagnose osteomyelitis, although some centers are using ^{99m}Tc-HMPAO leukocyte scans as an alternative method.[27,34,38,39] If septic arthritis is suspected, needle aspiration can be performed without causing subsequent false-positive bone scan results.[42]

Evaluation of foot and ankle pain of unknown cause also is a common indication for nuclear medicine bone scanning (Fig. 3–41).[23,29,32,34,35] This can detect

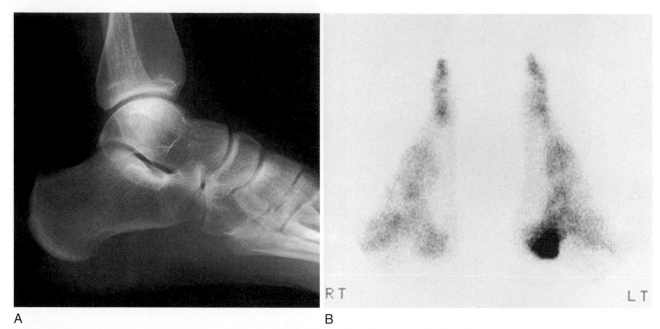

Figure 3–42 Occult fracture detection on bone scan. **A,** Normal initial radiograph of calcaneus. **B,** Increased metabolic activity in posterior calcaneus, consistent with stress fracture, which was confirmed on delayed radiographs.

osteoid osteomas, arthritis, occult fractures, and osteochondral injuries.[29] Reflex sympathetic dystrophy, now commonly referred to as *complex regional pain syndrome*, also can be diagnosed with three-phase bone scans.[25,29] Abnormal uptake in occult fractures even in patients with osteoporosis is detectable 72 hours after injury (Fig. 3–42).[31] The earliest that bone scan findings can return to normal after fracture is 6 months.[31] Reportedly, in 90% of uncomplicated fractures bone scans are normal by 2 years.[31]

It has been stated that a normal bone scan excludes injury.[26] There are, however, reports of normal planar bone scans with abnormal SPECT imaging, at least in the axial skeleton.[34,41] At many institutions, MRI has become the initial imaging technique used to evaluate pain of unknown cause in the foot and ankle because it can reveal both soft tissue and osseous abnormalities.

Potential future applications include development of new radiopharmaceutical agents and the further development of radioimmunoscintigraphy.[24,43,37,43] The latter depends on labeled monoclonal or polyclonal antibodies (immunoglobulin G) directed against certain tumor- or microbial-specific antigens. Accumulation of localized activity in the body would help detect specific pathologic processes.

COMPUTED TOMOGRAPHY

Computed tomography (CT) scan allows rapid evaluation of complex foot and ankle anatomy with thin-section imaging. The images allow three-dimensional appreciation of bone anatomy, allowing improved diagnostic accuracy and better definition of anatomy compared to plain radiographs. CT scanning plays a role in surgical planning because precise definition of bone loss or fracture planes can be appreciated by the treating surgeon. Modern software allows reconstruction in other two-dimensional planes with no additional radiation dose to the patient after initial thin-section acquisition. With some scanners, three-dimensional reconstruction can be used for preoperative surgical planning. Because of better definition of anatomy in tough cases, CT-directed diagnostic injection may be preferential to fluoroscopic imaging in cases where the anatomy is distorted.[64]

CT scanning has the disadvantage traditionally of being a non–weight-bearing investigation. This results in the foot's adopting a position that does not reflect the normal weight-bearing relationships. Researchers have as a result been trying to create simulated weight-bearing scans to better understand the pathology of flat foot deformity.[56] Simulated weight-bearing views have not as yet been performed routinely. However, the use of some form of splint to correctly align the foot in the scanner might aid understanding the pathologic process present.

Within the last few years many imaging departments have gone from using hard copy films to a picture archiving communication system (PACS), allowing access to imaged films. Because image storage is much cheaper, higher-resolution scans can be obtained and stored.[53]

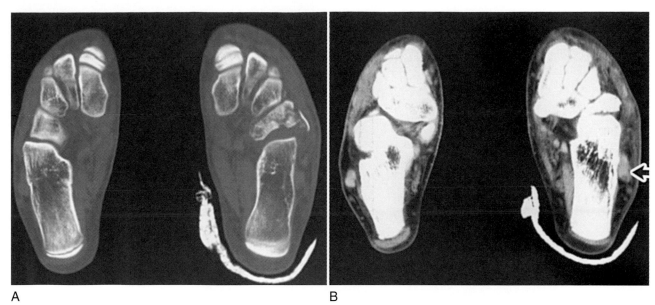

A   B

Figure 3–43 Axial computed tomographic (CT) scan of feet. **A,** Bone detail image using window width of 2000 and level of 400 details osseous abnormalities including comminuted cuboid fracture, widened calcaneocuboid articulation, and lateral fracture of lateral cuneiform indicating further Chopart's joint injury. **B,** Soft tissue detail image using window width of 350 and level of 50 demonstrates pathologically thickened left peroneal tendons in the same patient on adjacent scan level. On bone window images this abnormality could be missed *(arrow)*.

A CT scanner consists of a scanning gantry, an x-ray generator, a computerized data processing system, and an indexing movable patient table. In current CT scanners a fan shaped rotating x-ray beam is directed through the imaged body part. Older scanners obtain a slice at each indexed table interval with a short pause between images.

Modern scanners take continuous images as the table moves in a *helical* or *spiral scan.* This has the advantage of a shorter scan time. Earlier scanners had some loss of detail, limiting its use in the skeleton. Recent developments have allowed multidetector scans or helical scans using thin slices to obtain all of the raw data, allowing reformatting in multiple planes. The need for patient repositioning is obviated, and scans can therefore be obtained more rapidly. The resolution is improved to the point that hardware artifacts are reduced and nonunions can be diagnosed correctly. After passing through the imaged structure, the attenuated beam is detected by a fixed ring of detectors within the gantry. Attenuation or absorption of the x-ray beam reflects the density of the imaged tissue.

The computer analyzes the average attenuation in a three-dimensional volume, or voxel, of tissue. The attenuation is given a number based on a comparison with the attenuation of a similar voxel of water. The number is converted into a gray scale value and displayed on the screen as a pixel. Gray scale values are based Hounsfield units. (Water has a Hounsfield unit value of 0, air has a value of −1000 Hounsfield units, and bone has a value of +1000 Hounsfield units.) The range and center of gray scale value can be manipulated by altering the window width and window level, respectively. Narrow window widths and low window levels are used for soft tissue display. Wider widths and higher levels optimize bone detail (Fig. 3–43). Both soft tissue and bone images should be filmed to fully evaluate patients.[46,59,67]

The window widths need to be thin enough to prevent misdiagnosis by volume averaging. Helical scanning has now reached sufficient sophistication to allow enough tissue resolution. In the foot and ankle, 5-mm thick or thinner sections are required. If osseous detail is required, very thin contiguous sections (1.5 mm thick) or overlapping thin sections (3-mm thick sections obtained at 2-mm intervals) can be used (Fig. 3–44).[46,63,72]

The imaging planes are illustrated in Figure 3–45. Coronal and axial imaging planes have been occasionally misrepresented and may be a pitfall for the unwary reader.[65,69]

Patient positioning allows patient comfort and correct imaging. Axial images are obtained with the

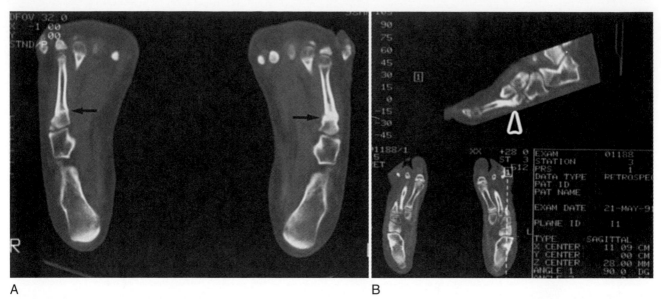

A   B

Figure 3–44 Two-dimensional reconstruction images on CT. **A,** Axial images of a foot demonstrate a complete stress fracture of the left fourth metatarsal and a clinically undiagnosed early right fourth metatarsal stress fracture (3-mm thick scan obtained at 2-mm intervals). **B,** Two-dimensional reconstruction from axial data has slightly decreased osseous detail but adequately demonstrates relationship of fracture fragments with apex plantar angulation *(arrowhead)*.

patient supine, with the knees extended, and with the feet in neutral position resting with mild pressure on a footboard. The gantry is angled to approximate a true axial plane with respect to bone structures (Fig. 3–46). Traditionally, coronal and coronal oblique images are obtained with the knees bent and the feet positioned flat on the table, on an angled foot wedge, or on a special table extension board (Fig. 3–47). The gantry is angled to approximate a coronal plane.

Helical scans now reconstruct the coronal planes from the axial images. The gantry angle can be varied to visualize specific anatomy. Incorrect gantry angles assessing a tarsal coalition can lead to a false-positive diagnosis.[61,72]

In the imaging of tarsal coalitions some authors recommend tilting the gantry toward the knee[46,69,71] (Fig. 3–48). Others disagree with this approach.[61] A paper by Heger and Wulff[58] illustrates the specific relationship of the talus and calcaneus . The medial facet and lateral portion of the posterior facet are almost parallel the long axis of the talus (Fig. 3–49). Scan angles not perpendicular to those joints fail to optimally

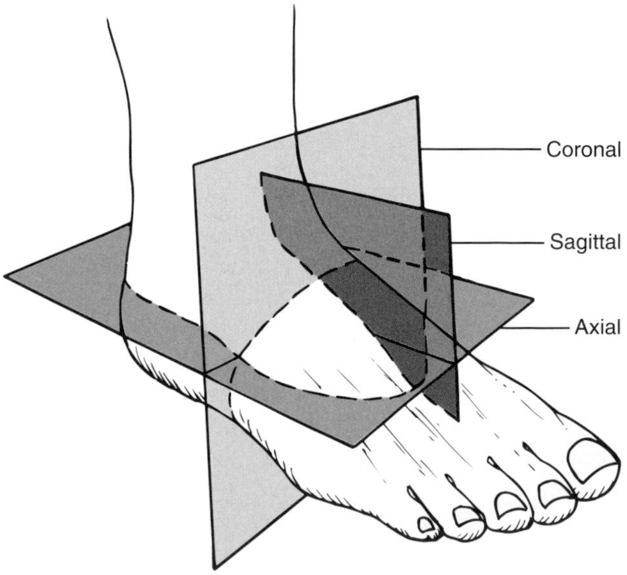

——— Coronal

——— Sagittal

——— Axial

Figure 3–45 Anatomic imaging planes of the foot and ankle. Erect anatomic position with coronal, axial, and sagittal planes is illustrated.

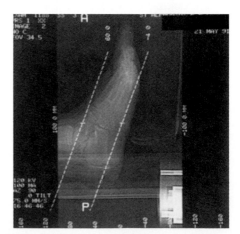

Figure 3–46 Gantry positioning for axial computed tomographic scan of the foot and ankle. Gantry is angled to produce and axial scan plane paralleling osseous structures of the foot.

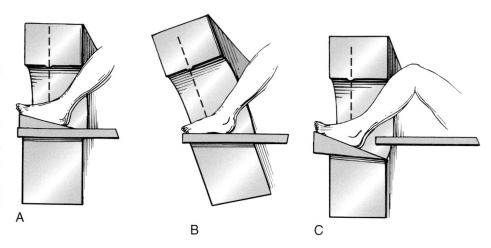

Figure 3–47 Coronal foot computed tomography positioning options. **A,** Feet positioned on angled foot wedge. **B,** Feet positioned flat on the table with an appropriate 20-degree gantry angulation for coalition evaluation. **C,** Feet positioned on a special table extension footboard. Note a foot wedge should be used or the gantry angled appropriately.

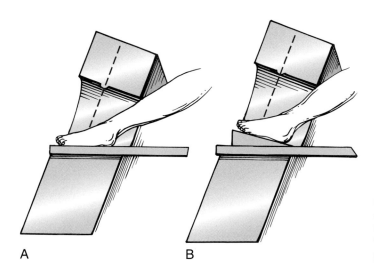

A   B

Figure 3–48 Inappropriate gantry angle for coronal coalition imaging. **A,** Feet positioned flat with the gantry inappropriately angled toward the knee. **B,** Feet positioned on an angled foot wedge with the gantry inappropriately angled toward the knee.

Figure 3–49 Anatomic orientation of subtalar joint. **A,** Sagittal reconstruction from coronal computed tomographic scan shows medial facet orientation paralleling long axis of the talus. Note that the gantry was tilted away from the knee to evaluate the medial facet in a true coronal plane. **B,** Sagittal reconstruction farther laterally illustrates lateral articular surface of posterior facet perpendicular to coronal scan plane.

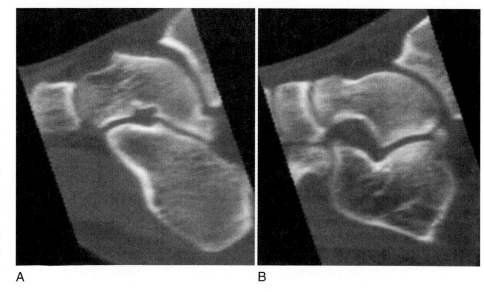

A   B

visualize the subtalar joint. This is particularly notable when lower-resolution 4- or 5-mm thick slices are used (Fig. 3–50).[71] CT scan with spiral imaging remains the imaging technique of choice for patients with tarsal coalition.[57]

The medial facet is the most common site of talo-calcaneal coalition and should be the focus of CT evaluation (Fig. 3–51). Thinner sections (3 mm or less) should be used, to image the medial facet and evaluate the medial portion of the posterior facet, obliquely oriented to the recommended scan plane.[72]

CT scan has been used to assess fractures, neoplasms, infections, foreign bodies, osteochondral injuries, tendons, avascular necrosis, arthritis, and congenital abnormalities (Fig. 3–52). CT is of use in evaluating traumatic injuries to the midfoot, and it can detect other occult fractures.[57] Some more complex fracture patterns have been identified via CT scan assessment, such as the posterior medial facet fracture.[55] MRI is preferred for evaluating soft tissue and marrow abnormalities. Soft tissue infections, osteomyelitis, avascular necrosis, tendon abnormalities, and soft tissue neoplasms usually are best evaluated by MRI.[50,51,66,73] However, the bone deficit is best analyzed on CT for patients with osteomyelitis during surgical planning. Early studies indicate that MRI can detect osteochondral injuries better than CT scan and in fact suggest that these injuries may be more common than previously suspected.[45]

CT scan remains the preferred method for evaluating fractures of the foot and ankle either after acute injury or after repetitive stress injuries. In the foot it is particularly useful in evaluating calcaneal fractures, talar fractures, midfoot fractures and dislocations, and navicular stress fractures. CT scan evaluation of calcaneal fractures illustrates the degree of posterior subtalar joint, sustentacular tali, and calcaneocuboid joint involvement (Fig. 3–53A to C).[52,68] Injuries to or impingement on adjacent soft tissue structures such as peroneal tendons may be identified (Fig. 3–53D).[54,67] Triplane, tillaux, pilon, and trimalleolar fractures are among the ankle fractures that can be evaluated by CT

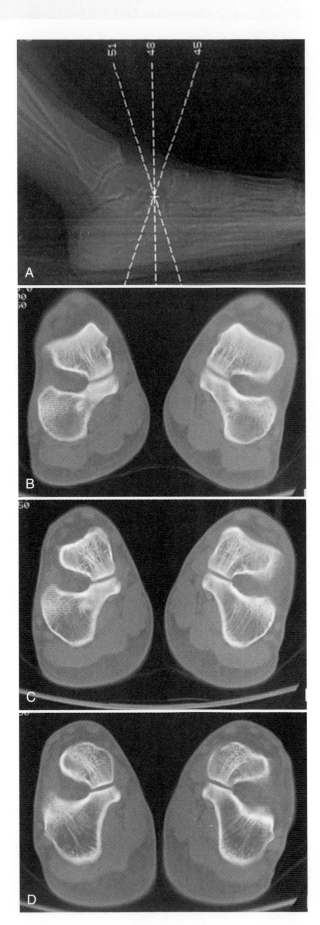

Figure 3–50 Scan plane in coronal imaging of the subtalar joint, allowing optimal imaging. **A,** Scout view illustrates gantry angles (51, 48, 45) used to obtain 5-mm thick scans obtained at the same level through the medial facet, varying scan angle. **B,** A gantry angled toward the knee produces a blurred appearance of the medial facets secondary to volume averaging along the oblique surface, preventing optimal evaluation (image angle 51). **C,** Gantry angle perpendicular to the tabletop shows improved visualization of the medial facet with less blurring (image angle 48). **D,** Appropriate gantry angle away from the knee perpendicular to the plane of the medial facet joint illustrates sharp osseous detail of a normal medial facet joint (image angle 45).

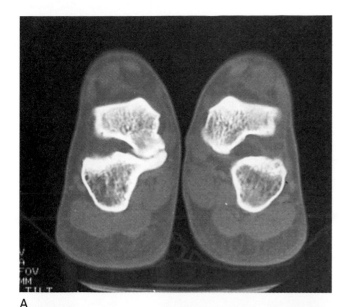

A

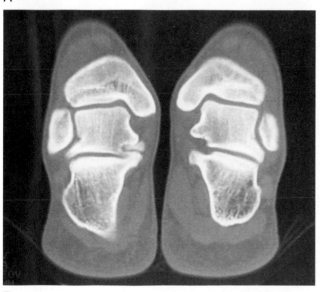

B

Figure 3–51 Talocalcaneal coalition. **A,** Abnormal orientation and morphology of partially fibrous and partially osseous right medial facet coalition. **B,** Posterior computed tomographic image in the same patient also demonstrates osseous bar bridging the medial portion of the posterior facet.

scan for preoperative planning[48,49,62] (Fig. 3–54). Two- and three-dimensional reconstruction is useful in preoperative surgical planning in complex injuries.[60] Multidetector row CT has recently improved the diagnosis of midfoot injuries.[57] In cases where stability of the midfoot needs to be assessed, the CT scan should be assessed with the standing radiographs because CT is a non–weight-bearing investigation. Stress radiography and MR may add additional information to the diagnosis.

Repetitive stress injuries, including navicular fractures, may be assessed by CT or MRI. Although the early diagnosis may be made by MRI, better definition of the anatomy and extent of the injury and its mechanical significance may be best assessed by CT scan.[47]

CT scan is the primary means for diagnosing adult tarsal coalitions, but MRI may be useful in some problem cases. CT scan can be used to assess arthritis, particularly in the subtalar joint.[65] Patients with persistent pain following silicone (Silastic) arthroereisis also can be evaluated with CT scan.[70]

MAGNETIC RESONANCE IMAGING

MRI advances are allowing better soft tissue imaging for musculoskeletal conditions. Benefits include soft tissue detail, contrast, and multiplanar imaging, allowing evaluation of the complex anatomy of the foot.

In reviewing the MRI literature, surgeons using the MRI should know the diagnostic ability of the scan to correctly define the pathologic process causing symptoms or disease. Test–retest reliability indicates the ability of two separate tests to reproduce the same result on the same condition.[84] For the MRI scan, this means the ability of two scans to correctly diagnose the same pathologic process in the same subject. Test retest–reliability may be performed using the same scanner and radiologist or a separate scanner and radiologist. No test–retest studies have been done, making it hard for surgeons to determine the diagnostic significance of their own scanners and radiologists compared to those reported in the literature.

Once the scan has been performed, the images may be reviewed by different observers (interobserver reliability) or the same observers (intraobserver reliability) on separate occasions.[103] The reliability of the test is usually quoted via a kappa statistic, where 1 is complete agreement and 0 is no agreement.

The results of the scan may then be compared to a gold standard (validity). The quality of the gold standard must be assessed when reviewing the paper. Usually this is a surgical confirmation of the disease process. The comparison is quoted as sensitivity (the ability of the test to correctly identify those with the disease), specificity (the ability of the test to correctly identify those without the disease), negative predictive value (the chance that a negative test is accurate), positive predictive value (the chance that a positive test is accurate), and accuracy.[103] Ideally the test is 100% sensitive and specific, meaning the study is normal when there is no disease and correctly picks up the disease when disease is present.

Many clinicians, patients, and insurance companies assume that MRIs are 100% accurate for most condi-

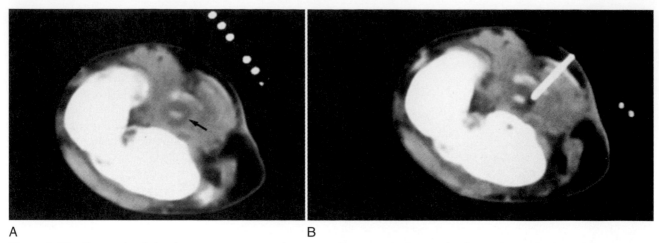

Figure 3-52   Foreign body localization on computed tomographic scan. **A,** Foreign bodies with surrounding abscess *(arrow)* are demonstrated with localizer grid placed on plantar foot surface with patient prone. **B,** Direct preoperative localization with needle placed to inject methylene blue. Wood fragments were successfully recovered at surgery.

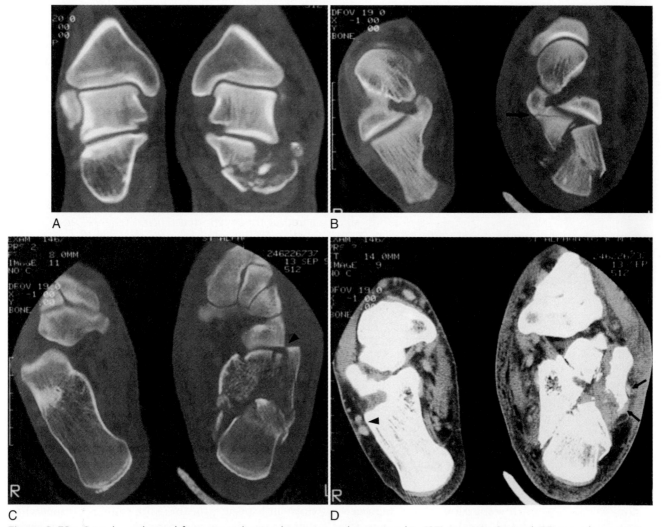

Figure 3-53   Complex calcaneal fracture evaluation by computed tomographic (CT) scan. **A,** Coronal CT scan demonstrates extensive comminution of the calcaneus involving the lateral third of the posterior facet. Note that the plaster splint present does not interfere with CT evaluation. **B,** Axial scan shows the position of the major calcaneal fragments and a coronal plane fracture of the sustentaculum *(arrow)* not suspected on coronal scans. **C,** Axial scan demonstrates degree of calcaneocuboid joint involvement *(arrowhead).* **D,** Axial scan illustrates laterally displaced calcaneal fragments impinging on the peroneal tendons *(arrows).* Note the normal contralateral peroneal tendons *(arrowhead).*

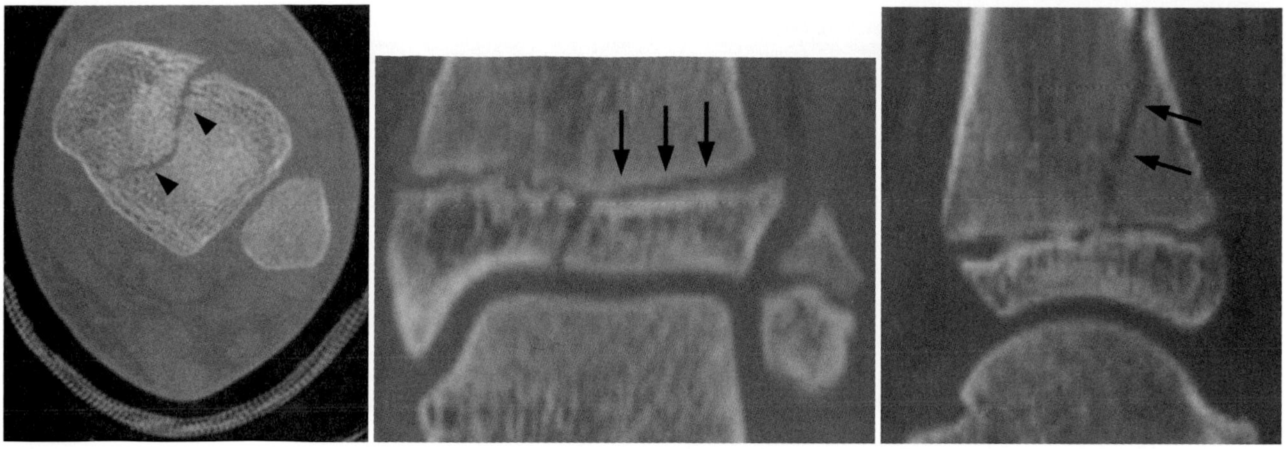

Figure 3–54 Triplane fracture with computed tomographic scan illustrating the three components extending along three planes. **A,** Axial image demonstrating the sagittally oriented vertical fracture bisecting the epiphysis (arrowheads). **B,** Coronal two-dimensional reconstruction image showing the horizontal fracture through the lateral aspect of the growth plate (arrows) and again demonstrating the vertical fracture through the epiphysis. **C,** Sagittal two-dimensional reconstruction image illustrating the coronal plane vertical fracture extending through the metaphysis (arrows).

tions in the foot and ankle. In fact, few conditions have been studied, and those that have been might not be clinically relevant. For example, a surgeon might not be so concerned about osteomyelitis in a diabetic patient but might be concerned about a deep abscess causing sepsis. The gold standard for osteomyelitis can also be called into question because the surgeon is often not blinded to the result of the MRI scan and the estimation and definition of osteomyelitis is not clear. Table 3–1 summarizes the studies to date reporting the diagnostic accuracy for MRI of foot and ankle disease involving infection; Table 3–2 summarizes the accuracy of MRI for disorders apart from infection.

The diagnostic accuracy of MRI for tendon disorders, soft tissue impingement, and chondral (as opposed to osteochondral) disorders is certainly not 100% in our practice. This might reflect the Hawthorne effect, a confounding factor in studies where the study center outperforms because a study is being performed.

As a result, the diagnostic accuracy of day-to-day MRIs might not be the same as those in study centers. Chondral injuries in isolation, soft tissue impingement, ligament tears, and tendon disorders in particular need to be interpreted in light of the clinical examination and physical exam: If there is a discrepancy, and the patient's report is consistent, then the MRI is more likely to be wrong and the patient correct in indication of pathology.

Hopefully more information on the diagnostic accuracy of MRI will become available for foot and ankle surgeons in time. If the surgeon bears in mind these limitations, MRI is a valuable tool for most soft tissue injuries, but it should never be interpreted without knowledge of the history and physical exam. This is

well illustrated in a paper assessing the diagnostic accuracy of MRI and ultrasound in diagnosing Morton's neuroma, where investigations were found to be inferior to the assessment by clinical examination.[132]

Basic Science

Current MRI scanners measure the response of ^{1}H protons in the body to a strong magnetic field. A number of these randomly aligned protons realign themselves parallel to the plane of the magnetic field (Z-plane), producing a net magnetization. They continue to precess or rotate around their axis in a nonuniform pattern. A radiofrequency pulse deflects these protons out of the field's alignment. The strength and combination of pulses determine the degree of deflection. The protons maintain this deflected angle and start to precess concordantly during the radiofrequency pulse. After the pulse is off, the protons return to their prior orientation in the field and gradually return to a random precession. This emits a radiowave signal, known as a T1 (spin-lattice [longitudinal] relaxation time) and T2 (spin-spin [transverse] relaxation time). The signal characteristics and subsequent image formation depend on the ratio of the T1 and T2 information plus proton density. Each tissue's composition has a unique T1 and T2 character. The relative contribution of tissue T1 and T2 image information can be controlled by the operator changing the scan parameters. Whiter areas on an image have higher signal intensity dependent on the radiowave emitted after excitation and relaxation.

An understanding of a tissue's T1 and T2 characteristics is of value. Anatomic features are best seen on T1

TABLE 3-1

Studies Reporting the Diagnostic Accuracy for MRI of Foot and Ankle Pathology for Infection*

Author	Journal	Date	Disease Process	Sens (%)	Spec (%)	PPV (%)	NPV (%)	Accuracy (%)	Number Pts
Al-Khawari et al[74]	Med Princ Pract	2005	Diabetic osteomyelitis	100	63	79	100	—	29
Cook et al[82]	Br J Surg	1996	Diabetic foot infection	91	77	77	91	—	25 infections
Craig et al[83]	Radiology	1997	Osteomyelitis	90	71	—	—	—	13
Croll et al[85]	J Vasc Surg	1996	Osteomyelitis	88	100	—	—	95	27
Enderle et al[89]	Diabetes Care	1999	Diabetic osteomyelitis	100	75	93	100	—	19 patients, histologic control
Levine et al[111]	Foot Ankle Int	1994	Osteomyelitis	77	100	—	—	90	29
Matowe and Gilbert[116]	Clin Radiol	2004	Osteomyelitis, meta-analysis	91	82	—	—	88	10 papers
Morrison et al[†]	Radiology	1993	Osteomyelitis, nonenhanced MR	79	53	—	—	—	51 cases
Morrison et al[†]	Radiology	1993	Osteomyelitis, enhanced MR	88	93	—	—	—	51 cases
Morrison et al[118]	Radiology	1995	Diabetic osteomyelitis	82	80	—	—	—	27
Nigro et al[‡]	J Am Podiatr Med Assoc	1992	Osteomyelitis	100	95	—	—	—	34
Wang et al[§]	Magn Reson Imaging	1990	Diabetic foot infections	99	81	—	—	94	61 cases

*Inclusion criteria were clinical studies of adult patients, more than 10 patients in the study, and the study outlines sensitivity and specificity.

[†]Morrison WB, Schweitzer ME, Bock GW, et al: Diagnosis of osteomyelitis: Utility of fat-suppressed contrast-enhanced MR imaging. *Radiology* 189(1):251-257, 1993.

[‡]Nigro ND, Bartynski WS, Grossman SJ, Kruljac S: Clinical impact of magnetic resonance imaging in foot osteomyelitis. *J Am Podiatr Med Assoc* 83:603-615, 1992.

[§]Wang A, Weinstein D, Greenfield L, et al: MRI and diabetic foot infections. *Magn Reson Imaging* 8(6):805-809, 1990.

MR, magnetic resonance; MRI, magnetic resonance imaging; NPV, negative predictive value; PPV, positive predictive value; Pts, patients; Sens, sensitivity; Spec, specificity.

(short relaxation time [TR], short echo time [TE]) and proton density (long TR, short TE) spin echo images. T1 images highlight tissue fat and T2 highlights water imaging. Tissues with short T1 relaxation times have highest signal intensity or brightness on T1 images. The speed of T1 relaxation is determined by the similarity of motion frequency of the tissue molecules compared to the resonant frequency of the scanner.[141] Fat molecules or triglycerides tumble at a rate similar to the resonance frequency of scanners currently in clinical use and have a very efficient T1 relaxation (Fig. 3–55A).[141] Molecules moving faster (e.g., water) or slower (e.g., protein) have inefficient T1 relaxation or long T1 relaxation, resulting in low image signal intensity (Fig. 3–55A).

Long T2 relaxation results in high signal intensity on T2-weighted images. T2 relaxation depends on the interaction between water molecules and other surrounding molecules.[141] Free motion of molecules in pure water results in a long T2 relaxation time (Fig. 3–55B). The motion of water molecules is slowed by adjacent macromolecules. The resulting T2 relaxation shortens, particularly in tissues with highly restricted molecular motion such as fibrous tissue or bone (see Fig. 3–55B).[141]

A number of other imaging sequences include short T1 inversion recovery (STIR), T2 fat-suppression spin-echo, fast-scan spin-echo, and gradient echo recall sequences.

Magnetic resonance scanners usually are low-field, mid-field, and high-field, depending on the strength of the magnets, measured in tesla (T). The most common magnetic resonance scanners in current use are mid-field 0.5 T, 1.0 T, and high-field 1.5 T. The high-field units offer improved resolution for small body parts. High-resolution imaging of the foot and ankle requires appropriate use of local coils in conjunction with small fields of view and thin imaging sections. A cir-

TABLE 3–2

Diagnostic Accuracy for Disorders Apart from Infection for MRI of Foot and Ankle Conditions*

Author	Journal	Date	Disease Process	Sens (%)	Spec (%)	PPV (%)	NPV (%)	Accuracy (%)	Number Pts
Breitenseher et al[†]	Rofo	1996	Acute ligament disruption, ATFL	100	100	—	—	—	12
Breitenseher et al[†]	Rofo	1996	Acute ligament disruption, FCL	64	100	—	—	—	12
De Smet et al[88]	Skeletal Radiol	1996	Stability of OCD lesions	97	100	—	—	—	40
Farooki et al[93]	Radiology	1998	Anterolateral ankle impingement	42	85	—	—	69	32
Gerling et al [94]	Invest Radiol	2003	Posterior tibial tendon tears (cadaver)	73	69	88	46	72	16 cadavers
Huh et al[96]	J Magn Reson Imaging	2004	Ankle synovitis	91.5	63.9	—	—	72.9	27
Huh et al[96]	J Magn Reson Imaging	2004	Ankle soft tissue impingement	76	96.9	—	—	94.4	15
Lamm et al[108]	J Foot Ankle Surg	2004	Peroneus brevis tears	83	75%	—	—	—	32
Lee et al[110]	Foot Ankle Int	2004	Ankle soft tissue impingement	91	84.4	—	—	—	38
Liu et al[113]	Am J Sports Med	1997	Anterior lateral impingement	39	50	—	—	—	22
Mintz et al[117]	Arthroscopy	2003	OCD of talus	95	100	88	100	—	14 controls 40 OCD lesions
Robinson et al[126]	Radiology	2001	Anterolateral ankle impingement	96	100	100	89	—	32
Rockett et al[127]	Foot Ankle Int	1998	Tendon disorders around foot and ankle	23	100	—	—	65.8	20
Rosenberg et al[157]	Radiology	1988	Posterior tibial tendon pathology	100	100	—	—	73	32
Saxena & Bareither[‡]	Foot Ankle Int	2000	Presence of plantaris tendon	92	100	100	—	—	18
Saxena & Wolf[128]	J Am Pod Med Assoc	2003	Peroneal tendonitis	82	50	100	—	—	40
Takao et al[134]	J Bone Joint Surg Br	2003	Syndesmosis tears of the ankle	100 ant 100 post	93 ant 100 post	—	—	96 ant 100 post	52
Verhaven et al[137]	Am J Sports Med	1991	Calcaneofibular ligament injury, acute	91	100	—	—	94	18
Verhaven et al[137]	Am J Sports Med	1991	ATFL injury, acute	100	50	—	—	94	18
Yao et al[139]	Skeletal Radiol	1999	Spring ligament disruption	54-77	100	—	—	—	13 cases 18 controls

*Inclusion criteria were clinical studies on adult patients with more than 10 patients in the study.
†Breitenseher MJ, Trattnig S, Kukla C, et al: [Injuries to the lateral ligaments of the ankle joint: Study technic and demonstration by means of MRI.] Rofo 164(3):226-32, 1996.
‡Saxena A, Bareither D: Magnetic resonance and cadaveric findings of the incidence of plantaris tendon. Foot Ankle Int 21(7):570-572, 2000.
ant, anterior; ATFL, anterior talofibular ligament; FCL, fibular collateral ligament; MR, magnetic resonance; MRI, magnetic resonance imaging; NPV, negative predictive value; OCD, osteochondritis dissecans; post, posterior; PPV, positive predictive value; Pts, patients; Sens, sensitivity; Spec, specificity.

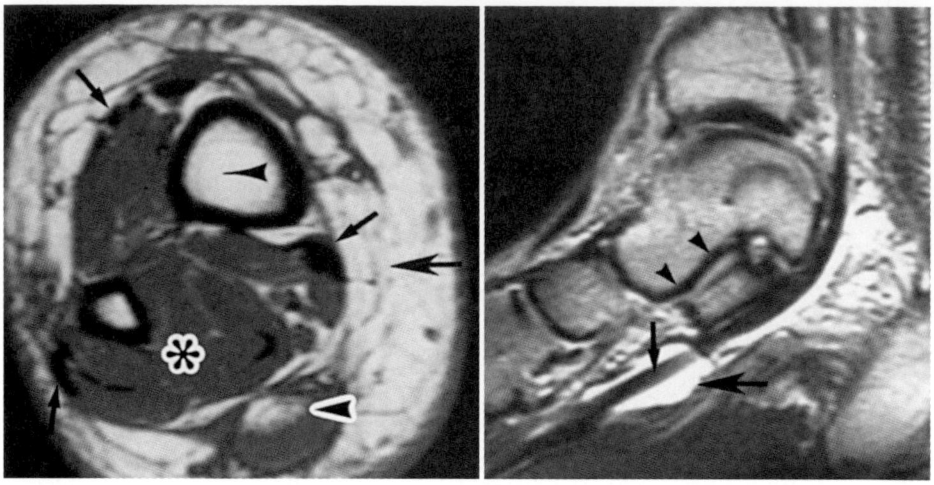

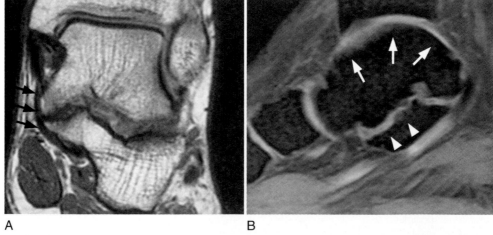

A   B

Figure 3–55   Tissue signal intensities on magnetic resonance imaging. **A,** Axial T1 (TR 600, TE 20) ankle image demonstrates typical high signal intensity *(white)* of subcutaneous fat *(large arrow)* and fatty marrow *(arrowhead)*. Hemorrhage often has high signal intensity, as demonstrated within a torn Achilles tendon *(bordered arrowhead)*. Low signal intensity *(black)* is seen in tendons *(small arrows)* and cortical bone. Muscle has intermediate signal intensity *(asterisk)*. **B,** Sagittal T2 (TR 2500, TE 80) ankle images demonstrate high signal intensity *(white)* due to long T2 relaxation of fluid in ganglion of the flexor hallucis longus *(large arrow)*. Very low signal intensity is seen in the adjacent tendon *(small arrow)* and cortical bone *(arrowheads)*.

cumferential whole volume coil or a partial volume coil of appropriate size is preferred for uniform evaluation of small structures. Surface or flat coils are used primarily for superficial structures.

Indications for MRI include trauma, neoplasms or masses, arthritis, inflammation or infection, osteonecrosis, sickle cell anemia, tarsal coalition, and reflex sympathetic dystrophy (Fig. 3–56).[77,105] It may be the imaging modality of choice in evaluation of soft tissue trauma[77,86] because MRI offers optimal visualization of soft tissue structures (Fig. 3–57).[104] Tendon disorders, both acutely injured and chronically diseased,

are well visualized for tears, partial tears, tenosynovitis, and postsurgical change.[86,112,114,125] The Achilles tendon is clearly demonstrated on MRI. The Achilles tendon is a common source of lower extremity complaints (Fig. 3–58).[98,129] The posterior tibialis and peroneal tendons, which are also important contributors to morbidity, are seen well on MRI. Anterior ankle impingement lesions are well seen on a preoperative MRI if a contrast-enhanced three-dimensional fast spoiled gradient recall (CE 3D FSPGR) sequence is used.[110]

Forefoot pain may be well assessed by MRI, particularly because the resolution of scans is improving.

A   B

Figure 3–56   Tarsal coalition on magnetic resonance imaging illustrating partially cartilaginous features. **A,** Coronal T1 (TR 800, TE 30) image demonstrates classic deformity medial facet talocalcaneal coalition *(arrows)*. **B,** Sagittal three-dimensional fat-suppressed spoiled gradient-echo (TR 24.5, TE 6, angle 40) image showing similar signal intensity in coalition *(white arrowheads)* and nearby articular cartilage *(white arrows)* in this sequence, which produces high signal intensity in hyaline cartilage.

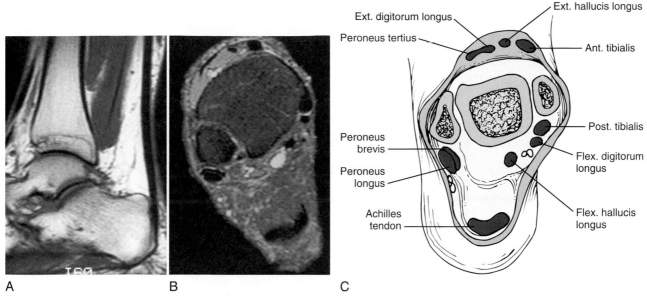

Figure 3–57 Normal ankle tendons on magnetic resonance imaging. **A,** Normal appearance of the Achilles tendon on sagittal proton density (TR 2500, TE 20) image. Note the normal morphology and low signal intensity *(black)*. **B,** Normal appearance of other ankle tendons on axial proton density (TR 4533, TE 30) image with fat suppression. **C,** Anatomic drawing for correlation illustrates location and relative size of ankle tendons in the axial plane.

Causes of forefoot pain include Morton's neuroma, stress fracture, plantar plate rupture, synovitis, Freiberg's infraction, tendon tears, and masses such as pigmented villonodular synovitis. For this reason, MRI may well be used to assess the causes of forefoot pain.[76]

Evaluation of recalcitrant hindfoot pain should include MRI imaging. Plantar fasciitis, plantar fascia rupture, and abnormalities in the heel pad may be only visualized by MR scans.[122] One MR study assessed the causes of ongoing pain after plantar fasciitis.[140] Causes include posterior tibial tendonitis, tarsal tunnel syndrome, and complete rupture. These changes might reflect a progression of flatfoot deformity after release.

Ligaments are well visualized on high-resolution MRI (Fig. 3–59).[92] Injured ligaments can be visualized,

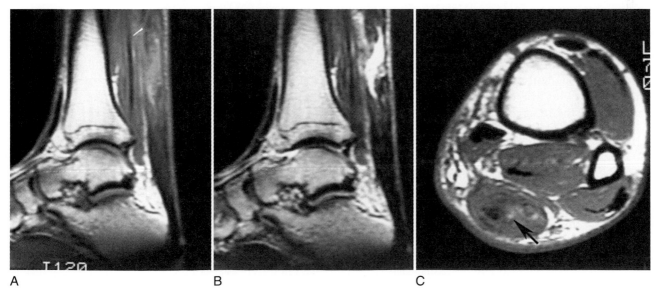

Figure 3–58 Achilles tendon tear on magnetic resonance imaging. **A,** Sagittal proton density (TR 2500, TE 20) image demonstrates thickened Achilles tendon with altered morphology and increased signal intensity beginning several centimeters proximal to its insertion. **B,** Sagittal T2 (TR 2500, TE 80) image illustrates very high signal intensity fluid spanning the gap between tendon remnants. **C,** Axial T1 (TR 600, TE 20) image shows increased signal intensity of the Achilles tendon relative to other ankle tendons. Areas of high signal intensity *(whiter areas)* in the Achilles tendon represent hemorrhage *(arrow)*.

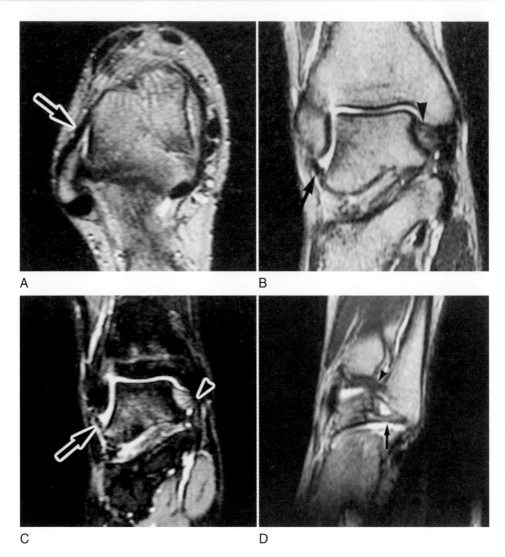

A

B

C

D

Figure 3–59 Normal ankle ligaments on magnetic resonance imaging. **A,** Anterior talofibular ligament on T2 (TR 2500, TE 80) axial image *(arrow)*. **B,** Normal anterior talofibular ligament *(arrow)* and deltoid ligament *(arrowhead)* on coronal T2 (TR 2500, TE 80) image. **C,** Normal deltoid ligament *(arrowhead)* and anterior talofibular ligament *(arrow)* on short T1 inversion recovery (STIR) (TR 2000, TI 160, TE 43) coronal image. **D,** Normal posterior talofibular ligament *(arrow)* and posterior tibiofibular ligament *(arrowhead)* on T2 (TR 2000, TE 80) coronal image.

but the exact role of MRI in evaluating ligamentous injuries is not clear, because the treatment is based on symptomatology and not imaging appearance. Many acute injuries resolve with nonoperative treatment regardless of the integrity assessed by imaging. Stress radiography is in common use, but early reports suggest noncontrast MRI in acute injuries and direct MR arthrography in chronic injuries may be more sensitive in detecting tears.[81,130,137] For acute midfoot injuries, MRI has a role in supplementing CT imaging in defining the anatomy of ligaments and fractures.[124] Osseous trauma requiring advanced imaging is best evaluated by CT scan and nuclear medicine except in the diagnosis of and possibly the staging of osteochondral lesions, in which case MRI may be the best noninvasive imaging modality.[75,87]

MRI is the technique of choice in evaluating soft tissue masses, particularly suspected malignancies.[80,101,138] MRI might suggest malignancy, in which case pathologic confirmation is required.[78,106,107,120,138] In some cases pathologic confirmation is required;

for example, 90% of plantar sole lesions are plantar fibromas. Benign masses such as pigmented villonodular synovitis (PVNS),[97] cysts, and lipomas have a characteristic MRI appearance and might merit follow-up scans alone. In most other cases, MRI probably is unable to differentiate between benign and malignant lesions in the foot and ankle* (Fig. 3–60). Histologic diagnosis is therefore required.

MRI can assist in the diagnosis of chronic regional pain syndrome (CRPS), previously known as reflex sympathetic dystrophy (RSD). However many of the changes are nonspecific, including bone marrow edema, fractures, and joint effusions.

MRI currently is the preferred investigation for detecting and evaluating avascular necrosis.[80,131] It is best used in conjunction with comparison radiographs.[77] Bone infarction can be clearly imaged, and MRI can aid in differentiating early infarction from malignancy or infection.[121]

---

*References 78, 100, 102, 106, 107, 119, and 120.

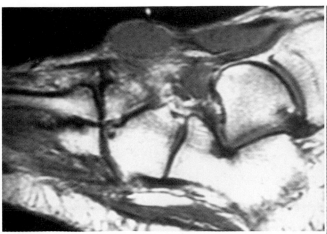

A

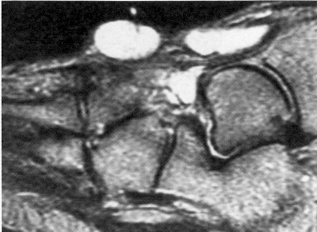

B

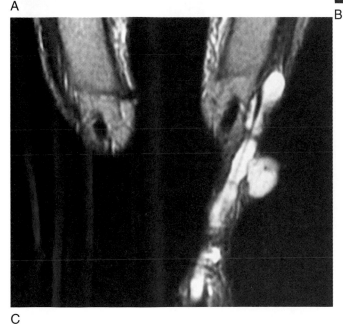

C

Figure 3–60 Soft tissue mass of foot on magnetic resonance imaging. **A,** Sagittal proton density (TR 2500, TE 20) image shows low signal intensity mass lying deep to skin marker, localizing palpable abnormality. **B,** Sagittal T2 (TR 2500, TE 80) image demonstrates high signal intensity in mass consistent with ganglion. Note deep component extending toward calcaneocuboid joint. **C,** Axial T2 (TR 2500, TE 80) image illustrates ganglion wrapping around extensor tendons and extending over greater than clinically suspected distance with appearance assisting in surgical planning.

MRI can accurately detect osteomyelitis and soft tissue abscesses. It is useful in preoperative planning of infection surgery because it provides detailed and accurate information regarding the extent of disease (Fig. 3–61).[91,95,115,118,135] Although osteomyelitis can be well defined by MRI, the surgeon must pay more attention to the clinical picture and treat the patient appropriately than wait for an MRI result.[116] MRI can detect changes of rheumatoid arthritis before they are clinically apparent.[123]

MRI has been used to evaluate stress fractures, growth plate fractures, reflex sympathetic dystrophy, and tarsal-tunnel syndrome (Fig. 3–62).[90,99,105,109] Other imaging may be better at diagnosing stress fractures or reflex sympathetic dystrophy.

The future of MRI not only includes further imaging advances but also probably includes spectroscopic and physiologic evaluation. This might allow evaluation of physiologic changes in muscles during exercise.[133] Spectroscopy can aid in evaluating viable tissue and bone marrow in ischemia.[77] These areas and others are being studied. The diagnostic accuracy of MRI needs to be evaluated further for test–retest reliability to allow surgeons to correctly apply weight to the investigation in the light of the clinical picture.

PRACTICAL ALGORITHMIC APPROACH TO CLINICAL PROBLEMS

The following sections each include a referenced short discussion and an imaging decision tree addressing common foot and ankle clinical problems. The brief discussions are not intended to fully review the subject. Rather, they introduce key concepts and some important decision-making points to aid in using the algorithms. The reader is encouraged to review the literature for further details.

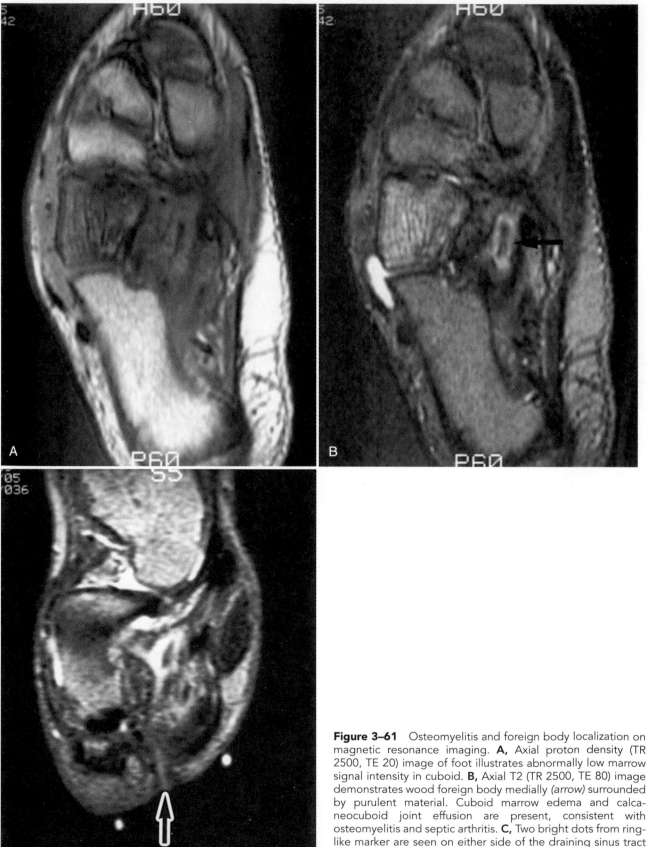

Figure 3–61 Osteomyelitis and foreign body localization on magnetic resonance imaging. **A,** Axial proton density (TR 2500, TE 20) image of foot illustrates abnormally low marrow signal intensity in cuboid. **B,** Axial T2 (TR 2500, TE 80) image demonstrates wood foreign body medially *(arrow)* surrounded by purulent material. Cuboid marrow edema and calcaneocuboid joint effusion are present, consistent with osteomyelitis and septic arthritis. **C,** Two bright dots from ringlike marker are seen on either side of the draining sinus tract leading up to the foreign body on this coronal T2 (TR 2000, TE 80) image *(arrow)*.

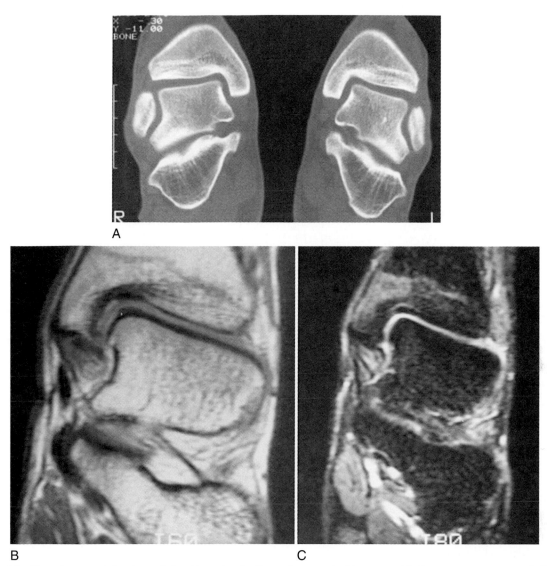

Figure 3–62 Chronic unexplained medial ankle pain. **A,** Coronal computed tomographic image appears normal. **B,** Coronal T1 (TR 600, TE 20) magnetic resonance image is normal, as were T2 coronal images. **C,** Coronal short T1 inversion recovery (STIR) (TR 2000, TI 160, TE 43) image demonstrates abnormal marrow edema in the left medial malleolus from a stress reaction in this athlete. STIR images increase the conspicuity of marrow abnormalities by suppressing the fat signal and increasing the contrast between normal and abnormal.

The algorithms are based on the imaging options currently thought to be the most efficacious in addressing a particular problem. The options are supported by the literature, but the choices also reflect our institutional experience and preferences. Where two options are currently thought to be equal, both options are listed. The reader might wish to use information in the discussion and from the previous advanced imaging sections to choose an alternative imaging method when appropriate to the specific clinical situation.

Therapeutic options appropriately are individualized to the particular patient and are included in the decision trees only when they are thought to alter the choices. It is assumed that all patients have had a complete clinical examination and the appropriate radiographs. Additional diagnostic information is obtained to guide the treatment plan.

Complex Regional Pain Syndrome

Complex regional pain syndrome is a complex disease process that is not fully understood.[144] It is the cause of considerable morbidity and can elude diagnosis. More importantly, it is often overlooked in the differential diagnosis (Fig. 3–63). Clinical examination remains the mainstay of diagnosis. Plain radiographs should be performed to rule out associated disorders. A three-phase nuclear medicine bone scan, although sometimes lacking the classic appearance described in

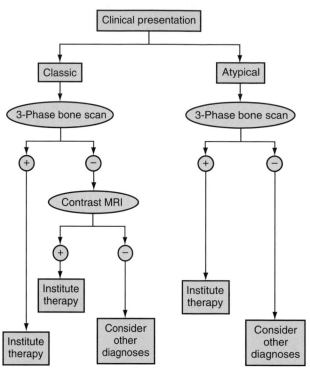

Figure 3–63   Algorithm for chronic regional pain syndrome. (From Resnick D, Niwayama G: *Diagnosis of Bone and Joint Disorders*, ed 2. Philadelphia, WB Saunders, 1988.)

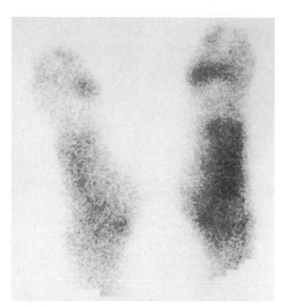

Figure 3–64   Bone scan appearance in chronic regional pain syndrome. Classic increased periarticular and osseous activity on delayed skeletal images. (From Resnick D, Niwayama G: *Diagnosis of Bone and Joint Disorders*, ed 2. Philadelphia, WB Saunders, 1988.)

the upper extremity, remains the primary diagnostic imaging modality (Fig. 3–64).[142,143]

Contrast-enhanced MRI focusing on soft tissue changes has shown promise in arriving at a definitive diagnosis even in stage 1 disease.[144,145]

Osteochondral Lesions

Osteochondral injuries are a significant problem in patients with ankle pain. Evaluation begins with standing AP, lateral, and mortise views of the ankle. Bone scans may be considered in patients with negative radiographs (Fig. 3–65).[146]

In patients without a radiographically visible anomaly, MRI is the next imaging method of choice.[146] A number of osteochondral abnormalities are visible on MRI that are not visible on CT scan.[146] If available, CT arthrography has a high diagnostic accuracy. When there is a radiographic abnormality without clear evidence for a detached fragment, an imaging technique should be chosen that is capable of determining whether a fragment is loose. This can involve combining double-contrast arthrography with a tomographic technique such as CT scan.[147,149,150] Detecting contrast surrounding a fragment confirms that it is loose or detached, and potentially unstable. MRI has also been successfully used to confirm loose fragments, offering a noninvasive alternative to CT arthrography.[148] This technique takes advantage of normal fluid and marrow

contrast differences on MRI[148] (Fig. 3–66). In difficult cases, it is likely that indirect or direct MR arthrography would be useful due to the improved contrast within the joints.[151]

Although MRI is sensitive with regard to osteochondral injury (combined bone and cartilage injury) it is not as sensitive at picking up isolated chondral injuries or soft tissue impingement. For lesions with a significant cystic component, CT scanning offers the added advantage of providing more accurate detail of the bone disorder.

Chronic Undiagnosed Post-traumatic Pain

Chronic undiagnosed post-traumatic pain is a clinical and imaging challenge (Fig. 3–67). Standing AP and lateral views of the affected part should be performed first. If no radiographic abnormality is detected, three-phase nuclear medicine might detect occult osseous abnormalities (Fig. 3–68).[155,156] CT scan is a useful adjunct for osseous evaluation when correlative radiographs are inconclusive in patients with abnormal metabolic activity on bone scan. CT scan is also used to better define bone disorder in patients in whom surgery is planned.

MRI is currently the primary means to evaluate soft tissue injuries in the foot and ankle (Fig. 3–69). Soft tissue trauma can be indicated by the nature of the injury or in patients with trauma and negative radiographs and CT scans.[152,153,155] It is important, however, for the clinician to realize that MRI is best used in a

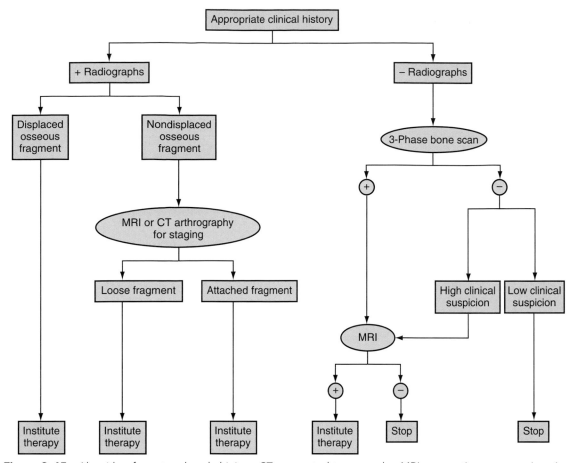

Figure 3–65 Algorithm for osteochondral injury. CT, computed tomography; MRI, magnetic resonance imaging.

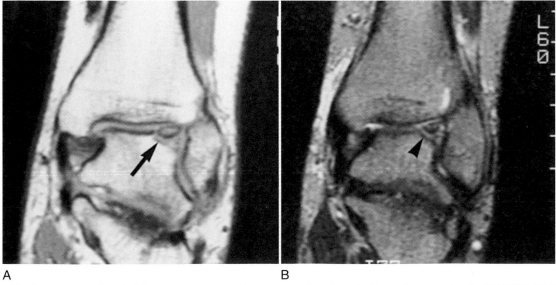

A   B

Figure 3–66 Loose osteochondral fragment on magnetic resonance imaging. **A,** Coronal proton density (TR 2500, TE 20) image demonstrates a lateral talar dome osteochondral lesion *(arrow)*. **B,** Coronal T2 (TR 2500, TE 80) image illustrates the presence of high signal intensity fluid surrounding a fragment consistent with loosening *(arrowhead)*.

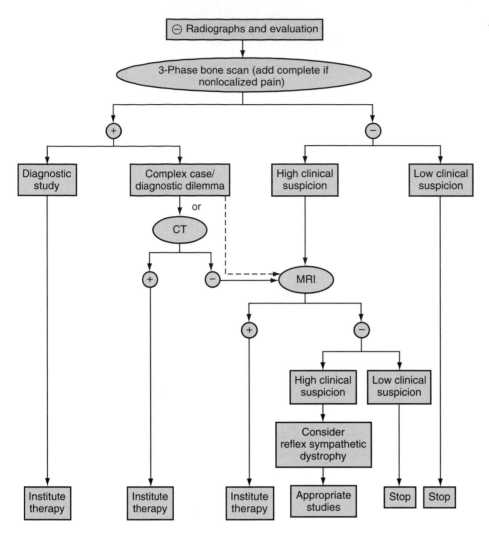

Figure 3–67 Algorithm for chronic undiagnosed post-traumatic pain. CT, computed tomography; MRI, magnetic resonance imaging.

problem-directed fashion, because of the complexity of lower extremity anatomy and the multiple MRI options available. Communication to the radiologist of the primary clinical concerns, such as tarsal tunnel syndrome or posterior tibial tendon injury, allows a portion of the examination to be specifically tailored to address that concern (Fig. 3–70).[152,157]

Unstable Ankle

Ligamentous tears and strains are common. Imaging evaluation usually is guided by the age of the injury (Fig. 3–71). Plain radiography is indicated based on the Ottawa ankle rules: In cases in which there may be a fracture present, plain radiographs should be performed at the time of presentation. Contrast arthrography is most useful in the acute setting, because 48 to 72 hours after an injury the ligamentous capsular tears often are sealed by fibrinous debris.[159-163] However these investigations are unlikely to change the management plan. Because of that, stress radiographs usually are substituted for arthrography in the subacute or chronic setting (Fig. 3–72).[164]

The role of MRI in ligament evaluation currently is not well established, although clearly some ligamentous tears can be visualized (Fig. 3–73).[158] Recent literature suggests that MRI and MR arthrography will play an important role in evaluation of suspected ligamentous injuries.[160,165] Peroneal tenography is the other major advanced imaging option for lateral ligamentous injuries, but it is not commonly used because it is painful and can be technically difficult.[161,164] The rate of associated injury to the cartilage surface or impingement lesions in the ankle with lateral ligament instability increases the need for diagnostic imaging via MRI.

Tendon Injury

The most exciting development in tendon imaging evaluation is the availability of MRI (Fig. 3–74).[166,167,172] Its multiplanar imaging capability and ability to evaluate internal tendon structure and peritendinous tissues make it the primary imaging option[169,170] (Fig. 3–75). Tenography is invasive and can be difficult to perform, so it is rarely used.[172,173] CT

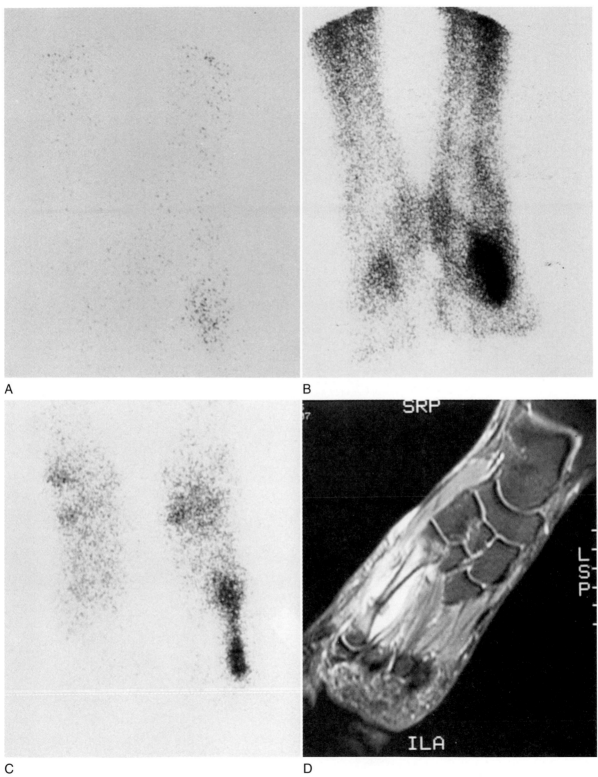

Figure 3–68 Evaluation of chronic undiagnosed post-traumatic pain. **A,** Perfusion. **B,** Blood pool. **C,** Delayed images from three-phase nuclear medicine bone scan demonstrate abnormal activity in the third metatarsal in a patient with an 8-week history of pain following an automobile accident. Pain was worsening over the past 2 weeks. **D,** Magnetic resonance imaging was performed because plain radiographs were normal and computed tomography had an equivocal cortical irregularity involving the distal third metatarsal in this patient with an abnormal bone scan. Axial short T1 inversion recovery (STIR) (TR 2000, TI 160, TE 43) shows soft tissue edema and marrow edema compared with fat-suppressed adjacent soft tissue and marrow spaces. Classic stress fracture with callus formation is demonstrated. Confirmatory radiographs were obtained 10 days later.

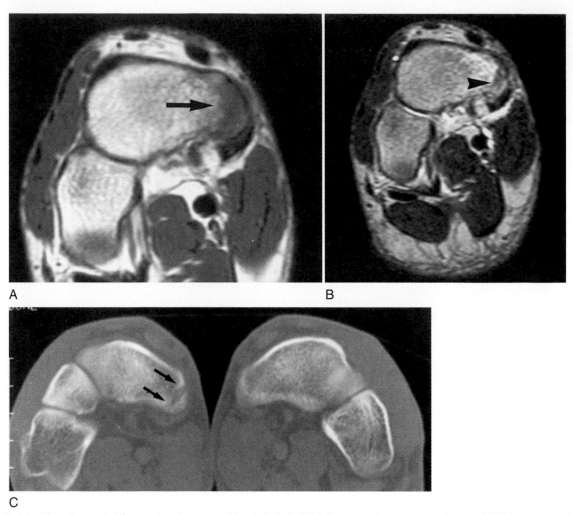

A

B

C

Figure 3–69 Chronic medial foot pain. **A,** Coronal T1 (TR 600, TE 20) magnetic resonance image (MRI) illustrates abnormal decreased marrow signal intensity deep to posterior tibialis tendon insertion *(arrow)*. **B,** Coronal T2 (TR 2500, TE 80) image demonstrates crescent of low signal intensity surrounded by high signal intensity edema *(arrowhead)*. Findings were thought to represent stress fracture. **C,** Confirmatory (no charge) computed tomographic scan was performed because this was early in our MRI experience. It confirms stress fracture of tarsal navicular *(arrows)*.

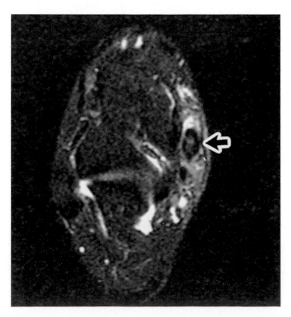

Figure 3–70 Chronic distal posterior tibialis tendon pain. Axial T2 (TR 2500, TE 80) fat-suppression magnetic resonance image demonstrates markedly thickened posterior tibialis tendon secondary to tendinosis and central partial tear *(arrow)*.

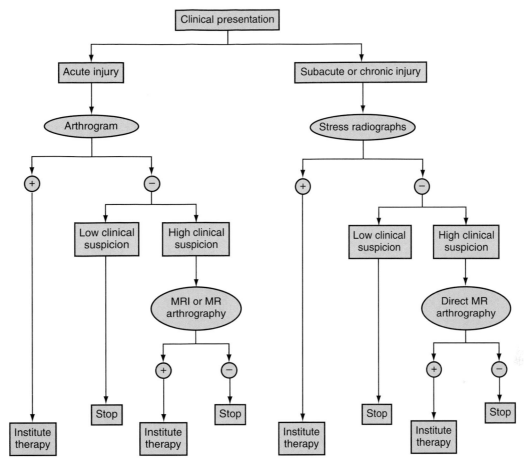

Figure 3–71 Algorithm for ligamentous injury. MR, magnetic resonance; MRI, magnetic resonance imaging.

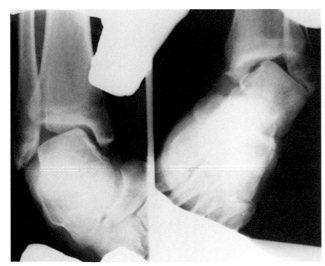

Figure 3–72 Chronic ankle injury. Abnormal varus stress ankle radiographs consistent with lateral ligamentous tears.

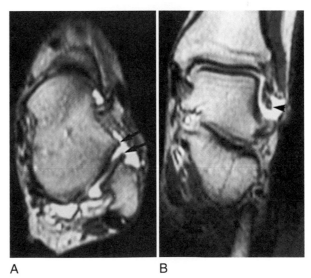

A   B

Figure 3–73 Anterior talofibular ligament tear on magnetic resonance imaging. **A,** Axial T2 (TR 2500, TE 80) image at expected location, anterior talofibular ligament (*arrows*). (See Fig. 3–55 for normal appearance.) **B,** Coronal T2 (TR 2500, TE 80) image illustrates retracted and thickened ligamentous remnant (*arrowhead*).

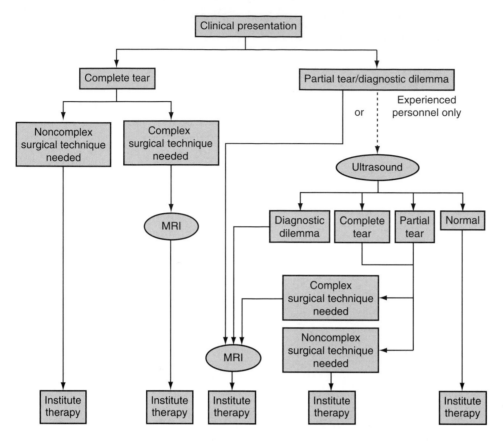

Figure 3–74 Algorithm for tendon injury. MRI, magnetic resonance imaging.

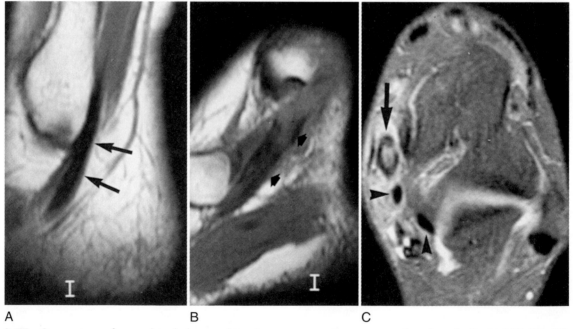

A   B   C

Figure 3–75 Comparison of normal and abnormal tendons on magnetic resonance imaging. **A,** Sagittal T1 (TR 600, TE 20) image demonstrates normal low signal intensity appearance of peroneal tendons *(arrows).* **B,** Sagittal T1 (TR 600, TE 20) image of abnormal posterior tibialis tendon shows that it is thickened and has higher signal intensity than normal *(arrowheads).* **C,** Axial proton density (TR 2500, TE 20) fat-suppression image illustrates partial tear and central degeneration of posterior tibialis tendon, explaining the abnormality demonstrated on the sagittal images *(arrow).* Note the normal adjacent flexor digitorum longus and flexor hallucis longus tendons *(arrowheads).*

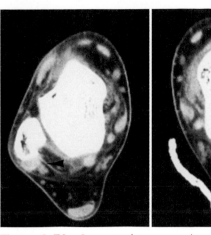
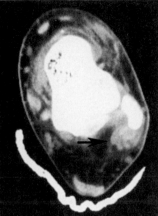

Figure 3–76 Computed tomography of peroneal tendon injury. Axial CT image demonstrates thickened appearance of left peroneal tendons and peritendinous tissue *(arrow)* compared with normal right ankle *(arrowhead)*. Note that CT scan does not optimally distinguish between tendinosis and partial tear.

scan or ultrasound, depending on the tendon in question, may be used as secondary imaging options[174] (Fig. 3–76).

Ultrasound as an option has limitations. It requires a high-frequency linear array transducer in the range of 7 to 10 MHz. The examination is technically demanding and requires experience to avoid false-positive examinations.[168] There have, however, been a number of technologic improvements, and in experienced hands, it is beginning to have a role not only in large straight tendons such as the Achilles but also in moderate-sized curved tendons such as the posterior tibial tendon.

In general we would recommend MRI for tendon evaluations, even for the Achilles (Fig. 3–77). Ultrasound may prove most useful as a less expensive screening examination to confirm a normal appearing Achilles tendon following injury. This has been shown to have a strong predictive value of a good outcome.[168,171]

Foreign Body Localization

Foreign body localization and removal can be a very frustrating process for both the patient and the clinician, particularly in the plantar aspect of the foot. The situation is complicated by the complex anatomy of the foot, the fact that many foreign bodies are radiolucent, and the disconcerting habit of foreign bodies to lie well away from the entry site.

Imaging is best approached first by routine radiography, with advanced imaging choices based on those results and the character of the injury (Fig. 3–78 and Fig. 3–79).[176-179]

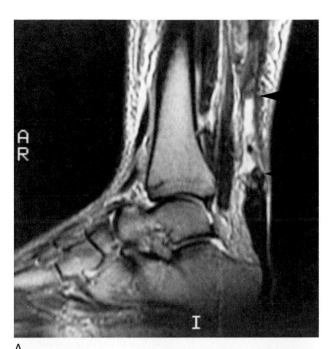

A

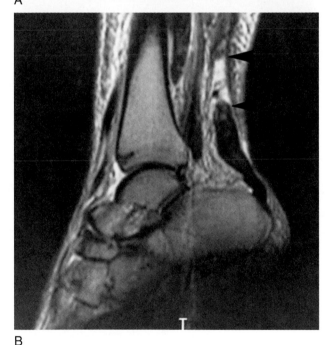

B

Figure 3–77 Achilles tendon tear evaluation with dorsiflexion and plantar flexion on magnetic resonance image. **A,** Dorsiflexion sagittal T2 (TR 2500, TE 80) image shows wide distraction of tendon fragments in patient with complete Achilles tendon tear *(arrows)*. **B,** Plantar flexion sagittal T2 (TR 2500, TE 80) image shows residual 2-cm gap between tendon fragments *(arrowheads)*. In patients in whom conservative therapy is being considered, knowledge of the degree of a persistent diastasis of tendon fragments can alter the therapeutic options.

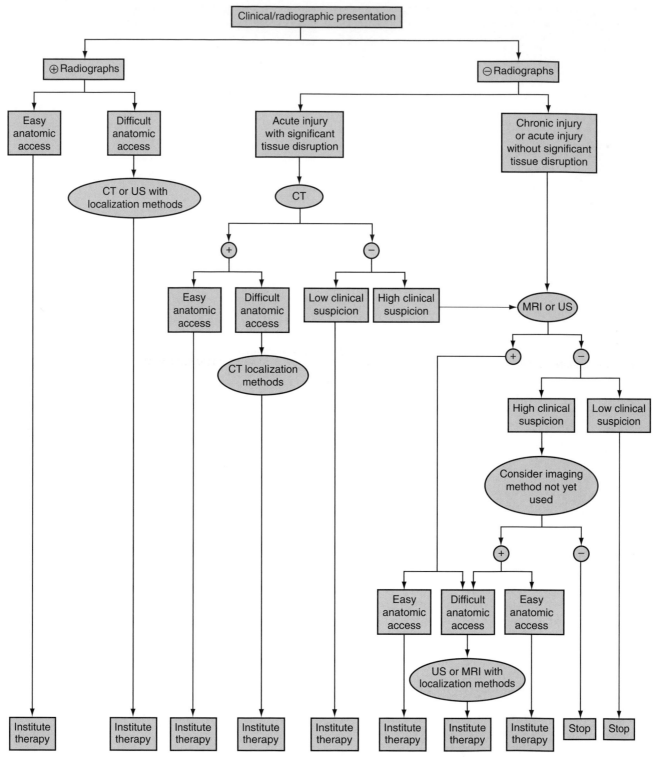

Figure 3–78   Algorithm for foreign body localization. CT, computed tomography; MRI, magnetic resonance imaging; US, ultrasound.

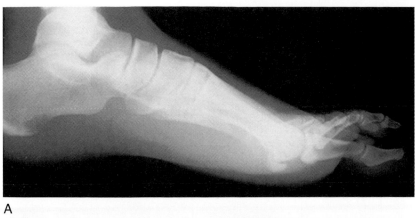

A

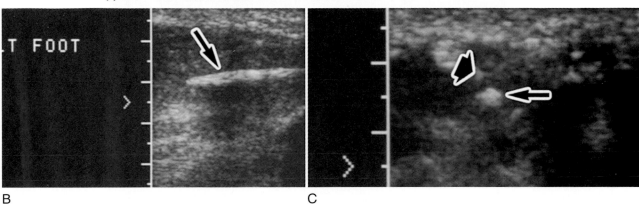

B   C

Figure 3–79 Foreign body localization. **A,** Soft tissue technique radiograph with markers bordering a palpable soft tissue mass. No foreign body is demonstrated. **B,** Long-axis view of echogenic, but radiolucent, foreign body demonstrated only on diagnostic ultrasound *(arrow)*. Foreign body is approximately 2 cm distal to the soft tissue mass, which was thought to represent an abscess. **C,** Short-axis view of the foreign body on ultrasound *(arrow)* with adjacent echogenic needle tip *(arrowhead)* placed percutaneously with ultrasound guidance. Methylene blue was injected at each end of the foreign body just prior to surgery, and a toothpick fragment was successfully removed.

Localized foreign bodies may be approached surgically. Despite excellent preoperative imaging and surgical technique, operative removal is often prolonged and unsuccessful (Fig. 3–80). If the initial surgery is unsuccessful, we have used interventional techniques to directly localize foreign bodies, resulting in a successful second operation. One may wish to consider direct preoperative localization initially to decrease operative time and improve the likelihood for successful foreign body removal.[175]

Avascular Necrosis

Avascular necrosis in the foot and ankle can occur in sesamoid, metatarsal, and tarsal bones.[180,182-186] The talus is the most common area of concern.[183-185] If routine radiographs are diagnostic, further imaging is necessary only to try to stage the abnormality and assess for additional abnormalities, such as articular surface collapse, subchondral cysts, loose bodies, and articular cartilage abnormalities, if that information will affect treatment (Fig. 3–81).

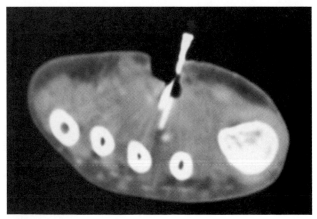

Figure 3–80 Successful foreign body direct localization following initially unsuccessful surgery. Multiple localization needles were placed under CT guidance through a patient incision following unsuccessful initial operation. Foreign body was successfully removed surgically after direct localization.

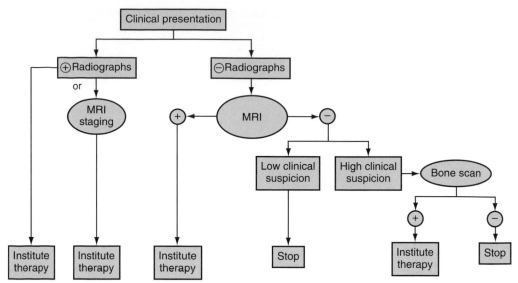

Figure 3–81   Algorithm for avascular necrosis. MRI, magnetic resonance imaging.

When routine radiographs are normal or inconclusive, MRI is recommended currently for detection (Fig. 3–82).[181] It is believed to be more sensitive than bone scan and has the added advantage of better resolution, which is helpful in small bones such as the talus.[181] There are a few case reports of false-negative MRI scans, so bone scans represent a second imaging option when clinical suspicion is high and the MRI is normal.[180]

Undiagnosed Mass

Evaluation of a mass or osseous lesion requires careful teamwork between the radiologist and clinician (Fig. 3–83).

Initial imaging decisions currently are usually decided by whether the abnormality is osseous or not. Plain radiographs remain the critical factor in developing a differential diagnosis for osseous lesions.[193] One should realize the importance of detecting a polyostotic process on nuclear medicine bone scan, because a more distant lesion might have characteristics on correlative radiographs that confirm a diagnosis.[189,191] Osseous abnormalities can be further staged by MRI or CT scan (Fig. 3–84).

Soft tissue lesions usually should be studied by MRI[188,193-195,197] (Fig. 3–85). Occasionally ultrasound is a reasonable alternative to confirm a suspected cystic lesion.[192] Even in cystic lesions, MRI can be helpful in preoperative planning, particularly in

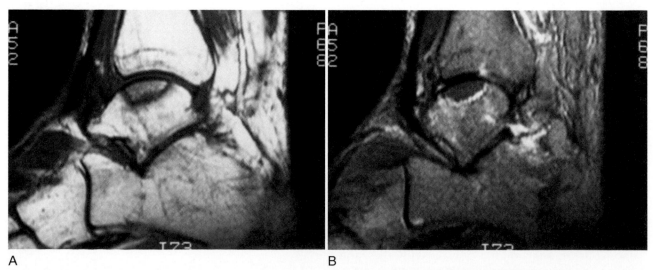

A   B

Figure 3–82   Avascular necrosis of talus on magnetic resonance imaging. **A,** Sagittal T1 (TR 600, TE 20) image demonstrates loss of normal fatty marrow signal intensity in a talar dome fragment. **B,** Sagittal T2 (TR 2500, TE 80) image shows low signal intensity in a fragment consistent with avascular necrosis with early changes of classic double-ring sign.

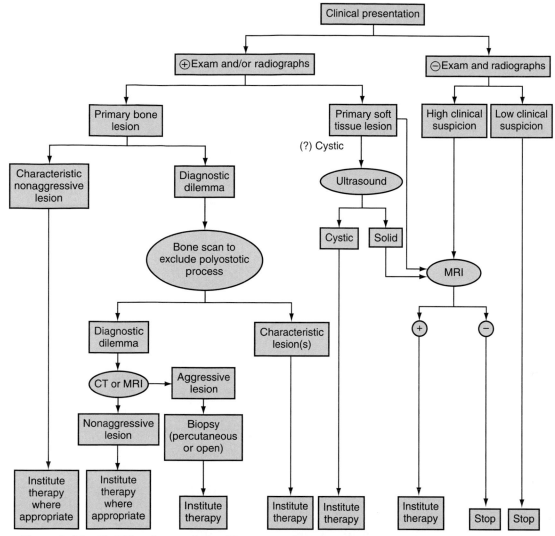

Figure 3–83 Algorithm for neoplasm. CT, computed tomography; MRI, magnetic resonance imaging.

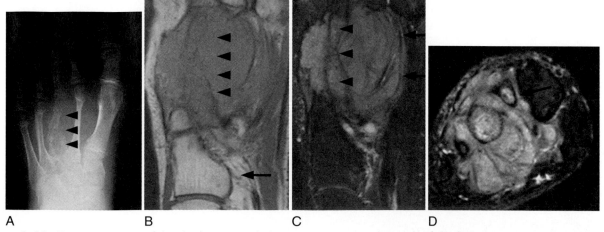

A   B   C   D

Figure 3–84 Ewing's sarcoma of the third metatarsal. **A,** Anteroposterior radiograph of the foot shows a permeative destructive process of third metatarsal *(arrowheads)* with mass effect suggested on adjacent bones. **B,** Axial T1 (TR 600, TE 30) image demonstrates complete replacement of fat signal intensity in the third metatarsal *(arrowheads)* compared to normal high fat signal intensity in the nearby cuboid *(arrow)*. **C,** Axial fast spin echo T2 (TR 2800, TE 75) image with fat suppression illustrates the marrow-replacing tumor *(arrowheads)* that has high signal intensity similar to the surrounding soft tissue mass *(arrows)*. **D,** Coronal fast spin echo T2 (TR 3800, TE 75) image with fat suppression demonstrates a mass enveloping the adjacent metatarsals, with some reactive marrow changes in the adjacent second metatarsal manifested by high signal intensity *(arrow)*.

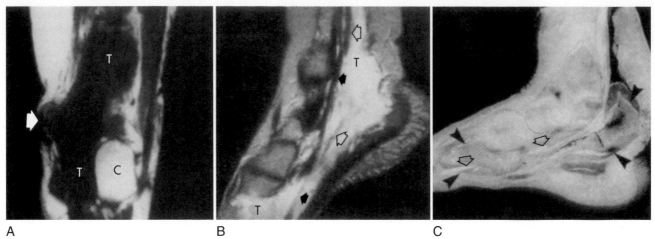

A   B   C

Figure 3-85   Magnetic resonance imaging appearance of synovial sarcoma with pathologic correlation. **A,** Coronal T1 (TR 500, TE 17) image shows large tumor *(T)* medial to the calcaneus *(C)* extending into the posterior compartment of the leg, which was not detected clinically in an obese patient. A small medial component *(arrow)* was palpable, and the initial clinical diagnosis was a ganglion cyst. **B,** Sagittal T2 (TR 2100, TE 90) image reveals longitudinal extent of tumor *(T)* with infiltrative margins and high signal intensity compared with fat. Note tumor growth along the flexor digitorum longus *(solid arrows)* and flexor hallucis longus *(open arrows)* tendons. **C,** Gross section of the specimen confirms the extent of neoplasm *(arrowheads)*, which was firmly adherent to the long flexor tendons in the foot *(open arrows)*. (From Wetzel L, Levine E: *AJR Am J Roentgenol* 155:1025-1030, 1990.)

recurrent lesions or in areas of complex anatomy (Fig. 3–86).

In some patients, despite normal findings on clinical and routine radiographic evaluation, further imaging is needed to exclude an occult neoplasm or neoplasm-like lesion. MRI is the best method for these patients.

Biopsy should be used judiciously by experienced radiologists and orthopaedic surgeons.[187,190,196] Care should be taken not to obtain biopsy specimens of malignancies in a manner that jeopardizes subsequent therapy, such as limb salvage. In addition, some nonaggressive lesions have a characteristic appearance

and should be left alone in the absence of complicating symptoms or pathologic findings.

Systemic Arthritis

Arthritis is an important consideration in patients with pain.[200] Pattern of onset can be variable, and diagnosis requires appropriate integration of clinical symptoms, laboratory test results, and imaging findings (Fig. 3–87).[199,201,202]

Character of radiographic findings and the distribution of abnormalities often leads to a diagnosis[199] (Fig. 3–88). Standing radiographs of both feet and

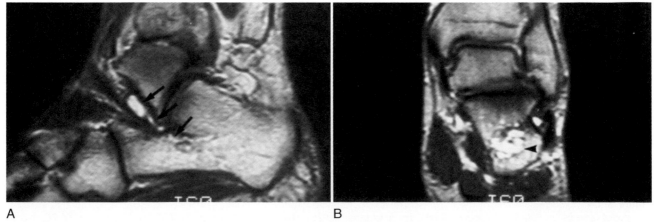

A   B

Figure 3-86   Recurrent ganglion with intraosseous extension. **A,** Sagittal T2 (TR 2500, TE 80) shows thin extension of clinically recurrent ganglion into the sinus tarsi, with entry into the calcaneus *(arrows)*. **B,** Coronal T2 (TR 2500, TE 80) best demonstrates the size of the intraosseous component *(arrowhead)*. Knowledge of the lesion's extent greatly affected preoperative planning.

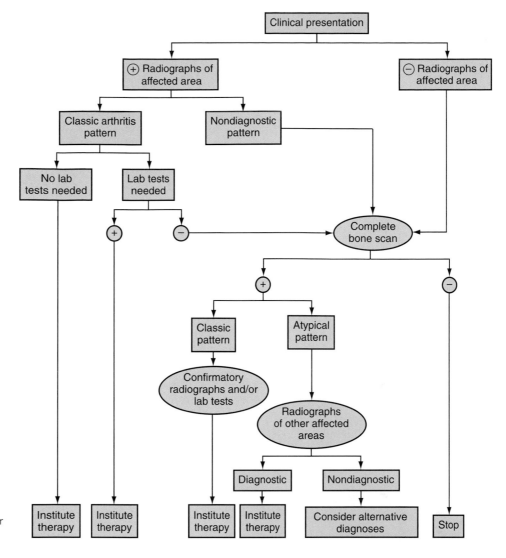

Figure 3–87 Algorithm for arthritis.

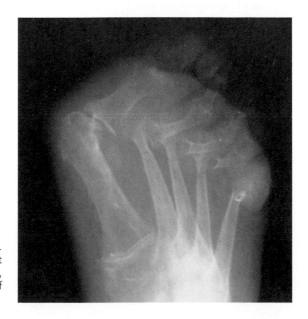

Figure 3–88 Characteristic foot radiograph in rheumatoid arthritis. Radiograph demonstrates soft tissue swelling, osteoporosis, joint space narrowing, erosions, and chronic changes of ulnar deviation, with dislocation at the metatarsophalangeal joints, representative of rheumatoid arthritis.

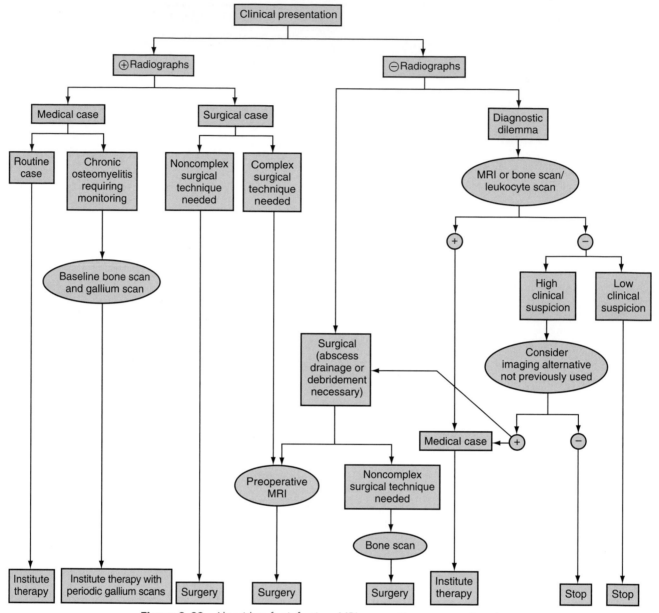

Figure 3–89 Algorithm for infection. MRI, magnetic resonance imaging.

both ankles should be performed as a baseline investigation. Deltoid ligament insufficiency can evade diagnosis in patients without a weight-bearing AP radiograph of the ankle. When radiographs are normal or nondiagnostic, a bone scan may be helpful in establishing the distribution of abnormalities.[203] If the distribution appears characteristic of a particular arthritis, one can consider laboratory tests or radiographs as options to complete the evaluation. Hand films commonly are used for correlation when multiple joints

are involved. If the distribution of disease is atypical, radiography of affected areas on the bone scan is suggested.

Other advanced imaging techniques usually are restricted for use in patients being considered for surgical therapy, in patients requiring further staging of their disease, or to exclude associated conditions such as tarsal coalition.[198,203] CT scan is a commonly used supplemental technique and is recommended to evaluate areas such as the subtalar joint.[200,203]

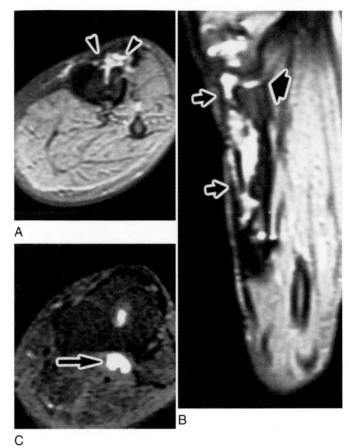

Figure 3–90 Preoperative demonstration of osteomyelitis with clinically unsuspected extraosseous extension in magnetic resonance images. **A,** Axial proton density (TR 2700, TE 20) fat-suppression image of the tibia illustrates changes of osteomyelitis primarily involving the ventral tibia and soft tissue *(arrowheads)*. **B,** Sagittal proton density (TR 2350, TE 20) fat-suppression image shows the extent of tibial involvement ventrally *(arrows)* and suggests fistula extending posteriorly *(arrowhead)*. **C,** Axial T2 (TR 2700, TE 80) demonstrates high signal intensity fluid collection posterior to proximal metaphyseal region of the tibia *(arrow)*. This clinically unsuspected abnormality was surgically confirmed and drained.

Infection

The role of imaging in infection is evolving.[208,214] Plain radiographs are the first step in evaluation (Fig. 3–89).[208,214] Factors such as whether the case is considered for surgical treatment help guide the imaging workup (Fig. 3–90).

The foot and ankle consist of a large number of small structures with a complex interrelationship. There are areas in the foot that require a more technical surgical approach when treating osteomyelitis, septic arthritis, or abscess. Understanding compartmental anatomy in the foot is key in these situations.[206] The high resolution of MRI and its proven ability to aid in surgical planning for treatment of infection make it the imaging modality of choice in these patients* (Fig. 3–91).

Other patients may be adequately evaluated by routine radiographs alone if findings are positive or by plain radiographs combined with three-phase nuclear medicine bone scan. It is important to recall that the bone scan will be positive well in advance of radiographic findings.[216,219] Leukocyte scan is a useful adjunct when results of bone scan are equivocal, particularly if symptoms are acute.[206,208,218] Gallium scans are less specific and no more sensitive in that situation.[210,212] Gallium scans have been suggested as a means to determine efficacy of treatment in patients receiving long-term antibiotic therapy.[204] This is primarily thought to be useful in patients with chronic osteomyelitis in whom initial therapy failed. It can be used periodically to monitor activity, with the expectation of gradual resolution of abnormal uptake if therapy is effective.[204]

---

*References 205, 208, 209, 211, 213, 215, and 217.

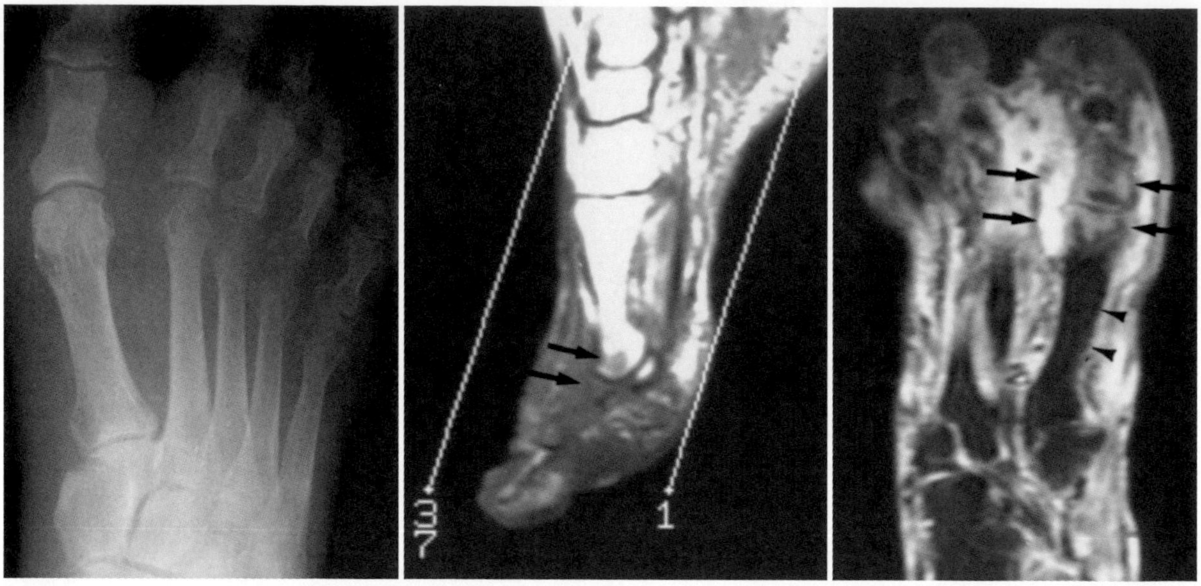

Figure 3–91 Magnetic resonance evaluation of osteomyelitis of the foot in a diabetic patient. **A,** Radiograph shows extensive soft tissue swelling involving the distal foot, consistent with cellulitis. No definite changes of osteomyelitis are identified. **B,** Sagittal T1 (TR 400, TE 20) localizer image for axial T2 series shows abnormal marrow involving the proximal phalanx and distal metatarsal at the first metatarsophalangeal joint *(arrows)*. **C,** Axial short T1 inversion recovery (STIR) (TR 2000, TI 160, TE 43) image shows changes of septic arthritis and osteomyelitis of the first metatarsophalangeal joint *(arrows)*. Note normal low signal intensity on the STIR image in the more proximal first metatarsal *(arrowheads)*.

REFERENCES

Routine Radiography

1. Anderson RB: Turf toe injuries of the hallux metatarsophalangeal joint. *Techniques in Foot and Ankle Surgery* 1(2):102-111, 2002.
2. Berquist TH, Bender CE, James EM, et al: Diagnostic techniques. In Berquist TH (ed): *Radiology of the Foot and Ankle.* New York, Raven Press, 1989, pp 35-98.
3. Berquist TH, Johnson KA: Trauma. In Berquist TH (ed): *Radiology of the Foot and Ankle.* New York, Raven Press, 1989, pp 99-212.
4. Brodén B: Roentgen examination of the subtaloid joint in fractures of the calcaneus. *Acta Radiol* 31:85, 1949.
5. Brostrom L: Sprained ankles. III. Clinical observations in recent ankle ruptures. *Acta Chir Scand* 130:560-569, 1965.
6. Canale ST, Kelly FB Jr: Fractures of the neck of the talus. Long-term evaluation of seventy-one cases. *J Bone Joint Surg Am* 60:143-156, 1978.
7. Cass JR, Morrey BF: Ankle instability: Current concepts, diagnosis, and treatment. *Mayo Clin Proc* 59:165-170, 1984.
8. Cobey JC: Posterior roentgenogram of the foot. *Clin Orthop Relat Res* 118:202-207, 1976.
9. Coughlin MJ, Saltzman CL, Nunley JA 2nd: Angular measurements in the evaluation of hallux valgus deformities: A report of the ad hoc committee of the American Orthopaedic Foot and Ankle Society on angular measurements. *Foot Ankle Int* 23:68-74, 2002.
10. DeLee JC: Fractures and dislocations of the foot. In Mann R (ed): *Surgery of the Foot,* ed 5. St Louis, Mosby, 1986, pp 592-808.
11. Feist JH, Mankin HJ: The tarsus. I. Basic relationships and motions in the adult and definition of optimal recumbent oblique projection. *Radiology* 79:250-263, 1962.

12. Gellman R, Beaman D: External fixation for distraction osteogenesis. *Foot Ankle Clin N Am* 9:489-528, 2004.
13. Isherwood I: A radiological approach to the subtalar joint. *J Bone Joint Surg Am* 43:566-574, 1961.
14. Johannsen A: Radiologic diagnosis of lateral ligament lesion of the ankle: A comparison between talar tilt and anterior drawer sign. *Acta Orthop Scand* 49:259-301, 1978.
15. Lindstrand A, Mortensson W: Anterior instability in the ankle joint following acute lateral sprain. *Acta Radiol* 18:529-539, 1977.
16. Norman A, Kleiger B, Greenspan A, et al: Roentgenographic examination of the normal foot and ankle. In Jahss M (ed): *Disorders of the Foot,* ed 2. Philadelphia, WB Saunders, 1990, pp 64-90.
17. Paley D: *Principles of Deformity Correction.* New York, Springer-Verlag, 2002.
18. Pinsky MJ: The Isherwood views: A roentgenologic approach to the subtalar joint. *J Am Podiatry Assoc* 69:200-206, 1979.
19. Sangeorzan BJ, Mosca V, Hansen ST Jr.: Effect of calcaneal lengthening on relationships among the hindfoot, midfoot, and forefoot. *Foot Ankle* 14:136-141, 1993.
20. Shereff MJ: Radiographic analysis of the foot and ankle. In Jahss MH (ed): *Disorders of the Foot,* ed 2. Philadelphia, WB Saunders, 1990, pp 91-108.
21. Shereff MJ, DiGiovanni L, Bejjani FJ, et al: A comparison of non–weight-bearing and weight-bearing radiographs of the foot. *Foot Ankle* 10: 306-311, 1990.
22. Steel MW, Johnson KA, DeWitz MA, et al: Radiographic measurements of the normal adult foot. *Foot Ankle* 1:151-158, 1980.

Nuclear Medicine

23. Anderson IF, Crichton KJ, Grattan-Smith T, et al: Osteochondral fractures of the dome of the talus. *J Bone Joint Surg Am* 71:1143-1152, 1989.

24. Datz FL: Radionuclide imaging of joint inflammation in the '90s (editorial). *J Nucl Med* 31:684-687, 1990.

25. Demangeat J-L, Constantinesco A, Brunet B, et al: Three-phase bone scanning in reflex sympathetic dystrophy of the hands. *J Nucl Med* 29:26-32, 1988.

26. Forrester DM, Kerr R: Trauma to the foot. *Radiol Clin North Am* 28:423-433, 1990.

27. Fox IM, Zeigler L: Tc-99m-HMPAO leukocyte scintigraphy for the diagnosis of osteomyelitis in diabetic foot infections. *J Foot Ankle Surg* 32:591-594, 1993.

28. Frank JA, Ling A, Patronas MJ, et al: Detection of malignant bone tumors: MR imaging vs. scintigraphy. *AJR Am J Roentgenol Am J Roentgenol* 155:1043-1048, 1990.

29. Holder LE: Clinical radionuclide bone imaging. *Radiology* 176:607-614, 1990.

30. Kim EE, Haynie TP: *Nuclear Diagnostic Imaging: Practical Clinical Applications.* New York, Macmillan, 1987.

31. Matin P: The appearance of bone scans following fractures, including immediate and long-term studies. *J Nucl Med* 20:1227-1231, 1979.

32. Maurice HD, Newman JH, Watt I: Bone scanning of the foot for unexplained pain. *J Bone Joint Surg Br* 69:448-452, 1987.

33. McAfee JG: What is the best method for imaging focal infections? (editorial). *J Nucl Med* 31:413-416, 1990.

34. McDougall IR, Rieser RP: Scintigraphic techniques in musculoskeletal trauma. *Radiol Clin North Am* 27:1003-1011, 1989.

35. Morrison WB, Schweitzer ME, Wapner KL, et al: Osteomyelitis in feet of diabetics: Clinical accuracy, surgical utility, and cost-effectiveness of MR imaging. *Radiology* 196:557-564, 1995.

36. Nussbaum AR, Treves ST, Micheli L: Bone stress lesions in ballet dancers: Scintigraphic assessment. *AJR Am J Roentgenol* 150:851-855, 1988.

37. Perentesis PJ, Yolles PS, Carrasquillo JA: Radioimmunoscintigraphy: A clinical perspective. *J Nucl Med Tech* 15:90-94, 1987.

38. Schauwecker DS, Park HM, Burt RW, et al: Combined bone scintigraphy and indium-111-leukocyte scans in neuropathic foot disease. *J Nucl Med* 29:1651-1655, 1988.

39. Seabold JE, Nepola JV, Conrad GR, et al: Detection of osteomyelitis at fracture non-union sites: Comparison of two scintigraphic methods. *AJR Am J Roentgenol* 152:1021-1027, 1989.

40. Tang JSH, Gold RH, Bassett LW, et al: Musculoskeletal infections of the extremities: Evaluation with MR imaging. *Radiology* 166:205-209, 1988.

41. Traughber PD, Havlina JM Jr: Bilateral pedicle stress fractures: SPECT and CT features. *J Comput Assist Tomogr* 15:338-340, 1991.

42. Traughber PD, Manaster BJ, Murphy K, et al: Negative bone scans of joints after aspiration or arthrography: Experimental studies. *AJR Am J Roentgenol* 146:87-91, 1986.

43. Vorne M, Soini I, Lantto T, et al: Technetium-99m-HMPAO–labelled leukocytes in detection of inflammatory lesions: Comparison with gallium-67-citrate. *J Nucl Med* 30:1332-1336, 1989.

44. Yuh WTC, Corson JE, Baraniewski HM, et al: Osteomyelitis of the foot in diabetic patients: Evaluation with plain film, Tc-99m-MDP bone scintigraphy and MR imaging. *AJR Am J Roentgenol* 152:795-800, 1989.

Computed Tomography

45. Anderson IF, Crichton KJ, Grattan-Smith T, et al: Osteochondral fractures of the dome of the talus. *J Bone Joint Surg Am* 71:1143-1152, 1989.

46. Berquist TH, Bender CE, James EM, et al: Diagnostic techniques. In Berquist TH (ed): *Radiology of the Foot and Ankle.* New York, Raven Press, 1989, pp 35-98.

47. Coris EE, Lombardo JA: Tarsal navicular stress fractures. *Am Fam Physician* 67(1):85-90, 2003.

48. Daffner RH: Ankle trauma. *Radiol Clin North Am* 28:395-421, 1990.

49. Dalinka MK, Boorstein JM, Zlatkin MB: Computed tomography of musculoskeletal trauma. *Radiol Clin North Am* 27:933-944, 1989.

50. Dalinka MK, Kricun ME, Zlatkin MB, et al: Modern diagnostic imaging in joint disease. *AJR Am J Roentgenol* 152:229-240, 1989.

51. Demas BE, Heelan RT, Lane J, et al: Soft tissue sarcomas of the extremities: Comparison of MR and CT in determining the extent of disease. *AJR Am J Roentgenol* 150:615-620, 1988.

52. Forrester DM, Kerr R: Trauma to the foot. *Radiol Clin North Am* 28:423-433, 1990.

53. Ghozlan R, Vacher H: Where is imaging going in rheumatology? *Baillieres Best Pract Res Clin Rheumatol* 14(4):617-633, 2000.

54. Giachino AA, Uhthoff HK: Intra-articular fractures of the calcaneus: Current concepts review. *J Bone Joint Surg Am* 71:784-787, 1989.

55. Giuffrida AY, Lin SS, Abidi N, et al: Pseudo os trigonum sign: Missed posteromedial talar facet fracture. *Foot Ankle Int* 24(8):642-649, 2003.

56. Greisberg J, Hansen ST Jr, Sangeorzan B: Deformity and degeneration in the hindfoot and midfoot joints of the adult acquired flatfoot. *Foot Ankle Int* 24(7):530-534, 2003.

57. Haapamaki V, Kiuru M, Koskinen S: Lisfranc fracture-dislocation in patients with multiple trauma: Diagnosis with multidetector computed tomography. *Foot Ankle Int* 25(9):614-619, 2004.

58. Heger L, Wulff K: Computed tomography of the calcaneus: Normal anatomy. *AJR Am J Roentgenol* 145:123-129, 1985.

59. Keyser KO, Gilula LA, Hardy DC, et al: Soft tissue abnormalities of the foot and ankle: CT diagnosis. *AJR Am J Roentgenol* 150:845-850, 1988.

60. Magid D, Fishman EK: Imaging of musculoskeletal trauma in three dimensions: An integrated two-dimensional/three-dimensional approach with computed tomography. *Radiol Clin North Am* 27:945-956, 1989.

61. Manaster BJ: Congenital anomalies. In Manaster BJ (ed): *Skeletal radiology.* St. Louis. Mosby, 1989, pp 320-377.

62. Mitchell MJ, Ho C, Resnick D, et al: Diagnostic imaging of lower extremity trauma. *Radiol Clin North Am* 27:909-928, 1989.

63. Newberg AH: Computed tomography of joint injuries. *Radiol Clin North Am* 28:445-460, 1990.

64. Newman JS: Diagnostic and therapeutic injections of the foot and ankle. *Semin Roentgenol* 39(1):85-94, 2004.

65. Pavlov H: Imaging of the foot and ankle. *Radiol Clin North Am* 28:991-1018, 1990.

66. Rosenberg ZS, Cheung Y: Diagnostic imaging of the ankle and foot. In Jahss M (ed): *Disorders of the Foot,* ed 2. Philadelphia, WB Saunders, 1990, pp 109-154.

67. Rosenberg ZS, Feldman F, Singson RD, et al: Peroneal tendon injury associated with calcaneal fractures: CT findings. *AJR Am J Roentgenol* 149:125-129, 1987.

68. Sanders R, Gregory P: Operative treatment of intra-articular fractures of the calcaneus. *Orthop Clin North Am* 26:203-214, 1995.

69. Sarno RC, Carter BL, Bankoff MS, et al: Computed tomography in tarsal coalition. *J Comput Assist Tomogr* 8:1155-1160, 1984.

70. Smith DK, Gilula LA, Totty WG: Subtalar arthrorisis: Evaluation with CT. *AJR Am J Roentgenol* 154:559-562, 1990.

71. Smith RW, Staple TW: Computerized tomography (CT) scanning technique for the hindfoot. *Clin Orthop Related Res* 177:34-38, 1983.

72. Solomon MA, Gilula LA, Oloff LM, et al: CT scanning of the foot and ankle. II. Clinical applications and review of the literature. *AJR Am J Roentgenol* 146:1204-1214, 1986.

73. Tang JSH, Gold RH, Bassett LW, et al: Musculoskeletal infection of the extremities: Evaluation with MR imaging. *Radiology* 166:205-209, 1988.

Magnetic Resonance Imaging

74. Al-Khawari HA, Al-Saeed OM, Jumaa TH, et al: Evaluating diabetic foot infection with magnetic resonance imaging: Kuwait experience. *Med Princ Pract* 14(3):165-172, 2005.

75. Anderson IF, Crichton KJ, Grattan-Smith T, et al: Osteochondral fractures of the dome of the talus. *J Bone Joint Surg Am* 71:1143-1152, 1989.

76. Ashman CJ, Klecker RJ, Yu JS: Forefoot pain involving the metatarsal region: Differential diagnosis with MR imaging. *Radiographics* 21(6):1425-1440, 2001.

77. Berquist TH: Magnetic resonance imaging of the foot and ankle. *Semin Ultrasound CT MR* 11:327-345, 1990.

78. Berquist TH, Ehman RL, King BF, et al: Value of MR imaging in differentiating benign from malignant soft-tissue masses: Study of 95 lesions. *AJR Am J Roentgenol* 155:1251-1255, 1990.

79. Breitenseher MJ, Trattnig S, Kukla C, et al: MRI versus lateral stress radiography in acute lateral ankle ligament injuries. *J Comput Assist Tomogr* 21(2):280-285, 1997.

80. Brody AS, Strong N, Babikian G, et al: Avascular necrosis: Early MR imaging and histologic findings in a canine model. *AJR Am J Roentgenol* 157:341-345, 1991.

81. Chandnani VP, Harper MT, Ficke JR, et al: Chronic ankle instability: Evaluation with MR arthrography, MR imaging, and stress radiography. *Radiology* 192:189-194, 1994.

82. Cook TA, Rahim N, Simpson HC, et al: Magnetic resonance imaging in the management of diabetic foot infection. *Br J Surg* 83(2):245-248, 1996.

83. Craig JG, Amin MB, Wu K, et al: Osteomyelitis of the diabetic foot: MR imaging—pathologic correlation. *Radiology* 203(3):849-855, 1997.

84. Crocker L, Algina J: *Introduction to Classical and Modern Test Theory.* Orlando, Harcourt Brace Jovanovich College Publishers, 1986.

85. Croll SD, Nicholas GG, Osborne MA, et al: Role of magnetic resonance imaging in the diagnosis of osteomyelitis in diabetic foot infections. *J Vasc Surg* 24(2):266-270, 1996.

86. Dalinka MK, Kricun ME, Zlatkin MB, et al: Modern diagnostic imaging in joint disease. *AJR Am J Roentgenol* 152:229-240, 1989.

87. DeSmet AA, Fisher DR, Burnstein MI, et al: Value of MR imaging in staging osteochondral lesions of the talus (osteochondritis desiccans): Results in 14 patients. *AJR Am J Roentgenol* 154:555-558, 1990.

88. De Smet AA, Ilahi OA, Graf BK: Reassessment of the MR criteria for stability of osteochondritis dissecans in the knee and ankle. *Skeletal Radiol* 25(2):159-163, 1996.

89. Enderle MD, Coerper S, Schweizer HP, et al: Correlation of imaging techniques to histopathology in patients with diabetic foot syndrome and clinical suspicion of chronic osteomyelitis. The role of high-resolution ultrasound. *Diabetes Care* 22(2):294-299, 1999.

90. Erickson SJ, Quinn SF, Kneeland JB, et al: MR imaging of the tarsal tunnel and related spaces: normal and abnormal findings with anatomic correlation. *AJR Am J Roentgenol* 155:323-328, 1990.

91. Erickson SJ, Rosengarten JL: MR imaging of the forefoot: Normal anatomic findings. *AJR Am J Roentgenol* 160:565-571, 1993.

92. Erickson SJ, Smith JW, Ruiz ME, et al: MR imaging of the lateral collateral ligament of the ankle. *AJR Am J Roentgenol* 156:131-136, 1991.

93. Farooki S, Yao L, Seeger LL: Anterolateral impingement of the ankle: Effectiveness of MR imaging. *Radiology* 207(2):357-360, 1998.

94. Gerling MC, Pfirrmann CW, Farooki S, et al: Posterior tibialis tendon tears: Comparison of the diagnostic efficacy of magnetic resonance imaging and ultrasonography for the detection of surgically created longitudinal tears in cadavers. *Invest Radiol* 38(1):51-56, 2003.

95. Gold RH, Hawkins RA, Katz RD: Bacterial osteomyelitis: Findings on plain radiography, CT, MR, and scintigraphy (pictorial essay). *AJR Am J Roentgenol* 157:365-370, 1991.

96. Huh YM, Suh JS, Lee JW, et al: Synovitis and soft tissue impingement of the ankle: Assessment with enhanced three-dimensional FSPGR MR imaging. *J Magn Reson Imaging* 19(1):108-116, 2004.

97. Iovane A, Midiri M, Bartolotta TV, et al: Pigmented villonodular synovitis of the foot: MR findings. *Radiol Med* (Torino) 106(1-2):66-73, 2003.

98. James SL, Bates BT, Osterling LR: Injuries to runners. *Am J Sports Med* 6:40-50, 1978.

99. Jaramillo D, Hoffer FA, Shapiro F, et al: MR imaging of fractures of the growth plate. *AJR Am J Roentgenol* 155:1261-1265, 1990.

100. Jelinek JS, Kransdorf MJ, Utz JA, et al: Imaging of pigmented villonodular synovitis with emphasis on MR imaging. *AJR Am J Roentgenol* 152:337-342, 1989.

101. Keigley BA, Haggar AM, Gaba A, et al: Primary tumors of the foot: MR imaging. *Radiology* 171:755-759, 1989.

102. Kirby EJ, Shereff MJ, Lewis MM: Soft-tissue tumors and tumor-like lesions of the foot: An analysis of 83 cases. *J Bone Joint Surg Am* 71:621-626, 1989.

103. Kirkwood BR, Sterne JAC: *Essentials of Medical Statistics,* ed 2. Malden, Mass, Blackwell Science, 2003.

104. Kneeland JB, Macranar S, Middleton WD, et al: MR imaging of the normal ankle: Correlation with anatomic sections. *AJR Am J Roentgenol* 151:117-123, 1988.

105. Koch E, Hofer HO, Sialer G, et al: Failure of MR imaging to detect reflex sympathetic dystrophy of the extremities. *AJR Am J Roentgenol* 156:113-115, 1991.

106. Kransdorf MJ: Malignant soft-tissue tumors in a large referral population: Distribution of diagnoses by age, sex, and location. *AJR Am J Roentgenol* 164:129-134, 1995.

107. Kransdorf MJ, Jelinek JS, Moser RP, et al: Soft-tissue masses: Diagnosis using MR imaging. *AJR Am J Roentgenol* 153:541-547, 1989.

108. Lamm BM, Myers DT, Dombek M, et al: Magnetic resonance imaging and surgical correlation of peroneus brevis tears. *J Foot Ankle Surg* 43(1):30-36, 2004.

109. Lee JK, Yao L: Stress fractures: MR imaging. *Radiology* 169:217-220, 1988.

110. Lee JW, Suh JS, Huh YM, et al: Soft tissue impingement syndrome of the ankle: Diagnostic efficacy of MRI and clinical results after arthroscopic treatment. *Foot Ankle Int* 25(12):896-902, 2004.

111. Levine SE, Neagle CE, Esterhai JL, et al: Magnetic resonance imaging for the diagnosis of osteomyelitis in the diabetic patient with a foot ulcer. *Foot Ankle Int* 15(3):151-156, 1994.

112. Liem MD, Zegel HG, Balduini FC, et al: Repair of Achilles tendon ruptures with a polylactic acid implant: Assessment with MR imaging. *AJR Am J Roentgenol* 156:769-773, 1991.

113. Liu SH, Nuccion SL, Finerman G: Diagnosis of anterolateral ankle impingement. Comparison between magnetic resonance imaging and clinical examination. *Am J Sports Med* 25(3):389-393, 1997.

114. Marcus DS, Reicher MA, Kellerhouse LE: Achilles tendon injuries: The role of MR imaging. *J Comput Assist Tomogr* 13:480-486, 1989.

115. Mason MD, Zlatkin MB, Esterhai JL, et al: Chronic complicated osteomyelitis of the lower extremity: Evaluation with MR imaging. *Radiology* 173:355-359, 1989.

116. Matowe L, Gilbert FJ: How to synthesize evidence for imaging guidelines. *Clin Radiol* 59(1):63-68, 2004.

117. Mintz DN, Tashjian GS, Connell DA, et al: Osteochondral lesions of the talus: A new magnetic resonance grading system with arthroscopic correlation. *Arthroscopy* 19(4):353-359, 2003.

118. Morrison WB, Schweitzer ME, Wapner KL, et al: Osteomyelitis in feet of diabetics: Clinical accuracy, surgical utility, and cost-effectiveness of MR imaging. *Radiology* 196:557-564, 1995.

119. Morrison WB, Schweitzer ME, Wapner KL, et al: Plantar fibromatosis: A benign aggressive neoplasm with a characteristic appearance on MR images. *Radiology* 193:841-845, 1994.

120. Moulton JS, Blebea JS, Dunco DM, et al: MR imaging of soft-tissue masses: Diagnostic efficacy and value of distinguishing between benign and malignant lesions. *AJR Am J Roentgenol* 164:1191-1199, 1995.

121. Munk PL, Helms CA, Holt RG: Immature bone infarcts: Findings on plain radiographs and MR scans. *AJR Am J Roentgenol* 152:547-549, 1989.

122. Narvaez JA, Narvaez J, Ortega R, et al: Painful heel: MR imaging findings. *Radiographics* 20(2):333-352, 2000.

123. Ostendorf B, Scherer A, Modder U, et al: Diagnostic value of magnetic resonance imaging of the forefeet in early rheumatoid arthritis when findings on imaging of the metacarpophalangeal joints of the hands remain normal. *Arthritis Rheum* 50(7):2094-2102, 2004.

124. Preidler KW, Peicha G, Lajtai G, et al: Conventional radiography, CT, and MR imaging in patients with hyperflexion injuries of the foot: Diagnostic accuracy in the detection of bony and ligamentous changes. *Am J Roentgenol* 173(6):1673-1677, 1999.

125. Quinn SF, Murray WT, Clark RA, et al: Achilles tendon: MR imaging at 1.5 T. *Radiology* 164:767-770, 1987.

126. Robinson P, White LM, Salonen DC, et al: Anterolateral ankle impingement: MR arthrographic assessment of the anterolateral recess. *Radiology* 221(1):186-190, 2001.

127. Rockett MS, Waitches G, Sudakoff G, et al: Use of ultrasonography versus magnetic resonance imaging for tendon abnormalities around the ankle. *Foot Ankle Int* 19(9):604-612, 1998.

128. Saxena A, Wolf SK: Peroneal tendon abnormalities. A review of 40 surgical cases. *J Am Podiatr Med Assoc* 93(4):272-282, 2003.

129. Schepsis AA, Leach RE: Surgical management of Achilles tendonitis. *Am J Sports Med* 15:308-315, 1987.

130. Schneck CD, Mesgarzdeh M, Bonakdarpour A: MR imaging of the most commonly injured ankle ligaments. II. Ligament injuries. *Radiology* 184:507-512, 1992.

131. Sebes JI: Diagnostic imaging of bone and joint abnormalities associated with sickle cell hemoglobinopathies. *AJR Am J Roentgenol* 152:1153-1159, 1989.

132. Sharp RJ, Wade CM, Hennessy MS, et al: The role of MRI and ultrasound imaging in Morton's neuroma and the effect of size of lesion on symptoms. *J Bone Joint Surg Br* 85(7):999-1005, 2003.

133. Shellock FG, Fukunaga T, Mink JH, et al: Acute effects of exercise on MR imaging of skeletal muscle: Concentric versus eccentric actions. *AJR Am J Roentgenol* 156:765-768, 1991.

134. Takao M, Ochi M, Oae K, et al: Diagnosis of a tear of the tibiofibular syndesmosis. The role of arthroscopy of the ankle. *J Bone Joint Surg Br* 85(3):324-329, 2003.

135. Tang GS, Gold RH, Bassett LW, et al: Musculoskeletal infection of the extremities: Evaluating with MR imaging. *Radiology* 166:205-209, 1988.

136. Theodorou DJ, Theodorou SJ, Resnick D: MR imaging of abnormalities of the plantar fascia. *Semin Musculoskelet Radiol* 6(2):105-118, 2002.

137. Verhaven EFC, Shahabpour M, Handelberg FWJ: The accuracy of three-dimensional magnetic resonance imaging in ruptures of the lateral ligaments of the ankle. *Am J Sports Med* 19:583-586, 1991.

138. Wetzel LH, Levine E: Soft-tissue tumors of the foot: Value of MR imaging for specific diagnosis. *AJR Am J Roentgenol* 155:1025-1030, 1990.

139. Yao L, Gentili A, Cracchiolo A: MR imaging findings in spring ligament insufficiency. *Skeletal Radiol* 28(5):245-250, 1999.

140. Yu JS, Spigos D, Tomczak R: Foot pain after a plantar fasciotomy: An MR analysis to determine potential causes. *J Comput Assist Tomogr* 23(5):707-712, 1999.

141. Zerhouni EA: Understanding tissue signals in MRI. presented at Society of Body Computerized Tomography, 1989.

Complex Regional Pain Syndrome

142. Demangeat J-L, Constantinesco A, Brunet B, et al: Three phase bone scanning in reflex sympathetic dystrophy of the hands. *J Nucl Med* 29:26-32, 1988.

143. Holder LE: Clinical radionuclide bone imaging. *Radiology* 176:607-614, 1990.

144. Koch E, Hofer HO, Sialer G, et al: Failure of MR imaging to detect reflex sympathetic dystrophy of the extremities. *AJR Am J Roentgenol* 156:113-115, 1991.

145. Schweitzer ME, Mandel S, Schwartzman RJ, et al: Reflex sympathetic dystrophy revisited: MR imaging findings before and after infusion of contrast material. *Radiology* 195:211-214, 1995.

Osteochondral Lesions

146. Anderson IF, Crichton KJ, Grattan-Smith P, et al: Osteochondral fractures of the dome of the talus. *J Bone Joint Surg Am* 71:1143-1152, 1989.

147. Brody AS, Ball WS, Towbin RE: Computed arthrotomography as an adjunct to pediatric arthrography. *Radiology* 170:99-102, 1989.

148. DeSmet AA, Fisher DR, Burnstein MI, et al: Value of MR imaging in staging osteochondral lesions of the talus (osteochondritis desiccans): Results in 14 patients. *AJR Am J Roentgenol* 154:555-558, 1990.

149. Heare MM, Gillesbey T III, Bittar ES: Direct coronal computed tomography arthrography of osteochondritis desiccans of the talus. *Skeletal Radiol* 17:187-190, 1988.

150. Resnick D: Arthrography, tenography, and bursography. In Resnick D, Niwayama G (eds): *Diagnosis of Bone and Joint Disorders*, ed 2. Philadelphia, WB Saunders, 1988, pp 302-440.

151. Vahlensieck M, Peterfy CG, Wischer T, et al: Indirect MT arthrography: Optimization and clinical applications. *Radiology* 200:249-254, 1996.

Chronic Undiagnosed Post-traumatic Pain

152. Berquist TH: Magnetic resonance imaging of the foot and ankle. *Semin Ultrasound CT MR* 11:327-345, 1990.
153. Dalinka MK, Kricun ME, Zlatkin MB, et al: Modern diagnostic imaging in joint disease. *AJR Am J Roentgenol* 152:229-240, 1989.
154. Erickson SJ, Quinn SF, Kneeland JB, et al: MR imaging of the tarsal tunnel and related spaces: Normal and abnormal findings with anatomic correlation. *AJR Am J Roentgenol* 155:323-328, 1990.
155. Forrester DM, Kerr R: Trauma to the foot. *Radiol Clin North Am* 28:423-433, 1990.
156. Maurice HD, Newman JH, Watt I: Bone scanning of the foot for unexplained pain. *J Bone Joint Surg* 69B:448-452, 1987.
157. Rosenberg ZS, Cheung Y, Jahss MH, et al: Rupture of the posterior tibial tendon: CT and MRI with surgical correlation. *Radiology* 169:229-235, 1988.

Unstable Ankle

158. Berquist TH: Magnetic resonance imaging of the foot and ankle. *Semin Ultrasound CT MR* 11:327-345, 1990.
159. Brostrom L, Liljedahl SO, Lindvall N: Sprained ankles. II. Arthrographic diagnosis of recent ligamentous ruptures. *Acta Chir Scand* 129:485-499, 1965.
160. Chandnani VP, Harper MT, Ficke JR, et al: Chronic ankle instability: Evaluation with MR arthrography, MR imaging, and stress radiology. *Radiology* 192:189-194, 1994.
161. Pavlov H: Imaging of the foot and ankle. *Radiol Clin North Am* 28:991-1018, 1990.
162. Olson RW: Ankle arthrography. *Radiol Clin North Am* 19:255-268, 1981.
163. Resnick D, Goergen TG, Niwayama G: Physical injury. In Resnick D, Niwayama G (eds): *Diagnosis of Bone and Joint Disorders*, ed 2. Philadelphia, WB Saunders, 1988, pp 2756-3008.
164. Rosenberg ZS, Cheung Y: Diagnostic imaging of the ankle and foot. In Jahss M (ed): *Disorders of the Foot*, ed 2. Philadelphia, WB Saunders, 1990, pp 109-154.
165. Vahlensieck M, Peterfy CG, Wischer T, et al: Indirect MR arthrography: Optimization and clinical applications. *Radiology* 200:249-254, 1996.

Tendon Injury

166. Berquist TH: Magnetic resonance imaging of the foot and ankle. *Semin Ultrasound CT MR* 11:327-345, 1990.
167. Dalinka MK, Kricun ME, Zlatkin MB, et al: Modern diagnostic imaging in joint disease. *AJR Am J Roentgenol* 152:229-240, 1989.
168. Kainberger FM, Engel A, Barton P, et al: Injuries of the Achilles tendon: Diagnosis with sonography. *AJR Am J Roentgenol* 155:1031-1036, 1990.
169. Khoury NJ, El-Khoury GY, Saltzman CL, et al: Peroneus longus and brevis tendon tears: MR imaging evaluation. *Radiology* 200:249-254, 1996.
170. Khoury NJ, El-Khoury GY, Saltzman CL, et al: MR imaging of posterior tibial tendon dysfunction. *AJR Am J Roentgenol* 167:675-682, 1996.
171. Mathieson JR, Connell DG, Cooperberg FL, et al: Sonography of the Achilles tendon and adjacent bursae. *AJR Am J Roentgenol* 151:127-131, 1988.
172. Pavlov H: Imaging of the foot and ankle. *Radiol Clin North Am* 28:991-1018, 1990.
173. Rosenberg ZS, Cheung Y: Diagnostic imaging of the ankle and foot. In Jahss M (ed): *Disorders of the Foot*, ed 2. Philadelphia, WB Saunders, 1990, pp 109-154.
174. Rosenberg ZS, Cheung Y, Jahss MH, et al: Rupture of the posterior tibial tendon: CT and MRI with surgical correlation. *Radiology* 169:229-235, 1988.

Foreign Body Localization

175. Bissonnette RT, Connell DG, Fitzpatrick DG: Preoperative localization of low-density foreign bodies under CT guidance. *J Can Assoc Radiol* 39:286-287, 1988.
176. Bodne D, Quinn SF, Cochran CF: Imaging foreign glass and wooden bodies of the extremities with CT and MR. *J Comput Assist Tomogr* 12:608-611, 1988.
177. Jarcke HT, Grossom LE, Finkelstein MS: Evaluation of the musculoskeletal system with sonography. *AJR Am J Roentgenol* 150:1253-1261, 1988.
178. Kaplan PA, Anderson JC, Norris MA, et al: Ultrasonography of post-traumatic soft-tissue lesions. *Radiol Clin North Am* 27:973-982, 1989.
179. Resnick D, Niwayama G: Soft tissues. In Resnick D, Niwayama G (eds): *Diagnosis of Bone and Joint Disorders*, ed 2. Philadelphia, WB Saunders, 1988, pp 4171-4294.

Avascular Necrosis

180. Berquist TH, Welch TJ, Brown ML, et al: Bone and soft tissue ischemia. In Berquist TH (ed): *Radiology of the Foot and Ankle*. New York, Raven Press, 1989, pp 316-348.
181. Brody AS, Strong M, Babikian G, et al: Avascular necrosis: Early MR imaging and histologic findings in a canine model. *AJR Am J Roentgenol* 157:341-345, 1991.
182. Haller J, Sartoris DJ, Resnick D, et al: Spontaneous osteonecrosis of the tarsal navicular in adults: Imaging findings. *AJR Am J Roentgenol* 151:355-358, 1988.
183. Hawkins LG: Fractures of the neck of the talus. *J Bone Joint Surg Am* 52:991-1002, 1970.
184. Manaster BJ: *Skeletal Radiology*, ed 1. St Louis, Mosby, 1989, pp 190-292.
185. Mindell ER, Cisek EE, Kartalian G, Dziob JM: Late results of injuries to the talus. *J Bone Joint Surg Am* 45:221-245, 1963.
186. Morrey BF, Cass JF, Johnson KA, et al: Foot and ankle. In Berquist TH (ed): *Imaging of Orthopaedic Trauma and Surgery*. Philadelphia, WB Saunders, 1986, pp 407-498.

Undiagnosed Mass

187. Berquist TH, Bender CE, James EM, et al: Diagnostic techniques. In Berquist TH (ed): *Radiology of the Foot and Ankle*. New York, Raven Press, 1989, pp 35-98.
188. Berquist TH, Ehman RL, King BF, et al: Value of MR imaging in differentiating benign from malignant soft-tissue masses: Study of 95 lesions. *AJR Am J Roentgenol* 155:1251-1255, 1990.
189. Frank JA, Ling A, Patronas MJ, et al: Detection of malignant bone tumors: MR imaging versus scintigraphy. *AJR Am J Roentgenol* 155:1043-1048, 1990.
190. Froelich JW, McKusick KA, Strauss HW, et al: Localization of bone lesions for open biopsy. *Radiology* 146:1549-1550, 1983.
191. Holder LE: Clinical radionuclide bone imaging. *Radiology* 176:607-614, 1990.
192. Jarcke HT, Grossom LE, Finkelstein MS: Evaluation of the musculoskeletal system with sonography. *AJR Am J Roentgenol* 150:1253-1261, 1988.
193. Keigley BA, Haggar AM, Gaba A, et al: Primary tumors of the foot: MR imaging. *Radiology* 171:755-759, 1989.
194. Kirby EJ, Shereff MJ, Lewis MM: Soft-tissue tumors and tumor-like lesions of the foot: An analysis of 83 cases. *J Bone Joint Surg Am* 71:621-626, 1989.

195. Kransdorf MJ, Jelinek JS, Moser RP, et al: Soft-tissue masses: Diagnosis using MR imaging. *AJR Am J Roentgenol* 153:541-547, 1989.
196. Murray WT, Mueller PR: Bone biopsy. In Athanasoulis CA, Pfister RC, Greene RE, et al (eds): *Interventional Radiology,* Philadelphia, WB Saunders, 1982, pp 753-763.
197. Wetzel LH, Levine E: Soft-tissue tumors of the foot: Value of MR imaging for specific diagnosis. *AJR Am J Roentgenol* 155:1025-1030, 1990.

Systemic Arthritis

198. Berquist TH, Bender CE, James EM, et al: Diagnostic techniques. In Berquist TH (ed): *Radiology of the Foot and Ankle.* New York, Raven Press, 1989, pp 35-98.
199. Manaster BJ (ed): *Skeletal Radiology.* St Louis, Mosby, 1989, pp 107-189, 320-377.
200. Maurice HD, Newman JH, Watt I: Bone scanning of the foot for unexplained pain. *J Bone Joint Surg Br* 69:448-452, 1987.
201. McLeod RA: Arthritis. In Berquist TH (ed): *Radiology of the Foot and Ankle.* New York, Raven Press, 1989, pp 213-246.
202. Resnick D: Articular disease. In Resnick D, Niwayama G, editors: *Diagnosis of Bone and Joint Disorders,* ed 2. Philadelphia, WB Saunders, 1988.
203. Rosenberg ZS, Cheung Y: Diagnostic imaging of the ankle and foot. In Jahss M (ed): *Disorders of the Foot,* ed 2. Philadelphia, WB Saunders, 1990, pp 109-154.

Infection

204. Alazraki N, Fierer J, Resnick D: Chronic osteomyelitis: monitoring by ^{99m}Tc phosphate and ^{67}Ga citrate imaging. *AJR Am J Roentgenol* 145:767-770, 1985.
205. Chandnani VP, Beltran J, Morris CS, et al: Acute experimental osteomyelitis and abscesses: Detection with MR imaging versus CT. *Radiology* 174:233-236, 1990.
206. Erickson SJ, Rosengarten JL: MR imaging of the forefoot: Normal anatomic findings. *AJR Am J Roentgenol* 160:565-571, 1993.
207. Fox IM, Zeigler L: Tc-99m-HMPAO leukocyte scintigraphy for the diagnosis of osteomyelitis in diabetic foot infections. *J Foot Ankle Surg* 32:591-594, 1993.
208. Gold RH, Hawkins RA, Katz RD: Bacterial osteomyelitis: Findings on plain radiography CT MR and scintigraphy (pictorial essay). *AJR Am J Roentgenol* 157:365-370, 1991.
209. Jaramillo D, Treves ST, Kasser JR, et al: Osteomyelitis and septic arthritis in children: Appropriate use of imaging to guide treatment. *AJR Am J Roentgenol* 165:399-403, 1995.
210. Larcos G, Brown ML, Sutton RT: Diagnosis of osteomyelitis of the foot in diabetic patients: Value of ^{111}In-leukocyte scintigraphy. *AJR Am J Roentgenol* 157:527-531, 1991.
211. Mason MD, Zlatkin MB, Esterhai JL, et al: Chronic complicated osteomyelitis of the lower extremity: Evaluation with MR imaging. *Radiology* 173:355-359, 1989.
212. McAfee JG: What is the best method for imaging focal infections? (editorial). *J Nucl Med* 31:413-416, 1990.
213. Morrison WB, Schweitzer ME, Wapner KL, et al: Osteomyelitis in feet of diabetics: Clinical accuracy, surgical utility, and cost-effectiveness of MR imaging. *Radiology* 196:557-564, 1995.
214. Rosenberg ZS, Chueng Y: Diagnostic imaging of the ankle and foot. In Jahss M (ed): *Disorders of the Foot,* ed 2. Philadelphia, WB Saunders, 1990, pp 109-154.
215. Tang GS, Gold RH, Bassett LW, et al: Musculoskeletal infection of the extremities: Evaluating with MR imaging. *Radiology* 166:205-209, 1988.
216. Traughber PD, Manaster BJ, Murphy K, et al: Negative bone scans of joints after aspiration or arthrography: Experimental studies. *AJR Am J Roentgenol* 146:87-91, 1986.
217. Unger E, Moldofsky P, Gatenby R, et al: Diagnosis of osteomyelitis by MR imaging. *AJR Am J Roentgenol* 150:605-610, 1988.
218. Vorne M, Soini I, Lantto T, et al: Technetium-99m-HMPAO-labelled leukocytes in detection of inflammatory lesions: Comparison with gallium-67-citrate. *J Nucl Med* 30:1332-1336, 1989.
219. Yuh WTC, Corson JE, Baraniewski HM, et al: Osteomyelitis of the foot in diabetic patients: Evaluation of plain film, Tc99mMDP bone scintigraphy, and MR imaging. *AJR Am J Roentgenol Am J Roentgenog* 152:795-800, 1989.

Conservative Treatment of the Foot

Keith L. Wapner

GENERAL CONSIDERATIONS

Office management of foot and ankle problems requires an understanding of the interaction of the foot and ankle and the shoe or device applied. The biomechanics of normal foot function and the effect of the disease entity being treated should be analyzed. The anatomy of the normal shoe, the function of each component, and the effect of modifying each of these components must be understood.[2-4, 13,14] The practitioner should have a thorough knowledge of the available orthoses and appliances and the effects of these devices on the foot and ankle.[5,9]

Most of the acquired forefoot deformities seen in the adult population are a consequence of poor-fitting footwear. These include hallux valgus deformity, hammer toes, hard corns, interdigital neuromas, and plantar keratoses. Educating the patient about the effects of improper shoes is the starting point of conservative management. This education is often met with resistance because ill-fitting shoes continue to be a hallmark of high fashion. It is often necessary to remind patients that there is no other part of the body they would consider putting in a container whose shape is so drastically different from that body part for daily dress. Comparing an outline of the patient's foot to his or her current footwear assists in conveying this

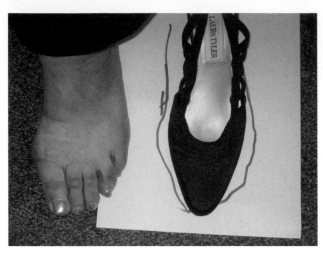

Figure 4–1 Comparing the outline of a foot to a woman's dress shoe demonstrates the disparity in shape.

point (Fig. 4–1). Unless the patient is willing to accept that a change in footwear is indicated, both conservative and operative intervention may be futile.

Proper fitting of the shoe should accommodate the variations in the person's foot.[11] A set of consumer guidelines has been developed by the National Shoe Retailers Association, the Pedorthic Footwear Association, and the American Orthopedic Foot and Ankle Society (Table 4–1). Foot width can expand up to two sizes and length by one-half size on weight bearing. For proper sizing of the shoe, the foot must be meas-

---

TABLE 4–1

10 Points of Proper Shoe Fit

1. Sizes vary among shoe brands and styles. Do not select shoes by the size marked inside the shoe. Judge the shoe by how it fits on your foot.
2. Select a shoe that conforms as nearly as possible to the shape of your foot.
3. Have your feet measured regularly. The size of your feet changes as you grow older.
4. Have both feet measured. For most persons, one foot is larger than the other. Fit to the larger foot.
5. Fit at the end of the day when the feet are largest.
6. Stand during the fitting process and check that there is adequate space (3/8 to 1/2 inch) for your longest toe at the end of each shoe.
7. Make sure the ball of your foot fits snugly into the widest part of the shoe.
8. Do not purchase shoes that feel too tight, expecting them to stretch.
9. Your heel should fit comfortably in the shoe with a minimum amount of slippage.
10. Walk in the shoe to make sure it fits and feels right.

National Shoe Retailers Association, the Pedorthic Footwear Association, and the American Orthopedic Foot and Ankle Society: *10 Points of Proper Shoe Fit.* Columbia, Md, National Shoe Retailers Association, 1995.

---

ured under weight bearing and late in the day because the foot expands in volume as much as 4% by the end of the day. Shoes should be fitted with the normally worn socks. There should be a full finger breadth at the tip of the shoe at the end of the longest toe with the toes fully extended.

The popularity of walking and jogging shoes has made proper-fitting shoes more socially acceptable. The breakdown of sexual stereotypes has allowed the redefinition of acceptable styles of footwear in many workplace environments. Acceptance of proper fit over trends in style often adequately relieves a patient's symptoms.

Deformity of the foot and ankle caused by progressive disease entities often requires modification of shoes or application of orthoses. The choice of the proper modification is based on a thorough understanding of the effects of the disease on the normal function of the foot. Disease can compromise motor function, joint function, skin integrity, sensation, and proprioception. Once the effects have been assessed, the proper modifications should be prescribed to try to restore normal function or protect the affected limb from further breakdown.

SHOE ANATOMY

Shoes can be broken down into various components. The upper is the part of the shoe that is seen from the top. The outsole and heel form the bottom of the shoe, which contacts the ground. The insole contacts the plantar aspect of the foot inside the shoe (Fig. 4–2).

The shank extends from the heel breast (the front of the heel) to the ball of the shoe. The ball is the area under the metatarsal heads. The forepart extends from the ball to the tip, or end of the shoe. The toe box describes the height of the shoe at this level. The vamp, part of the upper, extends from the tip back over the ball and instep to the quarters, which join in the back of the shoe at the back seam. The Balmoral, or Bal last, shoe has the quarters meeting at the front of the throat of the shoe, with the vamp extending as the tongue beneath them. The Blucher last has the quarters loose at the inner edge and is made to be laced over the vamp and tongue.

The last is the three-dimensional form that the upper of the shoe is made from (Fig. 4–3). Historically, all lasts were made by hand with no distinction between the left and right foot until about 1820. In the 1850s the ability to duplicate shoe lasts, mold the leather uppers, and attach them to the soles by machine allowed the shoemaker to progress from making 1 pair of shoes per day to more than 600 per day. Over the next century and a half, the technology

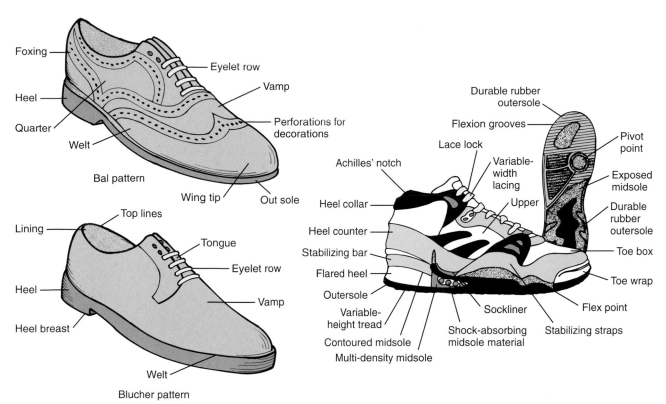

Figure 4–2 Structural components of the shoe.

of manufacturing has rapidly progressed, just as the materials available have.[9]

Lasting also describes the bottoming method that is employed to attach the upper to the sole. Many tech-

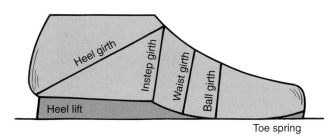

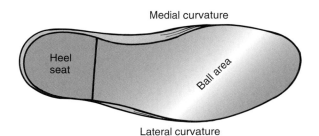

Figure 4–3 Diagram of the last, the form on which the shoe is made. (Adapted from Frey C: Shoe wear and pedorthic devices. In Lutter LD, Mizel MS, Pfeffer GB [eds]: *Orthopedic Knowledge Update: Foot and Ankle.* Rosemont, Ill, American Academy of Orthopaedic Surgeons, 1994.)

niques have been used, and one shoe can be lasted with more than one method, called *combination lasting.* *Slip lasting* involves sewing the upper pieces together moccasin style and gluing this to the midsole, giving a flexible construction. With *board lasting,* the upper is glued to a firm board, providing a stiff shoe; this method is often employed in athletic shoes to decrease pronation. A combination last can provide stability from a board-lasted heel and flexibility from a slip-lasted forefoot (Fig. 4–4).

Types of Uppers

Many different materials are available for constructing the upper of the shoe. Traditionally, leather has been employed because of its durability, moldability, and breathability. Athletic shoes are made from soft nylon, mesh nylon, and canvas reinforced at the counter, toe box, or vamp with leather, rubber, or plastics for added stability. This combination allows the shoe to be lighter but still stable. The nylon mesh shoe may be useful in accommodating deformities of the lesser toes.

Leather uppers can be stretched to accommodate forefoot deformities, but the extent of shoe deformation is limited. The toe box should have the height and width to properly fit the foot. If friction against the skin is a concern, as in a neuropathic foot, a

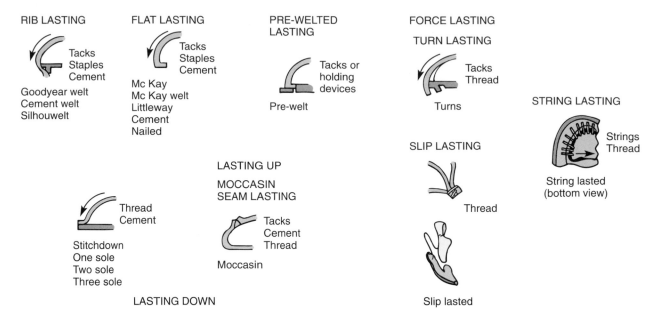

Figure 4–4   Lasting techniques used to attach the upper to the sole. (Adapted from Gould N: Footwear: Shoes and shoe modifications. In Jahss MH [ed]: *Disorders of the Foot and Ankle: Medical and Surgical Management,* ed 2, vol 3. Philadelphia, WB Saunders, 1991, p 2885.)

heat-moldable foam (Thermold) upper may be employed.

Several patterns of lace stays are available, and each has its own advantage (Fig. 4–5). The Blucher pattern, with no seam across the instep, has the advantage of allowing easier entry into the shoe. The Bal pattern can provide more stability, but the entry is limited and might not accept an orthotic device. The U-throat and lace-toe patterns allow the shoe to open even wider and may be useful in accepting an orthosis or allowing entry into the shoe after hindfoot fusion.

Many lacing patterns can secure a better fit of the shoe (Fig. 4–6). Athletic shoes often have multiple eyelets to allow for different lacing techniques. By changing the lacing to avoid crossing the dorsum of the foot, pressure can be relieved over bony

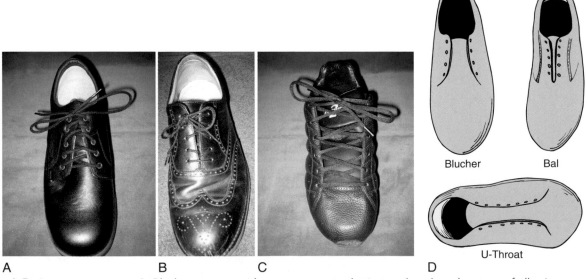

Figure 4–5   Lace stay patterns. **A,** Blucher pattern, with no seam across the instep, has the advantage of allowing easy entry into the shoe. **B,** Balmoral pattern may provide more stability, but the entry is limited and might not accept an orthotic device. **C,** The U-throat or lace-toe patterns allow the shoe to open even wider and may be useful in accepting an orthosis or allowing entry into the shoe after hindfoot fusion. **D,** Diagram of patterns of lace stays.

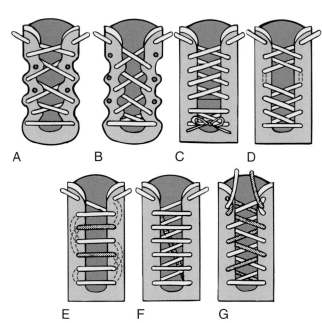

A B C D

E F G

Figure 4–6   Patterns of lacing. **A,** Variable for wide fit. **B,** Variable for narrow fit. **C,** Independent, using two laces. **D,** Crisscross to avoid bony prominences. **E,** High arch pattern to avoid lacing crossing top of foot. **F,** Pull-up pattern to allow relief of pressure on toes. **G,** Crisscross loop pattern to avoid heel blisters. (Adapted from Frey C: Shoe wear and pedorthic devices. In Lutter LD, Mizel MS, Pfeffer GB [eds]: *Orthopedic Knowledge Update: Foot and Ankle.* Rosemont, Ill, American Academy of Orthopaedic Surgeons, 1994, p 78.)

prominences or a high-arched foot. Wide or narrow feet can be secured by different lacing patterns.

Once the proper material, shape, and lacing pattern of the shoe have been determined, it may still be necessary to stretch the upper to avoid pressure over bony deformities. With the patient standing and bearing full weight on the affected foot, the area of impingement can be identified and marked. A shoemaker's wand can stretch the shoe at this area (Fig. 4–7).

Types of Lasts

Shoe manufacturers have many different lasts, and there is great variation in the fit of shoes that are labeled with the same size. A shoe manufacturer might have 30 to 60 active last styles with 80 to 90 sizes for as many as 5000 different lasts.[9] Thus it is difficult to define a normal last.

The concept of a *corrective last* is not accurate because the last cannot correct a deformity. Lasts come in several general categories (Fig. 4–8). A conventional last is made in right- and left-foot shapes. A straight last has a straight medial border from heel to toe without curving at the toe box. Women's dress shoes can simulate a straight last on the medial side and have the point of the toe box at the end of the great toe. The

outflare last, or reverse last, flares to the lateral side of the shoe and is often employed after treatment for metatarsus adductus. The inflare last curves medially and is used in athletic shoes, with a 7-degree curve to allow greater mobility of the foot.[6]

Types of Soles

Traditionally, soles of shoes were constructed of leather. In dress shoes this material is still commonly used. Soles in athletic, work, and recreational shoes are

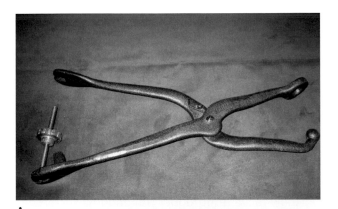

A

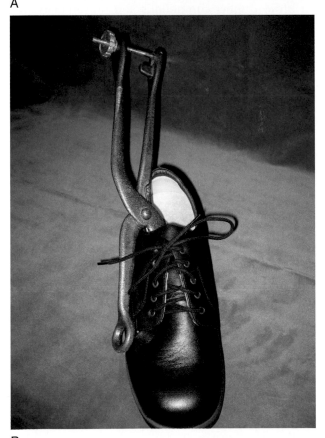

B

Figure 4–7   A, Shoemaker's wand. **B,** Stretching shoe with the wand.

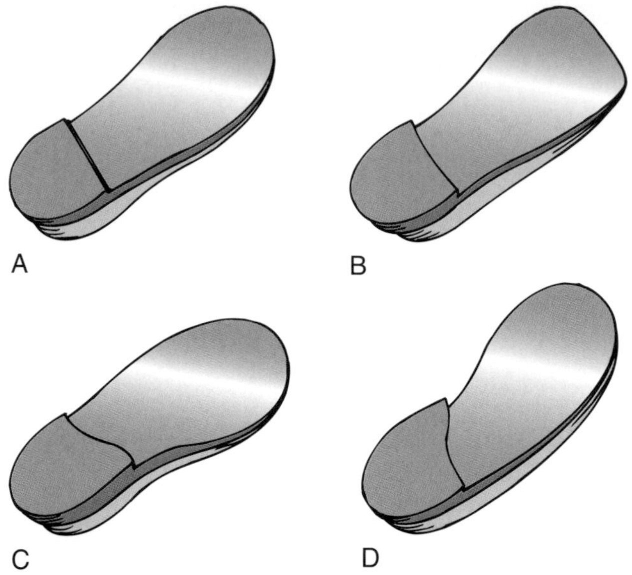

Figure 4–8 Lasts. **A,** Conventional. **B,** Straight. **C,** Outflare. **D,** Inflare. (Adapted from Gould N: Footwear: Shoes and shoe modifications. In Jahss MH [ed]: *Disorders of the Foot and Ankle: Medical and Surgical Management*, ed 2, vol 3. Philadelphia, WB Saunders, 1991, p 2903.)

generally made from rubber compounds. Microcellular blown rubber compounds and polyurethane are used for midsole and wedges. Black carbon rubber and styrene–butadiene are very hard-wearing compounds used for outsoles. Ethyl vinyl acetate is also commonly used in running shoes for its flexibility and impact-absorbing properties. Manufacturers often combine the blown rubber for impact resistance covered by black carbon rubber for wear on the outsole. The superior impact absorption of these rubber and synthetic materials can be used to decrease pressure and loading of the foot and ankle. As a result, many manufacturers now offer dress shoes with soles made of these materials.

Traction between the shoe and the floor can be influenced by the material of the sole and the pattern on the outsole. Various patterns have been developed for different sports (Table 4–2). The pattern and amount of friction can also influence how well a patient with balance or proprioceptive loss can tolerate a shoe. Too much friction can cause a patient to stumble, whereas loss of friction with a slick surface can be equally dangerous.

The outsole of the shoe can be modified (Fig. 4–9). A medial wedge can be used to decrease forefoot eversion, and a lateral wedge can be used to decrease forefoot inversion in a flexible foot.

Various metatarsal bars have been described for treating metatarsalgia. The principle is to have the bar placed proximal to the metatarsal heads to adequately relieve pressure under the area of greatest loading.

Rocker soles are often useful in unloading the forefoot and decreasing the need for metatarsophalangeal joint dorsiflexion. Rocker soles allow a better gait pattern when used with rigid bracing of the foot and ankle.

Types of Heels

The materials used for the heel are similar to those used for the sole. The decision about the material used should stem from the demands placed on the foot. Many modifications of the heel have been described (Fig. 4–10). The Thomas and Stone heels were used to help prevent pronation. Medial and lateral heel wedges help block heel eversion and inversion, respectively. These wedges should be used with a rigid heel counter to effectively grip the heel and produce the desired effect. External heel wedges have an advantage over inserts by not raising the heel out of the counter, which allows for a better grasp of the heel.

Flared and offset heels allow for a broader base of support in walking. These heels decrease the amount of subtalar motion in patients with arthritis. A lateral flare can help prevent ankle sprains in patients with chronic instability. The offset heel is often useful with bracing in patients with advanced hindfoot deformities.

The solid ankle cushion heel (SACH), or plantar flexion heel, is also useful with bracing when ankle motion is lost (Fig. 4–10G, H). It uses a wedge of soft compressible material within the heel. It may be combined with a rocker sole to compensate for decreased ankle dorsiflexion and plantar flexion. The degree of rocker-bottom effect is controlled by the height of the heel, thickness of the wedge, and position of the rocker bottom.

Heel lifts are used to compensate for leg-length discrepancy. These may be all external or combined with an internal device on the shoe. These are often useful

TABLE 4–2	
Outsole Options for Athletic Shoes	
Running Shoes	**Field Shoes**
Wear-area reinforcement	Multiclaw or stud designs
Cantilevered designs for shock absorption	Asymmetric studs
Court Shoes	**Hiking and Climbing Boots**
Pivot points	Traction and wear lugs
Herringbone pattern	
Suction-cup designs	
Radial edges	

Adapted from Frey C: Shoe wear and pedorthic devices. In Lutter LD, Mizel MS, Pfeffer GB (eds): *Orthopedic Knowledge Update: Foot and Ankle.* Rosemont, Ill, American Academy of Orthopaedic Surgeons, 1994, p 295.

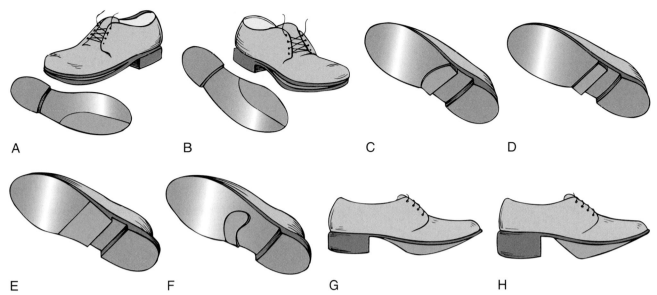

Figure 4–9 Outsole modifications. **A,** Lateral sole wedge. **B,** Medial sole wedge. **C,** Mayo's metatarsal bar. **D,** Flush's metatarsal bar. **E,** Denver's heel. **F,** Hauser's bar. **G,** Rocker sole. **H,** Extended rocker sole. (Adapted from Gould N: Footwear: Shoes and shoe modifications. In Jahss MH [ed]: *Disorders of the Foot and Ankle: Medical and Surgical Management,* ed 2, vol 3. Philadelphia, WB Saunders, 1991, p 2907.)

as a temporary device when the opposite extremity is placed in a prefabricated walking cast. These walking casts usually have a built-in rocker-bottom and are higher than the patient's normal shoe. Patients who have difficulty with this temporary leg-length discrepancy can be helped by application of a lift to the opposite shoe to compensate. A heel lift may also be used when a SACH and rocker bottom have been applied to the opposite shoe.

When the outsole and heel of the shoe for postural abnormalities are modified, the shank of the shoe should afford some flexibility to allow the foot to respond to the correction applied. When arthritic conditions of the midfoot and forefoot are treated, the shank should be stiffened to decrease the motion of the foot.

The advances in shoe manufacturing and materials have led to a new popularity of running and walking

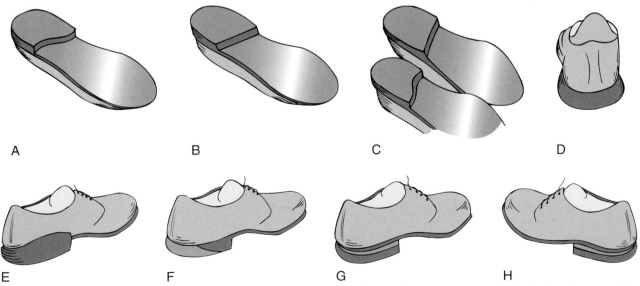

Figure 4–10 Heel modifications. **A,** Thomas heel. **B,** Stone heel. **C,** Reverse Thomas and Stone heel. **D,** Flare heel. **E,** Offset heel. **F,** Plantar flexion heel. **G,** Medial wedge heel. **H,** Lateral wedge heel. (Adapted from Gould N: Footwear: Shoes and shoe modifications. In Jahss MH [ed]: *Disorders of the Foot and Ankle: Medical and Surgical Management,* ed 2, vol 3. Philadelphia, WB Saunders, 1991, p 2906.)

shoes. In general, these shoes allow better fit of the forefoot and greater cushioning of the foot and ankle. The popularity of these shoes helps in the treatment of many foot and ankle problems without the need to prescribe the traditional orthopaedic oxford. Patient acceptance of this type of footwear affords greater compliance with treatment.

ORTHOSES

Orthoses are devices that can be placed inside a shoe to help accommodate anatomic abnormalities or to relieve pressure or stress at a specific site on the foot or ankle. They function by applying a force on the body in a controlled manner to achieve a desired result, that is, transfer of pressure or restriction of motion. Orthotic devices range from simple shoe inserts to braces. The popularity of shoe inserts for runners has led to many anecdotal claims about the efficacy of their use. There are few controlled studies to confirm these claims.

It should be remembered that orthoses are accommodative devices and not corrective devices. There is no evidence that an orthosis can correct or prevent the development of hallux valgus or other deformities or prevent knee, hip, or back arthritis. Given the correct indications, orthoses can be very effective in clinical management of many foot and ankle problems.

It is not always necessary to use a custom orthosis. For the accommodation of many forefoot- and heel-related problems, over-the-counter devices may be equally effective at a considerably lower cost. The abuse and overprescribing of custom inserts has led most medical insurance companies to deny payment for these inserts. Familiarity with the over-the-counter devices allows the treating physician to direct the patient on how to use these devices effectively.

Custom Orthoses

Custom orthoses can be rigid, semirigid, or soft. Rigid orthoses are generally used to diminish motion in the treatment of arthritis of the midfoot or forefoot. The device stiffens the shoe and functions similar to a steel shank within the shoe. Patients with plantar prominences or significant fat-pad atrophy might find these too uncomfortable to wear. A rigid orthosis has been prescribed to block pronation but may be no more effective than a semirigid device and may be more difficult to tolerate. Rigid orthoses offer no shock-absorbing properties and should be avoided in patients with impaired sensation.

Semirigid orthoses are the most commonly prescribed inserts. Unlike rigid orthoses, they offer shock absorption and some flexibility while still providing tensile strength and durability. They are used to support and stabilize flexible deformities and relieve pressure by weight transfer. Combinations of materials are often used; the inserts are generally thicker than rigid inserts and might require the patient to wear a deeper shoe. The materials used include leather, polyethylene compounds, closed or open cellular rubber compounds, cork, felt, and viscoelastic polymers.

Soft orthoses offer the most cushioning and impact absorption and reduce shear forces of friction in the insensate foot. They can be used to accommodate fixed deformities and may be combined with a semirigid material to gain better mechanical properties. These inserts are generally thicker than the rigid orthoses and require the use of an extra-depth shoe. The materials used are polyurethane foam, polyvinyl chloride foam, and latex foam.

There are several commonly prescribed foot orthoses made in accordance with these various rigidities (Fig. 4–11). Shaffer's orthosis, made of rigid or semirigid materials, incorporates a concave heel cup, convex longitudinal arch support, and medial heel wedge and is prescribed to control hindfoot pronation. Mayer's orthosis is a three-quarter-length inlay of semirigid material with a metatarsal pad to relieve pressure under the heads of the metatarsals. The Whitman orthosis is a rigid orthosis prescribed to block pronation. It consists of a concave heel cup, medial convexity under the navicular, and lateral wall flange at the cuboid. The pump, or cobra, insert allows the calcaneus to rest on the insole and uses a cupped heel and medial support to stabilize the hindfoot. Its low profile allows its use in a pump dress shoe. Morton's orthosis, of semirigid material, extends beyond the first metatarsal to redistribute weight bearing under the metatarsal head.

The Levy mold is a full-length orthosis that extends from the heel to the tip of the shoe. It is made from a positive mold of the foot in subtalar neutral position and can incorporate various corrections to accommodate fixed deformities and weight transfer. It can be made of a combination of rigid, semirigid, and soft materials and requires the use of an extra-depth shoe. The full-length cushioned inlay is made of compressible soft materials and reduces compression, friction, and impact on the foot.

Over-the-Counter Inserts

With the advances in material used in shoe manufacturing, it is often possible to accomplish many of the goals of orthosis without the expense of custommolded inlays. Several companies offer padded insoles for shock absorption and heel cushioning (Fig. 4–12).

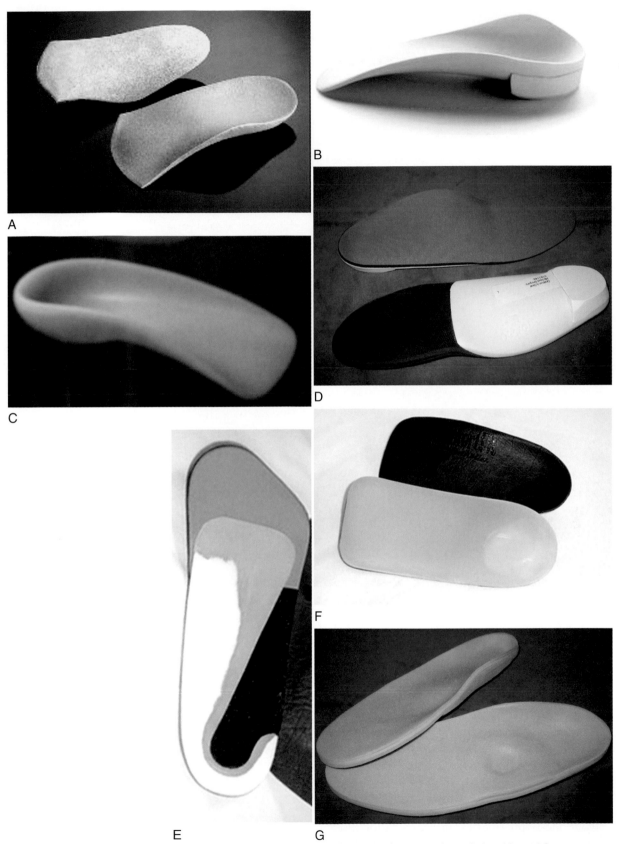

Figure 4–11 Types of orthoses. **A,** Shaffer, to reduce hindfoot pronation. **B,** Whitman with medial and lateral flange, to prevent heel valgus. **C,** Low profile University of California Biomechanics Laboratory (UCBL) insert, to control hindfoot motion. **D,** Semi-rigid full length. **E,** Cobra, or pump, insert for dress shoe. **F,** Three-quarter-length rigid with leather cover. **G,** Plastazote, PPT, Nora composite in sole.

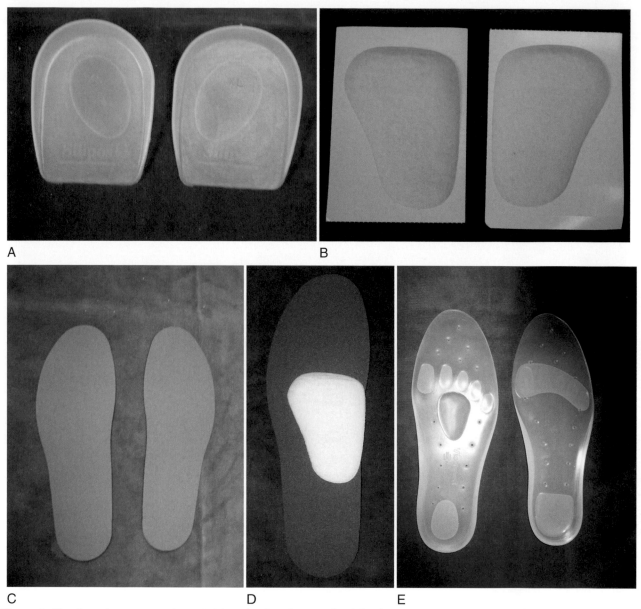

Figure 4–12   Over-the-counter inlays. **A,** Visco heel cushion and Tuli heel cup. **B,** Hapad longitudinal metatarsal support. **C,** Spenco liner. **D,** Combination Spenco liner and Hapad. **E,** Viscoped.

Spenco, Viscopeds, Dr. Scholl's, and other companies provide padded insoles and inlays that can be effective in providing relief for metatarsalgia and fat-pad atrophy. The addition of metatarsal supports, such as the Hapad longitudinal metatarsal pad on a cushioned inlay or in a shoe with a soft sole, can effectively relieve metatarsalgia or neuroma symptoms. Various heel inserts, such as Visco heels or Tuli heel cups, are often helpful in treating plantar heel pain. These devices are readily available through medical supply catalogs and are often found in pharmacies and athletic shoe stores. Patients should be educated on their proper placement and use.

Once the patient has been evaluated and the desired correction chosen, the proper footwear should be selected. In some instances, this may be all that is needed. If additional correction is needed, off-the-shelf items should be considered. The cost to the patient is considerable for custom orthoses, and more insurance companies now refuse payment for any orthosis that does not cross the ankle joint. If adequate correction cannot be accomplished, custom orthoses can be prescribed.

BRACES

Three types of braces that have proved useful in treating foot and ankle problems are the ankle–foot orthoses (AFO) of either molded polypropylene or

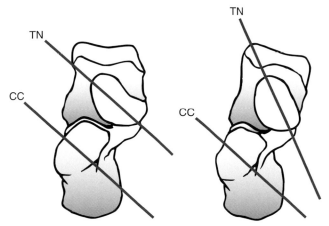

Figure 4–13 Function of the transverse tarsal joint, as described by Elftman, demonstrates that when the calcaneus is in eversion *(left)*, the resultant axes of talonavicular *(TN)* and calcaneocuboid *(CC)* joints are parallel. When the subtalar joint is in inversion *(right)*, axes are nonparallel, giving increased stability to the midfoot.

double-upright construction, Marzano braces, and University of California Biomechanics Laboratory (UCBL) inserts.

University of California Biomechanics Laboratory Inserts

The UCBL insert controls flexible postural deformities by controlling the hindfoot.[9] The brace should be molded with the heel in neutral position. To work successfully, the brace must be able to grasp the heel and prevent it from moving into valgus. By keeping the calcaneus in neutral position, the brace stiffens the transverse tarsal joints, and pronation and forefoot abduction can be diminished (Fig. 4–13). It may be necessary to add medial posting to the heel and front of the brace to keep the heel out of valgus. As medial

posting is added, it may be necessary to lower the medial trim line to avoid impingement on the medial malleolus.

In fixed deformities, such as arthritis of the midfoot, a UCBL insert can decrease motion and relieve pain. The manufacture of the brace is modified for this application. The foot is molded in situ, and the polypropylene should have a relief over the area of bony prominence. The brace can be lined with a material for pressure absorption such as polyurethane foam (PPT) in the relief, and then the entire brace can be covered with a material such as polyethylene foam (Plastazote) to resist shear forces (Fig. 4–14).

Marzano Braces

The Marzano brace (Fig. 4–15) combines a UCBL insert with an anterior shell and a hinged ankle. It has been employed to treat various foot conditions. It provides greater support than the UCBL and allows motion of the ankle.

Ankle–Foot Orthoses

AFOs can be made from double uprights attached to the shoe or molded polypropylene either as a posterior shell or incorporated into a leather lacer (Arizona brace) (Fig. 4–16). The molded AFO is more effective in most instances. The brace can be made with a fixed or hinged ankle. The brace is manufactured from a positive cast of the lower limb and can be lined with shear-resistant material such as Plastizote. Modifications can be made through reliefs over bony prominences to accommodate fit, and these can be lined with PPT under the Plastizote to afford pressure relief. These modifications of the brace allow better control of deformities and expand the use of these braces to rigid, as well as flexible, deformities.

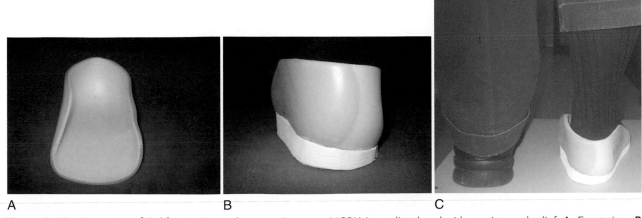

A   B   C

Figure 4–14 University of California Biomechanics Laboratory (UCBL) insert lined and with posting and relief. **A,** Front view. **B,** Rear view showing medial posting. **C,** UCBL insert controlling heel valgus.

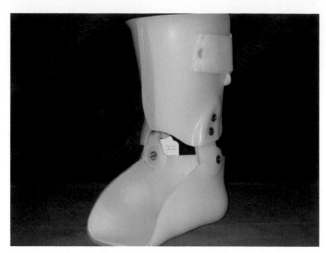

Figure 4–15 Marzano brace.

The molded AFO can provide stability to one or several joints of the foot and ankle complex. The trim line can be modified, depending on the rigidity desired. To diminish ankle motion, the trim lines should extend anteriorly to the midline of the malleoli, but the foot plate can end at the metatarsal heads. If one is controlling subtalar or transverse tarsal motion, the trim lines can be cut behind the malleoli to allow some ankle motion. If one is controlling midfoot arthritis, it may be necessary to use a full foot plate. A SACH heel can provide a smoother gait pattern for most patients. If a full foot plate is used, a rocker-bottom sole should be considered. In patients with a normal ankle joint, a hinged ankle may be employed to allow ankle motion.

The Arizona brace AFO can be constructed with either lace or hook-and-loop (Velcro) closures. It provides stability to the hindfoot through three-point fixation similar to a short-leg cast. It has the advantage of being lower than a standard molded AFO and might have better patient acceptance.

APPLIANCES

Various appliances have been developed for the treatment of forefoot deformities. Pads and cushions can be effective in relieving pain but will not correct deformities. Padding is effective only if the shoe is the correct shape and material. Pads take up additional space within the shoe and can increase pressure if the toe box is too small.

A toe crest can be effective in relieving pressure on the tips of the toes from hammer toe and mallet toe deformities. Corn and callus pads can also relieve pressure but are more effective if the overlying callus and corn tissue is removed and the shoe is stretched over the offending prominence or a wider toe box is employed. Foam or gel (Silipos) sleeves can also effectively relieve pressure (Fig. 4–17). Toe separators can be used, but lamb's wool can be equally effective between the toes and has the advantage of better absorption of moisture than the separators have.

TREATMENT

Arthritis

Bracing can be effective in the treatment of arthritis of the foot and ankle by decreasing the pressure and motion across the affected joint. Braces should be custom molded and padded appropriately over any bony deformity. The patient must understand that a brace does not cure the problem but can offer an effective means of controlling symptoms if he or she wishes to avoid surgery.

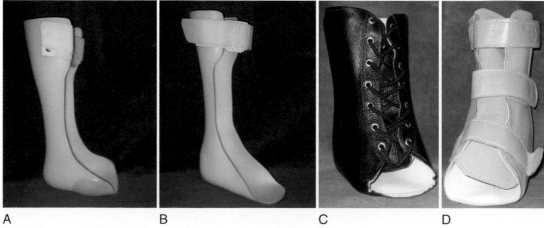

A   B   C   D

Figure 4–16 **A,** Molded ankle–foot orthosis (MAFO) with standard foot plate. **B,** MAFO with full foot plate. **C.** Arizona brace with lace closure. **D.** Arizona brace with hook-and-loop (Velcro) closure.

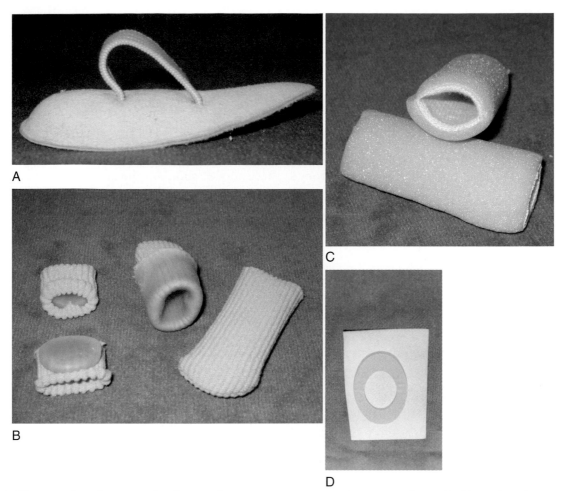

Figure 4–17 Examples of common forefoot appliances. **A,** Toe crest, to elevate tips of toes. **B,** Silipos digital cap, to relieve pressure on toes. **C,** Tube foam, to relieve pressure on toes. **D,** Callus pad.

For ankle and subtalar arthritis, a molded AFO with a fixed ankle or Arizona brace is most effective. In some patients with normal ankles and disease restricted to the subtalar joint, a molded AFO with a hinged ankle or a UCBL with high trim lines can be used. Often, these patients use the AFO for heavy activities and the UCBL for light activities of daily life.

For arthritis restricted to the transverse tarsal and tarsometatarsal joints, the same principles apply, but the success rate of the UCBL is much higher. A SACH and rocker-bottom sole can increase the effectiveness of the brace and afford the patient a more normal gait pattern. Patients often need to change the lacing pattern on their shoes to avoid pressure over dorsal spurs.

Tendon Dysfunction

Chronic tendon tears can lead to significant pain and deformity if left untreated. Although surgical reconstruction has proved successful, some patients are not candidates for surgery because of concomitant medical conditions, whereas others wish to undergo surgical intervention. For chronic dysfunction of the Achilles, peroneal, and anterior and posterior tibial tendons, a custom-molded AFO[4] or Arizona brace,[1] usually lined with Plastizote, can effectively control symptoms. These braces can be combined with a rocker bottom or SACH heel to give a better gait pattern, although a running shoe may be satisfactory.

Patients should understand that the purpose of the brace is to control the position of the foot and hopefully prevent progression of any deformity. If significant tendon damage is present, the brace will not be curative and the patient can decide between using a permanent brace or having reconstructive surgery.

In instances of tendinitis or early tendinosis, prolonged use of a molded AFO for ambulation can allow for healing. This has been successful in managing early tendinosis. Bracing is continued until the swelling, bogginess, and tenderness have resolved, and then progressive mobilization and physical therapy are prescribed. If the objective changes have not resolved within 6 months, bracing has proved not curative and the patient has the option of continuing with bracing as the elected form of treatment or choosing surgical correction.

In patients with complete tendon rupture, bracing can be effective for pain relief and providing increased, although not normal, function. With long-standing rupture there is often a fixed deformity of the foot and ankle complex. For bracing to be effective, the mold must incorporate reliefs and padding over bony prominences. An outflare heel may be needed to support the brace in the shoe and provide an adequate base of support in advanced deformities.

Heel Pain

The role of inserts in treating chronic heel pain remains controversial. It is an area with an abundance of anecdotal treatment but a paucity of scientific knowledge. Part of this problem comes from the difficulty in diagnosing a specific cause of heel pain. Recommendations for inserts for heel pain vary from the use of a rigid orthosis to soft pliable inserts.[12] Recent studies cast doubt on inserts being effective in the treatment of heel pain, but this might reflect the overprescription of these devices without the proper indications.[7,8]

In patients with atrophy of the heel fat pad, soft inserts and a well-padded shoe would be indicated. For chronic plantar fasciitis, soft inserts may be indicated for shock absorption if overuse is a causative factor. Over-the-counter devices and appropriate shoes can be as effective as custom devices at significantly less cost. This treatment should be combined with other treatment modalities.

Night splints for the treatment of chronic plantar fasciitis has been shown to be effective.[15] Although the original studies were performed using a custom-molded AFO with full foot plates, over-the-counter alternatives are now readily available and appear to be equally effective.

LESSER METATARSALS

Calluses And Corns

Callus and corn formation occurs in response to excessive pressure over a bony prominence. This may be the consequence of a loss of the normal fat pad without deformity, secondary to pressure developing in response to deformity, improper footwear causing pressure in an otherwise normal foot, or wearing improper shoes on an abnormal foot. Adequate man-

agement of these problems requires patient education and acceptance of appropriate shoes. Removal of the overlying hyperkeratotic tissue by paring the lesion produces significant relief of symptoms[16] (Fig. 4–18). To prevent recurrence of the lesion, the shoe must be modified to keep pressure off the affected area.

For plantar callosities, recurrence can be prevented by an appropriately sized metatarsal pad placed proximal to the lesion. The pad can be placed directly in the shoe or on a padded inlay that can be transferred from shoe to shoe. For dorsal corns, after the removal of the hyperkeratotic tissue, toe sleeves or toe crests may be effective (Fig. 4–19). Stretching the toe box above the affected toe also helps relieve pressure and decreases the rate and incidence of corn formation.

The commonly found corn over the dorsal and lateral aspects of the fifth toe without deformity is seen in patients wearing pointed dress shoes. Paring is initially effective; however, the lesion recurs if the footwear is not modified. If the patient is unwilling to change his or her footwear, the shoe should be prestretched with a shoemaker's wand over the affected toe to help decrease the pressure. Surgery in this instance is rarely successful if the patient is unwilling to change his or her shoe style. The success of shoe

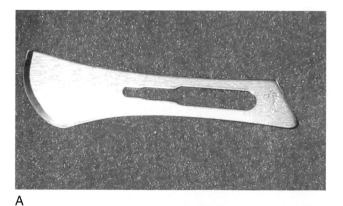

A

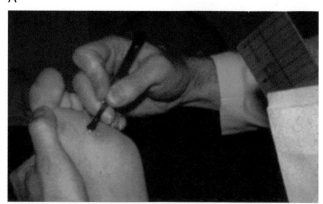

B

Figure 4–18 **A,** Number 17 blade for paring callus has no sharp points but rounded edges. **B,** Paring callus.

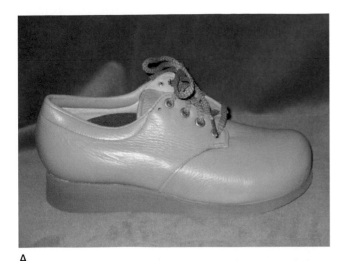

A

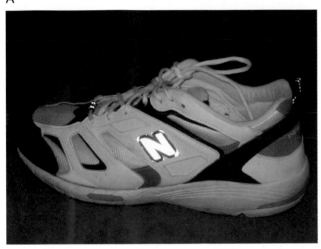

B

Figure 4-19 **A,** Extra-depth shoe to accommodate forefoot deformity or allow room for foot and insert or appliance. **B,** Running shoe with mesh top to accommodate forefoot deformity.

modifications when accepted by the patient makes surgery rarely indicated.

In some patients, a tongue pad can prevent the patient's foot from sliding forward in the shoe when walking and can increase the effectiveness of the other modalities (Fig. 4-20). This is also helpful when hammering has progressed from instability of the metatarsophalangeal joints to subluxation, dislocation, or crossover deformities. In these cases, the addition of a metatarsal pad is indicated to relieve plantar pain.

Taping can add stability to the metatarsophalangeal joint with a hammer toe deformity. A strip of 1/4-inch tape can be looped over the base of the toe to mimic the force of the intrinsic muscles and plantar plate (Fig. 4-21). This loop should be applied in the morning and removed at the end of the day. It can help patients with crossover deformities and subluxating hammer toe deformities.

Neuromas

Interdigital neuromas can often be successfully treated with appropriately placed and sized metatarsal supports (Fig. 4-22). A custom-molded orthosis is rarely indicated. If a custom orthosis is prescribed, rigid material at the distal end of the orthosis should be avoided. In my experience, a longitudinal metatarsal Hapad has proved most effective. When using these pads, the patient should be instructed to break in these devices gradually. A protocol starting with 4 hours the first day and then increasing by 1 hour per day is usually successful. In most instances, patients start with a small size and may increase the size of the pad if their symptoms have not been relieved once they are wearing the pad all day.

Bunionettes

Bunionettes can often be treated successfully by pre-stretching the shoe to avoid pressure over the bony prominence. A rounded or squared toe box can help prevent progression of the deformity.

FIRST METATARSOPHALANGEAL JOINT

Hallux Valgus

Hallux valgus deformities cannot be prevented or corrected by orthotic devices, and such devices should not be prescribed for that purpose. In patients with excessive pronation, an orthotic device to reduce pronation may be indicated and can relieve valgus stress on the great toe. Nonoperative treatment of hallux valgus revolves around the choice of proper footwear to accommodate the present deformity and prevent

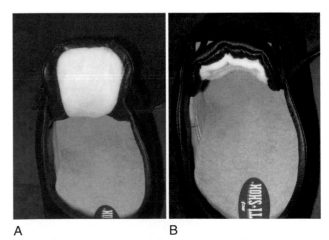

A   B

Figure 4-20 **A,** Tongue pad placement in shoe. **B,** Tongue pad keeps foot in rear of shoe to prevent forefoot pressure.

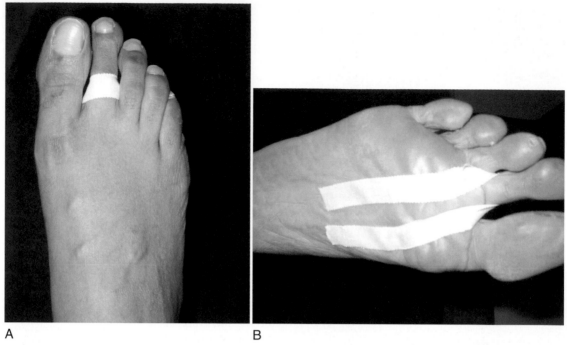

A   B

Figure 4–21   Toe taped for instability of the metatarsophalangeal joint. **A,** Dorsal view. **B,** Plantar view.

increased valgus pressure on the great toe to reduce progression. The choice of shoes is determined by the severity of the deformity. To prevent development of hallux valgus or to accommodate a mild deformity, the patient should wear a shoe built on a straight last. Prestretching of the shoe above the first metatarsophalangeal joint can be useful to relieve pressure.

In moderate-to-severe deformities, an extra-depth shoe may be required. The shoe can be prestretched over the bunion, and a soft leather upper or Thermold should be used. A tongue pad can also keep the foot seated in the shoe.

Hallux Rigidus

Hallux rigidus is an arthritic condition, and nonoperative management involves accommodating the dorsal exostosis and decreasing the motion at the joint. An

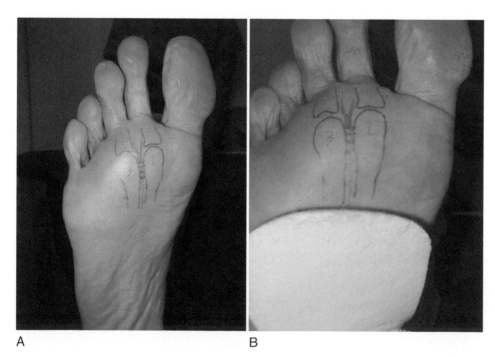

A   B

Figure 4–22 A, Diagram of location of Morton's neuroma at the level of the transverse metatarsal ligament. **B,** Pad placement to relieve pressure proximal to the neuroma.

extra-depth shoe with a steel shank and rocker bottom can be used. If significant dorsal exostosis is present, the toe box might need to be stretched. A full-length rigid orthosis can prevent motion at the metatarsophalangeal joint but should be used with a rocker-bottom shoe.

REFERENCES

1. Augustin JF, Lin SS, Berberian WA, Johnson JE: Nonoperative treatment of adult acquired flat foot with the Arizona brace. *Foot Ankle Clin* 8:491-502, 2003

2. Bordelon RL: Correction of hypermobile flatfoot in children by molded inserts. *Foot Ankle Int* 1:143-150, 1980.

3. Bordelon RL: Hypermobile flatfoot in children. Comprehension, evaluation, and treatment, *Clin Orthop Relat Res* 181:7-14, 1983.

4. Cavanagh PR, Ulbrecht JS, Zanine W, et al: A method for investigation of the effects of outsole modifications in therapeutic footwear. *Foot Ankle Int* 17:706-708, 1996.

5. Choa W, Wapner KL, Lee TH, et al: Nonoperative treatment of posterior tibial tendon dysfunction. *Foot Ankle Int* 17:736-741, 1996.

6. Frey C: Shoe wear and pedorthic devices. In Lutter LD, Mizel MS, Pfeffer GB (eds): *Orthopaedic Knowledge Update: Foot and Ankle*. Rosemont, Ill, American Academy of Orthopaedic Surgeons, 1994.

7. Gill LH, Kiebzak GM: Outcome of nonsurgical treatment for plantar fasciitis. *Foot Ankle Int* 17:527-532, 1996.

8. Gill LH: Plantar fasciitis: Diagnosis and conservative management. *J Am Acad Orthop Surg* 5:109-117, 1997.

9. Gould N: Footwear: Shoes and shoe modifications. In Jahss MH (ed): *Disorders of the Foot and Ankle: Medical and Surgical Management*, ed 2, vol 3. Philadelphia, WB Saunders, 1991, pp 73-88.

10. Henderson WH, Campbell JW: UCBL shoe insert: Casting and fabrication. *Univ Calif Biomech Lab Tech Rep*, Series 53, August 1967.

11. Janisse DJ: The art and science of fitting shoes. *Foot Ankle Int* 13:257-262, 1992.

12. Mizel MS, Marymount JV, Trepman E: Treatment of plantar fasciitis with a night splint and shoe modification consisting of a steel shank and anterior rocker bottom. *Foot Ankle Int* 17:732-735, 1996.

13. Perry JE, Ulbrecht JS, Derr JA, et al: The use of running shoes to reduce plantar pressures in patients who have diabetes. *J Bone Joint Surg* 77A:1819-1826, 1995.

14. Rozema A, Ulbrecht MB, Pammer SE, et al: In-shoe plantar pressures during activities of daily living: implications for therapeutic footwear design. *Foot Ankle Int* 17:352-359, 1996.

15. Wapner KL, Sharkey PF: The use of night splints for treatment of recalcitrant plantar fasciitis. *Foot Ankle Int* 12:135-137, 1991.

16. Young MJ, Cavanagh PR, Thomas G, et al: The effect of callus removal on dynamic foot pressures in diabetic patients. *Diabet Med* 9:55-57, 1992.

Ambulatory Surgery and Regional Anesthesia

Michael J. Coughlin • Greg A. Horton

Almost all operative procedures involving the foot and ankle require some type of anesthesia. The specific type of anesthetic varies and depends on the collective preference and experience of the patient, surgeon, and anesthesiologist. Variables of the surgical procedure itself, such as the realistic anticipated duration and patient positioning, can influence the choice of anesthetic. By their nature and location, surgical proce-

dures of the foot and ankle can typically be performed in the ambulatory (outpatient) setting. The complexity and types of procedures performed on an outpatient basis continue to expand. There are considerable benefits for both the patient and the surgeon. Without sacrificing patient safety, high-quality care can be provided with lower procedural costs and much greater efficiency than in a traditional hospital setting.

Hospital admission following foot and ankle surgery may be necessary for monitoring or management of a systemic illness, particularly in patients with multiple comorbid conditions. Brittle diabetic patients and patients with cardiac disease, renal insufficiency, and gastric motility problems are common examples.

There are many advantages in using regional anesthesia for foot and ankle surgery. Often the complications associated with general anesthesia, such as central nervous system depression, nausea, and dehydration, are avoided. Following a successful peripheral nerve block, a gradual onset of pain is expected as the anesthetic wears off. This slow emergence period allows the patient or the caregiver to titrate the level of orally administered analgesics for pain control as the effect of the block dissipates. The peak level of pain once the block wears off is rarely of the magnitude or duration seen in patients who awaken from an anesthetic that does not provide lasting analgesia. This allows a substantial reduction in the need for parenteral analgesics, which can cause oversedation and nausea. It can also have a benefit of higher patient satisfaction and confidence in the success of the procedure.

Although an anesthesiologist may attend the patient during the immediate perioperative period, it is most often the operative surgeon who addresses postsurgical issues of pain control. This includes prescribing the medication that the patient will use once discharged home. The relationship between the patient and the anesthesiologist is typically of a finite duration and rarely extends beyond the confines of the operative suite and postanesthesia recovery room. This is certainly the case in the setting of the ambulatory surgery center.

The relationship between the patient and the operative surgeon is distinctly different. Phone calls about postoperative pain, bleeding, wound management, and medication refills are directed to the operative surgeon and office staff. Therefore, it is in the surgeon's best interest to attempt to minimize potential problems. Knowledge and skill in peripheral anesthetic techniques can optimize the postoperative process.

The ability of a physician to communicate with the patient during and after surgery and the ability of a patient to cooperate before, during, and after a procedure complement peripheral anesthesia in an outpatient setting. These factors aid in patient comprehension of a procedure, help attain the goals of the procedure, and increase postoperative compliance.[64]

With increasing concern regarding the upward escalation of inpatient hospital costs, the use of ambulatory surgery has increased dramatically. In striving to decrease surgery expenses, the primary objective remains to maintain quality and safety of patient care. Although hospitalization is avoided with ambulatory surgery, routine surgical procedures are performed. A patient who undergoes an operative procedure and then is discharged within a few hours requires a different approach in the preoperative preparation and postoperative management to ensure a successful result.

PREOPERATIVE MANAGEMENT

After the decision is reached that surgical intervention is indicated for treating a specific foot and ankle problem, a preoperative patient assessment is performed. Much of a patient's past medical history can be elicited by a health information form (Fig. 5–1). Pertinent facts can include previous surgeries, serious medical illnesses, prior anesthetic difficulties, bleeding tendencies, current medications, medication allergies, and other important medical information. A review of major organ systems dysfunction can be incorporated into this form to screen for any significant problems.

Evaluation of the patient's overall medical condition will help the physician determine whether ambulatory surgery is feasible. Typically a patient scheduled for ambulatory surgery is in good health and is considered at low risk for problems with anesthesia. A systemic illness, if not incapacitating, does not rule out ambulatory surgery.

The history should identify all medications and supplements that the patient is taking. This includes both prescription and over-the-counter medication. Of particular importance is identification of medications that alter or interfere with blood clotting and hemostasis.[31] Warfarin is typically discontinued 4 or 5 days prior to a surgical procedure to normalize the prothrombin time (PT) and international normalized ratio (INR). Alternative administration of low-molecular-weight (LMW) heparin may be needed depending upon the underlying medical condition. LMW heparin can usually be given up to 24 hours prior to the procedure without significant bleeding complications. Clopidogrel (Plavix) is usually stopped at least 7 days prior to surgery and ticlopidine (Ticlid) 10 to 14 days prior to surgery. Discontinuation or alteration of anticoagulant regimens is often coordinated with or done by the patient's primary care physician. Aspirin and nonsteroidal antiinflammatory drugs (NSAIDs) can also affect hemostasis. Aspirin produces an irreversible inhibition of platelet aggregation that can take several days to normalize. Traditional COX-1 NSAIDs can also increase bleeding type by reversible platelet binding. These medications should be discontinued 7 to 10 days prior to elective surgery unless contraindicated.

Dr Update

PATIENT QUESTIONNAIRE
Michael J. Coughlin, M.D.

Pt Update

Name: _____   Date: _____

Please describe what brings you here today: _____

Where does it hurt? _____

How long have you had the problem? _____

What makes it better? _____   What makes it worse? _____

Please describe the type of pain you have (check all that apply)

☐ Sharp   ☐ Aching   ☐ Stabbing

☐ Dull   ☐ Cramping   ☐ Throbbing

☐ Pins and needles   ☐ Constant   ☐ Comes and goes

If it is an injury when did it happen? _____

How did it happen? _____

_____

On a scale of 1–10, how severe is the pain?
No pain 1 2 3 4 5 6 7 8 9 10 severe pain

Where did it occur?
☐ Home ☐ School ☐ Work ☐ Auto ☐ Other

Who is your primary care physician? _____

Do you see any other specialists? _____

Which pharmacy do you use? _____   Telephone: _____

Please list any medications you are now taking, prescription and over the counter

Name of medication	Dosage (example 10 mg.)	How often do you take it?

Social History

Do you get regular exercise?   ☐ No   ☐ Yes (what type and how often?)

Do you drink alcohol?   ☐ No   ☐ Yes (how many drinks per week?)

Do you smoke?   ☐ No   ☐ Yes—How many per day?   How long?

What is your occupation? _____

How many years of school? _____

Please continue on reverse side of this form!

A

Figure 5–1 Patient questionnaire. **A,** Front.   *Continued*

The COX-2 inhibitors do not routinely require discontinuation because the effect on bleeding time is less substantial.

The use of nonprescription medication is often not disclosed by the patient and not inquired about by the physician. This includes the use of increasingly popular herbal products and nutritional supplements. Many herbal preparations have side effects that can complicate a surgical procedure and the anesthetic.[35] Increased bleeding is associated with ingestion of

Your height: _____   **Your weight:** _____

Do you have any allergies? Please list and describe reaction

_____

_____

_____

_____

Past Family History – Please check any of the following medical problems anyone of your **immediate family**
(mother, father, brother, sister, grandparents) has had

☐ Arthritis	☐ Diabetes	☐ Heart problems	☐ Anesthesia problems
☐ Bleeding problems	☐ Blood clot	☐ Foot problems	

Review of Systems – Please check any of the following you have had

☐ Chest pain	☐ Palpitation or fluttering heart	☐ Cough	☐ Shortness of breath	☐ Extremity weakness
☐ Frequent rashes	☐ Joint pain	☐ Muscle pain	☐ Trouble walking	☐ Use cane or walker
☐ Extremity swelling	☐ Bruise easily	☐ Loss of sensation in feet	☐ Excessive thirst	☐ Excessive urination
☐ Burning with urination	☐ Difficulty swallowing	☐ Stomach pain or burning	☐ Frequent loose stools	☐ Frequent constipation
☐ Difficulty sleeping	☐ Fainting spells	☐ Troubled by depression	☐ Troubled by anxiety	☐ Severe headaches
☐ Trouble hearing	☐ Wear hearing aid	☐ Wear glasses or contacts		

Past Medical History – Please check any of the following you have had

☐ High blood pressure	☐ Heart problems	☐ Bleeding problems	☐ Blood clots (phlebitis)	☐ Irregular heartbeat
☐ Varicose veins	☐ Stroke	☐ Pneumonia	☐ Tuberculosis	☐ Asthma
☐ Emphysema	☐ Mitral valve prolapse	☐ Psoriasis	☐ Gout	☐ Rheumatoid arthritis
☐ Diabetes	☐ Kidney failure	☐ Urinary infections	☐ Gallbladder problems	☐ Colitis
☐ Hiatal hernia	☐ Ulcers	☐ Seizures	☐ Psychiatric problems	☐ Thyroid problems
☐ Cancer	☐ HIV / AIDS	☐ Other infections		

Please describe any of the problems you checked off from the above list

_____

_____

_____

_____

Please describe any past surgeries (and year)

_____

_____

_____

_____

_____

B

Figure 5–1—cont'd   B, Back.

feverfew, garlic, ginger, ginkgo, and ginseng. It is suggested that all herbal medications be discontinued 2 to 3 weeks before an elective surgical procedure.

Hematology and chemistry studies are often not required for the ambulatory surgery patient because low-risk patients are the norm. In some cases no tests are performed or only a hematocrit and hemoglobin values are obtained. A complete blood cell count (CBC) may be indicated in other patients. Electrolyte or potassium levels are obtained if the patient is receiving antihypertensive or cardiac medications. Electrocardiograms, chest radiographs, and multichannel chemistry screens are ordered infrequently for the low-risk patient.

Inasmuch as the patient is not hospitalized preoperatively, patient education is initiated in the outpatient setting. The normal expectations of a procedure, alternatives of treatment, operative risks, and common complications of the proposed procedures are reviewed before surgery as part of the informed consent process

When surgery is selected as the preferable choice of treatment, patient education involves a discussion of the intended procedure. In the case of commonly performed procedures, a patient information booklet or handout can expedite teaching and gives the patient material to review in the home environment. Information may also be disseminated by video tapes and anatomic models. A question and answer period in which a patient's concerns and questions are addressed can be quite helpful. This can improve patient comprehension, understanding, and retention of pertinent facts to be remembered in the perioperative period. The discussion with a patient in the preoperative setting with regard to the options for treatment, the benefits and risks of surgery, and possible complications is very important. The physician should remember, however, that this discussion occurs during a particularly stressful time.

On occasion, at the initial meeting, whether it occurs in a hospital emergency department or clinic examination room, a discussion of the procedure and the intended goals of treatment are coupled with a history and physical examination. Furthermore, at this time when the patient may be scheduled for surgery, the environment is complicated by a patient's concerns about work and insurance-related issues. Thus, it is important for the treating physician to attempt to ensure that the patient has a clear understanding of the goals of treatment and the risks of surgery.

Shurnas and Coughlin[54] evaluated informed consent in a group of patients scheduled to undergo elective forefoot surgery. Three months following surgery the patient's memory of the preoperative discussion and the recall of proposed risks was assessed.

Although patients expressed their complete satisfaction with the preoperative discussion, patients' recall of the discussion and the proposed risks was extremely poor. Less than 10% of discussed risks were routinely recalled by patients. Poor recall occurred despite of the use of a written description of the procedure and the use of patient educational videotapes. Thus, every effort should be made to ensure a patient has the opportunity to discuss the proposed treatment plan and ask appropriate questions. The discussion should be documented in the patient chart as well.

To minimize the risk of pulmonary aspiration secondary to impairment of upper airway protective reflexes, it is necessary to ensure that the stomach is empty. The American Society of Anesthesiologists has developed practice guidelines for preoperative fasting.[4] All healthy patients (adults and children) should refrain from ingesting solid food after midnight or for 6 hours prior to the anticipated procedure. For fried or fatty foods, a fasting period of 8 hours is recommended. The patient may take his or her necessary medication on the morning of surgery with a sip of water. The patient may have clear liquids up to 2 hours before arriving at the hospital or surgery center. Clear liquids include water, fruit juices without pulp, carbonated beverages, clear tea, and black coffee (no cream or milk is allowed). Patients with conditions that can alter gastric emptying should take nothing by mouth (NPO) after midnight or 6 hours prior to surgery (solids as well as liquids). Other patients who might have increased risk of altered gastric motility include those who are pregnant or obese or who have a hiatal hernia, gastroesophageal reflux, ileus or bowel obstruction, or gastroparesis.

Surgeons do need to have a realistic approach to the appropriateness of certain patients for outpatient surgery. Consultation with the facility anesthesia staff in questionable cases is preferable to canceling surgery on the day of the procedure. Many outpatient centers obtain screening information from patients before they arrive. In most cases, however, the anesthesiologist does not evaluate the patient until immediately before the surgical procedure. Some centers encourage preoperative evaluation at the facility by a nurse in consultation with the anesthesiologist for patients with more substantial medical conditions.

PERIOPERATIVE CONSIDERATIONS

It is without debate that wrong-site, wrong-procedure, and wrong-person surgery must be avoided. Although this seems to be an unthinkable possibility, a series of avoidable errors and omissions is a common thread for those who have had acquaintance with such a misadventure. Although the operative consent is certainly part of the process, it is inadequate to rely upon a single preventive measure. Participation by the patient, the operating surgeon, and other members of the surgical team helps to ensure accuracy.

Adherence to a standardized universal protocol is intended to eliminate wrong-side, wrong-procedure, and wrong-person errors. Labeling of extremities varies from institution to institution and region to region. Whereas some label the opposite extremity with the word "NO" (Fig. 5–2A), others prefer labeling the operative site with the word "YES" (Fig. 5–2B). Some institutions have implemented the recommendations of the American Academy of Orthopedic Surgeons (AAOS) and require surgeons to sign the operative site with their initials (Fig. 5–2C).[3] For organizations accredited by the Joint Commission on Accreditation of Healthcare Organizations (JCAHO), mandatory signing is one of the components of the "Universal Protocol for Eliminating Wrong Site, Wrong Procedure, and Wrong Person Surgery."[2] The AAOS has endorsed this protocol, urging surgeons along with other health care provider groups to play a cooperative role in implementing patient safety principles.[2]

In consultation with the patient, the surgeon should place an unambiguous mark in the area of the intended operative site. A permanent marking pen ensures the mark will be visible following the preparation and draping of the extremity. Some consider the use of an "X" to be ambiguous and inadequate for documentation or confirmation. On occasion, patients write words of endearment or encouragement on the extremity prior to an elective procedure. This is not a substitute for the necessary consistent institutional implementation of a prevention protocol and can actually add a confusing element to the labeling process.

A member of the operative team typically double checks the consent, medical records, and radiographs to ensure they are in agreement with the marked site. Likewise, review of the office chart and radiographs prior to surgery are important factors in ensuring the correct site and procedure. Immediately prior to the procedure, an active communication by the entire operative team should take place. This "time out" or "stop and pause" is carried out to confirm the identity, side, site, and procedure as a final verification before incision of the skin. Because of the limited exposure of the operating physician and nursing staff to the patient before surgery, all of these efforts help to minimize inadvertent surgical errors. The use of single-limb regional anesthesia is a further element that increases the safety factor in obtaining the correct surgical site and procedure.

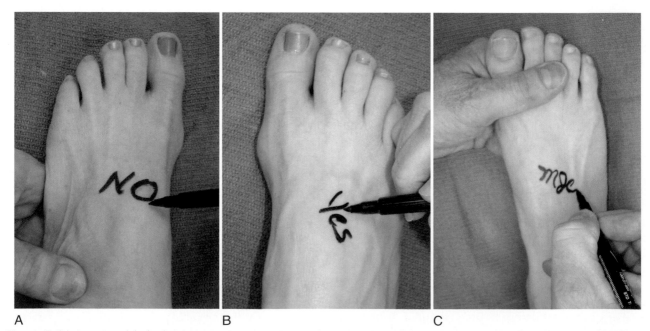

A　　　　　　　　　　　B　　　　　　　　　　　C

Figure 5–2　A patient labels the nonoperative extremity with "NO" **(A)** and the operative extremity with "YES" **(B). C,** The physician may also ■ mark the operative extremity with his or her initials.

POSTOPERATIVE MANAGEMENT

In the initial stage, postoperative management is concerned with the recovery process after anesthesia. After this, an educational process is begun to prepare the patient and family for continued recovery at home.

During this recovery period, it is important to have the nursing staff attuned to the postanesthesia recovery process. The use of short-acting analgesic agents that minimize postoperative sedation expedites this recovery process. The use of intravenous and intramuscular narcotic analgesics during the recovery process seems to prolong the recovery from anesthesia. An observation period after anesthesia is important for monitoring the patient's recovery from anesthesia.

As the recovery process progresses, education of the patient and family is directed toward the specific procedure that has been performed. The ambulatory philosophy is that the continued recovery process does not end at the time of discharge but is continued at home. Postoperative planning plays an integral role in preparation for discharge. The patient and family must be educated regarding signs and symptoms to watch for in the perioperative period. They should also be instructed whom to contact if complications arise.

After foot and ankle surgery, a postoperative shoe or cast-boot is fitted and gait training is initiated where indicated; for some patients, ambulation may be difficult. The choice of crutches, walker, wheelchair, or other ambulatory assistive devices are chosen depending upon the coordination and ability of the individual patient (Fig. 5–3). The patient is instructed regarding elevation of the extremity and the judicious use of ice and analgesics.

Family members are instructed regarding home nursing care. Responsibility for home care is transferred to the patient's family at discharge. A patient must be coherent or have family members who are able to recognize problems should they occur.[18]

If a patient is discharged to an isolated home environment, a home health referral for nursing care or a visiting nurse may be requested. Follow-up office appointments are scheduled. Oral analgesics are dispensed for pain control. Instructions in the use of analgesics before discharge allow the patient to adjust dosage and frequency depending on symptoms. Initially the use of a strong oral narcotic analgesic (e.g., oxycodone [Percodan] or controlled-release oxycodone [OxyContin], or sustained-release morphine [MS Contin, Oramorph SR]) may be used for significant pain as peripheral anesthesia diminishes several hours after surgery. NSAIDs may be added to supplement analgesia. With diminishing symptoms, orally administered analgesics including acetaminophen with codeine, hydrocodone (Vicodin, Norco), and

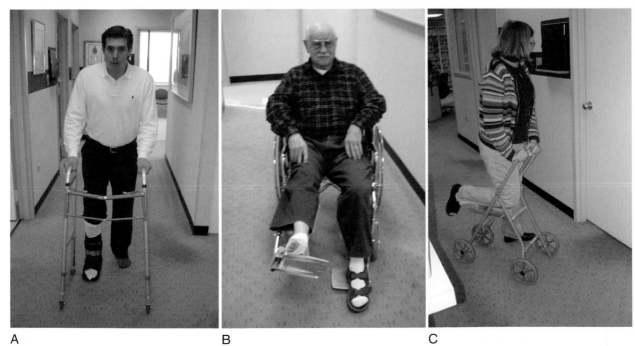

A   B   C

Figure 5–3 Instruction in postoperative gait training is important. Some patients demonstrate an inability to ambulate safely. **A,** Walker. **B,** Wheel chair with leg extension. **C,** Roller-type scooter used for operative extremity.

acetaminophen and propoxyphene napsylate (Darvocet) may be substituted for stronger oral narcotic analgesics. The postoperative assessment of a patient is important to assess patient compliance. The patient or family member must have an adequate understanding to be able to comply with postoperative instructions.

FOLLOW-UP CARE

Postoperative follow-up care by the operating physician usually is done soon after surgery. Inspection of the wound, dressing changes, assessment of pain control, evaluation of ambulatory capacity, and an inspection for other postoperative complications is performed. Nausea and vomiting, respiratory difficulties, and other residual effects of anesthesia can require further medical follow-up observation as well.

DISCUSSION

The success of ambulatory surgery also depends on an outpatient philosophy characterized by increased patient awareness and patient involvement in the recovery process. The involvement of the nursing staff from both the physician's office and the outpatient surgery center is important in providing adequate patient care and patient instruction. Preoperative preparation greatly reduces patient anxiety, and postoperative teaching likewise helps to prevent anxiety and difficulties for the patient. The promotion of "different" patient expectations is helpful in a successful ambulatory experience. A philosophy of wellness with positive expectations regarding successful ambulation and an uneventful recovery is part of the perioperative educational process. A patient can then look forward to recovering in the comfort of his or her own home.

Most physicians can recall the experience of admitting a patient after a minor surgical procedure because of an extenuating medical concern. The patient is then sedated with narcotics, given a sleeping medication, and is ambulated infrequently. The outcome often is a 3- to 4-day hospitalization after a minor procedure.

The ambulatory philosophy of using a peripheral anesthetic block, minimizing parenteral analgesics, performing aggressive nursing care, and providing education is oriented toward the patient's rapid recovery.

A wide variety of anesthetic techniques may be used alone or in combination to produce a satisfactory outcome. These can include spinal, epidural, general endotracheal, laryngeal mask airway, and monitored anesthesia care (MAC). Although each of these alternatives may be used in an ambulatory surgery setting,

the specific anesthetic techniques of spinal, epidural, and general anesthesia are not within the scope of this discussion. The factors considered when one is choosing the particular method of anesthesia depend on such variables as patient preference, age, medical condition, duration of the operative procedure, and the amount of time available for the anesthetic to take effect.[5,23]

The benefits of extended postsurgical analgesia are by no means limited to the outpatient ambulatory setting. Peripheral nerve blocks may be used as the sole anesthetic in some cases or used in concert with other anesthetic techniques. For instance, a spinal anesthetic may be chosen for intraoperative management. This does not preclude the addition of a regional technique such as a sciatic popliteal block by either the anesthesiologist or the surgeon. Depending on the agent used, the spinal anesthetic will wear off in an hour or two without any lasting analgesic effect. The addition of a popliteal block can offer an extended analgesic effect for 12 to 24 hours. This of course assumes a safe cumulative dose of local anesthetic for both procedures.

ANATOMY

Although the foot is demarcated by specific dermatomes, anastomotic branches may be present between nerves that alter expected dermatome distribution. The relationship of nerves and the respective area innervated in the foot and ankle may vary, necessitating anesthetic block of adjacent nerves to give adequate anesthesia for the proposed area of surgery. For example, if the sural nerve distribution extends medially into the third interspace, the area innervated by the intermediate dorsocutaneous nerve (branch of the superficial peroneal nerve) will contract. Likewise, expansion of the area of the superficial peroneal nerve laterally causes a simultaneous contraction of the area innervated by the sural nerve. The relationship of nerves and the respective area innervated in the foot and ankle can vary, necessitating anesthetic block of adjacent nerves to give adequate anesthesia for the proposed area of surgery. An understanding of the anatomy and potential anatomic variations is useful for surgical exposure, preventing iatrogenic nerve injury, and performing peripheral nerve blockade.

Sciatic Nerve in the Thigh and at the Knee

The sciatic nerve descends in the posterior thigh region, lying posterior to the adductor magnus. The nerve is positioned anterior to the hamstring muscles, namely the semimembranosus and semitendinosus (medially) and the biceps femoris (laterally). As these muscles separate into their respective tendinous insertions, the medial and lateral borders of the triangular popliteal fossa are formed. The transverse inferior border of the triangle is formed by the origin of the medial and lateral heads of the gastrocnemius muscle. In the proximal portion of the triangle, the sciatic nerve is located lateral and posterior to the accompanying popliteal vessels. The popliteal vein is medial to the nerve; the artery lies medial and anterior to the vein. The tibial nerve, along with the popliteal vessels, continues deep between the heads of the gastrocnemius muscle.

The common peroneal nerve separates 5 to 7 cm above the posterior knee flexion crease and courses in a lateral direction, following the biceps femoris muscle along the superior lateral margin of the popliteal fossa. It then travels around the head of the fibula, dividing into the superficial and deep peroneal divisions. The tibial and common peroneal divisions are usually within a common perineurium until division in the upper portion of the popliteal triangle. Some patients have a distinct separation of these divisions more proximally in the posterior thigh. These anatomic variations need to be taken into account when attempting block of both the divisions.

Tibial Nerve

Descending distally between the soleus and the posterior tibial muscle, the tibial nerve passes along the posterior aspect of the medial malleolus. The tarsal tunnel is a fibro-osseous tunnel bordered anteriorly by the tibia and laterally by the posterior process of the talus and calcaneus. The flexor retinaculum courses over the contents of the tarsal tunnel and can extend 10 cm above the level of the medial malleolus. The contents of the tarsal tunnel include the tibial nerve, the posterior tibial artery and vein, and the tendons of the posterior tibialis, flexor hallucis longus, and flexor digitorum longus. A complex venous plexus often accompanies the nerve and artery. Varicosities or hypertrophy of this venous plexus can result in increased pressure within the confines of the tarsal tunnel.[25]

As the tibial nerve descends behind the medial malleolus and exits the tarsal tunnel, several terminal branches are given off.[51] The two major branches of the posterior tibial nerve are the medial and lateral plantar nerves. Division into the medial and lateral plantar branches usually occurs in the retromalleolar area, although more proximal bifurcation up to 14 cm above the medial malleolus has been demonstrated. Cadaveric studies have revealed multiple calcaneal branches that can originate from both the medial and

lateral plantar nerves. One terminal branch of the lateral plantar nerve is the mixed sensory motor nerve branch to the abductor digiti quinti (Fig. 5–4).[15]

Medial Plantar Nerve

The most anterior branch of the posterior tibial nerve, the medial plantar nerve, is bordered on its medial aspect by the superior portion of the abductor hallucis muscle and the laciniate ligament (Fig. 5–4A). The nerve passes through the deep investing fascia of the abductor hallucis. The medial plantar nerve then courses deep to the tendons of the flexor hallucis longus and flexor digitorum longus and then occupies an interval between the abductor hallucis and the flexor digitorum brevis. Within the middle plantar compartment at the base of the first metatarsal, it then divides into two main branches, the medial and lateral terminal branches. The medial branch bifurcates, giving off the most medial branch (the proper digital nerve of the hallux), which provides sensation to the medial aspect of the great toe. The lateral branch of the medial terminal branch becomes the first common digital nerve, supplying sensation to the plantar aspect of the first web space.

The lateral terminal branch of the medial plantar nerve divides into the second and third common digital nerves. The second common digital nerve traverses the second intermetatarsal space and bifurcates, forming the lateral digital nerve of the second toe and the medial digital nerve of the third toe. The third common digital nerve traverses the third intermetatarsal space and bifurcates, forming the lateral digital nerve to the third toe and the medial digital nerve to the fourth toe. A communicating branch often occurs between the third common digital nerve and the fourth common digital nerve (Fig. 5–5).[26,34]

Lateral Plantar Nerve

The lateral plantar nerve, located posterior to the medial plantar nerve at the lower border of the tarsal tunnel, passes laterally beneath the fascia of the quadratus plantae. The first branch of the lateral plantar nerve has received attention as a potential source of heel pain, with potential entrapment between the deep fascia of the abductor hallucis muscle and the medial caudal margin of the medial head of the quadratus plantae muscle.[6] Several motor branches from the lateral plantar nerve innervate the lumbricals and the interossei of the second, third, and fourth interspaces. The lateral plantar nerve then divides into the fourth common digital nerve, which often gives off a communicating branch to the third common digital nerve before it terminates as the lateral digital nerve of

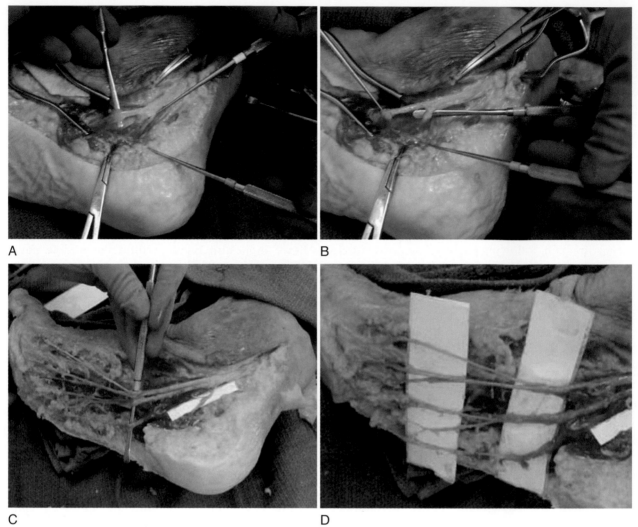

A

B

C   D

Figure 5–4   Anatomy of posterior tibial nerve. **A,** Medial plantar branch of the posterior tibial nerve. **B,** Lateral plantar branch of posterior tibial nerve. **C,** Posterior tibial nerve with both major branches demonstrated. **D,** Distal branches including proper digital nerves to the toes.

the fourth toe and the medial digital nerve of the fifth toe. The most lateral branch of the lateral plantar nerve, the proper digital nerve of the fifth toe, innervates the lateral plantar aspect of the fifth toe (Fig. 5–4B-D).

Sural Nerve

The sural nerve innervates the dorsolateral aspect of the foot and terminates as the dorsolateral cutaneous nerve of the fifth toe. The sural nerve is formed by two proximal branches: the median sural nerve (a branch of the tibial nerve) and an anastomotic branch of the common peroneal nerve. Emerging from between the

heads of the gastrocnemius, the median sural nerve is joined by the anastomosing branch of the common peroneal nerve on the posterior aspect of the midcalf (Fig. 5–6). The sural nerve then lies on the lateral border of the Achilles tendon in the lower calf. At the level of the ankle the nerve courses around the distal tip of the fibula, 1 to 1.5 cm beneath the lateral malleolus just distal to the peroneal tendons. The sural nerve gives off one or two calcaneal branches proximal to the lateral malleolus and several small cutaneous branches to the lateral aspect of the midfoot and ankle. As the sural nerve courses toward the base of the fifth metatarsal, it divides into its two terminal branches. The larger medial branch proceeds obliquely in a

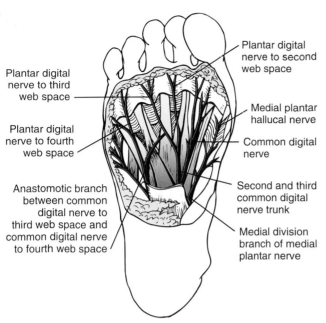

Figure 5–5 Communicating branch of plantar nerve.

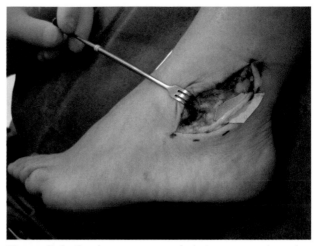

Figure 5–6 Sural nerve exposed during peroneal tendon reconstruction.

dorsomedial direction, providing sensation to the dorsolateral aspect of the fourth toe (the dorsolateral cutaneous nerve of the fourth toe and the dorsomedial cutaneous nerve of the fifth toe). A smaller lateral terminal branch, the dorsolateral cutaneous nerve of the fifth toe, provides sensation to the dorsolateral aspect of the fifth toe.

Superficial Peroneal Nerve

The superficial peroneal nerve (Fig. 5–7), also a branch of the common peroneal nerve, provides sensation to the anterior lateral ankle and the dorsum of the foot. The nerve is typically described as a single branch coursing in the lateral compartment deep to the peroneus longus. It then descends between the peroneus longus and brevis muscles and exits the crural fascia 10 to 15 cm above the level of the ankle, where it becomes subcutaneous. It often divides approximately

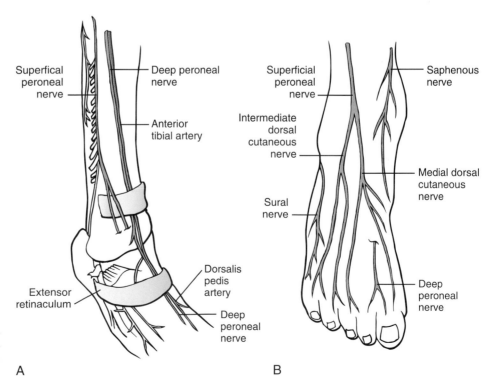

Figure 5–7 **A,** Peroneal nerve in calf, with branches. **B,** Superficial peroneal nerve with branches in foot.

A

B

6 cm above the level of the lateral malleolar into two main branches, the medial and intermediate dorsal cutaneous, which subsequently arborize to provide sensation to the dorsal aspect of the foot and toe, save for the first web space. The intermediate dorsal cutaneous nerve divides into a dorsolateral branch to the third toe and a dorsomedial branch to the fourth toe.

The medial dorsal cutaneous nerve proceeds superficially to the extensor retinaculum toward the medial border of the foot. It then trifurcates into a medial, a middle, and a lateral branch (Fig. 5–8). The medial branch becomes the dorsomedial cutaneous nerve to the hallux; the middle branch innervates the dorsomedial aspect of the second toe and the dorsolateral aspect of the hallux; the lateral branch divides into the dorsolateral cutaneous branch of the second toe and the dorsomedial cutaneous branch of the third toe. The medial terminal branch originates either lateral or dorsal to the extensor hallucis longus (EHL) tendon and then crosses over the EHL. Distal to the first tarsocuneiform joint, the nerve is consistently medial to the EHL.

Most commonly, the superficial peroneal nerve branches into the medial and intermediate dorsal cutaneous nerves after exiting the crural fascia. However in 25% to 30% of patients, the medial and intermediate dorsal cutaneous nerves arise independently from the superficial peroneal nerve and have unique exit sites from the lateral or even the anterior compartment. In some persons, the intermediate branch of the superficial peroneal nerve courses parallel to the posterior border of the fibula, crossing the fibula to reach the dorsum of the foot.

Deep Peroneal Nerve

The deep peroneal nerve (Fig. 5–9), another branch of the common peroneal nerve, lies between the tendons

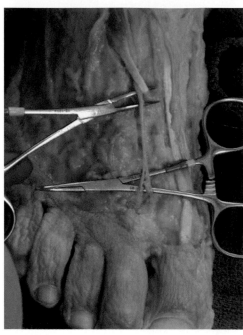

Figure 5–9   Deep peroneal nerve, which innervates the first web space.

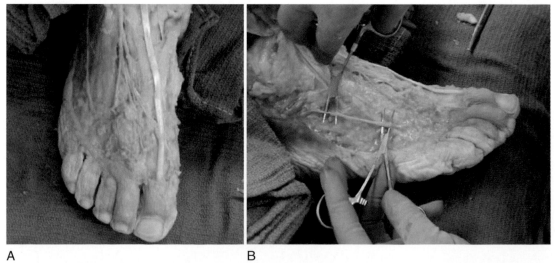

A   B

Figure 5–8   Anatomy of peroneal nerve. **A,** The skin has been removed. The veins and superficial branches of the peroneal nerve are just beneath the superficial fascia. **B,** The branches of the superficial peroneal nerve, including the intermediate dorsocutaneous nerve, are seen here in this dissection.

of the extensor digitorum longus and the extensor hallucis longus at the level of the ankle. It lies lateral to the anterior tibial artery and beneath the extensor retinaculum. One centimeter above the ankle joint, the deep peroneal nerve divides into its two terminal branches: a medial branch and a lateral branch. The larger medial branch lies lateral to the dorsalis pedis artery and courses on the lateral border of the extensor hallucis longus tendon until it terminates as the dorsolateral cutaneous nerve of the hallux and the dorsomedial cutaneous nerve of the second toe, innervating the first web space. The smaller lateral branch of the deep peroneal nerve terminates with several small branches innervating the metatarsophalangeal, interphalangeal, and tarsometatarsal joints and gives a small motor branch to the extensor digitorum brevis.

Saphenous Nerve

The saphenous nerve is the terminal branch of the femoral nerve. It becomes superficial between the gracilis and sartorius muscles. It extends distally on the medial aspect of the lower leg accompanying the saphenous vein and innervates the skin on the medial aspect of the leg and foot. It lies on the medial aspect of the tibia (Fig. 5–10) just posterior to the saphenous vein and terminates as two distinct branches. The larger branch passes anteriorly to the medial malleolus and provides sensation to the medial aspect of the foot and the medial aspect of the hallux; the smaller branch provides innervation to a cutaneous area on the medial aspect of the ankle.

PERIPHERAL NERVE BLOCKS OF THE FOOT

General Considerations

Although some surgeons choose not to enlist the services of an anesthesiologist or nurse anesthetist, most surgeons prefer their support. There are variable levels of interest and experience in regional anesthetic techniques among anesthesiologists, even within the same hospital. Likewise, the experience and comfort of the anesthesia staff in the use of peripheral anesthetic blocks plays a major role in the frequency of their use. Hadzik et al[29] have reported that peripheral blocks, especially in the lower extremity, are underutilized by anesthesiologists. With further experience, the popularity of peripheral anesthesia in an outpatient setting will undoubtedly increase.

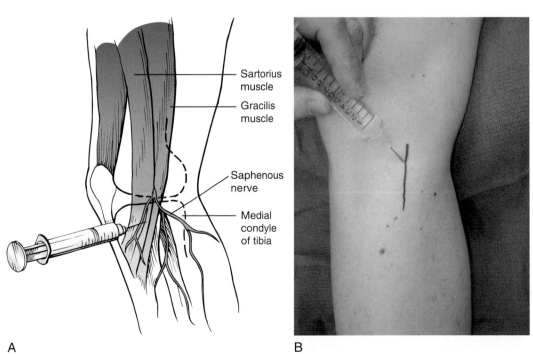

Sartorius muscle
Gracilis muscle
Saphenous nerve
Medial condyle of tibia

A   B

Figure 5–10 **A,** Location of the saphenous nerve at the knee. **B,** The anesthetic agent is injected into the subcutaneous region a fingerbreadth below the medial joint line in an anterior-to-posterior direction.

If the surgeon is experienced with the techniques of peripheral nerve block, a collaborative effort is possible. In some cases, the surgeon performs the block and the anesthesiologist supplies sedation or supplemental anesthesia. Other times the anesthesiologist blocks the next patient while the surgeon is operating. This can facilitate a quick turnover and better ensure an adequate block.

Both the surgeon and the patient need to reach a certain comfort level for the surgical procedure to be successful. Some patients are excessively anxious despite their desire to remain awake. Some surgeons don't have any interest in conversing with the patient during the procedure. If the patient cannot remain stationary or the surgeon is distracted, the surgical results might be compromised. With multiple personal, professional, and institutional variables, there is no one formula that is correct or optimal. The goal should be to create an environment that promotes safety and comfort for the patient pre-, intra-, and postoperatively.

Strict adherence to preoperative fasting guidelines is necessary for regional anesthetic techniques. If the peripheral block is unsuccessful or incomplete, additional sedation or conversion to a general anesthetic may be necessary. Prior to the anesthetic injection, an intravenous line is started so that a sedative may be administered. Preoperative sedation and intraoperative narcotics (fentanyl citrate [Sublimaze], midazolam [Versed], and diazepam [Valium]) can be used to achieve adequate patient relaxation. Prophylactic antibiotics may also be administered intravenously. Intravenous access is also important in case of hypersensitivity reactions, allergic reactions, or other complications.

Cardiopulmonary resuscitation equipment should be available in case of a severe complication. The operating physician and anesthesiologist must be prepared for an allergic reaction to the anesthetic agent, which can require rapid and definitive treatment. Seizures can occur after an intravascular injection or can occur later from high blood levels; peak absorption is usually approximately 30 minutes after injection.

Choice of Anesthetic Agent

The choice of local anesthetic agent depends on many factors, including the desired time of onset and the duration of anesthesia.

Bupivacaine

Sarrafian[52,53] recommends 0.5% bupivacaine (Marcaine). When 0.5% bupivacaine without epinephrine was used, Sarrafian injected an average volume of up to 25 mL in each foot but cautioned not to exceed a total of 40 mL of 0.5% bupivacaine when bilateral

blocks were performed. Beskin and Baxter[8] used a mixture of 1% lidocaine and 0.25% bupivacaine. When this mixture is used, they recommend a maximum dose of lidocaine of 3 mg/kg of body weight. With a 1:1 mixture, the maximum dose would be 50% or less of each medication, inasmuch as they are mixed in a combined ratio of 1:1. Adriani[1] has recommended a maximum dose of 500 mg of lidocaine within a 24-hour period. Epinephrine delays absorption of the anesthetic agent and can allow increased dosing at the time of injection but does not appear to lengthen the anesthetic time. A dilute concentration of epinephrine (1:200,000) added to bupivacaine reduces absorption, and thus a slightly larger total dose can be used. Casati et al[13] found that there was no difference in the anesthesia obtained with 20 mL of 0.5% bupivacaine or 0.5% levobupivacaine. The time of onset and duration of anesthesia were the same for each anesthetic. Routinely, we do not add epinephrine to the mixture for foot and ankle blocks.

Ribotsky et al[47] investigated mixing of anesthetic agents and the efficacy of anesthesia. In evaluating a 1:1 mixture of lidocaine and bupivacaine, they determined that there was no significant difference in the mean onset time of anesthesia and no significant difference in the duration of anesthesia between plain lidocaine and the mixture of bupivacaine and lidocaine. They concluded that there was no clinical advantage in using a mixture of lidocaine and bupivacaine. Ptaszek et al[46] concluded that a mixture of different anesthetic agents can produce unpredictable results. Hernandez et al,[32] in a similar study in which a combination of lidocaine and bupivacaine was used, observed that the onset was similar to that of bupivacaine, thus contradicting Ribotsky's findings.[47] Neither author recommended a mixture of anesthetic agents.

Myerson et al[43] recommended that if surgery were imminent, equal volumes of 0.5% bupivacaine and 1% lidocaine should be used. They recommended that the maximum safe dose of lidocaine without epinephrine should not exceed 4.5 mg/kg of body weight and in general did not recommend a maximum dose greater than 300 mg (i.e., for a 70-kg adult, 30 mL of 1% lidocaine). They also recommended that a maximum safe dose of bupivacaine without epinephrine should not exceed 2.5 mg/kg of body weight (i.e., for a 70 kg adult, a maximum dose of approximately 175 mg, or 35 mL of 0.5% bupivacaine). In our practice, we use a maximum of 2.0 mg/kg of body weight, or 3.0 mg/kg when mixed with epinephrine. The addition of epinephrine decreases systemic absorption so that higher doses are possible.

When using bupivacaine, we prefer to use a maximum dose of bupivacaine without epinephrine

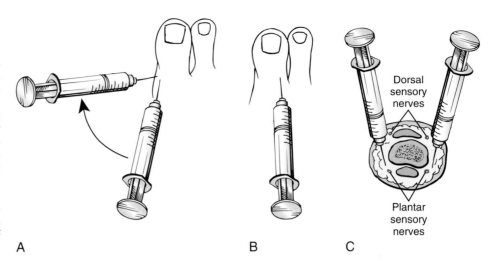

Figure 5–11 Digital block. Anesthesia of the toe usually is achieved with injection of 1% lidocaine hydrochloride. **A,** Initially a medial wheal is raised in the skin. The needle is advanced in a dorsoplantar direction. It is then turned horizontally, and the dorsum of the toe is blocked. **B,** The second wheal is raised on the lateral aspect of the toe, and then a dorsoplantar injection is performed. **C,** Cross section of the toe demonstrates the path of the needles.

not exceeding 2.0 mg/kg of body weight and 3.0 mg/kg when using bupivacaine with epinephrine. Myerson et al[43] suggested that a maximum safe dose of 1% lidocaine with epinephrine should not exceed 7 mg/kg of body weight (i.e., for a 70-kg adult, a dose of 50 mL of 1% lidocaine with epinephrine, or 500 mg). With a 1:1 ratio mixture of lidocaine and bupivacaine, they noted that a maximum safe dose would be limited to 15 mL of 1% lidocaine and 17.5 mL of 0.5% bupivacaine.

Ropivacaine

Ropivacaine (Naropin) has been used extensively in the clinical practice and investigations of popliteal sciatic block.* Compared with bupivacaine, ropivacaine has an anesthetic potency that is clinically equivalent with respect to sensory anesthesia but that is slightly less potent with respect to motor block when used in lower concentrations (0.2% or less).[21] The addition of epinephrine has not been shown to prolong the duration of ropivacaine. Adding clonidine (Duraclon) (0.1 μg/kg) to ropivacaine[15,21,49] can extend duration of anesthesia by 20%.[59] The onset of action is slightly longer than fast-onset local anesthetics such as mepivacaine.[57] The duration of anesthesia and analgesia is comparable to bupivacaine's and has been reported to last 16 to 19 hours.[13,14,24,49,55] The main advantage of ropivacaine is a more favorable toxicity profile than bupivacaine.

The dosage in adults for peripheral nerve block infiltration is 10 to 40 mL of 0.75% ropivacaine or 75 to 250 mg. Infiltration of 30 mL of 0.75% administers 225 mg of ropivacaine. Cumulative doses of up to 800 mg over a 24-hour period for surgery and postoperative pain have been well tolerated in adults in clinical studies.[41] The direct myocardial toxicity is substantially less than that of bupivicaine.[49] A dose of 30 mL of 0.75% ropivacaine has been shown to provide reliable extended analgesia with very low toxicity.[24,58] One identifiable disadvantage is the substantially increased cost over readily available and inexpensive agents.

Digital Block

Many toenail and lesser toe surgical procedures may be performed after administration of a digital 1% lidocaine HCl anesthetic block (Fig. 5–11).[39]

DIGITAL NERVE BLOCK

Technique

1. A small wheal is raised in the skin with the anesthetic agent on the dorsomedial aspect of the toe at its base. The dorsomedial and plantar medial sensory nerves are anesthetized as the needle is directed vertically from the dorsal to the plantar surface of the toe.
2. The needle then is withdrawn into the subcutaneous tissue and is turned in a horizontal lateral direction. The dorsal aspect of the toe is then infiltrated with the anesthetic agent.
3. The needle is withdrawn, and another wheal is raised on the dorsolateral aspect of the base of the toe. The dorsolateral and plantar lateral digital nerves are then anesthetized by a vertical injection on the lateral aspect of the toe.

---

*References 13, 16, 22, 24, 49, 57, 58, and 60.

Other Considerations

It is important to use an anesthetic agent without epinephrine (a vasoconstrictor agent). For the hallux, often 3 to 5 mL of 1% lidocaine is used for a complete toe block; for a lesser toe block, considerably less volume is used.[39] The onset of anesthesia is relatively rapid, depending on the anesthetic agent used.

Ankle Block

The number of peripheral nerves that need to be blocked depends on the location and the magnitude of the surgery. It may be reasonable to block only the nerves expected to innervate the operative field. The use of a tourniquet at the level of the ankle may be better tolerated with a complete ankle block. The success of an ankle block usually depends on satisfactorily anesthetizing the tibial nerve. The superficial peroneal, sural, and saphenous nerves all lie in the subcutaneous plane and can be easily anesthetized by a generous ring-type block about the anterior ankle. The failure of peripheral blocks often can be attributed to impatience in commencing an operative procedure in a situation where there has been inadequate time for the peripheral nerve block to take effect (see video clip 46).

POSTERIOR TIBIAL NERVE BLOCK

The posterior tibial nerve provides sensation to the plantar aspect of the foot.

Technique

1. For a posterior tibial nerve block, the patient is positioned on his or her side with the nonsurgical leg inferior. An alternative may be to externally rotate the leg to place the posterior medial ankle in a more accessible position. The surgical leg is positioned on a pillow or on two or three towels to improve the exposure of the injection site. The knee is flexed approximately 45 degrees, and the ankle is dorsiflexed slightly or held in a neutral position.
2. The tip of the medial malleolus is marked, and at a point two fingerbreadths proximal to the tip of the medial malleolus, a horizontal line is drawn to mark the level of the injection to anesthetize the posterior tibial nerve. At this level, the posterior tibial nerve is just posterior to the tibial shaft and is directly beneath the medial border of the Achilles tendon (Fig. 5–12).
3. A 25-gauge needle, 1½ inches (38 mm) long, is used for the anesthetic injection.[19] Paresthesias are elicited occasionally but not routinely. It is not mandatory that paresthe-

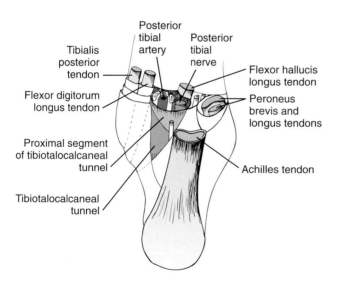

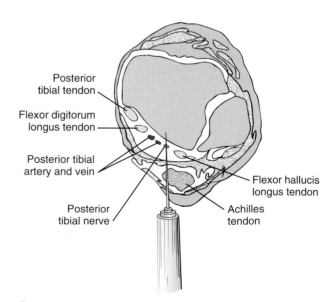

A

B

Figure 5–12   Proximal segment of tibial calcaneal tunnel. **A,** Injection site of posterior tibial neurovascular tunnel. **B,** Cross section of tibia at the level of the ankle shows the posterior tibial nerve to be in a direct line with the medial border of the Achilles tendon. It is 2 to 3 mm superficial to the posterior cortex of the tibia.

sias be elicited in order to proceed with the injection. A nerve stimulator may be used to locate the posterior tibial nerve (Fig. 5–13).[65] A nerve stimulator might not be helpful if used in a patient with prior nerve injury, motor dysfunction, or paralysis because it requires active motor function.[30,50] From a clinical standpoint, following a peripheral nerve block, the concomitant sympathetic block obtains both cessation of sweating and a vasodilation of the superficial skin with increased skin temperature.[40]

4. The needle is inserted on the medial border of the Achilles tendon and advanced perpendicular to the tibial shaft until the tip of the needle touches the posterior cortex of the tibia (Fig. 5–14). Then the needle is withdrawn 2 to 3 mm. Aspiration is attempted to ensure that the injection will not be made into an adjacent artery or vein. In the absence of blood return, the anesthetic agent is then injected. Five to 10 mL of 0.5% bupivacaine is injected into the region of the posterior tibial nerve.[52,53]

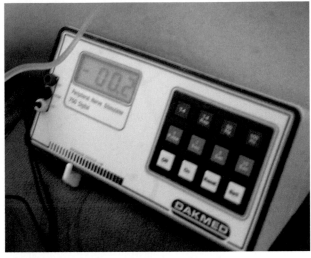

Figure 5–13 A peripheral nerve stimulator is attached to an insulated needle for use with the popliteal block.

SUPERFICIAL PERONEAL NERVE BLOCK

The superficial peroneal nerve supplies sensation to the dorsum of the foot. The branches of the superficial peroneal nerve are anesthetized with a superficial block in a ring fashion. Before the injection, if there is not significant subcuta-

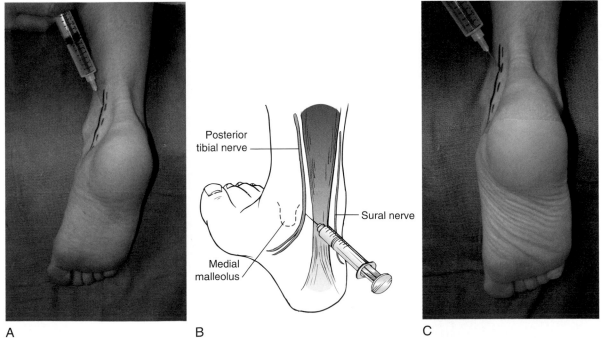

A   B   C

Figure 5–14 **A,** Injection technique of posterior tibial nerve. The needle is directed along the medial border of the Achilles tendon and directed toward the tibia. **B,** Schematic diagram of injection technique. **C,** Technique of posterior tibial nerve injection. *Colored area* on the foot marks the area of anesthesia.

neous adipose tissue, one may demonstrate the branches just beneath the skin by having the patient plantar flex and invert the foot.

Technique

1. A 25-gauge needle is used for the anesthetic injection. The needle penetrates the skin at a level two fingerbreadths proximal to the tip of the lateral malleolus (Fig. 5–15).
2. The anesthetic agent is infiltrated subcutaneously from lateral to medial. Often three or four injection sites are used to carry out the ring type of block. Five to 10 mL of 0.5% bupivacaine is used for the block.

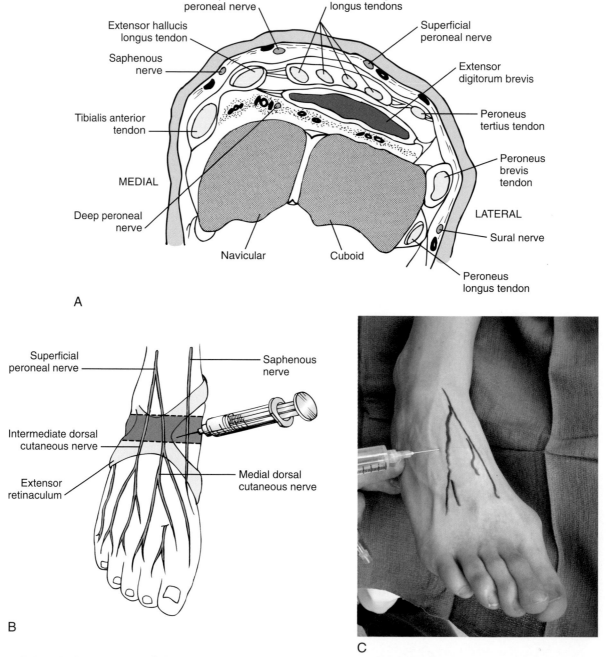

Figure 5–15 A, Cross section of the right foot passing through the navicular and cuboid joint demonstrates the anatomy encountered in a ring block of the midfoot. **B,** Technique of injection of the superficial peroneal nerve. **C,** Technique of injection of the superficial peroneal nerve. *Colored area* denotes area of anesthesia.

3. The injection is carried out deep to the sub-cutaneous veins but superficial to the long extensor tendons. Again, care must be taken to avoid an intravascular injection.

DEEP PERONEAL NERVE BLOCK

The deep peroneal nerve provides sensation to the first web space.

Technique

1. The patient is placed in a supine position for the injection. The patient is asked to dorsi-flex the hallux, and the tendon of the extensor hallucis longus is marked on the dorsum of the foot (Fig. 5–16). Then the patient is requested to dorsiflex the lesser toes, and the medial border of the extensor digitorum longus tendon is marked; the dorsalis pedis artery is palpated and marked as well.

2. In the interval between the extensor digitorum longus and the extensor hallucis longus on the lateral border of the dorsalis pedis artery lies the deep peroneal nerve. It is deep to the extensor retinaculum. A 25-gauge needle is used to anesthetize the nerve. The needle is advanced to the underlying tarsal bone and then withdrawn 2 mm.

3. Aspiration is attempted to ensure that the injection is not made into the adjacent artery or vein. Five milliliters of 0.5% bupivacaine is injected into this region.

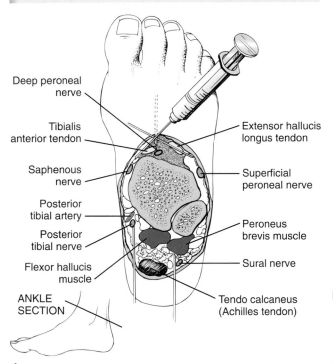

Deep peroneal nerve

Tibialis anterior tendon

Saphenous nerve

Posterior tibial artery

Posterior tibial nerve

Flexor hallucis muscle

ANKLE SECTION

Extensor hallucis longus tendon

Superficial peroneal nerve

Peroneus brevis muscle

Sural nerve

Tendo calcaneus (Achilles tendon)

A

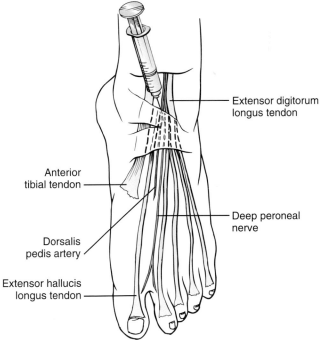

Extensor digitorum longus tendon

Anterior tibial tendon

Dorsalis pedis artery

Extensor hallucis longus tendon

Deep peroneal nerve

B

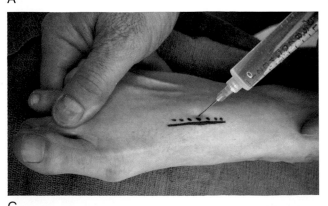

C

Figure 5–16 **A** and **B,** Technique of block of the deep peroneal nerve. The nerve is in the interval between the extensor hallucis longus tendon and the extensor digitorum longus tendon just to the lateral aspect of the dorsalis pedis artery. **C,** Technique of deep peroneal nerve block. The nerve is located just on the lateral border of the dorsalis pedis artery. *Colored area* denotes area of anesthesia.

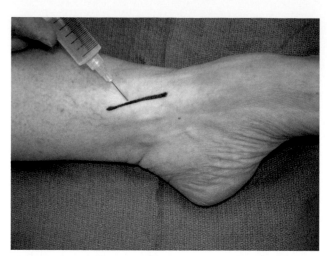

Figure 5–17   Technique of block of the saphenous nerve at the ankle. Often the saphenous nerve can be palpated just anterior to the medial malleolus. It is often blocked in a ring fashion when the superficial peroneal nerve is blocked. *Colored area* denotes area of anesthesia.

SAPHENOUS NERVE BLOCK AT THE ANKLE

The saphenous nerve provides sensation to the medial midfoot and the area adjacent to the medial malleolus.

Technique

1. The saphenous nerve is located two finger-breadths proximal to the tip of the medial malleolus and one fingerbreadth anterior to the medial malleolus (Fig. 5–17). The nerve often can be palpated just posterior to the saphenous vein.
2. A 25-gauge needle is used for infiltrating the anesthetic agent. Care is taken to avoid injection into the saphenous vein. Three milliliters of the anesthetic agent is injected into the subcutaneous tissue in a transverse fashion from posterior to anterior.

SURAL NERVE BLOCK

The sural nerve provides sensation to the lateral border of the forefoot. The sural nerve is found 1 to 1½ cm distal to the tip of the fibula[37] and can be palpated if there is not significant subcutaneous adipose tissue. If surgery is confined to the medial aspect of the foot, the sural nerve may not need to be anesthetized. If lateral fore-

foot surgery is contemplated, a sural nerve block is appropriate.

Technique

1. The sural nerve lies very superficially in the subcutaneous tissue. A 25-gauge needle is used for the anesthetic injection (Fig. 5–18).
2. An attempt is made to ensure that the injection is not made into an adjacent artery or vein. Three to 5 milliliters of the anesthetic agent is injected.

Alternative Site

Lawrence and Botte[37] found that the sural nerve was consistently located just adjacent to the peritenon of the Achilles tendon at a distance 7 cm proximal to the tip of the lateral malleolus, and this location is an alternative site for anesthetic injection for a sural nerve block.

Sciatic Nerve Block in the Thigh and the Leg

The sciatic nerve can be blocked in a number of areas as it descends posteriorly in the thigh.

POPLITEAL BLOCK

The *classic approach* to perform popliteal block posteriorly with the patient in a prone position. This can also be attempted with the patient in a lateral decubitus position. If the block is performed preoperatively, adjustment to a prone position is not usually difficult. If sedation is given, care must be taken that the airway can be accessed or managed while in a prone position. Turning a patient to a prone position postoperatively can be more challenging.

A *lateral approach* to blockade of the sciatic nerve in the region of the popliteal fossa is an alternative to the classic posterior approach. The efficacy of the lateral approach is clinically equivalent to the classic posterior approach. Although the onset of the block might be slower, the lateral approach has the advantage of supine positioning for the block.[57]

Blockade at the more proximal level is potentially advantageous because the common per-

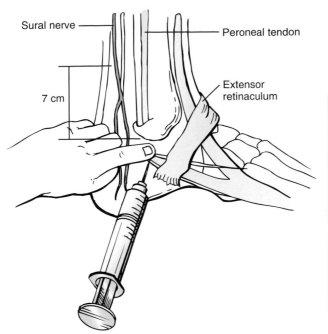

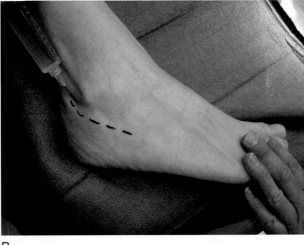

A   B

Figure 5–18 **A,** Technique of sural nerve block. The anesthetic agent is injected either one fingerbreadth below the tip of the fibula or 7 cm above the tip of the fibula. **B,** Technique of sural nerve block. *Colored area* denotes the area of anesthesia.

oneal and tibial nerves are either still within the common sheath or likely still in close proximity.[62] As one goes distal to the bifurcation in the popliteal fossa, separate injections of the tibial and peroneal components may be required to achieve a suitable anesthetic block. Anesthesiologists often employ the *subgluteal technique* for single injection blocks as well as catheter insertion for continuous sciatic nerve block. The insertion site for the subgluteal approach is posterior between the ischeal tuberosity and the greater trochanter. A *midfemoral approach* has also been described.

The sciatic nerve may be anesthetized in the *popliteal fossa* so that anesthesia is achieved in the distribution of both the common peroneal and tibial nerves and then over the posterior and anterior aspects of the ankle and the dorsal and plantar surfaces of the foot. This does not cover the distribution of the saphenous nerve, a terminal branch of the femoral nerve.[11,30] Procedures about the ankle and hindfoot require the saphenous nerve to be blocked separately. This can be done at the level of the ankle just medial and proximal to the medial malleolus (see Fig. 5–17). Alternatively, the saphenous nerve can be blocked at the level of the knee where it becomes superficial between the gracilis and

sartorius muscles along the pes anserine insertion (see Fig. 5–10)

The popliteal fossa is bordered superiorly by the semitendinous and semimembranous muscles on the medial aspect and the biceps femoris muscle on the lateral aspect. Inferiorly it is bordered medially and laterally by the muscle bellies of the gastrocnemius. At the knee flexion crease, a horizontal line bisects the popliteal space superiorly and inferiorly (Fig. 5–19). Bisecting this line again vertically in the midline creates four quadrants. The superior lateral quadrant is the area in which a popliteal sciatic block is placed. In this quadrant, the tibial and common peroneal nerves are present either separately or combined before bifurcation. The common peroneal nerve separates from the tibial nerve either at this level or more proximally in the popliteal fossa.

Classic Approach Technique

1. With the patient lying *prone* with the knee slightly flexed, a point is marked 5 cm superior to the posterior popliteal skin flexion crease and 1 cm lateral to the midline.
2. A 22-gauge insulated needle, 2 inches (5 cm) long, attached to a nerve stimulator is intro-

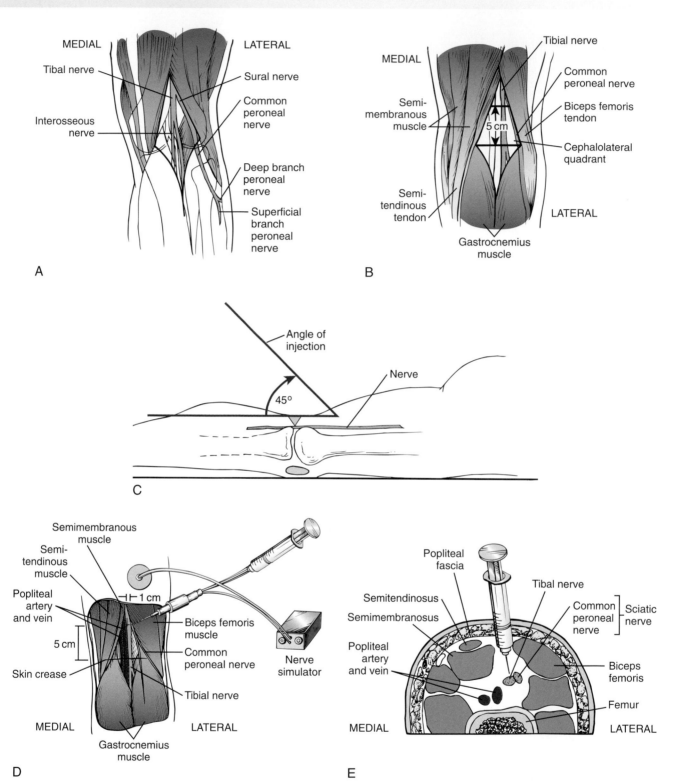

Figure 5–19 Technique of popliteal block. **A,** Anatomy of popliteal fossa. **B,** A horizontal line drawn at the posterior knee-flexion crease and a vertical line bisecting the popliteal fossa identify four quadrants. **C,** A needle is inserted at a 45-degree angle cephalad at a point 5 to 7 cm proximal to and 1 cm lateral to the midline. **D,** The common peroneal nerve may be anesthetized when anesthetic is injected more proximally or laterally in relation to the tibial nerve. **E,** Cross-sectional anatomic features of the popliteal fossa demonstrating the location of the tibial nerve and common peroneal nerve in the superior lateral quadrant.

duced and directed in an anterior superior direction at an angle of approximately 45 degrees. By angulating the needle at a 45-degree angle cephalad, one can place the nerve block in the region where the common peroneal nerve divides from the sciatic nerve. Thus, anesthesia of both terminal branches of the sciatic nerve can be achieved (Fig. 5–20).

3. The nerve is approached with output on the nerve stimulator of approximately 2 to 3 mA until either the toe flexors or the gastrocnemius and soleus twitch. The nerve stimulator intensity is then reduced to an output of 0.5 to 1.0 mA while the stimulator maintains muscle twitching. The use of a nerve stimulator allows accurate placement of a nerve block and decreases the need for additional

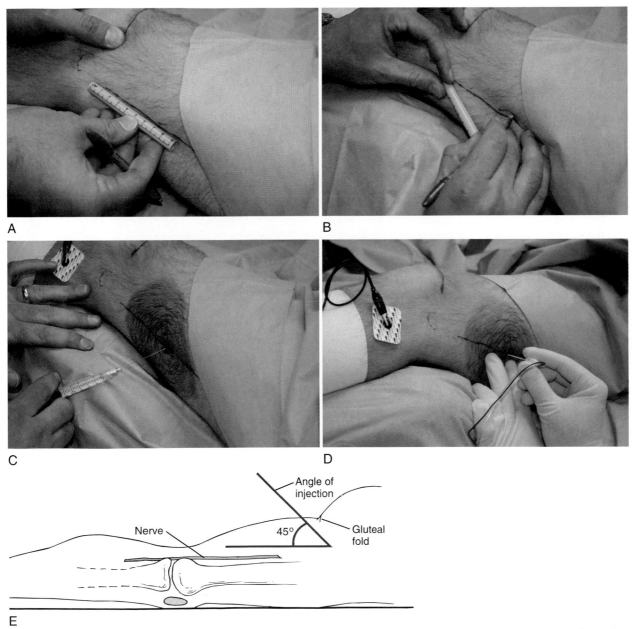

Figure 5–20 Sciatic block using lateral approach. **A** and **B,** The injection site is marked 9 to 10 cm above the femoral epicondyle. **C,** Local anesthesia prior to the nerve block. **D,** With the nerve stimulator attached to the needle, anesthetic is injected at the sciatic nerve. **E,** Alternatively, the sciatic nerve can be blocked more proximally at the gluteal crease (lateral decubitus position).

volume of the anesthetic agent. The lowest possible setting should be used to obtain a motor response so as to decrease the possibility of nerve damage.[61] Tibial nerve stimulation is a better predictor of a complete block than is peroneal stimulation alone.[7]

4. A double injection technique does not require an additional needle insertion; rather the stimulating catheter can be slightly redirected, withdrawn, or advanced. Aspiration of the syringe is necessary to ensure that an intravascular injection is avoided. Thirty milliliters of the chosen local anesthetic is then injected. Repeat aspiration should be performed if the needle has been repositioned.

Lateral Approach Technique

The landmark for insertion from the *lateral approach* is between the biceps femoris and the vastus lateralis muscles (Fig. 5–20 A-D). This can typically be palpated in line with the lateral femoral epicondyle.

1. The leg is extended or just slightly flexed. The long axis of the foot is positioned at 90 degrees to the table. The level of injection is approximately 7 cm cephalad to the most prominent point of the lateral femoral epicondyle.
2. The needle (with attached nerve stimulator) is directed posteromedially at an angle of approximately 30 degrees. The common peroneal nerve is encountered first, given the more lateral position. Further advancement or redirection, or both, of the needle more posteriorly will elicit tibial nerve stimulation. An effort should be made to elicit tibial nerve stimulation in preference to peroneal nerve stimulation because this, again, is a better predictor of a complete block of the foot.[7]
3. Ropivacaine or bupivacaine with epinephrine is then injected. Alternatively, separate injections of the tibial and peroneal branches can be performed with 10 to 15 mL of anesthetic agent.

Lateral Midfemoral Approach Technique

The landmarks for the *lateral midfemoral approach* are the posterior aspect of the greater trochanter and the lateral femoral epicondyle. An injection site halfway between the greater trochanter and the lateral femoral epicondyle allows stimulation of the sciatic nerve. The onset of anesthesia for this more proximal lateral approach may be faster and durations of the sensory and motor block may be similar.[60] Again, at this more proximal level, the tibial and common peroneal components are likely juxtaposed. Another potential advantage is that the risk of vascular puncture or injection is lower because the vessels are much farther medial at this level.

Lateral Decubitus Approach Technique

Alternatively, a sciatic nerve block can be performed with the patient in a lateral decubitus position. The sciatic nerve is localized 2 to 3 inches below the gluteal fold just lateral to the midline. A similar technique of localization and infiltration is used as described earlier (Fig. 5–20E).

Supine Approach Technique

Vloka and coworkers[63] and others[28,45] have blocked the sciatic nerve with the patient in a supine position and found this position to be easily used as well. When combined with a saphenous nerve block, this technique provides excellent anesthesia in the forefoot and hindfoot.

1. With the patient in the supine position, the leg is flexed both at the knee and the hip.
2. Following identification of the popliteal fossa landmarks, an insulated needle attached to a peripheral nerve stimulator is inserted 7 cm above the popliteal crease and directed 45 degrees cephalad.
3. The clinician injects 30 to 40 mL of local anaesthetica solution.

General Considerations After Peripheral Nerve Block

The average time from injection of a peripheral block to onset of anesthesia is 15 to 20 minutes.[48,52] The efficacy of the anesthetic block can be checked with a needle point or sharp pin (Fig. 5–21A). This technique, however, can break the skin surface, leaving numerous pinprick sites. A peripheral nerve stimulator (routinely used by anesthesiologists to check temporal muscle relaxation with general anesthesia before intubation)

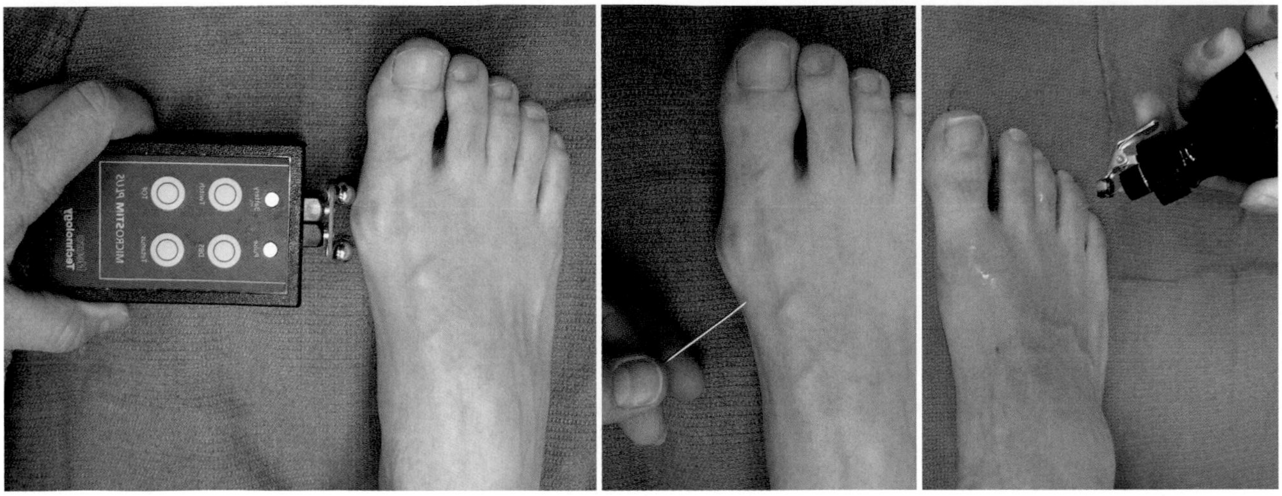

A   B   C

Figure 5–21 Method of checking efficacy of anesthesia. **A,** Peripheral nerve stimulator is used to check efficacy of anesthesia. **B,** Stimulator does not break the skin as a needle often does. **C,** Ethyl chloride spray can be used to test perception of cold and efficacy of nerve block.

provides an excellent stimulus to check the onset of anesthesia (Fig. 5–21B). The device emits a single impulse or continuous impulses that are sensed as a "shock" on unanesthetized skin. With successful sensory anesthesia, the patient does not detect the impulses. Ethyl chloride can also be used in an awake patient to test for perception of cold (Fig. 5–21C), because absence of cold sensation is also an indication of a successful peripheral block.

After a peripheral nerve block is administered, the patient is transported to the operating suite. After completion of the skin preparation and draping, adequate anesthesia is routinely obtained. Sarrafian et al[53] and others[43] have reported a 94% to 95% success rate with peripheral blocks using similar techniques. Depending upon the technique, a popliteal block can take some time to reach maximum anesthetic efficacy. This can, on occasion, occur after the patient leaves the postanesthetic recovery area.

Local anesthetic supplementation can be used intraoperatively to augment an incomplete or evolving peripheral nerve block. Assuming that the maximum dose of local anesthetic has not been met or exceeded, a local field block with bupivacaine can be used. For example, an intra-articular injection can be used at the completion of an ankle arthroscopy following closure of the portals. A supplemental ring block around the anterior aspect of the ankle can ensure anesthetic coverage of the saphenous nerve. For forefoot procedures, a superficial ring block across the midfoot, along with a dorsal intermetatarsal injection directed plantarly to block the common digital nerve in the adjacent rays, is effective. Proximal intermetatarsal injection allows instillation of a greater volume than could be safely achieved at the base of the toe. This helps to prevent unnecessary swelling of the toe or vascular embarrassment secondary to the volume of the injection. If the procedure has been performed with sedation or general anesthesia, it is important that the patient emerge with as little pain as possible. The addition of supplemental local anesthetic can prove to be the difference between an ambulatory experience and an unexpected admission for management of postoperative pain.

As an alternative to a peripheral block, or if a peripheral block has been ineffective, local anesthetic can be instilled in the wound before wound closure. Bourne and Johnson[10] instilled 0.5% bupivacaine into open wounds before closure after foot and ankle surgery. They reported effective pain relief that was long lasting after surgery. Pain was significantly reduced up to 24 hours after surgery following bathing of the open wounds with 0.5% bupivacaine.

Contraindications, Complications, and Results

The volume and dosage of an anesthetic agent should be carefully calculated before injection to prevent administering an excessive amount. Although foot blocks can require a significant volume of anesthetic agent, when 0.5% bupivacaine HCl is administered, the average volume injected is 20 to 25 mL per foot. When bilateral blocks are administered, the total volume of anesthetic agent should not exceed 40 mL for both feet.[52] In calculating the dose of bupivacaine or any other anesthetic agent, one should consider patients with known liver disease because many anesthetic agents are metabolized by the liver.

In a report by Myerson et al,[43] one case of lidocaine toxicity in 353 patients occurred. Adverse reactions after lidocaine injection include central nervous system irritation (restlessness, nervousness, dizziness, confusion, tremors, and convulsions). Cardiovascular manifestations include bradycardia, hypotension, and ventricular arrhythmias. Bupivacaine toxicity is similar to lidocaine toxicity, with central nervous system and cardiac irregularities. Sensitivity may be attributable to the local anesthetic agent or to methylparaben, an antimicrobial agent used to preserve the lidocaine in multiple-dose vials.

Rongstad, Mann, et al[48] reported on 86 patients who had a sciatic–popliteal block after major foot or ankle surgery. The duration of the block averaged 20 hours. No complications were noted, and 95% of patients were satisfied with the pain relief afforded. The authors noted that often a period of analgesia persists even after the return of sensation after a popliteal block. They recommended a dose of 30 mL of 0.5% bupivacaine for a popliteal block and noted this contained only 150 mg of bupivacaine, well below the recommended single maximum dose of 225 mg. They further noted that the recommended daily maximum dose of 400 mg of bupivacaine allowed a second popliteal block within a 24-hour period before discharge from the ambulatory care unit. The efficacy and safety of this technique has been confirmed by a number of investigators.[40,44,52] The reliability of obtaining a suitable block has been correlated with the concentration and volume of injection, double injection techniques, the type of evoked motor response, and the intensity at which stimulation can be achieved.

Sarrafian[52] suggests that foot and ankle edema may be a contraindication to peripheral anesthesia. In this situation and in patients with a large foot with significant subcutaneous tissue, a spinal needle may be necessary to block the posterior tibial nerve.

Needoff et al,[44] in a prospective randomized, controlled trial, evaluated the analgesia provided by an ankle block in a patient placed under general anesthesia to evaluate the postoperative pain relief after forefoot surgery. They observed that there was a significant difference in postoperative analgesia and concluded that an ankle block is a useful addition to general anesthesia. They used a solution of 0.5% bupivacaine and reported excellent pain relief at 6 hours but found that there was no significant difference at 24 hours after surgery. They reported no significant complications with an ankle block.

Mathies et al[40] reported their experience with a sciatic block in 340 patients undergoing surgery for rheumatoid forefoot deformity. A 92% success rate was reported. When blocks were unsuccessful, supplementary anesthesia was obtained with a femoral nerve block, local anesthetic, or reblocking of the sciatic nerve.

Singelyn et al[56] reported a 92% success rate using a popliteal sciatic block in 507 patients. The sciatic nerve was approached at the apex of the popliteal fossa in the midline using a peripheral nerve stimulator to isolate the sciatic nerve. Ninety-five percent of patients were completely satisfied with the technique of peripheral anesthesia.

Medicino et al[42] and others[30] have used a combination of sciatic popliteal blocks with a proximal saphenous nerve block. This technique appears to have several advantages because it achieves excellent anesthesia during the operation and for a mean duration of 10 hours postoperatively, it permits the use of a proximal calf tourniquet if the surgeon wishes, and it avoids the systemic complications sometimes associated with general , spinal, or epidural anesthesia.

Unless contraindicated, the surgical procedure is performed with an ankle tourniquet. An Esmarch bandage is used to exsanguinate the foot and is then used as a tourniquet. Sterile padding may be placed beneath the Esmarch tourniquet. Although initially the patient may complain of discomfort with an Esmarch tourniquet, this discomfort usually subsides over time. Intravenous sedation may be used to decrease discomfort.

TOURNIQUET USE

Bleeding into the local soft tissues can distort soft tissue dissection and lead to prolongation of the surgical procedure. A tourniquet is not intended as an alternative to surgical hemostasis. Liberal use of electrocautery or clamps in an attempt to achieve visualization can cause inadvertent injury to adjacent neurologic structures. When used properly and judiciously, neurovascular identification and safe hemostasis can be achieved. In the dysvascular extremity, a tourniquet is typically not needed nor advised. Caution should also be exercised in patients with known vasospasm or Raynaud syndrome.

If a tourniquet is to be used, the type employed varies depending on the nature of the surgical procedure, the type of anesthetic, and the surgeon's preference. For brief digital or toenail procedures, a small

5/16-inch Penrose drain can be applied at the base of the toe. Most procedures of the forefoot and midfoot can be performed with a tourniquet applied at the level of the ankle.

Certain procedures require tensioning of soft tissue or critical evaluation of foot position that could be altered or obscured with a tourniquet at the level of the ankle. Procedures of this nature as well as those around the ankle and hindfoot might require the use of a pneumatic tourniquet applied about the thigh. Patients with a limited regional nerve block of the lower extremity might not tolerate a tourniquet applied about the thigh without the use of supplemental analgesia or anesthesia.

Esmarch Bandages

Johann Friederich August von Esmarch described the use of a flat rubber bandage for use as a peripheral tourniquet in 1873.[27] Although Klenermann[36] and Bruner[12] have cautioned against the use of an Esmarch bandage, stating either that such bandages were unsafe or that pneumatic tourniquets were the treatment of choice, Biehl et al[9] found few or no problems with the use of an Esmarch tourniquet. In their evaluation of 3-inch and 4-inch Esmarch bandages wrapped circumferentially with both three and four wraps, they consistently demonstrated tourniquet pressures in the range of 200 to 300 mm Hg. They reported no significant difference in the magnitude or consistency of the pressure generated with the Esmarch bandage between experienced and inexperienced wrappers of the tourniquet. They concluded that generally safe and reliable pressures could be achieved with either 3-inch or 4-inch Esmarch bandages applied circumferentially around the ankle.

They recommended some form of padding between the tourniquet and limb and found that either stockinette, a sterile towel, or cast padding could be used. They also emphasized that resterilization of Esmarch bandages could change the efficacy as well as the pressure achieved. They advocated presterilized latex rubber Esmarch tourniquets designed for single use. They also noted that the leg diameter and amount of subcutaneous soft tissue can make a difference in the pressures achieved.

Grebing and Coughlin[27] reported on a comprehensive evaluation of the Esmarch bandage used as a supramalleolar tourniquet. In this study, 10 foot-and-ankle surgeons wrapped 4-inch and 6-inch bandages at the ankle. The average pressure beneath the tourniquet for the 10 surgeons over several trials using three circumferential wraps and a tuck was 222 mm Hg. With four circumferential wraps and a tuck, the average pressure beneath the tourniquet was 288 mm Hg. There was no

significant difference whether the surgeon stood or sat. When cast padding was used, there was no different in the tourniquet pressure; however, there was a significant pressure drop when a padded towel was used beneath the tourniquet. Biehl et al[9] emphasized that not all Esmarch bandages are the same. In fact, they may be white, brown, or blue and come in different thickness and apparent elasticity. Nonetheless, Grebing and Coughlin,[27] in evaluating several different types of these bandages, reported that there was no difference among different types of 6-inch Esmarchs.

Grebing and Coughlin[27] also collected data on the experience of the different surgeons in their study who used the Esmarch bandage as a tourniquet. When interviewed about complication rates, the 10 surgeons estimated they had performed almost 11,000 surgical procedures with a complication rate of 0.1%. Thus, the practice of using a 6-inch Esmarch bandage as a tourniquet at the ankle level for forefoot surgery is a safe and reliable method. Although pressures obtained varied among surgeons, the average pressure was noted to be in an effective and safe range.

POSTOPERATIVE PAIN CONTROL

Continuous popliteal block with the use of an indwelling catheter has become an alternative to single-injection popliteal blocks. This potentially expands the number and types of procedures that can be performed on an ambulatory basis. In addition to being used for postoperative analgesia in the hospital, continuous postoperative pain control at home with infusion devices has received attention. Improvements in technique, including the use of stimulating catheters, can help to encourage more widespread use of this technique. For procedures that require the use of a tourniquet about the thigh, more proximal placement of the catheter is likely to be required if it is to be placed preoperatively.

Macaire et al[38] reported on the use of continuous perineural analgesia following a popliteal sciatic block or posterior tibial nerve block at the ankle. The analgesic catheter was inserted prior to surgery with assistance of a nerve stimulator. Following an injection with mepivacaine, appropriate surgery was performed under regional anesthesia. Postoperatively, an elastomeric pump delivered 0.2% ropivacaine at a rate of 5 mL/h. Twenty-one posterior tibial nerve blocks and 24 popliteal sciatic blocks were performed. No major complications occurred, pain was dramatically reduced with the continuous infusion, and a high level of patient satisfaction was reported. The authors concluded that continuous postoperative perineural analgesia in an outpatient setting was safe and effective and less expensive than hospitalization.

Ilfeld et al[33] investigated the efficacy of regional analgesia administered using a sciatic perineural catheter in the popliteal fossa with the infusion of 0.2% ropivacaine administered with a portable infusion pump following lower extremity surgery. They reported marked relief of pain in comparison to a control group. di Benedetto et al[20] compared continuous sciatic blocks with an infusion catheter for both posterior popliteal blocks and a subgluteal approach. They reported that both approaches provided similar postoperative analgesia.

Clough et al[17] examined two groups of patients undergoing lower extremity surgery. Patients were assigned either to a group that only received general anesthesia or to a group that received general anesthesia and an anesthetic foot block. The researchers reported that although there was a delay in the onset of pain in the group that also received the peripheral block, there was no difference in either group in the number of pain pills taken, no difference in the pain score on the first or second postoperative day, and no difference in overall patient satisfaction. Thus, peripheral anesthesia might only delay the onset of eventual pain for many patients. On the other hand, it allows them to recover in the confines of a familiar environment, and the gradual onset or introduction of pain at the operative site allows them to commence the gradual introduction of time-release and rapid-onset oral analgesics.

SUMMARY

A peripheral anesthetic block can be advantageous in foot and ankle surgery. Preoperative evaluation and appropriate selection of patients for this technique are important. Careful preoperative and postoperative evaluation, planning, and organization are necessary to achieve patient comfort. The patient must be able to comply postoperatively in the management of his or her own care during the recovery process. Education of the patient regarding expectations as well as possible complications and routine postoperative treatment are important to ensure patient conformity and safety.

The use of peripheral nerve anesthesia is not difficult but does require that a surgeon or anesthesiologist be familiar with the pertinent neurovascular anatomy of the lower extremity. The prolonged anesthesia and analgesia that a peripheral nerve block provides can significantly diminish postoperative pain for many hours and afford significant patient comfort in the postoperative period.

Hadzic et al[29] reported in a survey of anesthesiologists in the United States that lower-extremity nerve blocks were underutilized. The success of peripheral anesthesia requires the interest and dedication of the anesthesia staff to achieve a routinely high success rate. Another alternative, although more time consuming, is for the foot and ankle surgeon to provide anesthesia for patients when the anesthesia staff is either uncomfortable with or not interested in providing peripheral blocks.

The use of peripheral anesthesia can improve the efficiency of the operating surgeon by diminishing the turnover time. Successful peripheral anesthesia requires the interest and cooperation of the involved anesthesiologist, though another option is for the operating surgeon to provide sedation and the anesthetic block without the involvement of an anesthetist or anesthesiologist.

REFERENCES

1. Adriani, J: Techniques and clinical applications. In Adriani J (ed): *Labat's Regional Anesthesia.* Philadelphia, WB Saunders, 1969.
2. American Academy of Orthopaedic Surgeons: JCAHO Universal Protocol for Eliminating Wrong Site, Wrong Procedure, Wrong Person Surgery. Available at http://www3.aaos.org/safety/protocol.htm (accessed February 20, 2006).
3. American Academy of Orthopaedic Surgeons: Advisory statement: Wrong-site surgery. Document number 1015. Rosemont, Ill, American Academy of Orthopaedic Surgeons, 2003. Available at http://www.aaos.org/wordhtml/papers/advistmt/1015.htm (accessed February 20, 2006).
4. American Society of Anesthesiologist Task Force on Preoperative Fasting: Practice guidelines for preoperative fasting and the use of pharmacologic agents to reduce the risk of pulmonary aspiration: Application to healthy patients undergoing elective procedures. *Anesthesiology* 90(3):896-905, 1999.
5. Barton D: Anesthesia for outpatients in outpatient surgery. In Hill G (ed): *Outpatient Surgery.* Philadelphia, WB Saunders, 1980.
6. Baxter DE, Thigpen CM: Heel pain—operative results. *Foot Ankle* 5(1):16-25, 1984.
7. Benzon HT, Kim C, Benzon HP, et al: Correlation between evoked motor response of the sciatic nerve and sensory blockade. *Anesthesiology* 87(3):547-552, 1997.
8. Beskin JL, Baxter DE: Regional anesthesia for ambulatory foot and ankle surgery. *Orthopedics* 10(1):109-111, 1987.
9. Biehl WC 3rd, Morgan JM, Wagner FW Jr, Gabriel RA: The safety of the Esmarch tourniquet. *Foot Ankle* 14(5):278-283, 1993.
10. Bourne MH, Johnson KA: Postoperative pain relief using local anesthetic instillation. *Foot Ankle* 8(6):350-351, 1988.
11. Brown D: Popliteal block. In Brown D: *Atlas of Regional Anesthesia.* Philadelphia, WB Saunders, 1992.
12. Bruner JM: Safety factors in the use of the pneumatic tourniquet for hemostasis in surgery of the hand. *J Bone Joint Surg Am* 33(A:1):221-224, 1951.
13. Casati A, Borghi B, Fanelli G, et al: A double-blinded, randomized comparison of either 0.5% levobupivacaine or 0.5% ropivacaine for sciatic nerve block. *Anesth Analg* 94(4):987-990, 2002.

14. Casati A, Chelly JE, Cerchierini E, et al: Clinical properties of levobupivacaine or racemic bupivacaine for sciatic nerve block. *J Clin Anesth* 14(2):111-114, 2002.

15. Casati A, Magistris L, Fanelli G, et al: Small-dose clonidine prolongs postoperative analgesia after sciatic–femoral nerve block with 0.75% ropivacaine for foot surgery. *Anesth Analg* 91(2):388-392, 2000.

16. Chelly JE, Greger J, Casati A, et al: Continuous lateral sciatic blocks for acute postoperative pain management after major ankle and foot surgery. *Foot Ankle Int* 23(8):749-752, 2002.

17. Clough TM, Sandher D, Bale RS, Laurence AS: The use of a local anesthetic foot block in patients undergoing outpatient bony forefoot surgery: A prospective randomized controlled trial. *J Foot Ankle Surg* 42(1):24-29, 2003.

18. Coughlin MJ: Ambulatory surgery of the foot. In Jahss MH (ed): *Disorders of the Foot and Ankle*, ed 2. Philadelphia, WB Saunders, 1991, pp 335-344.

19. Delgado-Martinez AD, Marchal-Escalona JM: Supramalleolar ankle block anesthesia and ankle tourniquet for foot surgery. *Foot Ankle Int* 22(10):836-838, 2001.

20. di Benedetto P, Casati A, Bertini L, et al: Postoperative analgesia with continuous sciatic nerve block after foot surgery: A prospective, randomized comparison between the popliteal and subgluteal approaches. *Anesth Analg* 94(4):996-1000, 2002.

21. Eledjam JJ, Ripart J, Viel E: Clinical application of ropivacaine for the lower extremity. *Curr Top Med Chem* 1(3):227-231, 2001.

22. Fanelli G, Casati A, Beccaria P, et al: A double-blind comparison of ropivacaine, bupivacaine, and mepivacaine during sciatic and femoral nerve blockade. *Anesth Analg* 87(3):597-600, 1998.

23. Ferguson LK (ed): *Surgery of the Ambulatory Patient*, ed 5. Philadelphia, Lippincott, 1974.

24. Fernandez-Guisasola J, Andueza A, Burgos E, et al: A comparison of 0.5% ropivacaine and 1% mepivacaine for sciatic nerve block in the popliteal fossa. *Acta Anaesthesiol Scand* 45(8):967-970, 2001.

25. Gould N, Alvarez R: Bilateral tarsal tunnel syndrome caused by varicosities. *Foot Ankle* 3(5):290-292, 1983.

26. Graham CE, Graham DM: Morton's neuroma: A microscopic evaluation. *Foot Ankle* 5(3):150-153, 1984.

27. Grebing BR, Coughlin MJ: Evaluation of the Esmarch bandage as a tourniquet for forefoot surgery. *Foot Ankle Int* 25(6):397-405, 2004.

28. Guardini R, Waldron BA, Wallace WA: Sciatic nerve block: A new lateral approach. *Acta Anaesthesiol Scand* 29(5):515-519, 1985.

29. Hadzic A, Vloka JD, Kuroda MM, et al: The practice of peripheral nerve blocks in the United States: A national survey [p2e comments]. *Reg Anesth Pain Med* 23(3):241-246, 1998.

30. Hansen E, Eshelman MR, Cracchiolo A 3rd: Popliteal fossa neural blockade as the sole anesthetic technique for outpatient foot and ankle surgery. *Foot Ankle Int* 21(1):38-44, 2000.

31. Harder S, Klinkhardt U, Alvarez JM: Avoidance of bleeding during surgery in patients receiving anticoagulant and/or antiplatelet therapy: Pharmacokinetic and pharmacodynamic considerations. *Clin Pharmacokinet* 43(14):963-981, 2004.

32. Hernandez PA, Lubitz JJ, Steinhart AN: Lidocaine and bupivacaine. Is a mixture effective? *J Am Podiatry Assoc* 73(10):510-513, 1983.

33. Ilfeld BM, Morey TE, Wang RD, Enneking FK: Continuous popliteal sciatic nerve block for postoperative pain control at home: A randomized, double-blinded, placebo-controlled study. *Anesthesiology* 97(4):959-965, 2002.

34. Jones JR, Klenerman L: A study of the communicating branch between the medial and lateral plantar nerves. *Foot Ankle* 4(6):313-315, 1984.

35. Kaye AD, Kucera I, Sabar R: Perioperative anesthesia clinical considerations of alternative medicines. *Anesthesiol Clin North Am* 22(1):125-139, 2004.

36. Klenerman L: Tourniquet paralysis. *J Bone Joint Surg Br* 65(4):374-375, 1983.

37. Lawrence SJ, Botte MJ: The sural nerve in the foot and ankle: An anatomic study with clinical and surgical implications. *Foot Ankle Int* 15(9):490-494, 1994.

38. Macaire P, Gaertner E, Capdevila X: Continuous post-operative regional analgesia at home. *Minerva Anestesiol* 67(9 Suppl 1):109-116, 2001.

39. Mann RA, Coughlin MJ: Nerve disorders. In Mann RA, Coughlin MJ (eds): *Video Textbook of Foot and Ankle Surgery*. St. Louis, Medical Video Productions, 1991.

40. Mathies B, Sjostrom K, Raunio P: Evaluation of 350 sciatic blocks in rheumatoid foot surgery. *Arch Orthop Unfallchir* 87(2):171-175, 1977.

41. McClellan KJ, Faulds D: Ropivacaine: An update of its use in regional anaesthesia. *Drugs* 60(5):1065-1093, 2000.

42. Mendicino RW, Statler TK, Catanzariti AR: Popliteal sciatic nerve blocks after foot and ankle surgery: An adjunct to postoperative analgesia. *J Foot Ankle Surg* 41(5):338-341, 2002.

43. Myerson MS, Ruland CM, Allon SM: Regional anesthesia for foot and ankle surgery. *Foot Ankle* 13(5):282-288, 1992.

44. Needoff M, Radford P, Costigan P: Local anesthesia for postoperative pain relief after foot surgery: A prospective clinical trial. *Foot Ankle Int* 16(1):11-13, 1995.

45. Pandin P, Vandesteene A, D'Hollander A: Sciatic nerve blockade in the supine position: A novel approach. *Can J Anaesth* 50(1):52-56, 2003.

46. Ptaszek AJ, Morris SG, Brodsky JW: Midfoot field block anesthesia with monitored intravenous sedation in forefoot surgery. *Foot Ankle Int* 20(9):583-586, 1999.

47. Ribotsky BM, Berkowitz KD, Montague JR: Local anesthetics. Is there an advantage to mixing solutions? *J Am Podiatr Med Assoc* 86(10):487-491, 1996.

48. Rongstad K, Mann RA, Prieskorn D, et al: Popliteal sciatic nerve block for postoperative analgesia. *Foot Ankle Int* 17(7):378-382, 1996.

49. Rudkin GE, Rudkin AK, Dracopoulos GC: Bilateral ankle blocks: A prospective audit. *Aust N Z J Surg* 75(1-2):39-42, 2005.

50. Sanchez-Tirado JA, Recio-Cabrero D, Carrion-Pareja JC, et al: [Constraints on the use of a nerve stimulator in peripheral conduction blocks when there is disturbance in the neuromuscular junction]. *Rev Esp Anestesiol Reanim* 47(1):39-42, 2000.

51. Sarrafian SK: Nerves. In Sarrafian SK (ed) *Anatomy of the Foot and Ankle*. Philadelphia, Lippincott, 1983.

52. Sarrafian SK: Regional anesthesia of the midfoot. In Jahss MH (ed): *Disorders of the Foot and Ankle*, ed 2. Philadelphia, WB Saunders, 1991, pp 329-334.

53. Sarrafian SK, Ibrahim IN, Breihan JH: Ankle–foot peripheral nerve block for mid and forefoot surgery. *Foot Ankle* 4(2):86-90, 1983.

54. Shurnas PS, Coughlin MJ: Recall of the risks of forefoot surgery after informed consent. *Foot Ankle Int* 24(12):904-908, 2003.

55. Sinardi D, Marino A, Chillemi S, et al: Static nerve block with lateral popliteal approach for hallux vagus correction. Comparison between 0.5% bupivacaine and 0.75% ropivacaine. *Minerva Anestesiol* 70(9):625-629, 2004.

56. Singelyn FJ, Gouverneur JM, Gribomont BF: Popliteal sciatic nerve block aided by a nerve stimulator: A reliable technique for foot and ankle surgery. *Reg Anesth* 16(5):278-281, 1991.

57. Taboada M, Alvarez J, Cortes J, et al: The effects of three different approaches on the onset time of sciatic nerve blocks with 0.75% ropivacaine. *Anesth Analg* 98(1):242-247, 2004.

58. Taboada M, Cortes J, Rodriguez J, et al: Lateral approach to the sciatic nerve in the popliteal fossa: A comparison between 1.5% mepivacaine and 0.75% ropivacaine. *Reg Anesth Pain Med* 28(6):516-520, 2003.

59. Thannikary L, Enneking K: Non-opioid additives to local anesthetics. *Tech Reg Anesth Pain Manag* 8:129-140, 2004.

60. Triado VD, Crespo MT, Aguilar JL, et al: A comparison of lateral popliteal versus lateral midfemoral sciatic nerve blockade using ropivacaine 0.5%. *Reg Anesth Pain Med* 29(1):23-27, 2004.

61. Vloka JD, Hadzic A: The intensity of the current at which sciatic nerve stimulation is achieved is a more important factor in determining the quality of nerve block than the type of motor response obtained. *Anesthesiology* 88(5):1408-1411, 1998.

62. Vloka JD, Hadzic A, April E, Thys DM: The division of the sciatic nerve in the popliteal fossa: Anatomical implications for popliteal nerve blockade. *Anesth Analg* 92(1):215-217, 2001.

63. Vloka JD, Hadzic A, Koorn R, Thys D: Supine approach to the sciatic nerve in the popliteal fossa. *Can J Anaesth* 43(9):964-967, 1996.

64. Wolf D, Ross W: The foot in outpatient surgery. In Hill G (ed): *Outpatient Surgery.* Philadelphia, WB Saunders, 1980.

65. Zahari DT, Englund K, Girolamo M: Peripheral nerve block with use of nerve stimulator. *J Foot Surg,* 29(2):162-163, 1990.

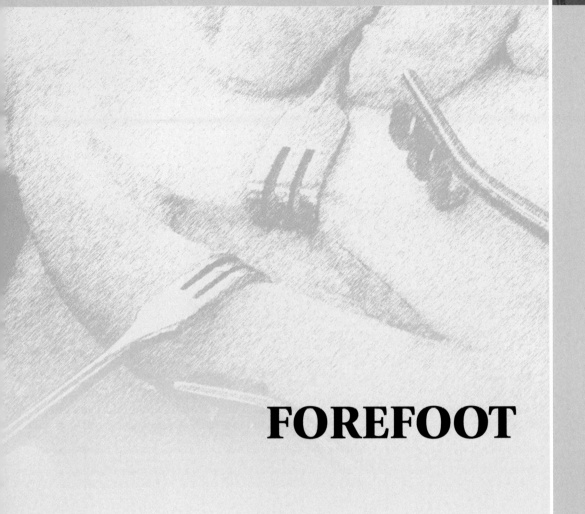

FOREFOOT

Hallux Valgus

Michael J. Coughlin • Roger A. Mann

INTRODUCTION

The term *bunion* is derived from the Latin word *bunio*, meaning turnip, which has led to some confusing misapplications in regard to disorders of the first metatarsophalangeal (MTP) joint. The word *bunion* has been used to denote any enlargement or deformity of the MTP joint, including such diverse diagnoses as an enlarged bursa, overlying ganglion, gouty arthropathy, and hallux valgus, as well as proliferative osseous changes that can develop secondary to MTP joint arthrosis (Fig. 6–1).

The term *hallux valgus* was introduced by Carl Hueter[164] to define a static subluxation of the first MTP joint characterized by lateral deviation of the great toe and medial deviation of the first metatarsal. It is now recognized, particularly in juvenile patients, that a hallux valgus deformity can originate due to lateral deviation of the articular surface of the metatarsal head without subluxation of the first MTP joint.[72,74,75]

A hallux valgus deformity can also be associated with abnormal foot mechanics, such as a contracted Achilles tendon, severe pes planus, generalized neuromuscular disease such as cerebral palsy or a cerebrovascular accident (CVA, stroke), or an acquired deformity of the hindfoot secondary to rupture of the posterior tibial tendon. It can likewise be associated with various inflammatory arthritic conditions, such as rheumatoid arthritis (Fig. 6–2).

ANATOMY

The specialized articulation of the first MTP joint of the great toe differs from that of the lesser toes in that it has a sesamoid mechanism. The head of the first metatarsal is round and covered by cartilage and articulates with the somewhat smaller, concave elliptical base of the proximal phalanx. A fan-shaped ligamentous band originates from the medial and lateral metatarsal epicondyles and constitutes the collateral ligaments of the MTP joint (Fig. 6–3). These ligaments interdigitate with ligaments of the sesamoids.

The strong collateral ligaments run distally and plantar-ward to the base of the proximal phalanx, whereas the sesamoid ligaments fan out plantar-ward to the margins of the sesamoid and the plantar plate. The two tendons of the flexor hallucis brevis, the abductor and adductor hallucis, the plantar aponeurosis, and the joint capsule condense on the plantar aspect of the MTP joint to form the plantar plate (Fig. 6–4A).

Located on the plantar surface of the metatarsal head are two longitudinal cartilage-covered grooves separated by a rounded ridge (the crista). A sesamoid bone is contained in each tendon of the flexor hallucis brevis and articulates by means of cartilage-covered convex facets on its superior surface, with the corresponding longitudinal grooves on the inferior surface of the first metatarsal head. Distally, the two sesamoids are attached by the fibrous plantar plate (sesamoid-phalangeal ligament) to the base of the proximal phalanx; thus, the sesamoid complex is attached to the base of the proximal phalanx rather than the metatarsal head. The sesamoids are connected by the intersesamoidal ligament, and this recess conforms to the crista on the plantar surface of the metatarsal head (Fig. 6–4B).

The tendons and muscles that move the great toe are arranged around the MTP joint in four groups. The dorsal group is composed of the long and short extensor tendons, which pass dorsally, with the extensor hallucis longus anchored medially and laterally by the hood ligament (Fig. 6–5). The extensor hallucis brevis inserts beneath the hood ligament into the dorsal aspect of the base of the proximal phalanx. The plantar group contains the long and short flexor tendons, which pass across the plantar surface, with the tendon of the flexor hallucis longus coursing through a centrally located tendon sheath on the plantar aspect of the sesamoid complex. This tendon is firmly anchored by this tunnel within the sesamoid complex. The last two groups are composed of the tendons of the abductor and adductor hallucis, which pass medially and laterally, respectively, but much nearer the plantar surface than the dorsal surface. Thus, the dorsomedial and dorsolateral aspects of the joint capsule are covered

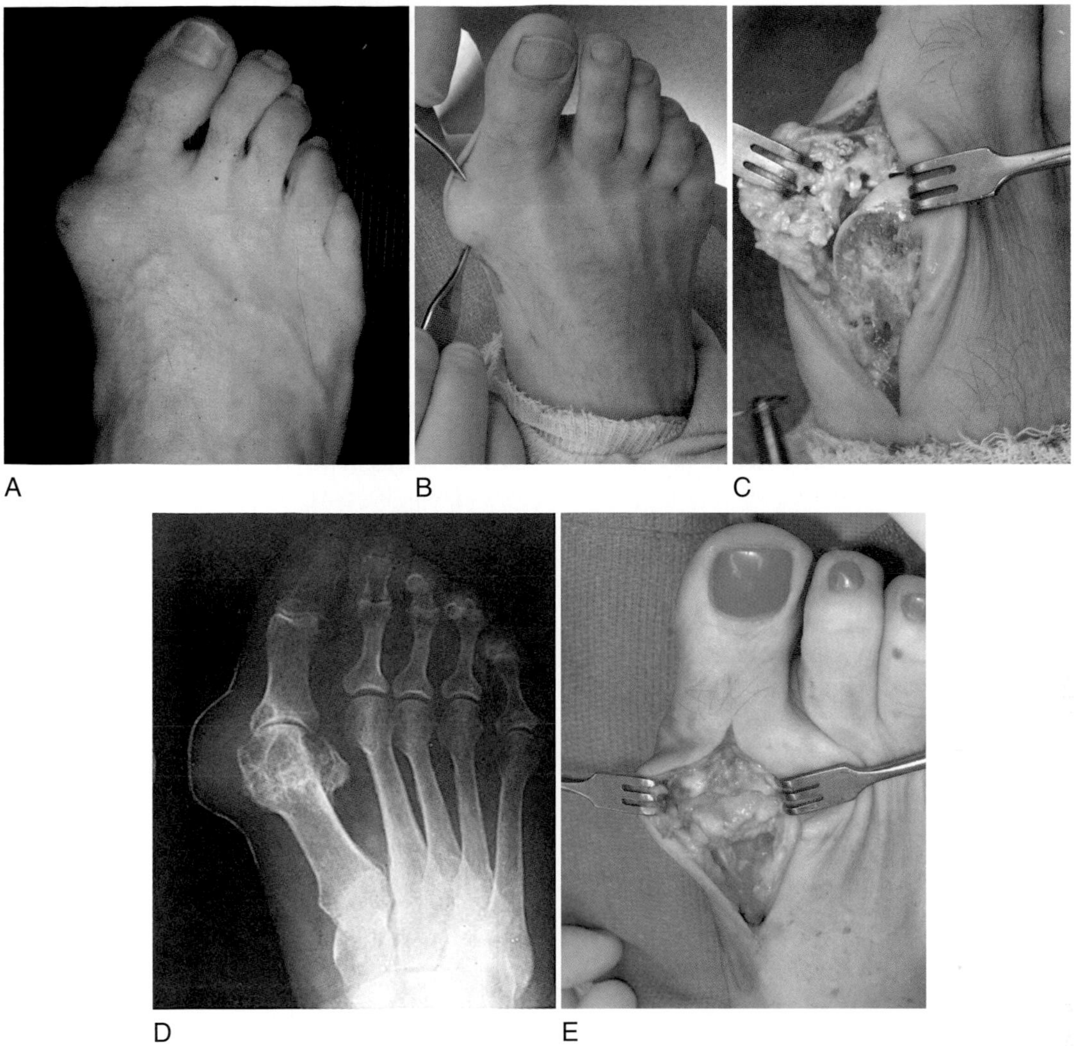

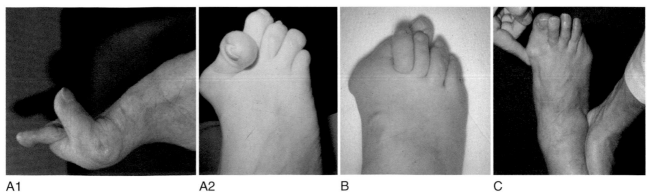

Figure 6–1   **A,** Appearance of hallux valgus deformity. **B,** Gouty arthropathy with a similar appearance. **C,** Intraoperative appearance with gouty tophi causing medial enlargement. **D,** Ganglion over the medial eminence causing enlargement. **E,** Enlargement due to hallux rigidus.

Figure 6–2   Hallux valgus deformity after a cerebral vascular accident (**A1** and **A2**), rheumatoid arthritis (**B**), and ruptured posterior tibial tendon (**C**).

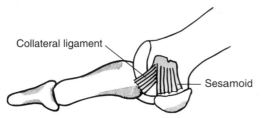

Figure 6–3 Collateral ligament structure around the first metatarsal head.

only by the hood ligaments, which maintain alignment of the extensor hallucis longus tendon.

The adductor hallucis, arising from the lesser metatarsal shafts, is made up of two segments, the transverse and the oblique heads, which insert on the plantar lateral aspect of the base of the proximal phalanx and also blend with the plantar plate and the sesamoid complex. The adductor hallucis balances the abductor forces of the abductor hallucis (Fig. 6–6). Acting in a line parallel to this bone and using the head of the first metatarsal as a fulcrum, the abductor hallucis pushes the first metatarsal toward the second metatarsal.

The base of the first metatarsal has a mildly sinusoidal articular surface that articulates with the distal articular surface of the first cuneiform. The joint has a slight medial plantar inclination. The medial lateral dimension is approximately half the length of the dorsoplantar dimension. The joint is stabilized by capsular ligaments and is bordered laterally by the proximal aspect of the second metatarsal, which extends more cephalad and offers a stabilizing lateral buttress to the first MTC articulation. In about 8% of cases, a facet may be present between the proximal first and second metatarsals (Fig. 6–7).[77] The orientation of the MTC joint may determine the amount of metatarsus primus varus, and the shape of the articulation may affect metatarsal mobility. A medial inclination of up to 8 degrees at the MTC joint is normal. Increased obliquity at this joint can increase the degree of metatarsus primus varus. The axis of motion of the MTC joint is aligned to permit motion in a dorsal-medial to plantar-lateral plane.

The tarsometatarsal articulation is quite stable in the central portion because of interlocking of the central metatarsals and cuneiforms (Fig. 6–8). This is not necessarily the case for the first and fifth metatarsals, where stability is determined not only by the inherent stability of the tarsometatarsal articulation but also by the surrounding capsular structures. Therefore, when ligamentous laxity is present, the first metatarsal may deviate medially and the fifth metatarsal laterally in the development of a splay foot deformity (Fig. 6–9).

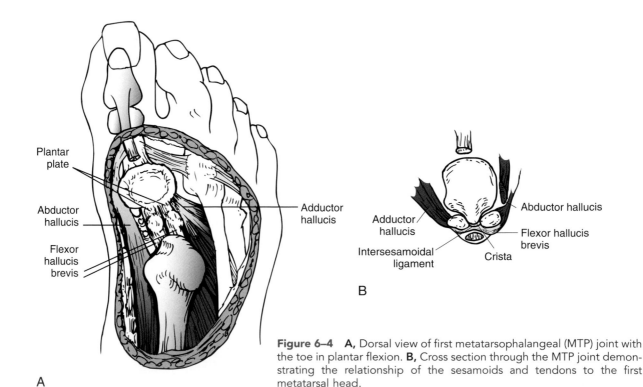

Figure 6–4 **A,** Dorsal view of first metatarsophalangeal (MTP) joint with the toe in plantar flexion. **B,** Cross section through the MTP joint demonstrating the relationship of the sesamoids and tendons to the first metatarsal head.

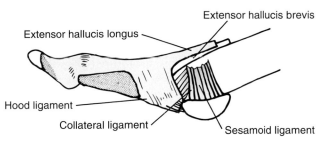

Figure 6–5 Collateral ligament structure and extensor mechanism around the first metatarsophalangeal joint.

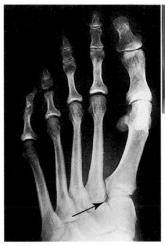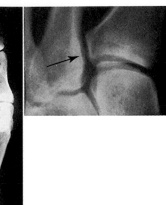

Figure 6–7 Radiographs demonstrating the first metatarsal maintained in varus position by a facet on its plantar lateral aspect.

PATHOANATOMY

Because no muscle inserts on the metatarsal head, it is vulnerable to extrinsic forces, in particular, constricting footwear. Once the metatarsal becomes destabilized and begins to subluxate medially, the tendons about the MTP joint drift laterally. The muscles that previously acted to stabilize the joint become deforming forces because their pull is lateral to the longitudinal axis of the first ray. The plantar aponeurosis and the windlass mechanism contribute significantly to stabilization of the first ray[303,309]; with progression of a hallux valgus deformity, their stabilizing influence is diminished[78,132] (Fig. 6–10). As the hallux valgus deformity progresses, the soft tissues on the lateral aspect of the first MTP joint become contracted, and those on the medial aspect become attenuated. The metatarsal head is pushed in a medial direction by the lateral

deviation of the proximal phalanx, thereby progressively exposing the sesamoids, which are anchored in place by the transverse metatarsal ligament and the adductor hallucis muscle. As the metatarsal head continues to deviate medially off the sesamoids, the crista, which normally acts to stabilize the sesamoids, is grad-

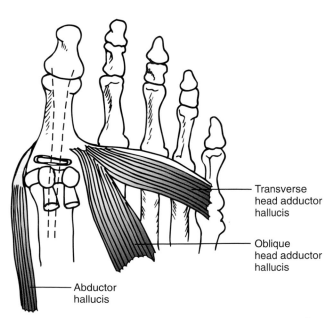

Figure 6–6 Normal anatomic configuration of the first metatarsophalangeal joint demonstrating the stabilizing effect of the abductor and adductor hallucis muscles.

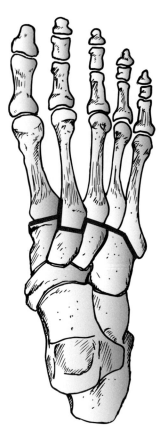

Figure 6–8 Stability of the tarsometatarsal articulation is maintained by interlocking of the central metatarsals.

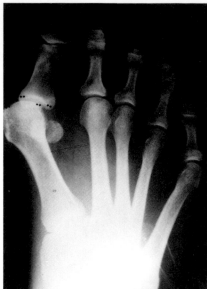

Figure 6–9 Ligamentous laxity may lead to medial deviation of the first metatarsal and lateral deviation of the fifth metatarsal.

ually eroded. As the sesamoid sling slides beneath the first metatarsal head, the hallux gradually pronates. As this dynamic joint deformity occurs, the medial eminence often becomes more prominent (Fig. 6–11).

The hallux and the first MTP joint play a significant role in the transfer of weight-bearing forces during locomotion. The plantar aponeurosis also plays a key role in this process by plantar flexing the first metatarsal as weight is transferred to the hallux. As the hallux is dorsiflexed at the first MTP joint, the first metatarsal is depressed, which results in increased weight bearing beneath the first metatarsal head and

A

B

Figure 6–10 A, Medial view of the plantar aponeurosis. **B,** From beneath, the insertion into the hallux stabilizes the first ray.

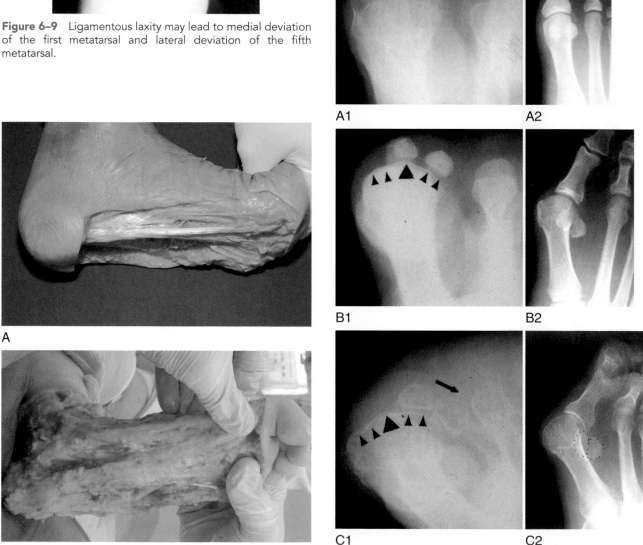

Figure 6–11 A1, Sesamoid view and, **A2,** anteroposterior (AP) view of a normal foot. **B1,** sesamoid view and, **B2,** AP view of moderate deformity. **C1,** sesamoid view and, **C2,** AP view of severe deformity.

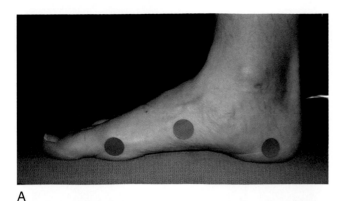

A

B

Figure 6-12 Dynamic function of the plantar aponeurosis. **A,** Foot at rest. **B,** Dorsiflexion of the metatarsophalangeal joints, which activates windlass mechanisms and brings about elevation of the longitudinal arch, plantar flexion of the metatarsal heads, and inversion of the heel.

stabilization of the medial longitudinal arch (Fig. 6-12). Certain pathologic conditions, either acquired or iatrogenic, diminish the ability of the first MTP joint and hallux to function as weight-bearing structures. This results in transfer of weight to the lateral aspect of the forefoot, which often leads to the development of a transfer lesion beneath the second or third metatarsal head. As less weight is borne by the first ray, transfer metatarsalgia and lesser toe deformities may develop. Coughlin and Jones[77] reported a 48% incidence of second MTP joint symptoms in a prospective study of adult patients undergoing repair of moderate and severe hallux valgus deformity.

PATHOPHYSIOLOGY

The dynamics of the hallux valgus deformity can best be understood by first examining the articulation where the deformity occurs, that is, the MTP and metatarsocuneiform (MTC) joints. The most stable MTP articulation has a flat articular surface, and conversely, the most unstable has a rounded head[65,99,108,237] (Fig. 6-13). A congruent MTP joint likewise is more stable than an incongruent or subluxated joint. A congruent joint tends to remain stable, whereas once a joint has begun to subluxate, the deformity tends to progress with the passing of time (Fig. 6-14).

A patient with more than 10 to 15 degrees of lateral deviation of the distal metatarsal articular surface may have a significant hallux valgus deformity that is symptomatic because of the presence of a prominent medial eminence, even though the joint is congruent and tends to be stable.

In some circumstances, alignment of the first MTP joint is normal but a valgus deformity is present because of a deformity within the proximal phalanx, and a hallux valgus interphalangeus deformity results (Fig. 6-15).

No muscle inserts into the first metatarsal head, and as a result its position is influenced by the position of the proximal phalanx. Because medial and lateral movement of the first metatarsal is to a great extent controlled by the position of the proximal phalanx, a certain degree of mobility at the MTC joint must exist for this to occur. A horizontal setting tends to resist an increase in the intermetatarsal angle, whereas an oblique setting is a less stable articulation.

The pathophysiology of a hallux valgus deformity varies, depending on the nature of the deformity. With a congruent hallux valgus deformity, the basic deformity consists of the prominent medial eminence (the bunion), which results in pressure against the shoe and thus a painful bursa or cutaneous nerve over the prominence. The MTP joint itself is stable and the deformity does not usually progress in adults.

With an incongruent or subluxated hallux valgus deformity, there is usually a progressive deformity. As the proximal phalanx moves laterally on the metatarsal head, it exerts pressure against the metatarsal head, which pushes it medially and results in an increased intermetatarsal angle. As this process occurs, there is progressive attenuation of the medial joint capsule, as well as a progressive contracture of the lateral joint capsule (Figs. 6-16 and 6-17).

While this deformity is occurring, the sesamoid sling, which is anchored laterally by the insertion of the adductor hallucis muscle and the transverse metatarsal ligament, remains in place as the metatarsal head moves medially and thereby creates pressure on the medial joint capsule. The weakest portion of the medial joint capsule lies just above the abductor hallucis tendon, and with chronic pressure this portion of the capsule gives way; as a result, the abductor hallucis muscle gradually slides beneath the medially deviating metatarsal head. As this process slowly progresses, atrophy of the crista occurs beneath the

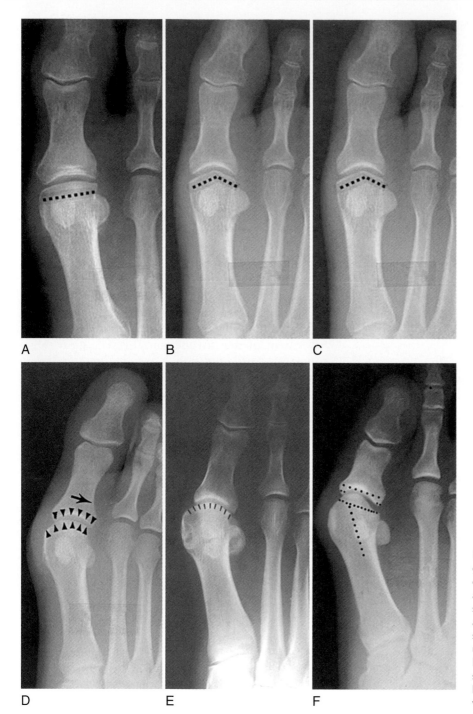

A

B

C

D

E

F

Figure 6–13 Anteroposterior radiographs demonstrating varying shapes of the metatarsophalangeal (MTP) articular surface. **A,** Flat MTP joint surface. **B,** Chevron-shaped surface in a juvenile and, **C,** in an adult without subluxation. **D** and **E,** A rounded articular surface is more prone to subluxation of the MTP joint (**D,** mild subluxation; **E,** moderate subluxation). **F,** Congruent MTP joint with hallux valgus.

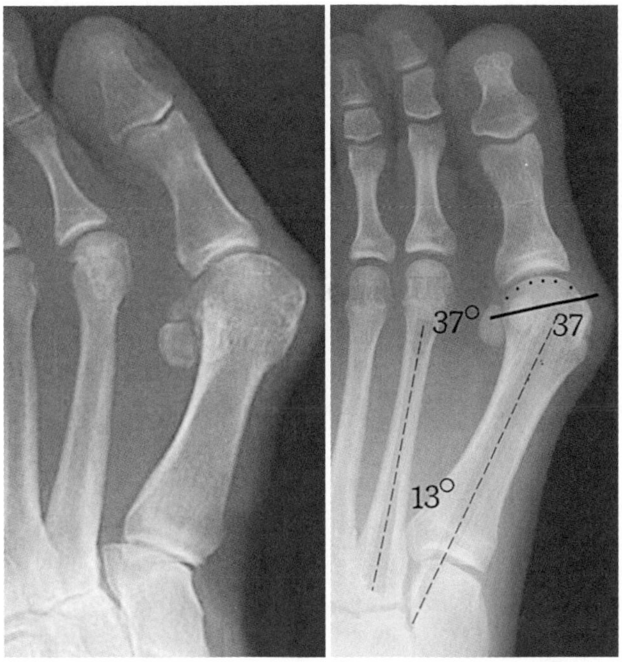

Figure 6–14 **A,** Subluxated metatarsophalangeal (MTP) joint with a hallux valgus deformity. **B,** Moderate metatarsus adductus with a congruent MTP joint (distal metatarsal articular angle, 37 degrees; hallux valgus angle, 37 degrees).

first metatarsal head, which normally helps stabilize the sesamoids (Fig. 6–18).

Once the abductor hallucis slides beneath the first metatarsal head, two events occur. First, the intrinsic muscles no longer act to stabilize the MTP joint but actually help enhance the deformity. Second, as the abductor hallucis rotates beneath the metatarsal head, because it is connected to the proximal phalanx, it will spin the proximal phalanx around on its long axis and give rise to varying degrees of pronation (Fig. 6–19). It has been well established that as the hallux valgus deformity progresses, so does the degree of pronation.[237,242]

Because of this abnormal rotation, calluses may develop along the medial aspect of the interphalangeal joint. Ultimately, as the MTP joint becomes less stable, the hallux carries less weight, body weight is transferred laterally in the forefoot, and callus may develop beneath the second, third, or both metatarsal heads. Increased pressure may lead to capsulitis, instability, or deviation of the second MTP joint as well.

With severe hallux valgus deformities, the extensor hallucis longus tendon is displaced laterally as the medial hood ligament and capsule become stretched. As a result, when the extensor hallucis contracts, it not only extends the toe but also tends to adduct it, thus further aggravating the deformity. The abductor

hallucis tendon, by migrating plantar-ward, loses its remaining abduction power. The flexor hallucis longus tendon, which retains its relationship to the sesamoids, moves laterally and also becomes a dynamic deforming force.

In rare circumstances, if the progressive deformity of the MTP joint continues unabated, dislocation of the MTP joint may occur over time, with the fibular and tibial sesamoids becoming dislocated into the first intermetatarsal space (Fig. 6–20).

Normally, a small eminence is present on the medial aspect of the first metatarsal head. The size of the medial eminence varies, and sometimes most of the enlargement is on the dorsomedial aspect of the head and is thus not apparent on anteroposterior (AP) radiographs. Thordarson and Krewer[347] and Coughlin and Jones[77] have both demonstrated that the overall width of the distal metatarsal head does not enlarge with progression of hallux valgus deformities. The medial eminence develops with lateral migration of the proximal phalanx, but it is not characterized by new bone formation or hypertrophy of the medial first metatarsal head. As the hallux valgus deformity develops, progressive medial deviation of the metatarsal head occurs and becomes symptomatic because of pressure against the shoe. Individuals who wear a broad, soft shoe or sandal are not usually bothered by the enlarged medial eminence, in contrast to persons who wear dress or high-heeled shoes. At times, an inflamed or thickened bursa may aggravate the problem. On rare occasions and usually in older patients, the skin over the medial eminence can break down and result in a draining sinus. On other occasions, a ganglion arising from the medial side of the joint can erode the joint capsule and make the eventual hallux valgus repair technically much more difficult (see Fig. 6–1D).

The splayed appearance of the forefoot in more severe cases of hallux valgus (see Fig. 6–9) occurs primarily because the first metatarsal head is no longer contained within the sesamoid sling and is displaced in a medially deviated position. The middle metatarsals do not splay because of the stable articulation at their tarsometatarsal joints. Occasionally, the fifth metatarsal lacks stability and drifts laterally, thereby completing the appearance of a splayed foot.

As the hallux drifts laterally, the lesser toes, particularly the second toe, are under increasing pressure. In response to this pressure, the second MTP joint may remain stable and the great toe may drift beneath the second toe or occasionally on top of it. At other times, progressive subluxation or complete dislocation of the second MTP joint occurs. Occasionally, no subluxation affects the second MTP joint; rather, all the lesser toes are pushed into lateral deviation or a

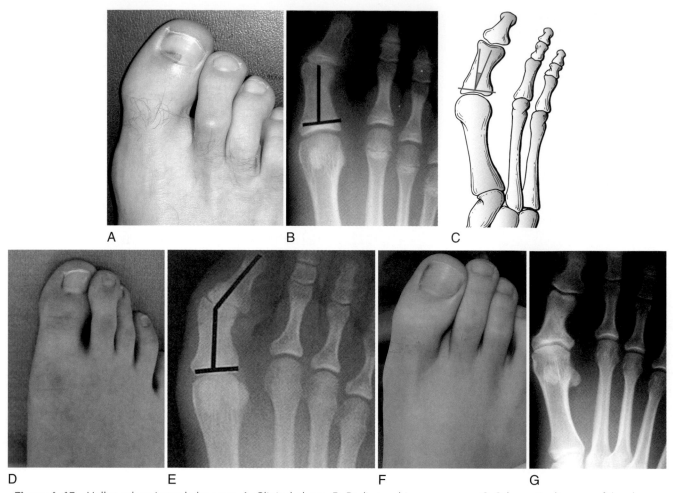

A B C

D E F G

Figure 6–15 Hallux valgus interphalangeus. **A,** Clinical photo. **B,** Radiographic appearance. **C,** Schematic diagram of the abnormality. **D,** Clinical appearance of the distal interphalangeus. **E,** Radiographic appearance. **F,** Clinical appearance. **G,** Radiographic appearance of the interphalangeus that developed after an epiphyseal injury in adolescence.

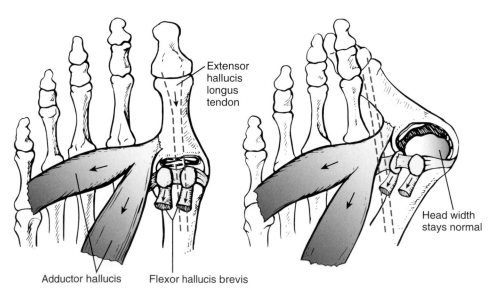

Extensor hallucis longus tendon

Adductor hallucis   Flexor hallucis brevis

Head width stays normal

Figure 6–16 Pathophysiology of hallux valgus deformity. Normally, the metatarsal head is stabilized within the sleeve of ligaments and tendons, which provide stability to the joint. As the proximal phalanx deviates laterally, it places pressure on the metatarsal head, which deviates medially. This results in attenuation of the medial joint capsule and contracture of the lateral joint capsule.

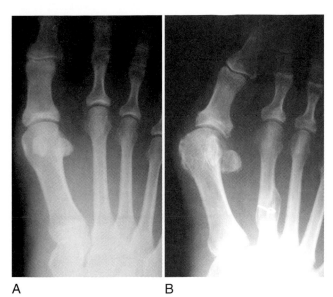

A   **B**

Figure 6–17 Progression of both hallux valgus and a 1-2 intermetatarsal angular deformity over a 5-year period. **A,** Initial radiograph. **B,** Twenty years later, a simultaneous increase in both angular deformities has occurred.

"wind-swept" appearance due to extrinsic pressure from the hallux.

DEMOGRAPHICS

Age of Onset

Piggott[281] reported on a series of adult patients evaluated for hallux valgus deformities. Fifty-seven percent of the patients interviewed recalled an onset of the deformity during their adolescent years, whereas only 5% recalled development of the bunion deformity after 20 years of age. In a long-term review of patients with hallux valgus deformities, Hardy and Clapham[143] reported that 46% of bunion deformities occurred

before the age of 20. Although Scranton[317] stated that a hallux valgus deformity rarely develops before 10 years of age, Coughlin[72] reported on a series of juvenile patients with bunions in whom the average age at onset was 12 years; 40% of these patients noted that the onset of their deformity occurred at the age of 10 years or younger. Thus, development probably occurs much earlier than has previously been appreciated.*

In contrast, Coughlin[68] reported onset by decade in a group of men and noted that 21 of 34 (62%) patients dated the development of their bunion to the third to fifth decade of life. Only 7 of 34 (20%) recalled onset in the adolescent years. Later, Coughlin and Jones[77] stated that 65% of adults reported the onset of their deformity in the third through fifth decades and only 4% in the first decade.

At what age a patient recognizes a hallux valgus deformity is obviously dependent on understanding the deformity, the symptoms, the magnitude of the deformity, the family history, and the keenness of a patient's observation skills. Many deformities can begin in the adolescent years but progress in magnitude in later decades when they become more symptomatic. The reported age at surgery after specific surgical techniques should not be confused with the age at onset. In a retrospective study, Coughlin and Thompson[86] reviewed more than 800 cases and reported the mean age at surgery to be 60 years. Of importance is the fact that late development after skeletal maturity occurs in a foot that at one point most likely had a normal structure, whereas an early onset in the juvenile years occurs before maturation in a foot that most likely "never had a normal structure." Coughlin[72] observed that early onset of hallux valgus (before 10 years of age) was associated with a much higher distal metatarsal articular angle (DMAA), a

---

*References 7, 43, 115, 136, 259, 317, and 318.

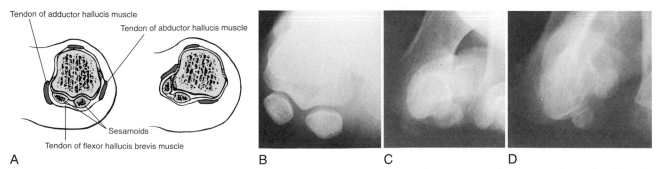

A   **B**   **C**   **D**

Figure 6–18 Relationship of the sesamoids to the metatarsal head. **A,** Diagram demonstrating the sesamoids stabilized by the crista, followed by atrophy of the crista as the metatarsal head deviates medially off the sesamoids. **B,** Normal relationship of the sesamoids to the crista. **C,** Moderate hallux valgus deformity. **D,** Severe hallux valgus deformity.

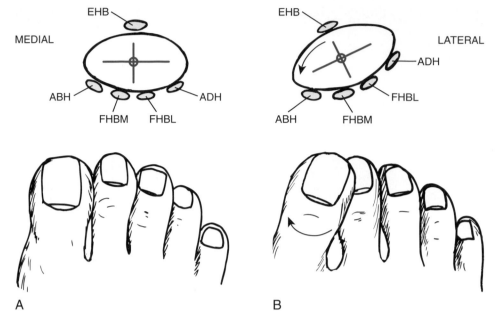

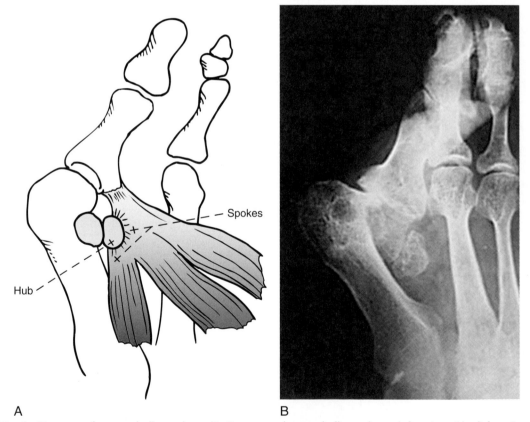

Figure 6–19 Schematic representation of tendons around the first metatarsal head. **A,** Normal articulation in a balanced state. **B,** Relationship of the tendons in hallux valgus deformity. ABH, abductor hallucis; ADH, adductor hallucis; EHB, extensor hallucis brevis; FHBL, flexor hallucis brevis lateral head; FHBM, flexor hallucis brevis medial head.

Figure 6–20 **A,** Diagram of severe hallux valgus. **B,** Severe end-stage hallux valgus deformity with dislocation of metatarsophalangeal joint and sesamoid mechanism into first web space.

finding that would probably change the choice of operative technique in these patients.

Gender

Although several studies have provided statistical data showing some predilection in the female population for the development of hallux valgus, this may be merely a reflection of a specific person's choice of footwear. Wilkins,[373] in a study of schoolchildren's feet, reported a female preponderance of 2:1. Hewitt et al[157] and Marwil and Brantingham,[247] in investigating male and female military recruits, found a predilection of approximately 3:1 in the female population. Creer[88] and Hardy and Clapham,[144] in reporting statistics from their surgical practices, found this ratio to be approximately 15:1 in adult patients. The reported incidence of females in the juvenile population undergoing surgical correction for hallux valgus deformities varies from 84% to 100%.* Several studies on adult patients report females to make up 90% or more of the patient population.† Coughlin and Jones[77] found that the proportion of females in their report on moderate and severe hallux valgus deformities was 92%. Certainly, shoes worn by women are generally less physiologic than those worn by men, and shoes of any type can lead to hallux valgus in susceptible persons; however, it is also likely that heredity plays a substantial role in the development of bunion deformities (Fig. 6–21).

Bilaterality

We previously believed that hallux valgus deformities commonly occurred as unilateral deformities.[234] This notion was based on reports of the results of surgical procedures in which a majority of patients underwent unilateral surgery.‡ However, this information does not truly document the incidence of bilaterality. Patients may have bilateral deformities yet have surgery performed on only one side. They may undergo bilateral surgery yet have only the index surgery performed during the period of study. Even though many reports cite unilateral occurrence, our prospective evaluation of moderate and severe hallux valgus deformities demonstrated that although 84% of patients had bilateral hallux valgus deformities, only 18% had both feet corrected during the study period.[77] Symptoms and varying magnitudes of deformity may

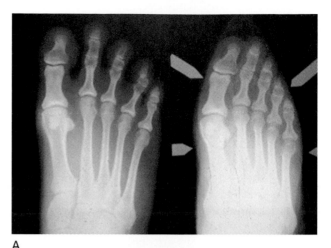

A

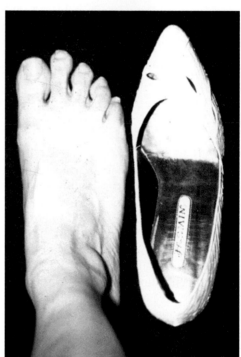

B

Figure 6–21 A, Normal foot on the *left*, foot in a fashionable shoe on the *right*. **B,** Photo of the foot on the *left* and shoe on the *right*.

lead a person to desire unilateral correction despite having bilateral hallux valgus deformities. We believe that the majority of patients have bilateral hallux valgus deformities of differing magnitude.

Handedness

Ninety percent of the population is right handed,[372] but how this translates to foot dominance is unknown.[371] Coughlin and Jones[77] reported that 91% of patients who underwent bunion surgery were right

---

*References 54, 153, 264, 344, 346, and 353.

†References 25, 27, 54, 55, 86, 144, 182, 215, 220, 237, 248, 264, and 281.

‡References 54, 100, 242, 246, 306, and 361.

handed and were unable to find a correlation between handedness and hallux valgus deformity. Although most series report the number of right and left feet involved, it is unknown whether handedness makes a difference in development of the deformity.

Frequency of Occurrence

Myerson[270] has suggested that hallux valgus deformities develop in 2% to 4% of the population. Although no published study has reported the frequency of development or the rate of surgical correction of hallux valgus deformities in the United States, Coughlin and Thompson[86,344] estimated that more than 200,000 hallux valgus corrections are performed in the United States each year. This figure is probably an underestimate of both the incidence of the deformity and the frequency of surgical correction.

ETIOLOGY

Extrinsic Causes

Footwear

Hallux valgus occurs almost exclusively in persons who wear shoes but does occasionally occur in unshod people (Fig. 6–22). The notion of footwear being the principal contributor to the development of hallux valgus was substantiated by a study of Sim-Fook and Hodgson[328] in which 33% of shod persons had some degree of hallux valgus as compared with 2% of unshod persons. Hallux valgus deformities were also extremely rare in the Japanese because of the nature of their traditional footwear, the tabi sandal (Fig. 6–23). When the manufacture of fashionable leather shoes greatly exceeded the manufacture of traditional sandals in the 1970s, the incidence of hallux valgus deformity increased substantially.[185] Conversely, physicians in France referred to the development of hallux valgus deformities as early as the 18th century. Before that time, the common footwear was a Greco-Roman style, flat-soled sandal. Studies by Maclennan[223] in New Guinea, Wells[370] in South Africa, Barnicot and Hardy[15] in West Africa, Engle and Morton[103] in the Belgian Congo, and James[170] in the Solomon Islands found some element of metatarsus primus varus and an occasional asymptomatic hallux valgus deformity in the indigenous populations (Fig. 6–24). One can

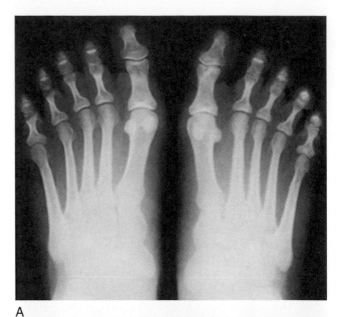

A

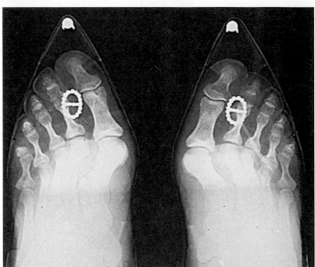

B

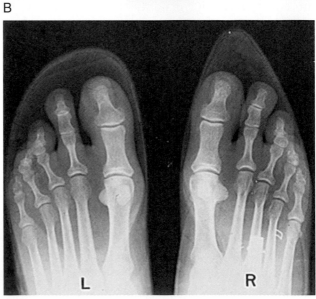

C

Figure 6–22 **A,** Normal feet of young woman during weight bearing. **B,** Feet in shoes during weight bearing. Note the developing hallux valgus. **C,** Effects of different types of shoes. The left shoe permits freedom of forefoot function; the right shoe restricts function of the four lesser toes.

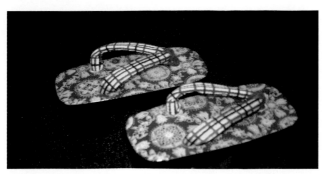

Figure 6–23 Traditional Japanese sandal.

conclude from these studies that an asymptomatic hallux valgus deformity in an unshod person may be attributed to hereditary causes. In shoe-wearing populations, however, a symptomatic and painful bunion would be expected to develop more commonly. A wide or splayed forefoot forced into a constricting shoe might thus lead to symptoms over the medial eminence.

Although shoes appear to be an essential extrinsic factor in the development of hallux valgus, the deformity does not develop in many people who wear fashionable footwear. Therefore, some intrinsic predisposing factors must make some feet more vulnerable to the effect of footwear and likewise predispose some unshod feet to the development of hallux valgus. Although high-fashion footwear has been implicated in the progression of hallux valgus deformities in adults,* Hardy and Clapham[144] and others[72,177] have suggested that in most cases a juvenile

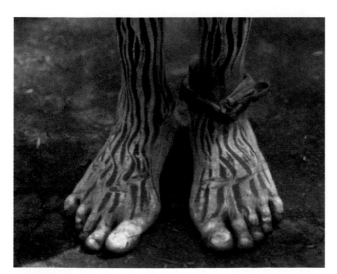

Figure 6–24 Kenyan tribesman with an asymptomatic hallux valgus deformity. (Courtesy of J. J. Coughlin, MD.)

*References 3, 80, 113, 256, 317, and 328.

hallux valgus deformity does not appear to be influenced by a history of constricting footwear. Poorly fitting shoes play a small role in juvenile hallux valgus. In a prospective study of adults with hallux valgus, Coughlin and Jones[77] reported that only 35% of patients undergoing surgical correction implicated constricting footwear as a cause of their deformity. In an earlier report, Coughlin[68] found that 60% of men with hallux valgus who had undergone surgical correction implicated ill-fitting shoes as a cause of their deformity.

Occupation

Cathcart[47] and Creer[88] have implicated occupation as a cause of hallux valgus. Again, objective evidence in the small percentage of patients who claim that their occupation contributed to their hallux valgus deformity is lacking. Coughlin and Jones[77] reported that patients considered occupation an infrequent cause of their deformity, with 17% implicating their job as a cause of their hallux valgus deformity.

Intrinsic Causes

Heredity

The notion that a hallux valgus deformity is inherited has indeed been suggested by many authors.* A positive family history of hallux valgus in 58% to 88% has been reported in five different series of adult patients.[54,127,144,264,287] Coughlin and Jones[77] stated that 86 of 103 adult patients (84%) reported a family history of hallux valgus deformities.

Johnston,[176] in 1956, reported an in-depth genetic history on subjects with hallux valgus. Based on a single-family case report, he proposed that this trait was autosomal dominant with incomplete penetrance. Juvenile hallux valgus deformities have been characterized by their familial tendency. Coughlin[72] reported a family history in 72% of patients in his retrospective study on juveniles and noted that a bunion was identified in 94% of 31 mothers of children with a family history of hallux valgus deformity. Of the 31 patients with a positive family history for the deformity, 4 females noted an unbroken four-generation history of hallux valgus transmission from maternal great-grandmother to maternal grandmother to mother to patient (Fig. 6–25). Eleven females reported a three-generation history of transmission from maternal grandmother to mother to patient, and 11 patients noted a two-generation history of mother-to-patient transmission. Of three males with hallux valgus in this

*References 27, 43, 85, 98, 101, 115, 127, 137, 139, 220, 318, and 346.

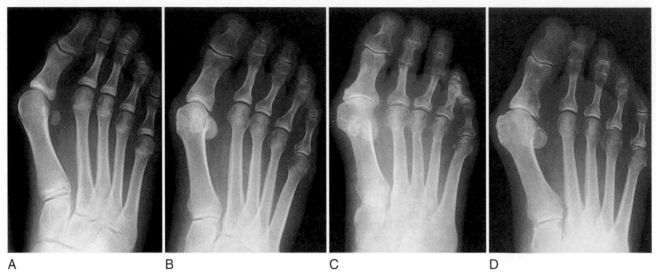

A   B   C   D

Figure 6–25   A family history of juvenile hallux valgus is common. **A,** Hallux valgus in a 16-year-old girl. **B,** Hallux valgus of long-standing duration in her 33-year-old mother. **C,** Hallux valgus in her 60-year-old grandmother. **D,** Hallux valgus in her 85-year-old great-grandmother present since her youth.

same series, two reported their mothers to have had a bunion and one reported a three-generation history of maternal transmission to the patient. Thus, 29 of 31 patients (94%) with a family history showed a pattern consistent with maternal transmission. The preoperative hallux valgus deformity in these patients was reported to be 5 degrees greater in those with a family history, although the average postoperative hallux valgus correction was similar in patients with and without a family history.

Both Bonney and Macnab[27] and Coughlin[72] observed an earlier onset of deformity in patients with a family history of hallux valgus. The high rate of maternal transmission noted in previous reports[72,144] makes it difficult to avoid a conclusion that there is a genetic predisposition for hallux valgus deformities in the female population. However, this trait can also be associated with X-linked dominant transmission, autosomal dominant transmission, or polygenic transmission.

Pes Planus

The association of pes planus with the development of a hallux valgus deformity is controversial. A low incidence of advanced pes planus in adults with hallux valgus led Mann and Coughlin to conclude that the occurrence of hallux valgus with pes planus is uncommon in patients without neuromuscular disorders.[237] The incidence of pes planus in the general population was defined in a review of normal adult military recruits by Harris and Beath.[146] They reported a 20% incidence of pes planus. Half of these cases represented an asymptomatic "simple depression of the longitudinal arch." In general, pes planus may be no more

common in those with hallux valgus than in the general population.* Pouliart et al[287] did not observe any relationship between the degree of pes planus and the severity of hallux valgus. Kilmartin and Wallace[192] found that the incidence of pes planus in the normal population and in those with a hallux valgus deformity was essentially the same. They concluded that pes planus in juveniles had no significant association either with the magnitude of the preoperative hallux valgus deformity or with the postoperative success or failure rate of a surgical repair. This finding was confirmed by Coughlin[72] and Trott,[353] who noted no increased incidence of pes planus in juvenile patients. Studies by Canale et al[43] and others[72,192] have reported no correlation between pes planus and the success rate of surgical repair of a hallux valgus deformity.

Arch height has been quantified by both Harris Mat imprints and radiographic measurements (Fig. 6–26).[85] Grebing and Coughlin[133] used Harris Mat imprints to assess arch height and demonstrated that a low arch was significantly more common in an adult group with hallux valgus than in a control group. They reported an 11% incidence of pes planus in a normal control group and a 24% incidence in a group with hallux valgus but also found no correlation between the hallux valgus angle and pes planus or between pes planus and first ray mobility. Saragas and Becker[308] did not find an increased incidence of pes planus when they examined the calcaneal pitch angle and found no association between the degree of pes planus and the severity of hallux valgus deformity. King and Toolan[193]

_____

*References 72, 77, 85, 192, 237, 308, and 353.

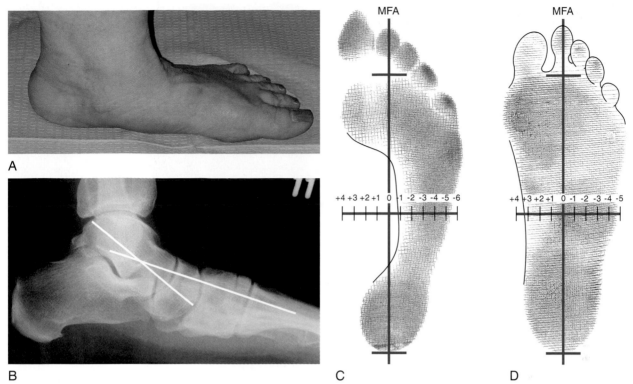

Figure 6–26   A, Pes planus deformity. **B,** Lateral talometatarsal angle demonstrating pes planus. **C,** Harris Mat imprint demonstrating a normal arch and, **D,** a pes planus deformity (MFA, midline foot axis, a line drawn from the middle of the second toe imprint to the center of the heel imprint. An imprint medial to the MFA represents a low arched foot or pes planus). (**C** and **D** with permission from Grebing B, Coughlin M: Evaluation of Morton's theory of second metatarsal hypertrophy. *J Bone Joint Surg Am* 86:1375-1386, 2004.)

observed an association between the hallux valgus angle and both Meary's line (lateral talometatarsal angle) and the AP talonavicular coverage angle in those with pes planus.

Other authors have suggested that a hallux valgus deformity tends to develop in a pronated foot.* Hohmann[161] was the most definitive and asserted that hallux valgus was always associated with pes planus and that pes planus is always a causative factor in hallux valgus. In attempting to resolve this contradiction, we believe that a patient with a pes planus deformity in whom hallux valgus develops will have more rapid progression of the deformity. However, hallux valgus does not develop in most patients with pes planus.

Models and radiographs can demonstrate the role of pronation in the pathophysiology of hallux valgus in a normal foot (Figs. 6–27 to 6–30). Though an excellent demonstration of the effect of pronation on the foot and hallux, it does not enable determination of

what initiates a hallux valgus deformity. In Figure 6–27, a pendulum has been attached to the nail of the great toe. As the foot is pronated, rotation of the first ray around its longitudinal axis is clearly seen. In Figure 6–28 a skeletal model has been photographed. With longitudinal rotation of the first metatarsal head, the fibular sesamoid becomes visible on the lateral side of the first metatarsal head. Figure 6–29 shows a dorsoplantar weight-bearing radiograph; with the pronated position of the sesamoids, they appear to have been displaced laterally. The fibular sesamoid is now visible in the interval between the first and second metatarsals, as would be anticipated from the skeletal model in Figure 6–30. Tangential or sesamoid views of the foot show that this appearance is caused solely by longitudinal rotation of the first metatarsal, not by actual lateral displacement; the sesamoids remain in a normal relationship with their facets located on the plantar surface of the metatarsal head (Fig. 6–30).

Pronation of the foot imposes a longitudinal rotation of the first ray (metatarsal and phalanges) that places the axis of the MTP joint in an oblique plane relative to the floor. In this position the foot appears to be less able to withstand the deforming pressures

---

*References 6, 21, 54, 66, 67, 87, 98, 104, 114, 141, 159, 166, 181, 182, 249, 250, 272, 299, 310, 314, 327, 339, and 360.

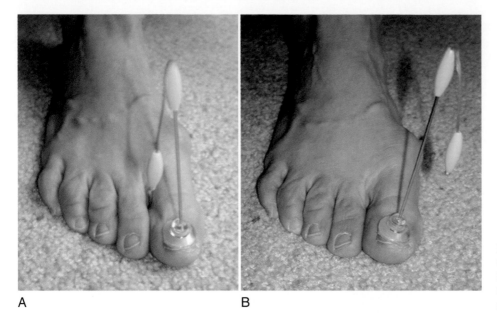

Figure 6–27 Longitudinal rotation of the first ray. **A,** Supination. **B,** Pronation. A pendulum is attached to the toenail of the great toe.

exerted on it by either shoes or weight bearing.[182] No data are available on the relationship between the degree of pes planus and the degree of hallux valgus in the small percentage of unshod persons in whom the condition develops. Furthermore, authors who have noted a relationship between pes planus and hallux valgus in shod people have presented no quantitative data.*

To discount pronation entirely, however, is not appropriate because in some cases it can play a sub-

stantial role in the development and progression of specific hallux valgus deformities. Pronation of the foot does alter the axis of the first ray.[184] With weight bearing, the first MTP joint assumes an oblique orientation with the ground. In some pronated feet, especially in patients with ligamentous laxity, pressure exerted on the medial capsule of the first MTP joint can lead to progression of a hallux valgus deformity because the soft tissue supporting structures are unable to withstand these deforming forces. In such pathologic situations, a physician should be aware of possible progression of deformity, as well as postoperative recurrence. The use of prefabricated or custom

*References 21, 54, 98, 141, 161, 166, and 314.

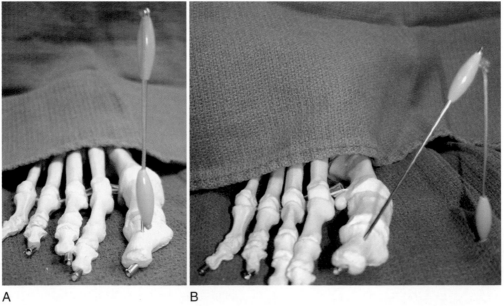

Figure 6–28 Skeletal model of the demonstration in Figure 6–27. **A,** Supination. **B,** Pronation.

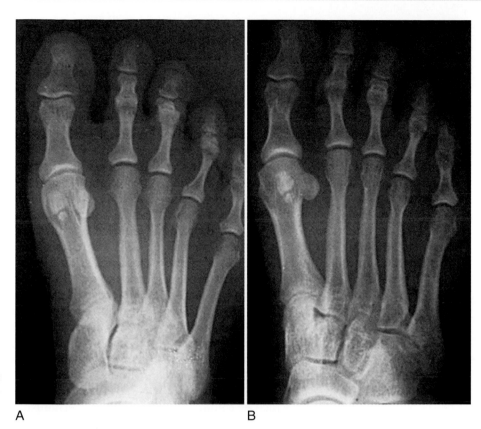

Figure 6–29 Foot during weight bearing. **A,** Supination. **B,** Pronation. Note the apparent lateral displacement of the sesamoids.

A   B

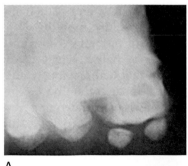

A

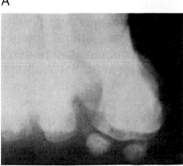

B

Figure 6–30 Tangential views of the sesamoids during weight bearing. **A,** Supination. **B,** Pronation. The degree of longitudinal rotation of the metatarsal is clearly demonstrated by the position of the sesamoids, which still retain a normal relationship to their facets beneath the metatarsal head.

orthoses in these patients may be beneficial. Persons with a mild hallux valgus deformity may experience rapid progression of the deformity if instability of the hindfoot secondary to rupture of the posterior tibial tendon, rear foot valgus secondary to rheumatoid arthritis, or instability of the first MTC joint develops. Therefore, pronation of the foot can be a factor predisposing to hallux valgus in certain conditions because the medial capsular structures offer limited resistance to the strong deforming forces.

Hypermobility of the Metatarsocuneiform Joint

The concept of hypermobility of the first ray was introduced by Morton in 1928.[267,268] Later, Lapidus[206-208] suggested an association between increased mobility of the first MTC joint and hallux valgus. Many reports dealing with correction of hallux valgus implicate first ray hypermobility as a cause yet offer no proof regarding the magnitude of preoperative or postoperative mobility.*

Others have disputed the significance of first ray mobility as a cause of hallux valgus.[85,97,132,143,302] In reports on series involving the treatment of hallux

---

*References 10, 21, 54, 65, 140, 141, 155, 197, 211, 271-273, 307, and 314.

valgus, Dreeben and Mann[97] and others[76,85] have found no evidence of first ray hypermobility after surgical correction of a hallux valgus deformity. Mann and Coughlin[234] estimated that the incidence of significant first ray hypermobility was 5% in patients with hallux valgus, and Wanivenhaus and Pretterklieber[368] reported a 7% incidence of MTC joint instability.

Clinical assessment of sagittal plane mobility of the first ray was described by Morton,[267,268] who suggested that with the ankle in neutral position, the examiner stabilize the lateral aspect of the forefoot with one hand and then grasp the first ray with the other hand (Fig. 6–31). The first ray was translated in a dorsal plantar direction until a soft end point was reached. First ray hypermobility was defined as excess motion on this examination. The biomechanical axis of the first MTC joint is obliquely placed, which permits motion of the metatarsal head to occur in a dorsomedial to plantar lateral direction (Fig. 6–32). This oblique motion of the joint can indeed be qualitatively observed on physical examination, but attempting to quantify it clinically has been difficult. Although Morton claimed that first ray hypermobility led to a multitude of foot problems,[267,268] he concluded that there was no reliable method by which he could quantify the magnitude of first ray hypermobility.[268] Efforts to quantify MTC mobility have proved difficult,[112,273,307] and surprisingly, no report of the results of first MTC joint arthrodesis has provided data on the preoperative and postoperative magnitude of first ray mobility.[273,307] Attempts to quantify first ray mobility have measured motion in either degrees[105,167,368] or millimeters of either dorsal displacement or total excursion[121-126] (Fig. 6–33). Efforts to accurately measure first ray mobility have evolved to the use of external calipers in recent years. Klaue, Hansen, and Masquelet[197] described a noninvasive caliper consisting of a modified ankle-foot orthosis and an external micrometer to quantify first ray mobility. The authors found measurable, repeatable values for both normal and hypermobile first rays and concluded that hypermobility was often associated with the development of hallux valgus. They reported that normal adult patients had approximately 5 mm of flexibility at the MTC joint and patients with hallux valgus had 9 mm or more of mobility. Although the applied force is not standardized when using this device, both the examination and the position of the foot and ankle are actually quite similar to the manual examination as originally described by Morton.[268,363] Jones and Coughlin have substantiated that the Klaue device is reliable and gives reproducible measurements of first ray excursion.[179] Glasoe et al[124,126] demonstrated comparability of both the Klaue device and the Glasoe device for external measurement of first ray mobility.

Other reports have also demonstrated that external calipers are reliable in quantifying first ray motion.[62,121-123,125] Klaue et al[197] and others[121,133] used external calipers to measure first ray mobility and reported greater mobility in patients with hallux valgus deformities than in control subjects. However, both Glasoe et al[122] and Cornwall et al[62] reported that the manual testing technique as described by Hansen[140] and others[21,54,140,271-273,307] was quite unreliable and not reproducible when compared with mechanical testing techniques. Using the Klaue device to assess postoperative first ray mobility after treatment with various hallux valgus surgical techniques, Coughlin et al[76] reported that the measured mobility was 4 mm after MTP arthrodesis and 5 mm after distal soft tissue reconstruction with proximal first metatarsal osteotomy.[85] In both series, no first ray hypermobility was observed after correction of the bunion. However, in neither of these studies were measurements made before correction of the hallux valgus.

Sarrafian[309] observed that the position of the ankle secondarily affects tension on the plantar aponeurosis (Fig. 6–34). Rush et al[303] suggested that first ray motion could affect tension on the plantar aponeurosis and windlass mechanism, thus secondarily diminishing first ray mobility.

It was Grebing and Coughlin[132] who defined the position of manual examination by investigating a group of patients with a modified Klaue device that enabled them to dorsiflex and plantar flex the ankle while measuring first ray mobility (Fig. 6–35). A control group (mean mobility, 5 mm), a group with moderate and severe hallux valgus (mean mobility, 7.0 mm), a group that had previously undergone first MTP arthrodesis (mean mobility, 4.4 mm), and a group that had previously undergone plantar fasciectomy (mean mobility, 7.4 mm) were studied. When the ankle was placed in 5 degrees of dorsiflexion, first ray mobility was significantly diminished in all four groups. When the ankle was placed in 30 degrees of plantar flexion, there was significantly increased mobility in the first three groups; however, the group that previously underwent plantar fasciectomy did not experience an increase in first ray mobility. Of interest is that in the hallux valgus group, when examined in neutral position, 21% were considered hypermobile, but when they were examined in plantar flexion, 92% were considered hypermobile. Thus, the position of the ankle substantially influences the perceived first ray mobility. When the ankle is plantar flexed 30 degrees, the amount of first ray mobility is increased almost twofold.

Coughlin et al,[78] in a cadaver study of specimens with hallux valgus, reported that first ray mobility as measured with the Klaue device was 11 mm

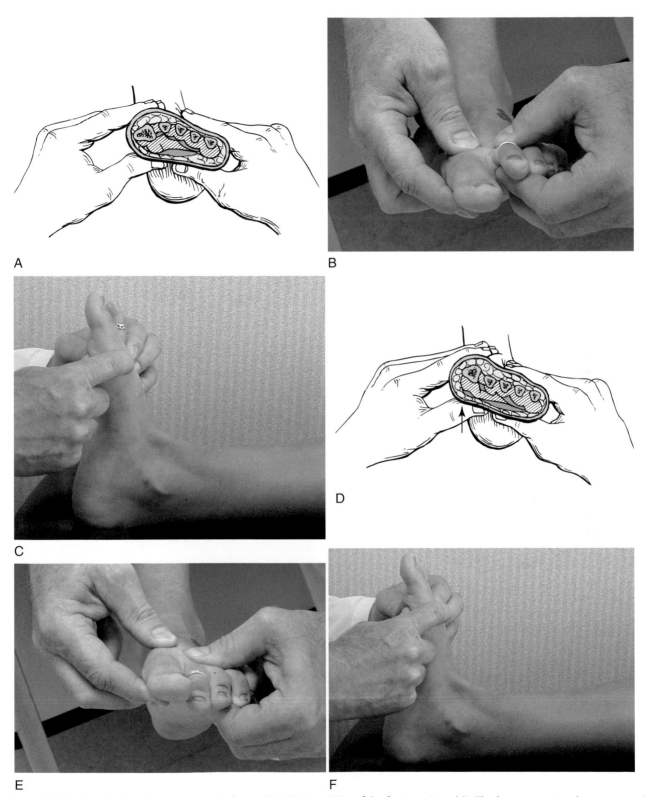

Figure 6–31 Examination for metatarsophalangeal (MTC) instability of the first ray. **A** and **B,** The lesser metatarsals are grasped between the index finger and the thumb of one hand, and the first metatarsal is grasped with the other hand. With the ankle in neutral position, the first metatarsal head is moved in the dorsoplantar direction. With a stable MTC joint, the distal ray does not become excessively elevated. **C** and **D,** With hypermobility, the first metatarsal head can be pushed in a dorsal direction above the sagittal plate axis of the lesser metatarsal heads. **E** and **F,** The ankle must be maintained in neutral position or "false hypermobility" may be diagnosed.

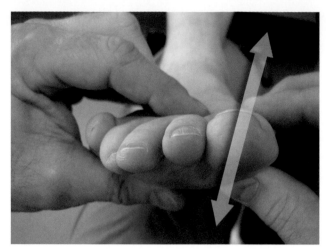

Figure 6–32 The mechanical axis of the first metatarso-cuneiform joint is from plantar lateral to dorsomedial.

preoperatively. After distal soft tissue repair and proximal osteotomy to correct the deformity, mean first ray mobility was 5 mm. In a follow-up prospective study in which a similar operative repair was performed on 122 feet with moderate and severe hallux valgus deformities, Coughlin and Jones[77] reported first ray mobility to have a preoperative mean of 7.3 mm that was reduced to a mean of 4.5 mm after surgical correction. Thus, with the ability to actually quantify first ray mobility, the authors concluded that first ray mobility is an effect of the hallux valgus deformity rather than a cause in most cases. The fact that it is reduced to a normal level after distal surgical realignment or proximal first metatarsal osteotomy that spares the MTC joint[77,78,85] makes a strong case for increased first ray mobility being a secondary rather than a primary cause. First ray stability is probably a function of first ray alignment and the effectiveness of the intrinsic and extrinsic muscles and the plantar aponeurosis and not an intrinsic characteristic of the first MTC joint.

Although Morton[268] claimed that first ray hypermobility was characterized by increased mobility on manual clinical examination, he concluded that the most notable structural feature of first ray hypermobility was hypertrophy of the second metatarsal diaphysis as demonstrated on an AP radiograph (1928). Prieskorn et al[289] attempted to relate mobility of the first MTC joint to thickening of the second metatarsal shaft and found no correlation. Grebing and Coughlin[133] analyzed second metatarsal shaft width and medial cortical hypertrophy and found no association with hallux valgus, first ray mobility, or first metatarsal length. They concluded that using second metatarsal cortical hypertrophy or shaft width was an inappropriate indication for first MTC arthrodesis in the treatment of a hallux valgus deformity (Fig. 6–36).

Myerson[270] and King and Toolan[193] suggested that a radiographic gap on the plantar aspect of the first MTC joint is associated with both hallux valgus and first MTC joint instability. The incidence of this finding is unknown. Coughlin and Jones,[77] in a prospective study of moderate and severe hallux valgus deformities, reported a 23% incidence of plantar gapping. Of those 122 cases, the average first ray mobility as measured by the Klaue device was 7.2 mm. The mean hallux valgus angle for these cases was 30 degrees.

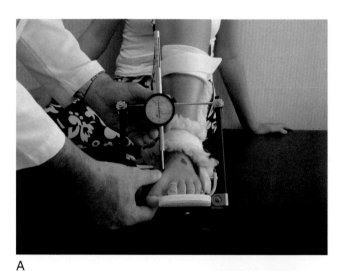

A

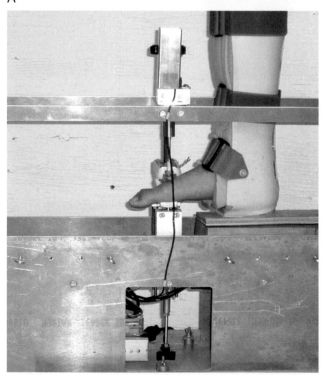

B

Figure 6–33 Two examples of external devices used to quantify first ray hypermobility. **A,** Klaue device. **B,** Glasoe device. (Courtesy of Ward Glasoe.)

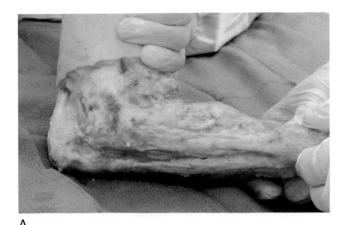

A

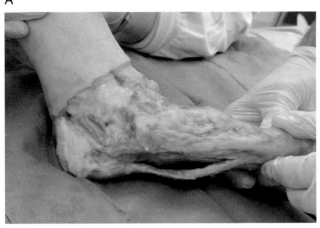

B

Figure 6-34 Plantar aponeurosis in neutral position (**A**) and plantar flexion of the ankle (**B**). Lax aponeurosis may play a significant role in first ray hypermobility when the examination is conducted with the ankle in plantar flexion.

King and Toolan[193] described the first metatarsal medial cuneiform angle (MMCA) as a reliable measure of dorsiflexion or plantar wedging of the first MTC joint (Fig. 6-37). All patients in King and Toolan's series were considered to have first ray instability when assessed by manual examination, although the magnitude of mobility was not quantified. They described increased dorsiflexion through the first MTC joint (hallux valgus patients, 2 degrees; controls, 0.2 degrees) and concluded that this demonstrated an association between the clinical and radiographic findings of first ray hypermobility and hallux valgus.

Ligamentous Laxity

Carl et al[44] observed mild generalized ligamentous laxity in a small series of patients with hallux valgus. Clark et al,[54] in a report on juveniles, noted that 69% of patients in their series had generalized laxity on physical examination. Others[65,237,272] have mentioned ligamentous laxity as an etiologic factor.

Beighton and Bird[22] defined ligamentous laxity with a 9-point scale in which 2 points were awarded for hyperextension of both elbows beyond 10 degrees (1 point for only one elbow), 2 points for hyperextension of both knees beyond 10 degrees (1 point for only one knee), 2 points for extension of the little finger beyond 90 degrees (1 point for each hand), 2 points for extension of the thumb flat with the wrist (1 point for each hand), and 1 point for the ability to place the hands flat on the ground with the knees extended. A total of 9 points can be accumulated on the examination. A score greater than 6 points indicated generalized ligamentous laxity or hypermobility. Beighton noted that most individuals (94% of males and 80% of females) score 2 or fewer points. Although studies[65,237,272] have correlated hyperflexibility of the thumb with hypermobility of the first ray, no study has documented the

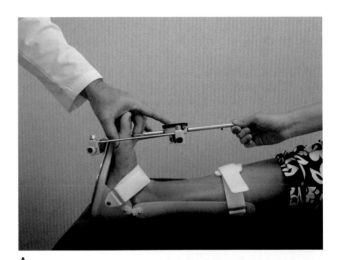

A

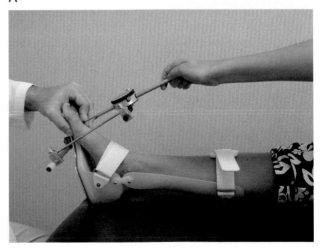

B

Figure 6-35 Modified Klaue device in dorsiflexion (**A**) and plantar flexion (**B**) demonstrating a substantial difference in first ray mobility.

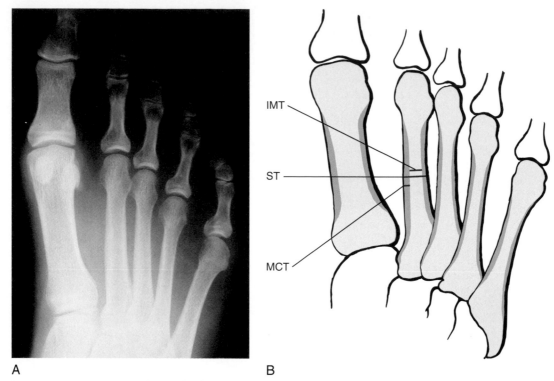

A   B

Figure 6–36   A, Anteroposterior radiograph of an asymptomatic foot with medial cortical hypertrophy. **B,** Measurements of medial cortical thickness (MCT), intramedullary thickness (IMT), and shaft thickness (ST) demonstrate no correlation with hypermobility of the first ray and hallux valgus. (**B,** Used with permission from Grebing B, Coughlin M: Evaluation of Morton's theory of second metatarsal hypertrophy. *J Bone Joint Surg Am* 86:1375-1386, 2004.)

preoperative and postoperative laxity of patients with Beighton and Bird's method. In one retrospective study[76] of a group of patients with moderate and severe hallux valgus deformities treated by first MTP arthrodesis (mean hallux valgus angle, 42 degrees), 17 of 19 patients demonstrated no evidence of any laxity on the 9-point examination (0 points). Attention should be addressed to ligamentous laxity in any evaluation before correction of hallux valgus. Although the finding of ligamentous laxity is probably uncommon in the typical adult patient with hallux valgus, patients with Ehlers-Danlos or Marfan's syndrome may be better treated conservatively because they may have an increased risk of postoperative recurrence.

Achilles Contracture

Morton[267] defined normal ankle dorsiflexion as requiring 15 degrees. Mann and Coughlin[237] and others[21,65,66,141] have suggested that on occasion, a contracted Achilles tendon is associated with the development of hallux valgus. In contrast, Coughlin and Shurnas[85] noted an absence of heel cord tightness in their series and found no correlation between ankle dorsiflexion and hallux valgus (Fig. 6–38).

DiGiovanni et al,[95] when using 10 degrees or less of ankle dorsiflexion as a guideline, noted that 44%

demonstrated "restricted dorsiflexion." When using 5 degrees or less of ankle dorsiflexion as a guideline for surgical intervention, they observed that 8 of 34 normal subjects (24%) had restricted dorsiflexion and recommended surgical lengthening of the Achilles complex.

Grebing and Coughlin[133] studied the incidence of ankle range of motion in normal subjects and patients with hallux valgus. In the control group the mean ankle dorsiflexion was 9 degrees, and in the hallux valgus group it averaged 11 degrees. They reported that 19% of normal patients had ankle dorsiflexion of 5 degrees or less. In a similarly sized group of patients with hallux valgus, 21% demonstrated ankle dorsiflexion of 5 degrees or less. Grebing and Coughlin noted that 81% of controls and 67% of those with hallux valgus had 10 degrees or less of ankle dorsiflexion. No correlation was found between ankle dorsiflexion and the magnitude of hallux valgus. In the report by Coughlin and Jones,[77] no correlation was demonstrated between ankle dorsiflexion and the hallux valgus angle.

Gastrocnemius lengthening has been recommended for patients with a limitation of 5 degrees or more.[140] However, none of the patients in the series reported by Grebing and Coughlin[133] were symptomatic, and no

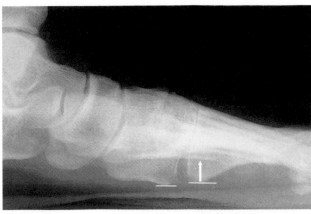

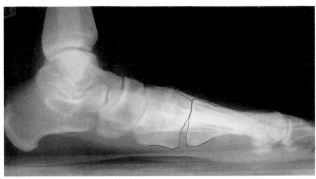

Figure 6–37 **A,** The first metatarsal lift is the difference in the perpendicular distance between the inferior border of the base of the first metatarsal and the inferior border of the first cuneiform. **B,** The first metatarsal–medial cuneiform angle (MMCA) is demonstrated on the lateral radiograph. (Courtesy of Chris Coetzee, MD.)

Achilles tendon lengthening was performed in the course of their treatment. An Achilles tendon contracture secondary to any cause can produce a gait pattern in which the person slightly externally rotates the foot or tends to roll off the medial border of the foot. This repetitive stress against the hallux has been postulated to lead to a hallux valgus deformity. This can be observed in patients with neuromuscular disorders (e.g., cerebral palsy, poliomyelitis) or patients who have had a CVA.

Although DiGiovanni et al[95] suggested that gastrocnemius lengthening be performed in patients undergoing foot surgery with dorsiflexion of less than 5 degrees, the fact that 81% of subjects demonstrated less than 10 degrees of ankle dorsiflexion suggests that this finding may not be abnormal. Furthermore, Coughlin and Jones[77] reported an incidence of 12% to 54% in patients with moderate and severe hallux valgus who had either less than 5 degrees (14 feet, 12%) or less than 10 degrees (66 feet, 54%) of ankle dorsiflexion. Of the 122 feet, in no case was an

Achilles tendon lengthening or gastrocnemius slide procedure performed in conjunction with the bunion correction. There was no correlation between the success of surgery and the tightness of the gastroc–soleus complex. Although on occasion a gastroc–soleus contracture may accompany a hallux valgus deformity, we believe this to be uncommon, and lengthening is recommended in the uncommon patients with substantial restriction in ankle dorsiflexion.

Miscellaneous Factors

Amputation of the second toe often results in a hallux valgus deformity, probably from loss of the support afforded by the second toe (Fig. 6–39). Mild hallux valgus may be seen after resection of the second metatarsal head.

Cystic degeneration of the medial capsule of the first MTP joint can occur. The resulting ganglion formation may sufficiently attenuate the capsule to permit the development of a hallux valgus deformity (see Fig. 6–1D).

ANATOMIC AND RADIOGRAPHIC CONSIDERATIONS

Angular Measurements

Radiographs of the foot should always be taken with the patient in the weight-bearing position. The basic studies should include AP, lateral, and oblique views. The AP radiographs are obtained with a tube-to-film distance of 1 m and the x-ray tube centered on the tarsometatarsal joint and angled 15 degrees toward the ankle joint relative to the plantar aspect of the foot.[81]

HALLUX VALGUS ANGLE

On an AP weight-bearing radiograph, axes are drawn on the first metatarsal and proximal phalanx so that they bisect metaphyseal reference points in the proximal and distal metaphyseal regions that are equidistant from the medial and lateral cortices of the proximal phalanx and the first metatarsal. The angle created by the intersection of these axes forms the hallux valgus angle. A normal angle is less than 15 degrees,[144] mild deformity is less than 20 degrees, moderate deformity is 20 to 40 degrees, and severe deformity is greater than 40 degrees[65] (Fig. 6–40).

1-2 INTERMETATARSAL ANGLE

On an AP weight-bearing radiograph, reference points are placed in the proximal and distal metaphyseal regions equidistant from the medial and lateral cortices of the first and second metatarsals.[81] The angle

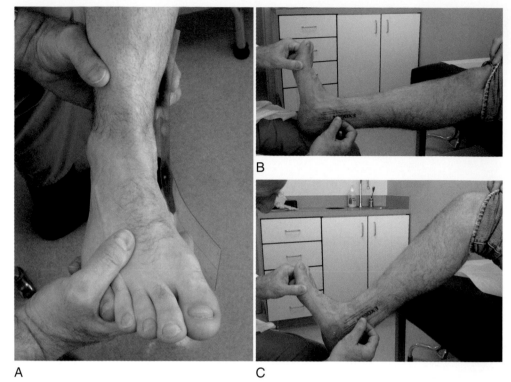

Figure 6–38 Ankle range of motion is quantified with the hindfoot in neutral position (**A**) and the knee both extended (**B**) and flexed (**C**).

created by the intersection of these axes forms the 1-2 intermetatarsal angle. Normal is less than 9 degrees,[144] mild deformity is 11 degrees or less, moderate deformity is greater than 11 and less than 16 degrees, and severe deformity is greater than 16 degrees[65] (Fig. 6–41).

HALLUX INTERPHALANGEAL ANGLE

On an AP weight-bearing radiograph, reference points are placed in the proximal and distal metaphyseal regions equidistant from the medial and lateral cortices of the proximal phalanx to create an axis of the proximal phalanx.[83] Reference points are placed at the

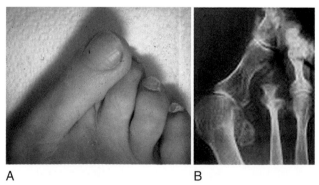

Figure 6–39 A, Clinical appearance. **B,** Radiograph of severe hallux valgus after amputation of the second toe.

center of the base of the distal phalanx and at the tip of the distal phalanx, and a second axis is drawn. The intersection of these two axes forms the hallux interphalangeal angle (Fig. 6–42).

DISTAL METATARSAL ARTICULAR ANGLE

On an AP weight-bearing radiograph, the DMAA defines the relationship of the distal first metatarsal articular surface to the longitudinal axis of the first metatarsal.[75] Points are placed at the most medial and lateral extent on the distal first metatarsal articular surface. A line connecting these points defines the lateral slope of the articular surface. Another line is drawn perpendicular to this articular line. The angle subtended by this perpendicular line and the longitudinal diaphyseal axis of the first metatarsal defines the DMAA. Normal is regarded as 6 degrees or less of lateral deviation[295] (Fig. 6–43).

METATARSOPHALANGEAL JOINT CONGRUENCY

On an AP weight-bearing radiograph, the congruency of the MTP joint is determined by inspecting the relationship of the articular surfaces of the base of the proximal phalanx and the first metatarsal head. Individual reference points are placed at the most medial and lateral extents of the phalangeal articular surface and the distal metatarsal articular surface.[75] With a subluxated (noncongruent) hallux valgus deformity,

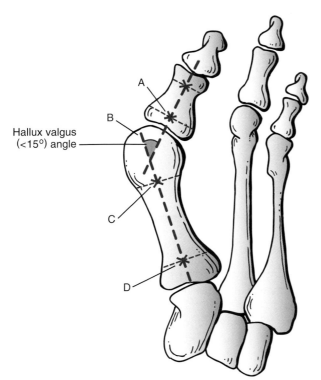

Figure 6–40 Hallux valgus angle. Marks are placed in the mid-diaphyseal region of the proximal phalanx and the first metatarsal at an equal distance from the medial and lateral cortices. The longitudinal axis of the proximal phalanx is determined by an axis drawn though points A and B, and the longitudinal axis of the first metatarsal is determined by a line drawn through points C and D. The hallux valgus angle is formed by the intersection of the diaphyseal axes of the first metatarsal (line CD) and the proximal phalanx (line AB).

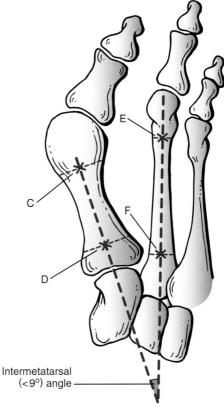

Figure 6–41 1-2 Intermetatarsal angle. Mid-diaphyseal reference points are placed equidistant from the medial and lateral cortices of the first and second metatarsals in both the proximal and distal mid-diaphyseal region. The longitudinal axis is drawn for both the first metatarsal (line CD) and the second metatarsal (line EF). The 1-2 intermetatarsal angle is formed by the intersection of these two axes (line CD and line EF).

the corresponding points on the proximal phalanx migrate laterally in relation to the corresponding points on the metatarsal head. With a nonsubluxated (congruent) hallux valgus deformity, concentric apposition of these points on the corresponding metatarsal and phalangeal joint articular surfaces occurs. No lateral shift of the proximal phalanx takes place with a congruent hallux valgus deformity[68] (Figs. 6–44 to 6–46).

Medial Eminence

One of the key components of a hallux valgus deformity is the size of the medial eminence. It is frequently this prominence that is the focus of pain and footwear intolerance by patients.[77] The size of the medial eminence is measured by drawing a line along the medial diaphyseal border of the first metatarsal. A perpendicular line is then drawn at the widest extent of the medial eminence and measured in millimeters[347] (Fig. 6–47).

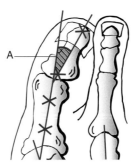

Figure 6–42 Hallux valgus interphalangeal angle. Mid-diaphyseal reference points are drawn on the proximal phalanx, and on the distal phalanx, a reference point is placed at the distal tip of the phalanx and at the midpoint of the articular surface of the distal phalanx. A line is drawn to connect the reference points for the axes of each phalanx. The intersection of the axis of the distal phalanx with the longitudinal axis of the proximal phalanx forms the hallux valgus interphalangeal axis (HVIP).

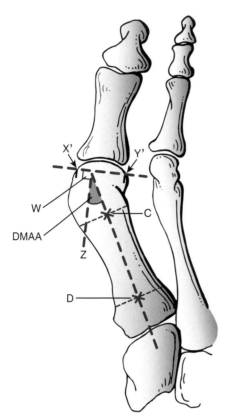

Figure 6–43 Distal metatarsal articular angle (DMAA). The DMAA defines the relationship of the articular surface of the distal first metatarsal with the longitudinal axis of the first metatarsal. Points are placed on the most medial and lateral extent of the distal metatarsal articular surface (X', Y'). A line drawn to connect these two points defines the "slope laterally of the articular surface." Another line through points (W, Z) is drawn perpendicular to the first line X'-Y'. A third line through points (C, D) defines the longitudinal axis of the first metatarsal. The angle subtended by the perpendicular line (W, Z) and the longitudinal axis of the first metatarsal (C, D) defines the DMAA.

Both Haines and McDougall[138] and Lane[205] suggested that the medial eminence was not a new growth, but merely a portion of the metatarsal that had become exposed with medial deviation of the proximal phalanx. The size of the articular surface diminishes as the sagittal sulcus migrates lateral-ward. The sagittal sulcus forms a border between the medial eminence and the remaining articular surface. Volkman[364] and Truslow[354] suggested that there was actually new bone formation with development of a bunion. Thordarson and Krewer[347] reviewed a series of feet and reported that the size of the medial eminence is similar in patients who undergo bunion surgery and those without a hallux valgus deformity (Fig. 6–48). They concluded that bone proliferation did not occur with bunion formation. Thordarson and Krewer[347] reported that the mean thickness of the measured

medial eminence was 4.4 mm in those with hallux valgus and 4.1 mm in those with normal feet. The mean difference was 0.2 mm. Coughlin and Jones[77] also concluded that the medial eminence does not reflect new bone formation. Resection of the medial eminence is a standard component of most hallux valgus repairs. Reducing a prominent medial eminence does aid in narrowing the forefoot; however, it is important to stress that the sagittal sulcus is not a reliable landmark for gauging resection of the medial eminence and may lead to excessive resection and subsequent hallux varus if a disproportionate amount of bone is removed.

Metatarsus Primus Varus

The simultaneous occurrence of hallux valgus and metatarsus varus has been noted frequently in the literature (Fig. 6–49). Hardy and Clapham[143,144] and others[77,85,133] have reported a correlation between the degree of hallux valgus and the size of the intermetatarsal angle. Of all the variables considered in their study, Hardy and Clapham[144] noted that the highest correlation was between metatarsus primus varus and hallux valgus ($p = 0.71$). The question of cause and effect between medial deviation of the first metatarsal and valgus of the great toe continues to be debated, but the findings indicate a combined

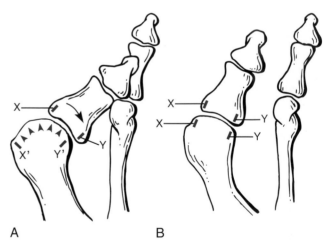

A   **B**

Figure 6–44 Congruency versus subluxation. **A,** Hallux valgus deformity with subluxation (noncongruent joint) is characterized by lateral deviation of the articular surface of the proximal phalanx in relation to the articular surface of the distal first metatarsal. **B,** Hallux valgus deformity with a nonsubluxated (congruent) metatarsophalangeal joint is caused most often by lateral inclination of the distal metatarsal articular surface. Points X and Y determine the medial and lateral extent of the articular surface of the proximal phalanx; points X' and Y' determine the medial and lateral extent of the metatarsal articular surface. Note the lateral slope of the distal metatarsal articular surface.

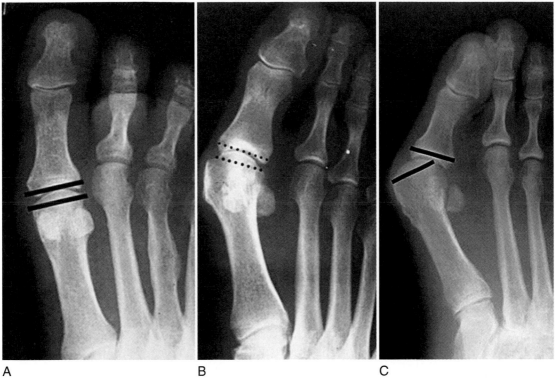

A   B   C

Figure 6–45   Relationship of the proximal phalanx to the metatarsal head. **A,** A congruent joint is one in which the articular surfaces are parallel. In this case, the distal metatarsal articular angle (DMAA) is normal. **B,** Congruent joint with DMAA increased to 27 degrees. **C,** With an incongruent or subluxated metatarsophalangeal joint, joint surfaces are no longer parallel, thus creating an unstable situation.

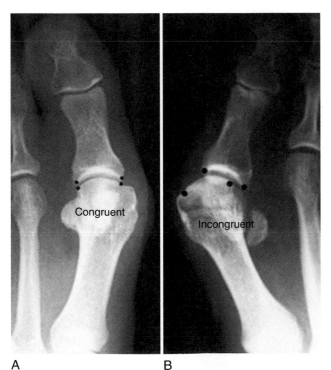

A   B

Figure 6–46   Examples of congruent (**A**) and incongruent (**B**) (subluxated) metatarsophalangeal joints. When a congruent joint is present, the proximal phalanx cannot be moved on the metatarsal head without creating an incongruent situation. An incongruent or subluxated joint can be corrected by rotating the proximal phalanx on the metatarsal head.

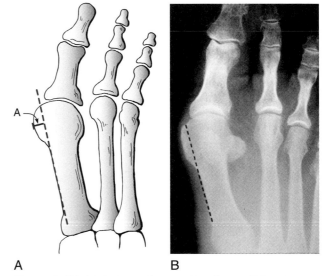

A   B

Figure 6–47   Technique of measuring the medial eminence. **A,** A longitudinal line is drawn along the medial diaphyseal shaft of the first metatarsal. A perpendicular line (A) is then drawn at the widest extent on the medial eminence and measured. **B,** Radiograph.

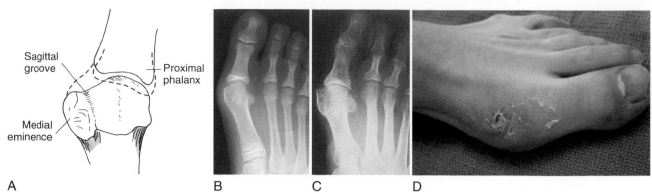

A

B   C   D

Figure 6–48   **A,** Schematic representation of the medial eminence and sagittal groove. **B,** Juvenile hallux valgus deformity with no significant medial eminence and no degenerative changes. Note the open epiphysis. **C,** Moderate hallux valgus deformity with a large medial eminence. **D,** Ulceration may develop over the medial eminence secondary to chronic pressure against the medial eminence and overlying bursa.

deformity to a greater or lesser extent in most patients. Truslow[354] proposed the term *metatarsus primus varus* to describe a congenital anomaly that if present, "inevitably resulted in hallux valgus" when the person was forced to wear shoes. Others have also supported his notion that the primary deformity is an increased 1-2 intermetatarsal angle.*

Studies by Hardy and Clapham[144] and Craigmile,[87] in contrast, indicate that metatarsus primus varus is

*References 27, 54, 104, 198, 208, 264, and 332.

secondary to the hallux valgus deformity. Others have supported this notion that lateral migration of the hallux leads to medial deviation of the first metatarsal.[143,181,237,248,253] A close relationship exists between the degree of metatarsus primus varus and hallux valgus, which must be considered in any corrective surgery. Metatarsus primus varus may predispose a foot at risk, and poor footwear may enhance the development of a hallux valgus deformity.

We believe that metatarsus primus varus is more frequently associated with the juvenile form of hallux valgus than the adult form and is probably a strong

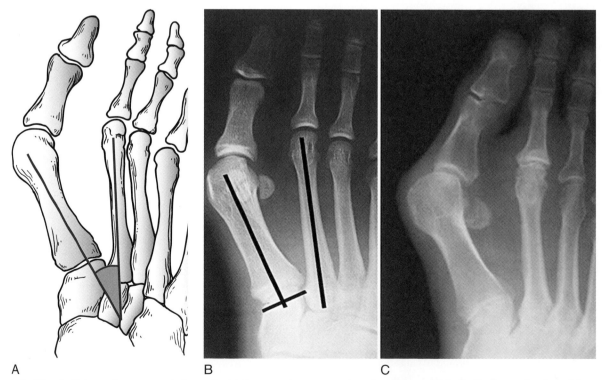

A   B   C

Figure 6–49   **A,** Schematic representation of metatarsus primus varus in a juvenile patient. **B,** Radiograph of an 18-year-old woman. **C,** Radiograph of a 55-year-old woman with metatarsus primus varus.

predisposing factor. In adults, metatarsus primus varus is probably more often a secondary change. Metatarsus primus varus can be associated with an adducted forefoot as well. Based on our analysis of available information, we are unable to conclude which is the primary deformity and can assert only the correlation between the two.

Hallux Valgus Interphalangeus

The relationship between the proximal and the distal phalanx of the hallux demonstrates that a line drawn perpendicular to the articular surface of the base of the proximal phalanx will usually not deviate laterally more than 10 degrees. When this line deviates more than 10 degrees laterally as it passes through the proximal phalanx, it gives rise to a hallux valgus interphalangeus deformity (see Fig. 6–15A-C). On occasion, the distal articular surface of the proximal phalanx deviates in a lateral direction, which creates a more severe hallux valgus interphalangeus deformity (see Fig. 6–15D and E). An epiphyseal injury can lead to deformity as well (see Fig. 6–15F and G). At times, a hallux valgus interphalangeus deformity coexists with a hallux valgus deformity and must be considered when correction of hallux valgus is carried out or the correction is incomplete.

Sorto et al[336] suggested that there is an inverse relationship between the hallux valgus angle and the hallux valgus interphalangeal (HVIP) angle. They concluded that an increased hallux valgus angle indicates MTP joint instability whereas a decreased angle indicates joint stability. Sorto et al[335] reported that in a normal foot the HVIP angle averages 13 degrees. They concluded that an increase in the HVIP angle is dependent on transverse plane stability at the MTP joint. An increase in the HVIP angle is associated with a low hallux valgus angle and increased transverse plane stability. Conversely, decreased stability (hallux valgus) is associated with a high hallux valgus angle and a low HVIP angle.

Barnett[14] reported that a normal value for the HVIP angle was 10 degrees or less. Bryant et al[38] reported that the average HVIP angle was 5 degrees for those with hallux valgus and 15 degrees for those with hallux rigidus. Coughlin and Shurnas[83] reported that the average HVIP angle was 18 degrees in those with hallux rigidus. They hypothesized that as the MTP joint becomes more resistant to a transverse plane deformity, the hallux becomes predisposed to an increase in the HVIP angle. In a report by Coughlin and Jones,[77] the average HVIP angle in this group with hallux valgus was 6.7 degrees. We suggest that in those with hallux valgus there is less resistance to transverse plane deformity, thus explaining the decreased HVIP angle.

First Metatarsal Length

The length of the first metatarsal in comparison to the second metatarsal with regard to a possible association with hallux valgus is controversial. Based on minimal supporting data, both a short[21,147,267,362] and a long* first metatarsal have been implicated as essential factors in the development of hallux valgus deformities. The method of metatarsal measurement appears to influence the measured frequency of a long or short first metatarsal. Morton[267] suggested drawing a transverse line between the distal extent of the first and second metatarsals to compare their relative lengths (Fig. 6–50A). Hardy and Clapham[144] thought that this method was influenced by angular deformities (hallux valgus, metatarsus primus varus, metatarsus adductus) (Fig. 6–50B). Using the arc method, Harris and Beath[147] reported 32% with short first metatarsals, 37% with equal lengths of the first and second metatarsals, and 31% with long first metatarsals in the general population. In his evaluation of juvenile patients with hallux valgus, Coughlin[72] reported short first metatarsals in 28%, first and second metatarsals of equal length in 42%, and long first metatarsals in 30%, data closely concurring with that previously reported by Harris and Beath.[147]

Mancuso et al[227] reported that 77% of patients with a hallux valgus deformity had a first metatarsal length equal to or longer than the second metatarsal. Mancuso et al[227] and others[133] recognized that Morton's method of measurement had inherent prob-

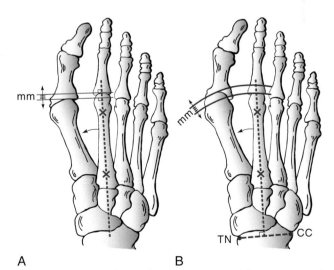

Figure 6–50 Method of measurement of first metatarsal length. **A,** Morton's method[267] using transverse lines. **B,** Hardy and Clapham's method[144] using arcs is not influenced by varying angular deformities.

---

*References 38, 138, 143, 227, 249, 250, 330, and 342.

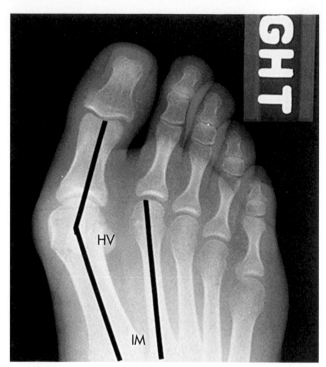

Figure 6–51 Note the long first metatarsal despite an increased hallux valgus and intermetatarsal angle.

Metatarsophalangeal Joint Shape

The shape of the head of the first metatarsal varies considerably from a round dome-shaped structure to a flat articular surface. The orientation and shape of the metatarsal and phalangeal articular surfaces have an important effect on the intrinsic stability of the first MTP joint. These respective articular surfaces may resist or predispose the hallux to deformity. The association of a curved metatarsal articular surface with hallux valgus has been proposed by several authors,[34,72,234,270] although the incidence of specific joint shapes in the general population is not known (Fig. 6–52). Schweitzer et al[316] reported no difference in the shape of the MTP joint when they compared patients with hallux valgus or hallux rigidus. DuVries[99] and others[65,234,237] have suggested that a curved surface is less stable and more prone to progressive hallux valgus deformity. Patients with hallux valgus have been shown to have a high incidence of rounded metatarsal heads varying in frequency from 71% to 91%.[77,108,227]

A flat or chevron-shaped MTP articulation (see Fig. 6–13A-C) is stable, tends to resist increased progressive valgus deformation, and is associated with hallux rigidus.[83] Coughlin and Shurnas[83] found that only 29 of 110 (26%) MTP joints in a group of patients with hallux rigidus had an oval or curved articular joint surface (see Fig. 6–13D and E). Coughlin and Jones[77] reported that a curved articulation was present in 71% of those with a moderate or severe hallux valgus deformity. We believe that a flattened or chevron-shaped articulation is more stable and tends to resist subluxation and that a curved joint shape is less resistant to

lems (Fig. 6–51). As the 1-2 intermetatarsal angle increases, there is apparent shortening of the first metatarsal. Grebing and Coughlin[133] compared the two methods of measurement in a control group and in a group with hallux valgus. In the control group, 30% were short with the arc method and 53% were short with Morton's method of measurement. In the group with hallux valgus, only 5% had a short first metatarsal with the arc method, whereas 63% were short when Morton's method was used. The normal group compared closely with results previously reported by Hardy and Clapham.[143] We believe that the notion of first metatarsal shortness as suggested by Morton[267] is largely an artifact based solely on his novel measurement technique. In fact, when the arc method of measurement is used, rarely is a short first metatarsal associated with a hallux valgus deformity.[133] The relationship between metatarsal length and the development of hallux valgus seems to be incidental, with decreased first metatarsal length playing essentially no role and increased length being of questionable significance.[72,147,237,308] Slight shortening of the first metatarsal typically occurs after many surgical procedures involving first metatarsal osteotomies. This may be an acceptable development due to the incidence of long first metatarsals in patients with hallux valgus.

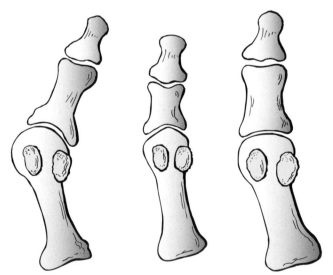

Figure 6–52 Schematic diagram demonstrating curved, chevron, and flat metatarsophalangeal articulations.

transverse plane deformity and predisposes to a hallux valgus deformity.

Joint Congruity

Congruity is the term used to describe the relationship of the metatarsal and phalangeal articular surfaces. A congruent hallux valgus deformity occurs when the corresponding articular surfaces of the metatarsal and phalanx are concentrically aligned.[65,72,281] When the proximal phalanx has migrated laterally off the metatarsal articular surface, the deformity is deemed a noncongruous or subluxated articulation (Fig. 6–53). Piggott[281] suggested that mild subluxation of the first MTP joint can progress to significant subluxation and leave the medial metatarsal articular surface uncovered (see Figs. 6–17, 6–39B, and 6–45C). Congruency of the first MTP joint was initially described by Piggott,[281] who noted that a congruous joint was typically stable and hallux valgus did not appear to increase with time (Fig. 6–54). Thus, the valgus orientation of the hallux can be caused by either joint subluxation or sloping of the metatarsal articular surface or the phalangeal articular surface in relation to the diaphyseal axis of their respective bones. With a congruent hallux valgus deformity, the magnitude of hallux valgus is determined by the magnitude of the DMAA. Piggott,[281] in

an analysis of 215 adult feet with hallux valgus, determined that 9% had a congruent joint (see Fig. 6–46A). Significant hallux valgus can occur with a congruent joint. In a patient with a symptomatic hallux valgus deformity and a congruent MTP joint who requires surgical intervention, intraarticular MTP joint realignment may create an incongruent joint.[8,52,69,152,153] This sloping of the joint articular surface may predispose the patient to a recurrent hallux valgus deformity[65,74,234] or the development of postoperative degenerative joint disease[3,52,69,152,153] (Fig. 6–55).

Chi et al[50] reported great difficulty in consistently and accurately assessing joint congruity, and Coughlin and Freund[75] found variable accuracy in their much larger study, with differing accuracy by some reviewers, and also found some radiographs more difficult to assess. Radiographs of the skeletally immature are much more difficult to assess regarding congruency. Although some feet are difficult to assess, others are clearly congruent, and it is these particular feet that warrant careful and specific surgical treatment (Fig. 6–56).

MTP joint congruity in a juvenile is believed to be a significant factor in a hallux valgus deformity[69,80,113,129,281] (Fig. 6–57). Coughlin[72] demonstrated that 47% of juveniles with hallux valgus were noted to have a congruent joint with a laterally sloping DMAA.

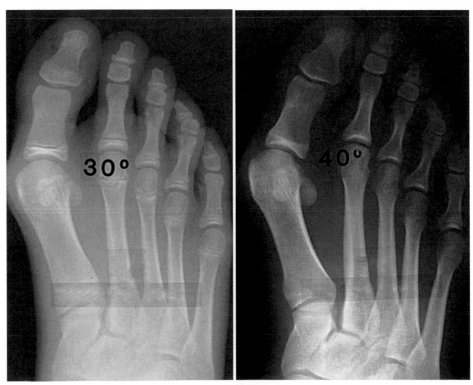

Figure 6–53 A, Moderate hallux valgus deformity in 10-year-old girl. **B,** At 19 years of age, before surgical correction, the deformity has increased, and the patient became much more symptomatic.

A   B

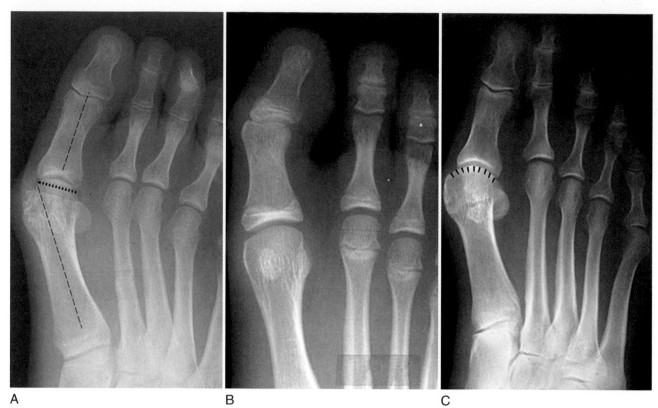

Figure 6–54 A, Radiograph demonstrating moderate hallux valgus deformity without subluxation of the first metatarsophalangeal (MTP) joint. The hallux valgus angle is caused primarily by 25 degrees of lateral angulation of the distal metatarsal articular angle. A sagittal sulcus has developed medial to the articular surface. There is a prominent medial eminence. The *dotted line* demonstrates the lateral slope of the distal metatarsal articular surface. **B,** Hallux valgus interphalangeus deformity. **C,** Subluxated MTP joint with a hallux valgus deformity caused primarily by subluxation of the first MTP joint.

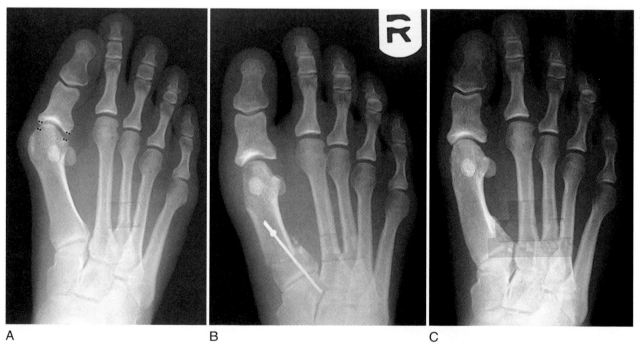

Figure 6–55 A, Preoperative radiograph demonstrating a hallux valgus deformity with a congruent metatarsophalangeal (MTP) joint. **B,** Radiograph after first metatarsal osteotomy and distal soft tissue repair. Note the lack of congruency at the MTP joint. **C,** Thirteen years later, a radiograph demonstrates incongruent MTP joint with narrowing of the medial joint space. The patient complained of greatly restricted MTP motion.

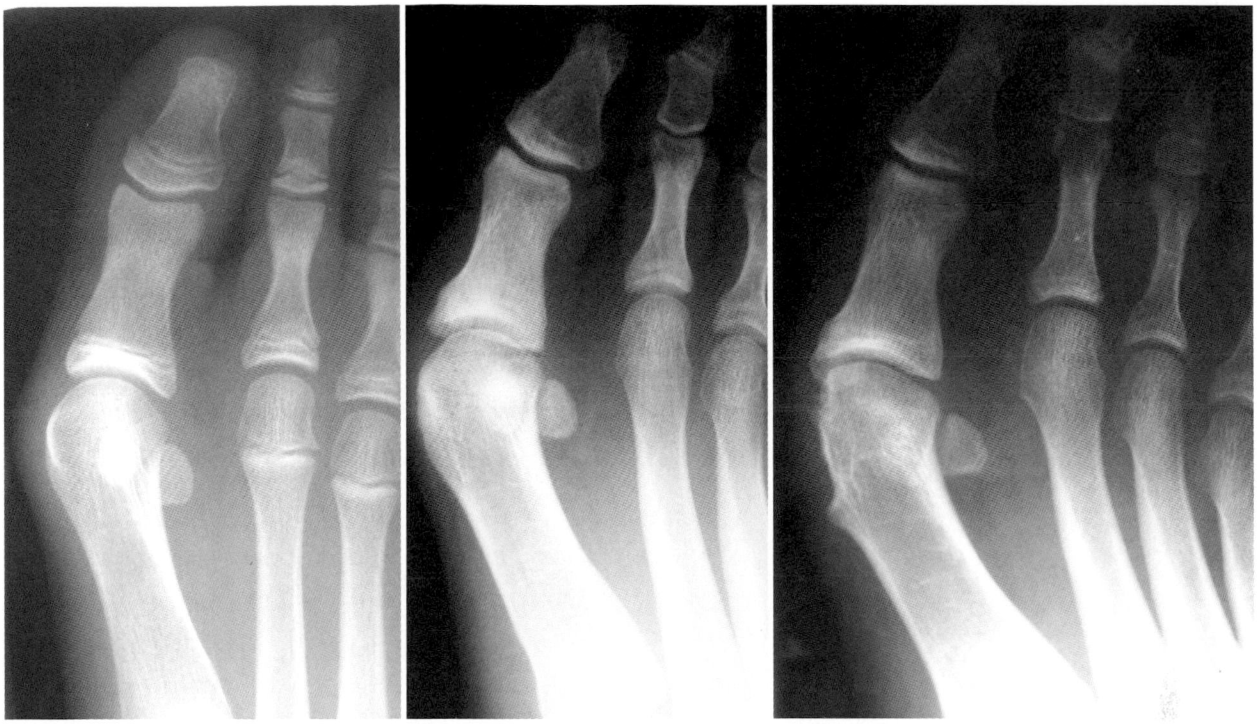

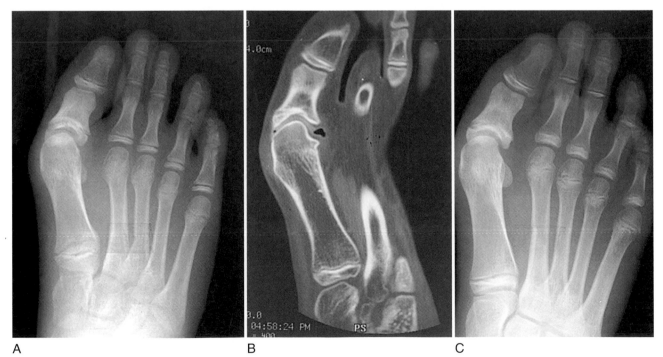

Figure 6–56 **A,** Juvenile hallux valgus deformity with a metatarsophalangeal (MTP) joint in which congruency is difficult to assess. **B,** Skeletally mature individual with a similar MTP joint that is difficult to assess. **C,** It is only with the unsuccessful surgical procedure that the congruent joint becomes more apparent.

Figure 6–57 **A,** Anteroposterior radiograph demonstrating a congruent metatarsophalangeal (MTP) joint with hallux valgus in a 10-year-old skeletally immature girl. **B,** Air computed tomographic arthrogram demonstrating congruent articular surfaces. **C,** Congruent MTP joint in a skeletally mature female.

For those with a subluxated first MTP joint, the average DMAA was 8 degrees. For congruent joints, the average lateral slope or DMAA was 15 degrees. The DMAA was noted to be significantly higher in patients with a positive family history, in those with early onset of hallux valgus (younger than 10 years), and in those with a long first metatarsal. The DMAA was not affected by the presence of metatarsus adductus. An increased DMAA is the defining characteristic of many juvenile hallux valgus deformities.

Coughlin[68] reported that a congruent joint was present in 37% of cases; the measured DMAA was twice as high (21 degrees) in congruent joints as in subluxated joints. When the postoperative hallux valgus angle was compared in the two groups, in those with a congruent joint the preoperative DMAA and postoperative hallux valgus angle were closely correlated.

Distal Metatarsal Articular Angle and Proximal Articular Set Angle

On an AP radiograph, the DMAA (or proximal articular set angle) defines the relationship of the articular surface of the distal first metatarsal to the axis of the first metatarsal (see Fig. 6–43). The radiograph may demonstrate that the articular surfaces of the distal first metatarsal and the proximal phalanx are not oriented at right angles to the long axis of the metatarsal and phalanx (see Figs. 6–45B and 6–46A). Slight valgus alignment allows lateral inclination of the great toe, and thus a hallux valgus angle of 15 degrees or less is considered normal.[144,163]

To measure the DMAA, a point is placed on the most medial extent of the metatarsal articular surface and a second point on the most lateral extent of the metatarsal articular surface. A line is then drawn connecting these two points. The angle subtended by the longitudinal axis of the first metatarsal and a line drawn perpendicular to the distal metatarsal articular surface defines the magnitude of the DMAA. The reported normal value of the DMAA in adults varies in the literature (6.3-18 degrees).[4,72,135,295,338] Lateral sloping of the articular surface of the distal first metatarsal or the base of the proximal phalanx may be the cause of a static valgus orientation of the great toe (see Fig. 6–54A). As the DMAA increases, the magnitude of the hallux valgus angle increases.

Piggott[281] stated that over time, this congruent orientation can lead to pain but that it is unusual for a deformity of this type to progress to a more severe abnormality. Measurement of this angle is extremely important when evaluating a patient with a hallux valgus deformity because it will in part determine what type of operative procedure should be performed.

Richardson et al[295] demonstrated in adults that the DMAA can be reliably quantified on an AP radiograph, whereas Pontious et al[284] observed that it is much more difficult to measure the DMAA in a young person before bone maturation. Coughlin[72] observed that in juvenile patients younger than 10 years with hallux valgus, the DMAA was 15 degrees, and in those older than 10 years, it averaged 9 degrees. Coughlin and Jones,[77] after eliminating all congruous hallux valgus deformities from their study, analyzed the remaining deformities, which were all deemed noncongruous or subluxated and measured the magnitude of the DMAA in these cases. The mean DMAA for these subluxated joints was 10.6 degrees. Coughlin[72] noted that the DMAA averaged 16 degrees in those with a long first metatarsal and 6.0 degrees in those with a short first metatarsal ($p = 0.002$). Of interest is that Breslauer and Cohen[35] observed that an increased DMAA greater than 15 degrees was associated with erosion of the plantar metatarsal articular surface.

The proximal phalangeal articular angle (PPAA, or the distal articular set angle) defines the orientation of the proximal phalangeal articular surface in relation to the long axis of the proximal phalanx (see Fig. 6–15). Although slight valgus inclination is often present in the proximal phalanx, it rarely exceeds 5 degrees. When this angle exceeds 5 degrees, a hallux valgus interphalangeus deformity occurs. Hallux valgus interphalangeus as a separate entity occurs infrequently (3%).[72]

A static hallux valgus abnormality can develop as a result of an abnormally large DMAA or PPAA, or a combination of both. Hallux valgus deformities caused by angulation of the articular surfaces are considered a static structural abnormality; although symptoms may develop, these deformities are unlikely to progress over time.[80,281] Coughlin and Shurnas[85] confirmed earlier findings that the preoperative DMAA measurement correlated with the magnitude of postoperative hallux valgus correction.

First Metatarsocuneiform Joint

The first MTC joint is a key factor in the development of both an enlarged 1-2 intermetatarsal angle and an increased hallux valgus angle. The shape of the MTC joint has a variable medial deviation. The orientation and flexibility of the MTC joint play an important role in development of the deformity at the MTP joint. On an AP radiograph, the angle formed by the intersection of the longitudinal axes of the first and second metatarsals defines the 1-2 intermetatarsal angle.[9,45,98,288] Metatarsus primus varus or a 1-2 intermetatarsal angle of 9 degrees or greater is considered abnormal[144] (see Fig. 6–41). The proximal articular

Figure 6–58 **A** and **B,** Flat metatarsocuneiform (MTC) joint. **C** and **D,** Curved MTC joint. **E,** Oblique MTC joint. **F,** Oblique MTC joint with severe metatarsus adductus and hallux valgus.

surface of the first metatarsal articulates with the distal articular surface of the first cuneiform. This elliptical concave joint surface is oriented in the transverse (coronal) plane.[138,309] Normally it is deviated medially, but in some cases it may have a marked degree of medial inclination, which is believed to result in joint instability. Both Ewald[104] and Berntsen[23] observed that when the first MTC joint was obliquely oriented, the first metatarsal was inclined medially and a hallux valgus deformity was much more prevalent. The MTC joint is difficult to visualize on plain radiographs. It is questionable whether a horizontal orientation, oblique orientation, or curved MTC articulation correlates with an increased 1-2 intermetatarsal angle (Fig. 6–58). Simon[330] and Brage et al[33] have questioned the "apparent orientation" of this joint and suggested that some of the apparent radiographic findings were indeed artifacts. After anatomic dissection of the MTC joint, Haines and McDougall[138] and Truslow[354] concluded that a hallux valgus deformity is often associated with an oblique orientation of the first MTC joint. Haines and McDougall[138] hypothesized that an abnormality in the first metatarsal base leads to a metatarsus primus varus deformity. First MTC joint orientation is the major factor associated with an increased magnitude of the 1-2 intermetatarsal angle. Mitchell et al[264] concluded that an increased 1-2 intermetatarsal angle is the result of an abnormal first MTC joint articulation.

Inman[166] and Piggott[281] suggested that with subluxation of the MTP joint, a simultaneous concomitant increase occurs in the 1-2 intermetatarsal angle (Fig. 6–59). DuVries[99] stated that in juveniles, the increased 1-2 intermetatarsal angle was responsible for the development of hallux valgus, whereas in adults, the increased 1-2 intermetatarsal angle was a secondary change following first MTP joint subluxation. The belief that in juveniles an increased 1-2 intermetatarsal angle is a primary deformity and the hallux valgus deformity is a secondary or acquired deformity is not new.*

When a hallux valgus deformity occurs with a concomitant increase in the 1-2 intermetatarsal angle, inherent flexibility at the first MTC joint may be present. In this situation, adequate correction of a hallux valgus deformity can be achieved by performing a distal soft tissue realignment without metatarsal osteotomy.[80,237] Antrobus[7] hypothesized that after a

---

*References 27, 45, 52, 98, 177, and 377.

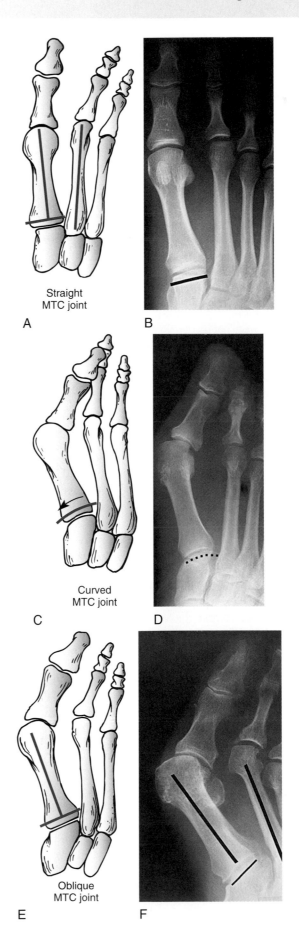

Straight
MTC joint

A

B

Curved
MTC joint

C

D

Oblique
MTC joint

E

F

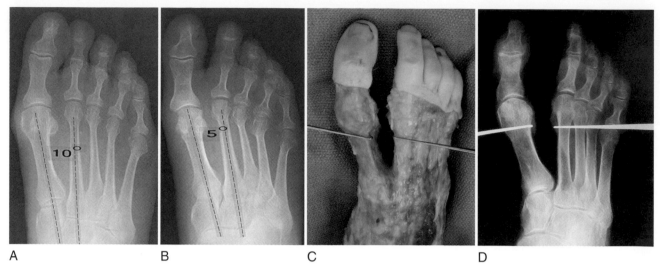

A   B   C   D

Figure 6–59 **A,** Mild to low-moderate hallux valgus deformity. **B,** Distal soft tissue repair. The hallux valgus deformity is corrected, but the 1-2 intermetatarsal angle is reduced because of distal soft tissue realignment. **C,** Anatomic specimen. **D,** Radiographic examination demonstrating the magnitude of MC joint mobility.

distal soft tissue repair (without a first metatarsal osteotomy) to correct a hallux valgus deformity, if the 1-2 intermetatarsal angle corrected to a normal range, the metatarsus primus varus deformity was secondary to the distal hallux valgus deformity. The inherent flexibility of the first MTC joint plays an integral role in the success of any hallux valgus surgical correction. MTC joint flexibility, however, can often be assessed only intraoperatively. Most distal first metatarsal osteotomies, MTP joint arthroplasties, and soft tissue realignments achieve correction of the 1-2 intermetatarsal angle by realignment of the MTP joint. Mann and Coughlin[237] reported an average decrease in the 1-2 intermetatarsal angle of 5.2 degrees after a modified McBride procedure in adults (without a first metatarsal osteotomy). Hawkins et al[150] reported an average 5.2-degree decrease in the 1-2 intermetatarsal angle after the Mitchell procedure. One can infer from these studies that sufficient flexibility often exists at the MTC articulation and allows a reduction in the 1-2 intermetatarsal angle after either a distal first metatarsal osteotomy or distal soft tissue realignment. This is an important issue because flexibility of the MTC joint can influence both the development of hallux valgus and the appropriate type of surgical repair used to achieve a successful outcome.

Intermetatarsal Facet/Os Intermetatarseum

An intermetatarsal facet located between the proximal lateral base of the first metatarsal and the proximal medial base of the second metatarsal (Fig. 6–60) may create a rigid MTC articulation that is resistant to surgical reduction after a distal osteotomy or distal soft

tissue procedure.[206,207,233,367] Likewise, the presence of an os intermetatarseum (Fig. 6–61) may create a rigid MTC articulation that resists correction of the 1-2 intermetatarsal angle.[233,354] The presence of an intermetatarsal facet or os intermetatarseum[234,237] in the proximal interval between the first and second metatarsals has been suggested to be incompatible with successful distal soft tissue repair because it is an impediment to diminution of the 1-2 intermetatarsal angle. Coughlin and Jones[77] demonstrated that the incidence of os intermetatarseum was 8% and that of an intermetatarsal facet was 8%.

Metatarsus Adductus

On an AP radiograph, the longitudinal axis of the lesser tarsus is used to measure the magnitude of metatarsus adductus.[102,209] A line is drawn on the lateral aspect of the foot between two points marking the most lateral extent of the calcaneocuboid joint and the most lateral extent of the fifth metatarsocuboid joint (Fig. 6–62). A second line is drawn along the medial lesser tarsus between two other points: the most medial extent of the talonavicular joint and the most medial extent of the first MTC joint. At the midpoint of these separate lines, a connecting line is drawn that bisects the lesser tarsus. Then a line is drawn perpendicular to the lesser tarsus bisection line. The angle that this line forms with the longitudinal axis of the second metatarsal determines the relationship of the forefoot to the lesser tarsus and thus the magnitude of metatarsus adductus. A normal value is 0 to 15 degrees, mild metatarsus adductus is 16 to 19 degrees, moderate metatarsus adductus is 20 to 25 degrees, and severe metatarsus adductus is greater than 25

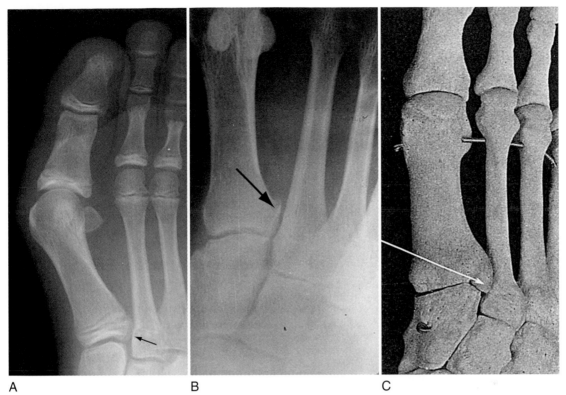

Figure 6–60   An intermetatarsal facet may limit correction of the 1-2 intermetatarsal angle if a first metatarsal osteotomy is not performed. **A,** Intermetatarsal facet associated with a juvenile hallux valgus deformity. **B,** Facet in an adult patient. **C,** Anatomic dissection demonstrating an intermetatarsal facet. (**C** from Dwight T: *Variations of the Bones of the Hands and Feet: A Clinical Atlas.* Philadelphia, JB Lippincott, 1907.)

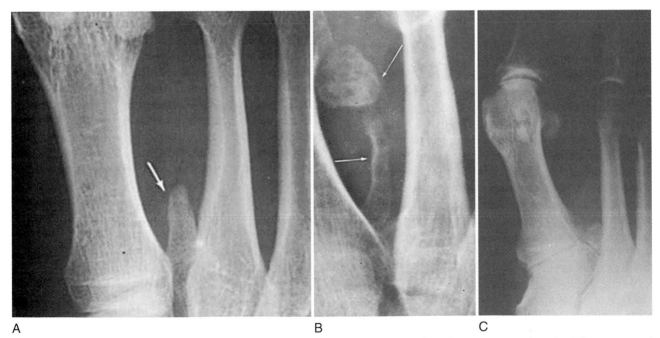

Figure 6–61   Os intermetatarseum. **A,** Os intermetatarseum with an increase in the 1-2 intermetatarsal angle. A first metatarsal osteotomy will be necessary to correct the intermetatarsal angle. **B,** Two examples of the variable appearance of an os intermetatarseum. (From Keats TE: *Atlas of Normal Roentgen Variants That Simulate Disease,* 4th ed. St. Louis, CV Mosby, 1987.) **C,** Hallux valgus deformity with an os intermetatarseum. This deformity will require a proximal osteotomy to achieve correction of the deformity.

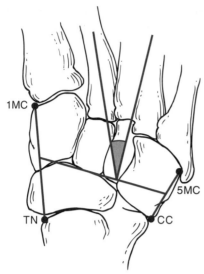

Figure 6–62 The magnitude of metatarsus adductus is determined by creating a longitudinal axis of the lesser tarsus and measuring its relationship to the longitudinal axis of the second metatarsal. A normal value is 0 to 15 degrees, mild metatarsus adductus is 16 to 19 degrees, moderate metatarsus adductus is 20 to 25 degrees, and severe metatarsus adductus is greater than 25 degrees. CC, most lateral extent of the calcaneocuboid joint; 5 MC, most lateral extent of the fifth metatarsal cuboid joint; TN, most medial extent of the talonavicular joint; 1 MC, most medial extent of the first metatarsocuneiform joint. A line connecting the midpoint of these two lines (1 MC–TN and 5 MC–CC) defines the axis of the lesser tarsus. The intersection of a line perpendicular to this axis forms an angle with the longitudinal axis of the second metatarsal and defines the magnitude of metatarsus adductus.

degrees.[12,72,102,209] In the presence of metatarsus adductus, a hallux valgus deformity is characterized by an abnormally low 1-2 intermetatarsal angle due to medial deviation of both the first and second metatarsals.[185]

The incidence of metatarsus adductus in the general population is 1 in 1000.[382] Griffiths and Palladino[135] found no relationship between hallux valgus and the metatarsus adductus angle with regard to gender. Ferrari and Malone-Lee[107] found that all women in their series with an abnormal metatarsus adductus angle had an increase in the hallux valgus angle. Men with metatarsus adductus, on the other hand, had a normal hallux valgus angle. Coughlin and Shurnas[85] and others[38,77,190] have found no association with hallux valgus in men (Fig. 6–63).

Whereas Staheli[337] suggested that there was no association of metatarsus adductus and juvenile hallux valgus, others have observed an increased incidence of hallux valgus and metatarsus adductus, mainly in the juvenile population.* Coughlin[72] reported a 22% inci-

---

*References 12, 72, 129, 135, 137, 139, 191, 209, 225, 284, and 353.

dence of metatarsus adductus in his series of patients with juvenile hallux valgus, and Banks et al[12] reported a linear correlation between an increasing hallux valgus angle and an increased incidence of metatarsus adductus. Mahan and Jacko[225] reported an increased recurrence rate after hallux valgus repair when metatarsus adductus was present, but Coughlin[72] was unable to substantiate this finding.

Metatarsus adductus associated with a hallux valgus deformity is a difficult condition to treat because there is little room to realign the first metatarsal laterally. Coughlin[72] reported no significant increase in the metatarsus adductus angle in patients with a positive family history of juvenile hallux valgus.

Blood Supply to the First Metatarsal Head

The blood supply to the first metatarsal passes through a nutrient artery traversing the lateral cortex of the midshaft of the metatarsal in a distal direction. The vessel divides within the medullary canal and sends branches both distally and proximally. Whereas the blood supply through the nutrient artery demonstrates little variation, the blood supply to the metatarsal head and to the base of the metatarsal does demonstrate variability (Fig. 6–64). According to Shereff et al,[322] the primary sources of circulation to the metatarsal head emanate from the first dorsal metatarsal artery, the first plantar metatarsal artery, and the superficial branch of the medial plantar artery. The majority of this blood supply penetrates the capsule in the general area along the dorsal and lateral aspects of the joint. Figure 6–65 shows the geographic distribution of the intraosseous blood supply to the metatarsal head. Proximally, the blood supply is centered around the area of the old epiphyseal plate region and seems to demonstrate a more uniform pattern. The surgical significance is that after medial capsulorrhaphy and distal metatarsal osteotomy, the vascular supply to the metatarsal head depends on the remaining metaphyseal vessels. Wide soft tissue dissection may imperil the circulation of the capital fragment and lead to avascular necrosis (AVN).

Open Epiphysis

A juvenile hallux valgus deformity may be further complicated by the presence of an open epiphysis at the base of the proximal phalanx and first metatarsal (Fig. 6–66). Postoperative recurrence of a hallux valgus deformity attributable to further epiphyseal growth has been speculated as a cause of recurrence and has led to the recommendation that surgical intervention

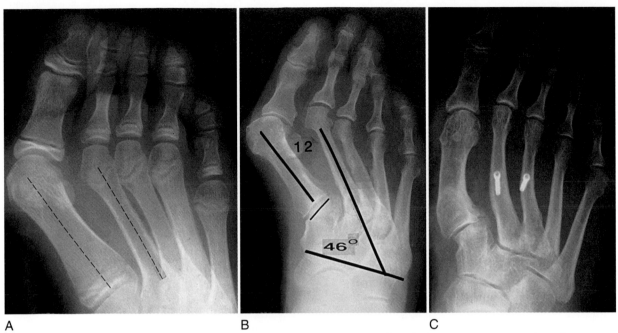

Figure 6–63 **A,** Juvenile hallux valgus with severe metatarsus adductus. Although the 1-2 intermetatarsal angle measures 2 degrees and parallelism exists between the first and second metatarsals, the 1-2 intermetatarsal angle would be approximately 35 degrees with a normal forefoot. **B,** Metatarsus adductus combined with metatarsus primus varus and a subluxated MTP joint. The metatarsus adductus angle measures 46 degrees, and the 1-2 intermetatarsal angle measures 12 degrees. With normal forefoot alignment, however, metatarsus primus varus might exceed 40 degrees. **C,** Correction of hallux valgus and osteotomies of the second and third metatarsals for metatarsus adductus. (Courtesy of Dr. Okuda.)

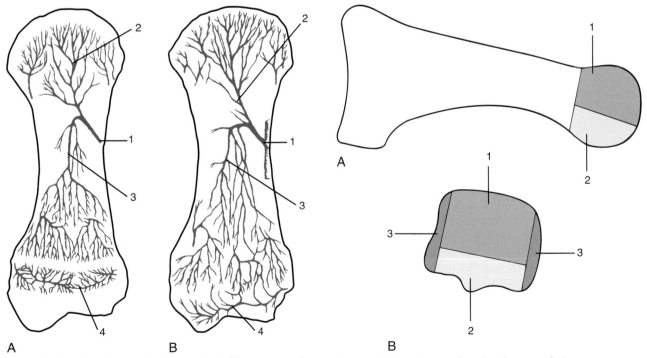

Figure 6–64 Blood supply to first metatarsal bone in an adolescent aged 12 to 13 years (**A**) and in adult (**B**). The nutrient artery (1) divides into a short distal branch (2) and a long proximal branch (3). The distal branch anastomoses with the distal metaphyseal and capital vessels. The proximal branch is longer and is directed proximally toward epiphysis, which in turn is supplied by arterial branches entering from its mediolateral side. 4, Epiphyseal vessels. (From Sarrafian SK: *Anatomy of the Foot and Ankle.* Philadelphia, JB Lippincott, 1983.)

Figure 6–65 Geographic distribution of the intraosseous blood supply to the metatarsal head. **A,** Lateral view. **B,** Axial view. Note the dorsal metaphyseal vessels (1), which supply the dorsal two thirds of the head; plantar metaphyseal vessels (2), which supply the plantar third of the head; and capital arteries (3), which supply the medial and lateral fourth of the head. (From Shereff MJ, Yang QM, Kummer FJ: Extraosseous and intraosseous arterial supply to the first metatarsal and metatarsophalangeal joints. *Foot Ankle* 8:81-93, 1987.)

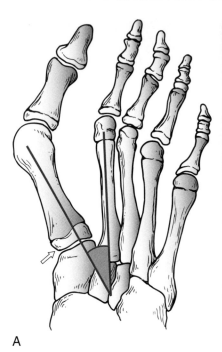

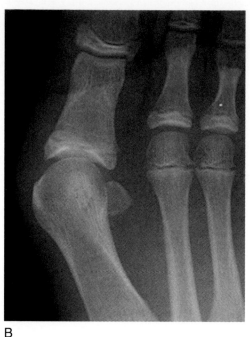

A   **B**

Figure 6–66 Epiphyses at the base of the proximal phalanx and first metatarsal present in a juvenile with hallux valgus must be protected at the time of surgery. **A,** Diagram. **B,** Radiograph.

be postponed until skeletal maturity has been achieved.* Helal[152] and Bonney and Macnab[27] have cautioned against early surgery because of the poor prognosis, but Goldner and Gaines[129] stated that "early surgery" may allow for remodeling of the articular cartilage. These authors and others[72,115,116,329] have noted no contraindications to early surgery. Coughlin[72] observed that patients who underwent surgical correction with an open epiphysis had greater correction of the hallux valgus angle.

The high recurrence rate in patients with an open epiphysis may be explained not only by a more severe deformity in those who undergo early surgery but also by a corresponding increased DMAA in younger patients with severe deformity. Coughlin[72] noted that in patients with an onset of hallux valgus before the age of 10, the average hallux valgus deformity was 32 degrees; in patients 10 years or older, the average preoperative deformity was 25 degrees. Significantly greater correction was achieved in patients with early onset of deformity. The average hallux valgus correction in the younger group was 24 degrees, and the average correction in the older group was 15 degrees ($p = 0.0001$).

The average DMAA of patients who underwent correction of hallux valgus in the presence of an open epiphysis was 21 degrees, whereas the average DMAA of those who underwent correction after the epiphysis was closed was 10 degrees. Greater deformity may have

been a factor influencing early correction of a hallux valgus deformity with an open epiphysis. The magnitude of the DMAA in these patients was two times greater than in those with a closed epiphysis. Luba and Rosman[221] hypothesize that medial inclination of the first metatarsal epiphysis causes tension forces to develop on the lateral aspect of the epiphysis and compression forces to develop on the medial aspect of the epiphysis, thereby leading to increased growth of the lateral epiphysis with subsequent increased medial inclination of the first metatarsal. They further hypothesized that the surgical correction achieved by a first metatarsal osteotomy distal to an open first metatarsal epiphysis may decrease with time because of lateral epiphyseal overgrowth. However, no evidence supports the premise that "epiphyseal overgrowth" of the proximal first metatarsal is the cause of recurrent hallux valgus in juvenile patients. A large DMAA in juvenile hallux valgus deformities treated by intraarticular correction (i.e., a distal soft tissue procedure) is associated with a high recurrence rate.[72] An increased DMAA may have led to the previous conclusion that surgery in the presence of an open epiphysis is contraindicated. Rather, in the presence of a large DMAA (often associated with severe deformity at a younger age), intraarticular correction is contraindicated.

A partial lateral first metatarsal epiphyseal arrest procedure in the early adolescent years may theoretically achieve gradual diminution of the 1-2 intermetatarsal angle. Ellis[101] and others[111,320,323] have proposed partial lateral epiphyseal arrest to achieve a gradual decrease in metatarsus primus varus. The efficacy of this tech-

*References 27, 52, 80, 139, 256, 259, 318, and 329.

nique remains hypothetical. Ellis,[101] in reporting on 20 cases of partial epiphyseal arrest, noted a high failure rate; others[107,323] report only anecdotal short-term experience with this technique.

The possibility of an epiphyseal injury at the base of either the first metatarsal or the proximal phalanx after an osteotomy must be considered when surgery is to be performed on a growing child, and this is probably the major reason for delaying surgical intervention. Anderson et al[5] analyzed the rate of growth in the female foot and determined that full foot growth is usually achieved by 14 years of age. At 12 years of age an average of less than 1 cm of total longitudinal foot growth remains. Less than 50% of this growth occurs at the proximal first metatarsal epiphysis, and thus a relatively small amount of growth occurs in the first ray after 12 years of age.[5] In adolescent boys, completion of growth tends to occur at an average age of 16 years. By age 12, however, boys still have almost 3 cm of total longitudinal foot growth remaining. Again, with an estimated 50% of the remaining longitudinal foot growth occurring at the first metatarsal epiphysis, approximately 1.5 cm of metatarsal growth remains.

The presence of an open epiphysis is not a contraindication to either surgical correction or an osteotomy in either the proximal phalanx or the proximal first metatarsal. At surgery it is important to determine the exact location of the phalangeal or metatarsal epiphysis to avoid causing an iatrogenic epiphyseal injury (Fig. 6-67). Correction of hallux valgus in a juvenile patient frequently requires an osteotomy to achieve complete correction. When either a phalangeal or a metatarsal osteotomy is planned in a patient 10 years or younger, it is important to ascertain the amount of growth that can be expected postoperatively, not only in the foot but also in the first metatarsal. If an iatrogenic epiphyseal injury does occur, one can then hypothesize its effect on ultimate phalangeal or metatarsal longitudinal growth. In an older juvenile patient, iatrogenic epiphyseal arrest or partial epiphyseal plate closure after surgery will have little effect on first ray length at this age. Surgery in a younger child is not contraindicated and may allow adaptation or remodeling of the MTP articular surfaces postoperatively.[129]

JUVENILE HALLUX VALGUS

To qualify as a juvenile hallux valgus deformity, the onset of the deformity must occur in the preteen or teenage years. Despite development during this period, however, a patient may choose to seek medical treatment later in life. Coughlin and Mann[80] and others[65,74] have observed that in adults, certain hallux valgus deformities are much more difficult to correct surgi-

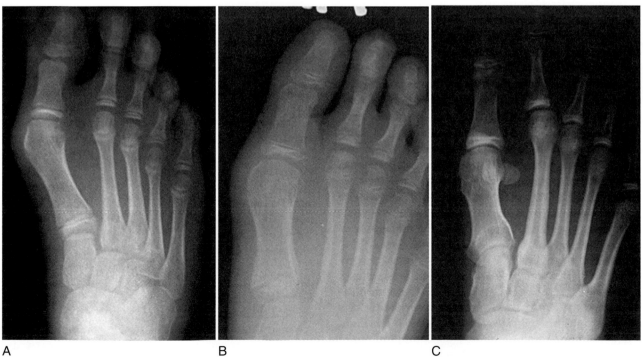

A   B   C

Figure 6–67 **A,** Radiograph before a proximal first metatarsal osteotomy with an open epiphysis. **B,** After proximal first metatarsal osteotomy, injury to the proximal first metatarsal epiphysis has occurred. **C,** A radiograph later demonstrates a shortened first metatarsal after an epiphyseal injury.

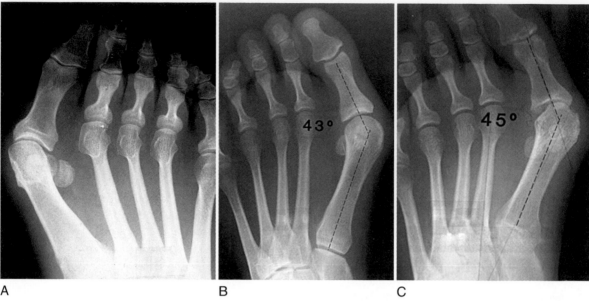

A   B   C

Figure 6–68 A, Postoperative recurrence in a patient with metatarsus adductus and a congruent metatarsophalangeal joint who underwent surgery in the teenage years. Hallux valgus deformity may develop in the adolescent years but can be surgically treated years later. Many juvenile deformities have pathologic elements that are extremely difficult to treat. **B** and **C,** Preoperative and postoperative radiographs in a juvenile who had rapid recurrence 8 weeks after surgical repair.

cally than others. These same patients appear to have a much higher risk of postoperative recurrence of deformity (Fig. 6-68). The authors hypothesized that these bunions occur in adults because of specific anatomic characteristics that developed during the juvenile and adolescent years.

Juvenile and adult hallux valgus deformities can be differentiated by several characteristics. Degenerative arthritis of the first MTP joint is rarely associated with a juvenile hallux valgus deformity but is more often associated with an adult bunion* (Fig. 6–69). Likewise, whereas bursal thickening over the medial eminence is typically found in older patients, it is rarely present in a juvenile with hallux valgus.* The epiphyseal growth plates at the base of the first metatarsal and proximal phalanges are frequently open in early adolescence.[80,259] In juveniles and adolescents with hallux valgus, the prominence of the medial eminence is of lesser magnitude[80,137,284,329] and the magnitude of the 1-2 intermetatarsal angle is often increased,[80] but the hallux valgus angle is typically of lesser magnitude.[80,137,139,259] Pronation of the hallux is much less common in juvenile patients.[137,284,321] Hypermobility of the first MTC articulation may be associated with a juvenile bunion.[54] However, a very rigid MTC joint articulation may also occur and make surgical repair resistant to correction without a metatarsal osteotomy.

*References 80, 139, 259, 284, 317, and 321.

CLASSIFICATION

The main purpose of a classification of hallux valgus deformities is to facilitate the decision-making process on how to treat the deformity. No one classification is perfect, and the numbers used to define a mild, moderate, or severe deformity are not "etched in stone." Classification should be used only as a general guide. With experience, the clinician will be able to appreciate which procedures can be "pushed" past these limits and which yield a satisfactory result when used for midrange conditions in the classification. As with any surgery, the finesse needed to carry out a good bunion procedure can be gained only through clinical experience.

With a mild bunion deformity the hallux valgus angle is less than 20 degrees, and part of the deformity may result from a hallux valgus interphalangeus deformity. The MTP joint is often congruent, and the intermetatarsal angle is usually 11 degrees or less (Fig. 6–70A). These patients typically complain of a painful medial eminence that frequently has a sharp ridge along the dorsomedial aspect. Radiographs generally demonstrate that the sesamoids are maintained in anatomic position. Occasionally, however, about 50% subluxation of the fibular sesamoid may be present.

A moderate hallux valgus deformity usually demonstrates subluxation of the MTP joint, unless the DMAA is abnormal. The hallux valgus angular deformity is 20

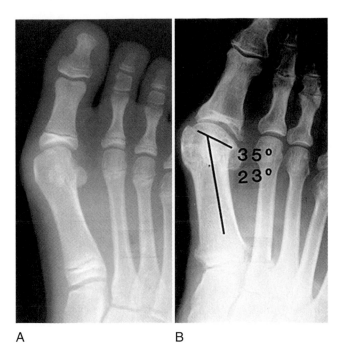

A   B

Figure 6–69 **A,** Juvenile hallux valgus deformity with no significant medial eminence and no degenerative changes. Note the open epiphysis. **B,** Hallux valgus deformity in an adult. Note the sagittal sulcus, degenerative changes at the first metatarsophalangeal joint, enlarged medial eminence, substantial subluxation of the sesamoids, and increased distal metatarsal articular angle (23 degrees).

to 40 degrees, and the great toe may exert some pressure against the second toe. The hallux is typically pronated. The intermetatarsal angle varies from 11 to 16 degrees (Fig. 6–70B). The fibular sesamoid is usually displaced 75% to 100%.

A severe hallux valgus deformity has greater than 40 degrees of lateral deviation of the hallux, and this often results in an underriding or overriding deformity of the second toe. The hallux is moderately or severely pronated. Because of the functional loss of the first MTP joint with a severe deformity, a painful transfer lesion may develop beneath the second metatarsal head. Radiographic examination demonstrates significant subluxation of the MTP joint and usually 100% lateral subluxation of the fibular sesamoid. The intermetatarsal angle is generally greater than 16 to 18 degrees (Fig. 6–70C).

PATIENT EVALUATION

History and Physical Examination

Evaluation of hallux valgus begins with a careful history of the patient's condition. This should include the chief complaint, which in our series of bunions is

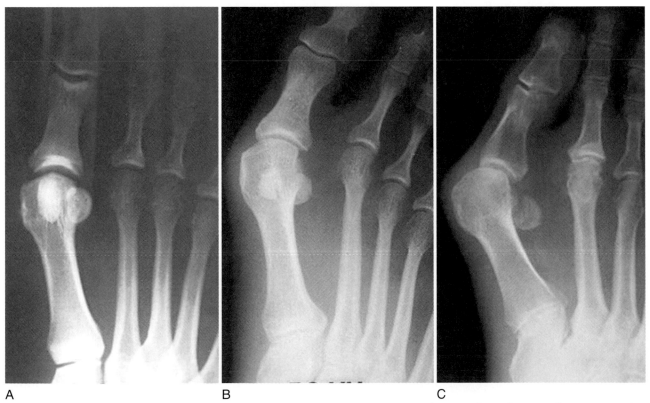

A   B   C

Figure 6–70 **A,** Radiograph of mild hallux valgus deformity, which has up to 20 degrees of angulation at the metatarsophalangeal joint. **B,** Radiograph of moderate hallux valgus deformity, which has between 20 and 40 degrees of angulation at the metatarsophalangeal joint. **C,** Radiographs of severe hallux valgus deformity demonstrate displacement of the metatarsal head off the sesamoids.

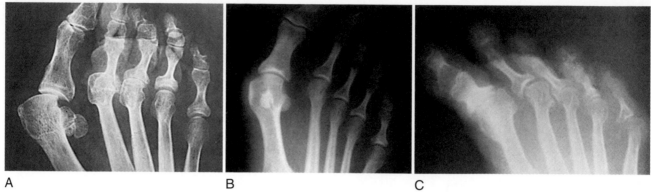

A   B   C

Figure 6–71   Deformities of lesser metatarsophalangeal (MTP) joints resulting from deviation of hallux. **A,** Dislocation of the second MTP joint and subluxation of the third MTP joint associated with hallux valgus deformity. **B,** Lateral deviation of all lesser MTP joints associated with hallux valgus deformity. **C,** Medial deviation of all lesser MTP joints associated with hallux varus deformity.

pain over the medial eminence in 70% to 75% of patients.[77,242] A symptomatic intractable plantar keratosis beneath the second metatarsal head was present in about 40% of patients in the earlier study.[242] Symptomatic metatarsalgia was present in 48% of patients in a later study.[77] Other associated problems include instability of the lesser MTP joints, interdigital neuromas, lesser toe deformities, corns, and calluses (Fig. 6–71). Information should be obtained regarding the patient's level of activity, occupation, athletic inclinations, preference for specific types of footwear, and reasons for choosing surgery. The patient's medical history should be obtained as well.

The physical examination is carried out by observing the patient's gait and then carefully observing the foot with the patient both standing and sitting. The magnitude of the deformity of the hallux and lesser toes is noted and the longitudinal arch and hindfoot position observed. The magnitude of pronation of the hallux is assessed (Fig. 6–72). Typically with more severe deformities, the magnitude of pronation increases.[85,237]

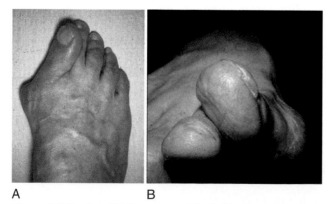

A   B

Figure 6–72   **A** and **B,** Pronation of the hallux is common with more severe deformities.

With the patient sitting, range of motion of the ankle, subtalar, transverse tarsal, and MTP joints is examined. Ankle range of motion is carefully assessed while the knee is both flexed and extended, with attention directed to gastroc–soleus muscle tightness (restricted ankle dorsiflexion) (see Fig. 6–38). Care is taken to ensure that the foot is held in neutral position (with the talonavicular joint reduced to eliminate transverse tarsal or subtalar motion)[28,133,146] with respect to the forefoot and hindfoot during assessment of the gastroc–soleus. Ankle joint motion is measured by placing a goniometer on the lateral aspect of the foot and ankle and using the fibula and plantar lateral border of the foot as landmarks for each limb of the goniometer. A right angle is considered a neutral position.

The posture of the forefoot is assessed (e.g., forefoot varus, valgus, neutral). The first MTP joint is carefully palpated for evidence of synovitis and crepitus, as well as for specific areas of pain.

Active and passive range of MTP joint motion is assessed with the patient sitting and measured with a goniometer by using the plantar aspect of the foot and the medial axis of the proximal phalanx as points of reference.[334] A neutral position is recorded as 0 degrees, and dorsiflexion and plantar flexion are measured from this point. Joseph[183] reported that the average passive range of motion of the first MTP joint in adults older than 45 years was 87 degrees (67 degrees of dorsiflexion and 20 degrees of plantar flexion).

Palpation over the dorsomedial cutaneous nerve often demonstrates irritability if there is a large medial eminence. While gently dorsiflexing and plantar flexing the first MTP joint, an attempt is made to manually reduce the deformity to determine how much correction can be achieved. At times, particularly with a long-standing hallux valgus deformity, a reduction in dorsiflexion occurs as the great toe is brought out of lateral deviation. This suggests that the distal metatarsal articular surface may be laterally deviated or that the articular cartilage has deteriorated to such an extent that dorsiflexion may be reduced after surgical realignment.

The mobility of the first MTC joint is also evaluated. This examination is performed with the patient sitting, the knee flexed, and the ankle positioned at a 90-degree angle or in neutral position.[132] The forefoot is stabilized with one hand and the first metatarsal is grasped between the thumb and index finger of the opposite hand. The first metatarsal is then moved from a dorsomedial to a plantar lateral direction and compared with the opposite side (see Figs. 6–31 and 6–32). In our experience, pathologic hypermobility exists in less than 5% of patients with a hallux valgus deformity. The plantar aspect of the foot is then examined for the presence of an intractable plantar keratosis, which most frequently is located beneath the second metatarsal head. Occasionally, one can form beneath the tibial sesamoid because of its centralized position beneath the metatarsal head. The intermetatarsal spaces are carefully palpated for evidence of neuritic symptoms. The lesser toes are then examined for evidence of lesser MTP joint instability, hammer toes, mallet toes, or interdigital corns.

Vascular evaluation includes palpation of the dorsalis pedis and posterior tibial pulses, observation of capillary filling of the toes, and assessment of the skin and hair pattern. If there is any question regarding the circulatory status of the foot, a Doppler evaluation is obtained.

The neurologic examination focuses on sensation, vibratory sense, and strength of the intrinsic and extrinsic muscles.

CONSERVATIVE TREATMENT

Conservative care in most patients with a bunion deformity is adequate to relieve symptoms. A symptomatic mild hallux valgus deformity should be periodically examined and radiographs obtained to evaluate any progression in the magnitude of the deformity. A custom or prefabricated orthotic device may assist in the treatment of a flexible flatfoot deformity or in a patient with ligamentous laxity and hallux valgus associated with pes planus (Fig. 6–73A).* Groiso[137] recommended the use of bunion night splints and exercises and noted a 50% improvement in hallux valgus deformities in a 7-year study of juvenile patients.

A physician should encourage the use of roomy footwear to reduce pressure over the medial eminence. A soft leather shoe with a wide toe box and preferably a soft sole may give significant relief of symptoms. A pedorthist can modify shoes by stretching and relieving pressure points over the bunion. Occasionally, custom-made footwear may help patients with severe hallux valgus deformities who are reluctant to undergo surgical correction. The use of bunion pads, night splints, bunion posts, and other commercial appliances may also help in relieving symptoms (Fig. 6–73B–D). Modification of footwear is probably the most important factor in achieving symptomatic relief of pain in a patient with a bunion deformity. It is difficult to achieve compliance in any patient with regard to wearing roomy footwear. Constricting footwear increases symptoms in patients with a hallux valgus deformity. Shoes with a low heel, an adequate toe box, and a soft upper tend to diminish symptoms.

The use of prefabricated or custom orthotics is controversial in the treatment of a patient with hallux valgus. It has not been demonstrated that orthotic devices prevent progression of the deformity. An orthotic device may be uncomfortable for a patient because it occupies space within the shoe. It may place increased pressure against the medial eminence and result in increased symptoms rather than relief of pressure on the first metatarsal head. Durman[98] and others[115,136,225,256,318] recommend their use postoperatively, but Canale et al[43] and others[72,189] have not used them. Kilmartin et al[189] curiously found that the hallux valgus angle increased more in patients who used orthotics and concluded that orthoses did not prevent progression of a hallux valgus deformity.

If conservative care has not led to a diminution of symptoms or the deformity has progressed, surgical correction can be considered.* Rapid progression of a hallux valgus deformity is unusual, and frequently, a hallux valgus deformity can be observed over a lengthy period (see Fig. 6–17). Although cosmesis is mentioned as a possible indication for surgery,[45,221,317,329,377] pain and discomfort should be the major considerations for surgical correction. It may be difficult on occasion to distinguish between a patient's concern for cosmesis and actual discomfort.[378]

Nonsurgical care should also be considered in patients with hyperelasticity, ligamentous laxity, or neuromuscular disorders because of the high recurrence rate. Surgery is not urgent. When contemplating surgery, careful decision making may decrease the incidence of postsurgical recurrence of a hallux valgus deformity.

---

*References 98, 136, 256, 259, 317, and 318.

*References 52, 72, 80, 115, 129, 281, 317, 318, and 329.

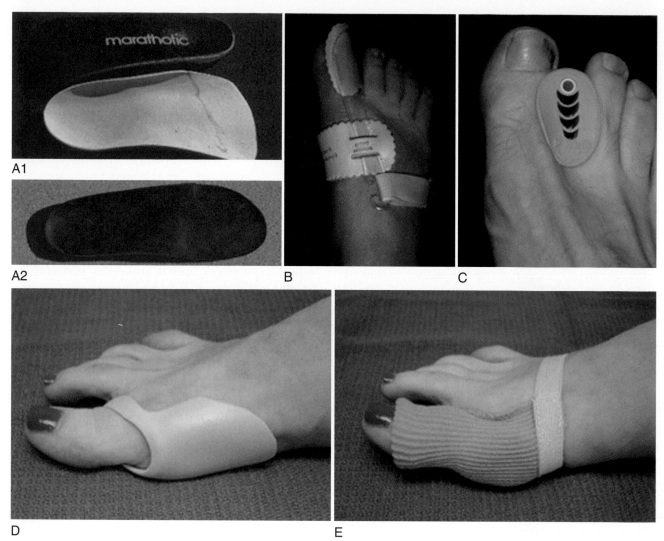

Figure 6–73 Conservative measures for the treatment of hallux valgus. **A1, A2,** Orthotics; **B,** night splint; **C,** bunion post; **D** and **E,** bunion pad.

SURGICAL TREATMENT

Decision Making

The decision-making process in hallux valgus surgery must begin with the understanding that not all hallux valgus deformities are equal. In the past, one repair was attempted for all types of hallux valgus deformity. Many different factors must be considered when evaluating a deformity. If a single procedure is used to correct all these various deformities, the possibility of success in most patients will be less than satisfactory.

The following issues should be considered in the decision-making process for hallux valgus surgery:

- The patient's chief complaint, occupation, and athletic interests
- Physical findings
- Radiographic evaluation, which should include the magnitude of the hallux valgus, intermetatarsal, and interphalangeal angles; the magnitude of the DMAA; the presence of a congruent or incongruent joint; the extent of MTP and MTC joint arthrosis; and the degree of pronation of the hallux
- The patient's age
- Neurovascular status of the foot
- The patient's expectations

Most of these issues can be quantified, but a patient's expectations of the procedure cannot. People who undergo bunion surgery often do not fully appreciate what outcome to expect. Many patients are unhappy after bunion surgery, mainly because they did not realize that they may not be able to return to their previous level of activity. They were not made fully aware of the potential postsurgical complications, or they fail to remember preoperative discussions.[325] A patient must fully understand that some residual stiffness, pain, or deformity may occur after surgery. Some patients have bunion surgery only because they believe that they will then be able to wear a more fashionable shoe and are subsequently disappointed when this goal cannot be achieved. In reviewing more than 300 bunion cases,[77,237,242] we have observed that a third of patients could wear the shoes that they wanted before surgery and that two thirds could after surgery. Unfortunately, this still leaves a third of patients unable to wear their shoe of choice, and this should be explained to the patient preoperatively.[325]

Another group of patients who pose a specific problem are those in professional sports or dance, who rely on their feet for their livelihood. Until it is no longer possible to perform in their chosen field, bunion surgery should probably be deferred.[67] If patients can eventually resume their previous level of activity after surgery, they will be much more satisfied with the outcome.[67]

With more than 100 surgical procedures described in the literature to correct a hallux valgus deformity, no procedure is adequate to correct all bunion deformities. We have developed an algorithm that gives the clinician a logical scheme with which to approach a patient with a hallux valgus deformity. The deformity is placed into one of three main groups according to the radiographic appearance: a congruent joint, an incongruent (subluxated) joint, or a joint with arthrosis (Fig. 6–74). Using these three basic groups, the algorithm correlates the radiographic appearance of the joint with procedures that provide optimal correction of the hallux valgus deformity. No algorithm is all-inclusive, nor can it include all operative procedures, but this algorithm helps organize the surgical considerations and uses proven surgical techniques that have been shown to withstand the test of time.

In using the algorithm, the clinician first must decide whether the hallux valgus deformity is accompanied by a congruent or incongruent (subluxated)

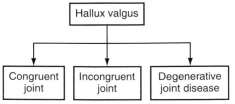

Figure 6–74 The initial algorithm for decision making divides hallux valgus deformities into those with a congruent joint, those with an incongruent joint, and joints with degenerative arthritis.

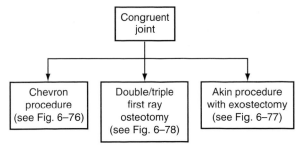

Figure 6–75 If a patient has congruent joint, these procedures will result in satisfactory correction.

MTP joint. A congruent MTP joint has no subluxation of the proximal phalanx on the metatarsal head. Therefore, the proximal phalanx, in theory, cannot be rotated back on the metatarsal head, or an incongruent situation might result. A surgical technique must respect a congruent joint when present, and no attempt should be made to alter joint congruency. Most patients with a congruent MTP joint will complain of pain over the medial eminence, although exceptions do exist when significant lateral deviation of the articular surface (increased DMAA) occurs and creates a hallux valgus deformity (see Figs. 6–55 to 6–57). For a mild hallux valgus deformity with a congruous MTP joint, an extraarticular repair (distal metatarsal osteotomy) is preferable because a distal soft tissue realignment may change a congruous joint into an incongruous joint. In patients with a congruent joint the following procedures will produce a satisfactory result (Fig. 6–75):

- Distal metatarsal osteotomy (Fig. 6–76)
- An Akin procedure with excision of the medial eminence (Fig. 6–77)
- Double/triple first ray osteotomy (Fig. 6–78)

An incongruent hallux valgus deformity (i.e., the proximal phalanx is subluxated laterally on the metatarsal head) requires a procedure that can move the proximal phalanx back onto the metatarsal head to reestablish a congruent joint. Because the degree of hallux valgus deformity varies, the procedure of choice depends on the severity of the deformity. We have divided severity into three groups: mild, moderate, and severe. These groups will obviously overlap, but the procedures described for each degree of deformity will probably produce the best overall results (Fig. 6–79).

With a **mild deformity**, the hallux valgus angle is **less than 20 degrees** and the intermetatarsal angle is **less than 11 degrees**. The following procedures are used:

- Distal metatarsal osteotomy (chevron, Mitchell) (Figs. 6–80 and 6–81)

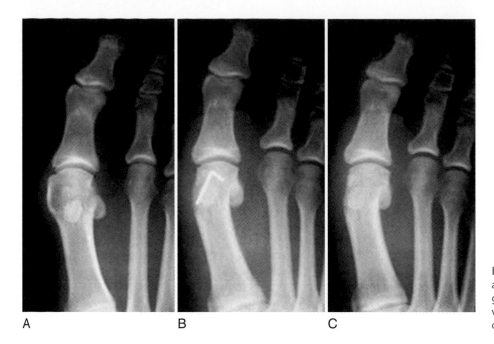

A   B   C

Figure 6–76 Preoperative (**A**) and postoperative (**B** and **C**) radiographs after correction of hallux valgus with a congruent joint. A chevron procedure was performed.

- Distal soft tissue procedure with or without proximal metatarsal osteotomy (Figs. 6–82 and 6–83)
- Midshaft osteotomy (scarf) (Fig. 6–84)

With a **moderate deformity**, the hallux valgus angle is **less than 40 degrees** and the intermetatarsal angle is **greater than 13 degrees**. The following procedures are recommended:

- Distal soft tissue procedure with a proximal metatarsal osteotomy (Fig. 6–85)
- Midshaft scarf osteotomy (see Fig. 6–84)
- Distal metatarsal osteotomy (the Mitchell procedure) (see Figs. 6–80 and 6–81)

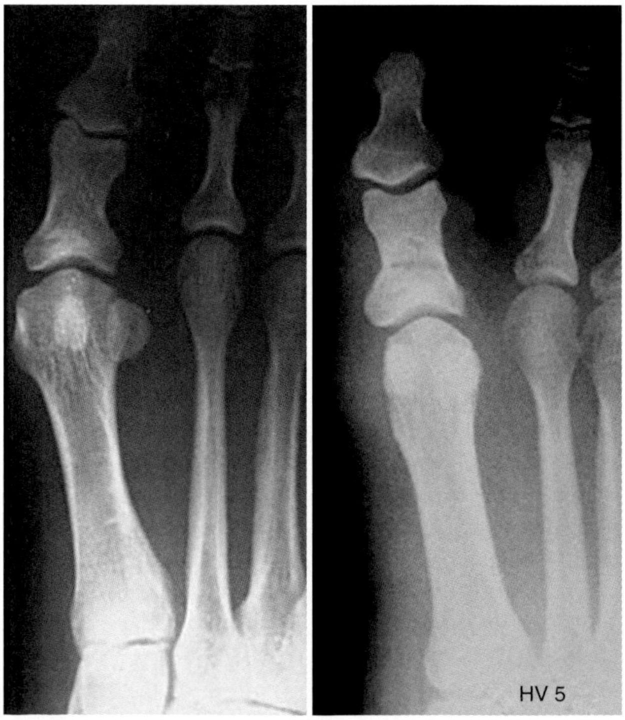

The chevron procedure is not included for treatment of moderate hallux valgus deformity because consistently reliable correction of the deformity in the upper ranges of the moderate group will often not occur. In the lower range of the moderate group, a chevron procedure may result in satisfactory correction.

With a **severe deformity**, the hallux valgus angle is **greater than 40 degrees** and the intermetatarsal angle is **greater than 20 degrees**. The following procedures are recommended:

- Distal soft tissue procedure with proximal metatarsal osteotomy (Fig. 6–85)
- Scarf osteotomy (see Fig. 6–84)
- A Lapidus procedure (Fig. 6–86)
- Arthrodesis of the first MTP joint (Fig. 6–87)

A distal osteotomy (Mitchell, chevron) is not recommended for a severe deformity because of its inability to consistently correct the deformity when the hallux valgus angle exceeds 40 degrees and the intermetatarsal angle exceeds 20 degrees. Severe deformities with or without associated first ray hypermobility can be treated with a distal soft tissue procedure and first MTC joint arthrodesis (the Lapidus procedure) (see Fig. 6–86).

HV 5

A   B

Figure 6–77 Preoperative (**A**) and postoperative (**B**) radiographs after correction of hallux valgus. An Akin procedure with excision of the medial eminence was performed.

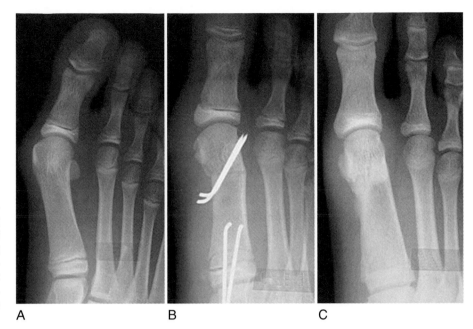

Figure 6–78 **A,** Anteroposterior radiograph of a 14-year-old girl demonstrating progression of deformity. **B,** After distal first metatarsal closing wedge osteotomy and proximal crescentic osteotomy, alignment is improved. **C,** A 2-year follow-up radiograph shows acceptable alignment.

A   B   C

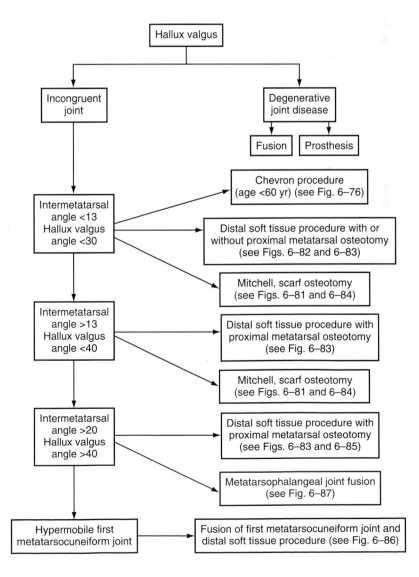

Figure 6–79 Algorithm for a patient with an incongruent joint. The procedure is based on the severity of deformity. For degenerative joint disease, we recommend fusion and rarely a prosthesis.

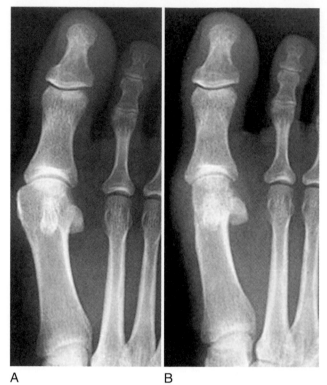

A   B

Figure 6–80 Preoperative (**A**) and postoperative (**B**) radiographs of a hallux valgus deformity with mild subluxation that was corrected with a chevron procedure.

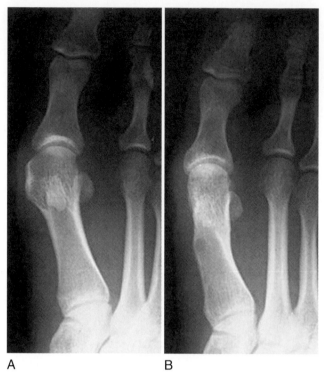

A   B

Figure 6–81 Preoperative (**A**) and postoperative (**B**) radiographs of a hallux valgus deformity with an incongruent joint that was corrected with a Mitchell procedure.

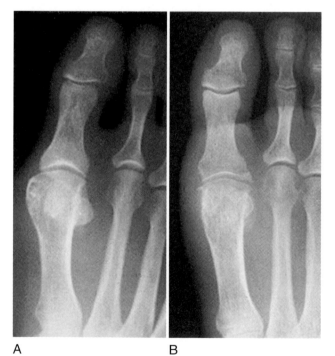

A   B

Figure 6–82 Preoperative (**A**) and postoperative (**B**) radiographs of a hallux valgus deformity with an incongruent joint that was corrected with a distal soft tissue procedure.

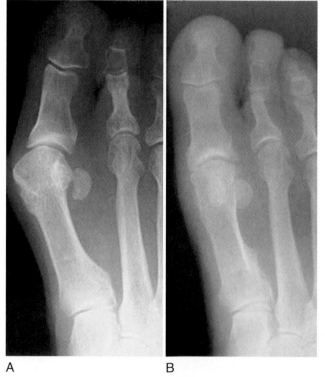

A   B

Figure 6–83 Preoperative (**A**) and postoperative (**B**) radiographs of a hallux valgus deformity with an incongruent joint that was corrected with a distal soft tissue procedure and proximal metatarsal osteotomy.

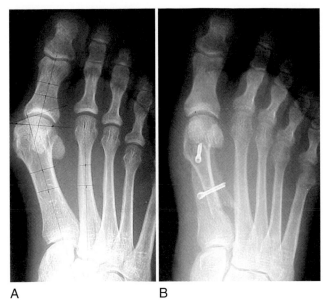

A B

Figure 6–84 **A,** Preoperative radiograph. **B,** After a scarf osteotomy.

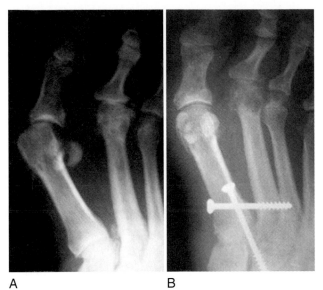

A B

Figure 6–86 Preoperative (**A**) and postoperative (**B**) radiographs of a severe hallux valgus deformity with an incongruent metatarsophalangeal joint and an unstable metatarsocuneiform (MTC) joint that was corrected with a distal soft tissue procedure and first MTC arthrodesis.

Significant arthrosis of the MTP joint negates the possibility of carrying out most realignment procedures because stiffness and pain of the MTP joint will usually result. Thus, we recommend performing an arthrodesis. This procedure produces a stable, painless joint that will not deteriorate over time. The use of an MTP joint prosthesis can be considered in a patient who does not place substantial stress on the foot. We believe that prostheses, in general, do not stand up to the test of time and frequently require revision or removal. At this time they are contraindicated in an active, sports-minded person.

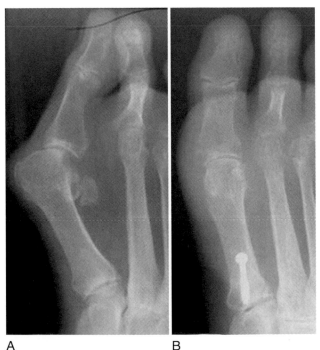

A B

Figure 6–85 Preoperative (**A**) and postoperative (**B**) radiographs of a severe hallux valgus deformity with an incongruent joint that was corrected with a distal soft tissue procedure and proximal metatarsal osteotomy.

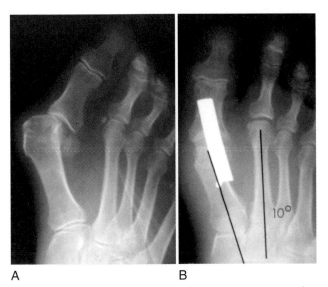

A B

Figure 6–87 Preoperative (**A**) and postoperative (**B**) radiographs of a severe hallux valgus deformity with incongruent joint corrected by arthrodesis of metatarsophalangeal joint. Note the dramatic reduction in the 1-2 intermetatarsal angle.

Surgical Procedures

Hallux valgus repair requires careful consideration of the surgical goals. The obvious objective is to correct the deformity anatomically so that a long-term satisfactory result is achieved. Thus, the ideal hallux valgus repair anatomically realigns the MTP joint without disrupting the biomechanics or normal weight-bearing function of the first MTP joint complex. Procedures that lead to excessive metatarsal shortening or dorsal displacement of the metatarsal head, that are associated with an excessive risk of AVN, or that use foreign materials that incite a local reaction or fail within the perioperative period should be avoided.

Most surgical procedures described here have been carefully reviewed in our own patient series and in some cases have been modified to enable us to achieve the best possible result.

The following procedures are described in detail:

- Distal soft tissue procedure
- Distal soft tissue procedure with proximal crescentic osteotomy
- The chevron procedure
- The Mitchell procedure (or other transverse distal osteotomy)
- The Akin procedure
- The Keller procedure
- Arthrodesis
- Scarf osteotomy
- Multiple first ray osteotomies

DISTAL SOFT TISSUE PROCEDURE

Distal soft tissue realignment as correction for a hallux valgus deformity has been advocated in several reports.* It was Silver,[327] however, who popularized the technique of medial capsulorrhaphy, medial exostectomy, and lateral capsular and adductor release. Later, McBride[251,252,254] modified this technique by removal of the lateral sesamoid and transfer of the conjoined adductor tendon to the lateral first metatarsal head. DuVries[99] and others[232,233,235,237,241] modified this procedure so extensively that the eponym "McBride" is no longer appropriate. Mann and Coughlin[237] and later Mann and Pfeffinger,[241] after reviewing the results of this procedure in

---

*References 96, 236, 251, 252, 254, and 262.

adults, recommended that the fibular sesamoid be preserved because of the high rate of hallux varus after sesamoid excision.

The basis of this procedure is that the contracted lateral joint structures (i.e., the adductor hallucis, lateral joint capsule, transverse metatarsal ligament) are released, thereby permitting the proximal phalanx to be realigned on the metatarsal head (video clip 26). The attenuated medial capsule is plicated after the medial eminence has been excised. The limiting factor with this technique is the magnitude of metatarsal primus varus present. Because this is only a soft tissue realignment, if there is a fixed malalignment with a 1-2 intermetatarsal angle of more than 10 degrees, long-lasting correction is unlikely. Therefore, the first MTC joint must have sufficient mobility to permit correction of the intermetatarsal angle from its preoperative position into a normal range postoperatively, or the hallux valgus deformity will recur.

Indications

A distal soft tissue procedure is indicated in a patient with an incongruent (or subluxated) joint, a hallux valgus deformity of less than 30 degrees, and an intermetatarsal angle of less than 11 degrees. If the indications for the procedure are pushed beyond this magnitude of deformity, sufficient mobility must exist at the MTC joint to allow reduction of the intermetatarsal angle. If the intermetatarsal angle does not reduce, the hallux valgus deformity often recurs, so a proximal metatarsal osteotomy is added to the distal soft tissue procedure to provide complete correction. This procedure is applicable to all age groups, from juvenile through octogenarian. An MTC arthrodesis can also be used in association with a distal soft tissue realignment.

Contraindications

The main contraindication to a distal soft tissue procedure is a deformity that exceeds the procedure's capability to gain adequate correction. If the hallux valgus angle is greater than 30 degrees and the intermetatarsal angle is greater than 11 degrees, this procedure will usually not result in a durable or predictable correction. In many cases, early recurrence often develops because the fixed intermetatarsal angle has not been adequately corrected. Another contraindication is the presence of a congruent joint with significant lateral deviation of the distal metatarsal articular surface (a DMAA greater than 15 degrees) (see Figs. 6–46, 6–55, and 6–56). In these circumstances a distal soft tissue procedure is contraindicated because it cannot correct the deformity and will transform a congruent into an incongruent joint. Other contraindications include advanced arthrosis of the MTP joint, spasticity of any type (e.g., cerebral palsy, CVA, head injury), and ligamentous laxity.

Technique

The surgical technique consists of three steps: release of the first web space, preparation of the medial aspect of the MTP joint with excision of the medial eminence, and subsequent reconstruction of the MTP joint.

Release of the First Web Space

1. A peripheral nerve block is used for anesthesia and a tourniquet is applied in the supramalleolar region. A 3-cm dorsal longitudinal incision is centered in the first intermetatarsal web space (Fig. 6–89A; see also Fig. 6–88A). The incision is deepened in the midline through the subcutaneous tissue and fat until the adventitious bursa is identified between the two heads. The dissection is made in the midline to protect the superficial branches of the deep peroneal nerve, which pass on either side of the web space.

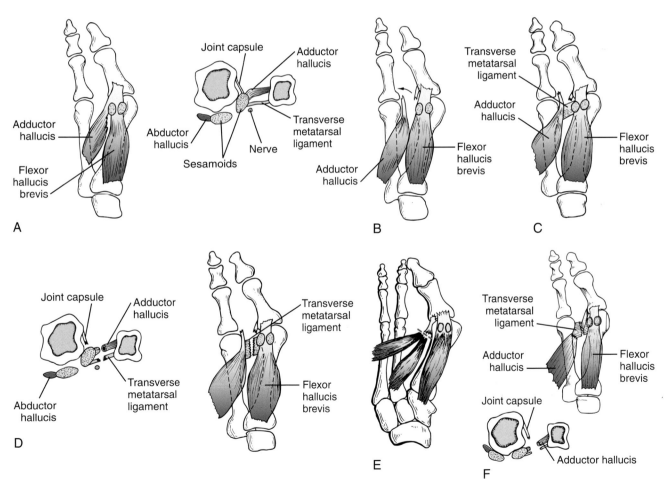

Figure 6–88 Technique for carrying out a distal soft tissue procedure. **A,** The adductor tendon inserts into the lateral aspect of the fibular sesamoid and into the base of the proximal phalanx. The *inset* demonstrates contracted tissue in cross section. **B,** The adductor tendon is released from its insertion into the lateral aspect of the fibular sesamoid and the base of the proximal phalanx. **C,** The transverse metatarsal ligament is noted to pass from the second metatarsal into the fibular sesamoid. **D,** The transverse metatarsal ligament has been transected. The *inset* demonstrates that at this point, contracted lateral structures (i.e., the lateral joint capsule, adductor hallucis, transverse metatarsal ligament) have been released. **E** and **F,** Alternative lateral release involving retention of a distal 2-cm stump of adductor tendon for the lateral capsular repair.

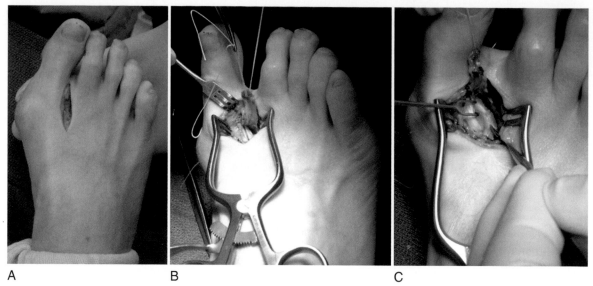

A   B   C

Figure 6–89   **A,** The initial skin incision is made in the web space between the first and second metatarsals. **B,** A Weitlaner retractor is used to expose the conjoined adductor tendon, which is released. **C,** The lateral sesamoid is freed up but not routinely excised.

2. A Weitlaner retractor or lamina spreader is inserted between the first and second metatarsal heads to facilitate exposure of the web space (Fig. 6–89B). The adductor hallucis tendon is identified along the dorsal aspect of the fibular sesamoid and the lateral aspect of the metatarsal head. The scalpel blade is inserted into this interval with the blade lying between the metatarsal head dorsally and the fibular sesamoid plantarward. The blade is directed distally until it strikes the base of the proximal phalanx; the knife is turned laterally against the adductor tendon and the tendon is released from the base of the proximal phalanx. The knife is then brought proximally in the same plane between the metatarsal head and sesamoid to cut the remainder of the capsule between the sesamoid and metatarsal (see Fig. 6–88B and C).

3. The distal end of the adductor tendon that was released from the base of the proximal phalanx is dissected from the lateral aspect of the fibular sesamoid until the junction of the flexor hallucis brevis and adductor hallucis muscle fibers is reached. The fibular sesamoid is inspected by pushing it plantarward with a Freer elevator. The fibular sesamoid is rarely excised unless significant degenerative changes are seen at the sesamoid-metatarsal articulation.

Alternative Technique[70]: The distal adductor tendon insertion is left attached to the base of the proximal phalanx, and the stump of the adductor tendon (2 cm in length) is left attached at its phalangeal insertion (Figs. 6–88E and 6–89B and C). The tendon is released at the level of the musculotendinous junction to allow the proximal adductor hallucis tendon to retract. The distal stump of the tendon is later sutured to the lateral aspect of the metatarsal capsule.

4. The self-retaining retractor is placed deeper into the wound, and the first and second metatarsals are spread apart to place tension on the transverse metatarsal ligament, which passes from the second metatarsal into the fibular sesamoid. The ligament is transected cautiously to prevent injury to the underlying common digital nerve and vessels in the first web space (Fig. 6–88D). Once the ligament is released, an elevator is passed along the plantar aspect of the fibular sesamoid to ensure that the sesamoids can be relocated beneath the metatarsal head. If the fibular sesamoid has been excised, the tendon of the flexor hallucis longus is inspected to ensure that it was not inadvertently transected.

5. The lateral capsule is perforated with several puncture wounds, and the toe is angulated medially to disrupt the remaining lateral capsule. (The purpose of this tearing tech-

nique is to leave some lateral capsular tissue present so that with healing it will stabilize the lateral MTP joint and minimize the risk of development of a postoperative hallux varus deformity.) Alternatively, a distally based capsular flap can be developed by detaching the lateral capsule from the lateral first metatarsal head. The stump of conjoined tendon that has been preserved is later sutured into the lateral metatarsal capsule and soft tissue for reinforcement of the lateral capsule to minimize varus inclination. If a distally based cuff of lateral capsule has been developed, it is later sutured into the proximal capsular tissue. If the lateral capsule has been released at the level of the MTP joint, three interrupted 2-0 absorbable sutures are used to approximate the first and second MTP joint capsules. These sutures are later tied at the conclusion of the procedure.

This completes release of the lateral contracture of the MTP joint, and attention is directed to its medial aspect (Fig. 6–88F).

Preparation of the Medial Aspect of the Metatarsophalangeal Joint

1. The medial incision is made in the midline and begins distally at the midportion of the proximal phalanx and continues proximally 1 cm beyond the medial eminence (Fig. 6–90A). The incision is deepened through the subcutaneous tissue to the joint capsule, and dissection is carried out along the capsular plane. It is important to create a full-thickness flap to prevent any possible skin slough. By reflecting the flaps dorsally and plantar-ward, the dorsal and plantar medial cutaneous nerves can be identified and retracted.
2. The dorsal and plantar flaps are retracted to expose the joint capsule. With a no. 11 blade, a vertical capsular incision is placed approximately 2 to 3 mm proximal to the base of the proximal phalanx. A second parallel incision is then made in the capsule, 4 to 8 mm more proximal, depending on the severity of the deformity (Fig. 6–90B and C).

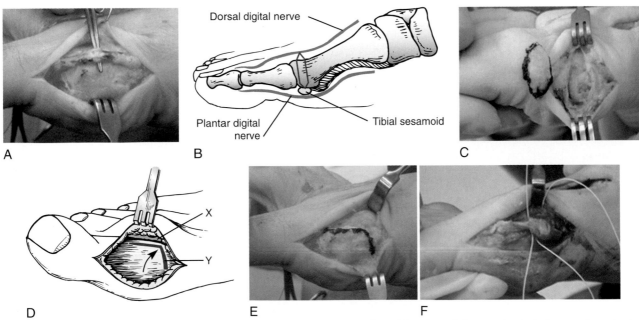

Figure 6–90 **A,** The medial incision is made in midline, beginning at the midportion of the proximal phalanx and continuing proximally 1 cm beyond the medial eminence. A clamp is used to elevate the dorsomedial cutaneous nerve, which must be protected. **B,** Diagram demonstrating the medial capsular incision, which begins 2 to 3 mm proximal to the base of the proximal phalanx. A second incision is made 3 to 8 mm more proximal to remove a flap of tissue. The size of the flap is determined by the severity of the deformity. **C,** Two parallel cuts in the medial capsule are shown. A wedge of tissue measuring approximately 6 mm has been removed. Note how the capsular cut is directed in a V configuration down through the abductor hallucis tendon, with the apex at the tibial sesamoid. Dorsally, the apex of the V is about 1 cm medial to the extensor tendon. **D** and **E,** An L-shaped capsulotomy releases the dorsal and proximal MTP joint capsule. **F,** A drill hole is made in the metaphysis to secure the dorsal proximal capsule.

The capsular incisions are connected dorsally by an inverted-V incision approximately 5 to 10 mm medial to the extensor hallucis longus tendon. The capsular flap is now exposed plantar-ward, where a V-shaped incision is made through the abductor hallucis tendon. When making this incision through the abductor tendon, the surgeon must keep the knife blade inside the joint to prevent any damage to the plantar medial cutaneous nerve, which passes just plantar to the sesamoid. If one attempts to make this incision from outside the capsule in, the plantar medial cutaneous nerve might be cut by the blade's tip. By working from the inside out, however, the sesamoid prevents the knife from passing too far plantar-ward, thereby protecting the plantar medial cutaneous nerve. (If by chance this nerve is transected, it should be freed up proximally and buried beneath the abductor hallucis muscle to prevent a neuroma from forming along the plantar medial aspect of the foot.) The medial eminence is exposed by creating a flap of capsule that is based proximally and plantar-ward. This is done by making an incision along the dorsomedial aspect of the capsule and carefully dissecting it from the medial eminence until it is exposed in its entirety. With a severe deformity, the dorsal portion of the joint capsule is often flimsy and could tear. This is not a cause for concern, however, because the plantar half of the capsule is the most important in the capsular repair.

Alternative Capsular Incision[70]: An L-shaped, distally based capsular flap is developed to release the capsular attachments on the dorsal and proximal aspects (Fig. 6–90D and E). If this capsular flap technique is used, a drill hole is then made on the dorsomedial aspect of the metaphysis of the first metatarsal. At the time of capsular repair, the proximal capsule is secured with interrupted absorbable suture through this drill hole (Fig. 6–90F). Several interrupted 2-0 absorbable sutures are used to repair the proximal as well as the dorsal capsular incision.

3. The MTP joint is inspected and the condition of the articular cartilage noted.

4. The sagittal sulcus is identified and the medial eminence removed, starting approximately 2 mm medial to the sagittal sulcus in

a line parallel with the medial diaphyseal cortex of the first metatarsal (Fig. 6–91). Care is taken to not remove an excessive amount of medial eminence to avoid narrowing the metatarsal head and creating medial instability that may lead to a hallux varus deformity. Before removing the medial eminence, the radiographs should be inspected; a line is projected along the medial aspect of the metatarsal distally through the medial eminence (Fig. 6–92D and E). This line provides a general idea about how much medial eminence should be excised. The osteotomized edges are smoothed with a rongeur, especially in the area of the dorsomedial corner of the metatarsal head, an area that often has a sharp prominence. This completes the preparation of the medial capsular structures.

Reconstruction of the Metatarsophalangeal Joint

1. After release of the soft tissue structures around the first metatarsal head, the mobility of the first MTC joint is assessed by pushing the first metatarsal head lateral-ward (Fig. 6–92A). If the first metatarsal head is easily translated medial-ward with little resistance or tendency to spread, one can assume that the intermetatarsal angle will probably reduce with only a soft tissue procedure. If, however, the first metatarsal head tends to "spring back" medially as though resisting realignment, a distal soft tissue procedure alone will probably be inadequate and a proximal metatarsal osteotomy should be performed as well. We tend to perform an osteotomy in approximately 95% of cases. If the first and second metatarsals tend to spring open, there will probably be residual widening of the intermetatarsal space and early recurrence of the deformity (Fig. 6–92B and C). As a general rule, if there is any question about whether to perform an osteotomy, it should probably be performed. The osteotomy technique is described later.

2. If an osteotomy is not necessary, the soft tissues on the lateral aspect of the MTP joint are repaired by identifying the adductor tendon in the plantar web space and placing two sutures between it and the remaining lateral capsular cuff of the first metatarsal head. These sutures secure the transferred

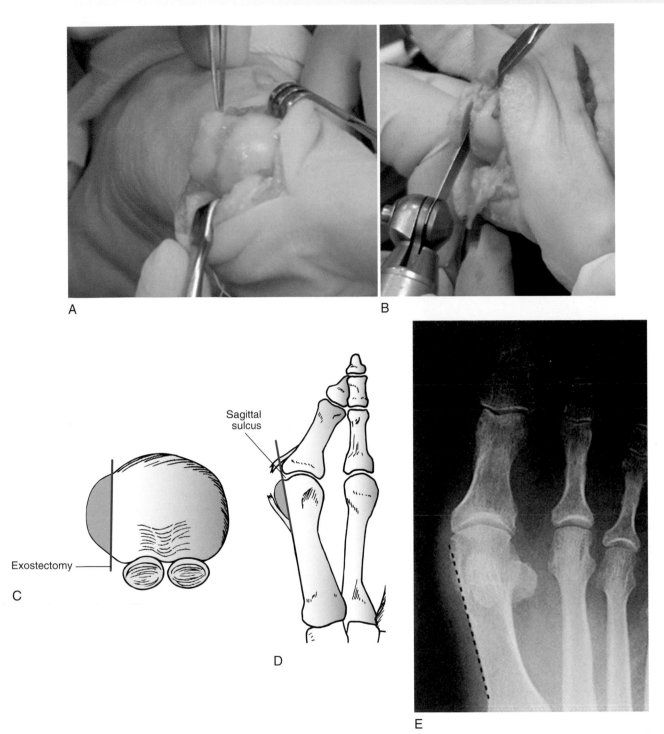

Figure 6–91 Excision of the medial eminence. **A,** Photograph demonstrating the medial aspect of the metatarsal head on end. **B,** Removal of the medial eminence is carried out on a line projected along the medial aspect of the first metatarsal shaft. **C,** Exostectomy should be carried out 1 to 2 mm medial to the sagittal sulcus. **D,** Excision of the medial eminence in line with the medial aspect of the metatarsal shaft. **E,** Radiograph demonstrating removal of the medial eminence in line with the medial aspect of the metatarsal shaft.

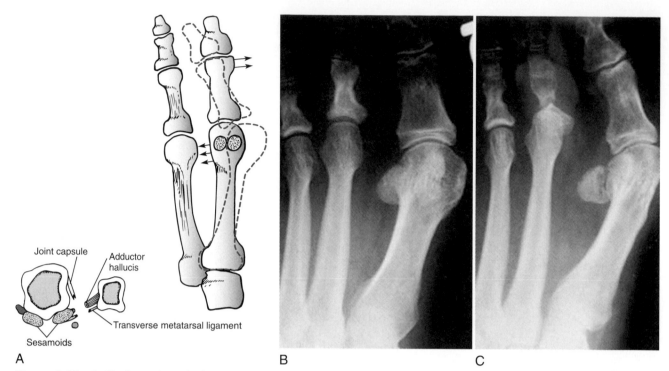

Joint capsule
Adductor hallucis
Transverse metatarsal ligament
Sesamoids

A   B   C

Figure 6–92 A, To determine whether an osteotomy is necessary after soft tissue releases have been carried out, the first metatarsal head is pushed laterally. If the metatarsal head tends to spring back medially, an osteotomy should be considered. We perform an osteotomy about 95% of the time. Preoperative (**B**) and postoperative (**C**) radiographs demonstrate a recurrent hallux valgus deformity from lack of correction of the intermetatarsal angle.

adductor tendon along the lateral aspect of the first MTP joint. We believe that the adductor tendon helps re-form the capsular tissue on the lateral aspect of the MTP joint (Fig. 6–93).

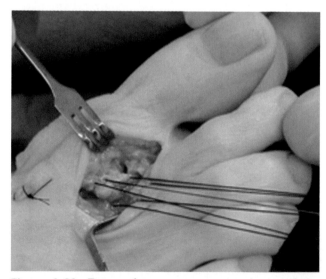

Figure 6–93 Two or three sutures are used to reef the capsule of the first and second metatarsophalangeal joints, with incorporation of the adductor tendon within the sutures.

3. The hallux is placed in correct alignment during repair of the medial joint capsule. This position consists of neither varus nor valgus. The base of the phalanx is aligned with the long axis of the first metatarsal. Any pronation is corrected by slightly supinating the hallux as the sutures are placed. The derotation of the phalanx ensures that the sesamoids, which are connected to the base of the proximal phalanx, are realigned beneath the first metatarsal head. The edge of the tibial sesamoid should be clearly visible in the base of the medial wound with the toe in a corrected position. (If such is not the case, release of any remaining lateral joint contracture is necessary so that the sesamoid sling can be rotated beneath the metatarsal head (Fig. 6–94).

4. The medial capsule is repaired with four or five interrupted sutures. The most important part of the capsular repair is the plantar half, which includes the abductor hallucis tendon and the thickest portion of the joint capsule. Before placing the sutures, the two edges of the capsule are brought into apposition to ensure that sufficient capsular tissue has

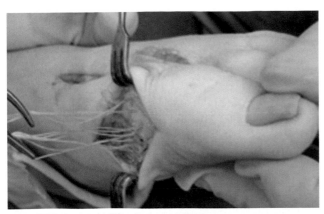

Figure 6–94 Plication of the medial joint capsule is carried out while the great toe is held in line with the first metatarsal, 2 to 3 degrees of varus, and rotated to place the sesamoids beneath the metatarsal head. The medial capsular flap then is approximated, and if redundant capsule still exists, more capsular tissue can be removed.

been removed. If there appears to be redundant capsule remaining, it is excised to allow the two capsular edges to be opposed with the capsular closure. On completion of the medial capsular repair, the hallux should be satisfactorily aligned. A slight degree of residual varus can usually be corrected with the postoperative dressings. If, however, the amount of correction is inadequate, that is, if there is residual valgus, the capsular sutures should be removed, more medial capsule resected, and the structures reapproximated.

5. The sutures in the first web space are tied.
6. The skin is approximated with fine interrupted suture, and a sterile compression dressing is applied for 12 to 24 hours.

Postoperative Care

The compression dressing is removed in the office 24 to 48 hours after the procedure, and a new dressing consisting of 2-inch Kling gauze and 1/2-inch adhesive tape is applied to hold the toe in anatomic alignment. The postoperative dressings are critical in obtaining satisfactory alignment after a hallux valgus repair. During the first 3 to 4 weeks after surgery, the dressings can influence the position of the toe. The purpose of the dressing is to bind the metatarsal heads tightly together, after which a spica-like dressing is placed around the hallux, either holding it in a neutral position or adjust-

ing it into slight varus or valgus, depending on the desired correction. To ensure that the sesamoids remain reduced beneath the metatarsal head, the gauze around the hallux of the right foot (when dressing the foot from the bottom of the bed) is wrapped in a counter-clockwise direction and that of the left foot in a clockwise direction (Fig. 6–95). This ensures that the correct rotational torque is placed on the hallux to maintain acceptable alignment of the sesamoids. After surgery the patient is permitted to ambulate as tolerated in a stiff-soled postoperative shoe. Initially, the patient ambulates on the heel and lateral aspect of the foot. It usually takes 2 to 4 weeks before the typical patient applies any significant pressure along the medial aspect of the foot.

The postoperative dressings are changed weekly for the first 4 weeks, and if the position of the hallux is satisfactory, they are changed every 10 days for the second 4 weeks. We do not believe that cast immobilization is necessary after this procedure. With the foot covered by a cast, the first MTP joint cannot be adequately observed, and thus fine adjustments to the alignment cannot be performed.

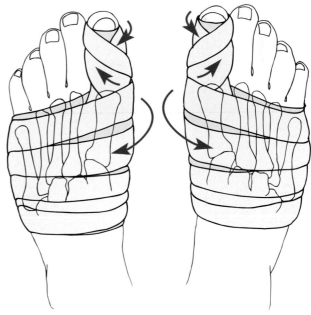

Figure 6–95 Postoperative dressings after correction of hallux valgus. Note that the metatarsal heads are firmly bound together with Kling bandage and that the great toe is rotated to keep the sesamoids realigned beneath the metatarsal head. This necessitates dressing the right toe in a counterclockwise direction and the left toe in a clockwise direction when one is standing at the foot of the bed.

At the second postoperative visit, approximately 7 to 10 days after surgery, an AP radiograph is obtained with as much weight bearing as possible. This identifies the alignment of the first MTP joint, and the toe is dressed into neutral, varus, or valgus alignment with the subsequent dressings. During the postoperative period, even with dressings in place, the patient is encouraged to perform active and passive range-of-motion exercises to reestablish dorsiflexion and plantar flexion (Fig. 6–96).

After 2 months of immobilization, the dressing is discontinued. As the swelling and thickening about the first MTP joint subside, the patient can progress from a sandal or broadtoed shoe eventually to fashionable footwear. The patient is encouraged to wear wide, soft shoes rather than narrow, high-heeled shoes. The time required for the swelling to adequately subside varies greatly from patient to patient and may exceed 3 months. If the toe is noted to drift into a slight valgus position after removal of the dressings, a night bunion splint may be indicated (see Fig. 6–73B).

Results

Although Silver[327] advocated resection of the medial eminence and release of the lateral soft tissues, he did not report his results with this procedure. In a review of simple bunionectomies with or without lateral capsulotomy in 33 adult patients, Kitaoka et al[195] reported a 5-degree increase in the hallux valgus angle postoperatively and a 2 degree increase in the 1-2 intermetatarsal angle at long-term follow-up. A failure rate of 24% was reported. Bonney and Macnab[27] reported generally poor results after simple exostectomy, with 37% of patients requiring additional treatment. Meyer et al[262] and others[173,237,241] have reported a high rate of success in the treatment of mild and moderate hallux valgus deformities in adults with a distal soft tissue realignment. Mann and Coughlin[237] reported an average 15-degree correction of the hallux valgus angle and an average 5.2-degree correction of the 1-2 intermetatarsal angle. However, with a severe hallux valgus deformity, distal soft tissue realignment alone achieves only a 50% correction of the deformity. Thus, the indications for distal soft tissue reconstruction alone are limited to a mild deformity (hallux valgus angle less than 30 degrees and intermetatarsal angle less than 11 degrees).

A high failure rate of the McBride procedure in juvenile patients that varies from 43% to 75% has been reported in the literature.[27,72,152,153,318] This technique in juveniles confirms the wider experience in the literature that this procedure has limited ability to correct a hallux valgus deformity with an increased DMAA. For a subluxated MTP joint with a moderate or severe hallux valgus deformity (hallux valgus angle requiring more than 20 degrees correction or an intermetatarsal angle greater than 15 degrees), proximal metatarsal osteotomy has been recommended in conjunction with distal soft tissue realignment.[99,129,380]

In a subsequent review of 72 feet in 47 patients undergoing distal soft tissue realignment, Mann and Pfeffinger[241] reported postoperative satisfaction in 92% of patients. The main reason for satisfaction was pain relief, decreased deformity, and diminution in bunion size. Unrestricted footwear was possible in 20% of patients preoperatively and 53% postoperatively. This still left 47% of patients unable to wear the shoes of their choice. The overall level of activity increased in 66% of patients and was unchanged in 34%.

Table 6–1 presents the preoperative and postoperative hallux valgus and intermetatarsal

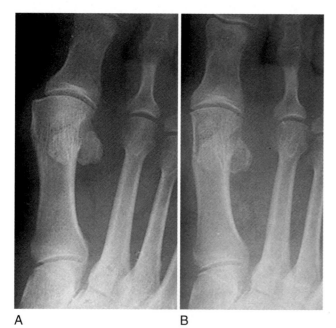

A   B

Figure 6–96 Results after correction of hallux valgus deformity with a distal soft tissue procedure.

TABLE 6–1

Summary of 72 Feet before and after a Distal Soft Tissue Procedure

Angle	Preoperative	Postoperative
Average hallux valgus	32.4°	15.9°
Average first/second intermetatarsal	14.3°	8.8°

angles for the entire group, and Table 6–2 lists the results by severity of the deformity. These results once again confirm that a satisfactory outcome can be obtained in the treatment of mild and moderate hallux valgus deformities. However, with a severe deformity, a distal soft tissue procedure alone will not usually result in a satisfactory outcome. Table 6–3 compares the results in patients with an intermetatarsal angle of less than 15 degrees and greater than 15 degrees and demonstrates that with severe deformity, a distal soft tissue procedure alone is routinely incapable of achieving satisfactory realignment. In the entire series, only 41% of feet had a residual hallux valgus angle of less than 16 degrees. This figure emphasizes that the reliability of this procedure, particularly for a more advanced deformity, is not good, and the procedure is indicated mainly for mild and low-end moderate deformity.

Complications

Recurrence of Deformity. Recurrence may be related to one or more of the following factors:

- Inadequate postoperative dressings
- Insufficient plication of the medial joint capsule
- Inadequate release of the lateral joint contracture, which may include the capsule, adductor hallucis tendon, or transverse metatarsal ligament
- Insufficient medial capsular tissues secondary to degenerative changes or cyst formation
- Failure to recognize and treat metatarsus primus varus
- Failure to recognize a congruent joint

Arthrofibrosis. Slight loss of motion occurred after surgery. Range-of-motion measurements demonstrated 67 degrees of dorsiflexion and 8 degrees of plantar flexion, as compared with 75 and 16 degrees, respectively, in the uninvolved foot. Arthrofibrosis may be caused by the following:

- Postoperative infection
- Unrecognized arthrosis of the MTP joint
- Unrecognized causes
- Realignment of a congruent joint

Peripheral Nerve Entrapment. Occasionally the dorsal or plantar cutaneous nerve to the great toe becomes injured or entrapped, which can cause pain if a large neuroma develops. Use of the incisions as described in this section reduces this complication to a minimum.

Hallux Varus. The major complication encountered in the series of Mann et al[242] was an 8% incidence of hallux varus deformity, which averaged 7.5 degrees (Fig. 6–97). The position of the proximal phalanx influenced the intermetatarsal angle; the intermetatarsal angle was corrected 12 degrees in feet with hallux varus versus 5 degrees in those without overcorrection. In all cases of hallux varus, the tibial sesamoid subluxated medially; however, in only

TABLE 6–2

Summary of Results of Distal Soft Tissue Procedures by Severity of Deformity

	Mild (<20°)	Moderate (21°–40°)	Severe (>40°)	Patients with Postoperative Hallux Varus
Number of feet	4	57	11	6
Mean age (y)	51	55	57	56
Mean hallux valgus angle				
Preoperative	18°	31°	46°	37°
Postoperative	11°	15°	19°	−7.5°
Mean first/second intermetatarsal angle				
Preoperative	10.7°	14°	17°	17°
Postoperative	8.5°	8.6°	10°	5°

TABLE 6–3

Postoperative Correction before and after Distal Soft Tissue Procedures

Hallux Valgus Angle	Preoperative Intermetatarsal Angle	
	<15°	>15°
Preoperative	28	38
Postoperative	11	18
Correction	17	20

half the feet with medial sesamoid subluxation did a hallux varus deformity develop. Preoperatively, the feet in which a hallux varus deformity developed were characterized by more severe deformities. Mann and Coughlin[237] recommended that release of the lateral MTP joint capsule be performed without a lateral sesamoidectomy. After this modification a reduced rate of hallux varus was reported.[233,236] Use of the stump of conjoined adductor tendon and cuff of the lateral MTP capsule to reinforce the lateral capsule at the time of surgical cor-

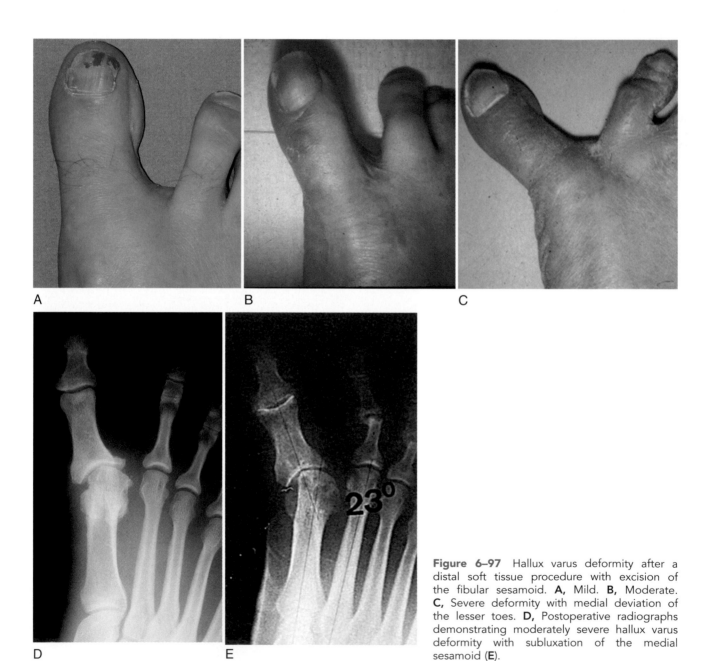

A   B   C

D   E

Figure 6–97 Hallux varus deformity after a distal soft tissue procedure with excision of the fibular sesamoid. **A,** Mild. **B,** Moderate. **C,** Severe deformity with medial deviation of the lesser toes. **D,** Postoperative radiographs demonstrating moderately severe hallux varus deformity with subluxation of the medial sesamoid (**E**).

rection may also help minimize the incidence of postoperative hallux varus.[70]

See page 345 at the end of this chapter for a discussion of hallux varus.

DISTAL SOFT TISSUE PROCEDURE WITH PROXIMAL CRESCENTIC OSTEOTOMY

Review of the experience with the distal soft tissue procedure in our series[237] led us to conclude that a soft tissue procedure alone is insufficient to completely and consistently correct a hallux valgus deformity when the intermetatarsal angle exceeds 12 degrees. We therefore added a proximal crescentic metatarsal osteotomy to correct the increased intermetatarsal angle. The results of this specific technique have since been reported in several studies (video clip 27).*

The crescentic osteotomy was chosen to minimize the loss of length when carrying out a metatarsal osteotomy and to create a broad stable osteotomy construct (Fig. 6–98). A proximal chevron osteotomy also produces results

---

*References 97, 100, 242, 278, 348, and 361.

similar to those of a proximal crescentic osteotomy.[30,100,246,306] Although a closing or opening wedge osteotomy is an alternative, substantial shortening or lengthening of the first ray is rarely necessary. In a study of more than 7000 feet, Harris and Beath[147] found that the first and second metatarsals were frequently of either equal length or within a few millimeters of each other in length. Although a lateral closing wedge osteotomy[292,318,367] has been proposed for reduction of the increased 1-2 intermetatarsal angle, it has an inherent problem that when the osteotomy is performed, more bone may be taken off dorsally than plantar-ward, which may lead to metatarsal dorsiflexion, as well as shortening, as the osteotomy is closed. This combination of shortening and dorsiflexion often leads to transfer metatarsalgia. Conversely, an opening wedge osteotomy of the first metatarsal has also been suggested*; typically, it is combined with an interposition graft. This osteotomy has the inherent problem of decreased stability at the osteotomy site. Furthermore, with more severe cases of hallux valgus, the extrinsic tendons and other soft tissue structures crossing the MTP joint are

---

*References 27, 48, 129, 215, 318, 329, and 353.

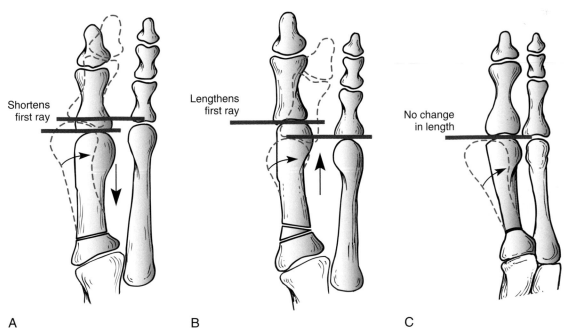

Shortens first ray

Lengthens first ray

No change in length

A   B   C

Figure 6–98   A, A closing wedge osteotomy shortens the first metatarsal. **B,** An opening wedge osteotomy lengthens the first metatarsal. **C,** A crescentic osteotomy tends to maintain first metatarsal length.

placed under greater tension. Goldner and Gaines[129] concluded that an opening wedge proximal first metatarsal osteotomy tightens the extensor mechanism and leads to postoperative recurrence of a hallux valgus deformity. A high rate of recurrence has been reported with opening wedge metatarsal ostetomies.[27,129,318] A crescentic osteotomy has thus been advocated as the means to correct an increased 1-2 intermetatarsal angle without significantly altering the length of the first metatarsal.[70,233] The osteotomy is located in the first metatarsal metaphysis because this area provides a broad contact area, which promotes rapid healing, and a relatively large surface area, which affords stability in a dorsoplantar direction.

Initially we performed the crescentic osteotomy with the concavity directed distally toward the great toe.[72,233] In a few cases, however, we noted that if the osteotomy site was inadvertently displaced medially and the metatarsal head was translated too far laterally, an incongruent MTP joint and, in some cases, hallux varus resulted (Fig. 6–99). This prompted us to reverse the direction so that the concavity was directed toward the heel (Fig. 6–100), a

technique now commonly reported by others as well.[100,242,278] From a biomechanical standpoint, with the concavity oriented proximally, the center of the rotational axis of the osteotomy is centered at the MTC joint,[304] thus making this correction much more anatomic. This permits the same degree of movement of the osteotomy, but the osteotomy also tends to compress with rotation, thereby lending stability to the osteotomy site. This also reduces the possibility of either displacing the metatarsal head too far laterally or creating a malunion.

Indications

A moderate or severe hallux valgus deformity with an incongruent (subluxated) MTP joint is the main indication for this procedure. As a general rule, the hallux valgus angle usually exceeds 30 degrees and the intermetatarsal angle is greater than 13 degrees. Although there is no specific upper limit to the deformity that this procedure can correct, complete correction is often not possible with a hallux valgus angular deformity in excess of 55 degrees or an

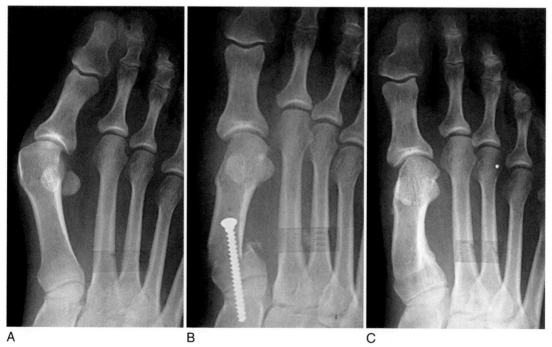

A   B   C

Figure 6–99 Overcorrection of a proximal osteotomy. **A,** Preoperative radiograph demonstrating a moderate hallux valgus deformity. **B,** Overcorrection of the 1-2 intermetatarsal angle with a proximal metatarsal osteotomy and resection of excessive medial eminence. **C,** Six-year follow-up radiograph demonstrating a mild hallux varus deformity. The patient had no symptoms, but progression of varus deformity is possible.

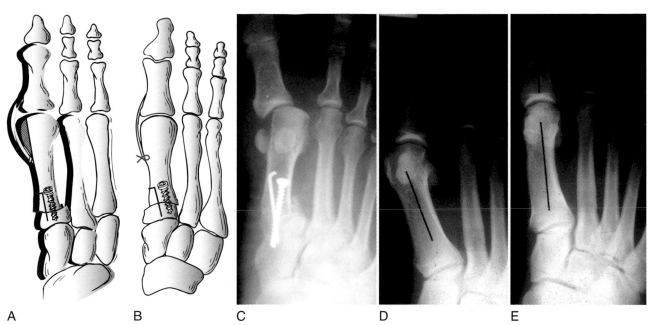

A   B   C   D   E

Figure 6–100   Proximal crescentic metatarsal osteotomies. **A,** With the concave surface oriented distally. **B,** With the concave surface oriented proximally. **C,** After osteotomy with the concavity oriented distally, overcorrection and hallux varus have resulted; medial displacement of the osteotomy results in excessive lateral displacement of the metatarsal head. **D,** Before and, **E,** after osteotomy with the concavity oriented distally. Note that this orientation prevents medial displacement of the osteotomy site and therefore prevents overcorrection of the metatarsal head. For this reason we now always carry out the crescentic osteotomy with the concavity directed (proximally) toward the heel.

intermetatarsal angle greater than 25 degrees. A deformity with an intermetatarsal angle less than 12 degrees will typically not require an osteotomy; if at surgery, however, there is resistance to reduction of the 1-2 intermetatarsal angle or if a lateral facet is present at the base of the first metatarsal (see Fig. 6–60), an osteotomy is indicated. The procedure is versatile and can be performed in patients of all ages, from juvenile to octogenarian.

Contraindications

Contraindications to distal soft tissue reconstruction with a proximal first metatarsal osteotomy include the presence of significant arthrosis, severe metatarsus adductus,[70] and spasticity of any type. Distal soft tissue reconstruction should also be avoided in the presence of a congruous MTP joint (with a DMAA greater than 15 degrees)[70,215,348] because recurrence, degenerative arthrosis, or postoperative stiffness could result. Coughlin[68] reported that the final angulation of the MTP joint mirrored the magnitude of the DMAA preoperatively; thus, with substantial sloping of the metatarsal artic-

ular surface, soft tissue realignment of the MTP joint is contraindicated.

Technique

Distal soft tissue reconstruction is typically performed in association with a proximal first metatarsal osteotomy. The MTP joint realignment is performed as described previously for the distal soft tissue procedure. After the lateral capsular tissues have been released, the medial capsule opened, and the medial eminence resected, the intermetatarsal angle is tested to see whether an osteotomy is indicated. The first metatarsal head is pushed laterally toward the second metatarsal. A tendency for these two metatarsals to spring apart indicates insufficient mobility at the MTC joint to permit reduction of the intermetatarsal angle, and an osteotomy is indicated (see Fig. 6–92C).

1. A third incision is made on the dorsal aspect of the base of the first metatarsal over the extensor hallucis longus tendon. The incision starts just proximal to the MTC joint and is carried distally for about 3 cm. It is deepened through the subcutaneous tissue to expose

the extensor tendon. The extensor tendon is retracted medially or laterally to expose the metatarsal shaft (Fig. 6–101A).

2. The MTC joint is identified with the tip of the knife blade, and the osteotomy site is located approximately 1 cm distal to the MTC joint (Fig. 6–101B). A screw (and Kirschner wire) is generally used for fixation of the osteotomy site and is inserted approximately 1 cm distal to the osteotomy site.

3. If a screw is used to fix the osteotomy, the initial glide hole is created at this time. A 3.5-mm drill bit is used to make a hole at an angle of about 45 to 50 degrees to the metatarsal shaft, with the bit passing into the metatarsal approximately 5 mm (see Fig. 6–104E). A countersink is used to lower the screw head. If a 4.0-mm cannulated screw is used, the guide pin is inserted and over-drilled later in the procedure.

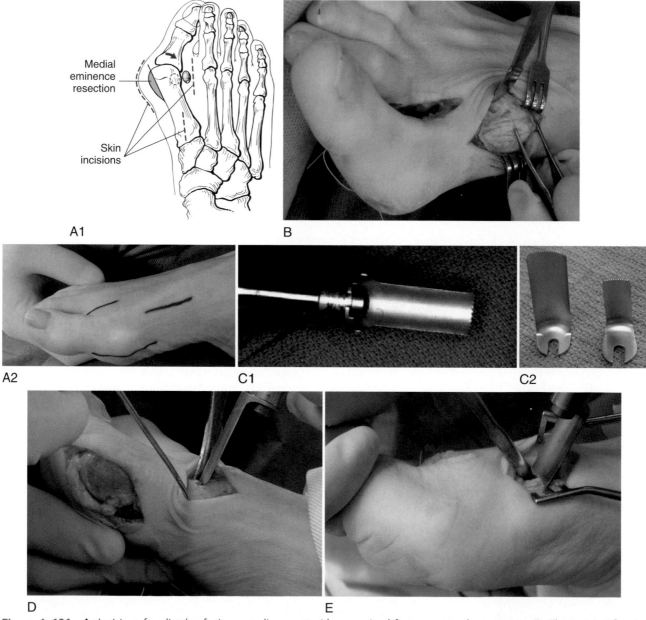

Figure 6–101 **A,** Incisions for distal soft tissue realignment with a proximal first metatarsal osteotomy. **B,** The incision for the osteotomy is made 1 cm distal to MTC joint. **C,** Saw blade used for crescentic osteotomy. **D,** Orientation of the saw blade with the concave surface oriented proximally. **E,** Orientation of the saw blade with the concave surface oriented distally.

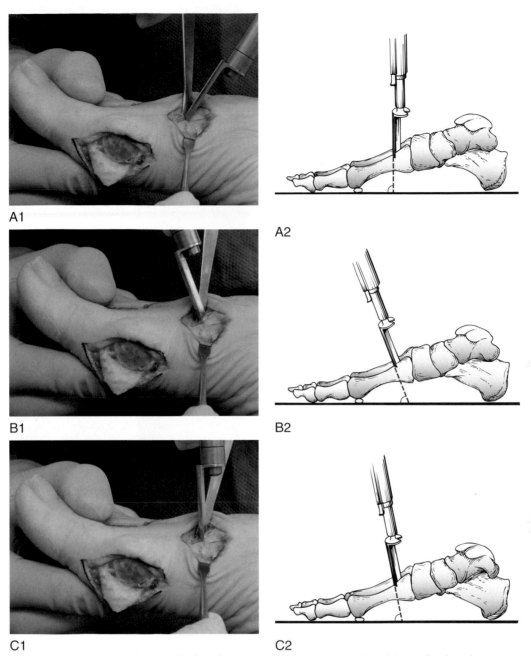

A1

A2

B1

B2

C1

C2

Figure 6–102 Errors in position of the saw blade. The crescentic osteotomy is placed 1 cm distal to the metatarsocuneiform joint or 8 mm distal to the open epiphysis in a juvenile. A lateral view of the osteotomy demonstrates the angle of the cut. The concave surface is proximal. **A,** This angle is incorrect because the blade is perpendicular to the floor. **B,** Incorrect angle of the osteotomy because the angle is too oblique. There is less contact at the osteotomy site. **C,** Correct angle of the osteotomy. The correct angle is neither perpendicular to the first metatarsal shaft nor perpendicular to the plantar aspect of the foot.

4. The osteotomy is created with a crescentic blade so that the concavity is directed proximally (Fig. 6–101C-E). The plane of the osteotomy is perpendicular to neither the first metatarsal nor the bottom of the foot; rather, it is halfway between (Fig. 6–102). In the coronal plane, it is critical that the saw blade be neither medially nor laterally rotated. Medial rotation can lead to elevatus (Fig. 6–103). Often, the leg of the patient externally rotates, and if care is not taken, inadvertent medial rotation of the saw blade occurs. To avoid this error, with the foot held in a plantigrade position, a vertical 0.045-

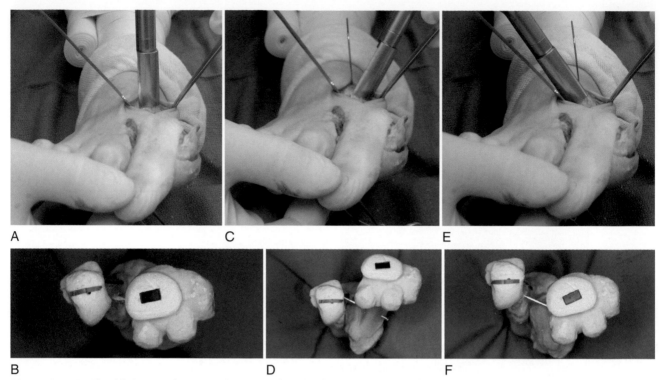

A   C   E

B   D   F

Figure 6–103   The blade must be correctly oriented to the first metatarsal shaft in the coronal plane. **A,** With the osteotomy oriented in the correct position, the first metatarsal is neither elevated nor depressed (**B**) as it is rotated laterally. **C,** If the saw blade is rotated medial-ward and the cut angled laterally, this leads to elevation (**D**) of the first metatarsal head as the first metatarsal is shifted laterally. **E,** If the saw blade is rotated lateral-ward, the first metatarsal head will be depressed (**F**) as the distal metatarsal is displaced laterally.

inch Kirchner wire is placed in the medial cuneiform as a guide. The saw blade is held parallel to the wire during the osteotomy, thus minimizing malrotation of the blade.[178] As the osteotomy is performed, the saw blade must exit the lateral aspect of the metatarsal shaft to ensure that the osteotomy is completed along this margin of the metatarsal. If it is not, it is difficult to complete the osteotomy in this narrow area, and the communicating artery may be damaged. If the osteotomy is not completed along the medial side, it is simple to finish the cut with a 4-mm osteotome. Once the osteotomy is complete, a Freer elevator is used to ensure that it is completely mobile and that any periosteal hinge that might prevent displacement of the osteotomy is released. The crescentic saw blade comes in two lengths, one 4 mm longer than the other. As the osteotomy is being performed, if the shoulder of the blade impinges on the skin just proximal to the osteotomy site, the longer

blade (no. 2296-31-416S7, 277-31-415, or 277-31-416S1, Stryker, Kalamazoo, MI, or no. 5053-176, Zimmer, Wausau, IN) is used. One should not undertake this osteotomy without having both blades available. Again, care must be taken to avoid either medial or lateral rotation of the saw blade because such rotation may lead to plantar flexion or dorsiflexion at the osteotomy site.

Reconstruction of Hallux Valgus Deformity

1. Having finished the osteotomy, attention is directed to the first web space, where two sutures are placed to approximate the adductor hallucis tendon to the lateral capsular tissues along the border of the first metatarsal head (see Fig. 6–93). If such approximation is not accomplished at this time, it is difficult to later expose the adductor tendon in the depths of the interspace after the osteotomy site has been displaced and stabilized.

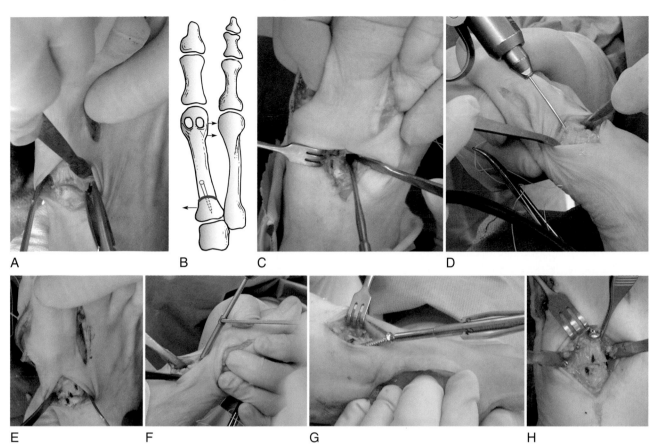

Figure 6–104 **A,** Exposure of the osteotomy site in the proximal portion of the metatarsal. A rongeur is used to remove the lateral spike of bone that frequently prevents displacement of the osteotomy. **B,** Diagram demonstrating that the proximal fragment is displaced medially as far as the metatarsocuneiform joint will permit while metatarsal head is pushed laterally against the second metatarsal. **C,** Intraoperative photograph demonstrating the Freer elevator pushing the proximal fragment medially and the surgeon's hand pulling the first metatarsal head laterally against the second metatarsal. **D,** Kirschner wire stabilizes the osteotomy site. **E,** Note that the osteotomy site is displaced 2 to 3 mm laterally. **F,** The hole is drilled at a 45-degree angle to the long axis of the metatarsal. **G,** The screw is placed approximately 1 cm distal to the osteotomy site. **H,** After placement of the wire and screw.

2. Returning to the osteotomy site, a Freer elevator is used to displace the proximal portion of the metatarsal base in a medial direction as far as possible (Fig. 6–104B and C). The index finger is used to push the metatarsal head in a lateral direction, which displaces the osteotomy site laterally. The displacement at the osteotomy site is usually only 2 to 3 mm because a small degree of translation proximally accounts for much movement distally. Care must be taken to not overcorrect the osteotomy site. If the osteotomy site does not move freely, some medial periosteum is still attached and must be released so that the osteotomy can be rotated laterally. Occasionally, a small spike of bone on the lateral aspect of the distal fragment must be removed to allow rotation of the osteotomy (Fig. 6–104A). At this point, the distal fragment can be slightly displaced plantar-ward (about 2 mm) to compensate for any possible dorsiflexion angulation at the osteotomy site. To ensure that the osteotomy site is not being held in a dorsiflexed position, the metatarsal head is pushed slightly plantar-ward until the osteotomy site just begins to open up.

3. While holding the osteotomy in a corrected position, the osteotomy is fixed with both a 0.062-inch Kirschner wire (Fig. 6–104D and E) and a 4.0-mm small-fragment compression screw to provide rotational stability, as well as compression (Fig. 6–104F-H). For placement of a lag screw, a 3.5-mm gliding drill

hole is made in the distal fragment, and a 2.0-mm drill hole is made into the proximal fragment; when placed, the compression screw stabilizes and compresses the osteotomy site. If a 4.0-mm cannulated screw is used, the dorsal cortex should be over-drilled with the 4.0-mm drill bit because the cannulated screw cannot usually penetrate the metatarsal at a 45-degree angle. The hole is also countersunk to lower the profile of the screw head and to prevent cracking the island of bone between the screw and osteotomy site.

4. Regardless of whether it is cannulated, as the screw is tightened, the osteotomy site is carefully observed so that once compression occurs, the screw is not overtightened, which can lead to fracture of the island of bone between the hole and the osteotomy site. If a fracture occurs and the osteotomy site is unstable, Kirschner wires can be driven across the osteotomy site to increase its sta-bility. The typical screw length is 26 to 30 mm but varies depending on the patient's size. If the bone is very osteopenic, at times we deliberately use a long screw to penetrate the MTC joint to gain greater stability at the osteotomy site. In about 5% of cases, the screw will penetrate the MTC joint because of the angle at which it is inserted. If joint penetration occurs, one should leave the screw if adequate fixation has been achieved

rather than remove it. Placement of a new screw may leave the construct with insuffi-cient stability. If the MTC joint is penetrated with internal fixation, the hardware can be removed after successful healing at the osteotomy site, typically 6 weeks after surgery. Coughlin and Shurnas[85] reported that internal fixation crossed the MTC joint in 13 of 35 cases. The hardware was removed 6 weeks after surgery, and at long-term follow-up they did not identify degenerative arthritis in the MTC joint. Intraoperative radi-ography or fluoroscopy (Fig. 6–105) may be beneficial to evaluate the correction of the intermetatarsal angle, as well as to evaluate the position of the internal fixation. Due to the increased incidence of infection with this method of internal fixation, we have in general discontinued the use of Steinmann pin fixation except for salvage situations (Fig. 6–106).

5. Once the osteotomy site is stabilized, the sutures in the first web space are tied and the medial capsular tissue is repaired as previ-ously described for the distal soft tissue pro-cedure. The skin is approximated in routine manner (Fig. 6–107).

6. Postoperatively, the foot is wrapped in a gauze-and-tape compression dressing to hold the hallux in correct alignment or in slight overcorrection if a severe deformity has been corrected (Fig. 6–108A).

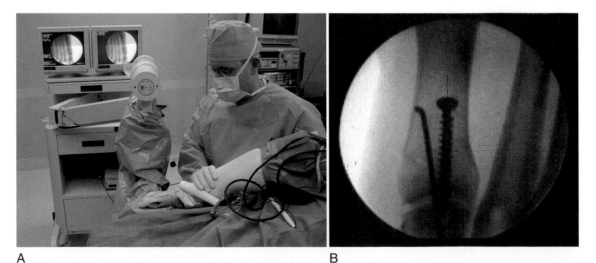

A   B

Figure 6–105 **A** and **B**, Intraoperative fluoroscopy can be helpful during the surgical procedure to check alignment of the osteotomy.

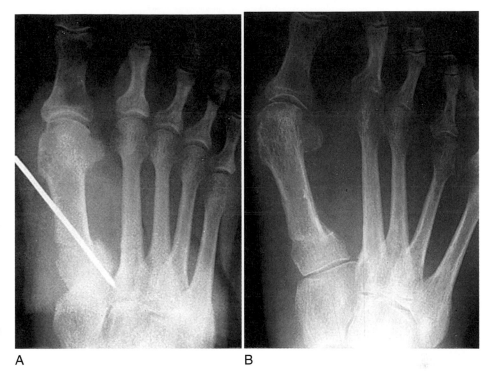

Figure 6–106 Fixation of the osteotomy site with an oblique 5/64-inch Steinmann pin. Owing to the high infection rate, this is rarely used except with unsuccessful internal fixation. **A,** Radiograph demonstrating the pin driven into the tarsal bones for added stability. Note that when the osteotomy site was reduced, the proximal fragment was not displaced medially on the cuneiform. **B,** After removal of the pin, the proximal fragment drifted in the medial direction on the cuneiform, which resulted in incomplete correction of the intermetatarsal angle and recurrence of the hallux valgus deformity owing to the lack of medial displacement of the proximal fragment.

A   B

Postoperative Care

As previously described for the distal soft tissue procedure, the foot is redressed weekly for 8 weeks (Fig. 6–108B). It is unusual to cast the foot postoperatively, although a cast may be necessary in an unreliable patient or one with precarious internal fixation. Radiographs are obtained at the first office visit after surgery. Based on this radiograph, the toe is dressed in a neutral position, varus, or valgus. The patient is allowed to ambulate in a stiff-soled postoperative shoe

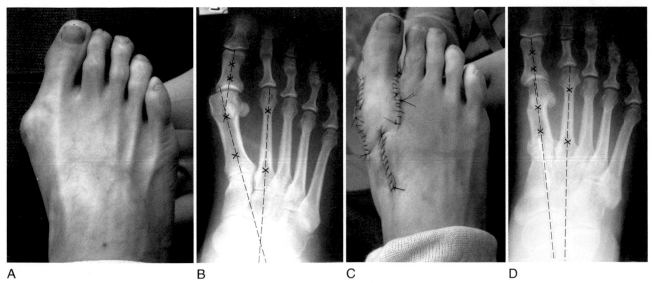

A   B   C   D

Figure 6–107 Distal soft tissue realignment with first metatarsal osteotomy. **A,** Preoperative clinical appearance and, **B,** radiograph demonstrating a moderate hallux valgus deformity with metatarsophalangeal (MTP) subluxation (hallux valgus angle, 34 degrees; 1-2 intermetatarsal angle, 15 degrees; DMAA, 10 degrees) and a subluxated MTP joint. **C,** Postoperative clinical appearance and, **D,** radiograph 5 years after a distal soft tissue procedure with a proximal metatarsal osteotomy. The alignment has been corrected (hallux valgus angle, 5 degrees; 1-2 intermetatarsal angle, 4 degrees).

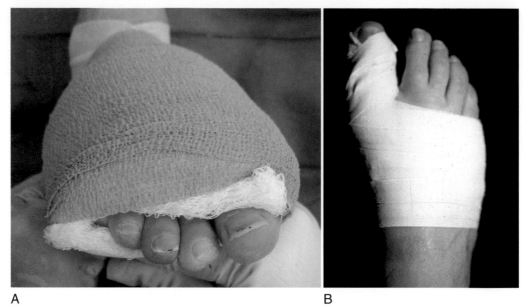

A   B

Figure 6–108   A, Immediate postoperative dressing. **B,** Dressing used for the remainder of treatment.

with weight bearing mainly on the heel and outer aspect of the foot for 8 weeks after surgery. After the final dressings are removed, the patient is permitted to ambulate as tolerated in a sandal or soft, wide shoe. Sutures are removed 2 to 3 weeks after surgery; when indicated, internal fixation is removed 6 weeks after surgery in an outpatient or office setting under local anesthesia. MTP joint range-of-motion exercises are initiated 3 to 4 weeks after surgery while the foot is still maintained in a postoperative dressing. An intensive walking program is begun 7 to 8 weeks after surgery.

The degree of swelling varies among patients, but usually within 4 to 5 months after surgery, the thickening about the joint and swelling of the foot have subsided.

Results

Reported patient satisfaction rates after proximal first metatarsal osteotomy vary from 78% to 93%.* Mann et al[242] reviewed 109 feet in which a distal soft tissue procedure and proximal crescentic osteotomy were performed. The major preoperative complaint was pain over the medial eminence in 75% of patients, around the first MTP joint or sesamoids in 7%, in the lesser toes in 7%, and from other causes in 11%.

*References 48, 77, 242, 292, 304, 306, 329, and 348.

Ninety-three percent of patients were satisfied postoperatively. Of the 7% dissatisfied, half complained of pain and half complained of the varus or valgus position of the hallux. At final follow-up, 39% of patients believed that they could perform more activities on their feet, 57% thought that their level of activity was unchanged, and 4% said that their level of activity was diminished. Preoperatively, 30% of patients could wear any shoe that they desired, and postoperatively, 59% could. Still, 41% were unable to wear the shoe of their choice.

The average correction of the hallux valgus angle is consistently reported to be 23 to 24 degrees,[97,233,242,292,348] with the degree of improvement being directly proportional to the severity of the preoperative deformity[30,245] (Fig. 6–109). Mann[232] reported that with more severe deformities, an average hallux valgus correction of 30 degrees was achieved. Average correction of the 1-2 intermetatarsal angle is 8 to 11 degrees after a crescentic osteotomy,[72,77,233,242,348] 3 to 6 degrees after a closing wedge osteotomy,[292,318] and 7 degrees after an opening wedge osteotomy.[215,329] Tables 6–4 and 6–5 summarize correction of the hallux valgus and intermetatarsal angles achieved in the series and by subgroups. Reporting on 33 cases of correction of a juvenile hallux valgus deformity with distal soft tissue reconstruction and proximal first metatarsal osteotomy,

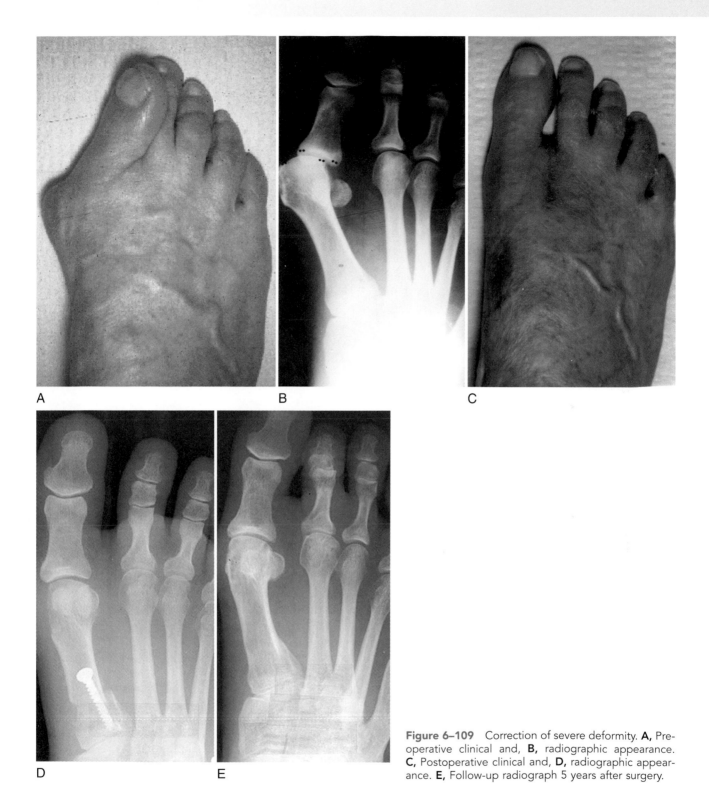

Figure 6–109 Correction of severe deformity. **A,** Preoperative clinical and, **B,** radiographic appearance. **C,** Postoperative clinical and, **D,** radiographic appearance. **E,** Follow-up radiograph 5 years after surgery.

TABLE 6–4

Summary of 109 Feet before and after Distal Soft Tissue Procedures with Proximal Crescentic Osteotomy

Angle	Preoperative	Postoperative
Average hallux valgus	30°	9°
Average first/second intermetatarsal	13°	5°

Coughlin[72] noted an average 23-degree correction of the hallux valgus angle and an average 8-degree correction of the 1-2 intermetatarsal angle, results identical to those reported by Mann[233] in adult patients. In the only prospective study of this procedure published, Coughlin and Jones[77] reported an average 20-degree correction of the hallux valgus angle and an average 10-degree correction of the intermetatarsal angle.

Mann et al[242] further observed that before surgery, 48 feet (44%) had a symptomatic callus beneath the second metatarsal head and that postoperatively, 30 of these calluses had resolved, 13 were unchanged but no longer painful, and 5 remained painful but no new lesions had developed. Coughlin and Jones[77] reported a 47% incidence of concomitant lateral

TABLE 6–5

Summary of Results by Severity of Deformity in Distal Soft Tissue Procedures with Proximal Crescentic Osteotomy

	Mild (<20°)	Moderate (21°–40°)	Severe (>40°)
Number of feet	9	87	13
Mean age (y)	48	52	59
Mean hallux valgus angle			
Preoperative	17°	30°	46°
Postoperative	3°	9°	13°
Mean first/second intermetatarsal angle			
Preoperative	11°	13°	16°
Postoperative	5°	6°	5°

Hallux varus
14 of 109 feet
 Mean deformity 5.4°
  <6°, 9 cases
  >6°, 5 cases (2 dissatisfied)

metatarsalgia in patients who were scheduled to undergo surgical correction for moderate and severe hallux valgus deformities. Overall, the first metatarsal was shortened an average of 2.2 mm, a finding identical to that in other reports in the literature on proximal first metatarsal osteotomies.[212,246,278,306]

As Easley et al[100] observed, in patients with moderate and severe hallux valgus deformities, evaluation of transfer lesions is hampered by the fact that forefoot problems are not isolated to the hallux and frequently involve the second and third MTP joints as well. Whereas some have suggested a relationship between first metatarsal shortening and metatarsalgia[367] or elevatus and metatarsalgia,[367] others have found no correlation.* When the metatarsal is already short before surgery, Schemitsch and Horne[311] found a positive correlation between further shortening of the first metatarsal and metatarsalgia.

Dorsiflexion at the osteotomy site should be avoided. Mann et al[242] observed on lateral weight-bearing radiographs that 28% of the feet demonstrated the first metatarsal to be slightly dorsiflexed, although the magnitude was not quantified. Saw position and rigid internal fixation, we believe, are import principles in avoiding elevatus.[65,70,216] Lippert and McDermott[216] found that medial or lateral rotation of the saw blade altered the eventual position of the distal first metatarsal head after the osteotomy was displaced. Medial rotation of the saw led to elevation, and lateral rotation led to plantar angulation after displacement of the osteotomy. Jones et al,[178] in a cadaveric and laboratory study, demonstrated a linear relationship between metatarsus elevatus and saw blade orientation. For every 10 degrees of saw blade angulation, a 2-mm change in the sagittal position of the distal first metatarsal was noted. They then used a Kirchner wire to help orient the saw blade to avoid malrotation of the saw and substantially improved the accuracy of the osteotomy in a cadaveric study.

Joseph[183] quantified MTP joint range of motion in normal subjects and reported total MTP motion of 87 degrees with an average dorsiflexion of 67 degrees and average passive plantar flexion of 20 degrees. In reports documenting postoperative MTP range of motion

_____

*References 130, 188, 242, 246, 264, 287, and 292.

after proximal osteotomy and distal soft tissue repair, total passive motion ranged from 64 to 86 degrees.[68,72,361] Coughlin[72] noted an average loss of 12 degrees when compared with the nonoperated side in juveniles and an average loss of 11 degrees in adults.[68] Mann et al[242] reported that patients demonstrated 55 degrees of dorsiflexion and 9 degrees of plantar flexion for a total range of 64 degrees at midterm follow-up after surgery. Veri et al[361] reported that preoperative total range of motion averaged 86 degrees; at a minimum 1-year follow-up, range of motion averaged 69 degrees; however, at a mean follow-up of 8 years, total motion averaged 86 degrees. In a cadaver study in which range of motion was measured immediately before and after a distal soft tissue procedure and proximal metatarsal osteotomy, Coughlin et al[78] reported that the total range of MTP joint motion decreased from 85 to 62 degrees. There was a significant loss of dorsiflexion motion but not plantar flexion motion. Thus, there appears to be an initial loss of motion after the realignment procedure that is probably due to intrinsic muscle tightness. Initiation of early range-of-motion activities may help diminish the eventual loss of motion, but patients should be counseled that it is not unusual to lose some motion as a consequence of the procedure (Fig. 6–110).

Two reports in the literature compared proximal crescentic osteotomy with proximal chevron osteotomy for the correction of hallux valgus (see Fig. 6–116).[100,246] In both reports the results were essentially the same with regard to correction of the hallux valgus deformity and intermetatarsal angle and relief of lateral metatarsalgia. The main difference was the lack of dorsiflexion at the osteotomy site, as noted occasionally after proximal crescentic osteotomy, but statistically it did not appear to affect either the incidence of new transfer lesions or the resolution of existing lesions. We believe that either procedure will result in satisfactory correction of the hallux valgus deformity, and it is the surgeon's preference which of these osteotomies should be used. Although Lian et al[214] reported proximal chevron and crescentic osteotomy to be of equal strength in resisting failure with dorsiflexion, criticism of the strength of the osteotomy and its fixation has been presented by McCluskey et al[255] and by Campbell et al.[42] They found both proximal chevron and

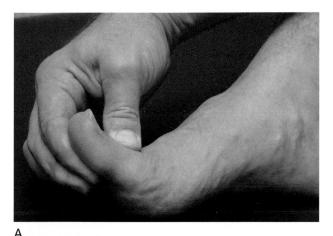

A

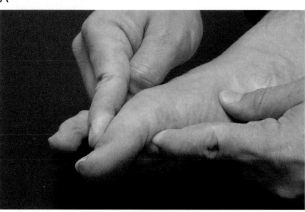

B

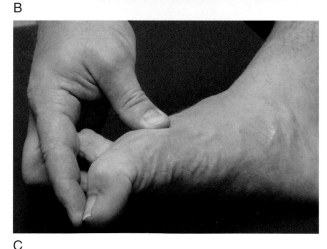

C

Figure 6–110 Passive dorsiflexion (**A**) and plantar flexion (**B**) range-of-motion exercises are important in regaining motion. Pressure placed on the proximal phalanx stretches the metatarsophalangeal (MTP) joint. **C,** Incorrect stretching places stress on the interphalangeal joint instead of the MTP joint.

oblique closing wedge osteotomy to be stronger constructs.

Coughlin[72] noted that this technique was less successful in correcting a congruent joint but, with a subluxated joint, had a relatively high success rate. Mild residual deformity or degenerative arthritis may develop if one fails to appreciate the presence of an increased DMAA (see Figs. 6–54 to 6–57). Mild degenerative arthritis has been reported at both the MTP joint[242,361,367] and the MTC joint,[77,367] although it is rarely symptomatic.

The important contribution of this procedure to bunion surgery is that the rate of correcting the hallux valgus deformity to a residual of 16 degrees or less was 72% (78 of 109 feet).[242] Proximal crescentic osteotomy is a more reliable procedure than a distal soft tissue procedure alone, which resulted in a residual hallux valgus deformity of 16 degrees or less in 42% (30 of 72 feet). It also provides a more satisfactory result in a wide spectrum of hallux valgus deformities, including moderate and severe subluxated hallux valgus deformities in juveniles and adults.

Complications

Potential complications after a distal soft tissue procedure have been listed previously. Complications after proximal osteotomy include shortening, metatarsalgia, failure of internal fixation, overcorrection (hallux varus) (Fig. 6–111), undercorrection (or recurrence) (Fig. 6–112), delayed union, and malunion (Figs. 6–113 and 6–115).

Shortening or dorsiflexion at the osteotomy site predisposes to the development of lateral metatarsalgia (Fig. 6–114), whereas lengthening the first metatarsal through an opening wedge osteotomy may lead to instability and malunion at the osteotomy site. Mann et al[242] reported a 28% incidence of dorsiflexion at the osteotomy site but used a single Steinmann pin for internal fixation. Various methods of internal fixation have been used to fix proximal osteotomies, including Steinmann pins,[131,233,242,292,361] a single screw,[106,246,278] a screw and pin,[70,100] and a dorsal plate.[300,359] Mann et al[242] noted that superficial inflammation around the pin site developed in approximately 10% of patients in whom the osteotomy site was fixed with an oblique Steinmann pin, a major reason why this method of fixation was discontinued (see Fig. 6–106).

Other alternatives to proximal osteotomies include a proximal oblique osteotomy[51,222,270] and a proximal chevron osteotomy[246,304,306] (see Fig. 6–116).

Chiodo el al[51] reported the results of 70 cases in which a Ludloff oblique osteotomy was

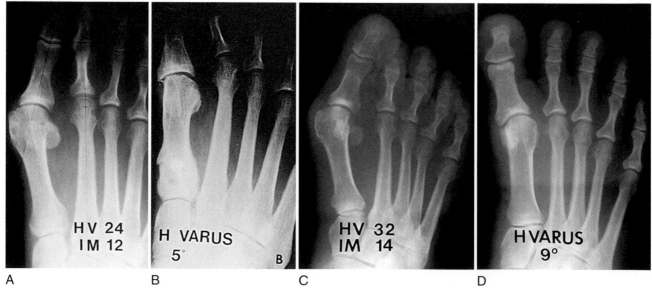

Figure 6–111 Hallux varus after a distal soft tissue procedure and proximal metatarsal osteotomy. **A** and **B,** Preoperative and postoperative radiographs demonstrating 5 degrees of varus. **C** and **D,** Preoperative and postoperative radiographs demonstrating 9 degrees of hallux varus. Hallux varus of this magnitude is rarely of clinical significance and represents mainly a radiographic finding.

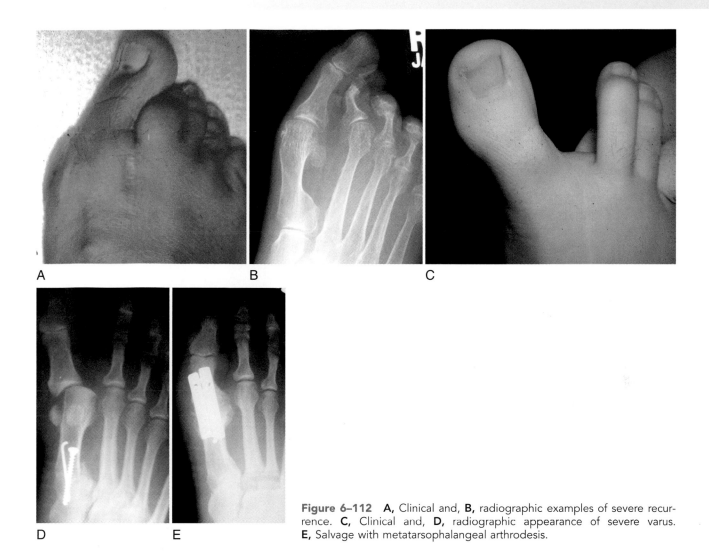

Figure 6–112 **A,** Clinical and, **B,** radiographic examples of severe recurrence. **C,** Clinical and, **D,** radiographic appearance of severe varus. **E,** Salvage with metatarsophalangeal arthrodesis.

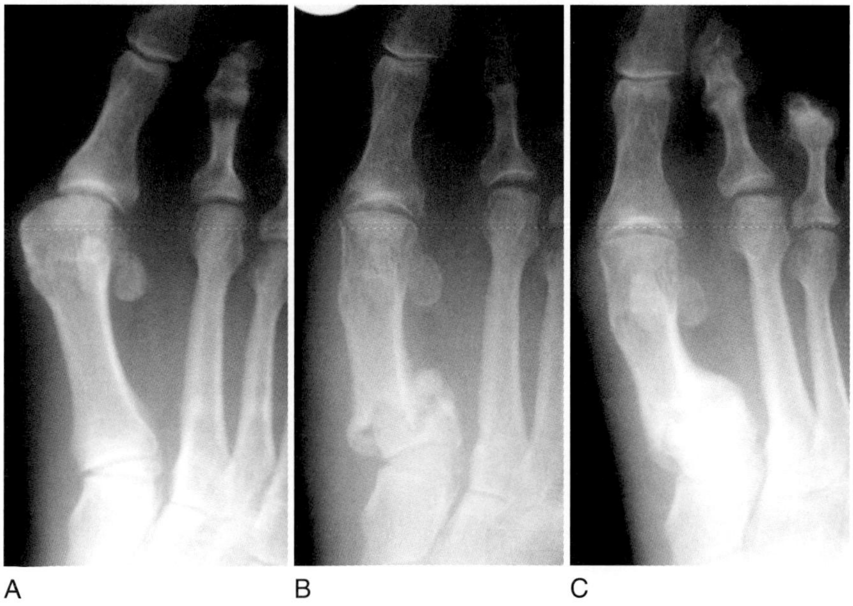

Figure 6–113 Delayed union after proximal crescentic osteotomy. **A,** Preoperative anteroposterior radiograph. **B,** Postoperative radiograph demonstrating delayed union. **C,** After below-knee casting for 6 weeks, successful union has occurred.

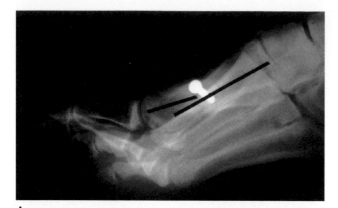

A

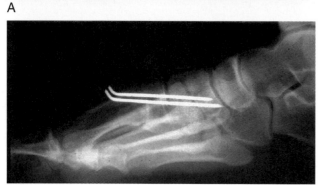

B

Figure 6–114 A, Elevatus after proximal osteotomy. **B,** Salvage with an opening wedge osteotomy and interposition dorsal graft.

performed for moderate and severe hallux valgus deformities. The average hallux valgus angle was corrected 20 degrees and the 1-2 intermetatarsal angle was corrected 9 degrees. In the sagittal plane, the first metatarsal was plantar flexed 1 mm. No transfer lesions were reported; varus occurred in 4 of 70 patients and delayed union in 3 of 70. The authors suggested that the plane of the osteotomy and the rigidity of the internal fixation placed the osteotomy site at minimal risk of dorsiflexion malunion.

Markbreiter and Thompson[246] and Sammarco et al[304] reported excellent correction with proximal chevron osteotomies of differing orientations. Complication rates were similar to those experienced with proximal crescentic osteotomy.

Rigid internal fixation appears to increase the stability at the osteotomy site. Thordarson and Leventen[348] reported less shortening with the use of a more stable internal fixation construct and emphasized that adequate internal fixation was vital to avoid dorsiflexion malunion. Malunion is an extremely difficult complication to

treat and may require extensive and complex salvage techniques (see Fig. 6–114).

Mann et al[242] reported that the most frequent complication of this procedure was hallux varus, which occurred in 14 (13%) of 109 feet and averaged 5.6 degrees. None of the patients complained of pain, and none had a cock-up deformity of the first MTP joint. Three patients were dissatisfied because of the position of

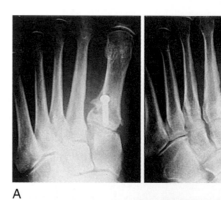

A

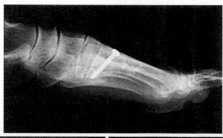

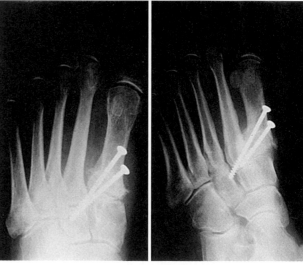

B

Figure 6–115 Nonunion after proximal crescentic osteotomy. **A,** Preoperative anteroposterior (left), oblique (right), and lateral (centered) radiographs demonstrating nonunion. **B,** Postoperative repair demonstrating satisfactory union after internal fixation and local bone graft.

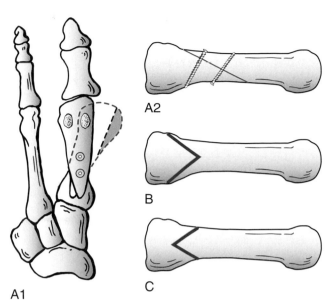

Figure 6–116 **A1** and **A2,** Ludloff osteotomy. **B,** Proximal chevron osteotomy (base proximal). **C,** Proximal chevron osteotomy (base distal).

the toe, whereas the others had essentially no functional complaints and were satisfied with the result. Simmonds and Menelaus[329] and Mann and Coughlin[237] cautioned that a lateral sesamoid should rarely if ever be removed. This amount of varus is typically a minimal deformity and is more a radiographic finding than a clinical entity (see Fig. 6–111). Frequently, a hallux varus deformity of less than 10 degrees is asymptomatic and is considered by patients to be a subjectively satisfactory result.[348]

Easley et al[100] reported a 12% (5 of 43 patients) incidence of hallux varus after proximal chevron osteotomy. In most cases, hallux varus develops due to lateral translation of the metatarsal head after medial displacement of the proximal osteotomy. This was a much more frequent occurrence for us before changing the osteotomy from being oriented concave distal to concave proximal[242] (see Figs. 6–99 and 6–112D and E). In a retrospective study, Trnka et al[352] presented a long-term follow-up of a group of patients in whom hallux varus developed (average deformity of 10 degrees of varus). In a series of 16 feet with a follow-up averaging 18 years, 12 (75%) of 16 patients still rated their result as excellent. Only those with a severe hallux varus deformity were dissatisfied or required further surgery. In most patients, the varus deformity was usually 15 degrees or less,

a finding similar to that reported by Mann et al[242] (see Fig. 6–111).

Nonunion is rarely reported after osteotomy in the proximal metaphyseal region. Cedell and Astrom[48] reported a 10% nonunion rate with an opening wedge osteotomy, and Sammarco and Russo-Alesi[306] reported three cases in a series of 72 operations involving a proximal chevron osteotomy. Although we[242] initially reported no nonunions of the osteotomy site, we have subsequently observed two nonunions in a series of 1500 cases. Both were corrected with an interposition bone graft and internal fixation (Fig. 6–115). Even though such treatment resulted in some shortening of the metatarsal, no symptomatic transfer lesion developed.

Epiphyseal injury can occur with a proximal first metatarsal osteotomy in the skeletally immature and lead to growth arrest and ultimately to a short first metatarsal (see Fig. 6–67). Care must be taken in an adolescent to protect the proximal first metatarsal epiphysis.

In the treatment of moderate and severe hallux valgus deformities with subluxation of the MTP joint, proximal first metatarsal osteotomy combined with distal soft tissue reconstruction can lead to a successful outcome. Although it is well recognized that this technique is technically difficult,[242,255,278] the attribute of crescentic osteotomy is that the powerful nature of this procedure allows correction of moderate and severe deformities.

DISTAL METATARSAL OSTEOTOMY (CHEVRON PROCEDURE)

The technique for a chevron osteotomy was initially described by Austin and Leventen[8,9] and Corless.[61] With a chevron osteotomy, resection of the medial eminence, distal metatarsal osteotomy, and medial capsulorrhaphy are used to realign the hallux, thereby producing some narrowing of the forefoot (video clip 25). Since its initial description, several modifications in the technical part of the procedure have been made, including the angle of the osteotomy and the use of various alternative methods of internal fixation. An Akin procedure has been added by some[265] to augment the angular correction.

Indications

A chevron osteotomy is indicated for mild and low-moderate hallux valgus deformities (hallux valgus angle less than 30 degrees or 1-2 intermetatarsal angle less than 13 degrees) with subluxation of the first MTP joint.[69,158,260] When used in patients with a greater deformity, the procedure's capability of achieving correction diminishes. A chevron osteotomy provides an extraarticular correction and can also be used for the treatment of a hallux valgus deformity with a congruous first MTP joint if the DMAA is 15 degrees or less. For the occasional patient with a DMAA greater than 15 degrees or in the presence of a congruent or minimally subluxated hallux valgus deformity, the end result can be enhanced by removal of a small wedge of bone from the medial aspect of the chevron cut to enable the articular surface to be rotated more perpendicular to the long axis of the metatarsal (see Fig. 6–119).[53] Likewise, moving the apex of the osteotomy slightly proximal tends to increase the angular correction that can be achieved. A chevron osteotomy does not correct hallux pronation and only partially corrects sesamoid subluxation. The indications for chevron osteotomy when combined with phalangeal osteotomy[265] include a hallux valgus deformity with a congruous first MTP joint (DMAA less than 20 degrees), as well as mild or moderate pronation of the hallux. Whereas Hattrup and Johnson[149] initially suggested that postoperative patient satisfaction seemed to decrease somewhat in patients older than 60 years, Trnka[350,352] reported high levels of satisfaction in even older age groups.

Contraindications

The main contraindication to a chevron osteotomy is a moderate to severe deformity with the hallux valgus angle exceeding 35 degrees, the intermetatarsal angle exceeding 15 degrees, and a congruous first MTP joint with a DMAA greater than 15 degrees. Moderate or severe pronation of the hallux is difficult to correct with the chevron procedure. Advanced age is only a relative contraindication, but it may be associated with decreased MTP motion. In patients with moderate or advanced joint arthrosis, stiffness usually develops after a chevron procedure and thus an alternative procedure should be considered.

Medial Approach and Exposure of the Metatarsal Head

1. A longitudinal incision is centered over the medial eminence beginning at the midportion of the proximal phalanx and extending 1 cm proximal to the medial eminence (Fig. 6–117A). The dissection is carried down to the joint capsule, and full-thickness dorsal and plantar skin flaps are created. As the dorsal flap is created, caution is exercised to avoid damage to the dorsomedial cutaneous nerve. As the plantar flap is created, one must avoid the plantar medial cutaneous nerve.

2. An L-shaped, distally based capsular flap is developed as previously described for a distal soft tissue procedure (Fig. 6–117B and C), with detachment of the dorsal and proximal capsular attachments.[212]
   Alternative Technique: A vertical capsular incision is made approximately 2 to 3 mm proximal and parallel to the base of the proximal phalanx. A second capsular incision is made 2 to 4 mm more proximal but parallel to the first cut. The two capsular incisions are joined dorsally by an inverted-V cut (see Fig. 6–90B and C). The capsular flap is then grasped with forceps and dissected plantarward, and a second V cut is made through the abductor hallucis tendon. With this inferior cut, the knife blade must remain inside the joint and come to rest against the tibial sesamoid at the apex of the plantar cut to prevent damage to the plantar medial cutaneous nerve. (Rarely is more than 4 mm of capsule removed.) An incision is made along the dorsomedial aspect of the metatarsal head to create a capsular flap, which when retracted exposes the medial eminence.

Technique of Osteotomy

1. The medial eminence is resected with an oscillating saw (or osteotome) in a line parallel with the medial border of the foot (Fig. 6–117D). The plane of the osteotomy through the medial eminence is not parallel to the metatarsal shaft but rather slightly oblique, which creates a broad base of the capital fragment that adds stability to the osteotomy site as it is displaced laterally. The cut begins at the lateral edge of the sagittal sulcus and is carried proximally (Fig. 6–118A).

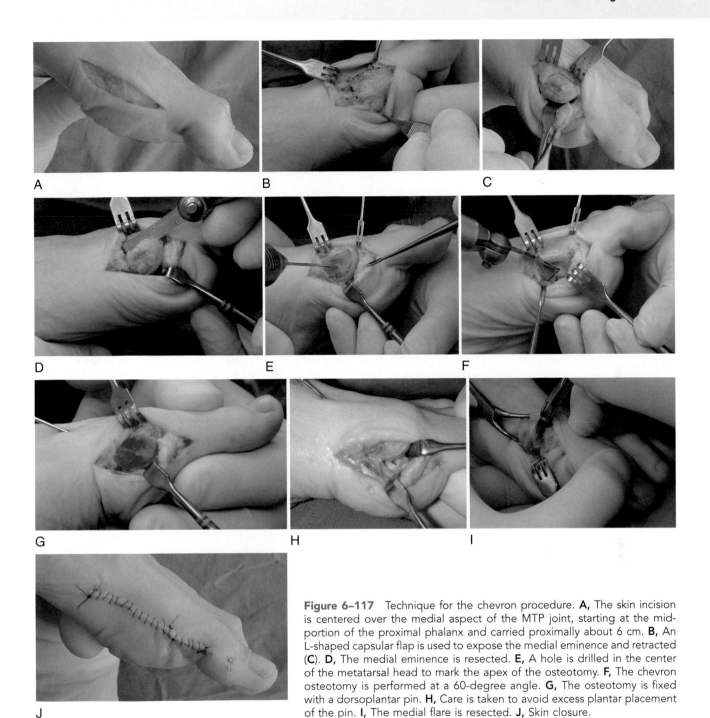

Figure 6–117 Technique for the chevron procedure. **A,** The skin incision is centered over the medial aspect of the MTP joint, starting at the midportion of the proximal phalanx and carried proximally about 6 cm. **B,** An L-shaped capsular flap is used to expose the medial eminence and retracted (**C**). **D,** The medial eminence is resected. **E,** A hole is drilled in the center of the metatarsal head to mark the apex of the osteotomy. **F,** The chevron osteotomy is performed at a 60-degree angle. **G,** The osteotomy is fixed with a dorsoplantar pin. **H,** Care is taken to avoid excess plantar placement of the pin. **I,** The medial flare is resected. **J,** Skin closure.

Any osteophytes, including the medial ridge of the sagittal sulcus, are removed with a rongeur.

2. Although we do not routinely release the adductor tendon and lateral capsular structures, others have successfully performed a release in conjunction with a chevron osteotomy.[134,199,279,283,350] Some surgeons reach across the joint and release the joint capsule,[340] whereas others choose an open exposure with a separate intermetatarsal dissection.* Excessive soft tissue stripping is avoided because it may endanger circulation to the metatarsal head. Most of the blood supply seems to emanate from the dorsal

---

*References 13, 134, 279, 312, 350, and 351.

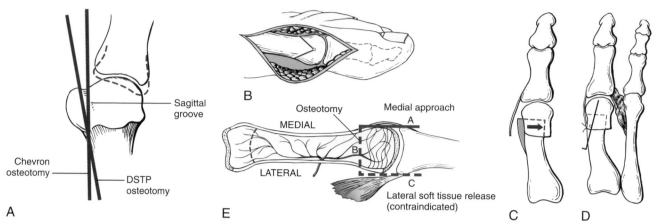

Figure 6–118   **A,** With a chevron osteotomy, resection of the medial eminence proceeds in line with the medial border of the foot. (With a distal soft tissue repair, the resection is in line with the medial border of the first metatarsal.) **B,** A drill hole is placed equidistant from the dorsal, distal, and plantar metatarsal articular surface. This point marks the apex of the osteotomy, with the chevron osteotomy oriented in a mediolateral plane. **C,** The capital fragment is translated laterally (*arrow*). **D,** The osteotomy is stabilized with a Kirschner wire, and the capsule is anchored by suture through the metaphyseal drill hole. **E,** Dorsal view of the first metatarsal demonstrating the vascular supply to the first metatarsal head. Distal metatarsal osteotomy (**B**) combined with extensive lateral soft tissue release (**C**) and medial capsulorrhaphy (**A**) may compromise the vascularity of the capital fragment.

and plantar aspects of the metatarsal head.[279] We believe, however, that if the deformity is too severe, rather than stretching the indications for a chevron osteotomy, another procedure might be preferable because the chance of vascular compromise would be eliminated.

3. The distal chevron osteotomy is carried out in the metaphyseal region because this area provides a large surface area for bone contact that is quite stable and aids in rapid healing (Fig. 6–118B). A 2-mm drill hole is useful to mark the apex of the osteotomy on the metatarsal head. The drill hole is placed at the center of an imaginary circle in which the radius is the distal articular surface (Fig. 6–117E). The hole is made in a lateral direction, parallel to the bottom of the foot and articular surface. A horizontal osteotomy is created with an oscillating saw that has a fine in-line tooth configuration. The angle of the chevron cut diverges at approximately a 60-degree angle; the base is oriented proximally (Fig. 6–117F). The plantar cut must exit proximal to the sesamoids, which places it just proximal to the synovial fold, thereby making it extraarticular. As the osteotomy is performed, one can feel the saw blade meet and penetrate the lateral cortex; care must be taken to not overpenetrate the cortex and enter the lateral soft tissues, which may damage the blood supply to the metatarsal

head[53] (Fig. 6–118E). Badwey et al[11] reported that the capital fragment can be displaced laterally up to 6 mm in males and 5 mm in females, which constitutes displacement of approximately 30% of the metatarsal's width. To displace the osteotomy, it is sometimes useful to hold the proximal portion of the metatarsal with a small towel clip while pushing the metatarsal head laterally (Fig. 6–118C).

4. *Alternative Technique:* We have also used a vertical distal osteotomy with a longitudinal plantar cut as an alternative to a chevron osteotomy. This enables placement of a dorsal plantar screw and is also more adaptable for a biplanar osteotomy (Fig. 6–120).

Reconstruction of the Joint

1. Once the osteotomy is displaced and the proximal phalanx centered on the articular surface of the metatarsal head, if a significant degree of valgus still remains, a biplanar chevron osteotomy is performed to produce a medial closing wedge osteotomy (Figs. 6–119 and 6–120). Two to 3 mm of bone can be removed from the medial aspect of the metatarsal cut to produce a medial closing wedge osteotomy. Rarely is it necessary to remove more than this amount of bone. After the initial chevron osteotomy, the surgeon retracts the capital fragment distally by

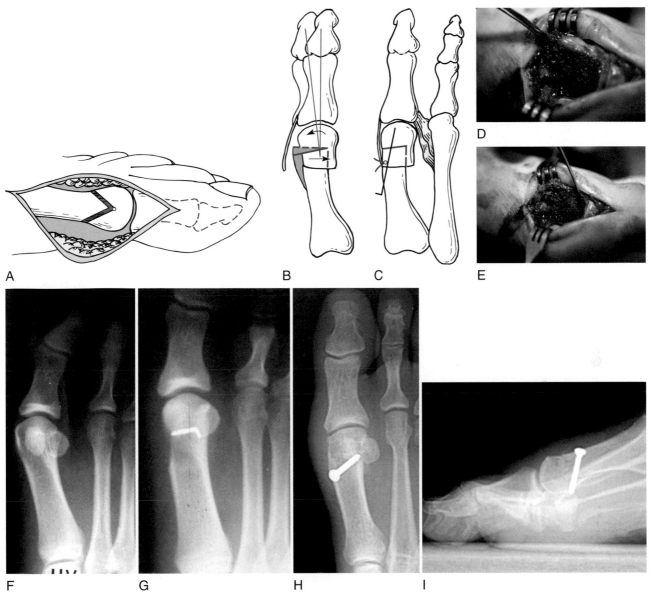

Figure 6–119 Biplanar chevron osteotomy. With an increased distal metatarsal articular angle, a biplanar chevron osteotomy is performed. A transverse chevron osteotomy is placed in a similar location. **A,** However, more bone is removed from the dorsomedial and plantar medial limb of the osteotomy to allow realignment (**B** and **C**) of a congruent metatarsophalangeal joint articulation with lateral translation of the capital fragment. **D,** Closing wedge osteotomy. **E,** Closure of the osteotomy site. **F,** Preoperative radiograph. **G,** Postoperative radiograph after a biplanar chevron osteotomy. **H** and **I,** With screw fixation.

grasping the osteotomized surface with a small, two-pronged bone hook. An oscillating saw is then used to resect a small medially based wedge of bone from the medial superior and medial inferior surfaces, with the resection beveled toward the lateral aspect of the metatarsal metaphysis. When the osteotomy site is closed, the capital fragment is angulated in a more medial direction than with a routine chevron osteotomy.

2. With either technique (standard or biplanar), the capital fragment is then impacted on the proximal fragment and fixed with a 0.062-inch Kirschner wire directed from a proximal dorsal to a distal plantar direction (see Figs. 6–117G and 6–118D). Care is taken to not penetrate the MTP joint with the Kirschner wire (Fig. 6–117H).
3. The prominent metaphyseal flare created by displacement at the osteotomy site

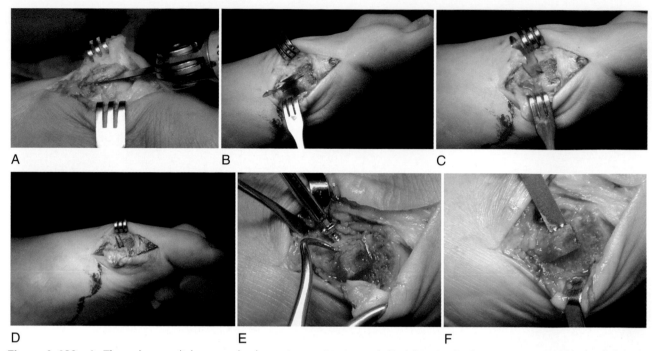

Figure 6–120   A, Through a medial approach, the eminence is resected. **B,** A longitudinal osteotomy is made parallel to the plantar surface of the foot, exiting above the sesamoid articulation. **C,** A vertical cut is made proximal to the articular surface. **D,** If biplanar correction is necessary, a single medial-based wedge is removed. **E,** A compression screw is placed. **F,** The medial flare is shaved with a saw.

is beveled with an oscillating saw (Fig. 6–117I).

4. The medial capsular flap is repaired with interrupted absorbable sutures with the toe held in neutral position. If correction is incomplete because of inadequate excision of capsular tissue, more capsule should be removed. When there is insufficient dorso-medial capsule with which to repair the capsular flap, a dorsal metaphyseal drill hole can be used to anchor the capsular repair (see Fig. 6–90F). The skin is closed in routine fashion (Fig. 6–117J).

5. Inadequate correction of valgus results from one of three anatomic problems: more capsular tissue may need to be removed from the medial joint capsule, the DMAA may be increased and should be corrected by the addition of a medial closing osteotomy at the chevron site, or a hallux valgus interphalangeus deformity may be present and require correction (Fig. 6–121).

6. Before placing a compression dressing, the foot is inspected to ensure that there is no excessive skin tension over the pin site. If

there is, a small incision should be made in the skin to release this tension.

Postoperative Care

The gauze-and-tape compression dressing applied at surgery is removed 1 to 2 days later, after which the foot is covered in a firm toe spica dressing consisting of 2-inch Kling gauze and 1/2-inch adhesive tape, similar to that used after a distal soft tissue procedure (see Fig. 6–108). If any pronation is present, the dressing must be wrapped in such a way that the toe is held in correct alignment to eliminate or minimize the pronation. The dressing is changed weekly. Sutures are removed 2 to 3 weeks after surgery. The patient is allowed to ambulate in a postoperative shoe with weight born on the heel and outer aspect of the foot. At initial follow-up, a radiograph is obtained to assess alignment of the first ray, and subsequent dressings are used to correct any residual varus or valgus deformity. The dressing is changed at 10-day intervals over an 8-week period after surgery, assuming that the alignment is satisfactory. The Kirschner wire

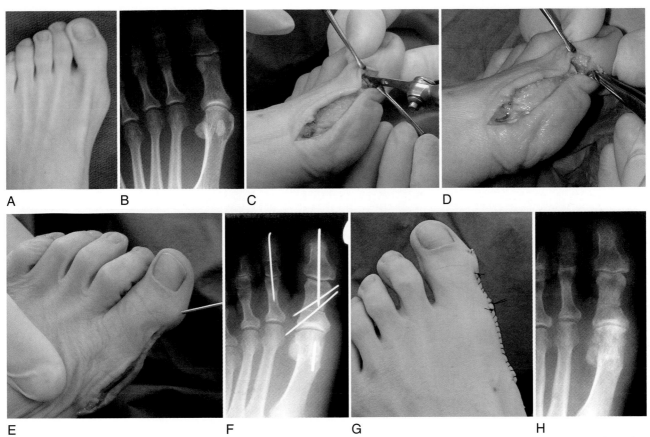

Figure 6–121 Combined chevron-Akin procedure. Preoperative clinical (**A**) and radiographic (**B**) appearance. **C** and **D**, Phalangeal osteotomy. **E**, Kirschner wire fixation. **F**, Internal fixation. **G**, Postoperative clinical appearance. **H**, Final radiographic appearance.

is usually removed 4 weeks after surgery in an office setting, and dressings are discontinued 6 to 8 weeks after the procedure. Patients are started on a program of active and passive range-of-motion exercises as pain permits; they are permitted to ambulate in a soft shoe 6 to 8 weeks after surgery.

Results

After a chevron osteotomy the satisfaction rate is relatively high, with the reported average correction of the hallux valgus angle being 12 to 15 degrees* and average correction of the 1-2 intermetatarsal angle varying from 4 to 5 degrees.† (Fig. 6–122). Reported postoperative narrowing of the forefoot varies from 3 to 6 mm after a chevron osteotomy. Zimmer et al[385]

---

*References 93, 149, 156, 158, 173, 213, 279, 283, and 350.
†References 149, 156, 158, 173, 212, 213, and 283.

published a report on the effectiveness of the chevron procedure in juvenile patients and reported a 20% recurrence rate. Extrapolating from these results, the limits of the procedure for a consistently reproducible outcome are a hallux valgus angle of less than 30 degrees and an intermetatarsal angle of less than 12 to 13 degrees. Expansion of the indications for this procedure to more severe deformities appears to increase the risk of patient dissatisfaction and complications. Reporting on 50 adults who underwent distal metatarsal osteotomy for hallux valgus, Meier and Kenzora[260] noted a 74% satisfaction rate when the 1-2 intermetatarsal angle was greater than 12 degrees and a 94% satisfaction rate when the 1-2 intermetatarsal angle was 12 degrees or less. As a rule, Harper[145] noted that 1 degree of correction is obtained for every 1 mm of lateral translation of the capital fragment. Greater correction has been achieved by Trnka et al[351] and Stienstra et

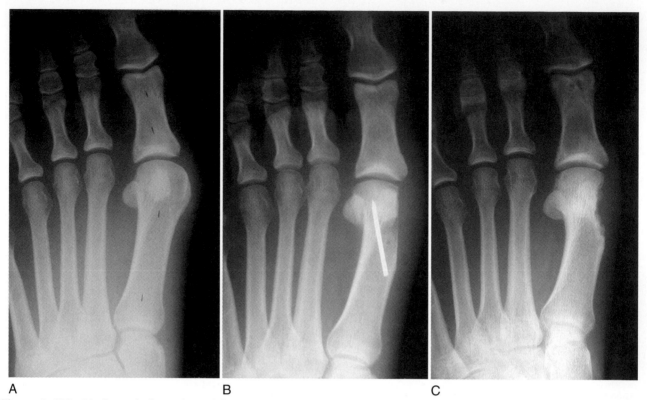

A   B   C

Figure 6–122 Moderate hallux valgus deformity. **A,** Preoperative radiographic appearance. **B,** Radiograph after a chevron osteotomy with correction of the hallux valgus angle. **C,** Twelve-year follow-up after the procedure.

al,[340] who reported 18 degrees of correction of the hallux valgus angle. In both studies, a lateral release was performed. Stienstra et al[340] reported that they translated the capital fragment almost 10 mm laterally. No cases of delayed union, nonunion, or AVN developed. Trnka et al[351] performed a retrospective study on 100 feet treated with a chevron osteotomy and translation of the capital fragment 3 to 6 mm and achieved 87% good or excellent results. They also released the lateral capsule, the adductor tendon, and the transverse intermetatarsal ligament. In a follow-up study,[350] there was no deterioration of the results or subjective satisfaction at 5-year follow-up.

In a series of 17 patients and 23 feet, Mann and Donatto[238] carefully analyzed the degree of correction of the hallux valgus angle, intermetatarsal angle, and the fibular sesamoid position to carefully define the true correction after a chevron procedure. They measured the hallux valgus and intermetatarsal angles by drawing lines that bisected the shafts of the first and second metatarsals and then compared the results with those from the center-of-head method, which measures the angle formed by a line drawn from the center of the first metatarsal head and middle of the metatarsal base and a line bisecting the second metatarsal shaft.[81] In the method in which both metatarsals were bisected, the preoperative and postoperative intermetatarsal angle was 11 degrees. In the center-of-head method, the intermetatarsal angle was 9 degrees preoperatively and 7 degrees postoperatively. When the hallux valgus angle was measured with one line through the longitudinal axis of the first metatarsal and the other through the proximal phalanx, as opposed to one line through the center of the first metatarsal head, the results demonstrated a correction of 5 degrees for the former and 8 degrees for the latter. Basically, this demonstrates that the degree of correction with the chevron procedure is quite small, which must be considered when selecting patients for this procedure. The position of the fibular sesamoid was essentially unchanged.

The chevron osteotomy has limited capability to correct a hallux valgus deformity with an increased DMAA.[72] Because of the limited cor-

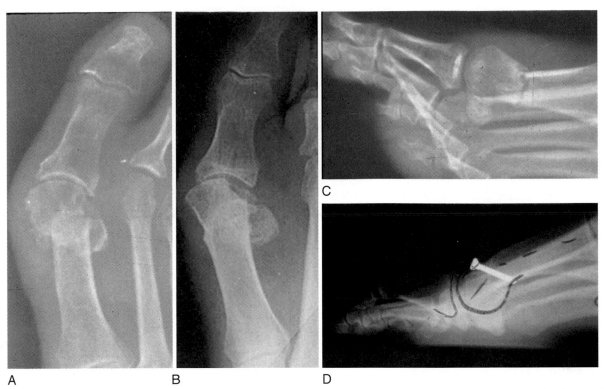

Figure 6–123 Malunion can occur in any plane. **A,** Medial, **B,** lateral, and **C,** dorsal displacement owing to lack of internal fixation. **D,** Plantar displacement with internal fixation.

rection achieved with a chevron osteotomy, it must be reserved for mild and moderate hallux valgus deformities. Chou et al[53] reported on 14 patients who had undergone a biplanar chevron osteotomy for mild and moderate hallux valgus deformities in which an average 7-degree correction of the DMAA was achieved.

Postoperative displacement of the osteotomy site varied from 1.8% in 225 cases reported by Hattrup and Johnson[149] to 12% reported by Johnson et al[172] and can lead to overcorrection or undercorrection[158] (Fig. 6–123). The incidence of postoperative displacement of the capital fragment medially or laterally or deviation dorsal or plantar-ward can be minimized by the use of some form of internal fixation rather than relying on impaction of the osteotomy site as was initially recommended,[9,173,351] especially in those for whom greater displacement of the osteotomy is desired (Fig. 6–124).

Early reports on internal fixation with absorbable implants demonstrated evidence of a foreign body reaction.[276] Recent reports using poly-L-lactic acid[13,39,93,158,276] demonstrated less common side effects of osteolysis or granuloma formation. Gill et al[118] reported a 10% incidence

of pin tract osteolysis when using PDS bioabsorbable pins to internally fix a chevron osteotomy.

Complications

Complications after the chevron procedure are similar to those noted with other procedures: pain, recurrence of the hallux valgus deformity, transfer metatarsalgia secondary to shortening, MTP joint arthrofibrosis, and postoperative neuritic symptoms secondary to entrapment of a cutaneous nerve. The most frequent complications reported with the chevron osteotomy are recurrence and undercorrection of a hallux valgus deformity, which vary in frequency from 10% to 20%[8,158,213] (Fig. 6–125).

Recurrence of hallux valgus deformity occurs in about 10% of cases.[4,113] The 10% recurrence rate can probably be significantly lessened if the indications for the procedure are not overextended. In the series reported by Hirvensalo et al,[158] the deformity recurred when the preoperative hallux valgus averaged 37 degrees and the intermetatarsal angle averaged 13 degrees. Hattrup and Johnson[149] noted recurrence of

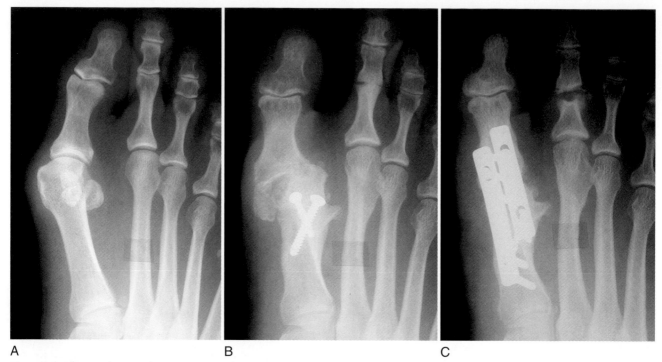

A   B   C

Figure 6–124   Malunion due to poor alignment of the osteotomy. **A,** Preoperative. **B,** Poor postoperative malalignment. **C,** Salvage with metatarsophalangeal joint arthrodesis.

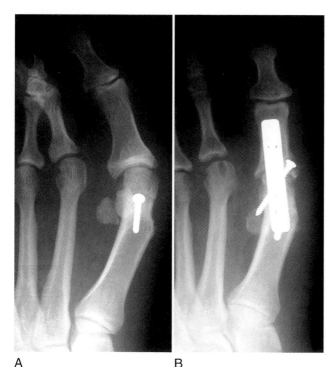

A   B

Figure 6–125   **A,** Recurrence after the chevron procedure. **B,** Salvage with metatarsophalangeal arthrodesis.

the deformity in 18 of 225 procedures; they reported that the average preoperative hallux valgus angle of 37 degrees was corrected to an average of 31 degrees postoperatively. Other authors have not documented the severity of the preoperative hallux valgus deformity when discussing recurrence.

Mean shortening of the first metatarsal averaged 2 to 2.5 mm in two series[158,238] and was as high as 6 mm in 28 cases reported by Pring et al.[290] Shortening can develop as a result of excessive bone loss[8,158,260] or be due to bone necrosis or resection at the osteotomy site. Klosok et al[199] reported the development of postoperative transfer lesions in 12% and postoperative metatarsalgia in 43% of patients after a chevron osteotomy (Fig. 6–126).

Although cutaneous nerve injury can occur with this procedure, the use of a medial midline surgical approach substantially reduces the incidence of nerve entrapment when compared with performance of the osteotomy through a dorsal or dorsomedial incision.

The location of the two limbs of the osteotomy, particularly the plantar limb, is critical. The plantar limb should be extraarticular, if

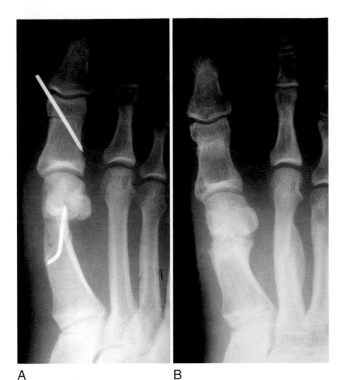

A   **B**

Figure 6–126   **A,** After a combined chevron-Akin procedure. **B,** Stress fracture of the second and third metatarsal 4 months after surgery.

possible, both to avoid injury to the sesamoids and to minimize the development of MTP joint adhesions between the sesamoids and the metatarsal head, which can lead to resultant loss of MTP joint motion. Trnka et al[350] noted that passive range of motion was 72 degrees preoperatively and 61 and 62 degrees at the 2-year follow-up after a chevron osteotomy. A patient should be counseled that decreased MTP range of motion may occur after the procedure (Fig. 6–127).

Hallux varus may develop due to lateral displacement of the capital fragment, medial subluxation of the tibial sesamoid, excessive excision of the medial eminence resulting in inappropriate narrowing of the metatarsal head, and AVN of the medial aspect of the capital fragment. Although these complications are uncommon, awareness of them may help in their prevention (Fig. 6–128).

The most serious complication after a chevron osteotomy is AVN (Fig. 6–129). The incidence of AVN varies from 4% to 20%.[134,162,172,279] In an early report, Meier and Kenzora[260] noted AVN in 20% of patients after a chevron osteotomy, and this figure increased to 40% when combined with an adductor tenotomy. Shereff et al[322] cautioned that lateral release increases the risk of

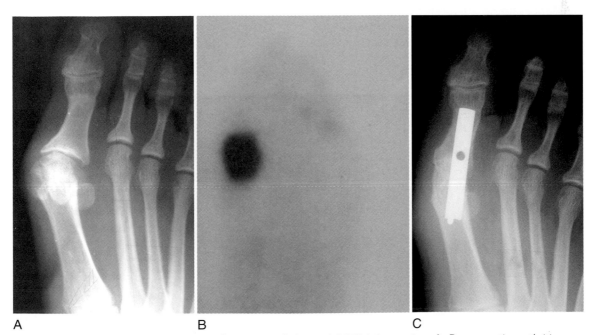

A   **B**   **C**

Figure 6–127   Patient with severe restriction of metatarsophalangeal (MTP) joint motion. **A,** Degenerative arthritis versus avascular necrosis 2 years after a chevron procedure. **B,** Increased uptake on bone scan at the MTP joint. **C,** Salvage with MTP joint arthrodesis.

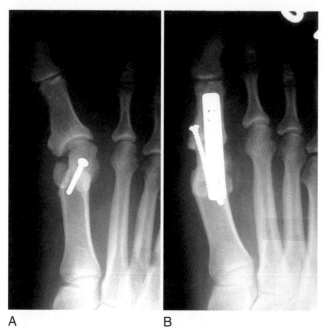

A   B

Figure 6–128 **A,** Hallux varus after a chevron procedure. **B,** Salvage with metatarsophalangeal arthrodesis. (Same patient as shown in Fig. 6–124 after recurrence on the contralateral side.)

AVN (Fig. 6–130). No AVN, however, was observed in a series of chevron procedures reported by Hattrup and Johnson.[149] More recently, Green et al[134] identified no evidence of first metatarsal AVN after release of the conjoined adductor tendon, sesamoidal ligament, and fibular sesamoid ligament through an intermetatarsal incision. Although excessive capsular

dissection has been implicated in the development of AVN, careful surgical technique and preservation of the distal vascular structures can help avoid AVN. Peterson et al[279] reported a case of AVN after lateral release. They suggested that a carefully performed chevron procedure preserves the dorsal and plantar blood supply and did not believe that a lateral capsular release above the sesamoids or an adductor tendon release interrupted the vascular supply. Trnka et al[351] performed a lateral release through a separate incision; after dissecting out and releasing the tarsometatarsal ligament and the lateral capsule, they reported no evidence of AVN at final follow-up. Trnka et al[350] then reviewed the combined series of Pochatko, Trnka, and Peterson[279,283,351,352] of 224 chevron procedures and found that only four cases of AVN developed (2%), and in three of these cases excessive stripping was documented.

AVN is a potential problem that may not be preventable in certain cases because of peculiarities in the blood supply to the capital fragment, but this does not necessarily preclude a successful end result. When performing a chevron procedure, however, excessive soft tissue stripping should be minimized. Excess lateral penetration of the saw blade should also be avoided because it can damage the lateral capsular circulation to the metatarsal head (Fig. 6–131). Release of the lateral structures may enable greater correction but, if done extensively, can increase the risk of AVN.[168,212,260,376]

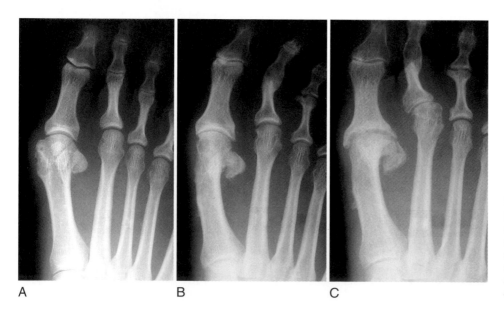

A   B   C

Figure 6–129 Avascular necrosis of the metatarsal head after distal osteotomy. **A,** Preoperative radiograph. **B,** After surgery. **C,** Five years after surgery, complete chondrolysis and avascular necrosis have developed.

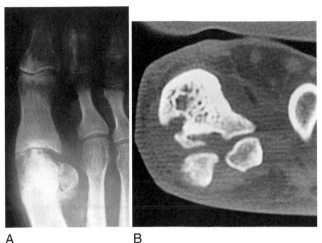

A   B

Figure 6–130 A, Avascular necrosis after a chevron procedure. **B,** Computed tomography scan demonstrating marked cystic degeneration.

The question of whether to release the lateral capsular structures when performing a chevron procedure depends on the perceived risk of AVN. Based on the literature,* careful, meticulous release of contracted lateral structures at the level of the joint is probably safe because it is distal to the blood supply to the metatarsal head. However, in the presence of a more severe deformity, it may be a better alternative to choose another procedure that does not have any risk of development of AVN. More extensive dissection along the lateral aspect of the metatarsal head, such as with excision of the fibular sesamoid, should be avoided because this dissection carries a higher risk of disturbing the blood supply along the lateral aspect of the metatarsal head.

*References 8, 199, 279, 283, 343, and 351.

Thomas et al[343] performed lateral soft tissue release and, frequently, fibular sesamoidectomy through a plantar incision. In a review of 80 of their chevron procedures, the radiographic changes suggested avascular compromise in 76% (61 of 80) of the feet, but at follow-up, none had progressed to AVN. Wilkinson et al[375] postoperatively evaluated 20 patients with magnetic resonance imaging after chevron osteotomy. Fifty percent had evidence of AVN, mostly in the dorsal metatarsal head, although none of the patients were symptomatic. The authors also performed McBride procedures as controls, and none showed evidence of decreased vascularity to the metatarsal head.

DISTAL METATARSAL OSTEOTOMY (MITCHELL, WILSON, BOESCH TYPES)

Correction of a hallux valgus deformity by means of a distal first metatarsal osteotomy was first described by Reverdin[293] in 1881 and later by both Peabody[277] and Hohmann.[161] However, it was Mitchell[150,264] who described and popularized the technique of a biplanar metaphyseal osteotomy, which achieves lateral and plantar displacement of the capital fragment, as well as shortening of the first metatarsal. Wilson[379] and

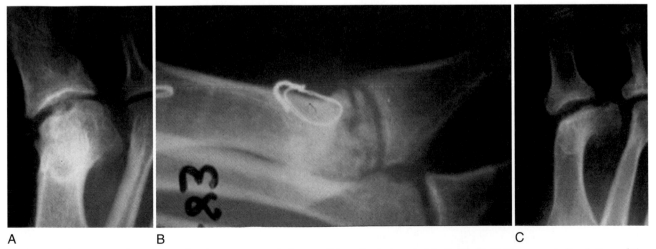

A   B   C

Figure 6–131 Avascular necrosis leading to varus deformity (**A**) and subchondral lysis (**B**). **C,** Collapse and dissolution of the metatarsal head.

others[130,266,311,357] described an oblique meta-physeal osteotomy; Bosch[31,32] and Kramer,[200] a transverse osteotomy; and Magnan,[19,228,229] a percutaneous osteotomy. The Mitchell procedure, as described by Hawkins et al,[150] is a double step-cut osteotomy through the neck of the first metatarsal. Several modifications have been made to this procedure through the years, including changes in the design of the medial capsulorrhaphy,[36,263,266,311] the osteotomy technique,* the method of internal fixation,† and postoperative care.[36,266,341] The changes described make the eponym Mitchell somewhat inadequate to describe the current procedure as now performed in many series. Nonetheless, Mitchell's important principles remain—that shortening should be kept to a minimum, plantar flexion of the capital fragment should consistently be achieved, and rotation of the capital fragment to realign the distal articular metatarsal surface is occasionally indicated.

Indications

Distal metatarsal osteotomy (whether oblique or transverse) is indicated for a moderate or moderately severe hallux valgus deformity with a subluxed MTP joint. If the DMAA is not substantial (less than 15 degrees), this osteotomy is still indicated. The upper limit is 35 to 40 degrees for hallux valgus angular deformity and 15 degrees for the 1-2 intermetatarsal angle. As a general rule, satisfactory results seem to diminish significantly with more severe deformities and in patients older than 60 years.[110] The location of the osteotomy in the proximal region of the distal metaphysis enables it to achieve slightly more correction than a chevron osteotomy does.

Contraindications

The procedure should not be used to treat patients with mild hallux valgus deformity, a short first metatarsal, lateral metatarsalgia, a DMAA greater than 20 degrees, or more than mild MTP joint arthrosis.

---

*References 31, 32, 36, 200, 228, 229, 263, 266, 286, 311, 357, and 379-381.
†References 36, 110, 204, 261, 266, 311, 341, 380, and 381.

Technique

The surgical technique for a distal metatarsal osteotomy is divided into the surgical approach, technique of the metatarsal osteotomy, and reconstruction of the osteotomy and MTP joint.

Surgical Approach

1. A longitudinal skin incision is made over the dorsomedial aspect of the first MTP joint. The incision begins distally at the midportion of the proximal phalanx and is carried proximally 6 cm over the metatarsal shaft. Care is taken to protect the dorsomedial and plantar medial cutaneous nerves of the hallux.
2. A distally based capsular flap[36] or a V/Y-shaped capsular flap[264] is developed over the medial aspect of the MTP joint to expose the medial eminence.
3. Subperiosteal dissection is carried out along the dorsomedial aspect of the distal metatarsal. Extensive dissection is avoided, especially in the area of the dorsal lateral capsular area. The adductor tendon and lateral capsular attachments are not released to avoid disrupting the blood supply to the metatarsal head.[260]
4. The medial eminence is exposed and excised in line with the medial aspect of the metatarsal shaft, starting about 1 mm medial to the sagittal sulcus.

Technique of First Metatarsal Osteotomy

1. A double osteotomy is performed in the distal first metatarsal metaphyses. The initial cut of the double osteotomy is an incomplete cut that is commenced 2 cm proximal to the distal metatarsal articular surface (Fig. 6–132A). The depth of this cut depends on the amount of correction desired. The wider the lateral shelf, the less correction obtained. Typically, a lateral bridge of bone measuring 4 to 5 mm is left. The plantar aspect of the metatarsal is inspected as the osteotomy is performed to ensure that the cut is proximal to the sesamoids.
2. Although in the classic description of the procedure by Mitchell et al[264] holes are drilled above and below the osteotomy for placement of cerclage suture, more rigid internal fixation is preferable. Either a 5/64-inch Steinmann pin or two Kirschner wires are

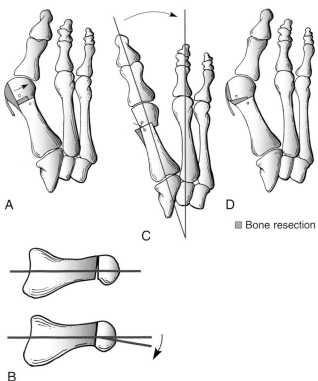

Figure 6–132 **A,** The proposed osteotomy for moderate hallux valgus deformity necessitates bone resection and shortening. The width of lateral shelf determines the amount of displacement of the capital fragment. The wider the shelf, the greater the lateral displacement. **B,** Slightly more bone is resected on the plantar aspect of the osteotomy site to decrease the prevalence of postoperative transfer lesions. **C,** After displacement and shortening, the capital fragment is translated laterally. The medial metaphyseal flare is removed. **D,** With an increased distal metatarsal articular angle, biplanar resection allows realignment of congruent metatarsophalangeal joint articulation.

commonly used to fix the shaft and the capital fragment.[12,110,204]

3. The second parallel osteotomy is cut completely through the metatarsal approximately 2 mm proximal and parallel to the initial cut in a medial-to-lateral direction. The magnitude of the deformity determines the amount of shortening desired, the thickness of the resection, and the width of the lateral shelf that is left. This cut is angled so that 2 mm more of bone is removed on the plantar aspect, thereby tilting the osteotomy site plantar-ward (Fig. 6–132C). The width of the lateral spike on the distal fragment depends on the magnitude of the intermetatarsal angle. With a severe deformity the spike may constitute approximately one third of the metatarsal shaft, whereas with a more

moderate deformity it consists of only about one sixth of the metatarsal's width. The degree of plantar tilting depends on the length of the first metatarsal and whether a plantar lesion is present under the second metatarsal.

Reconstruction of the Osteotomy and Metatarsophalangeal Joint

1. The osteotomy site is displaced laterally 4 to 5 mm until the lateral shelf locks over the edge of the proximal fragment, and the position is carefully checked to ensure that slight plantar flexion is present. Blum[25] reported that rather than removing more bone off the metatarsal's plantar aspect, the capital fragment was displaced plantar-ward 2 to 4 mm to compensate for this shortening (Fig. 6–132B). If the distal metatarsal articular surface is sloped laterally (increased DMAA), more bone can be removed from the medial aspect of the metatarsal, and the capital fragment is then rotated to align the articular surface more perpendicular to the metatarsal shaft (Fig. 6–132D).

2. The osteotomy site is stabilized with Kirschner wires,[110,158,163,204,341] screws,[380,381] staples,[36] or an oblique 5/64-inch Steinmann pin (Fig. 6–133).

3. The remaining medial metaphyseal flare created by the lateral displacement of the capital fragment is then resected with a power saw (Fig. 6–134).

4. The MTP joint is brought into a neutral or slight varus position, and the medial capsu-

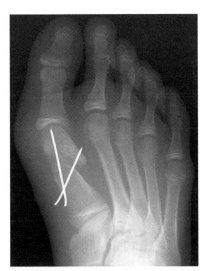

Figure 6–133 Internal fixation with two Kirschner wires.

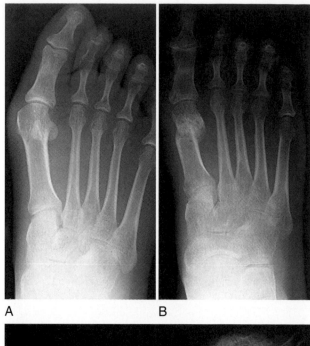

A   B

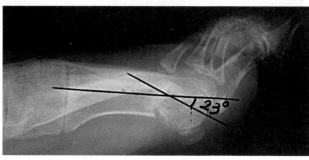

C

Figure 6–134 A, Preoperative radiograph demonstrating a moderate hallux valgus deformity. **B,** Radiograph after a Mitchell osteotomy. **C,** Lateral radiograph demonstrating plantar flexion of the capital fragment. (Courtesy of Kent Wu, MD.)

lar tissues are plicated with interrupted sutures.

5. The skin is closed with interrupted sutures and a firm compression dressing is applied.

6. Magnan et al[228,229] advocate a transverse osteotomy in the proximal metaphyseal region in which the metatarsal head is translated medial-ward without resection of the medial eminence. It is fixed with a longitudinal Steinmann pin (Fig. 6–135).

Postoperative Care

A gauze-and-tape compressing dressing is applied after completion of the surgical procedure. In the office 1 to 2 days after surgery, the compression dressing is removed and the patient placed in a firm spica-like dressing consisting of 2-inch Kling gauze and 1/2-inch adhesive tape dressing. Some authors will fashion a slipper cast to immobilize the hallux and forefoot. Most authors prefer that the patient remain non–weight bearing for 4 weeks after surgery because the osteotomy site is not as stable as some of the other osteotomies previously described. One to 3 weeks after surgery, the sutures are removed and a radiograph obtained with as much weight bearing as tolerated to assess alignment of the MTP joint. The dressing changes are then based on this radiograph. If pins are used, they are generally removed 4 to 6 weeks after surgery and the patient is then permitted to ambulate in either a postoperative shoe or a removable cast boot until the osteotomy site has healed, which typically occurs at approximately 6 to 8 weeks after surgery.

Results

The Mitchell procedure achieves high patient satisfaction and satisfactory correction of the hallux valgus and intermetatarsal angular deformities. The overall experience with both the Mitchell osteotomy and the modified Mitchell-type distal metatarsal osteotomies is that satisfactory correction is achieved in 82% to 97% of cases.* In two of the largest series, Blum[25] reported that 185 of 204 patients (91%) and Hawkins et al[150] reported that 182 of 188 patients (97%) were satisfied with the procedure. The average reported correction of the hallux valgus angle varies from 10 to 25 degrees,† and the average correction of the 1-2 intermetatarsal angle varies from 5 to 10 degrees.‡ Shortening of the first metatarsal is a key component in achieving correction of the hallux valgus deformity (see Fig. 6–137J); however, it places the patient at risk for postoperative metatarsalgia.[150] Excessive shortening is the most common cause of lesser MTP joint pain and callus formation after a distal first metatarsal osteotomy for correction of hallux valgus.§ Merkel et al[261] reported an average first metatarsal shortening of 7 mm. In patients who

---

*References 25, 45, 110, 127, 150, 204, 264, 380, and 381.
†References 25, 36, 110, 127, 194, 204, 380, and 381.
‡References 25, 36, 110, 127, 150, 194, 380, and 381.
§References 45, 110, 127, 150, 194, 263, 264, 311, and 379.

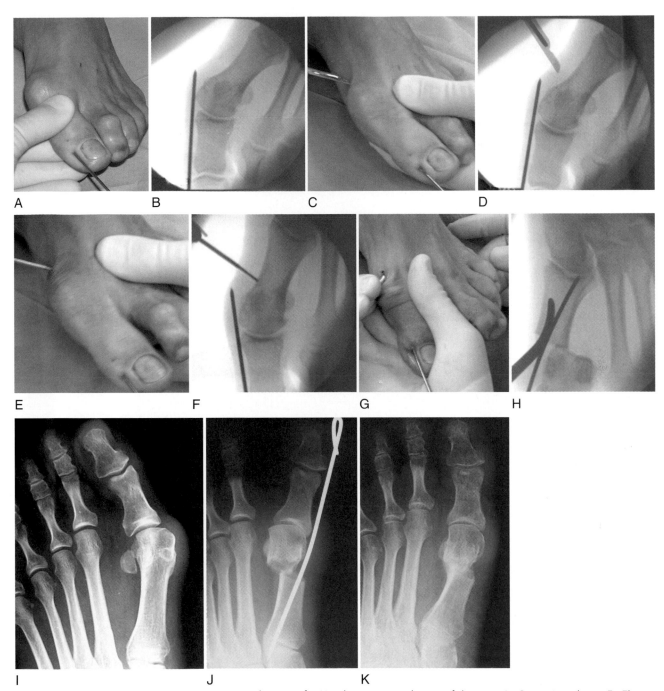

Figure 6–135 Percutaneous osteotomy: introduction of a Kirschner wire at the tip of the toe. **A,** Operative photo. **B,** Fluoroscopic view. **C,** Small incision. **D,** Fluoroscopic view. **E,** Osteotomy of the metaphysis. **F,** Fluoroscopic view. **G,** Reduction of the intermetatarsal angle. **H,** Fixation placed in the intramedullary canal. **I,** Preoperative radiograph. **J,** Intraoperative radiograph. **K,** Four months after surgery. (Courtesy of B. Magnan, MD.)

had more than 10 mm of shortening, a higher rate of dissatisfaction and a higher incidence of metatarsalgia were reported. Rates of postoperative metatarsalgia have been reported to vary from 10% to 40%,[150,194,204,380] with a 31% incidence reported by Hawkins et al[150] in the largest series. Plantar angulation[25,127,150,264] or plantar displacement[261,380,381] of the capital fragment has been advocated to diminish the ill effects of first metatarsal shortening. Dorsal angulation at the osteotomy site is associated with patient dissatisfaction because it tends

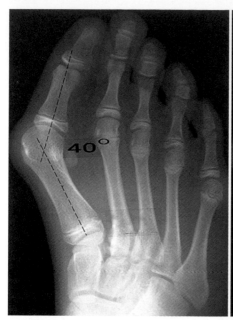

A

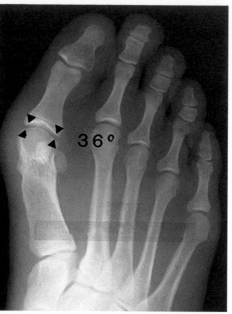

B

Figure 6–136 Complications after distal osteotomy. **A,** Preoperative radiograph of severe juvenile hallux valgus deformity with a congruent metatarsophalangeal joint (preoperative hallux valgus angle, 40 degrees). **B,** After a Mitchell osteotomy, the 1-2 intermetatarsal angle, hallux valgus angle, and distal metatarsal articular angle are uncorrected (postoperative hallux valgus angle, 36 degrees).

to compound the effects of first metatarsal shortening.[36,261,380,381]

Complications

Recurrence and undercorrection of hallux valgus deformity have also been recognized as complications after distal metatarsal osteotomy (Fig. 6–136). These complications have been reported to occur in approximately 10% of cases.* Use of a distal metatarsal osteotomy for more severe deformities increases the risk of recurrence, undercorrection, or malunion[110] (Fig. 6–137). Fokter et al[110] reported that results deteriorated with time: Subjective satisfaction rates of 97% at 10 years diminished to 64% with long-term follow-up.

The incidence of AVN with significant collapse of the metatarsal head is difficult to determine (Fig. 6–138). However, Meier and Kenzora[260] observed AVN in 1 of 12 patients, Das De and Hamblen[90] in 2 of 38 patients, Wu[380] in none of 100 patients, and Blum[25] in 5 of 204 patients, 1 of whom was symptomatic. Carr and Boyd[45] and others† have also reported the development of AVN after distal first metatarsal osteotomy. Wu[380,381] occasionally used a lateral soft tissue release in combination with the

*References 25, 127, 150, 264, 380, and 381.
†References 70, 130, 231, 260, 264, and 311.

osteotomy, whereas others have avoided lateral dissection.[45,150,265,357]

The main complication of shortening of the metatarsal is that it can lead to transfer metatarsalgia. The osteotomy should be avoided in an already short first metatarsal with a concomitant hallux valgus deformity. Plantar flexion of the head fragment is essential to prevent this complication. Loss of position at the osteotomy site into dorsal angulation or excessive medial or lateral deviation can result in a significant complication if not promptly recognized and corrected (Fig. 6–138). Arthrofibrosis, though not common, may occur as well due to the extensive soft tissue dissection.

The design of this type of transverse osteotomy renders it relatively unstable. Loss of correction,[194] delayed union,[261,263,264] nonunion,[261] and malunion[36,380,381] are all noted complications. The demanding technique with the high incidence of complications is the reason for the less frequent use of these types of procedures. If the hallux valgus deformity is mild, a distal chevron osteotomy, which is significantly more stable, is preferable; if the deformity is more severe, a distal soft tissue procedure with a proximal osteotomy may be advantageous. The Mitchell procedure is therefore used less commonly as more "user-friendly," proximal metatarsal osteotomies have become more refined.

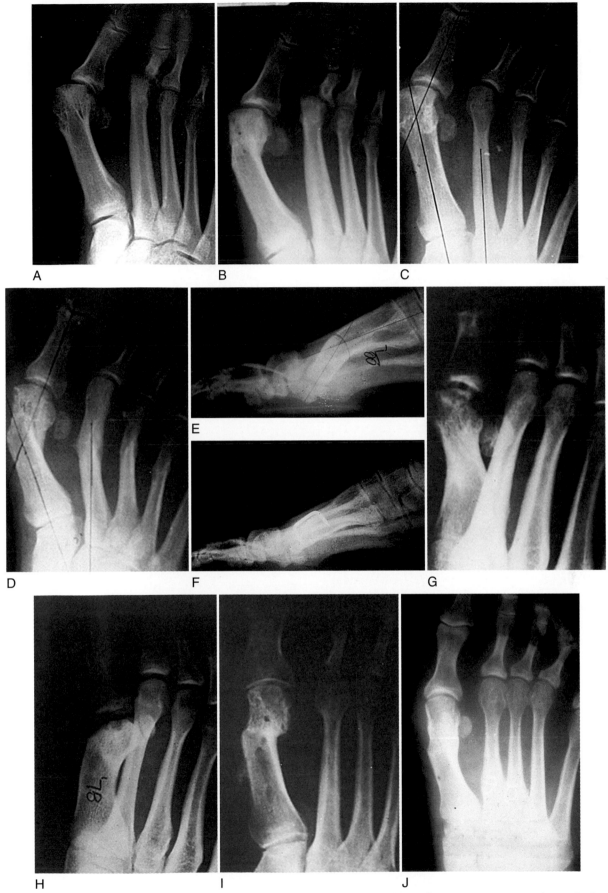

Figure 6–137 Complications after the Mitchell procedure. **A,** Preoperative radiograph. **B,** Postoperative radiograph showing incomplete correction because the deformity is too severe to be corrected by the Mitchell procedure. **C,** Preoperative radiograph. **D,** Postoperative radiograph showing lateral deviation of the capital fragment. **E,** Radiograph demonstrating plantar flexion of the capital fragment. **F,** Realignment after a dorsal closing wedge metatarsal osteotomy. **G,** Dorsiflexion of the distal fragment. **H,** Plantar flexion of the distal fragment. **I,** Avascular changes in the metatarsal head. **J,** Shortening of the first ray.

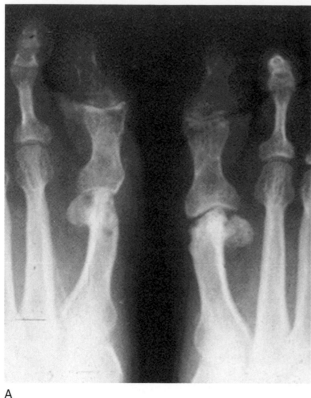

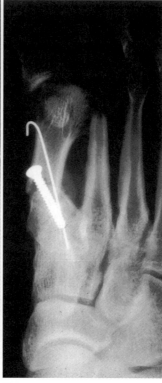

A   B

Figure 6–138 A, Avascular necrosis after a Mitchell-type osteotomy with loss of the entire head and collapse and severe shortening of the first ray. **B,** Malunion after a distal midshaft osteotomy is associated with very difficult salvage.

AKIN PROCEDURE

An Akin procedure[1] achieves correction of hallux valgus deformity by means of a medial capsulorrhaphy, resection of the medial eminence, and medial closing wedge phalangeal osteotomy (video clip 24).* This procedure can produce a satisfactory result in the treatment of specific types of deformities but is not indicated in the presence of MTP joint subluxation.

Indications

The primary indication for this procedure is a hallux valgus interphalangeus deformity[282] (Fig. 6–139). In the presence of a congruous MTP joint with a significant hallux valgus deformity and an increased intermetatarsal angle, extraarticular repair can be achieved by a combination of proximal phalangeal osteotomy and first metatarsal osteotomy[60,265] (see Fig. 6–122). The use of an extraarticular repair may prevent disturbance of a congruent MTP articulation.[74,129] It is also useful to achieve derotation of a

*References 60, 69, 128, 282, 319, and 326.

pronated hallux[301,315] and shortening in patients with a long proximal phalanx.[160,301]

After an initial surgical procedure complicated by recurrent deformity, if any residual lateral deviation of the hallux results in pressure against the second toe, a phalangeal osteotomy can angulate the hallux medially away from the adjacent second toe. The procedure can also be used in conjunction with almost any bunion

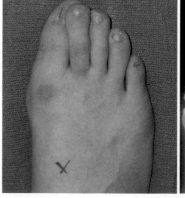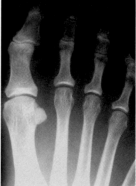

A   B

Figure 6–139   Hallux valgus interphalangeus: clinical (**A**) and radiographic (**B**) appearance.

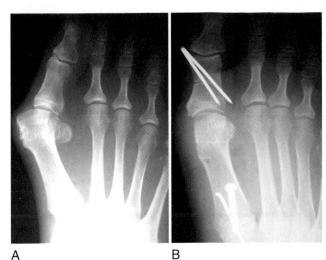

A   B

Figure 6–140   A, Preoperative radiograph. **B,** After a Mann-Akin procedure.

correction in which some valgus of the hallux is still present.[60,77,265] A phalangeal osteotomy can be combined with a more proximal first ray osteotomy[77] (Fig. 6–140). On occasion, phalangeal osteotomy can be used without medial eminence resection and medial capsular reefing if only an osteotomy is indicated to realign the great toe.

Contraindications

The Akin procedure is contraindicated as a primary procedure to correct a hallux valgus deformity if there is any subluxation of the MTP joint. An Akin procedure does not decrease the 1-2 intermetatarsal angle; therefore, with a significant metatarsus primus varus deformity, an Akin procedure alone is insufficient to correct the deformity. This procedure can actually lead to destabilization of the MTP joint if used as a primary procedure to correct a hallux valgus deformity characterized by a subluxated MTP joint.[282]

Technique

The surgical technique for the Akin procedure is divided into exposure, performance of the osteotomy, and reconstruction of the joint capsule and osteotomy.

Surgical Exposure

1. A medial longitudinal skin incision is centered over the medial eminence just proximal to the interphalangeal joint and extended 1 cm proximal to the medial eminence. Dorsal and plantar full-thickness skin flaps are created, with care taken to protect the dorsomedial and plantar medial cutaneous nerves.

2. An L-shaped, distally based capsular flap is created. With this L-shaped flap, the dorsal and proximal MTP joint capsular attachments are released while the distal and plantar capsular attachments remain intact. The capsule is carefully dissected off the medial eminence (see Fig. 6–90D).

3. Through this same exposure, subperiosteal dissection is used to expose the phalangeal metaphyseal region, with care taken to protect the distally based capsular flap. The soft tissue is not stripped past the dorsomedial and plantar medial surfaces of the proximal phalanx.
   Alternative to Step 2: A vertical capsulotomy is made with a no. 11 blade, starting 2 to 3 mm proximal to the base of the proximal phalanx. A second cut is made parallel to the first, with no more than 2 to 4 mm of capsular tissue removed. The amount of capsular excision depends on the size of the medial eminence (see Fig. 6–90B).

Technique of Resection of the Medial Eminence and Phalangeal Osteotomy

1. With an oscillating saw, the medial eminence is resected in line with the first metatarsal medial cortex. The osteotomy is begun slightly medial to the sagittal sulcus and extended proximally along the medial border of the first metatarsal. The remaining edges, particularly on the dorsomedial aspect of the metatarsal head, are smoothed with a rongeur.

2. A small, medially based wedge of bone is resected in the metaphyseal, diaphyseal-metaphyseal, or diaphyseal region. The location of the osteotomy depends on the site of maximal deformity, which in the proximal phalanx may be central, proximal, or distal[301] (Figs. 6–141A and B and 6–142). (A mini–image intensifier can be used to check the location of the phalangeal osteotomy site in reference to the location of the MTP joint, interphalangeal joint, and in a juvenile patient, open epiphysis.)

3. The lateral cortex of the phalanx is left intact (minimally), and the osteotomy site is closed.

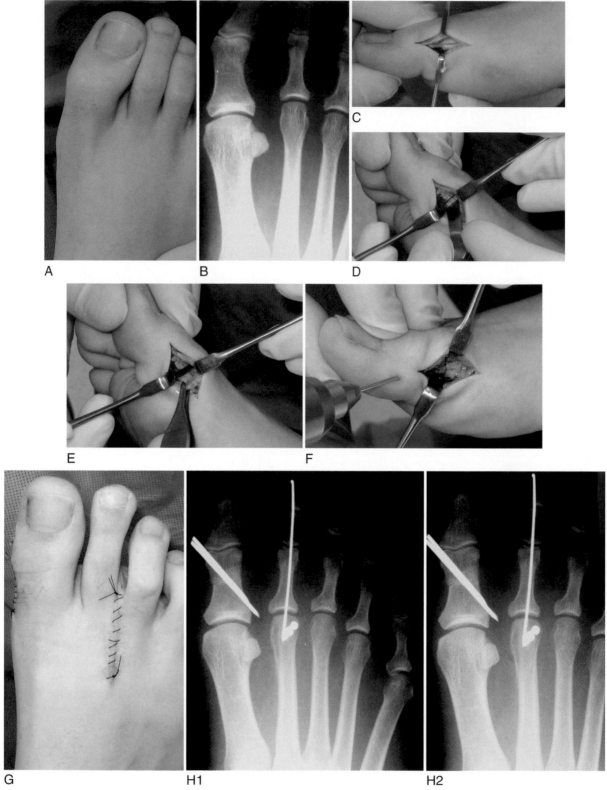

Figure 6–141   Technique of Akin phalangeal osteotomy. **A,** Preoperative clinical and, **B,** radiographic appearance. **C,** Operative incision for just phalangeal osteotomy. **D,** Two parallel cuts are made for the medially based closing wedge osteotomy. **E,** The wedge is removed. **F,** The osteotomy is closed and fixed with two Kirschner wires. **G,** Postoperative clinical and, **H,** radiographic appearance after osteotomy. (An interdigital neuroma and Weil osteotomy was performed as well.)

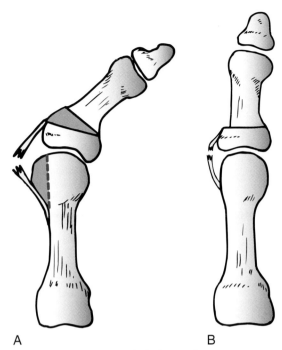

Figure 6–142 **A,** Proposed phalangeal osteotomy. **B,** After the osteotomy.

Routinely, a 2- to 3-mm-wide resection is performed with the apex at the lateral base; however, depending on the magnitude of the deformity, the closing wedge osteotomy may be smaller or larger (Fig. 6–141C and D). In addition, the surgeon must keep in mind that the phalangeal surface of the MTP joint is concave. When performing the initial osteotomy, there is a risk of penetrating the joint with the saw blade. A second cut is made slightly distal to the first, and usually 3 to 4 mm of bone is removed at the medial aspect of the osteotomy site. One should attempt to maintain a periosteal hinge laterally. If pronation of the hallux is present, the hallux can be derotated at the osteotomy site before placement of fixation to correct any remaining deformity (see Fig. 6–141E).

Reconstruction of the Joint Capsule and Osteotomy

1. The medial joint capsule is repaired because after this step, one can predict how much correction must be gained from the phalangeal osteotomy. The MTP capsule is repaired with interrupted absorbable suture. If insufficient capsule is present on the dorsal proximal aspect of the MTP joint, a small hole can be drilled in the metaphysis to anchor the capsular flap.

2. After capsular repair, the osteotomy site is approximated medially to assess alignment of the hallux. If the alignment is inadequate, more bone can be resected. The osteotomy site is stabilized with one or two 0.062-inch Kirschner wires (Fig. 6–141F-H). The pin or pins are placed obliquely from a distal medial location. Care is taken to avoid penetration of the interphalangeal and MTP joints. Intraoperative fluoroscopy or intraoperative radiography can be used to visualize the final position of the Kirschner wire. The pins are cut flush with the level of the skin to aid in later removal.

3. An alternative method of fixation of the osteotomy site can be achieved by using a staple, heavy suture, or wire placed through two pairs of medial drill holes, one on the dorsomedial aspect and one on the plantar medial aspect of the osteotomy site. This suture is passed through the drill holes and tied to stabilize the osteotomy (Fig. 6–143A). A compression staple can also be used (Fig. 6–143B).

4. The skin is approximated with interrupted sutures and a compression dressing applied.

Postoperative Care

A gauze-and-tape toe spica compression dressing is applied after surgery (see Fig. 6–108). The patient is permitted to ambulate in a postoperative shoe with weight borne on the outer aspect of the foot. The dressing is changed 1 to 2 days after surgery and then on a weekly basis. The toe is held in a neutral or slight varus position during this healing phase to allow the capsular tissues and osteotomy site to heal adequately. Rarely is casting necessary after a phalangeal osteotomy. The dressing is maintained until the osteotomy site has healed, which typically takes 6 to 8 weeks. If Kirschner wires were used for internal fixation, they are removed 3 to 6 weeks after surgery. Motion of the interphalangeal and MTP joints is initiated at this time.

Results

The best indication for the use of an isolated Akin phalangeal osteotomy is hallux valgus

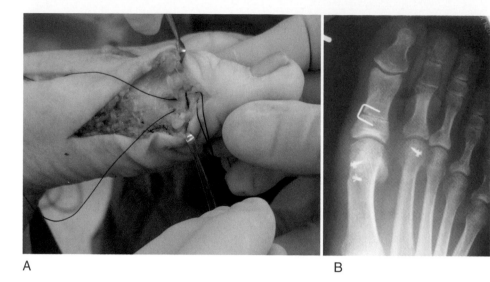

A

B

Figure 6–143 Alternative means of osteotomy fixation. **A,** Osteotomy site. Heavy suture material has been placed through drill holes on either side, after which the osteotomy site is closed and the sutures tied to secure the osteotomy in place. **B,** Small compression staple.

interphalangeus (Fig. 6–144). There are no studies that report the results of isolated Akin osteotomies for interphalangeal deformities alone. When used to correct a mild residual deformity after a previous hallux valgus correction, a phalangeal osteotomy can produce a satisfactory result, provided that the MTP joint is congruent and the residual valgus is caused by lateral sloping of the distal phalangeal articular surface (Fig. 6–145). The use of internal fixation is helpful in maintaining the operative correction and should achieve rigid stabilization of the osteotomy; malunion and nonunion are uncommon[319] (Fig. 6–146). The Akin procedure achieves little correction of the 1-2 intermetatarsal angle.[128,282] In reporting on a series of 22 adult patients, Plattner and Van Manen[282] initially observed an average 13-degree correction of the hallux valgus angle; however, at long-term follow-up, this correction diminished to only 6 degrees of correction. Seelenfreund et al[319] and Goldberg et al[128] reported high recurrence rates (16%-21%) and a high rate of postoperative dissatisfaction and concluded that

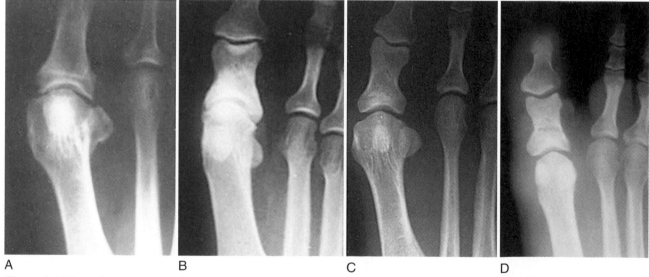

A   B   C   D

Figure 6–144 **A,** Preoperative radiograph demonstrating an irregularly shaped metatarsal head. This metatarsal head will not permit correction by medial displacement because an incongruent articular surface will result. **B,** Postoperative radiograph demonstrating satisfactory alignment after an Akin procedure with removal of the medial eminence without affecting the articular surface. Preoperative (**C**) and postoperative (**D**) radiographs of hallux valgus demonstrate correction with the Akin procedure and excision of the medial eminence.

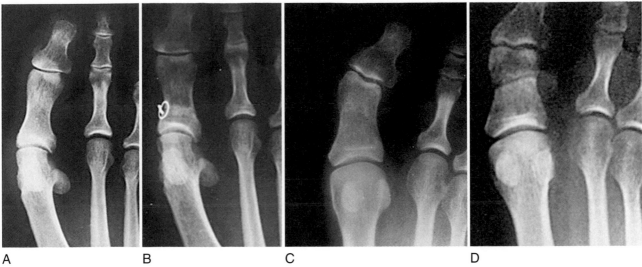

A   B   C   D

Figure 6–145 **A,** Preoperative radiograph of mild recurrence of hallux valgus deformity. **B,** Correction of recurrence with the Akin procedure. Preoperative (**C**) and postoperative (**D**) radiographs demonstrate correction of hallux valgus interphalangeus with the Akin procedure. Note that the osteotomy site is near the apex of the deformity, whereas in a routine Akin procedure, it is carried out in the proximal portion of the phalanx.

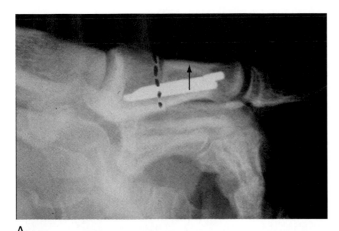

A

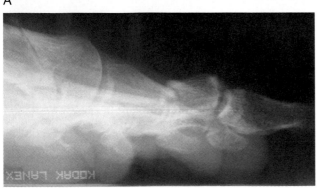

B

Figure 6–146 **A,** Rigid internal fixation holds the osteotomy. **B,** Dorsiflexion malunion due to early weight bearing.

isolated phalangeal osteotomy as treatment of a hallux valgus deformity does not have a sound biomechanical basis and is contraindicated as an isolated procedure (Figs. 6–147 and 6–148).

Although Akin[1] and Colloff and Weitz[60] advocated lateral MTP capsular release, we believe that in general, a wide capsular release should be avoided because it has the potential for devascularizing the proximal phalangeal fragment or the epiphysis in a younger patient. Extensive soft tissue stripping of the proximal phalanx should be avoided because it may lead to vascular compromise of the proximal fragment. Intra-articular extension of the osteotomy with subsequent arthritis occurs infrequently.[301]

Complications

The main complication of the Akin procedure is recurrence or progression of a deformity when the procedure was used to treat a deformity characterized by an incongruent or subluxated MTP joint (Fig. 6–147). Occasionally, when a phalangeal osteotomy is used to treat a hallux valgus deformity characterized by a congruent joint, the MTP joint may sublux postoperatively. Significant loss of interphalangeal joint plantar flexion of the great toe may occur, especially if the osteotomy is carried out distal to the midportion of the phalanx. If care is not taken, the

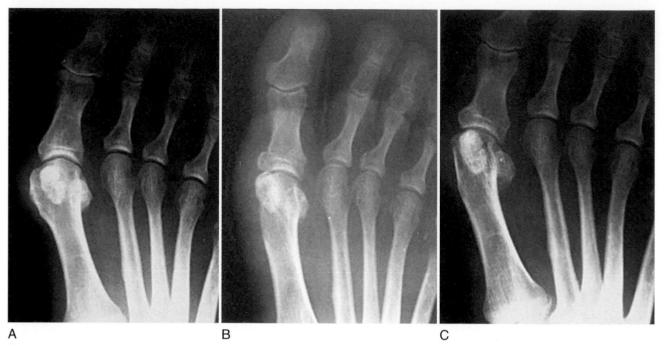

A   B   C

Figure 6–147   A, Preoperative radiograph demonstrating moderate hallux valgus deformity in a 25-year-old woman. **B,** After an Akin osteotomy and resection of the medial eminence, the 1-2 intermetatarsal angle has not been corrected. **C,** At final follow-up, the radiograph demonstrates recurrence of the deformity with subluxation of the MTP joint.

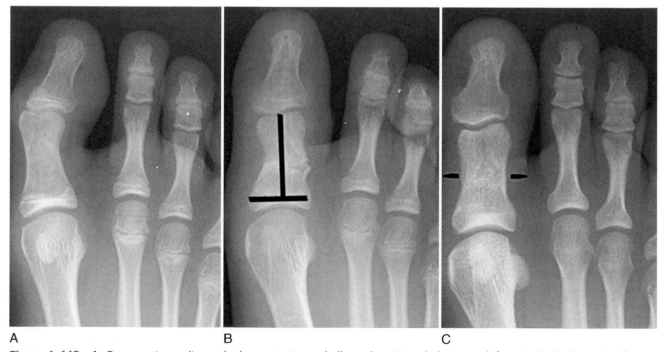

A   B   C

Figure 6–148   A, Preoperative radiograph demonstrating a hallux valgus interphalangeus deformity. **B,** Radiograph after an Akin phalangeal osteotomy. **C,** Seven years later, a radiograph demonstrates acceptable long-term alignment. (Note: medial capsulorrhaphy and medial eminence resection were not performed.)

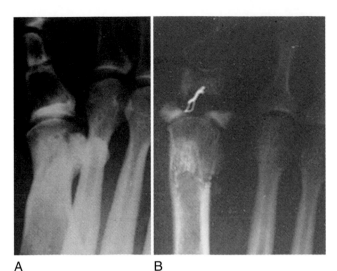

A   B

Figure 6–149 Complications after the Akin procedure. **A,** Delayed union or nonunion of the osteotomy site. **B,** Avascular necrosis.

tendon of the flexor or extensor hallucis longus could be inadvertently severed, particularly when the osteotomy is performed in the distal portion of the phalanx. AVN of the proximal phalanx may occur after excessive soft tissue stripping or excessive retraction of the soft tissues (Fig. 6–149). Other reported complications with this procedure include a poor cosmetic appearance and a high rate of subjective dissatisfaction postoperatively.[128,319]

KELLER PROCEDURE

Riedel[296] in 1886 was the first to perform a resection of the base of the proximal phalanx and arthroplasty of the MTP joint as treatment of hallux valgus. Davies-Colley[91] in 1887 described this same procedure for the treatment of hallux rigidus. It was popularized by Keller's reports in 1904 and 1912.[187] The purpose of the procedure in the treatment of hallux valgus is to decompress the MTP joint by resection of about a third of the proximal phalanx, thereby relaxing the contracted lateral structures (video clip 28). Although the Keller procedure was probably once the most widely used bunion procedure, with the development of other surgical techniques and critical clinical evaluation of results of the Keller procedure, its limitations and indications have been better defined.

Indications

The Keller procedure is indicated in an older patient in whom extensive surgery is contraindicated and who is essentially considered housebound ambulatory[358] or in an older patient with a severe hallux valgus deformity and marginal circulation that has resulted in chronic skin breakdown. It is often considered a salvage technique for treatment of a failed previous surgical procedure.[96,312,358] It is indicated for moderate hallux valgus deformities in which the hallux valgus angle is less than 30 degrees associated with degenerative arthritis of the MTP joint. The Keller procedure can also be used to treat hallux rigidus in patients in whom cheilectomy or arthrodesis cannot be performed. In this procedure, medial eminence resection, partial proximal phalangectomy, and medial capsulorrhaphy are performed to realign the hallux.[182,235,294,366]

Contraindications

This procedure is contraindicated in younger, more active individuals[220] in whom MTP joint mobility and function remain important because the stability of the first MTP joint is impaired by the Keller procedure.[79] Likewise, in older individuals in whom MTP joint function is important, who have substantial lateral metatarsalgia, or who have a severe deformity for which a subtotal correction is unacceptable, this procedure is contraindicated.

Technique

The surgical technique is divided into the surgical approach, resection of bone, and reconstruction of the MTP joint.

Surgical Approach

1. The first MTP joint is exposed through a medial approach that begins at the interphalangeal joint and extends proximally 1 cm beyond the medial eminence. A proximally based capsular flap is developed to create full-thickness dorsal and plantar skin flaps for exposure of the medial eminence (Figs. 6–150 and 6–151A and video clip 28).
2. The medial eminence is exposed by sharp dissection to create a flap of medial capsule based proximally.
3. The base of the proximal phalanx is exposed subperiosteally.

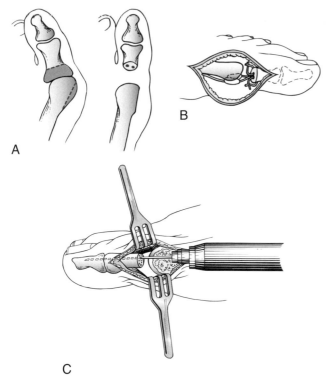

C

Figure 6–150 The Keller procedure. **A,** The medial eminence is removed in line with the medial aspect of the metatarsal shaft. The proximal third of the proximal phalanx is excised. **B,** An attempt is made to reapproximate the plantar and medial capsular structures to the remaining base of the proximal phalanx. **C,** Fixation of the metatarsophalangeal joint with a 5/64-inch Steinmann pin.

Resection of Bone

1. The medial eminence is removed in line with the medial aspect of the metatarsal shaft. Any osteophytes along the dorsal aspect of the metatarsal head are removed (Fig. 6–151B).
2. The proximal third of the phalanx is removed (Figs. 6–150A and 6–151C).
3. Resection of the lateral sesamoid is thought to release the lateral contracted structures, which aids in realignment of the hallux[96] (Fig. 6–151D).

Reconstruction of the Metatarsophalangeal Joint

1. To reestablish flexor function, an attempt is made to reapproximate the plantar aponeurosis and plantar plate to the proximal phalanx through two or three small drill holes in the remaining diaphyseal portion of the proximal phalanx.[65,366] Flexor function can also be enhanced by suturing the plantar aponeurosis to the flexor hallucis longus

tendon, which helps prevent a cock-up deformity of the MTP joint (see Fig. 6–153A).
2. A 5/64-inch Steinmann pin or two 0.062-inch Kirschner wires[96] are introduced at the joint and driven distally; they are then drilled in a retrograde direction across the joint into the metatarsal head to provide stability in the postoperative period and to create a 5-mm gap between the base of the phalanx and the metatarsal head. The tip of the pins should be bent to prevent proximal migration (Figs. 6–150C and 6–151E).
3. The medial capsular flap is sutured to the periosteum of the proximal phalanx and, in some cases, folded across the MTP joint to create an interposition arthroplasty (Fig. 6–151F).
4. The skin is closed with interrupted sutures and a compression dressing applied.

Postoperative Care

In the office 1 to 2 days after surgery, the compression dressing is removed and the patient placed in a firm dressing of 2-inch Kling gauze and 1/2-inch adhesive tape. The patient is permitted to ambulate in a postoperative shoe. The dressings are maintained for 6 weeks. The pins are removed 3 weeks after surgery, at which point gentle motion of the MTP joint is begun.

Results

After excision arthroplasty, the hallux valgus angle is typically reduced approximately 50% or less[226,357,358] and the 1-2 intermetatarsal angle is diminished very little.[294,299,357] Satisfactory results occur more reliably when the hallux valgus angle does not exceed 30 degrees so that correction can be achieved by resection of less than a third of the base of the proximal phalanx (Fig. 6–152). Reduction of pain after the procedure can be attributed to a diminution in size of the medial eminence, which enables the use of more comfortable shoes, as well as decompression of an osteoarthritic joint. Satisfaction rates after a Keller procedure judged mainly on the basis of relief of "bunion pain" as opposed to relief of metatarsalgia vary from 72% to 96%.[55] Rogers and Joplin[299] reported generally poor results with this procedure: marked improvement in 9%, no change in 71%, and postoperative deterioration in 20%. Bonney and Macnab[27] observed that the functional results tend to deteriorate with time. Henry et al[154] observed that after excisional arthroplasty, the hallux was

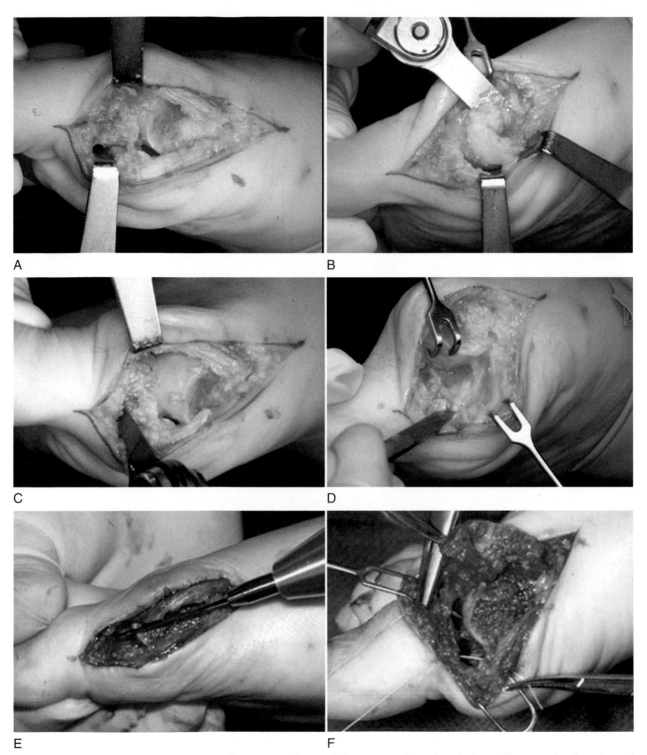

Figure 6–151 **A,** A midline incision is used to expose the medial eminence. Dorsal and plantar flaps are developed. **B,** The medial eminence is excised. **C,** The base of the proximal phalanx is resected with a power saw. **D,** The lateral sesamoid is excised. **E,** An intramedullary Kirschner wire is used to stabilize the toe. **F,** The medial capsule and intrinsics are reattached when possible to the base of the proximal phalanx. (Courtesy of E. Greer Richardson, MD.)

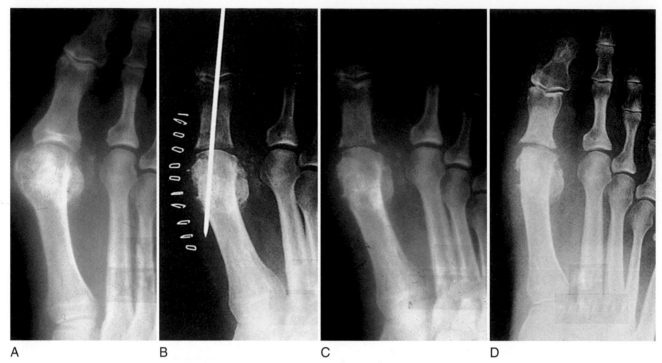

A   B   C   D

Figure 6–152   Results of the Keller procedure. **A,** Preoperative radiograph. **B,** Postoperative radiograph demonstrating pin fixation. **C,** Radiograph after pin removal. **D,** Position of the toe 9 months after surgery.

unable to bear weight, and resultant metatarsalgia developed.

Donley et al[96] and Richardson[294] both reported an average total MTP joint range of 40 to 50 degrees, most of which was dorsiflexion. Love et al[220] reported less than 10 degrees in 18 feet. When assessing the results of a Keller procedure, one must remember that for the procedure to be successful, it should be used in older patients, who by nature are less demanding of their feet. When the procedure is used in this group, a satisfactory result can be anticipated. If, however, the procedure is used in more active persons, dissatisfaction results because of the lack of push-off of the great toe, transfer metatarsalgia (usually beneath the second metatarsal head), cock-up deformity of the first MTP joint, and recurrence of the deformity. The Keller procedure cannot correct a significant hallux valgus deformity or intermetatarsal angle, and other procedures should be strongly considered.

Complications

Coughlin and Mann[79] and others* have reported a high incidence of metatarsalgia after exci-

---

* References 55, 96, 154, 182, 294, 299, and 357.

sional arthroplasty (Figs. 6–153 and 6–154). Postoperative varus and valgus deformity may occur due to lack of intrinsic control (Figs. 6–155 and 6–156). The magnitude of phalangeal resection appears to play a role in the level of satisfaction. Although excision of half of the phalanx has been recommended,[27,55,182] limited phalangeal resection is associated with higher rates of postoperative satisfaction.[358] Henry et al[154] reported an association between greater phalangeal resection and increased weight bearing beneath the lateral metatarsals, as well as an increased incidence of lateral metatarsalgia. On analyzing the length of the remaining phalanx, they noted that weight bearing on the hallux was present in 73% of feet from which a third or less of the proximal phalanx had been resected, whereas it was present in only 9% when more than a third of the phalanx was resected. In patients with more severe deformities, there is a tendency to resect a greater amount of the proximal phalanx to realign the hallux. Vallier et al[358] observed that excessive resection tended to leave a short, flail, functionless great toe (Figs. 6–157 and 6–158). Donley et al[96] reported that patients lost two thirds of plantar flexion and 40% lost plantar flexion power. Range of motion is often diminished after the Keller pro-

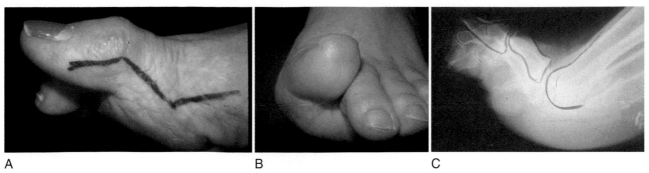

A   B   C

Figure 6–153 Cock-up deformity after the Keller arthroplasty. **A** and **B,** Clinical photos. **C,** Radiographic appearance.

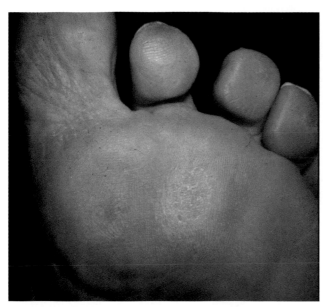

Figure 6–154 Intractable plantar keratosis beneath the second metatarsophalangeal joint after the Keller procedure.

cedure. Postoperative metatarsalgia has been reported in most series*; other reported complications include impaired control and function of the hallux,[79,154] diminished flexor strength,[79,226,324,357,358] marked shortening of the digit,[79,154] interphalangeal joint stiffness,[79,154] and cock-up deformity of the great toe.† Due to the high incidence of incomplete correction and the associated postoperative lateral metatarsalgia, excisional arthroplasty is recommended only for elderly sedentary patients with osteoarthritis of the first MTP joint in the absence of metatarsalgia preoperatively.[226] As Henry et al[154] concluded, "any operation for hallux valgus should attempt to restore (or at least not destroy) the ability of the big toe to bear weight." Salvage of a failed Keller arthroplasty can be a difficult procedure and may require an interposition bone graft[79] (Figs. 6–159 and 6–160).

*References 55, 154, 220, 294, 299, 324, and 358.
†References 79, 220, 226, 299, 324, and 357.

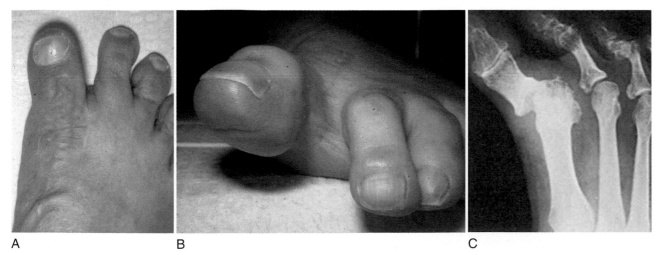

A   B   C

Figure 6–155 Varus deformity after the Keller procedure. **A** and **B,** Clinical photos. **C,** Radiographic appearance.

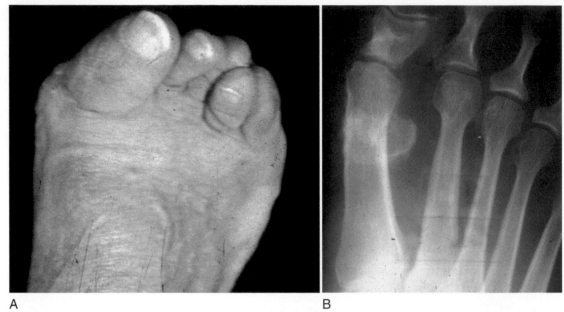

A   B

Figure 6–156   Valgus deformity after the Keller procedure: clinical (**A**) and radiographic (**B**) appearance. (**A** courtesy of E. Greer Richardson, MD.)

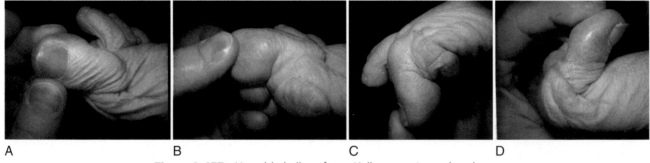

A   B   C   D

Figure 6–157   Unstable hallux after a Keller resection arthroplasty.

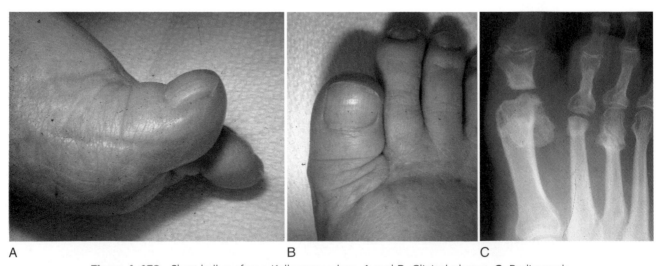

A   B   C

Figure 6–158   Short hallux after a Keller procedure. **A** and **B**, Clinical photos. **C**, Radiograph.

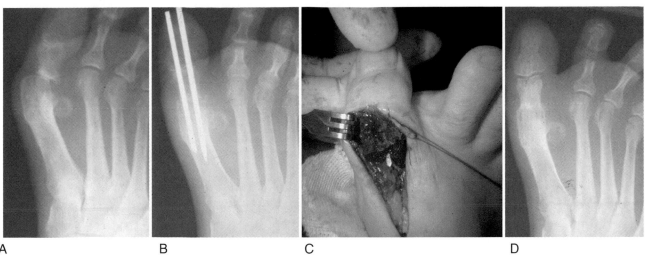

A   B   C   D

Figure 6–159 Failed Keller procedure—shortened and arthritic hallux. **A,** Clinical appearance. **B,** After arthrodesis with intramedullary Steinmann pins. **C,** Intraoperative photo. **D,** After successful fusion.

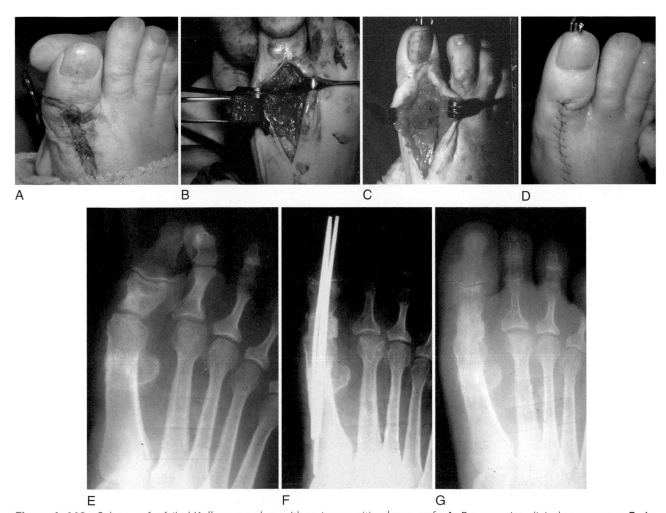

A   B   C   D

E   F   G

Figure 6–160 Salvage of a failed Keller procedure with an interposition bone graft. **A,** Preoperative clinical appearance. **B,** An iliac crest graft is harvested and inserted as an interposition graft. **C,** Graft placed between prepared surfaces. **D,** Placement of Steinmann pin fixation. **E,** Preoperative and, **F,** postoperative radiographs. **G,** After removal of internal fixation.

METATARSOCUNEIFORM ARTHRODESIS AND DISTAL SOFT TISSUE PROCEDURE

Arthrodesis of the first MTC joint in conjunction with a distal soft tissue procedure for correction of hallux valgus was popularized by Lapidus, although it was conceived by Albrecht,[2] Kleinberg,[198] and Truslow.[354] The procedure is predicated on the principle that metatarsus primus varus must be corrected to obtain satisfactory correction of the hallux valgus deformity. Initially, Lapidus[207] specified that a suitable patient preferably should be "young and robust," with an intermetatarsal angle of 15 degrees or greater and a "fixed" deformity of the MTC joint. In time, Lapidus[207] narrowed his indications substantially for the use of MTC joint fusion. If there was "adequate mobility of the first metatarsocuneiform joint to allow approximation of the first and second metatarsal heads," Lapidus indicated that a simple bunionectomy was sufficient treatment rather than MTC joint arthrodesis. Although Lapidus did not specifically use the procedure for the so-called hypermobile first ray, currently this appears to be one of the main indications.*

Indications

The major indication for this procedure is a moderate or severe hallux valgus deformity[140,307] (a hallux valgus angle of at least 30 degrees and a 1-2 intermetatarsal angle of at least 16 degrees). Other indications include juvenile hallux valgus,[21,54,117,129,271] recurrent hallux valgus,[271,307] severe deformity,[21,33,271,307] degenerative arthritis of the first MTC joint,[21,271] and a hallux valgus deformity in the presence of generalized ligamentous laxity.[21,271] Hypermobility of the first ray associated with a hallux valgus deformity is probably the most frequently listed condition for which the Lapidus procedure is indicated,† yet none of these reports give any objective data on the preoperative or postoperative quantification of first ray hypermobility. There remains continued difficulty in identifying patients who have substantial first ray instability.[132,133] We believe that this procedure is useful in about 5% of patients with an advanced hallux

---

*References 21, 54, 140, 141, 174, 218, 248, 271-273, 298, and 307.
†References 21, 33, 54, 140, 141, 174, 218, 271-273, and 298.

valgus deformity. The procedure is also used as a salvage procedure after failed repair of a previous hallux valgus deformity.[21,271,307]

Contraindications

The main contraindications are a short first metatarsal,[271] juvenile hallux valgus with an open epiphysis,[65] a moderate hallux valgus deformity without excessive first ray hypermobility,[65] and the presence of degenerative arthritis of the MTP joint.[224] There is probably a relative contraindication to using this procedure in a young person who is active in sports because of the stiffness that follows loss of first MTC joint function.

Technique

The surgical technique consists of a distal soft tissue procedure with lateral release of the first web space, excision of the medial eminence, and preparation of the medial joint capsule. Then the first MTC joint arthrodesis is performed, after which the first MTP joint is reconstructed.

Distal Soft Tissue Procedure

The distal soft tissue procedure is carried out in the same manner as discussed previously.

Metatarsocuneiform Joint Arthrodesis

1. The MTC joint is approached through a 5-cm dorsomedial, slightly curved incision centered over the first MTC joint.[58] The joint capsule is opened dorsally and medially to expose the joint (Figs. 6–161 and 6–162A).
2. With a small curet, ring curet, or osteotome, the articular cartilage is removed in its entirety from the MTC joint (Fig. 6–162B-D). This is a sinusoidal-shaped articular surface 30 mm in height, and it is important to remove the cartilage completely from the joint's plantar lateral aspect (Fig. 6–163). The inferior lateral portion of the medial cuneiform, as well as the lateral base of the first metatarsal, is resected with an osteotomy.[21] This allows correction of both excess valgus and mild plantar flexion. The adjoining lateral surfaces of the proximal first metatarsal and medial second metatarsal are denuded as well.[58] If a facet is present on the proximal lateral aspect of the base of the first metatarsal, it is also resected.

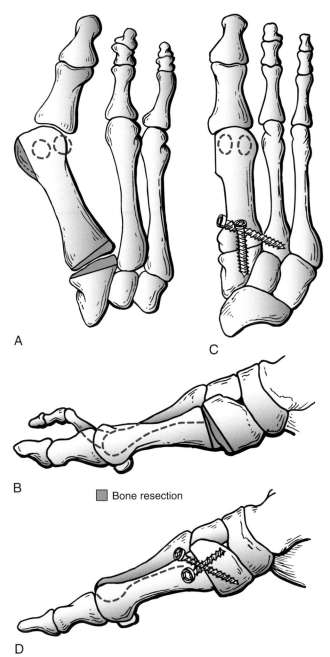

A

B

■ Bone resection

C

D

Figure 6–161 Technique of Lapidus (metatarsocuneiform [MTC]) fusion. **A,** Biplanar wedge resection of the MTC joint, anteroposterior (AP) plane. **B,** The lateral view demonstrates more plantar bone resection to plantar flex the first metatarsal. **C,** The AP view and, **D,** the lateral view after placement of internal fixation demonstrate plantar flexion of the osteotomy site. (A third screw can be placed from the first cuneiform through the first metatarsal in a proximal distal direction.)

3. The joint is gently manipulated from a dorsomedial to a plantar lateral position while bringing the first metatarsal head into a plantar lateral position (Fig. 6–162E-G). Moving the joint in this manner respects the joint's biomechanical axis. Placing the metatarsal head in a plantar lateral position corrects the intermetatarsal angle so that often little if any bone needs to be resected from the joint to achieve this alignment. Although some have advocated the use of an iliac crest bone block to realign the joint, we believe that this is rarely necessary and technically makes the procedure much more complex. On the other hand, placement of local bone graft obtained from the medial eminence into the interval between the first and second metatarsals may be advantageous.[21,58] Likewise, cutting a small dorsal slot and filling it with local bone graft is thought by some to aid the fusion process as well.[21,140,141]

4. Sutures are placed into the first web space to secure the adductor tendon into the lateral side of the first metatarsal.

5. The first MTC joint is "feathered" with a 4-mm osteotome to increase the bony surfaces. Alternatively, multiple small holes are drilled to perforate the subchondral plate on both adjoining surfaces. The first metatarsal is then reduced so that it is parallel with the second metatarsal to close the intermetatarsal angle. As this is done, the first metatarsal can be over-reduced into excess plantar direction or under-reduced and excessive dorsiflexion left. This is a key maneuver, and the surgeon must continuously assess the relationship of the first to the second metatarsal when displacing the first MTC joint. When proper alignment appears to be achieved, a guide pin is placed across the MTC joint, after which a 4.0-mm cannulated self-tapping screw is inserted from the first cuneiform into the first metatarsal and a second screw is placed from the first metatarsal into the cuneiform. Usually, two or three screws are used to gain rigid interfragmentary compression (Fig. 6–164). Fixation can also be achieved by placing a small plate along the joint's dorsomedial aspect that has been molded to hold the metatarsal in its corrected position. A derotational lag screw can be placed between the first and second

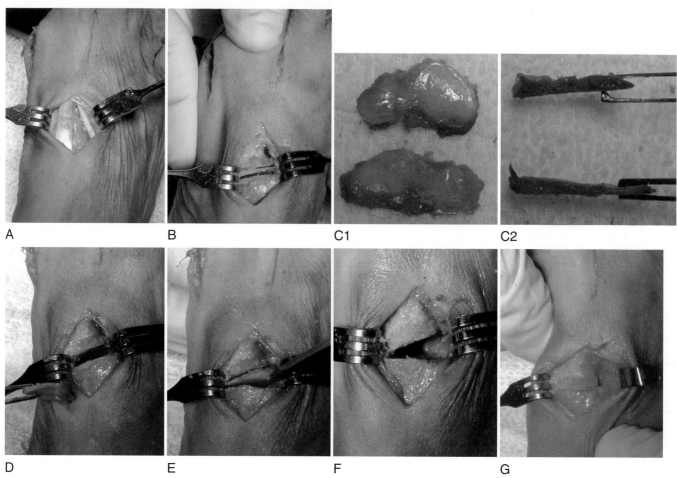

A   B   C1   C2

D   E   F   G

Figure 6–162   Technique for the Lapidus procedure. **A,** Operative incision. **B,** Resection of the articular surfaces. **C1, C2,** and **D,** Minimal resection of the articular surfaces. **E,** More extensive resection to reduce the intermetatarsal angle. **F,** After removal of the triangular resected segment. **G,** Closure of the arthrodesis site. (Courtesy of Chris DiGiovanni, MD.)

metatarsals.[21] If used, it is typically removed 12 weeks after surgery (Fig. 6–165).

Reconstruction of the Metatarsophalangeal Joint

1. The capsular tissues on the medial side of the MTP joint are plicated to place the hallux in satisfactory alignment. Any pronation is corrected when the sutures are placed along the joint's medial aspect.
2. The wounds are closed with interrupted sutures, and a compression dressing is applied.

Postoperative Care

In the office 1 to 2 days after surgery, the compression dressing is removed and another gauze-and-tape dressing applied, similar to that described for the distal soft tissue procedure. The patient is kept non–weight bearing on the affected extremity. This type of dressing is changed weekly for 8 weeks. The extremity is initially placed in a below-knee cast. One to 3 weeks after surgery the sutures are removed, a radiograph is obtained, and based on alignment of the hallux, a determination is made about how to align the MTP joint with the postoperative dressings. Weight bearing is allowed 4 weeks after surgery. After 8 weeks, if adequate fusion has occurred at the MTC joint, the patient is permitted to progress to ambulation in a sandal or shoe as tolerated. If the arthrodesis is not complete, the dressings are removed from the foot so that the patient can start range-of-motion exercises for the hallux. The patient is maintained in a short-leg removable cast until the fusion is complete.

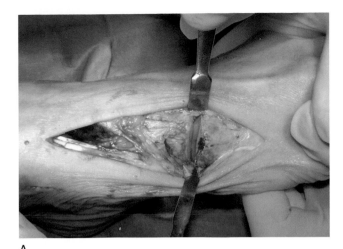

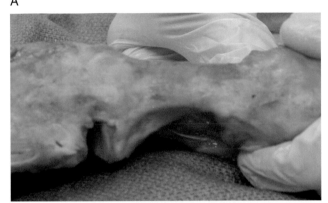

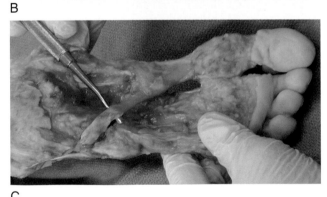

Figure 6–163 Exposure of the metatarsocuneiform joint. **A,** Wide exposure is necessary to prevent dorsiflexion malunion. **B,** Anatomic dissection demonstrates the depth of the joint. **C,** Care must be taken to avoid injury to the peroneus longus tendon on the plantar surface of the joint. (**A** courtesy of Chris Coetzee, MD.)

Results

Patient satisfaction rates vary from 74% to 92%.* Many of the reports on the Lapidus procedure are marked by no or little follow-up[129,224,318,354]; short-term follow-up of less than 1 year[54,198,208]; insufficient data on the demographics, method, or criteria of assessment or radiographic information[198,206-208,271]; inclusion of patients with varying preoperative diagnoses[21]; or use in combination with a silicon great toe implant.[10,31] The average correction of the hallux valgus angle varies from 10 to 22 degrees[21,58,248,271,272] and the 1-2 intermetatarsal angle from 6 to 9 degrees.†

---

*References 21, 41, 54, 58, 248, 257, 271, 272, and 307.
†References 21, 54, 58, 248, 257, 271, 272, and 307.

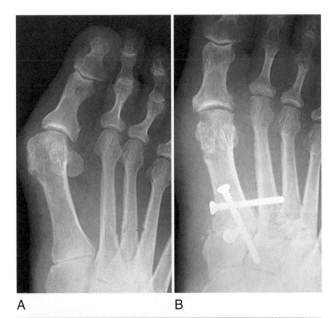

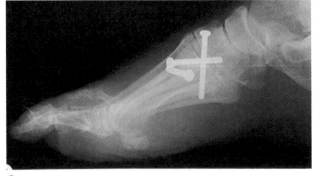

Figure 6–164 Lapidus procedure. **A,** Preoperative radiograph demonstrating a severe hallux valgus deformity. **B** and **C,** Postoperative correction has been achieved. Internal fixation is routinely removed 12-16 weeks after successful arthrodesis to avoid breakage of the intermetatarsal screw.

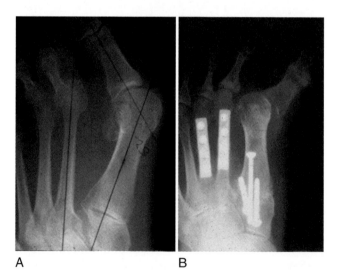

Figure 6–165 Preoperative (**A**) and postoperative (**B**) radiographs demonstrating the results of first metatarsocuneiform joint fusion with a distal soft tissue procedure.

Complications

Reported complications after the Lapidus procedure include a prolonged healing time,[307] malunion,[271,272,307] prolonged swelling,[271,307] continued pain,[307] nonunion,* stiffness,[21,208,271,272] recurrence,[21,58,208] and postoperative varus deformity[248] (Fig. 6–166). The pseudoarthrosis rate at the MTC joint varies from approximately

---

*References 58, 248, 271, 272, 275, and 307.

0% to 75%,* with symptoms in about half these patients (Fig. 6–167). The 5% to 24% pseudoarthrosis rate reported by most authors attests to the MTC being a difficult joint in which to obtain a satisfactory arthrodesis; however, Mauldin et al[248] reported a 74% incidence of nonunion.

Lombardi et al[218] noted a mean shortening of 8 mm after the procedure. Sangeorzan and Hansen[307] reported a 13% revision rate and a 20% overall failure rate. Mauldin et al[248] reported a 16% incidence of postoperative hallux varus, Myerson[271] and others[54,307] observed that the procedure was technically challenging, and Clark et al[54] noted a high rate of complications.

Most authors agree that first MTC joint arthrodesis with a distal soft tissue procedure is technically difficult and should not be used in patients with the typical bunion but rather in those with marked hypermobility of the first ray and significant medial angulation of the MTC joint or in salvage situations. Postoperative MTP range of motion was reported by McInnes and Bouche[257] to be 62 degrees. In a prospective study, Coetzee[57] observed preoperative dorsiflexion of 66 degrees and no significant diminution at almost 4 years' follow-up. Plantar flexion was not affected by the procedure. Rink-Brune[298] reported that it took longer than 3

---

*References 46, 54, 248, 257, 271, and 307.

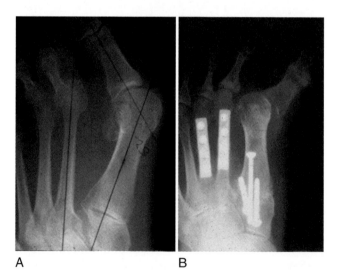

Figure 6–166 A, Severe hallux valgus deformity with metatarsalgia and instability of the metatarsocuneiform joint. **B,** After the Lapidus procedure, severe hallux varus deformity has resulted.

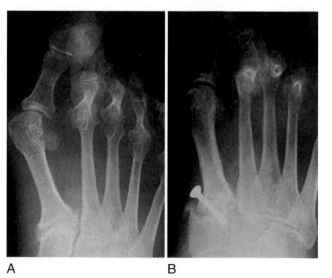

Figure 6–167 Preoperative (**A**) and postoperative (**B**) radiographs of painful nonunion after attempted metatarsocuneiform joint fusion.

months to resolve the swelling and subjective complaints in 16% of patients. McInnes and Bouche[257] reported that only 30% of athletes returned to their preoperative level of activity, whereas 75% of more sedentary patients achieved this goal. We believe that because of the stiffness that results after the procedure, it is rarely indicated in younger and more active individuals. When the procedure results in shortening because of bone resection, the metatarsal must be placed in sufficient plantar flexion to accommodate for this shortening. Myerson[271] noted, however, that 9% of the first metatarsals in his series were dorsiflexed, half of which resulted in transfer lesions beneath the second metatarsal.

With an overall failure rate reported to be as high as 28%,[307] this is not the procedure of choice for the occasional foot surgeon.

METATARSOPHALANGEAL ARTHRODESIS

Arthrodesis of the first MTP joint for treatment of hallux valgus deformity was described in 1852 by Broca[37] and subsequently by Clutton.[56] Many authors have recommended the use of first MTP joint arthrodesis as a primary procedure either to correct a severe hallux valgus deformity[76,171,291,349] or for rheumatoid arthritis (see video clip 51) (Fig. 6–168),* hallux rigidus,† or traumatic arthritis.[73,83] It can be used as a salvage procedure for failed bunion surgery or previous infection (see video clip 29).‡

First MTP joint arthrodesis is also useful in a patient with neuromuscular instability secondary to CVA, head injury, or cerebral palsy.[239,240,345,355] The rationale for the procedure is that the length of the first metatarsal is preserved and stability of the first ray is maintained, thereby allowing weight to be transferred to the hallux.

Indications

Arthrodesis is indicated in a patient with a severe hallux valgus deformity, usually with an angle greater than 50 degrees (Fig. 6–169); in a rheumatoid patient with hallux valgus; in an older patient with moderate or severe hallux valgus; in advanced cases of hallux rigidus; for primary arthritis or arthritis after trauma; and in a patient with a hallux valgus deformity after a CVA or head injury or with an underlying diag-

---

*References 20, 49, 64, 71, 73, 154, 240, 243, 244, 269, 345, 355, 356, 365, and 374.
†References 84, 109, 120, 245, 258, 305, 332, 333, 345, 355, 356, 365, 378, and 384.
‡References 79, 120, 245, 305, 355, and 365.

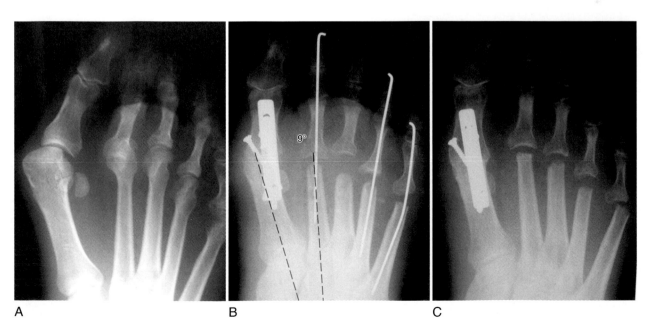

A   B   C

Figure 6–168 Rheumatoid arthritis with hallux valgus. **A,** Preoperative radiograph. **B,** Postoperative radiograph. **C,** Follow-up at 1 year. Note the diminution of the intermetatarsal angle as well.

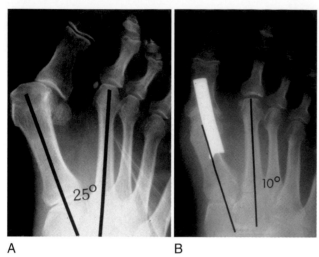

A   B

Figure 6–169 Severe hallux valgus. **A,** Preoperative radiograph with a widened intermetatarsal (IM) angle as well. **B,** After metatarsophalangeal arthrodesis, correction of both hallux valgus and the IM angle.

nosis of cerebral palsy. As a salvage procedure it is indicated for recurrent hallux valgus deformity, for a failed implant, and after unsuccessful cheilectomy.

Contraindications

Few contraindications to arthrodesis of the first MTP joint exist. Relative contraindications include arthrosis of the interphalangeal joint or an insensate foot. Another relative contraindication is lack of motion at the MTP joint, which in some cases is annoying to patients. A thorough discussion about the tradeoff between reduced MTP motion and realignment of the first ray is important preoperatively.

Technique

The surgical technique is divided into the surgical approach, preparation of the joint surfaces, and fixation of the arthrodesis.

Surgical Approach

1. The MTP joint is approached through a dorsal longitudinal incision just medial to the extensor hallucis longus tendon. The 5-cm incision extends from a point just proximal to the interphalangeal joint to above the MTP joint (Fig. 6–170A).
2. The incision is deepened through the extensor retinaculum, which is reflected along with the joint capsule. In this way the dorsomedial

cutaneous nerve is protected. The extensor tendon is usually retracted laterally. A complete synovectomy of the MTP joint is performed, after which the medial and lateral collateral ligaments are transected.

Preparation of Curved Concentric Surfaces

Curved concentric surfaces permit easy positioning and adjustment of the MTP joint surfaces for the arthrodesis. This process is less involved technically than cutting two flat surfaces. The following technique for preparation of congruous curved surfaces uses cup-shaped power reamers.[64,82,84]

1. After soft tissue release medially and laterally has been performed to expose the metatarsal and phalangeal articular surfaces, the medial eminence is removed with a small sagittal saw. A small wafer of bone can be resected from the base of the proximal phalanx and metatarsal head to decompress the joint or shorten the first ray if shortening is desired. If the procedure is being carried out in a rheumatoid patient and significant shortening is necessary, more of the metatarsal head can be removed at this time. If length is to be preserved, only the articular surface should be removed. On the other hand, preparation of the joint surfaces can be accomplished without initial bone excision, and one can proceed directly to the reaming process.
2. A 0.062-inch Kirschner wire is driven into the center of the first metatarsal head. The size of the metatarsal metaphysis is estimated and a corresponding reamer* of the appropriate size is chosen (Fig. 6–170B and C). (Reamers vary from 14 to 20 mm in size, although 14 to 16 mm is the most common diameter used.) A cannulated metatarsal head reamer is used to reduce the metatarsal head and metaphysis and to shape the articular surface area into a convex cup-shaped surface, after which the wire is removed.
3. The Kirschner wire is then driven into the base of the proximal phalanx. A convex male reamer is used to create a concave, cup-shaped surface. Typically, the smallest reamer is initially used. Reaming is continued with progressively larger reamers until the surface

---

*NewDeal, Inc., Lyon, France.

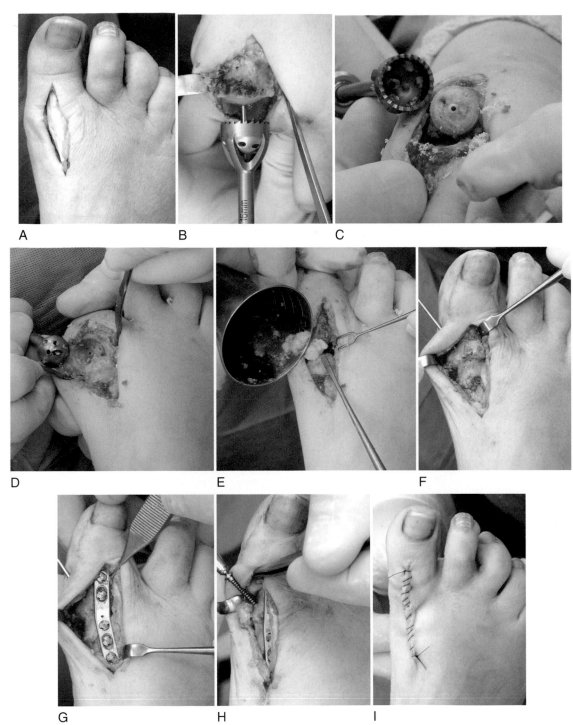

Figure 6–170 Technique of metatarsophalangeal arthrodesis. **A,** Longitudinal dorsal incision. **B,** A cannulated concave metatarsal head reamer (**C**) is used to prepare the metatarsal surface. **D,** Power-driven convex phalangeal reamers are used to prepare the phalanx. **E,** Bone slurry from the reamers is placed in the joint. **F,** Temporary fixation of the arthrodesis site with a Kirschner wire. **G,** Dorsal titanium plate fixation. **H,** Cross screw placement. **I,** Final appearance of the foot.

size matches the prepared metatarsal surface (Fig. 6–170D). The Kirschner wire is then removed.

4. The two curved congruent surfaces are rotated into proper alignment, which is 15 degrees of valgus and 15 to 20 degrees of dorsiflexion in relation to the first metatarsal shaft (Fig. 6–170E). The hallux is derotated so that there is no pronation. A 0.062-inch Kirschner wire is driven across the proposed arthrodesis site through a plantar medial stab wound and exits dorsolaterally (Fig. 6–170F).

Alternative Method of Joint Preparation

There are ways to create surfaces for the arthrodesis other than the curved surfaces just described.

1. The distal portion of the first metatarsal is cut with an oscillating saw, and only the articular surface is removed to create a flat surface that is angulated slightly dorsally and laterally. If the procedure is being carried out in a rheumatoid patient and significant shortening is necessary, more of the metatarsal head can be removed at this time, but if length is to be preserved, only the articular surface should be removed (Fig. 6–171A).

2. Longitudinal traction is placed on the hallux, and all the tissues inserting into the base of the proximal phalanx are released by sharp dissection.

3. The hallux is positioned with one hand holding it in approximately 15 degrees of valgus and 10 to 15 degrees of dorsiflexion in relation to the plantar aspect of the foot. The surgeon then carefully notes the relationship between the base of the proximal phalanx and the initial cut made in the metatarsal head. With the initial cut as a guide, another cut is made parallel to it to resect the entire articular surface and subchondral bone while leaving, if possible, the metaphyseal flare of the proximal phalanx intact (Fig. 6–171B).

4. The two parallel cuts are placed together, and their alignment is carefully observed. If the position is not correct, another cut is made, this time in the metatarsal head to adjust the alignment. If the procedure is being done in conjunction with a rheumatoid foot repair, no further shortening of the MTP joint should be undertaken until the metatarsal heads are resected and the final length of the first metatarsal can be determined.

5. The hallux is derotated so that there is no pronation. A 0.062-inch Kirschner wire is driven across the proposed arthrodesis site through a plantar medial stab wound and exits dorsolaterally.

Internal Fixation of the Arthrodesis

1. The prepared surfaces are apposed and the alignment carefully checked. Occasionally, if the lesser toes tend to deviate slightly medi-

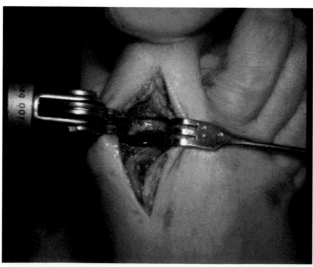 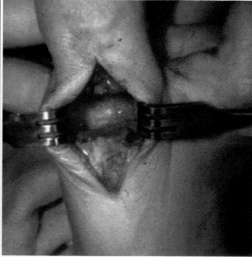

A   B

Figure 6–171   **A,** Phalangeal osteotomy to create flat surfaces. **B,** The joint is distracted before arthrodesis.

ally, the arthrodesis site is aligned in slightly more valgus. As a general rule, the desired alignment is 15 degrees of valgus, 15 to 20 degrees of dorsiflexion, and neutral rotation. With the curved congruous surfaces, these dimensions can be easily altered by merely changing the position of the hallux. With flat surfaces, further resection of the prepared surfaces is necessary to achieve the desired alignment. A 0.062-inch Kirschner wire is inserted as temporary fixation to hold the prepared surfaces (Fig. 6–170F). A second cross Kirschner wire can be placed if further stabilization is necessary before placement of internal fixation.

2. A dorsal six-hole titanium plate is then placed on the dorsal aspect of the distal first metatarsal and proximal phalanx (Fig. 6–170G). This preformed plate has 15 degrees of valgus and 20 degrees of dorsiflexion built into it to help align the first ray in the appropriate position. It is stabilized with six dorsal plantar bicortical screws. The Kirschner wire is removed and a cross screw placed to further fix the arthrodesis site (Fig. 6–170H and I).

3. Alternatively, an interfragmentary 4.0-mm cannulated screw can be inserted across the proposed arthrodesis site in a medial to lateral direction. The guide pin is placed slightly below the midline of the proximal phalanx and angled in a proximal to lateral direction. The cortex on the medial side of the phalanx is drilled and the hole countersunk. A 24- to 30-mm-long screw is inserted. As the screw is cinched down, the Kirschner wire, which is at a right angle to the screw, is removed to permit as much interfragmentary compression as possible.

4. Any remaining prominent bone or remnants of the medial eminence are resected with a rongeur.

5. The wound is closed in two layers with the capsule closed beneath the extensor tendon. The skin is closed with fine interrupted sutures, and a compression dressing is applied. The patient is permitted to ambulate in a postoperative shoe with weight bearing as tolerated.

Alternative Method of Fixation

Fixation of the arthrodesis site can be carried out in a variety of ways. Our philosophy is to obtain fixation that is as rigid as possible so that the patient can ambulate without a cast while achieving a satisfactory rate of fusion. At times, inadequate bone stock is present in the proximal phalanx when attempting to salvage a Keller procedure[79] or after removal of a prosthesis. Occasionally, in a rheumatoid patient with severe osteopenia, the plate-and-screw technique cannot be used. In these circumstances we prefer to use threaded Steinmann pins to gain fixation of the arthrodesis site (video clip 30).[63] These pins have the disadvantage of crossing the interphalangeal joint, although in two large series, this did not create a significant clinical problem.[240,244] The surgical technique follows.

1. The joint surfaces are prepared in the same manner as initially described or through the creation of congruous curved surfaces (Fig. 6–172; see also Fig. 6–171).

2. A 1/8-inch, double-pointed Steinmann pin is drilled in a proximal to distal direction out the tip of the hallux (Fig. 6–173A).

3. A second pin is drilled out parallel to the first one.

4. One of the pins protruding through the end of the proximal phalanx is cut about in half so that the chuck can be placed

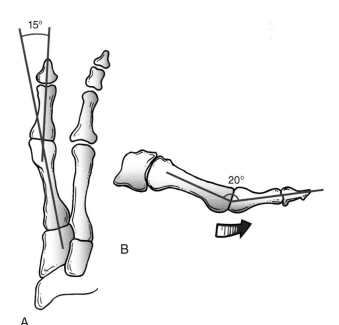

Figure 6–172 The fusion site is placed in 15 to 20 degrees of valgus (**A**) and about 20 degrees of dorsiflexion (**B**) in relation to the metatarsal shaft, which is approximately 10 to 15 degrees of dorsiflexion in relation to the floor.

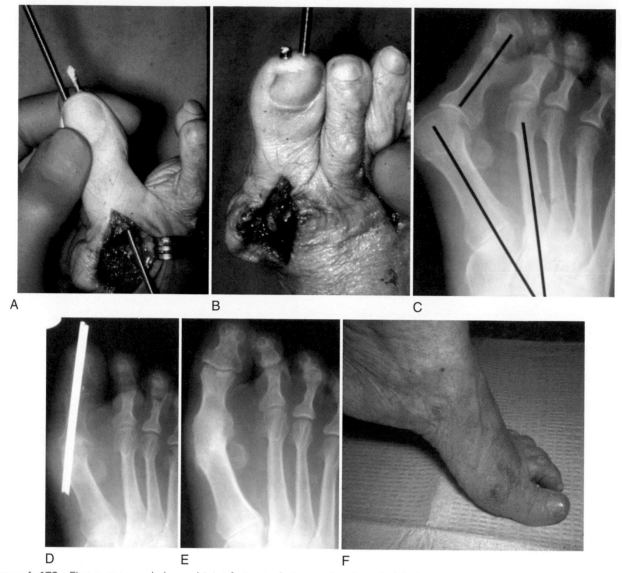

A   B   C

D   E   F

Figure 6–173 First metatarsophalangeal joint fusion technique using threaded Steinmann pins. **A,** A Steinmann pin is driven out through the tip of the great toe in retrograde manner. **B,** Pins are brought back across the attempted fusion site while manually compressing the bony surfaces together. **C,** Preoperative radiograph. **D,** After intramedullary Steinmann pin fixation. **E,** Fifteen years after surgery, a successful arthrodesis is observed. **F,** Fifteen years after surgery, the patient is able to walk on tiptoe.

onto the distal end of the longest Steinmann pin.

5. The MTP joint is reduced in proper alignment (varus/valgus, dorsiflexion/plantar flexion, rotation), and with the other hand holding the handle of the drill, the Steinmann pin is slowly drilled across the arthrodesis site into the metatarsal. It should be drilled in until the surgeon feels it penetrating the cortex of the proximal first metatarsal or until it reaches the proximity of the MTC joint. The first pin is then cut off approximately 5 mm from the tip of the skin; the second pin is drilled across the arthrodesis site in a similar manner (Fig. 6–173B).

6. The wound is closed with interrupted sutures and a compression dressing applied. The patient is permitted to ambulate as tolerated.

7. Postoperative care is the same as for other forms of arthrodesis (Fig. 6–173C-F).

On rare occasion, because of loss of significant bone stock, it becomes necessary to add an interposition bone graft to gain more length at the first MTP joint arthrodesis site. As a general rule, a slightly shorter great toe does not create a significant problem, but if circumstances indicate that a bone graft is needed, it can be placed between the proximal phalanx and the metatarsal head as a flat piece of tricortical iliac crest or an oval "football-type" graft (Fig. 6–174). Whenever a bone graft is added, the morbidity of the procedure increases substantially and the healing time is usually doubled 5 to 6 months. These patients should usually be kept non–weight bearing to avoid stress on the fixation device and to promote healing of the graft.

Postoperative Care

In the office 1 or 2 days after surgery, the compression dressing is removed and a firm 2-inch Kling gauze dressing with 1/2-inch adhesive tape is applied. The patient is permitted to ambulate in a postoperative shoe as tolerated with weight borne on the heel and lateral aspect of the foot.

The patient is evaluated with radiographs every 4 weeks until successful fusion occurs. At this time the postoperative shoe is discontinued. As a general rule, 10 to 12 weeks is required for complete fusion. If longitudinal Steinmann pins have been placed, they are easily removed under a digital block in an office setting.

Results

The reported rate of patient satisfaction after MTP arthrodesis varies from 78% to 93%.* In the only four studies reporting on the treatment of idiopathic hallux valgus by MTP arthrodesis,[76,165,291,349] subjective satisfaction was noted in more than 90% of patients (Fig. 6–175).

The rate of fusion varies, depending on the operative technique, the method of internal fixation, and the preoperative diagnosis. MTP joint fusion generally occurs in most patients between 10 and 12 weeks. Reported success rates vary from 77% to 100%, with an average rate of 90%.† Coughlin[63] reported a 10% failure

rate in a review of 1451 cases in the literature. In the largest series, Riggs and Johnson[297] reported a 91% fusion rate in 309 procedures. With the use of a dorsal compression plate, they reported a success rate ranging from 92% to 100%.[64,73,230,365] Coughlin and Abdo[73] reported subjective good and excellent results in 93% of cases. Inadequate fixation is the more commonly cited reason for nonunion,[119,291,297,356] but true failure of fixation is uncommon.[297] As McKeever[258] noted, an unsuccessful arthrodesis or pseudoarthrosis may still give a painless and successful result (Fig. 6–176).

The final alignment of the fusion is very important for patient satisfaction. The recommended angle of valgus ranges from 5 to 30 degrees with an average of 15 degrees.[79,109,244,291,297] Fitzgerald[109] warned that fusion in less than 20 degrees of valgus is associated with a threefold incidence of interphalangeal joint arthritis. The literature reports a 6% to 15% rate of degenerative arthritis of the interphalangeal joint after arthrodesis of the MTP joint[154,269,297] (Fig. 6–177). Coughlin, Grebing, and Jones[76] reported at an average 8-year follow-up and noted little progression of interphalangeal joint arthritis and negligible interphalangeal joint pain. Mann and Oates,[240] using Steinmann pins that crossed the interphalangeal joint for internal fixation, reported a 40% incidence of degenerative changes at the interphalangeal joint. Few of these patients had any clinical symptoms at final follow-up.

After arthrodesis, the increased 1-2 intermetatarsal angle associated with a severe hallux valgus deformity is routinely reduced,* and rarely if ever is a first metatarsal osteotomy necessary.[148,165,239] We do not believe that any attempt should be made to correct the intermetatarsal angle when carrying out an arthrodesis. If for some reason the intermetatarsal angle is unacceptable, it can be corrected with a basal osteotomy at another time rather than creating a situation in which besides attempting to obtain an arthrodesis at the MTP joint, one is simultaneously attempting to heal an osteotomy at the metatarsal's base.

In the sagittal plane, the recommended angle of dorsiflexion for the fusion varies from 10 to 40 degrees† (in relation to the shaft of the

---

*References 24, 79, 109, 119, 148, 165, 171, 230, 240, 244, 258, 291, 297, 355, 374, 378, and 379.
†References 24, 79, 109, 119, 148, 165, 171, 240, 244, 258, 291, 297, 355, 374, and 378.

*References 76, 165, 217, 239, 258, 269, 291, and 297.
†References 73, 79, 171, 240, 244, 266, 345, and 356.

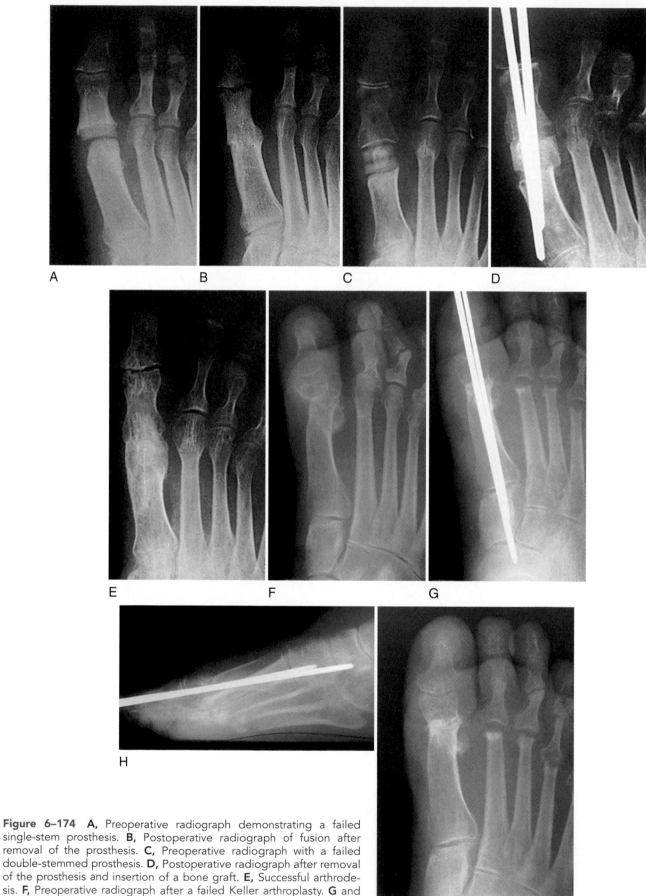

Figure 6–174 A, Preoperative radiograph demonstrating a failed single-stem prosthesis. **B,** Postoperative radiograph of fusion after removal of the prosthesis. **C,** Preoperative radiograph with a failed double-stemmed prosthesis. **D,** Postoperative radiograph after removal of the prosthesis and insertion of a bone graft. **E,** Successful arthrodesis. **F,** Preoperative radiograph after a failed Keller arthroplasty. **G** and **H,** After arthrodesis with the Steinmann pin technique. **I,** After removal of the pins.

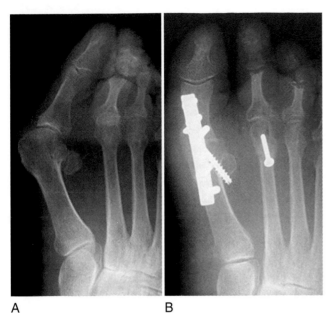

A   **B**

Figure 6–175   Correction of the intermetatarsal angle after first metatarsophalangeal joint arthrodesis. **A,** Preoperative radiograph. **B,** Postoperative radiograph demonstrating correction of the intermetatarsal angle from 18 to 10 degrees.

first metatarsal), with 20 to 25 degrees being the most commonly recommended position.[63] Coughlin[71] reported that there was a marked increase in interphalangeal joint arthritis when the dorsiflexion angle of fusion was less than 20 degrees. Fusion in excessive dorsiflexion leads to pressure beneath the sesamoids, whereas fusion in excess plantar flexion leads to pressure beneath the tip of the great toe.

Use of a dorsal mini-fragment or titanium compression plate is relatively easy and has been associated with reasonably high success rates of fusion. Whereas the larger and bulky small-fragment compression plates have frequently required removal,[64,230,365] the low-profile Vitallium plates[73] and titanium plates[82,84] have not required removal. Other reports on the use of compression screws for fixation have demonstrated their reliability as well and a high level of patient satisfaction.[171] The main advantage of rigid internal fixation is that it permits immediate ambulation with a postoperative shoe, thereby eliminating the need for a walking cast. In an older patient, particularly a rheumatoid patient, the ability to walk postoperatively without a cast is extremely important (Fig. 6–178).

The surgical technique used for MTP arthrodesis should be simple and achieve a predictable result (Fig. 6–179). Shaping of the curved congruous joint surfaces to enable the surgeon to easily adjust the metatarsal and phalanx to the desired position of valgus, extension, and rotation is a key part of this procedure. The use of rigid internal fixation is important in obtaining and maintaining the desired fusion until osseous fusion has occurred. As McKeever[258] said, however, "it is the [fusion] and its position that is important and not the method by which it is obtained."

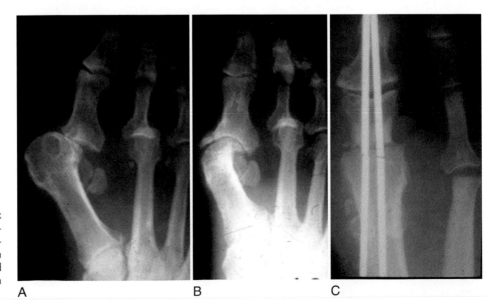

Figure 6–176   A, Severe hallux valgus associated with rheumatoid arthritis. **B,** Painful nonunion with a decrease in angular deformity in a satisfied patient. **C,** Broken Steinmann pins portend a nonunion.

A   **B**   **C**

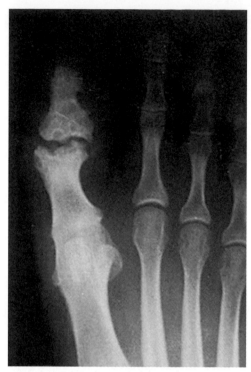

Figure 6–177 Degenerative arthritis of the interphalangeal joint is rarely symptomatic.

Complications

The main complications after MTP joint arthrodesis are nonunion, malalignment, and degenerative arthrosis of the interphalangeal joint of the great toe. With the use of an interfragmentary screw and dorsal plate, we believe that a fusion rate of 95% can probably be achieved. In some cases of hallux rigidus in which the bone ends are extremely sclerotic, the surgeon may anticipate difficulty in obtaining fusion, and possibly weight bearing should be delayed in these patients. In some cases we have found it necessary to make multiple drill holes through the sclerotic bone in an attempt to improve blood flow across the attempted arthrodesis site.

Nonunion, when it occurs, is often not painful.[258] If the patient has pain, repair is necessary, either by bone grafting if the fixation is adequate or by removal of the fixation device, bone grafting, and the application of new fixation if indicated.

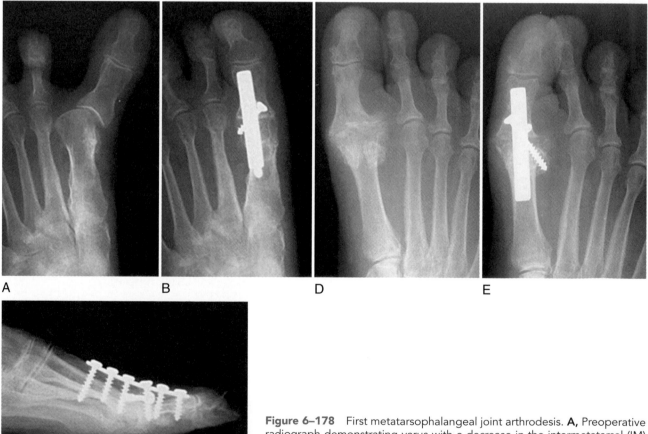

A   B   D   E

C

Figure 6–178 First metatarsophalangeal joint arthrodesis. **A,** Preoperative radiograph demonstrating varus with a decrease in the intermetatarsal (IM) angle. **B** and **C,** After arthrodesis the IM angle is actually increased to a normal value. **D,** Preoperative and, **E,** postoperative radiographs demonstrate fusion with advanced arthrosis.

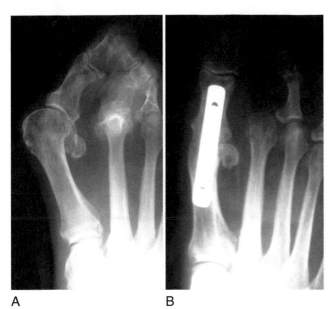

A   B

Figure 6–179 A, Preoperative radiograph demonstrating severe hallux valgus and a dislocated second metatarsophalangeal joint. **B,** Second toe amputation is possible with a fused hallux because there is no progression of deformity.

Malunion in any plane is poorly tolerated by patients. This emphasizes the importance of close attention to the final position of the arthrodesis. As Coughlin[65] said, "no bunion procedure requires a technique that is more exacting and unforgiving than that required in arthrodesis of the first metatarsophalangeal joint."

SCARF OSTEOTOMY

Meyer[177,202] (1926) is credited with first describing the longitudinal Z-type first metatarsal osteotomy, although both Burutaran[40] and Gudas[386] are also noted for early descriptions of this technique. However, Weil[29,369] and Barouk[16-18] popularized the procedure. It was Weil who coined the name scarf.[29] *Scarf* is a carpentry term that describes a joint made by notching or cutting the ends of two pieces of wood and then securely fastening them together in one continuous piece so that they lap over each other.

Weil[369] described three different types of scarf osteotomy determined by the length of the longitudinal osteotomy: a short scarf osteotomy (25 mm long) to treat hallux valgus with an intermetatarsal angle of 13 degrees or less, also used for those with a higher DMAA[18]; a medium-

length scarf osteotomy to treat an intermetatarsal angle of 14 to 16 degrees; and a long scarf osteotomy to treat an intermetatarsal angle of 17 to 23 degrees.

Many authors have recommended the use of a midshaft osteotomy combined with a distal soft tissue procedure as a primary procedure to correct moderate or severe hallux valgus.* Several others have added an Akin osteotomy to the technique.†

The rationale for the procedure is that the shaft of the first metatarsal is lateralized, thereby reducing the intermetatarsal angle; plantar displacement is achieved to increase load on the first ray; the metatarsal can be shortened or lengthened; and a DMAA of up to 10 degrees can be addressed as well.[369]

Indications

A scarf osteotomy is indicated for the treatment of a symptomatic hallux valgus deformity of moderate or severe nature characterized by a 1-2 intermetatarsal angle of 14 to 20 degrees,[16,94,202,331] a normal or slightly increased DMAA,[94] and adequate bone stock.

Contraindications

Although there is apparently no age limit to the procedure, osteopenia in an elderly patient may be a relative contraindication. Good bone density is important for stability of the osteotomy.[369] A scarf osteotomy is contraindicated for mild hallux valgus, for which a simpler, less complicated procedure is possible, and in the presence of joint arthrosis,[202,369] restricted MTP range of motion,[369] or an open epiphysis.[202]

Technique

The surgical technique is divided into the surgical approach, osteotomy and fixation, and postoperative care.

Surgical Approach

1. A 5- to 8-cm medial longitudinal incision is made at the junction of the dorsal and plantar skin (Fig. 6–180A). It is started from a point just proximal to the interphalangeal

---

*References 16-18, 29, 89, 92, 94, 180, 201, 202, 313, 331, 335, and 369.
†References 16, 89, 94, 180, 202, 331, and 369.

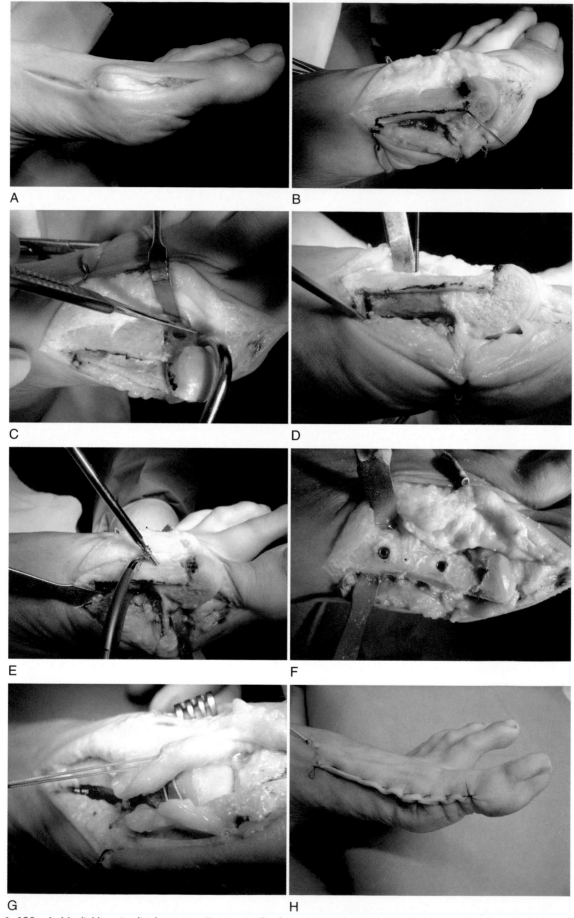

Figure 6–180 **A,** Medial longitudinal incision. **B,** Longitudinal osteotomy marked with Kirschner wires for orientation. **C,** Medial displacement and lateral release. **D,** Lateral displacement of the distal fragment. **E,** Lateral view. **F,** Dorsal view of internal fixation. **G,** Capsular closure. **H,** Skin closure.

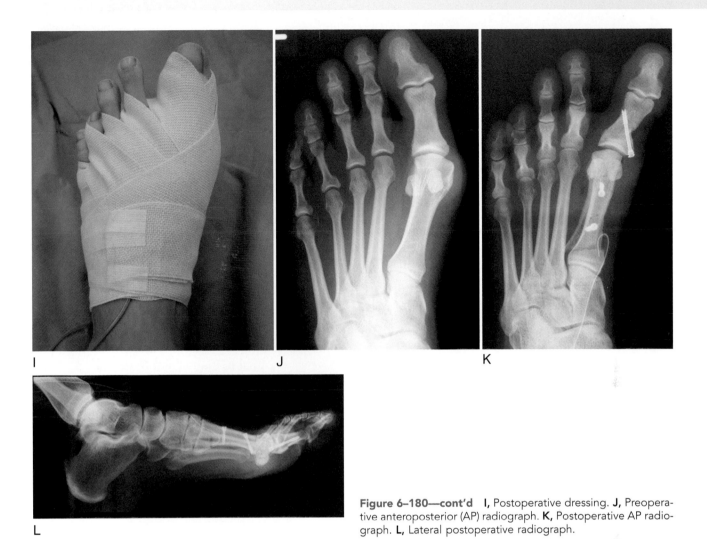

I

J

K

L

Figure 6–180—cont'd **I,** Postoperative dressing. **J,** Preoperative anteroposterior (AP) radiograph. **K,** Postoperative AP radiograph. **L,** Lateral postoperative radiograph.

joint and carried proximal to almost the MTC joint. The actual length of the proposed osteotomy determines the length of the actual skin incision.

2. A horizontal elliptical incision is used to excise redundant medial MTP joint capsule. The capsular flaps are developed with care taken to protect the dorsal and plantar sensory nerves. The small capillary network of plantar vessels just proximal to the sesamoids is protected, and release of the lateral metatarsal sesamoid ligament and lateral capsule is performed from the medial aspect. Rarely is the fibular sesamoid removed.

3. Alternatively, a separate interspace incision can be used for lateral capsular release. Care is taken to release the metatarsal sesamoid ligament and the lateral capsule as well.[196]

Preparation for the Osteotomy

1. A 0.045-inch Kirschner wire is drilled in a lateral direction into the upper third of the distal first metatarsal, 2 to 3 mm from the dorsal metatarsal surface and 5 mm from the proximal dorsal metatarsal articular surface. It is also directed 15 degrees plantar-ward and slightly proximal as well. A second guide pin is drilled at the proximal extent of the proposed osteotomy, 2 to 3 mm from the plantar surface of the first metatarsal, at a distance approximately 1 cm from the MTC joint. It is also directed slightly plantar-ward and slightly proximal (parallel to the first wire). The direction of these guidewires determines the eventual angle of the osteotomy. As the osteotomy is later displaced, it will shift laterally and plantar-ward (Fig. 6–180B).

2. A thin oscillating or sagittal saw blade is used to create a vertical dorsal cut in the dorsal distal metatarsal neck at a right angle to the shaft in line with the Kirschner wires. This osteotomy is located in the dense metaphyseal bone approximately 5 mm from the distal articular surface. It is inclined slightly proximally as the cut progresses in a medial to lateral direction (Fig. 6–180C and D).[17]

3. The saw guide is then rotated on the wire so that it is parallel with the longitudinal axis of the first metatarsal, but directed toward the inferior fourth of the proximal plantar cortex (where the second Kirschner wire is located) (Fig. 6–183).

4. A longitudinal cut is made with a 20-mm sagittal saw blade. The length of the osteotomy largely depends on the desired correction.[29,369] A longer osteotomy is used to correct larger deformities. A shorter osteotomy is used to correct smaller deformities with larger DMAAs. The typical length of the osteotomy is 30 to 35 mm, but the cut can extend almost the entire length of the metatarsal. As the osteotomy engages the lateral cortex, care is take to avoid overpenetration into the first intermetatarsal space because this may damage critical circulation to the metatarsal head and shaft. Barouk[16] suggests that the coronal level of the cut be located 2 to 3 mm from the dorsal surface distally and 2 to 3 mm from the plantar surface proximally (Fig. 6–181).

5. The third osteotomy is now performed. This cut exits the plantar aspect of the first metatarsal at a reverse 45-degree angle so that it acts as a locking mechanism as the osteotomy is translated. This cut is inclined slightly proximally as the cut progresses in a medial to lateral direction[16] so that it is parallel with the more distal cut.

6. The osteotomy is now complete and the distal fragment should be mobile. A clamp is placed on the proximal plantar fragment to both stabilize it and pull it medial-ward as the distal dorsal fragment is shifted lateral-ward. Lateral translation can be performed maximally to two thirds the width at the level of the metatarsal head. After displacement of the osteotomy, a bone clamp is placed to secure the reduction.

7. The osteotomy is internally stabilized with two screws directed from the dorsal medial aspect to the plantar lateral aspect of the diaphysis (see Fig. 6–184). Barouk[16] has advocated a self-compressing cannulated headless screw for internal fixation. Barouk suggests that an oblique distal screw should fixate the metatarsal metaphyseal-head region and a second dorsoplantar screw should stabilize the proximal osteotomy (Fig. 6–180E and F).

8. The excess bone remaining on the medial aspect of the metatarsal is then resected with a power saw. Although this entails removing a portion of the diaphysis and the medial eminence, care should be taken to preserve the plantar medial MTP joint articulation to avoid disturbing sesamoid function.

9. In more severe cases, an Akin osteotomy is added.[16,89,94,202,369]

Soft Tissue Repair

1. The medial capsule is repaired with interrupted absorbable suture to realign the hallux; however, overplication should be avoided (Fig. 6–180E). The subcutaneous tissue is also approximated along the course of the exposure, and the skin is closed in routine fashion.

2. A gauze-and-tape compression dressing is applied to protect the repair (Fig. 6–180F).

The patient is allowed to ambulate in a postoperative shoe with weight borne as tolerated on the heel and outer aspect of the foot.

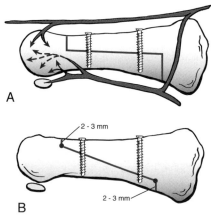

Figure 6–181 **A,** Dorsal and plantar circulation to the first metatarsal. **B,** After scarf osteotomy with internal fixation. The diagram also shows two techniques demonstrating variations in scarf osteotomy.

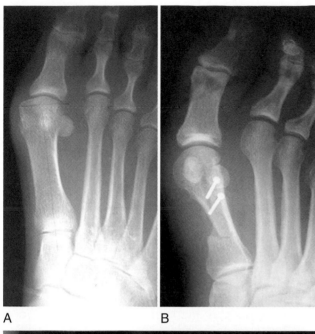

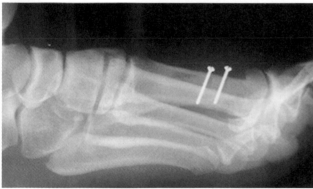

Figure 6–182 **A,** Preoperative radiograph. **B** and **C,** Postoperative radiographs after scarf osteotomy. (Courtesy of L. S. Weil, DPM.)

Key Points in the Technique

Displacement in a transverse plane: The distal fragment can be merely translated laterally in the case of a severe deformity or rotated medially with the translation to reduce an increased DMAA. When both transverse cuts are made parallel to each other, it is a pure translational displacement (Fig. 6–183).

Displacement in a frontal plane: To elevate the distal fragment in the case of a cavus foot, the longitudinal cut is made directly lateralward. To lower the head, the cut is made in a plantar direction inclined approximately 15 degrees plantar-laterally (Fig. 6–184).

Displacement in a sagittal plane: The osteotomy can be lengthened; however, lengthening may result in diminished MTP range of motion.[16] Shortening can be achieved by greater inclination of the transverse cuts, but it can also be achieved by resection of bone proximally and distally. This may have the effect of increasing range of motion of the MTP joint.

Complications

With the complexity of the scarf osteotomy come numerous possible complications, including undercorrection or recurrence,[16,58,89,202,369] overcorrection, hallux varus,[16,313,369] degenerative arthritis,[89,202] loss of fixation,[59,89,202] and delayed union.[59] Schoen et al[313] reported a 20% incidence of hallux varus in this series.

AVN has been reported after scarf osteotomy (Fig. 6–185).[313,369] Dereymaeker[94] makes the point that extensive soft tissue stripping should

Postoperative Care

The gauze-and-tape compression dressing is removed 1 week after surgery, radiographs are obtained, and the patient is instructed in postoperative range-of-motion exercises. At 1 week, Weil[369] allows patients to progress to a roomy athletic shoe as tolerated and dressings are discontinued. At 7 weeks after surgery, if radiographs demonstrate adequate healing, the patient is allowed to resume regular activities. Coetzee et al[58] suggest treatment with a below-knee cast for 2 weeks and partial weight bearing with dressings for an additional 4 weeks. Rehabilitation is then commenced (Fig. 6–180I-L).

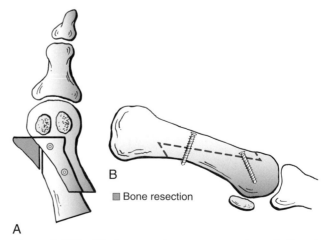

■ Bone resection

Figure 6–183 Displacement in a transverse plane. **A,** Dorsal view. **B,** Lateral view demonstrating the internal fixation.

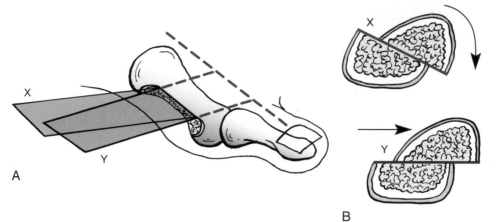

Figure 6–184 Displacement in a frontal plane. **A,** Different planes of the cut. "Y" is from a direct medial approach that does not change the elevation C of the capital fragment; "X" shifts the capital fragment downward (**B**).

be avoided with this procedure. Proximally, only the medial plantar surface is elevated; distally, the dorsal aspect of the distal metatarsal is exposed. In both areas, the vascular leash supplying the first metatarsal is protected (see Fig. 6–181).

Popoff et al[285] and Newman et al[274] found in laboratory studies that a scarf osteotomy was much stronger than other types of proximal osteotomies. Nonetheless, fractures can develop either acutely or in delayed fashion after surgery. Intraoperatively, if any of the cuts are not complete, twisting or translating the fragments may cause a fracture to develop[94,331]; Smith et al[331] also noted that fractures devel-

oped by overtightening the compression screws. A fracture places the osteotomy at high risk for elevatus and lateral metatarsalgia[16,369] or a subsequent stress fracture.[16,58,369] This usually occurs in the proximal metatarsal in the area of the transverse cut. If the remaining dorsal cortex is too thin, a stress fracture may occur. Weil[369] stressed the need to "plantarize" the transverse cut by placing it in the plantar third to fourth of the metatarsal. Pressure on the osteotomy leads to a fracture of the dorsal cortex, not the plantar cortex.[274,369] Barouk[16] reported a 3% incidence of stress fractures in his early experience.

Malunion of the osteotomy can develop as a result of shift and displacement of the diaphyseal segments. "Troughing" occurs when the cortices of the two halves of the metatarsal shaft wedge into the softer cancellous bone of the metatarsal shaft. Troughing is like roofing tiles that fit together in an overlapping fashion and occurs with lateral shift of the distal segment. It is more common in osteopenia.[94,369] Troughing causes dorsiflexion of the first ray and can lead to lesser MTP joint metatarsalgia or overload. Also with this displacement, rotation can occur, which leaves a very difficult situation to salvage.[58] To avoid this complication, the osteotomy must be kept in metaphyseal cancellous bone; the step cut should be only 2 to 3 mm into cancellous bone at the distal and proximal extent of the osteotomy (Fig. 6–186).

Weil[369] reported that diminished MTP range of motion occurs less often than in other bunion procedures, possibly due to the implementation of early exercise. Weil[369] reported average dorsiflexion of 70 degrees, but others have

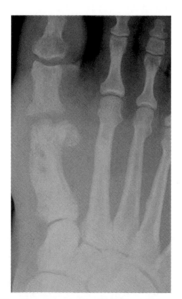

Figure 6–185 Osteonecrosis of first metatarsal head after scarf osteotomy. (Courtesy of C. Coetzee, MD.)

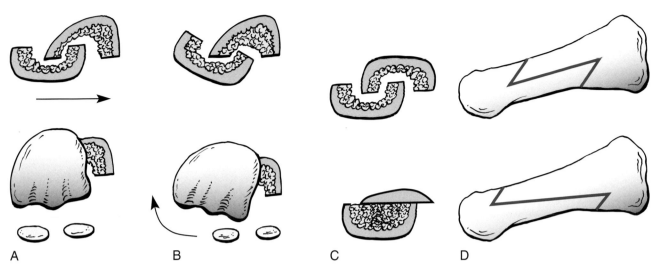

A   B   C   D

Figure 6–186 Complications of scarf osteotomy. **A,** Troughing. **B,** Troughing with malrotation. **C,** Troughing can occur as a result of making the osteotomy in the diaphyseal region. **D,** By maintaining the osteotomy in the dense bone of the metaphyses, troughing can often be avoided. (Adapted from the technique of L. S. Weil, DPM, and C. Coetze, MD.)

noted less motion.[89,313] Crevoisier et al[89] reported that 65% of patients in their series had diminished motion, which they attributed to the extensive exposure.

Results

Subjective satisfaction is reported to be routinely high and varies from 89% to 98%,[29,89,180,313,369] although Dereymaeker[94] reported that the results were slightly inferior when she compared scarf osteotomy with distal chevron osteotomy. Kundert and Fuhrmann[203] reported recurrence of the deformity in 25% of cases. Average correction of the hallux valgus angle varies from 15 to 19 degrees,[89,94,180,369] and average correction of the 1-2 intermetatarsal angle varies from 4 to 10 degrees.* Plantar displacement of the first ray varies from 1 to 3 mm.[29,94,369]

Dereymaeker[94] found that scarf osteotomy did not achieve adequate correction of the DMAA in her series. Barouk[17] suggested that this is the ideal situation for a "short scarf" (25 mm long) because it allows lateral rotation of the distal fragment to reduce the DMAA. A longer scarf osteotomy would not be able to rotate adequately into the intermetatarsal space.

_____

*References 29, 89, 92, 94, 180, 201, 369.

Day et al[92] subsequently reported using this technique and reduced the average DMAA from 20 to 4.5 degrees.

There is no question that the scarf technique is technically demanding,[29,202,364] and there is a difficult learning curve as well.[369]

MULTIPLE OSTEOTOMIES

The incidence of congruent hallux valgus deformities is unknown. Coughlin and Carlson[74] reviewed a series of 878 consecutive bunions over a 12-year period and determined that 18 patients (21 feet) qualified as having congruent deformities of such magnitude that they warranted extraarticular correction (2%). They noted that although 12 of the 18 patients underwent surgery before 20 years of age, they stressed that with deferred surgery, these deformities can occur during the adult years. Thus, congruent hallux valgus deformities, though decidedly uncommon (Fig. 6–187), may be seen and treated at any age. A soft tissue intraarticular reconstruction is contraindicated for repair of a hallux valgus deformity with a congruent MTP joint (DMAA greater than 15 degrees).[72] For this deformity, extraarticular correction can be achieved with either a double or triple first

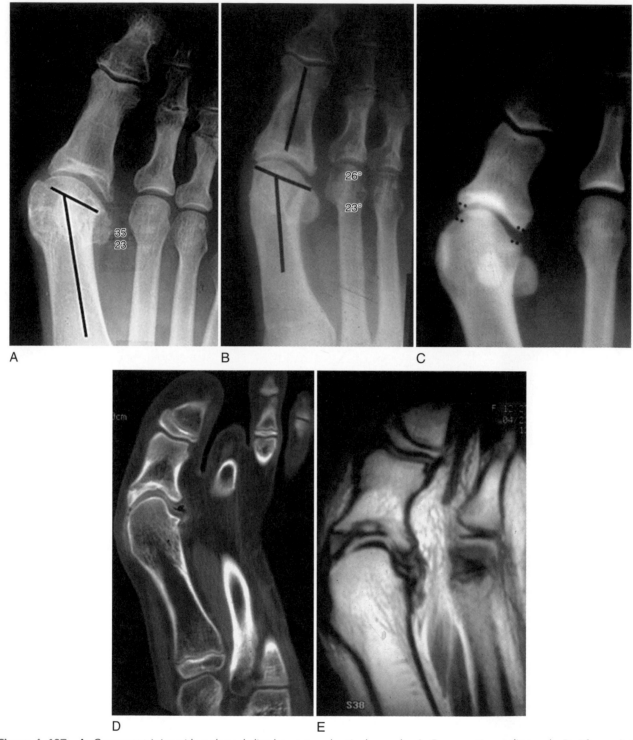

Figure 6–187   **A,** Congruent joint with a sloped distal metatarsal articular angle. **A,** Preoperative radiograph. **B,** After a distal soft tissue procedure, no improvement of the hallux valgus angle was achieved. **C,** Congruent joint as seen on a regular radiograph. **D,** Computed tomography scan. **E,** Magnetic resonance image.

ray osteotomy.[3,72,80,98,318] An Akin osteotomy can diminish phalangeal angulation because of an increased PPAA. A proximal first metatarsal osteotomy or cuneiform osteotomy can decrease an increased 1-2 intermetatarsal angle. In some situations, an increased DMAA requires a medial closing wedge osteotomy of the distal first metatarsal.[113,161,277,293] Mitchell and Baxter[265] reported on the combination of a chevron osteotomy and phalangeal osteotomy to achieve an extraarticular repair. The magnitude of the DMAA and the 1-2 intermetatarsal angle determines the necessity for multiple first ray osteotomies and the magnitude of realignment. In their radiographic analysis, Richardson et al[295] reported that the average normal DMAA was 6 to 7 degrees. Coughlin[72] has observed that this angle increases as the magnitude of the congruent hallux valgus deformity increases. Likewise, he has also reported that the final hallux valgus angle closely mirrors the underlying DMAA. Thus, any procedure that attempts to realign an MTP joint with an increased DMAA or lateral slope of the distal metatarsal articular surface has a substantial risk of reverting to the preoperative inclination determined by the underlying DMAA.[68]

First Cuneiform Osteotomy

Riedel[296] (1886), according to Kelikian,[186] first reported the use of a first cuneiform osteotomy for the correction of metatarsus primus varus. Young[383] used a first cuneiform osteotomy, and Bonney and Macnab[27] and Coughlin and Mann[69,80] reported on the use of a medial cuneiform osteotomy for realignment of the MTC joint to avoid disturbing an open proximal first metatarsal epiphysis. Up to now, no long-term series has been published on the use of this technique. All reports deal with individual case studies.

A medial cuneiform opening wedge osteotomy is most commonly indicated in a juvenile patient with an open proximal first metatarsal epiphysis and a hallux valgus deformity characterized by an abnormally widened 1-2 intermetatarsal angle. An opening wedge first cuneiform osteotomy is an alternative that can effectively reduce metatarsus primus varus or an increased 1-2 intermetatarsal angle without exposing the proximal first metatarsal epiphysis to an iatrogenic injury.

Technique

1. A medial longitudinal incision is centered over the first cuneiform. (The medial cuneiform is approximately 2 to 2.5 cm long, and the osteotomy is centered in the middle of the first cuneiform.)
2. The navicular-cuneiform and the MTC joints are identified.
3. The osteotomy is directed in a medial-lateral plane and carried to a depth of 1.5 cm. The osteotomy must transect both the dorsal and the plantar cortices.

   A vertical osteotomy is positioned in the center of the first cuneiform, and the osteotomy site is opened medially (Fig. 6–188A and B).

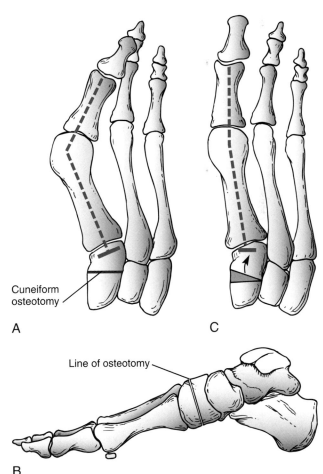

Cuneiform osteotomy

A   C

Line of osteotomy

B

Figure 6–188 Technique of cuneiform osteotomy. **A,** Anteroposterior diagram of a cuneiform osteotomy before distraction. **B,** Lateral diagram of a cuneiform osteotomy. **C,** After distraction of the osteotomy site and bone grafting, alignment has been improved. Internal fixation with Kirschner wires is typically used.

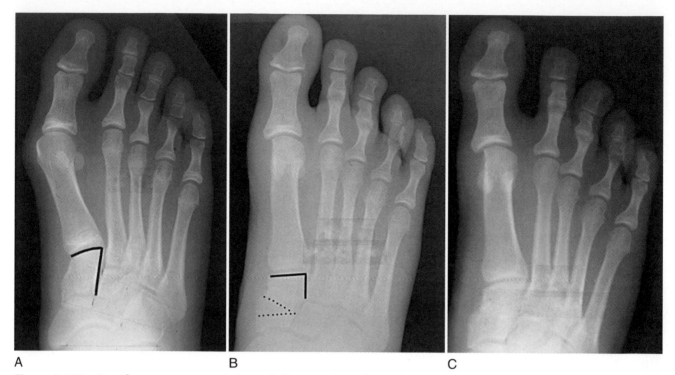

A   B   C

Figure 6–189 Cuneiform osteotomy technique. **A,** Preoperative radiograph demonstrating a juvenile hallux valgus deformity with metatarsus primus varus and an open epiphysis. **B,** Radiograph after opening wedge cuneiform osteotomy and distal soft tissue repair. **C,** Two-year follow-up radiograph after cuneiform osteotomy and distal soft tissue realignment.

4. Although the medial eminence can be used as an interposition graft, often little medial eminence remains with a juvenile bunion deformity. Therefore, it is best to use a wedge-shaped bicortical graft from the iliac crest. The iliac crest graft is removed in routine manner. Because of the height of the first cuneiform, a 2-cm-long graft is used. The base of the graft should be approximately 1 cm or less and should taper to a fine point at the apex. Once the osteotomy site has been distracted, a triangular bicortical iliac crest bone graft is impacted into place and stabilized with two 0.062-inch Kirschner wires (Fig. 6–188C).
5. With a hallux valgus deformity and a subluxated first MTP joint, a distal soft tissue realignment is performed with the cuneiform osteotomy (Fig. 6–189).
6. With a hallux valgus deformity and a congruent first MTP joint, a concomitant distal first metatarsal closing wedge osteotomy is an option (Fig. 6–190).
7. The wound is closed routinely.

Postoperative Care

A gauze-and-tape compression dressing or a below-knee cast is applied at surgery. Frequently, the osteotomy is combined with a distal soft tissue realignment or multiple other first ray osteotomies. The osteotomy will usually heal by 6 weeks after surgery. Internal fixation is removed after successful healing of the osteotomy site (Fig. 6–191).

Distal First Metatarsal Closing Wedge Osteotomy

First described by Reverdin[293] and later by Peabody[277] and others,[72,98,113,280] a distal first metatarsal closing wedge osteotomy can be used for the treatment of a juvenile hallux valgus deformity or in an adult with a congruent hallux valgus deformity. It is especially useful in the presence of an increased DMAA to reorient the metatarsal articular surface more perpendicular to the longitudinal axis of the first metatarsal.

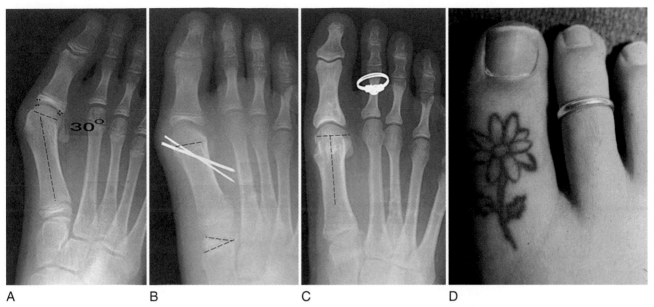

Figure 6–190 **A,** Juvenile hallux valgus with open epiphysis and DMAA of 30 degrees. **B,** Radiograph after opening wedge cuneiform osteotomy and closing wedge distal first metatarsal osteotomy. **C,** Eight-year follow-up radiograph demonstrating successful long-term repair. **D,** Clinical photograph at 8-year follow-up.

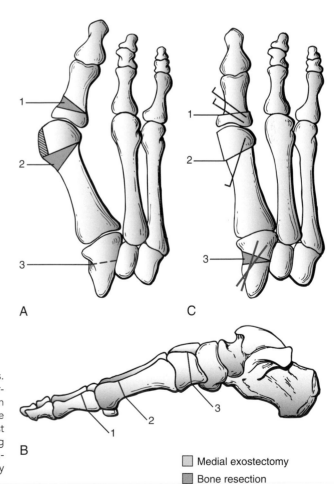

Figure 6–191 Technique of multiple first ray osteotomies. Multiple first ray osteotomies can be used to achieve extraarticular correction of a hallux valgus deformity, especially with an increased distal metatarsal articular angle. **A,** 1, Closing wedge osteotomy. 2, Closing wedge osteotomy of the distal first metatarsal with resection of the medial eminence. 3, Opening wedge osteotomy of the first cuneiform. **B,** Lateral view demonstrating the location of the osteotomies. **C,** A triple osteotomy improves the overall alignment of the first ray.

Medial exostectomy
Bone resection

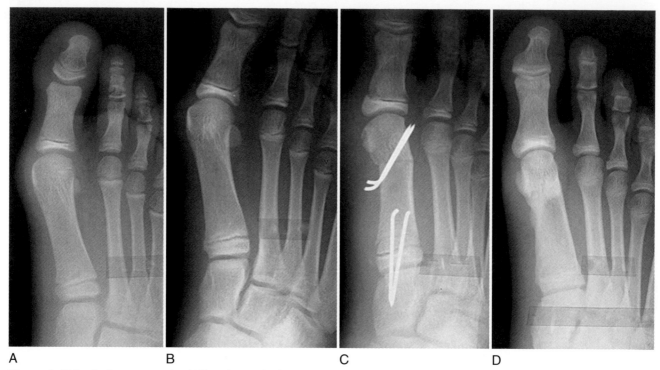

A   B   C   D

Figure 6–192 **A,** Anteroposterior (AP) radiograph demonstrating a mild hallux valgus deformity in an 11-year-old girl. **B,** AP radiograph of a 14-year-old girl demonstrating progression of the deformity. **C,** After distal first metatarsal closing wedge osteotomy and proximal crescentic osteotomy, alignment is improved. **D,** A 2-year follow-up radiograph shows acceptable alignment.

Technique

1. A medial longitudinal incision is centered over the MTP joint beginning at the mid-proximal phalanx and extending 2 cm above the medial eminence.
2. The medial MTP joint capsule is released on the dorsal proximal aspect with an L-shaped, distally based capsular flap (see Fig. 6–90D).
3. At a point 1.5 cm proximal to the MTP joint, an osteotomy of the proximal metatarsal metaphysis (just proximal to the sesamoids) is performed. A second osteotomy proximal to the first is located 6 to 10 mm proximal to the initial osteotomy. It converges at its apex at the lateral cortex with the distal osteotomy. The magnitude of the medial closing wedge osteotomy depends on the magnitude of the DMAA (1-mm resection = 5 degrees of correction of the DMAA) (Fig. 6–192).[210]
4. Care is taken to avoid injury to the sesamoid complex on the plantar aspect at the osteotomy site.
5. Once the wedge has been excised, the osteotomy site is closed. Medial translation of the capital fragment may be necessary. The osteotomy site is fixed with two oblique 0.062-inch Kirschner wires.
6. The medial eminence is resected with an oscillating saw.
7. The medial capsule is approximated and secured to the first metatarsal with suture placed through a medial metaphyseal drill hole. The dorsal and proximal capsular incisions are repaired with interrupted absorbable suture.
8. After completion of this osteotomy, the hallux should be oriented in slight varus because the articular surface now closely parallels the longitudinal axis of the first metatarsal shaft. This situation creates a need for a proximal first ray osteotomy to decrease the 1-2 intermetatarsal angle. An Akin osteotomy can also be added when necessary to create a triple osteotomy (Fig. 6–193).

Other Osteotomies

Another alternative is to combine a distal first metatarsal closing wedge osteotomy with a proximal crescentic osteotomy. Although this

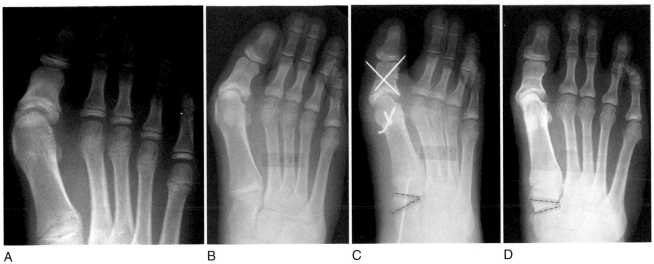

A   B   C   D

Figure 6–193 **A,** Preoperative radiograph demonstrating moderate hallux valgus deformity with a congruent MTP joint (see Fig. 7–10A for early preoperative radiographs when the patient was 10 years old). **B,** At skeletal maturity, a congruent MTP joint and moderate hallux valgus deformity are present. **C,** Triple osteotomy (closing wedge phalangeal osteotomy, closing wedge distal first metatarsal osteotomy, opening wedge cuneiform osteotomy) has achieved realignment. **D,** Four-year follow-up radiograph demonstrating excellent correction of a juvenile hallux valgus deformity with a congruent MTP articulation.

technique may be quite effective, careful dissection is necessary to protect the first metatarsal shaft from devascularization (Fig. 6–194). This interval may be rather small, thus increasing the risk of a vascular insult to the first metatarsal diaphysis. A better alternative may be to combine a distal first metatarsal osteotomy with a first cuneiform osteotomy, even though a first cuneiform osteotomy is more difficult. A proximal osteotomy of the first metatarsal may be considered but should be approached with caution because extensive soft tissue stripping of the first metatarsal can lead to AVN.

Alternative osteotomies have been described by Loretz et al[219] and Kramer et al.[201] Z-shaped osteotomies (scarf type) of the distal first metatarsal that both protect the sesamoid mechanism and allow realignment of the distal metatarsal articular angle are an alternative as well. Amarnek et al[3] used a crescentic distal phalangeal and a distal metatarsal crescentic osteotomy to realign the first ray.

Results

Funk and Wells[113] and others[161,277,293] have reported success with distal first metatarsal osteotomies, as have Durman[98] and Goldner and Gaines[129] with double first ray osteotomies.

Kramer et al[201] and Day et al[92] both reported an average 15-degree correction of the DMAA with a Z-shaped rotational osteotomy, and Loretz et al[219] reported similar correction of the hallux valgus deformity with an increase in the DMAA. Funk and Wells[113] reported an average 7.2-degree correction of the 1-2 intermetatarsal angle with a distal first metatarsal closing wedge osteotomy. Chou et al[53] used a biplanar distal chevron osteotomy to correct the DMAA 4 degrees with this procedure.

A variety of double osteotomies have been advocated, including proximal phalangeal and first metatarsal osteotomy,[3,72,74,129] double metatarsal osteotomy,[72,74,98] phalangeal and chevron osteotomy,[265] and phalangeal and cuneiform osteotomy.[142] Reporting on the use of double and triple osteotomies for the treatment of juvenile hallux valgus with congruous MTP joints, Coughlin[72] noted an average 23-degree correction of the hallux valgus angle and an average 8.3-degree correction of the 1-2 intermetatarsal angle. This correction occurred in the presence of an average DMAA of 19 degrees. These results are similar to those noted by Peterson and Newman,[280] who reported on 10 adolescent patients with an average 24-degree correction of the hallux valgus angle and an average 8-degree correction of the 1-2 intermetatarsal angle after double osteotomy. A high

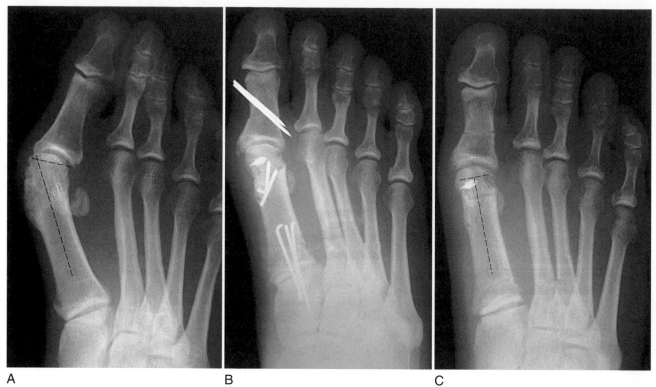

A   B   C

Figure 6–194 **A,** Preoperative radiograph in 40-year-old man who underwent unsuccessful juvenile hallux valgus correction. Note the congruent metatarsophalangeal joint (distal metatarsal articular angle of 30 degrees). **B,** Triple osteotomy (closing wedge phalangeal osteotomy, closing wedge distal first metatarsal osteotomy, crescentic proximal first metatarsal osteotomy) has achieved realignment of the first ray. **C,** One-year follow-up radiograph demonstrating improved alignment. (A suture anchor was used to stabilize a medial capsular disruption found at surgery.)

rate of subjective satisfaction was reported in both series. Coughlin and Carlson[74] reported on the results of 21 feet with congruent hallux valgus deformities (with an increased DMAA) treated by periarticular osteotomies. Both double and triple first ray osteotomies were performed in the series. The average correction of the hallux valgus angle was 23 degrees, the average correction of the intermetatarsal angle was 9 degrees, and the average correction of the DMAA was 14 degrees postoperatively.

In a laboratory study, Lau and Daniels[210] determined that the size of the wedge to be resected to reduce an abnormally high DMAA in a congruent hallux valgus deformity can be easily determined preoperatively. They suggested that for every 1 mm of bone resected from the distal metaphysis in the process of performing a closing wedge osteotomy, the DMAA was decreased by 4.7 degrees.

Complications

Complications after multiple metatarsal osteotomies may include loss of correction, malunion, loss of fixation, AVN, intraarticular injury from an associated fracture with the osteotomy, and degenerative arthrosis of the interphalangeal or MTP joints. These procedures are technically difficult and should be reserved for the occasional case of hallux valgus characterized by a congruent first MTP joint with a DMAA greater than 15 degrees. When possible, a simpler and technically easier procedure is preferable to a more complex and difficult technique. Degenerative arthritis has been reported by Bock et al,[26] who noted both metatarsal head and metatarsal sesamoid cartilaginous lesions, with increased occurrence related to the severity of the preoperative hallux valgus deformity.

Complications of Hallux Valgus Surgery

To discuss complications of bunion surgery, we should first clarify the goals of treatment of hallux valgus deformities. The main goal is to produce the most functional foot possible after surgery. This will vary, depending on the severity of the deformity and the functional capability of the patient. In a young patient with bunion pain secondary to a prominent medial eminence, a fully functional, painless foot is the goal; in a rheumatoid patient, a foot with satisfactory overall alignment that allows reasonable footwear and an ability to walk without pain is a realistic goal.

The algorithms that are found in Figures 6–74, 6–75, and 6–79 can help the clinician decide which type of surgical procedure will produce the best anatomic results. However, this does not address a patient's expectations. The patient and clinician must have the same goals in mind when surgery is being contemplated. We see many patients in consultation who have been misled regarding their surgery, and although the result obtained was within the normal spectrum for a specific procedure, the patient was extremely dissatisfied. If patients are made aware of the various complications associated with each specific procedure (e.g., loss of motion, residual joint pain, sensitivity about the scar), although they may not be totally satisfied, at least they faced no surprises. It is important to not "sell" a patient on a procedure but rather to be sure the patient believes that all types of conservative management have been attempted and that surgery will offer a realistic solution to the problem. If the patient has no pain, it is difficult to improve the situation.

To a certain extent, each age group has specific goals for correction of a foot problem. With the wide selection of leisure and sport shoes available today, people can wear a shoe that will not place excessive pressure over the painful area. Several age groups have specific problems. For example, women aged 25 to 35 years are prone to being dissatisfied with the results of bunion surgery. Their goal is usually to be able to fit into a more stylish shoe, but many of these women have a wide forefoot, so even after satisfactory correction of the deformity, they are still unable to wear their desired shoes. If they believed that the surgery would permit them to do so, they will often be quite dissatisfied. This is basically a problem in preoperative communication between the surgeon and patient. An athlete or dancer, particularly if professional, should always receive the most conservative treatment plan possible.[62] A general rule is that until such patients are significantly hampered in their ability to perform in their given profession, surgical intervention should be delayed because of the concern that after an unsuccessful surgical procedure, a painful foot will bring an end to their athletic career.

Causes of Surgical Failure

The following results represent an ideal hallux valgus repair:

- Correction of the hallux valgus and 1-2 intermetatarsal angles
- Creation of a congruent MTP joint with sesamoid realignment
- Removal of the medial eminence
- Retention of functional range of motion of the MTP joint
- Maintenance of normal weight-bearing mechanics of the foot

With this ideal type of repair in mind, we now examine some of the factors that result in failure of a hallux valgus repair.

If an inappropriate procedure is selected for the pathologic condition present, the outcome will often be suboptimal. As pointed out in the algorithms in Figures 6–74, 6–75, and 6–79, each hallux valgus deformity needs to be carefully analyzed before selecting the appropriate surgical procedure. If a patient has a congruent joint and an attempt is made to correct the hallux valgus deformity by realigning the proximal phalanx over the metatarsal head, an incongruent joint may result. This in turn can lead to either joint stiffness, if the phalanx does not slide back into its former congruent alignment, or recurrence of the deformity. If significant arthrosis is present in the joint and a realignment is carried out, restricted joint motion is a common result. Therefore, the first step in avoiding a complication is selection of the correct surgical procedure.

If the indications for a procedure are "stretched," a suboptimal result will be obtained. This may occur when choosing a "simple bunionectomy" when a metatarsal osteotomy should be performed as well. Although the hallux is initially well aligned, recurrence of the deformity quickly results. If a chevron procedure is used to correct a severe hallux valgus deformity, full correction is rarely achieved. When performing hallux valgus surgery, a surgeon must remember that a single procedure will not result in satisfactory correction of all deformities.

Inadequate or inappropriate postoperative management may result in failure even when technically the procedure was properly performed. Soft tissues need to be carefully and meticulously supported and protected after surgery to ensure a satisfactory result. After many orthopaedic procedures, meticulous postoperative management is unnecessary, but after most hallux valgus procedures, careful follow-up is necessary to ensure a successful result.

Other causes of failure that may result from soft tissue, neurologic, or bone problems are discussed in detail next. Postoperative sepsis, though infrequent, can be a cause of failure and result in significant joint stiffness, chronic swelling, and possibly even nonunion of the osteotomy.

Finally, unrealistic patient expectations may be the cause of a failed surgical procedure. If the patient does not understand the possible limitations of the procedure preoperatively, both the patient and the surgeon may be unhappy afterward.

In selecting the surgical procedure, the surgeon must consider the options for a salvage procedure if a complication develops. The following typical complications can occur after specific procedures: soft tissue realignment resulting in a hallux varus deformity; arthrodesis resulting in nonunion; proximal first metatarsal osteotomy resulting in nonunion or malunion; and distal metatarsal osteotomy resulting in malunion, nonunion, or AVN. In the treatment of a hallux varus deformity, adequate soft tissue realignment can usually be achieved frequently, but on occasion, an arthrodesis may be necessary. After nonunion of an arthrodesis, an interposition bone grafting procedure will frequently result in successful fusion. With malunion of a metatarsal osteotomy, a corrective osteotomy can often achieve satisfactory realignment. With AVN of the metatarsal head, an arthrodesis with an interposition bone block may be necessary to achieve a satisfactory result. We believe that patients should have a general understanding of the type of complication that may develop so that if a second procedure is required, they will have some basic knowledge of what may be necessary.

The more common complications of hallux valgus surgery are presented here to acquaint the surgeon with the various types of problems that may arise. It is hoped that with a familiarity with these problems, the surgeon will take precautions to prevent them. A certain degree of risk is associated with any type of surgical procedure, and complications can occur regardless of the precautions taken.

Soft Tissue Problems

INFECTION

A postoperative infection may be superficial or deep. The clinician must be constantly aware of the possibility of postoperative infection and treat it vigorously if it develops. It is very important to determine as quickly as possible whether an infection is superficial

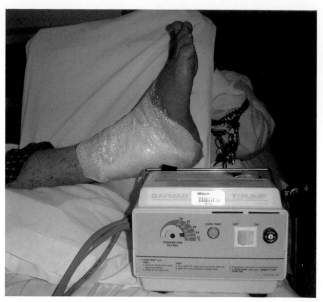

Figure 6–195 Infection after bunion surgery with ascending lymphangitis, treated with warm moist soaks and intravenous antibiotics.

to the MTP joint or whether it involves the joint itself (Fig. 6–195).

Generally speaking, a superficial infection is manifested by local cellulitis and, on occasion, evidence of ascending lymphangitis. The skin over the involved area may be red and warm, but motion of the joint will not usually cause significant pain. Attempts at aspiration of the MTP joint through an area of cellulitis are discouraged because of the risk of spreading a superficial infection into the joint space. Clinically, fever will usually develop in a patient with a superficial infection. Hematologic data may indicate an increase in the white blood cell (WBC) count with a left shift. Clinical judgment is important in choosing treatment, and the use of either oral or systemic antibiotics is indicated.

A deep infection involving the MTP joint is much more severe and is usually manifested as a marked increase in pain and swelling about the MTP joint. There may be evidence of purulent discharge from the wound. MTP joint motion will typically cause discomfort, as will palpation of the joint itself. Often a fever is present, and the WBC count and sedimentation rate are generally elevated. Management should be directed toward obtaining a specific culture and sensitivity of the offending organism. Prompt treatment with parenteral antibiotics is indicated. With purulent drainage, a decision must be made expeditiously regarding whether prompt irrigation and debridement of the joint are indicated.

After a severe joint space infection, marked intraarticular joint fibrosis and degenerative arthritis may ensue due to destruction of the articular cartilage. Changes in periarticular soft tissues after the infection may lead to recurrence of the original deformity.

DELAYED WOUND HEALING

Occasionally after foot surgery, the operative wound edges appear to be locally reddened and slightly separated. There is no evidence of surrounding cellulitis or purulent drainage. The joint itself is not usually particularly swollen, and motion of the joint does not cause increased discomfort. Such cases are often caused by a superficial fungal infection. Carbolfuchsin (Carfusin) painted on the wound on one or two occasions will generally result in prompt wound healing with no further sequelae. In the presence of increasing evidence of cellulitis, a more serious problem should be suspected and treated accordingly.

SKIN SLOUGH

Occasionally after surgery, a partial- or full-thickness slough about the wound may occur. Sloughing usually develops 7 to 14 days after surgery and, depending on its size, may create a significant problem. The cause of the sloughing is devascularization of the involved tissue, which can result from insufficient circulation secondary to a dysvascular foot, excessive retraction on the skin edge at surgery, placement of the skin under tension after correction of a severe deformity, or pressure from the postoperative dressing (Fig. 6–196).

Treatment varies depending on the severity of the tissue loss. In the case of a minor partial-thickness skin slough, local treatment and the passage of time usually result in a satisfactory outcome. Sloughing caused by a dysvascular foot may require revascularization of the extremity before satisfactory wound healing can occur. Other larger, full-thickness skin sloughs may eventually require skin grafting after a satisfactory granulating bed has been achieved or could even require amputation.

ADHERENT SCAR

Occasionally after a successful surgical procedure, a scar forms that is quite adherent to the underlying tissue. If a full-thickness dissection includes the underlying fatty tissue when skin flaps are developed at the time of the initial surgery, an adherent scar seldom occurs. As a general rule, an adherent scar may actually soften over time, thus rendering it less bothersome to the patient. Soft tissue and underlying fatty tissue are generally somewhat limited on the foot, and excision of a persistent, adherent scar will not usually result in significant improvement of the situation. Persistent massage of an adherent scar may in time help mobilize the restricted tissue.

PARESTHESIAS OF THE HALLUX

Entrapment or severance (partial or complete) of a cutaneous nerve may result in either dysesthesia or anesthesia distal to the involved nerve. Protection of sensory nerves at the time of surgery is paramount; however, once a nerve injury occurs, desensitization of the involved area is managed by frequent massaging, rubbing, or tapping. This will often produce a satisfactory result over a period of several months. Occa-

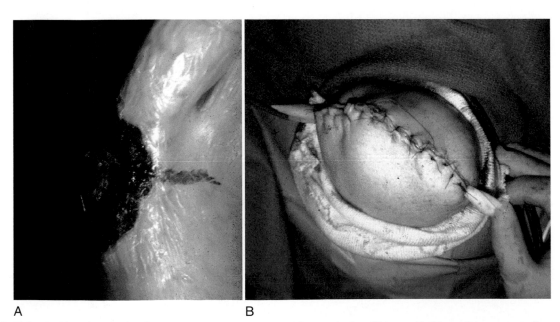

A   **B**

Figure 6–196 **A,** Skin slough after bunion surgery in a patient with vascular insufficiency. **B,** Above-knee amputation was eventually required.

sionally it is necessary to reexplore the injured nerve and further resect the nerve proximally to an area of soft tissue to diminish the symptoms. The use of a transcutaneous nerve stimulator may be effective if surgical intervention fails. On rare occasion, a regional pain syndrome may develop (see Chapter 33).

One of the most frequently involved nerves is the dorsomedial cutaneous nerve to the great toe (Fig. 6–197A-C). An incision on the dorsomedial aspect of the first MTP joint unfortunately overlies this cutaneous nerve. Occasionally, this nerve can be severed at the time of surgery or later become entrapped in scar tissue. As a general rule, neurolysis is rarely helpful, particularly if the nerve has been partially severed. Exploration of the injured nerve through a long, dorsomedial incision enables the identification of normal and injured nerve. After carefully freeing the nerve from surrounding scar tissue and sectioning the nerve more proximally, the nerve is then transferred beneath and sutured under minimal tension to the abductor hallucis muscle. In this way the nerve is transferred from an area of painful scar tissue to an area where there is little or no pressure. Although an area of numbness over the dorsomedial aspect of the great toe remains, the dysesthetic area is no longer present.

The plantar medial cutaneous nerve just plantar to the abductor hallucis tendon can also be injured. Symptoms develop with ambulation as the MTP joint dorsiflexes with plantar pressure over the neuroma, and often a patient transfers weight to the lateral border of the foot. Again, surgical treatment consists of exposing the plantar medial cutaneous nerve through a long medial incision just dorsal to the

weight-bearing surface. The nerve is identified and traced proximally to normal nerve tissue. After the nerve has been freed and sectioned, it is buried proximally beneath the abductor hallucis muscle. At the time of transposition, the sectioned nerve is sutured with a minimum of tension so that as the toes are brought into dorsiflexion, symptoms will not be exacerbated. After sectioning of the injured nerve, there is residual numbness along the plantar medial aspect of the great toe.

Occasionally, the common digital nerve to the first web space is partially or completely transected with exploration of the first web space. If a neuroma develops, there may be sensitivity on the plantar aspect of the foot, as well as dysesthesias on the plantar aspect of the first web space (Fig. 6–197B). Surgical treatment involves exposure through a dorsal first web space incision. The transverse metatarsal ligament is sectioned and the common digital nerve identified and carefully freed from surrounding tissue. If a significant neuroma is identified and transection of the nerve is necessary, it should be performed with as much length of the nerve left as possible. This ensures that the remaining stump can be elevated to an area alongside the first metatarsal so that the nerve end (where another neuroma will form) is removed from the plantar aspect of the foot. Proximal transection of the common digital nerve without elevation of the stump frequently results in a painful neuroma located more proximally in the foot. At times the common digital nerve can be freed from the adjacent soft tissue; if the nerve appears to be abnormal, it can be elevated off the plantar aspect of the foot and transferred above

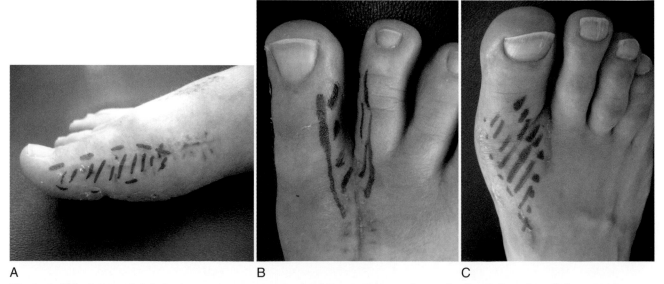

A   B   C

Figure 6–197 Iatrogenic injuries to nerves at surgery can lead to numbness and paresthesias. **A,** Dorsal medial cutaneous nerve to the hallux. **B,** Common digital nerve to the first web space. **C,** Injury to the superficial peroneal nerve.

a portion of the adductor hallucis muscle so that the nerve is not exposed to the trauma of weight bearing.

DELAYED WOUND BREAKDOWN

Occasionally after successful surgery and wound healing, the wound will once again become swollen and sensitive. This usually occurs 4 weeks or more postoperatively but may occur many months after surgery. Frequently the cause is a foreign body reaction to the underlying suture material. It frequently involves silk, but other suture materials (e.g., cotton, chromic, newer synthetic materials) may be involved. The area of the reaction forms a sterile abscess, the skin breaks down, and a suture granuloma develops. With time, the involved foreign material is usually extruded. Occasionally, exploration of the wound may be necessary to excise the foreign material. Once removed, prompt wound healing generally occurs, although cauterization of the remaining granulation material with silver nitrate is often required.

Complications Affecting the Metatarsal Shaft

After any metatarsal osteotomy, malposition or loss of position of the osteotomy site is possible. To avoid this problem, a broad stable osteotomy, rigid internal fixation, adequate postoperative immobilization, and protected ambulation are necessary. Some osteotomies are inherently more stable than others. Surgical judgment is required to determine which sites are sufficiently stable for ambulation and which are not.

The same surgical procedure in two different patients may require a different method of fixation and postoperative weight-bearing precautions.

The following are the most common types of problems seen after metatarsal osteotomy.

SHORTENING

Shortening occurs after most metatarsal osteotomies. After the chevron procedure an average shortening of 2.2 mm (range, 0-8) has been reported[158,290] (Fig. 6–198A). After the Mitchell procedure even more shortening has been reported* (Fig. 6–198B). The most shortening seems to follow the Wilson procedure, with an average of 11 mm[290] (Fig. 6–198C and D). After a distal soft tissue procedure and proximal osteotomy, approximately 2-mm shortening has been reported[77,242] (Fig. 6–198E and F). The main problem associated with shortening is the development of a transfer lesion beneath the second metatarsal head. It

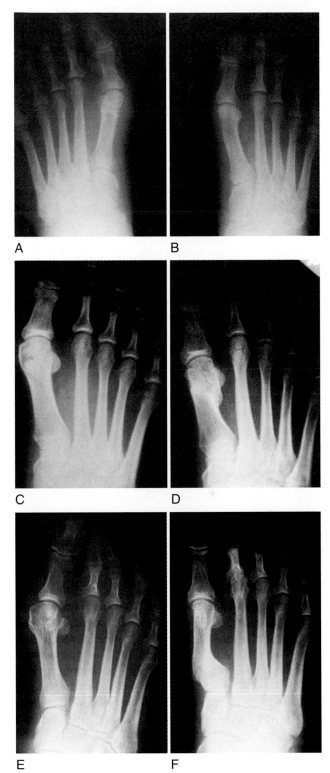

Figure 6–198 Shortening after hallux valgus surgery. **A,** Shortening after a chevron osteotomy. **B,** Shortening after a Mitchell procedure. **C,** Preoperative radiograph. **D,** Shortening after a Wilson procedure. **E,** Preoperative radiograph. **F,** Shortening after proximal metatarsal osteotomy. Shortening of first metatarsal may result in a transfer lesion.

---

*References 45, 110, 127, 150, 263, 264, 311, and 379.

is difficult to assign a specific amount of shortening that will produce metatarsalgia because a number of factors play a role, including the original length of the first metatarsal and whether dorsiflexion is associated with the shortening. The degree of hallux valgus correction, range of motion, and stability of the MTP joint are factors because weight is normally transferred to the great toe at the end of stance phase. This in turn unloads the second metatarsal head. With insufficient stability or inadequate correction of the hallux, the first metatarsal will not carry its share of the weight. After procedures that destabilize the MTP joint, such as the Keller procedure,[154] or with a prosthesis in which significant weight bearing no longer occurs beneath the great toe, the incidence of metatarsalgia is increased.

Certain procedures (e.g., Mitchell, Wilson, closing wedge proximal metatarsal osteotomy) have the potential for transfer metatarsalgia.[150,194,264,380] In these cases it is imperative that the length of the first and second metatarsals be carefully assessed when planning a surgical procedure to decide whether an alternative procedure that would produce less shortening should be used.

Those experienced with the Mitchell procedure emphasize that plantar flexion of the distal fragment should be carried out to help alleviate the potential for metatarsalgia.* However, if the first metatarsal is significantly short to begin with and more shortening ensues after surgery, metatarsalgia will inevitably result. Once shortening of the first metatarsal and metatarsalgia occur, further surgical treatment is often required. Surgical treatment of this condition is difficult, and the results are often less than optimal.

Lengthening of a metatarsal is difficult to achieve both anatomically and technically. Metatarsals do not "stretch" well, and even if an interposition bone block is used, some resorption may occur and subsequent tilting of the distal portion of the metatarsal may develop. If the second metatarsal is significantly longer than the first and third, shortening of the second metatarsal to achieve a normal weight-bearing pattern can be beneficial. On rare occasion, both the second and the third metatarsals can be shortened to realign the weight-bearing pattern of the foot. Occasionally, a plantar flexion osteotomy of the first metatarsal can be used to increase its weight-bearing function.

DORSIFLEXION

Dorsiflexion of the first metatarsal can occur after a proximal osteotomy of almost any type. It can also occur distally after a chevron, Mitchell, or Wilson

osteotomy. After MTC fusion, dorsiflexion of the metatarsal has been reported as well.[271,307]

Dorsiflexion, as with shortening of the metatarsal, should be avoided if possible. Unfortunately, dorsiflexion of an already short metatarsal only compounds the problem of transfer metatarsalgia. At times, dorsiflexion occurs with minimal shortening, and rarely does a problem result. Exactly how much dorsiflexion versus how much shortening can be tolerated after a surgical procedure varies from foot to foot. It probably depends on the overall rigidity of a foot, the relationship of the length of the first and second metatarsals, and a patient's activity level. When substantial dorsiflexion occurs, however, it creates a difficult management problem and is probably best handled by a plantar flexion first metatarsal osteotomy rather than by shortening or elevating the second metatarsal. Elevation of the second metatarsal often leads to a transfer lesion beneath the third metatarsal.

After a lateral closing wedge first metatarsal osteotomy, a dorsiflexion deformity usually develops because more bone is removed dorsally than plantarward at the osteotomy site. As the osteotomy is closed, the metatarsal moves laterally and dorsally. This combination of shortening and dorsiflexion can cause significant metatarsalgia. Furthermore, internal fixation must be adequate to maintain the desired position of the osteotomy (Fig. 6–199A and B).

If dorsiflexion of the first metatarsal results in a symptomatic transfer lesion beneath the first metatarsal or results in flattening of the longitudinal arch because of loss of support by the first metatarsal head, a plantar flexion osteotomy can be performed. There are many techniques with which to plantar flex the first metatarsal. We prefer to make a crescentic-shaped cut in the plantar half of the first metatarsal about 1 cm distal to the MTC joint. With this cut, the blade must exit plantar-ward. The top of the blade does not penetrate the dorsal surface, and the osteotomy is completed vertically with a sagittal saw (Fig. 6–199C).

After a proximal crescentic osteotomy, dorsiflexion can occur with inadequate internal fixation. This osteotomy offers a broad cancellous surface, which is quite stable with screw fixation. At times, if the bone is osteopenic or if a screw of inadequate length is chosen, dorsal angulation may develop. Mann et al[242] reviewed a series of 109 cases and reported postoperative dorsiflexion in approximately 28% of cases, although the magnitude of the deformity was not quantified. Some of the cases of dorsiflexion were quite minor. In none of these patients, however, did a transfer lesion develop. The explanation for this is that the first MTP joint was adequately realigned and, thus, the hallux continued to bear weight in a normal

---

*References 25, 127, 150, 261, 264, 380, and 381.

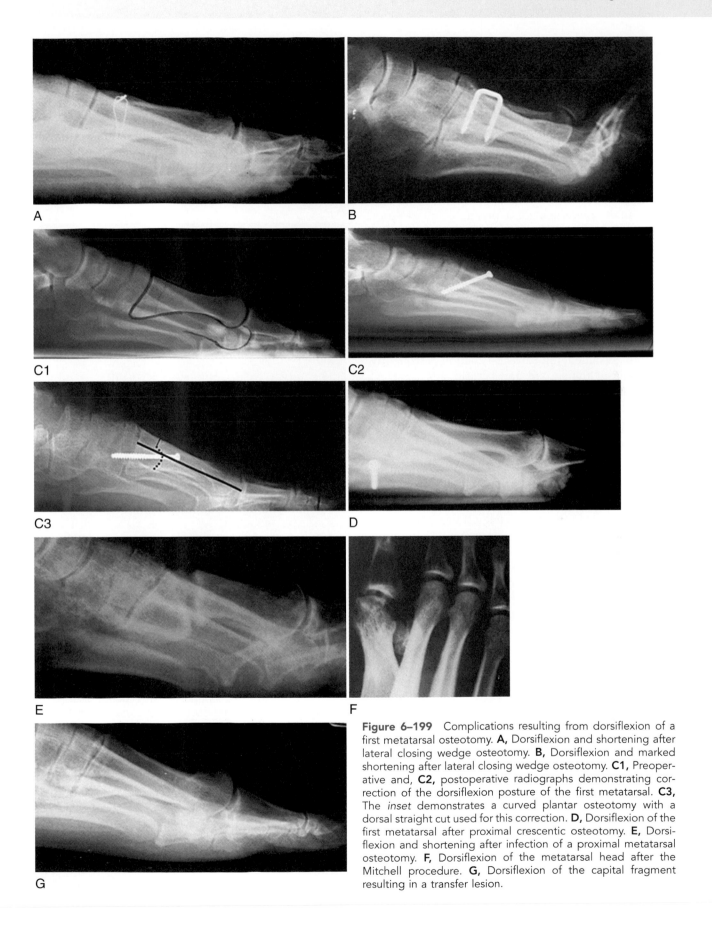

Figure 6–199 Complications resulting from dorsiflexion of a first metatarsal osteotomy. **A,** Dorsiflexion and shortening after lateral closing wedge osteotomy. **B,** Dorsiflexion and marked shortening after lateral closing wedge osteotomy. **C1,** Preoperative and, **C2,** postoperative radiographs demonstrating correction of the dorsiflexion posture of the first metatarsal. **C3,** The *inset* demonstrates a curved plantar osteotomy with a dorsal straight cut used for this correction. **D,** Dorsiflexion of the first metatarsal after proximal crescentic osteotomy. **E,** Dorsiflexion and shortening after infection of a proximal metatarsal osteotomy. **F,** Dorsiflexion of the metatarsal head after the Mitchell procedure. **G,** Dorsiflexion of the capital fragment resulting in a transfer lesion.

manner. This appears to compensate for the dorsiflex-ion that developed (Fig. 6–199D and E).

Shortening of the first metatarsal is an inherent part of the Mitchell procedure. The osteotomy is designed so that the shortening is compensated for by plantar flexion or plantar displacement (or both) of the distal fragment. Inadequate fixation of the distal fragment, however, can lead to postoperative dorsiflexion. With a dorsiflexed short first metatarsal, weight is trans-ferred to the lesser metatarsals. Prevention of this com-plication is far simpler than later treatment. Salvage often entails placement of a proximal interposition bone block to both plantar flex and lengthen the first metatarsal. If only dorsiflexion ensues, correction can be achieved with a bone graft placed in the distal third of the metatarsal, closer to the apex of the deformity (Fig. 6–199F).

After a distal oblique or Wilson-type osteotomy, both shortening and dorsiflexion occur because of inadequate fixation of the capital fragment. This presents a challenging salvage situation. Frequently, shortening of the second and occasionally the third metatarsal is necessary to relieve lateral metatarsalgia.

After a chevron osteotomy, dorsiflexion of the capital fragment may result in transfer metatarsalgia. Dorsal displacement of the capital fragment can be prevented by intraoperative internal fixation. When dorsiflexion of the distal fragment results in transfer metatarsalgia, it is preferable to treat the second metatarsal with a shortening osteotomy rather than attempt to realign the first metatarsal head due to the risk of AVN (Fig. 6–199G).

After MTC joint arthrodesis, dorsiflexion may develop at the MTC joint, particularly if a bone graft has been added to the procedure. When dorsiflexion is of such magnitude that a transfer lesion develops, a plantar flexion osteotomy of the first metatarsal can achieve realignment distal to the fused joint.

PLANTAR FLEXION

A plantar flexion deformity of the first metatarsal occurs infrequently and is caused by inadequate internal fixation of the osteotomy site. It frequently leads to increased weight bearing beneath the first metatarsal head with the subsequent development of a diffuse callus. An orthotic device that transfers weight laterally to the lesser metatarsal head region will often alleviate the symptoms. With a severe deformity, however, a corrective osteotomy to dorsiflex the first metatarsal can be performed (Fig. 6–200).

EXCESSIVE VALGUS (LATERAL DEVIATION) OF THE FIRST METATARSAL

Occasionally, the intermetatarsal angle will be over-corrected and a negative angle will be created (Fig.

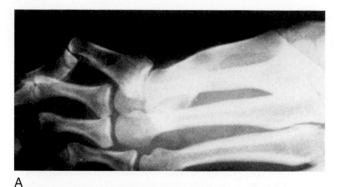

A

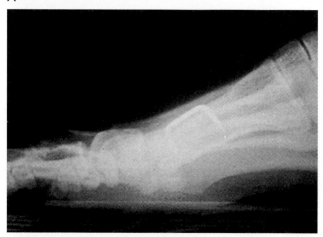

B

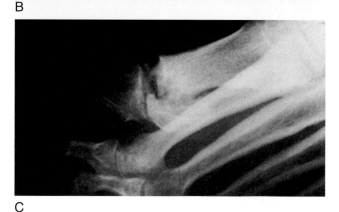

C

Figure 6–200 Complications after plantar flexion of a first metatarsal osteotomy. **A,** Plantar flexion deformity after the Mitchell procedure. **B,** Correction after dorsal osteotomy. **C,** Severe plantar flexion deformity after a chevron osteotomy.

6–201). If the deformity is minimal, no significant sequelae will develop. If the overcorrection is excessive, the articular surface slopes laterally, and as the proxi-mal phalanx is relocated on the metatarsal head, an incongruent joint surface is created. In time, the MTP joint will become painful and degenerative arthritis may develop.

After a proximal crescentic osteotomy, if the con-cavity of the saw blade faces distally, there is a ten-dency to displace the metatarsal shaft medial-ward as

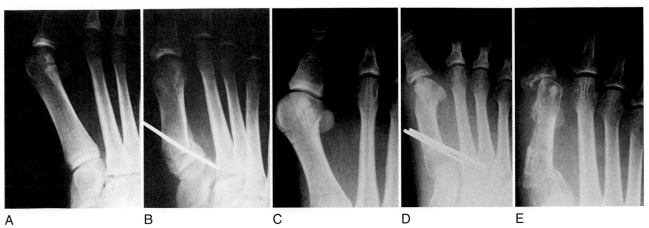

A   B   C   D   E

Figure 6–201 Complications associated with excessive adduction of the first metatarsal after proximal osteotomies. **A,** Hallux valgus associated with adduction of all metatarsals. **B,** Correction of hallux valgus with a proximal metatarsal osteotomy resulted in a negative intermetatarsal angle but a congruent MTP joint. To gain this correction, a negative intermetatarsal angle was necessary. **C,** Preoperative radiograph. **D,** Postoperative radiograph demonstrating the effects of a proximal metatarsal osteotomy with creation of an incongruent MTP joint. **E,** Creation of an incongruent joint from excessive lateral displacement of the proximal metatarsal osteotomy. When a congruent joint is present preoperatively, it must be resected. Any attempt to rotate the proximal phalanx on the metatarsal head will result in an incongruent joint.

the osteotomy is rotated. When this occurs, the metatarsal head may be translated too far laterally (Fig. 6–202). Concurrently, if the medial eminence is excessively resected, an unstable situation develops that is at risk for the development of a hallux varus deformity. Therefore, when a distal soft tissue procedure and proximal crescentic osteotomy are performed, the osteotomy to resect the medial eminence is performed

2 mm medial to the sagittal sulcus to leave a "medial buttress" so that the risk of overcorrection is reduced.

Correction of this complication, if long-standing, is difficult because degenerative arthritis of the MTP joint commonly develops. Prevention, if possible, is desirable, and the use of intraoperative fluoroscopy helps minimize this complication. On occasion it is necessary to revise the osteotomy of the metatarsal to realign the first ray. However, in most circumstances, correction of the first metatarsal must be combined with realignment of the soft tissues about the MTP joint. With advanced first MTP joint degenerative arthritis, an arthrodesis is sufficient to realign the joint and attain successful salvage.

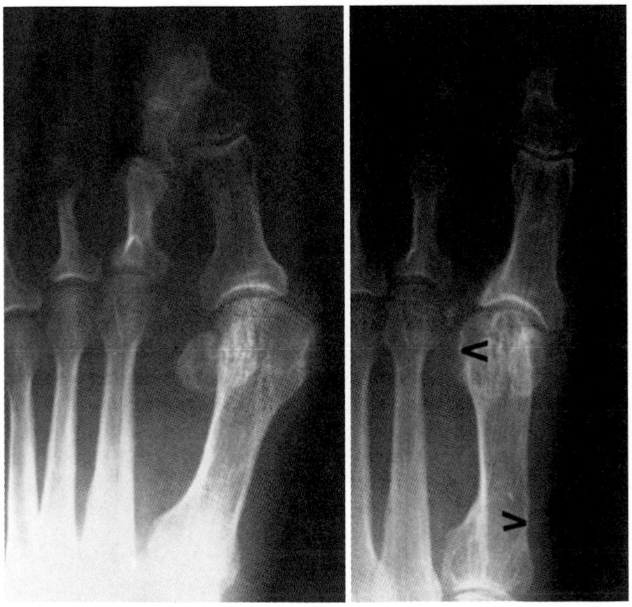

NONUNION OF THE FIRST METATARSAL

Nonunion of the first metatarsal (proximal or distal) can occur after any osteotomy. With the improved methods of internal fixation, this complication is not common. On occasion, delayed union develops. Given sufficient time (even 4-6 months), successful healing will usually occur with adequate immobilization.

Nonunion can generally be prevented by adequate preparation of the bone surfaces and adequate interfragmentary compression, which promotes rapid healing.

The problem that often arises as a result of nonunion is loss of position of the metatarsal shaft, shortening, or both. Treatment of this complication is determined by the nature of the problem and may vary from bone grafting the nonunion site to performing a corrective osteotomy and rigidly fixing the nonunion site (Fig. 6–203).

A   B

Figure 6–202 **A** and **B,** Excessive lateral displacement of the metatarsal head after a proximal crescentic osteotomy caused by medial deviation of the osteotomy site.

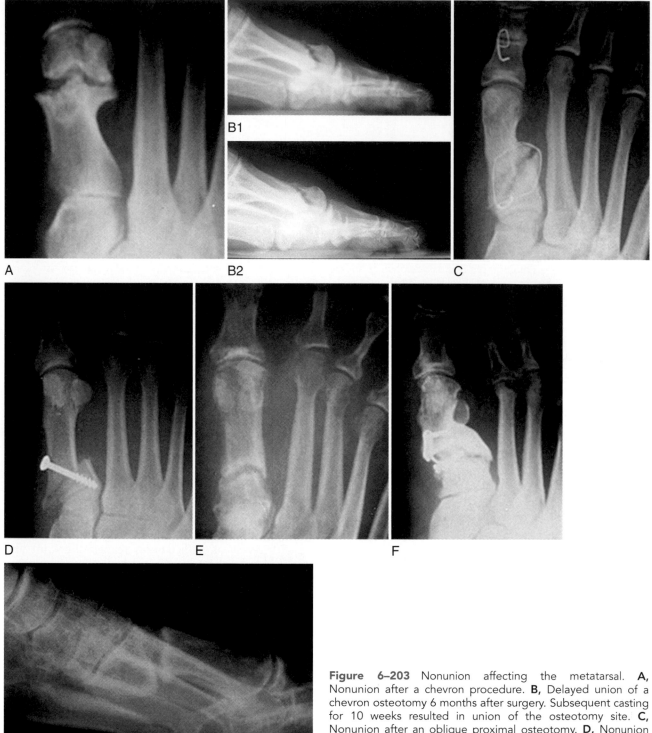

Figure 6–203 Nonunion affecting the metatarsal. **A,** Nonunion after a chevron procedure. **B,** Delayed union of a chevron osteotomy 6 months after surgery. Subsequent casting for 10 weeks resulted in union of the osteotomy site. **C,** Nonunion after an oblique proximal osteotomy. **D,** Nonunion after an oblique proximal metatarsal osteotomy. **E,** Anteroposterior and, **G,** lateral radiographs of nonunion of a proximal crescentic osteotomy. **F,** Nonunion of a proximal metatarsal osteotomy.

Complications Affecting the Metatarsal Head

EXCESSIVE EXCISION

When most bunion procedures are performed, the medial eminence is excised. When carrying out the distal soft tissue procedure, we advocate moving 1 to 2 mm medial to the sagittal sulcus to ensure that an adequate medial buttress is left in place to prevent a varus deformity. The absence of articular cartilage just lateral to the sagittal sulcus may invite further excision, but this will lead to the removal of an excessive amount of the metatarsal head and result in an unstable joint, which in turn can lead to a hallux varus deformity. Other times, excessive excision of the metatarsal head results in an incongruent articular surface, which leads to early degenerative arthritis (Fig. 6–204).

Treatment of excessive resection of the medial metatarsal head is difficult because insufficient metatarsal head remains to support the proximal phalanx. The most common means of salvage is an MTP arthrodesis to both realign the joint and eliminate the pain.

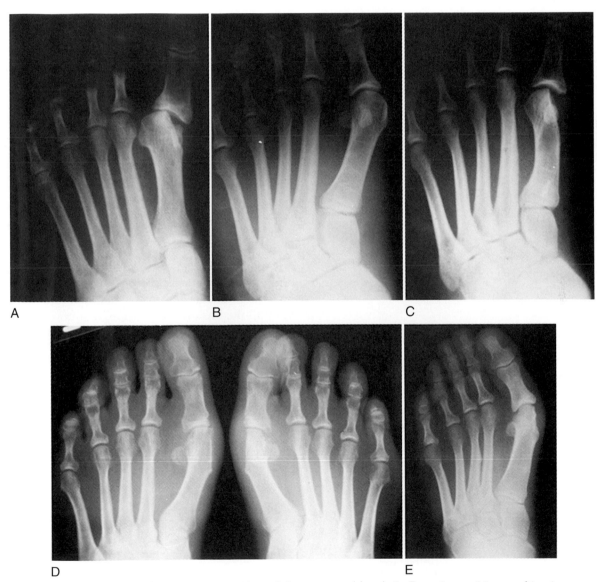

A   B   C

D   E

Figure 6–204 Complications after excessive excision of the metatarsal head. **A,** Excessive excision resulting in an unstable metatarsophalangeal (MTP) joint caused medial subluxation of the tibial sesamoid and a hallux varus deformity. **B,** Preoperative hallux valgus repair. **C,** Postoperative radiograph demonstrating excessive excision of the medial eminence, which resulted in a painful, unstable MTP joint. **D** and **E,** Excision of an excessive amount of metatarsal head resulted in an unstable, painful MTP joint.

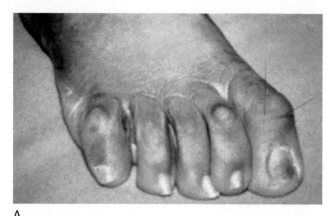

A

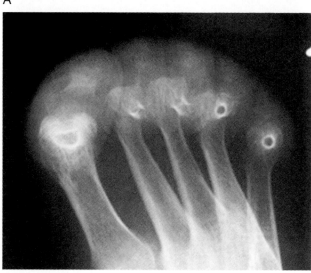

B

Figure 7–4   Photograph (**A**) and radiograph (**B**) of claw toe deformities involving hammer toe deformity associated with dorsiflexion of metatarsophalangeal joint.

mities of the forefoot in shoe-wearing societies (Fig. 7–8). DuVries[51] thought that shoes restrict the normal movement of the joints and impede the actions of the intrinsic muscles of the foot. It must be kept in mind, however, that anatomic predisposing factors vary extensively, and a large number of shoe wearers do escape deformities of the forefoot.

Mallet Toe

Other than its general relationship to pressure of the toe against the shoe, the specific cause of a mallet toe is unknown. Although most often idiopathic in nature, it can develop following a hammer toe repair or trauma,[28] or it can be associated with inflammatory arthritis.[28,29] The high incidence of mallet toe in the female population has led to speculation that a constricting toe box is a causative factor.[24,27,28] Female subjects constituted 84% of the patient population in

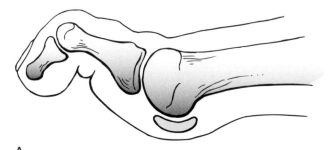

A

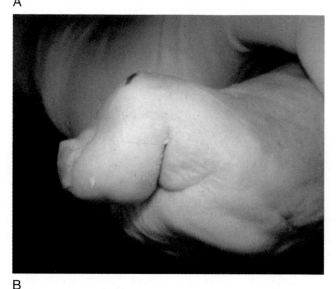

B

Figure 7–5   **A,** Hammered great toe. Note articulation of distal phalanx with plantar surface of the head of the proximal phalanx. **B,** Hammer toe deformity of hallux.

one reported series,[30] the gender difference being highly significant. Brahms[12] stated that a mallet toe is often limited to one toe, although Mann and Coughlin[100] noted that the deformity can occur in more than one toe. Coughlin[28] noted in his report (60 patients,

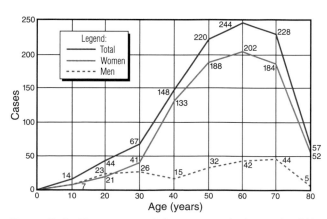

Figure 7–6   Hammer toe deformities peak during the fifth, sixth, and seventh decades in the female population. In the male population there is no increase in the frequency of hammer toe deformities with increasing age. (From Coughlin MJ, Thompson FM: *Instr Course Lect* 44:371-377, 1995.)

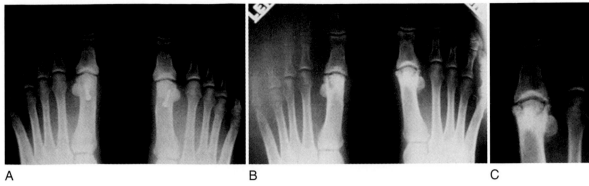

A   B   C

Figure 6–206 **A** and **B,** Sequence of radiographs demonstrating the development of central avascular necrosis (AVN) after placement of a screw for internal fixation. **C,** Close-up of AVN.

Adequate internal fixation of the osteotomy site can prevent most of these problems.

After a distal oblique osteotomy or Wilson bunion procedure where mild to moderate shortening of the first ray is permitted, the incidence of elevatus was reported to be as high as 20% in one series.[290] The pressure of weight bearing presents a significant risk to an osteotomy with inadequate internal fixation.

Realignment of a malunited distal metatarsal osteotomy is associated with many technical difficulties. Realignment of the osteotomy site may require extensive soft tissue stripping, which increases the risk of AVN. Successful realignment can be achieved, yet significant joint arthrofibrosis may develop due to soft tissue adhesions. MTP joint arthrodesis is probably the most reliable method to salvage this condition.

AVASCULAR NECROSIS

The blood supply to the metatarsal head must be protected with a distal osteotomy (see Figs. 6–64 and 6–65). Interruption of the vascular supply to the capital fragment after extensive dissection around the MTP joint with a distal metatarsal osteotomy can result in partial or complete AVN of the metatarsal head. The development of AVN does not necessarily mean that the joint will become symptomatic.

For some methods of distal osteotomy in which various techniques of internal fixation are used (i.e., screws instead of pins), more soft tissue stripping is necessary to gain adequate exposure for insertion of the fixation device. Although fixation is vitally important, the magnitude of soft tissue dissection should be minimized to prevent problems with AVN (Figs. 6–206 and 6–207).

The incidence of AVN, particularly after distal osteotomies, varies considerably. Meier and Kenzora[260] reported an incidence of 20% in 60 patients and pointed out that 40% of patients in whom AVN developed had also undergone some type of lateral release; however, only 15% of the patients were deemed symptomatic. Johnston[176] demonstrated cystic changes in 7 of 50 chevron procedures, along with 1 case of complete and 1 of partial AVN. Other authors of large series reported no cases of AVN.[134,149,279,283,350] Although it is difficult to determine the incidence of this complica-

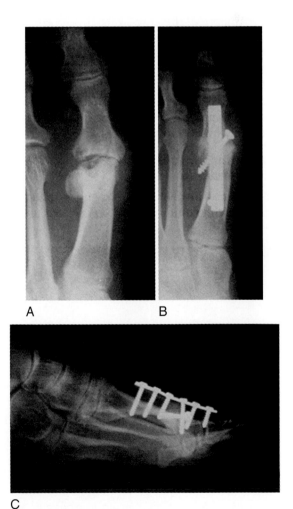

A   B

C

Figure 6–207 Treatment of avascular necrosis with arthrodesis of the metatarsophalangeal joint. **A** to **C,** Central avascular necrosis corrected by arthrodesis.

tion,[231] it is probably uncommon (see Figs. 6–129 to 6–131).

Three separate studies describe a lateral soft tissue release with the chevron procedure. Peterson et al[279] reviewed 58 cases and reported 1 case of AVN. Pochatko et al[283] reported on 23 cases with no AVN. Thomas et al[343] reviewed 80 cases in which lateral capsular release was carried out through a plantar incision along with excision of the fibular sesamoid and found no AVN. On the basis of these studies, a careful lateral release that respects the metaphyseal and capital blood supply should avoid damage to the vascularity of the metatarsal head.

AVN may be accompanied by marked pain and arthrofibrosis of the joint. Treatment of this complication usually requires MTP arthrodesis. When the arthrodesis is performed, every effort should be made to excise the avascular portion. This may leave the toe somewhat shortened, but it is preferable to placement of an interpositional bone graft, which may take a lengthy time to unite.

AVN is reported after the Mitchell procedure (see Fig. 6–137I). Blum[25] reported a 2% incidence of AVN. Salvage with MTP joint arthrodesis is the procedure of choice.

Of historic interest, after the LeLeivre bunion procedure, a 20% incidence of AVN has been reported.[169,293] Currently, this procedure is rarely performed due to the unacceptably high incidence of AVN.

Complications Involving the Proximal Phalanx

Complications involving a proximal phalangeal osteotomy are uncommon. Some are related to place-ment of the osteotomy, whereas others result from inadequate fixation of the osteotomy site.[282] When malunion or nonunion occurs, a salvage procedure may be technically difficult due to the small size of the phalanx.

NONUNION

Delayed union or nonunion of the phalanx seems to occur most frequently when the osteotomy is in the midshaft or distal phalanx rather than within the proximal third of the phalanx. The diaphyseal region may be at risk for delayed healing; however, with the passage of time, most phalangeal osteotomies do heal. In the presence of phalangeal nonunion, waiting for a period of 4 to 5 months may allow healing to occur (Fig. 6–208).

MALUNION

Malunion of the proximal phalanx usually occurs as a result of loss of fixation or inadequate internal fixation at the osteotomy site. Loss of position is not generally of sufficient magnitude to require corrective surgery (see Fig. 6–145B).

AVASCULAR NECROSIS

Although AVN generally occurs in the metatarsal head, occasionally it occurs in the proximal phalanx. After a proximal phalangeal osteotomy, AVN may develop due to excessive soft tissue and capsular stripping or excessive manipulation of the osteotomy site. AVN presents a difficult salvage situation; typically, a Keller procedure or arthrodesis is required to correct the problem.

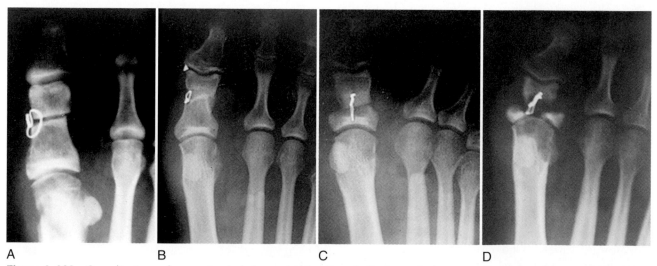

A   B   C   D

Figure 6–208 Complications after proximal phalangeal osteotomy. **A,** Radiograph demonstrating delayed union, which usually results because the osteotomy site is in the diaphysis rather than the metaphyseal portion of the bone. **B,** Sequence of radiographs demonstrating progressive avascular necrosis of the proximal phalanx after revision of the osteotomy site (**C**) and eventual complete collapse (**D**).

ADHESIONS OF THE FLEXOR HALLUCIS LONGUS

After a proximal phalangeal osteotomy, particularly if done in the midportion of the phalanx, the flexor hallucis longus tendon may be disrupted or become adherent to the osteotomy site. Flexion of the interphalangeal joint is either absent or significantly diminished. This complication can usually be avoided by adequately mobilizing and retracting the flexor hallucis longus tendon before performing the osteotomy to avoid inadvertent damage when the osteotomy is performed.

VIOLATION OF THE METATARSOPHALANGEAL JOINT

With a proximal phalangeal osteotomy, the osteotomy may inadvertently violate the MTP joint. The proximal phalanx has a concave articular surface. When the osteotomy is performed, care must be take to ensure that the proximal cut is distal to the articular surface. With this complication, arthrofibrosis or degenerative arthritis may develop and require MTP joint arthrodesis.

INSTABILITY AFTER RESECTION OF THE BASE (KELLER PROCEDURE)

With resection of the base of the proximal phalanx after a Keller procedure, the intrinsic muscle insertion to the toe is sacrificed. Attempts to restabilize the MTP joint involve reattachment of the intrinsic muscles to the proximal phalanx stump or suturing of the flexor hallucis longus tendon to the proximal phalanx. Although some procedures do help stabilize the joint, the forces involved in walking tend to over time force the remaining portion of the hallux into dorsiflexion and lateral deviation. With a fixed deformity, the toe pulp no longer strikes the ground. This creates a significant problem with footwear (Fig. 6–209; see also Figs. 6–153 to 6–156). The incidence of this complication can usually be diminished by adequate stabilization of the hallux with a Steinmann pin (for a period of 4 weeks) after the Keller procedure.

Another complication associated with instability of the proximal phalanx is that weight bearing of the great toe is greatly diminished. Weight is transferred to the lateral metatarsals, and either metatarsalgia or a transfer lesion develops (see Fig. 6–154).

Correction of instability of the hallux generally requires MTP joint arthrodesis. We prefer not to lengthen the toe but to accept some shortening.[79] The success rate of primary fusion without a bone graft is approximately 95%,[79] versus about 70% when a bone graft is added (see Fig. 6–159).

This salvage type of arthrodesis usually requires internal fixation with two intramedullary threaded Steinmann pins. Deficient bone stock or severe osteopenia in the proximal phalanx makes plate or screw fixation very difficult. Most patients are satisfied with the results of this salvage procedure.[79] The fusion increases the functional length of the first metatarsal and creates a lever arm that diminishes the stress placed on the second metatarsal head, which often relieves the metatarsalgia (see Fig. 6–160).

Complications Associated with Capsular Tissue of the First Metatarsophalangeal Joint

LOSS OF CORRECTION SECONDARY TO FAILURE OF MEDIAL JOINT CAPSULAR TISSUE

The etiology of recurrent hallux valgus is multifactorial. One cause is inadequate medial capsulorrhaphy, regardless of the procedure performed. This failure can result from an intrinsic problem within the capsule, such as ganglion formation or degeneration within the substance of the medial capsular tissue, or with a very severe hallux valgus deformity, it can result from

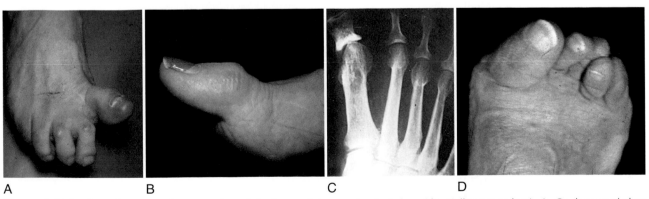

A   B   C   D

Figure 6–209 Complications after resection of the base of the proximal phalanx (the Keller procedure). **A,** Cock-up and claw toe deformity caused by loss of function of the intrinsic muscles inserting into the plantar aspect of the base of the proximal phalanx. **B,** Cock-up deformity. **C,** Hallux varus caused by excessive excision of the medial eminence. **D,** Recurrent hallux valgus after a Keller arthroplasty. (**D,** Courtesy of E. Greer Richardson, MD.)

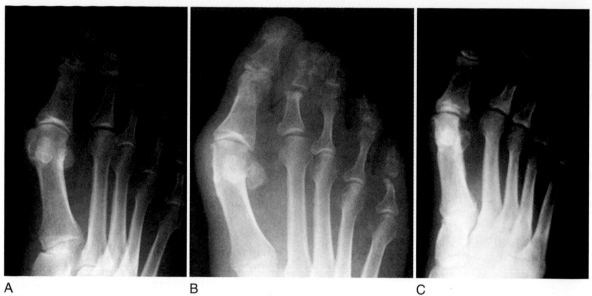

A   B   C

Figure 6–210 A-C, Recurrent hallux valgus deformity, probably caused by failure of the medial joint capsule to hold alignment of first metatarsophalangeal joint.

marked attenuation of the medial capsular tissue. When one of these conditions is encountered at surgery, it is preferable to imbricate the capsule rather than excise the medial capsule. A suture anchor can also be placed at the area of the defect to help stabilize the capsular deficiency. The formation of capsular fibrosis or scar tissue may prevent recurrence of the deformity (Fig. 6–210).

When the medial capsular flap is developed, it may be inadvertently detached at its proximal attachment. Anchoring the repair with metaphyseal drill holes may secure the proximal capsule. Postoperative dressings are crucial in this situation to afford adequate support while healing takes place. Likewise, inadequate postoperative dressings may allow capsular elongation or disruption of the capsular repair. This may necessitate a revision of the capsulorrhaphy, with substantial recurrence of the deformity.

FAILURE OF LATERAL JOINT CAPSULAR TISSUE

A significant lateral MTP joint contracture develops in most patients with a severe hallux valgus deformity. After lateral capsular release, a large gap is created that can be as long as 1 cm. With a defect of this size, it is uncommon for adequate tissue to re-form across this defect. This places the hallux at increased risk for a postoperative hallux varus deformity. Mann and Coughlin[237] observed that hallux varus occurred most commonly in feet in which a more severe deformity was corrected. To avoid this complication, the lateral joint capsule can be initially perforated with multiple small puncture incisions. Next, with varus pressure on

the hallux, the lateral capsule is gradually torn and the capsular tissue is "stretched out." This can lead to the formation of a large lateral capsular gap. Elevation and suturing of the adductor tendon to the lateral capsule aid in the re-formation of scar tissue in this area.

An alternative technique is to detach the capsule proximally and dorsally (L-shaped capsular release), which permits the lateral capsule to be slid distally as an entire unit, rather than incising it. The conjoined adductor tendon can actually be severed 3 cm proximal to its insertion and the stump sutured to the lateral capsule; this technique reinforces the lateral capsulorrhaphy as well.[70]

ARTHROFIBROSIS OF THE METATARSOPHALANGEAL JOINT

Marked arthrofibrosis of the MTP joint can occur after a hallux valgus reconstruction of any type. Restricted joint motion can be quite disabling if the toe is fixed in marked plantar flexion or dorsiflexion. If excessive stiffness around the joint is detected early during the postoperative period, early joint mobilization is initiated. When seen late, a vigorous course of physical therapy is instituted to mobilize the MTP joint. The arthrofibrosis will usually diminish in time and permit a functional but not normal range of motion. Joint manipulation may improve motion; however, repeat surgery in these patients rarely results in improved motion.

Complications Involving the Sesamoids

Repositioning of the sesamoids after hallux valgus surgery is difficult when the crista (which normally divides the plantar surface of the metatarsal head into two distinct articulating surfaces) is attenuated. Constant pressure by gradual migration of the metatarsal head off the sesamoid complex leads to erosion of the metatarsosesamoidal facets. Stabilization of the sesamoids is more difficult without a definite crista, and the sesamoids may assume a central rather than a medial position. Mann et al[242] were able to relocate the sesamoids from a medial to a normal or central location in 80% of cases; however, in the remaining cases the sesamoids remained in a lateral position.

Mann and Donatto[238] found no significant change in the tibial sesamoid position after a chevron osteotomy. Thus, a chevron procedure is contraindicated in a patient with preoperative pain attributed to the position of the tibial sesamoid beneath the metatarsal head.

Because the sesamoids are connected to the base of the proximal phalanx by the plantar plate, their location is determined in large part by the position and alignment of the proximal phalanx. If the sesamoids are not realigned adequately, more than likely the hallux valgus deformity has been undercorrected. In this situation, early recurrence is possible. Overcorrection of the position of the medial sesamoid leads to medial subluxation and a hallux varus deformity.

If the tibial sesamoid is located directly beneath the metatarsal crista, a plantar callus may develop. Shaving of the plantar half of the sesamoid will usually alleviate the problem (see Chapter 10).

UNCORRECTED SESAMOIDS

Inadequate correction of the position of the sesamoids generally results from failure to release the lateral MTP joint soft tissue contracture. This contracture is composed of several structures: the lateral joint capsule, the adductor tendon, and the transverse metatarsal ligament. The sesamoids cannot be mobilized and repositioned beneath the metatarsal head if this contracture is not released. The first metatarsal must be sufficiently mobile at the MTC joint to permit reduction of the metatarsal over the sesamoid complex. In the presence of fixed metatarsus primus varus or metatarsus adductus, unsuccessful relocation of the sesamoids requires a proximal osteotomy, or a recurrent hallux valgus deformity will develop.

MEDIAL SUBLUXATION OR DISLOCATION OF THE TIBIAL SESAMOID

Medial subluxation or complete dislocation of the tibial sesamoid may develop after a distal soft tissue procedure to correct a hallux valgus deformity. It may occur after an overcorrected proximal first metatarsal osteotomy or after lateral sesamoid excision, although it can occur even with the fibular sesamoid intact.

When the fibular sesamoid is excised, there is increased mobility of the sesamoid complex. A distal soft tissue realignment creates a situation in which medial displacement of the tibial sesamoid may occur. Subluxation or dislocation of the tibial sesamoid can also occur if the postoperative dressing holds the toe in excessive medial deviation or if a metatarsal osteotomy results in excessive lateral deviation of the metatarsal head.

Probably the most frequent cause of medial subluxation of the tibial sesamoid is excessive resection of the medial eminence. Although alignment of the sesamoids may not be too abnormal, absence of the plantar medial metatarsal articulation allows the tibial sesamoid to displace dorsally along the medial aspect of the metatarsal head. In time, this instability can lead to further medial migration of the sesamoid and a painful hallux varus deformity (Fig. 6–211).

Treatment of this complication must be individualized. A certain amount of medial subluxation of the sesamoid is often well tolerated. However, in very active persons, the medial sesamoid may become quite painful, even if a hallux varus deformity has not developed. Excision of the tibial sesamoid can be considered if it causes irritation along the medial aspect of the metatarsal head. Although excision of both sesamoids should be avoided, on occasion a painful tibial sesamoid is excised. If it has been a year or more since excision of the fibular sesamoid, the tibial

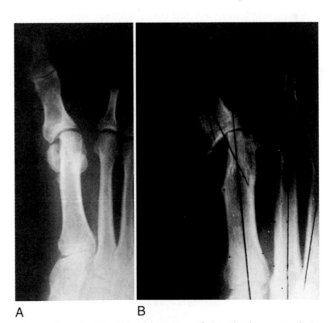

A   B

Figure 6–211 Medial subluxation of the tibial sesamoid. **A,** Excessive excision of the medial eminence and medial capsular plication resulting in medial subluxation of the sesamoid. **B,** Excessive excision of the medial eminence resulting in medial dislocation of the sesamoid.

sesamoid can be removed with only a small risk of a claw toe deformity developing. Medial dislocation of the tibial sesamoid is most commonly associated with a hallux varus deformity. When the hallux varus deformity is corrected, the tibial sesamoid is usually relocated beneath the metatarsal head.

With a severe hallux varus deformity, MTP joint arthrodesis is performed with excision of the dislocated tibial sesamoid.

COCK-UP DEFORMITY OF THE FIRST METATARSOPHALANGEAL JOINT

Plantar flexion of the first MTP joint is achieved primarily by the flexor hallucis brevis muscle, which inserts into the base of the proximal phalanx. With disruption of this mechanism, a muscle imbalance exists. The MTP joint is pulled into dorsiflexion by the unopposed force of the extensor hallucis brevis and the extensor hallucis longus. The flexor hallucis longus causes flexion of the interphalangeal joint. This deformity is often associated with hallux varus. After fibular sesamoid excision, the tibial sesamoid (which is the only connection between the flexor hallucis brevis and the proximal phalanx) is displaced medially. In this medially displaced position, no short flexor function is present at the MTP joint. Over time, soft tissue adhesions develop along with contracture of the abductor hallucis muscle, which leads to a fixed deformity (Fig. 6–212).

With previous tibial sesamoid excision, if a hallux valgus correction is performed with excision of the fibular sesamoid, a cock-up deformity can develop. Thus, under most circumstances, dual sesamoid excision, whether simultaneous or staged, should be avoided.

If a cock-up deformity of the hallux develops after removal of both sesamoids, treatment is tailored to the magnitude and rigidity of the deformity. In patients with a flexible MTP joint (with a minimum of 10 degrees of passive plantar flexion), an interphalangeal joint arthrodesis is performed. This procedure realigns the fixed flexion deformity of the interphalangeal joint and also permits the flexor hallucis longus tendon to function as a plantar flexor of the MTP joint. With a fixed extension contracture of the MTP joint, a "first-toe Jones procedure" is performed. This procedure involves transfer of the extensor hallucis longus tendon to the neck of the metatarsal. Transfer of this tendon provides the metatarsal head with a dorsiflexion force but also releases the dorsal contracture of the first MTP joint. A simultaneous interphalangeal joint arthrodesis realigns the interphalangeal joint and restores flexion power to the MTP joint (see Chapter 16). After a Keller procedure, a cock-up deformity is caused by loss of function of the flexor hallucis brevis

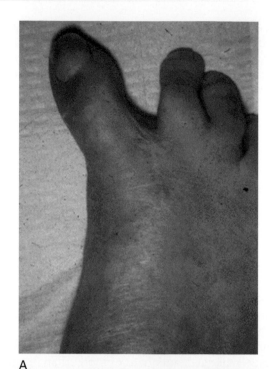

A

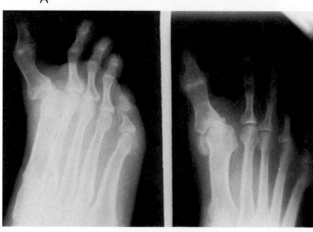

B

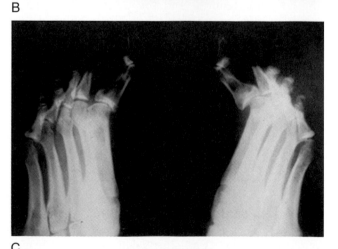

C

Figure 6–212 Cock-up varus deformity of the metatarsophalangeal joint after a McBride-type bunion repair. **A,** Clinical and, **B** and **C,** radiographic views.

muscle. This deformity is best treated by MTP joint arthrodesis rather than attempting to transfer a tendon to this small, unstable segment of the proximal phalanx (see Figs. 6–130 and 6–159).

INTRACTABLE PLANTAR KERATOSIS

After correction of a hallux valgus deformity, an intractable plantar keratosis may develop beneath the first metatarsal head. This lesion corresponds to the location of the tibial sesamoid, which at times is located in a central position directly beneath the metatarsal head. With progression of a hallux valgus deformity, the intersesamoidal ridge or crista is eroded by lateral pressure from the medial sesamoid. The crista is a major stabilizer of the sesamoid complex. With a relatively flat plantar metatarsal surface, the tibial sesamoid may be located centrally, which can be a source of pain for the patient.

Conservative treatment involves placing a metatarsal pad proximal to the sesamoid to relieve plantar pressure. Periodic trimming of the lesion is helpful. If the callosity continues to be painful, shaving the plantar half of the medial sesamoid usually produces a satisfactory clinical response (see Chapter 10). Excision of the tibial sesamoid should be avoided, especially if the lateral sesamoid has previously been removed. Dual sesamoid excision can result in a cock-up deformity of the first MTP joint because it disrupts the remaining short flexor function that stabilizes the first MTP joint. If the fibular sesamoid has not previously been removed, tibial sesamoidectomy is an option. Tibial sesamoid shaving, however, frequently alleviates the symptoms associated with a painful plantar callus in this area and is associated with much less morbidity than excision of the tibial sesamoid bone is.

Recurrent Hallux Valgus Deformity

Many factors need to be considered when evaluating a recurrent hallux valgus deformity. The characteristics of the initial deformity must be considered, as well as whether the correct surgical procedure was selected. Review of the postoperative management with the patient may provide information on the reason for failure.

The following broad categories need to be considered:

* Was selection of the surgical procedure appropriate?
* Were there technical problems during the course of the procedure that made it difficult to bring about complete correction?
* Was there a soft tissue problem, such as inadequate medial joint capsule secondary to capsular

attenuation or ganglion formation within the capsule?
* Was postoperative care inadequate?

These general questions are appropriate for the review of any recurrent hallux valgus deformity. For each general group of hallux valgus procedures, certain problems arise. They are briefly discussed in the following section.

Distal Soft Tissue Procedure

For a distal soft tissue procedure to succeed, adequate release of the distal soft tissues must be performed. The lateral capsular structures, including the adductor tendon insertion into the sesamoid and proximal phalanx, must be released along with the lateral joint capsule. The transverse metatarsal ligament must also be released from the sesamoid complex to allow the sesamoids to rotate beneath the metatarsal head. The medial joint capsule must be adequately plicated. If it has deteriorated secondary to cyst formation or a ganglion involving the capsular tissue, it will have insufficient strength to stabilize the joint.

The main reason for failure of a distal soft tissue procedure is failure to recognize that significant metatarsus primus varus is present. A distal soft tissue procedure cannot be used to correct a fixed bone deformity (see Fig. 6–92). A "simple bunionectomy" fails to release the lateral joint contracture, and recurrence is common.

Chevron Procedure

A frequent cause of recurrent hallux valgus after a chevron procedure is when it is selected to correct a deformity that is of greater magnitude than the procedure was intended for. Failure to appreciate joint congruency and a lateral slope of the distal metatarsal articular surface will prevent full correction with the chevron procedure. The DMAA should be measured before a chevron procedure. If it is greater than 15 degrees, a medial closing wedge chevron or an Akin procedure should be added (see Fig. 6–119). Inadequate capsular plication may also be another cause of recurrence. If the osteotomy is not stabilized with internal fixation, deformation may occur at the osteotomy site, with the capital fragment drifting medially and the toe laterally (see Fig. 6–197D and E).

Proximal Metatarsal Osteotomy

Recurrent deformity after a crescentic, closing wedge, or chevron-shaped proximal metatarsal osteotomy usually results from inadequate bone correction. This may be caused by failure to rotate the osteotomy site adequately or failure to remove enough bone to correct the metatarsus primus varus (Fig. 6–213).

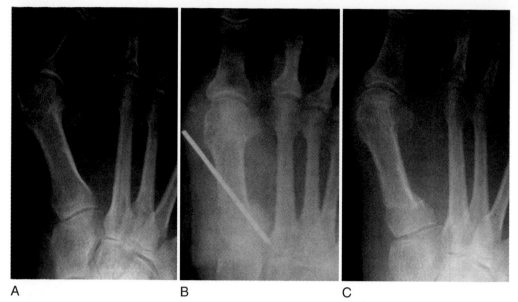

A   B   C

Figure 6–213   Recurrent hallux valgus deformity from inadequate medial displacement of the proximal metatarsal fragment at metatarsocuneiform joint after osteotomy. Preoperative radiographs (**A**) demonstrate lack of correction of the intermetatarsal angle after proximal metatarsal osteotomy (**B**), and recurrent hallux valgus develops (**C**).

Recurrence may also be caused by failure of the associated distal soft tissue procedure.

Akin Procedure

Recurrent deformities after an Akin procedure are generally the result of performing the procedure when it is not indicated. If there is incongruence or subluxation of the MTP joint, the Akin procedure rarely will bring about lasting correction of the deformity, and rapid recurrence may result (see Fig. 6–147). Likewise, an increased 1-2 intermetatarsal angle cannot be corrected with a phalangeal osteotomy and distal soft tissue repair.

Keller Procedure

After a Keller procedure, instability often develops at the MTP joint because the base of the proximal phalanx has been resected. As a result, the proximal phalanx may drift back into a valgus deformity and result in recurrent hallux valgus (see Fig. 6–209D). Typically, a Keller procedure corrects only about 50% of the angular deformity present with hallux valgus.

Preoperative Conditions

Certain underlying conditions associated with a hallux valgus deformity may preclude a satisfactory result. It is important to recognize these situations so that they can be addressed when performing the bunion procedure. At the very least, a patient should be alerted to the fact that the surgery may not be completely successful.

The following conditions, when present, may preclude obtaining a satisfactory result and should be considered in the preoperative planning:

- Lateral deviation of the distal articular surface will preclude complete correction of the MTP joint. This problem can be corrected with a medial closing wedge chevron procedure or a closing wedge metatarsal or phalangeal osteotomy.

- An underlying arthritic condition (hallux rigidus, rheumatoid arthritis) may be accompanied by inadequate capsular tissue to support a soft tissue repair. Likewise, articular cartilage degeneration may be present. In this situation, MTP joint arthrodesis should be considered for correction of the hallux valgus deformity.

- When joint hyperelasticity is present (Ehlers-Danlos syndrome), little can be done to increase stability of the joints other than MTP joint arthrodesis.

- With a severely pronated foot, rear foot surgery may be necessary to realign the foot and should be performed before a hallux valgus repair. If not corrected, the deformity may recur.

- If first ray hypermobility is present, MTC arthrodesis is performed in conjunction with the repair.

- When a significant equinus deformity at the ankle joint is present in conjunction with a hallux valgus deformity, the foot must be corrected to a plantigrade position before hallux valgus repair is attempted.

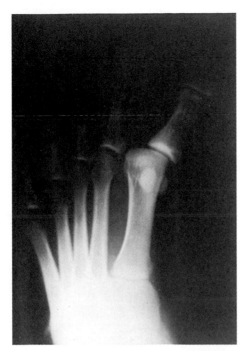

Figure 6–214 Congenital hallux varus deformity.

- If spasticity of any cause is present, an MTP joint soft tissue realignment is at high risk for failure, and an MTP joint arthrodesis is the procedure of choice.

HALLUX VARUS

Hallux varus is medial deviation of the great toe. Similar to hallux valgus deformities, hallux varus has varying degrees of severity and causes. This condition can occur on a congenital basis, although this is quite uncommon (Fig. 6–214). More frequently it is a defor-

mity acquired after either a surgical procedure or trauma in which the lateral collateral ligament of the hallux is ruptured. Hallux varus may occur after a distal soft tissue or McBride type of bunionectomy,[237,241] but it is also observed after the chevron, Mitchell, Keller, and Lapidus procedures.

The classic hallux varus deformity after the McBride procedure in which the fibular sesamoid is excised is characterized by MTP joint hyperextension, interphalangeal joint flexion, and medial deviation of the hallux (video clip 31). Anatomically, this deformity results from a muscle imbalance caused by medial dislocation of the tibial sesamoid, although other factors are involved as well (Fig. 6–215A).

The MTP joint is flexed by the flexor hallucis brevis muscle primarily through its pull on the sesamoid complex. After fibular sesamoid excision, the MTP joint hyperextends as the metatarsal head "buttonholes" through the soft tissue defect created by the deficiency in the flexor hallucis brevis. The medial deviation is aggravated by the detachment of the adductor tendon when the medial sesamoid is removed and compounded by the unopposed pull of the abductor hallucis muscle.

With time it becomes a fixed deformity that makes it difficult for the patient to obtain comfortable footwear. The interphalangeal joint of the great toe becomes flexed because the long extensor tendon can no longer effectively extend the interphalangeal joint. Simultaneously, the long flexor tendon is stretched around the metatarsal head, which creates a constant flexion force on the interphalangeal joint. In time this entire deformity becomes rigid. When the metatarsal head does not buttonhole through the soft tissue defect, the hallux varus deformity consists mainly of medial deviation of the proximal phalanx without any significant cock-up deformity of the MTP joint or flexion of the interphalangeal joint (Fig. 6–215B-D).

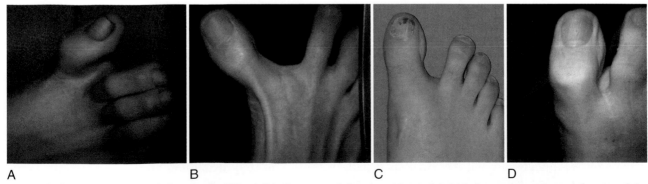

A   B   C   D

Figure 6–215 Hallux varus deformity. **A,** "Classic" hallux varus deformity with medial deviation and a cock-up deformity of the first metatarsophalangeal (MTP) joint after a distal soft tissue procedure. **B,** Hallux varus deformity with medial deviation of the MTP joint but no cock-up deformity of the joint. This type of varus may occur with both sesamoids intact. **C,** Mild hallux varus deformity. **D,** Mild varus associated with a mild cock-up deformity of the first MTP joint and flexion of the interphalangeal joint.

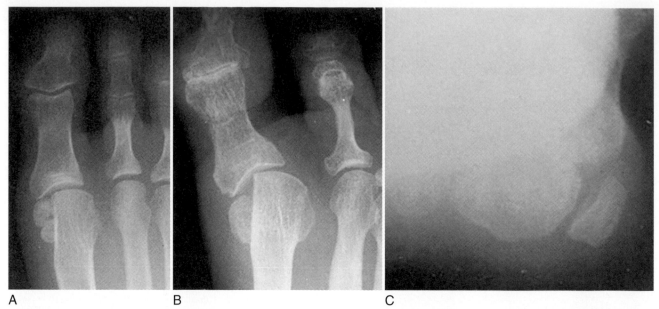

A   B   C

Figure 6–216   Various causes of hallux varus. **A,** Varus deformity, probably caused by overplication of the medial capsular structures. **B,** Medial displacement of the tibial sesamoid resulting in a varus deformity, probably caused by imbalance from lack of adequate lateral joint stability. **C,** Sesamoid view demonstrating medial displacement of the tibial sesamoid as a result of or resulting in a hallux varus deformity.

The following soft tissue factors can contribute to a hallux varus deformity:

- Overplication of the medial capsule (Fig. 6–216A)
- Medial displacement of the tibial sesamoid (Fig. 6–216B and C)
- Overpull of the abductor hallucis muscle against an incompetent lateral ligamentous complex (Fig. 6–217A-E)
- Overcorrection with a postoperative dressing holding the MTP joint in a varus position
- Excessive resection of the medial eminence (Fig. 6–217 F and G)

Hallux varus may occur after a proximal or distal metatarsal osteotomy when the metatarsal head is translated too far laterally, or if too much metatarsal head is resected, the potential exists for MTP joint instability and hallux varus.

With a chevron osteotomy, if the capital fragment is excessively displaced lateral-ward, a hallux varus deformity can develop (Fig. 6–218A). Likewise with a proximal osteotomy, the distal segment can be translated too far laterally (Fig. 6–218B-G). With a crescentic osteotomy, we initially directed the concavity distally toward the great toe. If the metatarsal osteotomy site is translated too far medially, excessive lateral translation of the metatarsal head occurs. Once this problem was recognized, the concavity was reversed so that it

faced proximally toward the heel. With this orientation, overtranslation rarely occurs because the distal metatarsal segment is locked into the proximal segment. Less commonly, a lateral closing wedge or proximal chevron osteotomy or Lapidus procedure can be overcorrected. This can create the dual deformity of overcorrection and shortening.

A hallux varus deformity must be carefully evaluated to determine which salvage procedure is appropriate.

If the varus deformity is caused by overplication of the medial capsule, release of the medial capsule may be effective. With a fixed deformity, however, a soft tissue capsular release is rarely effective. Plication of the lateral capsule can be added to the medial capsular release, but this does not generally produce a lasting result.

With medial displacement of the tibial sesamoid after excision of the fibular sesamoid or excessive resection of the medial eminence, a more aggressive surgical repair is necessary. In the initial determination, the question is whether sufficient articular surface remains to permit adequate joint function after realignment. In the presence of degenerative arthrosis, a soft tissue reconstruction is contraindicated because the MTP joint will only deteriorate further. Arthrodesis is the appropriate salvage procedure, although MTP joint motion is sacrificed.

In a hallux varus deformity with reasonable articular surface remaining, the extensor hallucis longus

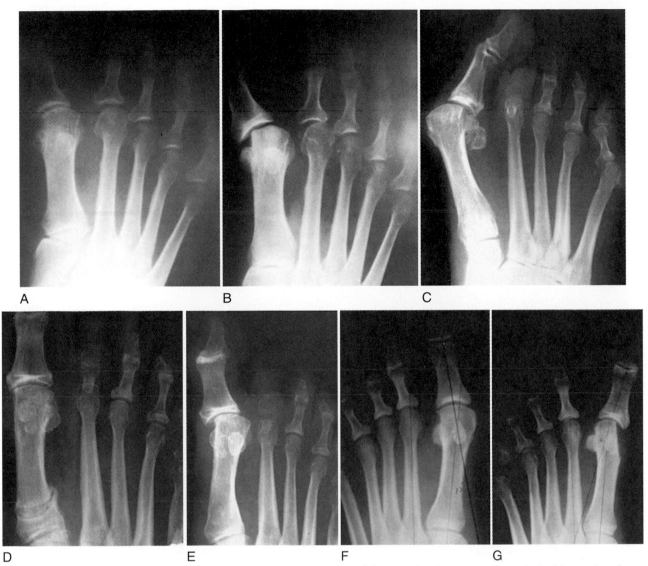

A   B   C

D   E   F   G

Figure 6–217 **A,** Immediately postoperatively. **B,** Progressive varus deformity developing over a period of 8 months after a distal soft tissue procedure. Note that both sesamoids are intact. This varus probably occurred because of lack of adequate lateral ligamentous stability. **C,** Preoperative radiograph. **D,** One month postoperatively, a radiograph demonstrates satisfactory alignment of the metatarsophalangeal joint. **E,** Two years postoperatively, a varus deformity has developed, probably from lack of reestablishment of the lateral ligamentous complex. Preoperative (**F**) and postoperative (**G**) radiographs demonstrate hallux varus caused by excessive excision of the medial eminence.

tendon can be used to create a dynamic correction of the deforming forces. Initially, the entire extensor hallucis longus tendon was transferred beneath the transverse metatarsal ligament and inserted into the base of the proximal phalanx of the great toe.[175] This was coupled with interphalangeal joint arthrodesis. Although this technique can produce a satisfactory result, if the interphalangeal joint does not have a fixed deformity (or can be straightened to within 10-15 degrees of full extension), it is not necessary to sacrifice interphalangeal joint function. Furthermore, if the extensor hallucis longus transfer fails and MTP joint arthrodesis is necessary, a mobile and functional interphalangeal joint is preferable. Therefore, we modified the original procedure and split the extensor hallucis longus tendon. A portion is transferred and a portion is left intact to control the interphalangeal joint of the hallux.

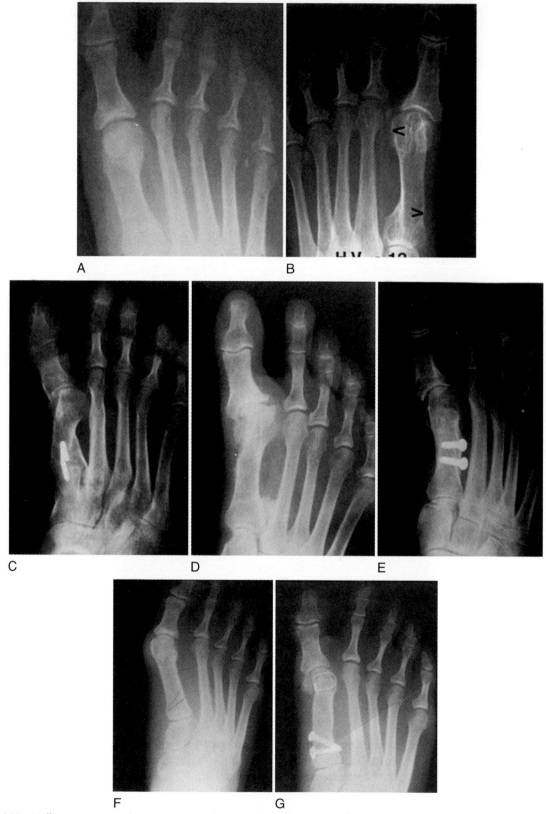

Figure 6–218   Hallux varus secondary to metatarsal osteotomies. **A,** Varus deformity after a chevron osteotomy. **B,** Varus deformity after a proximal crescentic osteotomy with excessive medial displacement of the base of the osteotomy leading to lateral translation of the metatarsal head. **C,** Varus deformity after an oblique metatarsal osteotomy resulting in excessive lateral translation of the metatarsal head. **D,** Varus deformity after metatarsophalangeal arthrodesis secondary to lateral displacement of the metatarsal head. **E,** Varus deformity secondary to midshaft metatarsal osteotomy with excessive lateral displacement of the metatarsal head. Preoperative (**F**) and postoperative (**G**) radiographs demonstrate a hallux varus deformity after proximal and distal metatarsal osteotomy.

EXTENSOR HALLUCIS LONGUS TRANSFER

The surgical technique for correction of hallux varus is divided into the surgical approach and preparation for the tendon transfer, release of the medial joint contracture, and reconstruction of the MTP joint.

Surgical Approach and Preparation for Tendon Transfer

1. A dorsal curvilinear incision is made starting just lateral to the insertion of the extensor hallucis longus tendon. The incision is carried laterally toward the first web space and follows the interval between the first and second metatarsals. It is then inclined medially and ends along the lateral aspect of the extensor hallucis longus tendon in the region of the first MTC joint (Fig. 6–219A).

2. The extensor hallucis tendon is dissected free of soft tissue attachments, and the lateral two thirds of the tendon is released from its insertion. Starting with the free end, the tendon is carefully "teased out" proximally to the level of the MTC joint (Fig. 6–219B and video clip 31). If when developing the lateral two thirds of the tendon the remaining portion of the tendon is inadvertently ruptured, it can be repaired by suturing the extensor hallucis brevis tendon to it.

3. The transverse metatarsal ligament is identified and a right-angle clamp or Mixner clamp is passed beneath it. Even if the transverse metatarsal ligament had been released at the time of the initial surgery, a sufficient amount of ligament usually re-forms. This remnant of the transverse metatarsal ligament is used as a pulley for the extensor tendon (Fig. 6–219C). A ligature is passed beneath the transverse metatarsal ligament to be used later in the procedure for pulling the extensor hallucis longus tendon beneath it.

Medial Joint Capsule Release

1. The medial aspect of the MTP joint is approached through a long midline incision beginning just proximal to the interphalangeal joint and ending at the midportion of the metatarsal shaft. Full-thickness dorsal and plantar skin flaps are developed, with care taken to avoid the cutaneous nerves. Too thin a skin flap can inadvertently result in sloughing of skin.

2. The medial joint capsule is cut obliquely starting at the plantar medial aspect of the base of the proximal phalanx where the abductor hallucis tendon inserts. The capsulotomy proceeds obliquely in a proximal and dorsal direction. This flap is dissected off the metatarsal head to permit the proximal phalanx to be brought out of its fixed varus deformity. A 5- to 7-mm gap is usually created in the capsular tissue.

3. The abductor hallucis tendon is identified beneath the cut in the capsule, and a long oblique cut releases the last remaining deforming force. At this point the proximal phalanx can be brought into a valgus position with no resistance. If resistance is still present, some residual medial structure has not been adequately released.

4. If the tibial sesamoid is displaced medially, the abductor hallucis tendon must be freed from its attachment to it to permit the sesamoid to be placed back beneath the metatarsal head. If too much of the metatarsal head was resected at the initial surgery and the sesamoid cannot be replaced beneath the metatarsal head or if the medial sesamoid is too prominent, excision of the sesamoid should be considered (Fig. 6–219D).

5. If an MTP joint dorsiflexion contracture is present, it is treated by releasing the dorsal capsule, which enables the MTP joint to be brought into approximately 10 degrees of plantar flexion.

6. A transverse drill hole in the base of the proximal phalanx is started in the midline. It is important that the hole be drilled distal enough so that it does not inadvertently penetrate the articular surface of the proximal phalanx (Fig. 6–219E).

Reconstruction of the Metatarsophalangeal Joint

1. A ligature is placed on the end of the extensor hallucis longus tendon and is used to pass the tendon beneath the transverse metatarsal ligament.

2. With the ankle joint in dorsiflexion (which relaxes the extensor hallucis longus), the extensor hallucis longus tendon is passed through the drill hole in the base of the proximal phalanx. It is pulled taut, and the hallux is brought into valgus. The tendon is sutured into the periosteum along the medial aspect

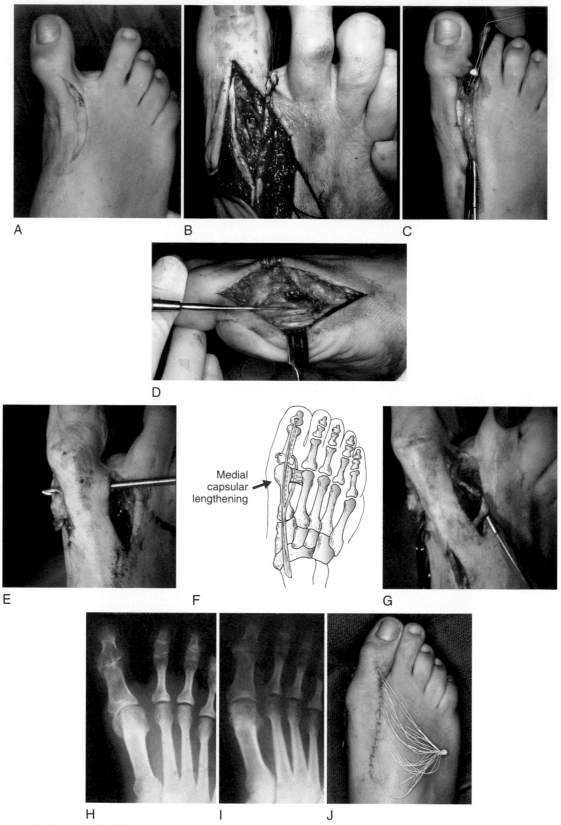

Figure 6–219 Technique of hallux varus correction. **A,** Initial skin incision. **B,** Detachment of the lateral two thirds of the extensor hallucis longus tendon and proximal split of the extensor tendon. **C,** The tendon is passed beneath the transverse metatarsal ligament. The ligature is pulled through and can be used later to pull the extensor tendon beneath the transverse metatarsal ligament. **D,** The medial joint capsule is released through a longitudinal incision. **E,** A transverse drill hole is made through the base of the proximal phalanx. **F,** Diagram demonstrating passage of the lateral two thirds of the extensor hallucis longus tendon beneath the transverse metatarsal ligament and across the proximal phalanx. Note that the medial capsular structures have been lengthened. **G,** The extensor tendon is pulled through the drill hole in the proximal phalanx as the ankle joint is held in dorsiflexion to gain added length of the tendon and the hallux is held in lateral deviation and slight plantar flexion. **H,** Preoperative radiograph. **I,** Postoperative radiograph demonstrating correction of the hallux varus deformity. **J,** Postoperative clinical appearance.

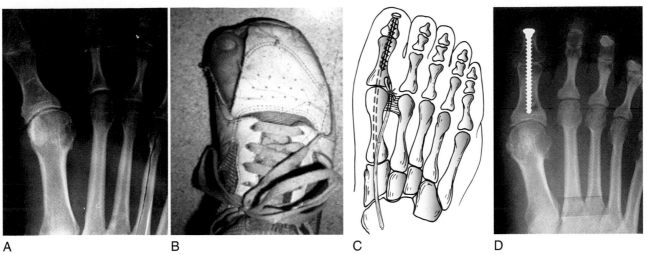

Figure 6–220 Complications after distal soft tissue repair. **A,** Hallux varus deformity after the McBride procedure. **B,** Footwear modified for the deformity. **C,** Schematic diagram of partial flexor hallucis longus transfer and interphalangeal joint fusion, which can be used to correct a hallux varus deformity. **D,** Postoperative radiograph after realignment.

of the proximal phalanx. At this point the toe should be aligned in approximately 10 to 15 degrees of valgus. If the toe still tends to drift into varus, either the soft tissue contracture on the medial side was inadequately released or the extensor hallucis longus tendon was not placed under sufficient tension (Fig. 6–219F and G).

3. The remaining medial third of the extensor hallucis longus tendon is plicated by weaving a suture through it to place it under tension.

4. The skin is closed with interrupted suture in routine manner, and a compression dressing is applied postoperatively (Fig. 6–125H and I).

Postoperative Care

The postoperative dressing is removed and replaced with a snug Kling dressing and adhesive tape to hold the toe in a slightly overcorrected valgus position. The patient is permitted to ambulate in a postoperative shoe. The dressings are changed weekly for 8 weeks. A postoperative shoe should be used for another 2 weeks to allow further maturation of the tendon transfer (Fig. 6–220).

This procedure will produce a satisfactory clinical result in about 80% of patients. Occasionally, slight overcorrection or undercorrection of the MTP joint occurs but is usually well tolerated. Typically, 50% to 60% of MTP joint motion is maintained after this procedure (Fig. 6–221).

If little or no motion is present at the MTP joint preoperatively, the patient should be advised that this procedure will not significantly improve range of motion but will improve the overall position of the hallux. Occasionally, minor skin slough develops in the skin along the medial side of the MTP joint or delayed wound healing occurs because of the tension created by pulling the toe into a valgus position from its previous varus position. We do not know how to avoid this problem because the medial incision cannot be placed in another location.

If the varus deformity develops after a resection arthroplasty (the Keller procedure), after excessive resection of the medial aspect of the metatarsal head, or in conjunction with MTP joint degenerative arthritis, MTP joint arthrodesis is the treatment of choice (see Figs. 6–159 and 6–160). Salvage with a silicone implant is contraindicated unless the deforming forces that led to the hallux varus deformity can be completely corrected. A joint replacement or silicone implant will maintain satisfactory joint alignment only if the surrounding soft tissues are well balanced.

A hallux varus deformity caused by nonunion of a metatarsal osteotomy is best corrected by MTP joint arthrodesis rather than an attempt at either tendon transfer or corrective metatarsal osteotomy. Although realignment osteotomy can occasionally be performed, complete balancing of the MTP joint soft tissues is crucial to obtain a successful and long-lasting correction.

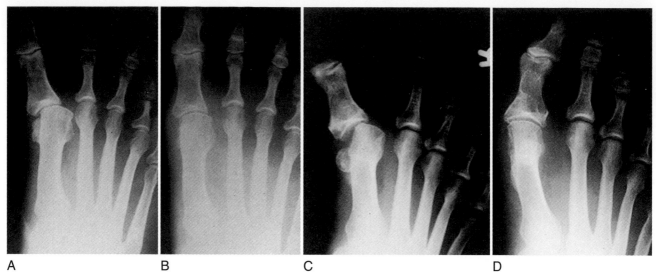

Figure 6–221 **A** and **C,** Hallux varus deformity resulting from a distal soft tissue procedure. **B** and **D,** Postoperative reconstructive procedure involving transfer of the extensor hallucis longus tendon.

PAIN AROUND THE FIRST METATARSOPHALANGEAL JOINT AFTER BUNION SURGERY

The most common complaint before bunion surgery is pain over the medial eminence.[242] Secondary problems include sesamoid pain, pain over the medial aspect of the great toe, pain from a transfer lesion beneath a lesser metatarsal head, and at times pain within the MTP joint. After hallux valgus surgery, regardless of the surgical procedure, most patients are satisfied with the reduction in pain over the medial eminence. Ten percent of patients continue to complain of pain around the first MTP joint area, and causes include nerve entrapment, degenerative MTP joint disease, sesamoid malalignment, and MTP joint arthrofibrosis. This discomfort is often poorly defined and rarely associated with clearly delineated intraarticular degenerative changes visible on radiographs. Although bone scans can define areas of arthritis, they are generally negative. Patients should be counseled preoperatively that they may have MTP joint discomfort after bunion surgery.[325]

PROSTHESES

The use of an MTP joint prosthesis in primary bunion surgery is rarely if ever indicated (Fig. 6–222). The occasional sedentary patient with advanced MTP joint degenerative arthritis who desires a prosthesis may be a candidate for the procedure. The use of a prosthesis in an active individual, regardless of age, is inadvisable because of the inherent problems of loosening, breakage, osteolysis, and synovitis and the high incidence of transfer metatarsalgia (Figs. 6–223 and 6–224).

The salvage procedure for a painful prosthesis entails removal of the prosthesis, complete joint synovectomy, placement of an intramedullary Kirschner wire to stabilize the joint, and soft tissue capsulorrhaphy. The Kirschner wire is removed 3 weeks after surgery and range-of-motion exercises are commenced.[196] After this technique, 70% to 80% of prostheses can be removed and the first ray salvaged without performing a simple arthrodesis or a much more extensive procedure entailing arthrodesis with an interposition bone block.[131,151]

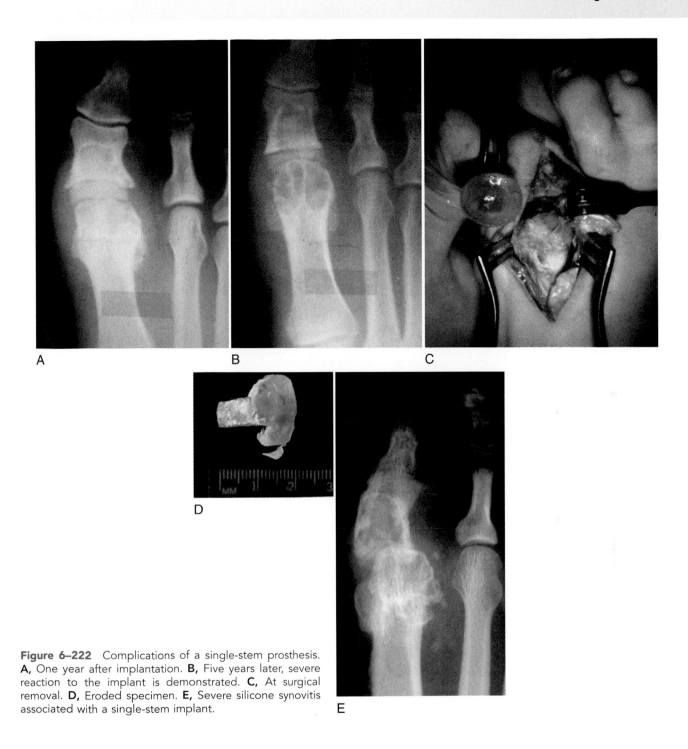

Figure 6–222 Complications of a single-stem prosthesis. **A,** One year after implantation. **B,** Five years later, severe reaction to the implant is demonstrated. **C,** At surgical removal. **D,** Eroded specimen. **E,** Severe silicone synovitis associated with a single-stem implant.

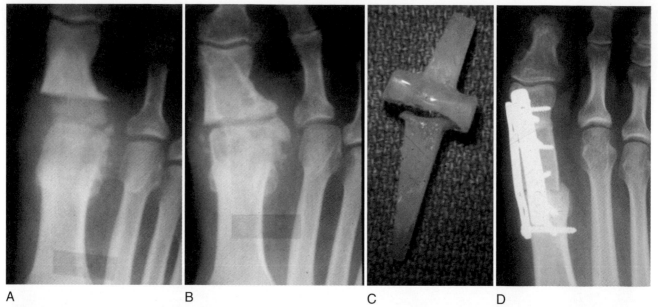

A   B   C   D

Figure 6–223 Complications of double-stem implants. **A,** Six months after implantation. **B,** Three years after surgery there is collapse and reaction surrounding the metatarsophalangeal joint. **C,** After removal later, the implant had fractured. **D,** A difficult salvage may involve an interposition bone graft. It is preferable to merely excise the reactive area and permanently remove the prosthesis when a severe reaction occurs.

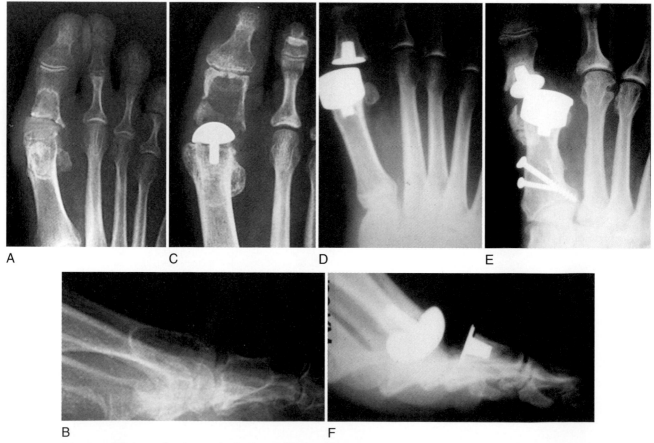

A   C   D   E

B   F

Figure 6–224 **A** and **B,** Lateral radiographs demonstrating settling and synovitis after implantation of a double-stemmed prosthesis. **C,** Severe osteolysis associated with loosening of components of a prosthetic replacement. **D-F,** Loosening of the metatarsal and phalangeal components with subluxation of the metatarsophalangeal joint.

REFERENCES

1. Akin O: The treatment of hallux valgus: A new operative procedure and its results. *Med Sentinel* 33:678-679, 1925.

2. Albrecht G: The pathology and treatment of hallux valgus. *Tussk Vrach* 10:14-19, 1911.

3. Amarnek DL, Jacobs AM, Oloff LM: Adolescent hallux valgus: Its etiology and surgical management. *J Foot Surg* 24:54-61, 1985.

4. Amarnek DL, Mollica A, Jacobs AM, Oloff LM: A statistical analysis on the reliability of the proximal articular set angle. *J Foot Surg* 25:39-43, 1986.

5. Anderson M, Blais MM, Green WT: Lengths of the growing foot. *J Bone Joint Surg Am* 38:998-1000, 1956.

6. Anderson R: Hallux valgus: Report of end results. *South Med J* 91:74-78, 1929.

7. Antrobus JN: The primary deformity in hallux valgus and metatarsus primus varus. *Clin Orthop* 184:251-255, 1984.

8. Austin DW, Leventen EO: A new osteotomy for hallux valgus: A horizontally directed "V" displacement osteotomy of the metatarsal head for hallux valgus and primus varus. *Clin Orthop* 157:25-30, 1981.

9. Austin DW, Leventen EO: *Scientific Exhibit: V-osteotomy of the First Metatarsal Head.* Chicago, American Academy of Orthopaedic Surgery, 1968.

10. Bacardi BE, Boysen TJ: Considerations for the Lapidus operation. *J Foot Surg* 25:133-138, 1986.

11. Badwey TM, Dutkowsky JP, Graves SC, Richardson EG: An anatomical basis for the degree of displacement of the distal chevron osteotomy in the treatment of hallux valgus. *Foot Ankle Int* 18:213-215, 1997.

12. Banks AS, Hsu YS, Mariash S, Zirm R: Juvenile hallux abducto valgus association with metatarsus adductus. *J Am Podiatr Med Assoc* 84:219-224, 1994.

13. Barca F, Busa R: Austin/chevron osteotomy fixed with bioabsorbable poly-L-lactic acid single screw. *J Foot Ankle Surg* 36:15-20; discussion 79-80, 1997.

14. Barnett CH: Valgus deviation of the distal phalanx of the great toe. *J Anat* 96:171-177, 1962.

15. Barnicot NA, Hardy RH: The position of the hallux in West Africans. *J Anat* 89:355-361, 1955.

16. Barouk LS: Osteotomie scarf du primier metarsien. *Med Surg Pied* 10:111-120, 1994.

17. Barouk LS: Scarf osteotomy of the first metatarsal in the treatment of hallux valgus. *Foot Dis* 2:35-48, 1991.

18. Barouk LS: Scarf osteotomy for hallux valgus correction. Local anatomy, surgical technique, and combination with other forefoot procedures. *Foot Ankle Clin* 5:525-558, 2000.

19. Bartolozzi P, Magnan BL: *Osteotomia Diatale Percutanea nella Chirurgia Dell'alluce Valgo.* Bologna, Italy, Timeo, 2000, pp 1-71.

20. Beauchamp CG, Kirby T, Rudge SR, et al: Fusion of the first metatarsophalangeal joint in forefoot arthroplasty. *Clin Orthop* 190:249-253, 1984.

21. Bednarz PA, Manoli A II: Modified Lapidus procedure for the treatment of hypermobile hallux valgus. *Foot Ankle Int* 21:816-821, 2000.

22. Beighton PGR, Bird H: *Hypermobility of Joints.* New York, Springer-Verlag, 1983, pp 10-12.

23. Berntsen A: De l'hallux valgus, contribution a son etiologie et a son traitement. *Rev Orthop* 17:101-111, 1930.

24. Bingold AC: Arthrodesis of the great toe. *Proc R Soc Med* 51:435-437, 1958.

25. Blum JL: The modified Mitchell osteotomy-bunionectomy: Indications and technical considerations. *Foot Ankle Int* 15:103-106, 1994.

26. Bock P, Kristen KH, Kroner A, Engel A: Hallux valgus and cartilage degeneration in the first metatarsophalangeal joint. *J Bone Joint Surg Br* 86:669-673, 2004.

27. Bonney G, Macnab I: Hallux valgus and hallux rigidus; a critical survey of operative results. *J Bone Joint Surg Br* 34:366-385, 1952.

28. Bordelon L (ed): *Surgical and Conservative Foot Care. A Unified Approach to Principles and Practice.* Thorofare, NJ, Slack, 1988, pp 13-14.

29. Borrelli AH, Weil LS: Modified scarf bunionectomy: Our experience in more than one thousand cases. *J Foot Surg* 30:609-612, 1991.

30. Borton DC, Stephens MM: Basal metatarsal osteotomy for hallux valgus. *J Bone Joint Surg Br* 76:204-209, 1994.

31. Bosch P, Markowski H, Rannicher V: Technik und erste Ergebnisse der subkutanen distalen Metatarsale-I-Osteotomie. *Orthop Praxis* 26:51-56, 1990.

32. Bosch P, Wanke S, Legenstein R: Hallux valgus correction by the method of Bosch: A new technique with a seven-to-ten-year follow-up. *Foot Ankle Clin* 5:485-498, v-vi, 2000.

33. Brage ME, Holmes JR, Sangeorzan BJ: The influence of x-ray orientation on the first metatarsocuneiform joint angle. *Foot Ankle Int* 15:495-497, 1994.

34. Brahm SM: Shape of the first metatarsal head in hallux rigidus and hallux valgus. *J Am Podiatr Med Assoc* 78:300-304, 1988.

35. Breslauer C, Cohen M: Effect of proximal articular set angle correcting osteotomies on the hallucal sesamoid apparatus: A cadaveric and radiographic investigation. *J Foot Ankle Surg* 40:366-373, 2001.

36. Briggs TW, Smith P, McAuliffe TB: Mitchell's osteotomy using internal fixation and early mobilisation. *J Bone Joint Surg Br* 74:137-139, 1992.

37. Broca P: Des difformities de la partie anterieure du pied produite par Faction de la chaussure. *Bull Soc Anat* 27:60-67, 1852.

38. Bryant A, Tinley P, Singer K: A comparison of radiographic measurements in normal, hallux valgus, and hallux limitus feet. *J Foot Ankle Surg* 39:39-43, 2000.

39. Burns AE, Varin J: Poly-L-lactic acid rod fixation results in foot surgery. *J Foot Ankle Surg* 37:37-41, 1998.

40. Burutaran H: Hallux valgus y cortedad anatomica del primer metatarsano (correction quinrugica). *Med Chir Pied* 13:261-266, 1976.

41. Butson AR: A modification of the Lapidus operation for hallux valgus. *J Bone Joint Surg Br* 62:350-352, 1980.

42. Campbell JT, Schon LC, Parks BG, et al: Mechanical comparison of biplanar proximal closing wedge osteotomy with plantar plate fixation versus crescentic osteotomy with screw fixation for the correction of metatarsus primus varus. *Foot Ankle Int* 19:293-299, 1998.

43. Canale PB, Aronsson DD, Lamont RL, Manoli A II: The Mitchell procedure for the treatment of adolescent hallux valgus. A long-term study. *J Bone Joint Surg Am* 75:1610-1618, 1993.

44. Carl A, Ross S, Evanski P, Waugh T: Hypermobility in hallux valgus. *Foot Ankle* 8:264-270, 1988.

45. Carr CR, Boyd BM: Correctional osteotomy for metatarsus primus varus and hallux valgus. *J Bone Joint Surg Am* 50:1353-1367, 1968.

46. Catanzariti AR, Mendicino RW, Lee MS, Gallina MR: The modified Lapidus arthrodesis: A retrospective analysis. *J Foot Ankle Surg* 38:322-332, 1999.

47. Cathcart E: Physiological aspect: Nature of incapacity. The feet of the industrial worker: Clinical aspect; relation to footwear. *Lancet* 2:1480-1482, 1938.

48. Cedell CA, Astrom M: Proximal metatarsal osteotomy in hallux valgus. *Acta Orthop Scand* 53:1013-1018, 1982.

49. Chana GS, Andrew TA, Cotterill CP: A simple method of arthrodesis of the first metatarsophalangeal joint. *J Bone Joint Surg Br* 66:703-705, 1984.

50. Chi TD, Davitt J, Younger A, et al: Intra- and inter-observer reliability of the distal metatarsal articular angle in adult hallux valgus. *Foot Ankle Int* 23:722-726, 2002.

51. Chiodo CP, Schon LC, Myerson MS: Clinical results with the Ludloff osteotomy for correction of adult hallux valgus. *Foot Ankle Int* 25:532-536, 2004.

52. Cholmeley JA: Hallux valgus in adolescents. *Proc R Soc Med* 51:903-906, 1958.

53. Chou LB, Mann RA, Casillas MM: Biplanar chevron osteotomy. *Foot Ankle Int* 19:579-584, 1998.

54. Clark HR, Veith RG, Hansen ST Jr: Adolescent bunions treated by the modified Lapidus procedure. *Bull Hosp Jt Dis Orthop Inst* 47:109-122, 1987.

55. Cleveland M, Winant EM: An end-result study of the Keller operation. *J Bone Joint Surg Am* 32:163-175, 1950.

56. Clutton H: The treatment of hallux valgus. *St Thomas Hosp Rep* 22:1-12, 1894.

57. Coetzee JC: Scarf osteotomy for hallux valgus repair: The dark side. *Foot Ankle Int* 24:29-33, 2003.

58. Coetzee JC, Resig SG, Kuskowski M, Saleh KJ: The Lapidus procedure as salvage after failed surgical treatment of hallux valgus. Surgical technique. *J Bone Joint Surg Am* 86(Suppl 1):30-36, 2004.

59. Coetzee JC, Wickum D: The Lapidus procedure: A prospective cohort outcome study. *Foot Ankle Int* 25:526-531, 2004.

60. Colloff B, Weitz EM: Proximal phalangeal osteotomy in hallux valgus. *Clin Orthop* 54:105-113, 1967.

61. Corless JR: A modification of the Mitchell procedure. *J Bone Joint Surg Br* 55/58:138, 1976.

62. Cornwall MW, Fishco WD, McPoil TG, et al: Reliability and validity of clinically assessing first-ray mobility of the foot. *J Am Podiatr Med Assoc* 94:470-476, 2004.

63. Coughlin MJ: Arthrodesis of the first metatarsophalangeal joint. *Orthop Rev* 19:177-186, 1990.

64. Coughlin MJ: Arthrodesis of the first metatarsophalangeal joint with mini-fragment plate fixation. *Orthopedics* 13:1037-1044, 1990.

65. Coughlin MJ: Hallux valgus. *J Bone Joint Surg Am* 78:932-966, 1996.

66. Coughlin MJ: Hallux valgus. Causes, evaluation, and treatment. *Postgrad Med* 75(5):174-178, 183, 186-187, 1984.

67. Coughlin MJ: Hallux valgus in the athlete. *J Sports Med Arthrosc Rev* 2:326-340, 1994.

68. Coughlin MJ: Hallux valgus in men: Effect of the distal metatarsal articular angle on hallux valgus correction. *Foot Ankle Int* 18:463-470, 1997.

69. Coughlin MJ: President's Forum: Evaluation and treatment of juvenile hallux valgus. *Contemp Orthop* 21:169-203, 1990.

70. Coughlin MJ: Proximal first metatarsal osteotomy. In Kitaoka H (ed): *The Foot and Ankle*, 2nd ed. Philadelphia, Williams & Wilkins, 2002, pp 71-98.

71. Coughlin MJ: Rheumatoid forefoot reconstruction. A long-term follow-up study. *J Bone Joint Surg Am* 82:322-341, 2000.

72. Coughlin MJ: Roger A. Mann Award. Juvenile hallux valgus: Etiology and treatment. *Foot Ankle Int* 16:682-697, 1995.

73. Coughlin MJ, Abdo RV: Arthrodesis of the first metatarsophalangeal joint with Vitallium plate fixation. *Foot Ankle Int* 15:18-28, 1994.

74. Coughlin MJ, Carlson RE: Treatment of hallux valgus with an increased distal metatarsal articular angle: Evaluation of double and triple first ray osteotomies. *Foot Ankle Int* 20:762-770, 1999.

75. Coughlin MJ, Freund E: Roger A. Mann Award. The reliability of angular measurements in hallux valgus deformities. *Foot Ankle Int* 22:369-379, 2001.

76. Coughlin MJ, Grebing BR, Jones CP: Arthrodesis of the metatarsophalangeal joint for idiopathic hallux valgus: Intermediate results. *Foot Ankle Int* 26:783-792, 2005.

77. Coughlin MJ, Jones CP: *Hallux valgus: Demographics, radiographic assessment and clinical outcomes. A prospective study.* Paper presented at the 21st annual summer meeting of the American Orthopaedic Foot and Ankle Society, July 17, 2005.

78. Coughlin MJ, Jones CP, Viladot R, et al: Hallux valgus and first ray mobility: A cadaveric study. *Foot Ankle Int* 25:537-544, 2004.

79. Coughlin MJ, Mann RA: Arthrodesis of the first metatarsophalangeal joint as salvage for the failed Keller procedure. *J Bone Joint Surg Am* 69:68-75, 1987.

80. Coughlin MJ, Mann RA: The pathophysiology of the juvenile bunion. *Instr Course Lect* 36:123-136, 1987.

81. Coughlin MJ, Saltzman CL, Nunley JA II: Angular measurements in the evaluation of hallux valgus deformities: A report of the ad hoc committee of the American Orthopaedic Foot & Ankle Society on angular measurements. *Foot Ankle Int* 23:68-74, 2002.

82. Coughlin MJ, Shurnas PS: Hallux rigidus. *J Bone Joint Surg Am* 86(Suppl 1):119-130, 2004.

83. Coughlin MJ, Shurnas PS: Hallux rigidus: Demographics, etiology, and radiographic assessment. *Foot Ankle Int* 24:731-743, 2003.

84. Coughlin MJ, Shurnas PS: Hallux rigidus. Grading and long term results of operative treatment. *J Bone Joint Surg Am* 85:2072-2088, 2003.

85. Coughlin MJ, Shurnas PS: Hallux valgus in men. Part II: First ray mobility after bunionectomy and factors associated with hallux valgus deformity. *Foot Ankle Int* 24:73-78, 2003.

86. Coughlin MJ, Thompson FM: The high price of high-fashion footwear. *Instr Course Lect* 44:371-377, 1995.

87. Craigmile DA: Incidence, origin, and prevention of certain foot defects. *BMJ* 4839:749-752, 1953.

88. Creer WS: The feet of the industrial worker: Clinical aspect; relation to footwear. *Lancet* 2:1482-1483, 1938.

89. Crevoisier X, Mouhsine E, Ortolano V, et al: The scarf osteotomy for the treatment of hallux valgus deformity: A review of 84 cases. *Foot Ankle Int* 22:970-976, 2001.

90. Das De S, Hamblen DL: Distal metatarsal osteotomy for hallux valgus in the middle-aged patient. *Clin Orthop* 218:239-246, 1987.

91. Davies-Colley N: Contraction of the metatarsophalangeal joint of the great toe (hallux flexus). *BMJ* 1:728, 1887.

92. Day MR, White SL, DeJesus JM: The "Z" osteotomy versus the Kalish osteotomy for the correction of hallux abducto valgus deformities: A retrospective analysis. *J Foot Ankle Surg* 36:44-50; discussion 80, 1997.

93. Deorio JK, Ware AW: Single absorbable polydioxanone pin fixation for distal chevron bunion osteotomies. *Foot Ankle Int* 22:832-835, 2001.

94. Dereymaeker G: Scarf osteotomy for correction of hallux valgus. Surgical technique and results as compared to distal chevron osteotomy. *Foot Ankle Clin* 5:513-524, 2000.

95. DiGiovanni CW, Kuo R, Tejwani N, et al: Isolated gastrocnemius tightness. *J Bone Joint Surg Am* 84:962-970, 2002.

96. Donley BG, Vaughn RA, Stephenson KA, Richardson EG: Keller resection arthroplasty for treatment of hallux valgus deformity: Increased correction with fibular sesamoidectomy. *Foot Ankle Int* 23:699-703, 2002.

97. Dreeben S, Mann RA: Advanced hallux valgus deformity: Long-term results utilizing the distal soft tissue procedure and proximal metatarsal osteotomy. *Foot Ankle Int* 17:142-144, 1996.

98. Durman DC: Metatarsus primus varus and hallux valgus. *AMA Arch Surg* 74:128-135, 1957.

99. DuVries H (ed): *Surgery of the Foot.* St Louis, CV Mosby, 1959, pp 346-442.

100. Easley ME, Kiebzak GM, Davis WH, Anderson RB: Prospective, randomized comparison of proximal crescentic and proximal chevron osteotomies for correction of hallux valgus deformity. *Foot Ankle Int* 17:307-316, 1996.

101. Ellis VH: A method of correcting metatarsus primus varus; preliminary report. *J Bone Joint Surg Br* 33:415-417, 1951.

102. Engel E, Erlick N, Krems I: A simplified metatarsus adductus angle. *J Am Podiatr Assoc* 73:620-628, 1983.

103. Engle ET, Morton DJ: Notes on foot disorders among natives of the Belgian Congo. *J Bone Joint Surg* 13:311, 1931.

104. Ewald P: Die Actiologie des Hallux valgus. *Dtsch Ztschr Chir* 114:90-103, 1912.

105. Faber FW, Kleinrensink GJ, Verhoog MW, et al: Mobility of the first tarsometatarsal joint in relation to hallux valgus deformity: Anatomical and biomechanical aspects. *Foot Ankle Int* 20:651-656, 1999.

106. Fadel GE, Rowley DI, Jain AS: Compression screw fixation for first metatarsal basal osteotomy. *Foot Ankle Int* 23:253-254, 2002.

107. Ferrari J, Malone-Lee J: A radiographic study of the relationship between metatarsus adductus and hallux valgus. *J Foot Ankle Surg* 42:9-14, 2003.

108. Ferrari J, Malone-Lee J: The shape of the metatarsal head as a cause of hallux abductovalgus. *Foot Ankle Int* 23:236-242, 2002.

109. Fitzgerald JA: A review of long-term results of arthrodesis of the first metatarso-phalangeal joint. *J Bone Joint Surg Br* 51:488-493, 1969.

110. Fokter SK, Podobnik J, Vengust V: Late results of modified Mitchell procedure for the treatment of hallux valgus. *Foot Ankle Int* 20:296-300, 1999.

111. Fox IM, Smith SD: Juvenile bunion correction by epiphysiodesis of the first metatarsal. *J Am Podiatr Assoc* 73:448-455, 1983.

112. Fritz GR, Prieskorn D: First metatarsocuneiform motion: A radiographic and statistical analysis. *Foot Ankle Int* 16:117-123, 1995.

113. Funk FJ Jr, Wells RE: Bunionectomy—with distal osteotomy. *Clin Orthop* 85:71-74, 1972.

114. Galland W, Jordan H: Hallux valgus. *Surg Gynecol Obstet* 66:95, 1938.

115. Geissele AE, Stanton RP: Surgical treatment of adolescent hallux valgus. *J Pediatr Orthop* 10:642-648, 1990.

116. Gerbert J: The indications and techniques for utilizing preoperative templates in podiatric surgery. *J Am Podiatr Assoc* 69:139-148, 1979.

117. Giannestras N: The Giannestras modification of the Lapidus operation. In Giannestras NJ (ed): *Foot Disorders: Medical and Surgical Management.* Philadelphia, Lea & Febiger, 1973.

118. Gill LH, Martin DF, Coumas JM, Kiebzak GM: Fixation with bioabsorbable pins in chevron bunionectomy. *J Bone Joint Surg Am* 79:1510-1518, 1997.

119. Gimple K, Anspacher J, Kopta J: Metatarsophalangeal joint fusion of the great toe. *Orthopedics* 1:462-467, 1978.

120. Ginsburg AI: Arthrodesis of the first metatarsophalangeal joint: A practical procedure. *J Am Podiatr Assoc* 69:367-369, 1979.

121. Glasoe WM, Allen MK, Saltzman CL: First ray dorsal mobility in relation to hallux valgus deformity and first intermetatarsal angle. *Foot Ankle Int* 22:98-101, 2001.

122. Glasoe WM, Allen MK, Saltzman CL, et al: Comparison of two methods used to assess first-ray mobility. *Foot Ankle Int* 23:248-252, 2002.

123. Glasoe WM, Allen MK, Yack HJ: Measurement of dorsal mobility in the first ray: Elimination of fat pad compression as a variable. *Foot Ankle Int* 19:542-546, 1998.

124. Glasoe WM, Yack HJ, Saltzman CL: Measuring first ray mobility with a new device. *Arch Phys Med Rehabil* 80:122-124, 1999.

125. Glasoe WM, Yack HJ, Saltzman CL: The reliability and validity of a first ray measurement device. *Foot Ankle Int* 21:240-246, 2000.

126. Glasoe WM, Grebing B, Beck S, et al: A comparison of device measures of dorsal first ray mobility. *Foot Ankle Int* 26:957-961, 2005.

127. Glynn MK, Dunlop JB, Fitzpatrick D: The Mitchell distal metatarsal osteotomy for hallux valgus. *J Bone Joint Surg Br* 62:188-191, 1980.

128. Goldberg I, Bahar A, Yosipovitch Z: Late results after correction of hallux valgus deformity by basilar phalangeal osteotomy. *J Bone Joint Surg Am* 69:64-67, 1987.

129. Goldner JL, Gaines RW: Adult and juvenile hallux valgus: Analysis and treatment. *Orthop Clin North Am* 7:863-887, 1976.

130. Grace D, Hughes J, Klenerman L: A comparison of Wilson and Hohmann osteotomies in the treatment of hallux valgus. *J Bone Joint Surg Br* 70:236-241, 1988.

131. Granberry WM, Noble PC, Bishop, JO, Tullos HS: Use of a hinged silicone prosthesis for replacement arthroplasty of the first metatarsophalangeal joint. *J Bone Joint Surg Am* 73:1453-1459, 1991.

132. Grebing BR, Coughlin MJ: The effect of ankle position on the exam for first ray mobility. *Foot Ankle Int* 25:467-475, 2004.

133. Grebing BR, Coughlin MJ: Evaluation of Morton's theory of second metatarsal hypertrophy. *J Bone Joint Surg Am* 86:1375-1386, 2004.

134. Green MA, Dorris MF, Baessler TP, et al: Avascular necrosis following distal chevron osteotomy of the first metatarsal. *J Foot Ankle Surg* 32:617-622, 1993.

135. Griffiths TA, Palladino SJ: Metatarsus adductus and selected radiographic measurements of the first ray in normal feet. *J Am Podiatr Med Assoc* 82:616-622, 1992.

136. Grill F, Hetherington V, Steinbock G, Altenhuber J: Experiences with the chevron (V-) osteotomy on adolescent hallux valgus. *Arch Orthop Trauma Surg* 106:47-51, 1986.

137. Groiso JA: Juvenile hallux valgus. A conservative approach to treatment. *J Bone Joint Surg Am* 74:1367-1374, 1992.

138. Haines RW, McDougall AM: The anatomy of hallux valgus. *J Bone Joint Surg Br* 36:272-293, 1954.

139. Halebian JD, Gaines SS: Juvenile hallux valgus. *J Foot Surg* 22:290-293, 1983.

140. Hansen ST: *Functional Reconstruction of the Foot and Ankle.* Philadelphia, Lippincott Williams & Wilkins, 2000, p 221.

141. Hansen ST Jr: Hallux valgus surgery. Morton and Lapidus were right! *Clin Podiatr Med Surg* 13:347-354, 1996.

142. Hara B, Beck JC, Woo RA: First cuneiform closing abductory osteotomy for reduction of metatarsus primus adductus. *J Foot Surg* 31:434-439, 1992.

143. Hardy RH, Clapham JC: Hallux valgus; predisposing anatomical causes. *Lancet* 1:1180-1183, 1952.

144. Hardy RH, Clapham JC: Observations on hallux valgus; based on a controlled series. *J Bone Joint Surg Br* 33:376-391, 1951.

145. Harper MC: Correction of metatarsus primus varus with the chevron metatarsal osteotomy. An analysis of corrective factors. *Clin Orthop* 243:180-183, 1989.

146. Harris R, Beath T: Hypermobile flat-foot with short tendo Achilles. *J Bone Joint Surg Am* 30:116-138, 1948.

147. Harris R, Beath T: The short first metatarsal: Its incidence and clinical significance. *J Bone Joint Surg Am* 31:553-565, 1949.

148. Harrison M, Harvey F: Arthrodesis of the first metatarsophalangeal joint for hallux valgus and rigidus. *J Bone Joint Surg Am* 45:471-480, 1963.

149. Hattrup SJ, Johnson KA: Chevron osteotomy: Analysis of factors in patients' dissatisfaction. *Foot Ankle* 5:327-332, 1985.

150. Hawkins F, Mitchell C, Hedrick D: Correction of hallux valgus by metatarsal osteotomy. *J Bone Joint Surg Am* 37:387-394, 1945.

151. Hecht PJ, Gibbons MJ, Wapner KL, et al: Arthrodesis of the first metatarsophalangeal joint to salvage failed silicone implant arthroplasty. *Foot Ankle Int* 18:383-390, 1997.

152. Helal B: Surgery for adolescent hallux valgus. *Clin Orthop* 157:50-63, 1981.

153. Helal B, Gupta SK, Gojaseni P: Surgery for adolescent hallux valgus. *Acta Orthop Scand* 45:271-295, 1974.

154. Henry AP, Waugh W, Wood H: The use of footprints in assessing the results of operations for hallux valgus. A comparison of Keller's operation and arthrodesis. *J Bone Joint Surg Br* 57:478-481, 1975.

155. Hernandez A, Hernandez PA, Hernandez WA: Lapidus: When and why? *Clin Podiatr Med Surg* 6:197-208, 1989.

156. Hetherington VJ, Steinbock G, LaPorta D, Gardner C: The Austin bunionectomy: A follow-up study. *J Foot Ankle Surg* 32:162-166, 1993.

157. Hewitt D, Stewart AM, Webb JW: The prevalence of foot defects among wartime recruits. *BMJ* 4839:745-749, 1953.

158. Hirvensalo E, Bostman O, Tormala P, et al: Chevron osteotomy fixed with absorbable polyglycolide pins. *Foot Ankle* 11:212-218, 1991.

159. Hiss J: Hallux valgus: Its causes and simplified treatment. *Am J Surg* 11:50-57, 1931.

160. Hodor L, Hess T: Shortening Z-osteotomy for the proximal phalanx of the hallux using axial guides. *J Am Podiatr Med Assoc* 85:249-254, 1995.

161. Hohmann G: Der Hallux valgus und die uebrigen Zchenverkruemmungen. *Egerb Chir Orthop* 18:308-348, 1925.

162. Horne G, Tanze, T, Ford M: Chevron osteotomy for the treatment of hallux valgus. *Clin Orthop* 183:32-36, 1984.

163. Houghton GR, Dickson RA: Hallux valgus in the younger patient: The structural abnormality. *J Bone Joint Surg Br* 61:176-177, 1979.

164. Hueter C: Klinik der Gelenkkrankheiten mit Einschluss der Orthopadie. Leipzig, Germany, Vogel, 1870-1871.

165. Humbert JL, Bourbonniere C, Laurin CA: Metatarsophalangeal fusion for hallux valgus: Indications and effect on the first metatarsal ray. *Can Med Assoc J* 120:937-941, 956, 1979.

166. Inman VT: Hallux valgus: A review of etiologic factors. *Orthop Clin North Am* 5:59-66, 1974.

167. Ito H, Shimizu A, Miyamoto T, et al: Clinical significance of increased mobility in the sagittal plane in patients with hallux valgus. *Foot Ankle Int* 20:29-32, 1999.

168. Jahss MH: Hallux valgus: Further considerations—the first metatarsal head. *Foot Ankle* 2:1-4, 1981.

169. Jahss MH: LeLeivre bunion operation. *Instr Course Lect* 21:295-309, 1972.

170. James C: Footprints and feet of natives of Soloman Islands. *Lancet* 2:1390, 1939.

171. Johansson JE, Barrington TW: Cone arthrodesis of the first metatarsophalangeal joint. *Foot Ankle* 4:244-248, 1984.

172. Johnson JE, Clanton TO, Baxter DE, Gottlieb MS: Comparison of Chevron osteotomy and modified McBride bunionectomy for correction of mild to moderate hallux valgus deformity. *Foot Ankle* 12:61-68, 1991.

173. Johnson KA, Cofield RH, Morrey BF: Chevron osteotomy for hallux valgus. *Clin Orthop* 142:44-47, 1979.

174. Johnson KA, Kile TA: Hallux valgus due to cuneiformmetatarsal instability. *J South Orthop Assoc* 3:273-282, 1994.

175. Johnson KA, Spiegl PV: Extensor hallucis longus transfer for hallux varus deformity. *J Bone Joint Surg Am* 66:681-686, 1984.

176. Johnston O: Further studies of the inheritance of hand and foot anomalies. *Clin Orthop* 8:146-160, 1956.

177. Jones A: Hallux valgus in the adolescent. *Proc R Soc Med* 41:392-393, 1948.

178. Jones C, Coughlin M, Pierce-Villadot R, Galano P: Proximal crescentic metatarsal osteotomy: The effect of saw blade orientation on first ray elevation. *Foot Ankle Int* 26:152-157, 2005.

179. Jones C, Coughlin M, Pierce-Villadot R, et al: The validity and reliability of the Klaue device. *Foot Ankle Int* 26:951-956, 2005.

180. Jones S, Al Hussainy HA, Ali F, et al: Scarf osteotomy for hallux valgus. A prospective clinical and pedobarographic study. *J Bone Joint Surg Br* 86:830-836, 2004.

181. Joplin RJ: Sling procedure for correction of splay-foot metatarsus primus varus, and hallux valgus. *J Bone Joint Surg Am* 32:779-785, 1950.

182. Jordan HH, Bordsky AE: Keller operation for hallux valgus and hallux rigidus. An end result study. *AMA Arch Surg* 62:586-596, 1951.

183. Joseph J: Range of movement of the great toe in men. *J Bone Joint Surg Br* 36:450-457, 1954.

184. Kalen V, Brecher A: Relationship between adolescent bunions and flatfeet. *Foot Ankle* 8:331-336, 1988.

185. Kato T, Watanabe S: The etiology of hallux valgus in Japan. *Clin Orthop* 157:78-81, 1981.

186. Kelikian H: *Hallux Valgus, Allied Deformities of the Forefoot and Metatarsalgia.* Philadelphia, WB Saunders, 1965, pp 136-235.

187. Keller W: Further observations on the surgical treatment of hallux valgus and bunions. *N Y Med J* 95:696, 1912.

188. Keogh P, Nagaria J, Stephens M: Cheilectomy for hallux rigidus. *Ir J Med Sci* 161:681-683, 1992.

189. Kilmartin TE, Barrington RL, Wallace WA: Metatarsus primus varus. A statistical study. *J Bone Joint Surg Br* 73:937-940, 1991.

190. Kilmartin TE, Barrington RL, Wallace WA: A controlled prospective trial of a foot orthosis for juvenile hallux valgus. *J Bone Joint Surg Br* 76:210-214, 1994.

191. Kilmartin TE, Flintham C: Hallux valgus surgery: A simple method for evaluating the first-second intermetatarsal angle in the presence of metatarsus adductus. *J Foot Ankle Surg* 42:165-166, 2003.

192. Kilmartin TE, Wallace WA: The significance of pes planus in juvenile hallux valgus. *Foot Ankle* 13:53-56, 1992.

193. King DM, Toolan BC: Associated deformities and hypermobility in hallux valgus: An investigation with weightbearing radiographs. *Foot Ankle Int* 25:251-255, 2004.

194. Kinnard P, Gordon D: A comparison between chevron and Mitchell osteotomies for hallux valgus. *Foot Ankle* 4:241-243, 1984.

195. Kitaoka HB, Franco MG, Weaver AL, Ilstrup DM: Simple bunionectomy with medial capsulorrhaphy. *Foot Ankle* 12:86-91, 1991.

196. Kitaoka HB, Holiday AD Jr, Chao EY, Cahalan TD: Salvage of failed first metatarsophalangeal joint implant arthroplasty by implant removal and synovectomy: Clinical and biomechanical evaluation. *Foot Ankle* 13:243-250, 1992.

197. Klaue K, Hansen ST, Masquelet AC: Clinical, quantitative assessment of first tarsometatarsal mobility in the sagittal plane and its relation to hallux valgus deformity. *Foot Ankle Int* 15:9-13, 1994.

198. Kleinberg S: Operative cure of hallux valgus and bunions. *Am J Surg* 15:75-81, 1932.

199. Klosok JK, Pring DJ, Jessop JH, Maffulli N: Chevron or Wilson metatarsal osteotomy for hallux valgus. A prospective randomised trial. *J Bone Joint Surg Br* 75:825-829, 1993.

200. Kramer J: Die Kramer-Osteotomie zur Behandlung des Hallux valgus und des Digitus quintus varus. *Operat Orthop Traumatol* 2:29-38, 1990.

201. Kramer J, Barry LD, Helfman DN, et al: The modified Scarf bunionectomy. *J Foot Surg* 31:360-367, 1992.

202. Kristen KH, Berger C, Stelzig S, et al: The SCARF osteotomy for the correction of hallux valgus deformities. *Foot Ankle Int* 23:221-229, 2002.

203. Kundert HP, Fuhrmann R: Personal communication, April 21, 2005.

204. Kuo CH, Huang PJ, Cheng YM, et al: Modified Mitchell osteotomy for hallux valgus. *Foot Ankle Int* 19:585-589, 1998.

205. Lane W: The causation, pathology, and physiology of several of the deformities which develop during young life. *Guy's Hosp Rep* 44:241, 1887.

206. Lapidus PW: The author's bunion operation from 1931 to 1959. *Clin Orthop* 16:119-135, 1960.

207. Lapidus PW: Operative correction of metatarsus varus primus in hallux valgus. *Surg Gynecol Obstet* 58:183-191, 1934.

208. Lapidus PW: A quarter of a century of experience with the operative correction of the metatarsus varus primus in hallux valgus. *Bull Hosp Jt Dis* 17:404-421, 1956.

209. La Reaux RL, Lee BR: Metatarsus adductus and hallux abducto valgus: Their correlation. *J Foot Surg* 26:304-308, 1987.

210. Lau JT, Daniels TR: Effect of increasing distal medial closing wedge metatarsal osteotomies on the distal metatarsal articular angle. *Foot Ankle Int* 20:771-776, 1999.

211. Lee KT, Young K: Measurement of first-ray mobility in normal vs. hallux valgus patients. *Foot Ankle Int* 22:960-964, 2001.

212. Leventen EO: The chevron procedure. *Orthopedics* 13:973-976, 1990.

213. Lewis RJ, Feffer HL: Modified chevron osteotomy of the first metatarsal. *Clin Orthop* 157:105-109, 1981.

214. Lian GJ, Markolf K, Cracchiolo A III: Strength of fixation constructs for basilar osteotomies of the first metatarsal. *Foot Ankle* 13:509-514, 1992.

215. Limbird TJ, DaSilva RM, Green NE: Osteotomy of the first metatarsal base for metatarsus primus varus. *Foot Ankle* 9:158-162, 1989.

216. Lippert FG III, McDermott JE: Crescentic osteotomy for hallux valgus: A biomechanical study of variables affecting the final position of the first metatarsal. *Foot Ankle* 11:204-207, 1991.

217. Lipscomb PR: Arthrodesis of the first metatarsophalangeal joint for severe bunions and hallux rigidus. *Clin Orthop* 142:48-54, 1979.

218. Lombardi CM, Silhanek AD, Connolly FG, et al: First metatarsocuneiform arthrodesis and Reverdin-Laird osteotomy for treatment of hallux valgus: An intermediate-term retrospective outcomes study. *J Foot Ankle Surg* 42:77-85, 2003.

219. Loretz L, DeValentine S, Yamaguchi K: The first metatarsal bicorrectional head osteotomy (distal "L"/Reverdin-Laird procedure) for correction of hallux abducto valgus: A retrospective study. *J Foot Ankle Surg* 32:554-568, 1993.

220. Love TR, Whynot AS, Farine I, et al: Keller arthroplasty: A prospective review. *Foot Ankle* 8:46-54, 1987.

221. Luba R, Rosman M: Bunions in children: Treatment with a modified Mitchell osteotomy. *J Pediatr Orthop* 4:44-47, 1984.

222. Ludloff K: Die Beseitigung des Hallux valgus durch die schrage planta dorsale Osteotomie des Metatarsus. *Arch Klin Chir* 110:364-387, 1918.

223. Maclennan R: Prevalence of hallux valgus in a Neolithic New Guinea population. *Lancet* 1:1398-1400, 1966.

224. Maguire WB: The Lapidus procedure for hallux valgus [abstract]. *J Bone Joint Surg Br* 55:221, 1973.

225. Mahan KT, Jacko J: Juvenile hallux valgus with compensated metatarsus adductus. Case report. *J Am Podiatr Med Assoc* 81:525-530, 1991.

226. Majkowski RS, Galloway S: Excision arthroplasty for hallux valgus in the elderly: A comparison between the Keller and modified Mayo operations. *Foot Ankle* 13:317-320, 1992.

227. Mancuso JE, Abramow SP, Landsman MJ, et al: The zero-plus first metatarsal and its relationship to bunion deformity. *J Foot Ankle Surg* 42:319-326, 2003.

228. Magnan B, Pezze L, Rossi N, Bartolozzi P: Percutaneous distal metatarsal osteotomy for correction of hallux valgus. *J Bone Joint Surg Am* 87:1191-1199, 2005.

229. Magnan B, Fieschi S, Bragantini A, et al: Trattamento chirurgico dell'alluce del primo metatarsale. *G Ital Ortop Traumatol* 24:473-487, 1998.

230. Mankey M, Mann RA: Arthrodesis of the first metatarsophalangeal joint utilizing a dorsal plate. Paper presented at the Summer Meeting of American Orthopaedic Foot and Ankle Society, July 1991, Boston.

231. Mann RA: Complications associated with the Chevron osteotomy. *Foot Ankle* 3:125-129, 1982.

232. Mann RA: Decision-making in bunion surgery. *Instr Course Lect* 39:3-13, 1990.

233. Mann RA: Hallux valgus. *Instr Course Lect* 35:339-353, 1986.

234. Mann RA, Coughlin MJ: Adult hallux valgus. In *Surgery of the Foot and Ankle*, 7th ed. St Louis, Mosby–Year Book, 1999, pp 150-269.

235. Mann RA, Coughlin MJ: The great toe. In *Video Textbook of Foot and Ankle Surgery.* St Louis, Medical Video Productions, 1991, pp 146-184.

236. Mann RA, Coughlin MJ: Hallux valgus and complications of hallux valgus. In Mann RA (ed): *Surgery of the Foot.* St Louis, CV Mosby, 1986, pp 167-296.

237. Mann RA, Coughlin MJ: Hallux valgus—etiology, anatomy, treatment and surgical considerations. *Clin Orthop* 157:31-41, 1981.

238. Mann RA, Donatto KC: The chevron osteotomy: A clinical and radiographic analysis. *Foot Ankle Int* 18:255-261, 1997.

239. Mann RA, Katcherian DA: Relationship of metatarsophalangeal joint fusion on the intermetatarsal angle. *Foot Ankle* 10:8-11, 1989.

240. Mann RA, Oates JC: Arthrodesis of the first metatarsophalangeal joint. *Foot Ankle* 1:159-166, 1980.

241. Mann RA, Pfeffinger L: Hallux valgus repair. DuVries modified McBride procedure. *Clin Orthop* 272:213-218, 1991.

242. Mann RA, Rudicel S, Graves SC: Repair of hallux valgus with a distal soft-tissue procedure and proximal metatarsal osteotomy. A long-term follow-up. *J Bone Joint Surg Am* 74:124-129, 1992.

243. Mann RA, Schakel ME II: Surgical correction of rheumatoid forefoot deformities. *Foot Ankle Int* 16:1-6, 1995.

244. Mann RA, Thompson FM: Arthrodesis of the first metatarsophalangeal joint for hallux valgus in rheumatoid arthritis. *J Bone Joint Surg Am* 66:687-692, 1984.

245. Marin GA: Arthrodesis of the metatarsophalangeal joint of the big toe for hallux valgus and hallux rigidus. A new method. *Int Surg* 50:175-180, 1968.

246. Markbreiter LA, Thompson FM: Proximal metatarsal osteotomy in hallux valgus correction: A comparison of crescentic and chevron procedures. *Foot Ankle Int* 18:71-76, 1997.

247. Marwil T, Brantingham C: Foot problems of women's reserve. *Hosp Corp Q* 16:98, 1943.

248. Mauldin DM, Sanders M, Whitmer WW: Correction of hallux valgus with metatarsocuneiform stabilization. *Foot Ankle* 11:59-66, 1990.

249. Mayo C: The surgical treatment of bunions. *Ann Surg* 48:300, 1908.

250. Mayo C: The surgical treatment of bunions. *Minn Med J* 3:326-331, 1920.

251. McBride ED: A conservative operation for bunions. *J Bone Joint Surg* 10:735-739, 1928.

252. McBride ED: The conservative operation for "bunions": End results and refinements of technic. *JAMA* 105:1164-1168, 1935.

253. McBride E: Hallux valgus, bunion deformity; its treatment in mild, moderate and severe stages. *J Int Coll Surg* 21:99-105, 1954.

254. McBride ED: The McBride bunion hallux valgus operation. *J Bone Joint Surg Am* 49:1675-1683, 1967.

255. McCluskey LC, Johnson JE, Wynarsky GT, Harris GF: Comparison of stability of proximal crescentic metatarsal osteotomy and proximal horizontal "V" osteotomy. *Foot Ankle Int* 15:263-270, 1994.

256. McHale K, McKay D: Bunions in a child: Conservative versus surgical management. *J Musculoskel Med* 3:56-62, 1986.

257. McInnes BD, Bouche RT: Critical evaluation of the modified Lapidus procedure. *J Foot Ankle Surg* 40:71-90, 2001.

258. McKeever DC: Arthrodesis of the first metatarsophalangeal joint for hallux valgus, hallux rigidus, and metatarsus primus varus. *J Bone Joint Surg Am* 34:129-134, 1952.

259. Meehan PL: Adolescent bunion. *Instr Course Lect* 31:262-264, 1982.

260. Meier PJ, Kenzora JE: The risks and benefits of distal first metatarsal osteotomies. *Foot Ankle* 6:7-17, 1985.

261. Merkel KD, Katoh Y, Johnson EW Jr, Chao EY: Mitchell osteotomy for hallux valgus: Long-term follow-up and gait analysis. *Foot Ankle* 3:189-196, 1983.

262. Meyer JM, Hoffmeyer P, Borst F: The treatment of hallux valgus in runners using a modified McBride procedure. *Int Orthop* 11:197-200, 1987.

263. Miller JW: Acquired hallux varus: A preventable and correctable disorder. *J Bone Joint Surg Am* 57:183-188, 1975.

264. Mitchell CL, Fleming JL, Allen R, et al: Osteotomy-bunionectomy for hallux valgus. *J Bone Joint Surg Am* 40:41-58; discussion 59-60, 1958.

265. Mitchell LA, Baxter DE: A chevron-Akin double osteotomy for correction of hallux valgus. *Foot Ankle* 12:7-14, 1991.

266. Mizuno K, Hashimura M, Kimura M, Hirohata K: Treatment of hallux valgus by oblique osteotomy of the first metatarsal. *Foot Ankle* 13:447-452, 1992.

267. Morton DJ: *The Human Foot*. New York, Columbia University Press, 1935.

268. Morton DJ: Hypermobility of the first metatarsal bone: The interlinking factor between metatarsalgia and longitudinal arch strains. *J Bone Joint Surg* 10:187-196, 1928.

269. Moynihan FJ: Arthrodesis of the metatarso-phalangeal joint of the great toe. *J Bone Joint Surg Br* 49:544-551, 1967.

270. Myerson MS: Hallux valgus. In *Foot and Ankle Disorders*. Philadelphia, WB Saunders, 2000, pp 213-289.

271. Myerson MS: Metatarsocuneiform arthrodesis for treatment of hallux valgus and metatarsus primus varus. *Orthopedics* 13:1025-1031, 1990.

272. Myerson M, Allon S, McGarvey W: Metatarsocuneiform arthrodesis for management of hallux valgus and metatarsus primus varus. *Foot Ankle* 13:107-115, 1992.

273. Myerson MS, Badekas A: Hypermobility of the first ray. *Foot Ankle Clin* 5:469-484, 2000.

274. Newman AS, Negrine JP, Zecovic M, et al: A biomechanical comparison of the Z step-cut and basilar crescentic osteotomies of the first metatarsal. *Foot Ankle Int* 21:584-587, 2000.

275. Patel S, Ford LA, Etcheverry J, et al: Modified Lapidus arthrodesis: Rate of nonunion in 227 cases. *J Foot Ankle Surg* 43:37-42, 2004.

276. Pavlovich R Jr, Caminear D: Granuloma formation after chevron osteotomy fixation with absorbable copolymer pin: A case report. *J Foot Ankle Surg* 42:226-229, 2003.

277. Peabody D: Surgical care of hallux valgus. *J Bone Joint Surg* 13:273-282, 1931.

278. Pearson SW, Kitaoka HB, Cracchiolo A, Leventen EO: Results and complications following a proximal curved osteotomy of the hallux metatarsal. *Contemp Orthop* 23:127-132, 1991.

279. Peterson DA, Zilberfarb JL, Greene MA, Colgrove RC: Avascular necrosis of the first metatarsal head: Incidence in distal osteotomy combined with lateral soft tissue release. *Foot Ankle Int* 15:59-63, 1994.

280. Peterson HA, Newman SR: Adolescent bunion deformity treated with double osteotomy and longitudinal pin fixation of the first ray. *J Pediatr Orthop* 13:80-84, 1993.

281. Piggott H: The natural history of hallux valgus in adolescence and early adult life. *J Bone Joint Surg Br* 42:749-760, 1960.

282. Plattner PF, Van Manen JW: Results of Akin type proximal phalangeal osteotomy for correction of hallux valgus deformity. *Orthopedics* 13:989-996, 1990.

283. Pochatko DJ, Schlehr FJ, Murphey MD, Hamilton JJ: Distal chevron osteotomy with lateral release for treatment of hallux valgus deformity. *Foot Ankle Int* 15:457-461, 1994.

284. Pontious J, Mahan KT, Carter S: Characteristics of adolescent hallux abducto valgus. A retrospective review. *J Am Podiatr Med Assoc* 84:208-218, 1994.

285. Popoff I, Negrine JP, Zecovic M, et al: The effect of screw type on the biomechanical properties of SCARF and crescentic osteotomies of the first metatarsal. *J Foot Ankle Surg* 42:161-164, 2003.

286. Portaluri M: Hallux valgus correction by the method of Bosch: A clinical evaluation. *Foot Ankle Clin* 5:499-511, vi, 2000.

287. Pouliart N, Haentjens P, Opdecam P: Clinical and radiographic evaluation of Wilson osteotomy for hallux valgus. *Foot Ankle Int* 17:388-394, 1996.

288. Price GF: Metatarsus primus varus: Including various clinico-radiologic features of the female foot. *Clin Orthop* 145:217-223, 1979.

289. Prieskorn DW, Mann RA, Fritz G: Radiographic assessment of the second metatarsal: Measure of first ray hypermobility. *Foot Ankle Int* 17:331-333, 1996.

290. Pring DJ, Coombes RRH, Closok JK: Chevron or Wilson osteotomy: A comparison and follow-up [abstract]. *J Bone Joint Surg Am* 67:671-672, 1985.

291. Raymakers R, Waugh W: The treatment of metatarsalgia with hallux valgus. *J Bone Joint Surg Br* 53:684-687, 1971.

292. Resch S, Stenstrom A, Egund N: Proximal closing wedge osteotomy and adductor tenotomy for treatment of hallux valgus. *Foot Ankle* 9:272-280, 1989.

293. Reverdin J: De la deviation en dehors du gros orteil et de son traitement chirurgical. *Trans Int Med Congr* 2:408-412, 1881.

294. Richardson EG: Keller resection arthroplasty. *Orthopedics* 13:1049-1053, 1990.

295. Richardson EG, Graves SC, McClure JT, Boone RT: First metatarsal head-shaft angle: A method of determination. *Foot Ankle* 14:181-185, 1993.

296. Riedel HL: Zur operativen Behandlung des Hallux valgus. *Zentralbl Chir* 44:573-580, 1886.

297. Riggs SA Jr, Johnson EW Jr: McKeever arthrodesis for the painful hallux. *Foot Ankle* 3:248-253, 1983.

298. Rink-Brune O: Lapidus arthrodesis for management of hallux valgus—a retrospective review of 106 cases. *J Foot Ankle Surg* 43:290-295, 2004.
299. Rogers WA, Joplin RJ: Hallux valgus, weak foot and the Keller operations: An end-result study. *Surg Clin North Am* 27:1295-1302, 1947.
300. Rosenberg GA, Donley BG: Plate augmentation of screw fixation of proximal crescentic osteotomy of the first metatarsal. *Foot Ankle Int* 24:570-571, 2003.
301. Roukis TS: Hallux proximal phalanx Akin-scarf osteotomy. *J Am Podiatr Med Assoc* 94:70-72, 2004.
302. Roukis TS, Landsman AS: Hypermobility of the first ray: A critical review of the literature. *J Foot Ankle Surg* 42:377-390, 2003.
303. Rush SM, Christensen JC, Johnson CH: Biomechanics of the first ray. Part II: Metatarsus primus varus as a cause of hypermobility. A three dimensional kinematic analysis in a cadaver model. *J Foot Ankle Surg* 39:68-77, 2000.
304. Sammarco GJ, Brainard BJ, Sammarco VJ: Bunion correction using proximal chevron osteotomy. *Foot Ankle* 14:8-14, 1993.
305. Sammarco GJ, Idusuyi OB: Complications after surgery of the hallux. *Clin Orthop* 391:59-71, 2001.
306. Sammarco GJ, Russo-Alesi FG: Bunion correction using proximal chevron osteotomy: A single-incision technique. *Foot Ankle Int* 19:430-437, 1998.
307. Sangeorzan BJ, Hansen ST Jr: Modified Lapidus procedure for hallux valgus. *Foot Ankle* 9:262-266, 1989.
308. Saragas NP, Becker PJ: Comparative radiographic analysis of parameters in feet with and without hallux valgus. *Foot Ankle Int* 16:139-143, 1995.
309. Sarrafian S: *Anatomy of the Foot and Ankle.* Philadelphia, JB Lippincott, 1983, pp 81-86.
310. Schede F: Hallux valgus, Hallux flexus und Fussenkung. *Z Orthop Chir* 48:564-571, 1927.
311. Schemitsch E, Horne G: Wilson's osteotomy for the treatment of hallux valgus. *Clin Orthop* 240:221-225, 1989.
312. Schneider W, Knahr K: Keller procedure and chevron osteotomy in hallux valgus: Five-year results of different surgical philosophies in comparable collectives. *Foot Ankle Int* 23:321-329, 2002.
313. Schoen NS, Zygmunt K, Gudas C: Z-bunionectomy: Retrospective long-term study. *J Foot Ankle Surg* 35:312-317, 1996.
314. Schoenhaus HD, Cohen RS: Etiology of the bunion. *J Foot Surg* 31:25-29, 1992.
315. Schwartz N, Hurley JP: Derotational Akin osteotomy: Further modification. *J Foot Surg* 26:419-421, 1987.
316. Schweitzer ME, Maheshwari S, Shabshin N: Hallux valgus and hallux rigidus: MRI findings. *Clin Imaging* 23:397-402, 1999.
317. Scranton PE Jr: Adolescent bunions: Diagnosis and management. *Pediatr Ann* 11:518-520, 1982.
318. Scranton PE Jr, Zuckerman JD: Bunion surgery in adolescents: Results of surgical treatment. *J Pediatr Orthop* 4:39-43, 1984.
319. Seelenfreund M, Fried A, Tikva P: Correction of hallux valgus deformity by basal phalanx osteotomy of the big toe. *J Bone Joint Surg Am* 55:1411-1415, 1973.
320. Seiberg M, Green R, Green D: Epiphysiodesis in juvenile hallux abducto valgus. A preliminary retrospective study. *J Am Podiatr Med Assoc* 84:225-236, 1994.
321. Selner AJ, Selner MD, Tucker RA, Eirich G: Tricorrectional bunionectomy for surgical repair of juvenile hallux valgus. *J Am Podiatr Med Assoc* 82:21-24, 1992.
322. Shereff MJ, Yang QM, Kummer FJ: Extraosseous and intraosseous arterial supply to the first metatarsal and metatarsophalangeal joint. *Foot Ankle* 8:81-93, 1987.
323. Sheridan LE: Correction of juvenile hallux valgus deformity associated with metatarsus primus adductus using epiphysiodesis technique. *Clin Podiatr Med Surg* 4:63-74, 1987.
324. Sherman KP, Douglas DL, Benson MK: Keller's arthroplasty: Is distraction useful? A prospective trial. *J Bone Joint Surg Br* 66:765-769, 1984.
325. Shurnas PS, Coughlin MJ: Recall of the risks of forefoot surgery after informed consent. *Foot Ankle Int* 24:904-908, 2003.
326. Silberman FS: Proximal phalangeal osteotomy for the correction of hallux valgus. *Clin Orthop* 85:98-100, 1972.
327. Silver D: The operative treatment of hallux valgus. *J Bone Joint Surg* 5:225-232, 1923.
328. Sim-Fook L, Hodgson AR: A comparison of foot forms among the non-shoe and shoe-wearing Chinese population. *J Bone Joint Surg Am* 40:1058-1062, 1958.
329. Simmonds F, Menelaus M: Hallux valgus in adolescents. *J Bone Joint Surg Br* 42:761-768, 1960.
330. Simon W: Der Hallux valgus und seine chirurgische Behandlung mit besonderer Berucksichtigung der Ludlof schen Operation. *Beitrage Klin Chir* 3:467-537, 1918.
331. Smith AM, Alwan T, Davies MS: Perioperative complications of the scarf osteotomy. *Foot Ankle Int* 24:222-227, 2003.
332. Smith NR: Hallux valgus and rigidus treated by arthrodesis of the metatarsophalangeal joint. *BMJ* 2:1385-1387, 1952.
333. Smith RW, Joanis TL, Maxwell PD: Great toe metatarsophalangeal joint arthrodesis: A user-friendly technique. *Foot Ankle* 13:367-377, 1992.
334. Smith RW, Reynolds JC, Stewart MJ: Hallux valgus assessment: Report of research committee of American Orthopaedic Foot and Ankle Society. *Foot Ankle* 5:92-103, 1984.
335. Sorto LA Jr, Balding MG, Weil LS, Smith SD: Hallux abductus interphalangeus: Etiology, x-ray evaluation and treatment. *J Am Podiatr Assoc* 66:384-396, 1976.
336. Sorto LA Jr, Balding MG, Weil LS, Smith SD: Hallux abductus interphalangeus. Etiology, x-ray evaluation and treatment. 1975. *J Am Podiatr Med Assoc* 82:85-97, 1992.
337. Staheli LT: Lower positional deformity in infants and children: A review. *J Pediatr Orthop* 10:559-563, 1990.
338. Steel MW III, Johnson KA, DeWitz MA, Ilstrup DM: Radiographic measurements of the normal adult foot. *Foot Ankle* 1:151-158, 1980.
339. Stein HC: Hallux valgus. *Surg Gynecol Obstet* 66:889-898, 1938.
340. Stienstra JJ, Lee JA, Nakadate DT: Large displacement distal chevron osteotomy for the correction of hallux valgus deformity. *J Foot Ankle Surg* 41:213-220, 2002.
341. Szaboky GT, Raghaven VC: Modification of Mitchell's lateral displacement angulation osteotomy. *J Bone Joint Surg Am* 51:1430-1431, 1969.
342. Tanaka Y, Takakura Y, Kumai T, et al: Radiographic analysis of hallux valgus. A two-dimensional coordinate system. *J Bone Joint Surg Am* 77:205-213, 1995.
343. Thomas RL, Espinosa FJ, Richardson EG: Radiographic changes in the first metatarsal head after distal chevron osteotomy combined with lateral release through a plantar approach. *Foot Ankle Int* 15:285-292, 1994.
344. Thompson FM, Coughlin MJ: The high price of high fashion footwear. *J Bone Joint Surg Am* 76:1586-1593, 1994.
345. Thompson F, McElveney R: Arthrodesis of the first metatarsophalangeal joint. *J Bone Joint Surg* 22:555-558, 1940.
346. Thompson GH: Bunions and deformities of the toes in children and adolescents. *Instr Course Lect* 45:355-367, 1996.
347. Thordarson DB, Krewer P: Medial eminence thickness with and without hallux valgus. *Foot Ankle Int* 23:48-50, 2002.
348. Thordarson DB, Leventen EO: Hallux valgus correction with proximal metatarsal osteotomy: Two-year follow-up. *Foot Ankle* 13:321-326, 1992.
349. Tourne Y, Saragaglia D, Zattara A, et al: Hallux valgus in the elderly: Metatarsophalangeal arthrodesis of the first ray. *Foot Ankle Int* 18:195-198, 1997.

350. Trnka HJ, Zembsch A, Easley ME, et al: The chevron osteotomy for correction of hallux valgus. Comparison of findings after two and five years of follow-up. *J Bone Joint Surg Am* 82:1373-1378, 2000.

351. Trnka HJ, Zembsch A, Wiesauer H, et al: Modified Austin procedure for correction of hallux valgus. *Foot Ankle Int* 18:119-127, 1997.

352. Trnka HJ, Zettl R, Hungerford M, et al: Acquired hallux varus and clinical tolerability. *Foot Ankle Int* 18:593-597, 1997.

353. Trott A: Hallux valgus in adolescent. *Instr Course Lect* 21:262-268, 1972.

354. Truslow W: Metatarsus primus varus or hallux valgus? *J Bone Joint Surg* 7:98-108, 1925.

355. Tupman S: Arthrodesis of the first metatarsophalangeal joint. *J Bone Joint Surg Br* 40:826, 1958.

356. Turan I, Lindgren U: Compression-screw arthrodesis of the first metatarsophalangeal joint of the foot. *Clin Orthop* 221:292-295, 1987.

357. Turnbull T, Grange W: A comparison of Keller's arthroplasty and distal metatarsal osteotomy in the treatment of adult hallux valgus. *J Bone Joint Surg Br* 68:132-137, 1986.

358. Vallier GT, Petersen SA, LaGrone MO: The Keller resection arthroplasty: A 13-year experience. *Foot Ankle* 11:187-194, 1991.

359. Venn A, LaValette D, Harris NJ: Re: Technique tip. Plate augmentation of screw fixation of proximal crescentic osteotomy of the first metatarsal. (Rosenbery, GA, Donley, BG: *Foot Ankle Int* 24:570-571, 2003.) *Foot Ankle Int* 25:605-606; author reply 606, 2004.

360. Verbrugge J: Pathogenie et traitement de l'hallux valgus. *Mem Bull Soc Delge Orthop* 3:40, 1933.

361. Veri JP, Pirani SP, Claridge R: Crescentic proximal metatarsal osteotomy for moderate to severe hallux valgus: A mean 12.2 year follow-up study. *Foot Ankle Int* 22:817-822, 2001.

362. Viladot A: Metatarsalgia due to biomechanical alterations of the forefoot. *Orthop Clin North Am* 4:165-178, 1973.

363. Voellmicke KV, Deland JT: Manual examination technique to assess dorsal instability of the first ray. *Foot Ankle Int* 23:1040-1041, 2002.

364. Volkmann A: Ueber die sogennante Exostose der grossen Zehe. *Virchows Arch Patgol Anat* 10:297, 1856.

365. von Salis-Soglio G, Thomas W: Arthrodesis of the metatarsophalangeal joint of the great toe. *Arch Orthop Trauma Surg* 95:7-12, 1979.

366. Wagner FW Jr: Technique and rationale: Bunion surgery. *Contemp Orthop* 3:1040-1053, 1981.

367. Wanivenhaus AH, Feldner-Busztin H: Basal osteotomy of the first metatarsal for the correction of metatarsus primus varus associated with hallux valgus. *Foot Ankle* 8:337-343, 1988.

368. Wanivenhaus A, Pretterklieber M: First tarsometatarsal joint: Anatomical biomechanical study. *Foot Ankle* 9:153-157, 1989.

369. Weil LS: Scarf osteotomy for correction of hallux valgus. Historical perspective, surgical technique, and results. *Foot Ankle Clin* 5:559-580, 2000.

370. Wells LH: The foot of the South African native. *Am J Phys Anthropol* 15:185, 1931.

371. Westbrook AP, Subramanian KN, Monk J, Calthorpe D: Best foot forward. Proceeding of the British Orthopaedic Foot Surgery Society. *J Bone Joint Surg Br* 85(Supp 3):249, 2003.

372. White LE, Lucas G, Richards A, Purves D: Cerebral asymmetry and handedness. *Nature* 368:197-198, 1994.

373. Wilkins EH: Feet with particular reference to school children. *Med Officer* 66:5, 13, 21, 29, 1941.

374. Wilkinson J: Cone arthrodesis of the first metatarsophalangeal joint. *Acta Orthop Scand* 49:627-630, 1978.

375. Wilkinson SV, Jones RO, Sisk LE, et al: Austin bunionectomy: Postoperative MRI evaluation for avascular necrosis. *J Foot Surg* 31:469-477, 1992.

376. Williams WW, Barrett DS, Copeland SA: Avascular necrosis following chevron distal metatarsal osteotomy: A significant risk? *J Foot Surg* 28:414-416, 1989.

377. Wilson DW: Treatment of hallux valgus and bunions. *Br J Hosp Med* 24:548-549, 1980.

378. Wilson JN: Cone arthrodesis of the first metatarso-phalangeal joint. *J Bone Joint Surg Br* 49:98-101, 1967.

379. Wilson JN: Oblique displacement osteotomy for hallux valgus. *J Bone Joint Surg Br* 45:552-556, 1963.

380. Wu K: Mitchell's bunionectomy and Wu's bunionectomy: A comparison of 100 cases of each procedure. *Orthopedics* 13:1001-1007, 1990.

381. Wu KK: Wu's bunionectomy: A clinical analysis of 150 personal cases. *J Foot Surg* 31:288-297, 1992.

382. Wynne-Davis R: Family studies and the causes of congenital clubfoot talipes equinovarus, talipes calcaneovalgus, and metatarsus varus. *J Bone Joint Surg Am* 46:445, 1967.

383. Young J: A new operation for adolescent hallux valgus. *Univ Penn Med Bull* 23:459, 1910.

384. Zadik FR: Arthrodesis of the great toe. *BMJ* 5212:1573-1574, 1960.

385. Zimmer TJ, Johnson KA, Klassen RA: Treatment of hallux valgus in adolescents by the chevron osteotomy. *Foot Ankle* 9:190-193, 1989.

386. Zygmunt KH, Gudas CJ, Laros GS: Z-bunionectomy with internal screw fixation. *J Am Podiatr Med Assoc* 79:322-329, 1989.

Lesser Toe Deformities

Michael J. Coughlin

LESSER TOE DEFORMITIES

Lesser toe deformities can be static or dynamic. They can occur as isolated entities or be associated with deformities of the hallux, midfoot, or hindfoot. Poor footwear is the most commonly attributed cause of lesser toe deformities, but they also can result from congenital and neuromuscular causes.[21,25,28,33,34]

The terms *hammer toe, mallet toe,* and *claw toe* have been used interchangeably by various authors in describing deformities of the toes, and their definitions have been confusing. The nomenclature adopted for this book is simple, and to a certain extent it follows that used to describe deformities of the fingers. A *mallet toe* involves the distal interphalangeal (DIP) joint; the distal phalanx is flexed on the middle phalanx (Fig. 7–1). A *simple hammer toe* involves the proximal interphalangeal (PIP) joint; the middle and distal phalanges are flexed on the proximal phalanx (Fig. 7–2A). A *complex hammer toe* involves typically one or two toes and consists of a flexion deformity of the PIP joint and hyperextension deformity of the metatarsophalangeal (MTP) joint. (Figs. 7–2B and 7–3). A *claw toe* involves a hammer toe deformity of the phalanges and dorsiflexion (extension) deformity at the MTP joint (Fig. 7–4). To some extent, there is an overlap in the definitions of complex hammer toes and claw toes; however, claw toes usually involve all of the lesser toes and often have an underlying neuromuscular cause.

With regard to the great toe, a hammer toe can involve the interphalangeal joint. No mallet toe deformity exists in the hallux (Fig. 7–5). A claw toe deformity, which is essentially synonymous with a cock-up deformity of the great toe, occurs when there is also hyperextension of the MTP joint.

These deformities of the lesser toes range in severity from a mild and easily correctable flexible deformity to a rigid and fixed contracture. In most cases these deformities are acquired. Both the mallet toe and the hammer toe deformities can occur in one or several toes of the same foot[28,33]; a claw toe deformity often

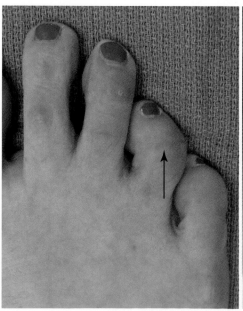
A

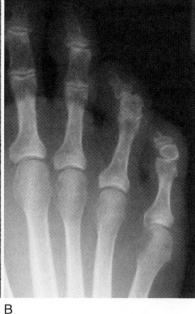
B

Figure 7–1 A, Mallet toe deformity involving distal phalangeal joint. **B,** Radiograph demonstrating mallet toe deformity.

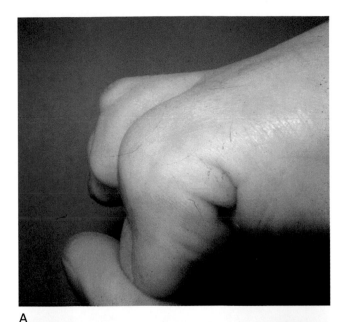

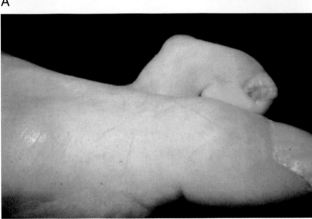

Figure 7–2 A, Simple hammer toe deformity with plantar flexion contracture of the PIP joint. **B,** Complex hammer toe with hyperextension deformity of the MTP joint and plantar flexion contracture of the PIP joint. Although this is similar to a claw toe, it typically involves only one digit. (**A** from Coughlin MJ: *Instr Course Lect* 52:421-444, 2003.)

involves multiple toes but can occur as an isolated entity.[27]

These deformities occur with varying frequency among different populations, but they are much more common in shoe-wearing societies. The literature dealing with deformities of the forefoot in populations who wear no shoes rarely mentions the mallet toe, hammer toe, or claw toe deformities.[4,54,79,171]

In various surveys regarding the incidence of these deformities among industrial workers[40,91] and wartime male recruits,[75] the incidence of hammer toe and claw toe deformities ranged from 2% to 20%. All of these studies seem to indicate, however, that the deformities develop slowly and insidiously and that their inci-

dence increases almost linearly with age, peaking in the sixth and seventh decades.* These deformities occur much more commonly in women than in men (4 to 5:1).[17,28,33,34,37] A hammer toe deformity rarely is seen in infants[74](Fig. 7–6).

Etiology

Footwear is generally considered to play an important role in the etiology of hammer toe and mallet toe deformities.[21,28,33] Placing the forefoot into the constricted confines of a pointed shoe no doubt plays a major role in the onset of these deformities. The toes, to conform to a small toe box, must of necessity buckle (Fig. 7–7). This fact explains why acquired mallet toes and hammer toes are among the most common defor-

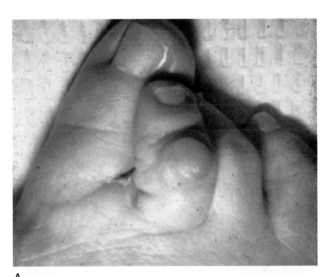

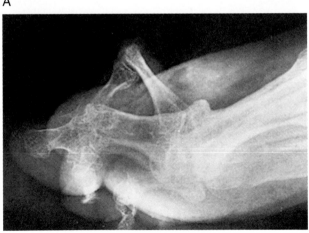

Figure 7–3 A, Complex hammer toe deformity involving metatarsophalangeal and proximal interphalangeal (PIP) joints. **B,** Lateral radiograph demonstrating severe flexion deformity of PIP joint.

---

*References 17, 24, 26, 37, 99, and 145.

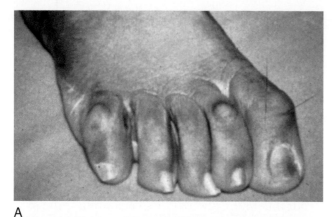

A

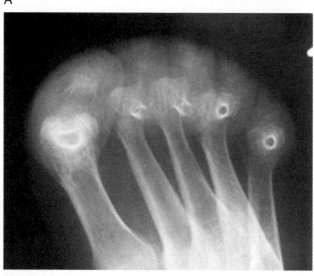

B

Figure 7–4   Photograph **(A)** and radiograph **(B)** of claw toe deformities involving hammer toe deformity associated with dorsiflexion of metatarsophalangeal joint.

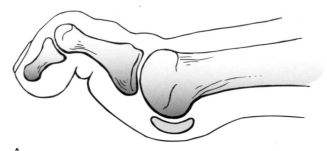

A

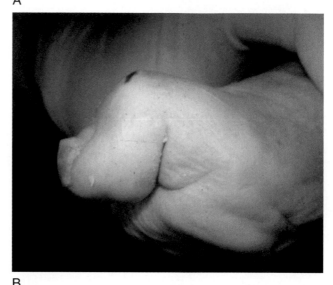

B

Figure 7–5   A, Hammered great toe. Note articulation of distal phalanx with plantar surface of the head of the proximal phalanx. **B,** Hammer toe deformity of hallux.

mities of the forefoot in shoe-wearing societies (Fig. 7–8). DuVries[51] thought that shoes restrict the normal movement of the joints and impede the actions of the intrinsic muscles of the foot. It must be kept in mind, however, that anatomic predisposing factors vary extensively, and a large number of shoe wearers do escape deformities of the forefoot.

Mallet Toe

Other than its general relationship to pressure of the toe against the shoe, the specific cause of a mallet toe is unknown. Although most often idiopathic in nature, it can develop following a hammer toe repair or trauma,[28] or it can be associated with inflammatory arthritis.[28,29] The high incidence of mallet toe in the female population has led to speculation that a constricting toe box is a causative factor.[24,27,28] Female subjects constituted 84% of the patient population in

one reported series,[30] the gender difference being highly significant. Brahms[12] stated that a mallet toe is often limited to one toe, although Mann and Coughlin[100] noted that the deformity can occur in more than one toe. Coughlin[28] noted in his report (60 patients,

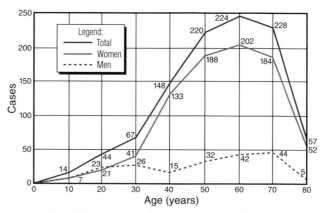

Figure 7–6   Hammer toe deformities peak during the fifth, sixth, and seventh decades in the female population. In the male population there is no increase in the frequency of hammer toe deformities with increasing age. (From Coughlin MJ, Thompson FM: *Instr Course Lect* 44:371-377, 1995.)

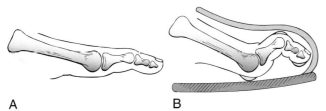

A   **B**

Figure 7–7 A, Phalanx extended to normal length. **B,** Buckling of the phalanx is caused by restriction of the toe box. The interphalangeal joints and metatarsophalangeal joints become subluxed. Over time, dislocation can occur.

86 toes) that although 65% of patients had single toe involvement, 18% of patients had multiple toe involvement, with three to five toes affected.

A mallet toe occurs with equal frequency in the second, third, and fourth toes,[28] but most often the involved toe is longer than the adjacent toes (Fig. 7–9). Because of pressure against the end of the shoe, the toe becomes plantar flexed at the DIP joint. Tightness of the flexor digitorum longus tendon in patients with a mallet toe deformity can be demonstrated, but whether this tightness is a primary cause or a secondary change is not known. In young children a tight flexor tendon can result in a flexion deformity of the PIP and DIP joint. This pediatric deformity has been termed a *curly toe*[8,70,122,139,155] and may also be associated with a delta-shaped phalanx.[44]

The major symptoms leading to surgical repair in the adult population include discomfort due to pressure on the tip of the toe, with callus formation or dorsal pain over the DIP joint.* Preoperative nail deformities occurred in 7% of toes in Coughlin's series, and 93% were noted to have dorsal pain or pain at the tip of the toe with callus formation (see Figs. 7–48B and F and 7–55C and D).

Hammer Toe

The causes of a hammer toe appear to be multifactorial. The high incidence of hammer toes in the female population has led some to suggest that a constricting toe box is also a causative factor of this deformity.[10,26,37,145] Coughlin[33] reported that 62% of the patients in his series considered ill-fitting shoes to be a cause of their hammer toe deformity. The high incidence of female involvement has been previously reported[17,37,135,145]; females constituted 85% of the patient population in a large series,[33] the gender difference being highly significant. The incidence of hammer toes is reported to occur with increasing age,[17,37,145] with the peak incidence in the fifth through seventh decades. Coughlin[33] noted in his report (67 patients; 118 toes) that 30% had only single toe involvement and 40% had three or more toes

---

*References 11, 12, 15, 27, 28, 116, and 138.

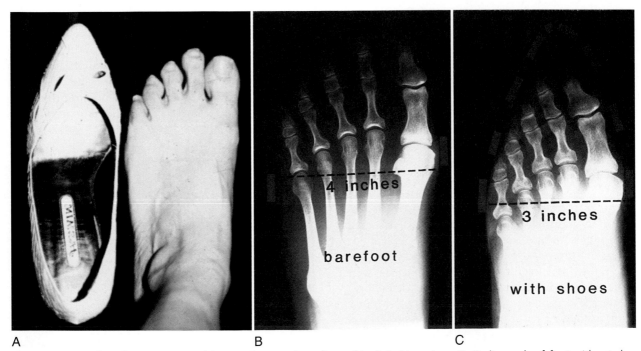

A   **B**   **C**

Figure 7–8 A, Clinical appearance of foot and pointed toe box of high-fashion shoe. **B,** Radiograph of foot without shoes showing width measuring 4 inches. **C,** Within high-fashion shoe, the forefoot width is compressed to 3 inches. Note constriction of toe box and lateral deviation of hallux.

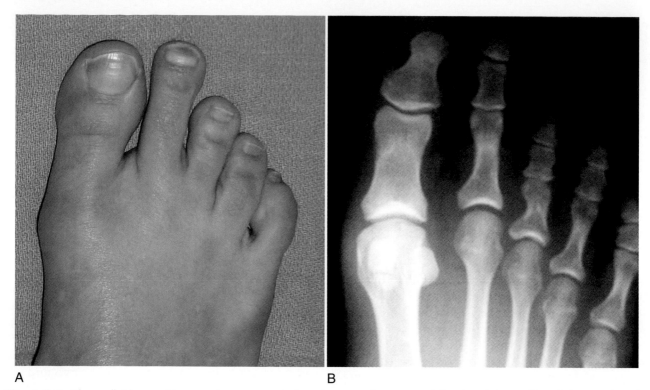

A   B

Figure 7–9 The mallet toe and hammer toe are most often the second toe, especially when it is significantly longer than the adjacent toes.

involved. Although Reece,[135] Coughlin,[33] and others[146,147,168] have reported the second toe to be the most commonly involved, Ohm[124] reported an equal frequency of occurrence in the second, third, and fourth toes. Coughlin[33] noted that increased length in comparison to adjacent digits might be a factor in hammer toe development, although this was not a factor in almost one half of cases.

A hammer toe deformity may be caused by a muscle imbalance in association with neuromuscular diseases such as Charcot–Marie–Tooth disease, Friedreich's ataxia, cerebral palsy, myelodysplasia, multiple sclerosis, and degenerative disk disease. The deformity also is seen in patients with an insensate foot associated with diabetes mellitus and Hansen's disease.[31] Patients with rheumatoid arthritis, psoriatic arthritis, and other types of inflammatory arthritis also can develop a hammer toe deformity.[26,27,31] Associated hallux valgus deformities have also been implicated as a cause of hammer toe formation.[13,31,146,147] Occasionally, following fractures of the tibia or other trauma,[55,147] a progressive hammer toe deformity is observed and is likely the result of nerve or muscle injury from elevated compartment pressures in the involved leg or foot.

Claw Toe

The cause of a claw toe deformity often is unclear, but it may be associated with the same neuromuscular dis-

eases, arthritic deformities, and metabolic diseases that cause hammer toe deformities (Fig. 7–10). In many patients with a severe claw toe deformity, no cause can be identified. A claw toe is a result of muscle imbalance between the intrinsic and extrinsic musculature.[115,147] Simultaneous contracture of the long flexors and extensors of the toe, without the modifying action of the intrinsic muscles of the foot, causes the typical deformity seen in this condition (Figs. 7–11 and 7–12).[145] Taylor,[157] however, found no abnormality of the intrinsic muscles in a series of 68 patients who had

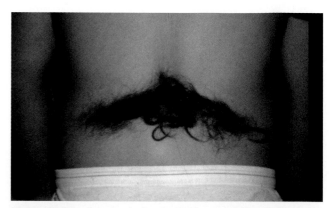

Figure 7–10 On physical examination, a patient with severe claw toe deformities is noted to have a hairy patch over the lumbosacral spine, a condition often associated with diastematomyelia.

claw toes and in whom the muscles were examined by gross inspection, stimulation, and histologic inspection.

A claw toe deformity usually involves multiple toes and often both feet (see Fig. 7–57).[25] The deformity may be either rigid or flexible. It is often associated with a cavus foot, with or without a contracted Achilles tendon. Claw toes are often made worse because the patient cannot find adequate shoes, and a painful bursa develops over the PIP joint. As the claw toe deformity becomes more rigid, the toes strike the top of the shoe and the metatarsal heads are forced plantarward. As the toes subluxate dorsally, the plantar fat pad is pulled distally and the metatarsal heads become more prominent on the plantar aspect of the foot. This deformity can result in the development of painful plantar callosities, which can ulcerate in severe cases, particularly if sensation of the foot is impaired.

Anatomy and Pathophysiology

An understanding of the anatomy and pathophysiology is helpful in selecting a treatment regimen. The most common deformity is the hammer toe, and this

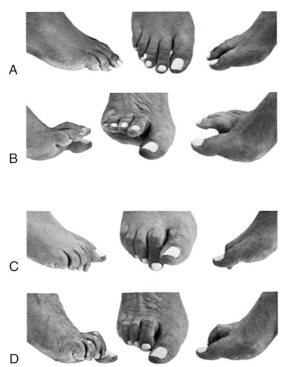

Figure 7–11 Action of muscles in claw toe deformity (from a fresh cadaver foot). **A,** At rest. **B,** Tension on the extensor digitorum longus alone. Note extension of the metatarsophalangeal joints and minimal extension of the interphalangeal joints. **C,** Tension on the flexor digitorum longus alone. Note that maximal flexion occurs at the interphalangeal joints. **D,** Tension simultaneously on the extensor digitorum longus and flexor digitorum longus. Note the resulting deformities in all but the great toe.

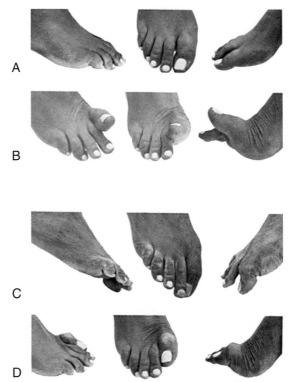

Figure 7–12 Action of muscles in a claw toe deformity of the hallux (from a fresh cadaver foot). **A,** At rest. **B,** Tension on the extensor hallucis longus alone. Note the extension of the metatarsophalangeal and interphalangeal joints. **C,** Tension on the flexor hallucis longus alone. Note the maximal flexion of the interphalangeal joints. **D,** Simultaneous tension on the extensor hallucis longus and flexor hallucis longus, with a resulting hammer toe deformity.

is used as the prototype in discussing the pathophysiology of all three deformities.

Extensor Digitorum Longus Muscle and Tendon

The central dorsal structure of the toe is formed by the tendon of the extensor digitorum longus, which divides into three slips over the proximal phalanx; the middle slip inserts into the base of the middle phalanx, and the two lateral slips extend over the dorsolateral aspect of the middle phalanx and converge to form the terminal tendon, which inserts into the base of the distal phalanx (Fig. 7–13).[142,143] The tendon is held in a central position dorsally by a fibroaponeurotic sling that anchors the long extensor to the plantar aspect of the MTP joint and to the base of the proximal phalanx. It is surprising that there is no dorsal insertion of the extensor digitorum longus into the proximal phalanx; rather, the phalanx is virtually suspended by the extensor digitorum longus tendon and its extensor sling (Fig. 7–14).

The main function of the extensor digitorum longus is to dorsiflex the proximal phalanx (Fig. 7–15). Only

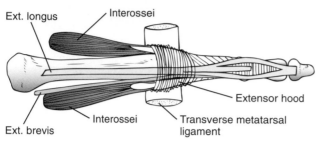

Figure 7–13 Diagram of dorsal view of the extensor mechanism of toes. (Redrawn from Sarrafian SK, Topouzian LK: *J Bone Joint Surg Am* 51[4]:669–679, 1969.)

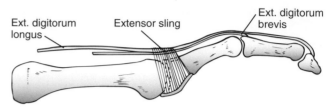

Figure 7–15 Lateral view of the extensor mechanism demonstrates the main function of the extensor digitorum longus, which is to dorsiflex the proximal phalanx.

when the proximal phalanx is held in flexion or in a neutral position at the MTP joint can this tendon become an extensor of the PIP joint. This concept is important because with a hammer toe deformity the long extensor tendon function on the PIP joint may be neutralized by extension of the proximal phalanx.[145]

The flexor digitorum longus tendon inserts into the distal phalanx and flexes the DIP joint, whereas the flexor digitorum brevis inserts into the middle phalanx, flexing the PIP joint. There is no insertion into the proximal phalanx, so the long flexor tendon influence on the proximal phalanx is minimal (Fig. 7–16A). Resistance to flexion at the MTP joint is maintained in the normal toe by the long extensor. Another important factor is the reactive force of the foot against the ground, which pushes the MTP joint into extension. As a result, with the proximal phalanx in an extended position, there are no major motor antagonists to the long and short flexors; thus the toe buckles, resulting in flexion of the DIP joint and the PIP joint. Over a long period of time, if this position becomes fixed, a hammer toe deformity occurs.

Interosseous Tendons

The interosseous tendons are located dorsal to the transverse metatarsal ligament, and the lumbricals are located plantar to this ligament (Fig. 7–16B). Both tendons of the intrinsic muscles, however, pass plantar to the axis of motion of the MTP joint, flexing the MTP

joint (Fig. 7–17), and pass dorsal to the axis of the PIP joint and DIP joint, extending these joints. This is an important concept to understand when performing a Weil osteotomy of the distal metatarsal; the center of MTP joint rotation is shifted plantarward, effectively making the intrinsic musculature MTP joint dorsiflex, which can lead to the development of a hyperextension deformity of the MTP joint (see Fig. 7–93).[165,169,170] The plantar and dorsal interossei have only a few fibers that reach the extensor sling and therefore are weak extensors of the interphalangeal joints. The lumbrical, with all of its fibers terminating in the extensor sling, is a stronger extensor of these joints. The interossei flex the proximal phalanx by their direct attachment to the base of the proximal phalanx, whereas the lumbrical achieves flexion by placing tension on the extensor sling (Fig. 7–18). With marked

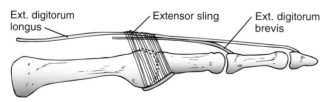

Figure 7–14 Lateral view of extensor mechanism of the lesser toe. Note that the extensor digitorum longus inserts only into the distal phalanx and secondarily suspends the metatarsophalangeal joint through the extensor sling mechanism.

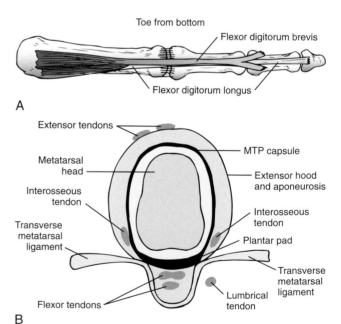

Figure 7–16 **A,** Plantar view of flexor tendon insertion. **B,** Cross section through the metatarsal head of the lesser toe demonstrates structures that pass through this region. Note that the interossei tendons are dorsal to the transverse metatarsal ligament, whereas the lumbrical is plantar to it. MTP, metatarsophalangeal.

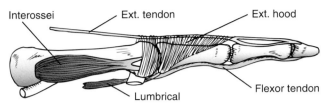

Figure 7–17 Lateral view of a lesser toe demonstrates that both tendons of the intrinsic muscles pass plantar to the axis of motion of the metatarsophalangeal joint, thereby flexing it. They pass dorsal to the axis of motion of the proximal and distal interphalangeal joints, thereby extending them. The lumbrical does not insert into the phalanx but into the extensor hood, and it is thus is a strong extensor of the interphalangeal joints.

dorsiflexion at the MTP joint, the lumbrical flexion power is quite limited because it is pulling at a 90-degree angle.

Plantar Plate and Collateral Ligaments

The most significant stabilizing factor of the MTP joint is the plantar plate, a combination of the plantar aponeurosis and plantar capsule.[31,130,145] During the walking cycle, varying degrees of dorsiflexion occur at the MTP joint. The static resistance of the

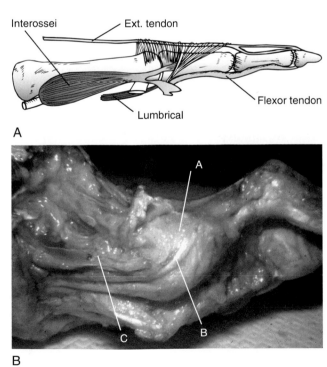

Figure 7–18 A, Lateral aspect of a lesser toe with portion of the extensor hood removed to demonstrate insertion of the interossei into the base of the proximal phalanx. This insertion permits the interossei to plantar flex the proximal phalanx on the metatarsal head. **B,** Anatomic dissection demonstrating extensor hood and intrinsics. *A,* Central axis of metatarsophalangeal joint; *B,* lumbrical; *C,* interossei.

plantar capsule combines with the dynamic force of the intrinsic flexors to pull the proximal phalanx back into a neutral position at the MTP joint (Fig. 7–19A). With chronic hyperextension forces on the proximal phalanx, the plantar plate can become stretched or attenuated and rendered less efficient (Fig. 7–19B).

The lesser MTP joint is stabilized by both the collateral ligaments and the plantar plate.[6,46,47] The plantar plate inserts on the base of the proximal phalanx, but it is attached to the metatarsal head by only a thin layer of synovial tissue that inserts just proximal to the articular surface.[46] The distal attachment of the plantar plate is composed of a medial and a lateral bundle. Proximally, the plantar plate forms the major attachment of the plantar aponeurosis. The plantar plate is the central stabilizing structure that determines the position of the flexor digitorum longus. The collateral ligaments are composed of two major structures: the phalangeal collateral ligament (PCL), which inserts onto the base of the proximal phalanx, and the accessory collateral ligament (ACL), which inserts onto the plantar plate.[46] The transverse metatarsal ligament attaches to the adjacent medial and lateral borders of the plantar plate.[83]

Pathophysiology

Fortin and Myerson[57] reported that the collateral ligaments were the primary stabilizers of the lesser MTP joint. When the collateral ligaments were sectioned in vitro, 48% less force was required to dislocate the

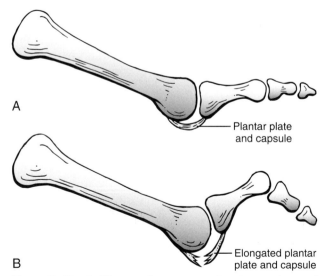

Figure 7–19 A, Diagram demonstrates the plantar plate and the capsule of the metatarsophalangeal (MTP) joint, which is sufficiently resilient to bring the MTP joint back into a neutral position after the joint has been dorsiflexed at lift-off. **B,** Diagram illustrates the effects of the elongated plantar plate and capsule. As a result of certain disease states, the capsular structures no longer are sufficient to restore the joint to its normal position following lift-off.

lesser MTP joint. When the researchers did an isolated release of the plantar plate, 29% less force was required to dislocate the MTP joint.

Deland and Sung[48] demonstrated a rupture of the lateral collateral ligament and attenuation of the lateral plantar plate in the dissection of a specimen of a crossover second toe. Associated with this deformity was a medial subluxation of the plantar plate. As tension was applied on the medially subluxated long flexor tendon, the proximal phalanx deviated medially. The stout attachment of the plantar plate to the proximal phalanx was observed to be intact.

Haddad et al[69] observed that the weakest area of the capsule is the thin synovial attachment of the plantar plate to the metatarsal neck. It either lengthens or ruptures, and patients often experience MTP joint pain long before observing any deviation of the digit. Incompetence of the lateral collateral ligament then allows unopposed pull of the first lumbrical, which allows medial deviation of the second toe.

The position of the proximal phalanx at the MTP joint is subject to the actions of the strong extensor digitorum longus through its sling mechanism, in opposition to the decidedly weaker antagonistic intrinsic muscles and the more static capsule and plantar aponeurosis complex. The positions of the middle and distal phalanges, on the other hand, are subject to the forces of the long and short flexors, which are directly opposed by the weaker intrinsic muscles. At each of these joints an obvious mismatch can occur, and in each case the extrinsic muscle overpowers the intrinsic muscle (Fig. 7–20).

The extensor digitorum longus helps extend the interphalangeal joints if the proximal phalanx is not hyperextended, and the flexor digitorum longus helps to flex the MTP joint if the proximal phalanx is not hyperextended. The hyperextended proximal phalanx, then, is definitely the key to the production of most hammer toe deformities. With a chronic hyperextended position of the proximal phalanx maintained throughout the entire walking cycle (by wearing high-heeled shoes), the plantar structures gradually become stretched and inefficient, and thus the proximal phalanx remains in a chronically dorsiflexed position. Therefore, with chronic extension of the proximal phalanx, the extensor digitorum longus tendon loses its tenodesing effect on the interphalangeal joints, allowing the distal phalanges to migrate into flexion. As the proximal phalanx extends, the intrinsic flexors are under greater tension, further increasing the flexion deformity at the PIP joint. The only counteracting forces to this flexion deformity are the lumbricals and the interossei, which are easily overpowered by the long flexor tendons.

Preoperative Evaluation

Physical Examination

When examining a foot with a lesser toe deformity it is important to assess the circulatory status of the lower extremity. Although some surgical procedures require limited exposure, other procedures require extensive dissection at the MTP joint, at the interphalangeal joints, and even along both the medial and lateral aspects of the phalanges. Whether an individual digit can withstand multiple procedures and extensive surgical exposure depends on the vascular status of the digit. Preoperative evaluation is necessary to assess not only the feasibility of an individual procedure but also whether multiple procedures can be performed if necessary.

The sensory status of a foot must be evaluated as well. An impaired sensory status can indicate a systemic disease such as diabetes, a peripheral neuropathy, or lumbar disk disease. Careful physical examination is necessary to differentiate MTP joint pain from an interdigital neuroma of the adjacent intermetatarsal space (Fig. 7–21).[35,36] Preoperative documentation of sensation is important because a surgical dissection can diminish postoperative sensation.

The plantar aspect of the foot is examined for development of intractable plantar keratoses. Callosities can develop in association with contractures of the lesser toes, the result of a buckling effect of the toes. A patient typically complains of pain caused by a callus over the distal aspect of the PIP joint but also can develop pain beneath the tip of the toe or a lesser metatarsal head (Fig. 7–22).[33,95] Realignment of the MTP joint and interphalangeal joints can decrease plantar pressure and help relieve symptomatic calluses.

The individual digits then are examined for callosities on the medial and lateral aspects, as well as over the interphalangeal joint and at the tip of the toe. With a fixed hammer toe deformity, callosities can develop

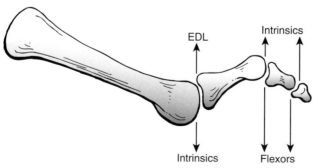

Figure 7–20 Diagram demonstrates the relationship of the intrinsic and extrinsic muscles about a lesser toe. The smaller intrinsics are overpowered by the extrinsics, leading to a hammer toe deformity. EDL, extensor digitorum longus.

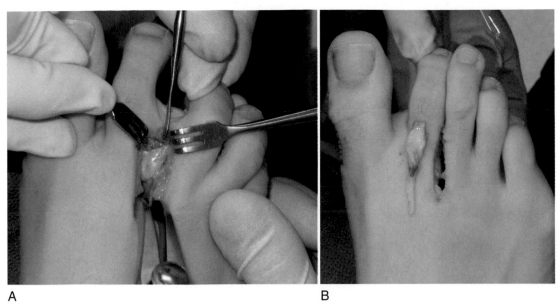

A   B

Figure 7–21   The diagnosis of combined metatarsophalangeal instability and an adjacent interdigital neuroma is uncommon and difficult to make. **A,** Medial deviation of the second toe with exposure of enlarged symptomatic interdigital neuroma. **B,** Following Weil osteotomy to realign the second toe and excise the interdigital neuroma.

over the contracted PIP joint as well as at the tip of the toe. Toenail deformities can develop as well.

The alignment of the MTP joint must be evaluated. Medial or lateral deviation of the toe should be noted, as well as an MTP joint hyperextension deformity.

Although the evaluation of a hammer toe deformity may be seen as relatively simple, certain factors must be carefully considered to fully appreciate the nature of the deformity. These include the rigidity of the toe

contractures (Fig. 7–23), the position of the MTP joint (Fig. 7–24A), and Achilles tendon tightness with the patient both sitting and standing. Tightness of the flexor digitorum longus tendon must be assessed along with examination of all of the lesser toes. Also, it is important to determine whether there is sufficient space for the involved toe when it is reduced to a normal position. The presence of prior surgical scars can influence the planned surgical exposure.

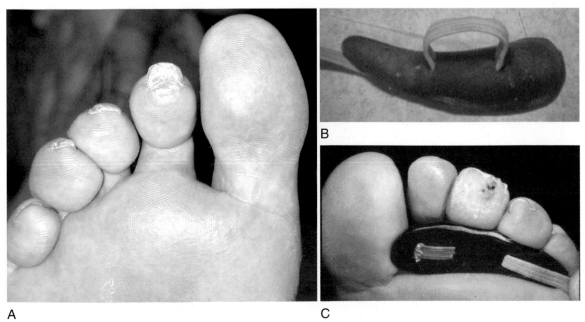

A   C

Figure 7–22   **A,** With a hammer toe deformity, a callus has developed at the tip of the second toe. **B,** A toe cradle. **C,** The cradle is used to decrease pressure beneath the tip of the lesser toe. (**C** from Coughlin MJ: *Instr Course Lect* 52:421-444, 2003.)

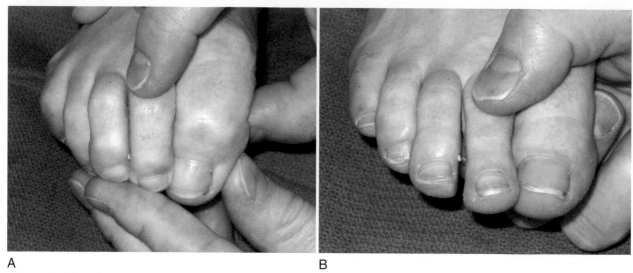

A   B

Figure 7–23   A hammer toe deformity is inspected to determine its flexibility. **A,** Fixed deformity. **B,** Flexible deformity.

Radiographic Examination

Although a physical examination is necessary to define the extent of a lesser toe deformity, radiographic examination is necessary to evaluate the magnitude of the bone deformity (Fig. 7–24B). On an anteroposterior (AP) projection, a severe hammer toe deformity can have the appearance of a gun barrel deformity (Fig. 7–24C) when the proximal phalanx is seen end on. Assessment of the interphalangeal joints is difficult on this projection. Diminution of the MTP joint space can indicate subluxation, and overlap of the base of the proximal phalanx in relation to the metatarsal head can indicate dislocation of the MTP joint (see Fig. 7–69). Medial or lateral deviation of the MTP joint can be determined as well. Subchondral erosion, flattening of the articular surfaces, or Freiberg's infraction can indicate the need for further radiographic or laboratory evaluation.

A lateral radiograph may be helpful to assess the magnitude of contracture of the interphalangeal joints (see Fig. 7–24B). Stress radiographs can help to determine subluxability of the MTP joint (see Fig. 7–65).

FIXED HAMMER TOE DEFORMITY

Preoperative Planning

A hammer toe deformity may be flexible, semiflexible, or rigid.[21,25,33,99-101] If the deformity is flexible, the toe may be passively corrected to a neutral position. However, if the deformity is rigid, joint contractures preclude passive correction. The rigidity of the deformity determines whether conservative or surgical treatment is indicated, as well as the specific surgical procedure that should be performed.

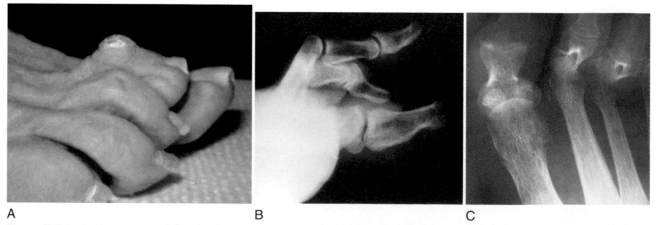

A   B   C

Figure 7–24   **A,** Hammer toe deformity demonstrates severe hyperextension. **B,** Lateral radiograph demonstrates hyperextension deformity of the proximal phalanx. **C,** Anteroposterior radiograph demonstrates the gun barrel sign. The proximal phalanx is seen end on, superimposed over the condyle. This conformation is pathognomonic of hyperextension deformity of the proximal phalanx.

The position of the MTP joint when the patient is standing must be carefully evaluated. If a hyperextension deformity is present, correction of only the hammer toe deformity will result in the toe sticking up in an extended position (Fig. 7–25), making shoe wearing difficult. If the MTP joint is subluxated or dislocated, this deformity should be corrected simultaneously with the hammer toe correction.[31,93,99,129]

Tightness of the flexor digitorum longus tendon should be carefully observed with the patient in a standing position. If the flexor digitorum longus tendon appears to be tight in the toe adjacent to the involved toe, the involved toe probably also has a contracture of the flexor digitorum longus tendon. In this case the tendon should be released in the deformed toe at surgery or the deformity will probably recur over time (Fig. 7–26).

Another consideration in the treatment of a hammer toe is that there must be sufficient space for the corrected toe to occupy (Fig. 7–27A). If a patient has a concomitant hallux valgus deformity that has diminished the interval between the first and third toes and forced the second toe into dorsiflexion, adequate space must be obtained for the corrected lesser toe or the deformity can recur.[100] An Akin phalangeal osteotomy may be used to create room for a second toe when a hammer toe correction is performed.[129] A hallux valgus repair may be necessary to obtain sufficient space between the first and third toes to realign the second toe successfully. At times the adjacent lesser toes can drift into medial or lateral deviation, again diminishing the interval that the corrected toe should occupy. These toes may need to be corrected to afford the corrected hammer toe adequate space.

A young patient with a nonfixed deformity is a candidate for conservative treatment. Likewise, an older

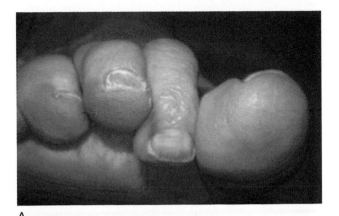

A

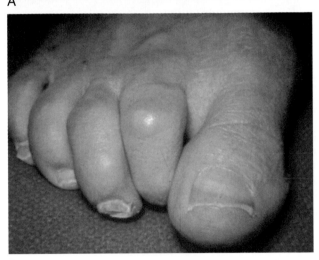

B

Figure 7–26 With a tight flexor tendon in an adjacent toe, a flexor tenotomy should be performed at the time of hammer toe repair. **A,** Contracture of just the second toe indicates a flexor tenotomy is possibly not necessary. **B,** A contracture is noted in all of the lesser toes. (**B** from Chapman M [ed]: *Operative Orthopaedics.* Philadelphia, JB Lippincott, 1988, pp 1765-1776.)

patient with multiple medical problems may be a poor surgical candidate as well. The most important conservative measure is for the patient to acquire roomy, well-fitted shoes.[37] The preferable characteristics of such shoes include a high and wide toe box and a soft sole with a soft upper portion of the toe box. This helps to prevent direct pressure against a hammer toe and subsequent development of painful callosities. Local treatment can consist of a doughnut-shaped cushion, foam toe cap (Fig. 7–27B), foam tube-gauze, or viscoelastic toe sleeves placed over the PIP joint (Fig. 7–27C-F).

The shoe itself might need to be modified if the patient has pain beneath the metatarsal head. Such a modification can consist of a soft metatarsal support, a metatarsal bar, or a comfortable orthosis that relieves pressure beneath the involved metatarsal head. At times patients modify their shoes to reduce pressure

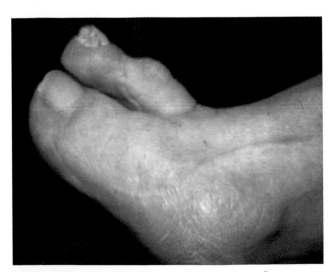

Figure 7–25 An isolated hammer toe repair or a flexor tenotomy can lead to hyperextension deformity of the involved toe.

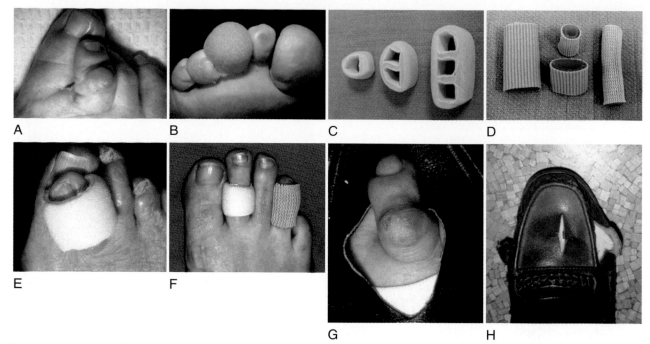

Figure 7–27   **A,** A hallux valgus deformity can reduce the space available for the second toe once the hammer toe has been corrected. **B,** A toe cap may be used to decrease pressure on the distal tip of the hammer toe. **C** and **D,** Various types of tube gauze may be used to pad a lesser toe deformity. **E** and **F,** Tube gauze is slid over the symptomatic toe to relieve pressure. **G,** Patient has modified footwear to make room for the prominent second toe. **H,** A shoe may be modified as in this case by a patient with a bunion, bunionette, and hammer toe deformity.

on a symptomatic hammer toe (Fig. 7–27G-H). A toe cradle can elevate the involved digit and reduce pressure on the tip of the toe (see Fig. 7–22B and C). In more advanced cases and with multiple toe involvement, an extra-depth shoe with a polyethylene foam (Plastazote) insole can help to distribute pressure more uniformly on the plantar aspect of the foot. A program with daily manipulation of the toes should be started to try to keep the toes flexible.

A traumatic boutonnière deformity can develop with a hammer toe deformity (Fig. 7–28). Rau and Manoli[134] initially reported on this rare deformity,

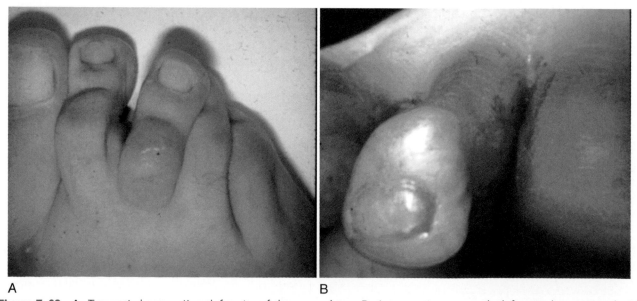

Figure 7–28   **A,** Traumatic boutonnière deformity of the second toe. **B,** A traumatic swan-neck deformity has occurred with development of a mallet toe as well as hyperextension of the PIP joint.

which is caused by a rupture of the central extensor slip. As the lateral bands displace, they become flexors of the PIP joint. A flexion deformity of the PIP joint occurs and is associated with a hyperextension deformity of the DIP joint. The authors recommended a direct repair of the central slip and recentralization of the lateral bands. Quebedeaux et al[132] reported on two cases of traumatic boutonnière deformity; one developed in association with chronic rheumatoid arthritis and was treated conservatively, and the other one developed following trauma. A delayed repair and PIP arthroplasty was performed.

If a deformity of the MTP joint exists along with a hammer toe deformity (a complex hammer toe deformity), surgical correction of this deformity also must be considered. In cases of a mild deformity, an extensor tenotomy or lengthening may be sufficient to achieve correction. In cases of a moderate hyperextension deformity of the MTP joint, an extensor tenotomy and MTP capsule release may be necessary.[49] Kirschner wire fixation also may be necessary to stabilize the arthroplasty site as well as the MTP joint. A flexor tendon transfer also may be necessary to achieve stability of the MTP joint. Where subluxation has progressed to frank dislocation of the MTP joint, the soft tissue procedures described are inadequate to achieve reduction, and a metatarsal osteotomy is necessary. (A complete discussion of the evaluation and treatment of MTP joint subluxation and dislocation is presented later in the chapter.)

With time, and even with appropriate conservative management, most of these deformities become fixed and often require surgical correction.[33,123] The algorithm presented in Figure 7–29 is a useful guide to treatment of the hammer toe deformity. If surgery is required, it is important that the procedure be carefully selected, depending on the specific cause and type of the deformity.

Indications

The DuVries arthroplasty is recommended for reduction of a fixed hammer toe deformity involving the middle three toes. This procedure does not necessarily achieve a joint fusion; it can achieve a fibrous union that usually allows approximately 15 degrees of motion. The arthroplasty may be performed under a digital anesthetic block if there is no MTP joint involvement. If there is an MTP joint deformity, more extensive anesthesia is necessary.

Contraindications

Contraindications include acute or chronic infection, vascular insufficiency, and flexible deformities for which a resection arthroplasty is not necessary. Relative contraindications include more severe deformities involving the MTP joint, for which more extensive surgery must be combined with the DuVries arthroplasty in order to realign the digit completely.

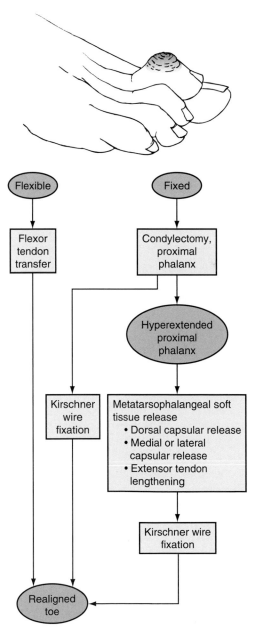

Figure 7–29 Algorithm for treatment of hammer toe deformity.

DUVRIES ARTHROPLASTY PROCEDURE

Surgical Technique

1. The patient is placed in a supine position on the operating room table. The foot is cleansed and draped in the usual fashion. The use of a 1/4-inch Penrose drain as a tourniquet is optional. If MTP joint surgery is performed, an Esmarch bandage can be used to exsanguinate the extremity and as an ankle tourniquet.[68] A digital block or ankle block is used for anesthesia depending upon the need for additional surgical procedures at the same time.

2. An elliptical or longitudinal incision is centered over the dorsal aspect of the PIP joint, excising the callus, extensor tendon, and joint capsule, thereby exposing the PIP joint (Figs. 7–30A and 7–31A and video clip 41).

3. The collateral ligaments on the medial and lateral aspects of the proximal phalanx are severed to allow the condyles of the proximal phalanx to be delivered into the wound (Figs. 7–30B and C and 7–31B and C). Care is taken to protect the adjacent neurovascular bundles.

4. The head of the proximal phalanx is resected just proximal to the flare of the condyles, and any prominent edges are smoothed with a rongeur (Figs. 7–30D and 7–31D).

5. At this point the toe should be brought into corrected alignment. If there still appears to be tension at the PIP joint, so that it is difficult to adequately correct the deformity, more bone should be resected. Also, consideration should be given to release of the flexor digitorum longus through this wound (Fig. 7–30E; see Fig. 7–26).

6. If a flexor tenotomy is performed, the plantar capsule of the PIP joint is carefully incised and the long flexor tendon is identified in the flexor tendon sheath. The tendon is transected and allowed to retract.

7. The articular surface of the base of the middle phalanx may be resected with a rongeur.[162] This is optional.[25,33]

8. A 0.045-inch Kirschner wire is introduced at the PIP joint and driven distally, exiting the tip of the toe. With the toe held in proper alignment, the pin is driven in a retrograde fashion to stabilize and align the toe. The wire is then bent at the tip of the toe and the excess pin removed (Figs. 7–30F and 7–31E).

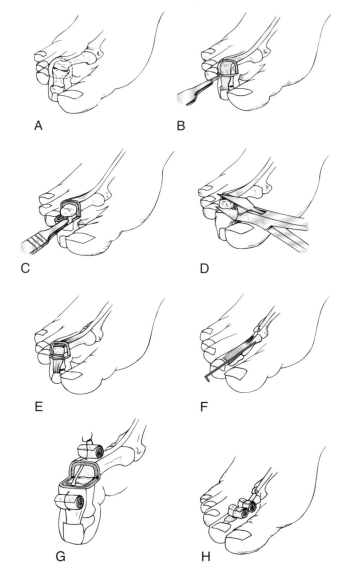

Figure 7–30   Technique for repair of a hammer toe deformity. **A,** Elliptical incision over the proximal interphalangeal (PIP) joint excises callus, if present, along with the extensor tendon and joint capsule. **B,** Removal of extensor tendon and joint capsule along lines of incision. **C,** When a knife blade is placed flat against the condyles, the collateral ligaments are cut, thereby delivering the head of the proximal phalanx into the wound. **D,** Excision of the head of the proximal phalanx proximal to the flare of the condyles. **E,** Condyles have been removed. At this time, a decision is made as to whether to perform a flexor tenotomy. If a flexor tenotomy is done, the plantar capsule is incised, and the long flexor tendon is incised in the depths of the wound. **F,** A 0.045-inch Kirschner wire is introduced at the PIP joint and driven distally, exiting the tip of the toe. The PIP joint is reduced, and the pin then is driven retrograde, stabilizing the repair. **G,** Alternate means of stabilization. Insertion of vertical mattress suture of 3-0 nylon. The deep portion of the suture approximates the extensor tendon, and the superficial portion of the suture coapts skin edges. The Telfa bolster is used to gain leverage to hold the toe in satisfactory alignment. **H,** The toe is held in satisfactory alignment after placement of sutures and bolsters.

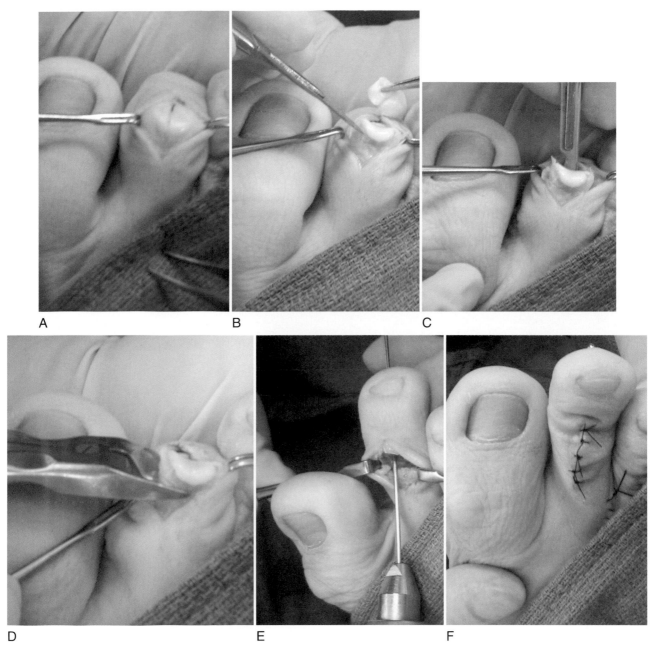

Figure 7–31 Hammer toe deformity of the second toe. **A,** Following skin excision, the dorsal capsule and extensor tendon are exposed. **B,** Removal of extensor tendon and joint capsule along the lines of the incision. **C,** The collateral ligaments and plantar capsule are released. **D,** Exposing the condyles of the proximal phalanx, which are excised. (After excision of the head of the proximal phalanx, a flexor tenotomy may be performed; also, the articular surface of the base of the middle phalanx may be resected.) **E,** Kirschner wire fixation. **F,** Following completion of repair.

9. The wound is closed with vertical interrupted mattress sutures of 3-0 nylon (Fig. 7–30F).

Alternative Fixation

A vertical mattress-type suture using 3-0 nylon and incorporating two Telfa bolsters is inserted. As the suture is tightened, a certain degree of leverage is placed on the toe to bring it into satisfactory alignment (Fig. 7–30G and H and Fig. 7–32).

Postoperative Care

A small compression dressing is placed around the toe, and the patient is allowed to ambulate in a postoperative wooden shoe. If Telfa bolsters have been used, the suture and bolsters are removed 1 week after surgery. The bolsters should not be left in place for more than 1 week because of the possibility of skin necrosis developing beneath them. If a Kirschner wire has been used, the sutures and wire are removed 3 weeks after surgery. In either case, it is important to support the toe with tape for the next 4 to 6 weeks after internal or external fixation has been removed. Localized trauma to the digit in the first few weeks after surgery can lead to recurrent deformity and must be avoided.

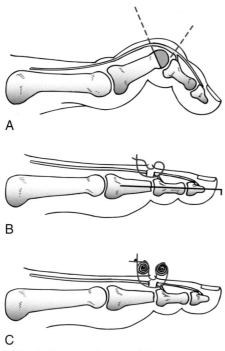

Figure 7–32 A, Proposed area of bone resection. **B,** Following bone resection, stabilization with intramedullary Kirschner wire. **C,** Stabilization with sutures and Telfa bolsters.

Results and Complications

Ohm et al[124] reported on 25 patients (62 hammer toe repairs); hammer toes were corrected with a digital fusion technique. An equal number of corrections were performed on the second, third, and fourth toes. At short-term follow-up, a 100% fusion rate was reported. Newman and Fitton[123] reported on results in 19 patients treated with a similar technique and surprisingly noted only 40% satisfactory results.

Coughlin et al[33] reported the largest study (67 patients, 118 toes). Patients were evaluated at an average of 5 years following proximal phalangeal condylectomy, middle phalangeal articular resection, and intramedullary Kirschner wire fixation. Fusion of the PIP joint occurred in 81% of cases, and subjective satisfactory results were observed in 84% of cases. Pain relief in 92% of patients was no different in those with a fibrous or a bony union, although many reports suggest that a fibrous union is consistent with a successful outcome.* Higgs[74] stated that a fibrous union placed the digit at risk for recurrent deformity. This notion was not confirmed by Coughlin's series. Although a PIP fusion is not necessarily the ultimate objective, increased stiffness or fusion of the PIP joint appears to help maintain alignment. Kelikian[87] observed that resection of both articular surfaces leads to a satisfactory result if it is followed by stiffness of the joint. The goal of surgery is to correct the deformity and maintain the correction.

Although some authors advocate attempted arthrodesis,[1,154,162,174] others have stated that a PIP joint resection suffices as treatment by achieving adequate alignment of the toe.[33,39,66,142] A fusion of the PIP joint or an arthrofibrosis succeeds by converting the pull of the flexor digitorum longus to flex the entire digit. A fusion also gives triplanar stability to the toe. The rate of pseudoarthrosis in attempted PIP joint fusions approaches 50% in some series, although some surgeons have obtained a high fusion rate (>90%) with a peg-and-dowel technique.[1,95,146] Pichney et al[129] used a V-type arthrodesis technique for correcting a hammer toe deformity with good success. Lehman and Smith[95] reported on PIP arthrodesis, noting a 50% satisfaction rate with a peg-and-dowel technique. Major reasons for postoperative dis-

*References 39, 74, 88, 123, 124, 147, 149, and 168.

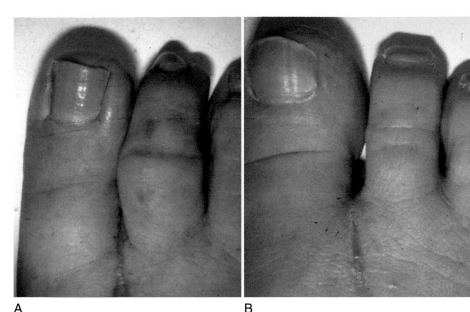

Figure 7–33 A, Postoperative swelling is common. **B,** With time, edema of the toe usually subsides. (From Coughlin MJ, Dorris J, Polk E: *Foot Ankle Int* 21[2]:94-104, 2000. Copyright © 2000 by the American Orthopaedic Foot and Ankle Society [AOFAS], originally published in *Foot and Ankle International*, Feb. 2000, Vol. 21, No. 2, pp 94-104 and reproduced here with permission.)

A   B

satisfaction were toe angulation and incomplete relief of pain. Because of the straight nature of the fusion, toe tip elevation was noted in 14% of cases. Transverse plane angulation was observed in 11%. Forty-four percent of patients developed flexion at the DIP joint, a finding also noted by Schlefman et al[146] in their series. Ohm et al[124] and Schlefman et al[146] noted that more bone resection was necessary for a peg-and-dowel technique. Shortening, however, is a common complaint following this technique of hammer toe repair.

Malalignment is often a major reason for dissatisfaction.[33] Malalignment can occur in any one of three planes—medial–lateral, dorsal–plantar, or rotational. Also, a hammer toe can develop in an adjacent nonoperated toe. A patient should be warned that there is a possibility of developing deformities in other toes.

The results of hammer toe repairs are in general most gratifying, and few, if any, complications are routinely reported. Swelling of the toe can persist for 1 to 6 months after the procedure.[95,124,130] Almost invariably, however, the swelling subsides if given sufficient time (Fig. 7–33). Coughlin[33] noted that no patient had digital swelling at long term follow-up.

Alternative treatments for hammer toe deformities include either a diaphysectomy or partial proximal phalangectomy (Fig. 7–34). McConnell[107,108] reported on a large series of patients treated with diaphysectomy of the proximal phalanx to correct a hammer toe deformity (Fig. 7–35). Satisfactory results were reported with this procedure. McConnell stated that "most cases heal by bony union." The actual alignment of the toe, complications, and rate of nonunion were not described in the report. A diaphysectomy is a useful procedure to treat a hammer toe and obtain shortening of a toe that is significantly longer than adjacent toes.

Partial proximal phalangectomy has been recommended by Johnson[82] and others[16,18,41] (see Figs. 7–98 and 7–99) as a treatment for a hammer toe deformity in association with MTP joint deformity. Cahill and Connor[16] reported on 78 patients (84 toes). They noted poor objective results in 50% of patients and concluded that partial proximal phalangectomy relieved symptoms but left a cosmetically poor end result (Fig. 7–36). Conklin and Smith[20] noted a 29% postoperative dissatisfaction rate; major complaints were shortening of the ray, floppiness of the toes, metatarsalgia, weakness, and stiffness.

A limited syndactylization may be combined with a partial proximal phalangectomy of adjoining phalanges. Daly and Johnson[41] reported 75% patient satisfaction with this procedure; however, 43% of patients had moderate footwear restrictions, 27% reported residual pain, 28% noted moderate or severe cosmetic problems, and 18% reported a recurrent cock-up deformity. In general, the treatment of a

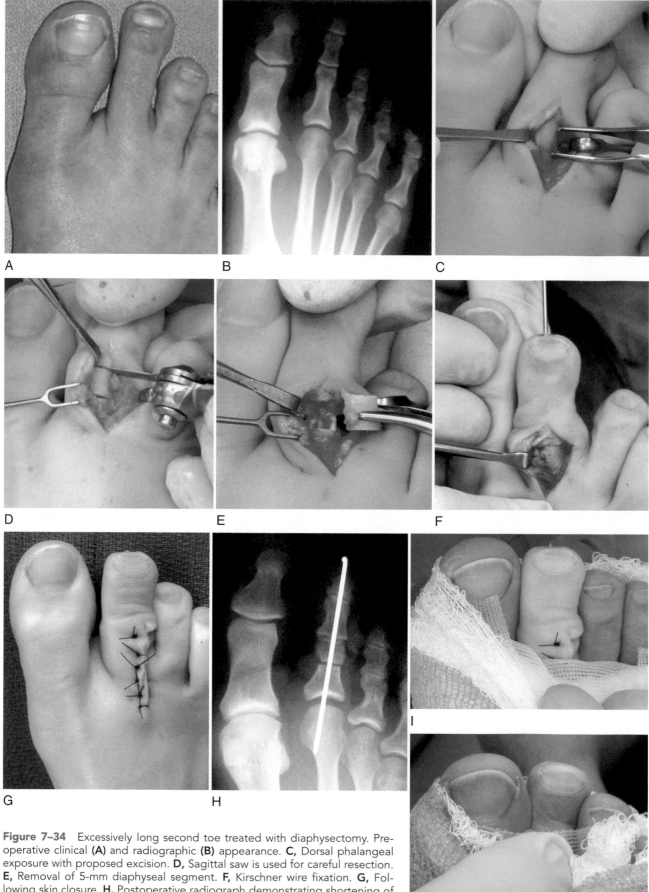

Figure 7–34 Excessively long second toe treated with diaphysectomy. Preoperative clinical (**A**) and radiographic (**B**) appearance. **C,** Dorsal phalangeal exposure with proposed excision. **D,** Sagittal saw is used for careful resection. **E,** Removal of 5-mm diaphyseal segment. **F,** Kirschner wire fixation. **G,** Following skin closure. **H,** Postoperative radiograph demonstrating shortening of digit. **I** and **J,** Evaluation of postoperative vascularity is important. Capillary filling may be slow and should be monitored.

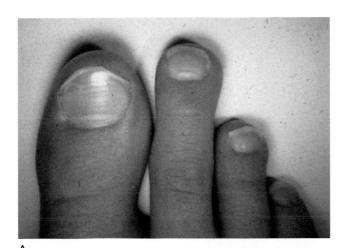

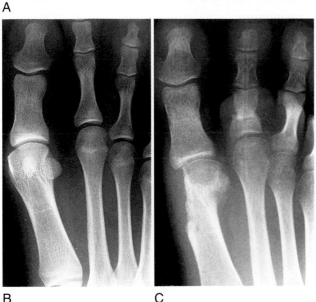

Figure 7–35 Preoperative clinical **(A)** and radiographic **(B)** views of patient with hammer toe symptoms and an unusually long second ray. **C,** Long-term radiographic follow-up.

hammer toe deformity by creating another deformity with a partial proximal phalangectomy and syndactylization should be discouraged except in a salvage situation.

Ely[53] believed a hallux valgus deformity would not progress after amputation of a second toe. Vander Wilde and Campbell[167] reported on 16 patients (22 feet) who underwent a second-toe amputation. They observed mild progressive drift of the hallux but believed that it was usually not significant. Despite these reports, it is generally accepted that removal of the second toe can place the patient at risk for a progressive hallux valgus deformity in time. Amputation of

the second toe may be an expeditious treatment for severe deformity in an elderly patient, but it is ill-advised in a younger patient because a hallux valgus deformity can progress (Fig. 7–37A, C, and D). Arthrodesis of the hallux MTP joint may be combined with a second-toe amputation to ensure that a hallux valgus deformity will not progress with time (Fig. 7–37E and F).

Implants in the lesser toes have been reported by a number of authors. Shaw and Alvarez[152] reported on 672 implants placed over an 11-year period for hammer toe deformities. Several implants were removed for pain, infection, or implant failure. The authors[38,58,62,110,150-153] noted that the only true function of an implant in the lesser toe was to act as a spacer, and they found no difference between implants left in permanently and those removed at least 6 weeks after surgery.

Reports of hinged silicone joint replacement for hammer toe deformities have also been reported by Gerbert and Benedetti[62] and others.[150-153] Although these series reported a high level of satisfactory results, it is doubtful that the long-term results of PIP joint implants are significantly different from results of excisional arthroplasty. The risk of implant placement in this relatively subcutaneous area and the cost of the implant and surgical procedure make its use questionable when similar results are obtainable with excisional arthroplasty.

Cracchiolo et al[38] and others[58,110,151,153] have reported on the use of silicone implant arthroplasty in the lesser MTP joints (Fig. 7–38). Sgarlato[151] proposed silicone arthroplasty of the lesser MTP joints for a dislocated MTP joint, arthritis, Freiberg's infraction, congenitally shortened toes, bunionette deformity, and failed resection arthroplasty. Cracchiolo et al[38] reported on lesser MTP replacement arthroplasty in 31 feet (28 patients), noting acceptable results in 63%. Transfer metatarsalgia was the most common postoperative complication, but other complications included lesser metatarsal stress fracture, soft tissue infection, and implant failure. Cracchiolo et al[38] concluded that the implant aided in maintaining the joint in a reduced position but that there were strict limitations in the indications for silicone replacement arthroplasty. Fox and Pro[58] reported on a similar success rate (70%) with lesser MTP implant arthroplasty. Silicone replacement arthroplasty of the lesser MTP joints or lesser

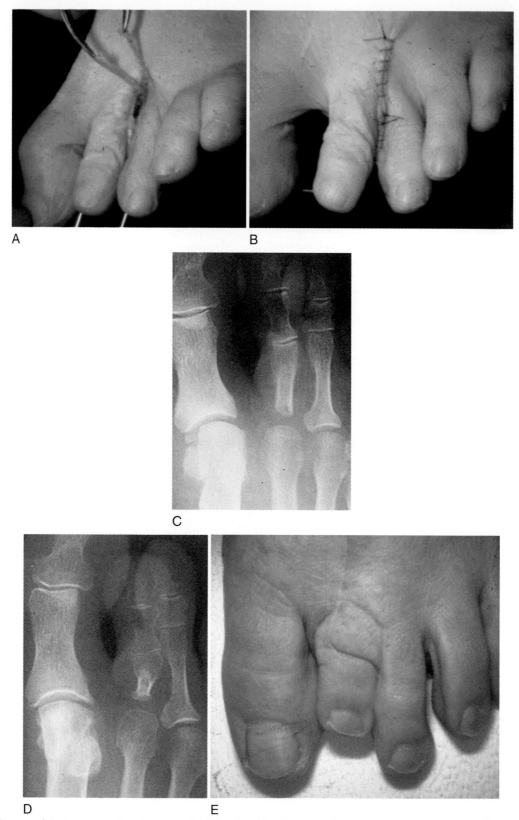

Figure 7–36   **A** and **B,** Intraoperative photographs following Kirschner wire fixation and syndactylization after partial proximal phalangectomy of the second toe deformity. **C,** Radiograph immediately following surgery. **D,** A radiograph 5 years postoperatively demonstrates severe shortening of the proximal phalanx with a varus deformity of the third toe. **E,** Cosmetically unacceptable syndactylization following partial proximal phalangectomy of only the second toe.

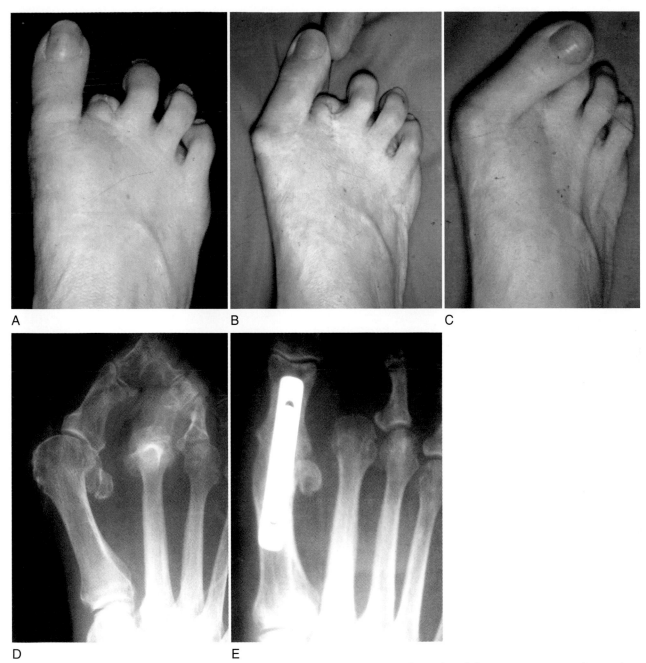

Figure 7–37 A, Following amputation of second toe. **B** and **C,** Progressive hallux valgus following amputation of second toe. **D,** Preoperative radiograph with hallux valgus and dislocated second metatarsophalangeal (MTP) joint. **E,** Following MTP fusion and second toe amputation.

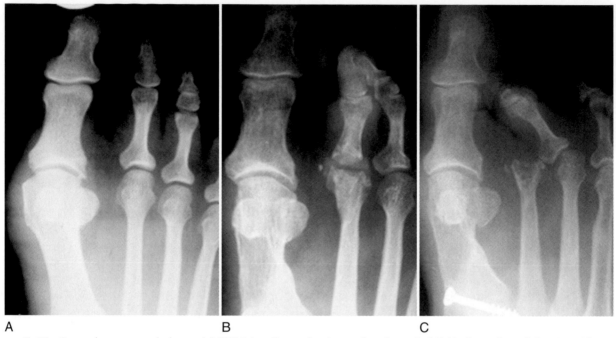

A   B   C

Figure 7–38   Second metatarsophalangeal (MTP) joint silicone implant arthroplasty. **A,** Mild hallux valgus deformity with painful second MTP joint. **B,** Following first metatarsal osteotomy and placement of second MTP joint double-stem silicone implant. (The implant went on to failure, with eventual salvage with a second-toe amputation.) **C,** At long-term follow-up, the lateral lesser toes have migrated medially.

toes is rarely indicated and should be reserved for the occasional salvage procedure when other more standard techniques either are contraindicated or have been unsuccessful.

Recurrence of a hammer toe deformity is one of the most frustrating complications following surgery. Although excessive resection of bone should be avoided because it leads to a floppy and unstable toe (Fig. 7–39A and B), adequate bone resection is necessary to decompress the toe in order to obtain an adequate correction. In the face of recurrence, a flexor tenotomy may be necessary to achieve adequate correction. If sufficient bone has been excised and the flexor digitorum longus has been released when indicated, recurrent deformity rarely occurs. Placing two pins for fixation and leaving Kirchner wires for 4 to 5 weeks can help to successfully stabilize a toe following redo surgery.

Following excessive bone resection, development of a flail toe is a most difficult complication to salvage.[60,97,109,129] Mahan[97,98] described a technique of bone graft stabilization of an iatrogenic flail second toe following unsuccessful hammer toe repair; however, this is an extensive reconstruction to perform on a lesser toe and should be reserved for a patient with significant symptoms (Fig. 7–39C-I). Friend[60] described a soft tissue repair using a V-Y skinplasty, soft tissue release, and partial metatarsal head resection to reconstruct an unstable flail lesser toe (Fig. 7–40).

The toe often assumes the shape of adjacent toes, a process termed *molding* (Fig. 7–41). Preoperative patient counseling about the possibility of molding usually alleviates postoperative concern on the part of the patient. If the great toe has an element of hallux valgus interphalangeus, the second toe will also probably have a slight lateral curvature. It is not possible for a repaired hammer toe to remain straight when a deforming force is applied by the great toe or an adjacent toe (Fig. 7–42).

Kirschner wire fixation of hammer toe repairs was introduced by Taylor in 1940[156] to stabilize the correction. This remains the most popular technique of digital stabilization due to the ease of placement and removal, the maintenance of

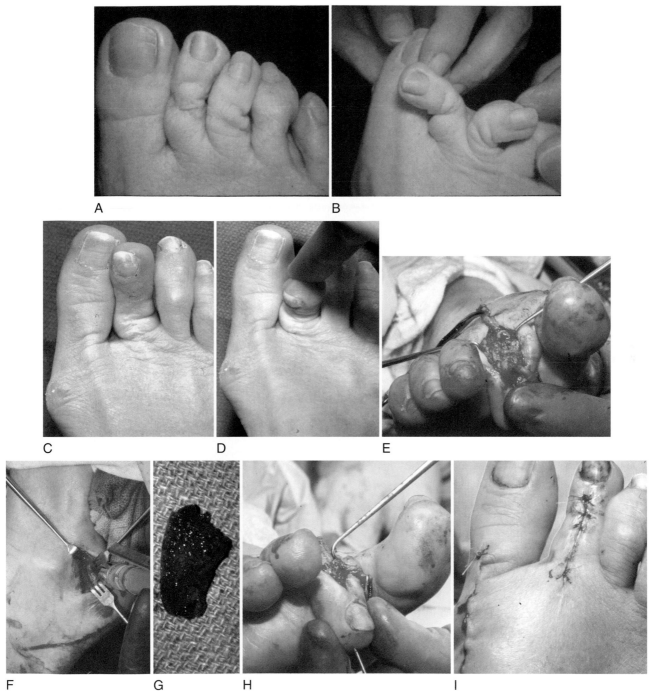

Figure 7–39 A and **B,** Excessive resection of bone can destabilize the lesser toes. **C** and **D,** Unstable second toe following excessive bone resection. **E,** Operative exposure of area of prior resection arthroplasty. **F,** Calcaneal exposure to obtain graft. **G,** Cylindrical donor graft. **H,** Placement of graft. **I,** Final clinical appearance following interposition graft. Note adequate vascularity of digit. (**C-I** courtesy of M.K. Mahan, DPM.)

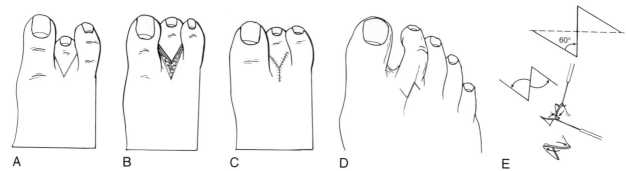

Figure 7–40 Soft tissue V-Y plasty for contracted lesser toe. **A,** Proposed V-shaped skin incision. **B,** Operative incision. **C,** Closure in Y fashion to lengthen the lesser toe. **D** and **E,** Z-plasty to correct contracted lesser toes.

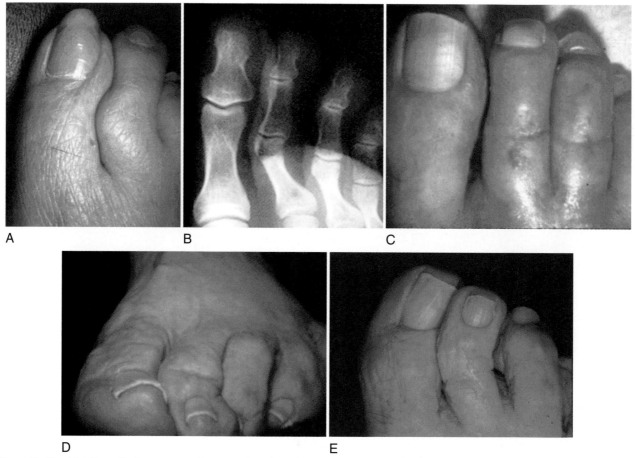

Figure 7–41 Molding of adjacent toes. Preoperative clinical examination **(A)** and radiograph **(B)** demonstrate molding of second toe. **C,** Molding of the second and third toes often occurs immediately after surgery but resolves with diminution of swelling. **D** and **E,** Molding of second toe following hammer toe repair. **(E** from Coughlin MJ: *Instr Course Lect* 52:421-444, 2003.)

Figure 7–42 Following hammer toe repair. **A,** Preoperative radiograph of second hammer toe with metatarsophalangeal joint subluxation. **B,** Following realignment. **C,** Lateral translation following hammer toe repair, with later development of interdigital corn. **D,** Mild medial angulation with satisfactory result; a successful arthrodesis resulted. **E** and **F,** Lateral deviation of the digit following hammer toe repair caused by pressure from an adjacent hallux valgus deformity. Both patients were dissatisfied. **G,** Medial deviation with fibrous union. **H,** A broken Kirschner wire at the MTP joint. Although the hammer toe repair was satisfactory, the MTP joint became malaligned. **I** and **J,** Hyperextension deformity following hammer toe repair. **(A, B, D, F, G,** and **I** from Coughlin MJ, Dorris J, Polk E: *Foot Ankle Int* 21[2]:94-104, 2000. Copyright © 2000 by the American Orthopaedic Foot and Ankle Society [AOFAS], originally published in *Foot and Ankle International*, Feb. 2000, Vol. 21, No. 2, pp 94-104 and reproduced here with permission.)

A   B   C

D   E   F

G   H   I

J

alignment,[136] and the increased stability following correction. Although complications such as pin tract infection (Fig. 7–43),[1,124,127-129,135,152] migration,[149,177] and breakage[1,31,124,146,177] have been observed (see Fig. 7–42G and H and Fig. 7–93), Zingas et al[177] reported a 2.5% failure rate when using 0.045-inch Kirschner wires for fixation of lesser toe deformities; however, they routinely left their Kirschner wires implanted for 6 weeks. A shorter period of implantation may in fact diminish the incidence of Kirschner wire failure. They noted the area of wire fracture occurred a few millimeters proximal to the metatarsal head but was rarely symptomatic. An 18% infection rate was reported by Reece[135] when Kirschner wires were left in place 6 weeks or more. In Coughlin's series,[33] only three of 118 toes developed a pin tract infection, and all resolved after pin removal. Kirschner wires were removed routinely 3 weeks after surgery.

Other uncommon complications include postoperative numbness caused by injury of an adjacent sensory nerve,[33,124] subsequent mallet toe deformity,[33,146] and decreased MTP range of motion.[124] On rare occasions, patients develop discomfort at the site where a pseudoarthrosis has developed. In these unusual cases, an injection of a corticosteroid usually gives lasting relief. If this is unsuccessful, revision hammer toe repair may be necessary to achieve bone union.

FLEXIBLE HAMMER TOE DEFORMITY

The patient with a flexible or dynamic hammer toe has a deformity when standing. Practically no deformity is present when the patient sits on the examining table with the foot in an equinus position. The deformity can then be reproduced by dorsiflexion of the ankle joint and with pressure placed beneath the metatarsal heads. These patients do not have the classic claw toe deformity because the MTP joint is not involved. The deformity appears to be caused by a contracture of the flexor digitorum longus tendon.

This deformity may be corrected by a flexor tendon transfer. Although Girdlestone[65] is often cited as the originator of the split flexor digitorum longus tendon transfer to the dorsum of the proximal phalanx, he did not report a surgical technique to correct clawed or hammered toes; rather, he discussed the concept of a loss of intrinsic muscle function that leads to clawing of the toes. Taylor[156] also is commonly credited with describing a flexor digitorum longus transfer; however, the surgical technique that he described has evolved significantly. The use of either of the eponyms Girdlestone or Taylor to describe this procedure as it is currently used is no longer appropriate.[159]

Preoperative Planning

The theory behind the flexor tendon transfer is that the transfer enables the flexor digitorum longus tendon to assume the function of the intrinsics (i.e., plantar flexion of the MTP joint and extension of the interphalangeal joints). Merely sectioning the flexor digitorum longus usually is not sufficient to straighten the toe in these patients and sacrifices a usable tendon. The flexor tendon transfer realigns the toe at the cost of prehensile action, which has been found to be an annoying problem for some patients. Often a patient has an absence or loss of active toe flexor power at the time of the flexor tendon transfer, and the patient commonly retains passive, but not active, toe function. Major complaints include restricted interphalangeal and metatarsophalangeal joint motion and loss of active flexor digitorum longus function to the other lesser toes.

Indications

A flexor tendon transfer is indicated for primary treatment of a flexible hammer toe. It may also be used in combination with other surgical techniques in the treatment of claw toes and toes that demonstrate instability of a lesser MTP joint.

Contraindications

A flexor tendon transfer is contraindicated as a primary treatment of a fixed hammer toe deformity.

TENDON TRANSFER PROCEDURE[25,31]

Surgical Technique

1. The foot is cleansed and draped in the usual fashion. The foot is exsanguinated with an Esmarch bandage. An Esmarch bandage may be used as a tourniquet above the level of the ankle (Fig. 7–44A and video clip 42).[68]
2. Under tourniquet control, a 5-mm transverse incision is made on the plantar aspect of the foot at the level of the proximal

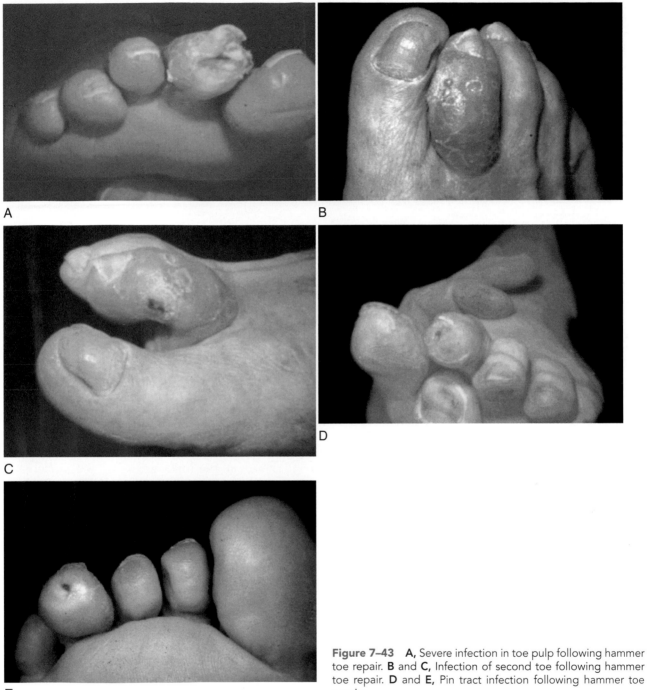

Figure 7–43 **A,** Severe infection in toe pulp following hammer toe repair. **B** and **C,** Infection of second toe following hammer toe repair. **D** and **E,** Pin tract infection following hammer toe repairs.

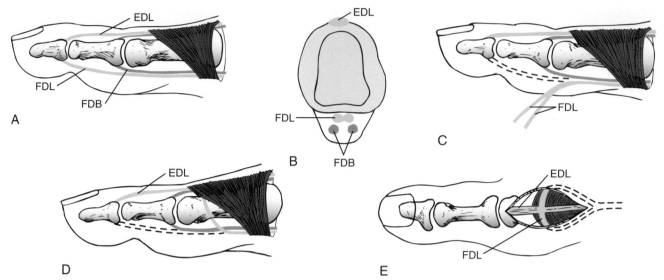

Figure 7–44   Technique for correction of dynamic hammer toe. **A,** Lateral view of lesser toe demonstrates the anatomy of flexor and extensor tendons. **B,** Cross-section anatomy through the metatarsal head region. Note that the flexor digitorum longus (FDL) is deeper than the flexor digitorum brevis (FDB). The FDL is characterized by a midline raphe. **C,** The FDL tendon has been detached from its insertion into the base of the distal phalanx and delivered into the plantar wound at the base of the toe. The tendon is then split longitudinally along its raphe, producing two tails. **D,** The FDL is delivered on either side of the extensor hood through a subcutaneous tunnel. **E,** The FDL is sutured into the extensor digitorum longus (EDL) tendon under moderate tension, and the metatarsophalangeal joint is held in approximately 20 degrees of plantar flexion.

plantar flexion crease of the toe. The soft tissue is spread and the flexor tendon sheath is identified.

3. The flexor tendon sheath is split longitudinally. Visualization of the contents of the sheath demonstrates three tendons. The flexor digitorum longus is the central of these three tendons, is larger, and is characterized by a midline raphe (Fig. 7–44B).

4. A small curved mosquito clamp is placed into the wound, and the flexor digitorum longus tendon is brought out under tension. Percutaneously, the long flexor tendon is released from its insertion into the plantar base of the distal phalanx (Fig. 7–44C, Fig. 7–45A).

5. The raphe or decussation in the flexor digitorum longus tendon is noted and the tendon is split longitudinally, creating two tails (Fig. 7–44C, Fig. 7–45B).

6. Attention is directed to the dorsal aspect of the toe, where a longitudinal incision is centered over the proximal phalanx. A mosquito hemostat is passed in a dorsal to plantar direction along the extensor hood, deep to the neurovascular bundle but superficial to the extensor hood, exiting at the plantar incision.

7. The tails of the flexor digitorum longus tendon then are passed dorsally on the medial and lateral aspects of the extensor hood in the midportion of the proximal phalanx (Fig. 7–44D, Fig. 7–45C).

8. With the toe placed in approximately 20 degrees of plantar flexion at the MTP joint, the flexor tendon is sutured to the extensor digitorum longus tendon under a slight degree of tension (Fig. 7–44E, Fig. 7–45D).

9. If a Kirschner wire is used to stabilize the toe, it should be used only to reinforce the repair. If it is used to realign the toe, the deformity can recur when the pin is removed. If a Kirschner wire is used, it is introduced into the MTP joint through a dorsal capsule incision made to expose the base of the proximal phalanx. The pin is driven distally and exits through the tip of the toe. The pin is then driven in a retrograde fashion across the MTP joint.

10. The wounds are closed and a gauze-and-tape compression dressing is applied.

Alternative Technique

Kuwada[89,90] has described a modification of the flexor tendon transfer. After the flexor digitorum

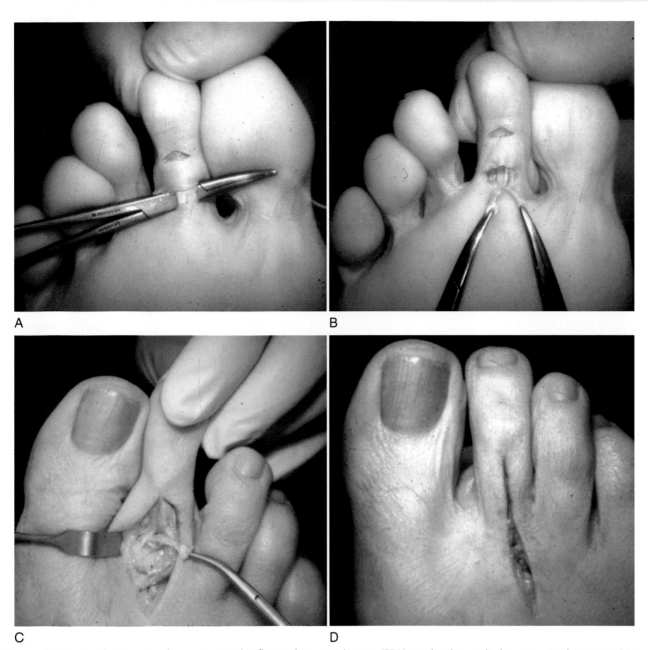

Figure 7–45 **A,** Plantar view demonstrates the flexor digitorum longus (FDL) tendon beneath the mosquito hemostat. Note the distal puncture wound releasing the long flexor tendon. **B,** The two limbs of the FDL tendon have been delivered through the more proximal plantar wound and split longitudinally. **C,** Each limb of the FDL is delivered on either side of the proximal phalanx and sutured to the extensor expansion with the toe in a corrected position. **D,** Final position of the corrected toe.

longus tendon is detached distally on the plantar aspect, it is transferred through a tunnel in the proximal phalanx and secured to the extensor digitorum longus tendon with interrupted sutures (Fig. 7–46). Gazdag and Cracchiolo[61] have reported no substantial difference between flexor tendon transfer techniques using circumferential tendon transfer or transfer through a central drill hole.

Postoperative Care

The patient is allowed to ambulate in a postoperative shoe. Dressing changes are performed weekly until the wound has healed. If a Kirschner wire has been placed, it is removed 3 weeks after surgery. Sutures are removed 3 weeks after surgery. The toe then is taped in correct alignment for an additional 3 to 6 weeks. Passive

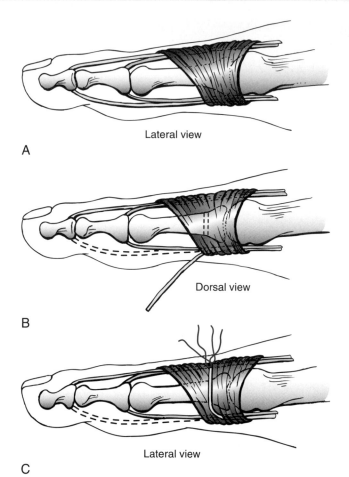

Lateral view

A

Dorsal view

B

Lateral view

C

Figure 7–46   Flexor tendon transfer through a drill hole in the proximal phalanx. **A,** Lateral view. **B,** Dorsal view. **C,** Following transfer of the flexor digitorum longus through a drill hole. The tendon is sutured to the extensor expansion of the extensor digitorum longus.

manipulation of the toe is begun 6 weeks after surgery and the patient is permitted to resume activities as tolerated.

Results and Complications

A flexor tendon transfer usually provides satisfactory correction not only for patients with an idiopathic flexible hammer toe but also for patients with cerebral palsy, patients who have had cerebral vascular accidents or a compartment syndrome, and patients with associated neuromuscular diseases such as Charcot–Marie–Tooth.[41] It is important for the surgeon to remember that if a fixed contracture is present, this procedure alone does not produce a satisfactory result. A flexor tendon transfer, however, may be used in association with other proce-

dures of the lesser toe to achieve realignment of the MTP joint.

Reports by Taylor,[156,157] Pyper,[131] and others[41,126] have noted inconsistent levels of satisfaction, with results ranging from 51% to 89%. (See the discussion of claw toe repair later in the chapter.) Thompson and Deland,[159] in reporting on results of a flexor tendon transfer, observed excellent postoperative pain relief; however, only 54% of those with a subluxated MTP joint had achieved complete correction at final follow-up.

Kuwada[89] and Barbari and Brevig[2] have reported a high level of satisfactory results (greater than 90%) in patients in their series following flexor tendon transfer. Barbari and Brevig[2] reported three cases where a fixed contracture of the interphalangeal joint developed postoperatively.

Complications experienced after this procedure are uncommon. Occasionally, swelling of varying degrees persists for a time, but it usually subsides. Transient numbness probably caused by stretching or contusion of the adjacent neurovascular bundles can occur, but this usually improves with time. Hyperextension of the DIP joint has been noted in a few patients with concomitant spasticity and is usually associated with recurrence of flexion at the PIP joint. This may be a result of concomitant tightness of the flexor digitorum brevis. Following a flexor tendon transfer, the ability to curl the toe is sacrificed. Often, at long-term follow-up after a flexor tendon transfer, stiffness develops in the PIP joint. A patient should be counseled preoperatively that there will be an absence of dynamic function of the involved toe and often the other lesser toes after a flexor tendon transfer. This does not tend to cause disability, but it can be annoying to the patient. They should be alerted to the trade-off of sacrificing flexor digitorum longus function for stability and realignment of the malaligned digit.

Occasionally the patient with a dynamic hammer toe also has an element of clawing. A release of the extensor digitorum longus tendon and simultaneous MTP capsulotomies may be performed at the same time as a flexor tendon transfer.

If a Kirschner wire has been placed across the MTP joint, the pin can break (see Fig. 7–42H).[135,177] Often the pin fractures just proximal to the articular surface of the metatarsal head, and in this case the distal fragment is

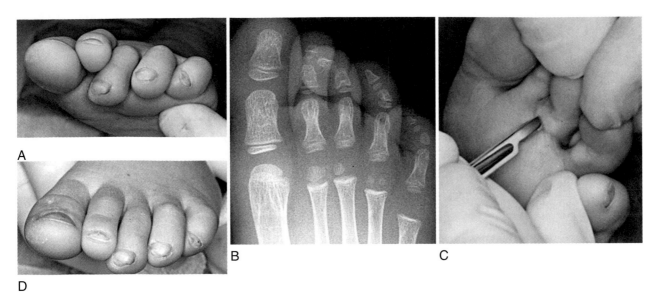

Figure 7–47 Repair of curly toe deformity. **A,** Curly toe deformity of third toe (similar to mallet toe deformity due to tight flexor digitorum longus tendon). **B,** Radiograph demonstrates curly toe deformity of third toe. **C,** Flexor tenotomy is performed to correct contracture. **D,** Frontal view after flexor tenotomy demonstrates correction of deformity.

removed and the proximal fragment is left within the metatarsal. If the distal aspect of the remaining pin penetrates the MTP joint or if it migrates, it may be surgically removed through an MTP joint arthrotomy.

Postoperative vascular insufficiency of a digit can require removal of the Kirschner wire. Other alternatives when there is slow capillary filling following surgery are avoiding ice or elevation, removing and rewrapping the dressing, and temporarily dropping the extremity over the side of the bed. When these methods are unsuccessful, topical nitroglycerin ointment (Nitropaste) along the borders of the involved digit can increase the capillary filling of the digit. Postoperative observation is important with this complication. Achievement of adequate alignment intraoperatively without the use of a Kirschner wire is important should the removal of internal fixation be necessary in the immediate postoperative period. Thus, the Kirschner wire is used to protect a flexor tendon transfer but not to achieve further realignment of the toe.

A curly toe deformity is often associated with a mallet toe. Typically, a curly toe occurs in a younger patient, is characterized by a flexion deformity of the PIP joint and DIP joint, and is caused by a contracture of the flexor digitorum longus tendon to a specific toe (Fig. 7–47A).[122]

Radiographs often demonstrate a deviation of the toe (Fig. 7–47B). Although some advocate stretching and taping to correct the deformity, Sweetnam[155] concluded that conservative treatment is rarely successful in straightening the toe. He found that there was a similar level of improvement in patients who were treated conservatively and in those who had no treatment, concluding that there was no progression or correction of deformity in either group.

A flexor tenotomy (Fig. 7–47C) often enables complete correction of the deformity (Fig. 7–47D). Ross and Menelaus[139] have noted no significant weakness of the involved toe at almost 10-year follow-up after flexor tenotomy. They reported 95% successful results following flexor tenotomy. Although a flexor tendon transfer may be performed, Hamer et al[70] examined patients who had either a flexor tenotomy or flexor tendon transfer for a curly toe deformity and noted no significant postoperative difference. Thus a simple flexor tenotomy appears to be sufficient treatment.

Boc and Martone[8] treated an adduction deformity of the distal digit with a laterally based elliptical arthroplasty. This procedure may indeed be necessary to correct a fixed bony deformity, but in most cases, a flexor tenotomy is adequate treatment for the flexible curly toe deformity in the younger child.

MALLET TOE DEFORMITY[27,28]

A mallet toe usually is a fixed deformity, but occasionally in a young patient it is flexible. Symptoms develop when the tip of the toe strikes the ground. This results in development of a callosity on the tip of the involved toe. This can be treated conservatively with a small felt pad placed beneath the toe to prevent the tip of the toe from striking the ground. A shoe with an adequate toe box must be worn to accommodate the toe with a felt pad beneath it.[27] A mallet toe occurs much less often than a hammer toe (ratio, 1:9).[28] It occurs in the longer toe in 75% of cases but with equal frequency in the second, third, and fourth toes (Fig. 7–48).[28]

Preoperative Planning

When the deformity is flexible, release of the flexor digitorum longus tendon percutaneously may be sufficient.[70,139] When the deformity is fixed (Fig. 7–49), which is more often the case, surgical intervention may be required. Bone decompression of the DIP joint with resection of the head of the middle phalanx and release of the flexor digitorum longus tendon results in satisfactory correction.

An algorithm, presented in Figure 7–50, describes the decision-making process for the treatment of a mallet toe.

Indications

The main indication for a surgical repair is a symptomatic mallet toe. Lateral or medial deviation of the digit at the DIP joint may be corrected with a mallet toe repair as well.

Contraindications

In the presence of a combined mallet toe and hammer toe, a decision must be made as to which deformity is more severe. A combined procedure for hammer toe and mallet toe is rarely if ever performed. When merely a flexor tenotomy is sufficient, a formal mallet toe repair can be avoided.

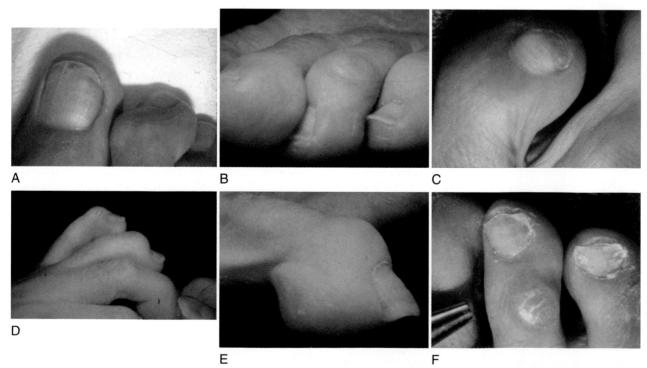

Figure 7–48 Types of mallet toe deformities. **A,** Plantar flexion and lateral deviation lead to overlapping of the third toe. **B,** Mallet toe deformity of the third toe leads to underlapping of the second toe. **C,** Curvature of the third toe impinges against the adjacent digit in the interspace. **D,** Multiple mallet toe deformities. **E,** Plantar flexion contracture of classic mallet toe. **F,** Callus formation on the dorsal aspect of the distal interphalangeal joint. (**D** from Coughlin MJ: *Instr Course Lect* 52:421-444, 2003.)

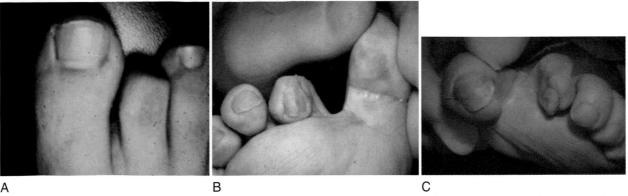

A   B   C

Figure 7–49   Mallet toe deformity. **A,** Dorsal view. **B,** View end on. **C,** Plantar view of another patient with severe mallet toe deformity.

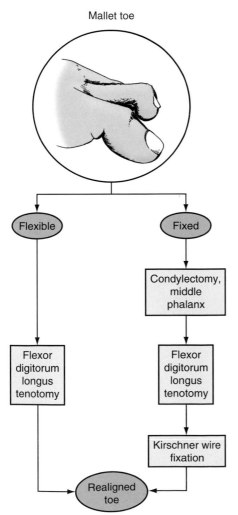

Figure 7–50   Algorithm for treatment of mallet toe.

MALLET TOE REPAIR[25]

Surgical Technique

1. The patient is placed in a supine position on the operating room table. If MTP joint surgery is performed, an Esmarch bandage may be used to exsanguinate the extremity and may also be used as an ankle tourniquet.[68] A digital block or ankle block is administered depending upon the necessity for additional surgical procedures.
2. The foot is cleansed and draped in the usual fashion. A 1/4-inch Penrose drain may be used as a tourniquet (Fig. 7–51A and video clip 40).
3. An elliptical incision is centered over the dorsal aspect of the interphalangeal joint. The dissection is carried down through the extensor tendon and joint capsule. The distal portion of the ellipse should be sufficiently proximal to avoid injuring the nail matrix (Fig. 7–51B, Fig. 7–52A).
4. The collateral ligaments are released on the medial and lateral aspects of the DIP joint. Care is taken to protect the adjacent neurovascular bundles (Fig. 7–51C).
5. The condyles of the middle phalanx are delivered into the wound. The bone is transected in the supracondylar region and the distal fragment is excised (Fig. 7–51D and E).
6. The plantar capsule is incised in the depths of the wound, and the flexor digitorum longus is identified and released under direct vision (Fig. 7–52B). The toe is brought into satisfactory alignment without tension. If the toe cannot be completely aligned, more bone is resected from the middle phalanx.

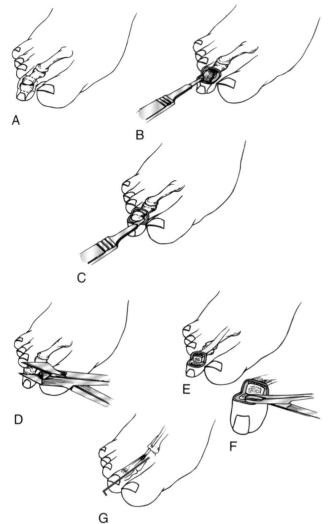

A

B

C

D

E

F

G

Figure 7–51 Technique for correction of mallet toe deformity. **A,** Elliptical skin incision centered over the distal interphalangeal joint. **B,** Excision of skin, extensor tendon, and capsule, exposing condyles of middle phalanx. **C,** The collateral ligaments are severed, exposing the condyles of the middle phalanx. **D,** Generous excision of the distal portion of the middle phalanx. **E,** Following resection of the condyle. **F,** The articular surface of the distal phalanx is removed with a rongeur. The flexor digitorum longus tendon is identified in the base of the wound and is released. **G,** Stabilization with intramedullary Kirschner wire. Vertical mattress sutures are used to coapt the skin.

7. The articular cartilage is removed from the base of the distal fragment (this is optional) (Fig. 7–51F, Fig. 52C).
8. A 0.045-inch Kirschner wire is introduced at the DIP joint and driven distally, exiting the tip of the toe (Fig. 7–51G, Fig. 52D). The toe is then aligned properly, and the Kirschner wire is driven in a retrograde fashion into the middle phalanx. The pin is bent at the tip of the toe, and the remaining pin is removed (Fig. 52E-G).

9. A gauze-and-tape compression dressing is applied at surgery and changed on a weekly basis until drainage has subsided.

Alternate Fixation

Interrupted vertical mattress sutures of 3-0 nylon are used to incorporate two Telfa bolsters (Fig. 7–53). They are inserted in a similar fashion for fixation of a hammer toe. As tension is applied to the suture, leverage is created to bring the toe into satisfactory alignment.

Postoperative Care

The patient is allowed to ambulate in a wooden-soled postoperative shoe. If bolsters have been placed, they are removed 1 week after surgery. If the bolsters are left longer than 1 week, there is risk of skin necrosis. If a Kirschner wire has been placed, the pin is removed 3 weeks after surgery. Sutures are removed at this time as well.

After removal of the pin or bolsters, the toe is held in a corrected position with a piece of tape for 6 weeks to ensure soft tissue healing.

Results and Complications

The expected results following this procedure have been routinely satisfactory. Using this procedure with resection of the condyles of the middle phalanx and the corresponding articular surface of the distal phalanx, Coughlin[28] reported successful fusion in 72% of cases (Fig. 7–54A). The satisfaction rate was only slightly higher in the group with a successful arthrodesis. Some 75% of those with a fibrous union were satisfied, although slightly less so than those with a successful DIP arthrodesis (Fig. 7–54B). Pain relief was noted by 97% and correction of the deformity by 91%. Although not performed in all cases, a flexor tenotomy appeared to be associated with a slightly higher rate of satisfaction and maintenance of the corrected position. Usually, correct alignment is maintained and complications are uncommon.

The few problems that have been observed postoperatively include the following:

• Swelling often persists for several months after the procedure, but it invariably resolves with time. At long-term follow-up, no patients were noted to have swelling.[28] Molding due to extrinsic pressure from adjacent toes can cause angulation or malalignment (Fig. 7–55A and B).

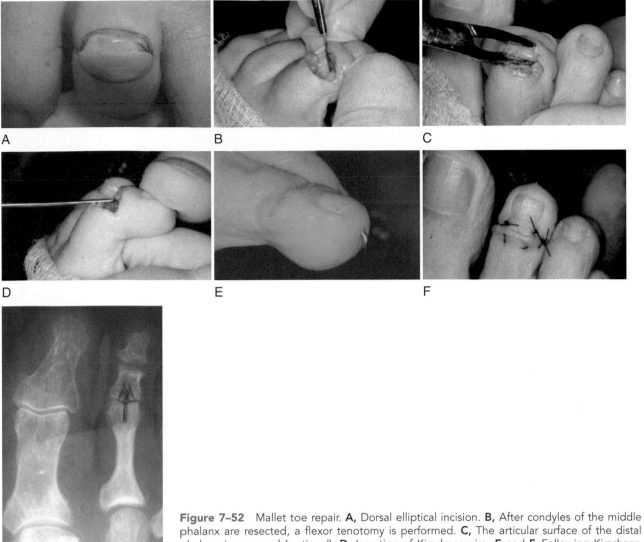

Figure 7–52 Mallet toe repair. **A,** Dorsal elliptical incision. **B,** After condyles of the middle phalanx are resected, a flexor tenotomy is performed. **C,** The articular surface of the distal phalanx is removed (optional). **D,** Insertion of Kirschner wire. **E** and **F,** Following Kirschner-wire insertion and closure. **G,** Radiograph with stable and painless fibrous union of corrected mallet toe deformity of the second toe.

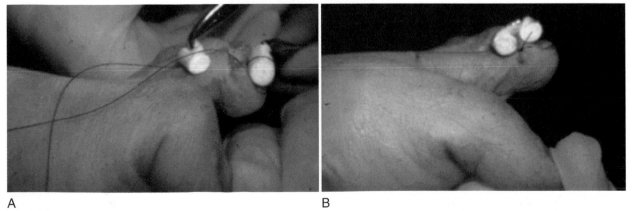

Figure 7–53 Alternative means of fixation for mallet toe repair. **A** and **B,** Placement of Telfa bolsters beneath 3-0 nylon vertical mattress suture.

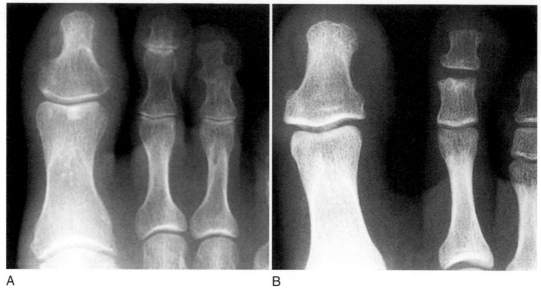

A   B

Figure 7–54   **A,** Arthrodesis of second toe distal interphalangeal (DIP) joint following mallet toe repair. **B,** Fibrous union of DIP joint of the second toe following mallet toe repair (asymptomatic).

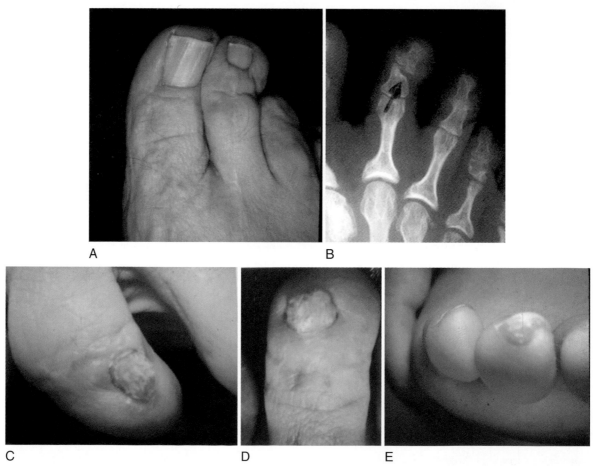

A   B

C   D   E

Figure 7–55   **A,** Molding of the toe following mallet toe repair. **B,** Lateral deviation following repair. **C** and **D,** Toenail deformity that preceded mallet toe repair does not improve following surgery. **E,** Callus at tip of toe usually resolves with time after surgical realignment.

- Occasionally recurrence of a mallet toe deformity is noted. This is usually because the flexor digitorum longus tendon was not released.

- Injury to an adjacent digital nerve can leave an area of numbness along either the medial or lateral border of the toe, although this is rarely a significant complaint.

- When a preoperative toenail deformity is associated with a mallet toe, this usually does not resolve following correction of the mallet toe (Fig. 7–55C-E). The patient should be warned that although the toe can be realigned, the toenail deformity will not be corrected.

CLAW TOE DEFORMITIES

A claw toe often develops in association with neurologic conditions in which a muscle imbalance occurs,[147] with weakness or loss of intrinsic muscle function.[115] It can also occur in arthritic conditions such as rheumatoid arthritis and other collagen deficiency syndromes. At times, a claw toe deformity is associated with a cavus foot deformity.[106]

In evaluating a claw toe deformity, every effort should be made to determine the specific diagnosis.[27] However, many of these cases are idiopathic.

What differentiates a claw toe from a hammer toe is the hyperextension deformity of the MTP joint.[122] A hammer toe may or may not be associated with hyperextension of the proximal phalanx, but a claw toe classically has a hyperextension deformity at the MTP joint.[59,73] In a claw toe, the DIP joint may be extended or flexed. The chronic hyperextended posture of the MTP joint forces the metatarsal heads plantarward and displaces the plantar fat pad, often resulting in symptomatic metatarsalgia over time. In patients with an insensate foot, ulcers can develop beneath the metatarsal heads.

Preoperative Planning

To successfully correct a claw toe deformity, the MTP joint must be brought into a neutral position so that the extensor tendon can function to extend the PIP joint and the intrinsic tendons can function as flexors of the MTP joint.

Treatment of a claw toe depends on the underlying condition. Figure 7–56 presents an algorithm for

treatment of a claw toe. If a significant pes cavus deformity is present, attention should be directed first to the midfoot and hindfoot deformities.[19,24,26,99,100] With a pes cavus deformity, the metatarsal heads are depressed as a result of the anatomic alignment of the foot, and the toes are extended by the contracted long extensors, creating the claw toe deformity (Fig. 7–57A).[73,75] When there is dynamic clawing without a significant cavus deformity, attention should be directed to the forefoot itself. If there is no clawing of the toes when the ankle is held in plantar flexion, and if clawing occurs with dorsiflexion of the ankle joint, a flexible claw toe deformity is present (Fig. 7–57B-E). This may be treated with a flexor tendon transfer.[2,131,155,157] This is the same type of procedure that is used to correct a flexible or dynamic hammer toe (see Figs. 7–44 and 7–45); however, release of the MTP joints (extensor tenotomies or MTP joint capsulotomies, or both) also may be necessary.[2]

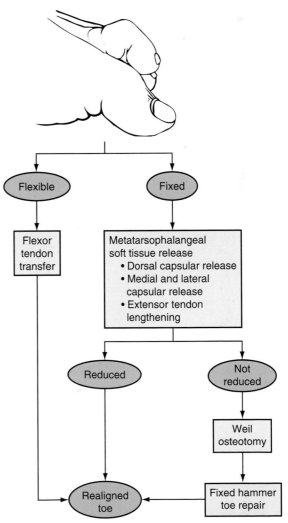

Figure 7–56 Algorithm for treatment of claw toe.

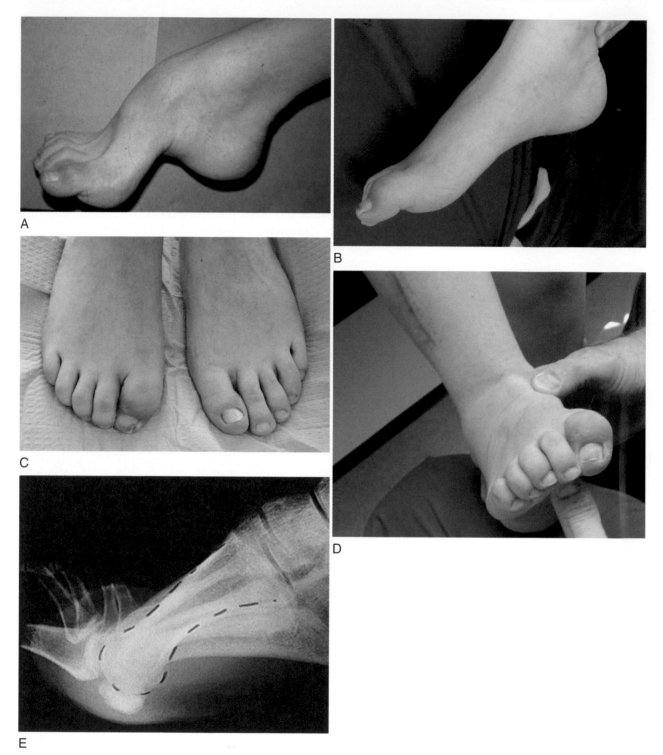

Figure 7–57   A, Lateral view of foot with claw toe deformities with diagnosis of Charcot–Marie–Tooth. **B,** Lateral view of another patient's foot; in equinus, the deformity is not obvious. The patient had had a previous compartment syndrome of calf. **C,** Frontal view of both feet demonstrates claw toe deformity of right foot and normal left foot. **D,** With dorsiflexion of the ankle, the deformity substantially increases. Note scar from previous compartment release laterally. **E,** Radiograph of claw toe deformity. Note articulation of base of lesser phalanges with dorsal aspect of metatarsal heads. Also note the plantar flexed first metatarsal due to contracted extensor hallucis longus tendon.

Feeney et al,[55] in treating patients with the sequelae of compartment syndromes following tibia fractures, have advocated selective proximal lengthenings of the flexor hallucis longus and flexor digitorum longus to relieve lesser toe contractures.

In the presence of a fixed contracture, a DuVries arthroplasty of the PIP joint is carried out, with concomitant release of the contracted structures at the MTP joint (see Fig. 7–76). In patients with severe contractures of the MTP and interphalangeal joints, release of both flexor tendons should be carried out at the time of the surgery. In patients with severe contractures, longitudinally placed Kirschner wires may be used to stabilize both the interphalangeal and MTP joints in satisfactory alignment.

Indications

In the presence of a fixed claw toe deformity, a condylectomy of the proximal phalanx is performed. Release of the extensor tendon and contracted capsule at the MTP joint depends on whether a fixed contracture is present. A fixed contracture at the interphalangeal joint of the hallux is treated with an interphalangeal joint fusion. With a contracture of the extensor hallucis longus tendon, a Jones tendon transfer is performed. An extensor tendon transfer to the distal metatarsal[59,73] and the midfoot[106] also has been advocated for treatment of claw toe deformity. A distal metatarsal osteotomy may also be an alternative in the treatment regimen of a severe claw toe deformity (discussed under Weil osteotomy).

Contraindications

In the presence of a flexible claw toe deformity, a flexor tendon transfer is performed identical to that for a flexible hammer toe deformity. Transfer of a flexor tendon as sole treatment of a fixed deformity is rarely successful.

DUVRIES ARTHROPLASTY PROCEDURE

Surgical Technique

1. The patient is placed in a supine position on the operating room table. A peripheral nerve block is typically used for anesthesia. The foot is cleansed and draped in the usual fashion. The foot is exsanguinated with an Esmarch bandage, which may be used as a tourniquet above the level of the ankle.
2. A longitudinal incision is centered over the PIP joint. The skin, extensor tendon, and

capsule are exposed and excised (Fig. 7–58A and B).

3. The toe is flexed and the collateral ligaments released on the medial and lateral borders of the condyle. The plantar capsule also is released (Fig. 7–58C and video clip 41).
4. The condyles of the proximal phalanx are resected with a bone-cutting forceps (Fig. 7–58D).
5. If an arthrodesis is desired, a rongeur is used to remove the base of the middle phalanx (Fig. 7–58E).
6. The toe is stabilized with a 0.045-inch Kirschner wire introduced at the interphalangeal joint and driven distally (Fig. 7–58F). A release of the flexor tendons may be necessary and may be performed in the depths of the wound from a dorsal approach.
7. With the toe aligned properly, the Kirschner wire is driven proximally, stabilizing the proximal phalanx. If an MTP joint capsule release is performed, the Kirschner wire may be driven across the MTP joint (Fig. 7–58G).
8. The skin is approximated with interrupted vertical mattress sutures.

CONTRACTURE RELEASE

In the presence of a hyperextension deformity of the MTP joint, a release of the contracted tissue and a tenotomy of the extensor tendon is performed (Fig. 7–59).

Surgical Technique

1. A 1.5-cm incision is centered over the MTP joint.
2. The dissection is deepened to the extensor tendon, which is released.
3. With retractors exposing the MTP joint capsule, the dorsal, medial, and lateral capsules and collateral ligaments are released. (This release must be carried down approximately 1 cm plantarward to allow reduction of the MTP joint.)
4. A 0.045-inch Kirschner wire is driven retrograde across the MTP joint, stabilizing the joint.
5. The pin is bent at the tip of the toe and the remainder of the pin is cut and removed.
6. A gauze-and-tape compression dressing is applied and is changed weekly until drainage has subsided.

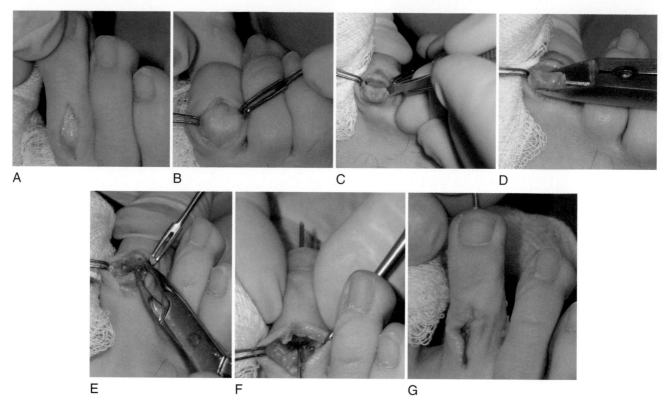

Figure 7–58   Repair of claw toe deformity. Longitudinal incision is centered over proximal interphalangeal joint **(A)** exposing the skin, extensor tendon, and capsule **(B)**, which is excised. **C,** The toe is flexed and the plantar capsule is released. The collateral ligaments are released from the medial and lateral border of condyles. **D,** The condyles of the proximal phalanx are removed with a bone-cutting forceps. **E,** If an arthrodesis is desired, the articular surface of the base of the middle phalanx is removed. **F,** A 0.045-inch Kirschner wire is introduced at the arthroplasty site and driven distally. **G,** With the toe reduced, the Kirschner wire is driven in a retrograde fashion, stabilizing the proximal phalanx. Following skin closure, the toe is adequately aligned.

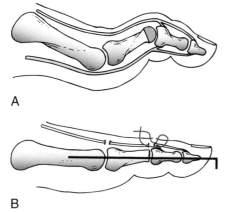

Figure 7–59   A, Claw toe deformity. **B,** Following proximal interphalangeal joint arthroplasty, metatarsophalangeal soft tissue release, and intramedullary Kirschner wire fixation.

INTERPHALANGEAL JOINT ARTHRODESIS

With a fixed contracture of the interphalangeal joint of the hallux, an interphalangeal joint arthrodesis is performed.

Surgical Technique

1. The foot is cleansed and draped in the usual fashion.
2. An elliptical incision is centered over the dorsal aspect of the interphalangeal joint. The skin, extensor tendon, and capsule are resected. The medial and lateral collateral ligaments and plantar capsule are released (Fig. 7–60A-C).

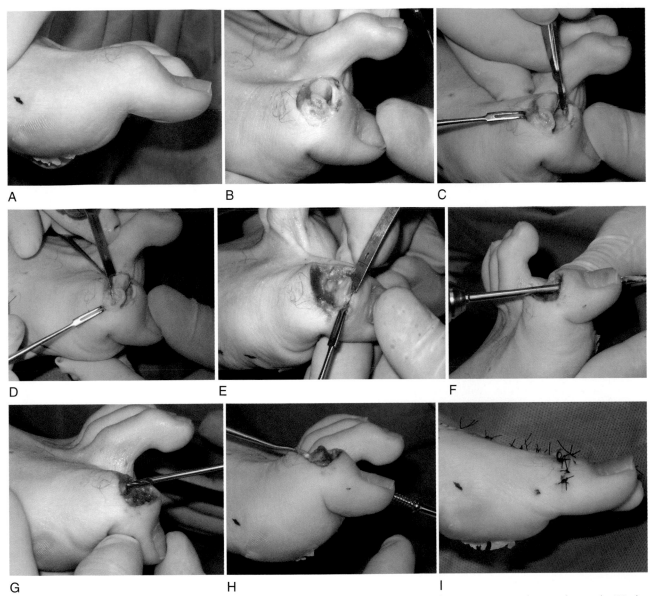

A

B

C

D

E

F

G

H

I

Figure 7–60 **A,** Repair of hammered great toe. After elliptical skin incision excises skin, extensor tendon, and capsule **(B)**, the collateral ligaments are released **(C)**. **D,** A power saw is used to remove the articular surface of the condyles of the proximal phalanx. **E,** The articular surface of the distal phalanx is removed with a power saw. **F,** A gliding hole is created through the distal phalanx. **G,** A fixation hole is created in the proximal phalanx. **H,** A lag screw is placed to stabilize the repair. **I,** Result following repair of all five toes.

3. A power saw is used to resect the articular surface of the condyles of the proximal phalanx (Fig. 7–60D).
4. The articular surface of the distal phalanx is also resected with the power saw (Fig. 7–60E).
5. A puncture wound is created in the skin (Fig. 7–60F). A 3.5-mm gliding hole is drilled through the distal phalanx. The drill is introduced at the interphalangeal joint and driven distally through the tip of the toe.
6. A 2.5-mm fixation hole is drilled in the proximal phalanx (Fig. 7–60G).
7. A lag screw is used to stabilize the fusion. Care must be taken not to place an excessively long screw that can penetrate the MTP joint (Fig. 7–60H).
8. A gauze-and-tape dressing is applied (Fig. 7–60I).

Postoperative Care

The patient is allowed to ambulate in a postoperative shoe. Sutures and Kirschner wires are removed 3 weeks after surgical repair of a fixed claw toe. The compression screw placed in the hallux to fuse the interphalangeal joint may be left in permanently, or if it causes discomfort it may be removed following administration of local anesthetic.

Results and Complications

Taylor[157] performed both soft tissue release and transfer of the long and short flexor tendons to the extensor hood. He reported that the operation restores "useful function to the toe at the cost of their prehensile action." In 68 patients (112 feet), 72% good results were reported. No resection arthroplasties were performed in this series.

Pyper[131] transferred both the long and short flexors to the extensor hood and reported 51% excellent and good results and 49% fair and poor results with this procedure. Suboptimal results were thought to result from uncorrected fixed flexion contractures of the lesser toes.

Parrish[126] transferred the flexor digitorum longus to the extensor hood in 23 patients. Transfer of the short flexor tendon was abandoned because of technical difficulties. Eighty-nine percent good and excellent results were reported.

Cyphers and Feiwell[40] reported their experience with flexor tendon transfer in patients with meningomyelocele and noted 60% good results.

Barbari and Brevig[2] reported on flexor tendon transfer for correction of a claw toe deformity. Satisfactory results were reported in 90% of cases, although one third of patients complained of metatarsalgia postoperatively. MTP motion was greater than 50 degrees in 33% of patients and less than 50 degrees in six patients. Twelve patients had no interphalangeal joint motion, 15 had reduced motion, and 12 had the same amount of motion at the interphalangeal joints. Continuing complaints were noted by patients who had a fixed claw toe deformity that might have been better treated with a resection arthroplasty. With refinement of this procedure and the use of just the flexor digitorum longus tendon, improved results have been noted, although Thompson and Deland[159] observed that only 54% of patients in their series achieved complete realignment of the MTP joint following flexor tendon transfer.

Heyman[73] advocated soft tissue release of the contracted capsular structures at the MTP and interphalangeal joints. No "excellent" results were noted, although no long-term evaluation was reported.

Lapidus[94] performed a dorsal capsule reefing at the interphalangeal joints coupled with a plantar capsulotomy and extensor tenotomy and reported uniformly good results.

Frank and Johnson[59] and McCluskey et al[106] advocated PIP joint arthroplasty to decompress the claw toe deformity and realign the toe.

Complications associated with repair of a claw toe deformity usually are related to recurrent deformity. In the presence of a flexible claw toe deformity, a flexor tendon transfer can adequately realign the deformed toes. Where a fixed contracture is present, a capital oblique osteotomy of the metatarsal may be necessary to achieve adequate realignment. (See the discussion of the Weil osteotomy later).

MTP joint capsule releases and an extensor tenotomy or lengthening may be combined to correct a significant hyperextension deformity.

Metatarsalgia may continue to be a complaint despite realignment of the lesser toes. An algorithm is helpful in the approach to differentiating forefoot problems (Fig. 7–61). Attention to midfoot and hindfoot deformities may be necessary to relieve symptoms of metatarsalgia. Treatment of the underlying problem leading to a claw toe deformity should be considered prior to lesser toe realignment. With extensive surgery, which can include an MTP joint release, a condylectomy of the proximal phalanx, and even a flexor tendon transfer, the vascular status of the toe or toes may be compromised. The patient must be monitored closely postoperatively, because it may be necessary to remove internal fixation (e.g., Kirschner wire) in the presence of vascular compromise.

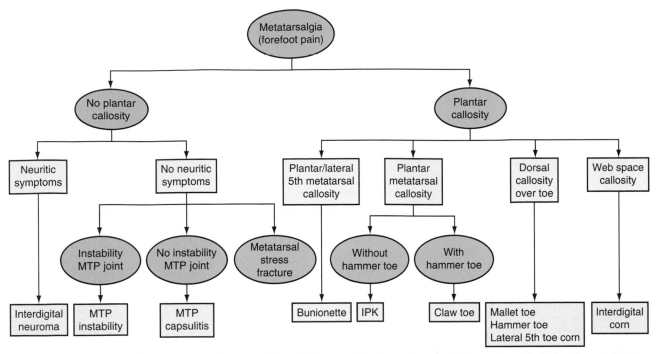

Figure 7–61   Algorithm for treatment of metatarsalgia. IPK, intractable plantar keratosis. (From Coughlin MJ: *J Bone Joint Surg Br* 82[6]:781-790, 2000.)

SUBLUXATION AND DISLOCATION OF THE SECOND METATARSOPHALANGEAL JOINT

Subluxation and dislocation of the second MTP joint occurs with relative frequency.[13,31,50] The MTP joint can be dislocated acutely after an injury, with disruption of the plantar capsule and MTP collateral ligaments. Chronic capsular insufficiency can develop in association with systemic arthritides (such as rheumatoid arthritis) and other connective tissue disorders as well as nonspecific synovitis.[102,103] Chronic synovitis eventually can lead to deterioration of the collateral ligaments and joint capsule, with subsequent instability of the MTP joint.[78,103]

Etiology

A traumatic episode can lead to dislocation of the second MTP joint (Fig. 7–62). Occasionally following a dorsiflexion injury to the second MTP joint, the joint is irreducibly dislocated.[119,133] The typical injury mechanism occurs with forced hyperextension and axial loading of the involved toe. The postinjury radiograph often demonstrates an increased MTP joint space, and an interposed plantar plate is often identified at surgery.

Brunet and Tubin[14] reported on 27 injuries (17 patients) to the lesser MTP joint associated with sport-

ing activities, motor vehicle accidents, and trauma. Invariably the plantar plate and capsule were torn from the metatarsal head and become interposed, preventing successful reduction. Occasionally, the transverse metatarsal ligament had to be sectioned to allow joint reduction.

Reis et al[137] have reported two cases of MTP dislocation following an intra-articular steroid injection and concluded that this can cause attenuation of the plantar capsule with subsequent dislocation. More commonly, dislocation occurs in older persons who have no history of injury or injection.

One reason for a traumatic dislocation of the second MTP joint is that the second ray (consisting of the second metatarsal and phalanges) is usually the longest in the foot.[22] Because of the pressure of the end of the toe against the toe box, the toe buckles and the proximal phalanx has a tendency to ride up onto the dorsal aspect of the second metatarsal head. Subluxation can eventually occur, and if untreated it can progress to dislocation. The longer the dislocation is present the greater the degree of change noted in the surrounding soft tissue and bone. The soft tissue contractures can include shortening of the extensor tendons and the dorsal, medial, and lateral capsule, with progressive elongation of the plantar capsule. Occasionally the dislocation is caused by degeneration or rupture of the plantar capsule, which then permits the MTP joint to subluxate dorsally.[25,46,47] During

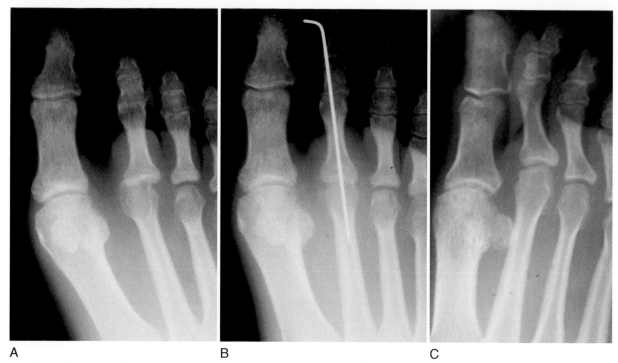

A   B   C

Figure 7–62 Traumatic dislocation of second metatarsophalangeal (MTP) joint following skydiving accident. **A,** Dislocated second MTP joint. **B,** Following open reduction and internal fixation. **C,** Follow-up shows adequately realigned second MTP joint.

walking, all of the forces across the MTP joint tend to hyperextend the joint. Therefore any imbalance about the MTP joint (i.e., capsular or tendinous) can result in progressive dorsal subluxation. In long-standing dislocations, an accessory facet can develop on the dorsal aspect of the metatarsal head.

With a marked hallux valgus deformity (Fig. 7–63A and B; see also Fig. 7–27A) it is not uncommon to see a subluxed or dislocated second MTP joint that deviates laterally (because of pressure from the hallux) or dorsally (with the hallux crossing under the second toe). Often, however, the second toe actually deviates medially, leaving a gap between the second and third toes. This can occur with or without a hallux valgus deformity. Often a long second ray[118] also is associated with this deformity[22] and is termed a *crossover toe deformity*. The toe may or may not be subluxed dorsally. Over time, erosion of the fibular collateral ligament of the second MTP joint and deterioration of the lateral joint capsule allow the toe to drift in a dorsomedial direction. Rarely a third or fourth toe also dislocates (Fig. 7–63C and D).

Hatch and Burns[71] suggested that an accessory medial head of the extensor digitorum brevis was associated with a crossover toe deformity and noted its presence in four of seven cadaver specimens. They

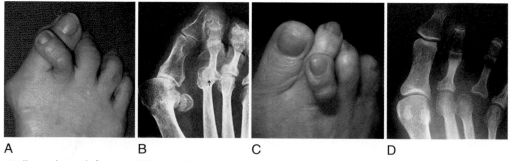

A   B   C   D

Figure 7–63 Hallux valgus deformity. Clinical **(A)** and radiographic **(B)** appearance of dislocation of second metatarsophalangeal (MTP) joint. The hallux has caused sufficient pressure against the second toe, which led to dislocation of the second MTP joint. **C,** Isolated dislocation of the third MTP joint due to synovitis. **D,** Radiographic appearance of dislocated third toe in a different patient.

speculated that the action of the extensor digitorum brevis to dorsiflex and adduct the second toe could be an underlying cause of a crossover second toe.

Preoperative Evaluation

Physical Examination

Synovitis of the second MTP joint on physical examination can be characterized by localized swelling in the joint or can involve the entire second toe.[103] Tenderness on palpation can be localized to either the medial or lateral aspect of the MTP joint or to the plantar aspect of the joint, depending on the exact location of the capsular disorder.

MTP joint subluxation and dislocation can lead to a subsequent hammer toe deformity.[22,30,32,100] With buckling of the second toe, an intractable plantar keratotic lesion can develop beneath the symptomatic metatarsal head. Likewise, a callus can develop over the dorsal aspect of the PIP joint as the toe impacts against the dorsal aspect of the toe box.

Often MTP joint subluxation develops insidiously. Complaints of pain in the intermetatarsal space are not uncommon with ambulation. The patient typically does not have pain at rest (Fig. 7–64). Palpation of the intermetatarsal space can cause pain, but the pain does not radiate to the toes. With dorsal dislocation of the second MTP joint, the typical symptoms result because the proximal phalanx lies dorsal to the second metatarsal, causing the toe to strike the top of the toe box, producing a painful lesion over the PIP joint. The shoe in turn forces the dislocated proximal phalanx downward against the metatarsal head, which can lead to development of a large, painful intractable plantar keratotic lesion. With dislocation of the toe, the prominent dorsal base of the proximal phalanx often is easily palpated. When a toe is subluxated, instability can be ascertained by dorsoplantar manipulation of the MTP joint. This *drawer sign*, described by Thompson and Hamilton[160] and others,[21,25,30] in which the toe is vertically subluxated, places pressure on the plantar capsule and often elicits characteristic pain (Fig. 7–65).[31] When testing MTP joint stability, the involved toe should be dorsiflexed 25 degrees at the MTP joint before the vertical stress test is performed.[47]

The specific diagnosis of MTP joint instability may be aided by local Xylocaine injections into the symptomatic areas. Differentiation of pain originating from a symptomatic interdigital neuroma or an unstable lesser MTP joint can be difficult. Coughlin[23] and others[36,114] have recommended sequential injections to help differentiate the specific area of pain.

Instability of the second MTP joint has been categorized by several authors into distinct grades.[69,159] We have also devised a subjective–objective clinical classification to characterize progressive deformity. Mendicino[112] and Yu[175] have both described a prodromal stage preceding subluxation characterized by MTP joint pain and swelling. Haddad et al[69] have suggested a four-stage description of second MTP joint instability. We have combined and modified these suggestions into a more comprehensive staging pattern, which is shown in the box on page 411.

The differential diagnosis of pain localized to the area of the second MTP joint includes MTP joint synovitis, capsule degeneration, Freiberg's infraction (video clip 38), metatarsal stress fracture, degenerative arthritis, systemic arthritis localized to the second MTP joint, synovial cyst formation, and interdigital neuroma (Figs. 7–66 and 7–67 and video clip 47).

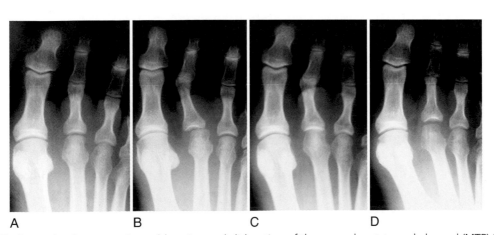

Figure 7–64 Radiographs demonstrating subluxation and dislocation of the second metatarsophalangeal (MTP) joint. **A,** Symptomatic second MTP joint without radiographic abnormality. **B,** Subluxation. **C,** Two months later, dorsal dislocation has occurred. **D,** Following surgical reconstruction, the second MTP joint is relocated and stabilized.

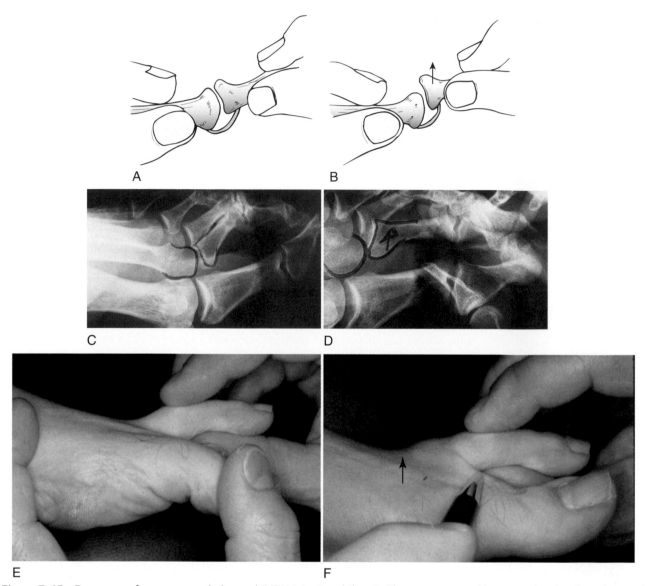

Figure 7–65 Drawer test for metatarsophalangeal (MTP) joint instability. **A,** The toe is grasped between the thumb and second finger. **B,** With dorsal force, an attempt is made to subluxate the MTP joint. With instability of the MTP joint, pain is elicited with stress on the plantar structures. **C,** Lateral radiograph of unstable second MTP joint prior to drawer test. **D,** Lateral radiograph following drawer test with the base of the proximal phalanx subluxed dorsally. **E,** Prior to dorsal subluxation of metatarsophalangeal joint with drawer test. **F,** Position of the base of the toe following dorsal subluxation.

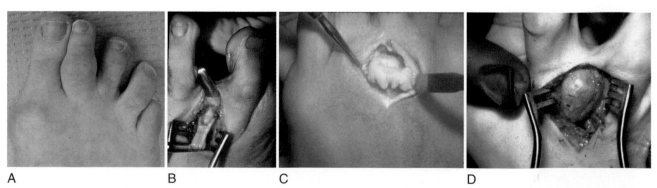

Figure 7–66 Causes of metatarsalgia. **A,** Nonspecific synovitis with swollen second toe and medial metatarsophalangeal (MTP) joint deviation. **B,** Interdigital neuroma can cause pain in this region. **C,** Freiberg's infraction of the second MTP joint. **D,** Synovial cyst causing deviation of the second and third toes.

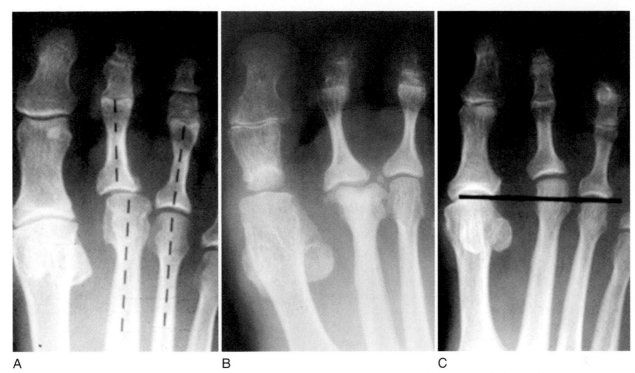

A   B   C

Figure 7–67 A, Anteroposterior radiograph demonstrating noncongruent second metatarsophalangeal (MTP) joint in early degenerative arthritis. **B,** Severe degenerative arthritis of the second MTP joint. **C,** A long second ray is often associated with a hammer toe or mallet toe deformity as well as instability of the second MTP joint.

Although a synovial cyst or interdigital neuroma may be associated with pain and deviation of the toe, intrinsic capsular instability more often is the cause of malalignment of the second MTP joint (Fig. 7–68).[22,30,32] It can be difficult to differentiate pain from MTP joint capsule instability and that from an adjacent interdigital neuroma[35,36,57]; however, typically a neuroma is associated with neuritic radicular pain to the involved toes as well as numbness. MTP joint

---

Grading System for Second Metatarsophalangeal Joint Subluxation

Grade 0: No instability. Joint pain, thickening or swelling of the MTP joint. Prodromal phase with pain but no deformity.

Grade I: Mild instability. Positive drawer sign, but no malalignment or deformity. Swelling of the MTP joint.

Grade II: Moderate instability. Positive drawer sign; medial, lateral, dorsal, or dorsomedial deformity at the MTP joint.

Grade III: Dislocated MTP joint. Positive drawer sign; fixed dorsomedial deformity. Severe deformity with overlapping of the hallux by the second toe.

Grade IV: Dislocated MTP joint. Fixed dorsomedial deformity.

---

instability typically is not associated with neuritic symptoms or numbness unless simultaneously there is a concomitant interdigital neuroma. Coughlin and Schenck[36] reported that 20% of the cases in which an interdigital neuroma was excised also demonstrated instability of the second MTP joint (see Fig. 7–21). With the progression of deformity, patients tend to lose the ability to curl the affected toe and can lose this ability in all the lesser toes (due to FDL dysfunction).

Johnson and Price[81] speculated that a pronation and adduction deformity of the midfoot and hindfoot was the contributing cause of a crossover second toe deformity; unfortunately, they failed to appreciate the significance of excessive second metatarsal length or capsule instability.

Radiographic Examination

Radiographic evaluation of the MTP joint may be less helpful than the clinical examination. Typically the lateral inclination of the lesser toes averages approximately 12 degrees.[22] With progressive deviation of the MTP joint, this orientation can increase or decrease. On the AP radiograph the diaphysis of the proximal phalanx may be hyperextended so that a gun barrel sign is seen (see Fig. 7–4B).[31] The diaphysis of the proximal phalanx projects as a round hole in the area

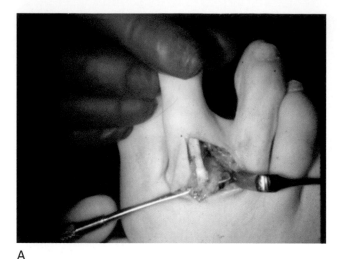

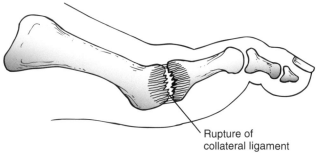

Rupture of
collateral ligament

A   B

Figure 7–68   A, Rupture of the lateral collateral ligament of the second metatarsophalangeal (MTP) joint in foot with crossover second toe deformity. **B,** With a crossover second toe deformity, the lateral collateral ligament can rupture, with subsequent medial deviation of the toe. With time, the rupture can extend plantarward, leading to hyperextension and dislocation of the MTP joint. Note excessive length of the second metatarsal compared to adjacent metatarsals. (**A** from Coughlin MJ: *Foot Ankle* 8[1]:29-39, 1987.)

of the distal condyle of the proximal phalanx. Radiographs may be helpful in evaluating the magnitude of the MTP joint deformity, assessing joint congruity (see Fig. 7–67A), ascertaining the presence of MTP joint arthritis (see Fig. 7–67B), and determining the length of the second metatarsal (see Fig. 7–67C).

Chondrolysis of the MTP joint may be associated with degenerative arthritis or Freiberg's infraction. In a typical radiograph the articular cartilage of the adjoining surface leaves a clear space of 2 to 3 mm (Fig. 7–69).[26] As hyperextension of the MTP joint develops, this clear space diminishes as the base of the proximal phalanx subluxates dorsally over the second metatarsal head. With frank dislocation, the base of the proximal phalanx can lie dorsally over the metatarsal head and is demonstrated as an overlapping of the adjacent bone on the AP radiograph (Fig. 7–70).

With progression of deformity, the second toe deviates medially or dorsomedially and gradually comes to rest above the hallux (Fig. 7–71). A hallux valgus deformity may be identified on examination, although association with a crossover toe is disputed.[3,22,81]

A lateral radiograph can demonstrate dislocation or hyperextension of the MTP joint (see Fig. 7–24B). The magnitude and the chronicity of the deformity appear to be related. With time, significant contractures of adjacent soft tissues can develop, with fixed dorsal dislocation at the MTP joint.

Karpman and MacCollum[86] and others[61] have described arthrography of the second MTP joint, which may be helpful in assessing capsule deterioration or instability of the MTP joint. Leakage of dye into the tendon sheath of the FDL tendon can indicate a

plantar plate rupture. A bone scan can help to differentiate ill-defined pain in the forefoot. Increased uptake can signify early intraarticular MTP joint instability (Fig. 7–72). Yao et al[173] have reported that magnetic resonance imaging is useful and reliable in the diagnosis of plantar plate abnormalities. In most cases, the diagnosis is made clinically.

Treatment

Conservative Treatment

A hammer toe may be managed conservatively with a comfortable well-fitted shoe with sufficient room in the toe box to accommodate the second toe deformity. Decreasing the heel height can alleviate plantar discomfort as well. A toe cradle prevents the toe tip from impacting against the ground, which also can decrease discomfort.[160] By taping the deformed toe in a neutral position, stability may be achieved over time, although this can require several months.[22,30] Prolonged taping does not correct the deformity but may achieve stabilization, with scarring at the MTP joint. However, once dislocation has occurred, taping is not helpful. The use of taping over a long period of time can lead to ulceration of the toe or chronic edema.

Placement of a metatarsal pad just proximal to a symptomatic metatarsal head can alleviate plantar discomfort by redistribution of weight on the plantar surface of the foot. Once an intractable plantar keratosis has developed, the use of an extra-depth shoe with a specialized liner or insert tends to relieve plantar discomfort. A roomy toe box accommodates both a fixed hammer toe deformity and a

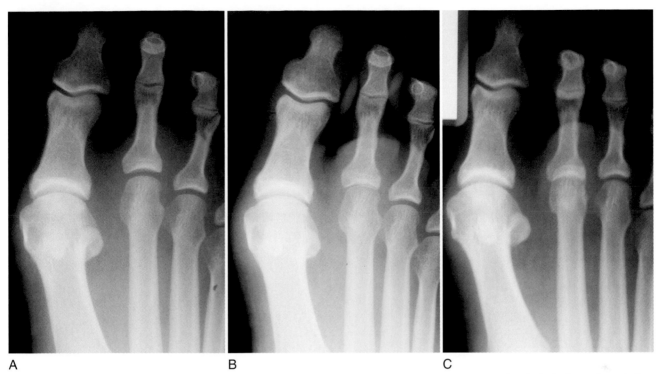

A   B   C

Figure 7–69 A, A 52-year-old man with pain at the second metatarsophalangeal (MTP) joint and a slight hallux valgus deformity. **B,** Six-month follow-up demonstrates narrowing of the joint space, pathognomonic of a hyperextension deformity. Often subluxation can occur insidiously. **C,** At 15-month follow-up, the second MTP joint has dislocated.

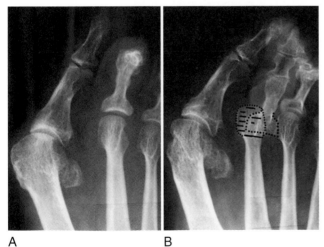

A   B

Figure 7–70 A, A 55-year-old woman with severe hallux valgus deformity. Note that the radiograph shows a hammer toe deformity of the second toe; however, the metatarsophalangeal (MTP) joint is well aligned. **B,** Three years following a simple bunionectomy, a recurrent hallux valgus deformity has occurred. There is now severe dislocation of the second MTP joint.

thickened insole. Padding over the tip of the contracted toe can help to decrease sensitivity of a callus either at the tip of the toe or overlying the hammer toe deformity.

The use of nonsteroidal anti-inflammatory drugs (NSAIDs) can decrease discomfort from inflammation at a symptomatic MTP joint. The judicious use of an intraarticular steroid injection may be considered. Trepman and Yeo[163] described nonsurgical treatment of second MTP joint synovitis with an intraarticular steroid injection and used a rocker sole to limit MTP joint dorsiflexion. At an average follow-up of 18 months, 60% of patients were asymptomatic and an additional 33% were improved. Mizel and Michelson,[117] reporting on a similar treatment with an intraarticular steroid injection and the use of a shoe modification with an extended steel shank, noted seven of nine symptomatic feet were asymptomatic at 6-year follow-up (Fig. 7–73).

Surgical Treatment

On the other hand, Fortin and Myerson[57] concluded that conservative care is usually unsuccessful and noted that an intraarticular steroid injection in their experience usually gave only temporary relief of 3 to 6 months, although occasionally a patient obtained permanent relief. Following an intraarticular steroid

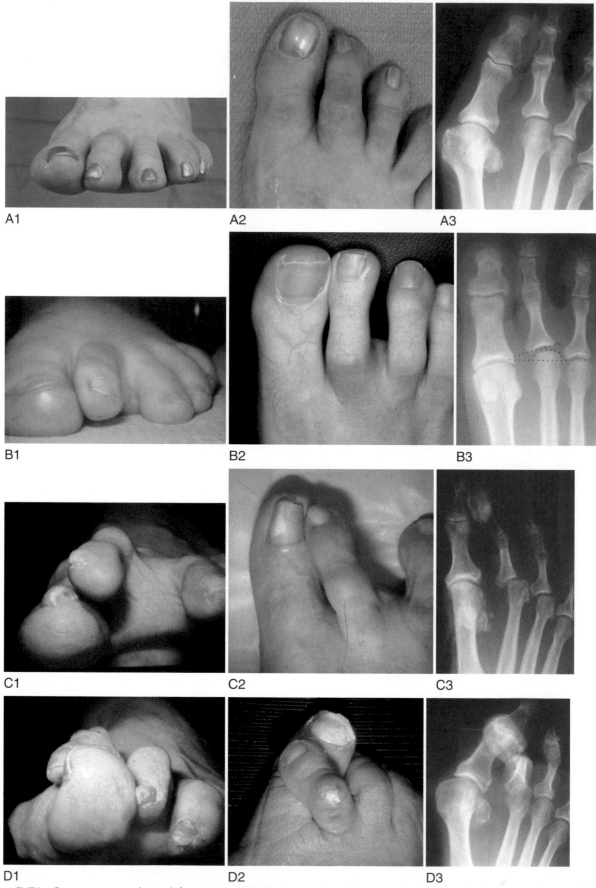

Figure 7–71 Crossover second toe deformity. **A,** Mild. **B,** Progressing deformity. **C,** Moderate deformity. **D,** Severe deformity beginning as mild subluxation of the metatarsophalangeal joint and finally progressing to frank dislocation. (**B1** from Coughlin MJ: *Instr Course Lect* 52:421-444, 2003.)

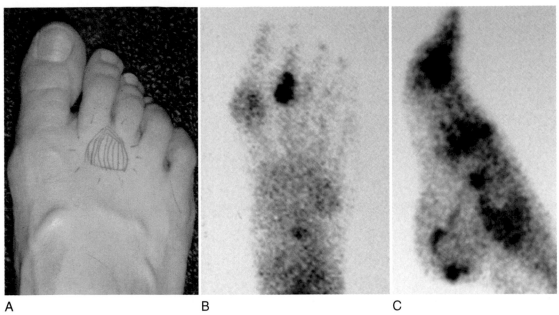

A   B   C

Figure 7–72 Patient with ill-defined forefoot pain. **A,** Clinical location of pain. ^{99}Tc bone scan, anteroposterior **(B)** and lateral **(C)** views, can demonstrate pathologic changes prior to radiographic changes. Note the increased uptake in the area of the second metatarsophalangeal joint.

injection, the affected toe is buddy taped to an adjacent toe for 6 to 12 weeks to reduce the incidence of MTP joint dislocation. When chronic pain is unrelieved by conservative methods or if progressive subluxation of the second MTP joint has developed, surgical intervention may be necessary.

Preoperative Planning

Certain factors must be appreciated in the development of the treatment plan for MTP joint subluxation or dislocation. The presence of a hallux valgus deformity may be a cause of or may have developed subsequent to the second toe abnormality. Although a hallux valgus deformity may be asymptomatic, surgical correction often is required to obtain adequate space for the corrected second toe once it has been realigned to a normal position. Mann and Mizel[103] reported on the treatment of seven patients (average age, 57 years) with generalized thickening of the second MTP joint, increased warmth and tenderness, and decreased range of motion. They were noted to have a positive vertical stress test in all cases. Six patients were treated with a synovectomy and 50% with resection of a second interspace interdigital neuroma. They reported generally good results with this treatment.

Figure 7–73 An intraarticular injection of lidocaine can temporarily relieve pain, aiding in the diagnosis of metatarsophalangeal joint instability. **A,** Injection. **B,** Fluoroscopic documentation of injection.

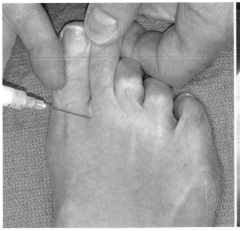

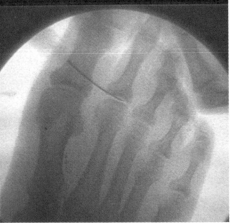

A   B

A second MTP joint abnormality often is associated with a hammer toe deformity. The rigidity and severity of the deformity determines the surgical correction that is necessary. When evaluating a hammer toe it is necessary to recognize the presence of a contracture of the flexor digitorum longus tendon. Hammering or clawing of an adjacent lesser toe can help the examiner to identify a contracture of the flexor digitorum longus (see Fig. 7–25). With this abnormality a tenotomy or release of the flexor digitorum longus in the involved toe is carried out at the time of surgery.

With progressive subluxation of the second MTP joint, deviation can occur medially, laterally, or dorsally. If surgery is indicated, the MTP joint is explored. An extensor tenotomy or lengthening of the extensor digitorum brevis and longus is performed. A dorsal capsulotomy is carried out. In the presence of dorsal subluxation at the MTP joint, an aggressive medial and lateral capsule release must be performed. This requires release of the capsule plantarward because a dorsal capsule release does not allow relocation of the MTP joint. In the presence of medial deviation,[46] a medial capsule release may be augmented by lateral capsule reefing to align a deviated toe. With a hyperextended MTP joint, it is not uncommon for adhesions to develop between the plantar capsule and the metatarsal head. Release of the plantar capsule may be necessary for reduction of the hyperextended MTP joint after a release of the dorsal structures.

Ford et al[56] and Jolly[84] have suggested a technique involving a direct repair of the plantar plate and believe this can offer the best stability and realignment of the malaligned lesser toe. Long-term follow-up is necessary to determine the efficacy of this suggested technique as well as associated complications with this plantar approach (Fig. 7–74).

Once an MTP joint capsule release has been performed, a flexor tendon transfer may be necessary to give plantar flexion stability to the proximal phalanx. With the progression of deformity and frank dislocation, a joint decompression may be necessary. An MTP joint arthroplasty in which a portion of the metatarsal head is resected may help to preserve some function while allowing relocation of the MTP joint. Often, internal fixation with a Kirschner wire is necessary after completion of any of these procedures.

The use of any of these procedures depends on the magnitude of the deformity of the MTP joint and the flexibility of the contracture of the interphalangeal joint. In the presence of a rigid deformity at the PIP joint, a fixed hammer toe repair is performed. With a rigid deformity of the MTP joint, a combination of a soft tissue release (extensor tendon lengthening, MTP capsule release), flexor tendon transfer, and bone

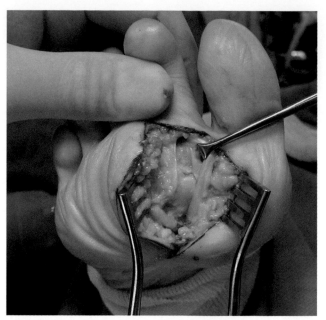

Figure 7–74 Direct repair of the plantar capsule. Note the longitudinal tear in the metatarsophalangeal capsule. (Courtesy of Dr. G. Jolly.)

decompression (either a shortening metatarsal osteotomy or an intraarticular bone resection) may be necessary to realign the toe. Treatment for a hammer toe deformity usually is performed simultaneously with MTP joint realignment. Early operative intervention prior to dislocation of the MTP joint can allow preservation of joint function. In the presence of severe deformity, the necessity for a resection arthroplasty limits the expected functional result.

In the initial evaluation, the vascular and neurologic status of the foot and lesser toes is important when planning surgery. Often multiple procedures are performed on the second toe to correct both a hammer toe and an MTP joint deformity. Numerous surgical procedures can impair the circulation to the toe, and occasionally surgery must be limited if the vascular integrity is compromised. It is not always easy to ascertain whether a toe will tolerate a few or many surgical procedures, and this may be determined only at the time of surgical intervention.

A step-by-step discussion of both fixed and flexible hammer toe repair is presented in the section on hammer toes. Often one of these procedures is performed in combination with MTP joint alignment.

MILD SUBLUXATION

The treatment of subluxation of the MTP joint should be approached in a progressive surgical fashion. Figure 7–75 presents an algorithm for treating mild and moderate subluxation of the MTP joint.

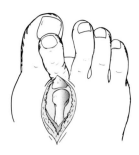

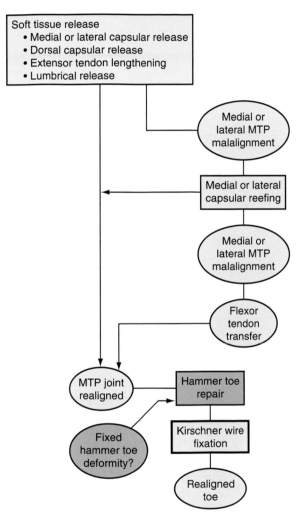

Figure 7–75 Algorithm for treatment of mild and moderate subluxation of the metatarsophalangeal joint.

SOFT TISSUE RELEASE

Indications

In the presence of a mild deformity, characterized by a soft tissue contracture of the MTP joint, a soft tissue release may be sufficient to realign the toe.

Contraindications

Where more severe deformities are present, characterized by fixed contractures, soft tissue releases are commonly unsuccessful in achieving a complete realignment of the digit. Care must always be taken in the presence of a digital deformity to avoid excessive surgery that could threaten the neurologic or vascular competency of the digit.

Surgical Technique[31]

1. The patient is placed in a supine position on the operating room table. The procedure is performed under a peripheral anesthetic block. The foot is cleansed and draped in the usual fashion. The foot is exsanguinated with an Esmarch bandage. The Esmarch bandage may be used as a tourniquet above the level of the ankle.
2. A dorsal lazy-S incision is centered over the second MTP joint.
3. The extensor tendon is exposed and released in a Z-type fashion. This release is later repaired in lengthened form with interrupted sutures.
4. The MTP joint dorsal capsule is released sharply, as are the medial and lateral capsules. Care is taken to release the collateral ligaments and capsule in a plantarward direction, from a dorsoplantar direction of about 2 to 3 cm in length, to avoid leaving any contracted tissue (Fig. 7–76A-D).
5. The first lumbrical on the medial aspect of the second toe may be a significant deforming force, and it should be released with the soft tissue release. Care is taken to protect the neurovascular bundle adjacent to the lumbrical.
6. In the presence of adhesions on the plantar aspect of the MTP joint between the plantar capsule and metatarsal head, a McGlamry elevator is advanced around the metatarsal head in a dorsoplantar direction. In this way, adhesions may be released, allowing

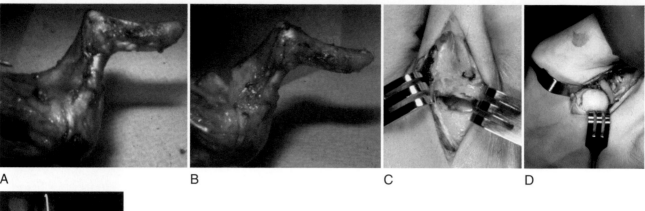

A　　　　　　　B　　　　　　　C　　　　　　　D

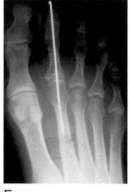

E

Figure 7–76　Soft tissue release and realignment. **A,** Lateral view of a cadaver dissection demonstrating a fixed hammer toe deformity and a fixed contracture of the metatarsophalangeal joint. Note the lumbrical pulling at a right angle. Also note the thickness of the lateral capsule. **B,** An extensor tenotomy and dorsal capsule release have been performed. This is an inadequate release to reduce the toe, as can be seen in this dissection. Note that a more extensive capsule release must be performed on the medial and lateral aspect in order to reduce the toe. **C,** Intraoperative photo demonstrating inadequate release. **D,** An adequate capsule release has been performed. **E,** Following metatarsophalangeal joint release, often intermedullary Kirschner-wire fixation is used to stabilize the repair.

reduction of the hyperextended proximal phalanx. A complete dorsal–medial and lateral synovectomy is performed.

7. Once the joint contractures have been released, a test for stability is performed. Repetitive passive dorsiflexion and plantar flexion of the ankle usually help determine whether the MTP joint will stay reduced. In an unstable situation, the MTP joint dislocates with intraoperative motion at the ankle (dorsoplantar flexion).

8. If the MTP joint is well aligned and stable, an intramedullary 0.045-inch Kirschner wire is introduced at the base of the proximal phalanx and driven in a distal direction exiting the tip of the toe (Fig. 7–76E). It is then driven retrograde across the MTP joint. It is bent at the tip of the toe, and the excess pin is removed. (If a fixed hammer toe repair has been performed, the pin is introduced at the PIP joint and driven distally. It is then driven in a retrograde fashion as described.)

9. After repair of the extensor tendon and routine skin closure, a compression gauze dressing is applied.

Postoperative Care

The patient is allowed to ambulate in a wooden-soled shoe. Sutures and the Kirschner wire are removed 3 weeks after surgery. The toe is then taped in a slightly plantar flexed position for 6 weeks. Passive range-of-motion exercises are initiated 3 weeks following surgery.

MODERATE SUBLUXATION

Preoperative Planning

In the presence of moderate MTP joint subluxation, a hyperextended proximal phalanx at the MTP joint is the most commonly seen deformity. There may be associated medial or lateral deviation of the second toe. On occasion, only medial or lateral deviation of the toe is noted. The degree and severity of the deformity and its direction determine the surgical repair (see Fig. 7–75).

Preoperative Evaluation

Initially the surgeon must determine if a fixed or flexible hammer toe deformity is present. If the hammer toe is fixed, a DuVries arthroplasty is performed (see the description of the technique of fixed hammer toe repair earlier in the chapter). If the hammer toe is flexible and is passively correctable, a flexor tendon transfer is performed. Often a fixed contracture of the MTP joint is present. With a pure hyperextension deformity at the MTP joint, a soft tissue release is performed (see the section on technique). A complete medial, lateral, and dorsal capsule release is performed in a sequential fashion to achieve complete reduction of the deformity.[57] With a hyperextension deformity, it often is necessary to release adhesions between the plantar capsule and the metatarsal head. A curved elevator is used to release these contractures. If there is residual medial deviation at the MTP joint, an extensor digitorum brevis transfer may be added to the capsule reefing.[57]

Placement of a Kirschner wire is optional. If a fixed hammer toe repair has been performed, or if the surgeon believes increased support for the surgical repair is necessary, a Kirschner wire should be placed. Placement of this pin may be somewhat difficult. Usually it is driven distally from the MTP joint and exits at the tip of the toe. The wire driver then is placed on the pin distally and the pin is driven in a retrograde fashion across the MTP joint. Occasionally some difficulty is encountered in transfixing the MTP joint. The pin can angle into the soft tissue adjacent to the MTP joint. Even if the pin does not transfix the MTP joint, it can provide significant stability to the repair. A Kirschner wire should not be used to achieve additional corrective alignment, because when the wire is removed the toe deformity can recur. The surgeon might find it easier to reef the capsule after the Kirschner wire has been advanced through the toe but before it is passed retrograde into the metatarsal.

Despite a soft tissue release and capsule reefing, often there remains an element of MTP joint hyperextension. A flexor tendon transfer must then be considered. A flexor tendon transfer removes the deforming force from the distal toe and adds a plantar flexion force to the proximal phalanx (Fig. 7–77). Whether this is a dynamic transfer or has a tenodesing effect is unclear, but the transfer typically depresses the proximal phalanx and achieves adequate alignment of the MTP joint (see the earlier discussion of flexor tendon transfer).

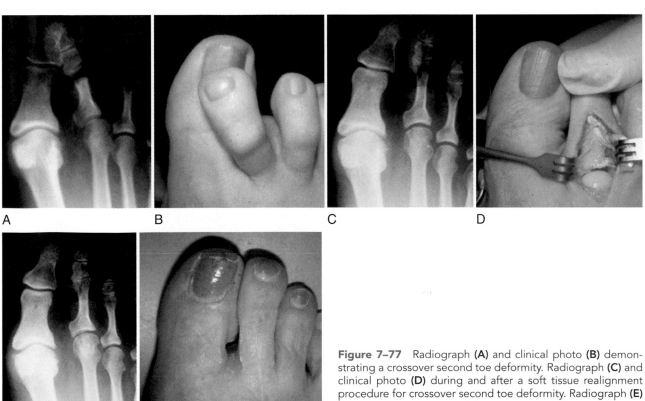

A   B   C   D

E   F

Figure 7–77 Radiograph **(A)** and clinical photo **(B)** demonstrating a crossover second toe deformity. Radiograph **(C)** and clinical photo **(D)** during and after a soft tissue realignment procedure for crossover second toe deformity. Radiograph **(E)** and clinical photo **(F)** at follow-up 9 years after a soft tissue release, lateral capsule reefing, and flexor tendon transfer. (From Coughlin MJ: *Foot Ankle* 8[1]:29-39, 1987.)

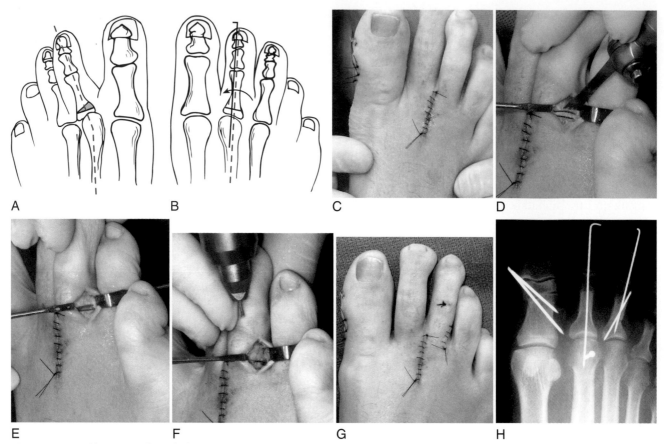

Figure 7–78 Closing wedge phalangeal osteotomy. **A,** Proposed lateral closing wedge proximal phalangeal osteotomy. **B,** Realignment following osteotomy. **C,** Following Weil osteotomy of second metatarsal, there is residual medial deviation of the third toe. **D,** Exposure of lateral proximal phalanx and closing wedge osteotomy. **E,** Removal of wedge. **F,** Closure of osteotomy. **G,** Following wound closure. **H,** Postoperative radiograph demonstrating realignment of proximal phalanx.

A distal metatarsal osteotomy may be necessary if the joint is not reducible (see the section on severe MTP joint instability). An osteotomy preserves some MTP joint function and is preferable. In the presence of joint instability when the MTP joint can be successfully reduced, a plantar condylectomy may be performed in conjunction with a soft tissue release to achieve stability; this succeeds by creating scarring of the MTP joint.

Davis et al[43] have described a closing wedge osteotomy at the base of the proximal phalanx to achieve axial alignment of a malaligned toe. No long-term follow-up on patients was reported regarding the durability of this procedure (Fig. 7–78). This procedure does not stabilize or realign the MTP joint, and the toe can redeform with time (Fig. 7–79).

Indications

In the presence of medial or lateral MTP joint deviation, release of the contracted capsule and reefing of the contralateral capsule can help to achieve realignment of the toe. A Weil osteotomy is preferable to a flexor tendon transfer if there is residual MTP joint malalignment following soft tissue release and reefing (see the section on technique).

Contraindications

In the presence of a severe deformity, a soft tissue release is ineffective in correcting the MTP joint malalignment.

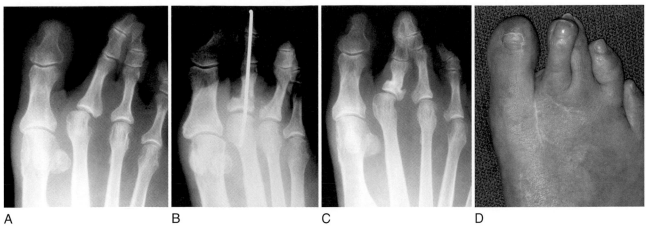

A   B   C   D

Figure 7–79 A, Preoperative radiograph demonstrating lateral deviation of the second toe at the metatarsophalangeal joint. **B,** Following medial closing wedge osteotomy of the proximal phalanx. Radiograph **(C)** and clinical photograph **(D)** at 8-year follow-up, demonstrating progressive lateral subluxation of metatarsophalangeal joint.

REEFING OF THE SECOND METATARSOPHALANGEAL JOINT CAPSULE[101]

Surgical Technique

1. The patient is placed in a supine position on the operating room table. The procedure is performed under a peripheral anesthetic block. The foot is cleansed and draped in the usual fashion. The foot is exsanguinated with an Esmarch bandage. The Esmarch bandage may be used as a tourniquet above the level of the ankle.
2. The extensor tendons are lengthened with a Z-type incision and are later repaired.
3. The MTP joint dorsal capsule is released.
4. If the digit is deviated medially, the tight contracted medial capsule is released in a dorsoplantar direction. This usually requires release of at least 1 cm of capsule to the plantar extent of the MTP joint.
5. When the second toe is deviated medially, release of the first lumbrical can remove a significant deforming force.
6. A suture is placed in the distal lateral MTP capsule, then directed into the region of the plantar metatarsal capsule in a more proximal direction. Usually a figure-of-eight suture is placed (Fig. 7–80A and B).
7. One or two sutures are placed and, with the toe held in a corrected position, are tied. Usually this achieves 5 to 10 degrees of axial realignment (Fig. 7–80C-E).
8. When a paucity of tissue is present in the area of the metatarsal head, the proximal suture may be anchored into the adjoining metatarsal capsule or, alternatively, a suture anchor may be placed in the lateral metatarsal head to secure the distal and plantar MTP capsule (Fig. 7–81).
9. Kirschner wire fixation may or may not be employed depending on whether a fixed hammer toe repair has been performed or based on the stability following MTP joint capsulorrhaphy.
10. The extensor tendon is repaired and the skin is approximated in a routine fashion.

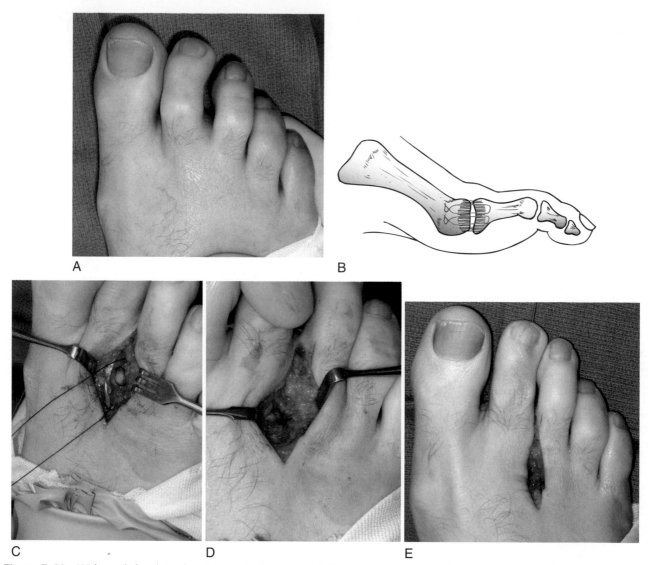

Figure 7–80   With medial or lateral metatarsophalangeal joint deviation, a release of the contracted capsule structures is performed in combination with reefing of the ligamentous structures on the contralateral or elongated side. **A,** Preoperative clinical photograph. **B,** Diagram. **C** and **D,** Intraoperative photo in which one or two interrupted sutures are used to reef the capsule; often this allows realignment of 5 to 10 degrees in an axial plane. **E,** Clinical photo following lateral capsule reefing to realign metatarsophalangeal joint.

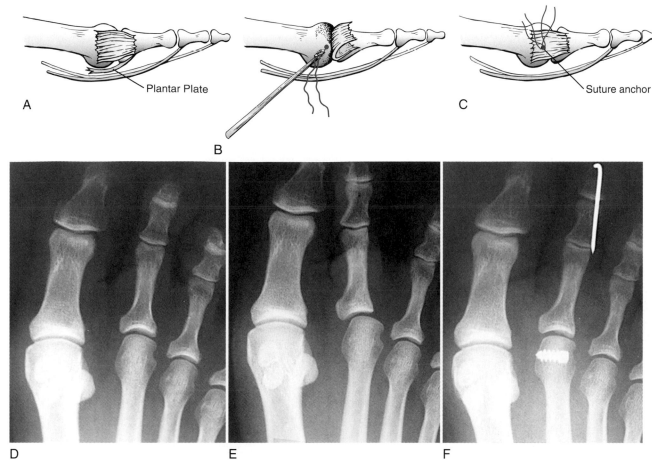

A — Plantar Plate

B

C — Suture anchor

D

E

F

Figure 7–81 A suture anchor may be helpful in reefing an elongated capsule. The capsule is detached from the metatarsal head and secured with a suture anchor. **A,** Normal lateral capsule. **B** and **C,** Lateral diagram of metatarsophalangeal (MTP) joint and plantar plate with placement of suture anchor. **D,** Radiograph demonstrating normal alignment with symptomatic second MTP joint. **E,** Preoperative radiograph demonstrating medial deviation. **F,** Following flexor tendon transfer and placement of suture anchor to secure lateral MTP capsule, successful realignment is achieved.

EXTENSOR DIGITORUM BREVIS TRANSFER[69]

Surgical Technique

1. The patient is placed in a supine position on the operating room table. The procedure is performed under a peripheral anesthetic block. The foot is exsanguinated with an Esmarch bandage. An Esmarch bandage may be used as a tourniquet above the level of the ankle. A dorsal longitudinal skin incision is centered over the MTP joint and second intermetatarsal space.

2. The MTP joint is released and the extensor digitorum brevis tendon is carefully dissected proximally (Fig. 7–82A-D).

3. Four centimeters proximal to the MTP joint, the extensor digitorum brevis tendon is severed and each end secured with an interrupted stay-suture (Fig. 7–82E-G).

4. The distal tendon stump is passed beneath the transverse metatarsal ligament from distal to proximal and passed lateral to the extensor hood. The distal attachment of the extensor digitorum brevis is carefully protected (Fig. 7–82H and I).

5. Prior to the tendon repair, a 0.065-inch Kirschner wire is inserted at the MTP joint and is driven distally and then retrograde across the MTP joint (Fig. 7–82J).

6. With the joint held in corrected alignment, the end of the distal stump is repaired to the

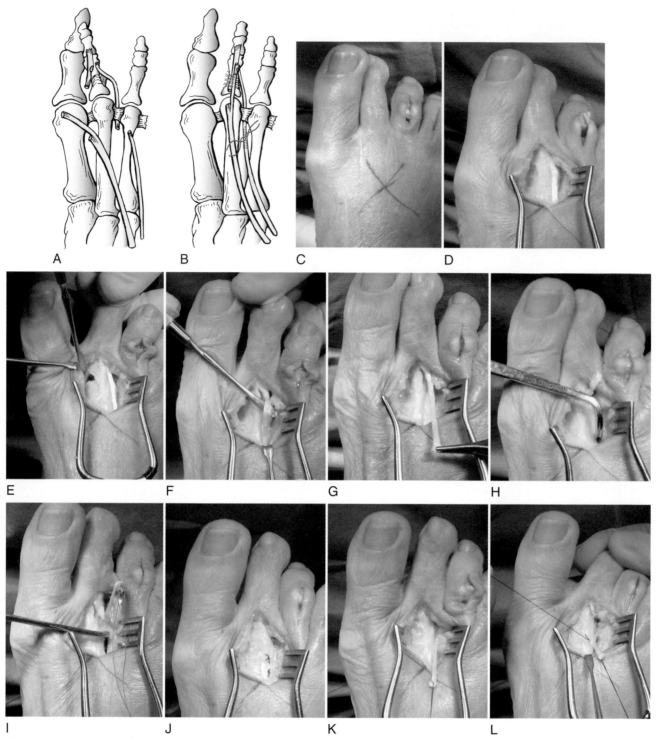

Figure 7–82 Extensor digitorum brevis transfer diagram. **A,** The distal stump of the extensor digitorum brevis is transferred beneath the transverse intermetatarsal ligament. **B,** It is reattached end to end with a Krakow suture, and the extensor digitorum longus is Z-lengthened. **C, D,** and **E,** Clinical photographs of transfer. **C,** Preoperative clinical appearance. **D,** Dorsal exposure. **E,** Release of medial capsule. **F,** Tension on extensor digitorum brevis tendon. **G,** Tendon is released proximally. **H,** Tendon passer develops tract beneath TML. **I** and **J,** Tendon is passed beneath ligament. **K** and **L,** Tendon is sutured with toe correctly aligned. (**I,** Courtesy of L.S. Weil, DPM.)

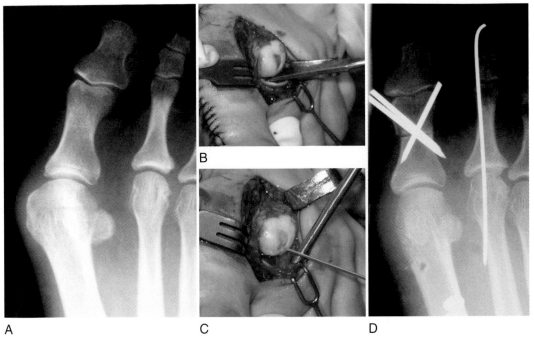

A   C   D

Figure 7–83 **A,** Preoperative radiograph demonstrating hallux valgus deformity with an unstable and painful second metatarsophalangeal (MTP) joint without obvious deformity. **B,** Intraoperative photograph demonstrating the osteochondral defect. The joint was unstable in the vertical plane. **C,** Plantar condylectomy. **D,** Postoperative radiograph demonstrating bunion repair and Kirschner-wire stabilization of second MTP joint after plantar condylectomy. Note that an Akin procedure has been performed on the hallux.

proximal stump with an end-to-end suture (Fig. 7–82K and L).

7. The soft tissue and skin are approximated in a routine fashion.

Postoperative Care

A gauze-and-tape dressing is applied postoperatively and changed weekly. Sutures are removed 3 weeks after surgery, and the toe is taped in appropriate alignment for 6 weeks after surgery.

PLANTAR CONDYLECTOMY

Surgical Technique

1. The foot is cleansed and draped in the usual fashion. The foot is exsanguinated with an Esmarch bandage. The Esmarch bandage may be used as a tourniquet above the level of the ankle.

2. A lazy-S incision is centered over the MTP joint. A soft tissue release is performed in which the extensor tendons are lengthened,

and the dorsal, medial, and lateral MTP capsules are released as well (Fig. 7–83A).

3. The metatarsal head is identified, and the proximal phalanx is plantar flexed to expose the plantar condyle. A McGlamry elevator is helpful is retracting the adjacent soft tissue.

4. A Hoke osteotomy is used to resect 3 to 4 mm of the plantar aspect of the metatarsal head. The distal metatarsal articular surface is left intact. The plantar portion is spun out from beneath the remaining metatarsal head. Care must be taken to minimize pressure on the metatarsal head to avoid a metaphyseal fracture (Fig. 7–83B-D).

5. A Kirschner wire is introduced at the MTP joint and driven distally out the tip of the toe. It is then advanced retrograde into the metatarsal to stabilize the MTP joint.

6. The extensor tendon is repaired and the skin is approximated with interrupted sutures.

Postoperative Care

A gauze-and-tape dressing is applied and changed weekly. The Kirschner wire and sutures are removed 2 to 3 weeks after surgery and the toe is then taped in corrected position for 6 weeks.

PHALANGEAL CLOSING WEDGE OSTEOTOMY ("AKINETTE")

Surgical Technique

1. The foot is cleansed and draped in the usual fashion. The foot is exsanguinated with an Esmarch bandage. The Esmarch bandage may be used as a tourniquet above the level of the ankle.
2. A longitudinal incision is centered over the dorsal aspect of the proximal phalanx of the involved digit (see Fig. 7–78A).
3. The extensor tendons are elevated and a closing wedge phalangeal osteotomy is performed in the region of the proximal phalangeal metaphysis (see Fig. 7–78B-E).
4. The osteotomy is closed and stabilized with one or two Kirschner wires (see Fig. 7–78F-H).
5. A Kirschner wire is introduced at the MTP joint and driven distally out the tip of the toe. It is then retrograded into the metatarsal, stabilizing the MTP joint.

Postoperative Care

A gauze-and-tape dressing is applied and changed weekly. The Kirschner wire and sutures are removed 3 weeks after surgery and the toe is then taped in corrected position for 6 weeks.

Results

Dhukaram et al[49] performed an extensive soft tissue MTP joint release and PIP joint arthroplasty for subluxated joint deformities. If a hyperextension deformity persisted following a careful soft tissue release, a Weil osteotomy was performed. In the evaluation of 69 patients (157 toes), 14% still had moderate or severe pain at the MTP joint, but only two cases demonstrated instability of the MTP joint. A patient should be forewarned that following surgery, pain might not totally resolve.

Coughlin[22] reported on the surgical correction of 15 toes (11 patients) with a variety of methods depending on the severity of the deformity. Extensor tenotomy or lengthening, MTP joint capsulotomy, flexor tendon transfer, Kirschner wire fixation, and occasionally metatarsal articular surface resection were used to treat these acute and chronic MTP subluxations. Findings at surgery demonstrated that 33% of second MTP joints had a rupture or complete erosion of the lateral MTP capsule and 40% had erosion with complete rupture of the joint capsule. In 27% a rupture could not be demonstrated, although the capsule was elongated. Some 90% were noted to have an elongated second metatarsal averaging 4 mm of increased length. Ninety-three percent good and excellent results were reported using this method of soft tissue reconstruction. Coughlin[30] later reported on a younger group of athletically active patients (9 patients, 11 toes). Using a similar soft tissue realignment procedure, 71% good and excellent results were reported.

Coughlin et al[36] reported on their experience in treating a series of 121 consecutive patients with an interdigital neuroma. Twenty percent of these patients had concurrent lesser MTP joint instability. They were treated with a correction of the joint instability and also neuroma excision. 85% rated their result good or excellent. Those with continued symptoms isolated their pain to the symptomatic MTP joint. Barca and Acciaro[3] have reported on the use of a flexor digitorum longus transfer combined with a medial soft tissue release in 27 patients (30 toes) and noted 83% good or excellent results.

If malalignment of the joint and a positive drawer sign was present, a joint injection was not necessary. Ill-defined forefoot pain in the area of the second MTP joint and second interspace may be difficult to differentiate, and sequential injections may be helpful in defining specific areas of pain (Fig. 7–84).

Haddad et al[69] reported on the results of 19 extensor digitorum brevis transfers for correction of mild to moderate crossover second toe deformity. At an average follow-up of almost 52 months, they noted successful realignment in 14 of 19 (74%) toes, two failures that were revised with a flexor digitorum longus transfer, and three toes with mild recurrent deformities that were asymptomatic. They noted an average postoperative passive range of motion of 78 degrees following flexor digitorum brevis transfer compared to a similar sized group in their study in which a flexor digitorum longus transfer was performed where there was an average of 62 degrees of passive motion at the MTP joint. The authors suggested that stiffness might not solely be due to the tendon transfer, because in fact deformities that were more severe were believed to develop more scarring following MTP joint realignment. However, they

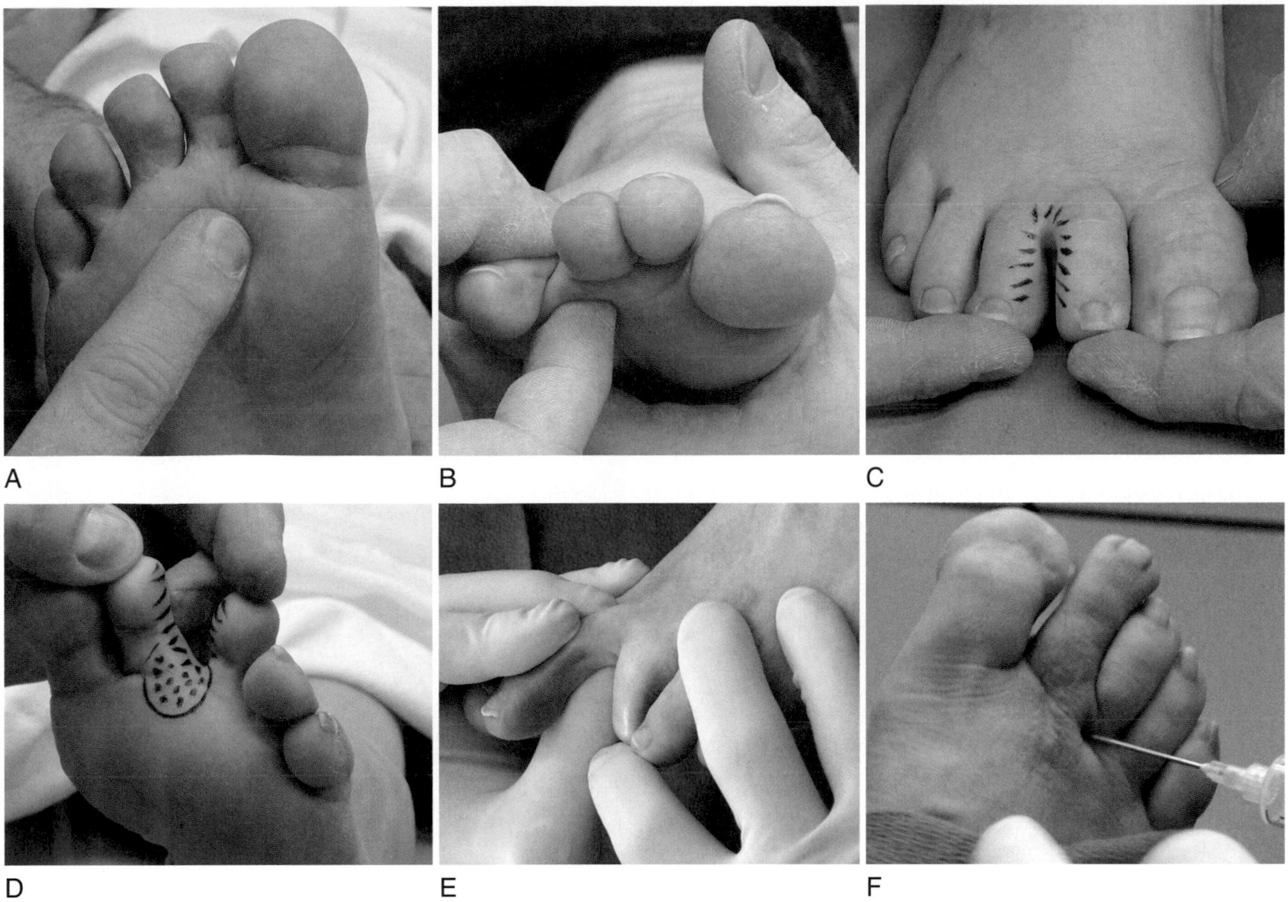

Figure 7–84 The examination to differentiate metatarsophalangeal joint pain from a neuroma can be difficult, especially in a patient who has had prior surgery. **A,** Pain is often localized to the plantar surface of the foot. **B,** Palpation for pain in the interspace can help to diagnose a neuroma. **C** and **D,** Areas of numbness or neuritic pain can occur with nerve irritation. **E,** A positive drawer sign is pathognomonic for capsular instability. **F,** Diagnostic injection may help to isolate the primary area of pain.

found that transferring the extensor digitorum brevis beneath the transverse metatarsal ligament was effective in controlling transverse plane abnormalities in the treatment of the crossover second toe deformity. They recommended short extensor tendon transfer for mild and moderate deformities that were flexible; they recommended long flexor tendon transfer for more severe deformities, for rigid deformities, and for patients with combined instability and concomitant interdigital neuromas of the second intermetatarsal space. Stiffness and continued pain were common following surgery, and complete satisfaction was noted by only 69% of patients. There are no reports on the long-term efficacy of the plantar condylectomy, although it has been used in combination with other procedures in several reports.[22,30,31]

SEVERE SUBLUXATION AND DISLOCATION

Dislocation of the MTP joint typically occurs insidiously (see Figs. 7–63, 7–69, and 7–70). An initial hyperextension deformity of the MTP joint can progress to severe subluxation, and over time dislocation can result. The dislocated toe may be a pure dorsal dislocation or have a dorsomedial or dorsolateral component.

Preoperative Planning

A step-by-step surgical approach is used to treat the toe. The algorithm presented in Fig. 7–75 describes the treatment of MTP joint subluxation and cases that have progressed to frank dislocation. A soft tissue dissection is performed with an extensive soft tissue release (tendon lengthenings and MTP capsule release). Any adhesions on the plantar aspect of the metatarsal head are released as well. In the presence of a recent dislocation, soft tissue releases can allow relocation of the MTP joint (Fig. 7–85). Often, a flexor tendon transfer is necessary, as is Kirschner wire stabilization for the relocated toe. In this situation, postoperative treatment is identical to that outlined for less severe deformities at the MTP joint (Fig. 7–86).

Indications

In the presence of a long-standing deformity, significant soft tissue contractures preclude adequate reduction of the toe with soft tissue procedures alone. In severe cases, bone decompression is necessary to realign the toe without creating significant tension on the neurovascular bundles. Although a partial proximal phalangectomy is an alternative, preservation of the trumpet-shaped base of the proximal phalanx affords significant stability to the MTP joint[57]; currently, a partial proximal phalangectomy is considered a salvage procedure. A DuVries arthroplasty also achieves joint decompression by excision of a small portion of the distal metatarsal articular surface. Although in the past I have favored this method of joint decompression, I now reserve a formal DuVries arthroplasty for salvage situations when other procedures have failed.

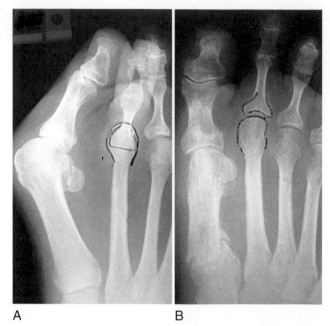

Figure 7–86 A, Preoperative radiograph demonstrates severe dislocation of second metatarsophalangeal joint, associated with a hallux valgus deformity. **B,** After a hallux valgus repair with a first metatarsal osteotomy, distal soft tissue release, and flexor tendon transfer, adequate realignment has been achieved.

Currently, joint preservation techniques that also provide joint decompression are preferred. Joint decompression, however, is mandatory when severe contractures are present. Excessive bone resection should be avoided because it can lead to a floppy, unstable toe. A distal metatarsal osteotomy preserves some MTP joint function and is preferable. Weil[169,170] has popularized a distal oblique osteotomy in the metatarsal metaphyseal region (Fig. 7–87). Proximal displacement of the distal metatarsal segment can achieve shortening of 2 to 6 mm. Internal fixation is recommended to stabilize the osteotomy site. The osteotomy may be translated or angled medially or laterally to improve axial realignment.

Contraindications

The main contraindication for a capital oblique distal metatarsal is severe deformity for which excisional arthroplasty is preferable. The limits of this procedure have yet to be defined, and although severe subluxation and dislocation may be reduced with a shortening osteotomy, the remaining forefoot and the possibility of transfer metatarsalgia must be considered when treating isolated metatarsophalangeal joints.

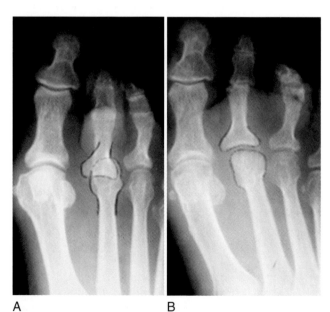

Figure 7–85 A, Relatively recent second metatarsophalangeal joint dislocation in a 60-year-old woman. **B,** Following soft tissue release and flexor tendon transfer, adequate realignment has been achieved.

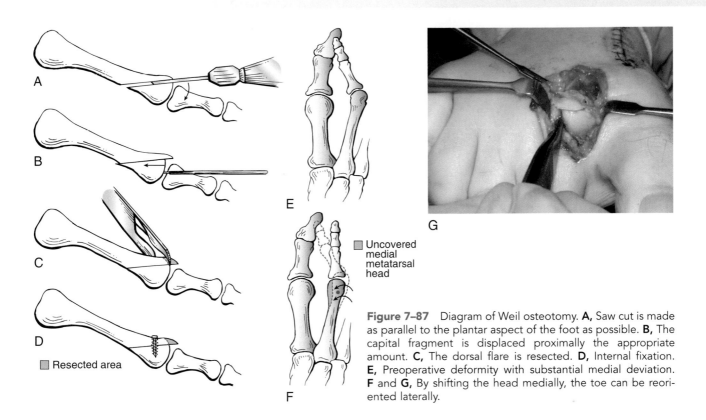

Uncovered medial metatarsal head

Figure 7–87 Diagram of Weil osteotomy. **A,** Saw cut is made as parallel to the plantar aspect of the foot as possible. **B,** The capital fragment is displaced proximally the appropriate amount. **C,** The dorsal flare is resected. **D,** Internal fixation. **E,** Preoperative deformity with substantial medial deviation. **F** and **G,** By shifting the head medially, the toe can be reoriented laterally.

Resected area

DISTAL OBLIQUE METATARSAL OSTEOTOMY[169]

Surgical Technique

1. The patient is placed in a supine position on the operating room table. The procedure is typically performed under a peripheral anesthetic block. An Esmarch bandage is used to exsanguinate the extremity and may be used as an ankle tourniquet.
2. A 3 to 4-cm longitudinal incision is centered either over the distal second metatarsal or in the second intermetatarsal space (Fig. 7–88A and video clip 37).
3. The metatarsal head and metaphysis are identified and the dorsal capsule is released. The medial and lateral collateral ligaments are not released unless shortening of more than 3 mm is desired. If more substantial shortening is desired, the collateral ligaments are released from the phalangeal attachment (Fig. 7–88B and C).
4. The subluxated or dislocated metatarsal head is reduced and the phalanx is plantar

flexed, exposing the metatarsal head. Occasionally a McGlamry elevator is used to expose the metatarsal head. It is used with care to prevent devascularization of the metatarsal metaphysis (Fig. 7–88D).
5. A longitudinal oblique distal metatarsal osteotomy is performed. The saw blade penetrates the distal superior metatarsal articular surface 2 mm inferior to the dorsal metatarsal surface. The plane of the osteotomy is parallel to the plantar surface of the foot and proceeds in a proximal direction until the saw blade has penetrated the proximal phalangeal cortex (Figs. 7–87A, 7–88E and F, and Fig.7–89A-C).
6. The distal fragment is then translated proximally the desired amount (2 to 6 mm) as planned preoperatively (Figs. 7–87B and 7–88G).
7. The osteotomy site is stabilized with a single dorsal plantar mini-fragment screw. Care must be taken not to place an excessively long screw, which can cause plantar symptoms. Occasionally two screws are

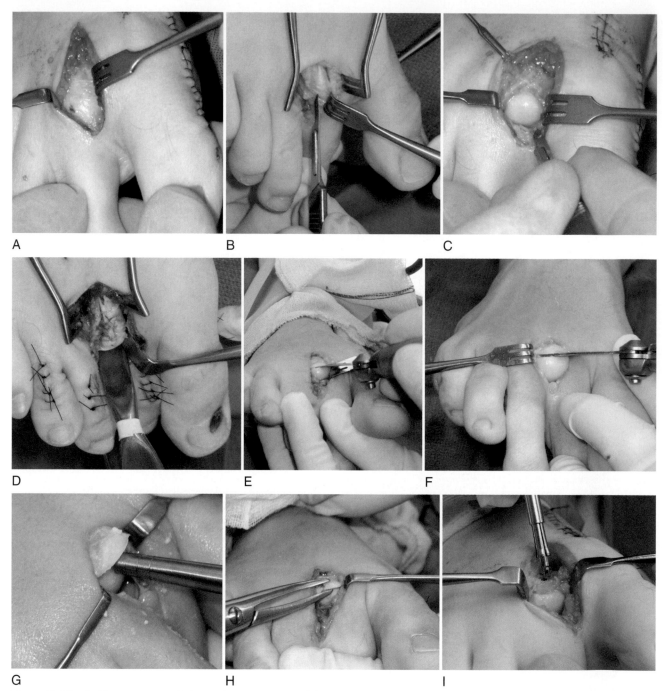

Figure 7–88 **A,** The metatarsophalangeal joint is exposed through a dorsal incision; the joint is freed up by releasing the distal ligamentous attachment and maintaining the metatarsal capsule. **B,** The capsule is released distally off of the phalanx, preserving the metatarsal head vascularity. **C,** Care must be taken when doing a proximal release not to strip the metatarsal vascular supply. **D,** An elevator may be used to free up the plantar capsule, but care must be taken to avoid disruption of the lateral capsular vascular supply. **E,** Proposed osteotomy. **F,** Stacked blades enable resection of more bone. **G,** The capital fragment is displaced proximally. A calibrated bone impactor is used to translate the capital fragment a measured amount. **H,** The dorsal ledge is resected. **I,** If a single screw does not adequately compress the ostotomy site, a second screw must be placed. (The screw must be long enough to engage the plantar fragment, but not excessively long. With shortening of more than 4 mm, two-screw fixation is often necessary.)

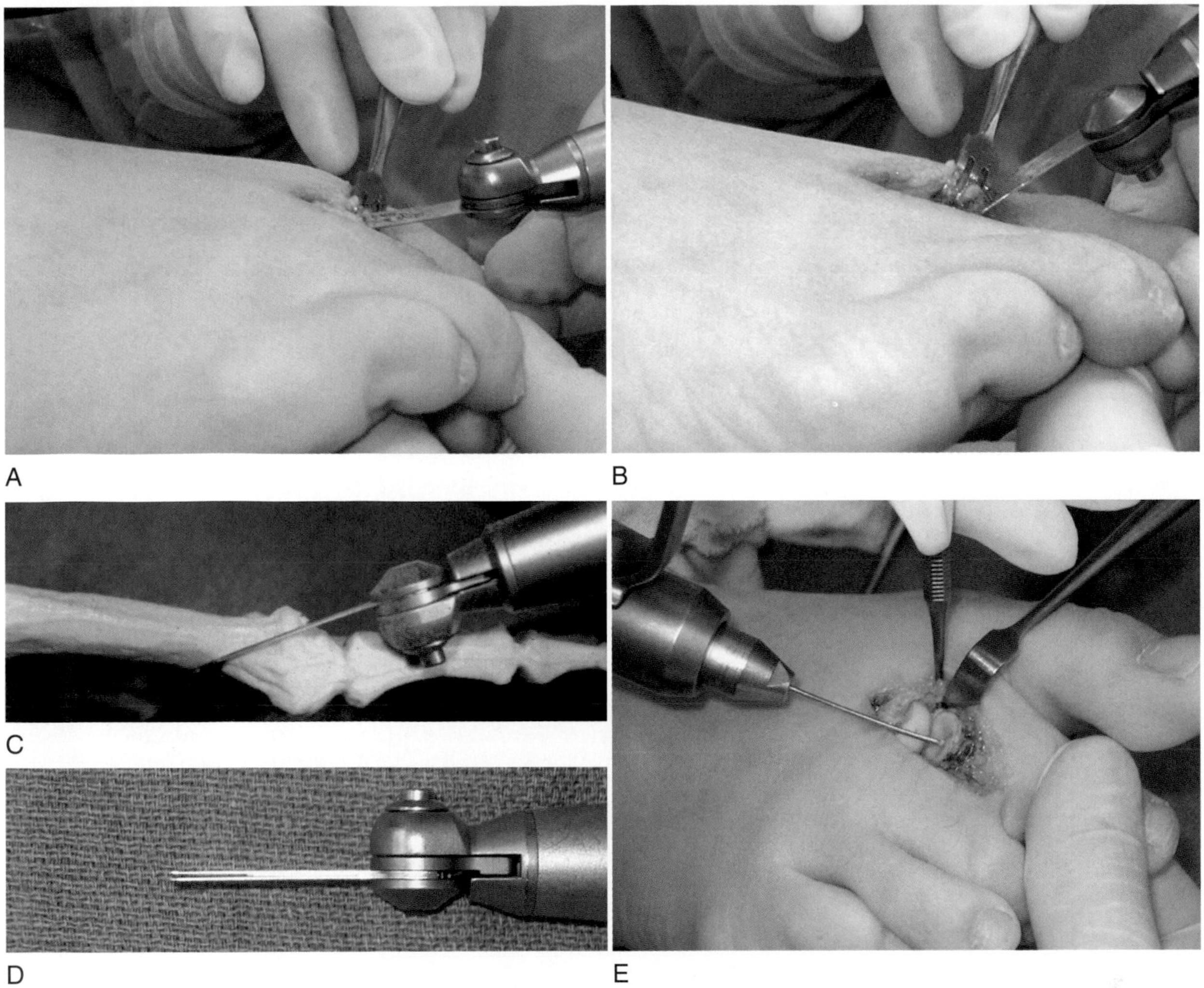

Figure 7–89 Tips for Weil osteotomy. **A,** Capital oblique osteotomy is performed with the saw plate parallel to the plantar aspect of the foot to minimize depression of the distal fragment as the osteotomy is translated proximal. **B** and **C,** Excessive plantar inclination of the saw blade can depress the translated capital fragment. (These examples shows excess plantar inclination of the saw blade.) **D,** To achieve less plantar displacement, stacked blades or a thicker blade can be used for the osteotomy. Note three blades are used here, which achieves a much wider cut. **E,** Often a Kirschner wire is used to stabilize the metatarsophalangeal joint, especially when substantial shortening has been achieved. Taping of the digit is another alternative.

necessary, especially when shortening of more than 4 mm is required (Figs. 7–87D and 7–88H and I).

8. The dorsal metatarsal surface that now extends beyond the articular surface is resected and beveled with a rongeur. Occasionally, two screws are necessary, especially when shortening of more than 4 mm is required (Fig. 7–87C).

9. The wound is closed in a routine fashion.

10. When shortening of more than 3 mm is required, a thin wafer of bone is removed to prevent plantar translation of the capital fragment.[169] Another alternative is to use stacked saw blades to make a thicker osteotomy (Fig. 7–89D). The capital fragment may be translated medially to help realign a severely angulated toe lateralward (Fig. 7–87).

11. The toe is stabilized with a .045-inch Kirschner wire that is driven out through the tip of the toe and then retrograded into the capital fragment (Fig. 7–89E). An alternative is to tape the toe securely to stabilize it during the postoperative period.

12. A flexor tendon transfer is used when the MTP joint is markedly unstable after the osteotomy (Fig. 7–90).

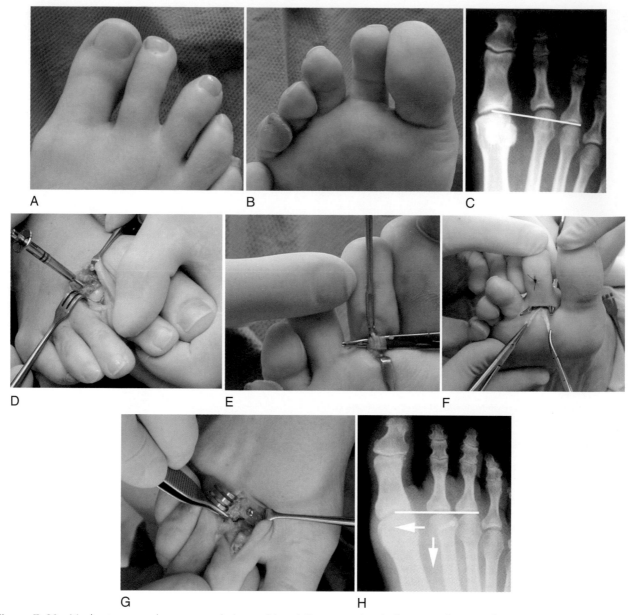

A   B   C

D   E   F

G   H

Figure 7–90   Moderate second metatarsophalangeal instability treated with flexor tendon transfer and Weil osteotomy. Preoperative clinical (**A** and **B**) and radiographic (**C**) presentation of deformity. **D,** Fixation following Weil osteotomy with shortening and medial translation. **E** and **F,** Harvest and transfer of the flexor tendon to the dorsal surface of the proximal phalanx. **G,** Dorsal view after flexor tendon transfer and Weil osteotomy. (The sutured tendon is at the inferior aspect of the wound.) **H,** Radiograph demonstrating shortening and medial translation of the capital fragment.

Postoperative Care

A gauze-and-tape compression dressing is applied at surgery and changed on a weekly basis. The toe is bandaged in five degrees of plantar flexion. Weight-bearing ambulation is permitted with weight borne on the heel and outer aspect of the foot. If a Kirschner wire has been placed, it is removed 2 to 3 weeks following surgery. Typically, 6 weeks following surgery, successful healing has occurred at the osteotomy site. A roomy shoe or sandal is then used for ambulation. The patient is encouraged to commence active and passive toe exercises 2 to 3 weeks following surgery. The toe is taped to the adjacent toe or to the forefoot for another 3 to 6 weeks after the pin is removed (Fig. 7–91).

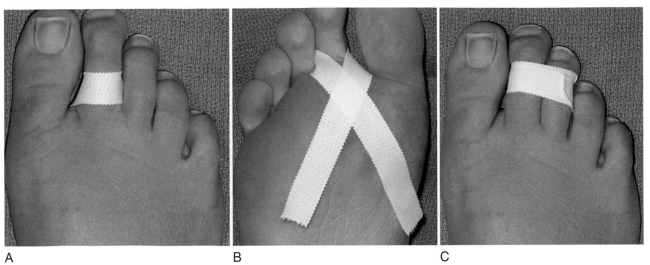

A   B   C

Figure 7–91 Postoperative taping technique. Taping is necessary in the postoperative period to stabilize the repair. **A,** Dorsal view. **B,** Plantar view. **C,** Buddy taping of adjacent toes can reduce pain as well.

Results and Complications

The capital oblique osteotomy was initially described by Barouk[5] and attributed by him to Weil.[169,170] The technique has been described in several reports.[21,25,42,164-166,170]

Davies et al[42] reported on the results of osteotomies in 39 patients. Eight of 39 patients had some continued pain, but a high level of satisfactory results were reported. No cases of avascular necrosis or nonunion were observed. O'Kane et al[125] reported on 17 patients in which a Weil osteotomy was performed. Shortening averaged 5.2 mm. Following surgery, 20% of the operated toes did not contact the ground, although the authors did not find this to be a source of patient dissatisfaction.

Trnka et al[164] reported on a comparison of the Helal and Weil osteotomies. In 15 patients (25 osteotomies), the second, third, and/or fourth metatarsals were osteotomized with Weil's technique as treatment for dislocation of the MTP joint and then were compared to results in a similar group for which Helal osteotomies were performed. Twelve of the patients who underwent Weil osteotomies were satisfied with their results. The major reason for dissatisfaction was pain associated with a prominent plantar screw. Although some of these patients had an asymptomatic callus beneath the involved metatarsal head, the authors reported no symptomatic transfer lesions. There were no reported cases of pseudoarthrosis, avascular necrosis,

nonunion, or transfer lesions following the Weil osteotomy. After the Weil procedure, four of the 25 dislocated MTP joints remained dislocated compared with eight of 22 MTP joints that remained dislocated after the Helal osteotomy. The authors concluded that the Weil osteotomy provided greater accuracy in metatarsal shortening and a high level of postoperative satisfaction. A limitation of plantar flexion following the osteotomy was thought to be caused by capsule scarring and weakening of the intrinsic musculature.

Aggressive physical therapy may be beneficial postoperatively. Early passive and active range-of-motion exercises of the involved digit help to regain toe function. Exercises should be performed several times a day. Although scarring of the plantar plate occurs following the osteotomy, vigorous manipulation does help to mobilize the joint.[165] Weil et al[170] reported on the results of 69 cases in which a capital oblique osteotomy was performed. The postoperative incidence of transfer metatarsalgia was 9%; plantar flexion range of motion was limited in 17% of patients, and a hammer toe developed in 5%. There were no cases of osteonecrosis or degenerative arthritis. Vandeputte et al[166] reported that MTP range of motion was reduced an average of 50% at final evaluation.

Weil[170] advocated angling the osteotomy at 25 degrees or less in relationship to the metatarsal to minimize depression of the metatarsal head. If it is necessary to shorten the metatarsal more than 5 mm, the possibility of increased plantar pressure necessitates bone resection at the osteotomy site to provide elevation in addition to shortening. This may be achieved by either resecting a thin slice of bone at the osteotomy site (3-5 mm) or stacking two or three saw blades in the sagittal saw to resect a greater thickness of bone (see Figs. 7–88F and 7–89D). Although the metatarsal declination angle determines the amount of plantar translation and varies from patient to patient, Weil concluded that at an osteotomy angle of 25 degrees, for each one millimeter of shortening there is one millimeter of metatarsal head depression.

Nonetheless, because of metatarsal head depression following an osteotomy, a dorsiflexion contracture can occur at the metatarsophalangeal joint following a Weil osteotomy.[113,125,165] Trnka[165] dissected two cadaver specimens and performed osteotomies at 25, 30, 35, and 40 degrees relative to the longitudinal axis of the metatarsal. Trnka[165] and O'Kane[125] both observed that the interossei tendons move dorsally with respect to the axis of the MTP joint due to depression of the plantar fragment and that the center of rotation is altered after the osteotomy, leading to MTP joint hyperextension (see Fig. 7–93). Trnka[165] suggested several alternatives to prevent a dorsiflexion contracture of the MTP joint: lengthening the extensor tendon, performing the osteotomy as parallel as possible to the plantar surface of the foot, transferring the FDL, and installing a temporary Kirschner wire across the MTP joint in five degrees of plantar flexion (see Fig. 7–89).

In another laboratory study, the amount of shortening and plantar translation was evaluated.[111] Osteotomies with angles of less than 25 degrees minimize plantar translation. With a 5-mm proximal shift, the plantar displacement with a 30-degree angle was 2 mm; with a 10-mm shift, it was 5 mm. With an osteotomy less than 25 degrees, the osteotomy exits the metatarsal shaft very proximally. Metatarsals do have differing inclination angles from patient to patient and even between other lesser metatarsals in the same foot. Modifying the Weil osteotomy by inclining the blade 15 to 20 degrees in reference to the metatarsal shaft and removing a slice of bone at the osteotomy site when substantial shortening is planned can reduce plantar displacement of the metatarsal head and help to reduce hyperextension deformities as well.

Weil[170] suggests taping the toe in five degrees of plantar flexion after surgery to minimize MTP joint hyperextension. A flexor tendon transfer may be required if the digit remains unstable (see Fig. 7–90)[25]; however, currently this appears to be a less popular alternative. Short-term intramedullary Kirschner wire fixation with the toe in slight plantar flexion controls alignment in both the sagittal and coronal planes and ensures an anatomic reduction. It minimizes the need for frequent dressing changes and allows early healing to stabilize the MTP joint capsule tissues, which promotes joint stability. The Kirschner wire is removed 2 to 3 weeks after the procedure, and range-of-motion exercises are commenced. With Kirschner wire stabilization, early weight bearing on the forefoot can displace the osteotomy site; a patient should be advised of the importance of protecting the forefoot region after a distal metatarsal osteotomy.

The results of distal metatarsal osteotomies performed without internal fixation have been mediocre. Idusuyi et al[76] noted a high incidence of MTP joint pain, limited motion, and unsatisfactory results. Trnka et al[164] reported a high rate of redislocation, transfer lesions, nonunions, and unsatisfactory results as well following distal metatarsal osteotomies that were not internally fixed. Davies et al[42] stressed that rigid internal fixation decreases the risk of transfer lesions. A shortening osteotomy of the second metatarsal may be performed proximal to the MTP joint. This decompresses the MTP joint by effectively lengthening the adjacent soft tissue structures. Giannestras[63] described a longitudinal oblique osteotomy of the diaphyseal portion of the metatarsal shaft (see Chapter 8). This is another technique that can be used to achieve shortening of the involved ray, but it is difficult and may be associated with delayed union, malunion, and transfer lesions (Fig. 7–92).

The obvious benefits of the Weil osteotomy are that the location affords a large area of bone contact, it is a relatively stable osteotomy, its design allows for controlled shortening, internal fixation is relatively easy to place, and the incidence of complications (other than MTP joint hyperextension) is low (Fig. 7–93). Postoperative nonunion, avascular necrosis, and degenerative arthritis are rare (Fig. 7–94). Although a certain amount of arthrofibrosis of the MTP joint develops following a Weil osteotomy, the decreased range of motion has a stabilizing effect on the

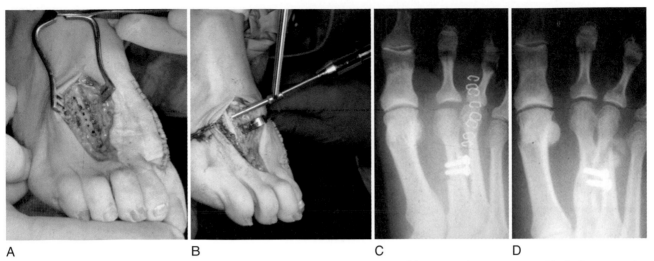

A   B   C   D

Figure 7–92 Longitudinal osteotomies require a long incision **(A)** and internal fixation with cross screws **(B). C,** Postoperative radiograph demonstrates shortening. **D,** Postoperative complications include delayed healing and stress fracture of the fourth metatarsal, with later synostosis of the adjacent metatarsals.

MTP joint. In general, patients with subluxation and dislocation of the MTP joint should expect a well-aligned toe that does not have normal dynamic function. The goal of surgery is to reduce plantar pain beneath the metatarsal

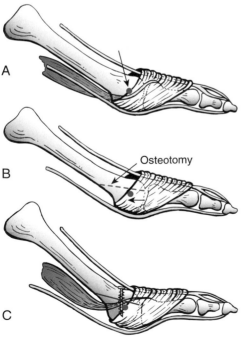

Figure 7–93 Axis of the metatarsophalangeal joint before and after Weil osteotomy. **A,** Lesser metatarsal prior to osteotomy; note intrinsics are plantar to the axis. **B,** Osteotomy is above the center of the metatarsal head. **C,** Following the osteotomy and proximal translation of the capital fragment, the intrinsics course dorsal to the axis of rotation. This can lead to metatarsophalangeal joint dorsiflexion.

head, to realign the toe, and to stabilize the MTP joint. Although generally there is significant improvement following these procedures, it should be explained to the patient that the involved toe will not have normal function.

With extensive surgery on a lesser toe, complications can result (Fig 7–94). The most severe complication of surgery is vascular compromise. Although it is difficult to give guidelines regarding the extent of surgery that is feasible for a second toe, occasionally the surgeon believes that sufficient surgery has been carried out and discontinues an attempt at further correction. In this situation, a second-stage procedure may be necessary at a later date. This is certainly preferable to vascular compromise of a lesser toe.

Occasionally the circulation to the toe is impaired after surgery. In this situation, if a Kirschner wire has been placed, it must be removed to decrease tension on the toe and relieve vascular spasm. Thus, it is important to use the Kirschner wire only as an augmentation of the surgical repair and not to achieve more alignment. If removal in the immediate postoperative period is necessary, the toe needs to be held in alignment with gauze-and-tape dressings until adequate healing has occurred.

Occasionally a Kirschner wire fatigues and breaks if the patient ambulates excessively. If a broken Kirschner wire interferes with MTP joint function, it should be removed. Typically the wire fatigues just proximal to the joint surface, and in this situation, removal of the proximal portion is unnecessary (Fig. 7–95).

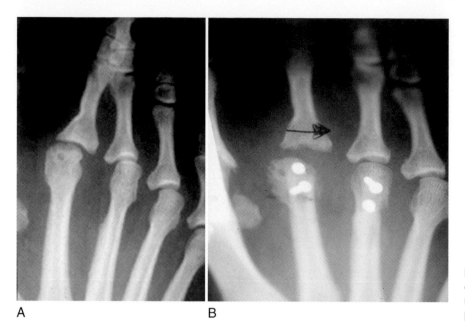

A   B

Figure 7–94 Complications of Weil osteotomy. **A,** Avascular necrosis of metatarsal head. **B,** Lateral subluxation postoperatively.

Excessive tension on the metatarsal head following relocation of a dislocated MTP joint may be complicated by avascular necrosis or degenerative arthritis. Scheck[144] has reported this occurrence following extensive soft tissue stripping in the reduction of a dislocated MTP joint.

Recurrence of an MTP joint deformity can be a complication of the subluxated and dislocated second toe. Adequate MTP soft tissue release is necessary at the initial surgery. Transfer of the long flexor tendon can remove one of the most significant deforming forces. Adequate bone decompression is necessary when a soft tissue release does not allow stable relocation of the MTP joint. The second toe must be completely realigned at surgery. Subtotal realignment that

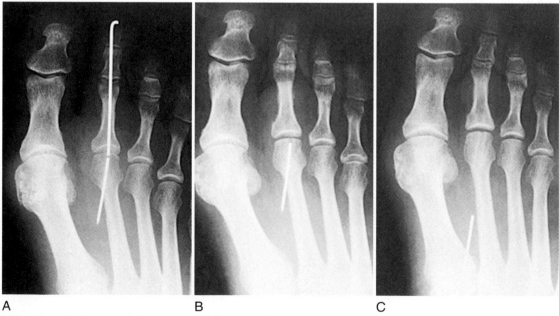

A   B   C

Figure 7–95 A, With placement of an intramedullary Kirschner wire across the metatarsophalangeal (MTP) joint, the pin can fracture. If a fractured pin compromises MTP joint function, it may be removed. **B,** Typically, the pin fractures 2 to 3 mm proximal to the articular surface, and in this case it may be left in the metatarsal shaft. **C,** Occasionally, migration of the proximal pin necessitates removal.

relies on the Kirschner wire to achieve the repair often results in redeformation once the Kirschner wire has been removed.

With numerous procedures being performed on the lesser toe, postoperative edema is common and can take months to subside (see Fig. 7–33). Likewise, molding of the second toe caused by extrinsic pressure from adjacent toes can occur (see Fig. 7–41). This is unavoidable, and it is important to inform the patient preoperatively about this possibility.

Postoperative pain at either the MTP joint arthroplasty site or the hammer toe site occurs occasionally. Although this pain should resolve with time, occasionally discomfort at the arthroplasty site continues. Often there is a moderate amount of restricted motion at the arthroplasty site as well. This restricted motion can afford joint stability, but it can make ambulation painful. In this situation a revision may be performed with a partial proximal phalangectomy[66,87]; this is an alternate procedure for MTP joint dislocation.

Decreased sensation occasionally occurs in the toe as a result of extensive surgery and injury to the digital nerves. Care must be taken not to injure the nerves when soft tissue procedures and tendon transfers are performed. Usually with the passage of time, sensation returns.

SALVAGE PROCEDURES

Indications

In the presence of severe deformities, recurrent deformity, avascular necrosis of the metatarsal head, or degenerative arthritis of the involved metatarsophalangeal joint, salvage procedures may be necessary. These include, but are not limited to, the DuVries metatarsophalangeal joint arthroplasty, partial proximal phalangectomy, and syndactylization of the lesser toes.

Contraindications

When possible, normal function of the lesser MTP joints should be preserved. Salvage procedures should be reserved for joints with severe arthritis, recurrent subluxation, or dislocation or following another unsuccessful surgical procedure with the goal of achieving a plantigrade, less painful foot and improving the ambulatory capacity of the patient.

DUVRIES METATARSOPHALANGEAL JOINT ARTHROPLASTY

Surgical Technique

1. The patient is placed in a supine position on the operating room table. The foot is cleansed and draped in the usual fashion. The foot is exsanguinated with an Esmarch bandage. The Esmarch bandage may be used as a tourniquet above the level of the ankle.
2. A lazy-S incision is centered over the MTP joint. A soft tissue release is performed in which the extensor tendons are lengthened, and the dorsal, medial, and lateral MTP capsules are released as well. (See the discussion of soft tissue release of the MTP joint.)
3. The metatarsal head is identified and the proximal phalanx is plantar flexed to expose the metatarsal articular surface. A McGlamry elevator can assist in the exposure.
4. An osteotomy is performed in a dorsoplantar direction, removing 3 to 4 mm of bone; the amount of overlap determines the amount of metatarsal head resected (Fig. 7–96A and B).
5. The medial and lateral edges are beveled with a rongeur, as are the dorsal and plantar condyles, achieving a somewhat rounded head to articulate with the concave base of the proximal phalanx.
6. After bone decompression, the second toe should be reducible. The ankle is dorsiflexed and plantar flexed, and if the MTP joint is stable, the phalanx remains reduced and does not dislocate.
7. Typically following a bone decompression, a flexor tendon transfer is performed to give stability to the proximal phalanx.
8. A Kirschner wire is introduced at the base of the proximal phalanx and driven distally, exiting the tip of the toe. It is then driven retrograde to stabilize the MTP joint. The pin is bent at the tip of the toe, and any excess pin is removed.
9. Myerson[121] has described a modification of the MTP arthroplasty in which the tendon of the extensor digitorum brevis and joint capsule is interposed in the joint space and anchored to the plantar aspect of the metatarsal head (Fig. 7–97). No results have been reported with this technique.

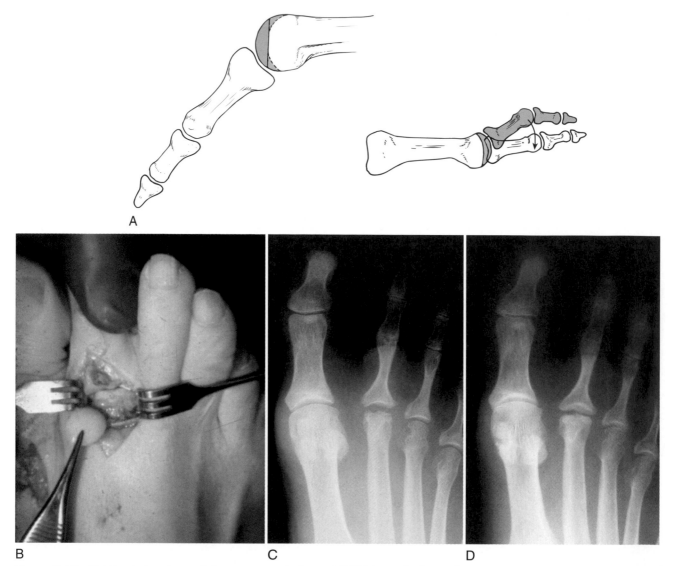

Figure 7–96   DuVries arthroplasty of the metatarsophalangeal (MTP) joint. **A,** Dorsoplantar osteotomy removes 2 to 3 mm of metatarsal head. The dorsoplantar and medial and lateral surfaces then are beveled to create a curved surface that will articulate with the trumpet-shaped base of the proximal phalanx. **B,** Intraoperative view of MTP arthroplasty demonstrates dorsoplantar osteotomy and removal of a wafer of metatarsal articular surface. **C,** Three years after arthroplasty of the second MTP joint. **D,** Five-year follow-up. Approximately 50% of joint motion is lost due to arthrofibrosis; however, this helps to maintain stability of the joint.

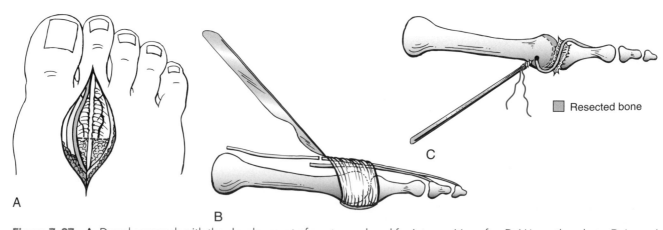

Figure 7–97   **A,** Dorsal approach with the development of a extensor hood for interposition after DuVries arthroplasty. **B,** Lateral view demonstrating area of release of extensor hood. **C,** The extensor hood is interposed between the base of the proximal phalanx and the resected surface of the metatarsal head and secured with a suture anchor (Myerson technique).

PARTIAL PROXIMAL PHALANGECTOMY AND SYNDACTYLIZATION[41]

Surgical Technique

1. The foot is cleansed and draped in the usual fashion. The foot is exsanguinated with an Esmarch bandage. With careful padding the Esmarch bandage may be used as a tourniquet above the level of the ankle.
2. The toes are distracted as a web-bisecting incision is made (Fig. 7–98A and B).
3. The web-bisecting incision is flanked by a pair of peridigital incisions. Plantar and dorsal flaps are developed and small triangles of skin are resected.
4. Adjacent partial proximal phalangectomies may be performed. Care is taken to protect the neurovascular bundles (Fig. 7–98C).
5. Adjacent dorsal and plantar flaps are apposed and closed with a running and interrupted suture (Fig. 7–98D-F).

Alternative Method

Following excision of the base of the proximal phalanx, an intramedullary Kirschner wire may be used to stabilize the repair until adequate healing is achieved (Fig. 7–99).

Postoperative Care

A gauze-and-tape dressing is applied and changed weekly. The patient is allowed to ambulate in a wooden-soled postoperative shoe. Sutures are removed 3 weeks after surgery. The adjacent toes are taped together for approximately 6 weeks to protect the surgical syndactylization.

Results and Complications

Conklin and Smith[20] reported 29% dissatisfaction following a proximal phalangectomy. Some 60% of patients had total relief of pain; however, shortening was the most common postoperative complaint (Fig 7–100).

Cahill and Connor[16] reported that proximal phalangectomy for a hammer toe or claw toe deformity relieved symptoms but gave a poor cosmetic end result. Objectively, poor results occurred in 50% of cases. (Fig. 7–100)

Daly and Johnson[41] reported a series of painful lesser toes characterized by subluxation and dislocation of the second and third MTP joints that were treated with partial proximal

phalangectomies and subtotal webbing. Some 28% had moderate or severe problems with cosmesis. Postoperatively, a recurrent cock-up deformity occurred in 18%, residual pain was noted in 27%, and excessive shortening was seen in 5% of cases. Some 75% of patients were satisfied or satisfied with reservations.

With degenerative arthritis of a lesser MTP joint, an interposition soft tissue arthroplasty can help to retain motion but diminish intractable pain (Fig. 7–101).

Karlock[85] has reported the use of second MTP joint arthrodesis to realign and stabilize a severely deformed second toe with subluxation or dislocation of the MTP joint (Fig 7–102). In 11 patients, 10 were noted to have a good or excellent results (see Fig. 7–98). Eight of the patients also had a first MTP arthrodesis for a severe hallux valgus deformity. Karlock[85] suggested second MTP arthrodesis as a salvage alternative to amputation of the severely deformed digit. This ensures the alignment of the first ray, while accomplishing a removal of the severely deformed second toe.

VanderWilde and Campbell[167] reported on the technique of amputation of the second toe for treatment of chronic painful deformity. Sixteen patients (23 amputations) were evaluated at long-term follow-up. Fifteen of 22 patients (68%) were satisfied. They noted that all patients experienced some progression of a preexisting hallux valgus deformity. The hallux valgus angle increased an average of 11.6 degrees on final radiographic follow-up, but only one patient came to first MTP arthrodesis.

Following multiple procedures to the second toe, soft tissue atrophy and chronic pain were associated with minimal MTP joint motion (Fig. 7–103). Although a metatarsal head excision may be considered, it rarely resolves a problem on a long-term basis and is associated with transfer metatarsalgia, which is quite difficult to salvage (Fig. 7–104).

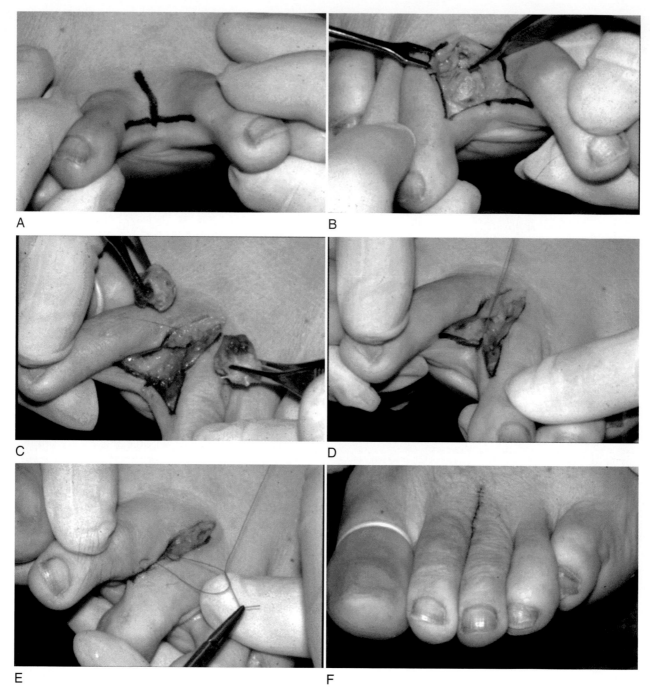

Figure 7–98   With a partial proximal phalangectomy, the base of the proximal phalanx is excised. Often adjacent partial prox-imal phalangectomies are performed in combination with syndactylization. **A** and **B,** An intramedullary web space incision is made to approach the adjacent metatarsophalangeal joints. **C,** The bases of the proximal phalanges of the second and third toes have been excised. **D-F,** Closure of deep and superficial tissue. (Courtesy of K. Johnson, MD.)

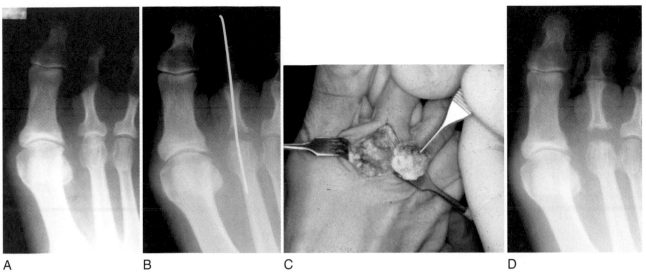

A   B   C   D

Figure 7–99 **A,** Painful degenerative arthritis of the second metatarsophalangeal joint. Radiograph demonstrates complete loss of the remaining joint space. **B,** Following excision of the base of the proximal phalanx of the second toe, an intramedullary Kirschner wire is used to stabilize the repair until adequate healing is achieved. **C,** Intraoperative photograph after partial proximal phalangectomy. **D,** Following removal of Kirschner wire.

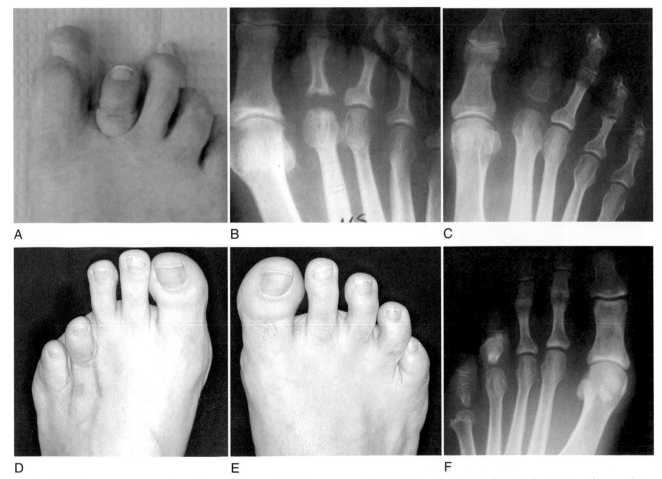

A   B   C

D   E   F

Figure 7–100 Long-term results of partial proximal phalangectomy. Clinical **(A)** and radiographic **(B)** shortening of second toe after partial proximal phalangectomy. **C,** Excessive resection of proximal phalanx. **D,** Postoperative left foot. **E,** Normal right foot. **F,** Radiographic appearance of left foot after partial proximal phalangectomy of fourth and fifth digits.

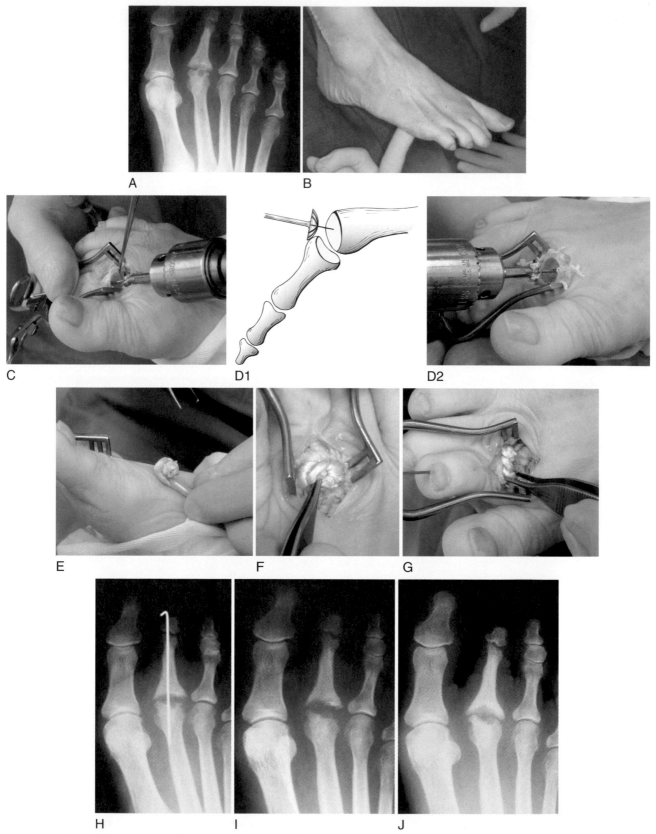

Figure 7–101 Soft tissue arthroplasty. **A** and **B,** Degenerative arthritis of the second metatarsophalangeal (MTP) joint associated with restricted range of motion. A flexion contracture of the MTP joint has occurred. Reaming of the base of the proximal phalanx **(C)** and the metatarsal head **(D). E,** Gracilis tendon bundle. **F** and **G,** Placement of an interposition tendon "anchovy." **H,** Intraoperative radiograph with Kirschner-wire fixation. **I,** Postoperative radiograph following treatment with a soft tissue arthroplasty. **J,** Two years following surgery, there is a 50% reduction in range of motion.

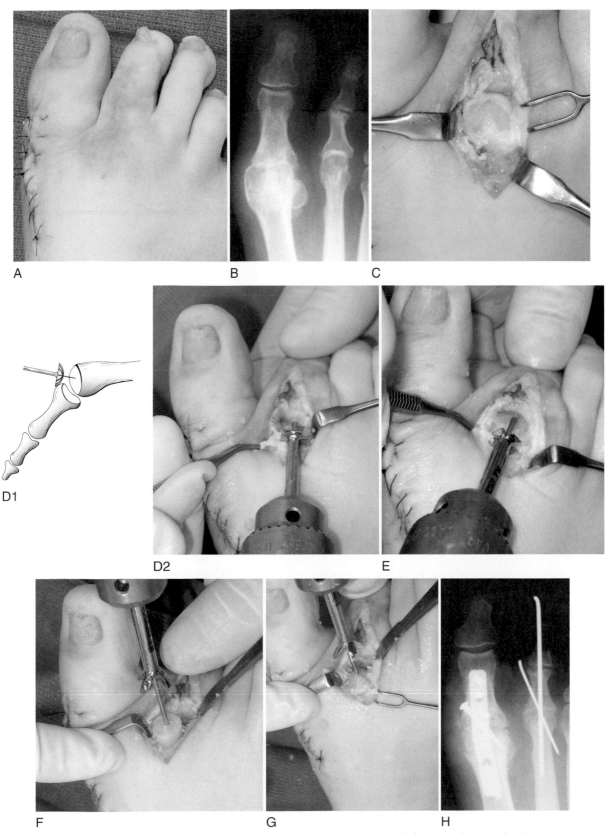

Figure 7–102 Lesser metatarsophalangeal (MTP) joint fusion. Preoperative clinical photograph **(A)** and radiograph **(B)** demonstrate end-stage arthritis of the first and second MTP joints. **C,** Clinical appearance of the metatarsal head with complete cartilage loss. **D** and **E,** Concave reaming of the base of the proximal phalanx. **F** and **G,** Convex preparation of the second metatarsal head. **H,** Following arthrodesis of the first and second MTP joints.

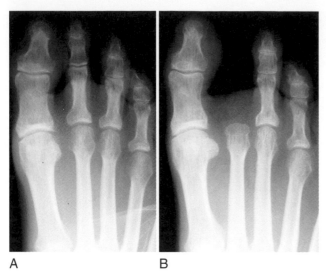

A   B

Figure 7–103 A, Following multiple procedures to the second toe, soft tissue atrophy and chronic pain were associated with minimal metatarsophalangeal joint motion. **B,** A 3-year follow-up following second metatarsophalangeal joint disarticulation for chronic pain.

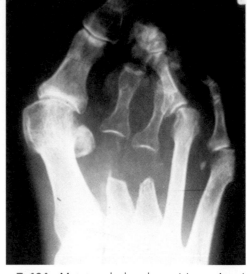

Figure 7–104 Metatarsal head excision. An isolated metatarsal head excision rarely solves a problem. Following a second head excision, later the third metatarsal head was excised. Note subluxation of the fourth metatarsophalangeal joint on the radiograph, denoting increased pressure.

FIFTH TOE DEFORMITIES

Etiology

Deformities of the fifth toe include hard corns, soft corns, and congenital or developmental MTP joint malalignment problems. Overlapping and underlapping of the fifth toe in general are congenital deformities, whereas a cock-up deformity often is associated with a hammer toe deformity. The surgical treatment of each deformity may be considerably different, and thus differentiation of the anatomic findings is important.

Anatomy

The overlapping fifth toe is a fairly common congenital deformity that can become uncomfortable because of pressure from footwear against the toe. The fifth toe is externally rotated and compressed in its AP plane. A dorsal contracture at the MTP joint is present and often is associated with a contracture of the extensor digitorum longus tendon. An underlapping fifth toe is externally rotated as it deviates beneath the fourth toe. Often a contracture of the flexor digitorum longus tendon is associated with an elongated extensor digitorum longus tendon. Trauma to the toenail of the fifth toe with ambulation can cause significant distortion of the toenail plate. Redundant capsule on the dorsal aspect of the MTP joint is associated with a contracted plantar medial MTP joint capsule.

With a severe cock-up deformity of the fifth toe (Fig. 7–105), the proximal phalanx articulates at nearly a right angle with the fifth metatarsal shaft. Often this deformity is associated with a fixed hammer toe deformity. Cockin[18] has described the presence of adhesions between the plantar capsule and the plantar aspect of the metatarsal head that can limit reduction at the MTP joint once a complete capsule release has been performed.

Preoperative Evaluation

Physical Examination

Preoperative evaluation of a deformed fifth toe necessitates appreciation of the axial rotational deformity,

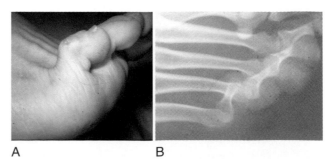

A   B

Figure 7–105 A, Cock-up deformity of the fifth toe. **B,** Radiograph demonstrates cock-up deformity of the fifth toe. Note that the subluxed proximal phalanx is almost at a right angle to the fifth metatarsal head.

as well as hyperextension or flexion at the MTP joint. The degree of varus or medial deviation of the fifth toe should be observed as well as the presence of a hammer toe deformity. A severe skin contracture can necessitate bone resection rather than a soft tissue realignment procedure. Attention to the neurovascular status preoperatively is important if a significant realignment procedure is necessary.

Conservative Treatment

When possible, shoe modifications and padding are preferable to surgical intervention. (See the section on hammer toes and padding.)

MILD OVERLAPPING FIFTH TOE DEFORMITIES

A mild overlapping fifth toe deformity may be treated in a number of ways, many of which give satisfactory results. The DuVries and the Wilson techniques are useful for a mild to moderate deformity; the Lapidus procedure, which involves a tendon transfer, is recommended for a more severe deformity.

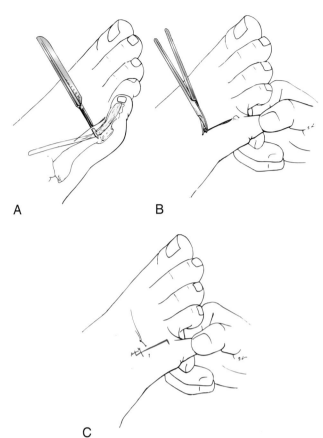

Figure 7–106 DuVries technique for repair of mild to moderate overlapping fifth toe. **A,** A longitudinal incision is made over the fourth web space. Tenotomy and capsulotomy of the fifth metatarsophalangeal joint are then performed. **B,** The fifth toe is plantar flexed to bring the fibular margin of the incision distal and the tibial margin proximal. This forms folds at each end of the incision, which are excised. **C,** The incision is sutured in the new position.

DUVRIES FIFTH TOE REALIGNMENT

Surgical Technique

1. A foot block or regional anesthesia, rather than a digital block, often is used for this procedure. The foot is cleansed in a routine fashion. The foot is exsanguinated with an Esmarch bandage. The Esmarch bandage may be used as a tourniquet above the level of the ankle.
2. A longitudinal incision is centered over the fourth interspace, beginning in the web space and extending proximally just past the fifth metatarsal head (Fig. 7–106A).
3. All MTP joint contractures are released on the dorsal and medial aspect. The extensor tendon is released, as well as the medial collateral ligament and MTP joint capsule.
4. The toe is placed into an overcorrected position by bringing it into plantar flexion with slight lateral deviation. If the soft tissue contracture has been adequately released, the toe tends to stay in this position and does not redeform.
5. When the toe is brought into the new position, the skin on the fibular margin is stretched distally and skin on the tibial

margin is displaced proximally. The puckered or dog-eared edges at the ends of these incisions are then excised (Fig. 7–106B).
6. The skin edges are approximated with interrupted sutures in this new position (Fig. 7–106C), and the fibular skin is advanced distally.

Postoperative Care

A gauze-and-tape compression dressing is used to hold the toe in an overcorrected position and is changed weekly for 8 weeks. The patient is allowed to ambulate in a wooden-soled shoe. Sutures are removed 3 weeks after surgery. The fifth toe is taped into plantar flexion for 3 to 6 weeks. Results are shown in Figure 7–107.

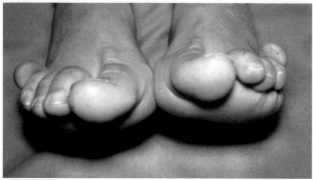

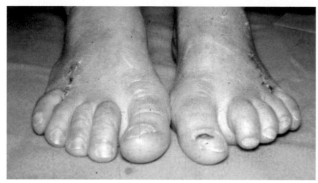

Figure 7–107 Preoperative **(A)** and postoperative **(B)** results following DuVries repair of overlapping fifth toes.

WILSON FIFTH TOE PROCEDURE[172]

Surgical Technique

1. A foot block or regional anesthesia, rather than a digital block, often is used for this procedure. The foot is cleansed in a routine fashion (Fig. 7–108A). The procedure is typically performed using an Esmarch ankle tourniquet with the patient in a slight lateral decubitus position.
2. A V-shaped incision is centered over the medial aspect of the fifth toe and extended into the fourth interspace (Fig. 7–108B).
3. The extensor tendons are sectioned (Fig. 7–108C) and the dorsal and medial MTP joint capsules are released. The toe is plantar flexed, which pulls the tongue of the incision distally, forming a Y-shaped skin flap. The toe is held in an overcorrected position and the skin is approximated with interrupted sutures (Fig. 7–108D).

Postoperative Care

A gauze-and-tape compression dressing is placed, holding the toe in an overcorrected

position, and changed weekly. The patient is allowed to ambulate initially in a wooden-soled shoe and later in a sandal. Sutures are removed 3 weeks after surgery. The fifth toe is taped to the adjacent toe for 3 to 6 weeks. Results are shown in Figure 7–108G.

Results of DuVries and Wilson Procedures

In general, the results from these procedures have been satisfactory. It is important to carry out a complete soft tissue release at the time of the surgical repair. When a more severe contracture is present, recurrence is more likely and a more aggressive surgical procedure, such as the Lapidus technique, should be considered.

SEVERE OVERLAPPING FIFTH TOE DEFORMITIES

LAPIDUS PROCEDURE[94]

The Lapidus procedure consists of tendon transfer of the extensor digitorum longus tendon into the abductor digiti quinti.[94]

Surgical Technique

1. Generally a peripheral nerve block or regional anesthetic is used rather than a digital block. The foot is cleansed in a routine fashion. A thigh tourniquet is used with the patient placed in a lateral decubitus position.
2. A curvilinear dorsal incision extends from the medial aspect of the fifth toe over the MTP joint, then laterally over the fifth MTP joint capsule (Figs. 7–109A and 7–110A and B).
3. Another incision approximately 2 to 3 cm proximal to the MTP joint capsule is used to release the extensor digitorum longus tendon (Fig. 7–109B, Fig. 7–110C and D).
4. With soft tissue dissection, the distal segment of the extensor tendon is preserved and is brought out through the distal wound. Through the distal exposure the dorsal, medial, and lateral MTP joint capsules are released.
5. With a curved elevator, any plantar adhesions between the plantar capsule and metatarsal head are released. This step is important because often there still is a hyperextension deformity of the MTP joint after the capsule

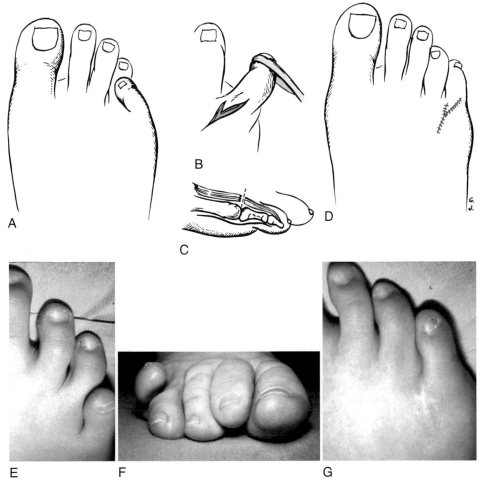

Figure 7–108 Wilson technique for correction of mild to moderate overlapping fifth toe. **A,** Preoperative appearance. **B,** V-shaped incision over the fifth metatarsophalangeal (MTP) joint. **C,** Sectioning of the extensor tendon and dorsal capsule of the MTP joint. **D,** Correction of the deformity and suturing of the skin. **E** and **F,** Preoperative appearance. **G,** Following Wilson procedure.

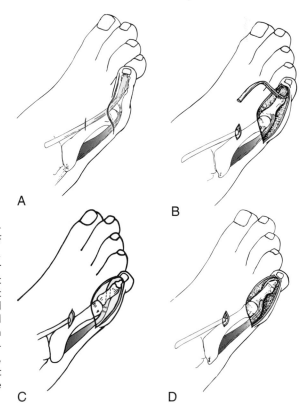

Figure 7–109 Lapidus technique for correction of a severe overlapping fifth toe. **A,** Curvilinear incision is placed over the dorsum of the fifth toe metatarsophalangeal (MTP) joint and metatarsal head. A second incision is placed over the midportion of the extensor tendon to the fifth toe. **B,** The extensor tendon is brought out through the more distal wound. Dorsal, medial, and lateral MTP joint capsules are released. The plantar capsule might need to be freed up with a curved elevator if any adhesions between the metatarsal head and the plantar capsule are present. **C,** The extensor tendon is transferred around the proximal phalanx and sutured to the periosteum or soft tissue or muscle proximal to the metatarsal head. **D,** The transferred tendon may be placed through the drill hole, but more often it is transferred extraosseously. This helps to reduce the toe and to derotate it.

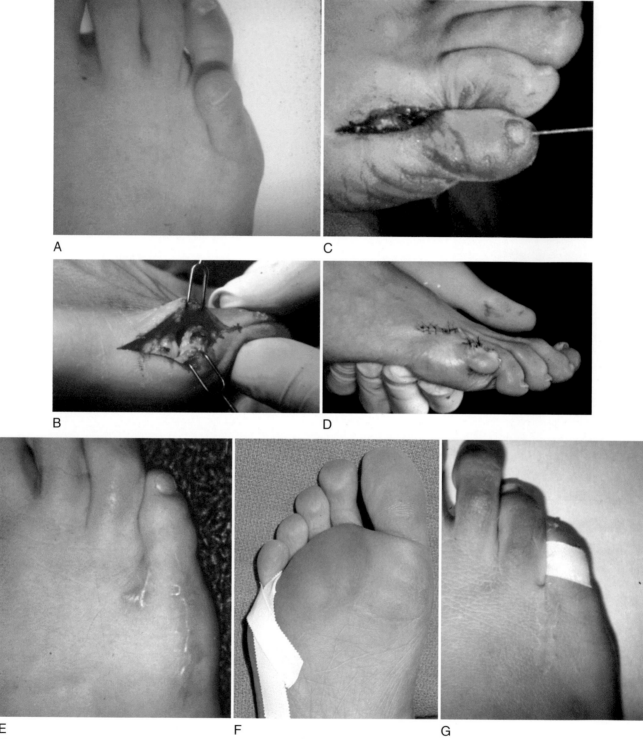

Figure 7–110   Modified Lapidus technique. **A,** Congenital overlapping fifth toe. **B,** Skin incisions are used to expose and release metatarsophalangeal joint. **C,** The extensor tendon is released through a proximal incision and brought distally into the main operative wound and transferred around the proximal phalanx, derotating and reducing the toe. Rarely is a drill hole through proximal phalanx used. **D,** At conclusion of the procedure, the toe is adequately aligned. **E,** Postoperative alignment of the fifth toe. **F** and **G,** Postoperative taping is used to protect the repair.

is released. Adhesions on the plantar aspect may be the cause of this remaining deformity.

6. With blunt dissection the soft tissue is spread around the medial, lateral, and plantar aspects of the proximal phalanx.

7. A suture is placed in the proximal end of the tendon stump and the tendon is delivered circumferentially around the proximal phalanx from medial to plantar to lateral (Fig. 7–109C). With the toe held in the corrected position, the tendon stump is sutured into the abductor digiti quinti muscle.

8. The toe is held in the corrected position and the skin edges are approximated with interrupted sutures.

Postoperative Care

A gauze-and-tape compression dressing is applied, holding the toe in the corrected position, and is changed weekly. The patient is allowed to ambulate in a wooden-soled shoe. Sutures are removed 3 weeks after surgery. The toe is taped in the corrected position for 6 to 8 weeks after surgery (Fig. 7–110F and G).

Results and Complications

In general this procedure has been effective in correcting a severe overlapping fifth toe deformity. If there is any doubt as to whether a more extensive procedure should be performed, preservation of the extensor digitorum longus tendon gives the surgeon a means for further correction of an overlapping fifth toe deformity if soft tissue release is not sufficient to achieve adequate alignment.

Whereas DuVries[51] suggested that a drill hole be placed in the proximal phalanx to aid in the tendon transfer, Lapidus[94] suggested a soft rerouting of the tendon, and this appears to be less complicated and equally successful (see Fig. 7–109D).

Lantzounis[92] described a soft tissue release and transfer of the extensor tendon into the fifth metatarsal neck. A soft tissue realignment was performed. Satisfactory results were reported. In general this technique does not differ significantly from the DuVries procedure.

Cockin[18] described the Butler procedure. A dorsal racquet incision is made, and extensive soft tissue dissection is performed. A dorsal capsulotomy and extensor tenotomy are performed. Attention should be directed to the plantar capsule because often adhesions are present between the plantar metatarsal head and the plantar capsule. A curved elevator is used to release these contractures, and often the toe then can be reduced. The skin is approximated with interrupted sutures. Cockin[18] and later Black et al[7] have both reported a high level of acceptable results with this procedure (greater than 91%). Although this procedure can achieve adequate realignment of the toe, the significant soft tissue dissection and required skin incisions can lead to prolonged postoperative edema. Black et al[7] reported two superficial wound infections that eventually led to unacceptable scar contractures with recurrence of the deformity.

Goodwin and Swisher,[67] Jahss,[78] Kelikian et al,[88] Leonard and Rising,[96] and Scrase[148] described a technique in which an MTP capsule release, extensor tenotomy, partial proximal phalangectomy, and syndactylization of the fourth and fifth toes were used to repair an overlapping fifth toe. Although adequate realignment may be achieved, the syndactylization procedure replaces one deformity with another. As a salvage procedure, a partial proximal phalangectomy and syndactylization may be considered.

UNDERLAPPING FIFTH TOE

In general, the deformities that occur with an underlapping fifth toe correspond to those in an overlapping fifth toe. Axial rotation, however, is associated with a redundant dorsal capsule and a contracted plantar MTP joint capsule. A redundant extensor digitorum longus is associated with a contracted flexor digitorum longus tendon. Thompson[158] has described an excisional arthroplasty to realign the underlapping fifth toe.

Surgical Treatment

THOMPSON REPAIR[158]

Surgical Technique

1. A peripheral anesthetic block or regional anesthesia is preferred to a digital block. The foot is cleansed in a routine fashion. The foot is exsanguinated with an Esmarch bandage. With careful padding, the Esmarch bandage

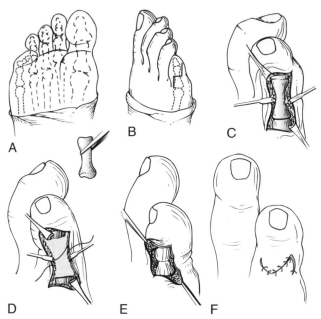

Figure 7–111 Thompson procedure. **A,** Plantar view of the preoperative deformity. **B,** Z-type incision is placed over the dorsal aspect of the proximal phalanx. **C,** The proximal phalanx is exposed. **D,** The proximal phalanx is resected in its entirety. **E,** The capsule is reefed with cerclage suture to diminish dead space. **F,** The Z-type incision is closed, with correction of deformity.

may be used as a tourniquet above the level of the ankle (Fig. 7–111A).

2. A Z incision is centered over the proximal phalanx with the distal limb oriented laterally and the proximal Z incision oriented medially. The extensor tendon is divided and the proximal phalanx identified (Fig. 7–111B).

3. The proximal phalanx is totally or partially excised, depending on the degree of deformity. The toe is then derotated and the capsule closed with interrupted sutures (Fig. 7–111C-E).

4. An intramedullary Kirschner wire may be used for stabilization of the toe as warranted. The Z incision is then rotated and closed with interrupted sutures (Fig. 7–111F).

Postoperative Care

A gauze-and-tape dressing is applied and is changed weekly until drainage has subsided. The patient is allowed to ambulate in a wooden-soled shoe and later in a sandal. Sutures and the Kirschner wire are removed 3 weeks after surgery. The toe is taped to the fourth toe for

approximately 6 weeks, until adequate healing has resulted.

Results and Complications

In general, results of this procedure are acceptable. Excessive resection can lead to an unstable toe or to a transfer keratotic lesion beneath the fourth metatarsal. Janecki and Wilde[80] recommended a Ruiz-Mora procedure for severe cock-up deformity of the fifth toe. Although this procedure with a plantar incision has been designed for the exact opposite of the Thompson excisional arthroplasty, Janecki stressed that a subtotal phalangectomy may be advantageous in retaining fifth toe stability. The extent of resection of the proximal phalanx depends on the degree of fifth toe deformity. A flail toe might require syndactylization as a salvage procedure.

COCK-UP FIFTH TOE DEFORMITY

Often a cock-up deformity of the MTP joint is associated with a fixed hammer toe deformity. With mild to moderate deformity, an extensor tenotomy or lengthening, MTP joint release, and fixed hammer toe repair may be considered. With a severe cock-up deformity, resection arthroplasty may be considered. Treatment must be directed toward bringing the toe into adequate alignment at both the MTP joint and the interphalangeal joint. The Ruiz-Mora procedure[140] as modified by Janecki and Wilde[80] is the preferred procedure.

Surgical Treatment

RUIZ-MORA PROCEDURE[52,80,140]

Surgical Technique

1. A peripheral block or regional anesthetic block is used in preference to a digital block. The foot is cleansed in a routine fashion. The foot is exsanguinated with an Esmarch bandage. The Esmarch bandage may be used as a tourniquet above the level of the ankle (Fig. 7–112A).

2. An elliptical incision is placed on the plantar aspect of the small toe and oriented along

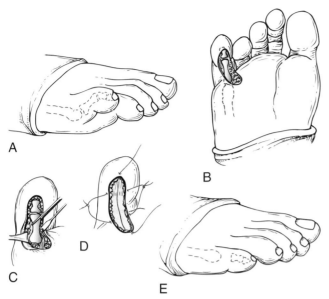

Figure 7–112 Technique for Ruiz-Mora procedure. **A,** Preoperative deformity. **B,** Radiograph of preoperative deformity. **C,** The proximal phalanx is removed through an elliptical plantar incision. **D** and **E,** Sutures are placed to reduce the skin defect, and the incision is closed so that the fifth toe is brought down into plantar flexion and slight medial deviation.

the longitudinal axis of the proximal phalanx, deviating slightly medially at the base of the toe (Fig. 7–112B).
3. An ellipse of skin is resected, after which the flexor tendon is incised. The proximal phalanx is resected (Fig. 7–112C). Janecki has recommended a subtotal resection of the proximal phalanx.
4. The skin incision is then closed at right angles to the long axis of the toe to enable the toe

to be corrected in a plantar–medial manner (Figs. 7–112D and E and 7–113).

Postoperative Care

A gauze-and-tape compression dressing is applied and is changed weekly. The patient is allowed to ambulate in a wooden-soled postoperative shoe and later in a sandal. Sutures are removed 3 weeks after surgery.

Results and Complications

In general, acceptable results have been reported with this procedure. Janecki and Wilde,[80] however, reported a 23% incidence of bunionette formation postoperatively. They also noted a 32% incidence of a hammer toe formation in the fourth toe. These authors thus recommended a subtotal resection of the proximal phalanx to avoid floppiness of the fifth toe. If floppiness of the fifth toe results, a syndactylization procedure may be necessary.

Dyal et al[52] reported on 12 patients who underwent a Ruiz-Mora procedure for severe contraction of the fifth toe. They found average shortening of the fifth ray of 12.8 mm but observed that this presented no functional problems and found it to be an effective procedure in dealing with a cock-up deformity of the fifth toe. Nine of the patients were satisfied with the procedure. They noted that only one fourth toe corn developed. No bunionettes were noted at long-term follow-up. A few patients were dissatisfied with severe shortening and the cosmetic result of the procedure. The authors concluded that the procedure was best reserved for iatrogenic cock-up fifth toe deformities, hard corns, and complicated cock-up fifth toe deformities (Fig. 7–114).

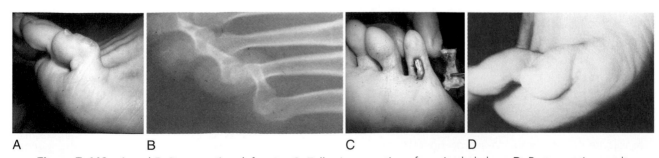

Figure 7–113 **A** and **B,** Preoperative deformity. **C,** Following resection of proximal phalanx. **D,** Postoperative result.

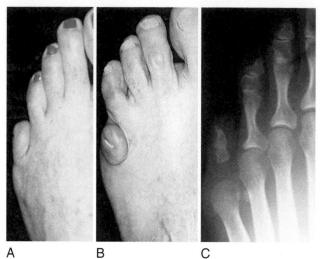

A   B   C

Figure 7-114 A, Acceptable cosmetic appearance after Ruiz-Mora procedure. **B,** Dorsal view of the foot with excessive shortening of the fifth toe. **C,** Anteroposterior radiograph following procedure. (From Dyal C, Davis W, Thompson F, Elonar SK: *Foot Ankle Int* 18:94-97, 1997. Copyright © 1997 by the American Orthopaedic Foot and Ankle Society [AOFAS] and reproduced here with permission.)

SYNDACTYLIZATION OF THE LESSER TOES

Surgical Technique

1. A foot block or regional anesthesia, rather than a digital block, often is used. The foot is cleansed in a routine fashion. An Esmarch bandage is used to exsanguinate the foot. The Esmarch may be used as a tourniquet as well.
2. The toes are distracted as a web-bisecting incision is made (Fig. 7-115A). The web-bisecting incision is flanked by a pair of peridigital incisions.
3. Plantar and dorsal flaps are developed and small triangles of skin are resected (Fig. 7-115B).
4. If adjacent partial proximal phalangectomies are to be performed, the bone decompression is carried out through this incision, with care to protect the neurovascular bundles (Fig. 7-115C and D).
5. The adjacent dorsal and plantar flaps are apposed and closed with running and interrupted sutures (Fig. 7-115E).

Postoperative Care

A gauze-and-tape dressing is applied and is changed weekly. The patient is allowed to ambulate in a wooden-soled postoperative

shoe. Sutures are removed 3 weeks after surgery. The adjacent toes are taped together for approximately 6 weeks to protect the surgical syndactylization.

Alternative Procedure

Thompson[158] suggested the use of a Z-plasty for a skin contracture associated with a fifth toe deformity. Myerson et al[120] has advocated this technique in treating an extension contracture of a lesser toe deformity in which mainly the skin is the contributing factor (see Fig. 7-40D and E). Thordarson[161] has recommended an MTP joint capsule release, extensor tendon lengthening, and Z-plasty of the overlying skin to correct the contracture.

Results and Complications

Kelikian et al[88] and others[41,105] have reported generally satisfactory results with this procedure. Although they found this to be a simple

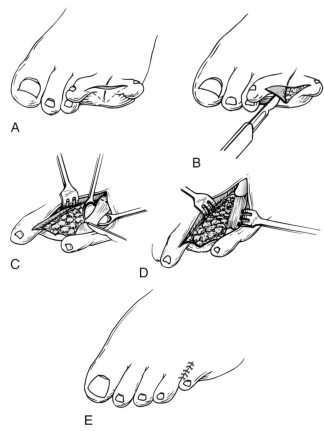

A   B   C   D   E

Figure 7-115 Syndactylization of fourth and fifth toes. **A,** Lines of incision for syndactylization. **B,** Skin is removed from two inferior triangles. **C,** Collateral ligaments of the proximal phalanx are incised. **D,** The proximal phalanx is resected. **E,** Skin is webbed inferiorly and superiorly.

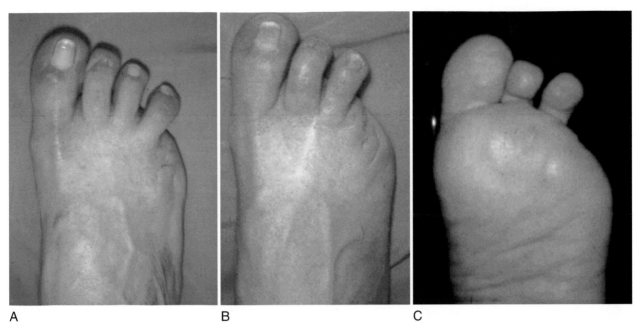

A   B   C

Figure 7–116 **A,** A 77-year-old woman who had an amputation of the fifth toe for a painful fifth toe hard corn. **B** and **C,** Five years later, her family physician had removed her fourth toe because of the development of a painful corn over the lateral aspect of the fourth toe.

and efficient procedure, syndactylization may be cosmetically unacceptable to some patients. Correcting a deformity by creating a second deformity might not be acceptable to the patient. Daly and Johnson[41] have described a relatively cosmetic syndactylization in which concomitant adjacent partial proximal phalangectomies have been performed. They reported an overall 80% subjective satisfaction in 52 patients who had undergone syndactylization procedures.

Syndactylization does not always stabilize the toes. After syndactylization, a deformity can develop in an adjacent toe (see Fig. 7–96).

Surgical realignment of abnormalities of the fifth toe can be difficult. Adequate alignment must be achieved at the time of surgery. If a soft tissue release is not sufficient, either tendon transfer or bone resection must be considered. Correction of severe deformities may be complicated by skin contractures or excessive tension on the neurovascular bundles. In this situation, bone decompression of the fifth toe may be necessary to achieve acceptable alignment.

Jahss[77] reported on 10 cases of chronic and recurrent dislocation of the fifth toe with instability of the PIP or MTP joint. Recurrent disloca-

tion developed as a result of excessive medial joint laxity and was accentuated on weight bearing. He found the simplest and most satisfactory surgical correction involved resection arthroplasty and syndactylization of the fourth and fifth toes. Marek et al[104] also advocated syndactylization as an effective and cosmetic salvage for an unstable fifth toe. Amputation of the fifth toe rarely solves a problem associated with the fifth toe on a long-term basis and can lead to a bunionette deformity or subsequent deformity of the fourth toe (Fig. 7–116).

KERATOTIC DEFORMITIES OF LESSER TOES

Etiology

A lateral fifth toe corn (Fig. 7–117) forms primarily on the exposed surfaces of the fifth toe[9] as a result of extrinsic pressure from footwear.[27,31] An interdigital corn forms over a condyle of the phalanx between the toes (Fig. 7–118).[105] It can form deep in the web space, where differentiation from a mycotic infection may be difficult, or along the distal surface of one of the lesser toes, in which case a firm keratosis is most common.

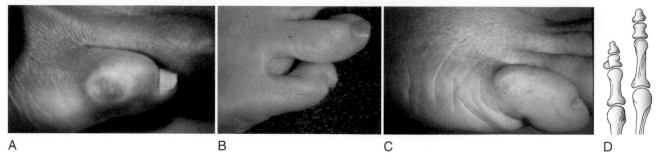

Figure 7–117   **A,** Lateral fifth toe corn over prominent condyles of the proximal phalanx. **B,** Rotation of the fifth toe can lead to a lateral fifth toe corn. **C,** Contracture of the fifth toe can lead to callus formation. **D,** Prominent condyle of either proximal or middle phalanges.

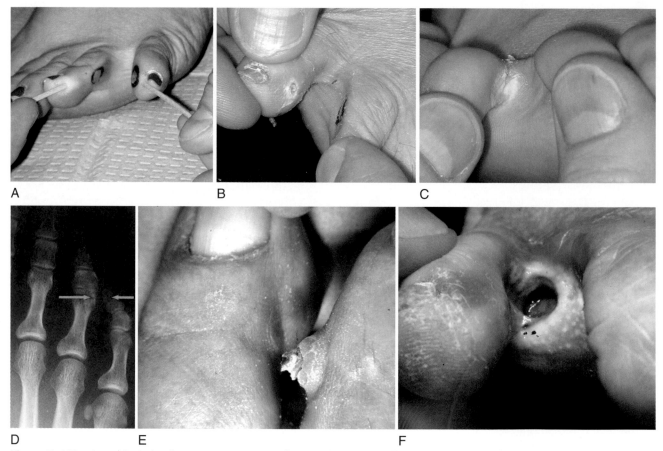

Figure 7–118   **A** and **B,** A distal interspace corn. **C,** Often a soft corn is confused with mycotic infection. **D,** Radiograph demonstrating impingement between the fourth and fifth toes. **E,** Keratotic buildup in first web space. **F,** Sinus tract in the fifth web space.

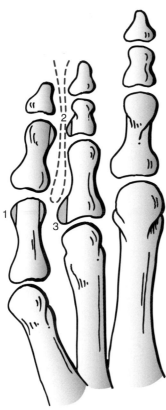

Figure 7–119 Nomenclature for corns. **A,** Lateral fifth toe corn. **B,** Interdigital corn. **C,** Web space corn. (From Coughlin M, Kennedy M: *Foot Ankle Int* 24:147-157, 2003. Copyright © 2003 by the American Orthopaedic Foot and Ankle Society [AOFAS] and reproduced here with permission.)

A soft corn can become extremely painful as a result of the pressure between adjoining bony prominences.[64]

Various terms have been used to describe a lateral fifth toe corn including *hard corn, heloma durum,* and *clavus durum* (Fig. 7–119). Terms used to describe a soft corn include *web space corn, heloma molle, clavus mollum, tyloma molle,* and *interdigital clavus.* Although it is common to refer to an interdigital corn as soft, in reality is often anything but soft. A *kissing corn* refers to the apposition of two prominent surfaces that have developed callosities; however, on occasion it can develop next to an adjacent toenail rather than a bony prominence. Thus, the use of Greek or Latin terminology is discouraged. Likewise, using terms that characterize the consistency and texture of the lesion is discouraged because the lesions are identical histologically. It is preferable to use the location of the callosity to describe the corn, and thus, the terms *lateral fifth toe corn* and *interdigital corn* are preferred.

A corn is an accumulation of keratotic layers of epidermis over a bony prominence. The bones of the foot have numerous projections over the condyles of the heads and the bases of the metatarsals and phalanges. The shoe exerts an extrinsic pressure on these prominent condylar processes, and the soft tissues over these prominences bear the brunt of the pressure and friction that the shoe exerts on the foot. Nature attempts to protect the irritated soft tissue by accumulations of thickened epithelium, but this accumulation also elevates the prominence so that the extrinsic pressure of the shoe exerts further pressure on the underlying soft tissues. With increased pressure, the skin sometimes breaks down rather than forming callus. This typically happens if pressure is applied rapidly rather than over a long period of time. In a patient with an insensate foot who is not aware of this increased pressure, often an ulceration, rather than keratotic changes, develops over a bony prominence because of the severity of pressure against the bony prominences as well. Occasionally when a callosity becomes too thick, a cleavage plane develops between the callus and the normal skin and can become secondarily infected.

Although many authors[51,176] have suggested that an underlying exostosis is a cause of corn formation, Kelikian[88] reported that in a review of 5000 radiographs, he rarely found evidence of osseous changes. Coughlin et al[34] observed the presence of an exostosis in only three of 62 cases. An enlarged condyle was not seen in any case.

Preoperative Evaluation

Physical Examination

A hard corn typically is found on the fibular aspect of the fifth toe. An obvious buildup of keratotic skin may be noted.[105] It usually is uncomfortable but not exquisitely tender to touch. Corns are common in this region because the fifth toe receives maximal pressure from the curvature of the outer border of the toe box of standard shoes. Ordinarily the head of the proximal phalanx of the fifth toe is the most prominent surface at this point, which is why a hard corn nearly always is located over the fibular condyle of the head of the proximal phalanx.

A corn or callus can form over the dorsal aspect of the PIP joint or DIP joint, and in this situation it is almost indistinguishable from a hammer toe or mallet toe deformity. With a significant hammer toe or mallet toe deformity, a keratotic lesion can develop on the tip of the involved toe due to pressure exerted with ambulation. Correction of the hammer toe or mallet toe deformity often is adequate treatment for the keratotic lesion.

Although a soft corn is essentially the same as a hard corn, its location between two of the lesser toes can result in maceration of the tissue, hence the term *soft corn*. On examination, a soft corn often manifests as a medial lesion overlying the condyle of the proximal phalanx of the fifth toe, abutting a lesion on the lateral base of the proximal phalanx of the fourth toe. When found distally on the toes, this typically is a firm keratotic lesion (see Fig. 7–118A); however, when found in a web space, the degree of maceration can make it difficult to differentiate from an ulceration of the skin or a mycotic infection (see Fig. 7–118C). Occasionally a sinus tract results, with secondary infection.

Radiographic Evaluation

Markers may be placed on the skin to identify the bony prominence associated with the keratotic lesion. Radiographs also are helpful in the case of an ulcerated lesion, to identify areas of possible osteomyelitis (see Fig. 7–118D).

Treatment

Conservative Treatment

Palliative measures such as reduction of the keratotic accumulation, changing the patient's footwear to broad-toed, soft-soled shoes with a larger toe box, and padding of the symptomatic area (Fig. 7–120A-C) to relieve pressure often give relief.[64] Many patients can be taught to care for the callus themselves by shaving the area or using a pumice stone after bathing (Fig. 7–120D and E).[11]

Surgical Treatment

TREATMENT OF LATERAL FIFTH TOE CORNS

The algorithm (Fig. 7–121) for treatment of a lateral fifth toe corn is helpful in defining a successful course. For a flexible deformity, a simple flexor tenotomy (Fig. 7–122) can allow reduction of the deformity and alleviation of discomfort. The following procedure may be used for a condylectomy of the proximal phalanx[11] beneath a corn on the fibular aspect of the fifth toe. This lesion usually involves the head of the proximal phalanx, but it can involve the lateral condyle of the middle phalanx as well.

Surgical Technique

1. The patient is placed is a slight lateral decubitus position. A digital block is applied, and the foot is cleansed in the usual fashion. Typically a tourniquet is not used.
2. A longitudinal skin incision is centered on the dorsal aspect of the fifth toe just dorsal to the hard corn (Figs. 7–123A and 7–124A and video clips 43 and 44). The incision extends

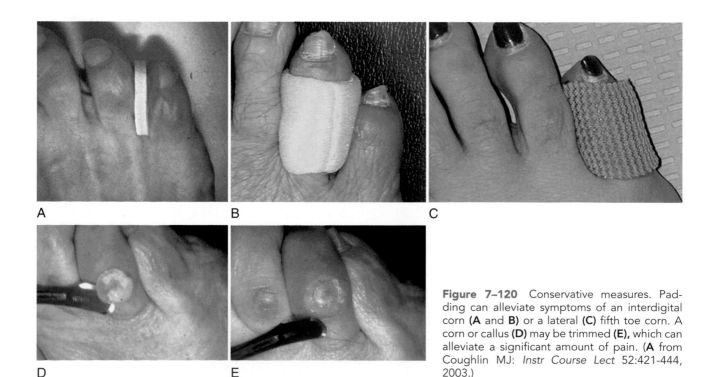

A   B   C

D   E

Figure 7–120 Conservative measures. Padding can alleviate symptoms of an interdigital corn (**A** and **B**) or a lateral (**C**) fifth toe corn. A corn or callus (**D**) may be trimmed (**E**), which can alleviate a significant amount of pain. (**A** from Coughlin MJ: *Instr Course Lect* 52:421-444, 2003.)

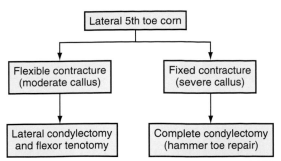

Figure 7–121 Algorithm for treatment of a lateral fifth toe corn. (Adapted from Coughlin M, Kennedy, M: *Foot Ankle Int* 24:147-157, 2003. Copyright © 2003 by the American Orthopaedic Foot and Ankle Society [AOFAS] and reproduced here with permission.)

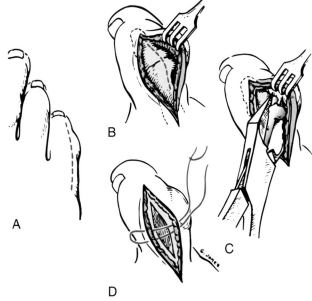

Figure 7–123 DuVries technique for condylectomy for fifth toe exostosis. **A,** Longitudinal incision over the dorsolateral aspect of the fifth toe. **B,** Skin and capsule are retracted. **C,** Fibular condyles of phalanges are excised. **D,** Skin and capsule are approximated.

from the midportion of the middle phalanx to the base of the proximal phalanx. (The corn itself is not excised, because this can lead to further friction postoperatively. The callus tends to be somewhat avascular, which can delay healing.)

3. The incision is deepened to the bone through the subcutaneous tissue and extensor tendon. (Fig. 7–124B)

4. The capsule and collateral ligaments are shaved off the prominent condyle superior-to-inferiorly (Fig. 7–1123B).
5. The prominent condyle is excised with a rongeur, leaving the remainder of the joint intact (Fig. 7–123C, Fig. 7–124C). (If both the distal portion of the proximal phalanx and the proximal portion of the middle phalanx are involved, the prominence on the middle phalanx should be excised as well.)
6. The remaining edges are smoothed with a rongeur.
7. Interrupted capsule closure is performed to stabilize the repair (Fig. 7–123D, Fig. 7–124D).
8. The skin is closed with interrupted nylon sutures. (Fig. 7–124E and F)

Postoperative Care

A bulky dressing is applied and changed weekly until drainage has subsided. The patient is allowed to ambulate in a wooden-soled shoe until dressings are discontinued. Sutures are removed 3 weeks after surgery. The toe is then taped to the fourth toe for approximately 6 weeks to increase stability of the soft tissues.

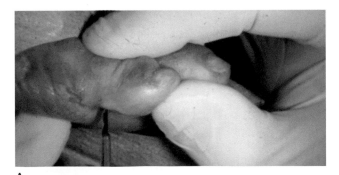

A

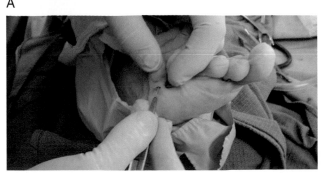

B

Figure 7–122 **A,** A flexor tenotomy can decrease a flexion deformity and diminish pain and callus formation for a lateral fifth toe corn. **B,** With the scalpel blade in place, hyperextension of the fifth toe simplifies the tenotomy.

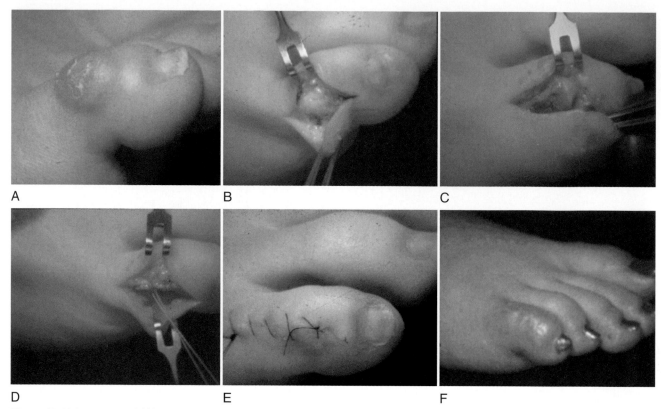

Figure 7–124   **A,** Lateral fifth toe corn. **B,** Dorsal exposure is used for resection of prominent condyle. **C,** Resection of the lateral condyle. **D,** Tight capsular closure tends to decrease the chance of later subluxation. **E,** Following skin closure. **F,** Swelling diminished with time. **(A, C,** and **D** from Coughlin, MJ: *J Bone Joint Surg Br* 82:781-790, 2000.)

TREATMENT OF INTERDIGITAL CORNS

For treatment of an extremely macerated soft corn, placement of lamb's wool, soft gauze, or a pad (see Fig. 7–118C) between the toes often allows desiccation of the area so that the tissues can heal. The use of a desiccating agent such as carbolfuchsin (Carfusin) (which is both an anti-fungal agent and an astringent) or rubbing alcohol often helps the tissue to heal more rapidly. Once the tissue has healed, surgical intervention may be considered. An algorithm (Fig. 7–125) is helpful in developing a treatment plan. The treatment consists of excising the condyles of the proximal phalanx in combination with excising a corresponding condyle of the middle phalanx. Whether a single or dual excision of corresponding lesions is performed is the surgeon's preference.[11] Usually the mag-

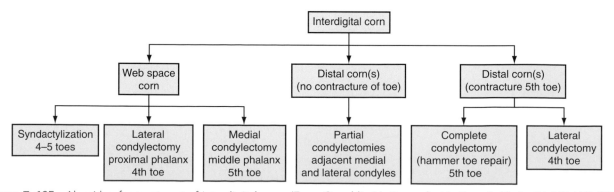

Figure 7–125   Algorithm for treatment of interdigital corn. (From Coughlin M, Kennedy, M: *Foot Ankle Int* 24:147-157, 2003.)

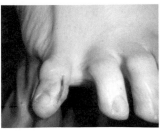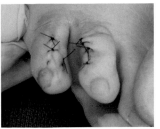

A   B

Figure 7–126 **A,** Shaving of single condyle. **B,** Shaving of adjacent condyles.

nitude of the deformity helps to elucidate whether a single or double excision is necessary. A soft corn can occur between any of the lesser toes over any bony prominence. Although soft corns tend to be common on the medial aspect of the fifth toe, they can occur in any web space.

Surgical Technique

1. After placing a digital block, the foot is cleansed in the usual fashion. Typically a tourniquet is not used. The patient is placed is a slight lateral decubitus position.
2. A small incision is centered dorsally over the keratotic lesion (Fig. 7–126A and video clip 45).
3. The incision is deepened to the capsule overlying the prominent exostosis. The capsule is stripped off the exostosis.
4. A rongeur is used to resect the exostosis, and roughened areas are smoothed.
5. A small concavity is produced in the area of the lesion. If possible, the interphalangeal joint capsule is repaired with interrupted sutures.
6. The skin is approximated with interrupted sutures.
7. If a simultaneous incision is made on a corresponding lesion, the exostosis is resected in a similar fashion. (Fig. 7–126B)

Postoperative Care

A gauze-and-tape compression dressing is applied and changed weekly. The patient is allowed to ambulate in a postoperative shoe. Sutures are removed 3 weeks after surgery. Often padding is placed between the involved toes for 3 to 6 weeks after surgery. At approximately 4 to 6 weeks after surgery the keratotic lesion can be gently lifted from its bed, and usually normal-appearing skin is noted beneath it.

Results and Complications

Patients generally do well after a simple condylectomy. In approximately 2% of patients the keratotic lesion tends to persist despite relief of the bony prominence beneath it. In these cases, frequent trimming usually results in eventual reduction of the keratotic lesion to a minimally symptomatic state. Where a lateral fifth toe corn has recurred after a condylectomy, a flexor tenotomy may be used to reduce a fifth toe contracture and can alleviate symptoms. For significant recurrence or a more severe hard corn deformity, a complete condylectomy is the treatment of choice (see the section on repair of hammered fifth toe). This procedure is performed identically to a fixed hammer toe repair.

Postoperatively it is imperative to keep the fifth toe taped to the fourth toe for 6 weeks to prevent it from becoming floppy or hanging up in stockings. An excision of a significant portion of the middle phalanx should be avoided because a floppy toe can result (see Fig. 7–100) and can become dislocated over time. With instability of the fifth toe, syndactylization of the fourth and fifth toes usually alleviates symptoms (Fig. 7–127).[77]

In the only comprehensive report of surgical repair of lateral fifth toe corns and interdigital corns, Coughlin et al[34] reported on the results of treatment of 31 lateral fifth toe corns over a 20-year period and 31 interdigital corns. Indications for surgery were intractable pain that was refractory to shaving or to shoe modifications. For lateral fifth toe corns, a lateral condylectomy was performed in 20 feet and a total condylectomy was performed in 11. For interdigital corns, a single or dual condylectomy was performed in 13, a complete condylectomy in 14, and a combination condylectomy and hammer toe repair in adjacent digits in four other feet for combined lateral and interdigital corns.

At an average follow-up of 92 months, overall satisfaction was excellent in 85%, good in 11%, and fair or poor in 4%. Pain was relieved in 47 of 51 patients (92%), and the average American Orthopaedic Foot and Ankle Society (AOFAS) score was 92 points. Two patients had significant callus reformation, but no chronic swelling was noted in any case. Toe stiffness was a common

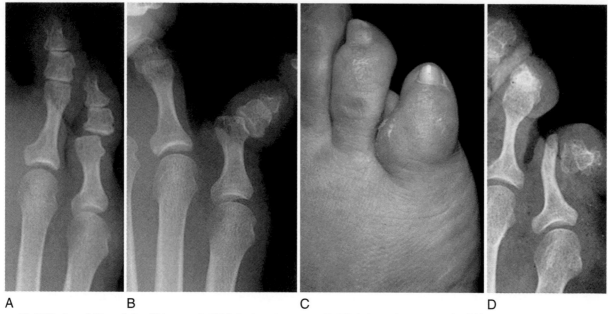

A   B   C   D

Figure 7–127   Instability of the fifth toe. **A,** Weight-bearing x-ray. **B,** With lateral stress to the fifth toe. **C,** Fracture dislocation of the lesser toe can lead to development of a soft corn. **D,** A flail fifth toe can result from excessive bone resection. Instability of the fifth toe may be treated with a PIP arthroplasty with Kirschner-wire fixation.

postoperative occurrence but was not associated with patient dissatisfaction. Subjective alignment was acceptable in 54 of 62 feet. Twenty-six of 62 feet had a hallux valgus deformity and 25 of 62 had a bunionette deformity.

This series supports the theory that a wide foot is predisposed to develop a corn. All patients were women and 73% associated the corn formation with constricting footwear. A lateral condylectomy was recommended for mild deformities and a complete condylectomy was recommended for more severe deformities characterized by fixed contractures and for combined interdigital and lateral fifth toe corns on the same digit. In the interdigital-corn subgroup, a dual condylectomy was recommended for moderate deformities; when the corn was associated with a contracted fifth toe, a fifth toe complete condylectomy was preferred. In general, satisfactory results follow an interdigital corn excision.

Zeringue and Harkless[176] retrospectively evaluated 30 patients treated for a web space corn between the fourth and fifth toes. Some 94% of the affected feet were noted to have rotation of the fifth toe. They were treated with a PIP joint arthroplasty of the fifth toe combined with a lateral-based condylectomy of the proximal phalanx of the fourth toe. A high level of satis-

faction was found at an average of 33 months follow-up.

Postoperative stiffness or fibrosis of the involved interphalangeal joints is experienced by some patients. Passive manipulation can help to alleviate such stiffness. The patient should be alerted that an interphalangeal joint arthroplasty can leave residual stiffness. Recurrence of deformity, however, is the most common complaint. Where a recurrent lesion develops, a more extensive resection should be considered. A complete condylectomy (see the discussion of hammer toe repair) may be necessary in the case of recurrence or in the presence of a severe deformity.[11,34] With a soft corn, a web space incision should be avoided, because it can lead to delayed healing, infection, or continued maceration.[12,34]

REFERENCES

1. Alvine FG, Garvin KL: Peg and dowel fusion of the proximal interphalangeal joint. *Foot Ankle* 1(2):90-94, 1980.
2. Barbari SG, Brevig K: Correction of clawtoes by the Girdlestone–Taylor flexor–extensor transfer procedure. *Foot Ankle* 5(2):67-73, 1984.
3. Barca F, Acciaro AL: Surgical correction of crossover deformity of the second toe: A technique for tenodesis. *Foot Ankle Int* 25(9):620-624, 2004.

4. Barnicot NA, Hardy RH: The position of the hallux in West Africans. *J Anat* 89(3):355-361, 1955.

5. Barouk LS: [Weil's metatarsal osteotomy in the treatment of metatarsalgia]. *Orthopade* 25(4):337-344, 1996.

6. Bhatia D, Myerson MS, Curtis MJ, et al: Anatomical restraints to dislocation of the second metatarsophalangeal joint and assessment of a repair technique. *J Bone Joint Surg Am* 76(9):1371-1375, 1994.

7. Black GB, Grogan DP, Bobechko WP: Butler arthroplasty for correction of the adducted fifth toe: A retrospective study of 36 operations between 1968 and 1982. *J Pediatr Orthop* 5(4):439-441, 1985.

8. Boc SF, Martone JD: Varus toes: A review and case report. *J Foot Ankle Surg* 34(2):220-222, 1995.

9. Bonavilla EJ: Histopathology of the heloma durum: Some significant features and their implications. *J Am Podiatry Assoc* 58(10):423-427, 1968.

10. Boyer A: *A Treatise on Surgical Diseases, and the Operations Suited to Them,* 2 vols, trans Alexander H. Stevens. New York, T and J Swords, 1815-1816, pp 383-385.

11. Brahms MA: Common foot problems. *J Bone Joint Surg Am* 49(8):1653-1664, 1967.

12. Brahms MA: The small toes. In Jahss M (ed): *Disorders of the Foot and Ankle.* Philadelphia, WB Saunders, 1991, p 1187.

13. Branch H: Pathological dislocation of the second toe. *J Bone Joint Surg Am* 19:977-984, 1937.

14. Brunet JA, Tubin S: Traumatic dislocations of the lesser toes. *Foot Ankle Int* 18(7):406-411, 1997.

15. Buggiani FP, Biggs E: Mallet toe. *J Am Podiatry Assoc* 66(5):321-326, 1976.

16. Cahill BR, Connor DE: A long-term follow-up on proximal phalangectomy for hammer toes. *Clin Orthop* 86:191-192, 1972.

17. Cameron HU, Fedorkow DM: Revision rates in forefoot surgery. *Foot Ankle* 3(1):47-49, 1982.

18. Cockin J: Butler's operation for an over-riding fifth toe. *J Bone Joint Surg Br* 50(1):77-81, 1968.

19. Cole WH: The classic. The treatment of claw-foot. By Wallace H. Cole. 1940. *Clin Orthop* (181):3-6, 1983.

20. Conklin MJ, Smith RW: Treatment of the atypical lesser toe deformity with basal hemiphalangectomy. *Foot Ankle Int* 15(11):585-594, 1994.

21. Coughlin MJ: Common causes of pain in the forefoot in adults. *J Bone Joint Surg Br* 82(6):781-790, 2000.

22. Coughlin MJ: Crossover second toe deformity. *Foot Ankle* 8(1):29-39, 1987.

23. Coughlin MJ: Lesser toe abnormalities. *Instr Course Lect* 52:421-444, 2003.

24. Coughlin MJ: Lesser toe abnormalities. In Chapman M (ed): *Operative Orthopaedics.* Philadelphia, JB Lippincott, 1988, pp 1765-1776.

25. Coughlin MJ: Lesser toe abnormalities. *J Bone Joint Surg Am* 84:1446-1469, 2002.

26. Coughlin MJ: Lesser toe deformities. *Orthopedics* 10(1):63-75, 1987.

27. Coughlin MJ: Mallet toes, hammer toes, claw toes, and corns. Causes and treatment of lesser-toe deformities. *Postgrad Med* 75(5):191-198, 1984.

28. Coughlin MJ: Operative repair of the mallet toe deformity. *Foot Ankle Int* 16(3):109-116, 1995.

29. Coughlin MJ: Rheumatoid forefoot reconstruction. A long-term follow-up study. *J Bone Joint Surg Am* 82(3):322-341, 2000.

30. Coughlin MJ: Second metatarsophalangeal joint instability in the athlete. *Foot Ankle* 14(6):309-319, 1993.

31. Coughlin MJ: Subluxation and dislocation of the second metatarsophalangeal joint. *Orthop Clin North Am* 20(4):535-51, 1989.

32. Coughlin MJ: When to suspect crossover second toe deformity. *J Musculoskel Med* 4:39-48, 1987.

33. Coughlin MJ, Dorris J, Polk E: Operative repair of the fixed hammer toe deformity. *Foot Ankle Int* 21(2):94-104, 2000.

34. Coughlin MJ, Kennedy MP: Operative repair of fourth and fifth toe corns. *Foot Ankle Int* 24(2):147-157, 2003.

35. Coughlin MJ, Pinsonneault T: Operative treatment of interdigital neuroma. A long-term follow-up study. *J Bone Joint Surg Am* 83A(9):1321-1328, 2001.

36. Coughlin MJ, Schenck RC Jr, Shurnas PS, et al: Concurrent interdigital neuroma and MTP joint instability: Long-term results of treatment. *Foot Ankle Int* 23(11):1017-1025, 2002.

37. Coughlin MJ, Thompson FM: The high price of high-fashion footwear. *Instr Course Lect* 44:371-377, 1995.

38. Cracchiolo A 3rd, Kitaoka HB, Leventen EO: Silicone implant arthroplasty for second metatarsophalangeal joint disorders with and without hallux valgus deformities. *Foot Ankle* 9(1):10-18, 1988.

39. Creer WS: Treatment of hammer toe. *BMJ* 1:527-528, 1935.

40. Cyphers SM, Feiwell E: Review of the Girdlestone–Taylor procedure for clawtoes in myelodysplasia. *Foot Ankle* 8(5):229-233, 1988.

41. Daly PJ, Johnson KA: Treatment of painful subluxation or dislocation at the second and third metatarsophalangeal joints by partial proximal phalanx excision and subtotal webbing. *Clin Orthop* (278):164-170, 1992.

42. Davies MS, Saxby TS: Metatarsal neck osteotomy with rigid internal fixation for the treatment of lesser toe metatarsophalangeal joint pathology. *Foot Ankle Int* 20(10):630-635, 1999.

43. Davis WH, Anderson RB, Thompson FM, Hamilton WG: Proximal phalanx basilar osteotomy for resistant angulation of the lesser toes. *Foot Ankle Int* 18(2):103-104, 1997.

44. Day MR, Hendrix CL, Gorecki GA, O'Malley D: Delta phalanx. *J Foot Ankle Surg* 35(1):49-53, 1996.

45. Deland JT: Anatomy of volar plate insufficiency. Presented at the 21st Annual Meeting of the American Orthopaedic Foot and Ankle Society, Anaheim, Calif, March 10, 1991.

46. Deland JT, Lee KT, Sobel M, and DiCarlo EF: Anatomy of the plantar plate and its attachments in the lesser metatarsal phalangeal joint. *Foot Ankle Int* 16(8):480-486, 1995.

47. Deland JT, Sobel M, Arnoczky SP, and Thompson FM: Collateral ligament reconstruction of the unstable metatarsophalangeal joint: An in vitro study. *Foot Ankle* 13(7):391-395, 1992.

48. Deland JT, Sung IH: The medial crossover toe: A cadaveric dissection. *Foot Ankle Int* 21(5):375-378, 2000.

49. Dhukaram V, Hossain S, Sampath J, and Barrie JL: Correction of hammer toe with an extended release of the metatarsophalangeal joint. *J Bone Joint Surg Br* 84(7):986-990, 2002.

50. DuVries HL: Dislocation of the toe. *J Am Med Assoc* 160:728, 1956.

51. DuVries HL (ed): *Surgery of the Foot.* St Louis, Mosby, 1959, pp 359-360.

52. Dyal CM, Davis WH, Thompson FM, Elonar SK: Clinical evaluation of the Ruiz-Mora procedure: Long-term follow-up. *Foot Ankle Int* 18(2):94-97, 1997.

53. Ely LW: Hammer toe. *Surg Clin North Am* 6:433-435, 1926.

54. Engle ET, Morton DJ: Notes on foot disorders among natives of the Belgian Congo. *J Bone Joint Surg Am* 13:311-319, 1931.

55. Feeney MS, Williams RL, Stephens MM: Selective lengthening of the proximal flexor tendon in the management of acquired claw toes. *J Bone Joint Surg Br* 83(3):335-338, 2001.

56. Ford LA, Collins KB, Christensen JC: Stabilization of the subluxed second metatarsophalangeal joint: Flexor tendon transfer versus primary repair of the plantar plate. *J Foot Ankle Surg* 37(3):217-222, 1998.

57. Fortin PT, Myerson MS: Second metatarsophalangeal joint instability. *Foot Ankle Int* 16(5):306-313, 1995.

58. Fox IM, Pro AL: Lesser metatarsophalangeal joint implants. *J Foot Surg* 26(2):159-163, 1987.

59. Frank GR, Johnson WM: The extensor shift procedure in the correction of clawtoe deformities in children. *South Med J* 59(8):889-896, 1966.

60. Friend G: Correction of iatrogenic floating toe following resection of the base of the proximal phalanx. *Clin Podiatr Med Surg* 3(1):57-64, 1986.

61. Gazdag A, Cracchiolo A 3rd: Surgical treatment of patients with painful instability of the second metatarsophalangeal joint. *Foot Ankle Int* 19(3):137-143, 1998.

62. Gerbert J, Benedetti L: Swanson design finger joint implant utilized in the proximal interphalangeal joints of the foot: A preliminary study. J Foot Surg 22(1):60-65, 1983.

63. Giannestras NJ: Shortening of the metatarsal shaft in the treatment of plantar keratosis: An end-result study. *J Bone Joint Surg Am* 40-A(1):61-71, 1958.

64. Gillet HG: Interdigital clavus: Predisposition is the key factor of soft corns. *Clin Orthop* 142:103-109, 1979.

65. Girdlestone GR: Physiotherapy for hand and foot. *J Chart Soc Physiother* 32:167-169, 1947.

66. Glassman F, Wolin I, Sideman S: Phalangectomy for toe deformity. *Surg Clin North Am* 29:275-280, 1949.

67. Goodwin FC, Swisher FM: The treatment of congenital hyperextension of the fifth toe. *J Bone Joint Surg Am* 25:193-196, 1943.

68. Grebing B, Coughlin MJ: Evaluation of the Esmarch bandage as a tourniquet for forefoot surgery. *Foot Ankle Int* 25(6):397-405, 2004.

69. Haddad SL, Sabbagh RC, Resch S, et al: Results of flexor-to-extensor and extensor brevis tendon transfer for correction of the crossover second toe deformity. *Foot Ankle Int* 20(12):781-8, 1999.

70. Hamer AJ, Stanley D, and Smith TW: Surgery for curly toe deformity: A double-blind, randomised, prospective trial. *J Bone Joint Surg Br* 75(4):662-663, 1993.

71. Hatch DJ, Burns MJ: An anomalous tendon associated with crossover second toe deformity. *J Am Podiatr Med Assoc* 84(3):131-132, 1994.

72. Hewitt D, Stewart AM, Webb JW: The prevalence of foot defects among wartime recruits. *BMJ* 4839:745-749, 1953.

73. Heyman CH: The operative treatment of clawfoot. *J Bone Joint Surg* 14:335-338, 1932.

74. Higgs SL: Hammer-toe. *Postgrad Med* 6:130, 1931.

75. Hoffman P: An operation for severe grades of contracted or clawtoes. *Am J Orthop Surg* 9:441-449, 1911.

76. Idusuyi OB, Kitaoka HB, Patzer GL: Oblique metatarsal osteotomy for intractable plantar keratosis: 10-year follow-up. *Foot Ankle Int* 19(6):351-355, 1998.

77. Jahss MH: Chronic and recurrent dislocations of the fifth toe. *Foot Ankle* 1(5):275-278, 1981.

78. Jahss MH: Miscellaneous soft tissue lesions. In Jahss M (ed):*Disorders of the Foot and Ankle.* Philadelphia, WB Saunders, 1991, pp 646-647, 843, 1982.

79. James CS: Footprints and feet of natives of the Solomon Islands. *Lancet* 2:1390-1393, 1939.

80. Janecki CJ, Wilde AH: Results of phalangectomy of the fifth toe for hammer toe. The Ruiz-Mora procedure. *J Bone Joint Surg Am* 58(7):1005-107, 1976.

81. Johnson JB, Price TWT: Crossover second toe deformity: Etiology and treatment. *J Foot Surg* 28(5):417-420, 1989.

82. Johnson K: Problems of the lesser toes. In Johnson K: *Surgery of the Foot and Ankle.* New York, Raven Press, 1989, pp 126-130.

83. Johnston RB 3rd, Smith J, Daniels T: The plantar plate of the lesser toes: An anatomical study in human cadavers. *Foot Ankle Int* 15(5):276-82, 1994.

84. Jolly G: Personal communication, San Diego, Calif, April 2004.

85. Karlock LG: Second metatarsophalangeal joint fusion: A new technique for crossover hammer toe deformity. A preliminary report. *J Foot Ankle Surg* 42(4):177-182, 2003.

86. Karpman RR, MacCollum MS 3rd: Arthrography of the metatarsophalangeal joint. *Foot Ankle* 9(3):125-129, 1988.

87. Kelikian H: Deformities of the lesser toes. In Kelikian H: *Hallux Valgus, Allied Deformities of the Forefoot, and Metatarsalgia.* Philadelphia, WB Saunders, 1965, pp 292-304.

88. Kelikian H, Clayton L, Loseff H: Surgical syndactylia of the toes. *Clin Orthop* 19:207-229, 1961.

89. Kuwada GT: A retrospective analysis of modification of the flexor tendon transfer for correction of hammer toe. *J Foot Surg* 27(1):57-59, 1988.

90. Kuwada GT, Dockery GL: Modification of the flexor tendon transfer procedure for the correction of flexible hammer toes. *J Foot Surg* 19(1):37-40, 1980.

91. Lamberinudi C: The feet of the industrial worker. *Lancet* 2:1480-1484, 1938.

92. Lantzounis LA: Congenital subluxation of the fifth toe and its correction by periosteocapsuloplasty and tendon transplantation. *J Bone Joint Surg* 22:147-150, 1940.

93. Lapidus PW: Operation for correction of hammer toe. *J Bone Joint Surg* 21:977-982, 1939.

94. Lapidus PW: Transplantation of the extensor tendon for correction of the overlapping of the fifth toe. *J Bone Joint Surg* 24:555-559, 1942.

95. Lehman DE, Smith RW: Treatment of symptomatic hammer toe with a proximal interphalangeal joint arthrodesis. *Foot Ankle Int* 16(9):535-541, 1995.

96. Leonard MH, Rising EE: Syndactylization to maintain correction of overlapping 5th toe. *Clin Orthop* 43:241-243, 1965.

97. Mahan KT: Bone graft reconstruction of a flail digit. *J Am Podiatr Med Assoc* 82(5):264-268, 1992.

98. Mahan KT, Downey MS, Weinfeld GD: Autogenous bone graft interpositional arthrodesis for the correction of flail toe. A retrospective analysis of 22 procedures. *J Am Podiatr Med Assoc* 93(3):167-173, 2003.

99. Mann RA, Coughlin MJ: Lesser toe deformities. In Jahss M (ed): *Disorders of the Foot and Ankle.* Philadelphia, WB Saunders, 1991, pp 1207-1209.

100. Mann RA, Coughlin MJ: Lesser toe deformities. *Instr Course Lect* 36:137-159, 1987.

101. Mann RA, Coughlin MJ: Lesser toe deformities. In Mann RA, Coughlin MJ (eds): *The Video Textbook of Foot and Ankle Surgery.* St Louis, Medical Video Productions, 1991, pp 47-49.

102. Mann RA, Coughlin MJ: The rheumatoid foot: Review of literature and method of treatment. *Orthop Rev* 8:105-112, 1979.

103. Mann RA, Mizel MS: Monarticular nontraumatic synovitis of the metatarsophalangeal joint: A new diagnosis? *Foot Ankle* 6(1):17-21, 1985.

104. Marek L, Giacopelli J, Granoff D: Syndactylization for the treatment of fifth toe deformities. *J Am Podiatr Med Assoc* 81(5):247-252, 1991.

105. Margo MK: Surgical treatment of conditions of the fore part of the foot. *J Bone Joint Surg Am* 49(8):1665-1674, 1967.

106. McCluskey WP, Lovell WW, Cummings RJ: The cavovarus foot deformity. Etiology and management. *Clin Orthop* 247:27-37, 1989.

107. McConnell BE: Correction of hammer toe deformity: A 10-year review of subperiosteal waist resection of the proximal phalanx. *Orthop Rev* 8:65-69, 1975.

108. McConnell BE: Hammer toe surgery: Waist resection of the proximal phalanx, a more simplified procedure. *South Med J* 68(5):595-598, 1975.

109. McGlamry ED: Floating toe syndrome. *J Am Podiatry Assoc* 72(11):561-568, 1982.

110. Mednick DL, Nordgaard J, Hallwhich D, et al: Comparison of total hinged and total nonhinged implants for the lesser digits. *J Foot Surg* 24(3):215-218, 1985.

111. Melamed EA, Schon LC, Myerson MS, Parks BG: Two modifications of the Weil osteotomy: Analysis on sawbone models. *Foot Ankle Int* 23(5):400-405, 2002.

112. Mendicino RW, Statler TK, Saltrick KR, Catanzariti AR: Predislocation syndrome: A review and retrospective analysis of eight patients. *J Foot Ankle Surg* 40(4):214-224, 2001.

113. Migues A, Slullitel G, Bilbao F, et al: Floating-toe deformity as a complication of the Weil osteotomy. *Foot Ankle Int* 25(9):609-613, 2004.

114. Miller SD: Technique tip: Forefoot pain: Diagnosing metatarsophalangeal joint synovitis from interdigital neuroma. *Foot Ankle Int* 22(11):914-915, 2001.

115. Mills GP: The etiology and treatment of claw-foot. *J Bone Joint Surg* 6:142-149, 1924.

116. Mizel MS: Anatomy and pathophysiology of the lesser toes. In Gould J (ed): *Operative Foot Surgery.* Philadelphia, WB Saunders, 1993, pp 84-85.

117. Mizel MS, Michelson JD: Nonsurgical treatment of monarticular nontraumatic synovitis of the second metatarsophalangeal joint. *Foot Ankle Int* 18(7):424-426, 1997.

118. Morton DJ: Metatarsus atavicus: The identification of a distinctive type of foot disorder. *J Bone Joint Surg* 9:531-544, 1927.

119. Murphy JL: Isolated dorsal dislocation of the second metatarsophalangeal joint. *Foot Ankle* 1(1):30-32, 1980.

120. Myerson MS, Fortin P, Girard P: Use of skin Z-plasty for management of extension contracture in recurrent claw- and hammer toe deformity. *Foot Ankle Int* 15(4):209-212, 1994.

121. Myerson MS, Redfern DJ: Technique tip: Modification of DuVries's lesser metatarsophalangeal joint arthroplasty to improve joint mobility. *Foot Ankle Int* 25(4):277-279, 2004.

122. Myerson MS, Shereff MJ: The pathological anatomy of claw and hammer toes. *J Bone Joint Surg Am* 71(1):45-49, 1989.

123. Newman RJ, Fitton JM: An evaluation of operative procedures in the treatment of hammer toe. *Acta Orthop Scand* 50(6 Pt 1):709-712, 1979.

124. Ohm OW 2nd; McDonell M, Vetter WA: Digital arthrodesis: An alternate method for correction of hammer toe deformity. *J Foot Surg* 29(3):207-211, 1990.

125. O'Kane C, Kilmartin TE: The surgical management of central metatarsalgia. *Foot Ankle Int* 23(5):415-419, 2002.

126. Parrish TF: Dynamic correction of clawtoes. *Orthop Clin North Am* 4(1):97-102, 1973.

127. Patton GW, Shaffer MW, Kostakos DP: Absorbable pin: A new method of fixation for digital arthrodesis. *J Foot Surg* 29(2):122-127, 1990.

128. Petrick M, Voos K, Suthers K, Smith M: Hammer toe correction using an absorbable pin. *Op Tech Orthop* 6:203-207, 1996.

129. Pichney GA, Derner R, Lauf E: Digital "V" arthrodesis. *J Foot Ankle Surg* 32(5):473-479, 1993.

130. Pontious J, Flanigan KP, and Hillstrom HJ: Role of the plantar fascia in digital stabilization. A case report. *J Am Podiatr Med Assoc* 86(1):43-47, 1996.

131. Pyper JB: The flexor-extensor transplant operation for claw toes. *J Bone Joint Surg Br* 40(3):527-533, 1958.

132. Quebedeaux T, Armstrong DG, Harkless LB: Acute and chronic pedal boutonniere deformity. *J Am Podiatr Med Assoc* 86(9):447-450, 1996.

133. Raó JP, Banzon MT: Irreducible dislocation of the metatarsophalangeal joints of the foot. *Clin Orthop* (145):224-226, 1979.

134. Rau FD, Manoli A 2nd: Traumatic boutonniere deformity as a cause of acute hammer toe: A case report. *Foot Ankle* 11(4):231-232, 1991.

135. Reece AT, Stone MH, Young AB: Toe fusion using Kirschner wire. A study of the postoperative infection rate and related problems. *J R Coll Surg Edinb* 32(3):157-159, 1987.

136. Reichert K, Caneva RG: The use of Kirschner wire fixation in forefoot surgery. *J Foot Surg* 22(3):217-221, 1983.

137. Reis ND, Karkabi S, Zinman C: Metatarsophalangeal joint dislocation after local steroid injection. *J Bone Joint Surg Br* 71(5):864, 1989.

138. Richardson E: Lesser toe abnormalities. In Crenshaw AH (ed): *Campbell's Operative Orthopaedics,* ed 8. St. Louis, Mosby, 1992, pp 2742-2744.

139. Ross ER, Menelaus MB: Open flexor tenotomy for hammer toes and curly toes in childhood. *J Bone Joint Surg Br* 66(5):770-771, 1984.

140. Ruiz-Mora J: Plastic correction of over-riding fifth toe. *Orthop Lett Club* 6, 1954.

141. Sarrafian SK: *Anatomy of the Foot and ankle.* Philadelphia, JB Lippincott, 1983.

142. Sarrafian SK: Correction of fixed hammer toe deformity with resection of the head of the proximal phalanx and extensor tendon tenodesis. *Foot Ankle Int* 16(7):449-451, 1995.

143. Sarrafian SK, Topouzian LK: Anatomy and physiology of the extensor apparatus of the toes. *J Bone Joint Surg Am* 51(4):669-679, 1969.

144. Scheck M: Degenerative changes in the metatarsophalangeal joints after surgical correction of severe hammer-toe deformities. A complication associated with avascular necrosis in three cases. *J Bone Joint Surg Am* 50(4):727-737, 1968.

145. Scheck M: Etiology of acquired hammer toe deformity. *Clin Orthop* 123:63-59, 1977.

146. Schlefman BS, Fenton CF 3rd; McGlamry ED: Peg in hole arthrodesis. *J Am Podiatry Assoc* 73(4):187-195, 1983.

147. Schnepp KH: Hammer toe and claw foot. *Am J Surg* 36:351-359, 1933.

148. Scrase WH: The treatment of dorsal adduction deformities of the fifth toe. *J Bone Joint Surg Br* 36:146, 1954.

149. Selig S: Hammer-toe. A new procedure for its correction. *Surg Gynecol Obstet* 72:101-105, 1941.

150. Sgarlato TE: Implants for lesser toes. *J Foot Surg* 22(3):247-250, 1983.

151. Sgarlato TE: Sutter double-stem silicone implant arthroplasty of the lesser metatarsophalangeal joints. *J Foot Surg* 28(5):410-413, 1989.

152. Shaw AH, Alvarez G: The use of digital implants for the correction of hammer toe deformity and their potential complications and management. *J Foot Surg* 31(1):63-74, 1992.

153. Silberman J, Kanat IO: Total joint replacement in digits of the foot. *J Foot Surg* 23(3):207-212, 1984.

154. Soule RA: Operation for the correction of hammer toe. *N Y Med J* 91: 649-650, 1910.

155. Sweetnam R: Congenital curly toes: An investigation into the value of treatment. *Lancet* 2(7043):397-400, 1958.

156. Taylor RG: An operative procedure for the treatment of hammer toe and claw-toe. *J Bone Joint Surg* 22:607-609, 1940.

157. Taylor RG: The treatment of claw toes by multiple transfers of flexor into extensor tendons. *J Bone Joint Surg Br* 33-B(4):539-542, 1951.

158. Thompson C: Surgical treatment of disorders of the fore part of the foot. *J Bone Joint Surg Am* 46:1117-1128, 1964.

159. Thompson FM, Deland JT: Flexor tendon transfer for metatarsophalangeal instability of the second toe. *Foot Ankle* 14(7): 385-388, 1993.

160. Thompson FM, Hamilton WG: Problems of the second metatarsophalangeal joint. *Orthopedics* 10(1):83-89, 1987.

161. Thordarson DB: Congenital crossover fifth toe correction with soft tissue release and cutaneous Z-plasty. *Foot Ankle Int* 22(6):511-512, 2001.

162. Threthowen WH: Treatment of hammer toe. *Lancet* 1:1312-1313, 1925.

163. Trepman E, Yeo SJ: Nonoperative treatment of metatarsophalangeal joint synovitis. *Foot Ankle Int* 16(12):771-777, 1995.

164. Trnka HJ, Muhlbauer M, Zettl R, et al: Comparison of the results of the Weil and Helal osteotomies for the treatment of metatarsalgia secondary to dislocation of the lesser metatarsophalangeal joints. *Foot Ankle Int* 20(2):72-79, 1999.

165. Trnka HJ, Nyska M, Parks BG, Myerson MS: Dorsiflexion contracture after the Weil osteotomy: Results of cadaver study and three-dimensional analysis. *Foot Ankle Int* 22(1):47-50, 2001.

166. Vandeputte G, Dereymaeker G, Steenwerckx A, Peeraer L: The Weil osteotomy of the lesser metatarsals: A clinical and pedobarographic follow-up study. *Foot Ankle Int* 21(5):370-374, 2000.

167. VanderWilde R, Campbell D: Second toe amputation for chronic painful deformity. Presented at the 23rd Annual Meeting of the American Orthopaedic Foot and Ankle Society, San Francisco, Calif, 1993.

168. Wee GC, Tucker GL: An improved procedure for the surgical correction of hammer toe. *Mo Med* 67(1):43-44, 1970.

169. Weil LS: Personal communication, April 29, 2004.

170. Weil LS, Borrelli A, Weil L, et al: Evaluation of the Weil metatarsal osteotomy. Long-term results. Presented at the Summer Meeting of the American Orthopaedic Foot and Ankle Society. Boston, Mass, 1998.

171. Wells LH: The foot of the South African native. *Am J Physiol Anthropol* 15:185-289, 1931.

172. Wilson JN: V-Y correction for varus deformity of the fifth toe. *Br J Surg* 41(166):133-135, 1953.

173. Yao L, Cracchiolo A, Farahani K, and Seeger LL: Magnetic resonance imaging of plantar plate rupture. *Foot Ankle Int* 17(1):33-36, 1996.

174. Young CS: An operation for the correction of hammer toe and clawtoe. *J Bone Joint Surg* 20:715-719, 1938.

175. Yu GV, Judge MS, Hudson JR, Seidelmann FE: Predislocation syndrome. Progressive subluxation/dislocation of the lesser metatarsophalangeal joint. *J Am Podiatr Med Assoc* 92(4):182-199, 2002.

176. Zeringue GN Jr, Harkless LB: Evaluation and management of the web corn involving the fourth interdigital space. *J Am Podiatr Med Assoc* 76(4):210-213, 1986.

177. Zingas C, Katcherian DA, Wu KK: Kirschner wire breakage after surgery of the lesser toes. *Foot Ankle Int* 16(8):504-509, 1995.

Keratotic Disorders of the Plantar Skin

Roger A. Mann • Jeffrey A. Mann

This chapter discusses the etiology and treatment of keratotic lesions of the plantar skin as a result of friction or pressure or both over a bony prominence. These must be distinguished from the intrinsic disorders of the skin such as verruca and dermatosis, especially tinea infestations (see Chapter 32).

Movement of the center of pressure along the plantar aspect of the foot illustrates the long period that the center of pressure dwells beneath the metatarsal heads during normal walking (see Chapter 1). After heel strike, the center of pressure moves very rapidly to the metatarsal head area, where it dwells for more than 50% of the stance phase, after which it moves toward the toes (Fig. 8–1). Because of this extended period of weight bearing in the metatarsal area, abnormal alignment of the forefoot, either localized or generalized, can result in a problem with a keratotic lesion.

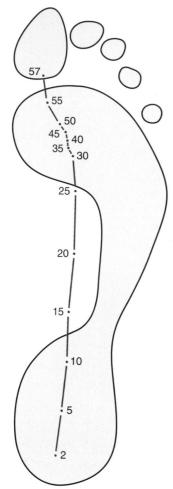

Figure 8–1 Movement of the center of pressure along the plantar aspect of the foot during walking. Note the way the center of pressure rapidly moves from the heel and dwells in the metatarsal region before moving distally to the great toe. (From Hutton WC, Stott JRR, Stokes JAF: In Klenerman L [ed]: *The Foot and Its Disorders.* Oxford, Blackwell Scientific, 1982, p 42.)

BOX 8–1   Causes of Plantar Keratoses

BONE CAUSES

Prominent fibular condyle metatarsal head

Long metatarsal

Morton's foot

Hypermobile first ray

Post-trauma effects

Abnormal foot posture (varus or valgus)

SYSTEMIC DISEASES

Rheumatoid arthritis

Psoriatic arthritis

DERMATOLOGIC LESIONS

Wart

Seed corn

Hyperkeratotic skin

SOFT TISSUE CAUSES

Atrophy of plantar fat pad

Crush injury sequelae

Plantar scar secondary to trauma

MECHANICAL CAUSES

Subluxed or dislocated metatarsophalangeal joint

Hallux valgus deformity resulting in transfer lesion

IATROGENIC CAUSES

Secondary to metatarsal surgery (e.g., plantar flexion)

Transfer lesion

Hallux valgus surgery (e.g., shortening or dorsiflexion of metatarsal)

PLANTAR KERATOSES

Examining the various causes of plantar keratoses (Box 8–1), one realizes that when the patient presents with a plantar callus, a significant differential diagnosis must be considered in the patient evaluation. As a rule the diagnosis is not difficult to make, but at times the diagnosis may not be clear-cut, and one needs to consider these various causes.

Anatomy

The usual pattern of the metatarsals demonstrates that the first metatarsal is shorter than the second approximately 60% of the time.[7] The mobility of the first metatarsocuneiform (MTC) joint or the first metatarsophalangeal (MTP) joint determines the degree of

weight bearing of the first ray. The plantar aponeurosis mechanism that brings about plantar flexion of the first metatarsal during the last half of stance phase becomes less functional as a hallux valgus deformity develops. As a result, plantar flexion of the first ray might not occur, which could result in a transfer of pressure to the second metatarsal head and subsequently a diffuse callus secondary to increased weight bearing. If the first MTC joint is hypermobile, which probably is pathologic in no more than 5% of patients, again the first metatarsal does not bear its share of the weight, and pressure is transferred to the lesser metatarsals, where a diffuse callus can develop beneath the second and possibly third metatarsal (Fig. 8–2). The second and third metatarsals are quite stable because of the rigidity of their tarsometatarsal articulations; therefore, if the first metatarsal is hyper-

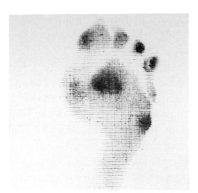

Figure 8–2 Harris mat print of a patient with hypermobility of the first metatarsal. Because the first metatarsal does not carry much weight, pressure is transferred to the second and third metatarsals as well as to the tip of the hallux.

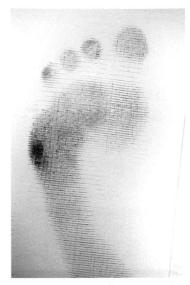

Figure 8–3 Harris mat print of patient with varus forefoot deformity. Note that pressure is borne on the lateral aspect of the foot with significantly decreased weight bearing beneath the medial aspect of the foot.

mobile or elevated from any cause, callus can form beneath these metatarsal heads. The fourth and fifth metatarsals are more mobile and therefore calluses rarely develop beneath them unless there is a problem with abnormal foot posture. A moderate degree of mobility also exists between the lateral two rays and medial three rays between the cuboid and lateral cuneiform.

The posture of the foot must always be considered in evaluating the patient with an intractable plantar keratosis (IPK). The IPK may be caused by the abnormal posture of the foot, and unless the posture is corrected by conservative or surgical treatment, the IPK will persist. Postures of the foot that can cause abnormal callus formation include an equinus deformity of the ankle joint, a cavus foot, a flatfoot, a varus forefoot deformity, a valgus flatfoot deformity, and an abnormal alignment of the MTP joints.

An equinus deformity of the ankle joint that results in localized weight bearing on the metatarsal head area usually results in a diffuse callus beneath the first, second, and third metatarsal heads. This can result in a painful condition, particularly in the older patient, who often develops atrophy of the fat pad. In the patient with an insensate foot, such as the patient with diabetes or a peripheral neuropathy, ulceration of the plantar aspect of the foot can occur.

The *cavus foot* is a rigid foot with a decreased area of weight bearing. In the cavus foot the calcaneus is usually in a dorsiflexed position and the forefoot in equinus, so the weight-bearing area is diminished, with a resultant diffuse callus beneath the metatarsal head area. Often this condition becomes more symptomatic as the patient ages and the fat pad atrophies more.

The *flatfoot* does not usually develop significant callus formation beneath the metatarsal heads. If it is associated with a hallux valgus deformity, however, the

patient can develop a callus along the plantar medial aspect of the great toe at the level of the interphalangeal joint.

A *varus forefoot deformity*, in which the lateral border of the foot is more plantar flexed than the medial border, often results in a diffuse type of callus beneath the fifth metatarsal area (Fig. 8–3).

A *valgus forefoot deformity*, in which the first metatarsal is more plantar flexed in relation to the lesser metatarsals, often results in a diffuse callus beneath the first metatarsal head region (Fig. 8–4). This is often associated with a cavus foot deformity.

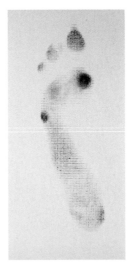

Figure 8–4 Harris mat print of patient with valgus forefoot deformity in which increased weight is borne along the medial side of the foot and, in particular, beneath the first metatarsal head.

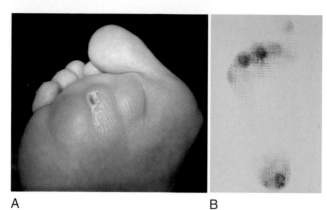

A   B

Figure 8–5   A, Foot in a patient with rheumatoid arthritis with large diffuse plantar calluses beneath the metatarsal heads and nonfunctional toes. **B,** Harris mat print demonstrating concentration of pressure beneath metatarsal heads and lack of weight bearing by lesser toes.

Abnormal alignment of the metatarsophalangeal joints secondary to either subluxation or dorsal dislocation results in a plantarward force on the metatarsal head that often develops into a diffuse callus beneath the involved metatarsal head. An extreme example is a patient with advanced rheumatoid arthritis (Fig. 8–5).

Diagnosis

The evaluation of a patient with a plantar keratotic lesion begins with a careful history of the condition and should include what type of footwear aggravates and relieves the pain as well as what type of treatment has been attempted in the past.

The physical examination begins with the patient standing. Careful observation should be made of the posture of the toes, characteristics of the MTP joints and longitudinal arch, and position and posture of the hindfoot. Then the range of motion of the ankle, subtalar, transverse tarsal, and MTP joints should be noted. The posture of the forefoot in relation to the hindfoot needs to be quantified. The neurovascular status of the foot is likewise evaluated.

The plantar aspect of the foot is carefully evaluated. The location of the lesion and its characteristics are observed. A plantar wart is usually localized but occasionally demonstrates a mosaic pattern. A wart is usually not specifically located beneath a metatarsal head, although it is usually present on the plantar aspect of the foot.

A keratotic lesion needs to be carefully evaluated to establish, first, which metatarsal head it is beneath and then its characteristics. The callus may consist of a localized seed corn, a discrete plantar keratosis beneath the fibular condyle of a metatarsal head, a diffuse callus beneath a metatarsal head, a diffuse callus beneath several metatarsal heads, or a localized callus beneath the tibial sesamoid.

To facilitate identification of the lesion and to be sure it is not a wart, the lesion is often trimmed with a no. 17 blade. Trimming enables the clinician to identify the margins of the callus, because in a well-localized plantar keratosis the callus itself has definite circumscribed edges, as opposed to a diffuse callus, which is a generalized thickening of the plantar skin without a defined margin. A wart, on the other hand, may have a small amount of hyperkeratotic skin overlying it, but very quickly one enters the warty material, which consists of multiple end arteries that bleed vigorously, as opposed to a true plantar keratosis, which has no blood supply (Fig. 8–6).

Weight-bearing radiographs should be obtained along with sesamoid views, if indicated. Occasionally

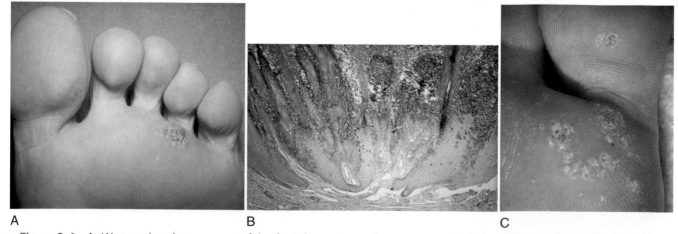

A   B   C

Figure 8–6   A, Wart on the plantar aspect of the foot does not usually occur on a weight-bearing area. **B,** Histologic features of the wart demonstrate considerable vascularity within the lesion. **C,** Mosaic wart has similar histology but is more widespread.

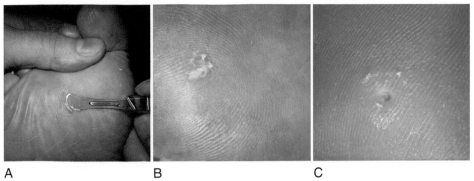

A   B   C

Figure 8–7 **A,** Debridement of callus with no. 17 blade. **B,** A seed corn is a small keratotic lesion on the plantar aspect of the foot that at times becomes symptomatic. **C,** Appearance of seed corn after debridement.

a small marker placed over the lesion helps to identify the offending structure.

Treatment

Conservative Treatment

The plantar callus is trimmed with a sharp knife. When trimming a callus, one should attempt to reduce the hyperkeratotic tissue, and if it is invaginated, this too should be trimmed. With a deep-seated lesion, however, it is not possible to remove all the keratotic lesion at the first trimming, and sometimes several trimmings are necessary to permit the deep-seated portion of the callus to surface. Occasionally a seed corn, which is a well-localized keratotic lesion usually 2 to 3 mm in diameter, can be removed at the first sitting, although it might require a second trimming (Fig. 8–7).

After debridement of the callus, a soft metatarsal support is used to relieve the pressure on the involved area (Fig. 8–8). The soft support can be used initially, provided that the patient's shoe is of adequate size. If the patient is wearing stylish women's dress shoes, there may not be sufficient volume for the foot and the metatarsal support. The patient with a significant keratotic lesion needs to be encouraged to wear a broad, soft, preferably low-heeled shoe to provide more cushioning for the plantar aspect of the foot. The metatarsal support is placed into the shoe just proximal to the area of the lesion (Fig. 8–9). When doing this, it is important to instruct the patient that initially this support may feel uncomfortable and may take a period of breaking in of a week to 10 days.

The patient is then seen periodically in the office for trimming of the lesion, adjustment of the metatarsal support, and possibly even placement of a larger one, as necessary. If the patient has a postural abnormality of the foot such as a forefoot varus or valgus, or pos-

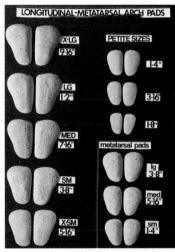

Figure 8–8 Various types of soft metatarsal supports that may be used to relieve pressure in the metatarsal area of the foot.

sibly a cavus foot, a well-molded soft orthotic device may be of benefit. The orthotic device, however, should not be used until one has experimented with the removable soft supports first to see whether the patient will respond to an orthosis.

If the callus persists and is symptomatic, surgical intervention can be considered.

Surgical Treatment
TYPES OF PLANTAR CALLOSITIES

Surgical management of a plantar keratosis is based on the characteristics of the callus.

A *discrete callus* with a central keratotic core is observed beneath the fibular condyle of the metatarsal head and beneath the tibial sesamoid (Fig. 8–10). When the patient with a localized lesion walks over a Harris mat, the imprint created is well localized beneath the prominence that has brought about the

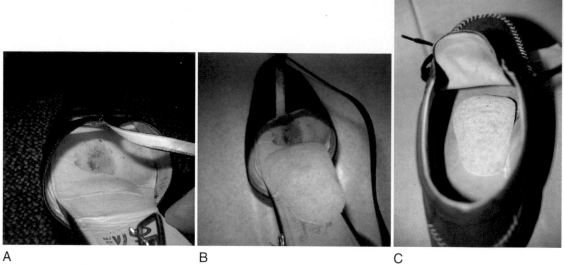

A   B   C

Figure 8–9 Placement of a soft metatarsal support in the shoe. **A,** Support is placed just proximal to the "smudge" on the insole. This is usually around the base of the tongue. **B and C,** The support can be moved medially or laterally, depending on the location of the plantar lesion.

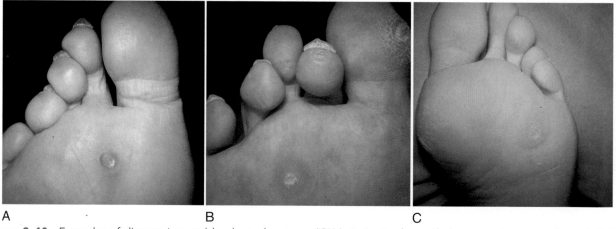

A   B   C

Figure 8–10 Examples of discrete intractable plantar keratoses (IPKs). **A,** Lesion beneath the second metatarsal head. **B,** Discrete keratosis beneath the third metatarsal head. **C,** Discrete keratosis beneath the fourth metatarsal head. (**B** from Mann RA: *Instr Course Lect* 33:289, 1984.)

callus (Fig. 8–11). Histologically this lesion is a dense, keratinized lesion with a central core (Fig. 8–12).

A *diffuse callus* is observed beneath a metatarsal head that does not have a prominent fibular condyle and is noted most often beneath the second metatarsal head. Occasionally a diffuse callus is noted beneath multiple metatarsal heads (Fig. 8–13). When this type of callus is present and is trimmed, although the material consists of hyperkeratotic skin, there is no central core as one observes in a discrete callus. When this patient walks over a Harris mat, the print that is observed is diffuse beneath the entire metatarsal head or beneath multiple metatarsal heads (Fig. 8–14). This

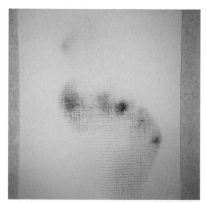

Figure 8–11 Harris mat print demonstrating well-localized area of pressure—a discrete plantar keratosis.

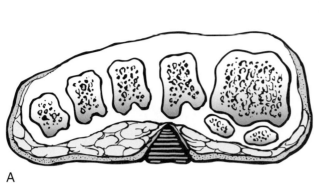
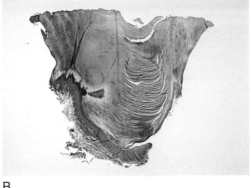

Figure 8–12 **A,** Location of a discrete plantar keratosis beneath a prominent fibular condyle. **B,** Histologic features of the keratotic lesion demonstrate layers of keratin with no blood vessels. Compare with Figure 8–6B.

type of diffuse lesion is occasionally observed beneath the first metatarsal head if it is plantar flexed. It is observed beneath the second metatarsal head when the first metatarsal is short or hypermobile or is functioning insufficiently because of instability brought about by an advanced hallux valgus deformity or possibly insufficiency after bunion surgery, if the joint has been destabilized. A diffuse callus beneath the second, third, and fourth metatarsal heads is usually observed in a patient with an extremely short first metatarsal, which results in increased weight bearing beneath the three middle metatarsals (Fig. 8–15). Occasionally a diffuse callus is present beneath the fifth metatarsal head in patients with a varus configuration of the forefoot, or it can be attributable to plantar flexion of the fifth metatarsal associated with a tailor's bunion.

A diffuse type of callus can result after trauma involving a metatarsal fracture that results in a metatarsal's becoming prominent if it is plantar flexed or, beneath an adjacent metatarsal, if it is dorsiflexed, with the normal metatarsal left to bear increased weight.

The importance of differentiating the type of the callus is that the nature of the callus determines the type of surgical procedure that will give the best result.

Localized Intractable Plantar Keratosis

A localized IPK, which is usually caused by the prominence of the fibular condyle, is treated by a DuVries metatarsal condylectomy. DuVries[3-5] initially described the procedure in which he carried out an arthroplasty of the MTP joint by removing a portion of the distal articular surface and the plantar condyle. Coughlin[1] and Mann[12] modified the procedure and removed only the plantar condyle, and both these procedures seem to result in satisfactory resolution of the problem.

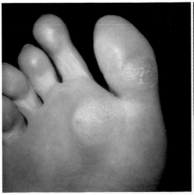
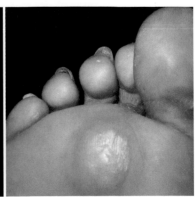

Figure 8–13 **A** and **B,** Examples of diffuse keratotic lesions. When these lesions are debrided, there is no central core, which distinguishes them from discrete keratotic lesions.

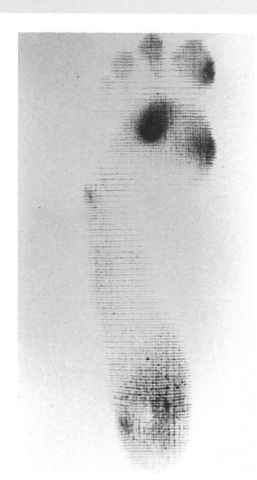

Figure 8–14 Harris mat print demonstrates diffuse keratotic lesion beneath second metatarsal head. Compare with Figure 8–13. (From Mann RA: *Instr Course Lect* 33:293, 1984.)

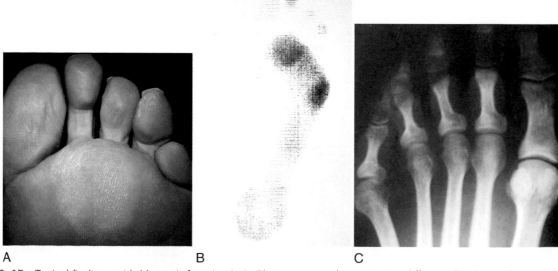

A   B   C

Figure 8–15 Typical findings with Morton's foot (toe). **A,** Plantar aspect demonstrates diffuse callus beneath second and third metatarsal heads. **B,** Harris mat print demonstrates increased weight bearing beneath the second and third metatarsals, with little or no weight bearing beneath the first metatarsal head. **C,** Radiograph demonstrates typical Morton's foot with short first metatarsal and relatively long second and third metatarsals.

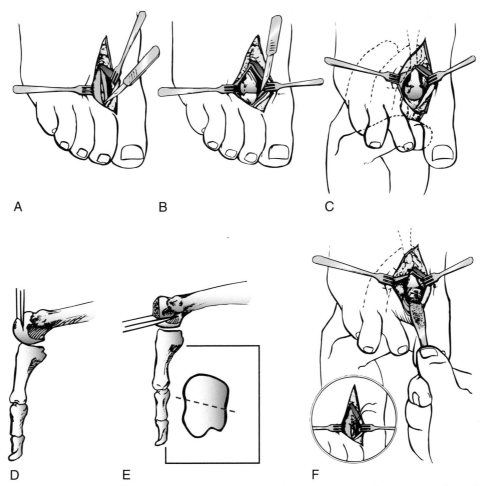

Figure 8–16 DuVries plantar metatarsal condylectomy. **A,** Hockey stick–shaped incision beginning in the web space is carried obliquely across the joint to about the middle of the metatarsal shaft. Skin and extensor tendons are retracted, and the capsule is incised longitudinally. **B,** Capsule and collateral ligaments on both sides of the metatarsal head are sectioned. **C,** The involved toe is plantar flexed with the left thumb while pressure is applied on the plantar aspect of the metatarsal shaft with the index finger. **D,** About 2 mm of articular cartilage is removed. **E,** Plantar 30% of the condyle is removed with an osteotome. Note angulation to facilitate removal of more of the fibular aspect. **F,** Edges of the metatarsal are smoothed, then the capsule and skin are closed.

DUVRIES METATARSAL CONDYLECTOMY

Surgical Technique

1. A hockey stick–shaped incision begins in the second web space and is carried across the metatarsal head proximally to about the distal third of the metatarsal shaft (Fig. 8–16A).
2. Passing medially and laterally to the extensor hood, the transverse metatarsal ligament is identified and released.
3. The interval between the two extensor tendons is opened and continued through the joint capsule to expose the MTP joint.

4. The collateral ligaments are transected, and the MTP joint is sharply plantar flexed while pressure is applied to the plantar aspect of the foot with the index finger of the same hand (Fig. 8–16B and C).
5. The distal 2 mm of articular cartilage is removed from the metatarsal head in a plane perpendicular to the metatarsal shaft. As this cut is made, the osteotome needs to be angled slightly proximally; otherwise it will skid off the cartilage and make an oblique cut (Fig. 8–16D).
6. The MTP joint is now sharply plantar flexed to bring into view the plantar condyle. The plantar 20% to 30% of the metatarsal head

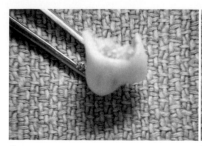
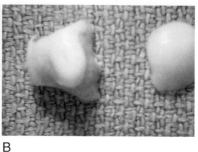

A   B

Figure 8–17 Excised plantar condyle. **A,** Note marked prominence of the fibular portion of the condyle in this specimen. **B,** Plantar view of the same specimen illustrating the large condyle. (**A** from Mann RA: *Instruct Course Lect* 33:292, 1984.)

is removed with a 10- to 12-mm thin osteotome. The osteotome must be angled slightly plantarward to avoid inadvertent splitting of the metatarsal shaft (Fig. 8–16E).

7. On completion of the osteotomy in the metatarsal head, the plantar condyle is delivered by use of a Freer elevator or thin rongeur in the adjacent interspace, and the condyle is removed. It is difficult to pull this fragment of bone out directly over the proximal phalanx, so it is pushed into the interspace and removed (Fig. 8–17).

8. The edges are carefully rongeured, and the joint is reduced (Fig. 8–16F). The skin is closed in a routine manner.

9. A compression dressing is applied for 12 to 18 hours, and the patient is permitted to ambulate in a postoperative shoe.

Postoperative Care

The bulky surgical dressing is changed after 18 to 24 hours, and the patient is placed into a snug compression dressing consisting of 2-inch conforming gauze (Kling) and adhesive tape. The patient is permitted to ambulate in the postoperative shoe, which is worn for 3 weeks. The shoe is removed and the patient encouraged to work on range-of-motion exercises.

Results

In a review of 100 patients surgically treated by Mann and DuVries,[13] there was 93% patient satisfaction. It was observed that 42% of the lesions were beneath the second metatarsal head, 31% beneath the third, 19% beneath the fourth, and 8% beneath the fifth. A transfer lesion occurred in 13% of the patients, and the original lesion failed to resolve in 5%.

The 5% complication rate included fracture of a metatarsal head, avascular necrosis of the metatarsal head, and clawing of the toe. There were no cases of dislocation of the MTP joint

after this procedure. Postoperative range of motion of the MTP joint rarely demonstrates more than 25% loss of motion. It has always been somewhat surprising that so little motion is lost after this type of arthroplasty, whereas when a similar procedure is carried out for a dislocated MTP joint, significantly more motion is lost.

COUGHLIN'S MODIFIED METATARSAL CONDYLECTOMY

The modification of the condylectomy by Coughlin is carried out in the same way as the DuVries metatarsal condylectomy except that the distal portion of the metatarsal is not removed (Fig. 8–18 and video clip 36).[1,12] This makes removing the plantar condyle a little more difficult. Up to now there has been no published report regarding the results of this modification of the DuVries procedure, although preliminary data indicate about a 5% incidence of transfer lesions.

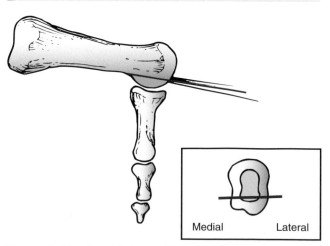

Medial   Lateral

Figure 8–18 Coughlin's modification of plantar condylectomy. Plantar 20% to 30% of the condyle is removed, and the distal portion of the metatarsal head is left intact.

VERTICAL CHEVRON PROCEDURE

A vertical chevron osteotomy of the metatarsal head has been described by Dreeben et al[2] for treatment of a painful callus beneath the metatarsal head. The article did not classify the callus into localized or diffuse categories. A vertical chevron osteotomy was performed in the metaphysis, and the metatarsal head was elevated approximately 3 mm.

Surgical Technique

1. A 2-cm dorsal incision is made over the metatarsal head and neck region. The incision is carried down, the extensor tendon moved aside, the metatarsal neck exposed subperiosteally, and the plantar periosteum left intact. The MTP joint is not entered.
2. A chevron-type cut with the apex based distally is produced with a power saw just proximal to the edge of the dorsal joint capsule. An attempt should be made to leave the plantar periosteum intact (Fig. 8–19 and video clip 39).
3. The metatarsal head is displaced dorsally by plantar pressure but not more than 3 to 4 mm.
4. The osteotomy site is stabilized with a 0.045-inch Kirschner wire introduced through a separate stab wound. The skin is closed in a routine manner.

Postoperative Care

The patient walks in a postoperative shoe with weight bearing as tolerated. The Kirschner wire is removed after 3 weeks, and gentle range of motion is begun at that time. The postoperative shoe is continued for a total of 6 weeks.

Results

The series reported by Dreeben et al[2] contained 45 patients. Complete relief of the symptoms was noted in 67%; 24% had residual pain, 9% demonstrated a transfer lesion, and in 4% the callus was unchanged. The authors pointed out that the metatarsal head should be elevated at least 3 mm but not more than 4.5 mm. Kitaoka and Patzer[11] used the same procedure on 21 feet—16 women and 3 men with a mean age of 59 years (32 to 85). They reported good results in 16, fair in two, and poor in three. In four patients (20%) the callosity persisted, and in three (14%) a transfer lesion developed.

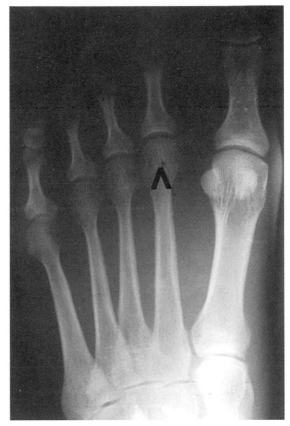

Figure 8–19 The vertical chevron procedure is carried out to create an osteotomy, as demonstrated in this radiograph. The metatarsal head should be elevated approximately 3 mm.

Discrete Callus Beneath Tibial Sesamoid

A discrete callus beneath the first metatarsal head lies under the tibial sesamoid. A localized lesion does not occur beneath the fibular sesamoid. A diffuse callus can be observed beneath the entire first metatarsal and is usually associated with a plantar-flexed metatarsal, often observed in the patient with a cavus foot or Charcot–Marie–Tooth disease.

The lesion beneath the tibial sesamoid can often be managed conservatively, although when it occurs after bunion surgery and the sesamoid is localized beneath the crista of the metatarsal head, surgical intervention is usually required (Fig. 8–20).

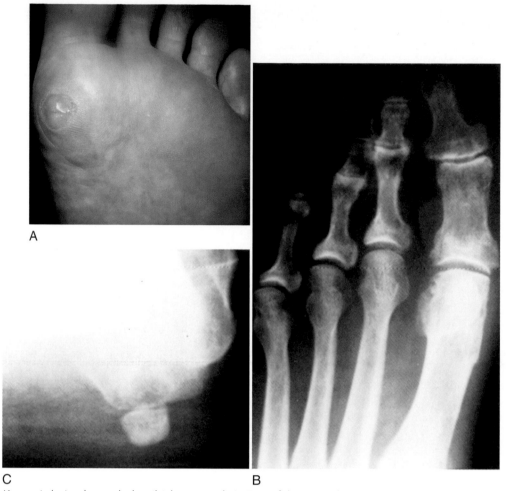

Figure 8–20   Keratotic lesion beneath the tibial sesamoid. **A,** Even if there is only a moderate amount of callus over the lesion, once it is trimmed, a discrete keratotic lesion is usually identified. **B,** Radiograph demonstrates a tibial sesamoid centered beneath the metatarsal head. **C,** Axial view demonstrates a sesamoid sitting beneath the crista.

TIBIAL SESAMOID SHAVING

The surgical procedure we prefer is tibial sesamoid shaving, in which the plantar half of the sesamoid is removed (video clip 34). In the past we advocated excision of the sesamoid for this problem, but after a review of our cases, we believe that tibial sesamoid shaving is a superior procedure with significantly less morbidity.[14]

Surgical Technique

1. The skin incision is made slightly plantar to the midline and centered over the medial aspect of the MTP joint. The incision is carried down to the capsular structures without undermining the skin (Fig. 8–21A).

2. Along the capsular plane the incision is developed in a plantar direction over the medial aspect of the tibial sesamoid. Great care is taken to identify the medial plantar cutaneous nerve, which often passes with a small vessel along the plantar aspect of the abductor hallucis tendon.

3. With the nerve identified and retracted plantarward, the periosteum over the tibial sesamoid is stripped to expose the plantar two thirds of the sesamoid. The plantar half of the tibial sesamoid is removed with a small oscillating saw, and the edges are smoothed (Fig. 8–21C and D).

4. The wound is closed in a routine manner and a compression dressing is applied (Fig. 8–21E and F).

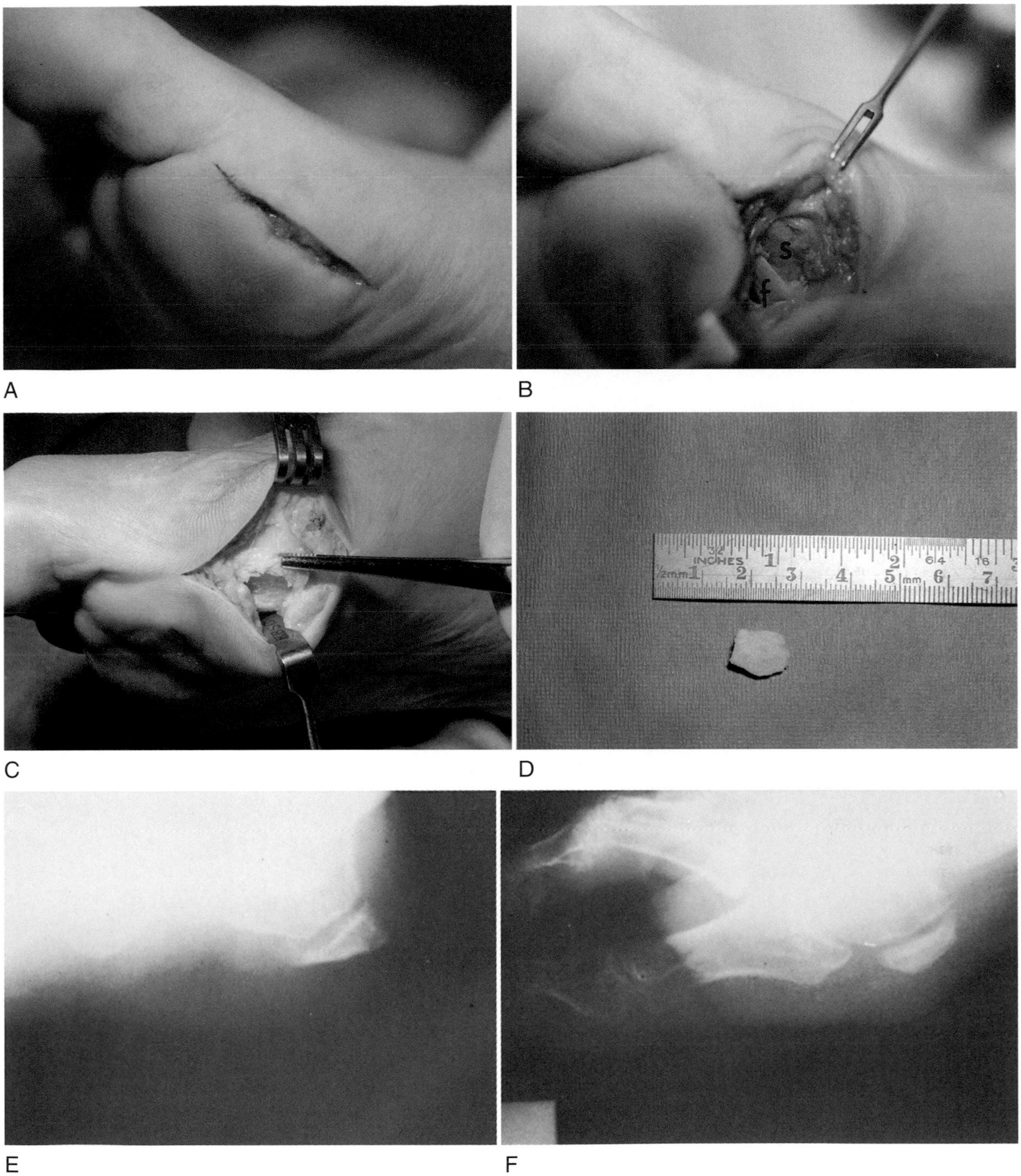

A

B

C

D

E

F

Figure 8–21   Tibial sesamoid shaving. **A,** Skin incision is made just below the midline and carried down to expose the joint capsule. The plantar medial cutaneous nerve is identified and retracted. **B,** After the tibial sesamoid is exposed, the plantar half is removed (s, sesamoid; f, flexor hallucis longus tendon). **C,** Appearance after excision of the plantar aspect of the tibial sesamoid. **D,** Excised piece of the tibial sesamoid. **E** and **F,** Axial and lateral radiographs demonstrate tibial sesamoid after removal of the plantar half. (**C** and **D** from Mann RA: *Instr Course Lect* 33:289, 1984.)

Postoperative Care

The patient is kept in a postoperative shoe with the foot in a firm dressing for 3 weeks and then is permitted to ambulate as tolerated.

Results

A follow-up study of 12 of our patients demonstrated that 58% had excellent results with no recurrent callus, 33% had good results with slight recurrence of the callus, and one patient (9%) had a fair result and required periodic trimming of the plantar callus.[14] All patients maintained full range of motion of the first MTP joint, and none had a painful scar.

Complications

The most significant complication after this procedure is injury to the medial plantar cutaneous nerve. If this occurs and is noted at surgery, one must consider freeing up the nerve more proximally and moving it away from the plantar aspect of the foot. If the damage to the nerve appears to be too severe, one must consider whether the nerve should be sectioned and buried beneath the abductor hallucis muscle to prevent a neuroma from forming on the plantar medial aspect of the foot.

Further discussion of tibial sesamoid shaving is presented in Chapter 10.

Diffuse Intractable Plantar Keratosis

At times the second metatarsal is long because of the anatomic pattern of the foot. Whether a true plantar-flexed metatarsal exists except after trauma has not been adequately demonstrated. A diffuse IPK beneath any lesser metatarsal head may be caused by a transfer lesion as a result of adjacent metatarsal osteotomy or trauma. A diffuse IPK beneath several metatarsal heads is mainly attributable to the lack of weight bearing by the first metatarsal and does not represent a surgical problem.

In attempting to be as precise as possible in the treatment of a diffuse IPK, if the offending metatarsal is long, it should be shortened to the level produced by a line connecting the two adjacent metatarsals (Fig. 8–22). This would mean that if the second metatarsal is long relative to the first and third, it should be shortened back to a line produced by connecting the first and third metatarsals. If a diffuse callus results because

of a transfer lesion and the metatarsal is not long, we prefer to carry out a basal osteotomy to bring the metatarsal head to the same level as the adjacent metatarsals.

When a metatarsal osteotomy of any type is considered, it is imperative that a contracture of the MTP joint is not present. An MTP joint fixed in a dorsiflexed position can cause a painful plantar callosity that should be managed by correction of the MTP joint and not the metatarsal. In general, metatarsal osteotomies are contraindicated in the patient with a fixed deformity of the MTP joint, unless one is treating an MTPS deformity.

OBLIQUE METATARSAL OSTEOTOMY

The concept of the oblique metatarsal osteotomy was described by Giannestras,[6] who produced a proximal step-cut osteotomy to shorten the symptomatic metatarsal. In his series of 40 patients, 10% developed a transfer lesion. Finding this surgical procedure technically difficult, we modified it to an oblique longitudinal osteotomy (Fig. 8–23). This is technically simpler and gives uniformly satisfactory results.[12]

Surgical Technique

1. The skin incision is a long dorsal incision centered over the involved metatarsal. It is developed through subcutaneous tissue and fat, with great caution taken to identify and retract the cutaneous nerves. The involved metatarsal is identified, an incision is made over its dorsal aspect down to the bone, and the metatarsal is exposed subperiosteally (Fig. 8–24A).

2. If more than 5 to 6 mm of shortening is required, the transverse metatarsal ligament needs to be sectioned, particularly when dealing with the third and fourth metatarsals. This is usually not necessary for the second metatarsal.

3. Before the osteotomy is performed, a transverse mark is etched in the metatarsal at the midportion of the osteotomy so that as the osteotomy site is displaced, the surgeon can measure precisely how much shortening is occurring. With a thin saw blade, an oblique osteotomy as long as possible is produced in the metatarsal shaft. When an osteotomy is performed in the second metatarsal, the

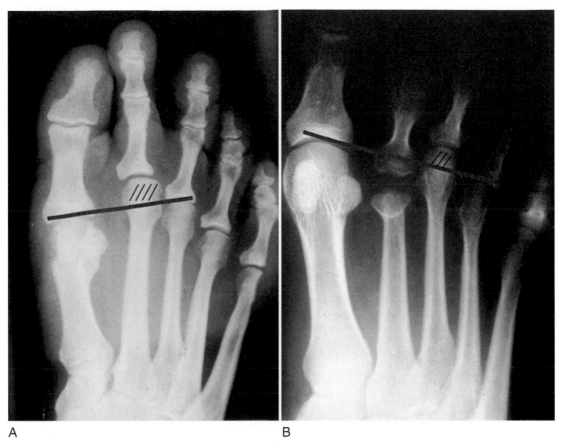

A   B

Figure 8–22   Metatarsal shortening. **A,** Line is drawn from first to third metatarsal head. This indicates the amount that the second metatarsal head needs to be shortened. **B,** Line is drawn between first and fourth metatarsal head to indicate the amount of shortening required to create a smooth metatarsal pattern.

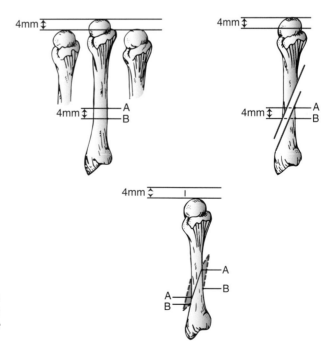

Figure 8–23   Diagram of oblique metatarsal osteotomy of a lesser metatarsal to correct the weight-bearing pattern. (From Mann RA, Coughlin MJ: *Video Textbook of Foot and Ankle Surgery.* St Louis, Medical Video Productions, 1991.)

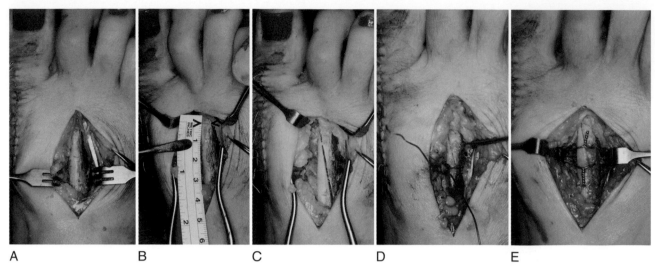

A   B   C   D   E

Figure 8–24 Surgical technique of oblique metatarsal osteotomy. **A,** Metatarsal is exposed through a longitudinal incision. Care is taken to avoid superficial nerves. Incision is made along the periosteum of the metatarsal, and muscle tissue is stripped from the metatarsal shaft. **B,** Mark is made on metatarsal *(arrows)*, then a ruler is used to mark a fixed distance on the metatarsal so the bone can be shortened accurately. **C,** Long oblique osteotomy has been made. When carrying this out on the second metatarsal, the osteotomy is made on this diagonal so as to avoid the artery in the first web space. **D,** Metatarsal is accurately shortened by using the marks on the bone as a guide. First the cerclage wire is passed through a drill hole after the metatarsal has been shortened. This helps to stabilize the length of the metatarsal. **E,** Second cerclage wire is placed to help increase stability of the osteotomy site.

base should be directed laterally to avoid bringing the saw blade into the interspace between the base of the first and second metatarsals where the communicating artery passes (Fig. 8–24B and C).

4. The osteotomy site can be fixated with cerclage wire, small-fragment screws, or a plate. We find that two cerclage wires produce satisfactory immobilization. One of the pieces of wire passes through the bone in its corrected length to control the length of the metatarsal (Fig. 8–24D and E). Small-fragment screws can be used, but technically this is difficult, and at times the bone splinters. The use of a mini-fragment plate would seem ideal, but we found a significant nonunion rate.

5. An attempt is made to repair the periosteum over the metatarsal shaft, and the skin is closed in a routine manner. A snug compression dressing is applied for the initial 18 to 24 hours.

Postoperative Care

Postoperatively the dressing is changed to a firm 2-inch Kling and tape dressing. The patient ambulates in a postoperative shoe if the fixation is adequate, and if not, the patient is placed into a short-leg walking cast. Healing usually occurs in 8 weeks. Although at times it appears that the healing is proceeding very slowly, in reality, clinically the osteotomy site has healed (Fig. 8–25).

Results

Although we have not specifically reviewed our series of cases, we have noted that the main complication is a transfer lesion, which occurs in about 10% of cases. This is usually not because the metatarsal was shortened too much but because the distal fragment dorsiflexes several millimeters. Better internal fixation using two oblique screws can alleviate this problem.

A recent study by Kennedy and Deland[10] used this procedure in 32 consecutive patients. Twenty-two patients had a single osteotomy of the second metatarsal and 10 had an osteotomy of the second and third metatarsals. Pain was relieved in 31 of 32 patients, and there were no transfer lesions. The median time to radiographic union was 10 weeks. The authors pointed out that they carefully adjusted the metatarsal length radiographically, as well as carefully palpating the plantar aspect of the foot to judge whether or not the correct amount of shortening had been achieved. The mean radiographic shortening was 3.4 mm (range, 1 to 5 mm).

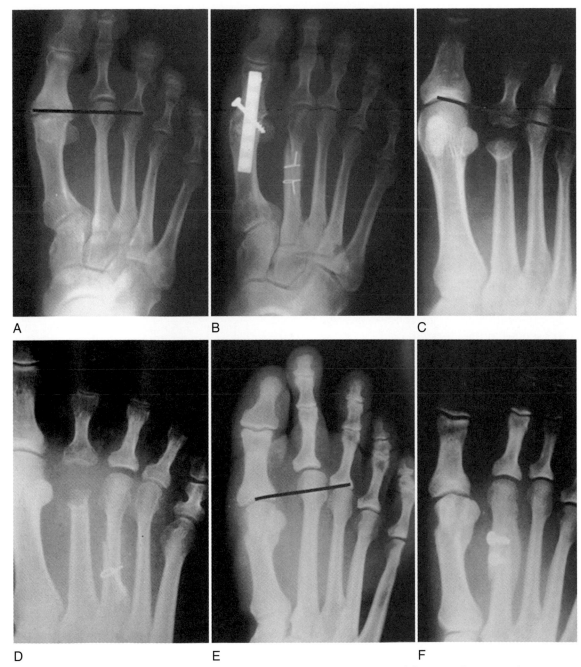

Figure 8–25 Preoperative **(A)** and postoperative **(B)** radiographs demonstrate shortening of the second metatarsal to create a smooth metatarsal arch. Preoperative **(C)** and postoperative **(D)** radiographs demonstrate shortening of the third metatarsal after resection of the second metatarsal head to create a smooth metatarsal pattern. Preoperative **(E)** and postoperative **(F)** radiographs demonstrate shortening of the second metatarsal by means of screw fixation.

DISTAL METATARSAL OSTEOTOMY (WEIL)

The usefulness of the distal metatarsal osteotomy (DMO) in the treatment of metatarsalgia has not been clarified in the literature.[16] Most of the articles that deal with the subject state that the DMO is used to reduce a subluxed or dislocated MTP joint, which, although producing metatarsalgia, might not result in an intractable plantar keratosis. Furthermore, the articles discussing this procedure do not say whether or not a keratotic lesion per se was present.[15,16] The DMO can produce shortening of up to about 1 cm, which would be useful in managing the patient with a diffuse IPK beneath the second metatarsal brought about by shortening of the first metatarsal. The DMO is also useful for a transfer metatarsalgia problem. Whether it would be useful for the treatment of the discrete IPK beneath the fibular condyle has yet to be presented in the literature.

The maximum shortening achieved by Kennedy and Deland[10] was 5 mm, which can be achieved by the DMO. Based upon our experience, we believe that up to 1 cm of shortening can be obtained with the DMO and may be preferred to the long oblique diaphyseal osteotomy in cases where a centimeter or less of shortening is necessary (video clip 37). The DMO can also be done on multiple metatarsals with less chance of producing elevation of one of the metatarsal heads as compared to the diaphyseal osteotomy.

BASAL METATARSAL OSTEOTOMY

The basal metatarsal osteotomy is used when a diffuse IPK is present and there is no metatarsal shortening. This condition usually occurs after previous metatarsal surgery or a fracture.

Surgical Technique

1. The skin incision is made over the dorsal aspect of the proximal half of the metatarsal and carried down through subcutaneous tissue and fat, with great caution taken to avoid the cutaneous nerves.
2. The dorsal aspect of the involved metatarsal is identified and an incision is made along the dorsal aspect of the metatarsal from about the midshaft area to the base. The periosteum is then stripped.
3. The site of the osteotomy should be just at the flare of the base of the metatarsal. If it is carried out much more proximal to this, the saw blade bounces off the adjacent metatarsals, and it is difficult to produce an accurate cut.
4. The size of the dorsally based wedge that is removed depends on the degree of depression of the metatarsal head. The involved metatarsal head usually needs to be elevated 2 to 4 mm, and thus the size of the base of the wedge should usually not exceed 2 to 3 mm. As the osteotomy is cut, an attempt is made to leave a plantar hinge intact.
5. We prefer to fix the osteotomy site by placing a 2.7-mm screw into the proximal portion of the base of the metatarsal, drilling a transverse hole distal to the osteotomy site, and then fixing these two points with a piece of 22-gauge wire. In this way the osteotomy site can be completely closed, with the metatarsal held in its precise position. There are other ways to fix the osteotomy site with a screw or pin, but we have found this technique to be the most reliable (Fig. 8–26).
6. The periosteum is closed, if possible, as is the skin. A compression dressing is applied.

Postoperative Care

The patient ambulates in a postoperative shoe until healing occurs in approximately 4 to 6 weeks. With the compression obtained by this method of fixation, we have had rapid healing of the osteotomy site and no nonunions. We have not tabulated our cases, but the postoperative incidence of transfer lesions is probably less than 5%, probably because in these cases, one can accurately produce the degree of dorsiflexion necessary to correct the problem. The only other potential problem with this procedure is entrapment of a dorsal cutaneous nerve, which can usually be avoided.

DORSIFLEXION OSTEOTOMY OF FIRST METATARSAL FOR PLANTAR-FLEXED FIRST METATARSAL

This procedure is described in Chapter 20.

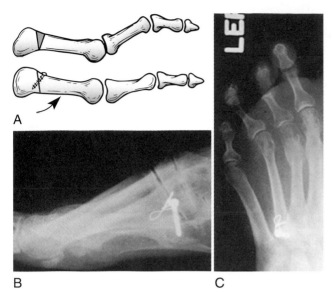

Figure 8–26 Technique of basal metatarsal osteotomy. **A,** Diagram demonstrates basal osteotomy in which a dorsally based wedge of bone is removed from the affected metatarsal. **B** and **C,** Radiographs demonstrate basal osteotomy with fixation done by using screw-and-wire tension band.

OTHER METATARSAL OSTEOTOMIES

Many types of osteotomies have been described for treating a plantar callus. Most authors have not attempted to define the type of callus (diffuse or discrete) that is being treated, as we have. The surgeon should attempt to apply the scientific method to the treatment of a plantar callus, carefully identifying the type of callus and then selecting a surgical procedure for the condition.

Helal[8] and Greiss[9] described a *distal oblique metatarsal osteotomy* of the three middle metatarsals to relieve metatarsalgia. In theory, the osteotomy permits the metatarsal head to slide proximally, and by early ambulation the "tread" would be leveled. In a follow-up study of this procedure, 77% of patients had good results. In a further follow-up study by Winson et al[18] of 94 patients (124 feet) who underwent this procedure, 53% had significant postoperative symptoms, including a nonunion rate of 13%, an incidence of transfer lesions of 32%, and a recurrence of the keratosis in 50% of patients. Multiple distal metatarsal osteotomies are not appropriate procedures and produce less than optimal results in the majority of patients.

Pedowitz,[15] using a distal oblique osteotomy and early ambulation for a single plantar callus of unspecified type, reported good results in 83% of patients. He did note a 25% incidence of either residual keratosis or transfer lesions. Treatment of a single IPK by resection of a metatarsal head should be avoided except when an infection or chronic ulcer has occurred. Resection of a metatarsal head only leads to significant problems, including development of a transfer lesion beneath an adjacent metatarsal head, shortening and contracture of the involved toe, and, in general, significantly more problems than are solved (Fig. 8–27).

When two adjacent metatarsals are significantly longer than the others, as is occasionally noted after significant shortening of the first metatarsal with a bunion procedure, shortening of the two metatarsals may be considered. As mentioned previously, if the three middle metatarsals are long because of a short first metatarsal, the problem should not be approached surgically. Osteotomies that allow the metatarsal heads to float or to level the tread should be discouraged (Fig. 8–28). Internal fixation to accurately elevate or shorten a metatarsal is important.

SUBHALLUX SESAMOID

At times a midline callus is present beneath the great toe at the level of the interphalangeal joint. This callus can become quite large and can occasionally even ulcerate. The callus is caused by a subhallux sesamoid, which is a sesamoid bone lying just dorsal to the flexor

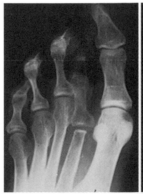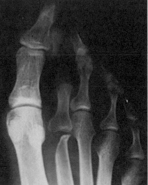

Figure 8–27 Resection of metatarsal head for intractable plantar keratosis should be avoided. After this procedure there is significant foreshortening of the toe, and a transfer lesion develops beneath the adjacent metatarsal head.

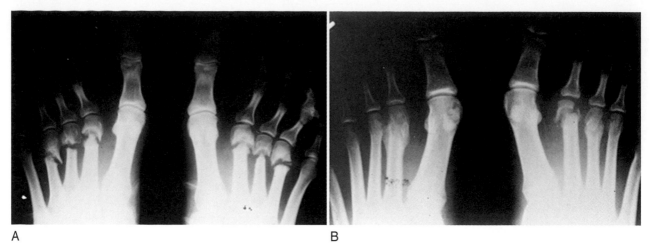

A   B

Figure 8–28 Complications after use of a high-speed bur to produce metatarsal osteotomies. **A,** Nonunions of six metatarsal necks. **B,** Radiograph of the left foot demonstrates abundance of new bone formation after the second metatarsal osteotomy. Radiograph of the right foot demonstrates nonunion through the second metatarsal head as well as joint involvement with osteotomy.

hallucis longus tendon before it inserts into the base of the distal phalanx. Radiographs demonstrate the sesamoid beneath the interphalangeal joint region (Fig. 8–29).

Conservative Treatment

Nonsurgical treatment involves placing a small felt pad just proximal to the lesion to keep the pressure off the callus area. If this fails, surgical intervention usually results in satisfactory resolution of the callus.

Surgical Treatment

REMOVAL OF SUBHALLUX SESAMOID

Surgical Technique

1. A longitudinal incision is made along the medial side of the hallux starting a little plantar to the midline. The incision starts at about the level of the MTP joint and is carried distally beyond the interphalangeal joint.
2. The skin flap is reflected plantarward, to the flexor tendon sheath, with some caution used because the plantar medial cutaneous nerve is in the plantar flap. The flexor hallu-

cis longus sheath is identified and opened to expose the flexor tendon up to its insertion into the base of the distal phalanx.
3. The flexor tendon is retracted plantarward, and the sesamoid is noted on the dorsal aspect of the tendon just before its insertion into the phalanx. The sesamoid is carefully shelled out, with care taken not to detach the tendon from its insertion.
4. The wound is closed in a single layer and a compression dressing is applied.

Postoperative Care

The patient ambulates in a postoperative shoe for approximately 3 weeks until the soft tissue has healed, after which activities are permitted as tolerated.

Results

The results after excision of a subhallux sesamoid are uniformly satisfactory. The callus rarely, if ever, reforms. The only possible significant complication would result from inadvertently detaching the flexor hallucis longus tendon when the sesamoid is excised. This can be avoided by careful surgical technique.

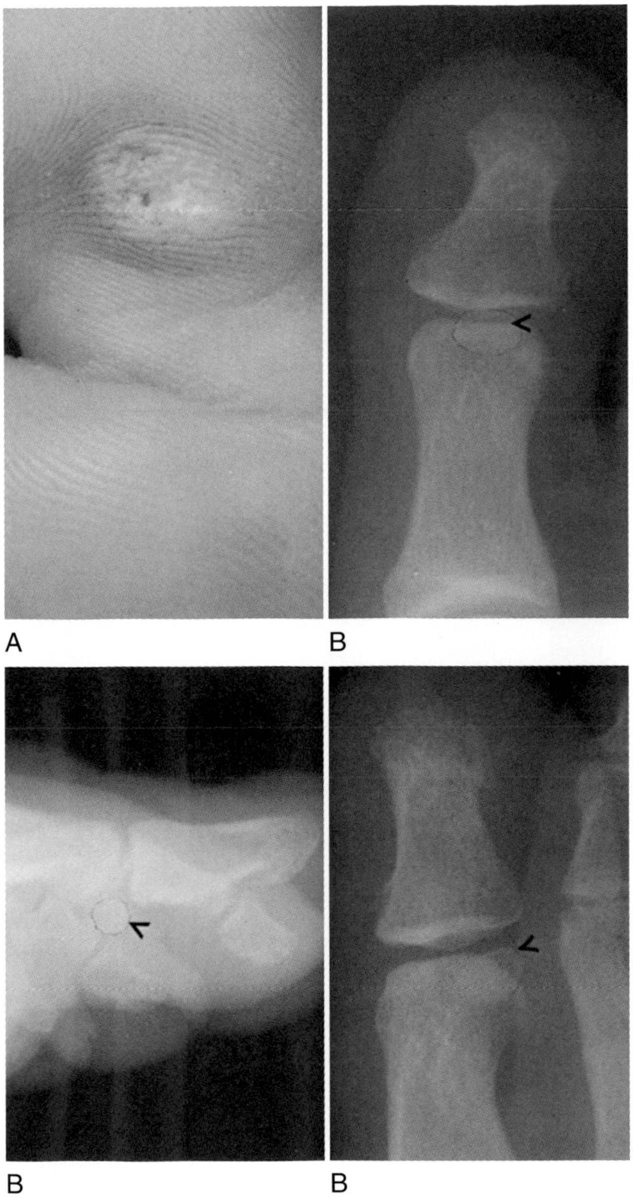

Figure 8–29 **A,** Subhallux sesamoid produces a midline callosity just proximal to the interphalangeal joint of the great toe. **B,** Radiographs demonstrate location of a subhallux sesamoid beneath the interphalangeal joint of great toe.

INTRACTABLE PLANTAR CALLUS ASSOCIATED WITH SIGNIFICANT SCAR TISSUE FORMATION

Occasionally a significant scar is present on the plantar aspect of the foot. This could result from burning of the plantar tissue by electrocautery, treatment of a wart with acid to produce a significant burn of the subdermal layers, radiation, or an infection. Under these circumstances, occasionally a painful keratotic lesion is present with little or no subcutaneous fat left to provide a cushion between the skin and metatarsal head (Fig. 8–30A).

Surgical Treatment

Despite frequent trimmings, these lesions present a significant disability for the patient. When such a problem occurs, an elliptical incision of the area, undermining of the surrounding tissue, and meticulous closure have been used to produce a satisfactory result.

SCAR EXCISION

Surgical Technique

1. The area to be excised is carefully mapped out. The criteria for the size of the lesion to be excised are based on attempting to reenter soft fatty tissue, which will provide an adequate cushion for the metatarsal region (Fig. 8–30B). A full-thickness ellipse of tissue is removed and all the scar tissue is excised (Fig. 8–30C).
2. The skin margins are undermined, and the skin is closed in layers.
3. The initial closure is carried out with 2-0 chromic suture placed in the subdermal layers to bring the skin edges together. Then a near-far/far-near stitch is used to support the skin edge by relieving tension on either side of it. After this, a fine running stitch is used to keep the skin edges in perfect apposition and minimize scar formation. A compression dressing is then applied (Fig. 8–30D).

Postoperative Care

The patient is kept non–weight bearing for approximately 4 weeks to allow the soft tissues to heal with minimal stress. Usually the sutures are left in place 2 to 3 weeks.

Results

Although this technique is used infrequently, the results have been satisfactory. Occasionally the patient develops a minor callosity along the area of the scar tissue, but the procedure usually significantly relieves the pain created by the previous scar tissue.

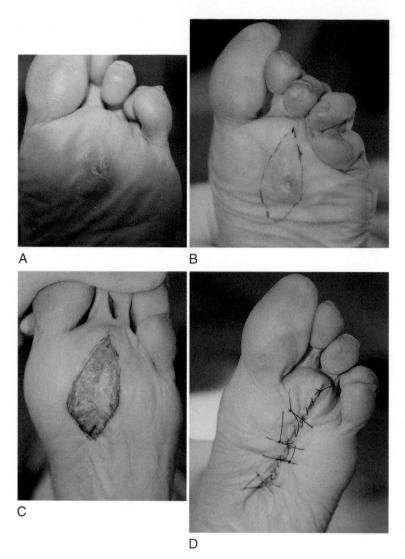

Figure 8–30 Surgical technique used to excise intractable plantar scar with callus formation. **A,** Keratotic scar. Note central hyperkeratotic lesion and surrounding adherent atrophic scar tissue. **B,** Outline of elliptic incision used to excise scar. **C,** Full-thickness removal of plantar skin, which is then undermined to mobilize it. **D,** Skin closure is carried out with retension sutures, a subdermal layer to minimize tension on the skin edge, and a fine, running cutaneous stitch to minimize scar formation.

SCARS ON THE PLANTAR ASPECT OF THE FOOT

Although plantar incisions for excision of an interdigital neuroma, procedures on the metatarsal head, and excision of the fibular sesamoid have been advocated in the literature, if an alternative incision is possible, it is preferable. Most plantar incisions heal benignly, but if a hypertrophic scar forms or the surrounding soft tissue atrophies, it can lead to an unsolvable problem. Most foot surgery can be carried out through a dorsal approach, and we strongly advise this, if possible. The fibular sesamoid can be removed through a dorsal incision in the first web space, which is preferable to the plantar incision. Interdigital neuromas and even recurrent neuromas can be removed through dorsal incisions rather than the plantar approach. At times the skin incision heals benignly, but the underlying fatty tissue unfortunately atrophies over a short period

and leaves the patient with inadequate cushioning on the plantar aspect of the foot (Fig. 8–31).

If a plantar incision is used, the incision must be placed between the metatarsal heads to avoid a scar directly under a metatarsal.

HYPERTROPHIC PLANTAR SKIN

Some patients have hyperkeratotic skin, and these patients might not respond to removal of a bony prominence. This is not because the procedure was done incorrectly but because the patient has some type of a congenital skin disorder. Although the pressure has been relieved on the skin, the hyperkeratotic lesion might remain. The clinician should carefully examine the feet of the patient with a keratotic lesion to be sure this condition is not present (Fig. 8–32).

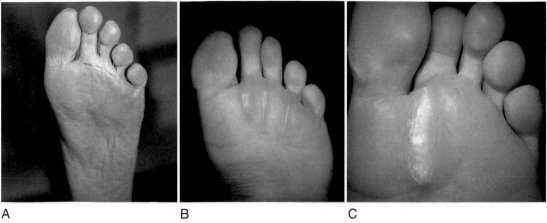

A   B   C

Figure 8–31 Painful plantar scars. **A** and **B,** Incisions that have been used to excise an interdigital neuroma. Unfortunately these scars often become quite painful, sometimes from keratoses along the scar and at other times from atrophy of the fat pad. These problems make it difficult for the patient to ambulate comfortably. **C,** Hypertrophic scar after plantar incision to remove a fibular sesamoid. There is no good remedy for this situation.

OSTEOCHONDROSIS OF A METATARSAL HEAD

Osteochondrosis of a metatarsal head (Freiberg's infraction) most often occurs in the second metatarsal head in adolescents and is most likely the result of an ischemic necrosis of the epiphysis. It is seen more often in girls.

The clinical complaint is usually pain and limitation of motion of the affected joint. The symptom complex is aggravated by activities and often relieved by rest. Physical examination demonstrates generalized thickening about the second MTP joint secondary to the synovitis. There is often some increased warmth. The joint demonstrates restricted motion secondary to pain.

Diagnosis

The diagnosis is confirmed by radiographs demonstrating osteosclerosis in the early stages and osteolysis with collapse in the later stages. At times in the early stages a central collapse is noted, and as the condition burns out, significant collapse often occurs with new bone formation (Fig. 8–33).

Treatment

Treatment is directed initially toward protection and the alleviation of discomfort. Early in the course of the disease, particularly if no significant distortion of the head has occurred, a short-leg walking cast or a stiff postoperative shoe to decrease the stress across the involved joint is indicated. As the disease process progresses or if the patient is seen after the acute phase has passed and the main problem is that of increased bone formation and restricted motion, surgical intervention may be of benefit. Surgery consists of debridement of the joint and excision of the proliferative bone (video clip 38).

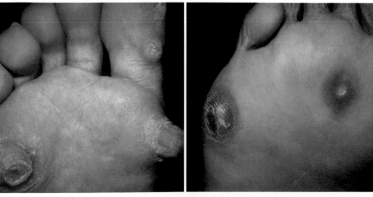

Figure 8–32 Examples of feet with hyperkeratotic skin.

A   B

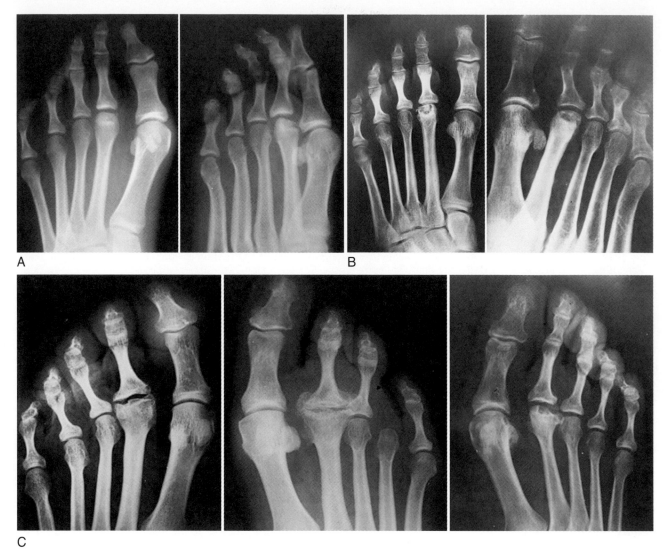

Figure 8–33 Radiographs of Freiberg's infraction. **A,** Early stages demonstrate osteolysis and central collapse. **B,** Later stages of Freiberg's infraction demonstrate central collapse and osteolysis.

EXCISION OF PROLIFERATIVE BONE

Surgical Technique

1. The joint is approached through a hockey stick–shaped incision starting in the second web space. The incision is carried obliquely across the metatarsal head and over the dorsal aspect of the metatarsal shaft (Fig. 8–34A).
2. The incision is deepened to expose the extensor tendons, which are split to enable one to dissect the extensor hood off the underlying synovial tissue. By sharp dissection, the synovial tissue is removed and the joint is inspected (Fig. 8–34B).
3. If proliferative bone is present around the metatarsal head, it is generally removed, similar to the procedure for cheilectomy to treat hallux rigidus. The mediolateral bone is removed in line with the sides of the metatarsal, and the dorsal 20% to 30% of the metatarsal head is resected (Fig. 8–34C and D). If necessary, new bone that has formed around the base of the proximal phalanx is excised, although this occurs infrequently.
4. At this time approximately 75 to 80 degrees of dorsiflexion should be possible at the MTP joint. If this has not been achieved, more bone probably needs to be resected.
5. The extensor mechanism is closed, the skin is closed in a single layer, and a compression dressing is applied.

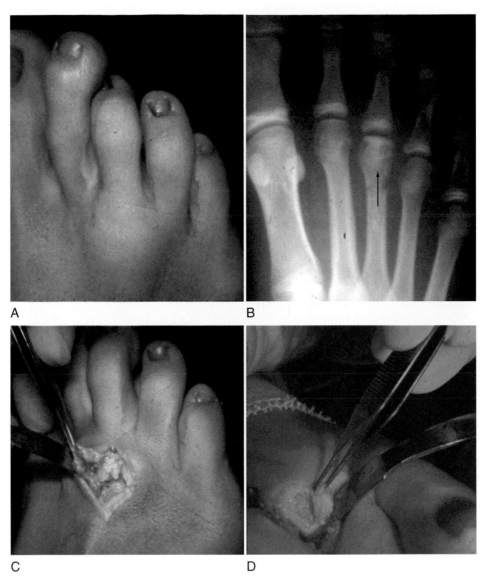

Figure 8–34 Surgical technique for debridement of Freiberg's infraction. Clinical photo **(A)** and radiograph **(B)** showing huge osteophyte formation *(arrow)* at the third metatarsophalangeal joint. **C,** Operative exposure. **D,** Removal of distal free fragment.

Postoperative Care

The patient is maintained in a firm dressing and postoperative shoe for approximately 10 days, until the wound has healed. The patient is then started on active and passive range-of-motion exercises to gain as much motion as possible.

Results

With this technique, satisfactory symptomatic relief can usually be achieved. In general, the patient will not regain as much active motion, but passively the MTP joint has sufficient flexibility that satisfactory function of the foot can be restored.

Although some have advocated excision of the metatarsal head or replacement with a prosthesis, we do not believe this procedure is indicated for this condition.

At times the only problem is a loose fragment, and this can be debrided without the necessity of excising any other bone.

REFERENCES

1. Coughlin MJ: Personal communication, Boise, Idaho, 1990.
2. Dreeben SM, Noble PC, Hammerman S, et al: Metatarsal osteotomy for primary metatarsalgia: Radiographic and pedobarographic study. *Foot Ankle* 9:214-218, 1989.
3. DuVries HL: Disorders of the skin. In DuVries HL (ed): *Surgery of the Foot*, ed 2. St Louis, Mosby, 1965, pp 168-169.
4. DuVries HL: New approach to the treatment of intractable verruca plantaris (plantar wart). *JAMA* 152:1202-1203, 1953.
5. DuVries HL (ed): *Surgery of the Foot*, ed 2. St Louis, Mosby, 1965, pp 456-462.
6. Giannestras NJ: Shortening of the metatarsal shaft in the treatment of plantar keratosis. *J Bone Joint Surg* 49:61-71, 1958.
7. Harris RI, Beath T: The short first metatarsal: Its incidence and clinical significance. *J Bone Joint Surg* 31:553, 1949.
8. Helal B: Metatarsal osteotomy for metatarsalgia. *J Bone Joint Surg Br* 57:187-192, 1975.
9. Helal B, Greiss M: Telescoping osteotomy for pressure metatarsalgia. *J Bone Joint Surg Br* 66:213-217, 1984.
10. Kennedy JG, Deland JT: Resolution of plantar pain following oblique osteotomy for central metatarsalgia; *in press*.
11. Kitaoka HB, Patzer GL: Chevron osteotomy of lesser metatarsals for intractable plantar callosities. *J Bone Joint Surg Br* 80B(3):526-518, 1998.
12. Mann RA, Coughlin MJ: Intractable plantar keratosis. In Mann RA, Coughlin MJ (eds): *Video Textbook of Foot and Ankle Surgery.* St Louis, Medical Video Productions, 1991.
13. Mann RA, DuVries MD: Intractable plantar keratosis. *Orthop Clin North Am* 4:67-73, 1973.
14. Mann RA, Wapner K: Tibial sesamoid shaving for treatment of intractable plantar keratosis under the tibial sesamoid. *Foot Ankle* 13:196-198, 1992.
15. Pedowitz WJ: Distal oblique osteotomy for intractable plantar keratosis of the middle three metatarsals. *Foot Ankle* 9:7-9, 1988.
16. Vandeputte G, Dereymaeker G, Steenwerckx A, Peeraer L: The Weil osteotomy of the lesser metatarsals: A clinical and pedobarographic follow-up study. *Foot Ankle Int* 21(5):370-374, 2000.
17. Weil LS: Weil head–neck oblique osteotomy: Technique and fixation. Presented at Techniques of Osteotomies of the Forefoot, Bordeaux (France), October 20-22, 1994.
18. Winson IG, Rawlinson J, Broughton NS: Treatment of metatarsalgia by sliding distal metatarsal osteotomy. *Foot Ankle* 9:2-6, 1988.

Bunionettes

Michael J. Coughlin • Brett R. Grebing

A bunionette deformity, or tailor's bunion, is characterized by a painful prominence of the lateral eminence of the fifth metatarsal head. Davies[12] observed that pressure over the lateral condyle of the fifth metatarsal head led to chronic irritation of the overlying bursa. The position of a tailor sitting in a cross-legged position has given rise to the term *tailor's bunion*.[62] Friction between an underlying bony prominence and constricting footwear can lead to the development of a keratosis over the lateral aspect[18,27,36] (Fig. 9–1A) or the plantar lateral aspect[25] of the fifth metatarsal head (Fig. 9–1B, Fig. 9–2A). The fifth toe deviates in a medial direction at the fifth metatarsophalangeal (MTP) joint (Fig. 9–2B) and the fifth metatarsal deviates laterally with respect to the fourth metatarsal.

ANATOMY

Kelikian[29] described a prominent fifth metatarsal lateral eminence of a bunionette deformity as being "analogous to the medial eminence of the first metatarsal head" in a hallux valgus deformity. DuVries[18] described several anatomic variations in the fifth metatarsal head that can lead to a symptomatic bunionette. Thus the etiology and anatomic variations that occur with a bunionette deformity are much more complex than what was originally described by Kelikian[29] and Davies.[12] Although painful symptoms can be localized to the fifth MTP joint region, an abnormal alignment of the fifth metatarsal may be associated with a bunionette deformity.

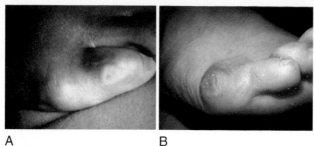

Figure 9–1 A, Lateral keratosis combined with lateral fifth toe corn. **B,** Plantar lateral keratosis overlying the fifth metatarsal head. This is the most common presentation of a symptomatic bunionette.

Recognition of the specific anatomic variation present is important in the preoperative evaluation and can influence the specific procedure chosen to correct the bunionette deformity. The radiographic analysis of a bunionette deformity is important in defining the magnitude and type of abnormality present.

CLINICAL SYMPTOMS

The major subjective complaints of a patient with a symptomatic bunionette deformity are pain and irritation caused by friction between constricting footwear and an underlying bony abnormality. On physical examination an inflamed bursa,[25,57,58] a lateral keratosis (see Fig. 9–1),[16] a plantar keratosis (see Fig. 9–2),[24,25,42] or a combined plantar lateral keratosis[16,27]

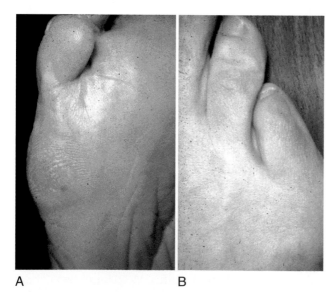

Figure 9–2 A, Plantar keratosis associated with bunionette deformity. **B,** Abduction deformity of the fifth toe.

may be present. Diebold and Bejjani[16] noted that two thirds of the patients in their series had significant pes planus. They reported that a third of the patients in their series developed a plantar keratosis, whereas half had a lateral keratotic lesion. The remaining had a combined plantar and lateral keratosis. Coughlin[10] noted that 10% of the patients in his series had developed a plantar keratosis, 70% had developed a lateral keratosis, and 20% had developed a combined plantar and lateral keratosis.

In general, a bunionette is a static deformity. Repeated activities such as running or jogging can lead to thickening or inflammation of the overlying bursa.

PHYSICAL EXAMINATION

The examination of the patient with a symptomatic bunionette is performed with the patient sitting and standing. The presence of pes planus, an Achilles tendon contracture, or other forefoot abnormalities must be recognized and treated appropriately if they are symptomatic. A key to preoperative planning is the recognition of a plantar keratosis in combination with a lateral keratosis because this differentiation can affect the choice of surgical procedure. In examining the bunionette deformity, an abducted fifth toe, as well as a digital rotational component to the axial deformity, must be recognized. A hammer toe deformity of the fifth toe might also be present. A bunionette can develop as an isolated deformity, but it can also develop in combination with a hallux valgus deformity. An increased angle between the fourth and fifth metatarsals (4-5 intermetatarsal angle), in combination with an increased angle between the first and second metatarsals, results in a very wide splayed-foot abnormality.[2,12,25,28,54] Likewise, the need for other forefoot surgical procedures affects the ambulatory capacity of a patient and must be considered as well. A neurovascular examination is important for determining the suitability of the patient for surgical correction.

DIAGNOSTIC AND RADIOGRAPHIC EXAMINATION

Radiographic evaluation of a symptomatic bunionette deformity includes standing anteroposterior (AP) and lateral radiographs. The significant angular measurements that define a bunionette deformity are the angle of the fifth metatarsophalangeal joint (MTP-5 angle) (Fig. 9–3) and the 4-5 intermetatarsal angle. The MTP-5 angle allows one to calculate the magnitude of medial deviation of the fifth toe in relation to the longitudinal axis of the fifth metatarsal shaft. Nestor et al[44]

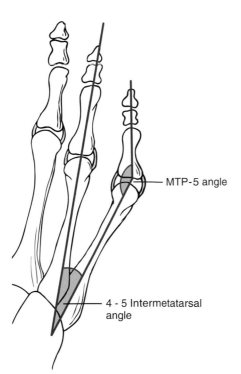

Figure 9–3 The metatarsophalangeal-5 (MTP-5) angle and the 4-5 intermetatarsal angle. The MTP-5 angle is that subtended by the axis of the proximal phalanx and fifth metatarsal. The 4-5 intermetatarsal angle is that subtended by the intersecting axis of the fourth and fifth metatarsals.

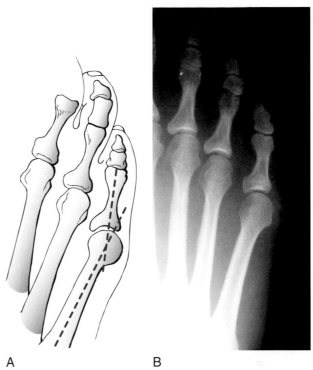

A   B

Figure 9–4 Type 1 bunionette deformity is characterized by an enlarged fifth metatarsal head.

reported that in normal feet the MTP-5 angle averaged 10.2 degrees, and Steele et al[55] noted that in 90% of normal cases, the angle was 14 degrees or less. Nestor et al[44] and Coughlin[10] have reported that in feet with bunionettes the MTP-5 angle averaged 16 degrees.

The 4-5 intermetatarsal angle is a measure of the divergence of the fourth and fifth metatarsals and is the angle measured by the intersection of lines bisecting the axis of the fourth and fifth metatarsals.[50] Divergence of the fourth and fifth metatarsals leads to pressure over the lateral eminence of the fifth metatarsal head.[14,28,33] Fallat and Buckholz[20] stated that the 4-5 intermetatarsal angle in normal feet averaged 6.2 degrees (range, 3 to 11 degrees). Although some[2,3,19,28,50] have noted that a 4-5 intermetatarsal angle greater than 8 degrees can be considered abnormal, Fallat[20] and Coughlin[10] have reported the 4-5 intermetatarsal angle on average to be greater than 9 degrees. In general, however, angular measurements serve only to describe a bunionette deformity; it is the symptoms and not the magnitude of deformity that necessitates specific surgical treatment.

A prominent lateral condyle of the fifth metatarsal head can lead to a type 1 bunionette deformity (Fig. 9–4).[18,20,57] Hypertrophy of the lateral condyle has been reported by DuVries[18] and others.[20,58,59] The inci-

dence of a type 1 deformity is reported to vary in incidence from 16 to 33%.[3,10,34] Zvijac et al[62] noted a variance in width of the fifth metatarsal from 11 mm at the smallest to 14 mm at the widest, and Fallat[20] stated that the normal width of the fifth metatarsal head was 13 mm. Throckmorton and Bradlee[58] and Fallat and Buckholz[20] both reported that with excessive pronation of the foot, the lateral plantar tubercle of the fifth metatarsal head rotated laterally to create the radiographic impression of an enlarged fifth metatarsal head. Fallat and Buckholz[20] also reported a 3-degree increase in the 4-5 intermetatarsal angle in the presence of a pes planus deformity. Whether true hypertrophy of the fifth metatarsal head occurs or prominence of the fifth metatarsal head results from pronation of the foot, a prominent lateral condyle of the fifth metatarsal head can become symptomatic without an increase in the 4-5 intermetatarsal angle.

Lateral bowing of the diaphysis of the fifth metatarsal shaft can lead to the development of a symptomatic prominence of the lateral condyle of the fifth metatarsal head[3,7,18-20,41,61] and is classified as a type 2 bunionette deformity (Fig. 9–5). Although the proximal fifth metatarsal shaft maintains a normal intermetatarsal alignment, a lateral curvature develops in the diaphysis of the fifth metatarsal that leads to a

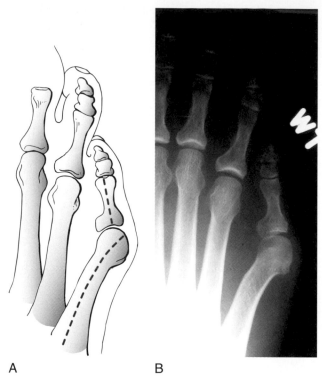

A   B

Figure 9–5 Type 2 bunionette deformity is characterized by lateral bowing of the fifth metatarsal head.

symptomatic bunionette deformity. A prominent lateral condyle of the fifth metatarsal head can also be caused by divergence of the fourth and fifth metatarsals, which is classified as a type 3 bunionette deformity (Fig. 9–6).

Kitaoka et al[33] in evaluating a series of patients with a symptomatic bunionette deformity, reported that an increase in the 4-5 intermetatarsal angle was most often associated with a symptomatic bunionette deformity. Fifth metatarsal bowing or an enlarged fifth metatarsal head was observed to be a cause in less than 10% of these cases, but Coughlin[10] noted the incidence of lateral bowing of the fifth metatarsal to be 23%.

Koti[35] has suggested an additional type that involves two or more components of the other three types. This adds unnecessary complexity and does not aid in defining a treatment plan.

Regardless of the underlying MTP joint orientation and fifth metatarsal angulation, the common symptom in all patients with a bunionette deformity is increased pressure over the lateral aspect of the fifth metatarsal head caused by constricting footwear. The female-to-male ratio is reported to vary from 3:1 to 10:1[5,7,22,44] in series of patients with symptomatic bunionettes that required surgical intervention. The increased frequency of occurrence of a bunionette deformity in the female population is most likely

attributable to their predilection for high-fashion footwear. With time, the development of a hypertrophic keratosis or a thickened bursa can lead to increased symptoms.

Harris mat studies can help in the assessment of increased pressure beneath a symptomatic fifth metatarsal head in association with a plantar keratosis (Fig. 9–7).

TREATMENT

Conservative Treatment

It is important for a patient to recognize that the use of constricting footwear is a significant cause of symptoms and places increased pressure on a prominent fifth metatarsal head.[11] Chronic irritation, pain, and swelling of the bursa overlying the fifth metatarsal head can be reduced by roomy, well-fitted shoes (Fig. 9–8).[12,29,36]

Shaving of a hypertrophic callus and padding of a prominent fifth metatarsal head[44] can reduce symptoms significantly. A prefabricated or custom orthotic device may be used to diminish pronation and as a result reduce discomfort over a prominent fifth metatarsal head (see Chapter 4) (Fig. 9–9).

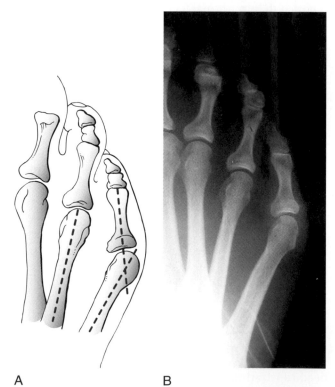

A   B

Figure 9–6 Type 3 bunionette deformity is characterized by an abnormally wide 4-5 intermetatarsal angle.

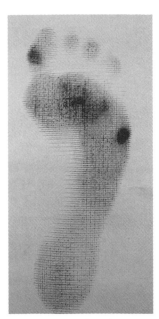

Figure 9–7 Harris mat study demonstrating increased plantar pressure beneath the fifth metatarsal head.

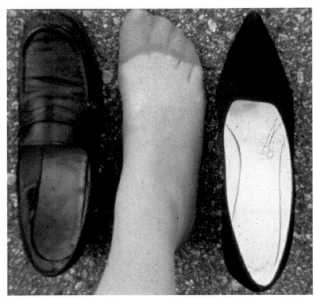

Figure 9–8 Constricting shoe *(right)* compared with roomy shoe *(left)*.

Conservative methods can be effective in a large number of patients. However, as painful plantar and lateral keratoses develop, surgical intervention may be necessary to relieve symptoms (Fig. 9–10). Various reported techniques are presented in this section. Preferred surgical methods are noted and discussed later in the chapter.

Surgical Treatment

Preoperative Evaluation

The preoperative evaluation of a patient with a painful bunionette begins with a comprehensive history and physical examination. An AP weight-bearing radiograph typically demonstrates the characteristics of the deformity, but it also helps the surgeon to assess the status of the MTP joint. Pain and swelling of the fifth MTP joint can be caused by degenerative or inflammatory arthritis. Laboratory evaluation is occasionally helpful in diagnosing such underlying causes as gout, early rheumatoid arthritis, and infection or cellulitis.

The presence of a concomitant hammer toe deformity or a sagittal plane deformity of the MTP joint requires treatment with the correction of the bunionette.

Assessment of both the circulatory status of the involved extremity as well as the neurologic status is important, especially in those with early peripheral vascular disease, diabetes, or neuropathy. Although surgery is not necessarily contraindicated, adequate protective sensation and adequate peripheral circulation are necessary for successful healing.

Preoperative Planning

The preoperative assessment determines the underlying cause of symptoms in the patient with a painful bunionette. Likewise, the radiographic findings help to

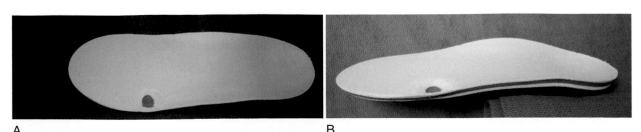

A   B

Figure 9–9 Conservative treatment may consist of relieving pressure beneath the fifth metatarsal head. **A** and **B,** Orthotics can be successful in alleviating symptoms.

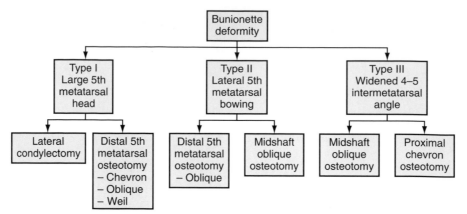

Figure 9–10 Algorithm for treatment of bunionette deformities.

determine the preferred surgical technique. A plantar–lateral callosity requires a surgical correction that reduces the size of the lateral eminence as well as elevating the fifth metatarsal head. The radiographic findings of a mild deformity or mainly an enlarged fifth metatarsal head make a distal fifth metatarsal osteotomy a feasible alternative. A moderate or severe deformity—typically a curved fifth metatarsal shaft or a widened 4-5 intermetatarsal angle—makes a midshaft diaphyseal osteotomy preferable. Thus, a careful correlation of the physical findings and radiologic information allow the physician to select the appropriate surgical procedure with which to correct a bunionette deformity.

Surgical Techniques

Numerous surgical techniques have been described to correct a symptomatic bunionette deformity. These include lateral condylectomy,* fifth metatarsal head resection,[†] fifth metatarsal implant arthoplasty,[1] fifth ray resection,[4] distal metatarsal osteotomy,[‡] diaphyseal osteotomy,[§] and proximal fifth metatarsal osteotomy.[¶] Correction of the underlying disorder is necessary for preventing a recurrence of deformity. Likewise, preservation of the function of the fifth MTP joint can prevent such complications as recurrence, subluxation, dislocation, or development of a transfer lesion.

---

*References 14, 18, 24, 35, 37, 41, and 57.
†References 17, 29, 31, 42, and 60.
‡References 3, 6, 7, 8, 13, 14, 25, 26, 28, 32, 33, 34, 43, 51, 54, 56, and 62.
§References 9, 10, 22, 23, 27, 39, and 59.
¶References 2, 15, 16, 20, 27, 38, 45, and 47.

LATERAL CONDYLECTOMY

With an isolated enlargement of the fifth metatarsal head or a prominent fifth metatarsal lateral condyle without an increased 4-5 intermetatarsal angle, a lateral condylectomy may be performed. The presence of pes planus or a pronated fifth ray is not necessarily a contraindication to a lateral condylectomy if the prominent lateral condyle is the only deformity present.

Indications

The main indication for a lateral condylectomy is an enlarged lateral condyle. In this situation a condylectomy can produce an adequate repair, although a distal metatarsal osteotomy might still be the procedure of choice. A second indication is for the treatment of localized infection overlying the lateral fifth metatarsal head.[35] Although lateral condylectomy might not achieve MTP joint realignment, it might alleviate the acute or chronic infection.

Contraindications

Preoperative radiographs are important in the evaluation of a bunionette deformity. With lateral angulation of the fifth metatarsal shaft in relationship to the fourth metatarsal shaft (increased 4-5 intermetatarsal angle; type 3 deformity) or with lateral bowing of the fifth metatarsal shaft (type 2 deformity), a condylectomy does not effectively reduce a prominent fifth metatarsal lateral eminence. With an enlarged 4-5 intermetatarsal angle, a fifth metatarsal osteotomy is necessary to correct this divergence.[38]

The significant recurrence rate after lateral condylectomy is attributable to the use of a lateral condylectomy when a fifth metatarsal osteotomy is indicated. Kelikian[29] noted that "at best a lateral condylectomy is a temporizing measure like simple exostectomy on the medial side of the foot; in time deformity will recur."

Surgical Technique

1. The patient is positioned in a semilateral decubitus position.
2. The extremity is cleansed in a normal fashion.

3. A longitudinal skin incision is centered over the lateral condyle of the fifth metatarsal head and extends from the interphalangeal joint to 1 cm proximal to the fifth metatarsal condyle. The dorsal cutaneous nerve of the fifth toe is protected (Fig. 9–11A and B).
4. An inverted-L capsular incision is used to detach the dorsal and proximal fifth metatarsal capsule. The weakest portion of the capsule is detached, and the strongest capsular attachments to the proximal phalanx and plantar capsule are maintained (Fig. 9–11C and D).
5. A sagittal saw (or osteotome) is used to resect the lateral condyle of the fifth metatarsal head (Fig. 9–11E-G).

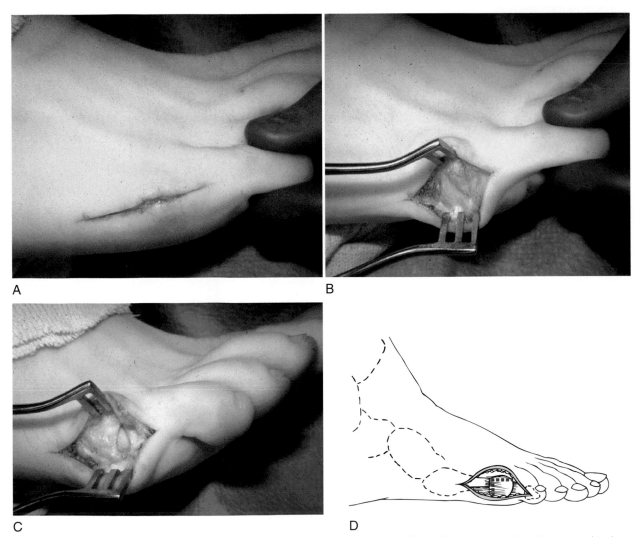

A

B

C

D

Figure 9–11 Lateral condylectomy. **A,** Skin incision. **B,** Capsular exposure. **C,** Elliptical capsular incision. **D,** Inverted L-shaped capsular incision is used to expose the fifth metatarsal head. Dorsal and proximal capsule, the weakest area of capsular attachment, is released, and the stronger plantar and distal attachments are left intact. *Continued*

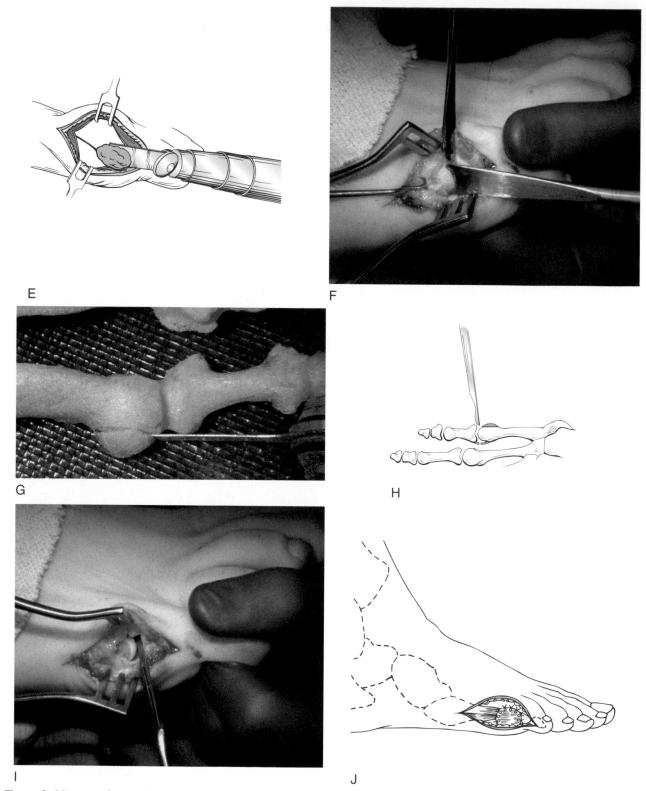

Figure 9–11—cont'd **E** and **F,** Lateral condyle is resected in line with the shaft of the fifth metatarsal. **G,** Sawbone model used to demonstrate condylar excision. **H** and **I,** Medial capsule is released by distracting the toe and cutting the medial capsule. **J,** Lateral capsule is reefed with interrupted absorbable sutures. The proximal capsule is reefed to the abductor digiti quinti muscle, and the dorsal capsule is approximated to the dorsal periosteum. (Where insufficient tissue is present, drill holes may be placed into the metaphysis of the fifth metatarsal to secure this capsular repair.)

6. The fifth metatarsal head is exposed, and with traction placed on the fifth toe, the MTP joint is distracted and the medial capsule is released with a scalpel (Fig. 9–11H and I).

7. The MTP capsule is closed by approximating it to the fifth MTP metatarsal metaphyseal periosteum and to the abductor digiti quinti muscle proximally (Fig. 9–11J). (For improved fixation, a drill hole in the fifth metatarsal dorsolateral metaphysis may be used to anchor the capsule repair.) A meticulous capsule repair is necessary to prevent recurrence of the deformity or lateral subluxation of the MTP joint.

8. The skin is closed routinely, and a compression dressing is applied.

Postoperative Care

A gauze-and-tape compression dressing is applied at surgery and is changed weekly for 6 weeks. The patient is allowed to ambulate in a postoperative shoe for 3 weeks and in a sandal for 3 weeks. Skin sutures are removed 3 weeks after surgery.

Results and Complications

Although this procedure has been frequently recommended for the repair of a bunionette deformity,* in general, only anecdotal follow-up has been published for series using a lateral condylectomy. Reported postoperative complications include subluxation of the MTP joint,[27,40,54] recurrence of deformity (Fig. 9–12),[†] and poor weight bearing with excessive resection.[36]

Kitaoka and Holiday[30] reported on 16 patients (21 feet) who had undergone a lateral condylar resection for a symptomatic bunionette (average follow-up, 6.4 years). Seventy-one percent of the patients were satisfied with their result. Twenty-three percent reported some element of forefoot pain, although half these patients considered it mild. The average preoperative 4-5 intermetatarsal angle measured 12.3 degrees and postoperatively it measured 11.1 degrees, for an average correction of 1.2

*References 12, 14, 18, 24, 35, 37, 40, and 42.
†References 25, 29, 36, 37, 42, 54, and 61.

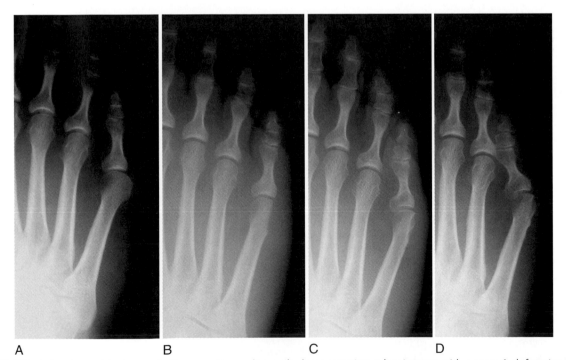

A   B   C   D

Figure 9–12 Lateral condylectomy. **A,** Preoperative radiograph demonstrating a bunionette with a type 1 deformity. **B,** After lateral condylectomy, adequate correction is achieved. **C,** Recurrence of deformity after 1 year. **D,** Recurrence of deformity after 10 years.

degrees. Much of this correction can be accounted for by the measurement techniques. The metatarsal-5 angle averaged 17.0 degrees preoperatively and 14.6 degrees postoperatively. This correction was not significant on statistical analysis. Furthermore, the authors concluded that no correlation existed between the amount of correction and the level of patient satisfaction. In two feet the MTP joint subluxated postoperatively as the fifth toe displaced medially. A tight capsule closure with excision of redundant MTP joint capsule was recommended to minimize this postoperative complication. The authors also concluded that although only a limited degree of correction of the deformity was possible with this procedure, a lateral condylectomy was often successful in relieving symptoms. No transfer lesions were reported in this series. With an intractable plantar keratotic lesion beneath the fifth metatarsal head, the authors believed that a simple condylectomy was contraindicated. Although a lateral condylar resection is a simple treatment for a bunionette deformity, the authors recognized the significant limitations of the procedure.

A meticulous fifth metatarsal capsule repair can prevent subluxation and recurrence of a bunionette deformity.[40,54] Attention to repair of the abductor digiti quinti muscle and fifth metatarsal capsule can prevent later dislocation of the MTP joint.[27]

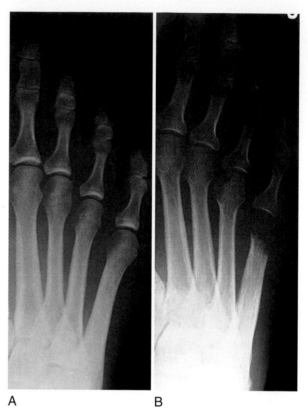

A   B

Figure 9–13 Fifth metatarsal head resection. **A,** Preoperative radiograph of 55-year-old man with diabetes and intractable ulceration beneath the fifth metatarsal head. **B,** Postoperative radiograph after fifth metatarsal head excision with successful healing of lesion.

FIFTH METATARSAL HEAD RESECTION

The failure of a lateral condylectomy as an effective treatment of a bunionette deformity has resulted in the recommendation for more extensive resection procedures. Excision of the fifth metatarsal head (Fig. 9–13),[1,17,18,31] resection of the distal half of the fifth metatarsal (Fig. 9–14),[42] and fifth ray resection (Fig. 9–15)[4] have all been advocated as treatment for a symptomatic bunionette deformity. McKeever[42] advocated excision of the fifth metatarsal head and one half to two thirds of the fifth metatarsal shaft; Brown[4] found that resection of almost the entire fifth ray and a fifth toe amputation adequately narrowed the foot and relieved symptoms. Kelikian[29]

recommended McKeever's technique but syndactylized the fourth and fifth toes to avoid a symptomatic flail fifth toe deformity.

Indications

Ray resection, extensive fifth metatarsal diaphyseal resection, and fifth metatarsal head resection should be reserved as a salvage procedure for intractable ulceration, severe deformity, and infection, as well as in rheumatoid arthritis when multiple metatarsal head resections are performed. Fifth metatarsal head resection may also be considered in the presence of recurrent deformity with a significant soft tissue contracture.

Contraindications

As a primary procedure in the treatment of a bunionette deformity, less radical procedures that preserve function of the fifth ray should be

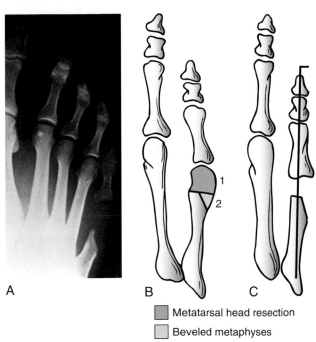

■ Metatarsal head resection

□ Beveled metaphyses

Figure 9–14 A, Fifth metatarsal head excision with resection of the distal half of the fifth metatarsal (McKeever technique) after osteomyelitis. **B,** Dorsal view of osteotomy of the fifth metatarsal. Shading denotes both resection and beveling necessary after osteotomy is performed. **C,** Intramedullary Kirschner wire fixation may be used to stabilize toe if neither infection nor plantar ulceration is present.

considered instead of resection arthroplasty. Implant arthroplasty is to be discouraged at the fifth MTP joint. No evidence indicates that it offers improved postoperative function over resection arthroplasty, and on occasion significant complications are associated with this procedure.

Surgical Technique

1. The patient is positioned in a semilateral decubitus position.
2. The extremity is cleansed in a normal fashion.
3. A longitudinal incision is centered over the lateral eminence, extending from the mid portion of the proximal phalanx to 1 cm above the lateral eminence. (With plantar ulceration, a dorsal incision may be used. With rheumatoid arthritis when multiple metatarsal heads are excised, a longitudinal intermetatarsal incision may be placed in the fourth intermetatarsal space.)

4. The capsular structures are released, and the fifth metatarsal head is exposed.
5. The fifth metatarsal shaft is transected in the metaphyseal region with a sagittal saw or a bone-cutting forceps (see Fig. 9-14A and B).
6. The prominent lateral and plantar aspects of the metatarsal shafts are beveled with a rongeur.
7. A 0.045-inch Kirschner wire is introduced at the base of the proximal phalanx and driven distally through the tip of the toe (see Fig. 9-14C). It is then driven in a retrograde manner into the metatarsal diaphysis to align and stabilize the fifth toe. With plantar ulceration or infection, Kirschner wire stabilization is contraindicated.
8. The capsule is plicated with interrupted absorbable suture. The skin edges are approximated in a routine manner.

Postoperative Care

A gauze-and-tape compression dressing is used for alignment of the fifth toe and changed weekly for 6 weeks. Ambulation is permitted in a postoperative shoe. Sutures and the Kirschner wire are removed 3 weeks after surgery.

Results and Complications

Although fifth metatarsal head resection has been recommended for treating a symptomatic bunionette deformity, in general only anecdotal experience has been reported. McKeever[42] reported success in the treatment of 60 cases, but no specific criteria were used for the postoperative evaluation, and no complications were noted. Extensive metatarsal head resection can lead to retraction of the fifth toe,[17,31,36] subluxation of the fifth toe,[27,31] and development of a transfer lesion beneath the fourth metatarsal head.[17,31,36] The development of a flail fifth toe deformity might require syndactylization to the fourth toe.

With fifth metatarsal head resection in seven patients (11 feet) at an average 8-year follow-up, Kitaoka and Holiday[31] reported 82% fair or poor results. Complications, which occurred in 64% of cases, included severe shortening of the toe (36%), transfer lesions or unresolved plantar callosities (75%), stiffness (25%), and continued symptoms (27%). The preoperative 4-5 intermetatarsal angle, which averaged 11 degrees, was noted to increase to 15.5 degrees after

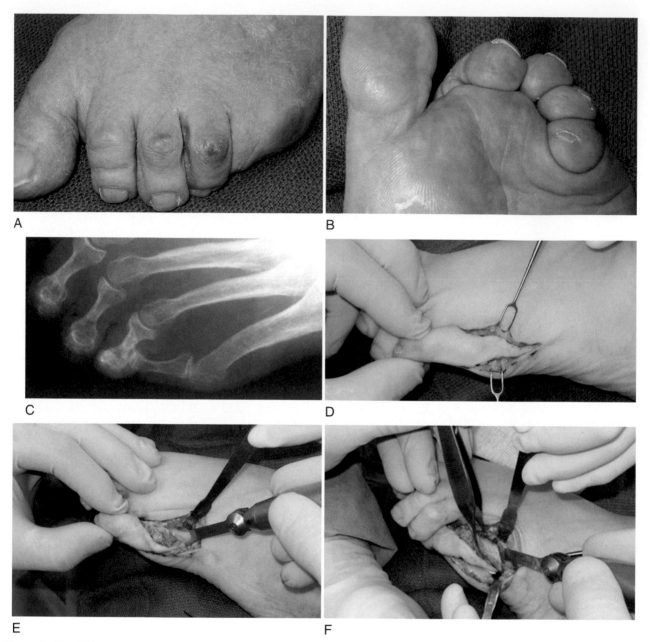

Figure 9–15   Fifth ray resection in a patient with rheumatoid forefoot deformity. **A** and **B**, Preoperative deformity. **C**, Preoperative radiograph demonstrating subluxation of the fifth metatarsophalangeal joint. **D**, Skin incision **E**, Oblique fifth metatarsal osteotomy. **F**, Transection of metatarsal.

surgery. Fifth ray shortening averaged 10 mm. Because of such complications as fifth ray shortening, transfer metatarsalgia, malalignment of the fifth toe, and loss of MTP joint function of the fifth ray, Kitaoka and Holiday[31] concluded that excisional arthroplasty was not indicated as a primary procedure. In 21 patients who underwent fifth metatarsal head excision (average follow-up, 17 months), Dorris and Mandel[17] reported malalignment of the fifth toe in 59% of patients. Although 84% of patients were satisfied with the results at postoperative evaluation, limited short-term follow-up of as little as 3 months raises a question as to the long-term efficacy and durability of this procedure in light of the report of Kitaoka and Holiday.[31]

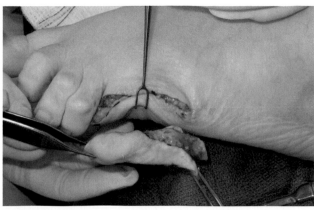

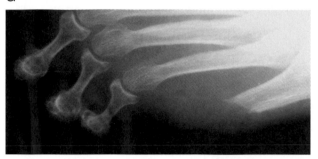

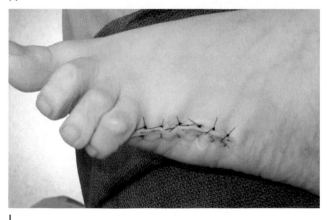

Figure 9–15—cont'd G, Specimen removed. **H,** Final postoperative radiograph. **I,** Following wound closure.

Addante et al[1] reported on 35 patients (50 cases) after fifth metatarsal head resection and placement of silicone spheric implants. They reported an 84% success rate. Complications occurred in 16% of cases and included traumatic dislocation of the implant, chronic subluxation, silicone inflammatory reaction, wound dehiscence, abscess formation, IPK, and transfer metatarsalgia.

DISTAL FIFTH METATARSAL OSTEOTOMY

An osteotomy of the fifth metatarsal may be used to correct alignment of the fifth metatarsal. Davies[12] stated that it was "unnecessary and unsatisfactory" to perform a fifth metatarsal osteotomy. Lelievre,[37,38] however, recognized that an increased 4-5 intermetatarsal angle should be corrected as a part of a bunionette repair. Kelikian[29] cautioned that delayed healing can occur after a fifth metatarsal osteotomy.

The location of the osteotomy and the surgical technique performed have a significant effect on the ultimate success of a metatarsal osteotomy. Distal, diaphyseal, and proximal metatarsal osteotomies have all been recommended in the treatment of symptomatic bunionette deformities. Many types of distal fifth metatarsal osteotomies have been recommended for the treatment of symptomatic bunionettes.* Although less correction of an increased 4-5 intermetatarsal angle is achieved than with more proximal osteotomies, a distal fifth metatarsal osteotomy achieves significantly more correction than with a lateral condyle resection. Instability of some types of distal metatarsal osteotomies has caused concern regarding the loss of alignment,[8,27] development of a subsequent transfer lesion, and recurrence of deformity (Fig. 9–16).[28]

Hohmann[26] and later Steinke[56] described a distal fifth metatarsal osteotomy, reporting on the use of a transverse osteotomy of the fifth metatarsal neck. Kaplan et al[27] advocated a distal closing wedge fifth metatarsal osteotomy that was internally fixed with a Kirschner wire. They suggested internal fixation because the distal osteotomy was unstable and might rotate postoperatively, with resulting loss of correction. Haber and Kraft[25] used a distal fifth metatarsal crescentic osteotomy. They did not use internal fixation to stabilize the osteotomy site and reported excessive callus formation at the osteotomy site and delayed healing. Catanzariti et al[8] performed a distal oblique fifth metatarsal osteotomy without internal fixation and reported a 26% recurrence rate and transfer lesions in 35% of cases.

Throckmorton and Bradlee[58] and others[3,6,9,32] described a distal fifth metatarsal transverse

*References 3, 8, 21, 26, 28, 32-34, 39, 43, 45, 48, 49, 54, 58, and 62.

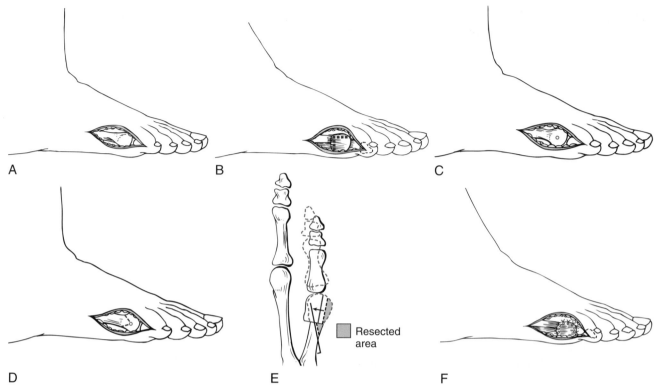

Figure 9–16 Distal chevron osteotomy. **A,** Lateral incision is centered over the fifth metatarsal head. **B,** An L-shaped capsular release is performed. Exostectomy is performed to remove the lateral condyle in line with the lateral border of the foot. **C,** Lateral-to-medial drill hole marks the apex of the chevron osteotomy. **D,** Osteotomy is performed (base proximal) at an angle of approximately 60 degrees. Distal capital fragment is displaced in a medial direction. Remaining bone is beveled around the osteotomy site. **E,** A 0.045-inch Kirschner wire is used to stabilize the capital fragment to the proximal metatarsal shaft. **F,** An interrupted capsular repair is carried out. Where insufficient capsular tissue is present, drill holes in the metaphysis may be used to secure the capsule repair.

chevron osteotomy. Because of the stable shape of this osteotomy, Throckmorton did not use internal fixation. Boyer and DeOrio[3] have used an absorbable fixation pin for internal fixation of a chevron osteotomy. A reverse Mitchell procedure,[36,54] distal chevron osteotomy,[3,22,32,43,58] distal transverse osteotomy,[26,27,56] distal crescentic osteotomy,[25] scarf,[13,51] and oblique distal osteotomy* have all been recommended as distal fifth metatarsal osteotomy techniques. Nonetheless, a distal fifth metatarsal osteotomy might help to achieve adequate correction of a symptomatic bunionette deformity.

Indications

With a type 1 deformity (enlarged head) or a moderate type 2 or type 3 deformity, a distal fifth metatarsal osteotomy may be employed to achieve adequate surgical correction. The choice of a specific type of osteotomy depends on the experience of the surgeon and the anatomic variation present. Internal fixation is often preferable because it stabilizes the correction obtained at surgery. Usually the Kirschner wire used for internal fixation can be removed without difficulty in an office setting a few weeks after surgery. An absorbable pin fixation has been used with success and provides an alternative to later hardware removal.[3,22]

Contraindications

The main contraindication to a distal metatarsal osteotomy is a moderate or severe angular deformity for which a distal metatarsal osteotomy is inadequate to correct the angular deformity. A chevron osteotomy is not effective in correcting a bunionette deformity characterized by a plantar keratosis; in this case, a distal osteotomy that elevates the fifth metatarsal head is preferable (distal oblique osteotomy, capital oblique osteotomy).

*References 7, 8, 28, 33, 34, 39, 48, 49, and 54.

DISTAL CHEVRON OSTEOTOMY (AUTHOR'S PREFERRED TECHNIQUE)

1. The patient is positioned in a semilateral decubitus position.
2. The extremity is cleansed in a normal fashion.
3. A longitudinal incision is centered directly over the lateral eminence and extended 1 cm above the lateral eminence. Care is taken to protect the dorsal and plantar neurovascular bundles (Figs. 9–16A and 9–17A and video clip 21).

4. The capsule of the MTP joint is incised along the dorsal and proximal border to create an inverted L-shaped capsule release. This flap is detached from the periosteum dorsally as well as the abductor digiti quinti muscle proximally (Figs. 9–16B and 9–17B).
5. The flap is turned downward to expose the lateral eminence, which is resected with a power saw (Fig. 9–17C).
6. A 0.045-inch Kirschner wire is drilled through the center of the metatarsal head in a lateral-to-medial direction. This drill

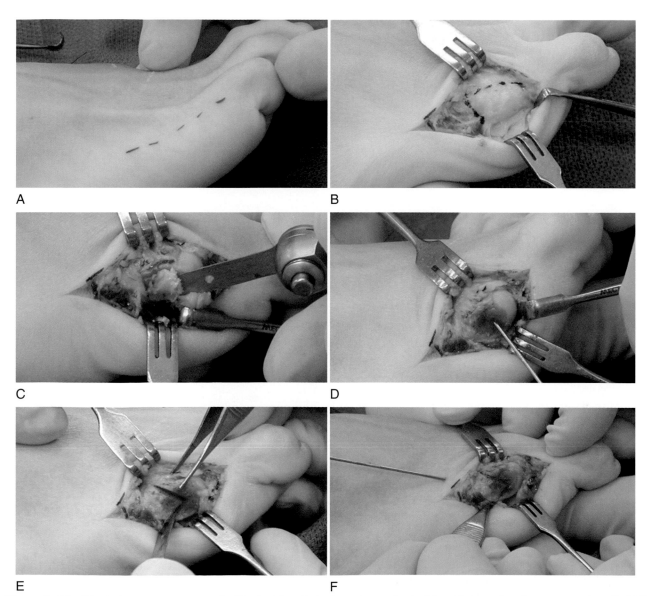

Figure 9–17 Distal chevron osteotomy. **A,** Skin incision. **B,** L-shaped capsular incision. **C,** Lateral eminence resection. **D,** Drill hole marks apex of the chevron osteotomy. **E,** Following chevron osteotomy. **F,** Following medial translation of capital fragment.

Continued

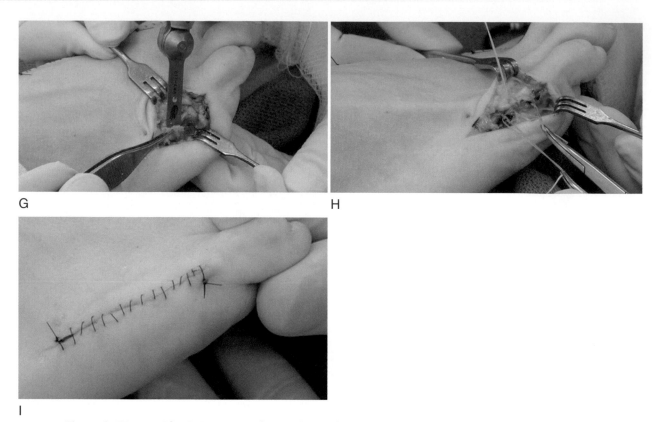

Figure 9–17—cont'd   **G,** Resection of metaphyseal flare. **H,** Capsular closure. **I,** Following skin closure.

hole marks the apex of the osteotomy (Figs. 9–16C and 9–17D).

7. A sagittal saw with in-line teeth is used to create the osteotomy. This saw blade configuration minimizes shortening at the osteotomy site (Figs. 9–16D and 9–17E).

8. The osteotomy cut is made from a lateral-to medial direction at an angle of approximately 60 degrees.

9. Care is taken to avoid excessive soft tissue stripping, because the remaining vascular supply to the fifth metatarsal is from the medial aspect of the capital fragment.

10. The metatarsal diaphysis is grasped with a towel clip, and the capital fragment and toe are displaced in a medial direction. The displacement is approximately 33% to 50% of the width of the metaphysis (Fig. 9–17F). The remaining metaphyseal flare is shaved with a power saw (Fig. 9–17G).

11. The capital fragment is stabilized with a 0.045-inch Kirschner wire (Fig. 9–16E).

12. The MTP joint capsule is repaired with interrupted absorbable suture. The capsule flap may be secured to the metatarsal metaph-ysis by drill holes placed in the metaphysis. The capsule is also secured to the dorsal periosteum of the fifth metatarsal and the abductor digiti quinti. A secure capsule closure helps to prevent recurrence of the deformity (Figs. 9–16F and 9–17H).

13. The skin is closed with interrupted sutures (Figs. 9–17I and 9–18).

Postoperative Care

The foot is wrapped with a gauze-and-tape compression dressing that is changed weekly for 6 weeks. The sutures and Kirschner wire are removed 3 weeks following surgery. The patient is allowed to ambulate in a postoperative shoe with weight bearing on the inner border of the foot for 6 weeks. The postoperative shoe is discontinued 3 weeks postoperatively (Fig. 9–18).

Results and Complications

Throckmorton and Bradlee[58] initially reported the use of a chevron osteotomy to correct a bunionette deformity. No long-term series were reported. Campbell[6] reported on nine patients

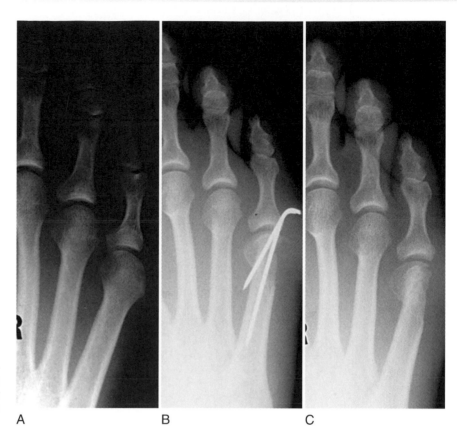

Figure 9–18 A, Preoperative radiograph demonstrates bunionette deformity. **B,** After chevron osteotomy with Kirschner wire fixation. **C,** Chevron osteotomy achieves adequate repair.

A   B   C

(12 chevron osteotomies) and noted that all patients were satisfied postoperatively. Leach and Igou[36] reported on a reverse Mitchell procedure on 11 feet. The average preoperative 4-5 intermetatarsal angle of 11.7 degrees was corrected to 4.9 degrees; thus an average 6.8-degree correction of the intermetatarsal angle was achieved. They noted no nonunions in this series.

Kitaoka et al[32] reported on the results of a distal chevron osteotomy in 13 patients (19 feet) treated for symptomatic bunionette deformities. At an average follow-up of 7.1 years, 12 of 19 feet (63%) were reported to have good or excellent results. Complications included a postoperative keratosis over the bunionette in one patient and transfer metatarsalgia in another. Radiographic analysis found the 4-5 intermetatarsal angle preoperatively measured 11.8 degrees and postoperatively 9.2 degrees, for an average correction of 2.6 degrees. The average MTP-5 angle measured 20.7 degrees preoperatively and 12.8 degrees postoperatively, for an average correction of 7.9 degrees. The average forefoot width was decreased by 3 mm. The

authors concluded that although a limited degree of correction is possible with a chevron osteotomy, this procedure reliably achieves subjective relief of symptoms. Although they used cast immobilization for 3 weeks after surgery, they observed that immobilization with a soft compression dressing and ambulation in a postsurgical shoe was an alternative. For an unreliable patient, they suggested cast immobilization. Although Kirschner wire internal fixation was not advocated, the authors noted that it could be used if the osteotomy site was not stable.

Pontious et al[46] reported on eight chevron osteotomies and noted no dorsal displacement, indicating that this was a very stable osteotomy. Excessive soft tissue stripping on the dorsal and plantar aspect of the distal metatarsal osteotomy does, however, increase the risk of instability at the osteotomy site and also predisposes to nonunion or avascular necrosis of the fifth metatarsal head. Reporting on 12 patients (16 osteotomies), Moran and Claridge[43] stressed that there was a low margin of error with this osteotomy but also a risk of recurrence or overcorrection. They suggested that the osteotomy site be stabilized with Kirschner wire internal fixation.

Boyer and DeOrio[3] reported the results of 10 patients with 12 osteotomies fixed with an absorbable pin (Fig. 9–19). At an average follow-up of 48 months, there was no evidence of avascular necrosis, displacement of the osteotomy, or osteolysis. All osteotomies healed by 6 weeks and the postoperative American Orthopaedic Foot and Ankle Society (AOFAS) score averaged 93 points. The 4-5 inter-metatarsal angle was diminished from 9.1degrees to 1.4 degrees postoperatively. The MTP-5 angle was corrected from 11.8 degrees preoperatively to 6.2 degrees postoperatively. No transfer lesions were noted. The technique of a modified chevron (scarf) osteotomy has been described by Dayton[13] and Seide.[51] Seide and Petersen[51] reported successful results in a follow-up of 10 feet and noted an average reduction in the 4-5 intermetatarsal angle of 4.5 degrees (Fig. 9–20).

DISTAL OBLIQUE OSTEOTOMY

Surgical Technique

1. The patient is positioned in a semilateral decubitus position.
2. The extremity is cleansed in a normal fashion.
3. A longitudinal incision is made directly over the lateral eminence beginning at the mid-portion of the proximal phalanx and extend-ing 1 cm above the lateral eminence. Care is taken to protect the dorsal and plantar neurovascular bundles.
4. The capsule of the MTP joint is incised along the dorsal and proximal border to create an inverted L-shaped capsular release. This flap is detached from the dorsal periosteum as well as the abductor digiti quinti muscle proximally (Fig. 9–21A).
5. After the lateral eminence of the fifth metatarsal head is exposed, the prominent condyle is resected with a sagittal saw.
6. An oblique osteotomy of the fifth metatarsal neck is carried out with the same sagittal saw. The osteotomy is oriented in a distal-lateral to proximal-medial direction (Fig. 9–21B and video clip 23).
7. The proximal fragment is grasped with a towel clip, and the capital fragment is dis-placed medially and impacted on the prox-imal fragment.
8. The osteotomy site is fixed with a 0.045-inch Kirschner wire, which may be left protruding through or buried just beneath the skin (Fig. 9–21C).
9. The MTP joint capsule is repaired with inter-rupted absorbable suture. The capsule flap may be secured to the metatarsal metaph-ysis by drill holes placed in the metaphysis. The capsule is also secured to the dorsal area of the periosteum of the fifth metatarsal and the abductor digiti quinti; a secure capsule closure helps to prevent recurrence of the deformity (Fig. 9–21D).
10. The skin is closed with interrupted sutures.

Postoperative Care

The foot is wrapped in a gauze-and-tape com-pression dressing that is changed weekly for 6 weeks. Sutures and the Kirschner wire are removed 3 weeks after surgery. The patient is allowed to ambulate in a postoperative shoe with weight bearing on the inner border of the foot for 6 weeks. At this time, use of the post-operative shoe is discontinued.

CAPITAL OBLIQUE OSTEOTOMY (MODIFIED WEIL)

Surgical Technique

1. The patient is positioned in a semilateral decubitus position.
2. The extremity is cleansed in a normal fashion.
3. A longitudinal incision directly over the lateral eminence is made beginning at the midportion of the proximal phalanx and extended 1 cm above the lateral eminence. Care is taken to protect the dorsal and plantar neurovascular bundles (Fig. 9–22A-C).

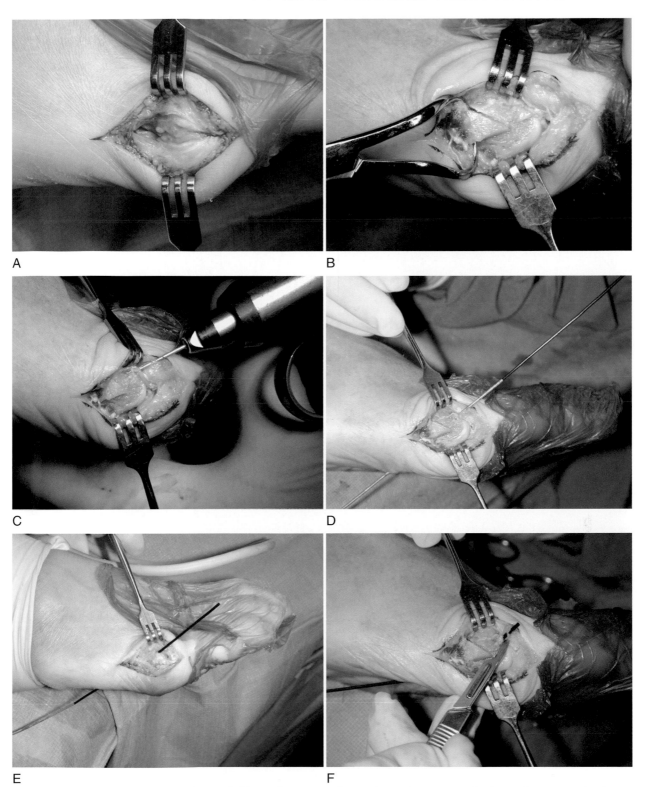

Figure 9–19 Chevron osteotomy with resorbable pin fixation (DeOrio technique). **A,** Longitudinal capsular incision. **B,** The proximal fragment is grasped with a towel clip as the capital fragment is translated medially. **C,** Fixation drill hole. **D,** Sheath with resorbable pin fixation. **E,** Sheath removed. **F,** Pin severed at the edge of the dorsal and plantar bone surfaces. (Courtesy of J. DeOrio, MD.)

Continued

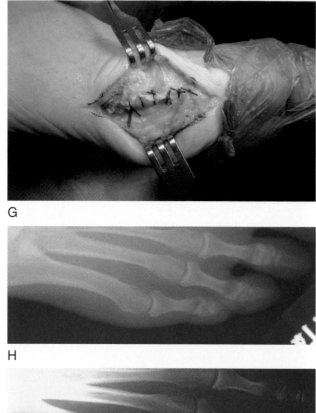

G

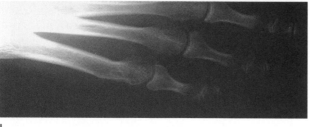

H

I

Figure 9–19—cont'd **G,** Capsular closure. Preoperative **(H)** and postoperative **(I)** radiographs.

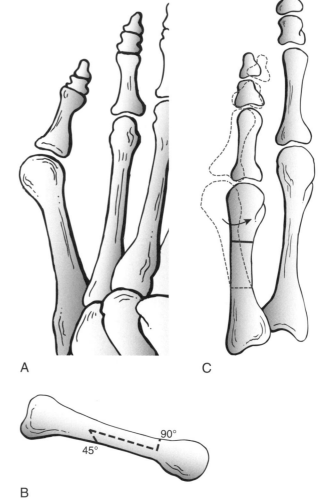

A

B

C

Figure 9–20 **A,** Diagram of preoperative angular deformity. **B,** Diagram of longitudinal scarf fifth metatarsal osteotomy. **C,** Following rotation and realignment of the osteotomy.

4. The capsule of the MTP joint is incised along the dorsal and proximal border to create an inverted L-shaped capsule release. This flap is detached from the dorsal periosteum as well as the abductor digiti quinti muscle proximally (Fig. 9–22D).
5. The lateral eminence of the fifth metatarsal head is exposed, and the prominent condyle is resected with a sagittal saw (Fig. 9–22E).
6. A longitudinal osteotomy of the fifth metatarsal is performed starting 2 to 3 mm plantar to the dorsal extent of the metatarsal articular cartilage. The osteotomy is usually parallel to the plantar aspect of the foot, although if a plantar cal-

losity is present, the saw blade may be tipped so that the capital fragment elevates as it is translated in a medial direction (Fig. 9–22F).
7. The capital fragment is then displaced in a medial direction 2 to 4 mm; care is taken not to shorten the fifth ray at the osteotomy site (Fig. 9–22G).
8. The osteotomy site is fixed with a dorsal–plantar mini-fragment screw; the dorsal metaphyseal flare is resected with a sagittal saw (Fig. 9–22H and I).
9. The MTP joint capsule is repaired with interrupted absorbable suture. The capsule flap may be secured to the metatarsal metaphysis by drill holes placed in the metaphysis.

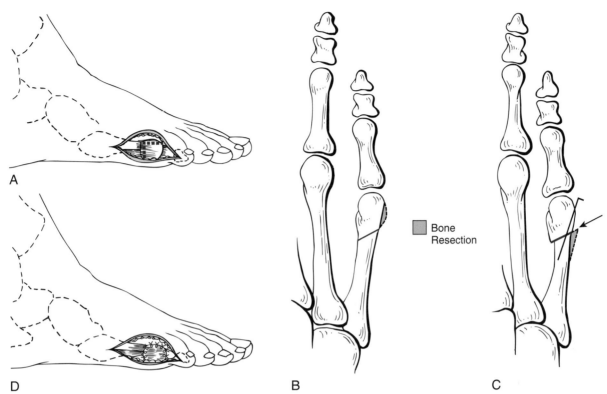

Figure 9–21 Distal oblique osteotomy. **A,** Lateral skin incision is centered over the fifth metatarsal head. L-shaped capsular release detaches the dorsal and proximal capsules (weakest area of capsular attachment). **B,** Oblique osteotomy is performed from a distal–lateral to proximal–medial direction. **C,** The capital fragment is displaced in a medial direction. Internal fixation with Kirschner wire stabilizes the osteotomy. **D,** The capsule is repaired with interrupted suture. In the presence of insufficient proximal capsule, drill holes may be placed in the metaphysis to secure the capsular repair.

The capsule is also secured to the dorsal area of the periosteum of the fifth metatarsal and the abductor digiti quinti (a secure capsule closure helps to prevent recurrence of the deformity) (Fig. 9–22J).

10. The skin is closed with interrupted sutures (Fig. 9–22K-M).

Postoperative Care

The foot is wrapped in a gauze-and-tape compression dressing that is changed weekly for 6 weeks. Sutures and the Kirschner wire are removed 3 weeks after surgery. The internal fixation is rarely removed unless it becomes symptomatic. The patient is allowed to ambulate in a postoperative shoe with weight bearing on the inner border of the foot for 6 weeks. At this time use of the postoperative shoe is discontinued.

Results and Complications

Sponsel[54] advocated an oblique distal fifth metatarsal osteotomy. The capital fragment was allowed to float because internal fixation was not used. An 11% delayed union rate was reported. Keating et al[28] also used an oblique distal fifth metatarsal osteotomy without internal fixation. Transfer lesions were reported in 75% of patients, and a 12% recurrence rate was noted. The authors attributed complications such as recurrent deformity and transfer keratotic lesions to medial displacement and dorsiflexion of the distal fragment after the osteotomy. They noted a success rate of 56%. Diebold and Bejjani[16] and Frankel et al[21] suggested that after distal fifth metatarsal osteotomies there may be a high dissatisfaction rate because of the instability of the osteotomy site and the difficulty in obtaining adequate fixation (Figs. 9–23 and 9–26).

Pontious et al[46] compared distal fifth metatarsal osteotomies that were internally fixed to those not fixed. They stressed that internal fixation controls dorsal displacement of the capital fragment, producing less shortening and fewer complications. In a report on 46 patients

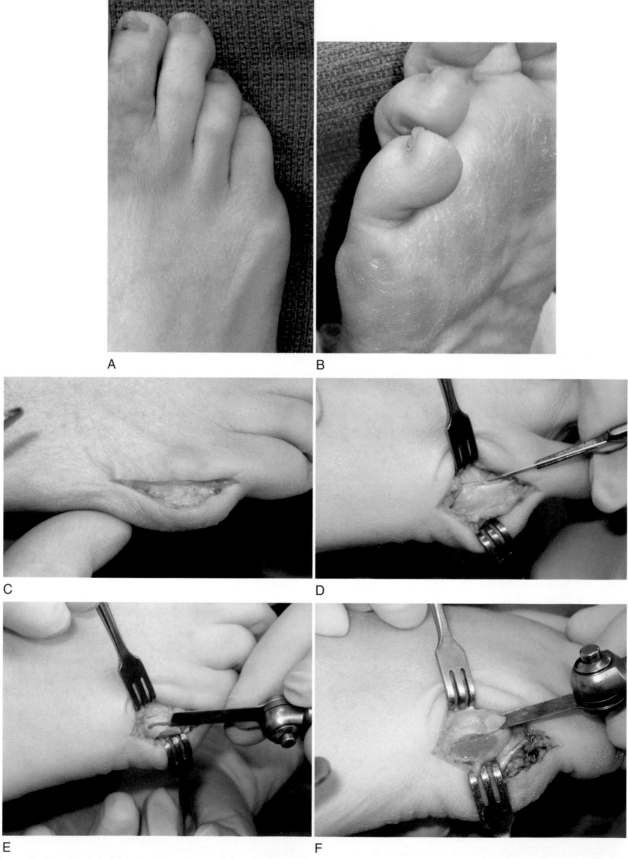

Figure 9–22 Capital oblique osteotomy. **A,** Preoperative deformity. **B,** Plantar view. **C,** Skin incision. **D,** L-shaped capsular incision. **E,** Lateral eminence resection. **F,** Capital oblique osteotomy. This cut can be rotated to elevate the capital fragment as it is translated in a medial direction.

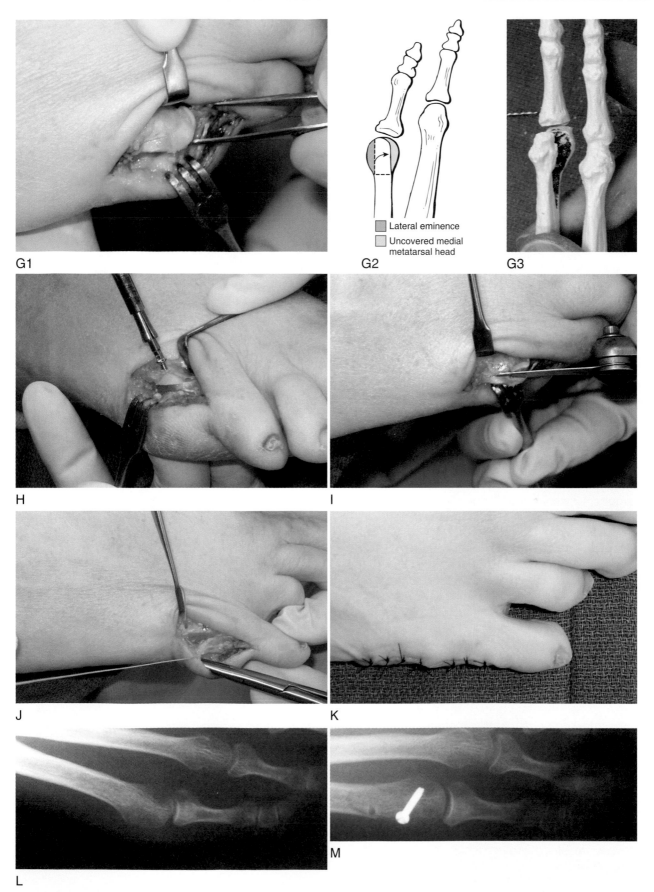

Lateral eminence

Uncovered medial
metatarsal head

Figure 9–22—cont'd   G1, The distal fragment is grasped with a forceps and pushed medially. **G2,** Diagram of medial translation of the capital fragment. **G3,** Demonstration of translation with sawbones model. **H,** Oblique screw fixation. **I,** Lateral flare of metaphysis is shaved. **J,** Capsule closure. **K,** Skin closure. **L,** Preoperative radiograph. **M,** Postoperative radiograph.

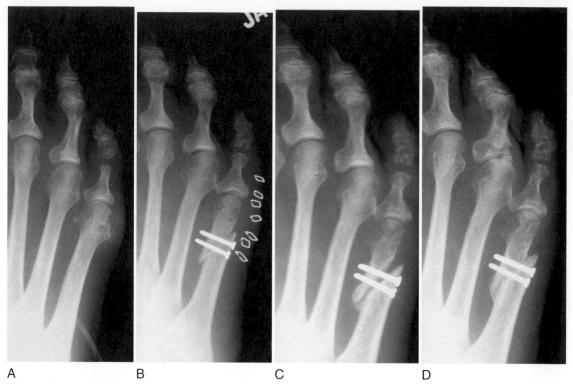

A   B   C   D

Figure 9–23   Oblique osteotomy. **A,** Preoperative radiograph. **B,** Following oblique osteotomy with double screw fixation. **C,** With premature weight bearing, the patient displaced the osteotomy. **D,** With time, successful union was achieved.

(56 feet) they noted that the average healing time was 8 weeks in osteotomies that were internally fixed and 11 weeks in those that were not. They concluded that osteotomies that were internally fixed healed more predictably and that fixation prevented displacement, making it possible to maintain the corrected osteotomy position. Kitaoka and Holiday[30] and Frankel et al[21] concluded that floating fifth metatarsal osteotomies that seek their own level in an uncontrolled manner have a significant incidence of transfer metatarsalgia (see Fig. 9–40).

Kitaoka and Leventen[33] performed a distal oblique osteotomy in 16 patients (23 feet) (Fig. 9–24). The orientation of this osteotomy was proximal–lateral to distal–medial. The fifth metatarsal head was displaced medially and impaled on the medial spike of the diaphyseal segment. The average 4-5 intermetatarsal angle was decreased from 13 to 8 degrees (average 5 degrees of correction). Forefoot width was diminished an average of 4 mm postoperatively. Eighty-seven percent of patients reported satisfactory results. One nonunion was reported (Fig. 9–24).

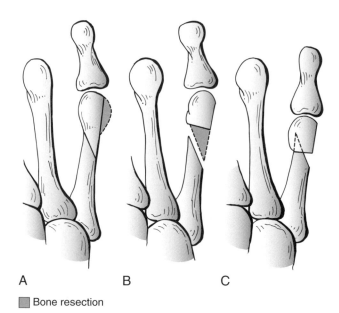

A   B   C

■ Bone resection

Figure 9–24   Leventen-type osteotomy, or oblique osteotomy in reverse direction. **A,** Proposed osteotomy. **B,** Shaded area marks metaphyseal resection. **C,** Capital fragment is impaled on a spike of proximal fragment.

Experience with distal metatarsal osteotomies demonstrates an average reduction in the 4-5 intermetatarsal angle of approximately 4 to 5 degrees.[49,51,62] Whether a chevron osteotomy,[6,43,58] distal transverse osteotomy,[21,34] or oblique osteotomy[28,33,48,49,54] is performed depends on a surgeon's preference. Less correction of the 4-5 intermetatarsal angle is obtained with an osteotomy located in the distal fifth metatarsal than with a more proximal osteotomy. The small area of metaphyseal bone in this region places the osteotomy at risk for delayed union, malunion, or nonunion regardless of the specific type of procedure (Fig. 9–25).

Although a lateral condylectomy may be used to correct a bunionette deformity characterized by an enlarged fifth metatarsal head, a distal oblique osteotomy or a chevron osteotomy appears to achieve more correction than a lateral condylar resection does alone. The potential complications of a distal osteotomy, such as delayed union, malunion, and development of an intractable plantar keratotic transfer lesion, make internal fixation or a stable osteotomy advisable.[8,21,49] In the presence of a bunionette deformity with formation of a lateral keratosis, either a chevron osteotomy or an oblique osteotomy, can achieve adequate correction. Because a chevron osteotomy does not allow elevation of the capital fragment, this procedure is contraindicated in the presence of a bunionette deformity with a plantar–lateral or plantar keratosis. A capital oblique or oblique osteotomy allows elevation by altering the plane of the osteotomy. No series has yet been reported on this variation of Weil's technique also used for the central lesser metatarsals.

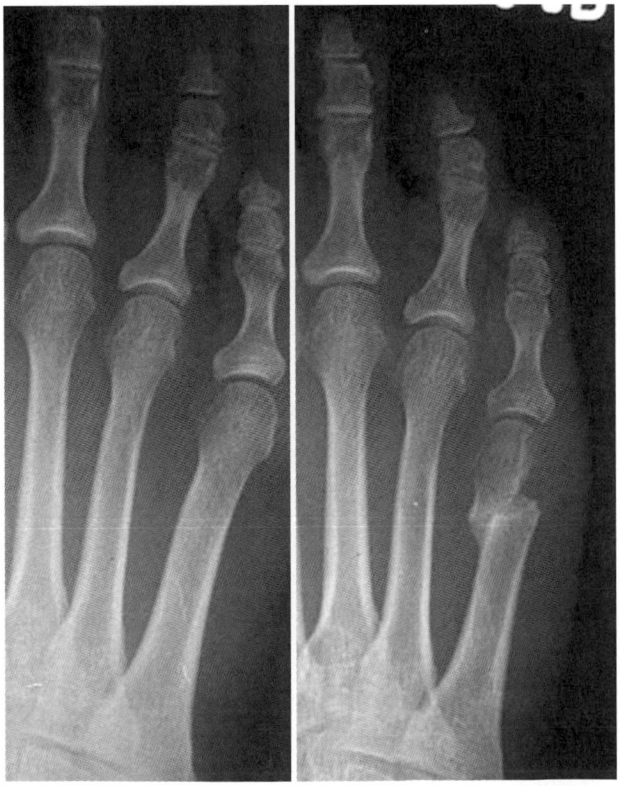

MIDSHAFT (DIAPHYSEAL) OSTEOTOMIES

An osteotomy in the diaphyseal region of the fifth metatarsal also has been recommended for the correction of a bunionette deformity. Yancy[61] described a double transverse closing wedge osteotomy in the diaphysis to correct a type 2 bunionette deformity characterized by lateral bowing of the fifth metatarsal. Okuda et al[45] have described a crescentic osteotomy in the diaphyseal region. Voutey[59] also advocated a transverse diaphyseal osteotomy but reported several complications, including delayed union, pseudarthrosis, and angulation at the osteotomy site. The transverse nature of this osteotomy rendered it relatively unstable.

Gerbert et al[23] and Shrum et al[53] described a closing wedge diaphyseal osteotomy that was internally fixed with a cerclage wire. They suggested that with a plantar or plantar lateral keratotic lesion, a biplanar osteotomy might be advisable to achieve medial and dorsal displacement of the distal fragment. Unfortunately, no long-term follow-up was reported in either study.

Mann[40] initially described an oblique fifth metatarsal diaphyseal osteotomy for the treatment of bunionette deformities characterized by diffuse keratotic lesions on the plantar or plantar lateral aspect of the fifth metatarsal head. The oblique nature of the metatarsal osteotomy allowed not only medial but also dorsal translation of the distal fragment with rotation at the

Figure 9–25 A, Preoperative radiograph demonstrates bunionette deformity. **B,** Postoperative radiograph demonstrates distal oblique osteotomy.

osteotomy site. Mann[40] advocated internal fixation with a wire loop, Kirschner wire, or small-fragment screw, or all three. The fifth MTP joint was not realigned in this procedure. Although no series was reported, Mann did report a case of nonunion. We have had extensive experience with this procedure and have encountered one other nonunion (Fig. 9–31 and video clip 22).

Indications

In the presence of a widened 4-5 intermetatarsal angle associated with a bunionette deformity (type 3) or with substantial lateral bowing of the fifth metatarsal shaft (type 2), a diaphyseal osteotomy combined with a distal soft tissue realignment affords an excellent means of correction. With a combined plantar–lateral keratotic lesion, the plane of the osteotomy can be altered to achieve elevation of the distal fragment.

Contraindications

For type 1 bunionette deformities, the magnitude of a longitudinal osteotomy is rarely nec-

essary, and a distal osteotomy is preferable. With an unreliable patient, a more stable distal osteotomy may be preferable, although it can sacrifice some magnitude of angular correction.

Midshaft Oblique Osteotomy (Author's Preferred Technique)

1. The patient is positioned in a semilateral decubitus position.
2. The extremity is cleansed in a normal fashion.
3. A mid lateral longitudinal incision is made from the mid portion of the proximal phalanx, extending in a proximal direction to the proximal aspect of the fifth metatarsal. The dorsolateral cutaneous nerve is isolated and protected (Figs. 9–27A and 9–28A).
4. The abductor digiti minimi muscle is reflected plantarward to expose the fifth metatarsal diaphysis. The periosteum on the medial aspect of the fifth metatarsal is not stripped to maintain vascular attachments.

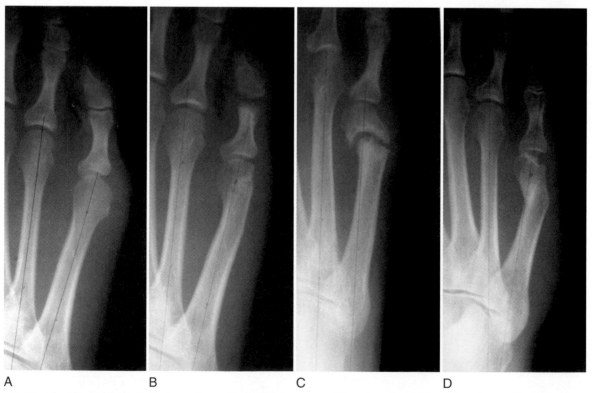

A   B   C   D

Figure 9–26   Modified L-shaped diaphyseal osteotomy. Preoperative **(A)** and postoperative **(B)** radiographs. **C,** Asymptomatic nonunion. **D,** Malunion following correction of type 3 deformity. (From Friend G, Grace K, Stone HA: *J Foot Ankle Surg* 32[1]: 14-19, 1993.)

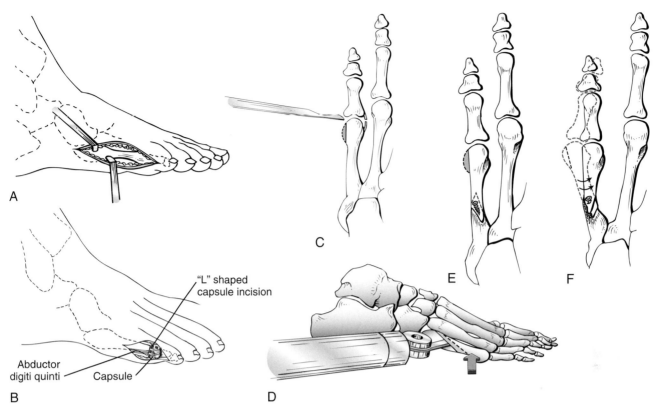

Figure 9–27 Diaphyseal oblique osteotomy. **A,** Longitudinal incision is centered over the lateral aspect of the fifth metatarsal beginning at the midportion of the proximal phalanx and extending to a point 2 cm below the base of the fifth metatarsal. **B,** L-shaped capsular incision releases dorsal and proximal aspects of the metatarsophalangeal joint capsule, the weakest area of capsular attachment. The stronger plantar and distal attachments are left intact, and the medial capsule is released. **C,** Lateral fifth metatarsal condyle is removed with a sagittal saw; the medial capsule is released with a scalpel. **D,** Orientation of diaphyseal oblique osteotomy is in a lateral-to-medial plane. **E** and **F,** Osteotomy site is rotated and fixed with a small-fragment screw. Kirschner wire fixation may be added to give rotational stability.

5. The MTP joint capsule is exposed and incised along the dorsal and proximal aspect with an L-shaped incision to expose the lateral eminence (Figs. 9–27B and 9–28B).
6. The fibular condyle of the fifth metatarsal head is resected with a sagittal saw in a line parallel with the metatarsal shaft (Fig. 9–28C). A drill hole is placed in the metaphysis for later capsule repair (Fig. 9–28D).
7. The fifth toe is grasped and distracted, and the fifth MTP joint is released on the medial aspect to allow its realignment at the conclusion of the procedure (Figs. 9–27C and 9–28E).
8. With a lateral keratosis, a horizontal osteotomy is begun. The osteotomy is directed in a dorsoproximal to plantar distal direction. The saw blade is oriented in a direct lateral-to-medial direction (Figs. 9–27D and 9–28F).
9. Before completing the osteotomy, a 3.5-mm drill hole is placed in the distal fragment (Fig. 9–28G). A 2.5-mm fixation drill hole is placed in the proximal fragment and tapped. The holes are drilled before completion of the osteotomy because this osteotomy can render the site quite unstable.
10. The osteotomy is completed, and the distal fragment is rotated to a point parallel with the fourth metatarsal (Fig. 9–27E and F).
11. A small-fragment fixation screw is used to stabilize the osteotomy site. A Kirschner wire may be used as well to stabilize and prevent rotation around the screw (Fig. 9–28H). (Multiple Kirschner wires

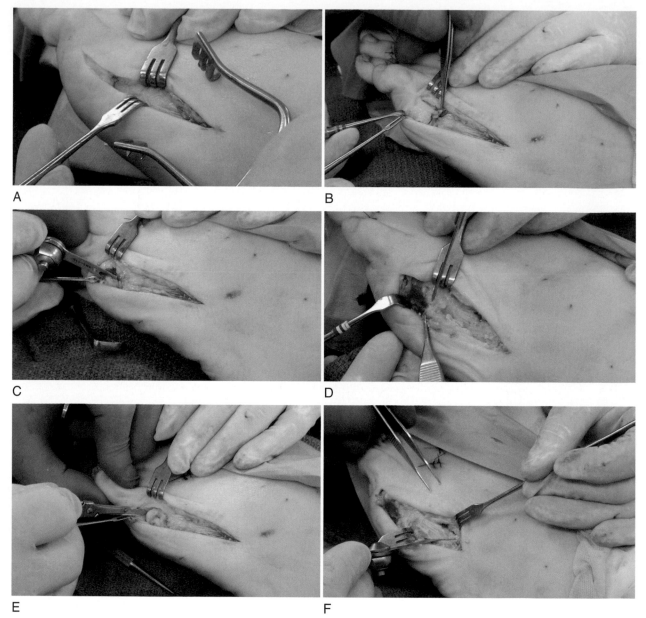

Figure 9–28   Diaphyseal oblique osteotomy. **A,** Longitudinal incision is centered over the lateral aspect of the fifth metatarsal beginning at the midportion of the proximal phalanx and extending to a point 2 cm below the base of the fifth metatarsal. **B,** L-shaped capsular incision releases the dorsal and proximal aspects of the MTP joint capsule, the weakest area of capsular attachment. **C,** Lateral eminence resection in line with the lateral cortex. **D,** Vertical drill hole in the metaphysis for later capsular repair. **E,** Medial capsular release. **F,** Longitudinal oblique osteotomy.

may be placed as an alternative to screw fixation, although this alternative is less desirable.)

12. Prominent bone at the osteotomy site is resected with a sagittal saw.

13. The fifth MTP joint capsule is repaired, and the fifth toe is brought into proper alignment. The abductor digiti quinti muscle is approximated to the capsule proximally, and dorsally the capsule is secured to the adjacent periosteum (Fig. 9–28I).

14. If necessary, the capsule may be attached through drill holes on the dorsoproximal aspect of the metaphysis (Fig. 9–28D).

15. The skin is closed with interrupted sutures or staples (Fig. 9–28J).

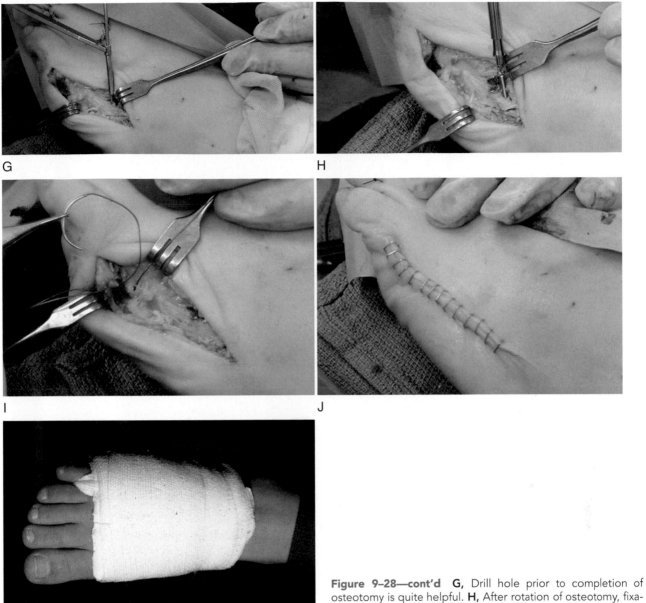

Figure 9–28—cont'd G, Drill hole prior to completion of osteotomy is quite helpful. **H,** After rotation of osteotomy, fixation with two mini-fragment screws. **I,** Capsular repair. **J,** Skin closure. **K,** Gauze-and-tape compression dressing.

Postoperative Care

A gauze-and-tape compression dressing is applied at surgery and changed weekly (Fig. 9–28K). An unreliable patient may be treated with a below-knee walking cast for 6 weeks. Sutures are removed at 3 weeks after surgery. Internal fixation may be removed at 6 weeks with radiographic proof of successful healing of the osteotomy (Fig. 9–29). The internal fixation is, however, rarely removed unless it becomes symptomatic. The patient is allowed to ambulate in a postoperative shoe with weight bearing on the inner border of the foot for 6 weeks. At this time use of the postoperative shoe is discontinued.

Variation

If a combined plantar–lateral keratosis is present, the orientation of the oblique diaphyseal osteotomy is altered. Although a

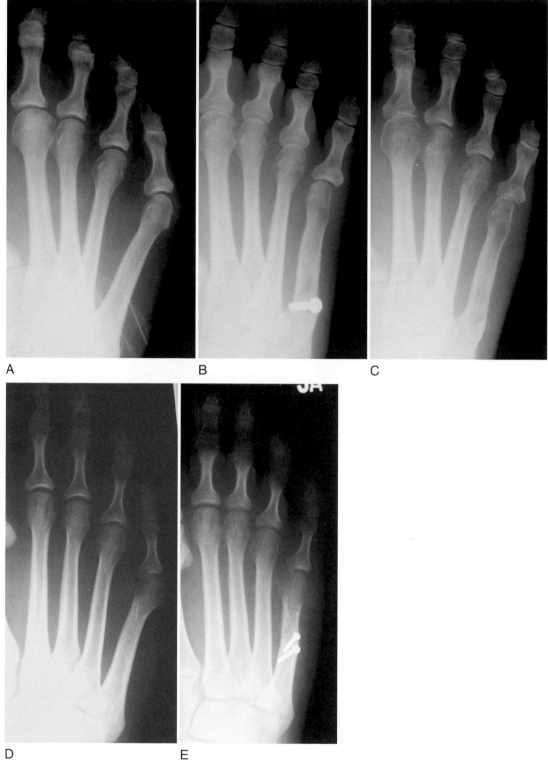

Figure 9–29 **A,** Preoperative radiograph of a type 3 deformity. **B,** Following midshaft oblique osteotomy. **C,** Five-year follow-up. **D,** Type 2 preoperative deformity. **E,** Following midshaft oblique osteotomy.

dorsal–proximal to plantar–distal cut is made, the orientation of the cut is changed from a direct lateral-to-medial direction to a more cephalad direction. The surgeon drops his or her hand and cuts in an upward direction (Fig. 9–30). Thus, as the osteotomy site is rotated, there is an elevating effect on the distal fragment. This relieves pressure on the plantar aspect of the fifth metatarsal head. The fifth MTP joint is realigned and the osteotomy is fixed as previously described. Postoperative management is similar to that described earlier.

Results and Complications

Most descriptions of fifth metatarsal diaphyseal osteotomies include little long-term follow-up. Coughlin[10] reported on a longitudinal diaphyseal osteotomy with MTP joint realignment and lateral condylectomy (Fig. 9–31). Twenty patients (30 feet) underwent surgical correction and were evaluated at an average 31 months of follow-up. No nonunions were reported. The average preoperative 4-5 intermetatarsal angle of 10.6 degrees was improved to 0.8 degrees, for an average correction of 9.8 degrees. The MTP-5 angle, noted to average 16 degrees preoperatively, was reduced to 0.5 degrees, for an average correction of 15.5 degrees. No symptomatic transfer lesions were reported. Patients had a 93% satisfaction rate. The average foot width was reduced by 6 mm (range, 2-15 mm).

The average fifth metatarsal shortening was 0.5 mm. No infections or incisional neuromas occurred.

Postoperative evaluation showed that one patient with a preoperative plantar keratosis had a mild, asymptomatic residual callus that was characterized as 75% reduced, one patient with a preoperative lateral IPK had a slight plantar keratosis, and one patient with a combined plantar and lateral keratosis had a remaining plantar keratosis that was characterized as 50% less than its preoperative size. All three patients characterized their subjective results as excellent or good. One other patient developed a mild transfer lesion that was asymptomatic, and her result was rated excellent. Three patients developed mild fifth hammer toe deformities that did not require further treatment, and all rated their results excellent.

Internal fixation included a single screw in 4 feet and a screw and Kirschner wire in 10 feet. When screw fixation was unsuccessful, multiple Kirschner wires (6 feet) were used. No loss of fixation occurred postoperatively at the osteotomy site. Because of the subcutaneous nature of the hardware, easy removal under local anesthesia can be performed in an office setting. Eighty-seven percent of patients underwent hardware removal.[10] Currently two mini-fragment screws are used to fix the osteotomy site. The initial screw serves as the center of rotation for the osteotomy. Once the osteotomy has been

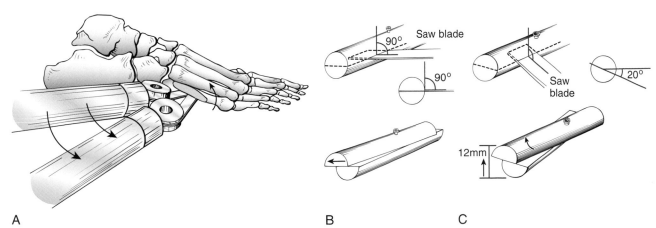

A   B   C

Figure 9–30 **A,** When an intractable plantar keratotic lesion is present, the saw blade is directed cephalad. The hand is dropped as the saw cut is created so that when the osteotomy site is rotated, the fifth metatarsal head is elevated. **B,** Schema illustrating the effect of horizontal osteotomy. With the saw blade oriented in a lateral-to-medial direction, the osteotomy site is rotated and does not elevate the distal metatarsal. **C,** Schema illustrating effect of oblique osteotomy. With the saw blade oriented in medial-lateral but also superior direction, as the osteotomy site is rotated, the distal fragment elevates. (**B** and **C** modified from Lutter L [ed]: *Atlas of Adult Foot and Ankle Surgery.* St Louis, Mosby, 1997, pp 110-111.)

aligned, a second screw is placed to further stabilize the osteotomy site.

London[39] performed a longitudinal oblique osteotomy at an angle reverse (dorsal–distal to plantar–proximal) to that described by Coughlin.[10] Although radiographs were only obtained up to 6 weeks following surgery, and telephone interviews were used to evaluate the clinical success, he hypothesized that this was a more stable osteotomy with this orientation. Only adequate follow-up will allow an evaluation of his theoretical concerns.

Okuda et al[45] reported on eight patients (10 feet) in whom a crescentic diaphyseal osteotomy was performed (Fig. 9–32). Three of the 10 developed a delayed union, which occurred in those cases in which the osteotomy was more proximally located (Fig. 9–33). The authors stressed that the osteotomy should not be performed at the base of the fifth metatarsal. Radiographic healing in the series averaged 11 weeks.

PROXIMAL FIFTH METATARSAL OSTEOTOMY

Indications

The rationale for a proximal fifth metatarsal osteotomy is that it achieves correction at the actual site of the deformity, not unlike a first ray bunion deformity. For a widened 4-5 intermetatarsal angle, the theoretical advantage of a proximal fifth metatarsal osteotomy is understandable. A proximal fifth metatarsal osteotomy has been advocated as a means to correct a widened 4-5 intermetatarsal angle.[15,16,20,27] Although a proximal osteotomy does achieve correction of the widened 4-5 intermetatarsal angle at the actual site of the deformity, some controversy surrounds this procedure. Lelievre[38] advocated a transverse osteotomy in the region of the styloid process. Diebold and Bejjani[16] noted that there was an increased "risk of disruption of the transverse metatarsal joint" with a proximally placed fifth metatarsal osteotomy.

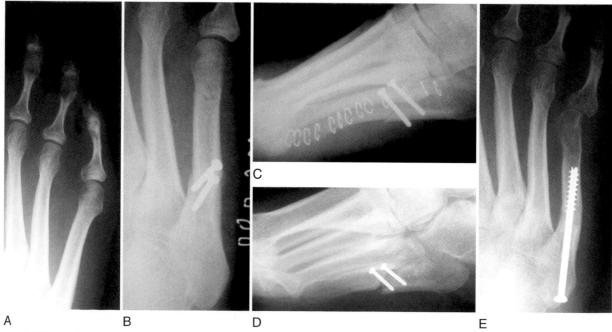

A   B   D   E

Figure 9–31 A, Preoperative radiograph demonstrates bunionette deformity with widened 4-5 intermetatarsal angle. **B,** Diaphyseal osteotomy with distal soft tissue repair achieves correction of deformity. Two mini-fragment screws are used for fixation. **C,** Lateral radiograph demonstrating fixation. **D,** Early weight bearing led to displacement and nonunion. **E,** Salvage with bone graft and intramedullary screw fixation.

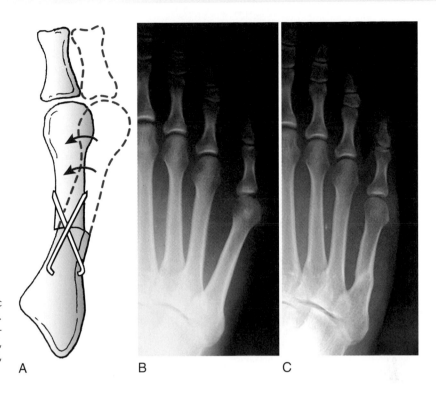

Figure 9–32 A, Midshaft crescentic osteotomy. **B,** Preoperative radiograph. **C,** Following crescentic osteotomy and hardware removal. (From Okuda R, Kinoshita M, Morikawa J, et al: *Clin Orthop* 396:179-183, 2002.)

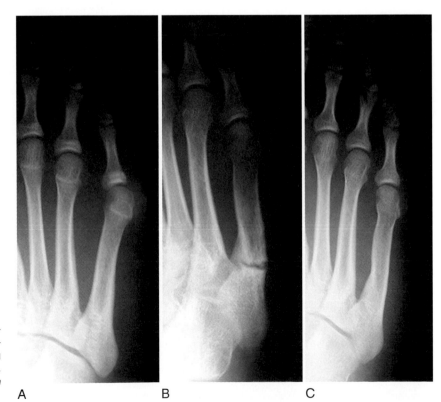

Figure 9–33 A, Preoperative radiograph. **B,** Delayed union following midshaft crescentic osteotomy. **C,** Following successful healing. (From Okuda R, Kinoshita M, Morikawa J, et al: *Clin Orthop* 396:179-183, 2002.)

Contraindications

Shereff et al[52] investigated the extraosseous and intraosseous arterial vascular supply of the proximal fifth metatarsal (Fig. 9–34). The intraosseous supply originates from a periosteal plexus, a nutrient artery, and metaphyseal and epiphyseal vessels. The extraosseous supply emanates from a dorsal metatarsal artery and several branches of the lateral plantar artery. The authors suggested that an osteotomy or fracture in the proximal 2 cm of the fifth metatarsal can injure both the extraosseous and the intraosseous supply, leading to delayed union or nonunion. Thus, although an osteotomy in the proximal fifth metatarsal can achieve maximal correction of a widened 4-5 intermetatarsal angle, the potential for delayed union, nonunion, or tarsometatarsal joint instability makes this area somewhat less optimal for surgical correction.

Gerbert et al[23] stated that the anastomosing arterial branches in the fourth intermetatarsal space may be vulnerable to injury with a proximal fifth metatarsal osteotomy. This observation is consistent with delayed healing of Jones-type

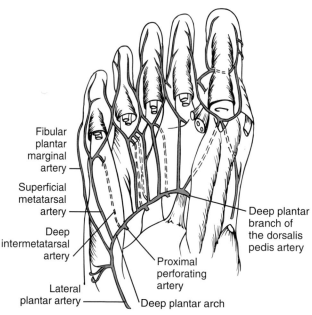

Fibular plantar marginal artery

Superficial metatarsal artery

Deep intermetatarsal artery

Lateral plantar artery

Deep plantar branch of the dorsalis pedis artery

Proximal perforating artery

Deep plantar arch

Figure 9–34 Plantar circulation is provided by the deep plantar arch, which is the source of several smaller arteries: superficial metatarsal artery, deep plantar metatarsal artery, deep plantar intermetatarsal artery, and fibular plantar marginal artery. From these vessels, numerous discrete branches supply the proximal fifth metatarsal. Area of convergence of these vessels in the proximal 1 to 2 cm of the proximal fifth metatarsal appears to be vulnerable to delayed union, with interruption of arterial circulation at this level.

fractures within the proximal 2 cm of the fifth metatarsal. Diebold and Bejjani[16] recognized that there was indeed a poor healing capacity for fractures in this region. Estersohn et al[19] emphasized the importance of the metaphyseal branch to the proximal fifth metatarsal region that enters on the medial aspect of the fifth metatarsal, and they cautioned that this important vascular supply should not be interrupted at surgery.

Surgical Technique

1. The patient is positioned in a semilateral decubitus position.
2. The extremity is cleansed in a normal fashion.
3. A 4-cm incision is made on the lateral aspect of the fifth metatarsal, beginning at its base and extending distally to the level of the distal metaphysis. A fifth MTP joint realignment is not usually performed (Fig. 9–35A).
4. The abductor digiti quinti muscle is retracted plantarward, taking care to protect the dorsal sensory nerve, a branch of the sural nerve.
5. A lateral-to-medial drill hole is created with a 0.062-inch Kirschner wire at a point 1 cm distal to the tip of the fifth metatarsal. This forms the apex of the chevron osteotomy (Fig. 9-35B).
6. A sagittal saw with "in-line" teeth is used to create the medial-to-lateral chevron with its base oriented in a distal direction (Fig. 9–35C).
7. The sagittal saw is used to create the two limbs of the chevron. The distal fifth metatarsal fragment is then rotated in a medial direction and stabilized to the fourth metatarsal with small Steinmann pins placed in the diaphysis in a lateral-to-medial direction (Fig. 9–35D and E). The pins are left extending through the skin.
8. Any prominent bone at the site of the osteotomy is beveled with a power saw.
9. The soft tissue is approximated with interrupted absorbable sutures, and the skin is closed with interrupted sutures.
10. A below-knee cast is applied.

Postoperative Care

Sutures are removed at 3 weeks, and the Steinmann pins that transfix the fourth and fifth

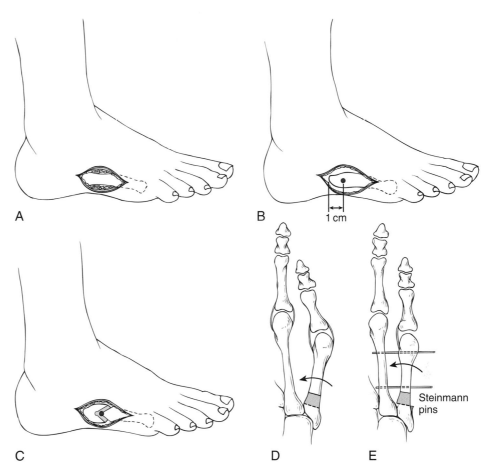

Figure 9–35 Proximal fifth metatarsal osteotomy. **A,** A 4-cm incision is centered over the base of the fifth metatarsal. **B,** After exposure of the fifth metatarsal, a drill hole is placed 1 cm distal to the fifth metatarsal base, marking the apex of the osteotomy site. **C,** Lateral-to-medial chevron osteotomy is performed with a sagittal saw. **D** and **E,** The osteotomy site is rotated and stabilized with two Steinmann pins, which transfix the fourth and fifth metatarsals. Excess bone is shaved at the osteotomy site.

metatarsals are removed at 6 weeks. Weight bearing is allowed in the cast at 3 weeks, and the cast is removed 6 weeks after surgery. At this time the patient is allowed to ambulate in a roomy sandal.

Results and Complications

In a series of 72 patients who underwent an opening wedge osteotomy of the proximal fifth metatarsal, Bishop et al[2] reported a diminished 4-5 intermetatarsal angle. Estersohn et al[19] performed a similar procedure in four cases. No long-term results were reported regarding the correction of the 4-5 intermetatarsal angle or the development of complications, including delayed union, nonunion, or transfer lesions. Regnauld[47] performed a proximal closing wedge osteotomy and stabilized it with a cerclage wire between the fourth and fifth metatarsals. Again, no results were reported.

In the only series in which significant follow-up study was reported after a proximal fifth metatarsal osteotomy, Diebold and Bejjani[16] performed a horizontal chevron osteotomy 1 cm

distal to the base of the fifth metatarsal. Steinmann pin fixation was used to immobilize the osteotomy by transfixation of the fourth and fifth metatarsals for 4 to 6 weeks. In 12 patients (average follow-up, 1 year), they reported excellent results in 90% of cases. No nonunions were reported. The 4-5 intermetatarsal angle was decreased from 17 to 7 degrees. Later in a follow-up report, Diebold and Bejjani[15] reported on 22 osteotomies that all successfully healed. The 4-5 intermetatarsal angle was diminished from 12 degrees to 1 degree postoperatively. They recommended removing the parallel Steinmann pins 5 weeks postoperatively with evidence of radiographic healing at the osteotomy site.

Although Kaplan et al[27] observed that both proximal and distal fifth metatarsal osteotomies heal adequately because of an abundant vascular supply, the experience with delayed healing of fractures in the proximal 2 cm of the fifth metatarsal should make the treating physician wary of an osteotomy in this area (Figs. 9–36, 9–37, and 9–38).

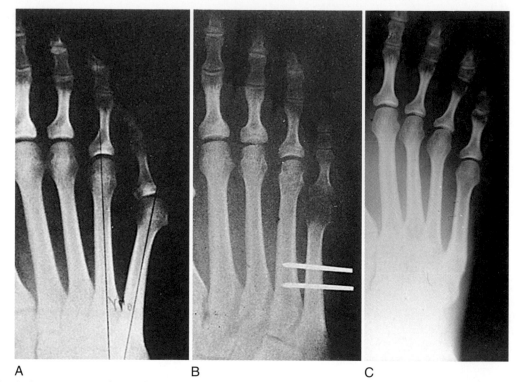

A   B   C

Figure 9–36 A, Preoperative radiograph demonstrates bunionette deformity. **B,** Proximal chevron osteotomy achieves correction of widened 4-5 intermetatarsal angle. **C,** After removal of internal fixation. (From Diebold PF, Bejjani FJ: *Foot Ankle* 8:40-45, 1987.)

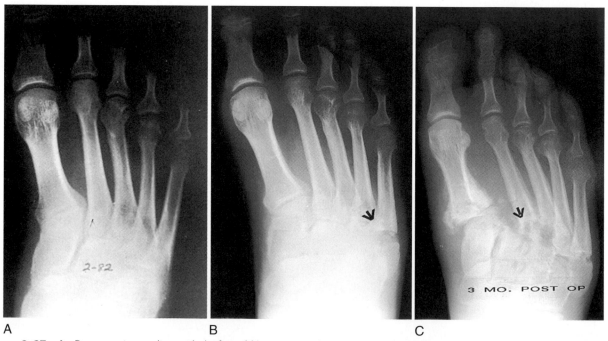

A   B   C

Figure 9–37 A, Preoperative radiograph before fifth metatarsal osteotomy. **B,** Radiograph after osteotomy demonstrates destabilization of tarsometatarsal joint. **C,** Further progression of Charcot arthropathy of the Lisfranc joint.

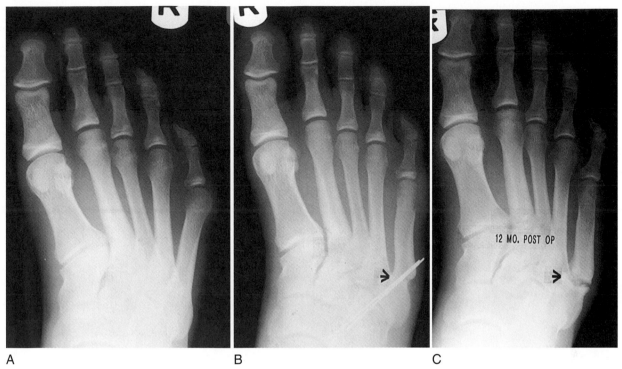

A   B   C

Figure 9–38 **A,** Preoperative radiograph demonstrates bunionette deformity. **B,** Radiograph after proximal fifth metatarsal osteotomy. **C,** After proximal fifth metatarsal osteotomy, delayed union has occurred. Osteotomy in this adolescent took approximately 12 months to heal.

AUTHOR'S PREFERRED METHOD OF TREATMENT

Conservative Treatment

Early conservative management of a symptomatic bunionette includes shaving the keratotic lesion, padding the lesion, and wearing roomy footwear. Most patients with symptomatic mild bunionette deformities can be successfully treated with shoe modifications and modified insoles or orthoses that relieve pressure over a painful lateral eminence. Often, conservative methods are effective in reducing symptoms; however, in the presence of chronic bursal thickening, development of symptomatic keratoses, and intractable pain, surgical intervention may be warranted. When a bursa becomes inflamed or infection occurs, a sandal or postoperative shoe may be necessary to completely relieve pressure. Plantar pain associated with an intractable keratotic lesion can often be relieved with a prefabricated or custom insole as well.

Surgical Treatment

When intractable symptoms are refractory to nonsurgical treatment, operative intervention may be neces-

sary. More than 30 different surgical techniques have been recommended for the surgical correction of a bunionette deformity. Excision of the lateral condyle, resection of the metatarsal head and fifth ray, and osteotomies of the fifth metatarsal (distal, diaphyseal, and proximal) with or without MTP arthroplasty have been described. In most cases the paucity of follow-up study with these procedures and the anecdotal reports of success with various techniques should raise a question as to their long-term efficacy. Likewise, the wide range of anatomic variations manifesting with bunionette deformities tends to make the choice of technique for surgical correction somewhat complicated.

An enlarged fifth metatarsal head or lateral condyle (with or without excessive pronation of the foot) may be treated either with a lateral condyle resection and fifth MTP joint realignment or with a distal metatarsal osteotomy. Realignment of the MTP joint and meticulous closure of the capsule are important to prevent lateral subluxation or dislocation of the fifth MTP joint (Fig. 9–39). The high recurrence rate with condyle resection tends to make this technique a less desirable procedure. With a pure lateral keratotic lesion, a distal chevron osteotomy or capital oblique osteotomy are preferable because of their inherent stability. Kirschner

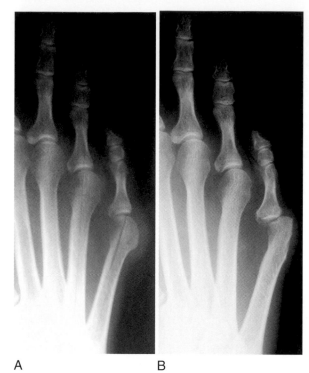

A   B

Figure 9–39 **A,** Preoperative radiograph. **B,** Dislocation of fifth metatarsophalangeal joint after lateral condylectomy.

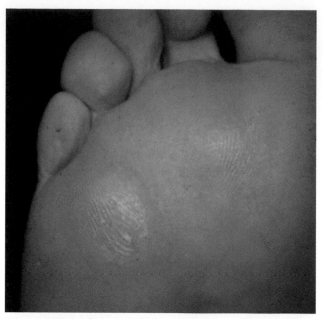

Figure 9–40   After distal fifth metatarsal osteotomy, a transfer lesion has developed beneath the fourth metatarsal.

wire or screw fixation tends to ensure stability of the osteotomy site until adequate healing has occurred. With a plantar or plantar–lateral keratosis, without an increase in the 4-5 intermetatarsal angle or without lateral fifth metatarsal deviation, a capital oblique osteotomy may be the procedure of choice. A diaphyseal or distal metaphyseal biplanar osteotomy may also be considered in this situation.

In the presence of a widened 4-5 intermetatarsal angle associated with a bunionette deformity (type 3) or with substantial lateral bowing of the fifth metatarsal shaft (type 2), a diaphyseal osteotomy combined with a distal soft tissue realignment affords an excellent means of correction. Midshaft diaphyseal osteotomies allow greater correction than distal metatarsal osteotomies and do not appear to threaten the tenuous vascular supply in the region of the proximal fifth metatarsal. With internal fixation, this osteotomy appears to allow correction without a significant risk of a transfer lesion. Understanding of the extraosseous and intraosseous vascular supply to the proximal fifth metatarsal as well as reports of delayed healing with fractures in this region make the possibility of vascular compromise after proximal metatarsal osteotomy a worrisome complication. A diaphyseal fifth metatarsal osteotomy appears to offer a less vulnerable area for a bunionette correction.

Although considerable disagreement exists regarding the need for internal fixation after a fifth metatarsal osteotomy, the frequently reported complications of malunion, nonunion, and transfer keratotic lesions after floating osteotomies indicate the need for either internal fixation or the use of an inherently stable fifth metatarsal osteotomy (Fig. 9–40). The principles of internal fixation where a fifth metatarsal osteotomy has been performed should be equally applied to the foot as well as elsewhere in the musculoskeletal system.

Preoperative radiographic evaluation of a bunionette deformity is important in analyzing the disorder present. Correlation of radiographic abnormalities with physical findings, including the location of the keratotic lesions, will help to define the appropriate surgical procedure.

Treatment of a symptomatic bunionette requires surgical versatility. Adapting the surgical repair to the underlying disorder will help to determine whether a condylectomy with a distal soft tissue repair, a distal metatarsal osteotomy, or a diaphyseal metatarsal osteotomy offers the best solution for a painful bunionette deformity.

REFERENCES

1. Addante JB, Chin M, Makower BL, et al: Surgical correction of tailor's bunion with resection of fifth metatarsal head and Silastic sphere implant: An 8-year follow-up study. *J Foot Surg* 25(4):315-320, 1986.
2. Bishop J, Kahn A 3rd, Turba JE: Surgical correction of the splayfoot: The Giannestras procedure. *Clin Orthop* 146:234-238, 1980.

3. Boyer ML, DeOrio JK: Bunionette deformity correction with distal chevron osteotomy and single absorbable pin fixation. *Foot Ankle Int* 24(11):834-837, 2003.

4. Brown JE: Functional and cosmetic correction of metatarsus latus (splay foot). *Clin Orthop* 14:166-170, 1959.

5. Buchbinder IJ: DRATO procedure for tailor's bunion. *J Foot Surg* 21(3):177-180, 1982.

6. Campbell D: Chevron osteotomy for bunionette deformity. *Foot Ankle* 2:355-356, 1982.

7. Castle JE, Cohen AH., Docks G: Fifth metatarsal distal oblique wedge osteotomy utilizing cortical screw fixation. *J Foot Surg* 31(5):478-485, 1992.

8. Catanzariti AR, Friedman C, DiStazio J: Oblique osteotomy of the fifth metatarsal: A five year review. *J Foot Surg* 27(4):316-320, 1988.

9. Coughlin MJ: Etiology and treatment of the bunionette deformity. *Instr Course Lect* 39:37-48, 1990.

10. Coughlin MJ: Treatment of bunionette deformity with longitudinal diaphyseal osteotomy with distal soft tissue repair. *Foot Ankle* 11(4):195-203, 1991.

11. Coughlin MJ, Thompson FM: The high price of high-fashion footwear. *Instr Course Lect* 44:371-377, 1995.

12. Davies H: Metatarsus quintus valgus. *Br Med J* 1:664-665, 1949.

13. Dayton P, Glynn A., Rogers WS: Use of the Z osteotomy for tailor bunionectomy. *J Foot Ankle Surg* 42(3):167-169, 2003.

14. Dickson FD, Diveley RL: *Functional Disorders of the Foot*, ed 3. Philadelphia, JB Lippincott, 1953, p 230.

15. Diebold PF: Basal osteotomy of the fifth metatarsal for the bunionette. *Foot Ankle* 12(2):74-79, 1991.

16. Diebold PF, Bejjani FJ: Basal osteotomy of the fifth metatarsal with intermetatarsal pinning: A new approach to tailor's bunion. *Foot Ankle* 8(1):40-45, 1987.

17. Dorris MF, Mandel LM: Fifth metatarsal head resection for correction of tailor's bunions and sub–fifth metatarsal head keratoma: A retrospective analysis. *J Foot Surg* 30(3):269-275, 1991.

18. DuVries H: *Surgery of the Foot*, ed 2. St. Louis, Mosby, 1965, pp 456-462.

19. Estersohn F, Scherer P, Bogdan R: A preliminary report on opening wedge osteotomy of the fifth metatarsal. *Arch Podiatr Med Foot Surg* 1:317-327, 1974.

20. Fallat LM, Buckholz J: An analysis of the tailor's bunion by radiographic and anatomical display. *J Am Podiatry Assoc* 70(12):597-603, 1980.

21. Frankel JP, Turf RM., King BA: Tailor's bunion: Clinical evaluation and correction by distal metaphyseal osteotomy with cortical screw fixation. *J Foot Surg* 28(3):237-243, 1989.

22. Friend G, Grace K, Stone HA: L-Osteotomy with absorbable fixation for correction of tailor's bunion. *J Foot Ankle Surg* 32(1):14-19, 1993.

23. Gerbert J, Sgarlato TE., Subotnick SI: Preliminary study of a closing wedge osteotomy of the fifth metatarsal for correction of a tailor's bunion deformity. *J Am Podiatry Assoc* 62(6):212-218, 1972.

24. Giannestras NJ: Other problems of the foot. In Giannestras NJ (ed): *Foot Disorders: Medical and Surgical Management*. Philadelphia, Lea & Febiger, 1973, pp 420-421.

25. Haber JH, Kraft J: Crescentic osteotomy for fifth metatarsal head lesions. *J Foot Surg* 19(2):66-67, 1980.

26. Hohmann F: *Fuss und Bein*. Munich, Bergman, 1951, pp 172-173.

27. Kaplan EG, Kaplan G, Jacobs AM: Management of fifth metatarsal head lesions by biplane osteotomy. *J Foot Surg* 15(1):1-8, 1976.

28. Keating SE, DeVincentis A, Goller WL: Oblique fifth metatarsal osteotomy: A follow-up study. *J Foot Surg* 21(2):104-107, 1982.

29. Kelikian H: Deformities of the lesser toe. In Kelikian H (ed): *Hallux Valgus, Allied Deformities of the Forefoot, and Metatarsalgia.* Philadelphia, WB Saunders, 1965, pp 327-330.

30. Kitaoka HB, Holiday AD Jr: Lateral condylar resection for bunionette. *Clin Orthop* (278):183-192, 1992.

31. Kitaoka HB, Holiday AD Jr: Metatarsal head resection for bunionette: Long-term follow-up. *Foot Ankle* 11(6):345-349, 1991.

32. Kitaoka HB, Holiday AD Jr, Campbell DC 2nd: Distal chevron metatarsal osteotomy for bunionette. *Foot Ankle* 12(2):80-85, 1991.

33. Kitaoka HB, Leventen EO: Medial displacement metatarsal osteotomy for treatment of painful bunionette. *Clin Orthop* (243):172-179, 1989.

34. Konradsen L, Nielsen PT: Distal metatarsal osteotomy for bunionette deformity. *J Foot Surg* 27(6):493-496, 1988.

35. Koti M, Maffulli N: Bunionette. *J Bone Joint Surg Am* 83(7):1076-1082, 2001.

36. Leach RE, Igou R: Metatarsal osteotomy for bunionette deformity. *Clin Orthop* 100:171-175, 1974.

37. Lelievre J: [Exostosis of the head of the fifth metatarsal bone; tailor's bunion]. *Concours Med* 78(46):4815-4816, 1956.

38. Lelievre J: *Pathologie du Pied*, ed 5. Paris, Masson, 1971, pp 526-528.

39. London BP, Stern SF, Quist MA, et al: Long oblique distal osteotomy of the fifth metatarsal for correction of tailor's bunion: A retrospective review. *J Foot Ankle Surg* 42(1):36-42, 2003.

40. Mann RA: Keratotic disorders of the plantar skin. In Mann RA (ed): *Surgery of the Foot*, ed 5. St. Louis, Mosby, 1986, pp 194-198.

41. McGlamry ED, Butlin WE., Kitting RW: Metatarsal shortening: Osteoplasty of head or osteotomy of shaft. *J Am Podiatry Assoc* 59(10):394-398, 1969.

42. McKeever DC: Excision of the fifth metatarsal head. *Clin Orthop* 13:321-322, 1959.

43. Moran MM, Claridge RJ: Chevron osteotomy for bunionette. *Foot Ankle Int* 15(12):684-688, 1994.

44. Nestor BJ, Kitaoka HB, Ilstrup DM, et al: Radiologic anatomy of the painful bunionette. *Foot Ankle* 11(1):6-11, 1990.

45. Okuda R, Kinoshita M, Morikawa J, et al: Proximal dome-shaped osteotomy for symptomatic bunionette. *Clin Orthop* (396):173-178, 2002.

46. Pontious J, Brook JW, Hillstrom HJ: Tailor's bunion. Is fixation necessary? *J Am Podiatr Med Assoc* 86(2):63-73, 1996.

47. Regnauld B: *Technique Chirurgicales du Pied*. Paris, Masson, 1974, p 23.

48. Sakoff M, Levy AI, Hanft JR: Metaphyseal osteotomy for the treatment of tailor's bunions. *J Foot Surg* 28(6):537-541, 1989.

49. Schabler JA, Toney M, Hanft JR, Kashuk KB: Oblique metaphyseal osteotomy for the correction of tailor's bunions: A 3-year review. *J Foot Surg* 31(1):79-84, 1992.

50. Schoenhaus H, Rotman S, Meshon AL: A review of normal intermetatarsal angles. *J Am Podiatry Assoc* 63(3):88-95, 1973.

51. Seide HW, Petersen W: Tailor's bunion: Results of a scarf osteotomy for the correction of an increased intermetatarsal IV/V angle. A report on ten cases with a 1-year follow-up. *Arch Orthop Trauma Surg* 121(3):166-169, 2001.

52. Shereff MJ, Yang QM, Kummer FJ, et al: Vascular anatomy of the fifth metatarsal. *Foot Ankle* 11(6):350-353, 1991.

53. Shrum DG, Sprandel DC., Marshall H: Triplanar closing base wedge osteotomy for tailor's bunion. *J Am Podiatr Med Assoc* 79(3):124-127, 1989.

54. Sponsel KH: Bunionette correction by metatarsal osteotomy: Preliminary report. *Orthop Clin North Am* 7(4):809-819, 1976.

55. Steel MW 3rd; Johnson KA, DeWitz MA, Ilstrup DM: Radiographic measurements of the normal adult foot. *Foot Ankle* 1(3):151-158, 1980.

56. Steinke MS, Boll KL: Hohmann-Thomasen metatarsal osteotomy for tailor's bunion (bunionette). *J Bone Joint Surg Am* 71(3):423-426, 1989.

57. Stewart M: Miscellaneous affections of the foot. In Edmonson A, Crenshaw AH (eds): *Campbell's Operative Orthopaedics*. St. Louis, Mosby, 1980, p 1733.

58. Throckmorton JK, Bradlee N: Transverse V sliding osteotomy: A new surgical procedure for the correction of tailor's bunion deformity. *J Foot Surg* 18:117-121, 1978.

59. Voutey H: Manuel de chirurgie orthopaedique et de reeducatioin du pied. Paris, Masson, 1978, pp 149-151.

60. Weisberg MH: Resection of fifth metatarsal head in lateral segment problems. *J Am Podiatry Assoc* 57(8):374-376, 1967.

61. Yancey HA Jr: Congenital lateral bowing of the fifth metatarsal. Report of two cases and operative treatment. *Clin Orthop* 62:20320-5, 1969.

62. Zvijac JE, Janecki CJ, Freeling RM: Distal oblique osteotomy for tailor's bunion. *Foot Ankle* 12(3):171-175, 1991.

Sesamoids and Accessory Bones of the Foot

Michael J. Coughlin

SESAMOIDS

Galen is reported to have first coined the term *sesamoid* because of the resemblance of these small rounded bones to the sesame seed.[37] The anatomic location of several of the sesamoids is constant, but the frequency of occurrence of other sesamoids is quite variable.[34]

The sesamoids function to alter the direction of muscle pull, diminish friction, and modify pressure. Sesamoids occur in the substance of their corresponding tendon. They may be totally or partially contained within the tendinous structure. Some sesamoids totally ossify, some remain entirely cartilaginous, and some partially ossify with a fibrocartilaginous interface between the ossified fragments. This variability in ossification might explain the radiographic absence or presence of various sesamoids, as well as the incidence of bipartism of sesamoids.[71]

The sesamoids in the foot and ankle region are contained within the plantar plates of the interphalangeal and metatarsophalangeal (MTP) joints and in the tendons of the flexor hallucis brevis, the intrinsic tendons of the lesser toes, the tibialis anterior tendon, the tibialis posterior tendon, and the peroneus longus tendon.

SESAMOIDS OF THE FIRST METATARSOPHALANGEAL JOINT

The sesamoids of the first MTP joint play an important role in the function of the hallux. Contained within the tendons of the flexor hallucis brevis, the sesamoids of the first MTP joint have many functions: to absorb the majority of the weight of the first ray; to protect the tendon of the flexor hallucis longus, which courses over the rather exposed plantar surface of the first metatarsal head; and to help increase the mechanical advantage of the intrinsic musculature of the first ray. Although sesamoid dysfunction is uncommon, it can occur with arthritis, trauma, infection, osteochondritis, and sesamoiditis.

First MTP sesamoid abnormalities are uncommon, but degeneration or isolated injury can cause pain and significant dysfunction. To understand the nature of the clinical problems and to appreciate appropriate indications for surgical intervention, an understanding of the function of the sesamoid mechanism and of the pertinent anatomy is necessary.

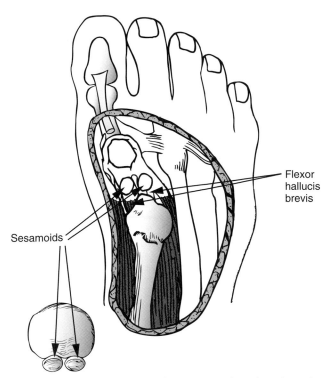

Figure 10–1 The sesamoids are enveloped within the double tendon of the flexor hallucis brevis.

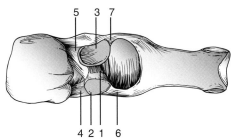

Figure 10–3 Metatarsophalangeal (MTP) joint from a dorsal exposure showing the intersesamoidal ligament *(1)*, the lateral sesamoid *(2)*, medial sesamoid *(3)*, lateral metatarsosesamoid ligament (plantar plate) *(4)*, medial metatarsosesamoid ligament (plantar plate) *(5)*, lateral joint capsule *(6)*, medial joint capsule with extension into the distal plantar plate *(7)*.

Anatomy

Location, Function, and Size

The sesamoid mechanism and intrinsic musculature of the hallux differentiate the first ray from the lateral toes. The hallucal sesamoids, enveloped within the double tendon of the flexor hallucis brevis (Fig. 10–1), articulate on their dorsal surface with the plantar facets of the first metatarsal head. A crista, or intersesamoid ridge (Fig. 10–2), separates the medial and lateral metatarsal facets. This intersesamoid ridge provides intrinsic stability to the sesamoid complex. In severe cases of hallux valgus with substantial subluxation of the sesamoid complex in relation to the first metatarsal head, the intersesamoid ridge atrophies and at times is obliterated (see Fig. 10–29).

The sesamoids are connected to the plantar base of the proximal phalanx through the plantar plate (Fig. 10–3), which is an extension of the flexor hallucis brevis tendon. The inferior surface of the sesamoids is covered by a thin layer of the flexor hallucis brevis tendon, whereas the superior surface is articular in nature. These sesamoids are entirely intratendinous except dorsally, where they articulate with the first metatarsal head. The sesamoids are suspended by a slinglike mechanism composed of the collateral ligaments of the MTP joint and the sesamoid ligaments (Fig. 10–4) on both the medial and lateral aspects of the MTP joint. The flexor hallucis brevis, through its sesamoid mechanism, provides a significant plantar flexion force at the MTP joint. The sesamoids also have an insertion into the joint capsule and the plantar aponeurosis; this provides both stabilization and a static plantar flexion force at the MTP joint.

On the medial aspect of the MTP joint, the abductor hallucis tendon (Fig. 10–5) inserts into the plantar–medial base of the proximal phalanx as well as the medial sesamoid and functions to stabilize the sesamoid mechanism medially. On the lateral aspect,

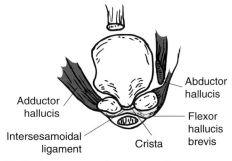

Figure 10–2 A cross section of the first metatarsal head demonstrates the sesamoid and the intersesamoidal ridge.

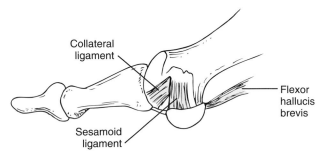

Figure 10–4 The sesamoids and collateral ligaments provide medial and lateral stability to the metatarsophalangeal joint.

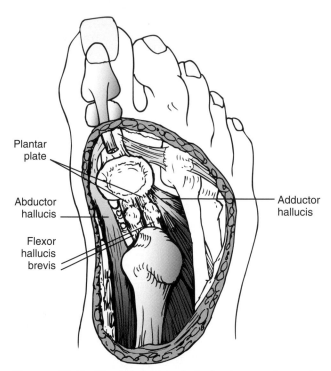

Figure 10–5 The abductor hallucis inserts into the plantar–medial base of the proximal phalanx, while the adductor hallucis inserts into the plantar–lateral base of the proximal phalanx. Both these intrinsic muscles also insert into their respective sesamoids.

the adductor hallucis tendon inserts into the lateral base of the proximal phalanx and into the lateral sesamoid to stabilize the sesamoid mechanism laterally. The medial and lateral sesamoids are connected by the intersesamoidal ligament that forms the base of the tendinous canal enveloping the tendon of the flexor hallucis longus.

Distal to the sesamoids, the phalangeal–sesamoid ligament is a thin layered structure that interdigitates with the collateral ligaments, extension of the plantar aponeurosis, and tendons of the flexor hallucis brevis to form the plantar plate. These structures are not individually distinguishable but rather coalesce to form the plantar plate.

When a person is in a standing position, the sesamoids are located posterior to the metatarsal head; however, with dorsiflexion of the hallux, the sesamoids move distally, thereby protecting the otherwise exposed plantar surface of the first metatarsal head. When a person rises onto the toes, the sesamoids (especially the medial sesamoid) act as the main weight-bearing focus for the medial forefoot.

Kewenter[45] noted that the medial sesamoid is located slightly more distal than the lateral sesamoid and is slightly larger. Orr[60] quantitated sesamoid size and reported that the tibial sesamoid averaged 9 to 11

mm in width and 12 to 15 mm in length. The fibular sesamoid was noted to have an average width of 7 to 9 mm and an average length of 9 to 10 mm.

Ossification

Although ossification of the hallucial sesamoids is variable, Kewenter reported that ossification usually occurs between the sixth and seventh years. Ossification of the sesamoids often occurs from multiple centers, and this may be the reason for the development of multipartite sesamoids.[45]

Circulation

The arterial circulation of the sesamoids was evaluated by Pretterklieber and Wanivenhaus.[62] In dissections of 29 cadavers that were studied arteriographically, three different types of arterial circulation were noted. The most common type (52%), type A, was characterized by arterial circulation derived from the medial plantar artery and the plantar arch. The less common type B (24%) was characterized by a pattern predominantly from the plantar arch, and in type C (24%) circulation was derived only from the medial plantar artery (Fig. 10–6). They concluded that the course and distribu-

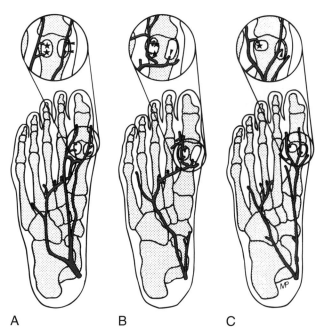

A   B   C

Figure 10–6 Circulation to the sesamoids. **A,** The most common pattern of arterial circulation to the sesamoids (52% of cases) involves a direct branch from both the medial plantar artery and the plantar arch. **B,** In 24% of cases, the sesamoid arterial supply is predominantly from the plantar arch. **C,** In 24% of cases, the major arterial supply is from only the medial plantar artery. When there is only one blood vessel supplying a sesamoid, a fracture may be at greater risk for avascular necrosis or nonunion. (Courtesy of Michael L. Pretterklieber, MD, and Axel Wanivenhaus, MD.)

tion of the arterial circulation to the sesamoids might have a bearing on the development of avascular necrosis following injury.

The number of arterial branches can affect healing of fractures as well as the incidence of avascular necrosis following trauma.[10] Multiple arterial branches can protect an injured sesamoid, whereas a single arterial branch to a damaged sesamoid may be interrupted by a fracture or injury and lead to delayed healing or a nonunion.

Sobel et al,[77] in their evaluation of sesamoid vascularity, mapped the vascular supply of both the medial and lateral sesamoids. The major vascular supply enters the sesamoids from the proximal and plantar aspect, with a minor arterial supply entering through the distal pole of the sesamoids (Fig. 10-7A). The distal vascular supply originates through distal capsular attachments providing, in most cases, a limited arterial supply. The proximal arterial supply, through the flexor hallucis brevis, supplies one third to two thirds of the proximal sesamoid. Vascular anastomoses occur between the proximal supply and that derived from the plantar surface to the body of the sesamoid (Fig. 10-7B). The distal portion of the sesamoid has the most tenuous vascular supply, and this can lead to delayed or unsuccessful healing following injury.

The sesamoids not only absorb weight-bearing forces on the medial aspect of the forefoot but also increase the mechanical advantage of the intrinsic musculature in plantar flexing the proximal phalanx. The tendon of the flexor hallucis longus is protected in its tendon sheath by the medial and lateral sesamoids and provides a plantar flexion force to the distal phalanx of the great toe.

Preoperative Evaluation

Physical Examination

Patients with a symptomatic sesamoid often complain of pain and discomfort during the toe-off phase of gait. Objective clinical findings include restricted range of MTP motion, pain on direct palpation, pain with motion of the first MTP joint, swelling of the first MTP joint, and diminished plantar or dorsiflexion strength. Synovitis of the first MTP joint may be noted as well on physical examination. Occasionally, an intractable plantar keratotic lesion develops beneath either the tibial or fibular sesamoid.

The orientation of the hallux must be inspected for lateral (hallux valgus) or medial (hallux varus) deviation or for clawing of the hallux. Progressive insidious deviation of the hallux can develop with sesamoid disruption caused by trauma or fracture. Progressive hallux valgus or hallux varus can also develop as a result of a previous sesamoid resection. Hyperextension of the hallux due to discontinuity of the sesamoid complex can occur following traumatic rupture of the plantar plate (Fig. 10-8).

Examination of the sensory nerves of the first ray is important in order to diagnose a compressed digital nerve,[33] which can manifest with isolated neuritic symptoms or numbness. With compression of either the medial or lateral digital nerve by either the tibial or fibular sesamoid, a Tinel sign can be elicited along the border of the sesamoid.

Radiographic Examination

Routine dorsoplantar and lateral radiographs (Fig. 10-9A and B) can provide limited information in the evaluation of a painful sesamoid. On the dorsoplantar view, the metatarsal head overlies both the medial and lateral sesamoid and often obscures detail; on the lateral projection, the medial and lateral sesamoids overlap each other. The fibular sesamoid is best demonstrated in a lateral oblique radiograph (Fig. 10-9C), where it can be seen between the first and second metatarsal heads. The tibial sesamoid is best seen on a medial oblique radiograph (Fig. 10-9D).[65] With the MTP joint dorsiflexed approximately 50 degrees, the roentgen beam is directed 15 degrees cephalad from a lateral position and is centered over the first metatarsal head. Often, however, the most useful radiograph is the axial sesamoid view (Fig. 10-9E).[36,51] Where radiographs appear normal in spite of a patient's subjective symptoms, a ^{99}Tc bone scan may be useful (Fig. 10-10). A bone scan can demonstrate increased uptake prior to the development of any significant radiographic change such as sclerosis, fragmentation, or disintegration.

BIPARTITE SESAMOIDS AND FRACTURES

The incidence of partite sesamoids as well as their cause has been the subject of substantial discussion in

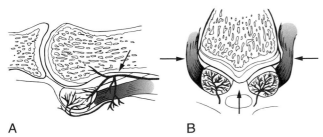

Figure 10-7 A, The major vascular supply enters the sesamoid proximally. An anastomosis occurs between the distal and proximal surface. **B,** The plantar vascular supply to the sesamoid is significant. (Adapted from Sobel M, et al: *Foot Ankle* 13:359-363, 1992.)

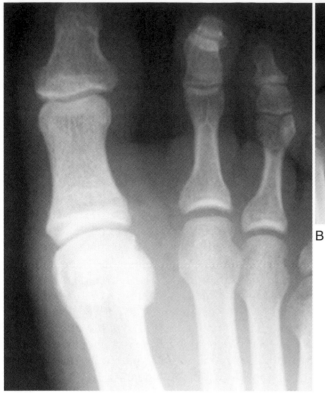

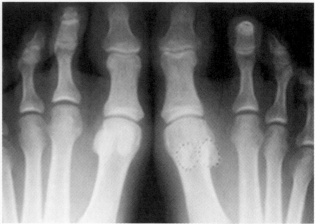

Figure 10–8   A, Anteroposterior (AP) radiograph immediately following hyperextension injury of the first metatarsophalangeal joint. **B,** AP radiograph of both feet one year later, demonstrating retraction of the sesamoid complex following disruption of the plantar plate.

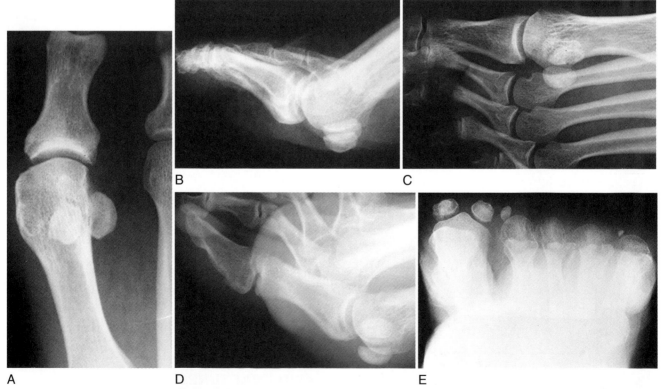

Figure 10–9   A, Dorsoplantar radiograph demonstrating the metatarsophalangeal sesamoids. The view is partially obstructed by the overlying metatarsal head. **B,** Lateral radiograph of the sesamoids. The medial and lateral sesamoids overlie one another and somewhat obscure the view of each individual sesamoid. **C,** A lateral oblique radiograph can best visualize the fibular sesamoid. **D,** A medial oblique radiograph shows more clearly the tibial sesamoid. **E,** An axial sesamoid radiograph presents the sesamoids without being obstructed by the overlying first metatarsal.

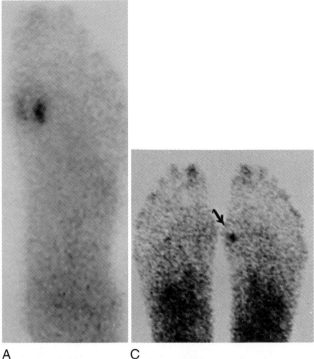

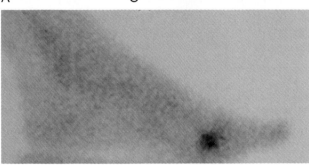

Figure 10–10 Anteroposterior **(A)** and lateral **(B)** [99]Tc bone scan demonstrating increased uptake in the lateral sesamoid. **C,** A bone scan may be helpful in diagnosing an abnormality when a routine radiograph appears normal. A fractured medial sesamoid *(arrow)* is demonstrated.

the literature (Table 10–1). Kewenter[45] examined 800 feet and found a 31% incidence of bipartite tibial sesamoids (Fig. 10–11), and Dobas and Silvers[19] examined radiographs of 1000 feet and found a 19% incidence of combined tibial and fibular sesamoid

TABLE 10–1

Proportion of Tibial and Fibular Division in Representative Series of Cases		
Authors	Number of Cases	Tibial Division (%)	Fibular Division (%)
Kewenter[45]	800	30.6	1.3
Dobas & Silvers[19]	1000	16.8	2.5
Burman & Lapidus[12]	1000	7.2	0.6

bipartism (Fig. 10–12). Dobas and Silvers reported that 80% of bipartite sesamoids involve the tibial sesamoid. Rowe[68] noted a 6% to 8% frequency of bipartite sesamoids and stated that 90% of these were bilateral. Dobas and Silvers[19] stated that approximately 25% of partite tibial sesamoids had an identical bipartite tibial sesamoid on the contralateral side, whereas the remaining sesamoids were asymmetric as far as division was concerned. Jahss[39] noted that bipartism was 10 times more common in the medial sesamoid. Giannestras[26] stated that the occurrence of bipartite sesamoids was typically symmetric, but this is obviously not the case. The medial sesamoid is often divided into two, three, or four parts, whereas the lateral sesamoid is rarely divided into more than two parts (Fig. 10–13).

Inge and Ferguson[37] reported that 85% of the bilateral partite sesamoids had asymmetric divisions. They also reported that the incidence of division decreased with time, thus implying that osseous union occurs with time in the divided sesamoid. They further reported that histologic evaluation of congenital bipartite sesamoids demonstrated that articular cartilage tended to dip down between the two osseous fragments. This can predispose a bipartite sesamoid to fracture or disruption of the synchondrosis with minimal injury (see Fig. 10–11D). They speculated that the medial sesamoid has a higher frequency of bipartism than the lateral sesamoid because it is more often traumatized, a result of its greater weight-bearing capacity. It has not been determined whether continued trauma with ambulation prevents the union of divided sesamoids or whether some of these partite sesamoids are actually nonunions of fractures.

The incidence of irregular ossification with bipartism in the medial sesamoid is well recognized. Kewenter[45] examined a series of sesamoids in cadavers and found that congenitally divided sesamoids fracture with much less force than normal sesamoids when experimental trauma was introduced. Although fractures of sesamoids are relatively rare, numerous cases have been reported in the literature.* Substantial trauma with MTP joint dislocation and simultaneous fractures of both sesamoids have been reported[18]; in general, the most frequently reported mechanism of injury is a fall onto the forefoot, sudden loading of the forefoot, or a crush injury.

It can be difficult to distinguish between a fractured sesamoid (see Fig. 10–13) and a symptomatic bipartite sesamoid.[25,81] With a divisionary line between two segments of a sesamoid, a careful physical examination and history must be correlated with radiographic findings to differentiate between a partite sesamoid

*References 1, 8, 11, 12, 25, 27, 35, 38, 47, 61, 66, and 81.

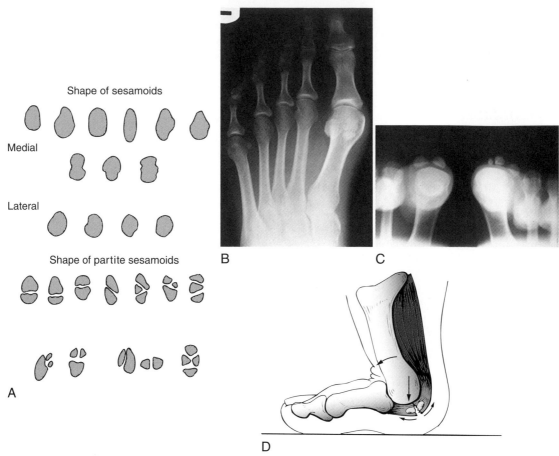

Figure 10–11 Many variations can occur in ossification of sesamoids of the metatarsophalangeal joint of the hallux. **A,** Various shapes of medial and lateral sesamoids. **B,** An anteroposterior (AP) radiograph demonstrates a bipartite medial sesamoid. **C,** An axial radiograph demonstrates a longitudinal bipartite medial sesamoid. **D,** Hyperextension injury mechanism resulting in disruption of the sesamoid complex.

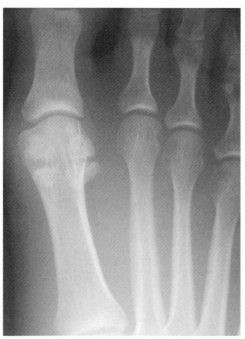

Figure 10–12 Anteroposterior radiograph demonstrating asymptomatic bipartite medial and lateral sesamoids.

and a superimposed fracture.[25] With a sesamoid fracture, pain is localized to the region of the specific sesamoid. Symptoms are typically exacerbated with ambulation and reduced with rest. Often the patient ambulates with weight bearing on the lateral aspect of the foot to avoid motion and loading of the sesamoid complex.

On physical examination, forced passive dorsiflexion and plantar flexion can cause discomfort. Synovitis or nonspecific swelling on the plantar aspect of the sesamoid complex may be observed. The development of pain following minimal trauma in the presence of a bipartite sesamoid should alert the examiner to the possibility of a superimposed fracture of a bipartite sesamoid. An acute fracture may be noted on a radiograph with a sharp radiolucent line (Fig. 10–14); however, Inge and Ferguson[37] suggested that a fracture should not be diagnosed unless callus is present. Delay in diagnosis of a sesamoid fracture is therefore common because of the difficulty of confirming the fracture by radiography.[80,84]

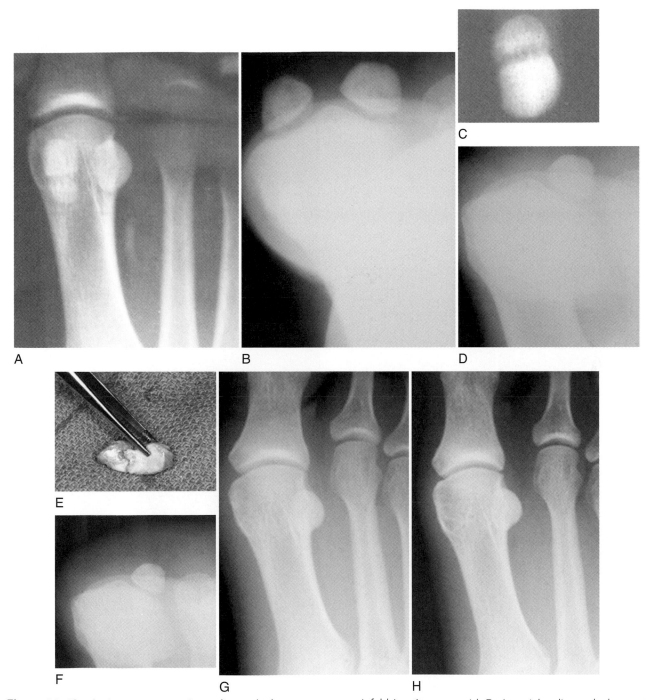

Figure 10–13 A, An anteroposterior radiograph demonstrates a painful bipartite sesamoid. **B,** An axial radiograph does not show evidence of a fracture or bipartite sesamoid. **C,** Radiograph of a pathology specimen showing rounded edges pathognomonic of a bipartite sesamoid. **D,** Axial view following excision of medial sesamoid. **E,** Gross pathology of a specimen. **F** and **G,** Immediately following surgery. **H,** At 19-year follow-up after medial sesamoid excision. Alignment of the first metatarsophalangeal joint is well maintained.

Although rarely is a preinjury film available in helping to differentiate a partite sesamoid and a fracture, increased separation between fragments can be a definitive finding in the presence of a disruption of a partite sesamoid (Fig. 10–15). Richardson[65] recommends a bone scan to aid in diagnosis of a fracture in the presence of a bipartite sesamoid.

Hobart[34] recommended non–weight bearing and casting until the sesamoid fracture had healed, which usually occurred in 6 to 8 weeks (Fig. 10–16). Anderson and McBryde[2] reported on 21 patients treated with bone grafting for symptomatic tibial sesamoid nonunions (Fig. 10–17). They curetted and bone grafted the diastasis, which was typically 1 mm wide. All patients were noted to have a positive bone scan prior to surgery. In two cases where articular surface deterioration was noted, a sesamoidectomy was performed. Three other patients had excessive motion at the diastasis site and were not considered candidates for bone grafting. Through an inferior extra-articular approach, they curetted and bone grafted the diastasis "nonunion site." No internal fixation was used. The patients were placed in a below-knee cast and kept non–weight bearing for 4 weeks. At final follow-up, 19

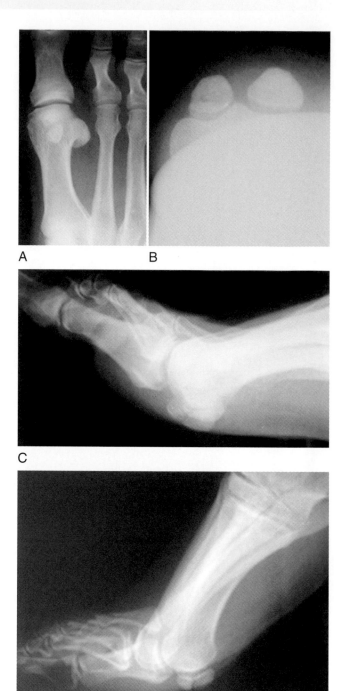

Figure 10–15 **A,** Anteroposterior radiograph demonstrating a multipartite medial sesamoid. **B,** Axial view demonstrating defect. **C,** Lateral radiograph demonstrating alignment of proximal and distal fragments. **D,** With dorsiflexion of the hallux, the alignment of the fragments changes, demonstrating motion consistent with a fracture of a partite sesamoid.

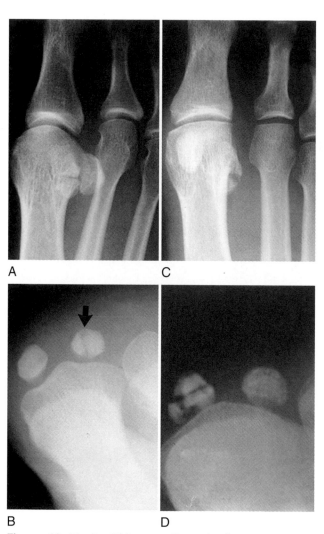

Figure 10–14 **A,** Oblique radiograph demonstrating an acute fracture of the medial sesamoid. **B,** Axial radiograph demonstrating a longitudinal fracture *(arrow)* of the lateral sesamoid. This fracture was only demonstrated on this particular view. **C,** Anteroposterior radiograph demonstrating a comminuted fracture of the lateral sesamoid. **D,** Axial radiograph demonstrating a comminuted fracture of the medial sesamoid.

of 21 sesamoids had healed. Two patients had a persistent nonunion.

Rodeo et al[66] reported on four cases of injuries to the hallux with progressive diastasis of bipartite sesamoids. The patients were treated with a distal

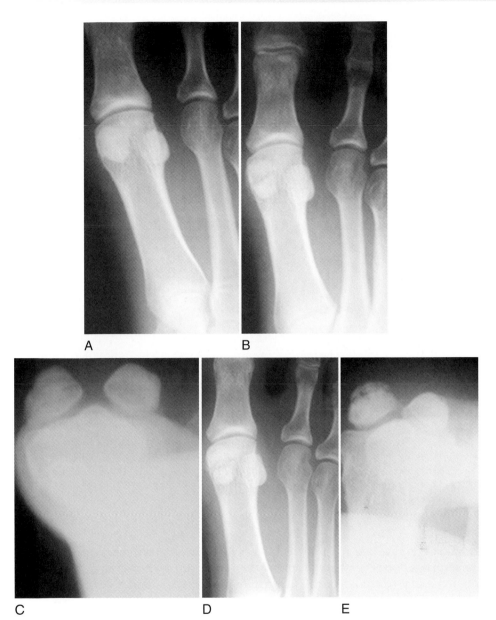

Figure 10–16 **A,** Anteroposterior (AP) radiograph of normal contralateral foot. **B,** AP radiograph of symptomatic bipartite medial sesamoid. **C,** Axial view. The patient was treated with a below-knee cast for 6 weeks, unweighting the sesamoids, and symptoms resolved. **D** and **E,** 15-year follow-up. AP radiograph **(D)** and axial view **(E)** demonstrating no radiographic changes. Patient remains completely asymptomatic.

resection of a smaller fragment and repair of the sesamoid mechanism.

Biedert and Hintermann[7] reported on five athletes who developed stress fractures of the medial sesamoids. Surgical excision of the proximal fragment and repair of the flexor hallucis brevis were performed. After casting for 6 weeks following surgery, full return to sports activity was allowed at 8 weeks.

Brodsky et al[10] retrospectively reviewed a series of 37 patients with fractured sesamoids. Avascular necrosis secondary to fracture was noted in nine cases, 16 cases were diagnosed as stress fractures, and 12 cases were related to direct trauma. Following surgical excision of the fractured sesamoid, an average postoperative AOFAS (American Orthopaedic Foot and Ankle Society) score of 93 was achieved.

Saxena and Krisdakumtorn[73] reported on 24 patients at a mean follow-up of 86 months following sesamoidectomy. There were 10 fibular and 16 tibial sesamoidectomies. Eleven patients were professional or varsity athletes and returned to activity in 7.5 weeks. The other patients returned to normal activities in 12 weeks. Complications included one varus deformity, one valgus deformity, and two cases of neuroma formation associated with fibular sesamoidectomy. Patients took longer to recover from surgery for tibial sesamoidectomy, which the authors surmised was probably due to increased weight bearing. Patients with fibular

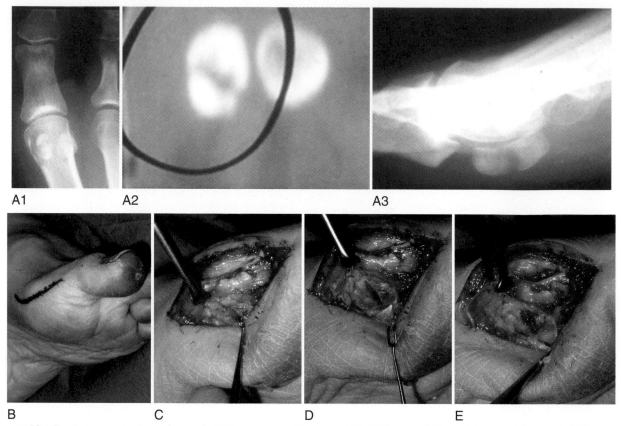

Figure 10–17 Anteroposterior radiograph **(A1)**, computed tomographic (CT) scan **(A2)**, and lateral radiograph **(A3)** demonstrating nondisplaced fracture of tibial sesamoid. **B,** Incision used to approach metatarsal sesamoid articulation for bone grafting. **C,** Extraarticular approach exposing plantar surface of sesamoid. Following curettage, the nonunion is identified, debrided **(D),** and bone grafted **(E).** (Courtesy of R. Anderson, MD, Charlotte, NC.)

sesamoidectomies had an earlier return to activity. They noted that a dorsolateral approach may be more difficult for fibular sesamoidectomy and that the two nerve problems both occurred with a dorsolateral approach.

Custom and prefabricated orthotics and scaphoid and metatarsal pads can relieve pressure in the sesamoid region, diminishing symptoms. Taping of the toe to reduce dorsiflexion can also relieve symptoms. If conservative methods fail, surgical removal of the involved sesamoid may be necessary.

Rosenfield and Trepman[67] have described the use of a rocker-soled walking shoe with a full-length steel shank. An orthotic insole is added with a recess beneath the sesamoid region (Fig. 10–18).

CONGENITAL ABSENCE OF THE SESAMOIDS

Congenital variations in regard to ossification of the tibial and fibular sesamoids are common. Congenital absence of a sesamoid has been infrequently reported; however, it is probably more prevalent than is realized.[48] Jeng et al[41] noted that only 11 cases of absent hallucal sesamoids have been reported in the literature. Patients are typically asymptomatic with absent sesamoids. Inge and Ferguson[37] reported two cases of congenital absence of the tibial sesamoid. Goez and DeLauro[29] and Zinsmeister and Edelman[85] have reported absence of the tibial sesamoids as well. Jeng et al[41] reported a case of an absent fibular sesamoid.

Although absence of a sesamoid can be asymptomatic, following removal of a sesamoid for painful plantar keratosis, pain can develop postoperatively beneath the remaining sesamoid. The absence of a tibial sesamoid can produce a clawing of the hallux or development of a progressive postoperative hallux valgus deformity (Fig. 10–19A and B).[29,85]

Jahss[40] has reported that congenital absence of both sesamoids is extremely rare (Fig. 10–19C).

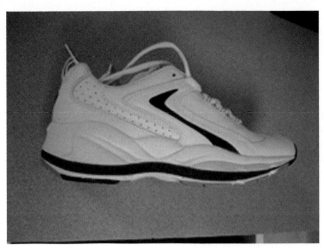

Figure 10–18 Rocker-soled walking shoe with a full-length steel shank and a custom orthotic insole may be used to relieve sesamoid pain. (Courtesy of E. Trepmann.)

DISTORTED OR HYPERTROPHIED SESAMOIDS

Congenital variations of the sesamoids can lead to localized discomfort if the plantar surface of the sesamoid is irregular. Hypertrophy of a sesamoid can create an extraordinarily large or thickened projection on the plantar surface and lead to development of a hyperkeratotic lesion (Fig. 10–20). Mowad et al[58] described an osteochondroma of the tibial sesamoid manifesting with a painful plantar mass and a hypertrophic plantar keratosis (Fig. 10–21A and B).

Acquired irregularities of a sesamoid can result from a congenital anomaly in the shape of the sesamoid, from previous injury, or from a rotational deformity of the great toe. Although the sesamoids normally articulate with the plantar metatarsal facets (see "Anatomy"), pronation of the hallux with adduction of the first metatarsal tends to lead to a rotational deformity in the metatarsal sesamoid articulation. This distortion can lead to hypertrophy of the sesamoid. If the hypertrophy occurs in a plantar direction, excess bone formation can lead to a symptomatic keratotic lesion that can ultimately ulcerate because of weight-bearing pressure.

Unrelenting pain with ambulation is the most common presenting symptom of a hypertrophied or distorted sesamoid. Although a thickened keratotic lesion may be mistaken for a verruca plantaris, trimming of the keratosis helps to differentiate the two lesions.

The soft tissue directly beneath the sesamoids can ulcerate, leading to secondary infection and

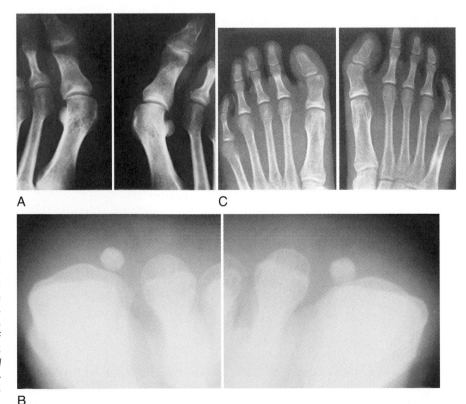

Figure 10–19 Congenital absence of both tibial sesamoids. The hammering of the hallux occurred with development of pain beneath the first metatarsal head. **A,** Anteroposterior radiograph. **B,** Axial radiograph. **C,** Congenital absence of both sesamoids. (From Jahss MS [ed]: *Disorders of the Foot and Ankle: Medical and Surgical Management,* ed 2. Philadelphia, WB Saunders, 1991.)

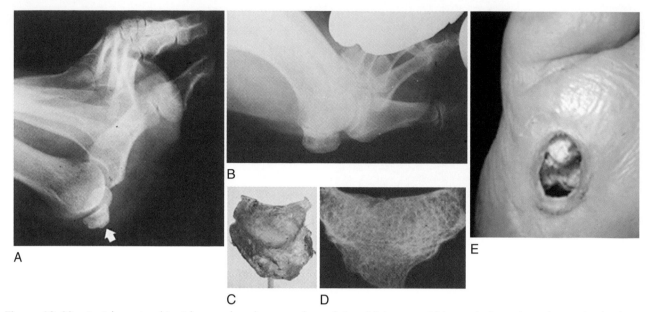

Figure 10–20   A, A hypertrophic ridge on the plantar surface of the tibial sesamoid is producing a hyperkeratotic skin lesion *(arrow).* **B,** Unusually thick tibial sesamoid that induced a deep-seated callus beneath the tibial sesamoid. **C,** Extensive hypertrophy of an excised sesamoid. A chronic ulcer developed under the first metatarsal head and sesamoid. **D,** Radiograph of the medial sesamoid, demonstrating a large plantar exostosis. **E,** Plantar ulcer beneath hypertrophic sesamoid.

osteomyelitis. A misshapen or hypertrophied fibular sesamoid is infrequently associated with a keratotic skin lesion because normally there is minimal weight bearing on the fibular sesamoid. Nonetheless, a patient can experience pain in the first intermetatarsal space due to local irritation (Fig. 10–22A-C), and occasionally an exostosis develops on the fibular sesamoid (Fig. 10–22D). Saxby et al[72] have reported that a case of coalition of the tibial and fibular sesamoids with plantar pain was treated successfully with a custom orthotic device used to relieve pressure beneath the symptomatic sesamoid coalition (Fig. 10–23).

Treatment

Shaving of the symptomatic keratoses and the use of a metatarsal pad, scaphoid pad, or prefabricated or custom orthotic device can redistribute the weight-

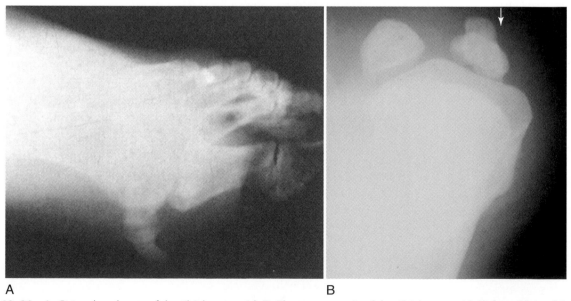

Figure 10–21   A, Osteochondroma of the tibial sesamoid. **B,** Plantar exostosis of the tibial sesamoid. (**A** from Mowad S, Zichichi S, Mullin R: *J Am Podiatr Med Assoc* 85:765-766, 1995.)

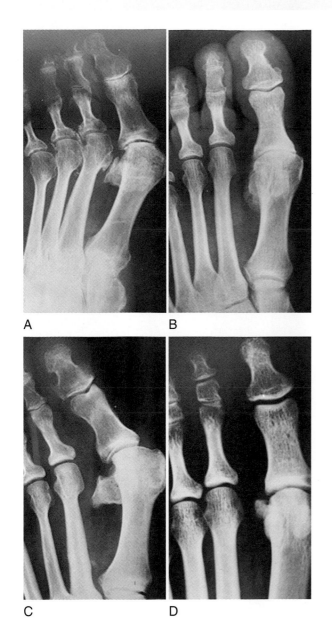

A   B

C   D

Figure 10–22 A to **C,** Hypertrophic changes in a fibular sesamoid with development of pain in the first intermetatarsal space. **D,** Exostosis of the fibular sesamoid.

bearing pressures and relieve symptoms (Fig. 10–24). With protracted symptoms, sesamoid shaving or sesamoidectomy may be necessary.

INTRACTABLE PLANTAR KERATOSES

An intractable plantar keratotic lesion can develop beneath the tibial sesamoid without significant hypertrophy or previous injury. Because of the position of the tibial sesamoid and its increased weight-bearing status, it is the tibial sesamoid that is often associated with an intractable plantar keratosis. A keratotic lesion

can develop with a cavus foot deformity or with a plantar flexed first ray, and this anatomy must be considered when evaluating a keratosis beneath the first metatarsal head. An osseous deformity of the sesamoid can lead to development of a symptomatic plantar keratotic lesion.

A more diffuse keratosis beneath the entire metatarsal head is usually associated with a plantar flexed first ray or cavus deformity. A more localized callus is usually associated with a prominent sesamoid.

Treatment

Often a keratotic lesion may be debrided or shaved. A custom-molded orthosis or a soft pad placed just proximal to the symptomatic lesion often alleviates symptoms. An extra-depth shoe (increased vertical volume) with a prefabricated or custom insole can provide relief of symptoms (Fig. 10–24D). With continued symptoms, sesamoid shaving can alleviate symptoms without impairing joint function.

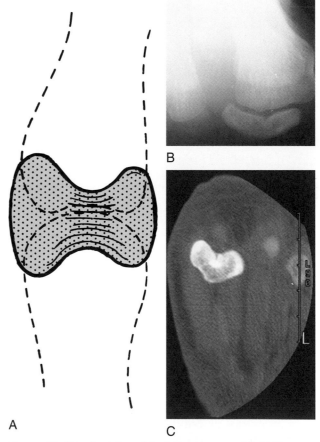

A   C

B

Figure 10–23 Coalition of the hallucal sesamoid. **A,** Diagram of sesamoid coalition. **B,** Axial radiograph. **C,** CT scan demonstrating coalition of tibial and fibular sesamoids. (**A** and **B** from Saxby T, Vandemark R, Hall R: *Foot Ankle* 13:355-358, 1992.)

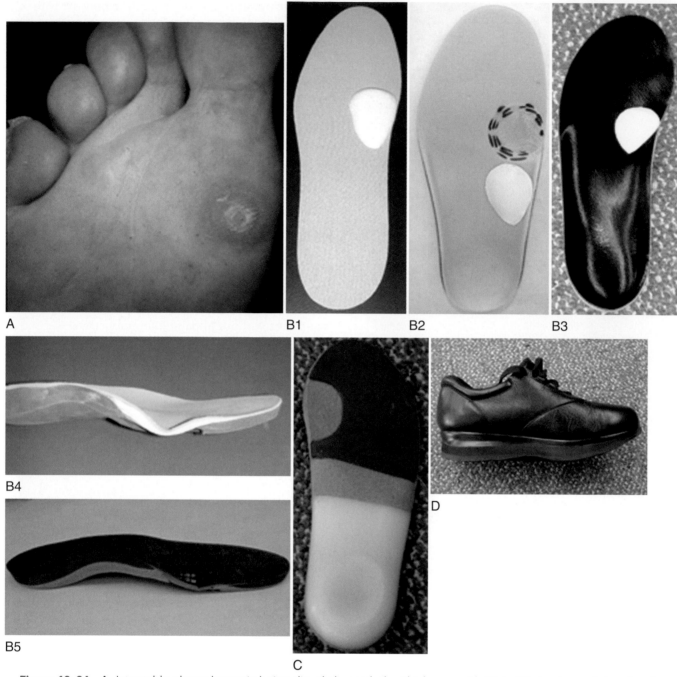

A

B1

B2

B3

B4

B5

C

D

Figure 10–24   A, Intractable plantar keratotic lesion directly beneath the tibial sesamoid. **B1** to **B5,** Insoles and shoe inserts. **B1,** Insole with Hapad placed just proximal to the sesamoids, relieving pressure. **B2,** Plastazote insert with proximal Hapad and area beneath sesamoid relieved. **B3,** Custom insert with proximal Hapad. **B4** and **B5,** Custom insert with sesamoid region molded to diminish pressure. **C,** Insert (see **B5**) shown from plantar aspect, with area beneath sesamoids decompressed. **D,** An extra-depth shoe might be necessary to accommodate the specific insert used to relieve sesamoid pain.

Occasionally a sesamoidectomy is necessary for an intractable lesion. Resection of a sesamoid in the presence of a cavus deformity or a plantar-flexed first ray is often associated with the recurrence of a plantar keratotic lesion. In this situation, a closing wedge dorsiflexion metatarsal osteotomy is preferable (see Fig. 10–39).

BURSITIS

Jahss[40] estimates that a bursa exists under the first metatarsal in 30% of normal feet (Fig. 10–25). With a cavus foot, a plantar-flexed metatarsal, or just excessive ambulation or standing, a subacute or chronic

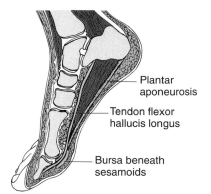

Figure 10–25 A bursa exists beneath the first metatarsal head and sesamoids in approximately 30% of normal feet.

Plantar aponeurosis

Tendon flexor hallucis longus

Bursa beneath sesamoids

sesamoid bursitis can develop. Chronic bursitis may be associated with a hypertrophied or arthritic medial sesamoid as well. Kernohan et al[44] reported a case of painful calcific bursitis of the sesamoid treated successfully with surgical debridement.

Treatment

Redistribution of weight bearing with the use of a custom orthotic device or metatarsal pad placed just proximal to the symptomatic sesamoid often diminishes discomfort (see Fig. 10–24). When symptoms are refractory to conservative treatment, surgery should be tailored to the underlying cause. A bursectomy sometimes gives long-lasting relief when a plantar-flexed first metatarsal or cavus foot is the underlying cause of symptoms. When the medial sesamoid is the cause of continued symptoms, surgical excision with resection of the overlying bursa often relieves symptoms.

NERVE COMPRESSION

The plantar–medial digital nerve and plantar–lateral digital nerve are located adjacent to the medial and lateral sesamoids (Fig. 10–26). Impingement of either of these branches may be a source of pain in the area of the sesamoids. Helfet[33] reported compression of the lateral plantar cutaneous nerve to the hallux. The plantar medial digital nerve can also be compressed by the medial sesamoid in a similar fashion. Often pain is difficult to differentiate from pain localized to the adjacent sesamoid. Occasionally a Tinel sign can be detected at the site of nerve compression. Patients might or might not appreciate decreased sensation distal to the nerve compression.

Treatment

A metatarsal pad or custom orthosis can relieve symptoms of a compressed nerve. Continued symptoms in spite of conservative care can necessitate surgical intervention. Surgical excision of the involved sesamoids may be used to relieve pain; however, a surgeon must isolate and protect the involved nerve in order to avoid injury. A postoperative neuroma following surgery

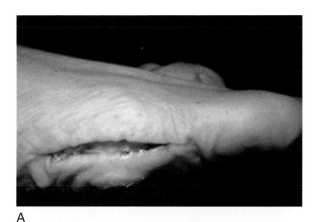

A

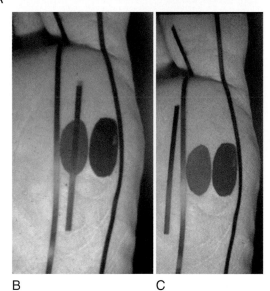

B   C

Figure 10–26 **A,** Medial view demonstrating the dorsal and plantar common digital nerves of the hallux. Note the proximity of the plantar digital nerve to the medial sesamoid. A medial incision exposure of the sesamoids is made dorsal to the medial digital nerve. **B,** A plantar view of the foot demonstrating the common digital nerves to the hallux. Note the proximity of each nerve (red lines) to the medial and lateral sesamoids (blue circles). (An incision directly over a sesamoid should be avoided.) **C,** The plantar incision (blue line) advocated by Jahss to expose the lateral sesamoid is made between the first and second metatarsal heads just lateral to the lateral common digital nerve. Red lines indicate nerves, and blue circles indicate the medial and lateral sesamoids.

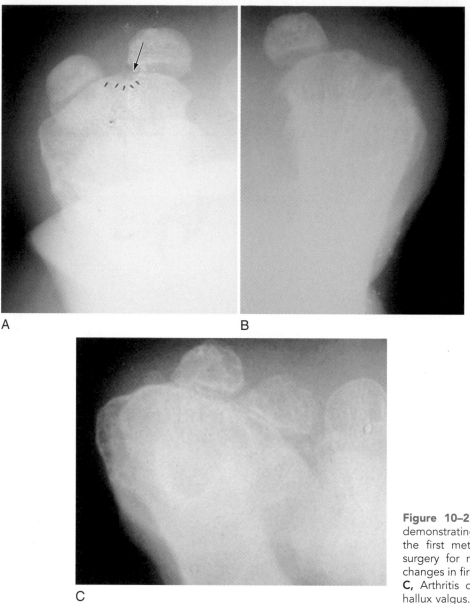

Figure 10–27 A, Axial view of a sesamoid demonstrating cystic degenerative changes in the first metatarsal head. **B,** One year after surgery for medial sesamoid resection, cystic changes in first metatarsal head remain present. **C,** Arthritis of the sesamoids associated with hallux valgus.

may be more symptomatic than a patient's original complaint.

ARTHRITIS

Degenerative arthritis of the first metatarsal sesamoid articulation has been reported by several investigators.* Subchondral cyst formation can develop as a secondary change.[50] Symptoms may be associated with rheumatoid arthritis, hallux rigidus, psoriatic arthritis,

or other systemic arthritides. Local degenerative arthritis of one or more of the sesamoids can occur. Diffuse idiopathic skeletal hyperostosis (DISH) can involve the sesamoids and lead to osteophyte formation.[40] Rupture of either the abductor hallucis or the adductor hallucis can result in the development of progressive hallux valgus or hallux varus. Complete rupture of the plantar plate can lead to clawing of the hallux.

Scranton and Rutkowski[75] reported erosion of articular cartilage in cases of progressive sesamoid chondromalacia that eventually required surgical excision. Degenerative arthritis of the metatarsal sesamoid articulation can develop as a progression of localized trauma, chondromalacia, or sesamoiditis (Fig. 10–27).

*References 31, 37, 39, 45, 50, 64, and 74.

Initial symptoms include swelling, synovitis, and erythema and can be demonstrated on physical examination. Restricted MTP joint motion, pain with forced dorsiflexion, and pain on localized palpation may be noted as well.

Treatment

The goal of conservative care is to relieve discomfort with ambulation. A stiff insole, extended shank, rocker outer sole, and custom orthosis or metatarsal pad that relieves pressure beneath the first metatarsal head or reduces MTP joint motion often eliminates symptoms. NSAIDs can also decrease inflammation.

Surgical resection of the involved sesamoid may also be considered for isolated arthritis of either the lateral or medial sesamoid. In the presence of long-standing arthritis, MTP joint motion often fails to improve with surgical resection of a sesamoid, although pain may be significantly relieved.[15] When both the medial and lateral sesamoids are involved, a combined resection is contraindicated because it will destroy the intrinsic insertion of the flexor digitorum brevis and lead to clawing of the great toe. An MTP joint arthrodesis may be necessary to relieve pain. A Keller resection arthroplasty is another alternative, although it can lead to postoperative clawing of the hallux as well (Fig. 10–28).[16]

SUBLUXATION AND DISLOCATION OF THE SESAMOIDS

As the magnitude of a hallux valgus deformity increases, pronation of the great toe occurs. As the hallux migrates into valgus, the first metatarsal deviates medially. As the deformity increases, the first metatarsal head progressively subluxates off of the sesamoid mechanism. Although the term "sesamoid subluxation" is associated with a hallux valgus deformity, the sesamoid migration occurs solely in relation to the first metatarsal head.[22] The sesamoid mechanism retains its relationship anatomically to the second metatarsal because it is tethered by the transverse metatarsal ligament and the conjoined adductor hallucis tendon.[41] Increased weight-bearing forces are transmitted through the first metatarsal head and tibial sesamoid. The fibular sesamoid, however, becomes displaced into the first intermetatarsal space, where weight-bearing forces are diminished.

Weil and Hill,[82] in an evaluation of 500 normal radiographs, noted a 15% incidence of bipartite tibial sesamoids in the general population. In contrast, in the examination of 500 radiographs of feet with hallux

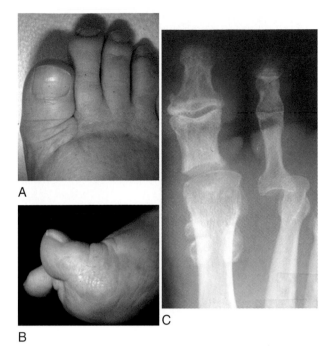

Figure 10–28 **A** and **B,** Photographs demonstrating postoperative clawing following the Keller procedure. **C,** Anteroposterior radiograph demonstrating postoperative retraction of the sesamoids following resection arthroplasty. Note also the dislocated second metatarsophalangeal joint.

valgus they observed a 32% incidence of hallux valgus associated with bipartite tibial sesamoids and concluded that multipartite sesamoids can predispose the first ray to a hallux valgus deformity.

As sesamoid displacement develops, the intersesamoid ridge erodes (Fig. 10–29). Axial radiographs often show gradual attrition of the intersesamoid ridge with a mild and moderate hallux valgus deformity. With a severe deformity, complete erosion of the crista occurs. Insertion of the conjoined adductor tendon into the plantar–lateral base of the proximal phalanx and lateral sesamoid leads to a pronation or rotational force on the great toe as the hallux valgus deformity increases.

Treatment

Following correction of a hallux valgus deformity, the alignment of the sesamoids may be undercorrected, adequately corrected, or overcorrected. Although the goal is to realign the sesamoids with the first metatarsal plantar facets, it may be necessary to achieve this correction through release of the conjoined adductor tendon and lateral capsular structures. On occasion a lateral sesamoidectomy is performed. Although such procedures allow relocation of the tibial sesamoid to the plantar–medial facet of the first

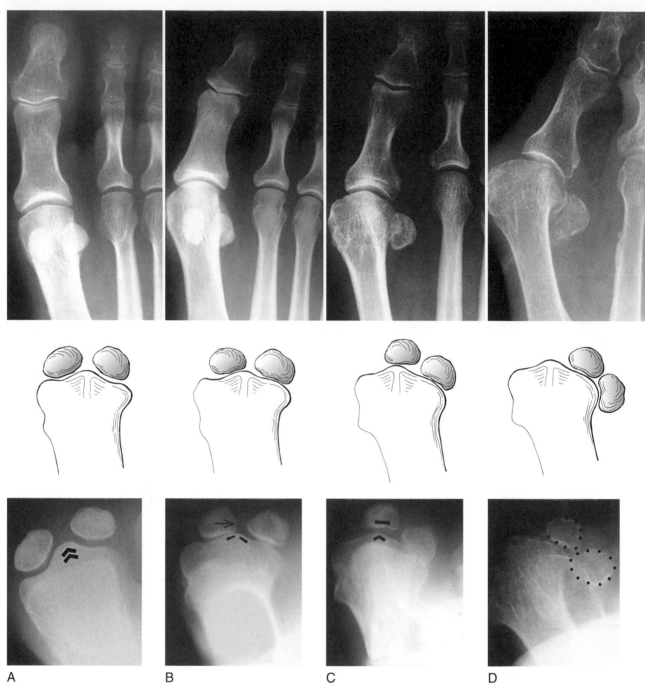

Figure 10–29 **A,** Normal axial position of the sesamoids centered on either aspect of the cristae. An anteroposterior (AP) radiograph demonstrates the normal position of the sesamoids. **B,** Mild hallux valgus deformity with mild subluxation. **C,** Moderate hallux valgus deformity associated with moderate sesamoid subluxation. An AP radiograph demonstrates moderate sesamoid subluxation. **D,** Severe hallux valgus associated with severe subluxation of the sesamoids. An AP radiograph demonstrates a hallux valgus angle of 60 degrees.

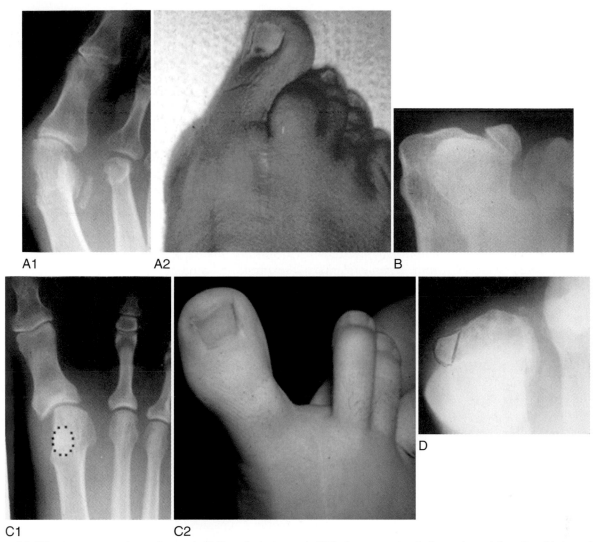

A1   A2   B

C1   C2   D

Figure 10–30   Anteroposterior radiograph **(A1)** and photograph **(A2)** demonstrating hallux valgus deformity with lateral sub-luxation of the lateral sesamoid following medial sesamoid excision. **B,** Axial radiograph demonstrating lateral subluxation of the lateral sesamoid. Anteroposterior radiograph **(C1)** and photo **(C2)** demonstrating hallux varus deformity with dislocation of the medial sesamoid following lateral sesamoid excision. **D,** Axial radiograph demonstrating medial dislocation of the medial sesamoid.

metatarsal, an unstable situation occasionally develops because of erosion of the intersesamoid ridge. In this case the medial facet is no longer a stable articulating surface. Recurrent lateral sesamoid migration with the development of a recurrent hallux valgus deformity or medial migration of the tibial sesamoid with a resultant hallux varus deformity can occur (Fig. 10–30). The use of semirigid dressings in the acute postoperative period can help to maintain the surgical correction until the sesamoid mechanism becomes stabilized.

Although McBride[55] recommended excising the fibular sesamoid to achieve adequate release of the lateral capsular contracture, we believe a fibular

sesamoid should rarely be removed in the correction of a hallux valgus deformity. After a complete lateral soft tissue release has been performed, if a significant contracture remains or if significant degenerative changes of the lateral sesamoid restrict adequate MTP joint motion with realignment of the hallux, a fibular sesamoid resection may be contemplated.

An 8% incidence of postoperative hallux varus after a McBride procedure has been reported where a fibular sesamoid has been removed.[52] A postoperative hallux varus deformity is associated with the correction of hallux valgus deformities of a more severe nature (hallux valgus angle greater than 40 degrees).[52] Complete erosion of the intersesamoid ridge coupled with a contracted intrinsic musculature can lead to this potentially unstable situation. Overaggressive medial capsulorrhaphy and an excessive medial exostectomy can predispose to a postoperative hallux varus deformity.

INFECTION

Infections of the sesamoids are not common; however, several cases have been reported in the orthopaedic literature.* Osteomyelitis of the sesamoid can develop following trauma, a puncture wound, or breakdown of the plantar skin with chronic neuropathic ulceration. Often osteomyelitis of the sesamoid progresses to infection of the MTP joint. A gram-negative bacterial infection is often associated with chronic plantar ulceration.

On physical examination, the MTP joint becomes swollen and erythematous. Manipulation of the hallux causes pain. Often a delay in diagnosis occurs because of the insidious nature of the infection. Radiographic changes can be very slow to develop. Patients with decreased sensation because of diabetic neuropathy, sciatic nerve injury, myelodysplasia, and peripheral neuropathy are at risk for skin breakdown and sesamoid infection. Hypertrophic callus formation beneath the sesamoids can develop due to increased pressure. Skin breakdown and trophic ulceration can develop with subsequent osteomyelitis.

Treatment

Early conservative treatment may be used to reduce pressure beneath the sesamoids. A molded insole or metatarsal pad can reduce pressure beneath the sesamoids, and paring of abundant callus can relieve symptoms.

In the case of a diabetic patient who has an ulcer beneath the first metatarsal head, measures to ensure that the ulceration does not recur should be undertaken after the acute infection has subsided. Use of extra-depth shoes with a polyethylene foam (Plastizote) liner (see Fig. 10–24B2) can significantly reduce the recurrence of ulceration.

Where osteomyelitis of the sesamoid has developed, surgical excision may be necessary. In the case of acute infection, an attempt should be made to make a bacteriologic diagnosis at the time of the surgical debridement of the sesamoid. Excision of either or both sesamoids may be necessary depending upon the extent of the infection.[28] Irrigation, aggressive debride-

ment, and localized wound care are often necessary to achieve control of the wound. Although a double sesamoidectomy should be routinely avoided, advanced osteomyelitis with involvement of both sesamoids can necessitate their removal (Fig. 10–31). Preservation of the tendons of the abductor and adductor hallucis and subperiosteal resection of the sesamoids can help to prevent a cock-up deformity of the hallux. An interphalangeal arthrodesis might eventually be necessary following dual sesamoid excision to treat a clawing of the interphalangeal joint of the hallux. Postoperatively, restricted range of motion and decreased strength of the hallux are noted following sesamoidectomy; however, often the scarring that develops following infection prevents the claw toe deformity that typically develops after a bilateral sesamoid resection.

OSTEOCHONDRITIS OF THE SESAMOIDS

Osteochondritis of the sesamoids is a rare condition that can affect either sesamoid. It is characterized by pain, tenderness to palpation, and osseous fragmentation or mottling on radiographic examination.[24,36,46,70] Ilfeld and Rosen[36] described osteochondritis of the sesamoid and noted it occurred infrequently. Although the cause is unclear, Helal[32] and Brodsky[10] have suggested that osteochondritis develops after trauma or a crush injury. Kliman et al[46] hypothesized that the development of a sesamoid stress fracture and the subsequent reparative process lead to osteochondritis. Although trauma is likely to be the most common cause, Jahss[39] has associated osteonecrosis with diminished vascularity. He noted that osteonecrosis tends to occur in women around the age of 25 years, but it can occur in both sexes from 13 to 80 years of age. Jahss[40] reports that the tibial and fibular sesamoids are equally involved. Julsrud[42] reported simultaneous osteonecrosis in a 22-year-old woman. An interphalangeal joint fusion was combined with a sesamoid excision to prevent later clawing of the hallux.

The circulation of the sesamoids can play a role in the development of osteonecrosis. Pretterklieber and Wanivenhaus[62] and Sobel et al[77] (see Figs. 10–6 and 10–7) have described the arterial circulation of the sesamoids. Individual arterial patterns can predispose a sesamoid to degeneration following injury. An injury pattern that disrupts the interosseous circulation can predispose an injured sesamoid to osteonecrosis. Often, however, a patient gives no history of injury. On physical examination, pain and tenderness are localized to the involved sesamoid. The metatarsal head is usually nontender.

*References 14, 31, 49, 68, 76, and 79.

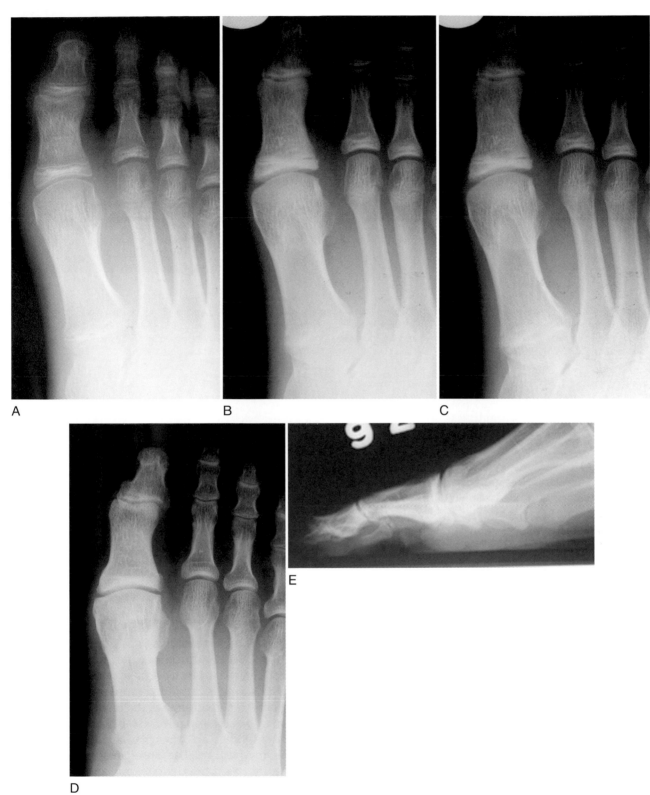

A

B

C

D

E

Figure 10–31   **A,** Osteomyelitis of the medial sesamoid in a skeletally immature person. **B,** Following excision of both sesamoids as treatment for sesamoidal osteomyelitis. **C,** Two years after surgery, due to postoperative scarring, a cock-up deformity did not develop. Anteroposterior **(D)** and lateral **(E)** radiographs at 13 years' follow-up demonstrate no subsequent deformity in spite of dual sesamoid excision.

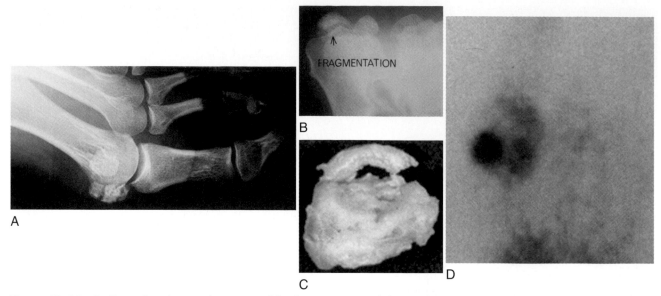

Figure 10–32 A, Osteochondritis is characterized by fragmentation of the medial sesamoid. **B,** Chondrolysis of the medial sesamoid as seen on an axial radiograph. **C,** Pathologic specimen demonstrating fragmentation of the sesamoid. **D,** Osteochondritis of the medial sesamoid as characterized by increased uptake on a technetium bone scan. (From Coughlin MJ: *Instr Course Lect* 39:23-25, 1990.)

The diagnosis of osteochondritis is usually made by an axial radiograph depicting the sesamoid in profile (Fig. 10–32A-C). Often radiographic findings are negative for 9 to 12 months. In time, lysis and resorptive changes in the involved sesamoid are combined with areas of sclerosis. Mottling, fragmentation, flattening, and elongation of the sesamoid can develop. A high-resolution technetium bone scan can help to make the diagnosis of osteochondritis in the absence of radiographic findings. With a bone scan, typically the sesamoid demonstrates increased uptake without significant involvement of the MTP joint (Fig. 10–32D).

Treatment

Conservative care includes reducing weight-bearing stress on the involved sesamoid. A metatarsal pad placed just proximal to the sesamoids or a custom-molded orthosis that diminishes weight bearing on the involved sesamoid might afford some relief. Although Fleischli and Cheleuitte[24] proposed casting as a treatment modality, they showed no evidence of any efficacy of this method. Indeed it is relatively difficult to immobilize the great toe in a below-knee cast. NSAIDs can relieve symptoms.

Although conservative care can help to diminish some symptoms, fragmentation or collapse of the sesamoid usually indicates the need for surgical resection of the involved sesamoid. Fleischli and Cheleuitte[24] discussed the use of a silicone implant, which was also proposed by Helal.[32] No long-term studies have been reported on this experimental procedure, and its use should be discouraged. An intraarticular steroid injection in the presence of osteonecrosis, although not contraindicated, is unlikely to provide long-term relief and is discouraged. It can temporarily reduce swelling and discomfort, allowing increased activity, which ultimately may lead to further degeneration of the involved sesamoid.

SESAMOIDITIS

The diagnosis of sesamoiditis is a diagnosis of exclusion. Often this condition occurs in teenagers and young adults and may be associated with trauma. Pain on weight bearing is a typical complaint. Often there is tenderness to palpation over the involved sesamoid, which may be accompanied by inflammation or a bursal thickening on the plantar aspect of the sesamoid mechanism. The onset may be sudden or gradual, with pain on weight bearing and dorsiflexion of the great toe. Although radiographic findings are typically normal, a high-resolution technetium bone scan might demonstrate increased blood flow to the involved sesamoid.[65]

Some types of trauma associated with sesamoid injuries include jumping from a height, excessive walking or dancing, excessive dorsiflexion of the MTP joint, or the chronic use of high-fashion footwear.[69] The tibial sesamoid is more often involved because of increased weight bearing in this area of the first metatarsal head.

Dobas and Silvers[19] defined sesamoiditis as an inflammation and swelling of the peritendinous structures involving the sesamoids. Apley[5] referred to "chondromalacia of the sesamoids" and described a condition similar to sesamoiditis. Apley dissected the medial sesamoid and found remarkable similarities between the articular cartilage and the degeneration seen with sesamoiditis and that of chondromalacia of the patellofemoral joint.

Treatment

Decreased walking activities and the use of metatarsal pads and custom foot orthoses may reduce weight-bearing pressure and relieve symptoms. A stiff-soled shoe or a graphite insole can diminish MTP joint motion and relieve pain (Fig. 10–33). Taping of the great toe in some degree of plantar flexion also helps to relieve pressure on the sesamoids (Fig. 10–34). Decreasing shoe heel height can reduce pressure on the involved sesamoid and relieve symptoms. NSAIDs are also efficacious at times. In the presence of continuing symptoms, surgical excision may be necessary.

Conservative Treatment

Often sesamoid problems can be treated effectively with conservative management. A decrease in activity

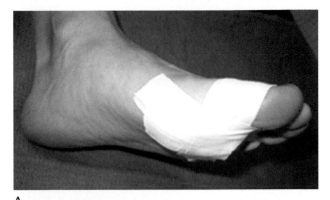

A

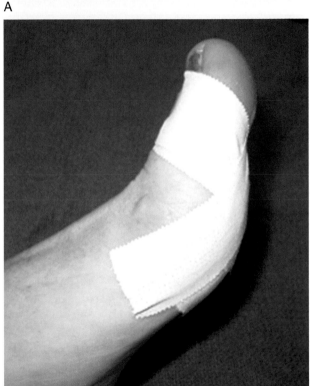

B

Figure 10–34 Taping of the hallux prevents excessive dorsiflexion.

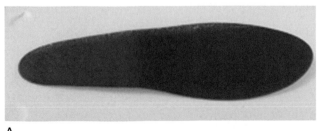

A

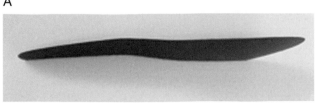

B

Figure 10–33 Graphite insole can diminish metatarsophalangeal joint motion. **A,** Top view. **B,** Side view.

in both athletes and sedentary patients can help to diminish symptoms. The use of low-heeled shoes reduces pressure on the sesamoids and often relieves discomfort. When a fracture has occurred, a below-knee walking cast or wooden-soled shoe may be used to decrease stress on the sesamoid and MTP joint, although typically it is extremely difficult to control the hallux and sesamoid mechanism with a below-knee cast unless the cast is extended to the tips of the toes. A custom-molded insole or metatarsal pad placed just proximal to the symptomatic area can help to

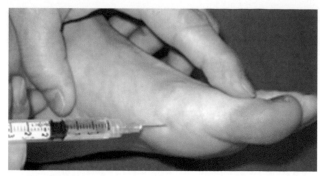

Figure 10–35 Injection for the sesamoid complex may be achieved from the medial aspect. The needle is directed between the medial sesamoid and the plantar metatarsal surface. Plantar flexion of the proximal phalanx aids in the injection by relaxing the capsular structures.

decrease pressure in the sesamoid region. Any of these modalities may be effective in treating fractures, sesamoiditis, or localized inflammation. They can also help to relieve discomfort from an intractable plantar keratotic lesion. Taping of the hallux in a neutral or slightly plantar-flexed position helps to reduce dorsiflexion with ambulation and can reduce localized irritation in the MTP joint. NSAIDs can also relieve symptoms. The infrequent judicious use of an intraarticular steroid injection can relieve inflammation or sesamoiditis (Fig. 10–35), but an injection in the presence of osteonecrosis or a sesamoid fracture is contraindicated.

Decision Making in the Excision of a Sesamoid

Either a tibial or fibular sesamoid may be excised if conservative care is ineffective in relieving symptoms. It is uncommon for a significant deformity to develop following isolated excision of either of these sesamoids, assuming that the patient does not have a hallux valgus or hallux varus deformity. Because the flexor digitorum brevis inserts into the base of the proximal phalanx after passing around the sesamoids, this attachment may be disrupted if both sesamoids are excised. Because the flexor digitorum brevis stabilizes and plantar flexes the proximal phalanx, a cockup deformity can develop. Thus only one sesamoid should be excised. If one sesamoid has previously been resected, it is preferable that the remaining sesamoid be protected to minimize the risk of a postoperative claw toe deformity. In the presence of an isolated intractable plantar keratotic lesion beneath the remaining sesamoid, shaving the plantar half of the remaining sesamoid is preferable to resection.

Surgical excision of a chronically painful sesamoid has been advocated when conservative treatment has failed.* Giurini et al,[28] in reporting on sesamoidectomy for the treatment of chronic neuropathic ulceration beneath the first metatarsal head in diabetic patients, noted two of 13 patients developed clawing, although there was minimal follow-up on these patients. Abraham et al[1] reported one case of dual sesamoid excision following trauma, and Julsrud[42] reported simultaneous osteonecrosis in a 22-year-old woman. In both reports, an interphalangeal joint fusion was combined with a dual sesamoid excision. Dual sesamoid excision should in general be avoided.[15,32,37] Scranton and Rutkowski[75] reported on simultaneous medial and lateral sesamoid excision and recommended a reapproximation of the defect created by surgery to minimize postoperative disability. Jahss[39] likened the repair of the defect in the flexor hallucis brevis to a repair of the quadriceps mechanism following a patellectomy.

The surgical approach used for sesamoid excision depends on which sesamoid is to be removed. The medial sesamoid can be approached through either a plantar–medial incision or a medial approach. Kliman et al[46] cautioned against using a plantar approach because of the proximity of the plantar digital nerves, and Mann et al[53] noted the possibility of the development of a painful plantar scar (see Fig. 10–42).

Mann and Coughlin[52] and Ferris et al[23] have advocated a dorsolateral approach to resect the fibular sesamoid in cases of hallux valgus; others[15] have advocated this approach for isolated fibular sesamoidectomy as well. Van Hal et al,[80] Helal,[32] and Jahss[40] recommended a longitudinal plantar incision adjacent to the fibular sesamoid for resection of a fibular sesamoid. Jahss found the dorsal approach for sesamoidectomy "almost impossible." Indeed, the use of a direct plantar approach to excise a symptomatic lateral sesamoid makes sense; however, a painful plantar scar can be an extremely difficult complication to resolve. In the case of a normally aligned first ray, I believe a plantar approach is technically easier; however, in the presence of a hallux valgus deformity, a dorsal approach is equally easy and avoids a plantar incision.

---

*References 5, 13, 14, 20, 21, 30-32, 34, 37, 39, 43, 46, 53, 59, 63, 74, 76, 78-80, and 84.

EXCISION OF THE TIBIAL SESAMOID

Excision of the medial sesamoid (Fig. 10–36) is much simpler than excision of the lateral sesamoid.

Surgical Technique

1. The tibial sesamoid is approached through a mid-medial 3-cm incision from a point just proximal to the first metatarsal head and extending distally toward the base of the proximal phalanx (Fig. 10–37A). The incision is carried down to the joint capsule. Care is taken to isolate and protect the medial plantar cutaneous nerve, which courses just over the medial border of the tibial sesamoid (Fig. 10–37B).
2. By incising the medial capsule (Fig. 10–37C) and retracting it plantarward, the articular surface of the sesamoid can be visualized (Fig. 10–37D).
3. The tibial sesamoid is then resected subperiosteally (Fig. 10–37E). In the case of a transverse fracture of the medial sesamoid, if the surgeon chooses to resect just the proximal pole of the sesamoid, it is excised sharply along the fracture line.
4. In the depths of the wound, the tendon of the flexor hallucis longus should be identified (Fig. 10–37F). Care should be taken to avoid injury to this structure.
5. An attempt is made to close the surgical defect created by excision of the sesamoid. Usually a purse-string closure helps to approximate or reduce the remaining defect (Fig. 10–37G and H). Care must be taken to avoid injury to the adjacent sensory nerve during this dissection.
6. The skin is approximated (Fig. 10–37I), and a gauze-and-tape compression dressing is applied. The patient is allowed to ambulate in a postoperative shoe for approximately 3 weeks.

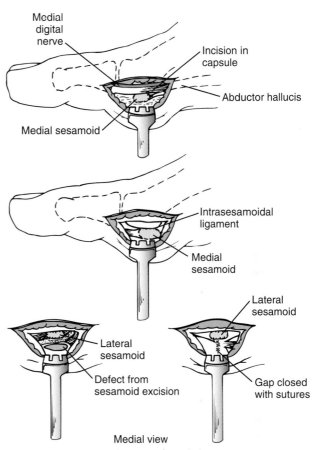

Figure 10–36 Technique of medial sesamoid excision.

SHAVING A PROMINENT TIBIAL SESAMOID[54]

Although surgical excision of a prominent tibial sesamoid may be used to treat an intractable plantar keratotic lesion, an alternative is to shave the plantar half of the tibial sesamoid (video clip 34). Resecting and beveling the plantar half of the tibial sesamoid can reduce a prominent tibial sesamoid enough to substantially relieve or reduce a plantar keratotic lesion.

Surgical Technique

1. A longitudinal plantar–medial incision is made similar to that used for a medial sesamoidectomy (see Fig. 10–37A).

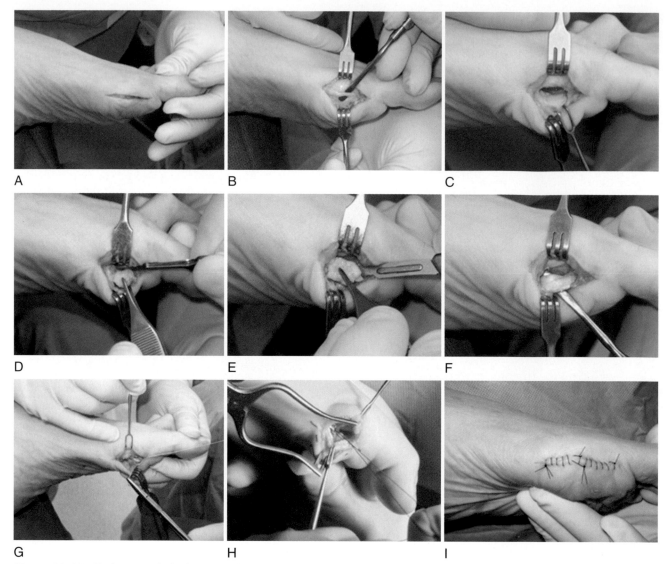

A   B   C

D   E   F

G   H   I

Figure 10–37   Technique of tibial sesamoid excision. **A,** A midline skin incision is made. **B,** Surgical dissection demonstrates the medial plantar sensory nerve just dorsal to the medial sesamoid. **C,** The capsule is incised just dorsal to the medial sesamoid to expose the medial sesamoid articulation. **D,** The sesamoid is retracted downward to improve visualization. **E,** The tibial sesamoid has been excised. **F,** The flexor hallucis longus tendon is inspected to ensure continuity. **G** and **H,** The defect is reduced or closed with 2-0 absorbable suture. Note the medial plantar sensory nerve overlying the repair site. **I,** Wound closure.

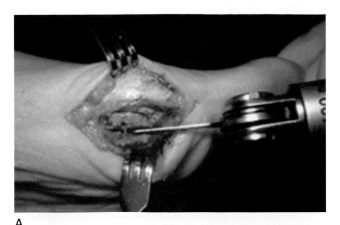

A

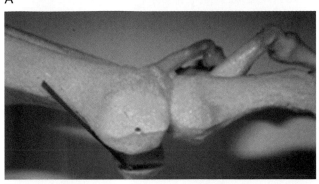

B

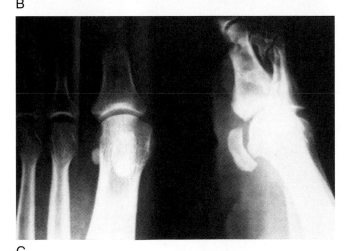

C

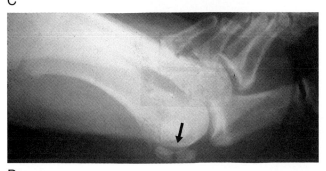

D

Figure 10–38 Technique of tibial shaving. **A,** A power saw is used to remove the plantar half of the tibial sesamoid. **B,** Model demonstrating 50% shaving of medial sesamoid. **C,** Following shaving of the tibial sesamoid, a flat plantar surface is achieved. **D,** Fracture following medial sesamoid shaving.

2. Care is taken to isolate the medial plantar digital nerve, which courses over the medial border of the tibial sesamoid (see Fig. 10–37B).
3. The metatarsal sesamoid ligament is incised to define the superior extent of the sesamoid (see Fig. 10–37C).
4. The plantar fat pad is retracted and a sagittal saw is used to resect the plantar half of the sesamoid (Fig. 10–38A and B).
5. Care is taken to protect the flexor digitorum longus tendon, which lies immediately lateral to the tibial sesamoid.
6. Once the tibial sesamoid has been shaved, the sharp edges are beveled with a rongeur.
7. The skin is approximated in a routine fashion (see Fig. 10–37I).
8. The toe is protected in a gauze-and-tape dressing, and the patient is allowed to ambulate in a postoperative shoe for 3 weeks following surgery.

Usually MTP motion returns quickly, and strength is unimpaired following surgery.

Postoperative Results

Aquino et al[6] reported their results in the evaluation of 26 feet that had undergone tibial sesamoid shaving for intractable plantar keratoses. An 89% subjective success rate was reported with this procedure. Because the intrinsic musculature was not disrupted, there was a negligible increase in the hallux valgus angle at final follow-up. The authors found minimal weakness at the first MTP joint postoperatively following this procedure. This procedure, however, is contraindicated in the presence of a plantar-flexed first metatarsal (Fig. 10–39). In this situation, a dorsiflexion osteotomy is the treatment of choice for an intractable plantar keratotic lesion. If the first metatarsal is plantar-flexed more than 8 degrees in relation to the lesser metatarsals, a sesamoid planing procedure is contraindicated.

Mann and Wapner[54] reported on 14 patients (16 feet) who underwent tibial sesamoid shaving. They noted no functional limitations, and at final follow-up, patients were reported to have a normal range of motion. Excellent or good results were reported in 15 feet. There was one case of recurrent callus formation and four cases of slight recurrence of callosity. The authors reported fracture of the remaining sesamoid as a possible complication, although none occurred.

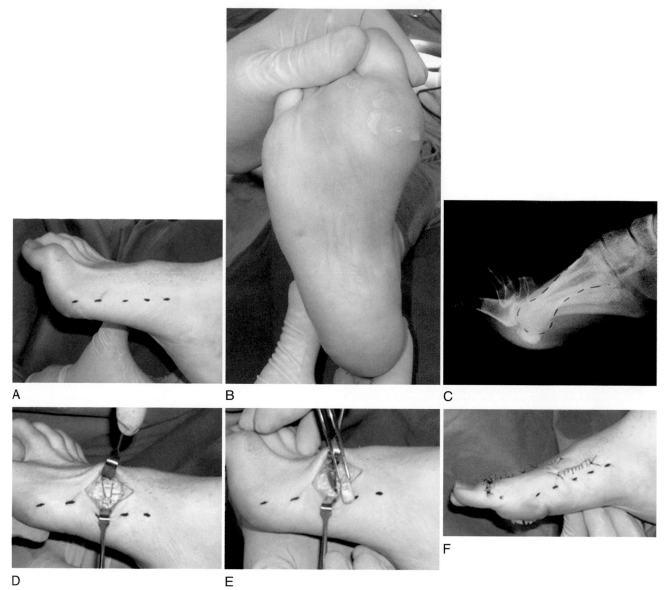

Figure 10–39   A sesamoidectomy is contraindicated with a plantar-flexed first metatarsal because symptoms usually continue postoperatively. A dorsal wedge closing osteotomy of the first metatarsal can reduce the pressure beneath the first metatarsal head. **A,** Preoperative photograph demonstrating plantar flexion of the first metatarsal. **B,** Intractable plantar keratotic lesion beneath the first metatarsal head. **C,** Lateral radiograph demonstrating a plantar-flexed first metatarsal. **D,** Outline of a closing wedge first metatarsal osteotomy. **E,** The wedge has been excised and the osteotomy closed. **F,** Appearance of the foot after closing dorsiflexion osteotomy of the first metatarsal.

EXCISION OF THE FIBULAR SESAMOID

Dorsal Approach

The fibular sesamoid may be approached through a dorsal incision in the first intermetatarsal space.

Surgical Technique

1. A 3-cm dorsal incision is made in the first intermetatarsal space (Fig. 10–40A).
2. A Weitlaner retractor or lamina spreader is used to spread the first and second metatarsals. With the tendon of the adductor hallucis as a guide, the adductor tendon is detached from the lateral joint capsule, and the fibular sesamoid is exposed. The adductor tendon is then dissected off of the lateral aspect of the sesamoid, and the intersesamoidal ligament is severed (Fig. 10–40B).
3. Care is taken to avoid damage to the common digital nerve in the first web space, which lies just beneath the transverse intermetatarsal ligament.
4. The sesamoid is firmly grasped with a toothed forceps and is excised in its entirety. Another alternative is to drill a threaded Kirschner wire into the lateral sesamoid, which can then be grasped as the sesamoid is excised.[23] It is very difficult to complete a partial sesamoid excision through a dorsal approach.
5. The plantar aspect of the wound is inspected to ensure that the flexor hallucis longus tendon has not been inadvertently severed.
6. If the adductor hallucis tendon has been detached, it should be reapproximated to the base of the proximal phalanx or the lateral MTP joint capsule.
7. The skin is approximated with interrupted sutures. A gauze-and-tape compression dressing is applied and the patient is allowed to ambulate in a postoperative shoe for 3 weeks.

The use of a dorsal incision for excision of a fibular sesamoid may be difficult. It is somewhat more demanding than a plantar approach but avoids significant postoperative morbidity. It avoids the possibility of a painful or hypertrophic plantar scar (Fig. 10–41).

Plantar Approach

If a plantar incision is used to approach the fibular sesamoid, an intermetatarsal incision is preferred to an incision directly beneath the first metatarsal head (see Fig. 10–26, C). Postoperative scarring or keloid formation directly

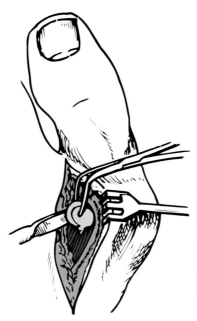
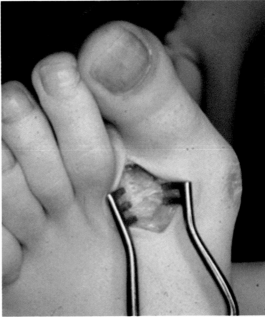

Figure 10–40 **A,** A 3-cm dorsal incision is made in the first interspace to resect the lateral sesamoid. **B,** A Weitlaner retractor aids in spreading the first and second metatarsals to expose the lateral sesamoid for resection.

A

B

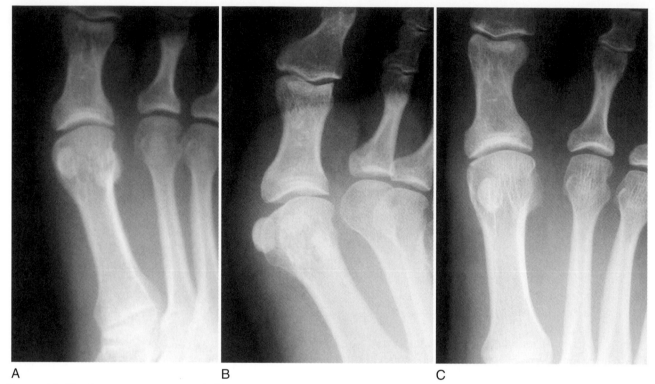

A   B   C

Figure 10–41   Anteroposterior **(A)** and oblique **(B)** radiographs of avascular necrosis of the lateral sesamoid. **C,** Following excision of the lateral sesamoid through a dorsal interspace incision, adequate alignment is maintained.

beneath a metatarsal or sesamoid can cause intractable pain (Fig. 10–42).

Surgical Technique

1. A slightly curved longitudinal incision is made on the lateral edge of the first metatarsal fat pad (Figs. 10–43 and 10–44A).
2. Care is taken to isolate and protect the lateral plantar digital nerve to the hallux, which can course directly over the lateral edge of the fibular sesamoid.
3. The metatarsal fat pad is retracted medially with the digital nerve.
4. The lateral sesamoid is covered by a thin layer of fascia from the conjoined tendon but can be palpated in the depths of the wound. It is carefully excised with a no. 15 blade (Fig. 10–44B and C). The adductor hallucis tendon is preferably left intact.
5. The tendon of the flexor hallucis longus is inspected to ensure its continuity.
6. The fascial defect left by the excised sesamoid is approximated, if possible, with 2-0 absorbable suture and an interrupted suture technique or a purse-string closure (Fig. 10–44D and E).

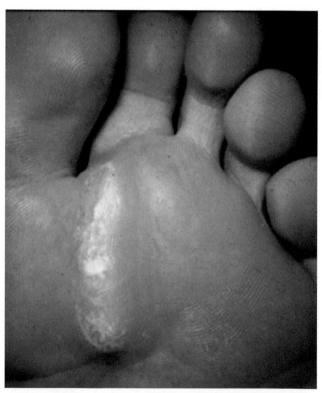

Figure 10–42   A painful plantar scar has developed after a plantar approach to resect a fibular sesamoid. (From Coughlin MJ: *Instr Course Lect* 39:23-25, 1990.)

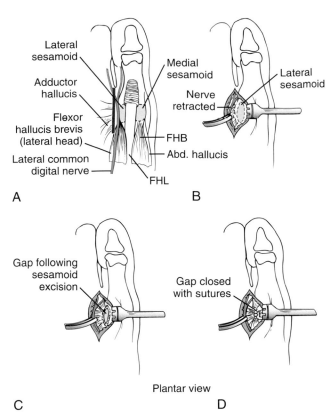

Plantar view

C   **D**

Figure 10–43 Technique of lateral sesamoid excision through the plantar approach. **A,** A longitudinal plantar incision is made between the first and second metatarsal heads just lateral to the common digital nerve. **B,** With the nerve retracted, the lateral sesamoid is identified and excised. **C** and **D,** The capsule is closed with 2-0 absorbable suture to minimize the surgical defect. FHB, Flexor hallucis brevis; FHL, flexor hallucis longus.

7. The skin is approximated with interrupted 5-0 nylon suture, with care taken to evert the skin edges to minimize postoperative scarring (Figs. 10–44F and 10–45).

Postoperative Results

An isolated excision of a sesamoid can lead to a muscle imbalance of the MTP joint. The development of a hallux varus deformity after fibular sesamoidectomy was noted by Mann and Coughlin,[52] who reported an 8% incidence of hallux varus in a postoperative review of the treatment of hallux valgus deformities with the McBride procedure. Nayfa and Sorto[59] reported a 2.2-degree increase in the intermetatarsal angle after tibial sesamoidectomy and a 6.2-degree valgus drift of the hallux following tibial sesamoidectomy. Jahss[39] noted that a wide medial excision of the tibial sesamoid could disrupt the medial MTP joint capsule and lead to a hallux valgus deformity. Likewise, a wide lateral excision with disruption of the adductor hallucis tendon can lead to a hallux varus deformity (see Fig. 10–30C and D).

Mann et al,[53] reporting on a series of sesamoidectomies, noted a valgus or varus drift of the hallux in 10% of the patients (see Fig. 10–30A and B); Saxena[73] reported varus or valgus drift in 8% of patients following sesamoidectomy. Maintenance of the integrity of the medial capsule and abductor hallucis when a tibial sesamoidectomy is performed and maintenance of the integrity of the adductor hallucis and lateral capsule when a fibular sesamoidectomy is performed are important in diminishing migration of the hallux postoperatively. When possible, it is advantageous to repair the defect left by the sesamoid excision. Following tibial sesamoidectomy, a lateral capsule release, medial capsule reefing,[15,59] and even metatarsal osteotomy may be considered if there appears to be an increased risk of a hallux valgus deformity after tibial sesamoid excision.

Surgical excision of a sesamoid is recommended when conservative care has proved unsuccessful. Little information, however, is available regarding postoperative results. Although some[74,80,84] have reported complete relief of pain and resumption of normal activities, Inge and Ferguson[37] noted that only 41% of patients achieved complete relief (Fig. 10–46). Mann et al[53] reported complete relief of pain in 50% of their patients.

The reports from many series suggest that surgical excision can lead to significant MTP joint stiffness.* Mann et al[53] reported restricted range of motion in one third of their cases. Of 14 patients with a full range of motion, 10 had tibial and four had fibular sesamoidectomies. In seven patients with restricted range of motion, three fibular sesamoidectomies and four tibial sesamoidectomies had been carried out. There does not appear to be a predilection for restricted range of motion following either tibial or fibular sesamoidectomy. Saxena et al[73] reported a shorter recovery period following fibular sesamoidectomy. Biedert[7] reported successful return to athletic activity in a small group

---

*References 14, 40, 46, 53, 74, and 79.

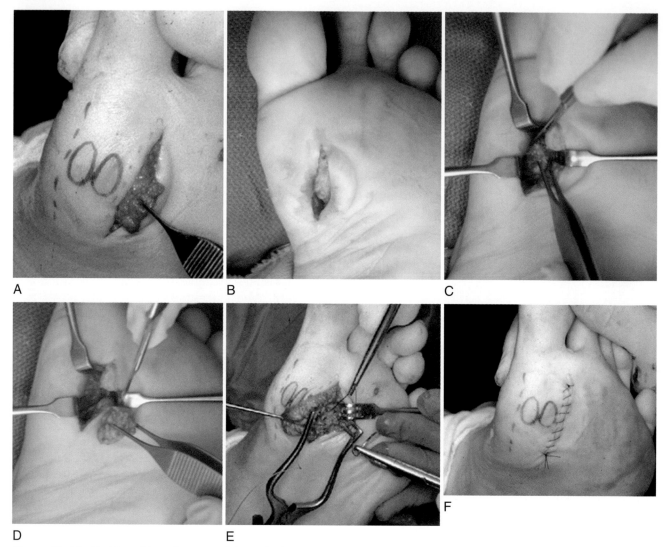

Figure 10–44 Excision of lateral sesamoid through plantar approach. **A** and **B,** Plantar longitudinal incision is centered between first and second metatarsal heads. Lateral sesamoid is freed from surrounding ligamentous attachments **(C)** and excised **(D). E,** Closure of adjacent soft tissue; care is taken to protect the common digital nerve as the defect is repaired. **F,** Skin closure.

of patients following excision of only the proximal pole of the symptomatic sesamoid.

Van Hal et al[80] noted no diminution in plantar flexion strength and reported no cock-up deformities of the hallux following sesamoid excision. Inge and Ferguson,[37] however, found a 17% incidence of clawing of the hallux postoperatively. They also noted that 58% of their patients had restricted MTP joint range of motion, clawing, or continued pain postoperatively. Mann et al[53] reported a 60% incidence of plantar flexion weakness. A lengthy period of preoperative conservative treatment in Mann's series may have contributed to the latter postoperative restricted motion and weakness.

Inge and Ferguson[37] reported on 31 patients (41 feet) following sesamoid excision. Twenty-five patients underwent dual sesamoidectomy. A medial sesamoid was excised in 15 and a fibular sesamoid was excised in one. Only 41.5% of patients noted normal function and complete relief of pain following surgery. The 17% incidence of a postoperative claw toe deformity was likely due to the dual sesamoid excision.

Aper et al[3] reported on their laboratory investigation regarding first ray strength of the hallux following medial and lateral sesamoidectomy and dual sesamoidectomy. They reported that following only medial sesamoidectomy, it is unlikely that the mechanical advantage of the

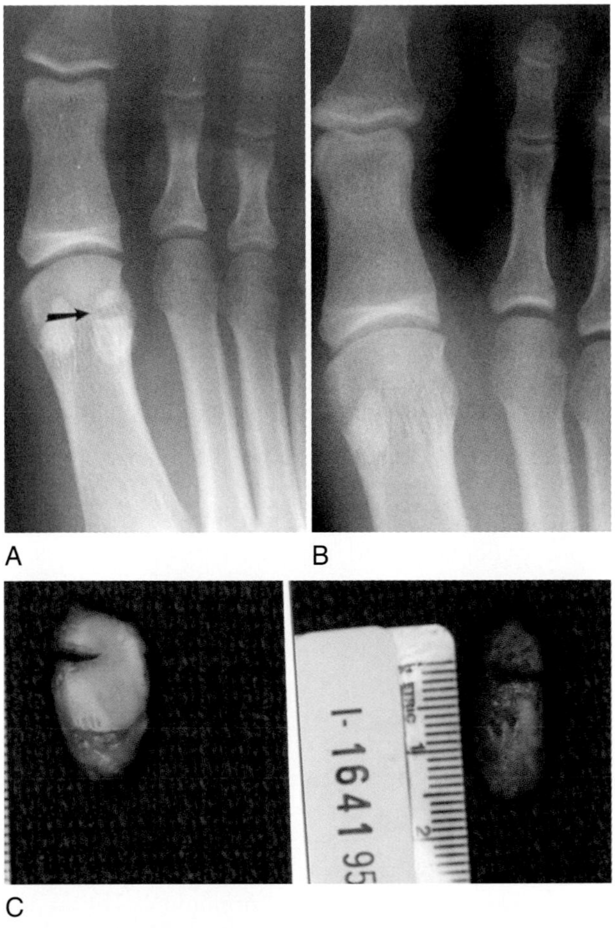

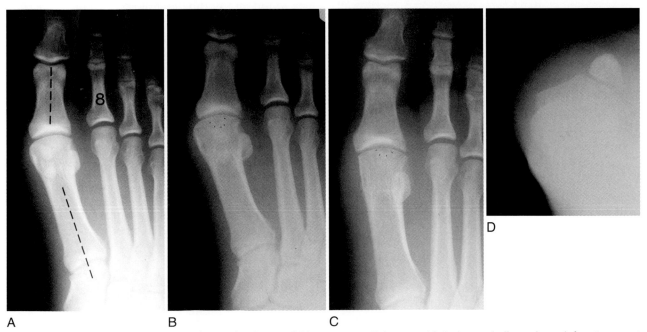

Figure 10–45 **A,** Preoperative anteroposterior radiograph demonstrating a painful lateral sesamoid suspected to be a fracture of a partite lateral sesamoid. **B,** Following lateral sesamoid excision through a plantar approach. **C,** Operative specimen demonstrating evidence of disruption of the partite sesamoid.

Figure 10–46 **A,** Anteroposterior radiograph of a painful bipartite medial sesamoid; 8-degree hallux valgus deformity associated with a multipartite medial sesamoid. **B,** Five years later, the valgus deformity has increased. A lengthy period of conservative care may be associated with degenerative arthritic changes of the first metatarsophalangeal (MTP) joint. Note the cyst in the first metatarsal head. There has been gradual separation of the sesamoid fragments, and increasing pain had developed. **C** and **D,** Five years following surgery, with medial capsulorrhaphy to stabilize the first MTP joint.

flexor hallucis brevis is compromised. In a follow-up study, Aper et al[4] reported that excision of either the medial or lateral sesamoid causes a significant decrease in the moment arm of the flexor hallucis longus. Their explanation was that removal of a sesamoid allows the flexor hallucis longus to move closer to the center of rotation, weakening the moment arm.

Mann et al,[53] in reporting on the surgical excision of sesamoids in 21 patients, found that the average age was 41 years and that 66% of their patients were women. Thirteen tibial and eight fibular sesamoids were excised. Only 50% of patients noted complete relief of pain. Of those who were still symptomatic, 75% noted only occasional or mild symptoms. Sixty percent (12 patients) noted plantar flexion weakness. One third of the patients noted restricted range of motion. There appeared to be no difference in the postoperative results of tibial or fibular sesamoid excision. In 10% of cases there was a mild drift of the hallux into either varus or valgus following surgery. Although the subjective level of patient satisfaction was high, the postoperative objective limitations noted were significant.

Brodsky[9] reported on 23 sesamoid fractures that went on to chronic nonunion. Thirteen medial and 10 lateral sesamoids were involved. The mean time to surgery was 38.8 months. Although 21 of 23 patients had satisfactory results following surgical excision, two patients had postoperative weakness of the hallux, two had neuritic symptoms, and six had mild to moderate pain following surgery. In a follow-up report, Brodsky et al[10] reported on 37 patients (18 male and 19 female) with painful fractured sesamoids that were treated operatively. Avascular necrosis secondary to a sesamoid fracture was observed in 9 patients, 16 were noted to have sesamoid stress fractures, and 12 were related to direct trauma. Following surgical excision, the average AOFAS score was 93 points. Several cases of post-traumatic arthritis developed.

The first MTP joint sesamoids play an integral role in the dynamic function of the first MTP joint. Deterioration of function due to trauma, inflammation, fracture, or surgery can lead to significant disability. Although surgical intervention may be necessary in the treatment of a chronically painful sesamoid, the sesamoid complex should be preserved whenever possible. When conservative care is ineffectual and a sesamoidectomy is performed, care should be taken to maintain the integrity of the remaining intrinsic muscles and capsule to maintain stability and function of the first MTP joint. A single diseased sesamoid can be removed with acceptable postoperative results; however, the resection of both sesamoids should be avoided unless absolutely necessary.

INTERPHALANGEAL SESAMOID OF THE HALLUX

A subhallux sesamoid can occur as an accessory bone beneath the head of the proximal phalanx of the hallux (Fig. 10-47). This accessory bone is located on the dorsal aspect of the flexor hallucis longus tendon and articulates within the interphalangeal joint. A subhallux sesamoid is found superior to or within the tendon of the flexor hallucis longus[83] and typically is located in the midline or oriented slightly to the fibular aspect of the flexor hallucis longus tendon. It varies in size from 3 to 5 mm in diameter.[56]

Miller and Love[57] have described a cartilaginous sesamoid located in the plantar ligament of the interphalangeal joint. Trolle,[263] in sectioning 508 embryo feet, found an interphalangeal sesamoid in 56%. Typically it is unilateral, but it can occur bilaterally. Its occurrence has been reported by Bizarro[8] to be 5% (radiographic study) and by Jahss[39] to be 13%.

If the subhallux sesamoid is large or if it is associated with hyperextension of the interphalangeal joint, pressure can be exerted against the sesamoid. Occasionally in patients with a mild hallux flexus deformity, increased pressure is exerted on the plantar skin beneath the sesamoid. A painful hyperkeratotic lesion, and in some cases ulceration, can develop, particularly in an insensitive foot.

The diagnosis of a subhallux sesamoid is confirmed with a lateral radiograph of the hallux. The radiograph demonstrates the sesamoid just beneath the interphalangeal joint (Fig. 10-48).

Treatment

Treatment should be directed toward relieving the pressure on the subhallux sesamoid. The keratotic lesion may be shaved, and a pad may be placed just proximal to this area, which can decrease localized pressure. When conservative treatment is unsuccessful, surgical excision may be considered.

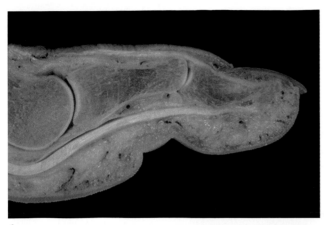

A

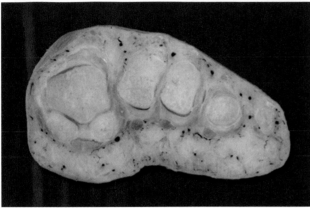

B

Figure 10–47 Subhallux sesamoid and metatarsophalangeal sesamoids as demonstrated in anatomic dissection. **A,** Lateral cross-section. **B,** Coronal cross-section. (Courtesy of Pau Golano, MD, University of Barcelona, Spain.)

longus is inadvertently detached from its insertion into the base of the proximal phalanx, it should be reattached by placing a suture through drill holes in the distal phalanx.

4. The wound is closed in a single layer.

Postoperative Care

A gauze-and-tape compression dressing is applied at surgery and changed on a weekly basis. The patient ambulates in a postoperative shoe for approximately 3 weeks until soft tissue healing has occurred, after which activities are permitted as tolerated.

Results

The results following excision of a subhallux sesamoid are routinely satisfactory. The callus rarely, if ever, re-forms. The significant major complication is an inadvertent detachment of the flexor hallucis longus tendon at the time of the sesamoid excision. If detachment is recognized, repair of the tendon can be accomplished without residual deficit. A less common complaint is reduced sensation or a postoperative neuroma along the medial border of the hallux due to interruption or injury to the small sensory branches of the plantar medial digital nerve; however, this is rarely a problem.

EXCISION OF A SUBHALLUX SESAMOID

Although a midline plantar incision can be used,[56,83] a medial incision is preferred.

Surgical Technique

1. Through a longitudinal medial incision centered over the interphalangeal joint, the dissection is carried plantarward to the flexor hallucis longus tendon (Fig. 10–48D).
2. The flexor hallucis longus tendon is incised on the dorsal aspect of the tendon near its insertion. The subhallux sesamoid is embedded within the tendon. By slightly plantar flexing the interphalangeal joint, exposure is improved and the excision is made easier.
3. The subhallux sesamoid is carefully shelled out, but the flexor hallucis longus tendon is protected. If the tendon of the flexor hallucis

ACCESSORY BONES OF THE FOOT AND THE UNCOMMON SESAMOIDS

Accessory bones of the foot are considered developmental anomalies.[219] Accessory bones can develop as subdivisions of normal bones or as a prominence of an ordinary tarsal bone that is abnormally separated from the main tarsal bone. Accessory ossicles can occur either bilaterally or unilaterally but are more commonly found in only one foot. Therefore, comparison radiographs might not be helpful in differentiating accessory bones from trauma. When multiple accessory bones occur in a single foot, O'Rahilly[219] has noted that they are unilateral in 50% or more of cases.

Pfitzner,[224] Dwight,[126] Trolle,[263] and O'Rahilly[219] have studied accessory bones in great detail. Trolle[263] studied serial microscopic sections from 108 feet of 254 embryos between 6 and 27 weeks of fetal age. He demonstrated that in nearly 80%, accessory bones were preformed in hyaline cartilage. The high incidence of accessory bones in embryonic feet does not

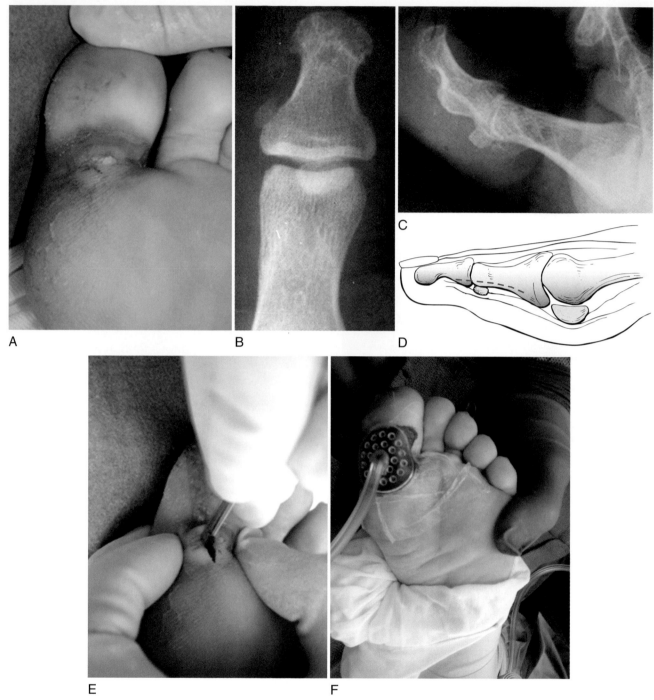

Figure 10–48   A, An interphalangeal sesamoid can produce a midline plantar callus and in time an infection as demonstrated here beneath the interphalangeal joint. **B,** Interphalangeal sesamoid on anteroposterior radiograph. **C,** Lateral radiograph demonstrating a large subhallux sesamoid beneath the interphalangeal joint, which on occasion may result in chronic ulceration. **D,** Lateral incision technique for simple excision of subhallux sesamoid. **E,** Direct plantar incision for infection. **F,** Wound vacuum-assisted closure application following infection beneath subhallux sesamoid.

correlate with their incidence in adult feet. Trolle[263] was unable to find an os trigonum in any of the embryonic feet he studied, although it is common in adults. Conversely, in 13% of embryonic feet he found anlagen of the os paracuneiforme in spite of a much lower incidence in adult feet. He concluded that accessory bones can develop from an independent element preformed in cartilage, can develop from an independent ossification center, can be explained as tendon bones, and can be caused by unrecognized pathologic lesions. Thus it would seem that there are several explanations for the presence of these abnormalities.

O'Rahilly[219] catalogued 38 tarsal and sesamoid bones and stated that the bones may have been incomplete fusions, accessory bones, or bipartitions. Henderson[159] has shown heritable causation of accessory bones in some instances. From a clinical standpoint, only two accessory bones, the accessory navicular and the os trigonum, cause symptoms with any frequency.

INCONSTANT SESAMOIDS

Accessory or inconstant sesamoids can occur beneath any weight-bearing surface of the foot, especially beneath the lesser metatarsal heads, beneath any of the phalanges, and at times beneath all of the metatarsal heads. Accessory sesamoids vary widely in shape and size. Although ordinarily they are asymptomatic, they can become painful when an ossicle is extraordinarily large or a keratotic lesion develops. Rarely is surgery necessary to excise a symptomatic inconstant sesamoid of the forefoot.

The incidence of accessory bones of the foot varies significantly depending on the method used to assess their individual incidence (Fig. 10–49). This information is most readily obtained by radiographic examination. Even here, however, the number, variety, and technique of the radiographic projection can influence the frequency of occurrence of accessory bones. Kewenter,[175] for example, obtained radiographs from three different aspects of the forefoot to evaluate the first MTP joint sesamoids. By correlating these views, he obtained a much higher frequency of bony abnormalities in these bones than had previously been reported. Trolle[263] used a similar method, and his work is still considered a classic in assessing the radiographic incidence of accessory bones.

Another technique for investigating the frequency of accessory bones is through anatomic dissection or assessment of skeletal remains retained in archives. This is an extremely time-consuming process. Pfitzner[224] examined 425 feet, and much of his work

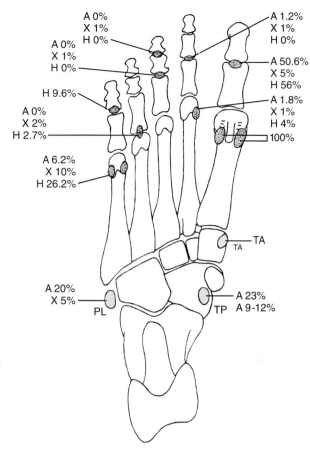

Figure 10–49 Sesamoids of the foot. Frequency of occurrence based on anatomic evaluation (A), histoembryologic investigation (H), and radiographic investigation (X). PL, peroneus longus; TP, tibialis posterior.

still forms the basis for information we use today. Mann[197,198] more recently has investigated specific bones by reviewing archive specimens as well.

Sesamoids occur uncommonly in the posterior and anterior tibial tendons, being much more common in the peroneus longus (os peroneum). Uncommon accessory bones include the os subtibiale, os subfibulare, os trigonum, os calcaneus secundarius, os calcaneus accessorius, os sustentaculi, os subcalcis, os aponeurosis plantaris, os cuboides secundarium, os talonaviculare dorsale, os supratalare, os intercuneiforme, os cuneometatarsale, os intermetatarseum, and os vesalianum.

The accessory navicular is a much more common accessory bone. Partition of the navicular and first cuneiform has also been described. Accessory bones are relatively unusual and rarely of clinical significance. Their presence can create a diagnostic dilemma, and it is important for a physician to be able to differentiate them from an acute fracture or injury. They are often identified in radiographs obtained for other

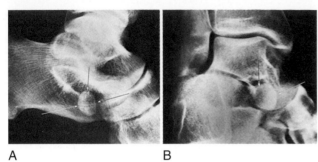

Figure 10–50 A, Lateral radiograph demonstrating large sesamoid in tibialis posterior tendon. **B,** Mortise view of the ankle demonstrating a sesamoid in the posterior tibial tendon. (From Keats TE: *Atlas of Normal Roentgen Variants That Simulate Disease,* ed 4. St Louis, Mosby, 1987.)

reasons, such as following trauma or for complaints of pain unrelated to the accessory bone.

SESAMOID OF THE TIBIALIS POSTERIOR TENDON

Anatomy and Incidence

This sesamoid lies within the tibialis posterior tendon, where it crosses the inferior border of the spring ligament. It lies on the plantar aspect of the navicular tuberosity (Fig. 10–50).[171,263] Its occurrence has been reported to vary from 9.2%[224] to 23%[255] (Fig. 10–51). Storton[255] reported that a sesamoid of the posterior tibial tendon was paired in 52% and unpaired in 47%

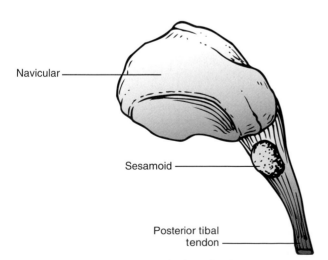

Navicular

Sesamoid

Posterior tibal tendon

Figure 10–51 The posterior tibial tendon has a sesamoid in 23% of anatomic dissections.

of feet examined in his anatomic study. Delfaut et al[17] demonstrated a fibrocartilaginous nonossified sesamoid in seven of eight anatomic specimens. They also reported that with magnetic resonance imaging (MRI) examination of 33 asymptomatic patients, 36% demonstrated a fibrocartilaginous sesamoid adjacent to the spring ligament. Although an ossified sesamoid of the posterior tibial tendon is uncommon, a thickening or fibrocartilaginous sesamoid appears to be relatively common.

Clinical Significance

The sesamoid of the posterior tibial tendon should be differentiated from both an accessory navicular and a fracture (see Fig. 10–55); it is often more proximal than the former, and its rounded nature should help differentiate it from the latter.

A classification scheme has been used to describe various types of accessory naviculars.[144,190,244] A type I accessory navicular is truly a sesamoid in the substance of the posterior tibial tendon. Type II is more typical of the accessory navicular commonly seen and is characterized by a synchondrosis (Fig. 10–52A). Type III is a cornuate navicular (see discussion of os tibiale externum) (Fig. 10–52B). Lepore et al[190] stated that type I (a sesamoid within the posterior tibial tendon) occurs in 30% of cases, although Grogan et al[144] noted no occurrence in 25 patients (39 feet). Bareither et al[94] examined 165 cadavers. When the accessory bone was within the posterior tibial tendon (Fig. 10–53), it was separated from the navicular tuberosity by 3 to 6 mm. The accessory bone was completely or partially imbedded within the superior or deep portion, or both, of the posterior tibial tendon.

SESAMOID OF THE TIBIALIS ANTERIOR TENDON

The sesamoid of the tibialis anterior tendon is located within the substance of the tibialis anterior near the insertion into the first cuneiform. The sesamoid lies on the anteroinferior corner of the medial surface of the first cuneiform and articulates with a facet on the medial surface of the medial cuneiform. Described by Zimmer,[286] its occurrence is very rare (Fig. 10–54).

The major clinical significance of this sesamoid is to differentiate it from a fracture on the medial aspect of the first cuneiform. A lack of tenderness in this region should alert the examiner to the possibility that this is a sesamoid within the tendon of the tibialis anterior.

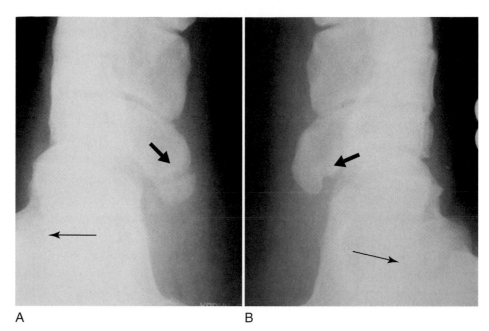

Figure 10–52 A, Type II accessory navicular with synchondrosis between the navicular and the accessory fragment. **B,** Type III accessory navicular with cornuate navicular.

A   B

OS PERONEUM

The sesamoid of the peroneus longus (the os peroneum) is located within the substance of the peroneus longus tendon and articulates with the lateral wall of the calcaneus, the calcaneocuboid joint articulation, or the inferior aspect of the cuboid in the region of the cuboid tunnel.[126,200,252] The sesamoid often lies where the tendon angles around the inferior cuboid on the plantar–lateral aspect of the foot (Fig. 10–56).

Sobel et al[252] described four soft tissue structures that stabilize the os peroneum: a cuboid band, a fifth metatarsal band, a plantar fascial band, and a band to the peroneus brevis, each of which attaches the

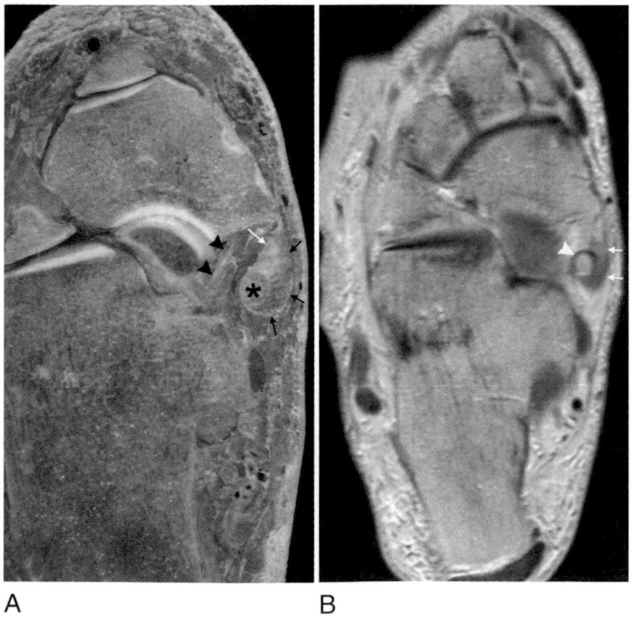

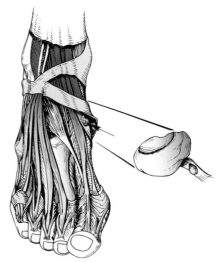

A   B

Figure 10–53 A, Anatomic cross section demonstrating sesamoid embedded in the posterior tibial tendon. **B,** Magnetic resonance (MR) image demonstrating same cross section. (Courtesy of A. Cotton.)

Figure 10–54 A sesamoid in the tibialis anterior tendon is located near the tendon insertion on the anterior inferior corner of the medial cuneiform.

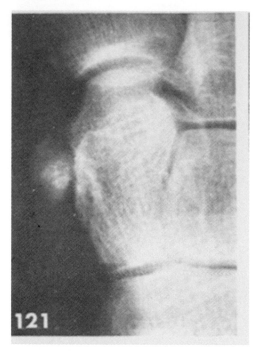

Figure 10–55 Sesamoid in the posterior tibial tendon.

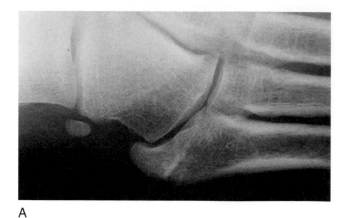

A

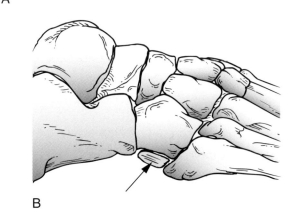

B

Figure 10–56 **A,** Radiograph demonstrating os peroneum. **B,** Os peroneum articulating with cuboid *(arrow)*. A more proximal location can denote a ruptured tendon.

sesamoid to those respective structures (Fig. 10–57). In the region of the lateral calcaneal wall, the sesamoid comes in contact with two osseous processes, the peroneal tubercle and the anterior calcaneal peroneal facet. The peroneus longus tendon is encompassed by a synovial sheath, which extends from a point proximal to the lateral malleolus to the region of the cuboid tunnel.

Sarrafian[236] notes that the sesamoid is always present but may be in an ossified, cartilaginous, or fibrocartilaginous state. Pfitzner,[224] in reporting on a series of anatomic dissections, noted its frequency to be 8.5%. Trolle,[263] in his histologic–embryologic examination of 500 feet, noted the frequency to be 0.4%. Numer-

ous radiographic studies have found the frequency to vary between 2.3% and 8.3%.* On anatomic dissection, the fully ossified os peroneum occurs in 20% and the less than fully ossified os peroneum occurs in 75%.

---

*References 87, 90, 101, 136, 157, 167, and 188.

Figure 10–57 The os peroneum (OP) has four soft tissue attachments. **A** and **B,** The os peroneum is shown with its attachment to a plantar fascial band, a fifth metatarsal band, and a band to the peroneus brevis. The fourth band (not seen in this diagram) attaches the os peroneum to the cuboid. (Redrawn from Sobel M, Pavlov H, Geppert M, et al: *Foot Ankle* 15:112-124, 1994.)

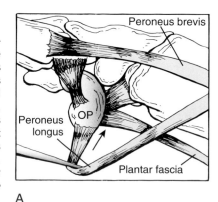

A

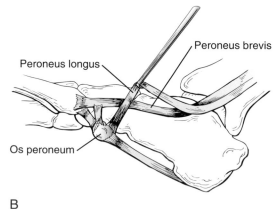

B

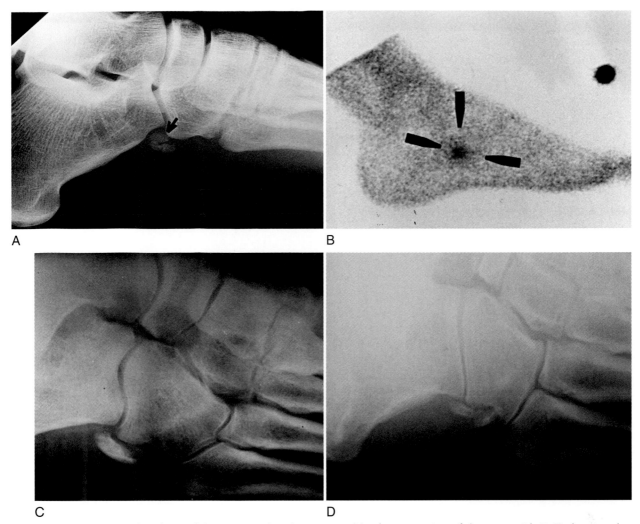

Figure 10–58 **A,** Osteochondritis of the sesamoid is demonstrated by fragmentation of the sesamoid. **B,** Technetium bone scan demonstrates increased uptake in the os peroneum. **C,** Osteochondritis of the os peroneum as demonstrated by a sclerotic appearance of sesamoid. **D,** Fracture of the os peroneum.

The os peroneum may be multipartite, and this must be differentiated from an acute fracture.*

Occasionally this sesamoid bone becomes symptomatic due to arthritic deterioration.[110] Osteochondritis dissecans of the os peroneum can lead to painful symptoms as well (Fig. 10–58). Okazaki et al[217] have described a stress fracture of the os peroneum treated with excision and primary end-to-end repair (Fig. 10–59). Thompson and Patterson[262] and others[221,275] have reported on the isolated rupture of the peroneus longus as demonstrated by the proximal migration of the os peroneum (Fig. 10–60) (see Chapter 22).

---

*References 143, 163, 177, 195, 204, 221, 223, 260, 265, 275, and 280.

Clinical Significance

Awareness of the presence of the os peroneum can help a clinician to differentiate between a fracture and an accessory bone. Although this accessory bone is not common, the appearance on a radiograph of rounded edges can help to differentiate it from a fracture of the cuboid (Fig. 10–61). This accessory bone is often unilateral, and comparison films might not aid differentiating it from a fracture.

A painful os peroneum can present a diagnostic dilemma. Pain may be due to an acute fracture or disruption of a multipartite sesamoid, a chronic diastasis of a multipartite sesamoid, a degenerative tear of the peroneus longus distal or proximal to the os peroneum, an acute disruption of the peroneus longus tendon, or an enlarged peroneal tubercle (Fig. 10–62) that can entrap the peroneus longus tendon or os

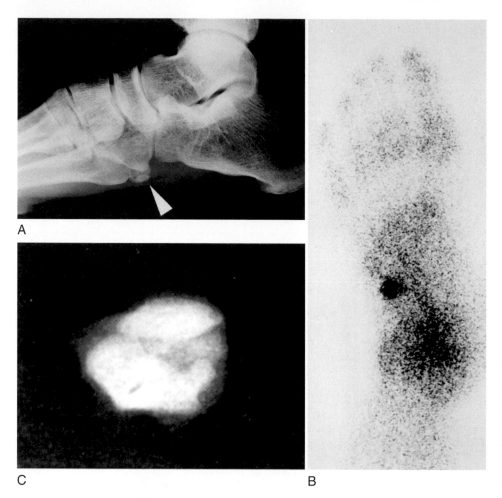

Figure 10–59 A, Lateral radiograph demonstrates fracture of the os peroneum. **B,** Increased uptake on bone scan. **C,** Radiograph of operative specimen demonstrating fractured os peroneum. (From Okazaki K, Nakashima S, Nomura S: *J Orthop Trauma* 17:654-656, 2003; used by permission.)

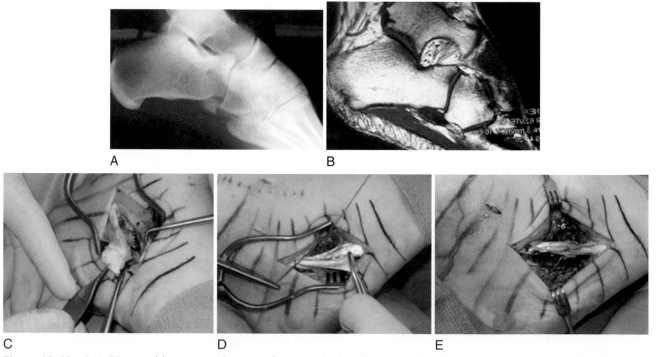

Figure 10–60 A, A 55-year-old woman with onset of pain on the lateral aspect of the foot and ankle with os peroneum slightly proximal to the normal position. **B,** MRI of hindfoot demonstrating abnormality of the os peroneum. **C,** Intraoperative photograph demonstrating the os peroneum and discontinuity of the peroneus longus tendon. **D** and **E,** Tenodesis with Pulvertaft weave of the peroneus longus into the peroneus brevis tendon.

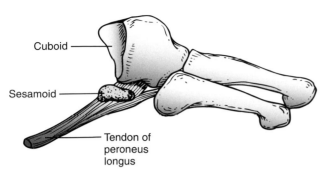

Cuboid

Sesamoid

Tendon of peroneus longus

Figure 10–61 Storton demonstrated a 26% incidence of an os peroneum on anatomic dissection.

peroneum, limiting excursion.[252] Ruiz et al[234] described the major anatomic functions of the peroneal tubercle as providing an insertion of the inferior peroneal retinaculum, separating the tendons of the peroneus brevis and longus in a common peroneal tendon sheath and providing a fulcrum for excursion of the peroneal tendon. An enlarged peroneal tubercle that entraps the peroneus longus tendon or os peroneum can lead to tenosynovitis[98,225] and require surgical excision. Berenter and Goldman[98] and Pierson and Inglis[225] described surgical resection to reduce the size of an enlarged and symptomatic peroneal tubercle.

When an os peroneum fractures, there may be disruption due to direct trauma, a violent muscle contraction, or an inversion injury associated with an ankle sprain.[99,223] Symptoms of edema and pain may be associated with either a partial or total rupture of the peroneus longus. Perlman[223] reported a case of an entrapped sural nerve associated with fracture of the os peroneum. With injury to the os peroneum and disruption of the peroneus longus at or distal to the sesamoid, proximal migration of the os peroneum or a fragment may be demonstrated on oblique radiograph[262,265] due to retraction of the tendon.[275]

Thompson and Patterson[262] reported a disruption of the peroneus longus tendon occurring distal to the os peroneum. Various treatment modalities include casting and nonsurgical treatment[163,265]; excision of the degenerated or fractured os peroneum, leaving the tendon in continuity[143,223,280]; or excision and tendon repair or tenodesis with a disrupted peroneus longus (see Chapter 22).[221,262,275]

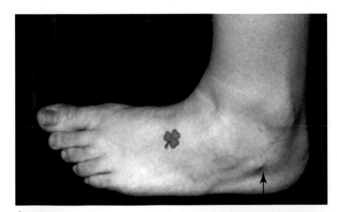

A

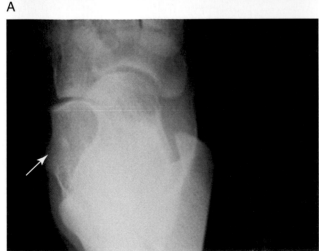

B

Figure 10–62 Clinical appearance **(A)** and radiographic appearance **(B)** of enlarged peroneal process.

EXCISION OF THE OS PERONEUM AND TENODESIS OF THE PERONEUS LONGUS

1. The involved foot is exsanguinated and a calf or thigh tourniquet is used for hemostasis. The foot is cleansed in the usual fashion.
2. A 4- to 6-cm longitudinal incision is centered over the lateral aspect of the cuboid and os peroneum.
3. Care is taken to identify and protect the sural nerve, which lies in close proximity to the peroneal tendon sheath.
4. The peroneus longus tendon is identified and the os peroneum is excised. If the tendon is intact, the os peroneum may be excised and the tendon reinforced with interrupted sutures. If the tendon is ruptured and retracted, the os peroneum is excised.
5. A tenosynovectomy of the peroneus longus tendon sheath is performed.
6. The tendon sheath of the peroneus brevis is incised, and a tenodesis of the peroneus longus to the peroneus brevis is performed with the foot in dorsiflexion and eversion.

The proximal segment of the peroneus longus is woven through the peroneus brevis with a Pulvertaft weave. Several interrupted nonabsorbable sutures are used to secure the tenodesis.

7. The tendon sheaths are left open to prevent constriction at the area of the tenodesis.

8. The wound is closed with interrupted sutures. Care is taken to protect the sural nerve.

Postoperative Care

A below-knee posterior splint is applied to immobilize the foot and ankle. The patient is permitted to ambulate in a non–weight-bearing cast for 2 weeks following surgery. Then a below-knee walking cast is applied, and the patient is allowed to ambulate with weight bearing as tolerated for 4 weeks. Following this, a removable cast or ankle brace is used for another 4 weeks. Peroneal strengthening exercises are commenced after removal of the below-knee cast.

OS SUBTIBIALE

Anatomy and Incidence

The os subtibiale is located beneath the medial malleolus.* It is a rare accessory bone appearing as a rounded, well-defined ossicle on the posterior aspect of the medial malleolus. In the younger patient it is important to differentiate this accessory bone from a second ossification center of the medial malleolus.[166,229] Ossicles related to the anterior aspect of the medial malleolus are smaller; Coral[119,120] found them to be present in approximately 2.1% of ankle radiographs. He hypothesized that this anterior accessory bone represents an unfused secondary ossification center. Likewise, posttraumatic ossification might explain some of the other small accessory bones and less well defined fragments in the area of the medial malleolus. Coral found accessory bones related to the medial malleolus in 4.6% of the 700 radiographs examined, but only one example was found of a true os subtibiale.

The os subtibiale was first described by Bircher in 1918,[263] and there have been isolated case reports of this accessory bone since that time. Arho[90] reported a

*References 108, 130, 141, 184, 219, 235, 264, 271, 276, 278, and 284.

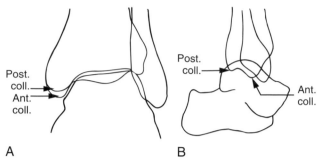

Figure 10–63 **A,** On an anteroposterior radiograph, the posterior colliculus is a flat line seen through the shadow of the more distal anterior colliculus. **B,** On a lateral radiograph, the anterior and posterior colliculi are seen in profile.

0.7% incidence of the os subtibiale, Holle[167] reported a 1.2% incidence, and Leimbach[188] reported a 0.2% incidence. In the area of the medial malleolus, a groove separates the anterior and posterior colliculi (Fig. 10–63). On an anteroposterior (AP) radiograph, the anterior colliculus is normally seen as the pointed tip of the medial malleolus because it extends more distally. The posterior colliculus is demonstrated as a sclerotic shadow overlying the anterior colliculus. A lateral radiograph demonstrates the anterior and posterior colliculi more clearly. Radiographs of the ankle can demonstrate abnormal ossification that may be accessory ossification centers, post-traumatic ossification, or avulsion fractures, and these should not be confused with an os subtibiale.

An accessory ossification center can occur at the distal tip of the medial malleolus (Fig. 10–64). Selby[243] evaluated serial radiographs in healthy children. He reported that in his series of 151 children, an accessory ossification center of the tip of the medial malleolus occurred more often in girls (47%) than in boys (17%). It typically appears during the eighth and ninth

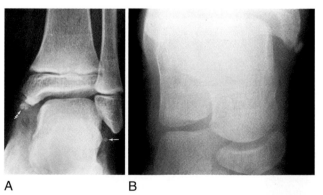

Figure 10–64 **A,** The secondary ossification center is seen at the tip of the medial malleolus. **B,** Secondary ossification center on anterior aspect of medial malleolus. (**A** from Keats TE: *Atlas of Normal Roentgen Variants That Simulate Disease,* ed 4. St Louis, Mosby, 1987.)

years of age (mean age for girls, 7.65 years; mean age for boys, 8.76 years). Bilaterality was reported in 90% of the girls but only 27% of the boys. The incorporation of the accessory ossification center with the medial malleolus is usually complete by the eleventh year.

Powell[228] in a radiographic study of 100 children (aged 6 to 12 years) found an accessory ossification center of the medial malleolus in 20% of cases. He also examined 50 adults with no previous ankle injury and found a 4% incidence of submalleolar ossicles.

In 1918, Bircher[263] described the os subtibiale as a large, rounded accessory bone with a well-defined cortex. Coral[119] reported a large os subtibiale with a diameter of 15 mm. He reported that the lateral radiograph showed this accessory bone and its relationship to the posterior colliculus. Coral[120] suggested that the characteristics of an os subtibiale are a rounded ossicle with a diameter greater than 4 mm and well-defined margins in relation to the posterior colliculus of the medial malleolus. If a rounded ossicle with well-defined margins is related to the anterior colliculus, one should suspect an unfused ossification center. An accessory bone with poorly defined margins in this region can suggest trauma and a partial or complete avulsion of the deltoid ligament.

Clinical Significance

The rounded nature of an accessory bone at the tip of the medial malleolus tends to indicate a chronic condition. Rarely is surgical excision indicated. The differentiation of an os subtibiale from an acute fracture is the major diagnostic objective, although it may be necessary to differentiate it from an unfused ossification center. The relationship to the anterior or posterior colliculus can help to differentiate an unfused ossification center from an os subtibiale. Even in the case of acute trauma overlying such an accessory bone, conservative treatment usually results in successful relief of symptoms.

OS SUBFIBULARE

Anatomy and Incidence

The os subfibulare is located beneath the lateral malleolus.* Trolle[263,264] suggested that this was a sesamoid within the peroneus longus tendon. It can be as large as 5 to 10 mm and is often well seen on an AP radiograph of the ankle joint. Trolle[263,264] reported its incidence as 0.2%, as did Leimbach,[188] who reviewed 500 radiographs of the ankle.

Abnormalities of the distal fibula including the presence of an apophysis of the lateral malleolus are less commonly reported than those of the medial malleolus, according to Goedhard.[140] de Cuveland[124] described the apophysis of the lateral malleolus as lying anterior to the lateral malleolus (Fig. 10–65A). Goedhard[140] evaluated radiographs of 200 normal children aged 7 to 12 years to evaluate the apophysis of the lateral malleolus. He found four unilateral ununited apophyses and three bilateral ununited apophyses. He concluded that a contralateral radiograph is not necessarily helpful, because in more than 50% of the cases the apophysis was only unilateral. In adults this apophysis is much less common.

Although the more common ununited apophysis is an oval accessory bone anterior to the tip of the fibula, another smaller accessory bone may be seen at the tip of the lateral malleolus (Fig. 10–65B). Bjornson[102] reported that it was rare that a persistent secondary center of ossification was present in the lateral malleolus. He noted that this persistent ossification center is quite different from the os subfibulare as described by Leimbach.[188] Bowlus et al,[107] reporting on a review of 300 ankle radiographs, found 20 instances of os subfibulare for an incidence of 6.67%. Maffulli et al[194] observed that it was one of the rarest accessory bones of the foot, and Shands and Wentz[246] reported it occurred in only two cases in 850 children (0.2%).

Bowlus et al[107] reported on two patients who presented with painful symptoms that required surgical excision. In both cases the anterior talofibular ligament was attached to the ossicle. Mancuso et al[196] reported on a similar case of lateral ankle instability in which the anterior talofibular ligament inserted solely onto the os subfibulare. Surgical reconstruction of the lateral ankle reestablished ankle stability. The ossicle was differentiated from an avulsion fracture by its rounded, even appearance and well-defined cortical margins.

The os subfibulare is located posterior to the tip of the lateral malleolus and thus can be differentiated from the more anterior accessory ossification center (Fig. 10–65C). Kohler and Zimmer[178] have reported several cases in adults. This accessory bone can be oval or elongated and can have a well-defined articulation with the lateral malleolus. It may be difficult to differentiate from a secondary ossification center or from a traumatic injury to the tip of the lateral malleolus. It should also be differentiated from other accessory bones on the lateral aspect of the hindfoot such as a calcaneus secundarius and an os peroneum (see Fig. 10–56).

---

*References 142, 147, 196, 212, 219, and 278.

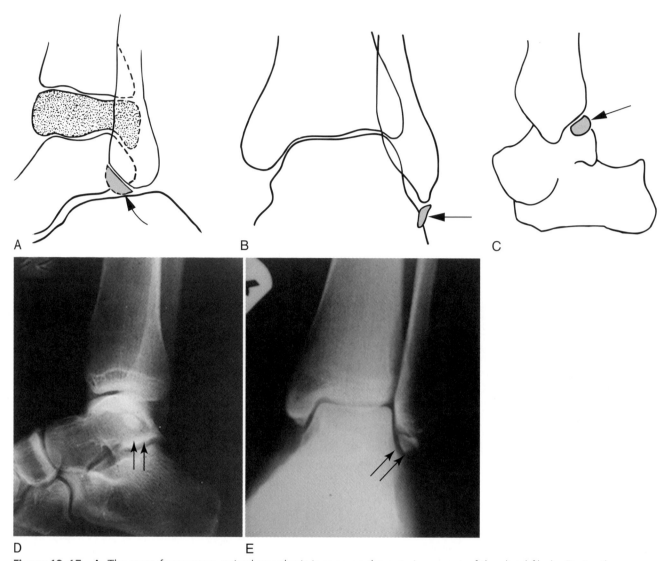

Figure 10–65   A, The more frequent un-united apophysis is seen on the anterior aspect of the distal fibula. **B,** Another accessory bone at the tip of the fibula. **C,** A true os subfibulare is located on the posterior aspect of the lateral malleolus. **D,** Lateral radiograph of un-united apophysis. **E,** True os subfibulare *(arrows).*

Champagne et al[115] had suggested the os subfibulare is contained in the tendon of the peroneal tendons based on their anatomic dissection, although most others consider the os subfibulare to be intimately associated with the distal fibula. Callanan et al[112] have described an accessory bone on the lateral aspect of the subtalar joint, heretofore unreported, that might have been secondary to trauma or actually a true accessory subtalar ossicle.

Clinical Significance

Usually the rounded nature of an accessory bone at the tip of the lateral malleolus indicates a chronic condition. Rarely is surgical excision indicated. Differentiation of an os subfibulare from acute trauma is a major diagnostic goal, and a bone scan may be helpful if trauma is suspected. Even in the case of acute trauma overlying an accessory bone, conservative treatment usually alleviates the symptoms.

Gruber[146] described an accessory bone in the area of the distal third of the fibula that he termed the *os retinaculi* (Fig. 10–66). This bone is found overlying the bursa of the lateral malleolus in the area of the peroneal retinaculum. This is typically a flat-shaped bone that is visible on an AP radiograph of the ankle. Although extremely rare, it should be differentiated from an accessory ossification center or trauma.

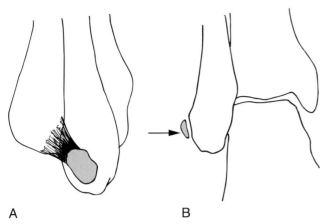

Figure 10–66 **A,** The os retinaculi is situated over the area of the bursa overlying the fibular malleolus. **B,** On the anteroposterior view, the os retinaculi is seen in profile.

OS TRIGONUM

Anatomy and Incidence

The os trigonum was first described by Rosenmuller.[233] In 1822 Shepherd[248] described it as a fracture of the posterolateral tubercle of the talus. The os trigonum varies greatly in size and shape and appears at the pos-

terior process of the talus (Fig. 10–67).* It may be an actual part of the body of the talus or develop as a separate bone that may or may not be adherent to the talus by a cartilaginous articulation.

Typically the ossicle is asymptomatic and detected only during routine radiographic examination. Often mistaken as a fracture of the posterior process of the talus, it arises as a separate ossification center and appears between 8 and 11 years of age.[207] It is present in 1.7% to 7% of radiographs of normal feet.[101] Ossicles that are separated from the talus can become painful on plantar flexion of the foot. Distinguishing between an articulating ossicle and a fracture of the posterior process of the talus can be difficult (Fig. 10–68).

According to Mann and Owsley[199] there was no apparent side predominance, and the lateral tubercle of the talus varied greatly in size. A free os trigonum probably represents a normal anatomic variant resulting from an unfused secondary center of ossification. The lateral tuberosity of the talus varies from a mild extension behind the posterior tubercle to an elongated thumb-shaped projection (Stieda's process) that could reach 1 cm in length, and the accessory bone

---

*References 86, 90, 96, 97, 100, 103, 108, 129, 130, 136, 152, 154, 157, 158, 165-167, 186, 192, 205, 215, 219, 220, 224, 233, 256, 266, 267, 273, 278, and 281.

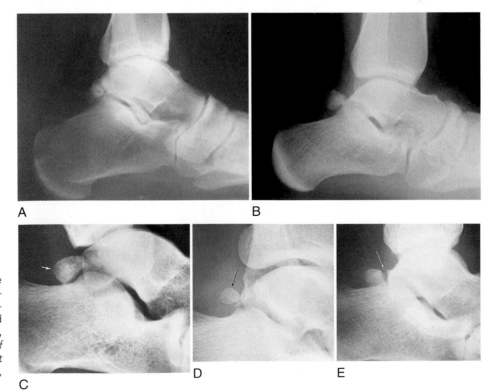

Figure 10–67 Variations in the os trigonum. **A,** This appearance may be mistaken for a fracture. **B to E,** Varying sizes and shapes of the os trigonum. (**C, D,** and **E** from Keats TE: *Atlas of Normal Roentgen Variants That Simulate Disease,* ed 4. St Louis, Mosby, 1987.)

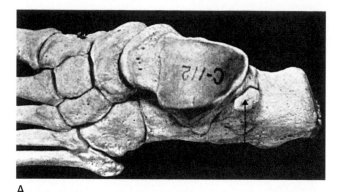

A

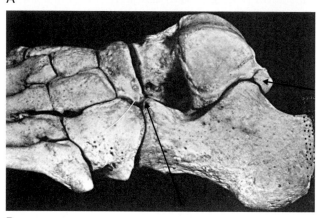

B

Figure 10–68 Calcaneus secundarius is demonstrated. **A,** Dorsal view demonstrating os trigonum. **B,** Lateral anatomic specimen demonstrating os trigonum. (**B** from Dwight T: *Clinical Atlas of Variations of the Bones of the Hand and Foot.* Philadelphia, JB Lippincott, 1907.)

occurs just lateral to the talar groove of the flexor hallucis longus tendon (Fig. 10–69).

Clinical Significance

The os trigonum can cause pain in the retrocalcaneal space; the pain is aggravated on walking and especially

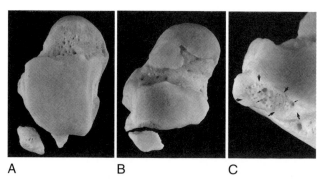

A   B   C

Figure 10–69 Os trigonum. **A,** Dorsal view of the left talus and free os trigonum (33-year-old white man). **B,** Plantar view of the left talus and free os trigonum. **C,** Semilunar concavity for attachment of the os trigonum (photo taken posterolateral). (Courtesy of Robert Mann, PhD.)

when the foot is placed in plantar flexion (Fig. 10–70). The os trigonum syndrome usually affects young athletes such as ballerinas and others whose activities involve forced plantar flexion. This forced plantar flexion can lead to a fracture of the trigonal process of the talus or impingement of the os trigonum against the posterior tibial plafond. Flexor hallucis longus tendinitis can develop because the tendon and tendon sheath can become inflamed secondary to compression in this region. When pressure is applied with the thumb and index finger against the posterior lip of the talus, pain may be exacerbated.

Except with a sudden fracture of the os trigonum (Shepherd's fracture),[248,249] the onset of symptoms is typically gradual. The symptoms can become worse, and the condition must be differentiated from retrocalcaneal bursitis. Likewise, differentiation must be made from a fracture of the posterior facet of the talus.[279] Giuffrida et al[139] has reported six cases of a fracture of the posterior talus, several of which were misdiagnosed. A subtalar dislocation occurred with these injuries; the authors stressed that a CT scan helps to differentiate an os trigonum from a posterior process fracture. Also, with accompanying swelling and substantial pain, there should be a high index of suspicion for a talar fracture and subtalar subluxation.

With retrocalcaneal bursitis, the symptoms are acute and are generally associated with swelling and tenderness overlying the retrocalcaneal space just posterior to the insertion of the Achilles tendon instead of at the anterior aspect of the retrocalcaneal space. Symptomatic cases can require removal of the os trigonum.

Conservative Treatment

Conservative treatment includes reduced range of motion and limitation of activity, casting,[103] and nonsteroidal antiinflammatory medications. Local steroid injection is generally discouraged because it can lead to a tendon rupture.[203]

Karasick and Schweitzer[172] have stated that pain can develop as a result of disruption of the cartilaginous synchondrosis between the os trigonum and the lateral talar tubercle. Also, part of the differential diagnosis is flexor hallucis longus tenosynovitis.

Wakeley et al[273] demonstrated that MRI was helpful in evaluating the cause of painful os trigonum syndrome. An os trigonum should be differentiated from a bipartite talus (Fig. 10–71).[240,280] On occasion, differentiation between a large os trigonum and a bipartite talus may be difficult (Fig. 10–72).

Surgical Treatment

A painful os trigonum may be approached through a medial exposure[103,154,281] or a lateral exposure.[103]

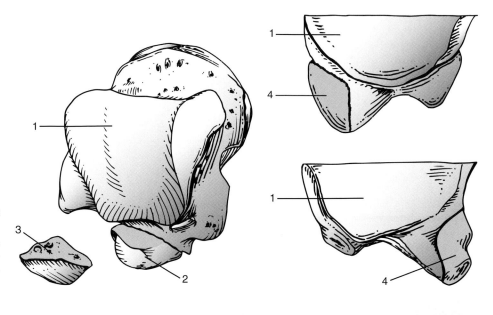

Figure 10–70 Dorsal view of talus and os trigonum. *1,* Dorsal talar articular surface; *2,* os trigonum; *3,* articular interface of os trigonum; *4,* articulated os trigonum.

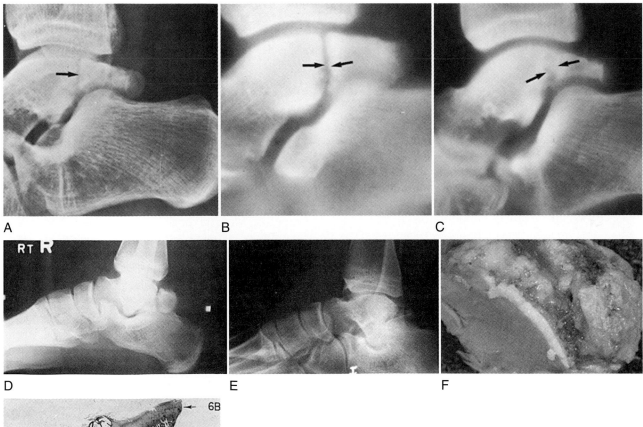

Figure 10–71 **A,** Lateral radiograph demonstrating talus partitus. This unusual anomaly is not a true os trigonum and should be appreciated and differentiated from a fracture. **B** and **C,** Tomograms of right ankle. **D,** A similar radiograph demonstrating talus partitus. **E,** Postoperative radiograph after resection of talus partitus. **F,** Surgical specimen following removal. **G,** Pathologic sectioning of resected fragment. (**A** to **C** from Schreiber A, Differding P, Zollinger H: *J Bone Joint Surg Br* 67:430-431, 1985. **D** to **G** from Weinstein S, Bonfiglio M: *J Bone Joint Surg Am* 57:1161-1163, 1975.)

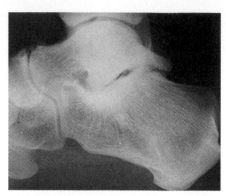

Figure 10–72 Os trigonum as an actual part of the posterior talus.

REMOVAL OF THE OS TRIGONUM (LATERAL APPROACH)

Surgical Technique

1. A thigh tourniquet is applied with the patient carefully positioned in a lateral decubitus position. The foot and lower part of the leg are cleansed and draped in the usual fashion.
2. A longitudinal incision approximately 5 cm in length is made over the retrocalcaneal space posterior to the distal aspect of the fibula.
3. The skin is retracted and the fascia incised. Care is taken to protect the sural nerve. The anterior margin of the fascia will be contiguous with the sheath of the peroneal tendons, which are readily retracted to expose the retrocalcaneal space.
4. The os trigonum is denuded of all attachments. A separated os trigonum can usually be delivered in one piece from the wound. An ossified os trigonum may be resected with an osteotome.
5. The remaining articular surface is smoothed with a rongeur and rasp.
6. The tendon of the flexor hallucis longus is inspected.
7. The fascia and skin are closed in layers.

Postoperative Care

A compression dressing is applied, and the patient ambulates with crutches. Touch-down weight bearing is allowed. Usually full weight bearing is tolerated within 1 week after surgery. Immobilization is usually discontinued 3 weeks after surgery.

Results

Wredmark et al[281] reported on a series of ballerinas treated for symptoms of impingement pain in the hindfoot with plantar flexion of the ankle. Surgery involved excision of the os trigonum or prominent lateral posterior process with division of the flexor hallucis longus tendon sheath. On physical examination, deep palpation in the posterior ankle region elicited pain, although only one third of patients complained of pain with passive plantar flexion. They positioned the patient supine and used a medial approach with a 5 cm vertical incision anterior to the Achilles tendon. The neurovascular bundle was identified and retracted. The tendon sheath of the flexor hallucis longus was incised longitudinally. The os trigonum was identified and excised. In half of the cases, a thickening of the flexor hallucis longus tendon or tendon sheath was observed and the tendon sheath was released. No casting was used and rehabilitation was started immediately with non–weight-bearing range of motion for 2 weeks. They recommend the medial approach because of the common finding of flexor hallucis longus tendon disease.

Marotta and Micheli[203] reported on 16 patients who underwent excision of an os trigonum through a posterolateral approach. Preoperative symptoms included pain localized to the posterior ankle, limitation of ankle motion, weakness, swelling, or neurologic changes associated with athletic activity. Eight of 16 still had occasional symptoms and the postoperative recovery time averaged 3 months. Marotta and Micheli stated that this condition is twice as common unilaterally as bilaterally. Differential diagnosis included peroneal tendinitis, Achilles tendinitis, retrocalcaneal bursitis, ankle joint arthritis, or an acute fracture of the talar tuberosity.

Hedrick and McBryde[154] reported on 30 cases of os trigonum, all developing after plantar flexion injury. An os trigonum was present in 63% of cases, and an intact posterior process was symptomatic in 36%. Some 60% of cases were treated nonoperatively, and 40% required operative excision.

OS CALCANEUS SECUNDARIUS

Anatomy and Incidence

The os calcaneus secundarius is located on the dorsal beak of the calcaneus in an interval between the anteromedial aspect of the os calcis, the proximal

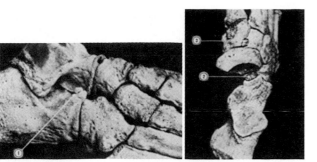

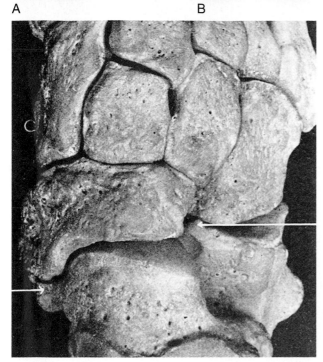

Figure 10-73 **A,** Os calcaneus secundarius, lateral view. **B,** Os calcaneus secondarius, oblique view. An os intercuneiforme is also present. **C,** Enlarged tuberosity or fused os calcaneus secondarius. This borders on being a tarsal coalition and can result in decreased subtalar motion. (From Dwight T: *Clinical Atlas of Variations of the Bones of the Hand and Foot.* Philadelphia, JB Lippincott, 1907.)

referred to this accessory bone as the os calcaneus secundarius. Mann[197,198] has studied anatomic collections and found the incidence in early twentieth century U.S. samples to be approximately 2%, whereas the incidence for more prehistoric groups was approximately 4.4% (Fig. 10-74). Its reported incidence in radiographic and anatomic studies varies among Pfitzner,[224] anatomic, 3.1%; Stieda,[254] anatomic, 2.5%; Geist,[136] radiographic, 2%; Holle,[167] radiographic, 1.7%; Arho,[90] radiographic, 1%; Bizarro,[101] radiographic, 1%; Leimbach,[188] radiographic, 0.4% (Fig. 10-75); and Trolle,[263] histoembryologic examination, 0%. Hoerr et al[162] evaluated radiographs in adolescents and found this accessory bone to be more frequent in boys (7% to 11%) than girls (6% to 7%).

Geist[136] noted this condition to be extremely rare and observed that the calcaneus secundarius can

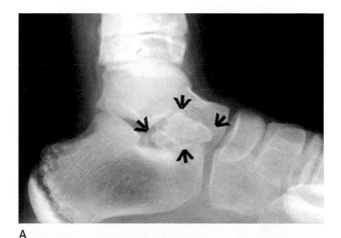

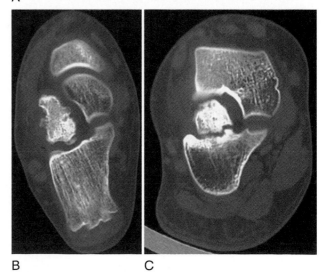

Figure 10-74 Large os calcaneus secundarius. **A,** Lateral radiograph. **B** and **C,** Appearance on CT examination. Restricted subtalar motion preoperatively was dramatically improved following resection. (The os calcaneus secundarius demonstrated here did not involve either the anterior or posterior subtalar facets.)

aspect of the cuboid and navicular, and the head of the talus (see Fig. 10-68).* It can be round or triangular (Fig. 10-73), is typically 3 to 4 mm in diameter, and is visible on a lateral oblique radiograph of the hindfoot.

First described by Stieda,[254] the earliest known specimen of a calcaneus secundarius is reported by Holland[166] to have been found in a mummy from Thebes. Pfitzner[224] reported the first comprehensive anatomic study, and it was Dwight[128] in 1907 who first

---

*References 88, 100, 108, 130, 173, 177, 182, 183, 210, 242, and 278.

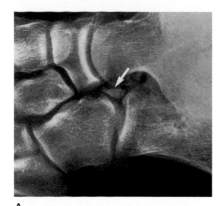

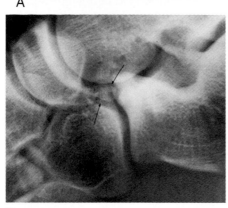

Figure 10–75 **A,** Oblique radiograph demonstrating small os calcaneus secundarius. **B,** Lateral radiograph demonstrating a small calcaneus secundarius. (From Keats TE: *Atlas of Normal Roentgen Variants That Simulate Disease,* ed 4. St Louis, Mosby, 1987.)

simulate a fracture of the beak of the calcaneus. Other conditions to be differentiated are a tarsal coalition or a fibrous tarsal coalition.[150]

Clinical Significance

Differentiation of an os calcaneus secundarius from an acute fracture of the tuberosity of the calcaneus is the main objective (Fig. 10–76).[160] Some patients complain of restricted subtalar motion and pain localized to this region. Differentiation from a partial or fibrous calcaneonavicular coalition must be made as well, because both may be associated with restricted hindfoot motion (Fig. 10–77). Wagner[272] reported excision of the anterior tuberosity of the calcaneus for chronic pain. Krida[180] reported a case of excision of an os calcaneus secundarius for pain, with a successful outcome. The differentiation of a fracture of the anterior tuberosity of the calcaneus from an os calcaneus secundarius may be delineated by a bone scan. Callanan et al[112] have described an accessory bone in the sinus tarsi that may be secondary to trauma or an atypical os calcaneus secundarius (Fig. 10–78).

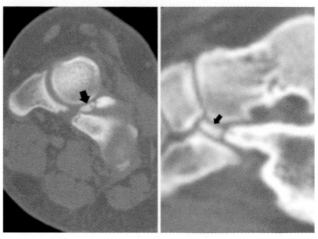

Figure 10–76 Computed tomographic scan demonstrates an os calcaneus secundarius. (From Stauss J, Connolly L, Perez-Rossello J, Treves S: *Clin Nucl Med* 28:424-425, 2003. Used by permission.)

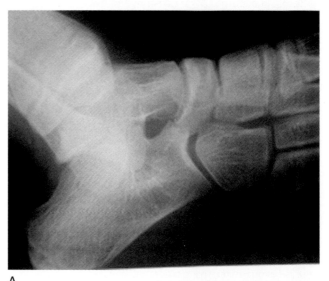

A

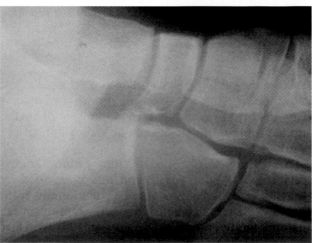

B

Figure 10–77 A complete **(A)** and partial **(B)** calcaneonavicular coalition must be differentiated from the os calcaneus secundarius.

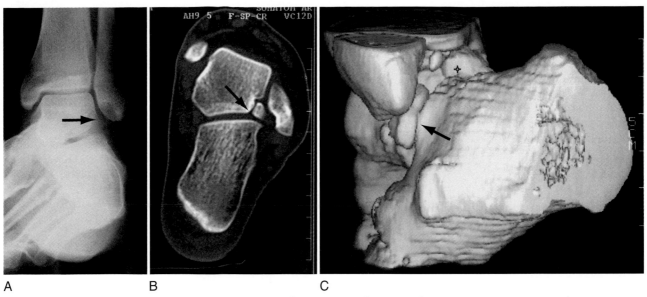

Figure 10–78   A, Normal anteroposterior radiograph of ankle. **B,** Axial CT scan demonstrating accessory ossicle in sinus tarsi. **C,** Reconstruction of CT demonstrating what may be an old fracture of a true accessory bone. (From Callanan I, Williams L, Stephens M: *Foot Ankle Int* 19:475-478, 1998. Used by permission.)

CALCANEUS ACCESSORIUS

Anatomy and Incidence

The calcaneus accessorius was first described by Pfitzner.[224] This accessory bone approximates the trochlear process of the calcaneus on the fibular aspect just distal to the fibular malleolus.[161,166,210] At its largest extent it is approximately 5 mm in diameter. This has also been referred to as the "os talocalcaneare laterale" by O'Rahilly (Fig. 10–79A).[219] Because it is a very rare accessory bone,[236] Trolle[263] is the only one to note its incidence, reported in his histoembryologic examination as 0.6%. He observed that it is rarely larger than "the size of a pea."

In 1860, Hyrtl[263] first described an enlarged calcaneal tuberosity in this area as the processus trochlearis (Fig. 10–79B). It had been seen radiographically on a dorsoplantar view of the foot with the ankle in hyperextension.

Clinical Significance

The calcaneus accessorius must be differentiated from an os subfibulare or an avulsion fracture. A bone scan can be used to differentiate a fracture from a calcaneus accessorius. Uhrbrand and Jensen[268] reported a large calcaneus accessorius that became symptomatic in a 5-year-old boy. This led to varus malalignment of the hindfoot, and the enlarged bone was excised with excellent results.

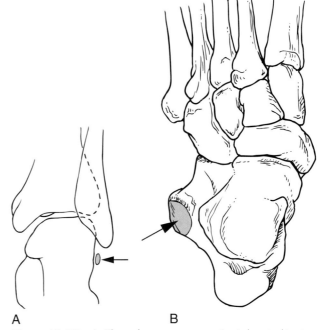

Figure 10–79   A, The calcaneus accessorius is located just to the lateral aspect of the trochlear process of the calcaneus (*arrow*). **B,** The trochlear process of the calcaneus (*arrow*) may be enlarged and occasionally symptomatic.

OS SUSTENTACULI

Anatomy and Incidence

The os sustentaculi is located on the posterior aspect of the sustentaculum tali (Fig. 10–80).* Pfitzner[224] first described this accessory bone. He noted that it occurred in fewer than 1% of cases and observed that it is often connected by a fibrocartilaginous or fibrous tissue interface with the sustentaculum. Neither Dwight[126] nor Trolle[263] reported this as a separate accessory bone. Holle[167] described its incidence as 1.5% in a review of 1,000 radiographs. Hoerr et al[162] reported that 2% to 3% of boys and 0% of girls presented with this accessory bone in his radiographic review of 501 patients.

Clinical Significance

The os sustentaculi (Fig. 10–81), which is found on the medial aspect of the calcaneus, should be differentiated from the calcaneus accessorius, which is found on the lateral aspect of the talocalcaneal articulation. Harris and Beath[151] suggested that an os sustentaculi

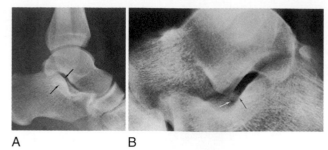

A   B

Figure 10–81   A and **B,** Two examples of the os sustentaculi seen in lateral projections simulating a fracture of the articular surface of the calcaneus. (From Keats TE: *Atlas of Normal Roentgen Variants That Simulate Disease,* ed 4. St Louis, Mosby, 1987.)

may be associated with a tarsal coalition and peroneal spastic flatfoot. Its presence may be demonstrated on routine radiography (Fig. 10–82). A computed tomographic (CT) scan of the hindfoot can help to differentiate this accessory bone from a tarsal coalition (Fig. 10–83). A tarsal coalition can require surgical intervention, whereas an os sustentaculi rarely requires surgical excision.

OS SUBCALCIS AND OS APONEUROSIS PLANTARIS

Anatomy and Incidence

Accessory bones on the plantar aspect of the calcaneus include the os subcalcis[263] (Fig. 10–84) and the os aponeurosis plantaris (Fig. 10–85).[111] O'Rahilly[219] described an accessory bone in the plantar aponeurosis

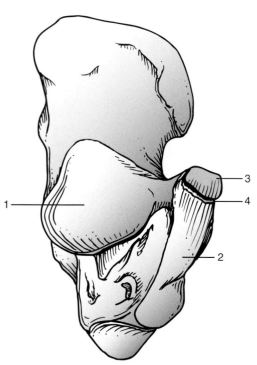

Figure 10–80   Os sustentaculi. *1,* The posterior facet of the calcaneus; *2,* the sustentaculum tali, *3,* os sustentaculi; *4,* fibrocartilaginous interface between the sustentaculum tali and os sustentaculi.

*References 100, 104, 109, 166, 202, 209, and 219.

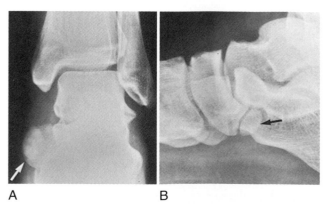

A   B

Figure 10–82   Os sustentaculi. This accessory bone is found at the posterior aspect of the sustentaculum tali on the superior aspect. **A,** Anteroposterior projection. **B,** Lateral projection. This anomalous bone may be incorporated in an accessory joint between the sustentaculum tali and the talus. (From March HC, London RI: *AJR Am J Roentgenol* 76:1114, 1956.)

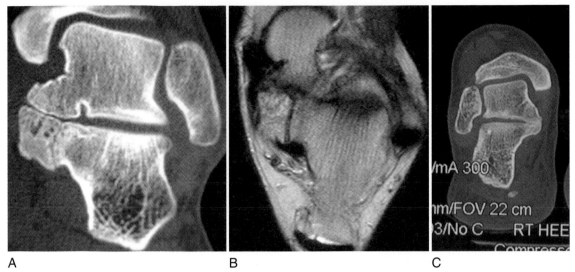

A   B   C

Figure 10–83   A and **B,** Axial scans demonstrating os sustentaculi. **C,** Talocalcaneal coalition should be differentiated from an os sustentaculi. (**A** and **B** from Mellado J, Salvado E, Camins A, et al: *Skeletal Radiol* 31:53-56, 2002. Used by permission.)

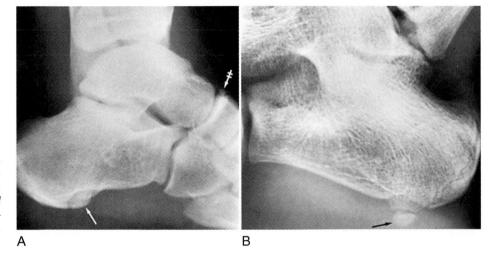

Figure 10–84   A and **B,** The os subcalcis occurs beneath the body of the calcaneus. (From Keats TE: *Atlas of Normal Roentgen Variants That Simulate Disease,* ed 4. St Louis, Mosby, 1987.)

A   B

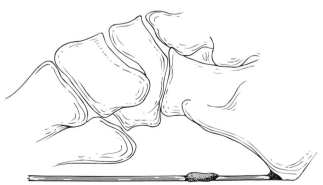

Figure 10–85   The os aponeurosis plantaris is oblong and flat and can vary significantly in size.

close to but not adjoining the medial tubercle of the calcaneus. This should be differentiated from a calcaneal spur or a fracture of a calcaneal spur. The os aponeurosis plantaris lies enclosed in the plantar aponeurosis and can vary significantly in size. It is usually oblong and flat and can best be seen in a lateral radiograph. The os subcalcis is found on the plantar aspect of the calcaneus slightly posterior to the insertion of the plantar fascia. This bone can reach a diameter of 10 mm. There is no reported incidence of either bone.

Clinical Significance

It may be necessary to differentiate an os subcalcis from a traumatic fracture. Rarely is surgery indicated for either of these conditions unless they are associated with chronic intractable pain.

OS CUBOIDES SECUNDARIUM

Anatomy and Incidence

The os cuboides secundarium is a rare ossicle located between the calcaneus, talus, navicular, and cuboid (Fig. 10–86).* Located on the plantar aspect of the foot, it was first described by Pfitzner[224] who recognized it to occur in two different locations: fused with the cuboid and articulating with the talus (Fig. 10–87A) and fused with the navicular and articulating with the talus (Fig. 10–87B and C). This ossicle can be as large as 5 to 10 mm and is seen radiographically in both a dorsoplantar and a lateral oblique view. Although Pfitzner[224] and Dwight[126] reported the

---

*References 100, 126, 128, 166, 171, 263, 278, and 285.

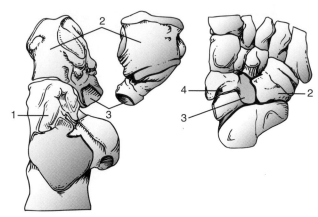

Figure 10–86 The os cuboides secundarium. *1*, The calcaneus; *2*, the cuboid; *3*, the os cuboides secundarium; *4*, the navicular.

occurrence of this accessory bone, Hoerr et al[162] in their evaluation of radiographs in 501 adolescent feet noted this accessory bone occurred in 1% to 3% of adolescents (Fig. 10–87D and E). Gaulke et al[135] described the excision of this bone in a nine-year-old boy and

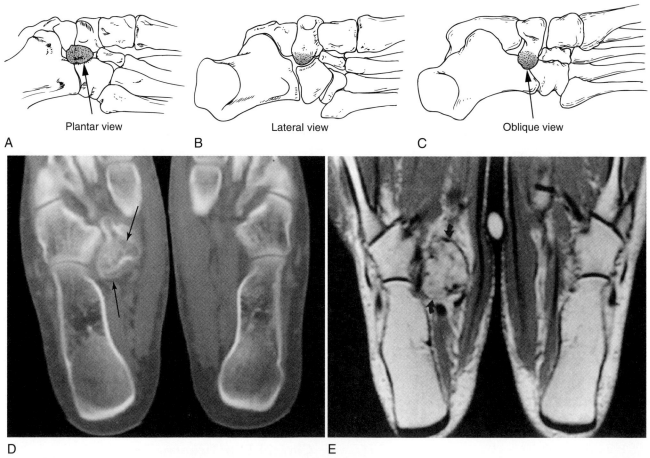

Plantar view

Lateral view

Oblique view

A

B

C

D

E

Figure 10–87 **A,** Os cuboides secundarium articulating with the cuboid and calcaneus (plantar view). **B** and **C,** Os cuboides secundarium arising from the navicular. **D,** Transverse CT scan demonstrates os cuboides secundarium (*arrows*). **E,** MRI demonstrates bowing of the abductor hallucis adjacent to the os cuboides secundarium (*arrows*). (**D** and **E** courtesy of M. Logan, MD.)

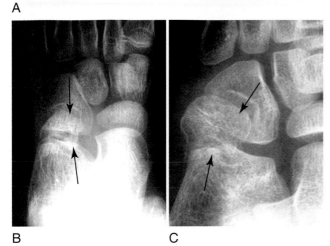

B   **C**

Figure 10–88 Lateral **(A)** and anteroposterior **(B)** radiographs and close-up view **(C)** demonstrating large os cuboides secundarium. (From Gaulke R, Schmitz H: *J Foot Ankle Surg* 42:230-234, 2003. Used by permission.)

found the accessory bone bisected the tendon of the flexor digitorum brevis (Fig. 10–88).

Clinical Significance

Most commonly this ossicle is asymptomatic and is indeed difficult to visualize on routine radiographs. Logan et al[193] demonstrated this accessory bone on both CT scan and MRI as well. In general, it is uncommon for this accessory bone to be symptomatic.

This is a rare bone of doubtful clinical significance except in the differentiation of it from a fracture. Although it has been suggested that an os cuboides secundarium might represent a variant of a cubonavicular coalition, the CT scan and MRI performed by Logan et al[193] demonstrated no coalition of the cuboid, the navicular, or the os cuboides secundarium.

OS TALONAVICULARE DORSALE, OS SUPRATALARE

Anatomy and Incidence

The os talonaviculare dorsale (Fig. 10–89) (also referred to as Pirie's bone, os supranaviculare, talonavicular ossicle, os supratalare) describes accessory bones of varying size and shape in the area of the talonavicular joint. Pirie[226,227] reported 14 cases of an os talonaviculare dorsale, four of which were bilateral. Pfitzner[224] hypothesized that this accessory bone was really an avulsed exostosis. Hoerr et al,[162] in a radiographic study of 134 adolescents, reported a 15% incidence of this accessory bone in boys and an 11% incidence in girls (Figs. 10–90 and 10–91).

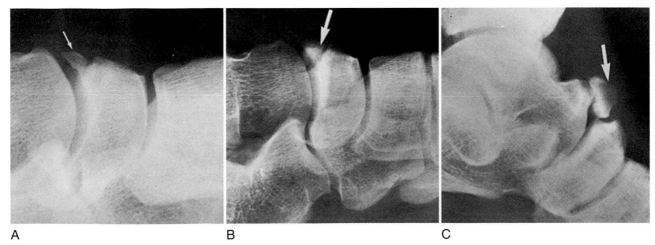

A   **B**   **C**

Figure 10–89 **A** and **B**, *Arrows* indicate os talonaviculare dorsale. **C**, Large os talonaviculare dorsale *(arrow)* with articulation with both the navicular and the talus. (From Keats TE: *Atlas of Normal Roentgen Variants That Simulate Disease*, ed 4. St Louis, Mosby, 1987.)

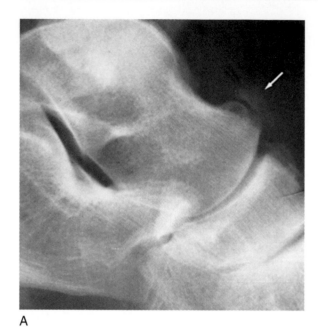

A

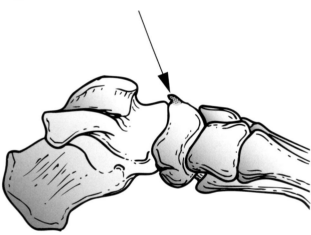

B

Figure 10–90   A, Os supratalare *(arrow).* The os supratalare emanates from the talus, whereas the os talonaviculare dorsale or supranaviculare emanates more commonly from the navicular. **B,** Diagram of os talonaviculare dorsale *(arrow).* (**B** from Keats TE: *Atlas of Normal Roentgen Variants that Simulate Disease,* ed 4. St Louis, Mosby, 1987.)

Osteoarthritic degeneration (Fig. 10–92) of the talonavicular joint should be differentiated from this accessory bone. The ossicle may be fused with the talus or with the navicular. The os supratalare (talus secundarius) is located on the dorsum of the talus between the ankle and talonavicular joints and may be fused with the talus or remain as a free accessory bone. It is rarely larger than 4 mm.

Clinical Significance

Accessory bones in the area of the talonavicular joint are uncommon. They should be differentiated

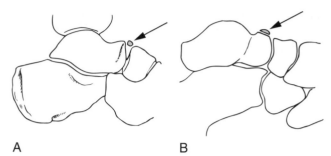

A   B

Figure 10–91   A, The os talonaviculare dorsale *(arrow)* can lie in the talonavicular joint on the dorsal aspect. **B,** An accessory ossicle on the dorsal surface of the talus *(arrow)* is called an *os supratalare.*

from degenerative arthritic spurs, avulsion fractures, or other traumatic conditions. Miller and Black[213] reported a case of impingement of the deep peroneal nerve due to an os supranaviculare, which was treated with surgical excision. In an exploration of this area, a surgeon must protect the deep peroneal nerve and dorsalis pedis artery and vein during the dissection.

When acute pain has developed in this region, a bone scan can help to differentiate one of these accessory ossicles from an acute injury.

ACCESSORY NAVICULAR

Anatomy and Incidence

In 1605 Bauhin[136] first described the accessory navicular. Since that time, numerous names have been suggested in the literature for this accessory bone including accessory scaphoid, accessory navicular, prehallux, and os tibiale externum.[231] Grogan et al[144] have stated that up to 13% of the population might have an accessory navicular.

An accessory navicular is a congenital anomaly in which the tuberosity of the navicular develops from a secondary center of ossification. It is located on the medial aspect of the arch in association with the

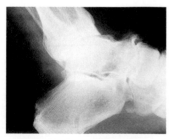

Figure 10–92   Degenerative arthritis of the talonavicular joint may be confused with an os talonaviculare dorsale or an os supratalare.

navicular.* Geist[137] reported a 14% incidence of this ossicle in supposedly normal feet, and Harris and Beath[150] reported a 4% incidence in young men; however, other authors have reported a varying frequency of occurrence. In radiographic evaluations, Hoerr et al,[162] in a study of 501 adolescents, showed an incidence of 3% to 8% in girls and 4% to 9% in boys; Bizarro[101] reported a 2% incidence, and Holland[166] demonstrated a 10% to 12% incidence. Pfitzner,[224] in an anatomic study of 425 feet, reported an 11.5% incidence, and Dwight,[128] in an anatomic study, reported a 10% incidence of an accessory navicular. Trolle,[263] in a histoembryologic study, noted a 6.4% incidence. McKusick[208] lists an accessory navicular as being inherited as an autosomal dominant trait and reports an incidence of 5%.

Three distinct types of accessory navicular are described.[190,231,244] Type 1 is a small accessory bone without attachment to the body of the navicular but formed in a well-defined round or oval shape (Fig. 10–93A). This most probably represents the sesamoid of the tibialis posterior tendon, and it is located on the plantar aspect of the tendon at the level of the inferior calcaneonavicular ligament. (See discussion on the sesamoid posterior tibial tendon.) It is almost always asymptomatic.

---

*References 89, 90, 94, 100, 105, 121, 129-131, 144, 148, 149, 153, 157, 164, 165, 171, 186, 190, 192, 201, 214, 215, 220, 222, 237, 244, 257, 261, 269, 274, 278, and 285.

The second type (type 2) of accessory navicular is a definite part of the body of the navicular, but the tuberosity is separated by a fibrocartilaginous plate of irregular outline (Fig. 10–93B and C) less than 2 mm in width.[94] This type often becomes symptomatic and is occasionally mistaken for a fracture of the tuberosity of the navicular (Figs. 10–94 and 10–95). The remaining discussion concerns this type. Sella and Lawson[244] have differentiated type 2 accessory naviculars into two separate entities. A type 2A accessory navicular is connected with the talar process by a less acute angle, and a Type 2B accessory navicular is situated more inferiorly. The main force on a type 2A is a tension force, whereas type 2B develops a shearing force. The two types can only be distinguished radiographically. Type 2A is more at risk for an avulsion injury. There is a great deal of controversy over whether an accessory navicular is the cause of a pes planus deformity. Sella[244] has stated that increased pronation can cause more stress to the synchondrosis. Only type 2 accessory naviculars are characterized by a synchondrosis.

Type 3 accessory naviculars are united by a bony ridge, producing a cornuate navicular. Type 2 and type 3 accessory naviculars constitute 70% of these deformities.[190]

A symptomatic accessory navicular is often caused by an injury. This can be due to tension, shearing, or compression forces transmitted through the posterior tibial tendon to the fibrocartilaginous interface.

Zadek[282] studied 14 cases of symptomatic accessory navicular. Radiographically, he noted definite fusion

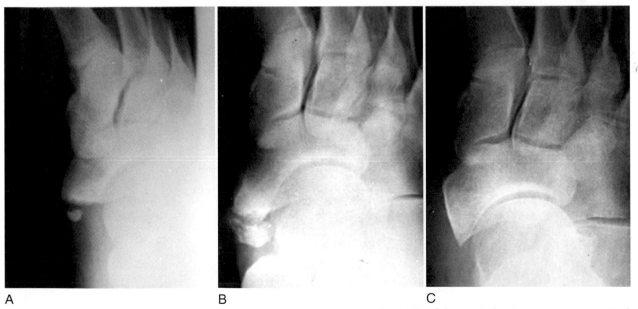

A   B   C

Figure 10–93 A, Small accessory navicular bone without attachment to the body of the navicular. Large accessory navicular seen **(B)** preoperatively and **(C)** 1 year postoperatively following excision of accessory navicular and excision of large medial tuberosity.

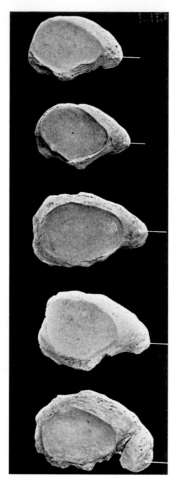

Figure 10–94 Variation in five naviculars showing varying development of the accessory navicular. These are all characteristic of type 3 accessory naviculars. (From Dwight T: *Clinical Atlas of Variations of the Bones of the Hand and Foot.* Philadelphia, JB Lippincott, 1907, pp 14-24.)

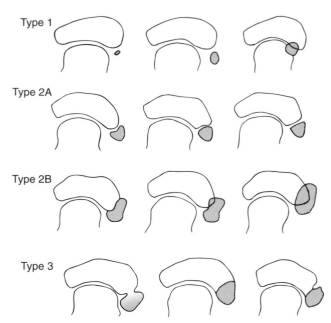

Figure 10–95 Variations in radiographic form of accessory navicular from large free fragment to small accessory fragment.

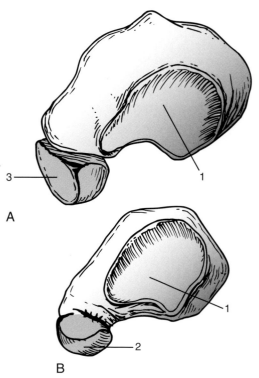

Figure 10–96 A, Type 2A accessory navicular. **B,** Type 3 accessory navicular. *1,* Proximal articular surface of navicular; *2,* incomplete segmentation of accessory navicular; *3,* accessory navicular.

with the body of the navicular in five cases, partial fusion in three, and complete separation in six. Zadek and Gold[283] studied the microscopic articulation of the accessory navicular to the body of the navicular. They reported that these structures were composed of hyaline cartilage, dense fibrocartilage, or both and sometimes showed ossification as well. This study of adolescents as they aged demonstrated that bony union definitely occurred in a large portion of cases. Of 14 accessory naviculars studied,[282] five later went on to fuse, three partially fused, and six failed to fuse. The authors concluded that many accessory naviculars do unite with the body of the navicular, but some can persist into adult life (Figs. 10–96 and 10–97).

Kidner[176] studied the relationship of pes planus in the presence of an accessory navicular and hypothesized that flatfoot deformity had one of three causes: alteration of the line of pull of the posterior tibial

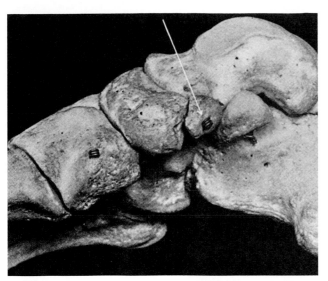

Figure 10–97 Accessory navicular demonstrated on anatomic specimen *(arrow)*. (From Dwight T: *Clinical Atlas of Variations of the Bones of the Hand and Foot.* Philadelphia, JB Lippincott, 1907, pp 14-23.)

tendon as a result of the prominence created by the accessory navicular; forcing of the posterior tibial tendon by the accessory navicular to become more of an adductor than a supinator of the forefoot, thereby decreasing support for the longitudinal arch; and impingement of the accessory navicular against the medial malleolus as the foot adducts, which tends to keep the foot in an abducted position and thus partially flattens the longitudinal arch.

Evaluation and Treatment

The accessory navicular should be differentiated from the os paracuneiforme (Fig. 10–98), which is found on the tibial aspect of the foot in close relationship to the naviculocuneiform joint. Also to be considered is the os cuneometatarsale I tibiale, which is located in proximity to the first metatarsocuneiform joint. Trolle[263] reported the os paracuneiforme to have a 13% incidence.

An accessory navicular can become symptomatic in childhood or early adulthood. In children the symptoms are usually caused by pressure of the accessory bone against the shoe. At times the condition is associated with progressive flattening of the longitudinal arch. In adults, symptoms usually develop after trauma to the foot, often resulting from a twisting injury. Physical examination often reveals tenderness over the prominence on the medial aspect of the instep. Radiographs demonstrate the accessory navicular. A tech-

netium bone scan can help to differentiate a fracture from an accessory navicular.

In the asymptomatic case of an accessory navicular, reassurance of the patient is usually adequate. In cases that have become acutely symptomatic following an injury, immobilization in a below-knee walking cast followed by the use of a longitudinal arch support often diminishes symptoms.[144] Initial treatment should consist of casting or an orthosis, although in the majority of cases Grogan et al[144] have observed that nonoperative treatment is not successful and surgical treatment is eventually necessary. When symptoms are caused by pressure over the navicular, a shoe that avoids pressure over this area should be worn. The occasional judicious use of a corticosteroid injection into the symptomatic area gives relief. When symptoms become intractable, surgical intervention may be necessary.

The Kidner procedure may be successful in alleviating symptoms. When a Kidner procedure is performed in a young patient with a pes planus deformity, excision of the accessory navicular should be accompanied by rerouting of the tibialis posterior tibial tendon through the navicular to increase the tension on the

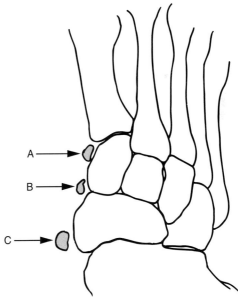

Figure 10–98 Accessory bones on the medial aspect of the boot may be confusing. An accessory bone adjacent to the first metatarsocuneiform joint is termed the *os cuneometatarsale I tibiale (A)*. An accessory bone adjacent to the naviculocuneiform joint is termed the *os paracuneiforme (B)*, and a bone adjacent to the proximal pole of the navicular *(C)* is termed *accessory navicular*. An os paracuneiforme is found just medial to the first cuneiform and distal to the location of the accessory navicular. With a larger distance between the accessory bone and the body of the navicular, a sesamoid of the anterior tibial tendon might be considered.

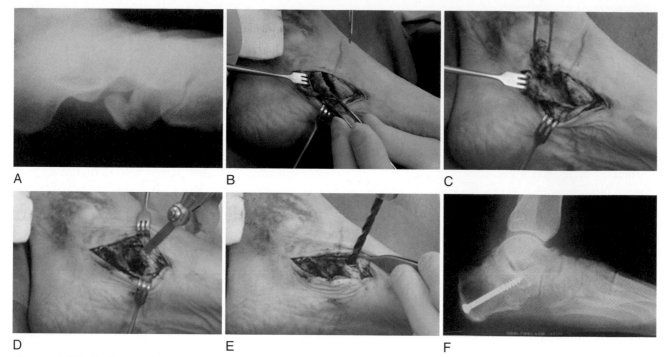

A   B   C

D   E   F

Figure 10–99   Radiograph **(A)** and intraoperative photograph **(B)** of large accessory navicular. **C,** Excision of navicular. **D,** Shaving of prominent navicular tuberosity. **E,** Drill hole for transfer of posterior tibial tendon. **F,** Following calcaneal osteotomy in conjunction with modified Kidner procedure.

tendon. When the accessory navicular is not associated with a pes planus deformity, simple excision of the accessory navicular and plication of the tendon are sufficient. In an adult patient with a symptomatic accessory navicular with or without an associated flatfoot, the accessory navicular is excised and the tendon sutured to the side of the medial aspect of the navicular. No attempt is made to shorten or plicate the posterior tibial tendon. A calcaneal osteotomy may be performed in the presence of increased pes planus (Fig. 10–99).

KIDNER PROCEDURE

Surgical Technique

1. A thigh tourniquet is applied with the patient in a supine position. The foot is cleansed and draped in the usual fashion. The foot and leg are exsanguinated and the tourniquet is inflated.
2. A longitudinal skin incision parallel to the upper border of the tibialis posterior tendon starts 1 cm anterior to the tip of the medial malleolus and extends to the medial cuneiform.
3. The dissection is carried down to the superior border of the tibialis posterior tendon along the length of the incision until the tendon courses plantarward beneath the navicular.
4. The accessory navicular is identified within the substance of the tendon and is excised with sharp dissection.
5. If the tibialis posterior tendon is to be rerouted through the navicular, it is detached as distally as possible.
6. If there is a significant prominence to the medial tuberosity of the navicular, it is osteotomized and resected.
7. If the tibialis posterior tendon is to be advanced, a dorsal–plantar drill hole is placed through the navicular. The foot is placed in maximal inversion and equinus. The tendon is then passed in a plantar-to-dorsal direction through the drill hole with a tendon passer, and the tendon is sutured back to itself or to the surrounding periosteal tissue.
8. If the tibialis posterior tendon is not advanced, it is sutured to the raw medial surface of the navicular with a no. 0 nonabsorbable suture. Alternatively, a suture

anchor may be placed in the navicular (on the plantar–medial aspect) and the tendon is secured to the plantar aspect of the navicular. The periosteum that has been elevated from the navicular before the excision of the tuberosity is now plicated over the tendon.

Optional Procedure

In the presence of increased pes planus associated with an accessory navicular, a calcaneal slide osteotomy is performed. Through a small vertical incision inferior to the tip of the fibula and peroneal tendons, the calcaneus is exposed with care taken to protect the sural nerve. An osteotomy of the calcaneus is performed just behind the posterior facet. The proximal calcaneal fragment is translated medially 8 to 10 mm and fixed temporarily with a Steinman pin introduced through a separate puncture incision at the tip of the heel. In the younger patient with an open calcaneal apophysis, internal fixation with a compression screw is discouraged.

Postoperative Treatment

The foot is placed in a non–weight-bearing below-knee cast for 3 weeks, and then a below-knee walking cast is used for 3 weeks. In the case of a patient on whom a tendon transfer has been performed, the foot is placed in an equinus adducted position for 4 weeks in a non–weight-bearing cast and then in a plantigrade walking cast for the final 4 weeks.

Results

Grogan et al[144] reported on 17 of 22 patients who underwent excision of an accessory navicular for a total of 39 excisions, 75% of which were type 2 and type 3 accessory naviculars. Grogan noted that excision of the accessory navicular without reimplantation of the posterior tibial tendon was routinely successful. Of 17 patients (25 feet) who underwent surgical excision, all but one reported excellent results and improvement from preoperative symptoms.

Ray and Goldberg[231] described management of the accessory navicular using a similar procedure in 29 feet. They excised the accessory navicular, sutured the fibers of the posterior tibial tendon to the anterior surface of the navicular, and reported good or excellent results in 26 of the cases.

In a review of 20 patients (age range, 7 to 40 years), all with an accessory navicular, Chater[116] reported similar successful results. Twelve patients were treated successfully by nonoperative means. Of the remaining eight, six children underwent excision of the ossicle, and two underwent a Kidner procedure (excision of the accessory navicular, detachment and reinsertion of the posterior tibial tendon into a drill hole into the navicular). Chater[116] noted that the Kidner technique appeared to have two advantages over a simple excision: it reinforced the spring ligament, and it helped to counteract and to correct sagging of the talonavicular joint. Leonard et al[189] reported on 13 patients (25 feet) with an accessory navicular associated with a pes planovalgus deformity treated with a Kidner procedure. They reported satisfactory restoration of the longitudinal arch and correction of heel valgus. Giannestras[138] observed on the contrary that pes planovalgus was only occasionally associated with an accessory navicular. He advocated simple surgical excision of the ossicle.

Harris and Beath[150] found a 4% incidence of an accessory navicular in 3619 Canadian army recruits. In a follow-up study of 77 of these men, only four developed significant symptoms, and the authors concluded that rarely was an accessory navicular symptomatic and that the need for surgical treatment was uncommon.

BIPARTITE NAVICULAR

Anatomy and Incidence

A bipartite navicular has also been reported by several authors.* Initially Volk[270] reported two cases. Zimmer[285] reported a case of a bipartite navicular in a 19-year-old patient. Typically the navicular is segmented into tibial and fibular segments that are well seen on a dorsoplantar radiograph. The fragments can be of varying size. Sarrafian[236] notes that on a dorsoplantar radiograph, the smaller fragment is wedge-shaped with a medially directed base. On the lateral radiograph, the same fragment is wedge-shaped in appearance, with the apex in a plantar direction. The smaller fragment is typically more dorsal in direction and may be superimposed over the first and second cuneiforms.

---

*References 118, 164, 206, 215, 220, and 278.

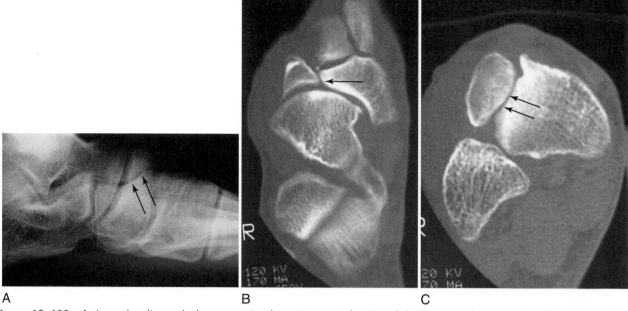

Figure 10–100 A, Lateral radiograph demonstrating bipartite navicular. **B** and **C,** CT scans demonstrating bipartite navicular. *Arrows* mark line of segmentation. (Courtesy Dr. Anik Shawdon.)

Shawdon et al[247] have demonstrated the bipartite navicular on CT scanning to be clearly evident on both axial and coronal planes. In the axial scan, the navicular appears wedge-shaped, with tapering interval margins (Fig. 10–100). On CT evaluation, the appearance is distinctly different from that demonstrated with a fracture or stress fracture of the navicular. A bipartite navicular should be differentiated from an asymptomatic stress fracture or an acute fracture of the navicular. In a patient with no history of trauma who has presented with medial midfoot pain and an abnormal but nondiagnostic radiograph, a CT scan may be helpful in differentiating the diagnosis of a bipartite navicular.

Clinical Significance

A bipartite navicular should be differentiated from an asymptomatic stress fracture or an acute fracture of the navicular.

OS INTERCUNEIFORME

Anatomy and Incidence

The os intercuneiforme is a very rare accessory bone located on the dorsum of the midfoot in an interval between the first and second cuneiforms just distal to the navicular (Fig. 10–101). Often an intercuneiform

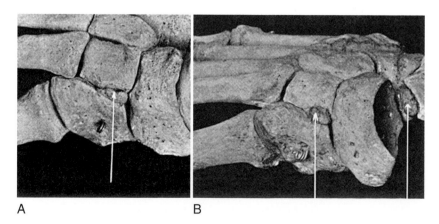

Figure 10–101 A, Dorsal view demonstrating os intercuneiforme *(arrow).* **B,** An oblique view demonstrating os intercuneiforme *(left arrow)* and os cuboides secundarium *(right arrow).* (From Dwight T: *Clinical Atlas of Variations of the Bones of the Hand and Foot.* Philadelphia, JB Lippincott, 1907, pp 14-23.)

A   B

fossa is present. It is typically triangular in appearance. Dwight[126,127] initially reported this accessory bone, and Hoerr et al[162] stated that the incidence of the os inter-cuneiforme was 1% in his radiographic evaluation of 367 adolescents. Geist[136] reported this accessory bone was present in 2% of cases.

Clinical Significance

This is a rare accessory bone, and the major clinical importance is that it should be distinguished from an acute fracture or a chronic nonunion of a fracture of the first or second cuneiforms. In the presence of pain localized to this region, a bone scan can help to differentiate this uncommon accessory bone from an acute fracture.

OS CUNEO-I METATARSALE-I PLANTARE, OS CUNEO-I METATARSALE-II DORSALE

Anatomy and Incidence

The os cuneo-I metatarsale-I plantare occurs on the plantar aspect of the foot at the base of the first metatarsal (Fig. 10–102).[219] It articulates with the

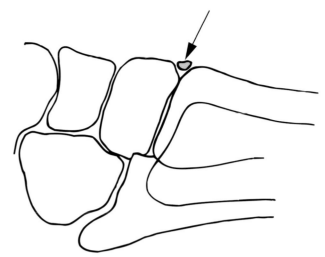

Figure 10–103 The os cuneo-I metatarsale-II dorsale *(arrow)* lies dorsally between the middle cuneiform and the second metatarsal.

plantar base of the first metatarsal and the first cuneiform. Pfitzner[224] first described this very rare accessory bone. Trolle[263] estimated its diameter as the size of a "cherrystone." It is not often seen on a dorsoplantar radiograph but can be seen in a lateral oblique view.

The os cuneo-I metatarsale-II dorsale lies on the dorsal aspect of the articulation of the second metatarsal and second cuneiform (Fig. 10–103).[239] It is wedge-shaped with the base oriented dorsally. Trolle[263] characterized it as "peppercorn" in size. This is also difficult to identify on a radiograph but can be seen in a lateral or lateral oblique view.

Clinical Significance

These are rare accessory bones that may be noted radiographically in a symptomatic or an asymptomatic patient. When present, they should be differentiated from an acute injury. Where this differentiation is difficult, a technetium bone scan can help to distinguish this from a fracture.

BIPARTITE FIRST CUNEIFORM

Anatomy and Incidence

Although first described by Morel (1797),[263] Pfitzner[224] reported the incidence of the bipartite first cuneiform as 0.5% in his series of anatomic specimens. Gruber (1877) reported an incidence of 0.33%, and Trolle[234] reported an incidence of 2.4%. Gruber (1877)[263] noted 10 complete segmentations of the first cuneiform and

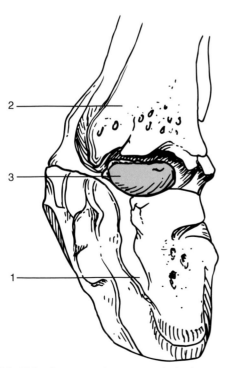

Figure 10–102 Os cuneo-I metatarsale-I plantare. *1,* First cuneiform, plantar aspect; *2,* first metatarsal, plantar aspect; *3,* os cuneo-I metatarsale-I plantare.

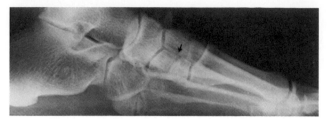

Figure 10–104 Horizontal bifurcation *(arrow)* of the first cuneiform.

five incomplete ones in his evaluation of 2500 anatomic specimens (Fig. 10–104).

The first cuneiform is often segmented horizontally into a larger dorsal and smaller plantar segment.*

The dorsal segment articulates distally with the dorsal aspect of the first metatarsal base and proximally with the navicular (Fig. 10–105). The lateral surface articulates with the middle cuneiform and with the base of the second metatarsal. The plantar segment articulates as well with the base of the first metatarsal and proximally with the navicular. The inferior surface has a prominent tubercle for insertion of the posterior tibial tendon. Together, the two segments of the bipartite first cuneiform amass a volume slightly larger than the undivided medial cuneiform (Fig. 10–106). The partition can be difficult to view on a dorsoplantar radiograph and may be better visualized on an oblique radiograph or CT scan.[125]

Clinical Significance

A bipartite first cuneiform is typically nonpainful and rarely if ever requires surgery. With trauma to the

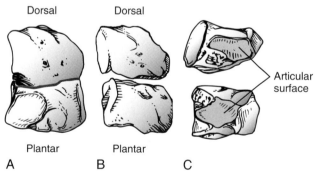

Figure 10–105 Bipartite first cuneiform. **A,** Articulated bipartite first cuneiform. **B,** Slightly separated view of first cuneiform. **C,** Disarticulated specimen showing the dorsal and plantar articular surfaces.

---

*References 91, 93, 95, 100, 101, 106, 125, 133, 155, 171, 191, 215, 218, 251, and 278.

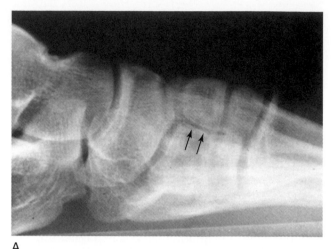

A

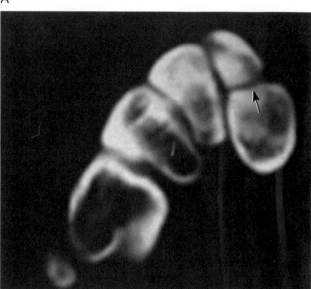

B

Figure 10–106 Bilateral bipartite medial cuneiform. **A,** Lateral radiograph demonstrating bipartite medial cuneiform *(arrow)*. **B,** Computed tomographic scan demonstrating bilateral bipartite medial cuneiforms *(arrows)*. (From Dellacorte M, Lin P, Grisafi P: *J Am Podiatr Med Assoc* 82:475-478, 1992.)

medial aspect of the foot, it may be necessary to distinguish a fracture from a bipartite first cuneiform[218] and from a tarsal coalition (Fig. 10–107).[181] In evaluation of pain in this region, a segmented first cuneiform can be identified on CT or MRI scan. On the other hand, Kumai et al[181] have described synostosis or coalition and the medial and intermediate cuneiform, which can only be identified on CT or MRI scan. Chiodo et al[117] have described excision of the medial aspect of the bipartite medial cuneiform, and Azurza et al[91] have described internal fixation of the fragment.

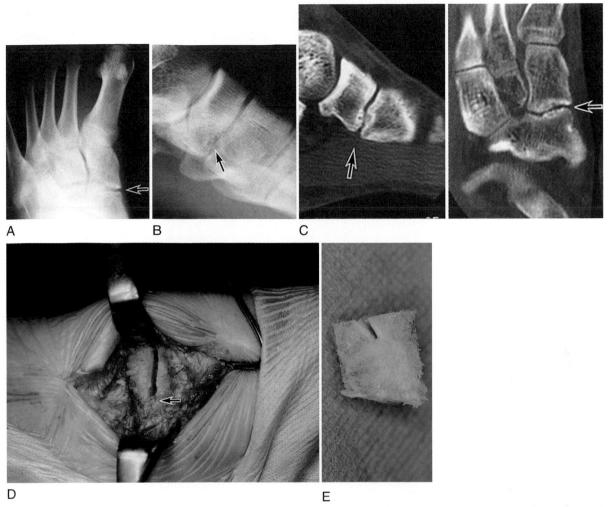

A   B   C   D   E

Figure 10–107   **A** and **B,** Anteroposterior and lateral radiographs demonstrating area of first naviculocuneiform joint coalition *(arrows).* **C,** Computed tomographic scan demonstrating first naviculocuneiform joint coalition *(arrow).* **D,** Operative appearance demonstrating coalition. **E,** Resected bone block shows fibrous and cartilaginous coalition. (From Kumai T, Tanaka Y, Takakura Y, et al: *Foot Ankle Int* 17:635-640, 1996.)

METATARSOCUNEIFORM COALITION

Anatomy and Incidence

Coalitions of the first metatarsocuneiform joint are rare. Day[123] and others[134,168,258] have described osseous coalitions. Tanaka et al[259] have described a fibrous coalition in which resection was performed successfully in a 32-year-old man (Fig. 10–108), and Takakura and Nakata[258] fused the joint to relieve pain (Fig. 10–109).

Clinical Significance

Although rare, first metatarsocuneiform coalition must be differentiated from intraarticular fractures and degenerative arthritis.

OS INTERMETATARSEUM

The os intermetatarseum is observed between the medial cuneiform and the base of the first and second metatarsals.* It was first described by Gruber in 1856,[264] but Pfitzner[224] and Dwight[128] gave the first comprehensive description of the variations of the os intermetatarseum. The os intermetatarseum (Fig. 10–110) is a spindle-shaped bone that originates from the distal corner of the medial cuneiform, tapers distally, and projects between the first and second metatarsals. It may be fused to either the first or second metatarsal or can articulate with the first and second metatarsals (Fig. 10–111) and the medial cuneiform.

_____

*References 101, 114, 132, 179, 216, 263, and 277.

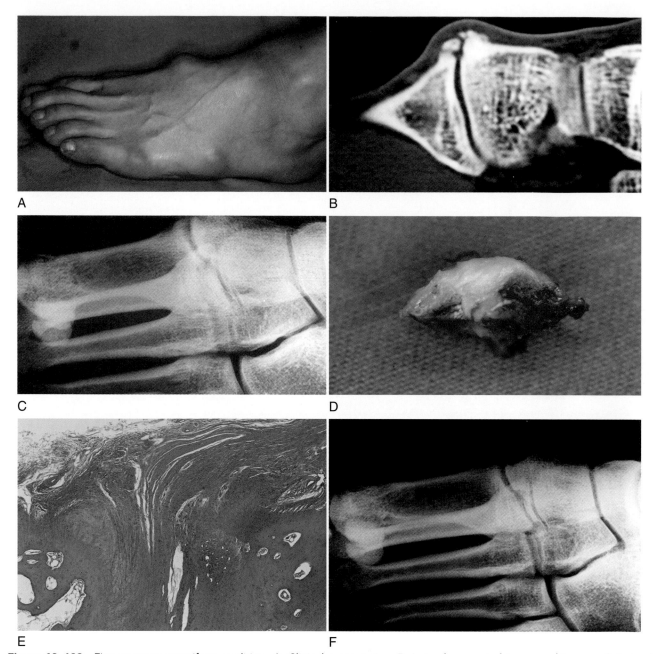

Figure 10–108 First metatarsocuneiform coalition. **A,** Clinical presentation. **B,** Lateral computed tomographic scan. **C,** Lateral radiograph. **D,** Resected dorsal coalition. **E,** Histology of resected specimen. **F,** Lateral radiograph following the resection. (From Tanaka Y, Takakura Y, Sugimoto K, Kumai T: *Foot Ankle Int* 21:1043-1046, 2000. Used by permission.)

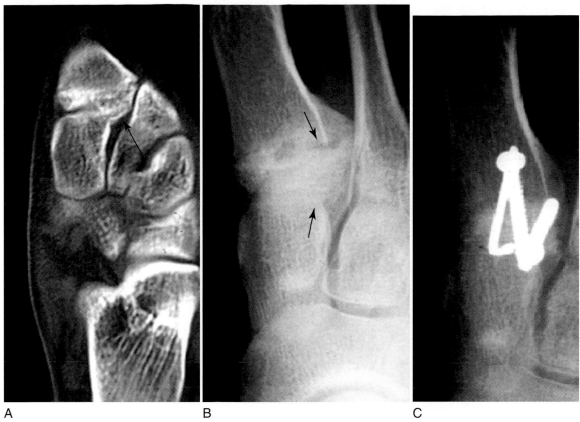

A   B   C

Figure 10–109 Metatarsocuneiform coalition. Computed tomographic scan **(A)** and radiograph **(B)** demonstrating first metatarsocuneiform fibrous coalition. **C,** Following arthrodesis. (From Tanaka Y, Takakura Y, Sugimoto K, Kumai T: *Foot Ankle Int* 21:1043-1046, 2000. Used by permission.)

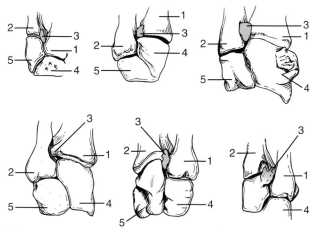

Figure 10–110 Os intermetatarseum. The os intermetatarseum may be a separate ossicle, or it can arise from the first or second metatarsal or from the first cuneiform. It may be incorporated or may be a free ossicle. *1,* First metatarsal; *2,* second metatarsal; *3,* os intermetatarseum; *4,* first cuneiform; *5,* second cuneiform.

Henderson[159] reported four cases of bilateral os intermetatarseum. All were associated with hallux valgus, and three cases were familial (Fig. 10–112). He noted a tendinous structure extending from the tip of the accessory bone through the muscle belly of the first dorsal interosseous that attached to the base of the proximal phalanx on the lateral aspect of the hallux. Burman and Lapidus[108] reported a 3.3% incidence of os intermetatarseum in a review of 1000 cases. Only four were reported to be painful. It was noted that the os intermetatarseum may be attached to either the first or second metatarsal (or both) (Fig. 10–113) or the first cuneiform or may be a completely unattached accessory bone and can appear as either a single bone or in several pieces.

Reichmister[232] reported a series of three cases in which two instances of painful os intermetatarseum were excised and one was treated conservatively. Reichmister noted that this accessory bone can cause pressure and pain by compression of the superficial peroneal nerve. Noguchi et al[216] reported on a soccer player who developed deep peroneal nerve symptoms

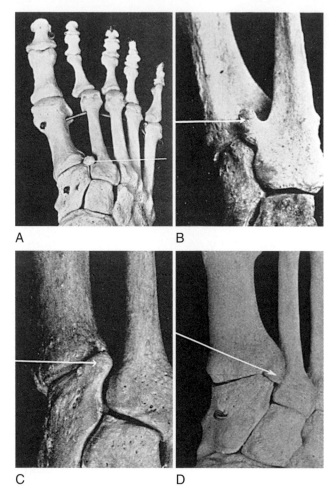

A   B
C   D

Figure 10–111   A, Os intermetatarseum, a separate ossicle. **B,** Os intermetatarseum *(arrow)* arising from the second metatarsal. **C,** Os intermetatarseum *(arrow)* off of first cuneiform. **D,** Os intermetatarseum *(arrow)* at the base of the first metatarsal. This can create a rigid articulation and when associated with a hallux valgus deformity may be resistant to correction without a metatarsal osteotomy. (From Dwight T: *Clinical Atlas of Variations of the Bones of the Hand and Foot.* Philadelphia, JB Lippincott, 1907, pp 14-23.)

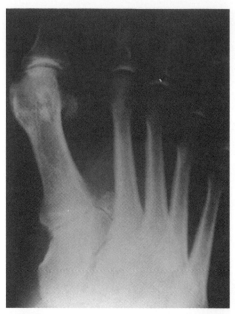

Figure 10–112   Os intermetatarseum with deviated first and second metatarsals. A first metatarsal osteotomy will be necessary to correct the intermetatarsal angle.

adjacent metatarsal or cuneiform, and post-traumatic osteophyte formation.

Clinical Significance

Typically this accessory bone is asymptomatic (Fig. 10–114). Its presence may be associated with hallux valgus, and in the decision-making process for correcting a hallux valgus deformity, the first metatarso-

due to impingement from an os intermetatarsum, with symptoms consistent to an anterior tarsal tunnel syndrome.

Kohler and Zimmer[177] reported two cases of fracture of the os intermetatarseum, one of which healed and one of which went on to nonunion. The incidence of the os intermetatarseum has ranged from 1.2% (Faber,[263] radiologic examination; Shands,[245] radiologic examination) to 10% (Dwight,[128] anatomic). Scarlet et al[238] reported this condition to be more often bilateral and to have a familial tendency.

An os intermetatarseum IV has been reported to lie between the fourth and fifth metatarsals.[263]

The differential diagnosis includes a calcified dorsalis pedis artery, a ligamentous avulsion of the

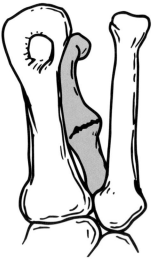

Figure 10–113   A huge os intermetatarseum links the first and second metatarsals.

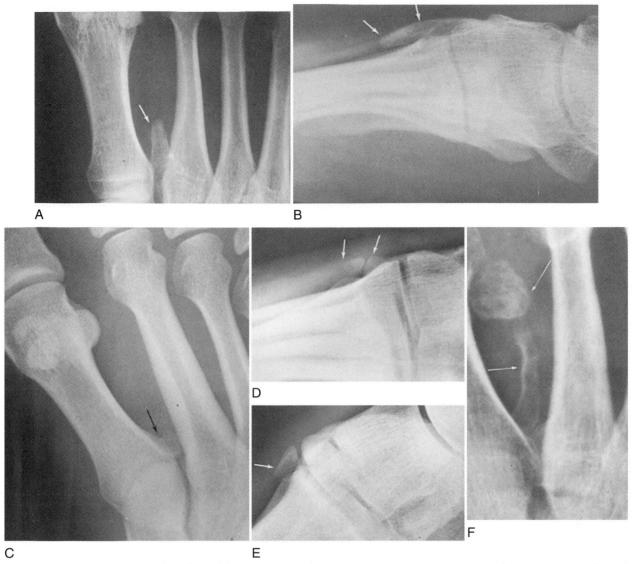

Figure 10–114 **A** to **F,** Examples of variable appearance of os intermetatarseum *(arrows).* Note the accessory ossicle at the distal end of the os intermetatarseum **(F).** (From Keats TE: *Atlas of Normal Roentgen Variants That Simulate Disease,* ed 4. St Louis, Mosby, 1987.)

cuneiform joint must be evaluated. The presence of an os intermetatarseum or a facet between the first and second metatarsal and medial cuneiform can indicate the necessity for a first metatarsal osteotomy in order to correct an increased angle between the first and second metatarsals. Tanaka et al[259] and others[123,168,259] have described a fibrous coalition at the first metatarsal cuneiform joint that can also restrict motion, which also may be pertinent in treating a hallux valgus deformity. Rarely if ever, is elective surgical resection required for an os intermetatarseum. Scarlet et al[238] and Reichmister[232] have both reported cases where a symptomatic os intermetatarseum has been excised.

OS VESALIANUM

Anatomy and Incidence

The os vesalianum is a rare accessory bone located at the proximal extent of the fifth metatarsal (Fig. 10–115).* Geist[136] found one case in 100 feet examined radiographically, and Dameron,[122] in a radiographic study of 1000 feet, noted only one case of an os vesalianum. Trolle,[263] Pfitzner,[224] and Holle[167] in

---

*References 92, 100, 108, 129, 145, 146, 165, 166, 170, 174, 185, 192, 215, 220, 250, 253, and 278.

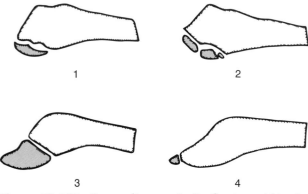

Figure 10–115 Os vesalianum. *1,* Ossification within the apophysis of the fifth metatarsal base; *2,* fragmentation within the ossification of the fifth metatarsal apophysis; *3,* un-united apophysis of the fifth metatarsal base; *4,* position of os vesalianum (note different orientation of articulation).

histoembryologic, anatomic, and extensive radiographic studies found no evidence of an os vesalianum. Heimerzheim[156] found a 0.9% incidence of this accessory bone in an evaluation of 1800 radiographs.

Trolle[263] noted that the os vesalianum can attain the size of an almond and is visible on both dorsoplantar and lateral oblique radiographs (Fig. 10–116A and B). On the dorsoplantar view, a small bone can be visualized within the tuberosity of the fifth metatarsal.

Clinical Significance

The major objective in diagnosis is to differentiate an os vesalianum from an ossifying apophysis of the fifth metatarsal base, an apophysitis of the fifth metatarsal

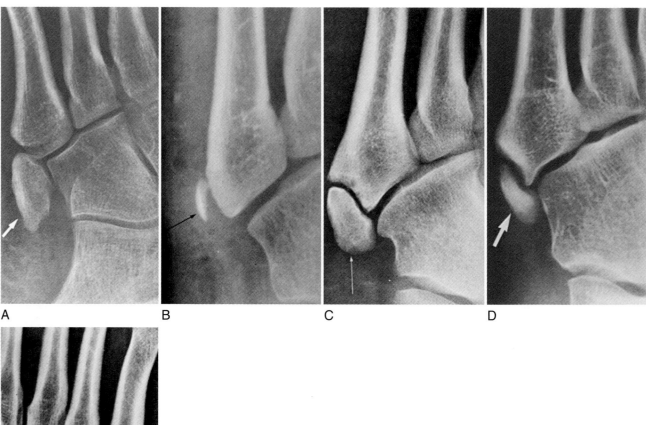

A   B   C   D

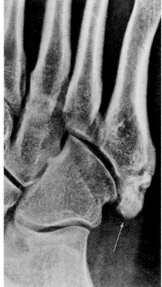

E

Figure 10–116 **A,** Os vesalianum. **B,** Apophysis of the base of the fifth metatarsal. **C,** Failed union of the apophysis at the base of the fifth metatarsal. **D,** Unfused apophysis of fifth metatarsal in a 19-year-old man. **E,** Failed union of the apophysis at the base of the fifth metatarsal. (From Keats TE: *Atlas of Normal Roentgen Variants That Simulate Disease,* ed 4. St Louis, Mosby, 1987.)

base,* a fracture of the tuberosity of the fifth metatarsal, a nonunion of a tuberosity fracture of the fifth metatarsal, an ununited apophysis of the fifth metatarsal base (Fig. 10–116C-E), and an os peroneum (see Fig. 10–56). Iselin[169] described an apophysitis of the base of the fifth metatarsal in teenagers. Fewer than 10 cases have been reported in the world literature. The apophysis is located within the flare of the proximal fifth metatarsal in the area where the peroneus brevis inserts.

Reported successful treatment includes rest and casting.[113,187] Canale[113] reports that bony union usually occurs with time. Ralph et al[230] reported excision of the painful fragment without disruption of the peroneus brevis tendon with complete resolution of symptoms.

Sarrafian[236] noted the following characteristics that aid in differentiating an os vesalianum: a fracture of the apophysis or base of the fifth metatarsal is transverse in direction; the ossification center of the apophysis is linear initially and longitudinally oriented parallel to the metatarsal shaft; an os vesalianum is located just proximal to the tip of a well-developed fifth metatarsal tuberosity; and with an os vesalianum, the opposing surfaces may be sclerotic and denote a chronic condition.

Iselin[169] described an apophysitis of the proximal fifth metatarsal (Fig. 10–117). It has been recognized by Canale et al[113] and others[187,230] as a condition in which the ossification center undergoes aseptic necrosis followed by gradual resorption of the fragment. It must be differentiated from a fracture and may be caused by repetitive trauma. When symptomatic, it can be successfully treated with rest, limited weight bearing, and occasionally casting. With apophysitis of the fifth metatarsal, a traumatic episode can occur, resulting in avulsion of a portion of the apophysis.

Typically the localized pain and tenderness resolve in time, because this is a self-limiting disorder in which conservative treatment can be used. Following apophysitis, there may be a residual irregularity of the proximal fifth metatarsal and prominence, but this typically does not interfere with function.[241]

REFERENCES

Sesamoids

1. Abraham M, Sage R, Lorenz M: Tibial and fibular sesamoid fractures on the same metatarsal: A review of two cases. *J Foot Surg* 28:308-311, 1989.
2. Anderson R, McBryde A: Autogenous bone grafting of hallux sesamoid nonunions. *Foot Ankle Int* 18:293-296, 1997.
3. Aper R, Saltzman C, Brown T: The effect of hallux sesamoid resection on the effective moment of the flexor hallucis brevis. *Foot Ankle Int* 15:462-470, 1994.
4. Aper R, Saltzman C, Brown T: The effect of hallux sesamoid excision on the flexor hallucis longus moment arm. *Clin Orthop Relat Res* 325:209-217, 1996.
5. Apley AG: Open sesamoid: A reappraisal of the medial sesamoid of the hallux. *Proc R Soc Med* 59:120, 1966.
6. Aquino M, DeVincentis A, Keating S: Tibial sesamoid planing procedure: An appraisal of 26 feet. *J Foot Surg* 23:226-230, 1984.
7. Biedert R, Hintermann B. Stress fractures of the medial sesamoids in athletes. *Foot Ankle Int* 24:137-141, 2003.
8. Bizarro AH: On the traumatology of the sesamoid structures. *Ann Surg* 74:783-791, 1921.
9. Brodsky J: Sesamoid excision for chronic nonunion. 21st Annual Meeting of the American Orthopaedic Foot and Ankle Society, Anaheim, Calif, March 10, 1991.
10. Brodsky J, Krause J, Robinson A, Watkins D: Hallux sesamoidectomy for painful chronic fracture: Histological and radiographic characteristics and clinical outcome. 29th Annual Meeting of the American Orthopaedic Foot and Ankle Society, Anaheim, Calif, February 7, 1999.
11. Brown TIS: Avulsion fracture of the fibular sesamoid in association with dorsal dislocation of the metatarsophalangeal joint of hallux. *Clin Orthop Relat Res* 149:229-231, 1980.
12. Burman MS, Lapidus PW: The functional disturbances caused by the inconstant bones and sesamoids of the foot. *Arch Surg* 22:960-964, 1931.
13. Cartlidge IJ, Gillespie WJ: Haematogenous osteomyelitis of the metatarsal sesamoid. *Br J Surg* 66:214-216, 1979.
14. Colwill M: Osteomyelitis of the metatarsal sesamoids. *J Bone Joint Surg Br* 51:464-468, 1969.
15. Coughlin MJ: Sesamoid pain: Causes and treatment. *Instr Course Lect* 39:23-35, 1990.
16. Coughlin MJ, Mann RA: Arthrodesis of the first metatarsophalangeal joint as a salvage for the failed Keller procedure. *J Bone Joint Surg Am* 69:68-75, 1987.
17. Delfaut E, Demondion X, Bieganski A, et al: The fibrocartilaginous sesamoid: A cause of size and signal variation in the normal distal posterior tibial tendon. *Eur Radiol* 13:2642-2649, 2003.

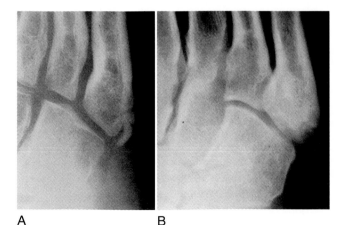

Figure 10–117 A, Iselin's disease. **B,** Following passage of time and consolidation of apophysis. (Courtesy of S. Terry Canale, MD, Memphis, Tenn.)

*References 113, 169, 187, 211, 230, and 240.

18. DeLuca FN, Kenmore PI: Bilateral dorsal dislocation of the metatarsophalangeal joints of the great toes. *J Trauma* 15:737-739, 1975.

19. Dobas DC, Silvers MD: The frequency of the partite sesamoids of the first metatarsophalangeal joint. *J Am Podiatr Assoc* 67:880-882, 1977.

20. DuVries HL: *Surgery of the Foot,* ed 2. St Louis, Mosby, 1965, pp 259-278.

21. Enna CD: Observations on the hallucal sesamoid in trauma to the denervated foot. *Int Surg* 53:97-107, 1970.

22. Esemenli T, Yildirim Y, Bezer M: Lateral shifting of the first metatarsal head in hallux valgus surgery: Effect on sesamoid reduction. *Foot Ankle Int* 24:922-926, 2003.

23. Ferris D, Thomas J, Owens J: Extirpation of the fibular sesamoid simplified. *J Foot Surg* 24:255-257, 1985.

24. Fleischli J, Cheleuitte E: Avascular necrosis of the hallucal sesamoids. *J Foot Ankle Surg* 34:358-365, 1995.

25. Frankel J, Harrington J: Symptomatic bipartite sesamoids. *J Foot Surg* 29:318-323, 1990.

26. Giannestras NJ: *Foot Disorders: Medical and Surgical Management.* Philadelphia, Lea & Febiger, 1973, p 426.

27. Giannikas A, Papachristou G, Papavasiliou N, et al: Dorsal dislocation of the first metatarsophalangeal joint. *J Bone Joint Surg Br* 57:384-386, 1975.

28. Giurini J, Chrzan J, Gibbons G, et al: Sesamoidectomy for the treatment of chronic neuropathic ulcerations. *J Am Podiatr Med Assoc* 81:167-173, 1991.

29. Goez J, DeLauro T: Congenital absence of the tibial sesamoid. *J Am Podiatr Med Assoc* 85:509-510, 1995.

30. Golding C: The sesamoid of the hallux. *J Bone Joint Surg Br* 42:840-843, 1960.

31. Gordon SL, Evans C, Greer RB: *Pseudomonas* osteomyelitis of the metatarsal sesamoid of the great toe. *Clin Orthop Relat Res* 99:188-189, 1974.

32. Helal B: The great toe sesamoid bone: The lus or lost souls of Ushaia. *Clin Orthop Relat Res* 157:82-87, 1981.

33. Helfet A: Pain under the head of the metatarsal bone of the big toe. *Lancet* 267:846, 1954.

34. Hobart MH: Fracture of sesamoid bones of the foot. *J Bone Joint Surg* 11:298-302, 1929.

35. Hubay CA: Sesamoid bones of the hands and feet. *Am J Roentgenol* 61:493-505, 1949.

36. Ilfeld FW, Rosen V: Osteochondritis of the first metatarsal sesamoid. *Clin Orthop Relat Res* 85:38-41, 1972.

37. Inge GAL, Ferguson AB: Surgery of the sesamoid bones of the great toe. *Arch Surg* 27:466-488, 1933.

38. Jahss M: Traumatic dislocations of the first metatarsophalangeal joint. *Foot Ankle* 1:15-20, 1980.

39. Jahss ML: The sesamoids of the hallux. *Clin Orthop Relat Res* 157:88-97, 1981.

40. Jahss MS (ed): *Disorders of the Foot and Ankle: Medical and Surgical Management,* ed 2. Philadelphia, WB Saunders, 1991, pp 1062-1075.

41. Jeng C, Maurer A, Mizel M: Congenital absence of the hallux fibular sesamoid: A case report and review of the literature. *Foot Ankle Int* 19:329-331, 1999.

42. Julsrud M: Osteonecrosis of the tibial and fibular sesamoids in an aerobics instructor. *J Foot Ankle Surg* 36:31-35, 1997.

43. Kaiman ME, Piccora R: Tibial sesamoidectomy: A review of the literature and retrospective study. *J Foot Surg* 22:286-289, 1983.

44. Kernohan J, Dakin P, Helal B: Dolorous calcification of the lateral sesamoid bursa of the great toe. *Foot Ankle* 5:45-46, 1984.

45. Kewenter Y: Die Sesambeine des 1. Metatarsophalangealgelenks des Menschen. *Acta Orthop Scand Suppl* 2:1-113, 1936.

46. Kliman ME, Gross AE, Pritzker KP, et al: Osteochondritis of the hallux sesamoid bone. *Foot Ankle* 3:220-223, 1983.

47. Konkel KF, Muehlstein JH: Unusual fracture-dislocation of the great toe. *J Trauma* 15:733-736, 1975.

48. Lapidus P: Congenital unilateral absence of medial sesamoid of the great toe. *J Bone Joint Surg Am* 21:208-209, 1939.

49. Lavery L, Haase K, Krych S: Hallux hammertoe secondary to pseudomonas osteomyelitis. *J Am Podiatr Med Assoc* 81:608-612, 1991.

50. Lemont H, Khoury M: Subchondral bone cysts of the sesamoids. *J Am Podiatr Med Assoc* 75:218-219, 1985.

51. Leonard MH: The sesamoids of the great toe—The pedal polemic. *Clin Orthop Relat Res* 16:295-301, 1960.

52. Mann RA, Coughlin MJ: Hallux valgus—Etiology, anatomy, treatment, and surgical considerations. *Clin Orthop Relat Res* 151:31-41, 1981.

53. Mann RA, Coughlin MJ, Baxter D, et al: Sesamoidectomy of the great toe. 15th Annual Meeting of the American Orthopaedic Foot and Ankle Society, Las Vegas, January 24, 1985.

54. Mann RA, Wapner K: Tibial sesamoid shaving for treatment of intractable plantar keratosis. *Foot Ankle* 13:196-198, 1992.

55. McBride E: Hallux valgus bunion deformity. *J Bone Joint Surg* 9:334-346, 1952.

56. McCarthy D, Reed T, Abell N: The hallucal interphalangeal sesamoid. *J Am Podiatr Med Assoc* 76:311-319, 1986.

57. Miller W, Love B: Cartilaginous sesamoid or nodule of the interphalangeal joint of the big toe. *Foot Ankle* 2:291-293, 1982.

58. Mowad S, Zichichi S, Mullin R: Osteochondroma of the tibial sesamoid. *J Am Podiatr Med Assoc* 85:765-766, 1995.

59. Nayfa TM, Sorto LA: The incidence of hallux abductus following tibial sesamoidectomy. *J Am Podiatr Assoc* 72:617-620, 1982.

60. Orr TG: Fracture of great toe sesamoid bones. *Ann Surg* 67:609-612, 1918.

61. Parra E: Stress fractures of the sesamoid. *Clin Orthop Relat Res* 18:281-285, 1960.

62. Pretterklieber M, Wanivenhaus A: The arterial supply of the sesamoid bones of the hallux: The course and source of the nutrient arteries as an anatomical basis for surgical approaches to the great toe. *Foot Ankle* 13:27-31, 1992.

63. Renander A: Two cases of typical osteochondropathy of the medial sesamoid bone of the first metatarsal. *Acta Radiol* 3:521-527, 1924.

64. Resnick D, Niwayama G, Feingold ML: The sesamoid bones of the hand and feet: Participators in arthritis. *Diagn Radiol* 123:57-62, 1977.

65. Richardson EG: Injuries to the hallucal sesamoids in the athlete. *Foot Ankle* 7:229-244, 1987.

66. Rodeo S, Warren R, O'Brien S, et al: Diastasis of bipartite sesamoids of the first metatarsophalangeal joint. *Foot Ankle* 14:425-434, 1993.

67. Rosenfield J, Trepman E: Technique tip: Treatment of sesamoid disorders with a rocker shoe modification. *Foot Ankle Int* 21:914-915, 2000.

68. Rowe MM: Osteomyelitis of metatarsal sesamoid. *BMJ* 2:1071-1072, 1963.

69. Salamon PB, Gelberman RH, Huffer JM: Dorsal dislocation of the metatarsophalangeal joint of the great toe. *J Bone Joint Surg Am* 56:1073-1075, 1974.

70. Salvi V, Tos L: L'osteochondrosi die sesamoidi. *Arch Ortop* 75:1294-1304, 1962.

71. Sarrafian SK: Osteology. In *Anatomy of the Foot and Ankle,* Philadelphia, JB Lippincott, 1983, pp 83-87.

72. Saxby T, Vandermark R, Hall R: Coalition of the hallux sesamoids: A case report. *Foot Ankle* 13:355-358, 1992.

73. Saxena A, Krisdakumtorn T. Return to activity after sesamoidectomy in athletically active individuals. *Foot Ankle Int* 24:415-419, 2003.

74. Scranton PE: Pathologic anatomic variations in the sesamoids. *Foot Ankle* 1:321-326, 1981.

75. Scranton PE, Rutkowski R: Anatomic variations in the first ray. *Clin Orthop Relat Res* 151:256-264, 1980.

76. Smith R: Osteitis of the metatarsal sesamoid. *Br J Surg* 29:19-22, 1941.

77. Sobel M, Hashimoto J, Arnoczky S, et al: The microvasculature of the sesamoid complex: Its clinical significance. *Foot Ankle* 13:359-363, 1992.

78. Speed K: Injuries of the great toe sesamoids. *Ann Surg* 60:478-480, 1913.

79. Torgerson WR, Hammond G: Osteomyelitis of the sesamoid bones of the first metatarsophalangeal joint. *J Bone Joint Surg Am* 51:1420-1421, 1969.

80. Van Hal ME, Keene JS, Lange TA, et al: Stress fractures of the great toe sesamoids. *Am J Sports Med* 10:122-128, 1982.

81. Ward W, Bergfeld J: Fluoroscopic demonstration of acute disruption of the fifth metatarsophalangeal sesamoid bones. *Am J Sports Med* 21:895-897, 1993.

82. Weil L, Hill M: Bipartite tibial sesamoid and hallux abducto valgus deformity: A previously unreported correlation. *J Foot Surg* 31:104-111, 1992.

83. Yu G, Nagle C: Hallux interphalangeal joint sesamoidectomy. *J Am Podiatr Med Assoc* 86:105-111, 1996.

84. Zinman H, Keret D, Reis ND: Fractures of the medial sesamoid bone of the hallux. *J Trauma* 21:581-582, 1981.

85. Zinsmeister B, Edelman R: Congenital absence of the tibial sesamoid: A report of two cases. *J Foot Surg* 24:266-268, 1985.

Accessory Bones of the Foot and Uncommon Sesamoids

86. Albrecht P: Das os intermedium tarsi der Saugetiere. *Zoolog Anz* 139:419-420, 1883.

87. Anatomical Society Collective Investigation: Sesamoids in the gastrocnemius and peroneus longus. *J Anat Physiol* 32:182, 1897.

88. Anderson T: Calcaneus secundarius: An osteo-archaeological note. *Am J Phys Anthropol* 77:529-531, 1988.

89. Anspach W, Wright EB: The divided navicular of the foot. *Radiology* 29:725-728, 1937.

90. Arho AO: Raajojen ylilukuiset luut rontgenkuvissa. *Duodecim* 56:399-410, 1940.

91. Azurza K, Sekellariou A: Osteosynthesis of a symptomatic bipartite medial cuneiform. *Foot Ankle Int* 22:499-501, 2001.

92. Baastrup CI: Os vesalianum tarsi and fracture of tuberositas ossis metatarsi. *Acta Radiol* 1:334-350, 1921.

93. Barclay M: A case of duplication of the internal cuneiform bone of the foot (cuneiforme bipartitum). *J Anat* 67:175-178, 1932.

94. Bareither D, Muehlman C, Feldman N: Os tibiale externum or sesamoid in the tendon of tibialis posterior. *J Foot Surg* 34:429-434, 1995.

95. Barlow TE: Os cuneiforme I bipartitum. *Am J Phys Anthropol* 29:95-111, 1942.

96. Bennett EH: On the ossicle occasionally found on the posterior border of the astragalus. *J Anat Physiol* 21:59-65, 1887.

97. Bentzon PGK: Bilateral congenital deformity of the astragalo-calcanean joint: Bony coalescence between os trigonum and the calcaneus. Communication from the Orthopaedic Clinic, Copenhagen, to the Northern Orthopaedic Association, 1930, pp 359-364.

98. Berenter J, Goldman F: Surgical approach for enlarged peroneal tubercles. *J Am Podiatr Med Assoc* 79:451-454, 1989.

99. Bessette B, Hodge J: Diagnosis of the acute os peroneum fracture. *Singapore Med J* 39:326-327, 1998.

100. Bierman MI: The supernumerary pedal bones. *Am J Roentgenol* 9:404-411, 1922.

101. Bizarro AH: On sesamoid and supernumerary bones of the limbs. *J Anat* 55:256-268, 1921.

102. Bjornson R: Developmental anomaly of the lateral malleolus simulating fracture. *J Bone Joint Surg Br* 38:128-130, 1956.

103. Blake R, Lallas P, Ferguson H: The os trigonum syndrome: A literature review. *J Am Podiatr Med Assoc* 82:154-161, 1992.

104. Bloom RA, Libson E, Lax E, et al: The assimilated os sustentaculi. *Skeletal Radiol* 15:455-457, 1986.

105. Bocker W: Zur Kenntnis der Varietaten des menschlichen Fußskeletts. *Berl Klin Wochenschr* 45:499-502, 1908.

106. Boker H, Muller W: Das Os cuneiform I bipartitum, eine fortschreitende Umkonstruktion des Quergewölbes im menschlichen Fuß. *Anat Anz* 83:193-204, 1936.

107. Bowlus T, Korman S, Desilvio M, et al: Accessory os fibulare avulsion secondary to the inversion ankle injury. *J Am Podiatr Assoc* 70:302-303, 1980.

108. Burman MS, Lapidus PW: The functional disturbances caused by the inconstant bones and sesamoids of the foot. *Arch Surg* 22:936-975, 1931.

109. Burman MS, Sinberg SE: An anomalous talo-calcaneal articulation: Double ankle bones. *Radiology* 34:239-241, 1940.

110. Burton S, Altman M: Degenerative arthritis of the os peroneum: A case report. *J Am Podiatr Med Assoc* 76:343-345, 1986.

111. Caffey J: *Pediatric X-ray Diagnosis*, ed 8. St Louis, Mosby, 1985, p 469.

112. Callanan I, Williams L, Stephens M: Os post pernei and the posterolateral nutcracker impingement. *Foot Ankle Int* 19:475-478, 1998.

113. Canale S, Williams K: Iselin's disease. *J Pediatr Orthop* 12:90-93, 1992.

114. Case D, Ossenberg N: Os intermetatarsum: A heritable accessory bone of the human foot. *Am J Phys Anthropol* 107:199-209, 1998.

115. Champagne I, Cook D, Kestner S, et al: Os subfibulare. Investigation of an accessory bone. *J Am Podiatr Medical Assoc* 89:520-524, 1999.

116. Chater EH: Foot pain and the accessory navicular bone. *Ir J Med Sci* 442-471, 1962.

117. Chiodo C, Parentis M, Myerson M: Symptomatic bipartite medial cuneiform in an adult athlete: A case report. *Foot Ankle Int* 23:348-351, 2002.

118. Clausen A: Os naviculare bipartitum pedis. *Nord Med* 23:1802-1804, 1944.

119. Coral A: Os subtibial mistaken for a recent fracture. *BMJ* 292:1571-1572, 1986.

120. Coral A: The radiology of skeletal elements in the subtibial region: Incidence and significance. *Skeletal Radiol* 16:298-303, 1987.

121. Cravener EK, MacElroy DG: Supernumerary tarsal scaphoides. *Surg Gynecol Obstet* 71:218-221, 1940.

122. Dameron TB Jr: Fractures and anatomical variations of the proximal portion of the fifth metatarsal. *J Bone Joint Surg Am* 57:788-794, 1975.

123. Day F, Naples J, White J: Metatarsocuneiform coalition. *J Am Podiatr Med Assoc* 84:197-199, 1994.

124. de Cuveland E: Über Beziehungen zwischen vorderer Aussenknochelapophyse und Os subfibulare mit differentialdiagnostischen Erwagungen. *Fortschr Rontgenstr* 83:213-221, 1955.

125. Dellacorte M, Lin P, Grisafi P: Bilateral bipartite medial cuneiform: A case report. *J Am Podiatr Med Assoc* 82:475-478, 1992.

126. Dwight T: Description of a free cuboides secundarium, with remarks on that element and on the calcaneus secundarius. *Anat Anz* 37:218-224, 1910.

127. Dwight T: Os intercuneiforme tarsi, os paracuneiforme tarsi, calcaneus secundarius. *Anat Anz* 20:465-472, 1902.

128. Dwight T: *Variations of the Bones of the Hands and Feet: A Clinical Atlas.* Philadelphia, JB Lippincott, 1907, pp 14-23.

129. Fischer H: Beitrag zur Kenntnis der Skelettvarietaten (uberzahlige Karpalia und Tarsalia, Sesambeine, Kompaktainseln). *Fortschr Nyklearmed Gebiete Rontgenstr* 19:43-66, 1912.

130. Francillon MR: Beitrag zur Klinik und Röntgenologie inkonstanter Skelettelemente des Fusses. *Dtsch Med Wochenschr* 60:1097-1100, 1934.

131. Francillon MR: Untersuchungen zur anatomischen und klinischen Bedeutung des Os tibiale externum. *Z Orthop Chir* 56:61-85, 1932.

132. Friedl E: Das Os intermetatarseum und die Epiphysenbildung am Processus Trochlearis Calcanei. *Dtsch Z Chir* 188:150-160, 1924.

133. Friedl E: Divided cuneiform I in childhood. *Rontgenpraxis* 6:193-195, 1934.

134. Fujishiro T, Nabeshima Y, Yasue S, et al: Coalition of bilateral first cuneometatarsal joints: A case report. *Foot Ankle Int* 24:793-797, 2003.

135. Gaulke R, Schmitz H: Free os cuboideum secundarium: A case report. *J Foot Ankle Surg* 42:230-234, 2003.

136. Geist ES: Supernumerary bones of the foot—A roentgen study of the feet of one hundred normal individuals. *Am J Orthop Surg* 12:403-414, 1914.

137. Geist ES: The accessory scaphoid bone. *J Bone Joint Surg* 7:570-574, 1925.

138. Giannestras NJ: *Foot Disorders: Medial and Surgical Management.* Philadelphia, Lea & Febiger, 1973, pp 233-234, 583-588.

139. Giuffrida A, Lin S, Abidi N, et al: Pseudo os trigonum sign: Missed posteromedial talar facet fracture. *Foot Ankle Int* 24:642-649, 2003.

140. Goedhard G: The apophyses of the lateral malleolus. *Radiol Clin Biol* 39:330-333, 1970.

141. Grasmann M: Zur Kenntnis des Os subtibiale. *Munch Med Wochenschr* 79:824-825, 1932.

142. Griffiths J, Menelaus M: Symptomatic ossicles of the lateral malleolus in children. *J Bone Joint Surg Br* 69:317-319, 1987.

143. Grisolia A: Fracture of the os peroneum: Review of literature and report of one case. *Clin Orthop Relat Res* 28:213-215, 1963.

144. Grogan D, Gasser S, Ogden J: The painful accessory navicular: A clinical and histopathological study. *Foot Ankle* 10:164-169, 1989.

145. Gruber W: Auftreten der Tuberositas des Os metatarsale V sowohl als persistirende Epiphyse, als auch mit einer an ihrem ausseren Umfange aufsitzenden persistirenden Epiphyse. *Arch Pathol Anat Physiol Klin Med* 99:460-471, 1885.

146. Gruber W: Über den Fortsatz des Seitenhockers—Processus tuberositatis lateralis—des Metatarsale V und sein Auftreten als Epiphyse. *Arch Anat Physiol Wissenschaft Med* 48-58, 1875.

147. Gruber W: Über einem am Malleolus externus articulirenden Knochen. *Arch Pathol Anat Physiol Klin Med* 27:205-206, 1863.

148. Guntz E: Os tibiale and Unfall (Abriss des Os tibiale). *Arch Orthop Ungall Chir* 34:320-326, 1934.

149. Haglund P: Ueber Fraktur des Tuberculum ossis navicularis in den Jugendjahren und ihre Bedeutung als Ursache einer typischen Form von Pes valgus. *Z Orthop Chir* 16:347-353, 1906.

150. Harris RI, Beath T: Army Foot Survey, vol 1. Ottawa, National Research Council of Canada, 1947, p 52.

151. Harris RI, Beath T: Etiology of peroneal spastic flat foot. *J Bone Joint Surg Br* 30:624-634, 1948.

152. Hasselwander A: Über die Entwickelung des Processus posterior tali und des Os trigonum tarsi. *Z Morphol Anthropol* 18:553-578, 1914.

153. Hatoff A: Bipartite navicular bone as a cause of flatfoot. *Am J Dis Child* 80:991-992, 1950.

154. Hedrick M, McBryde A: Posterior ankle impingement. *Foot Ankle* 15:2-8, 1994.

155. Heidsieck E: Os cuneiforme I bipartitum. *Rontgenpraxis* 8:712-715, 1936.

156. Heimerzheim A: Über einen seltsamen Knochenbefund am Calcaneus. *Dtsch Z Chir* 187:281-283, 1924.

157. Heimerzheim A: Über einige akzessorische Fusswurzelknochen nebst ihrer chirurgischen Bedeutung. *Dtsch Z Chir* 190:96-112, 1925.

158. Henderson MS: Fractures of the bones of the foot—except the os calcis. *Surg Gynecol Obstet* 64:454-457, 1937.

159. Henderson RS: Os intermetatarseum and a possible relationship to hallux valgus. *J Bone Joint Surg Br* 45:117-121, 1963.

160. Hermann N: An unusual example of a calcaneus secundarius. *J Am Podiatr Med Assoc* 82:623-624, 1992.

161. Hirschtick AB: An anomalous tarsal bone. *J Bone Joint Surg Am* 33:907-910, 1951.

162. Hoerr NL, Pyle DI, Francis CC: *Radiographic Atlas of Skeletal Development of the Foot and Ankle: A Standard of Reference.* Springfield, Ill, Charles C Thomas, 1962, pp 41-44.

163. Hogan J: Fractures of the os peroneum: Case report and literature review. *J Am Podiatr Med Assoc* 79:201-204, 1989.

164. Hohmann G: Über Frakturen und andere traumatische Storungen am Os naviculare des Fusses. *Arch Orthop Unfall Chir* 43:12-19, 1944.

165. Holland CT: On rarer ossifications seen during x-ray examinations. *J Anat* 55:235-248, 1920.

166. Holland CT: The accessory bones of the foot. In *The Robert Jones Birthday Volume.* London, Oxford University Press, 1928, pp 157-182.

167. Holle F: Über die inkonstanten Elemente am menschlichen Fussskelett (Inaugural-Dissertation). Munich, 1938.

168. Horinouchi T, Kinoshita M, Okuda R, et al. Coalition between the medial cuneiform and the first metatarsal. A case report. *J Jpn Soc Surg Foot* 20:93-96, 1999.

169. Iselin H: Wachstumsbeschwerden zur Zeit der Knochernen entwicklung der Tuberositas metatarsi quinti. *Deutsche Z Fur Chirurgie* 117:529-535, 1912.

170. Johansson S: Os vesalianum pedis. *Z Orthop Chir* 42:301-307, 1922.

171. Jones FW: *Structure and Function as Seen in the Foot,* ed 2. London, Bailliere, Tindall, & Cox, 1949, pp 83-100.

172. Karasick D, Schweitzer M: The os trigonum syndrome: Imaging features. *AJR Am J Roentgenol* 166:125-129, 1996.

173. Kassianenko W: Calcaneus secundarius, talus accessorius und os trigonum tarsi beim Pferde. *Anat Anzeiger* 80:1-10, 1935.

174. Keats T: *An Atlas of Normal Roentgen Variants That May Simulate Disease,* ed 3. St Louis, Mosby, 1984.

175. Kewenter Y: Die sesambeine des I. metatarsophalangealgelenks des menschen. *Acta Orthop Scand* Suppl 2:1-113, 1936.

176. Kidner FC: The prehallux (accessory scaphoid) in its relation to flat foot. *J Bone Joint Surg* 11:831-837, 1929.

177. Kohler A, Zimmer E: *Borderlands of the Normal and Early Pathologic in Skeletal Roentgenology,* ed 3. New York, Grune & Stratton, 1968, pp 245, 460, 464-468, 489, 502-527.

178. Kohler A, Zimmer E: *Grenzes des Normalen and Anfange des Pathologischen im Rontgenbilde des Skelettes,* ed 9. Stuttgart, Georg Thieme, 1953.

179. Kricun M: *Imaging of the Foot and Ankle.* Rockville, Md, Aspen, 1988, p 113.

180. Krida A: Secondary os calcis. *JAMA* 80:752-753, 1923.

181. Kumai T, Tanaka Y, Takakura Y, et al: Isolated first naviculo-cuneiform joint coalition. *Foot Ankle Int* 17:635-640, 1996.

182. Laidlaw PP: The os calcis. Part II. *Anat Physiol* 39:161-176, 1905.

183. Laidlaw PP: The varieties of the os calcis. *J Anat* 38:133-143, 39:161-177, 1904.

184. Lapidus PW: Os subtibale: Inconstant bone over the tip of the medial malleolus. *J Bone Joint Surg* 15:766-771, 1933.

185. Laquerriere D: On the vesalian bone. *J Radiol Electrother* 21:395-400, 1916.

186. Latten W: Histologische Beziehungen zwischen Os tibiale und Kahnbein nach Untersuchungen an einem operierten Falle. *Dtsch Z Chir* 205:320-327, 1927.

187. Lehman R, Gregg J, Torg E: Iselin's disease. *Am J Sports Med* 14:494-496, 1986.

188. Leimbach G: Beitrage zur Kenntnis der Inkonstanten Skeletele-mente des Tarsus, (Akzessorische Fusswurzelknochen). *Arch Orthop Trauma Surg* 38:431-448, 1938.

189. Leonard MH, Gonzalez S, Breck LW, et al: Lateral transfer of the posterior tibial tendon in certain selected cases of pes plano valgus (Kidner operation). *Clin Orthop Relat Res* 40:139-144, 1965.

190. Lepore L, Francobandiera C, Maffulli N: Fracture of the os tibiale externum in a decathlete. *J Foot Surg* 29:366-368, 1990.

191. Lichte E: On bipartite os naviculare pedis. *Acta Radiol* 22:377-382, 1941.

192. Lilienfeld A: Über die sogenannten Tarsalia, die inkonstanten accessorischen Skelettstucke des Fusses und ihre Beziehungen zu den Frakturen, im Rontgenbild. *Z Orthop Grenz Chir* 18:213-238, 1907.

193. Logan M, Connell D, Janzen D: Painful os cuboideum secundarium: Cross-sectional imaging findings. *J Am Podiatr Med Assoc* 86:123-125, 1996.

194. Maffulli N, Lepore L, Francobandiera C: Traumatic lesions of some accessory bones of the foot in sports activity. *J Am Podiatr Med Assoc* 80:86-90, 1990.

195. Mains D, Sullivan R: Fracture of the os peroneum. *J Bone Joint Surg Am* 55:1529-1530, 1973.

196. Mancuso J, Hutchison P, Abramow S, et al: Accessory ossicle of the lateral malleolus. *J Foot Surg* 30:52-55, 1991.

197. Mann RW: Calcaneus secundarius: Description and frequency in six skeletal samples. *Am J Phys Anthropol* 81:17-25, 1990.

198. Mann RW: Calcaneus secundarius: Variation of a common accessory ossicle. *J Am Podiatr Med Assoc* 79:363-366, 1989.

199. Mann RA, Owsley D: Os trigonum: Variation of a common accessory ossicle of the talus. *J Am Podiatr Med Assoc* 80:536-539, 1990.

200. Manners-Smith T: A study of the cuboid and os peroneum in the primate foot. *J Anat Physiol* 42:397-414, 1908.

201. Manners-Smith T: A study of the navicular in the human and anthropod foot. *J Anat Physiol* 41:255-279, 1907.

202. March HC, London RI: The os sustentaculi. *Am J Roentgenol* 76:1114-1118, 1956.

203. Marotta J, Micheli L: Os trigonum impingement in dancers. *Am J Sports Med* 20:533-536, 1992.

204. Marti T: Die Skeletvarietaten des Fusses. Ihre klinische und unfallmedizinische Bedeutung. In Debrunner H, Francillon MR (eds): *Praktische Beitrage zur Orthopädie,* vol 2. Bern, H Huber, 1947, pp 27-118.

205. Martin B: Posterior triangle pain: The os trigonum. *J Foot Surg* 28:312-318, 1989.

206. Mau H: Zur Kenntnis des Naviculare bipartitum pedis. *Z Orthop* 93:404-411, 1960.

207. McDougall A: The os trigonum. *J Bone Joint Surg* 37:257-265, 1955.

208. McKusick V: Mendelian inheritance in man: Catalogs of Autosomal Dominant, Autosomal Recessive, and X-Linked Phenotypes, ed 2. Baltimore, Johns Hopkins University Press, 1978, p 147.

209. Mellado J, Salvado E, Camins A, et al: Painful os sustentaculi: Imaging finding of another symptomatic skeletal variant. *Skeletal Radiol* 31:53-56, 2002.

210. Mercer J: The secondary os calcis. *J Anat* 66:84-97, 1931.

211. Micheli L: The traction apophysitis. *Clin Sports Med* 6:389, 1987.

212. Michelson G: Zur Frage der sogenannten Stiedaschen Fraktur. *Rontgenpraxis* 2:896-898, 1930.

213. Miller G, Black J: Symptomatic os supra naviculare: A case report. *J Am Podiatr Med Assoc* 80:248-250, 1990.

214. Monahan JJ: The human pre-hallux. *Am J Med Sci* 160:708-720, 1920.

215. Mouchet A, Moutier G: Osselets surnumeraires du tarse. *Presse Med* 23:369-374, 1925.

216. Noguchi M, Iwata Y, Miura K, Kusaka Y: A painful os inter-metatarseum in a soccer player: A case report. *Foot Ankle Int* 21:1040-1041, 2000.

217. Okazaki K, Nakashima S, Nomura S: Stress fracture of an os peroneum. *J Orthop Trauma* 17:654-656, 2003.

218. O'Neal M, Ganey T, Ogden J: Fracture of a bipartite medial cuneiform synchondrosis. *Foot Ankle Int* 16:37-40, 1995.

219. O'Rahilly R: A survey of carpal and tarsal anomalies. *J Bone Joint Surg Am* 35:626-642, 1953.

220. Paal E: Fehlbeurteilungen bei Rontgenbildern. *Arch Orthop Unfall Chir* 33:153-158, 1933.

221. Peacock K, Resnick E, Thoder J: Fracture of the os peroneum with rupture of the peroneus longus tendon. *Clin Orthop Relat Res* 202:223-224, 1986.

222. Peh W, Gilula L: A 37-year-old man with left foot pain: Symptomatic accessory navicular synchondrosis. *Ortho Rev* 23:958-961, 1994.

223. Perlman M: Os peroneum fracture with sural nerve entrapment neuritis. *J Foot Surg* 29:119-121, 1990.

224. Pfitzner W: Beitrage zur Kenntmiss des Menschlichen Extremitatenskelets: VII. Die Variationen in Aufbau des Fusskelets. In Schwalbe G (ed): *Morphologische Arbeiten.* Jena, Gustav Fischer, 1896, pp 245-527.

225. Pierson J, Inglis A: Stenosing tenosynovitis of the peroneus longus tendon associated with hypertrophy of the peroneal tubercle and an os peroneum. *J Bone Joint Surg Am* 74:440-442, 1992.

226. Pirie AH: A normal ossicle in the foot frequently diagnosed as a fracture. *Arch Radiol Electrother* 24:93-95, 1919.

227. Pirie AH: Extra bones in the wrist and ankle found by roentgen rays. *AJR Am J Roentgenol* 569-573, 1921.

228. Powell HDW: Extra centre of ossification for the medial malleolus in children. *J Bone Joint Surg Br* 43:107-113, 1961.

229. Puhl H, Lindemann K: Über die Entstehung freier Körper im Talocruralgelenk. *Arch Orthop Unfall Chir* 38:726-739, 1938.

230. Ralph B, Barrett J, Kenyhercz C, DiDomenico LA: Iselin's disease: A case presentation of nonunion and review of the differential diagnosis. *J Foot Surg* 38:409-416, 1999.

231. Ray S, Goldberg V: Surgical treatment of the accessory navicular. *Clin Orthop Relat Res* 177:61-66, 1983.

232. Reichmister JP: The painful os intermetatarseum: A brief review and case reports. *Clin Orthop Relat Res* 153:201-203, 1980.

233. Rosenmuller J: *De mon nullis musculorum corpus humani varietatibus.* Leipzig, 1804.

234. Ruiz J, Christman R, Hillstrom H: Anatomical considerations of the peroneal tubercle. *J Am Podiatr Med Assoc* 83:563-575, 1993.

235. Sandor L: Zur traumatischen Genese des Os subtibiale. *Beitr Orthop Traumatol* 24:558-563, 1977.

236. Sarrafian SK: Osteology. In Sarrafian SK: *Anatomy of the Foot and Ankle.* Philadelphia, JB Lippincott, 1983, pp 35-106.

237. Saupe E: Malazieartige Veranderungen am schmerzhaften os tibiale externum. *Rontgenpraxis* 11:533-536, 1939.

238. Scarlet JJ, Gunther R, Katz J, Schwartz H: Os intermetatarseum-one: Case report and discussion. *J Am Podiatr Assoc* 68:431-434, 1978.

239. Schoen W: Seltenere akzessorische Knochen am Fussrucken. *Rontgenpraxis* 7:775-776, 1935.

240. Schreiber A, Differding P, Zollinger H: Talus partitus. *J Bone Joint Surg Br* 67:430-431, 1985.

241. Schwartz B, Jay R, Schoenhaus H: Apophysitis of the fifth metatarsal base: Iselin's disease. *J Am Podiatr Med Assoc* 81:128-130, 1991.

242. Seddon HJ: Calcaneo-scaphoid coalition. *Proc R Soc Med* 26:419-424, 1932.

243. Selby S: Separate centers of ossification of the tip of the internal malleolus. *AJR Am J Roentgenol* 86:496-501, 1961.

244. Sella E, Lawson J: Biomechanics of the accessory navicular synchondrosis. *Foot Ankle* 8:156-163, 1987.

245. Shands A: Accessory bones of the foot. *South Med Surg* 93:326, 1931.

246. Shands A, Wentz I: Congenital anomalies, accessory bones, and osteochondritis in the feet of 850 children. *Surg Clin North Am* 33:1643, 1953.

247. Shawdon A, Kiss Z, Fuller P: The bipartite tarsal navicular bone: Radiographic and computed tomography findings. *Australa Radiol* 39:192-194, 1995.

248. Shepherd FJ: A hitherto undescribed fracture of the astragalus. *J Anat Physiol* 17:79-81, 1883.

249. Shepherd FJ: Note on the ossicle found on the posterior border of the astragalus. *J Anat Physiol* 21:335, 1887.

250. Smith AD, Carter JR, Marus RE: The os vesalianum: An unusual cause of lateral foot pain. *Orthopedics* 7:86-89, 1984.

251. Smith T: A foot having four cuneiform bones. *Trans Pathol Soc* 17:222-223, 1865.

252. Sobel M, Pavlov H, Geppert M, et al: Painful os peroneum syndrome: A spectrum of conditions responsible for plantar lateral foot pain. *Foot Ankle* 15:112-124, 1994.

253. Spronck CH: Auftreten der ganzen Tuberositas (lateralis) des Os metatarsale V als ein für sich bestechendes, am Metatarsale und Cuboides artikulierendes Skelett-Element. *Anat Anz* 2:734-739, 1887.

254. Stieda L: Der M. peroneus longus und die Fussknochen. *Anat Anz* 4:600-607, 624-640, 1889.

255. Grant JCB (ed): *Grant's Atlas of Anatomy,* ed 5. Baltimore, Williams & Wilkins, 1972, p 356.

256. Sutton JB: A case of secondary astragalus. *J Anat Physiol* 21:333-334, 1887.

257. Swenson PC, Wilner D: Unfused ossification centers associated with pain in the adult. *AJR Am J Roentgenol* 61:341-353, 1949.

258. Takakura Y, Nakata H: Isolated first cuneometatarsal coalition: A case report. *Foot Ankle Int* 20:815-816, 1999.

259. Tanaka Y, Takakura Y, Sugimoto K, Kumai T: Non-osseous coalition of the medial cuneiform–first metatarsal joint: A case report. *Foot Ankle Int* 21:1043-1046, 2000.

260. Tehranzadeh J, Stoll D, Gabriele O: Diagnosis: Posterior migration of the os peroneum of the left foot, indicating a tear of the peroneal tendon. *Skeletal Radiol* 12:44-47, 1984.

261. Thews K: Fehldeutung und behandlung auf Grund von Varietaten der Handwurzel und Fusswurzel im Rontgenbilde. *Rontgenpraxis* 11:184-186, 1939.

262. Thompson F, Patterson A: Rupture of the peroneus longus tendon. *J Bone Joint Surg Am* 71:293-295, 1989.

263. Trolle D: Accessory bones of the human foot: A radiological, histoembryological, comparative anatomical and genetic study. Copenhagen, Musksgaard, 1948, pp 20-53.

264. Trolle D: De to accessoriske knogler: Os subtibiale og os subfibulare i relation til diagnosen af malleolarfracturer. *Nord Med* 25:247-249, 1945.

265. Truong T, Dussault R, Kaplan P: Fracture of the os peroneum and rupture of the peroneus longus tendon as a complication of diabetic neuropathy. *Skeletal Radiol* 24:626-628, 1995.

266. Turner W: A secondary astragalus in the human foot. *J Anat Physiol* 17:82-83, 1883.

267. Turner W: Note of another case of secondary astragalus. *J Anat Physiol* 21:334-335, 1887.

268. Uhrbrand B, Jensen T: A case of accessory calcaneus. *Acta Orthop Scand* 57:455, 1986.

269. Uhrmacher F: Varietaten des Fussskeletts als Grundlage von Fussbeschwerden. *Z Orthop Chir* 61:180-186, 1934.

270. Volk C: Zwei Falle von os naviculare pedis bipartitum. *Z Orthop* 66:396-403, 1937.

271. Volkmann J: Das Os subtibiale. *Fortschr Geb Rontgenstrahlen Neven Bildgeb Verfahr Erganzungsbd* 48:225-227, 1933.

272. Wagner W: Personal communication, 1989.

273. Wakeley C, Johnson D, Watt I: The value of MR imaging in the diagnosis of the os trigonum syndrome. *Skeletal Radiol* 25:133-136, 1996.

274. Waldeyer W: Bemerkungen uber das "Tibiale externum." In *Sitzungesberichte der königlich preussischen Akademie der Wissenschaft.* 1904, pp 1326-1332.

275. Wander D, Galli K, Ludden J, et al: Surgical management of a ruptured peroneus longus tendon with a fractured multipartite os peroneum. *J Foot Ankle* Surg 33:124-128, 1994.

276. Waschulewski H: Os subtibiale I and II. Os subfibulare. *Rontgenpraxis* 13:468, 1941.

277. Waters L: Os intermetatarseum: Case study and report. *J Am Podiatr Assoc* 48:252-254, 1958.

278. Watkins WW: Anomalous bones of the wrist and foot in relation to injury. *JAMA* 108:270-274, 1937.

279. Weinstein SL, Bonfiglio M: Unusual accessory (bipartite) talus simulating fracture. *J Bone Joint Surg Am* 57:1161-1163, 1975.

280. Wilson R, Moyles B: Surgical treatment of the symptomatic os peroneum. *J Foot Surg* 26:156-158, 1987.

281. Wredmark T, Carlstedt C, Bauer H, et al: Os trigonum syndrome: A clinical entity in ballet dancers. *Foot Ankle* 11:404-406, 1991.

282. Zadek I: The significance of the accessory tarsal scaphoid. *J Bone Joint Surg* 24:618-626, 1926.

283. Zadek I, Gold AM: The accessory tarsal scaphoid. *J Bone Joint Surg Am* 30:957-968, 1948.

284. Zerna M: Das sogenannte Os subtibiale—eine seltene Anomalie. *Zentralbl Chir* 95:1481-1487, 1970.

285. Zimmer EA: Krankheiten, Verletzungen und Varietaten des Os naviculare pedis. *Arch Orthop Unfall Chir* 38:396-411, 1938.

286. Zimmer EA: Skelettelemente medial des Cuneiforme. *Acta Radiol* 34:102-114, 1950.

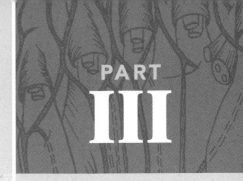

PART
III

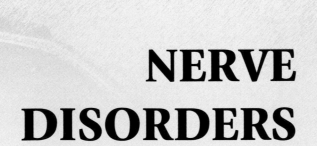

NERVE
DISORDERS

Diseases of the Nerves

Lew C. Schon • Roger A. Mann

The diagnosis and treatment of diseases of the peripheral nerves in the foot and ankle usually are quite straightforward, but at other times they present a very complex clinical and surgical problem. Nerve problems can result from overuse injuries (due to repetitive stresses) or from one-time traumatic events. Nerve disorders in many patients resolve uneventfully and do not require much, if any, treatment. Some nerve disorders resolve as a more recognizable condition receives treatment, such as in a patient with a grade 3 ankle sprain and a mild traction injury to the superficial peroneal nerve.

The more challenging diagnostic cases are dynamic and occur only with mechanical stresses such as walking, running, or wearing certain shoes. Some nerve disorders occur as a *double-crush syndrome.* In the double-crush syndrome, a more proximal nerve dysfunction (radiculopathy), which may be subclinical, causes impairment of axoplasmic flow and diminishes the threshold for distal nerve symptoms from focal disease.[38,196] The role of metabolic, endocrinologic, chemical, pharmacologic, or rheumatologic conditions in nerve physiology and function must be recognized as creating or enhancing nerve dysfunction. Occasionally the clinical problem has been aggravated by surgery, and the preoperative condition must be distinguished from the postoperative condition. The foot and ankle specialist is challenged to elucidate the differences between the symptoms from mechanical nonneurologic symptoms and those that arise from the nerves. Awareness of these features and manifestations of these conditions will help the specialist design an effective treatment plan and anticipate the outcome of the interventions.

INTERDIGITAL PLANTAR NEUROMA

The history of the interdigital neuroma has been long and colorful. Kelikian's detailed chronology of the history[29] is briefly summarized here. The condition was first described in 1845 by the Queen's Surgeon–Chiropodist Lewis Durlacher.[16] He described a "form of neuralgic affection" involving "the plantar nerve between the third and fourth metatarsal bones." In 1876 T.G. Morton[36] related the problem to the fourth metatarsophalangeal (MTP) joint and suspected a neuroma or some type of hypertrophy of the digital branches of the lateral plantar nerve (LPN). In 1877 Mason[34] reported a case of pain around the second MTP joint and suspected involvement of a digital branch of the medial plantar nerve. In 1893 Hoadley[25] actually explored the digital nerves under the painful area, "found a small neuroma," excised it, and claimed that he obtained a "prompt and perfect cure." In 1912 Tubby[51] reported observing on two occasions that the plantar digital nerves were congested and thickened. In 1940 Betts[8] stated that "Morton's metatarsalgia is a neuritis of the fourth digital nerve." In 1943 McElvenny[35] stated that it was caused by a tumor involving the most lateral branch of the medial plantar nerve. In 1979 Gauthier[18] speculated that the condition was a nerve entrapment, an idea supported anatomically by others.[21,30]

Etiology

In discussions of interdigital neuroma, it must first be pointed out that the subject is not a neuroma per se, but rather a painful clinical entity involving the common digital nerve. Thus, the best terminology for the condition should perhaps be *interdigital neuralgia* based on the complexity and variability of the cause. The term *neuritis* is a less favorable descriptor because the suffix "-itis" implies inflammation. Because the condition can occur as an entrapment without inflammatory cells or mediators, the suffix "-algia," used to describe pain, is more accurate.

Studies by Lassmann[30] and Graham and Graham[21] have demonstrated that most if not all of the histologic changes in the nerve occur beyond the transverse metatarsal ligament and that the nerve proximal to the ligament appears to be normal. These authors demonstrated quantitatively that there was a decrease in the number of thick myelinated fibers, decreased diameter in the individual nerve fibers as a result of attenuation of their myelin sheaths, and increased nerve and vesicular width. Alterations in the interdigital arteries could not be correlated with the alterations found in the nerves. Hyalinization of vessel walls has been observed in patients with interdigital neuroma, but it has also been observed in control material in patients without interdigital neuroma. In a study of 133 patients with a clinical diagnosis of Morton's syndrome, light and electron microscopic investigations revealed that in the early stages of the disease the histologic findings are dominated by certain alterations of the nerves independent of alterations of the interdigital vessels. These alterations include sclerosis and edema of the endoneurium, thickening and hyalinization of the walls of the endoneurial vessels caused by multiple layers of basement membrane, thickening of the perineurium, deposition of an amorphous eosinophilic material built up by filaments of tubular structures, demyelination and degeneration of the nerve fibers without signs of Wallerian degeneration, and local initial hyperplasia of unmyelinated nerves followed by degeneration. These authors concluded that Morton's syndrome is probably caused by an entrapment neuropathy predominantly characterized by the deposition of an amorphous eosinophilic material followed by a slow degeneration of the nerve fibers.

Giannini et al[19] reported on the histopathology in 63 cases and found intraneural (epineurium and perineurium) fibrosis and sclerohyalinosis and an increase of the elastic fibers in the stroma. They also found hyperplasia of the muscle layer, very evident internal elastic lamina, and proliferation of small vessels in the muscle layer and adventitia in the vessels.

Although these studies seem to support the theory that the main cause for an interdigital neuroma is an entrapment neuropathy beneath the transverse metatarsal ligament, other factors should be considered in the origin of this condition, including anatomic, traumatic, and extrinsic factors.

Anatomic Factors

From an anatomic standpoint, the medial plantar nerve (MPN) has four digital branches (Fig. 11–1). The most medial branch is the proper digital nerve to the medial aspect of the great toe. The next three branches are the first, second, and third common digital nerves and are distributed to both the medial and the lateral aspects of the first, second, and third interspaces, respectively. The LPN divides into a superficial branch (which splits into a proper digital nerve to the lateral side of the small toe) and a common digital nerve to the fourth interspace. The common digital nerve often has a communicating branch that passes to the third digital branch of the MPN in the third interspace.

Researchers have speculated that because the common digital nerve to the third interspace consists of branches from the medial and lateral plantar nerves, the common digital nerve has increased thickness and is therefore more subject to trauma and possible neuroma formation[28] (Fig. 11–2). In an anatomic dissection of 71 feet, Levitsky et al[32] observed that a communicating branch to the nerve to the third web space was present in only 27% of specimens and was absent in 73%. This anatomic finding seems to indicate that the communicating branch has little relation to the cause of interdigital neuroma. The authors did observe, however, that the second and third interspace was significantly narrower than the first and fourth and postulated that this further indicated the possibility of

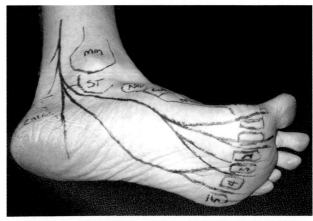

Figure 11–1 Illustration of nerves on the plantar aspect of the foot. Note the third toe has mixed innervation from the medial and lateral plantar nerves.

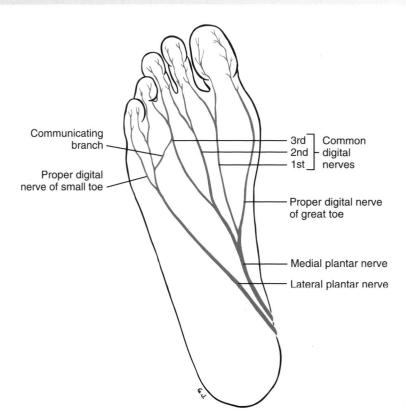

Communicating branch

Proper digital nerve of small toe

3rd
2nd   Common digital nerves
1st

Proper digital nerve of great toe

Medial plantar nerve

Lateral plantar nerve

Figure 11–2   Plantar nerves of the right foot.

an entrapment. The frequency of the communicating branch was confirmed by Govsa et al.[20] They studied the anatomy of the communicating branches of the common plantar digital nerves between the fourth and third nerves in 50 adult male cadavers and found it in 28% of the feet.

Some variation exists in the distribution of the common digital nerves to the plantar aspect of the foot and their relationship to the metatarsal heads. At times when an interdigital neuroma is resected, an accessory nerve branch appears to pass obliquely beneath the metatarsal head and joins the common digital nerve before its bifurcation into the digital branches. Because these accessory branches appear to come from beneath the metatarsal head region, when they are transected, the nerve end can retract beneath the metatarsal head and result in a recurrent neuroma.

The mobility that occurs between the medial three rays and the lateral two rays may be a reason for the increased incidence of neuromas in the third web space. The medial three rays are firmly fixed at the metatarsocuneiform joints, whereas the fourth and fifth metatarsals are fixed to the cuboid, which is more mobile. This anatomic fact results in increased mobility in the third web space, and the increased motion can result in trauma to the nerve or possibly the development of an enlarged bursa, which can secondarily place pressure on the nerve. The significant number of neuromas found in the second web space in part negates this as the main cause for the development of a neuroma.[33]

During normal gait, dorsiflexion of the MTP joints along with the action of the plantar aponeurosis causes plantar flexion of the metatarsal heads and, in theory, exposes the nerve to increased trauma (Fig. 11–3). The incidence of interdigital neuromas is eight to 10 times more common in women, whose toes are often hyperextended at the MTP joint by high-fashion footwear, and this is probably a significant factor. Rather than increased trauma to the nerve itself resulting from long-term hyperextension of the MTP joints, the nerve may be tethered beneath the transverse metatarsal ligament, which results in the entrapment neuropathy previously discussed (Fig. 11–4).

Traumatic Causes

Acute trauma resulting from a fall from a height, a crush injury, or stepping on a sharp object occasionally results in a traumatic origin of an interdigital neuroma. Runners, persons who spend many hours on their feet at work, or people who engage in certain athletic endeavors such as racquet sports or dance and place much stress on the metatarsal region do not demonstrate an increased incidence of neuroma formation. The precise cause of neuroma development in one person but not in another exposed to essentially the same level of activity or inactivity remains an enigma. Even patients with atrophy of the plantar fat

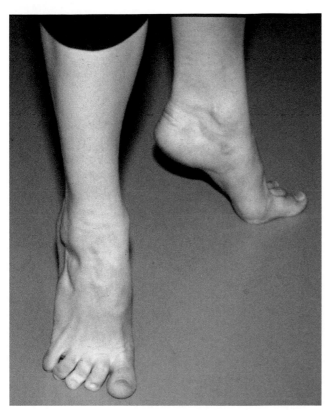

Figure 11–3 The demi-pointe position can increase the stretch on the common digital nerve.

pad with resultant metatarsalgia rarely, if ever, report focal neuritic symptoms isolated to a single web space.

Extrinsic Factors

Extrinsic pressure against the nerve can result from a mass above the transverse metatarsal ligament or below the ligament. Anatomically a bursa is normally present between the metatarsal heads and is located above the transverse metatarsal ligament. Bossley and Cairney[10] studied this bursa by injecting dye in cadaver feet and demonstrated extension of the bursa distal and proximal to the transverse metatarsal ligament in the third web space. They did not observe extension of the bursa in the fourth web space. They hypothesized that the bursa can cause inflammation resulting in secondary neurofibrosis of the nerve but did not believe that the bursa caused a compressive force against the nerve. Awerbuch and Shephard[3] noted similar findings of an inflamed intermetatarsal bursa in patients with rheumatoid arthritis, which they believed resulted in an alteration in the interdigital nerve, as well as some direct compressive effect on the nerve by the enlarged bursa.

Degeneration of the capsule of the MTP joint from unknown causes can result in a localized inflammatory response, but the nerve is not usually involved

because it is above the transverse metatarsal ligament. Such deterioration of the capsule, however, can cause deviation of the proximal phalanx, usually of the third toe, in a medial direction. This in turn results in lateral deviation of the third metatarsal head against the fourth. The pressure can result in compression of bursal material present above the ligament and subsequently pressure against the underlying nerve. The deviation of the toe or instability of the MTP joint could also result in traction on the nerve, which could lead to disease (Fig. 11–5). Clinical symptoms of a neuroma are observed in approximately 10% to 15% of patients with deviation of the MTP joint, which may be accounted for by this anatomic malalignment (Fig. 11–6).

Occasionally the transverse metatarsal ligament itself is thickened or contains an aberrant band that causes pressure against the common nerve. We have seen a few patients in whom this was present in the second web space, but we have not observed it in any other web space. In these cases, release of the transverse metatarsal ligament resulted in relief of the neuritic problem. A ganglion or synovial cyst can arise from the MTP joint, either as a primary entity or

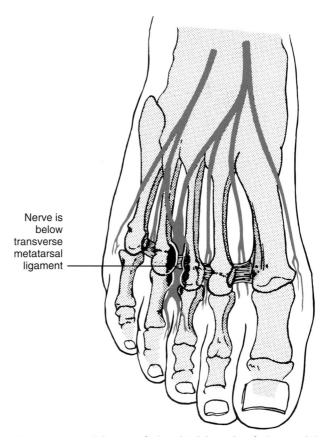

Nerve is below transverse metatarsal ligament

Figure 11–4 Schema of the third branch of the medial plantar nerve. Note that the nerve courses plantarward, under the transverse metatarsal ligament.

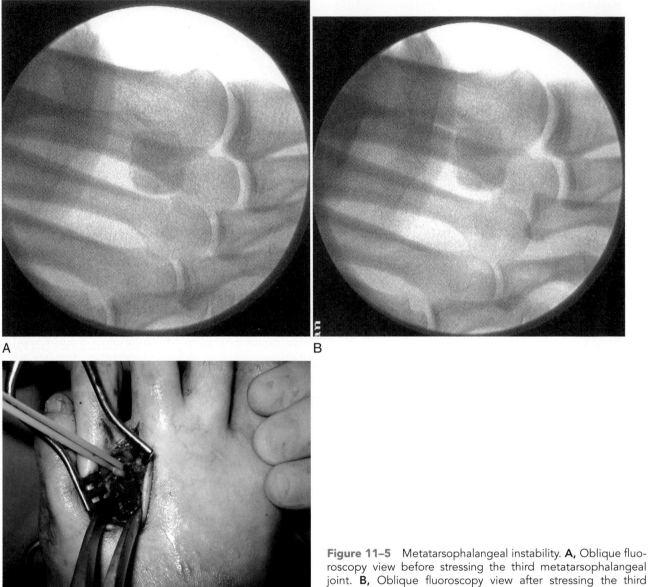

A

B

C

Figure 11–5   Metatarsophalangeal instability. **A,** Oblique fluoroscopy view before stressing the third metatarsophalangeal joint. **B,** Oblique fluoroscopy view after stressing the third metatarsophalangeal joint. **C,** Neuroma identified next to unstable joint.

possibly in association with degeneration of the plantar plate. This lesion can cause direct pressure against the nerve as it passes beneath the transverse metatarsal ligament. A lipoma on the plantar aspect of the foot can result in similar compression against the nerve.

Fracture of the metatarsal from stress or a single traumatic event can result in altered loading of the metatarsal, with resultant interdigital neuralgia. In these cases, deviation of the malunion in any plane can cause traction or compression from the bone or any anchored soft tissues. For example, alteration in the length or function of the tendons directly from the callus or indirectly from malunion with shortening of the bone can lead to a claw toe or deviated toe with

development of nerve symptoms. This can be further complicated in a traumatically induced fracture by a direct insult to the nerve by the causative mechanism (e.g., crush, twist) at the time of bone injury.

Symptom Complex

Mann and Reynolds[33] performed a critical analysis of 56 patients in whom 76 neuromas were excised. There were 53 women and three men. This represents a greater female-to-male ratio than that observed by Bradley et al[11], who reported a ratio of 4 : 1. The average age of the patient in the Mann and Reynolds[33] series was 55 years (range, 29 to 81 years).

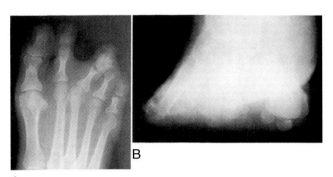

Figure 11–6 Increased pressure is created in the web space as a result of deviation of lesser toes, forcing metatarsal heads together. **A,** Anteroposterior radiograph shows lateral deviation of third toe, resulting in narrowing of second interspace. **B,** Axial view demonstrates narrowing of second interspace.

TABLE 11–1

Preoperative Symptoms of Interdigital Neuroma

Symptom	Patients Affected (%)
Plantar pain increased by walking	91
Relief of pain by resting	89
Plantar pain	77
Relief of pain by removing shoes	70
Pain radiating into toes	62
Burning pain	54
Aching or sharp pain	40
Numbness in toes or foot	40
Pain radiating up foot or leg	34
Cramping sensation	34

An interdigital neuroma is usually unilateral, although bilateral neuromas were observed in 15% of the patients. The development of two neuromas simultaneously in the same foot rarely occurs; in a review of 89 neurectomies, Thompson and Deland[50] concluded that the incidence was probably less than 3%. The majority of the literature reports that the neuroma usually involves the third interspace, but an equal number of neuromas in the second and third interspaces have been noted. This same distribution was subsequently noted by Hauser[24] but was not supported by Graham et al,[22] who noted that there were twice as many neuromas in the third web space as the second. An interdigital neuroma of the first or fourth interspace is rare and probably does not exist as a clinical entity.

The most common symptom of an interdigital neuroma is pain localized to the plantar aspect of the foot between the metatarsal heads. The pain is usually characterized as burning, stabbing, tingling, or electric and radiates to the toes of the involved interspace in approximately 60% of cases. On occasion the patient feels something "moving around" in the plantar aspect of the foot that periodically gets "caught" and results in an acute, sharp pain that radiates to the toes. This symptom complex is probably because the nerve is trapped beneath the metatarsal head, which, when body weight is applied, causes the acute pain. Occasionally, patients observe that the pain radiates toward the dorsum of the foot or more proximally along the plantar aspect of the foot.

The symptom complex is aggravated by activities on the foot, and most often the pain occurs when the patient puts on a tight-fitting high-heeled shoe. This pain is often relieved by removing the shoe and rubbing the forefoot. Often the patient finds that the pain during gait can be limited by voluntarily curling the toes or by avoiding rolling through the ball of the feet. The patient often notes no symptoms when walking barefoot on a soft surface, only to feel pain when a high-heeled shoe is worn again. At times, wearing a broad, soft walking or jogging shoe results in a significant decrease in the symptom complex. Nonetheless, prolonged walking can induce symptoms regardless of shoe type.

Table 11–1 lists the preoperative symptoms by percentage in patients with interdigital neuroma.[33]

Diagnosis

The diagnosis of an interdigital neuroma is based on the patient's history and the physical findings. No electrodiagnostic studies are useful unless a peripheral neuropathy or radiculopathy is suspected. Radiographs are helpful to assess the foot in general and to identify an underlying bone or joint disease. Magnetic resonance imaging (MRI) may be useful in some cases to rule out other pathologies but is not warranted for establishing the diagnosis (Fig. 11–7). Similarly, ultrasound may be helpful in some situations, but the rate of false positives and negatives is too high to depend on the test. In some cases it may be necessary to reevaluate the patient several times before one makes the diagnosis of an interdigital neuroma if the patient's symptoms are atypical.

Physical Examination

The physical examination begins by having the patient stand, with the physician carefully observing the foot for evidence of deviation of the toes, subluxation or clawing of the toes, or evidence of fullness in the involved web space or fullness of a web space not observed in the uninvolved foot. Then the range of motion of the MTP joints is observed. The MTP joints

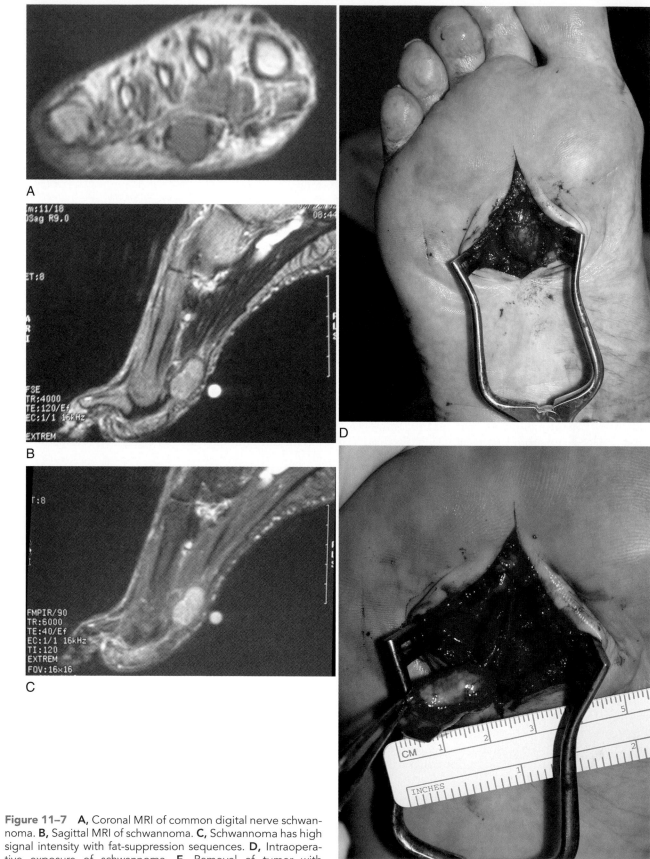

Figure 11–7   A, Coronal MRI of common digital nerve schwannoma. **B,** Sagittal MRI of schwannoma. **C,** Schwannoma has high signal intensity with fat-suppression sequences. **D,** Intraoperative exposure of schwannoma. **E,** Removal of tumor with intrafascicular dissection from the common digital nerve.

are carefully palpated on their dorsal and plantar aspects to look for evidence of synovitis of the joint, pain in the plantar pad area indicating early degeneration of the plantar pad, and evidence of pain around the joint. The patient with an interdigital neuroma does not have pain over the dorsal metatarsal heads. Typically there is no pain over the plantar metatarsal head but the presence of some tenderness here should be considered relative to the tenderness in the web space. Thus, if there is more pain in between the metatarsals, especially if it reproduces the character of the patient's symptoms of burning, shooting, radiating pain, then a neuroma is suspected.

Next, the physician carefully palpates the interspaces, starting just proximal to the metatarsal heads and proceeding distally into the web space. This usually reproduces the patient's pain, which often radiates out toward the tips of the toes. It is important when performing this test to ensure that there is no inadvertent compression of the dorsal tissues as a counterforce to the plantar pressures that are directed dorsally. The physician should press the web space with one finger plantarly, using the other hand to stabilize the foot over a broad area of the midfoot or forefoot or against the resistance of the patient's foot alone (Fig. 11–8). Concomitant dorsal pressure can lead to discomfort from other etiologies that must be distinguished from interdigital neuralgia.

The web spaces are reexamined, and pressure is applied in a mediolateral direction with one hand to increase pressure on the tissue between the metatarsal heads. This maneuver often results in a significant crunching or clicking feeling (Mulder's sign[37]), most

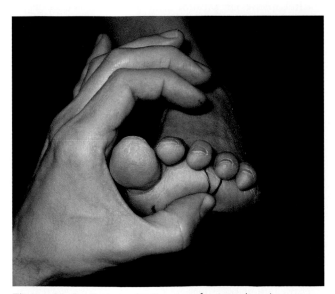

Figure 11–8 Deep palpation test for interdigital neuroma. The examiner should press from plantar to dorsal, avoiding inadvertent dorsal palpation.

often in the third web space and occasionally in the second web space. The maneuver can reproduce the patient's pain and, if so, is diagnostic of an interdigital neuroma. The presence of only a crunching or clicking feeling in the web space without reproduction of the patient's pain does not indicate a neuroma. Examination of a normal foot can demonstrate a crunching or clicking feeling, particularly in the third web space and occasionally in the second. It is unusual to elicit this crunch or click in the first and fourth web spaces. This test is not as helpful following a prior neuroma resection. When the plantar aspect of the foot is palpated, occasionally a mass representing a small synovial cyst or ganglion is observed. Usually this mass is less than 1 cm in diameter and can be rolled beneath the examiner's fingers. When the mass is associated with a web space, pressure against the mass often reproduces the patient's symptoms. A sensory examination rarely demonstrates any deficit in the patient with a neuroma.

A more complete neurologic exam should include palpation of all the web spaces and along the course of the tibial nerve branches. The tibial nerve itself should be palpated and percussed with palpation in the posterior leg, the popliteal space, and behind the femur. Other nerves should be examined including the sural, saphenous, deep peroneal, and superficial peroneal nerves. A straight leg maneuver should be performed to rule out radiculopathy when clinically indicated. A quick motor exam including eversion, inversion, dorsiflexion, and plantar flexion of the toes, foot, and ankle is useful. When warranted, an examination of reflexes is performed. Checking the patient's hands for evidence of intrinsic atrophy or tremor can help identify systemic neurologic conditions.

At times the patient's physical examination is not conclusive, and the patient needs to be reevaluated on several occasions to ensure that the symptom complex indeed indicates a neuroma. If there is pain around an MTP joint as well as in the web space, caution is advised in making the diagnosis of a neuroma, because early degeneration of the plantar pad, early synovitis of the MTP joint, or some degeneration of the plantar fat may be present. It is useful to stress the MTP joint by checking for a dorsal drawer sign and instability of the MTP and induction of symptoms. When undertaking this maneuver, the physician must secure the base of the toe at the proximal phalanx without inadvertently pressing on the nerve. With the other hand securing the foot at the metatarsals, slight traction is applied to the toe and an attempt is made to translate the base of the proximal phalanx dorsally. The adjacent and contralateral toes should be checked to determine the baseline joint laxity for the patient (Fig. 11–9). This test may be positive with instability or

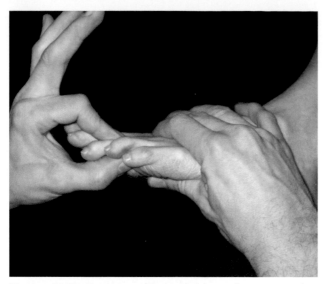

Figure 11–9 A provocative evaluation of metatarsopha-langeal joint instability or inflammation is important because these can be either contributing factors or the primary cause of the patient's pain. The metatarsals are stabilized by one hand while the other secures the toe at the base of the proximal phalanx. A dorsal thrust in the sagittal plane can reveal subluxation or dislocation and can induce pain. The patient's symptoms may be either mechanical or neuritic depending on the pathology.

synovitis, which can coexist with neuralgia, but if the pain is not reproduced with the symptoms, then instability or synovitis is not triggering the neuralgia or the patient's forefoot pain may be coming from another condition.

The physical findings from an analysis of patients in one (RAM) practice are as follows: plantar tenderness, 95%; radiation of pain into the toes, 46%; palpable mass, 12%; numbness, 3%; and widening of the interspace, 3%.

Diagnostic Studies

A radiograph of the foot during weight bearing should always be obtained in an evaluation of the patient with a suspected interdigital neuroma. The purpose of the radiographic study is to observe any abnormalities within the osseous structures; subluxation, dislocation, or arthritis of the MTP joint; or possibly evidence of a foreign body.

In the opinion of one of us (LCS), MRI has not been demonstrated to be effective in the diagnosis of an interdigital neuroma. This has been substantiated by a study by Bencardino,[5] who found a lack of correlation of an MRI finding of a neuroma and symptoms in 33% of patients. If there is a question about the presence of other etiologies of the patient's pain, an MRI may be performed in a prone position[52] using a combination

of contrast enhancement and fat suppression.[49] One study by Biasca et al[9] suggested that a more favorable result could be achieved after neuroma resection when the nerve has a transverse measurement larger than 5 mm on MRI scans.

Ultrasound is operator dependent,[45] and although there are proponents of this imaging technique,[31,40,41] we do not find it a useful modality.[42,43] This impression has been substantiated in a report by Sharp et al.[47] These authors looked at the accuracy of preoperative clinical assessment, ultrasound, and MRI and compared these findings to intraoperative histology and the clinical outcome. They found the accuracy of the ultrasound and MRI was similar and dependent on lesion size. Small lesions were not well visualized on ultrasound. There was no correlation among the size, the pain score, or the change in pain score following surgery. Reliance on either ultrasound or MRI would have led to an inaccurate diagnosis in 18 of 19 cases. The predictive values attained by clinical assessment surpass imaging with one or both modalities.

No reliable electrodiagnostic studies are available to document the presence of an interdigital neuroma. However these studies are useful to help identify a proximal entrapment, radiculopathy, or neuropathy when their presence is suspected.

Lidocaine can be injected into the suspected web space for diagnostic purposes. The recommended dose is 2 mL of anesthetic placed below the transverse metatarsal ligament. Although complete relief of symptoms can be obtained, caution is advised in interpreting this as confirming an interdigital neuroma because this injection also relieves pain from local pathologic conditions such as degeneration of the joint capsule or plantar plate. Younger et al[54] performed a study to determine the role of a diagnostic block in predicting the results of surgery. In 37 patients with 41 excisions (7 patients with revisions) 24% of the primary procedures were failures despite relief with a block and 43% of the 7 revision procedures were failures.

Administration of cortisone can be useful in about one third of patients, but cortisone can cause deterioration of the joint capsule or possibly the plantar fat. Only infrequently should more than one hydrocortisone injection be made into the web space. In some patients, medial or lateral deviation of the adjacent MTP joint has developed after multiple steroid injections, presumably from damage to a collateral ligament (Fig. 11–10). Decreasing the volume effect of the injection can help diminish the risk of damage to the MTP joint capsule, ligament, or tendon. This can be accomplished by injecting proximal to the MTP joint below the intermetatarsal ligament as opposed to

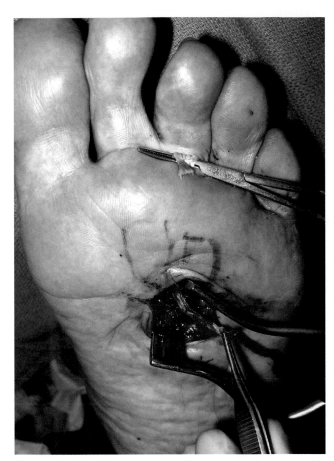

Figure 11–10 Ruptured flexor digitorum brevis tendon following cortisone injections with resultant instability of the metatarsophalangeal (MTP) joint. The patient required neuroma excision and reconstruction of the tendon and the MTP joint.

more distally. Additionally if during the injection the toes begin to spread apart, the injection should be stopped. If the deviation is noted following an injection, the toes should be supported by taping.

Differential Diagnosis

Many other conditions can mimic interdigital neuroma. Box 11–1 provides a differential diagnosis to assist physicians regarding this condition.

Treatment

Conservative Treatment

Conservative management consists of fitting the patient with a wide, soft, laced shoe, preferably with a low heel. This type of shoe allows the foot to spread out and thereby relieves some of the pressure on the metatarsal head region and eliminates the chronic hyperextension of the MTP joints. Thicker compressi-

---

BOX 11–1   Differential Diagnosis of Interdigital Neuroma

Arthrosis of MTP joint
Degeneration of plantar pad or capsule
Degenerative disk disease
Freiberg's infraction
Lesion of medial or lateral plantar nerve
Lesions of plantar aspect of foot
Metatarsal stress fracture
Metatarsophalangeal joint disorders
Pain of neurogenic origin unrelated to interdigital neuroma
Peripheral neuropathy
Soft tissue tumor (e.g., lipoma)
Soft tissue tumor not involving MTP joint (e.g., ganglion, lipoma, synovial cyst)
Subluxation or dislocation of MTP joint
Synovial cysts
Synovitis of MTP joint caused by nonspecific synovitis or rheumatoid arthritis
Tarsal tunnel syndrome
Tumor of metatarsal bone

MTP, metatarsophalangeal.

ble rubber soled shoes can also make a big difference by providing shock attenuation to the forefoot region. A soft metatarsal support is added to the shoe just proximal to the metatarsal head region, which further relieves the pressure from the involved area and helps to spread the metatarsal heads to relieve pressure on the nerves (Fig. 11–11). Occasionally a soft metatarsal support can be added to a high-heeled shoe, provided sufficient room exists in the toe box area for both the

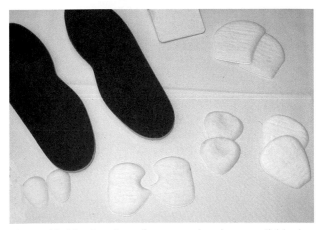

Figure 11–11 A variety of metatarsal pads are available that can be applied to the insole of the shoe or to a generic purchased insole.

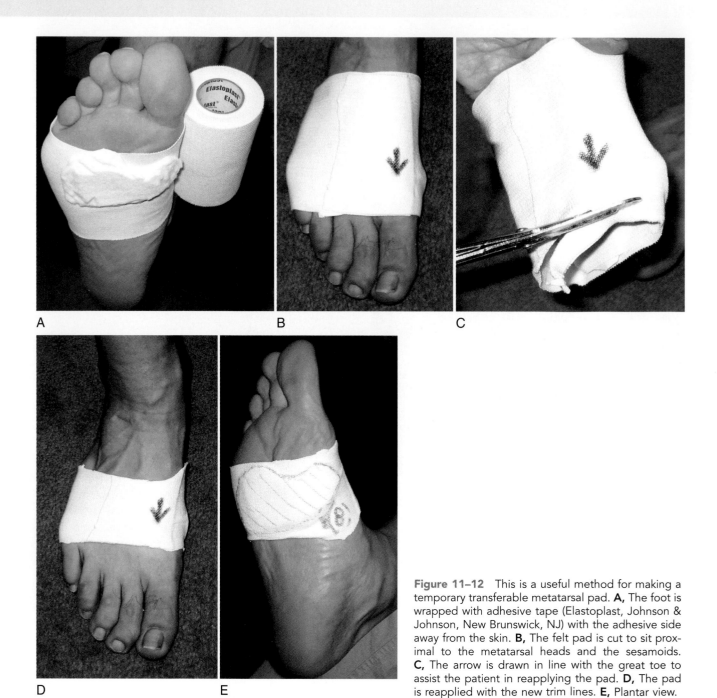

Figure 11–12   This is a useful method for making a temporary transferable metatarsal pad. **A,** The foot is wrapped with adhesive tape (Elastoplast, Johnson & Johnson, New Brunswick, NJ) with the adhesive side away from the skin. **B,** The felt pad is cut to sit proximal to the metatarsal heads and the sesamoids. **C,** The arrow is drawn in line with the great toe to assist the patient in reapplying the pad. **D,** The pad is reapplied with the new trim lines. **E,** Plantar view.

support and the foot (Fig. 11–12). When the patient has synovitis, instability, or deviation of the MTP, a Budin splint (Fig. 11–13) or canopy toe strapping (Fig. 11–14) can be useful to decrease secondary neuralgia. Shoe modifications such as a metatarsal bar or rocker sole can be also helpful (Fig. 11–15).

Injection of the interspace with a local anesthetic may be useful as a diagnostic tool, particularly if there is tenderness in two interspaces of the same foot. However, the effectiveness of the injection depends on the use of a small quantity of anesthetic agent that

must be carefully directed to the common digital nerve. If the area is flooded with a large quantity of anesthetic agent, the patient might feel a relief of symptoms, but the test is not very specific for pathologic conditions caused by the nerve.

Steroids can occasionally be helpful but rarely produce long-lasting relief. In a study of 76 cases of suspected interdigital neuroma, Greenfield et al[23] noted significant relief with a series of steroid injections; 30% of patients had relief that lasted more than 2 years. Injection of corticosteroids into the area

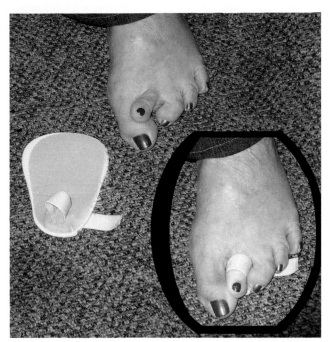

Figure 11–13 The medially deviated toe caused neuritic symptoms in this patient. The Budin splint helped secure the toe in a better position *(inset)* and minimized the traction on the nerve.

can occur. One of the more serious problems is disruption of the joint capsule adjacent to the injection site, with resultant deviation of the toe medially or laterally, depending on which capsule has been involved. This is a very unfortunate consequence of steroid injections and one that then creates a significant new problem for the patient.

Other nonsurgical management options include oral vitamin B6 100 mg bid; anti-inflammatory medications and tricyclic antidepressants (TCAs) such as imipramine (Tofranil), nortriptyline (Pamolar), desipramine (Norpramin), and amitriptyline (Elavil); selective serotonin reuptake inhibitors such as sertraline (Zoloft); paroxetine (Paxil); other antidepressants such as venlafaxin (Effexor) or duloxetine (Cymbalta); or antiseizure medications such as gabapentin (Neurontin), pregabalin (Lyrica), topiramate (Topomax), and carbamazepine (Tegretol). This use of these drugs is off label, but they have been useful to lessen the severity of nerve-related symptoms. For a more complete discussion of the various medications for chronic pain, consult the American Chronic Pain Association's Medications and Chronic Pain Supplement.[1] One of us (LCS) recommends considering these medications for diffuse or atypical forefoot neuralgia or when there is a history of a more proximal nerve lesion.

of the suspected neuroma is associated with some problems, and so the injections must be used with a certain degree of caution. Atrophy of the subcutaneous fat and discoloration of the skin can occur and be quite disturbing to the patient. If the injection is placed beyond the nerve, some atrophy of the plantar fat pad

Radiofrequency ablation and alcohol nerve injections have been proposed as less traumatic, more conservative methods of treating neuromas. Fanucci et al[17] reported their results with 40 interdigital neuroma injections with alcohol (70% carbocaine-adrenaline and 30% ethylic alcohol) under ultrasound guidance.

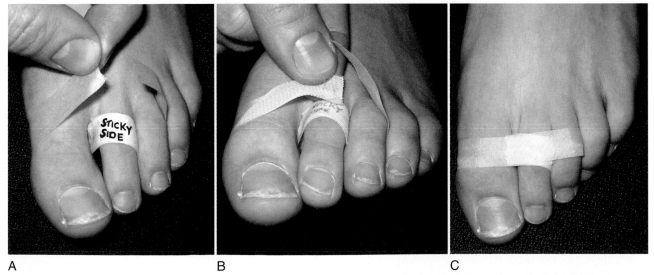

A   B   C

Figure 11–14 **A,** Canopy toe taping is applied with the adhesive side upward around the second toe. **B,** The tape goes underneath the first and third toes with the adhesive side against the skin. Enough tension is applied to secure the second metatarsophalangeal joint in neutral position. **C,** The final appearance.

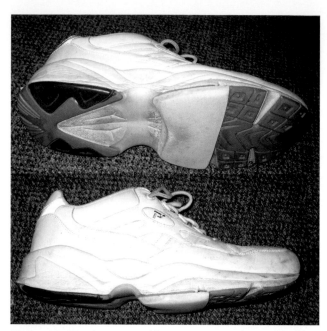

Figure 11–15 A metatarsal bar is constructed onto the outer sole of the shoe.

Total or partial symptomatic relief was obtained in 90% of cases without complications. There was temporary plantar pain in 15%. Although the authors claimed the technique was feasible and cost-efficient and had high rates of therapeutic success, further investigation is warranted.

Most patients seem to respond fairly well to initial conservative management in that they obtain some relief of their clinical symptoms. Occasionally the physical findings of localized pain in the involved interspace improve, but as a general rule they do not. The majority of patients continue to have symptoms, and, in time, 60% to 70% elect excision of the neuroma. Not infrequently, this choice of surgical management is made because of the patient's desire to be able to wear high-heeled shoes even though they are often comfortable in their low, soft shoes.

Surgical Treatment

SURGICAL EXCISION

An interdigital neuroma may be excised through a dorsal or a plantar approach. The main advantage of the dorsal approach is prevention of scar formation on the plantar aspect of the foot. With a dorsal approach, if the incision is not kept in the midline or is made too proximal, one of the dorsal cutaneous nerves to the web space may be disrupted or become painful, but this is an

unusual complication. The plantar approach, although it sounds simple, must be accurately placed in the interspace so that it does not pass directly beneath the metatarsal head. When this incision is made, it is important that it be carried deeply down through the thick plantar fat to expose the nerve and the web space. Dissection performed medially or laterally only creates scarring of the fatty tissue; as a result, the scar can become somewhat puckered, or the fat pad beneath a metatarsal head can become atrophic (Fig 11–16).

Alternative plantar approaches include either longitudinal or transverse incisions proximal to the metatarsal head. These can avoid the painful scar in the weight-bearing area of the foot. Exposure of the nerve is usually quite easy but for the surgeon who is unfamiliar with the anatomy from this perspective, it can be a challenge. If a keloid develops from any plantar incision, the symptoms can become very difficult to rectify. Thus, for treatment of a primary interdigital neuralgia, the dorsal approach is preferred.

Surgical Technique

1. With or without tourniquet control an incision is made in the dorsal aspect of the foot, starting in the web space between the involved toes. The incision is carried proximally for about 3 cm to the level of the metatarsal

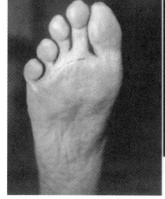
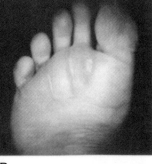

B

A

Figure 11–16 Examples of scars from plantar incisions used to excise interdigital neuroma. **A,** Transverse scar at the base of the toes can remain painful. Because of the location of the scar, the nerve is not resected proximally enough and often becomes symptomatic once again. **B,** Multiple longitudinal incisions resulted in atrophy of fat pad and some mild hyperkeratosis of scars. This results in chronic metatarsal plain.

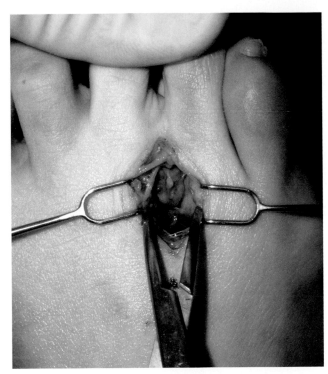

Figure 11–17 The dorsal nerve branches can be encountered—here on the medial side of the incision—during the exposure of the interdigital neuroma.

head. It is important to keep the incision directly in the midline because deviation to either side can result in cutting one of the dorsal digital nerves, which could cause a painful neuroma (Fig. 11–17 and video clip 47).

2. The incision is deepened through the soft tissue to the level of the metatarsal heads. A Weitlaner retractor or laminar spreader is placed between the metatarsal heads to gain optimal exposure (Fig. 11–18). This places the transverse metatarsal ligament under significant tension. If there is difficulty inserting the spreader or retractor, a hemostat can be inserted between the metatarsals first to facilitate its placement.

3. Use of a neurologic Freer elevator to dissect the contents of the interspace allows the transverse metatarsal ligament to be identified and transected (Fig. 11–19).

4. The retractor or spreader is removed, set deeper between the metatarsal heads, and spread. This allows visualization of the contents of the web space. The neurologic Freer elevator allows the common digital nerve to be identified in the proximal portion of the

wound, and it is traced distally to its bifurcation. Digital pressure under the web space from the plantar aspect pushes the nerve more dorsally and facilitates visualization.

5. Once the bifurcation is reached, a significant amount of soft tissue, sometimes almost appearing bursa-like, may be around the nerve. If possible, this tissue should be removed so that the nerve can be followed past the bifurcation. However, if the adhesions are too great, all this material is removed along with the nerve rather than taking the time to carefully dissect it. When the interspace is explored, the surgeon should look carefully for any accessory branches that might be coming out from beneath the adjacent metatarsal head to identify them and alter the treatment plan, if necessary. Whenever possible, preservation of the vascular structures is advantageous.

6. In the proximal portion of the wound, the common digital nerve is cut proximal to the metatarsal head, dissected out distally past the bifurcation, and excised (Fig. 11–20). As little plantar fat as possible should be

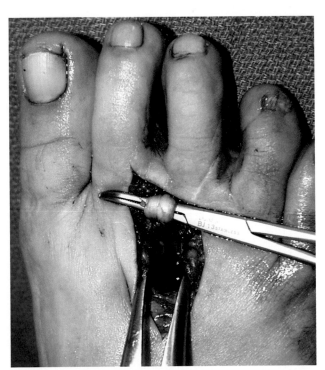

Figure 11–18 The laminar spreader between the metatarsals facilitates exposure.

removed (Fig. 11–21). If a significant accessory nerve trunk passing to the common nerve either medially or laterally is observed, the consequences of cutting this nerve and allowing it to retract under the metatarsal head area must be considered. If the nerve trunk appears to be larger than 2 mm, rather than resecting the neuroma proximal to the metatarsal heads, the common nerve should be cut just proximal to its bifurcation, which is also just proximal to the thickening usually observed in the nerve distal to the transverse metatarsal ligament. The distal portion of the nerve is removed. The cut end is sutured to the side of the metatarsal or one of the intrinsic muscles so that it will not drop onto the plantar aspect of the foot. By placing the nerve alongside the metatarsal off the bottom of the foot when the stump neuroma forms, it will not be in a weight-bearing position. When this is carried out, it is important that the nerve not be under any tension when it is sutured.

7. The skin is closed in a single layer, and a comfortable compression dressing is applied.

Postoperative Care

The patient is permitted to ambulate in a postoperative shoe. The sutures are removed between 7 and 14 days. A compressive wrap is used for 2 to 5 weeks, after which the patient is encouraged to work on active and passive range-of-motion exercises.

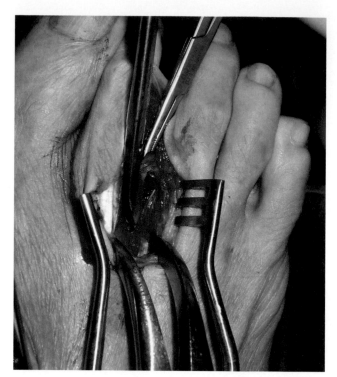

Figure 11–20   The proximal aspect of the nerve is transected beyond the metatarsal heads.

Uncommon Findings

Excision of an interdigital neuroma usually is a straightforward procedure. Occasionally a large bursa is found between the metatarsal heads and, in particular, the third interspace and must be removed to expose the underlying nerve. This is carried out by sharp dissection, with care taken not to remove any plantar fat. An accessory nerve trunk may be encountered, as mentioned earlier; if it is greater than 2 mm in diameter, the nerve distal to it can be excised and the nerve sutured to the side of the metatarsal to prevent formation of a recurrent neuroma beneath the metatarsal head. We estimate that this accessory nerve is noted in about 10% of neuromas.

Occasionally a cyst, which usually consists of material that appears to be degenerated fat, is identified adjacent to a metatarsal head. This does not appear to be a true cyst but does have a somewhat irregular lining. When present, it should be unroofed, but again, as little fat as possible is removed to prevent atrophy of the fat pad beneath a metatarsal head.

Results

An analysis of patients in Mann and Reynolds' series after excision of an interdigital neuroma

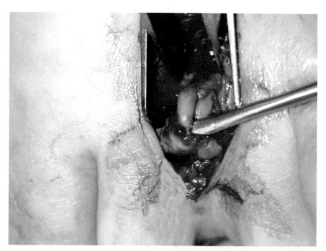

Figure 11–19   The Freer elevator is used to help identify the nerve and dissect the contents of the interspace.

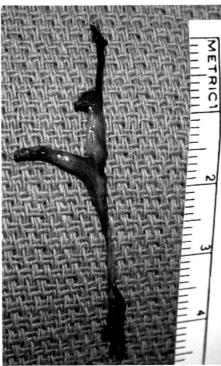
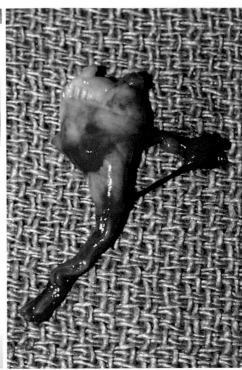

Figure 11–21 Two examples of neuromas. **A,** A thin neuroma is noted with its bifurcation. **B,** A large bulbous neuroma with a thickened bifurcation.

A   B

demonstrated the following results: 71% essentially asymptomatic, 9% significantly improved, 6% marginally improved, and 14% failure.[33]

The patients who had marginal improvement with surgical failure were carefully reevaluated, with no evidence of other pathologic findings that would account for the persistent pain, such as synovitis of the MTP joint, subluxation of the MTP joint, or the presence of a neuroma in an adjacent web space. Obviously, a certain group of patients have a condition similar to an interdigital neuroma, which clinically is not fully understood at this time. The results for those patients in whom a neuroma was removed from the second web space and third web space were the same. Other follow-up studies of patients after excision of an interdigital neuroma have demonstrated similar results.[11]

Physical examination of the satisfied patient population demonstrated the following postoperative findings: local plantar pain, 65%; numbness in the interspace, 68%; and area of plantar numbness adjacent to the interspace, 51%.

Not infrequently, although the patient believed that the neuritic pain was gone, some discomfort was still noted on the plantar aspect of the foot. At times this was described as a feeling as if the sock was wrinkled under the foot or a feeling of stepping on a piece of cotton. The fact that 32% of the patients still had normal sensation in the web space after complete excision of their interdigital neuroma indicates the degree of overlap that is present in the innervation of the area. It is also important to consider this when one is evaluating a patient with a recurrent neuroma, because the presence of sensation does not necessarily mean that the neuroma has not been adequately excised. About half the patients noted some numbness on the plantar aspect of the foot adjacent to the interspace. This probably results from the plantar innervation that comes off the common digital nerve and is disrupted when the nerve is excised.

Coughlin and Pinsonneault[13] reported on 66 patients with an average of 5.8 years' follow up. Overall satisfaction was rated as excellent or good by 85%, but 65% were pain free with minor or major footwear restrictions. Major activity restrictions following surgery were uncommon. Subjective numbness was present but variable in pattern in half the patients' feet. The numbness was bothersome in 4 of 71 feet. Patients with bilateral neuroma excision or adjacent neuroma resection had a slightly lower level of satisfaction, but this difference was not significant.

Giannini et al[19] reported on 60 patients (three bilateral) who were treated with excision of interdigital neuroma. The clinical results were excellent or good in 49 (78%) feet, fair in 12 (19%), and poor in two (3%). Of these patients, 62% had normal sensation and no paresthesias and the remaining 38% had numbness; 57% had no difficulty with footwear and 40% had some limitation.

Benedetti et al[6] reported on fifteen patients (19 feet) who underwent simultaneous surgical excision of two primary interdigital neuromas in adjacent web spaces with an average follow-up of 68.6 months. Ten feet (53%) had complete resolution of symptoms, six feet (31%) had minimal residual symptoms, and three feet in two patients (16%) continued to have significant pain. The authors reported a dense sensory loss of the plantar aspect of the third metatarsal head to the tip of the third toe and proximal dorsal sensory loss to the second, third, and fourth toes. Although the numbness did not cause disability, the patients reported some awkwardness with nail care.

Hort and DeOrio[26] described another approach for adjacent web space neuralgia using a single incision with excision of one nerve and release of the adjacent nerve. Twenty-three patients were studied with a mean follow-up of 11 months. Of the patients, 19 (90%) had resolution of all or most of their pain, 20 (95%) had no or only minimal activity limitation, and 20 (95%) were completely satisfied with their outcome. Of 19 patients examined, none had pain with compression of the interspace of the excised nerve, although two (11%) had discomfort with compression of the interspace of the nerve that was only released.

Stamatis and Myerson[48] reported on re-exploration in 60 interspaces (49 patients, 49 feet) for recurrence or persistent symptoms after one or more previous procedures for excision of an interdigital neuroma with an average follow-up of 39.7 months. Ten patients had a simultaneous excision of an adjacent primary neuroma and 19 underwent additional forefoot surgery. Fifteen patients (30.7%) were completely satisfied, 13 (26.5%) were satisfied with minor reservations, ten (20.4%) were satisfied with major reservations, and 11 (22.4%) were dissatisfied with the outcome. Twenty-nine (59.2%) had moderate or severe restriction of footwear and eight (16.3%) had moderate restriction of activity after revision surgery.

A few complications deserve mention. In cases where patients had multiple steroid shots followed by surgery, there is an additional risk of wound complications such as delayed healing or infection. When adjacent web space neuromas have been resected, the loss of sensation in the tip of the middle toe possibly coupled with some vascular compromise can increase the risk of frostbite in the winter. Stress fracture or damage to the MTP capsule can occur if the retraction is too vigorous or the tissue or bone is incompetent. Rarely a patient can develop complex pain syndrome type 2 (causalgia) following a neuroma resection.

PLANTAR INCISION FOR RESECTION OF THE ATYPICAL NEUROMA

When the patient has a very proximal focal tender trigger point for the neuralgia, one of us (LCS) uses a transverse approach proximal to the metatarsal plantar fat. This permits a more direct exposure of the nerve that lies plantar to the intermetatarsal ligament and just beneath the plantar fascia and next to the flexor digitorum tendon. It allows the nerve resection to be performed off of the weight-bearing surface of the forefoot as well as resection more proximal to the level of the transverse metatarsal ligament. It permits identification of anomalous nerve branches that can anastomose with the site of the neuroma and provides for easier access to adjacent digital nerves with minimal dissection through soft tissues. Finally, there is a better ability to avoid the artery and vein, which is advantageous for patients with vascular compromise. Disadvantages primarily are the potential for development of painful plantar scars or plantar keratosis.

There are two types of incisions: transverse and longitudinal. Transverse incision permits greater exposure for multiple nerve dissections. Transverse incision made 1 cm proximal to the weight-bearing region allows for exposure of the adjacent interdigital nerve. It also facilitates identification of accessory or aberrant nerve branches. Avoidance of the artery, vein, and tendon is easier because the dissection is proximal to where these structures are more intermingled. The incision is within the skin fold lines, making the scar cosmetic and well tolerated. Because the exposure is proximal to the disease, the surgeon must be comfortable that nothing in the web space requires resection. Some experience is necessary to be comfortable with this approach and the orientation. The longitudinal incision is also reported to be cosmetic because it runs parallel to the lines of the connective tissue fibers. It can be continued distally between the metatarsal heads or proximally into the midfoot or hindfoot. This permits identification and resection of distal disease as well as higher transection with or without nerve burial (transposition).

Surgical Technique: Transverse Approach

1. The incision should be made 1 cm proximal to the weight-bearing area of the metatarsal heads (Fig. 11–22).
2. Dissection should be performed straight down through the subcutaneous fat and then immediately through the plantar fascia to avoid creating soft-tissue planes.
3. The interdigitial nerve will be exposed immediately deep to the plantar fascia within the fatty tissue between the flexor digitorum longus tendons.
4. Aberrant or accessory nerve branches can be identified in this area.
5. The nerve can be transected proximally.
6. Adjacent interdigital neuromas can be approached by widening the incision (Fig. 11–23).
7. The wound is closed with 4-0 nylon suture.
8. A compression dressing is applied for 10 to 14 days until sutures are removed.
9. A wrap is recommended for 1 to 2 more weeks as the patient is allowed to progress with weight bearing.

Surgical Technique: Longitudinal Approach

1. The incision should be centered directly over the intermetatarsal space so that any subsequent scarring will not take place directly under the metatarsal head. Typically the incision should be made approximately 1 to 2 cm proximal to the proximal end of the metatarsal head.
2. Dissection should be performed straight down through the subcutaneous fat and then

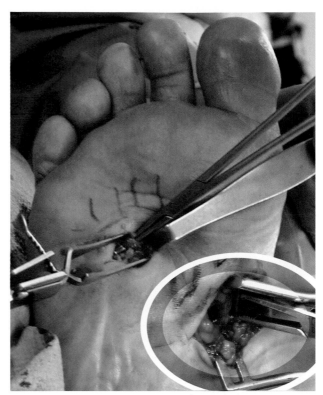

Figure 11–22 A transverse incision is made 1 cm proximal to the weight-bearing area of the metatarsal heads. The plantar fascia is cut, and the hemostat is used to spread between the long flexor tendons. As the hemostat is spread, the nerve is apparent as demonstrated in the *inset*.

immediately through the plantar fascia to avoid creating soft-tissue planes.
3. The interdigitial nerve will be exposed immediately deep to the plantar fascia within the fatty tissue between the flexor digitorum longus tendons (Fig. 11–24).
4. Aberrant or accessory nerve branches can be identified in this area.
5. The nerve can be transected as proximally as possible or kept slightly longer to permit transposition into muscle (Fig. 11–25).
6. When a transposition is performed, the end of the transected nerve's epineurium can be held with a 4-0 Vicryl suture. The suture is fed through a straight needle (Keith needle), and the needle is passed through muscles between the metatarsal. It then penetrates the dorsum of the foot. With the nerve end within the muscle belly, the suture can be tied on the dorsum to help keep the nerve in place during the first 10 to 14 days.

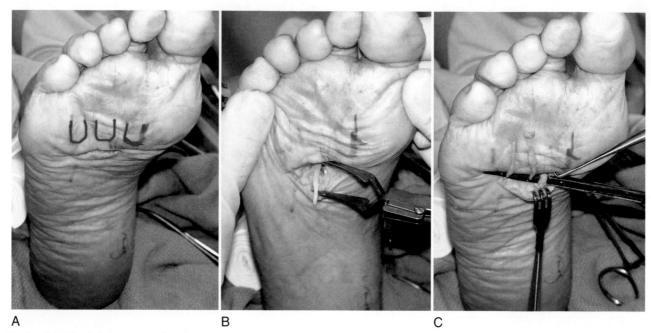

A   B   C

Figure 11–23   Adjacent interdigital neuroma can be approached by widening the incision. **A,** The incision is made 1 cm proximal to the metatarsal heads. **B,** A thin second web space nerve is found distally traveling underneath the third metatarsal head. **C,** The third web space nerve is found going between the third and fourth metatarsal heads. With further dissection in the second web space, a larger nerve is found traveling between the second and third metatarsal heads.

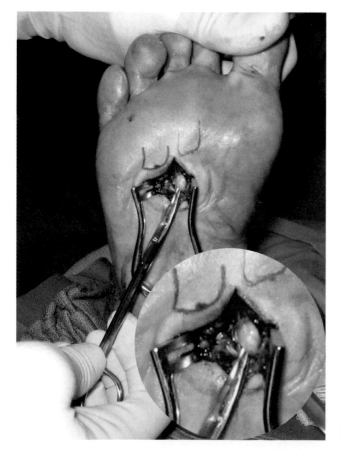

Figure 11–24   The plantar longitudinal incision is made over the intermetatarsal space so that any subsequent scarring will not take place directly under the metatarsals. *Inset,* the bulbous neuroma.

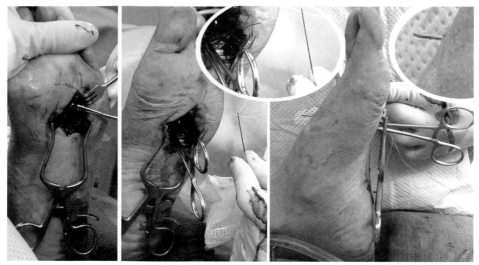

Figure 11–25 This patient had a recurrent neuroma and a history of a postoperative infection and complex regional pain syndrome type II. The nerve is transected more proximally in this operation *(left)*. The transected nerve's epineurium can be held with a 4-0 Vicryl suture. The suture is fed through a straight needle (Keith needle) *(center; inset* shows close-up). The needle is passed through muscles between the metatarsals and out the dorsum of the foot *(right; inset* shows close-up of dorsum). The suture is loosely tied on the dorsum to help keep the nerve ending in place within the muscles. This dorsal suture is removed in 10 to 14 days.

7. The wound is closed with 4-0 nylon suture.
8. A compression dressing is applied for 10 to 14 days until sutures are removed.
9. A wrap is recommended for 1 to 2 more weeks as the patient is allowed to progress with weight bearing.

NEUROLYSIS OF THE COMMON DIGITAL NERVE AND ITS TERMINAL BRANCHES

The notion that an interdigital neuroma is caused by entrapment of the plantar digital nerve by the intermetatarsal ligament and bursa was initially discussed by Gauthier.[18] Okafor et al[39] also believed that it was a nerve entrapment and recommended neurolysis of the interdigital nerve 1 cm distal to the transverse metatarsal ligament and 3 cm proximal to it. Several other reports have discussed the techniques and outcomes of either an open or endoscopic release of the nerve. Further middle-term and long-term studies are needed to determine the results and the best candidates for these procedures.[4,15,35,44,46]

Surgical Technique

1. With or without tourniquet control, an incision is made in the web space and carried proximally approximately 3 cm. It is important that the incision is made in the midline to avoid cutting one of the dorsal digital branches, which could result in a painful neuroma.
2. The incision is deepened through the soft tissues to the level of the metatarsal heads. A Weitlaner retractor or laminar spreader is placed between the metatarsal heads to spread them apart; this places the transverse metatarsal ligament under tension.
3. Using a neurologic Freer elevator to dissect out the contents of the interspace, the surgeon identifies and transects the transverse metatarsal ligament.
4. The retractor is removed and set deeper between the metatarsal heads and spread. This permits the surgeon to visualize the contents of the web space. A neurologic Freer elevator is used to identify the common digital nerve in the proximal portion of the wound and trace it distally to its bifurcation.
5. At this point, a neurolysis is performed, first by carefully excising any bursal material that may be present about the bifurcation of the common digital nerve. The presence of bursal material proximal to the transverse metatarsal ligament is rare. Then any adhesions between the nerve and the surrounding tissues are carefully released. Caution is necessary, because plantar-directed nerve branches pass from the plantar aspect of the

nerve into the tissue on the bottom of the foot.[2] Transection of these nerves can result in a painful plantar neuroma.

6. Once the nerve is freed from approximately 3 cm proximal to the intermetatarsal ligament and 1 cm distal to it, an adequate dissection has been achieved. If the nerve is inadvertently damaged during dissection, it should be excised in the usual manner as far proximal to the metatarsal heads as possible, dissected distally, and removed at the level of the bifurcation.

7. The wound is closed in a routine manner with interrupted nylon sutures.

8. A sterile compression dressing is applied, and the foot is kept wrapped for a period of 2 to 3 weeks to allow the soft tissues to heal.

9. After 3 weeks the patient can progressively increase the level of activities.

Results

In describing their results in a series of 35 patients, Okafor et al[39] noted that if the patient had no foot disorder other than the interdigital neuroma, 13 (72%) of 18 patients noted 100% relief of symptoms after neurolysis. If the patient had a common foot disorder such as a hallux valgus or hammer toe, 5 (30%) of 17 had complete relief and 12 (70%) of 17 still had some symptoms. In 20 of their patients who underwent a lidocaine (Xylocaine) block before surgery with complete relief, 15 (75%) of 20 patients noted complete relief postoperatively, and 5 (25%) of 20 had significant relief.

RECURRENT NEUROMAS

Recurrent symptoms after resection of an interdigital neuroma are very disheartening for both the patient and the surgeon. In a review of 39 patients with recurrent neuromas, Beskin and Baxter[3] noted that two thirds had symptoms within 12 months of the original surgery and one third had symptoms 1 to 4 years after the initial surgery. The problem of a recurrent neuroma may be viewed in two ways. Patients in whom the clinical picture is similar to an interdigital neuroma, but unfortunately is not, and who continue to have symptoms in the foot after the initial surgery probably represent the two thirds of the patients noted by Beskin and Baxter[7] who had recurrence of their symptoms within 12 months of the original surgery. In most the initial symptoms probably never subside.

In the second group of patients, the symptoms are caused by the bulb neuroma that forms at the end of the common digital nerve. In most cases it probably takes at least a year or more for the neuroma to be of sufficient size for symptoms to develop. This probably represents the one third of the patients in the series who had symptoms 1 to 4 years after the initial surgery. The recurrent neuroma could develop because the resection of the nerve initially was not sufficiently proximal to the metatarsal head. Then a neuroma formed beneath the metatarsal head, possibly because of an aberrant branch, as noted earlier, and in some cases for reasons that are not understood.

In discussing an anatomic basis for a recurrent neuroma, Amis et al[2] noted that plantar-directed nerve branches tether the common digital nerve to the plantar skin. These branches are concentrated about the bifurcation of the proper digital nerve, and therefore the cut end of the nerve can fail to retract. The authors observed that no plantar branches occurred 4 cm proximal to the transverse metatarsal ligament. Therefore an effort should be made to cut the nerve 4 cm proximal to the transverse metatarsal ligament to ensure that the nerve adequately retracts. Another way to ensure that the nerve will retract is to dorsiflex the ankle joint after the nerve has been transected, thereby pulling the nerve into a more proximal position. The surgical site can be examined to see whether the nerve has indeed retracted, and if not, the more proximal resection can be considered.

In approximately three fourths of patients with a recurrent neuroma, the cause is either inadequate resection of the nerve or the formation of an adherent neuroma beneath a metatarsal head.

Johnson et al[27] reviewed a series of 39 patients with recurrent interdigital neuroma. In 67% of cases they observed a retained primary interdigital neuroma because it was not adequately resected initially, and in 33% a true amputation stump neuroma was the cause of the recurrent symptoms.

Clinical Symptoms

The main symptom of patients with a recurrent neuroma is pain on the plantar aspect of the foot. The pain may be similar to the initial preoperative pain, or an extremely painful area can develop that, when stepped on, causes significant electric-like pain. The symptom complex is aggravated by activity and diminished by rest.

Some patients who have persistent pain after excision of a neuroma report that the pain is almost identical to what they experienced before their initial surgery. Other patients note that the new pain is different, well localized, and electric-like in quality.

Diagnosis

Physical examination in this group of patients must be carefully performed in the same manner as that for a primary neuroma. The MTP joints should be carefully palpated to look for other disorders, along with careful palpation of the web spaces. As a general rule, the patient with a recurrent neuroma demonstrates a well-localized area of tenderness, usually either beneath a metatarsal head or just adjacent to it. When this area is palpated by the examiner, it usually elicits a significant electric-like pain, and the patient states that this is similar to the symptomatic pain.

At times the pain is along the medial or lateral aspect of a metatarsal head and can represent either a stump neuroma that has become adherent to the metatarsal head or possibly an accessory branch that sometimes passes obliquely beneath the metatarsal head. It is possible that the recurrent symptoms represent an activated adjacent web space neuroma. This can be confusing to both the surgeon and the patient based on symptoms and findings and can require a nerve block for final distinction. Unfortunately, response to a nerve block is helpful but not reliably conclusive. Rarely the neuritic symptoms are coming from a damaged dorsal nerve branch.

Patients who have well-localized findings and demonstrate a Tinel sign in a small area usually respond best to repeat surgery. The response to the diagnostic block is also helpful to predict a success. After the physical examination, a radiographic study of the foot should be obtained to look for any osseous pathologic conditions or changes around the MTP joints.

The differential diagnosis presented for a virgin interdigital neuroma should be once again considered in a patient with a recurrent neuroma. Careful examination of the posterior tibial nerve and its terminal branches should be carried out to rule out a tarsal tunnel syndrome as the cause of the recurrent symptoms. One of us (LCS) has seen several patients with growing or recurrent neurilemomas or ganglions involving the tibial nerve or its branches that were thought to be forefoot neuromas that were mistaken for recurrent neuromas.

Treatment

Conservative Treatment

Conservative management of recurrent neuroma is similar to that for the virgin neuroma. The patient should wear a broad-toed, soft-soled, laced shoe with a soft metatarsal support to relieve pressure on the metatarsal head region and interspace. The medications to help diminish nerve excitation (e.g., tricyclic antidepressants, antiepilepsy medications) discussed under the conservative treatment of interdigital neuromas deserve more consideration here because a subgroup of these patients have severe symptoms and underlying nerve sensitivity. If conservative measures fail and the symptoms persist, reexploration of the interspace may be indicated.

Occasionally the use of a transcutaneous nerve stimulator or ultrasound is useful in helping to break up the patient's pain pattern. These modalities are useful in only about 10% to 20% of cases but merit a try.

Surgical Excision

Before reexploration of an interspace, the foot should be carefully examined to attempt to localize the neuroma as accurately as possible. This helps to direct the surgeon to the area where the patient experiences maximum pain and sometimes can save needless searching in the interspace.

The question arises at times as to whether the recurrent neuroma should be explored from a plantar or a dorsal approach. The web space can be adequately explored from a dorsal approach, although the incision must be extended proximally slightly more (1 cm) than when removing a virgin neuroma. Advocates of a plantar approach to a recurrent neuroma believe that the neuroma should be approached through a longitudinal plantar incision centered between the metatarsal heads and the nerve identified and resected proximally to the metatarsal head. They point out that it is easier to find the nerve in most cases.

The other school of thought is that because so much scarring is present around the area where the nerve had been previously excised, it is better to approach the common digital nerve proximal to the metatarsal heads and section the nerve in this region without exploring the interspace distally. In a study with this approach, 86% of 39 patients obtained significant improvement of 50% of their discomfort, but fewer than half the patients were completely symptom free. Fifty-eight percent had difficulty wearing certain shoes, and 88% had discomfort in high heels.[3]

An analysis of seven patients with 11 recurrent neuromas excised through a dorsal incision demonstrated that 81% of the patients were essentially asymptomatic, 9% had marginal improvement, and 9% had no improvement. Bradley et al[11] noted that only two of eight patients had improvement after surgery.

Wolfort and Dellon[53] reported their results with 17 recurrent neuromas in 13 patients. At a mean of 33.8 months, 80% had excellent relief with a plantar longitudinal approach and implantation of the nerve ending into muscle. The authors also identified deficits along the tibial nerve territory by quantitative sensory exam in 54% of their patients.

Colgrove et al[12] performed a prospective, randomized study comparing the treatment of an interdigital neuroma by the standard resection operation with a transection distal to the neuroma and transposition into muscle. The follow-up was by blinded telephone interview. In the resection group, the average pain level was slightly lower through the first 6-month period, but at the 12-month review the resection group had a slightly higher average pain level . At the 36- to 48-month review the resection group again reported a greater average pain level and fewer asymptomatic patients. The authors concluded that it is unnecessary to excise the interdigital neuroma to obtain excellent relief of pain. They also concluded that intermuscular transposition of the neuroma produced significantly better long-term results than did the standard resection operation.

Overall, reexploration for a recurrent neuroma through either a dorsal or a plantar incision results in less than complete satisfaction in 20% to 40% of cases. This fact should be very carefully explained to the patient before surgery.

Because choosing the approach can present a dilemma for the surgeon, we recommend primarily proceeding with the technique that is most familiar. If there is no bias based on experience, we suggest the following algorithm that is based on whether the primary neuroma excision was sufficiently proximal and whether there is an adjacent neuralgia. If there is a small dorsal incision, it is possible that the resection was not adequate and a repeat transection can be made through a longer dorsal incision. If there is an adjacent neuralgia in this scenario, either a release or resection is performed via the dorsal approach. If the incision was long enough or the primary surgeon felt that the nerve was taken back sufficiently, then a plantar approach is considered. If there is an adjacent primary neuroma as well, then a plantar transverse approach is to be considered. If the same nerve is the site of the recurrent neuroma, then a plantar longitudinal incision can permit a more proximal transection and burial.

EXCISION OF RECURRENT NEUROMA

Surgical Technique

1. The skin incision is made in the dorsal aspect of the web space, usually passing through the previous scar for a distance of 4 cm. If there is evidence of entrapment of a superficial nerve adjacent to the scar, an attempt should be made to identify it and excise it. The incision is carried down through the scar tissue in the web space by staying as much in the midline as possible.
2. A Weitlaner retractor is placed between the two metatarsals to pry them apart. In a recurrent neuroma this is sometimes difficult to do until the dissection has been carried down through the transverse metatarsal ligament. A neurologic Freer elevator usually can be used to break up the scar tissue between the two metatarsals to identify the transverse metatarsal ligament.
3. Although the transverse metatarsal ligament might have been transected initially, it almost invariably re-forms and needs to be identified and sectioned again.
4. After the transverse metatarsal ligament is cut, the Weitlaner retractor should be reinserted more plantarward and is used to separate the metatarsal heads. If the metatarsal heads cannot be adequately separated, a portion of the transverse metatarsal ligament is still intact or some dense scar tissue has not been transected.
5. By using a neurologic Freer elevator and starting as proximal as possible in the wound, preferably in tissue that was not previously involved, one can identify the common digital nerve. As mentioned, before surgery the examination should reveal the approximate location of the neuroma, and this is very helpful at surgery. Occasionally, if the nerve cannot be identified, the skin incision is extended proximally another centimeter, and more tissue is separated in the web space to enhance the exposure. On rare occasions a Gelpi retractor is used to gain greater access to the web space.
6. Careful dissection allows the common digital nerve to the web space to be identified and traced distally. Once this is accomplished and the tip of the nerve is excised from the surrounding scar tissue, the nerve is cut as far proximal to the metatarsal head as possible.
7. The ankle is dorsiflexed to help pull the nerve more proximally into the foot.
8. The skin is closed with interrupted sutures and a compression dressing is applied.

For recurrent neuroma from a plantar transverse or longitudinal approach, please see techniques under the heading for a primary resection.

Postoperative Care

Postoperative management consists of re-dressing the foot in 18 to 24 hours with a firm compression dressing. The foot is kept dressed for 3 weeks, during which time the patient ambulates in a postoperative shoe. After 3 weeks the shoe is removed and the patient is started on active and passive range-of-motion exercises; the level of activity is progressively increased as tolerated. Running is restricted for approximately 2 months after excision of a recurrent neuroma to permit adequate healing to occur.

Uncommon Findings

Occasionally, reexploration of the web space reveals a quantity of thick, bursa-like material that requires excision. This material usually lies dorsal to the transverse metatarsal ligament. When the web space is explored, dense scar tissue is present about the end of the nerve, but proximal to this the nerve appears to be almost normal. When the muscle wraps itself around the end of the nerve, identification of the nerve requires meticulous dissection of the tissues to locate it.

TARSAL TUNNEL SYNDROME

The tarsal tunnel syndrome is an entrapment neuropathy involving the posterior tibial nerve within the tarsal canal or one of its terminal branches after the nerve leaves the tarsal canal. The earliest description of the syndrome was by Kopell and Thompson[72] in 1960, and it was named "tarsal tunnel syndrome" by Keck[68] in 1962 and Lam[74] in 1967. The condition is somewhat analogous to the carpal tunnel syndrome in the wrist, but it occurs much less often.

The tarsal canal is located behind the medial malleolus, and it becomes the tarsal tunnel as a result of the flexor retinaculum's passing over the structures and creating a closed space. The tarsal tunnel is a fibro-osseous structure created by the tibia anteriorly and the posterior process of the talus and calcaneus laterally. The flexor retinaculum that creates the tarsal tunnel is intimately attached to the sheaths of the posterior tibial, flexor hallucis, and flexor digitorum longus tendons (Fig. 11-26).

The posterior tibial nerve, which is a branch of the sciatic nerve, enters the canal proximally, and in 93% of cases the nerve branches into its three terminal branches—medial plantar nerve, lateral plantar nerve, and medial calcaneal nerve within the tunnel. The medial calcaneal nerve arises off the posterior aspect of the posterior tibial nerve about 75% of the time and off the LPN about 25%. It is a single branch in 79% of specimens and multiple branches in 21%. The calcaneal branches originate proximal to the tarsal tunnel in 39% of cases, within the tunnel in 34%, and distal to the tunnel in 16%.[66]

In another study, Davis and Schon[60] confirmed that the tibial nerve bifurcates within 2 cm of the medial malleolar calcaneal axis in 90% of cadaveric specimens (Fig. 11-27). In contrast to Havel's study,[66] they found 60% had multiple calcaneal nerve branches and 20% of specimens had aberrant innervation of the abductor hallucis muscle. Dellon et al [62] confirmed this finding in a study of the calcaneal nerve as observed during 85 tarsal tunnel releases. In this report 37% of feet had one calcaneal nerve, 41% had two, 19% had three, and 3% had four. They found that the MPN gave origin to a calcaneal nerve in 46% of feet. The topographic anatomy of the nerve is also useful to help understand the position of the various branches before they ramify. This helps to localize damaged nerve fascicles within the trunk of the nerve.[77]

In approximately 60% of patients with tarsal tunnel syndrome, a specific cause could be identified.[78] Some were associated with a significant specific injury, such as a severe ankle sprain, crush injury, fracture of the distal end of the tibia, dislocation of the ankle, or calcaneal fracture, and others were caused by a space-occupying lesion, such as lipoma, varicosities, ganglion, synovial cyst, or exostosis. In a review of 24 reports in the literature, Cimino[58] noted that a specific cause could be identified in about 80% of patients with a tarsal tunnel syndrome (Table 11-2).

TABLE 11-2

Causes of Tarsal Tunnel Syndrome Presented in the Literature: Summary of 24 Reports

Causes	Cases
Idiopathic	25
Traumatic	21
Varicosities	16*
Heel varus	14
Fibrosis	11
Heel valgus	10
Ganglion	3
Diabetes	3
Obesity	3
Tight tarsal canal	3
Hypertrophic abductor hallucis	3
Rheumatoid arthritis	3
Lipoma	2
Anomalous artery	1
Acromegaly	1
Ankylosing spondylitis	1
Regional migratory osteoporosis	1
Flexor digitorum accessorius longus	1
SUBTOTAL	122
Causes not reported	64
TOTAL	186

*Represents 14% of the cases.
From Cimino WR: *Foot Ankle* 11:47-52, 1990.

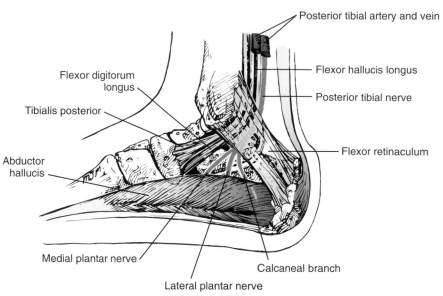

Posterior tibial artery and vein

Flexor hallucis longus

Posterior tibial nerve

Flexor digitorum longus

Tibialis posterior

Flexor retinaculum

Abductor hallucis

Medial plantar nerve

Calcaneal branch

Lateral plantar nerve

A

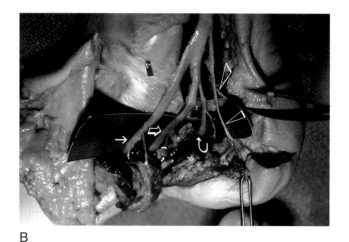

B

Figure 11-26 A, The schematic anatomy of the tibial nerve. **B,** An anatomic dissection of the tibial nerve and its branches demonstrates the medial plantar nerve *(solid arrow)*, the lateral plantar nerve *(open arrow)*, the first branch of the lateral plantar nerve *(curved arrow)*, and the calcaneal nerve *(open triangular arrows)*.

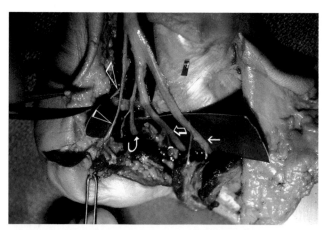

Figure 11-27 The tibial nerve is shown with its branches. The *triangular arrows* indicate the calcaneal branches, the *curved arrow* indicates the first branch of the lateral plantar nerve, the *open arrow* indicates the lateral plantar nerve, and the *solid arrow* indicates the medial plantar nerve.

Certain local causes can result in a tarsal tunnel syndrome and include the following:

• Ganglion of one of the tendon sheaths passing adjacent to the tarsal canal or one of the terminal branches of the posterior tibial nerve (Fig. 11-28).

• Lipoma within the tarsal canal exerting pressure against the posterior tibial nerve.

• Exostosis or fracture fragment from the distal end of the tibia or calcaneus.

• Medial talocalcaneal bar that protrudes into the inferior aspect of the tarsal canal (Fig. 11-29).

• Enlarged venous complex surrounding the posterior tibial nerve within the tarsal canal.

• Neurilemoma of the posterior tibial nerve within the tarsal canal (Fig. 11-30).

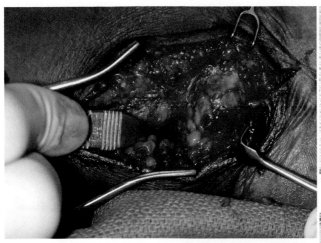

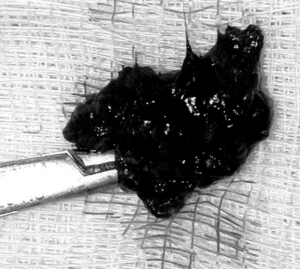

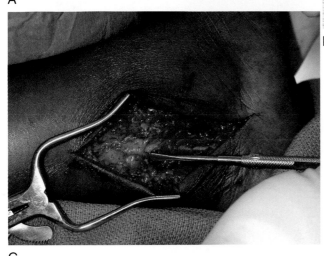

Figure 11–28 **A,** A large ganglion is noted posterior and deep to the tibial nerve. **B,** The ganglion has been removed. **C,** The tibial nerve is shown after removal but before a proximal release of the tarsal tunnel.

- Severe pronation of the hindfoot that results in stretching or compressing of the posterior tibial nerve.
- Accessory muscle within the tarsal tunnel, such as an accessory soleus or accessory flexor digitorum longus (Fig. 11–31).

The role of postural deformities or mechanical abnormalities in tarsal tunnel syndrome should not be underestimated. A study of 56 feet in 28 patients with pes planus showed abnormalities in their electrodiagnostic tests.[57] Treppman et al[88] demonstrated increased pressures in the tarsal tunnel with inversion or eversion. Daniels et al[59] demonstrated increased tibial nerve tension in an unstable foot versus a stable one in eversion, dorsiflexion, and cyclical load. Lau and Daniels[75] demonstrated that tibial nerve tension was increased after a tarsal tunnel release during eversion, dorsiflexion–eversion, and cyclical load in the unstable versus the stable foot. This supported the notion that structural deformity plays a critical role in resolving tarsal tunnel syndrome in an unstable foot.

Labib et al[73] reported on the combination of plantar fasciitis, posterior tibial tendon dysfunction, and tarsal tunnel syndrome in 14 patients. They postulated that the failure of the fascia and posterior tibial tendon resulted in traction on the tibial nerve. In their series, 12 of 14 patients responded to tarsal tunnel and plantar fascia release in conjunction with correction of the hindfoot deformity. Hindfoot correction included hindfoot fusion, medial displacement osteotomy of the calcaneus, and/or tendon transfer. We have often noted that when patients with tibial neuralgia and structural deformity undergo surgical correction of the malalignments, their neuritic symptoms improve or totally resolve.

Clinical Symptoms

Whereas the patient with an interdigital neuroma is usually able to localize the area of maximum

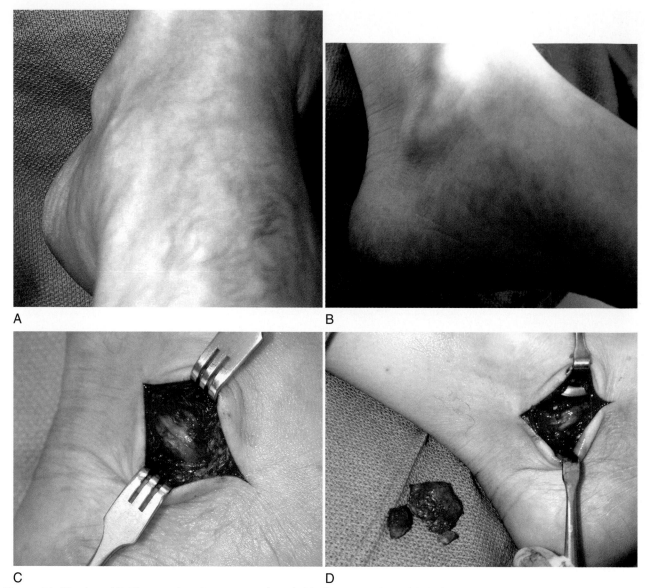

Figure 11–29   A and **B,** The tarsal coalition created medial bulk against the medial plantar nerve (MPN) and gave this patient tarsal tunnel symptoms. **C,** The coalition is approached and the MPN and flexor digitorum longus tendons are exposed. **D,** The medial talocalcaneal coalition is resected, decompressing the nerve.

tenderness on the plantar aspect of the foot, the patient with a tarsal tunnel syndrome usually has difficulty describing the nature of the pain. When questioned, however, the patient usually states that the pain is diffuse on the plantar aspect of the foot and at the medial ankle. The pain is characterized as a burning, shooting, searing, electric, shocking, stabbing, tingling, numbing type that is usually aggravated by activities on the feet and relieved by rest. However, certain patients report that the pain is worse in bed at night and they actually obtain relief by arising and moving around. About a third of the patients with

tarsal tunnel syndrome note proximal radiation of pain along the medial aspect of the leg to the midcalf region (Valleix's phenomenon).

As with all the nerve disorders, the type of activity and the specific movements or positions that exacerbate the pain should be identified. Any history of systemic disorders that can affect nerves must be noted (e.g., rheumatologic disorders, Lyme disease, diabetes, thyroid disease). A review of medications, chemical exposure, alcohol abuse, or low back pain with radiculopathy should be documented to rule out other nonfocal causes of tibial neuralgia.

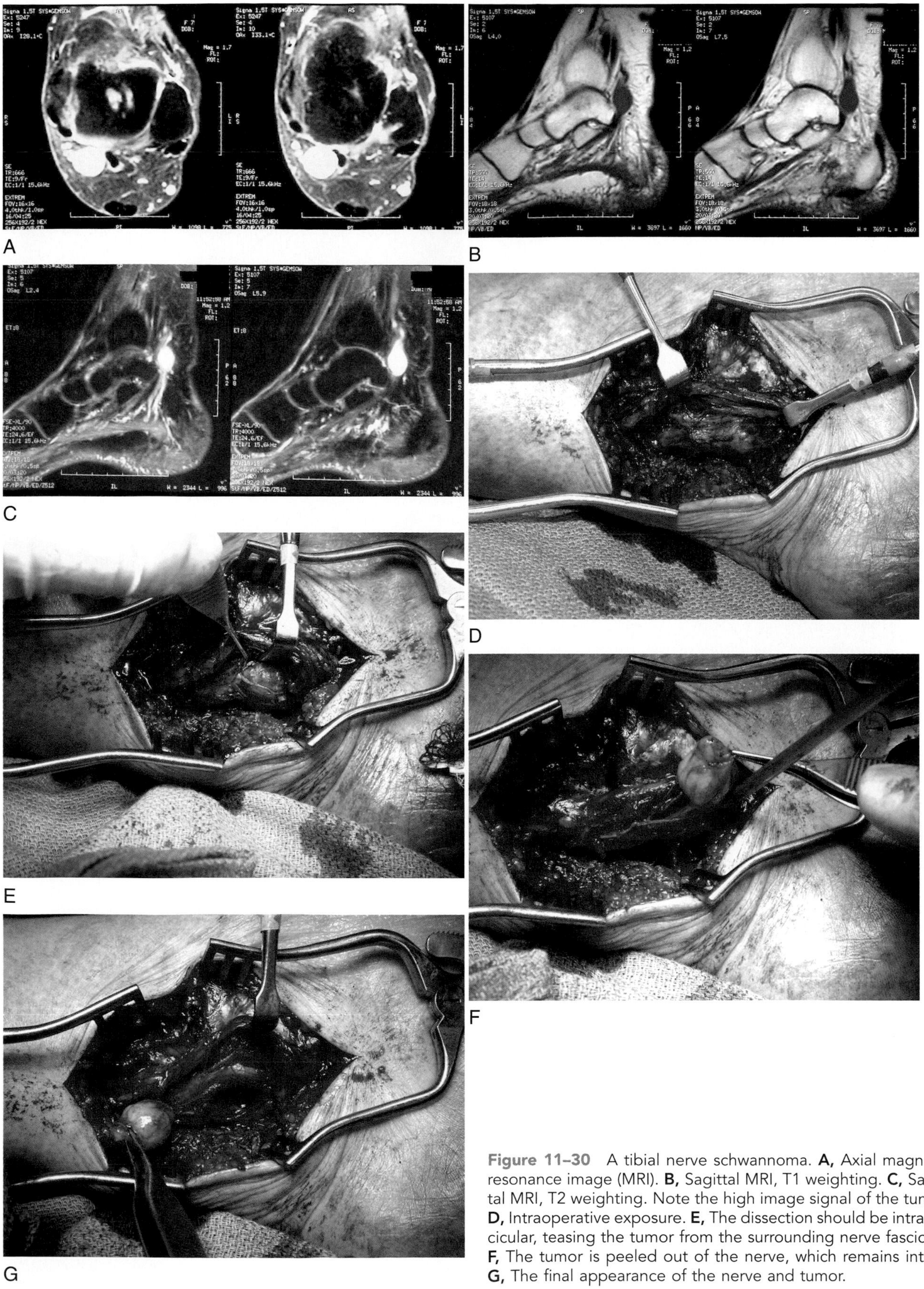

Figure 11–30 A tibial nerve schwannoma. **A,** Axial magnetic resonance image (MRI). **B,** Sagittal MRI, T1 weighting. **C,** Sagittal MRI, T2 weighting. Note the high image signal of the tumor. **D,** Intraoperative exposure. **E,** The dissection should be intrafascicular, teasing the tumor from the surrounding nerve fascicles. **F,** The tumor is peeled out of the nerve, which remains intact. **G,** The final appearance of the nerve and tumor.

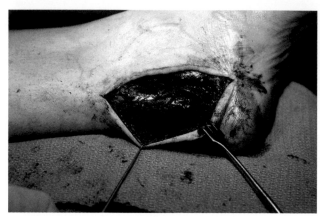

Figure 11–31 An accessory soleus is encountered during this tarsal tunnel release. A small calcaneal nerve branch is seen coursing over the muscle mass, explaining the patient's neuritic heel pain.

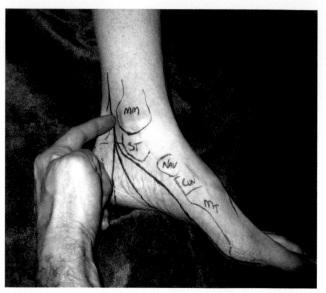

Figure 11–32 The tibial nerve and its branches are palpated and percussed.

Diagnosis

Physical Examination

The physician begins the physical examination by having the patient stand and observing the overall posture of the foot. Any significant varus or valgus deformity of the hindfoot should be noted. Claw toe deformities or intrinsic wasting can indicate advanced nerve compromise. The range of motion of the ankle, subtalar, and transverse tarsal joints is observed next to detect any restriction of motion that can indicate a previous injury, coalition, or possibly arthrosis. The posterior tibial tendon function should be carefully tested with a side-to-side comparison of inversion power across the midline from the neutral position and from the abducted position. Watching the patient walk can also be revealing of subtle weaknesses, malalignments, or neurologic abnormalities. If a specific task brings on the pain, observing the patient performing that movement or simulating the provocative stresses can be helpful.

The entire course of the posterior tibial nerve is percussed, starting proximal to the tarsal tunnel and proceeding distally along its terminal branches to look for evidence of irritability of the nerve, as manifested by tingling or discomfort (Fig. 11–32). Percussion over the area of the entrapment can cause radiation of pain along the distribution of the medial or lateral plantar nerve. After percussion of the nerve, the nerve and its terminal branches should be carefully palpated to look for evidence of thickening or swelling, which can indicate a space-occupying lesion such as a ganglion, synovial cyst, or lipoma. On rare occasions, a bony ridge is noted along the course of the posterior tibial nerve.

Sensory examination of the foot is usually not revealing. Although patients often complain of dyses-

thesias and numbness, it is difficult to demonstrate actual areas of numbness on the bottom of the foot. If there is specific involvement of the medial or lateral plantar nerve, occasionally it is possible to detect a sensory loss in the foot. Sensory testing of distal sensory branches using the Semmes–Weinstein monofilaments or two-point discrimination can reveal tibial nerve deficits (Fig. 11–33).

Motor weakness is also difficult to evaluate in such patients. Muscle weakness is difficult to detect, although at times atrophy of the abductor hallucis or abductor digiti quinti muscle may be observed when one foot is compared with the other.

The literature has mentioned that the dysesthesias in the foot can be brought on when the hindfoot is

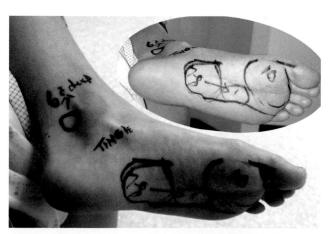

Figure 11–33 The patient had a Tinel sign at the tarsal tunnel in conjunction with severe pain and zones of subtle decreased sensation along the branch of the medial plantar nerve. The numbers indicate the level of pain in that region.

held in an inverted or everted position, but this can be difficult to reproduce. A recent study by Kinoshita et al[71] reported success with a maneuver that passively dorsiflexed the ankle , everted the heel, and dorsiflexed all the toes. In their study, symptoms were induced after a few seconds. They also found tibial nerve tenderness and a positive percussion sign (Tinel's sign).

Radiographic evaluation of the foot and ankle should be obtained to evaluate for stress fractures, fracture sequelae, bone lesions, or arthritis. If a space-occupying lesion is suspected, an MRI scan should be obtained.

Frey and Kerr[63] conducted a study in which 35 feet with suspected tarsal tunnel syndrome were evaluated with MRI. In 88% of patients a pathologic condition was identified. The diagnosis included flexor hallucis longus tenosynovitis (11 cases), dilated veins (9), focal mass (5), fracture or soft-tissue injury (5), fibrous scar tissue (3), posterior tibial tenosynovitis (1), and hypertrophied abductor hallucis muscle (1). Of the 20 patients in this group who had a positive Tinel sign, 17 (85%) had positive MRI findings. These findings included flexor hallucis longus tenosynovitis (7), venous dilation (4), focal mass (3), fibrous scar tissue (2), posterior tibial tenosynovitis (1), and negative scan (3). When an MRI scan of the contralateral limb was obtained in these 20 patients, five (25%) were positive. Three scans demonstrated dilated veins, and two showed flexor hallucis longus tenosynovitis. In the series, 21 patients had surgery, and the MRI finding was confirmed in 19 patients.

Ultrasound has been performed for tarsal tunnel syndrome. In a study by Nagaoka and Matsuaki[79] 17 patients with tarsal tunnel syndrome were evaluated, and the cause of the syndrome was identified and confirmed intraoperatively. The authors reported in their series 10 ganglia, 1 talocalcaneal coalition , 3 talocalcaneal coalitions associated with ganglia, and 3 varicose veins in patients with tarsal tunnel syndrome. Although ultrasound in experienced hands can be useful, we have not found it practical in our centers and prefer MRI for a more detailed analysis of soft tissues, joint and bony abnormalities.

Electrodiagnostic Studies

Electrodiagnostic testing should be performed in all patients to make the diagnosis of a tarsal tunnel syndrome or to rule out other neuropathies or proximal nerve lesions. The specific technique and the relevance of the findings have been debated in the literature.[64,82,83] In general, the electrodiagnostic tests fall into three categories: nerve conduction studies of the medial and lateral plantar nerve, measurement of the amplitude and duration of the motor-evoked potentials and seeking the presence of fibrillation potentials,

and sensory conduction velocities. The conduction velocity of the common peroneal nerve should be obtained to determine whether a peripheral neuropathy is also present.

The terminal latency of the MPN to the abductor hallucis muscle should be less than 6.2 ms, and that of the LPN to the abductor digiti quinti muscle should be less than 7 ms. If the difference in terminal latency to the abductor hallucis and abductor digiti quinti is greater than 1 ms, it can indicate a tarsal tunnel syndrome. Some electromyographers believe that this is one of the less sensitive tests for this study. A study of the motor evoked potentials, which demonstrate a decreased amplitude and increased duration in patients with a tarsal tunnel syndrome, is considered more sensitive than a study of distal motor latencies.[67] When this study is performed, a search for fibrillation potentials should also be conducted. The sensory nerve conduction velocity is probably the most accurate study, although differing views exist as to the ease and reproducibility of these measurements. Proponents of this test believe that the sensitivity is about 90%.[81]

Patel et al[82] recently performed an evidence-based review to evaluate the utility of nerve conduction studies (NCSs) and needle electromyography (EMG) in the diagnosis of tarsal tunnel syndrome. A total of 317 articles published in English from 1965 through April 2002 were reviewed on the basis of six selection criteria. Four articles met inclusion criteria and were considered to meet Class III level of evidence. These papers examined the use of electrodiagnostic studies for the evaluation of patients with clinically suspected tarsal tunnel syndrome and found that NCSs were abnormal in some patients. Sensory NCSs were more likely to be abnormal than motor NCSs, but given the available data, the actual sensitivity and specificity could not be determined. The sensitivity of needle EMG abnormalities could not be determined. NCSs may be useful for confirming the diagnosis of tibial neuropathy at the ankle. The authors concluded that better studies are needed to more definitively evaluate electrodiagnostic techniques in tarsal tunnel syndrome.

It is obvious that the diagnosis of tarsal tunnel syndrome cannot be made solely on the basis of electrodiagnostic results, but these must be correlated with the history given by the patient and with the physical findings.

Differential Diagnosis

Box 11–2 presents the differential diagnosis of the tarsal tunnel syndrome.[90] When making the diagnosis of tarsal tunnel syndrome, the examiner must be alert to many other clinical entities that can mimic this diagnosis. For this reason the diagnosis must be based

---

BOX 11–2   Differential Diagnosis of Tarsal Tunnel Syndrome

REMOTE CAUSES

Interdigital neuroma
Intervertebral disk lesion
Plantar fasciitis
Plantar fibromatosis

INTRANEURAL CAUSES

Peripheral neuritis
Peripheral vascular disease
Diabetic neuropathy
Leprosy
Neurilemoma
Neuroma

EXTRANEURAL CAUSES

Ganglion
Nerve tethering
Fracture (callus, malunion, nonunion, displaced fragment)
Blunt trauma
Valgus hindfoot
Rheumatoid arthritis
Venous varicosities
Tenosynovitis
Ligament constriction
Abductor hallucis origin constriction
Tarsal coalition (middle or posterior facet)
Lipoma

Modified from Wilemon WK: *Orthop Rev* 8:111, 1979.

on a strong history by the patient of neuritic symptoms in the foot in the distribution of the tibial nerve or its branches, or both, definite physical findings as demonstrated by percussion-induced tingling along the posterior tibial nerve or its terminal branches, and supportive NCS. If all three criteria are not met, the examiner should strongly consider a diagnosis other than the tarsal tunnel syndrome. If only one criterion is met, the diagnosis of tarsal tunnel syndrome should be viewed with skepticism. If two of the three criteria are met, the patient is carefully monitored, and if the findings are reproducible, the diagnosis of a tarsal tunnel syndrome may be considered.

Treatment

Conservative Treatment

The conservative management of tarsal tunnel syndrome is based partially on the diagnosis. If a space-occupying lesion is present, one should excise it rather than treating the patient conservatively. If a lesion is not present, conservative management is indicated. Conservative management involves administration of nonsteroidal anti-inflammatory drugs (NSAIDs), oral vitamin B_6 100 mg bid, and tricyclic antidepressants such as imipramine (Tofranil), nortriptyline (Pamolar), desipramine (Norpramin), or amitriptyline (Elavil). Selective serotonin reuptake inhibitors (SSRIs) such as sertraline (Zoloft) and paroxetine (Paxil), other antidepressants such as venlafaxin (Effexor) or duloxetine (Cymbalta), or antiseizure medications such as gabapentin (Neurotin), pregabalin (Lyrica), topiramate (Topomax), or carbamazepine (Tegretol) can also be used.

One of us (LCS) recommends using NSAIDs, vitamin B_6 100 mg bid, and either amitriptyline (starting at 10 or 25 mg at night and gradually increasing to up to 75 mg at night over several months), pregabalin (starting at 75 mg bid and progressing to 150 mg bid over 2 to 3 weeks), or gabapentin (starting at 100 or 300 mg at night and progressing to a tid routine and then increasing the dose to up to 900 mg tid if not effective at the lower dosages). Occasionally narcotic medications are warranted to enhance pain control. The dosing and increases depend on the patient's medical history, symptomatic response, and tolerance of side effects. An orthopaedist who is not comfortable with the nature of the medications, the drug interactions, their risks, or their side effects, should refer the patient to a neurologist, physiatrist, or pain specialist.

Infrequently an injection of a steroid preparation adjacent to the posterior tibial nerve can be helpful. Often, placing the extremity in a stirrup brace, off-the-shelf boot brace, or short-leg walking cast provides relief. If the patient has a postural abnormality, an orthotic device (foot orthosis or ankle–foot orthosis) to hold the foot in the neutral position may be of benefit. If the patient has edema, an elastic stocking may be used to control the swelling. If conservative management fails and the clinical symptoms are of sufficient magnitude, tarsal tunnel release should be considered.

Surgical Treatment

If the patient has a symptomatic identifiable space-occupying lesion involving the tibial nerve, surgical release should include resection of the lesion with care to minimize traumatizing the nerve. When a structural deformity is identified, correction of the deformity should be adequate to resolve the symptoms. At times, the nerve release is required in addition to the realignment procedure.[73] When there is an adjacent pathologic structure that can account for the patient's tarsal tunnel symptoms, addressing the structure (debriding a synovitic tendon, fusing an arthritic joint, reconstructing a fracture malunion or nonunion, resecting a tarsal coalition) can provide relief even without direct tibial nerve release.

When no underlying nonneurologic disease is identified, the tibial nerve release should be performed following reasonable conservative treatment as outlined above. The role of tibial nerve release as well as other concurrent nerve releases for the treatment of diabetic neuropathy has been proposed by Dellon.[55,56,61,76] The indications for this procedure are being confirmed but include decreased sensation in the plantar aspect of the foot as determined by two-point discrimination, the presence of a positive tibial percussion test (Tinel's sign), and pain in the territory of the tibial nerve. The procedure is contraindicated in patients with vascular disease.

Prior to surgery the patient should be advised of the complications of tibial nerve release including but not limited to a lack of response of the symptoms to the release, increased symptoms, numbness dysesthesias, persistent tenderness or paresthesias over the tarsal tunnel, swelling, nerve damage, vascular damage, infection, wound healing problems, difficulty with footwear, and causalgia or complex regional pain syndrome type 2.

TIBIAL NERVE RELEASE

The course of the tibial nerve and its branches should be determined prior to surgery to identify potential compression sites. Careful palpation for focal tender spots or positive percussion signs (Tinel's sign) will help direct the surgeon to areas of disease. Depending on the experience of the surgeon, loupe magnification may be useful. The use of bipolar cautery assists in achieving atraumatic hemostasis.

The procedure can be performed with or without a tourniquet. Placing the patient in a mild Trendelenburg position can assist in maintaining a clear field when the tourniquet is not used. There are several advantages of not using the tourniquet: The artery and veins can be well visualized during the exposure; as the neurovascular structures are released, the surgeon can observe the unrestricted pulsations of the artery and filling of the veins; the vaso nervorum (the small vessels on the nerve) can be observed to determine adequacy of the decompression; and hemostasis can be achieved as the case proceeds, minimizing the search for random surprise bleeders.

Surgical Technique

1. The tarsal tunnel is approached through a curved incision that begins about 10 cm proximal to the tip of the medial malleolus and 2 cm posterior to the posterior margin of the tibia. It is carried distally parallel to the tibia to the level of the medial malleolus and then gently curves distally and plantarward to end at about the level of the talonavicular joint and over the midportion of the abductor hallucis muscle.

2. The incision is deepened through the subcutaneous tissue and fat to expose the flexor retinaculum. All the vessels encountered are carefully identified and cauterized (Fig. 11–34A and video clip 48).

3. The proximal portion of the flexor retinaculum is identified. Usually, the posterior tibial tendon is in its own sheath immediately behind the posterior margin of the tibia, after which the flexor digitorum longus and posterior tibial nerve, artery, and vein are within the next sheath. At times, however, each structure has its own sheath. When the sheath is opened proximally, it should be carefully explored to be sure that it is the sheath containing the posterior tibial nerve. The retinaculum is then carefully released (Fig. 11–34B). Distally around the area of the medial malleolus and distal to it, the retinaculum may be extremely taut and dense. In dissection of this area, a curved clamp should be placed between the retinaculum and the underlying tissues so as not to injure a vital structure inadvertently.

4. Once the retinaculum has been released, again, starting proximally, the posterior tibial nerve is carefully identified by blunt dissection. It is traced distally and through the tarsal tunnel, where branching into the three terminal branches occurs.

5. The MPN is traced distally around the malleolus and is followed along beneath the abductor hallucis until it passes through a fibrous tunnel at the level of the talonavicular joint. As this dissection is carried around the medial malleolus, it may be difficult to follow the nerve, and it is sometimes necessary to identify the nerve distally and trace it back proximally underneath the leash of vessels that is covering it. Infrequently it is necessary to ligate some of the large veins if they are regarded as a factor in compression

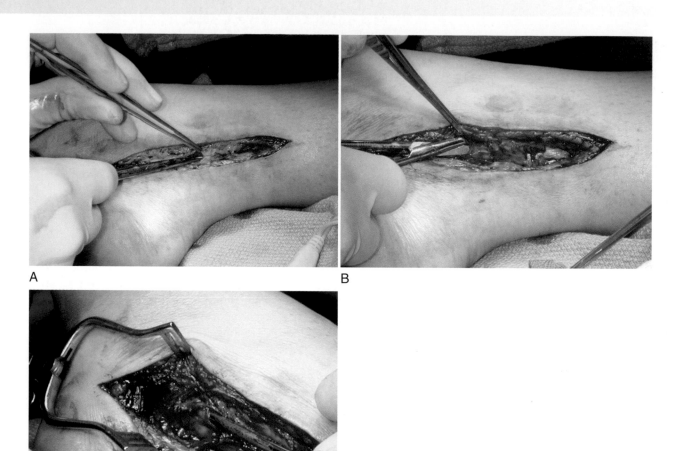

A

B

C

Figure 11–34 A, Tarsal tunnel release exposure of the retinaculum. **B,** The retinaculum is carefully released. **C,** The medial plantar nerve through its fibrous tunnel in the abductor hallucis should be observed and released.

of the nerve. The passage of the MPN through its fibrous tunnel in the abductor hallucis should be observed, and the nerve should be released (Fig. 11–34C).

6. The LPN is traced distally by blunt dissection as it passes distal to the medial malleolar calcaneal axis (a line that can be drawn between the tip of the medial malleolus and the posterior inferior aspect of the heel); it may be difficult to trace due to local vessels. The nerve can be identified more distally at the edge of the abductor hallucis. The superficial fascia over the muscle is released, and either the muscle is reflected inferiorly or a portion of the dorsal half of the origin from the calcaneus is taken down. This exposes the deep fascia of the abductor, which can then be released. This fascia has a concave orientation and can readily compress the nerve here.

7. The first branch of the LPN is a posterior branch off the LPN that runs to the inferior aspect of the calcaneus just dorsal to the location of the typical plantar heel spur. Because it has a separate compartment distinct from the LPN, it should be released by sectioning the deep fascia of the abductor muscle.

8. By carefully following along the posterior aspect of the LPN, the medial calcaneal branch or branches should be identified. As these pass distally, care should be taken to ensure no bands of fibrous tissue are constricting them.

9. Once the posterior tibial nerve and its terminal branches have been released, the tourniquet, if one was used, should be deflated. The nerve is then carefully observed to determine whether capillary filling is adequate

along the course of the nerve. Occasionally the nerve does not pink up in certain areas, which can represent an area of constriction. If constriction is present, release of the epineurium overlying the nerve may be considered. This observation is made in about 5% of cases. Neurolysis is not typically performed because doing so can make the nerve more vulnerable to scarring by disrupting its surrounding bed and damaging the vaso nervosum. Any bleeding must be controlled, after which the wound is closed in layers without closing the retinaculum. If there appears to be any significant oozing around the wound, it may be closed over a drain. A compression dressing incorporating a plaster splint is applied.

Postoperative Care

Postoperative care consists of keeping the patient relatively immobilized for 2 to 3 weeks, with no weight bearing on crutches. If the wound is healing adequately at 10 days, the sutures can be removed and gentle range of motion is encouraged to limit adhesions. After another 2 to 3 weeks, weight bearing is permitted as tolerated, and more aggressive active and passive range-of-motion exercises are initiated.

Results

When a well-localized lesion is present, such as a ganglion, lipoma, or even a neurilemoma, the clinical response is usually satisfactory, with complete relief of symptoms.

If no specific cause can be identified, approximately 75% of patients obtain significant relief from the surgery, and 25% obtain little or no relief. A small group of patients have increased symptoms after tarsal tunnel release. After surgery, a subgroup of patients experience satisfactory relief of symptoms for a varying period (6 to 12 months) only to have their symptom complex recur.

Cimino[58] reviewed 24 articles and reported that 84 of 122 (69%) patients had good results, 27 of 122 (22%) were improved, 8 of 122 (7%) had poor results, and 3 of 122 (2%) had a recurrence of symptoms (Table 11-3). Pfeiffer and Cracchiolo[83] noted better results earlier in 32 feet but reported a decline with further follow-up at an average of 31 months. Thirty-

TABLE 11-3

Results of Tarsal Tunnel Treatment: Summary of 24 Reports

Results	Number of Patients
Surgery	
Good (resolution of symptoms)	84
Improved (mild residual symptoms)	27
Poor (symptoms unchanged or worse)	8
Recurrent (symptoms return)	3
PERCENTAGE OF GOOD AND IMPROVED	91%
Orthoses	
Good (resolution of symptoms)	10
Poor	0
Refused treatment or pending	12
Other methods	
Injection, resolution	3
Spontaneous resolution	4
Results not reported	35
TOTAL	186

From Cimino WR: *Foot Ankle* 11:47-52, 1990.

eight percent were dissatisfied with the result and had no long-term relief of the pain. In six feet (19%), the pain was decreased but the patients still had some pain and disability (a fair result). There were four wound complications (13%): three infections and one delayed healing.

Takakura et al[86] reported on 50 feet with tarsal tunnel syndrome and noted that the poorest results were in patients who had a traumatic or idiopathic cause. The hemorrhage and crush of the nerve during the trauma can lead to more adhesions and intraneural disease. Increased duration of symptoms was also correlated with a worse outcome. In another report, Takakura et al[87] had a talocalcaneal coalition and a ganglion in six patients with pain, sensory disturbance in the sole, and a positive Tinel sign. After resection, despite early pain relief, sensory changes and paresthesias persisted. The results were excellent in one patient, good in four, and fair in one.

Better results were reported by Nagaoka and Satou,[80] who operated on 29 patients. Of these patients, 21 had excellent and 8 had good results with a ganglion excision for tarsal tunnel symptoms. Five of the patients had an associated tarsal coalition.

Kinoshita et al[70] treated 41 patients (49 feet) with tarsal tunnel syndrome. In seven patients (eight feet) there was an accessory muscle. An accessory flexor digitorum longus muscle was identified in six patients and an accessory soleus muscle in one patient (both feet). The patients with an accessory muscle had a history of trauma or strenuous athletics. After decompression of the tibial nerve and excision of the muscle, signs and symptoms improved at an average of 4.1 months. At final follow-up (24 to 88 months), no functional deficit was observed.

Sammarco and Chang[84] reviewed 62 patients with tarsal tunnel findings and positive electrodiagnostic tests who underwent release. Symptom duration was 31 months. Postoperatively, the average time for return to usual activity was 9 months. Average length of follow-up was 58 months. The authors reported that the most common surgical findings included arterial vascular leashes indenting the nerve and scarring about the nerve. The outcome of surgery was not affected by the history of trauma. The lack of a discrete space-occupying lesion and prolonged preoperative symptoms were not associated with a poor outcome.

Gondring et al[65] studied 60 patients (68 feet) who underwent tarsal tunnel release. All of the patients demonstrated both a positive Tinel sign and an abnormal motor nerve conduction velocity measurement. Despite an objectively assessed 85% complete symptomatic relief, there was only 51% symptom relief subjectively, according to a questionnaire. There was improvement in the quality of work in 51%, in job productivity in 47%, and in interpersonal relationships in 46% of these patients.

Urguden et al[89] assessed 12 patients (13 feet) who underwent surgery for tarsal tunnel syndrome with a mean follow-up of 83 months. The symptoms had resolved in six feet, were improved in four, were unchanged in two, and recurred after five years in one. As in other studies, better results were obtained in patients with a space-occupying lesion than in those with idiopathic or post-traumatic cause. In their 4 cases with foot deformities (three pes planus and one splay foot) there were two good results, one fair and one poor. It was not clear whether these patients had any additional reconstruction to correct their underlying structural issues.

Kim et al[69] performed a retrospective study of 33 years of clinical and surgical experience with 135 tibial nerve lesions to review operative techniques and their results and to provide management guidelines for the proper selection of surgical candidates at the Louisiana State University Health Sciences Center. Of the 135 cases, traumatic injury accounted for 71, tarsal tunnel syndrome for 46, and nerve sheath tumor for 18. Of 22 lesions not in continuity, good to excellent functional recovery was achieved in four (67%) of six patients who required end-to-end suture repair and 11 (69%) of 16 patients who required graft repair. There were 113 tibial nerve lesions in continuity, which underwent primarily external or internal neurolysis or resection of the lesions. Among the 113 patients with lesions in continuity, 76 (81%) of 94 patients receiving neurolysis had good or excellent results. Five of six (83%) receiving suture repair and 11 of 13 (85%) receiving graft repair recovered good to excellent function. Repair results were best in patients with recordable nerve action potentials treated by external neurolysis. Results were poor in a few patients with very lengthy lesions in continuity and in reoperated patients with tarsal tunnel syndrome.

FAILED TARSAL TUNNEL RELEASE

Overview and Etiology

Persistent or recurrent pain after previous tarsal tunnel release is a clinical challenge and a management dilemma. Failure of the patient to respond to the primary release suggests the possibilities of an incomplete release, an incorrect diagnosis (nerve not entrapped in the tarsal tunnel, more proximal cause, neuroma in continuity, true neuroma, systemic neuropathy, or radiculopathy) or poor technique (excessive nerve trauma during surgery). Analyzing what has occurred and speculating about what needs to be rectified can be difficult.

The underlying failure may be due to either intrinsic nerve damage or extrinsic nerve damage. Where there is intrinsic nerve damage, the axons have been disrupted. The failure after tarsal tunnel release occurs in this scenario when the initial nerve disease was too extensive to respond to a release (i.e., nothing was compressing or tethering the nerve to begin with or the nerve was disrupted partially or completely either initially or subsequently). When there is extrinsic nerve damage, an external process affects the nerve. In these cases, a failure to respond to release may be due to incompletely addressing the compression or tethering in the first place or there was too much damage to the environment around the nerve to permit successful release. Occasionally, the nerve bed was not damaged before the procedure, but after the procedure, extensive scarring occurred. This can be triggered by extensive postoperative bleeding, a wound complication, or infection. In the cases of external nerve compromise, there may be little to no primary axonal damage. Although some cases have both internal and external issues, considering these two etiologies may be helpful.

In the cases of external nerve compromise after prior release, the symptoms and signs can be labeled "adhesive neuralgia" or, as Gould prefers, "traction neuritis." In theses cases, the patient has a release and might temporarily have relief but then suffers a recurrence. The pain is typically exacerbated by movement or postural changes. On examination, there is a tender, often thickened scar that when palpated induces the patient's symptoms. Range of motion also induces the patient's pain syndrome.

In the event of internal nerve damage, there are two types of symptom complexes. The first is ectopic neuralgia, in which the patient's nerve symptoms occur spontaneously without provocation. This can be thought of as a peripheral nerve seizure and represents electrochemical imbalance within the nerve. The second type of symptom complex is nociceptive neuralgia. Here the patient experiences nerve pain with mechanical provocation. A physical event, such as a certain position of the foot or an irritation from a shoe or brace, triggers the pain. This latter situation is commonly seen with a neuroma that is lying in a vulnerable location.

It is useful to separate the cases into three categories, facilitating management and permitting a more predictable outcome. The categories (A, B, C) are based on the presence of scar tissue around the tibial nerve and the adequacy of decompression of the trunk and the affected distal branches. The first group (A) comprises nerves encased in scar tissue but an adequate distal release based on operative report or length of scar. This group can be subdivided into patients who never experienced relief after the first surgery (A1), patients who experienced temporary relief but then recurrence (A2), and patients who became worse and developed new symptoms (A3). The second group (B) consists of a combination of tibial nerve branches encased in scar tissue and inadequate release of a portion of the nerve and its branches. The third group (C) has no tibial nerve scarring and an incomplete release.[85,91,94,104-106,114]

Evaluation

The history and physical examination are the cornerstone of the evaluation. The history is usually consistent with recurrent or new symptoms or an intensification of prior manifestations of the tarsal tunnel syndrome. Knowledge of the mechanism of injury can also be helpful. If there was a space-occupying lesion (an external or nonintraneural lesion) or there had been repetitive trauma, external nerve compression or an entrapment might have been the primary diagnosis. However, if a crush or stretch injury was noted, the primary problem might not have been an external nerve problem but rather an internal nerve disorder that might never respond to a fascia release. An important component of the history is to explore the nature, duration, and intensity of the symptoms before the previous tarsal tunnel release. A review of the prior operative report may be useful in

defining incomplete previous release or incorrect diagnosis. A history of wound compromise or infection after the initial release suggests new entrapment of the nerve or adhesive neuralgia.

Although pain may be poorly localized, physical examination should attempt to find foci of maximum involvement, specifically with regard to proximal or distal areas of symptoms. Percussion paresthesias over the scar of the tibial nerve release often indicate scar formation around the nerve, whereas similar findings more distal or proximal to the old incision suggest incomplete decompression. A more focal point of paresthesias might indicate a neuroma or neuroma in continuity. A zone of numbness surrounded by increased nerve sensitivity with proximal trigger points suggests a deafferentation phenomenon, a sign of nerve transection. Anesthesia dolorosa or a numb zone that is painful to touch also indicates nerve transection and neuroma. Decreased and painful range of motion and a thickened scar are consistent with adhesive neuralgia.

Occasionally, recurrent or persistent symptoms indicate complex regional pain syndrome (CRPS) type II. These include vasomotor instability; changes in extremity temperature, skin color, or hair quality; and sweating or dryness that are manifestations of sympathetically mediated pain. Other features of CRPS II include spontaneous or evoked pain, allodynia (painful response to a stimulus that is not usually painful), hyperalgesia (exaggerated response to a stimulus that is usually only mildly painful), pain that is disproportionate to the inciting event, and evidence of autonomic dysregulation (e.g., edema, alteration in blood flow, hyperhidrosis).

As in primary tarsal tunnel syndrome, electrodiagnostic studies may be of benefit, especially to localize the nerve disease, to identify transected nerve branches, and to distinguish between external nerve entrapment and internal nerve damage (especially unrecognized peripheral neuropathy or a more proximal area of disease). When conduction delays are found, the diagnosis of external entrapment is supported. Evidence of axonal damage and muscle denervation supports intraneural damage (i.e., neuroma or neuroma in continuity).[85,105] Although only limited data are available, MRI shows promise in identifying factors leading to failed tarsal tunnel release (Fig. 11–35).[117]

Injections can help isolate the involved nerve or branch. A series of injections beginning distally and progressing more proximally can find the damaged structure. It is also worthwhile to inject suspicious adjacent structures such as tendon sheaths (e.g., posterior tibial tendon), joints (e.g., the ankle or subtalar joint) or bony sites (e.g., nonunion sites). In cases of

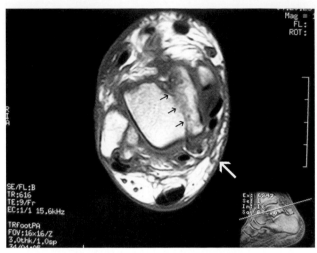

Figure 11–35 Coronal magnetic resonance image through the talus and tarsal tunnel in a patient who failed to respond to nerve release demonstrated the persistent talus nonunion (*small black arrows*). There were signal abnormalities around the tibial nerve and changes from the previous tarsal tunnel release (*white arrow*).

CRPS II, medications and injections aimed at interfering with the sympathetic component of the pain can be both diagnostic and therapeutic. Perhaps the best method of blocking the autonomic dysfunction is to perform a lumbar sympathetic injection. Another useful strategy is to administer an intravenous phentolamine infusion. A patient who responds to the infusion may be a good candidate for trying phenoxybenzamine orally to control sympathetic dystrophy. We have also used intravenous lidocaine as a nerve membrane stabilizer. We have administered it under close monitoring and found it diagnostic and therapeutic. If a benefit is noted, then mexiletine, an oral version of lidocaine, can be considered to control the neuralgia.

Treatment

Conservative Treatment

Nonoperative management of persistent or recurrent tarsal tunnel syndrome may be extremely challenging. With persistent or recurrent symptoms, the patient has typically failed nonoperative measures before primary release, and thus it is unlikely that nonoperative measures will alleviate continued symptoms. However, NSAIDs, TCAs, antiepileptic medications, ketamine, an N-methyl-D-aspartate (NMDA) receptor antagonist, pain creams (e.g., Lidoderm patches) or custom compounded medications, orthotics, physical therapy, or desensitization by transcutaneous electrical nerve stimulation (TENS) should be attempted before performing revision surgery. Input by pain specialists,

who can provide insight into other effective means of pain control, should be considered. A multimodality approach is often warranted.

Surgical Treatment

The goal of revision surgery is to achieve pain relief and improve function. Options for revision surgery include revision release, revision release with barrier procedure, revision release with transection and burial of a neuroma, and peripheral nerve stimulation (PNS) or spinal cord stimulator. The best indications for revision release are usually limited to inadequate previous release with focal areas of nerve irritability. It is useful to separate the cases into the three categories (A, B, C) described earlier.[85]

REVISION NEUROLYSIS

Revision neurolysis is indicated for category C patients (the prior release was inadequate based on the location of the scar, the operative record, conversation with the original surgeon, and location of the symptoms and signs). For example, if the patient had a tarsal tunnel release and did not specifically have a release of the MPN but has no symptoms and signs referable to the MPN, this tarsal tunnel release should be redone, including releasing the MPN. In this scenario, the patient has a good likelihood of a positive outcome. A revision that includes a more proximal or distal release or attention to specific branches is generally worthwhile for the patient.[85,105]

On the other hand, if the patient is in category A and has had a prior tarsal tunnel release through what appears to be an adequate surgical approach, but the patient has little or no relief of the dysesthesias and pain, reexploration of the tarsal tunnel and revision neurolysis alone has rarely been beneficial. For the patient in category B, the revision release has had some success because the nerve was not adequately released. However, in this group the tibial nerve scarring was found to be associated with a less-favorable prognosis.

Skalley et al[85] studied 12 patients (13 feet) who underwent release of a recurrent tarsal tunnel after unsuccessful surgery. They noted that nine patients had abnormal electromyographic results and four patients normal test results. The results comprised three groups: four feet with encasement of the tibial nerve in scar and an adequate initial release had poor results; five feet with scarring and an inadequate release had equivocal results; and four feet with no scarring and an inadequate initial release had good results. We also concluded that the clinical history and physical examination rather than the electromyographic studies helped define the problem with regard to the extent of the lesion and its location.

REVISION NEUROLYSIS AND VEIN WRAP

This procedure is best indicated for patients in category B: those with histories of prior release who had temporary relief and those with adhesive neuralgia. Early on we had found that the revision neurolysis alone did not provide control for scar tissue recurrence. To address this problem with the tissue bed, the vein wrap was developed as a barrier method to block scar tissue from growing into the re-released nerve. The wrap has been shown to be effective in the laboratory and in several series.*

The vein is typically harvested from the ipsilateral saphenous vein in the lower leg. The vein is wrapped in a barber-pole fashion around the re-released nerve. The vein, with its endothelial side against the nerve, provides a barrier to inhibit scar tissue growth. It will not, however, provide a gliding surface for the nerve. Our study of removed sections of previously vein-wrapped nerve branches found a separable junction between the two structures,[91] with apposition of the two without any capacity for gliding. The procedure was successful in cases where the internal nerve damage was not extreme relative to the external scarring.

Surgical Technique

Prior to surgery, the patient is examined to identify areas of focal increased tenderness to ensure that all affected branches are addressed (Fig. 11–36A). Additionally, while the patient is standing, a rubber tourniquet is applied to the mid leg and the saphenous vein is palpated and marked for ease of subsequent intraoperative identification (Fig. 11–36B).

1. The tibial nerve and its branches are circumferentially released over the entire course of the suspected disease (determined by scarring or tenderness to palpation) (Fig. 11–36C).
2. The saphenous vein is harvested, anticipating that for every 1 cm of nerve to be wrapped, 3 cm of vein is needed (Fig. 11–36D and E).
3. The small branches of the vein are occluded with vascular clips on both sides before cutting, providing hemostasis and later permitting reinflation of the vein.

4. Care is taken not to damage the two or more associated branches of the saphenous nerve (Fig. 11–36F).
5. Once sufficient length is obtained, the vein is clamped, tied off, and removed.
6. A bulb-tipped heparin needle is inserted into the distal end of the vein and sealed with a suture to prohibit fluid leakage. The vein is then inflated with 1% lidocaine without epinephrine and maintained in a distended fashion for at least 20 minutes to block the sodium channels. This keeps the vein attenuated (wider and thinner) for greater surface area during wrapping.
7. The external surface of the vein is marked with a surgical marker to help distinguish it from the endothelial side (Fig. 11–36G).
8. The vein is cut longitudinally (Fig. 11–36H).
9. The nerve is typically wrapped in a barber-pole fashion to encase the nerve and affected branches (Fig. 11–36I). If only a portion of the nerve is scarred, the nerve is not skeletonized and the vein can be opened and place over the released nerve (Fig. 11–36J).
10. 6-0 nylon is used from one edge of the graft to the other whenever a spiral is completed. This helps contour the vein covering to the surface of the nerve and keeps it from bunching up. If the procedure is done without a tourniquet, the wrap can be laid on the nerve without constriction. If the tourniquet is used, the surgeon should anticipate a 15% volume increase in the nerve and therefore wrap the nerve more loosely.
11. The wrap should cover any nerve or branch that was scarred to its bed. Any small neuromas should be included, if possible, into the wrap.
12. Meticulous hemostasis should be achieved with the tourniquet down.
13. The soft tissue is reapproximated without closing the fascia
14. The skin is sutured.

Postoperative Care

Postoperatively, the leg is placed in a well-padded splint with the ankle in neutral. The sutures are removed at 10 to 14 days. The limb is placed into a removable off-the-shelf boot brace and the patient is allowed to progressively apply weight during ambulation. The patient

*References 94, 95, 100, 101, 106, 109, 113, and 116.

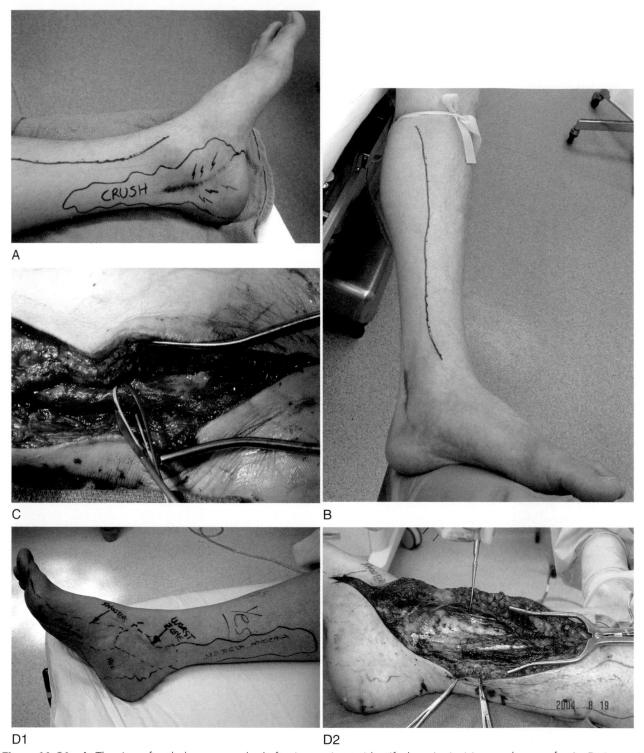

Figure 11–36   **A,** The sites of pathology are marked after inspection to identify the prior incisions and areas of pain. **B,** A tourniquet applied around the leg preoperatively facilitates tracing and marking the saphenous vein. **C,** The nerve was found to be totally encased in scar tissue. **D1** and **D2,** The vein can be harvested from the leg beginning just proximal to the tarsal tunnel.

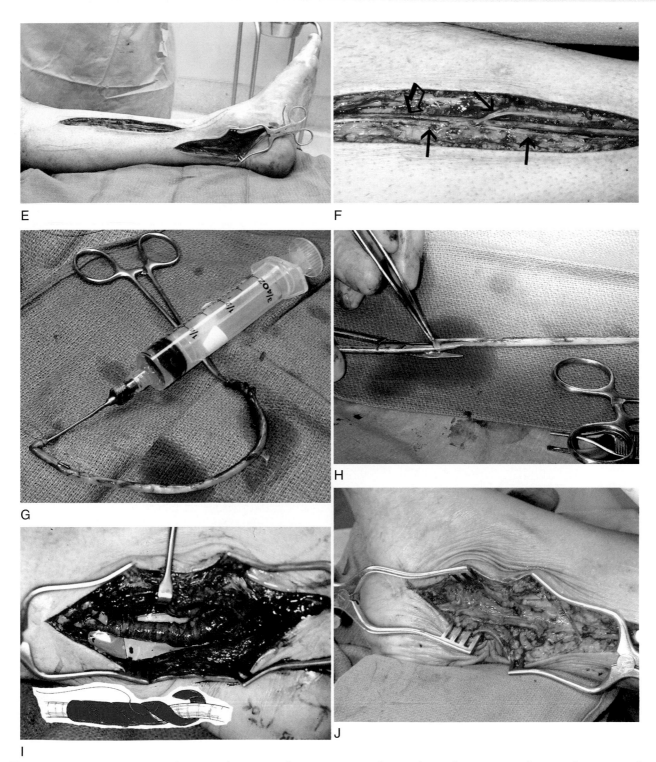

Figure 11-36—cont'd **E,** An alternative harvest can begin anterior to the tarsal tunnel exposure as shown in this case. **F,** The saphenous vein *(open arrow)* is shown with a branching saphenous nerve *(black arrows)*. **G,** The vein is distended with lidocaine and then marked to facilitate wrapping the correct side, the endothelial side, toward the nerve. **H,** The vein is cut longitudinally. **I,** The endothelial side of the vein (unmarked) is placed on the released nerve in a barber-pole fashion. **J,** If only a portion of the nerve is scarred, then the nerve is not skeletonized and the vein can be opened and placed over the released nerve.

should use elastic wraps or support stockings for 3 to 12 months to minimize complications from the vein harvest.

Results

Gould et al[95] studied 64 patients at an average of 31 months of follow-up. Of those 64 patients, 63% had an excellent or good outcome and 25% reported an increase in symptoms. However, that study had a mixed population: Not all patients had primarily adhesive neuralgia.

In our series,[106] of 58 consecutive limbs (51 with tibial nerve involvement), all had adhesive neuralgia that was a result of a combination of the original nerve insult (primary compression or entrapment, traction or stretch injury, crush injury, transection, idiopathic cause, deep infection, compartment syndrome, and injection injury) and subsequent surgery (such as postoperative scarring). Duration of symptoms before vein wrapping averaged 62 months (range, 11 to 353 months). The number of previous surgeries for the same nerve problem averaged 2.5 (range, one to seven procedures). All limbs had undergone at least one neurolysis procedure, which had provided a period of complete or partial pain relief. Sixteen had previous intentional or unintentional transection of a branch of the nerve. Other complications of previous surgery that might have contributed to the adhesive neuralgia included two deep-space infections and six wound dehiscences.

Retrospective follow-up was available for all patients. Follow-up averaged 48.6 months. Pain scores improved from a preoperative average of 8.8 points (range, 6 to 10 points) to a postoperative average of 5.1 points (range, 0 to 10 points). Dysfunction scores improved from a preoperative average of 7.4 points (range, 3 to 10 points) to a postoperative average of 4.4 points (range, 0 to 9 points). Time to maximum improvement in this group averaged 12 months (range, 3 to 30 months). Fifty-five percent of the patients were satisfied, 14% were satisfied with reservations (gaining mild or minimal relief of symptoms), and 31% had unsatisfactory results. No patient reported worsening of the symptoms after a suitable recovery from the surgical procedure.

Thirty-eight of the 58 had an autograft saphenous vein and 20 had an allograft umbilical vein (Fig. 11–37). In 7 of 38 saphenous vein patients,

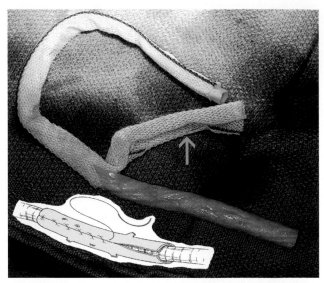

Figure 11–37 An alternative to the saphenous vein autograft is a preserved umbilical vein. The Dacron mesh *(green arrow)* that surrounds the umbilical vein is removed. The *inset* shows the method of wrapping the longitudinally split vein around the nerve.

there were complications from the vein harvest: 3 of 38 limbs had mild saphenous nerve symptoms, 3 of 38 had mild wound healing problems, 2 of 38 had swelling from the vein harvest incisions, and 2 of 38 had prolonged donor site pain. All but 2 of 38 had resolution of the symptoms. Of the 58 limbs with the 20 umbilical veins, there were no infections, rejections, or wound complications. Unfortunately, only 7 of 20 patients were satisfied and 11 of 20 were dissatisfied in the umbilical vein subgroup compared with 25 of 38 satisfied and 7 of 38 dissatisfied in the saphenous vein subgroup. Thus, we no longer use the umbilical vein.

Interestingly Ruch et al[103] studied 24 Sprague-Dawley rats and performed vein wraps with autograft versus glutaraldehyde-preserved allografts. They found that the allograft vein wraps incited a marked inflammatory response, with epineural scarring and adherence to the underlying nerve, whereas autograft vein wraps did not.

Varitimidis et al[113] studied the vein autogenous saphenous wrap in 19 patients with recurrent carpal tunnel and cubital tunnel syndrome. The average number of surgeries before vein wrapping was 3.3, and the mean follow-up period was 43 months. All patients reported reduction in pain, improvement in the sensory disturbances, and better electrodiagnostic findings.

PERIPHERAL NERVE STIMULATION FOR FAILED TARSAL TUNNEL RELEASE

For patients who fail to get temporary relief (group A1) or who are worse after release (group A3), especially if they have ectopic neuralgia, anesthesia dolorosa, or deafferentation phenomenon, neurostimulation should be considered. Those whose symptoms are along the tibial nerve are possible candidates for PNS. For a patient who has diffuse nerve symptomatology, with more than two nerves involved, and especially one who does not respond to a nerve block, spinal cord stimulation is preferable to peripheral neurostimulation.

Patients with a suspected combination of nerve branches encased in scar tissue and inadequate release of a portion of the nerve (group B) can undergo another revision nerve release with a vein wrap. If a major component of sympathetically mediated pain is apparent or if the patient has CRPS II, then surgery and postoperative management should include a continuous sympathetic block via epidural catheter.

Diagnostic criteria for CRPS II include:

- Continuing pain, allodynia, or hyperalgesia after a nerve injury, not necessarily limited to the distribution of the injured nerve.

- Evidence of edema, changes in skin blood flow, or abnormal sudomotor activity in the region of the pain.

- Diagnosis excluded by conditions that account for the degree of pain and dysfunction.

All three criteria must be satisfied.[110]

Although some have suggested tibial nerve grafting for patients with traumatic tibial nerve transection,[92] we have not seen therapeutic benefit with tibial nerve transection for chronic pain. Over the course of 16 years in one (LCS's) practice, nine patients who have had a tibial nerve transection for chronic tibial nerve pain did poorly.

The PNS procedure can be technically challenging and permanently leaves the patient with restrictions (inability to use local ultrasound, prohibition from obtaining an MRI, difficulty with electronic security systems). The device is subject to electronic malfunction (generator power depletion, alteration due to electromagnetic field interference) and mechanical malfunction (fluid leaks with loss of pattern of stimulation, wire breakage, lead migration, generator malposition, wire malposition with local soft tissue irritation, short circuits).

TECHNIQUE FOR PERIPHERAL NERVE STIMULATION

When the pain is due to a lesion of one or two nerves, the procedure should be considered. Although benefit from TENS is not an indication that the patient will do well, a patient who experiences more pain with TENS is typically a poor candidate for neurostimulation. Failure of spinal cord stimulation is not a contraindication to PNS because the ability to get specific coverage in the tibial nerve territory is generally better with PNS. Previous infection or wound complications are not contraindications to PNS, but a history of recurrent infections in the extremity or elsewhere (e.g., dental or bladder infections) are a relative contraindication for PNS. Patients with idiopathic or systemic neuropathies are poor candidates for the procedure.

A meeting with the representative of the company or discussion with another patient is helpful prior to surgery. The patient is instructed to mark the leg, ankle, and foot with the zones of numbness, worst pain, trigger points, and so on.

1. The entire limb from the pelvis distal is prepped and draped
2. The nerve trunk (or trunks) proximal to the level of the disease is circumferentially exposed.
3. The wound is anesthetized, carefully avoiding nerve injection. The patient is then reversed from general anesthesia (Fig. 11–38A).
4. A trial stimulation is performed, with the patient giving feedback about the location and quality of the pain relief while the lead from an external pulse generator is moved around the nerve (Fig. 11–38B).
5. Paraesthesia in the zone of pain typically indicates good placement of the lead on the nerve. If this zone can be palpated or percussed during the stimulation with reduced or absent pain, the lead placement is complete.
6. If there are still other zones of uncontrolled pain, the lead is moved around the nerve to improve the paresthesias and pain relief. If there are still zones of uncontrolled pain, intraoperative nerve blocks are then performed. A decision is made regarding additional nerve trunk stimulation versus

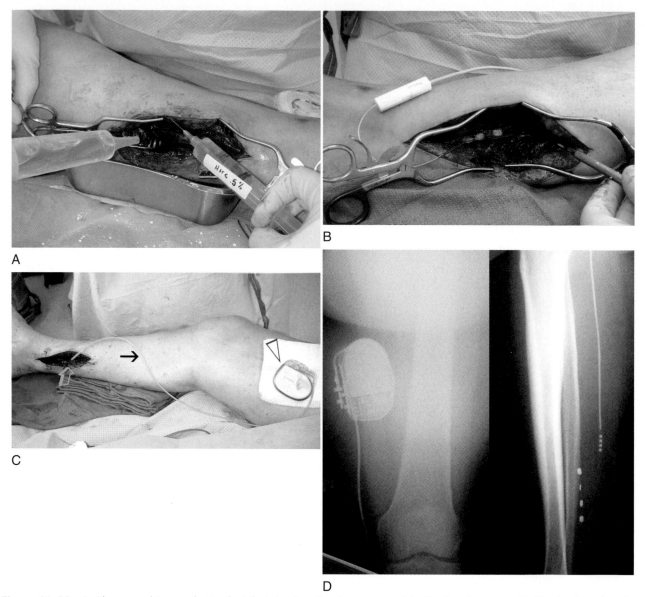

Figure 11–38 A, The wound is anesthetized while irrigating the tissues to avoid affecting the nerve. **B,** The lead is placed on the nerve. **C,** The lead *(green open arrow)* will be attached to the extension wire *(black solid arrow),* which is connected to the pulse generator *(red arrowhead).* **D,** The wire will be tunneled under the tissues with special tools.

additional nerve procedures (e.g., transection, transposition, or additional nerve stimulation) in conjunction with the primary stimulation.

7. Once the placement of the lead (or leads) is finalized, the lead is sutured onto the epineurium with 5-0 proline suture. The lead should lie on the nerve without undue stress and with the four electrodes flush with its surface. The sutures should not pinch the nerve fibers because this can induce pain.

Securing the lead with the patient's immediate feedback prevents creating new problems inadvertently.

8. If paresthesia (stimulation) in the zone of pain is obtained with minimal relief to palpation or percussion, a trial using a temporary external generator connected to the internal lead is then instituted. After 4 to 5 days, if the pain is controlled with adjustment of the stimulator, an internal generator is implanted. If the pain has not decreased, a series of nerve blocks is

performed to identify the nerve that produces or carries the pain signal. Once this is determined, a second-stage procedure is performed to adjust the leads, add another lead to the other nerve(s), or perform additional nerve procedures (for example, transection, translocation, or containment procedures).

9. If the stimulation is adequate, the patient is reanesthetized with general anesthesia, and the PNS generator and extension wires are implanted. It is important to route the lead and extension wires so that they do not impinge on other structures (tendons, arteries, veins, other nerves) because mechanical stress on either the wires or the tissues can require revision. The extension wire placement is performed using special tunneling tools. The pulse generator is placed in the medial thigh (Fig. 11–38C).

Postoperative Care

The leg is placed in a splint for 2 weeks. Compression wraps are applied around the thigh. Sutures are removed at 10 to 14 days. The compression wraps are used for 4 to 6 weeks.

Results

In 62 consecutive limbs, the duration of symptoms before PNS averaged 46 months (range, 13 to 96 months). [94,105,106] Of the 62 limbs, 58 (94%) had undergone at least one previous peripheral neurosurgical procedure for treatment of the neuropathic pain. The number of previous peripheral neurosurgical surgeries averaged 2.8 (range, 0 to 12) and included neurolysis (57), revision neurolysis (24), vein wrapping after unsuccessful neurolysis (16), transection (47), and centrocentral anastomosis (three). Thirty-eight limbs had stimulation of a single nerve trunk. The remaining had stimulation of two to four nerves. The nerves stimulated included the tibial (28 limbs), the tibial and the sural (4 limbs), the tibial and the saphenous (3 limbs), the tibial and the superficial peroneal nerves (4 limbs), the superficial peroneal and the sural nerves (2 limbs), the superficial peroneal and the deep peroneal nerves (3 limbs), the sural (3 limbs), superficial peroneal (8 limbs), the saphenous nerve (1 limb), the deep peroneal nerve (1 limb), the femoral nerve (1 limb) and the tibial nerve with at least 2 other nerves (four limbs).

Pain scores improved from a preoperative average of 9 points (range, 7 to 10 points) to a postoperative average of 5.1 points (range, 0 to 8 points), and dysfunction scores improved from a preoperative average of 8 points (range, 7 to 10 points) to a postoperative average of 6.4 points (range, 3 to 10 points). The average overall percentage improvement reported by the patients was 42%. Time to maximum improvement after PNS averaged 5.2 months (range, 1 to 10 months). Satisfaction was reported in 38 of 62 (61%) limbs, satisfaction with reservations in 13 of 62 (21%) limbs and dissatisfaction in 11 of 62 (18%). In the 48 (of 58, 83%) patients who were satisfied, only one patient had complete relief of symptoms and at 2.5 years' follow-up no longer uses the PNS. In these 48 patients there were improvements in hours of sleep per night, hours of uninterrupted sleep, and average walking distance. They generally felt that their quality of life and psychological well-being had improved.

Twenty-nine of 62 limbs required revisions over the five-year study period. Major revisions with lead replacements were performed in 21 of 29 limbs. Ten of the 21 required another nerve to be stimulated at a later surgery. Eight of the 21 had revisions of the pulse generator for battery depletion during a lead revision. New pulse generators were inserted in 2 of 29 limbs. Four of the 29 limbs have had minor hardware revisions.

Six patients had postoperative infections. Four of 29 limbs had revisions for postoperative infections (3 of these limbs are already counted in the 21 of 29 major revisions) within 6 months of implantation; one patient had a previous history of osteomyelitis. Two of 29 limbs had late infections—one at 1.5 years and one at 3 years—requiring removal of some or all of the implanted components. The patient with infection at 3 years had undergone additional lead insertion within 3 months postoperatively. Four of the six patients had resolution of the infection with intravenous antibiotics and subsequently had reimplantation of the PNS with satisfactory results. One of the patients who had had the osteomyelitis did not have adequate relief with the initial implantation and requested an amputation. The other patient who was initially satisfied with his relief of pain for 1.3 years did not feel that there was adequate functional improvement. This patient ultimately decided to undergo transtibial amputation. Following his amputation, he had further improvement of pain and function.[94,105,106]

Other series have reported improvement of pain symptoms in the upper extremity of 53% to 84%.*

About the lower extremities there is a paucity of literature, but Hassenbusch et al[97] reported on 30 patients who underwent PNS, 12 for lower extremity nerve pain. In this subgroup, all had stimulation of a single nerve; 7 had stimulation of the posterior tibial nerve and 5 had stimulation of the common peroneal nerve. Of the 12 patients, only 2 had good results; both of these had stimulation of the posterior tibial nerve. The lack of success in this study might have represented problems with inclusion criteria or technical factors.

Failure of response to re-release, vein wrap, neuroma resection and burial, or PNS does occur. The options for these patients grow more limited and include continued pain management with medications and activity modifications. Options include spinal cord stimulation (SCS), an internally implanted pain pump, and, as a last resort in select patients, amputation.

*References 96, 97, 99, 102, 111, and 115.

SPINAL CORD STIMULATION

SCS provides neurostimulation by direct lead application to the spinal cord and may be effective in relieving limb pain.[108,112]

Trial stimulation can be performed percutaneously, usually with only local anesthesia, and is similar to an epidural catheter insertion. The zone of stimulation tends to be broader than PNS but might not cover the distal tibial nerve territory as adequately. Regardless, if lead placement adequately covers the pain, a surgical procedure is then warranted to insert the pulse generator.

Disadvantages of the SCS include the variable acceptance by patients of the need for a spinal procedure to control limb pain. In addition, the broad coverage at times introduces abnormal sensations to normal, nonpainful zones, which may be a limiting factor in the patient's ability to increase the stimulation to the painful zones. Finally, lead positional change or migration with flexion and extension of the spine can occur and can require limits in the patient's function to prevent fluctuations in stimulation intensity.

Both PNS and SCS are end-stage salvage procedures that should only be explored after all conventional treatment alternatives have been exhausted but before considering amputation. Appropriate patient selection is critical to the success of PNS and SCS, and better-defined patient selection criteria are needed. Our prospective experience with a group of 60 patients with PNS with a minimum of 3-year follow-up has been good. Although the middle-term results of PNS and SCS are encouraging, long-term follow-up is required to assess the long-term results for the management of intractable lower extremity neuropathic pain.

AMPUTATION

With intractable neurogenic pain that has failed all limb-salvage procedures, proximal amputation may be the ultimate end-stage option. One of us (LCS) uses a proximal compression test to help determine if the patient might do well with an amputation. The test is performed by circumferentially squeezing the leg at the level of proposed amputation. If the patient does not experience any pain or neuralgia at this level, our experience with amputation has been good.

In our prospective review of patients who had a transtibial amputation and a prefabricated prosthesis, the Airlimb (Aircast, Summit, NJ), a subgroup of 5 patients underwent the procedure because of chronic pain. We (LCS) have had 11 additional patients who underwent transtibial amputation for chronic nerve pain since this publication. Of these 16 patients, 12 are doing well and able to wear a custom prosthesis. One is better than before, wears a prosthesis, and no longer needs pain medication, but still has a only a fair result. One is better than before surgery but is unable to tolerate a custom prosthesis, and two are doing poorly with residual stump neuropathic pain and need of further revision surgery. Some of the patients had a standard recovery for a transtibial amputation and some had resolution of their pain only after 2 to 3 years (unpublished data). This procedure is only used for situations when all other possible alternatives have been exhausted.[107]

There is little published on the results of amputation in the treatment of intractable nerve pain. Dielissen and colleagues[93] reviewed their results in 28 patients who underwent amputations in limbs with complex regional pain syndrome (CRPS; also called *reflex sympathetic dystrophy*). Amputations were performed for untenable pain (5), recurrent infection (14), or to improve residual function (15). Although only two patients were relieved of pain, nine of 15 had improvement of residual function. They reported that the CRPS recurred in the stump and that only two patients could wear a prosthesis. Despite this, 24

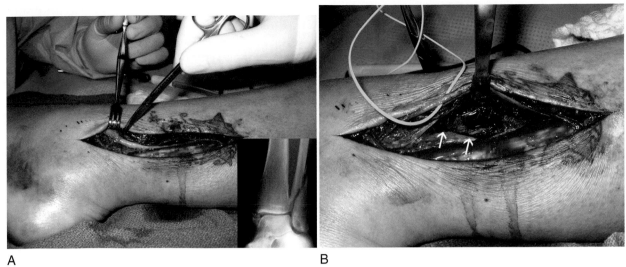

A   **B**

Figure 11–39   A, The superficial peroneal nerve is identified during exposure of this fibula fracture. *Inset,* Preoperative radiograph of fibula fracture. **B,** The nerve is released prior to performing open reduction and internal fixation.

patients were satisfied with their results. The authors recommended against amputation for pain relief in CRPS.

Honkamp et al[98] reported on 18 patients with chronic pain (not just from chronic nerve pain) who underwent amputation. Of these 18, 16 would have amputation again and are satisfied with the outcome. In this study, the visual analogue scale (VAS) improved in pain frequency (9.8 to 1.7) and in pain intensity (8.4 to 2.6). Walking distance improved. Ten patients were able to stop their narcotics, and 7 decreased their level or dosage, or both. Prior to amputation three patients continued to work, and eight patients returned to work after amputation. Although this was not a select group of intractable tibial neuralgia cases, it does give some sense of potential results in select cases.

TRAUMATIC AND INCISIONAL NEUROMAS

A neuroma in the region of the dorsum of the foot can result in significant disability because little soft tissue covers the dorsum, and footwear causes constant irritation of the painful site. Traumatic neuromas result from lacerations or crushing injuries of the foot and are usually not under the surgeon's control, but incisional neuromas are and therefore should be avoided. This is particularly true with arthroscopic procedures that use 3- to 5-mm incisions in areas where the small sensory nerves or branches are vulnerable. In a review or 612 arthroscopies, nerve injuries occurred in 4.4% of cases: 15 superficial peroneal, six sural, five saphenous, and one deep peroneal.[125]

Nerve injuries are also often seen in common foot and ankle procedures such as open reduction and internal fixation of ankle fractures. For example, one study of 120 ankle fractures found symptomatic superficial peroneal nerve injury with (21%) and without surgery (9%), and the nerve injury was associated with worse results (Fig. 11–39).[137] Other percutaneous or minimal incision surgeries such as a fascial compartment release can increase the risk of nerve injury as well.[130]

Although surgeons are well aware of the general neuroanatomy of the foot and ankle, the pattern and distribution of nerves can vary. Whenever an incision is made on the foot or ankle, great care needs to be exercised in the dissection to identify the less common anatomic patterns that might be present.

In a study by the Anatomical Society of Great Britain and Ireland,[118] 229 foot examinations demonstrated that in 55% of specimens the nerve distribution to the dorsum of the foot follows the pattern cited in most anatomy textbooks. The main variation noted in 24% of specimens was the increased distribution of the sural nerve to the lateral three toes instead of only the small toe. In the remaining 21% of the specimens, 10 different patterns of distribution were identified. This varying pattern of distribution must be noted in an evaluation of the patient with a neuroma, because the distribution of the dysesthesias or numbness can extend over a larger or smaller area than normally expected from a specific nerve trunk. The greater sensory distribution of the sural nerve was also identified by Solomon et al,[139] who found that it supplied the lateral half of the foot and toes in 40% of 68 specimens.

Clinical Symptoms

The clinical history of the patient with a neuroma is quite typical in that the patient either recalls the specific laceration or notices the symptoms after a surgical incision. The patient usually has fairly well localized pain and might point to the site of the neuroma. At times the patient is fairly comfortable when ambulating without shoes but feels significant dysesthesias and paresthesias when shoes are worn. Sometimes patients try treating themselves with various types of padding, but unfortunately this is rarely successful in relieving pressure on the involved area.

Diagnosis

Physical examination demonstrates a scar, and usually a painful neuroma within it can be palpated or at least percussed (Fig. 11–40). At times the neuroma is adjacent to the scar rather than within it. A small blunt instrument such as the end of a pen can be used to carefully percuss along the nerve trunk to define the involved area if palpation of the neuroma is difficult. As a general rule there is decreased sensation distal to the area of the neuroma, although the anatomic

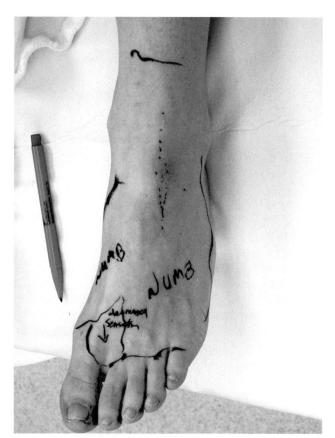

Figure 11–40 Preoperative photograph of foot with superficial and deep peroneal neuromas.

pattern can vary greatly because of nerve distribution variability.

The diagnosis can be verified and the degree of clinical response demonstrated by injection of a small amount (2 to 3 mL) of local anesthetic into the area just proximal to the neuroma. At times this also indicates whether there has been complete transection of the nerve or if it is only a neuroma in situ. If the nerve is completely transected, the area of anesthesia will be the same as when the nerve is injected, whereas in cases of neuroma in situ, the area of anesthesia will probably be greater than that mapped out during nerve percussion.

Treatment

Conservative Treatment

The conservative management of neuromas is difficult. Shoes or braces can be specially purchased or customized that prevent contact with the vulnerable area. Various types of pads may be placed or the shoe may be expanded to help avoid pressure over the involved area. The pad or pads can be fashioned to create a channel through which the nerve can pass without pressure from the shoe.

Cortisone injections may be helpful but carry the risk of thinning the skin, making future conservative or surgical management more challenging. Other agents such as alcohol have been injected to damage the nerve with the hope of interrupting the pain. These agents can also cause local tissue damage that limits their effect. Furthermore, at times the neurotrauma from the chemicals induces more pain. Perhaps the best treatment is lidocaine patches or various compounded pain creams. Although they have been an effective treatment in some cases, rarely do they completely improve the pain in an active patient.

Surgical Treatment

Neuromas in the foot have two forms: a bulb type of neuroma that occurs when the nerve has been transected or a spindle neuroma that results from a nerve that is still in continuity.[140]

In the treatment of neuromas on the dorsum of the foot, the surgical approach should be carefully planned to avoid placing a scar, if possible, in an area that is subject to pressure from the shoe, such as directly over the dorsum of the foot. The other area that must be carefully avoided is the anterior aspect of the ankle joint, particularly in a worker whose boot will cut across this area.

My (LCS) current approach is to consider transection and burial for patients with either neuromas or severe intraneural damage with nociceptive neuralgia. If the posterior tibial nerve or other major mixed motor and sensory nerve (e.g., sciatic, common peroneal) is involved, I routinely offer the patient a trial of peripheral nerve stimulation before transection. Although there have been reports of successful transection and interposition reconstruction of major nerves (e.g., tibial),[124,135] we have not experienced good outcomes and do not recommend this procedure.

When performing revision transection and burial procedures, I suggest dissection to the affected nerve from proximal to distal toward the trigger spot. Clinically, this is more successful than an isolated proximal nerve transection and burial without distal nerve dissection. It is hypothesized that distal communication between nerves can result in the noxious stimulus coursing along an adjacent nerve, despite the proximal transection.

NERVE TRANSECTION AND BURIAL

Surgical Technique

1. The surgery may be carried out with or without tourniquet control. Loupe magnification should be used so that excellent visualization is possible.

2. The nerve trunk must be carefully identified and dissected from the surrounding soft tissues (Fig. 11–41). As a general rule, unless one of the larger nerve trunks over the dorsum of the ankle area (e.g., intermediate dorsal cutaneous nerve, medial dorsal cutaneous nerve) is involved, resection of the nerve is recommended over attempted repair or dissection of a spindle neuroma from it. Often the resulting dysesthesias tend to be more bothersome than the anesthesia that may be created by transection of the nerve. Typically, there is sufficient overlap in the foot that an area of anesthesia is usually not too bothersome to the patient, although an area of dysesthesia can be.

3. After the nerve has been identified and traced proximally, an adequate bed must be found for it. Any possible depression in the foot (e.g., area of the sinus tarsi) should be sought, but in other areas the nerve needs to be traced proximally and buried beneath the extensor digitorum brevis muscle (Fig. 11–42).

4. It is useful to secure the nerve ending within the zone of protective tissue. This can be

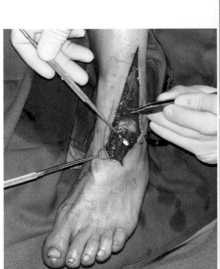 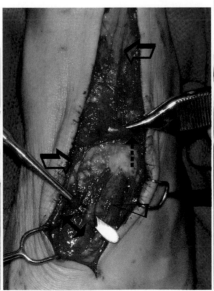 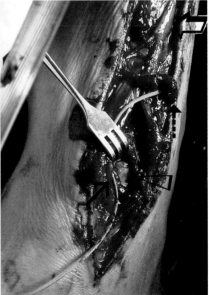

A B C

Figure 11–41 Operative photographs of patient shown in Figure 11–40. This patient had a prior ganglion resection over the anterior ankle. The patient had postoperative numbness in the territory of the superficial nerve (SPN) and decreased sensation to the deep peroneal nerve (DPN). **A,** The superficial peroneal nerve is exposed. **B,** The SPN is identified *(open arrow)*, and two branches are found to be transected. The *dotted arrow* indicates the proximal end and the *double-headed arrow* indicates the distal nerves. The deep peroneal nerve was identified over the dorsal capsule of the talonavicular joint *(open triangular arrow)*. **C,** The capsule of the talonavicular joint is opened, and the DPN is released *(open triangular arrow)*. The vessel loop is around the main trunk of the DPN *(solid arrow)*. The *dotted arrow* indicates the neuroma of the SPN.

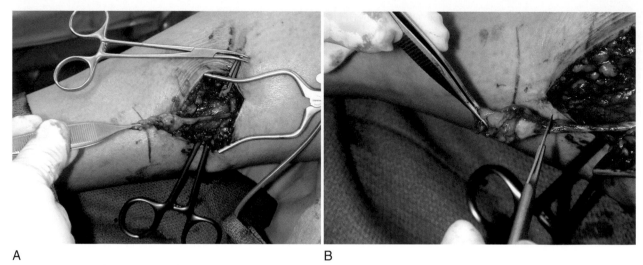

A   B

Figure 11–42 A, The neuroma of the sural nerve is identified in the posterior aspect of the leg. A curved hemostat is buried into the muscle and will be used to pass the nerve end once it is cut. **B,** The bulbous neuroma will be transected and then pulled through the muscle belly.

achieved by placing an epineural suture of 4-0 Vicryl and using it for passing the nerve and then tying it to fascia or periosteum without undue tension. Another alternative is to bury the nerve end into bone.

Postoperative Care

The patient is treated with a compression dressing, possibly incorporating plaster splints for the first 10 days after surgery. The sutures are then removed, and a compression dressing, usually an elastic bandage, is maintained for another 3 to 4 weeks, with ambulation permitted as tolerated.

Results

Results of neurectomies *without* burial of painful neuromas in the foot have been successful in 65% to 83% of patients in primary situations.[131,141] The concern with performing simple transection is that the response of the nerve is unpredictable; occasionally, a more proximal nerve transection results in greater disability for the patients than was previously present. As described in terms of pathophysiology, disruption of the peripheral pain pathway can lead to deafferentation pain or anesthesia dolorosa. The results of revision transection are typically less favorable than those reported for primary neurectomy, with satisfactory relief of pain.

To optimize results, transection has been combined with several other procedures

designed to contain or translocate the new nerve stump. The containment procedures are categorized into physical, synthetic, and physiologic types, all with the goal of limiting axonal regeneration and relocating the new stump away from noxious stimuli.

Physical containment by sealing of the distal nerve ending has been attempted by techniques involving freezing, cauterization, electrocoagulation, chemical sclerosis, mechanical crush or ligation, and nonsynthetic capping (i.e., fascia). Results of ligation techniques, chemical sclerosis, or mechanical crushing of transected nerve endings have been variable and might sometimes increase the pain.[121,141]

Synthetic containment has been attempted using methyl methacrylate, cellophane, collodium, silicone, glass, tin, tantalum, and silver and gold foils. Problems include an inability to fully seal the nerve endings with these materials and stimulation of foreign-body reactions, leading to greater neuroma formation.[123,136,138,143]

Physiologic containment methods include excision and retraction into proximal normal tissue,[141] implantation into muscle,[123] and implantation into bone.*

The results of translocation of a transected nerve to limit exposure to mechanical stimuli have been variable. In a large series by Tupper and colleagues,[141] 78% of patients had a suc-

*References 122, 126, 128, 129, 133, 134, and 142.

cessful outcome with repeat neurectomy. Crush injuries had a better prognosis than sharp injuries. Dellon and Aszmann[123] presented an approach to the treatment of dorsal foot pain of neuroma origin with translocation of the appropriate nerves into the muscles of the anterolateral compartment away from the joint. With this approach they reported excellent results in 9 of the 11 patients with a mean follow-up of 29 months. Miller described significant pain improvement with proximal transection and burial into bone of the dorsomedial cutaneous nerve after iatrogenic primary injury.[134] Chiodo and Miller[122] reported an average perceived pain relief of 75% with transection and burial into bone for treatment of superficial peroneal neuroma. Their study demonstrated a significant improvement in results for symptomatic superficial peroneal neuromas when treated with transection with transposition of the proximal nerve stump into bone as compared with transposition into muscle. Other physiologic containment techniques include end-to-end repair and centrocentral nerve anastomosis. These procedures decrease the likelihood of painful neuroma by containing or controlling rejuvenant nerve growth after transection.[119,120,127,132,138]

Transection and containment procedures are advantageous because of the good reported results, technical ease, and the minimal requirements for complex postoperative treatments. The ideal patient for revision transection is one with a focal neuroma who experiences nociceptive neuralgia (severe pain with palpation or physical provocation at the trigger end of the nerve). Such patients for whom other therapies have failed are best treated with more proximal transection and burial because this method removes the irritated or irritable nerve from the zone of physical stress.

There are several potential problems with nerve transection: deafferentation pain or anesthesia dolorosa, motor denervation (which can result in muscle imbalance and deformities), vulnerability to ulcers and infections from insensate plantar aspect of the foot, loss of essential nerve function (i.e., tibial nerve), and ectopic or spontaneous neuralgia.[106]

In patients who demonstrate ectopic neuralgia and not nociceptive neuralgia, more proximal transection and burial might not provide relief. When these cases are associated with the deafferentation phenomenon or anesthesia dolorosa, there is a particularly poor prognosis according to our experience. For these patients, PNS may be a better alternative than transection and burial. In my (LCS) retrospective review of patients undergoing PNS,[106] 47 of the 62 patients had previously undergone transection and burial before PNS. Of these, eight did not respond adequately to PNS and had poor results. The remainder all had allodynia that responded to some degree to PNS. These results suggest that for patients who fail transection techniques, PNS is still a viable option.

LATERAL PLANTAR NERVE ENTRAPMENT

First Branch

Although heel pain can occur from many conditions such as plantar fasciitis, calcaneal stress fracture, or subcalcaneal bursitis, the diagnosis of entrapment of the first branch of the LPN should be entertained in chronic cases (Fig. 11–43).

Anatomy

Anatomic dissections have helped unravel the complexity of this region. The posterior tibial nerve divides into three branches: the medial calcaneal nerve, the lateral plantar nerve, and the medial plantar nerve. The medial calcaneal nerve branches off the posterior tibial nerve and penetrates or passes below the laciniate ligament to innervate the posterior and posteromedial aspect of the skin of the heel. In the retromalleolar region the posterior tibial nerve then branches into the LPN and the MPN. The LPN is separated from the MPN by a fibrous septum originating from the calcaneus and inserting on the deep fascia of the abductor hallucis muscle. The first branch of the LPN courses between the abductor hallucis muscle and the quadratus plantae in an oblique direction. It then changes direction and courses laterally in a horizontal plane. This branch then further ramifies into three major branches. One innervates the periosteum of the medial process of the calcaneal tuberosity, one innervates the flexor digitorum brevis as it passes dorsal to this muscle, and the terminal branch innervates the abductor digiti minimi muscle. The branch that innervates the periosteum of the calcaneal tuberosity often supplies branches to the long plantar ligament and occasionally provides a branch that innervates the quadratus plantae muscle.[144,160,168]

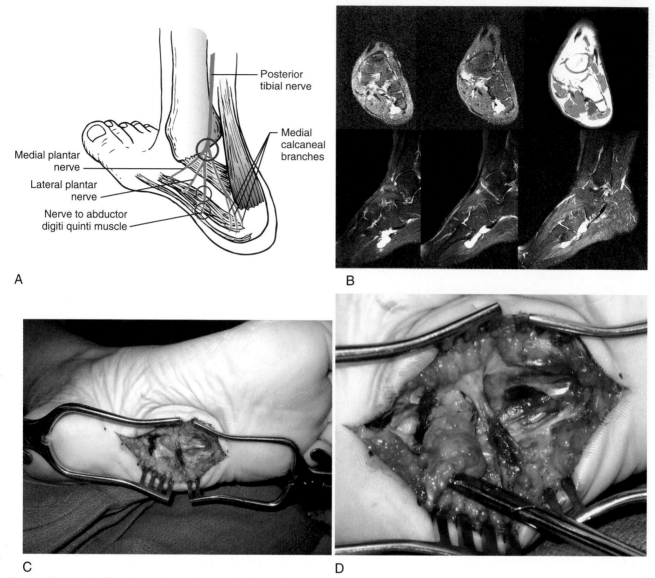

Figure 11–43 **A,** Tarsal tunnel syndrome. *Circles* indicate areas of impingement. The lateral plantar nerve can be trapped in several locations along the medial ankle: at the trifurcation of the tibial nerve, below the deep fascia of the abductor, and where the nerve changes course heading plantarly in a longitudinal fashion to traveling laterally between the quadratus plantae and the flexor digitorum brevis. **B,** The lateral plantar nerve (LPN) can be compressed in the arch of the foot after giving off the first branch of the LPN. Here the patient had numbness and tingling in the lateral aspect of the forefoot and no heel pain. The magnetic resonance image demonstrated a ganglion beneath the cuboid. **C** and **D,** At surgery the ganglion is found and removed underneath the LPN in the midfoot region.

Incidence

Approximately 5% to 15% of patients with chronic unresolving heel pain have entrapment of the first branch of the LPN (Fig. 11–44).[73,105,147,148,150-153] The condition occurs in athletes and nonathletes. Although runners and joggers account for the majority of cases, entrapment has been reported in athletes who participate in soccer, dance, tennis, track and field events, baseball, and basketball.[144,160,165] The average age in athletes in the series reported by Baxter and Pfeffer[144] was 38 years, and 88% were men. In

Henricson and Westlin's series[146] of international and national athletes, the average age was approximately 26 years, and 90% were men.

Etiology

According to several recent anatomic and clinical studies, entrapment of this branch of the LPN occurs between the deep fascia of the abductor hallucis muscle and the medial caudal margin of the quadratus plantae muscle. Inflammation from chronic pressure can also occur as the nerve courses over the plantar side of the

monic finding in these patients is tenderness over the first branch of the LPN deep to the abductor hallucis muscle. Pressure on this point causes reproduction of the symptoms and radiation of pain proximally and distally.

Surgical Treatment

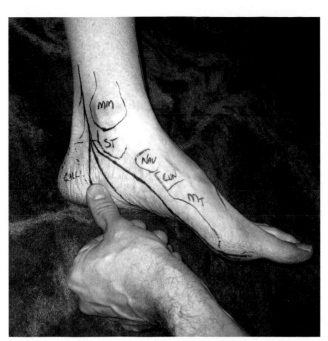

Figure 11–44 The tender spot in plantar fasciitis coincides with the first branch of the lateral plantar nerve.

long plantar ligament or the osteomuscular canal between the calcaneus and the flexor digitorum brevis. Athletes with hypermobile pronated feet may be particularly susceptible to chronic stretching of the nerve.[167] Hypertrophy of the abductor hallucis muscle or the quadratus plantae muscle might also explain the occurrence of this condition. Accessory muscles, abnormal bursae, and phlebitis in the calcaneal venous plexus have also been implicated.[144,167,172]

Clinical Symptoms

Patients with entrapment of the first branch of the LPN report chronic heel pain. Often the pain is increased by walking or running. Pain radiates from the medial inferior aspect of the heel proximally into the medial ankle region of the foot. The pain can radiate across the plantar aspect to the lateral aspect of the foot. Often the pain is worse in the morning. Unless more proximal entrapment of the nerve occurs, patients do not usually describe numbness in the heel or the foot. The average duration of symptoms was 22 months in Baxter and Pfeffer's series.[144] The patient often gives a history of having already tried stretching programs, heel cups, NSAID administration, and injections.

Diagnosis

The physical examination must be performed with a thorough knowledge of the anatomy of this region. More proximal and distal nerve entrapments must be excluded by palpation along the entire course of the posterior tibial nerve and its branches. The pathogno-

RELEASE OF THE FIRST BRANCH OF THE LATERAL PLANTAR NERVE

Surgical Technique

1. The patient should be in the supine position on the operating table. An ankle block is used most often, and no tourniquet is required, although an ankle tourniquet MAY be used.
2. A 4-cm oblique incision is made on the medial aspect of the heel over the proximal abductor hallucis muscle. The incision is centered over the course of the first branch of the LPN. The incision is oblique and placed distal to the medial calcaneal sensory nerves (Fig. 11–45A).
3. The superficial fascia of the abductor hallucis muscle is divided with a No. 15 blade and the muscle is retracted superiorly with a small retractor (Fig. 11–45B and C).
4. The abductor muscle is reflected inferiorly and the deep fascia is released (Fig. 11–45D). The muscle is reflected distally and the deep fascia is released (Fig. 11–45E).
5. The abductor muscle is reflected proximally and the deep fascia is released directly over the area where the nerve is compressed between the taut fascia and the medial border of the quadratus plantae muscle (Fig. 11–45F).
6. The muscle is reflected proximally and the deep fascia is released. A small portion of the medial plantar fascia may be removed to facilitate exposure and clearly define the plane between the deep abductor fascia and the plantar fascia (Fig. 11–45G).
7. The heel spur, if present, is exposed with a Freer elevator, with care taken to protect the nerve that runs superiorly. The abductor hallucis muscle belly and its superficial fascia are left intact.
8. An extensive plantar fascia release is not performed unless direct visualization shows evidence of a pathologic condition in the entire proximal portion of the plantar fascia.

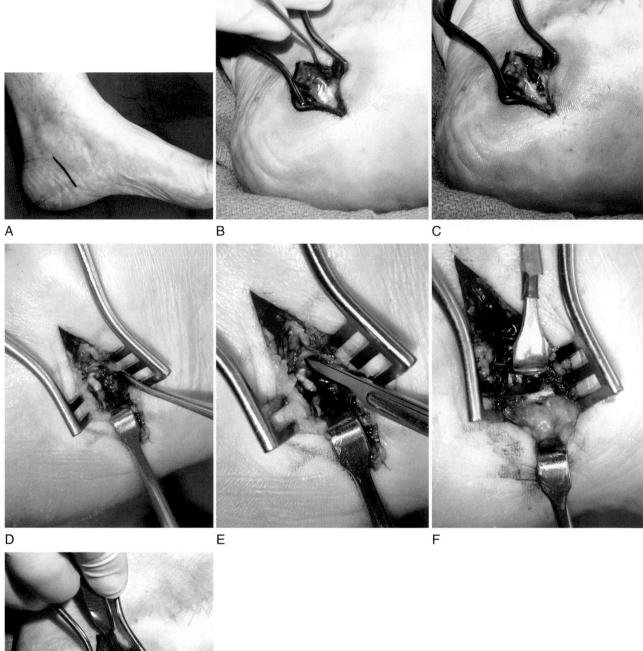

Figure 11–45 **A,** The incision is oblique along the course of the first branch of the lateral plantar nerve. **B,** The incision deepened to the superficial fascia of the abductor. **C,** The fascia is incised. **D,** The muscle is reflected distally and the deep fascia is released. **E,** Next, the abductor muscle is reflected proximally and the deep fascia is released directly over the area where the nerve is compressed between the taut fascia and the medial border of the quadratus plantae muscle. **F,** The muscle is reflected proximally, and the deep fascia is released. A small portion of the medial plantar fascia may be removed to facilitate exposure and clearly define the plane between the deep abductor fascia and the plantar fascia. **G,** A portion of the plantar fascia is released.

9. The wound is closed with interrupted sutures.
10. A bulky dressing is applied.

Postoperative Care

The sutures are removed at 10 to 14 days. The patient is allowed to bear weight on the heel at 10 days. We do not routinely use a boot brace or a cast, but if patients are having difficulty progressing, one can be used.

Results

Baxter and Pfeffer[144] reported on 61 heels; they had excellent or good results in 89% and complete resolution of pain in 83%. Watson et al[153] reported 88% good and excellent results. They found that MRI findings consistent with plantar fasciitis were associated with good and excellent results. The authors strongly advocated nonoperative treatment for 12 to 18 months prior to surgery and noted that 52% of patients required more than 6 months to reach maximum improvement.

Calcaneal Branches

Overview, Etiology, and Anatomy

The medial calcaneal branches of the tibial nerve provide sensation on the medial aspect of the heel. Anatomic studies have demonstrated a proximal origin of the medial calcaneal branches from the tibial nerve and the existence of multiple medial calcaneal branches.[14,66] One study showed that 70% of medial calcaneal nerves originated proximal to the tarsal tunnel and that 60% of specimens had multiple branches.[14] Compromise of the medial calcaneal nerve branches might contribute to chronic heel pain (Fig. 11–46). The medial calcaneal nerve branches do exhibit a considerable amount of variation in terms of location, origin, and course. A medial calcaneal nerve occasionally originates from the MPN.[62,152]

Calcaneal neuromas can produce a painful heel syndrome; however, most likely such a painful heel syndrome secondary to medial calcaneal nerve compromise occurs only when a true medial calcaneal nerve neuroma resulted from a transection injury during previous surgery (Fig. 11–47).[152] With an accessory muscle (soleus or flexor hallucis longus), we have seen symptomatic tenting of the medial calcaneal nerve over the bulky muscle.

Evaluation

Confirmation of medial calcaneal nerve compression cannot be achieved by standard electrodiagnostic studies because the medial calcaneal nerve is a sensory nerve. Testing methods that rely on the patient's sensing and expressing skin sensitivity to two-point stimulation or irritation can help objectify the findings. An accessory muscle or space-occupying lesion can be appreciated on computed tomography or MRI scan.

Management

As with other syndromes, nonoperative techniques can be used. When these fail, surgical management may be

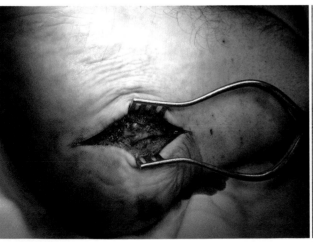
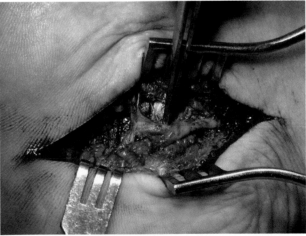

A   B

Figure 11–46 This police officer had sustained a high-energy impact injury to his medial heel with a steel bar. He had persistent pain and dysesthesias of the medial heel that did not respond to local and systemic modalities. He underwent exploration of the medial calcaneal nerves. **A,** The calcaneal nerve was enlarged and found entrapped in dense scar tissue. **B,** After release, his pain and function improved.

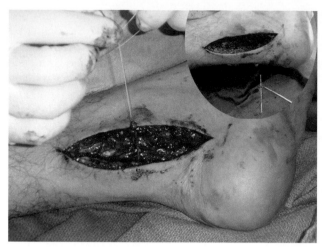

Figure 11–47 A traumatic calcaneal neuroma is identified during surgery in a patient who had a medial ankle laceration or crush. *Inset*, the neuroma is transected and buried into the posterior soft tissue with the assistance of a Keith needle.

Results

In the authors' experience with a limited number of cases of medial calcaneal nerve entrapment, good to excellent results have been obtained 75% of the time.[105,145,149]

MEDIAL PLANTAR NERVE ENTRAPMENT

After the MPN travels underneath the flexor retinaculum, it courses deep to the abductor hallucis muscle. The nerve runs along the plantar surface of the flexor digitorum longus tendon and passes through the knot of Henry. It continues along the medial border of the foot and ramifies into branches that lie on the medial and lateral aspects of the flexor hallucis longus tendon. This condition should be easy to distinguish based on history of a neuroma from transection or severe crush injury of the MPN. Although transient neuralgia is more common than a transection injury, surgery for the jogger's foot is less common (Figs. 11–49 and 11–50).

Incidence

Medial plantar nerve entrapment classically affects joggers (jogger's foot). Although it has been reported most often in men, there is no gender predilection. No specific age distribution has been encountered.[155,182]

Etiology

Medial plantar nerve entrapment occurs in the region of the knot of Henry. Most patients are found to walk

considered. Typically, release of the tarsal tunnel with careful release of the medial calcaneal nerve is performed. It is advisable to identify the tibial nerve and then trace it distally into the heel. The medial and LPNs dive deep to the fascia of the abductor, and the calcaneal nerve(s) are found superficial to the muscle. Rarely the nerve pierces the superficial fascia of the abductor and then travels in the subcutaneous fat. The nerve, which can range in diameter from 1 mm to 4 mm, ramifies into the skin of the medial and medial plantar heel (Fig. 11–48). When there is an accessory muscle, resection of the bulky distal portion is suggested.

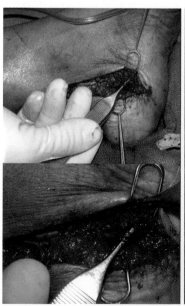
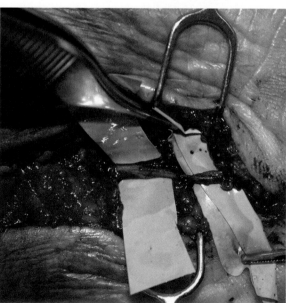

Figure 11–48 The patient had atypical medial heel neuralgia following a twisting injury. With percussion over the tibial nerve, the patient had tingling of the medial heel but not into the plantar aspect of the midfoot and forefoot. *Upper left* and *lower right* (close-up), the calcaneal nerve and two branches are identified after releasing the inferior fascia of the tarsal tunnel. The nerve was constricted by the flexor retinaculum where it penetrated the fascia. *Right*, the blue background is underneath the main trunk of the large calcaneal nerve and its more posterior branch.

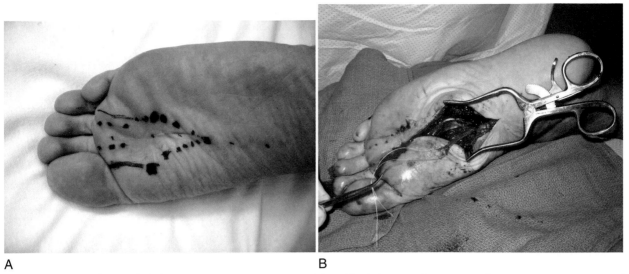

A

B

Figure 11–49 **A,** The medial plantar nerve territory was painful and had decreased sensation after a transection injury to the arch of the foot. **B,** The medial plantar nerve formed a neuroma where it was injured. This was transected more proximally and the end buried into muscle.

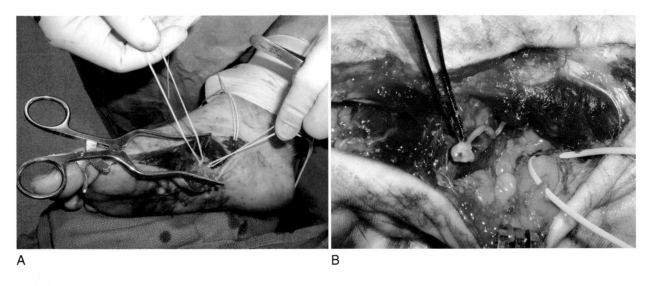

A

B

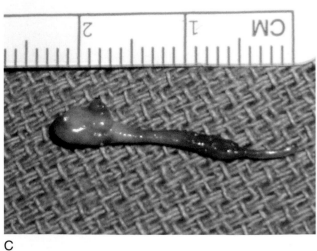

C

Figure 11–50 The patient complained of chronic recalcitrant medial plantar foot pain and dysesthesias after a bunion surgery with a proximal metatarsal osteotomy. The medial plantar nerve was identified proximally deep to the abductor muscle. Distally the medial plantar nerve divides into two branches held by vessel loops inferior to the abductor muscle. **B,** The smaller branch is found to have a bulbous neuroma in the area of maximal preoperative tenderness. **C,** The neuroma is resected and the end buried into the muscle.

or run with excessive heel valgus or with hyperpronation of the foot. Arch supports, especially those that are built up, can compress the nerve. Kopell and Thompson[154] described the entity associated with hallux rigidus. They postulated that overactivity of the tibialis anterior, caused by the patient's attempting to lift the arch of the foot to avoid pain, contributed to the syndrome. They also believed that MPN denervation resulted in increased stress in the first MTP joint, which ultimately led to arthrosis.[154] An avid walker who had a long history of rigidus subsequently had medial plantar neuralgia. This was believed to be caused by abductor hallucis and flexor brevis muscle spasm, which was her unconscious attempt to splint the first MTP joint against dorsiflexion.

Clinical Symptoms

The patient describes aching or shooting pain in the medial aspect of the arch. The pain often radiates distally into the medial three toes and can radiate proximally into the ankle. The pain is worse with running on level ground but may be induced by workouts on stairs (Fig. 11–51). The patient might report onset of the syndrome associated with the use of a new orthosis or shoes.

Diagnosis

The patient should be examined in a weight-bearing position to identify hindfoot valgus, which triggers this condition. The patient should also be examined standing on his or her orthotic device to identify any areas of external compression. Palpation along the MPN usually reproduces symptoms consisting of medial arch tenderness with radiation, dysesthesia, or paresthesia to the medial three toes. Symptoms may be increased with

tightening of the adductor hallucis brevis muscle, which can be accomplished with a heel rise or eversion of the heel. Because of the close proximity of the MPN and the medial tendons, it can be difficult to distinguish between neuralgia and tendinitis. Occasionally it is necessary to have a patient run on a treadmill for several minutes to identify symptoms. Decreased sensation is usually present only after the patient has been running or walking for a prolonged period.

Surgical Treatment

MEDIAL PLANTAR NERVE RELEASE

Surgical Technique

1. Under ankle block anesthetic with or without tourniquet and loupe magnification, the patient is positioned in a supine manner.
2. A 7.5-cm (3-inch) longitudinal incision is made just inferior to the talonavicular joint.
3. The superficial fascia over the abductor muscle is released and the muscle is reflected plantarly.
4. The deep fascia is released and the naviculocalcaneal ligament is released just inferior to the talonavicular joint (knot of Henry). In addition to the MPN, the flexor digitorum longus tendon crosses the flexor hallucis longus tendon at the location of entrapment.
5. Care is taken to avoid stripping the nerve of any fatty tissue.
6. After wound irrigation, the skin is closed with interrupted sutures and a compression dressing applied.

SUPERFICIAL PERONEAL NERVE ENTRAPMENT

The superficial peroneal nerve is a branch of the common peroneal nerve. It courses through the anterolateral compartment and innervates the peroneus brevis and peroneus longus. Traveling between the anterior intermuscular septum and the fascia of the lateral compartment, it pierces the deep fascia approximately 8 to 12.5 cm above the tip of the lateral malleolus (Fig. 11–52). The nerve then becomes subcutaneous, and approximately 6.4 cm above the lateral malleolus it divides into two branches (the intermediate and the medial dorsal cutaneous nerves). The intermediate dorsal cutaneous nerve usually provides sensation to the dorsal aspect of the lateral dorsal aspect

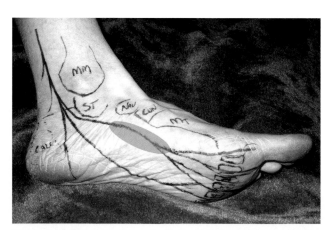

Figure 11–51 The jogger's foot with compression of the medial plantar nerve in the arch as demonstrated by the *shaded oval.*

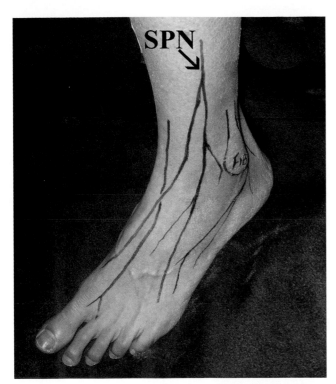

Figure 11–52 The superficial peroneal nerve (SPN) is drawn here after it penetrated the lateral fascial compartment.

of the ankle as well as the fourth toe and portions of the third and fifth toes. The medial dorsal cutaneous nerve provides sensation to the dorsomedial aspect of the ankle as it extends toward the medial aspect of the hallux as well as to the second and third toes.[170]

Incidence

The average age of patients is approximately 36 years (range, 15 to 79 years). Among the athletic population, the average age is 28 years. In both the general and the athletic populations, the syndrome occurs equally in men and women. Most athletes are runners, although several are soccer players. This syndrome also has been described in hockey, tennis, and racquetball players.[161-164,171,174]

Etiology

According to clinical and anatomic studies, the site of entrapment of the peroneal nerve occurs at its exit point from the deep fascia. In most cases the fascial edge impinges on the exiting nerve. Fascial defects with muscle herniation exacerbate the impingement. Such herniations might only occur in the dynamic state and be part of a localized anterior exertional compartment syndrome.

Styf[173] described a short fibrous tunnel between the anterior intermuscular septum and the fascia of the lateral compartment. In almost half his cases he described a fibrotic, low-compliance tunnel that can predispose to a local compartment syndrome. Rosson and Dellon[169] retrospectively reviewed the location of the superficial peroneal nerve in a consecutive series of 35 limbs in 31 patients with entrapment of the superficial peroneal nerve. They found the location of the superficial peroneal nerve in the anterior compartment in 47% of the patients.

Chronic ankle sprains, a major underlying factor, subject the nerve to recurrent stretching (Fig. 11–53). A previous anterior compartment fasciotomy causes shifting of the fascia with resultant stretch and impingement of the nerve.[147,151,170] Peroneal nerve entrapment can occur idiopathically, or it can be associated with direct trauma (with ganglion) (Fig. 11–54), fibular fracture, exertional compartment syndrome (and previous fasciotomy), muscle herniation, syndesmotic sprains, lower extremity edema, and (rarely) mass effects such as tumors.[173,174]

Clinical Symptoms

Patients report a several-year history of pain over the outer border of the distal portion of the calf and the dorsum of the foot and ankle. About one third have numbness and paresthesias along the distribution. Occasionally, patients report pain only at the junction of the middle and distal thirds of the leg, with or without local swelling (Fig. 11–55). The pain is typically worse with physical activity ranging from

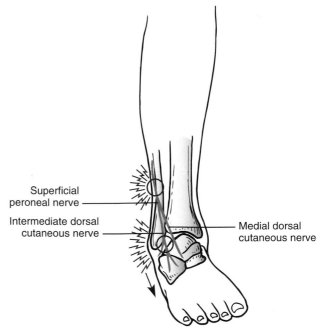

Figure 11–53 Superficial peroneal nerve entrapment. *Circles* indicate areas of impingement.

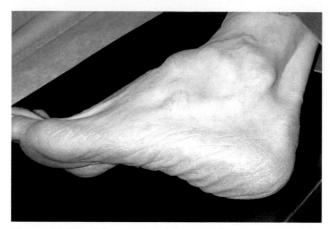

Figure 11–54 A large multilobular ganglion compresses the superficial peroneal nerve.

walking, jogging, and running to squatting. Nocturnal pain is uncommon. Relief by conservative measures is uncommon.[157,161-164,171,174]

Approximately 25% of patients with the syndrome have a history of prior trauma to the extremity, most commonly an ankle sprain. The syndrome has been reported after anterior compartment fasciotomy.

Diagnosis

Physical examination must include an evaluation of the lower part of the back for sciatic nerve pain. The region where the common peroneal nerve sweeps around the neck of the fibula must also be examined to exclude proximal entrapment. Point tenderness is usually elicited where the nerve emerges from the deep fascia, approximately 8 to 12.5 cm above the tip of the distal end of the fibula. Paresthesias and numbness are often noted. Approximately 60% of the patients described in the literature have a palpable fascial defect.

Styf[173] describes three provocative tests to suggest a diagnosis. In the first test, the patient actively dorsi-

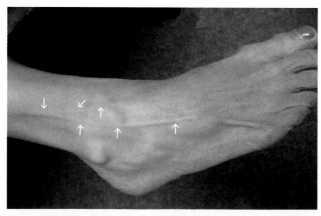

Figure 11–55 The superficial peroneal nerve is easily seen in this foot and ankle. The *white arrows* are emphasizing the course of the nerve.

flexes and everts the foot against resistance while the nerve impingement site is palpated. In the second and third tests, the physician plantar flexes and inverts the foot, first without pressure over the nerve and then with percussion along the course of the nerve.

Treatment

Conservative Treatment

Conservative treatment of superficial peroneal nerve injuries includes strengthening the lateral muscles of the leg, wearing a supportive ankle brace to prevent inversion of the ankle, and wearing a lateral heel and sole wedge in the shoe to prevent inversion. A boot brace may be helpful during the day. For the atypical patients who have some nocturnal symptoms, a night splint can be used to hold the ankle in dorsiflexion.

Surgical Treatment

SUPERFICIAL PERONEAL NERVE RELEASE

Surgical Technique

1. The patient is placed supine on the operating table. A beanbag or bump is useful to help tilt the patient in to a 30- to 45-degree lateral position.
2. A regional anesthetic is used to block the area proximal to the entrapment of the superficial peroneal nerve. This block needs to be carried out approximately 15 cm proximal to the tip of the fibula.
3. A 7.5-cm incision is made in the area of maximum symptoms.
4. Once the superficial peroneal nerve is identified, the nerve is released by incising the fascia proximal and distal to its exit point from the compartment (Fig. 11–56).
5. Often the nerve is compressed at a localized area where the muscle herniates. No attempt is made to repair or close this hernia. When the patient had previous surgery along the course of the superficial peroneal nerve, the cause of the pain could be a compression from a fascial edge or a more distal entrapment (Fig. 11–57).
6. If there is a tunnel of compression before the nerve leaves the fascia, care must be taken to release the entire fascial sheath until the nerve lies within the muscles proximally.
7. After irrigating the wound, the skin is closed with interrupted sutures and a compression

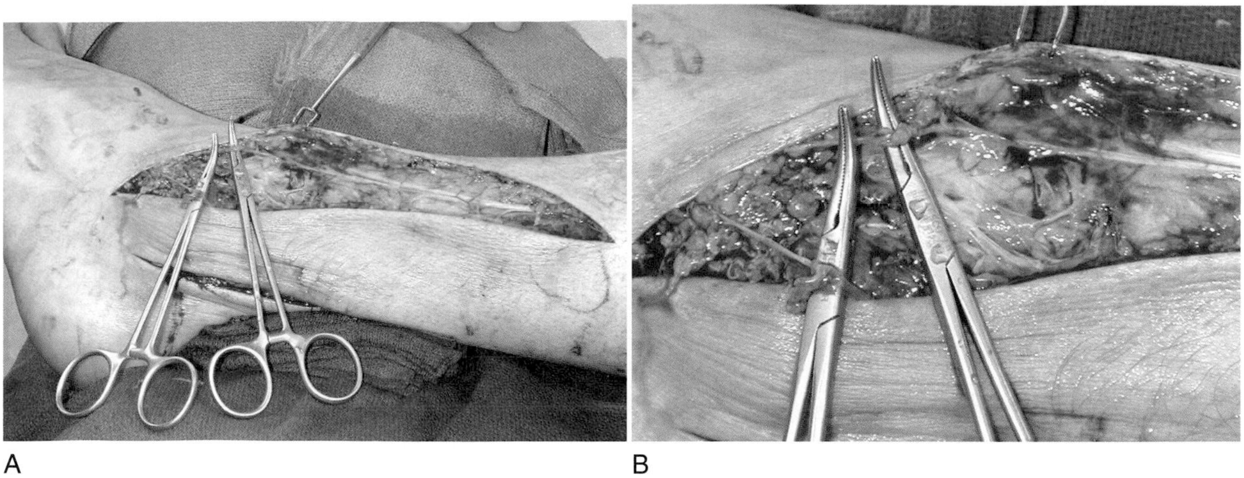

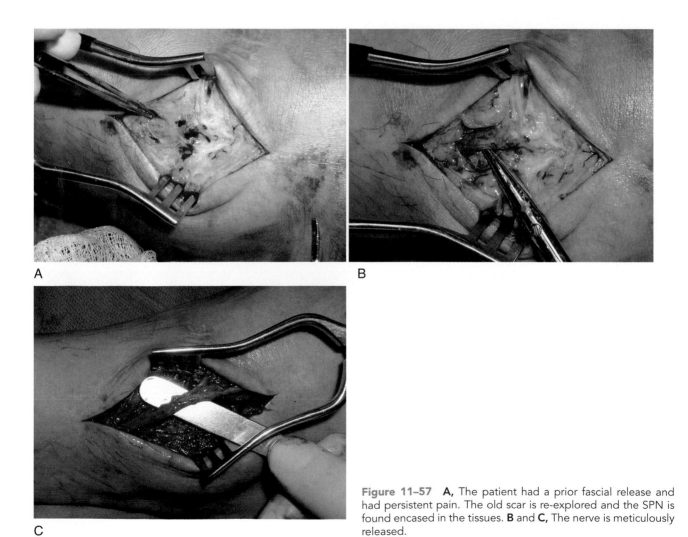

Figure 11–56 **A,** The superficial peroneal nerve is seen here, after release, piercing the lateral fascia. The nerve branches and is traced distally to the zone of trauma. **B,** The nerves become thin and are found in scar tissue in this case.

Figure 11–57 **A,** The patient had a prior fascial release and had persistent pain. The old scar is re-explored and the SPN is found encased in the tissues. **B** and **C,** The nerve is meticulously released.

dressing is applied. In cases of extensive release, a splint might be applied as well.

Postoperative Care

Postoperatively the patient wears a compressive wrap or splint. Ambulation is allowed as tolerated after 3 to 4 days. The sutures are removed at 2 weeks, and activities can be resumed 3 weeks after surgery if symptoms permit.

Results

A larger series of superficial peroneal nerve decompressions suggests that improvement of

symptoms can be anticipated in 75% of cases, but the author warned that results are less predictable in athletes.[173] Schepsis et al[171] looked at eight of 18 (44%) patients who had symptoms, signs, and surgical findings of entrapment of the superficial peroneal nerve after surgery for exertional anterior compartment syndrome of the lower leg. All eight patients with documented peroneal nerve entrapment had a satisfactory outcome. Other series of superficial peroneal nerve release have demonstrated effective relief of symptoms.[162,163,165,169] When the nerve has been released and the symptoms remain, the nerve can be re-explored, and transection and burial into muscle may be considered (Fig. 11–58).

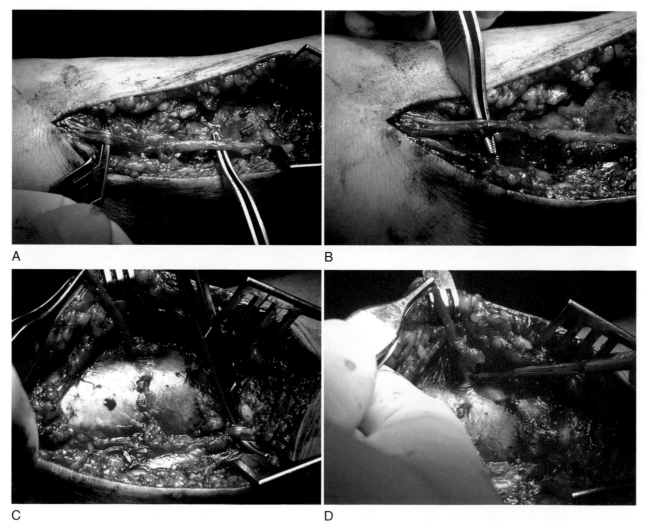

Figure 11–58   A, The superficial peroneal nerve is lifted by forceps more distally. The nerve was found to be frayed, flattened, and irregular in appearance in the zone of trauma. Proximal to where the nerve is lifted by the hemostat, the nerve is bound down by scar tissue. **B,** The nerve has been freed from constriction, but the amount of damage was thought to be too extensive for recovery given the magnitude of pain and the chronicity. **C,** Transection was performed, followed by transposition. The nerve, seen over the hemostat, had been passed deep into the anterior compartment and pulled out medially to ensure deep burial. **D,** The nerve is gently pulled and cut where it pierces the fascia. It is allowed to retract into the deep musculature of the anterior compartment.

DEEP PERONEAL NERVE ENTRAPMENT

The deep peroneal nerve lies between the extensor digitorum longus and the tibialis anterior muscles in the proximal third of the leg (Fig. 11–59). The nerve travels between the extensor digitorum longus and the extensor hallucis longus in the region approximately 3 to 5 cm above the ankle joint, just below the inferior edge of the superior extensor retinaculum. Approximately 1 cm above the ankle joint, the nerve divides to give off a lateral branch that innervates the extensor digitorum brevis muscle. This division occurs in the region underneath the oblique superior medial band of the inferior extensor retinaculum. The medial branch of the deep peroneal nerve continues alongside the dorsalis pedis artery underneath the oblique inferior medial band of the inferior extensor retinaculum. The nerve can be compressed in this region between the retinaculum and the ridges of the talonavicular joint. The nerve continues distally between the extensor hallucis brevis and the tendon of the extensor hallucis

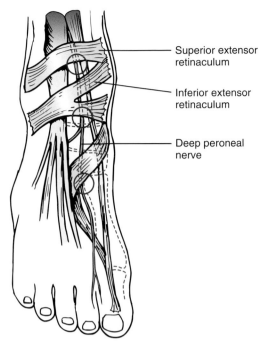

Figure 11–60 Deep peroneal nerve entrapment. *Circles* indicate areas of impingement.

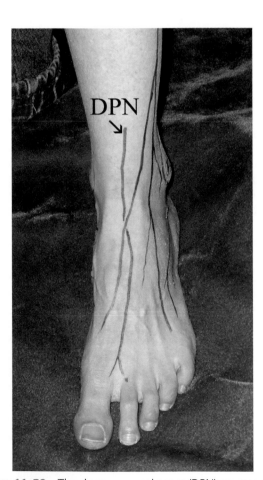

Figure 11–59 The deep peroneal nerve (DPN) courses along the lateral face of tibia.

longus. The nerve supplies sensation to the first web space in the adjacent borders of the first and second digits.[38]

Etiology

Deep peroneal nerve entrapment was initially described by Kopell and Thompson[72] in 1960 and was designated an anterior tarsal tunnel syndrome by Marinacci[155] in 1968. Krause et al[180] described a partial anterior tarsal tunnel syndrome in which only the motor or sensory component was involved.

The deep peroneal nerve can become entrapped in several locations. The most frequently described entrapment is the anterior tarsal tunnel syndrome. This syndrome refers to entrapment of the deep peroneal nerve under the inferior extensor retinaculum. Entrapment can also occur as the nerve passes under the tendon of the extensor hallucis brevis.[72] Additionally, entrapment has been described under the superior edge of the inferior retinaculum, where the extensor hallucis longus tendon crosses over the nerve.[72,155,177] Compression by underlying dorsal osteophytes of the talonavicular joint and an os intermetatarseum (between the bases of the first and second metatarsals) has previously been described in runners[156] (Fig. 11–60).

Trauma often plays a role in this syndrome. Many patients have a history of recurrent ankle sprains. As the foot plantar flexes and supinates, the nerve is placed under maximum stretch, especially over the talonavicular joint.[177] Thus, with repetitive ankle sprains, nerve entrapment can occur. Tight-fitting shoes or ski boots have been implicated as an inciting factor.[155,178,180,182] Occasionally a jogger ties a key into the lacing of the shoe, and the external compression of this key can cause localized pressure on the deep peroneal nerve. External compression can also occur in athletes who do sit-ups with their feet hooked under a metal bar. Fracture residuals or osteophytes in the region of the distal tip of the tibia, talus, navicular, cuneiforms, or metatarsal bases place undue stress on the nerve as well. Pressure from edema or a ganglion can result in a deep peroneal neuropathy.

Akyuz et al[177] reported on 14 of 300 patients with deep peroneal nerve symptoms that were correlated with abnormalities on nerve conduction velocity and EMG. In their study from Turkey, they identified that *namaz*, or Islamic prayer in the kneeling position, caused prolonged stretching of the nerve.

Incidence

Entrapment of the deep peroneal nerve occurs most often in runners, but it can also be seen in other athletes, dancers, and people whose feet are subjected to pressure or stretch.

Evaluation

History

Patients with deep peroneal neuralgia complain of dorsal foot pain that can radiate to the first web space. As with other nerve symptoms of the foot and ankle, a history of low back pain should be documented. If the symptoms are aggravated by activity or exercise, then consideration must be given to exertional compartment syndrome. Symptoms related to tight footwear or particular activities (such as sit-ups with the anterior aspect of the ankles under a metal restraint) should be noted. A history of foot and ankle trauma or chronic ankle instability is also important.

Physical Examination

Palpation along the course of the deep peroneal nerve can identify an area of maximum nerve irritation, which is usually in the area of the inferior extensor retinaculum. Palpation can also locate dorsal ankle and foot osteophytes and rarely a ganglion related to previous trauma or degenerative change. Sensation in the first web space may be diminished. Areas of more proximal nerve compromise should be ruled out with examination of the lower spine, sciatic nerve, and common peroneal nerve. Weakness or atrophy,

or both, of the extensor digitorum brevis muscle suggests a complete anterior tarsal syndrome or more proximal disease. However, patients can have symptoms consistent with an anterior tarsal tunnel syndrome with both motor and sensory nerve compression despite a lack of extensor digitorum brevis atrophy. This situation is secondary to an accessory extensor digitorum brevis innervation from the superficial peroneal nerve, noted in approximately 22% of patients.[179,181]

When symptoms are reported to occur in the dynamic state, the evaluation should include dorsiflexion and plantar flexion of the ankle and testing for ankle instability. If the history is consistent with an anterior compartment syndrome, then examination should also be performed after exacerbation of symptoms on a treadmill, with measurements of compartment pressures.

Diagnostic Studies and Tests

Plain radiographs are useful in identifying exostoses or osteophytes that can contribute to nerve compression. Electrodiagnostic studies can reveal areas of distal entrapment but are typically more helpful in identifying areas of more proximal nerve compression or peripheral neuropathies. Akyuz et al[183] reported prolonged distal nerve conductions velocities, distal latencies, and decreased amplitude of the deep peroneal nerve. They also had needle EMG findings in the extensor digitorum brevis muscle.

Occasionally, nerve conduction studies assist in distinguishing between distal and proximal deep peroneal nerve compression within the anterior tarsal tunnel. A diagnostic nerve block can confirm clinical findings, and compartment pressures should be measured if anterior compartment syndrome is suspected.

Treatment

Conservative Treatment

Nonoperative measures include use of accommodative footwear that eliminates external compression on the dorsal ankle and foot and activity modification to avoid activities that exacerbate symptoms. As for superficial peroneal neuralgia, ankle braces can alleviate nerve pain related to ankle instability but can potentially worsen symptoms if external pressure is created. Vitamin B_6, NSAIDs, tricyclic antidepressants, and gabapentin or other antiepileptic medications should be considered. Because the nerve is rather superficial, Lidoderm patch and topical compounded pain creams can reduce symptoms as mentioned earlier in other sections. Corticosteroid injection at the site of nerve irritation might also be beneficial.

Surgical Treatment

DEEP PERONEAL NERVE RELEASE

Surgical Technique

1. The patient is placed on the operating table in the supine position.
2. Regional anesthesia is induced at the ankle, with the anesthetic injected proximal to the area of compression.
3. The area of compression is located before surgery. This area of compression could be at the anterior ankle joint, dorsal talonavicular joint, or first metatarsal–tarsal joint area. The area is opened by making a 5- to 7.5-cm incision.
4. Care is taken to release only a portion of the retinacular ligament, just in the area of compression. Preferably, only half rather than the entire retinacular ligament should be released to avoid bowstringing of the tendons. If more of the retinaculum needs to be released, it should be cut in a Z fashion to facilitate closure in a lengthened position.
5. The nerve and fatty tissue are retracted. If a localizing bony exostosis or an area of compression is present, this area is resected. Occasionally, when the compression is at the base of the metatarsals and there is no bony prominence to remove, the extensor hallucis brevis tendon must be released.
6. If ankle instability is diagnosed as a major contributing factor to deep peroneal neuralgia, then ankle ligament reconstruction might need to be considered. When anterior compartment syndrome has been identified, fasciotomy is also considered.
7. The wound is irrigated and the retinaculum is closed in the lengthened position if it was completely released. The skin is closed with interrupted sutures.
8. A compressive dressing is applied. If the retinacular closure was necessary a splint is recommended.

Postoperative Care

The patient uses crutches for 4 to 5 days and gradually resumes weight bearing as tolerated. If surgery is extensive, a splint is used for 2 weeks followed by a boot brace for 2 to 4 additional weeks. If the retinaculum was not released completely, training is gradually resumed as tolerated beginning 4 to 6 weeks postoperatively.

Results

The experience of Dellon[61] with 20 deep peroneal nerve entrapments managed with surgical decompression suggests an 80% satisfactory outcome. Poor results were typically related to internal nerve damage or neuropathies contributing to nerve compromise, in which case simple neurolysis usually proved ineffective.[61] My (LCS) experience with this nerve release has been the best when there is a bony prominence or osteophyte. When the lesion occurred from a crush injury, the results have been less satisfactory.

SURAL NERVE ENTRAPMENT

The medial sural nerve runs between the heads of the gastrocnemius muscle and penetrates its deep aponeurosis approximately halfway up the leg. Subsequently, it anastomoses with the peroneal communicating nerve and travels along the border of the Achilles tendon next to the short saphenous veins. The nerve runs along the midline of the calf; then, at a mean distance of 9.8 cm from the calcaneus, it crosses over the edge of the Achilles tendon (Fig. 11–61).[188]

Two centimeters above the ankle, it gives off branches: one supplies sensation to the lateral aspect of the heel, and the other often anastomoses with the lateral branch of the superficial peroneal nerve. After giving off the branches to the heel, the nerve runs inferior to the peroneal sheaths in a subcutaneous position. As it reaches the tuberosity of the fifth metatarsal, the nerve ramifies to provide sensation to the lateral aspect of the fifth toe, the fourth web space, and often the third and fourth toes. Thus this network of branches supplies sensation to the posterior lateral lower leg and ankle, the lateral foot and heel, and the lateral two or three toes.[171,183,187]

Etiology

Sural nerve entrapment can occur anywhere along its course. Several cases have been described in runners who sustained fractures of the base of the fifth metatarsal after severe plantar flexion and inversion injuries.[185,186] Recurrent ankle sprains can lead to fibrosis and subsequent nerve entrapment.[186] Ganglions of the peroneal sheath or calcaneocuboid joint have also been reported.[186] An interesting case reported by Husson et al[167] developed after compression by an area

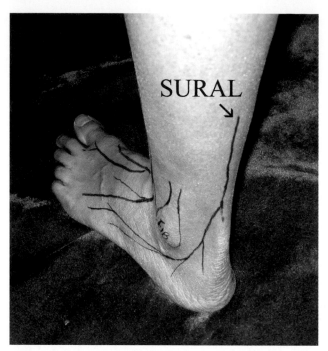

Figure 11–61   The sural nerve crosses the lateral border of the Achilles tendon.

of myositis ossificans circumscripta at the musculo-tendinous junction of the Achilles.

Surgery about the posterior calf, such as the Strayer procedure, can result in scarring around the sural nerve proximally. Achilles tendon reconstructions, calcaneal fracture open reduction and fixation, calcaneal osteotomy (Dwyer procedure), the approaches for lateral ligamentous reconstructions or peroneal tendon repairs, and the exposure for subtalar fusion can lead to sural nerve injury by transection, traction, or encasement in scar tissue (Fig. 11–62).

Clinical Symptoms

Most patients with sural nerve disorders recall a history of ankle injuries, typically acute or recurrent ankle sprains. Patients with persistent pain after ankle sprains might note radiating symptoms or paresthesias associated with instability. Although the pain pattern may be poorly localized, occasionally a focus of pain allows for identification of a specific area of nerve compromise along the course of the sural nerve. Previous surgery on the posterior calf, lateral heel ankle, and foot should be documented, including preoperative and postoperative symptoms.[147,151]

Diagnosis

Examination of the entire course of the sural nerve should be performed from the popliteal fossa and pos-

terior aspect of the proximal fibula to the toes.. If the pain occurs only during certain activities, the patient should walk, run, or move the foot excessively before examination. Local tenderness and a positive Tinel sign are characteristic after running activities. Occasionally numbness is noted. The patient should be examined for coexisting disease such as Achilles or peroneal tendinosis, ankle instability, subtalar arthritis, calcaneal fracture residua, and fifth metatarsal nonunions.

Plain radiographs should be obtained to rule out bone or joint abnormality that can contribute to nerve compression. An MRI may be helpful when soft-tissue masses are suspected. Electrodiagnostic studies can occasionally confirm a clinical suspicion of limited sural nerve conduction, but these tests are typically most useful in diagnosing more proximal sites of nerve compromise. Diagnostic nerve blocks are of some use in defining sural nerve entrapment symptoms. If the nerve block fails to relieve symptoms, injection of the superficial peroneal nerve may be warranted. Select injection into the tendon sheath or joints can also help identify contributory disease.

Treatment

Conservative Treatment

Nonoperative management of sural neuralgia requires identification of the cause of nerve compromise. Isolated sural neuralgia might respond to the medications previously discussed: vitamin B_6, NSAIDs, tricyclic antidepressants, and gabapentin or other antiepileptic medications. The Lidoderm patch and topically compounded pain creams have been particularly useful

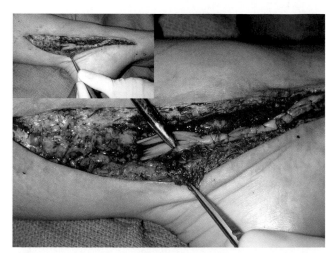

Figure 11–62   The sural nerve (draped over scissors) was released during an exposure for a peroneal tendon transfer for chronic lateral ankle ligament reconstruction. After failing rerelease, the nerve was wrapped with an umbilical vein. *Inset*, wide view of the exposure.

because the nerve is rather superficial. If nerve compromise is secondary to traction from chronic ankle instability, then bracing, orthotics, or shoe modifications can be effective, as for superficial peroneal neuralgia. Caution with bracing is advised because external compression can aggravate sural nerve symptoms..

Surgical Treatment

SURAL NERVE RELEASE

Surgical Technique

1. The patient is placed on the operating table in the supine position with a beanbag positioner or a roll under the hip of the affected leg. This internally rotates the leg so that the sural nerve can be better visualized.
2. A regional anesthetic is used with the block proximal to the area of compression. A tourniquet may or may not be used.
3. The area of compression is located before surgery, and only a small area of the skin is incised over the area of compression.
4. The sural nerve is identified at the area of compression and an appropriate release carried out.
5. If necessary, the nerve is moved in one direction or the other so that it will not be in an area of compression.
6. If any bony exostoses rub on the nerve, these are removed carefully, and excessive dissection or resection of fat away from the nerve is avoided.
7. Care is taken to cover the nerve and to suture the skin with interrupted suture.
8. A compressive dressing is applied.

Postoperative Care

The patient uses crutches for 3 to 4 days after surgery. If the area of release is in a joint, a boot brace is used for 2 to 4 weeks. Activity is resumed as tolerated. Usually physical activities are not resumed until 4 weeks postoperatively.

Results

Fabre et al[184] described 13 athletes (18 limbs) who had sural nerve entrapment by the superficial sural aponeurosis in the calf. Neurolysis was performed by incising the aponeurosis and the fibrous band where the nerve exited. Their results were excellent in 9 limbs (2 bilateral), good in 8 limbs (2 bilateral), and fair in 1 case.

Surgical decompression of mass effects (such as scar entrapment, ganglions, and avulsion fractures) typically results in satisfactory symptomatic relief.[147,185,186] When the cause was prior surgery, release of the nerve is not as predictable. When performing a nerve release, if a branch neuroma is encountered, resecting that damaged nerve branch with burial into a healthy bed can improve symptoms. It has been our experience that sural neuralgia due to ankle instability is managed effectively with lateral ankle stabilization, without directly addressing the sural nerve.

SAPHENOUS NERVE ENTRAPMENT

Overview, Etiology, and Anatomy

Saphenous nerve entrapment or neuralgia is not common. Typically, entrapment of this nerve occurs about the knee, but because its terminal distribution is at the medial ankle and foot, patients can present with medial distal lower extremity pain secondary to compromise of this nerve. The saphenous nerve courses with the superficial femoral artery after originating from the femoral nerve. It penetrates the subsartorial fascia approximately 10 cm proximal to the medial femoral condyle and then divides into the infrapatellar and sartorial or distal saphenous branches. The sartorial component descends along the medial tibial border with the greater saphenous vein. Approximately 15 cm proximal to the medial malleolus, the sartorial or distal saphenous nerve separates into two branches: one that supplies sensation to the medial aspect of the ankle and one that innervates the medial foot. Although entrapment or compression can occur anywhere along the nerve's course, the most likely site of compromise is at the subsartorial fascia, just proximal to the medial femoral condyle.

Evaluation

History

Because the nerve compromise may be proximal, it is important to identify any history of knee injury, knee or bypass surgery, or pain. Direct trauma anywhere along the course of the nerve may be responsible for entrapment within scar tissue. A history of saphenous vein stripping, medial compartment release, or medial malleolar fracture may be an indication that the nerve is damaged from the injury or surgical approach.

Garland et al,[190] in a retrospective survey of patients with saphenous vein harvest following coronary bypass, found related numbness or tingling in 61%, of whom 37% improved within 3 months. There was persistent numbness beyond 2 years in 41%. Although pain was common, most improved by 3 months and only 10% had pain persisting beyond 2 years.

In another study, Morrison et al[192] documented that 40% of patients reported symptoms of saphenous nerve injury after operation, but these symptoms affected quality of life in only 6.7%.

Hutchinson et al[191] reported on a technique of endoscopically assisted leg compartment fascial release. They found a reduced risk of saphenous vein injury (30% to 100%), comparing a blind percutaneous release through a 2- to 3-cm incision versus an endoscopically assisted technique.

Physical Examination

Although the patient might complain of medial ankle and foot pain, point tenderness is typically located over the subsartorial canal proximal to the medial femoral condyle. Occasionally, hyperextension of the knee produces distal symptoms. In isolated saphenous nerve compromise, no motor deficits will be present. The entire course of the nerve should be palpated to identify any other sites of possible nerve compromise. Obviously sites of prior surgical exploration should be carefully palpated.

Diagnostic Studies

Rarely, plain radiographs can demonstrate a bony abnormality responsible for the saphenous nerve compression, but typically physical examination will prompt radiographic evaluation. Soft-tissue masses may be assessed with MRI or ultrasound. Selective injection at the site of nerve compromise in the subsartorial canal or along the medial border of the tibia or medial malleolus can be useful. Some clinicians have demonstrated that somatosensory evoked potentials might aid in diagnosing saphenous nerve entrapment.[189,197]

Treatment

Conservative Treatment

Nonoperative management can involve activity modification if symptoms have a dynamic component. The medications discussed earlier and the topical patches and creams can be useful, especially in a thin patient where the nerve is more superficial. Cortisone added to the diagnostic nerve block noted previously can prove therapeutic. Treating saphenous nerve entrapment with therapeutic blocks has resulted in satisfactory relief of symptoms in 38% to 80% of patients.[193,194]

Surgical Treatment

Surgical management of the more proximal entrapments requires release of the anterior aspect of Hunter's canal and dissection of the saphenous and sartorial nerve fibers from the surrounding fascia.[72,195]

For the more distal entrapments, the nerve release is performed locally. It is useful to identify the saphenous vein because the two nerve branches distally can be difficult to find.

Release of the focal entrapment can yield good results, especially when the entrapment is associated with a space-occupying lesion. Often there has been a transection of one of the branches, and a more proximal transection and burial is needed. Rarely patients continue to have pain and require revision nerve transection or peripheral nerve stimulation.

SUMMARY

Nerve entrapments can occur frequently, but they can be underdiagnosed when the presentation is atypical. Because pain is a subjective experience, the symptoms can be vague and may be referred. Thus, the examiner must have an awareness of these syndromes in obtaining a history. A thorough knowledge of peripheral nerve anatomy is essential in establishing the diagnosis. Radiographs might reveal bony abnormalities that are causing the problems. The presence of more proximal lesions (double crush) and metabolic conditions should not be overlooked. Electrodiagnostic test results may be normal, but it can be useful to find these other systemic or more proximal pathologies.

In some patients, changing the shoes, wearing an orthosis, or modifying activity can result in relief. Use of oral medications and topical agents can be helpful in controlling the symptoms. In certain cases injections may be both diagnostic and therapeutic. For recalcitrant cases, surgery may be indicated and usually gives satisfactory results. In performing surgery, the risks of poor response remain. When a patient fails nerve release, revision release and transection of damaged nerves can be helpful. For those unfortunate patients who continue to suffer intractable nerve pain, the options include further nerve transection, vein wrap or other nerve-containment procedures, peripheral nerve stimulation, or spinal cord stimulation.

REFERENCES

Interdigital Plantar Neuroma

1. American Chronic Pain Association: Medications and Chronic Pain Supplement 2005. PDF available for download at http://www.theacpa.org/cp_01.asp (accessed March 31, 2006).

2. Amis JA, Siverhus SW, Liwnicz BH: An anatomic basis for recurrence after Morton's neuroma excision. *Foot Ankle* 13:153-156, 1992.

3. Awerbuch MS, Shephard E, Vernon-Roberts B: Morton's metatarsalgia due to intermetatarsophalangeal bursitis as an early manifestation of rheumatoid arthritis. *Clin Orthop Relat Res* 167:214-221, 1982.

4. Barrett S, Pignetti TT: Endoscopic decompression for intermetatarsal nerve entrapment—the EDIN technique: Preliminary study with cadaveric specimens and early clinical results. *J Foot Ankle Surg* 33:503-506, 1994.

5. Bencardino J, Rosenberg ZS, Beltran J, et al: Morton's neuroma: Is it always symptomatic? *AJR Am J Roentgenol* 175:649-653, 2000.

6. Benedetti RS, Baxter DE, Davis PF: Clinical results of simultaneous adjacent interdigital neurectomy in the foot. *Foot Ankle Int* 17:583, 1996.

7. Beskin JL, Baxter DE: Recurrent pain following interdigital neurectomy—a plantar approach. *Foot Ankle* 9:34-39, 1988.

8. Betts LO: Morton's metatarsalgia: Neuritis of the fourth digital nerve. *Med J Aust* 1:514, 1940.

9. Biasca N, Zanetti M, Zollinger H: Outcomes after partial neurectomy of Morton's neuroma related to preoperative case histories, clinical findings, and findings on magnetic resonance imaging scans. *Foot Ankle Int* 20:568-575, 1999.

10. Bossley CJ, Cairney PC: The intermetatarsophalangeal bursa: Its significance in Morton's metatarsalgia. *J Bone Joint Surg Br* 62:184-187, 1980.

11. Bradley N, Miller WA, Evans JP: Plantar neuroma analysis of results following surgical excision in 145 patients. *South Med J* 69:853, 1976.

12. Colgrove RC, Huang EY, Barth AH, Greene MA: Interdigital neuroma: Intermuscular neuroma transposition compared with resection. *Foot Ankle Int* 21:206-211, 2000.

13. Coughlin MJ, Pinsonneault T: Operative treatment of interdigital neuroma. A long-term follow-up study. *J Bone Joint Surg Am* 84:1276-1277, 2002.

14. Davis TJ, Schon LC: Branches of the tibial nerve: Anatomic variations. *Foot Ankle Int* 16:21-29, 1995.

15. Dellon AL: Treatment of Morton's neuroma as a nerve compression: The role for neurolysis. *J Amer Pod Med Assoc*, 82:399-402, 1992.

16. Durlacher L: *A Treatise on Corns, Bunions, the Disease of Nails and the General Management of the Feet.* London, Simpkin, Marshall, 1845.

17. Fanucci E, Masala S, Fabiano S, et al: Treatment of intermetatarsal Morton's neuroma with alcohol injection under US guide: 10-month follow-up. *Eur Radiol* 14:514-518, 2004.

18. Gauthier G: Thomas Morton's disease: A nerve entrapment syndrome. *Clin Orthop Relat Res* 142:90, 1979.

19. Giannini S, Bacchini P, Ceccarelli F, Vannini F: Interdigital neuroma: Clinical examination and histopathologic results in 63 cases treated with excision. *Foot Ankle Int* 25:79-84, 2004.

20. Govsa F, Bilge O, Ozer MA: Anatomical study of the communicating branches between the medial and lateral plantar nerves. *Surg Radiol Anat* 27:377-381, 2005.

21. Graham CE, Graham DM: Morton's neuroma: A microscopic evaluation. *Foot Ankle* 5:150-153, 1984.

22. Graham CE, Johnson KA, Ilstrup DM: The intermetatarsal nerve: A microscopic evaluation. *Foot Ankle* 2:150-152, 1981.

23. Greenfield J, Rea J Jr, Ilfeld FW: Morton's interdigital neuroma: Indications for treatment by local injections versus surgery. *Clin Orthop Relat Res* 185:142-144, 1984.

24. Hauser ED: Interdigital neuroma of the foot. *Surg Gynecol Obstet* 133:265-267, 1971.

25. Hoadley AE: Six cases of metatarsalgia. *Chicago Med Rec* 5:32-37, 1893.

26. Hort KR, DeOrio JK: Adjacent interdigital nerve irritation: Single incision surgical treatment. *Foot Ankle Int* 23:1026-1030, 2002.

27. Johnson JD, Johnson KA, Unni KK: Persistent pain after excision of an interdigital neuroma. *J Bone Surg Am* 70:651-657, 1988.

28. Jones JR, Klenerman L: A study of the communicating branch between the medial and lateral plantar nerves. *Foot Ankle* 4:313-315, 1984.

29. Kelikian H: *Hallux Valgus, Allied Deformities of the Forefoot and Metatarsalgia.* Philadelphia, WB Saunders, 1965.

30. Lassmann G: Morton's toe: Clinical, light, and electron microscopic investigations in 133 cases. *Clin Orthop Relat Res* 142:73-84, 1979.

31. Levine SE, Myerson MS, Shapiro PP, et al: Ultrasonographic diagnosis of recurrence after excision of an interdigital neuroma. *Foot Ankle Int* 19:79-84, 1998.

32. Levitsky KA, Alman BA, Jesevar DS, Morehead J: Digital nerves of the foot: Anatomic variations and implications regarding the pathogenesis of the interdigital neuroma. *Foot Ankle* 14:208-214, 1993.

33. Mann RA, Reynolds JD: Interdigital neuroma: A critical clinical analysis. *Foot Ankle* 3:238, 1983.

34. Mason E: A case of neuralgia of the second metatarsophalangeal articulation: Cured by resection of the joint. *Am J Med Sci* 74:445, 1877.

35. McElvenny RT: The etiology and surgical treatment of intractable pain about the fourth metatarsophalangeal joint (Morton's toe). *J Bone Joint Surg* 25:675-679, 1943.

36. Morton TG: A peculiar and painful affection of fourth metatarsophalangeal articulation. *Am J Med Sci* 71:37-45, 1876.

37. Mulder JD: The causative mechanism in Morton's metatarsalgia. *J Bone Joint Surg Br* 33:94-95, 1951.

38. Nemoto K, Mikasa M, Tazaki K, Mori Y: Neurolysis as a surgical procedure for Morton's neuroma. *Nippon Seikeigeka Gakkai Zasshi* 63:470-473, 1989.

39. Okafor B, Shergill G, Angel J: Treatment of Morton's neuroma by neurolysis. *Foot Ankle Int* 18:284-287, 1997.

40. Quinn TJ, Jacobson JA, Craig JG, et al: Sonography of Morton's neuromas. *AJR Am J Roentgenol* 174:1723-1728, 2000.

41. Read JW, Noakes JB, Kerr D, et al: Morton's metatarsalgia: Sonographic findings and correlated histopathology. *Foot Ankle Int* 20:153-161, 1999.

42. Redd RA, Peters VJ, Emery SF, et al: Morton's neuroma: Sonographic evaluation. *Radiology* 171:415-417, 1989.

43. Resch S, Stenstrom A, Jonsson A, et al: The diagnostic efficacy of magnetic resonance imaging and ultrasonography in Morton's neuroma: A radiological–surgical correlation. *Foot Ankle Int* 15:88-92, 1994.

44. Rosson G, Dellon AL: Surgical approach to multiple interdigital nerve compressions. *J Foot Ankle Surgery* 44:70-73, 2005.

45. Shapiro PP, Shapiro SL: Sonographic evaluation of interdigital neuromas. *Foot Ankle Int* 16:604-606, 1995.

46. Shapiro SL: Endoscopic decompression of the intermetatarsal nerve for Morton's neuroma. *Foot Ankle Clin* 9:297-304, 2004.

47. Sharp RJ, Wade CM, Hennessy MS, Saxby TS: The role of MRI and ultrasound imaging in Morton's neuroma and the effect of size of lesion on symptoms. *J Bone Joint Surg Br* 85:999-1005, 2003.

48. Stamatis ED, Myerson MS: Treatment of recurrence of symptoms after excision of an interdigital neuroma. A retrospective review. *J Bone Joint Surg Br* 86:48-53, 2004.

49. Terk MR, Kwong PK, Suthar M, et al: Morton neuroma: Evaluation with MR imaging performed with contrast enhancement and fat suppression. *Radiology* 189:239-241, 1993.

50. Thompson FM, Deland JT: Occurrence of two interdigital neuromas in one foot. *Foot Ankle* 14:15-17, 1993.

51. Tubby AH: *Deformities, Including Diseases of the Bones and Joints*, vol 1, ed 2. London, Macmillan, 1912.

52. Weishaupt D, Treiber K, Kundert HP, et al: Morton neuroma: MR imaging in prone, supine, and upright weight-bearing body positions. *Radiology* 226:849-856, 2003.

53. Wolfort SF Dellon AL: Treatment of recurrent neuroma of the interdigital nerve by implantation of the proximal nerve into muscle in the arch of the foot. *J Foot Ankle Surg* 40: 404-410, 2001.

54. Younger AS, Claridge RJ: The role of diagnostic block in the management of Morton's neuroma. *Can J Surg* 41:127-130, 1998.

Tarsal Tunnel Syndrome

55. Aszmann O, Tassler PL, Dellon AL: Changing the natural history of diabetic neuropathy: Incidence of ulcer/amputation in the contralateral limb of patients with a unilateral nerve decompression procedure. *Ann Plast Surg* 53:517-522, 2004.

56. Biddinger KR, Amend KJ: The role of surgical decompression for diabetic neuropathy. *Foot Ankle Clin* 9:239-254, 2004.

57. Budak F, Bamac B, Ozbek A, et al: Nerve conduction studies of lower extremities in pes planus subjects. *Electromyogr Clin Neurophysiol* 41(7):443-446, 2001.

58. Cimino WR: Tarsal tunnel syndrome: review of the literature. *Foot Ankle* 11:47-52, 1990.

59. Daniels TR, Lau JT, Hearn TC: The effects of foot position and load on tibial nerve tension. *Foot Ankle Int* 19:73-78, 1998.

60. Davis TJ, Schon LC: Branches of the tibial nerve: Anatomic variations. *Foot Ankle Int* 16:21-29, 1995.

61. Dellon AL: Diabetic neuropathy: Review of a surgical approach to restore sensation, relieve pain, and prevent ulceration and amputation. *Foot Ankle Int* 25(10):749-755, 2004.

62. Dellon AL, Kim J, Spaulding CM: Variations in the origin of the medial calcaneal nerve. *J Am Podiatr Med Assoc* 92:97-101, 2002.

63. Frey C, Kerr R: Magnetic resonance imaging and the evaluation of tarsal tunnel syndrome. *Foot Ankle* 14:159-164, 1993.

64. Galardi G, Amadio S, Maderna L, et al: Electrophysiologic studies in tarsal tunnel syndrome. Diagnostic reliability of motor distal latency, mixed nerve and sensory nerve conduction studies. *Am J Phys Med Rehabil* 73:193-198, 1994.

65. Gondring WH, Shields B, Wenger S: An outcomes analysis of surgical treatment of tarsal tunnel syndrome. *Foot Ankle Int* 24:545-550, 2003.

66. Havel PE, Ebraheim NA, Clark SE, et al: Tibial branching in the tarsal tunnel. *Foot Ankle* 9:117-119, 1988.

67. Kaplan PE, Kernahan WT: Tarsal tunnel syndrome: An electrodiagnostic and surgical correlation. *J Bone Joint Surg Am* 63:96-99, 1981.

68. Keck C: The tarsal tunnel syndrome. *J Bone Joint Surg Am* 44:180-182, 1962.

69. Kim DH, Ryu S, Tiel RL, Kline DG: Surgical management and results of 135 tibial nerve lesions at the Louisiana State University Health Sciences Center. *Neurosurgery* 53:1114-1124, 2003.

70. Kinoshita M, Okuda R, Morikawa J, Abe M: Tarsal tunnel syndrome associated with an accessory muscle. *Foot Ankle Int* 24:132-136, 2003.

71. Kinoshita M, Okuda R, Morikawa J, et al: The dorsiflexion–eversion test for diagnosis of tarsal tunnel syndrome. *J Bone Joint Surg Am* 83:1835-1839, 2001.

72. Kopell HP, Thompson WAL: Peripheral entrapment neuropathies of the lower extremity. *N Engl J Med* 262:56-60, 1960.

73. Labib SA, Gould JS, Rodriguez-del-Rio FA, Lyman S. Heel pain triad (HPT): The combination of plantar fasciitis, posterior tibial tendon dysfunction and tarsal tunnel syndrome. *Foot Ankle Int* 23:212-220, 2002.

74. Lam SJS: Tarsal tunnel syndrome. *J Bone Joint Surg Am* 49:87-92, 1967.

75 Lau JT, Daniels TR: Effects of tarsal tunnel release and stabilization procedures on tibial nerve tension in a surgically created pes planus foot. *Foot Ankle Int* 19(11):770-777, 1998.

76. Lee CH, Dellon AL: Prognostic ability of Tinel sign in determining outcome for decompression surgery in diabetic and nondiabetic neuropathy. *Ann Plast Surg* 53:523-527, 2004.

77. Lumsden DB, Schon LC, Easley ME, et al: Topography of the distal tibial nerve and its branches. *Foot Ankle Int* 24:696-700, 2003.

78. Mann RA: Tarsal tunnel syndrome. *Orthop Clin North Am* 5:109-115, 1974.

79. Nagaoka M, Matsuzaki H: Ultrasonography in tarsal tunnel syndrome. *J Ultrasound Med* 24:1035-1040, 2005.

80. Nagaoka M, Satou K: Tarsal tunnel syndrome caused by ganglia. *J Bone Joint Surg Br* 81(4):607-610, 1999.

81. Oh SJ, Savaria PK, Kuba T, et al: Tarsal tunnel syndrome: Electrophysiologic study. *Ann Neurol* 5:327-330, 1979.

82. Patel AT, Gaines K, Malamut R, et al; American Association of Neuromuscular and Electrodiagnostic Medicine: Usefulness of electrodiagnostic techniques in the evaluation of suspected tarsal tunnel syndrome: An evidence-based review. *Muscle Nerve* 2005 Aug;32(2):236-40.

83. Pfeiffer WH, Cracchiolo A 3rd: Clinical results after tarsal tunnel decompression. *J Bone Joint Surg Am* 76:1222-1230, 1994.

84. Sammarco GJ, Chang L: Outcome of surgical treatment of tarsal tunnel syndrome. *Foot Ankle Int* 24:125-131, 2003.

85. Skalley TC, Schon LC, Hinton RY, Myerson NS: Clinical results following revision tibial nerve release. *Foot Ankle Int* 15:360-367, 1994.

86. Takakura Y, Kitada C, Sugimoto K, et al: Tarsal tunnel syndrome. Causes and results of operative treatment. *J Bone Joint Surg Br* 73:125-128, 1991.

87. Takakura Y, Kumai T, Takaoka T, Tamai S: Tarsal tunnel syndrome caused by coalition associated with a ganglion. *J Bone Joint Surg Br* 80:130-133, 1998.

88. Trepman E, Kadel NJ, Chisholm K, Razzano L: Effect of foot and ankle position on tarsal tunnel compartment pressure. *Foot Ankle Int* 20:721-726, 1999.

89. Urguden M, Bilbasar H, Ozdemir H, et al: Tarsal tunnel syndrome—the effect of the associated features on outcome of surgery. *Int Orthop* 26:253-256, 2002.

90. Wilemon WK: Tarsal tunnel syndrome, *Orthop Rev* 8:111, 1979.

Failed Tarsal Tunnel Release

91. Campbell JT, Schon LC, Burkhardt LD: Histopathologic findings in autogenous saphenous vein graft wrapping for recurrent tarsal tunnel syndrome: A case report. *Foot Ankle Int* 19:766-769, 1998.

92. Dellon AL, Mackinnon SE: Results of posterior tibial nerve grafting at the ankle. *J Reconstr Microsurg* 7(2):81-83, 1991.

93. Dielissen PW, Claassen AT, Veldman PH, Goris RJ: Amputation for reflex sympathetic dystrophy. *J Bone Joint Surg Br* 77:270-273, 1995.

94. Easley ME, Schon LC: Peripheral nerve vein wrapping for intractable lower extremity pain. *Foot Ankle Int* 21:492-500, 2000.

95. Gould JS, Hart TS, O'Brien TS, Winkler MV: Outcome analysis of vein wrapping for intractable painful nerves in continuity. Presented at the 12th Annual Summer Meeting of the American Foot and Ankle Society, Hilton Head, SC, June 28, 1996.

96. Gybels J, Van Calenbergh F: The treatment of pain due to peripheral nerve injury by electrical stimulation of the injured nerve. *Adv Pain Res Ther* 13:217-222, 1990.

97. Hassenbusch S J, Stanton-Hicks M, Schoppa D, et al: Long-term results of peripheral nerve stimulation for reflex sympathetic dystrophy. *J Neurosurg* 84:415-423, 1996.

98. Honkamp N, Amendola A, Hurwitz S, Saltzman CL: Retrospective review of 18 patients who underwent transtibial amputation for intractable pain. *J Bone Joint Surg Am* 83(10): 1479-1483, 2001

99. Law JD, Swett J, Kirsch WM: Retrospective analysis of 22 patients with chronic pain treated by peripheral nerve stimulation. *J Neurosurg* 52:482-485, 1980.

100. Masear VR, Colgin S: The treatment of epineural scarring with allograft vein wrapping. *Hand Clin* 12:773-779, 1996.

101. Masear VR, Tulloss JR, St. Mary E, Meyer RD: Venous wrapping of nerves to prevent scarring [abstr]. *J Hand Surg Am* 15: 817-818, 1999.

102. Nashold, BS Jr, Goldner JL, Mullen JB, Bright DS: Long-term pain control by direct peripheral-nerve stimulation. *J Bone Joint Surg Am* 64:1-10, 1982.

103. Ruch DS, Spinner RM, Koman LA, et al: The histological effect of barrier vein wrapping of peripheral nerves. *J Reconstr Microsurg* 12(5):291-295, 1996.

104. Schon LC, Anderson CD, Easley ME, et al: Surgical treatment of chronic lower extremity neuropathic pain. *Clin Orthop Relat Res* 389:156-164, 2001.

105. Schon LC, Easley ME: Chronic pain. In Myerson MS (ed): *Foot and Ankle Disorders*. Philadelphia, WB Saunders, 2000, pp 851-881.

106. Schon LC, Lam PW, Easley ME, et al: Complex salvage procedures for severe lower extremity nerve pain. *Clin Orthop Relat Res* 391:171-80, 2001.

107. Schon LC, Short KW, Soupiou O, et al: Benefits of early prosthetic management of transtibial amputees: A prospective clinical study of prefabricated prosthesis. *Foot Ankle Int* 23:509-514, 2002.

108. Shealy CN, Mortimer JT, Reswick JB: Electrical inhibition of pain by stimulation of the dorsal columns: Preliminary clinical report. *Anesth Analg* 46:489-491, 1967.

109. Sotereanos DG, Giannkopoulos PN, Mitsionis GI, et al: Vein graft wrapping for the treatment of recurrent compression of the median nerve. *Microsurgery* 16:752-756, 1995.

110. Stanton-Hicks M, Burton AW, Bruehl SP, et al: An updated interdisciplinary clinical pathway for CRPS: Report of an expert panel. Pain Practice 2:1-16, 2002.

111. Strege DW, Cooney WP, Wood MB, et al: Chronic peripheral nerve pain treated with direct electrical nerve stimulation. *J Hand Surg Am* 19:931-939, 1994.

112. Turner JA, Loeser JD, Bell KG: Spinal cord stimulation for chronic low back pain: A systematic literature synthesis. *Neurosurgery* 37:1088-1096, 1995.

113. Varitimidis SE, Vardakas DG, Goebel F, Sotereanos DG: Treatment of recurrent compressive neuropathy of peripheral nerves in the upper extremity with an autologous vein insulator. *J Hand Surg Am* 26:296-302, 2001.

114. Vora AM, Schon LC: Revision peripheral nerve surgery. *Foot Ankle Clin* 9(2):305-318, 2004.

115. Waisbrod H, Panhans C, Hansen D, Gerbershagen HU: Direct nerve stimulation for painful peripheral neuropathies. *J Bone Joint Surg Br* 67:470-472, 1985.

116. Xu J, Sotereanos DG, Moller AR, et al: Nerve wrapping with vein grafts in a rat model: A safe technique for the treatment of recurrent chronic compressive neuropathy. *J Reconstr Microsurg* 14(5):323-328, 1998.

117. Zeiss J, Fenton P, Ebraheim N, Coombs RJ: Magnetic resonance imaging for ineffectual tarsal tunnel surgical treatment. *Clin Orthop Relat Res* 264:264-266, 1991.

Traumatic and Incisional Neuromas

118. Anatomical Society of Great Britain and Ireland: Report of Committee of Collective Investigation on the Distribution of Cutaneous Nerve on the Dorsum of the Foot. *J Anat Physiol* 26:89, 1891/1892.

119. Barbera J, Albert-Pamplo R: Centrocentral anastomosis of the proximal nerve stump in the treatment of painful amputation neuromas of major nerves. *J Neurosurg* 79:331-334, 1993.

120. Barbers J, Gonzalez J, Gil JL: The quality and extension of nerve fibre regeneration in the centrocentral anastomosis of the peripheral nerve. *Acta Neurochir Suppl* (Wien) 43:205-209, 1988.

121. Bauer RD, Eft AL: Clinical effect of nitrogen mustard on neoplastic diseases. *Am J Med Sci* 219:216, 1950.

122. Chiodo CP, Miller SD: Surgical treatment of superficial peroneal neuromas. *Foot Ankle Int* 10:689-694, 2000.

123. Dellon AL, Aszmann OC: Treatment of superficial and deep peroneal neuromas by resection and translocation of the nerves into the anterolateral compartment. *Foot Ankle Int* 19:300-303, 1998.

124. Dellon Al, MacKinnon SE: Susceptibility of the superficial sensory branch of the radial nerve to form painful neuromas. *J Hand Surg Br* 9:42-45, 1984.

125. Ferkel RD, Heath DD, Guhl JF: Neurological complications of ankle arthroscopy. *Arthroscopy* 12:200-208, 1996.

126. Goldstein SA, Sturim HS: Intraossoeus nerve transposition for treatment of painful neuromas. *J Hand Surg Am* 10:270-274, 1985.

127. Gorkisch K, Boese-Landgraf J, Vaubel E: Treatment and prevention of amputation neuromas in hand surgery. *Plast Reconstr Surg* 73:293-299, 1984.

128. Herndon JH, Hess AV: Neuromas. In Green DP, Hotchkiss RN (eds): *Operative Hand Surgery*. New York, Churchill Livingstone, 1982, p 939.

129. Herndon JH, Hess AV: Neuromas. In Gelberman RH (ed): *Operative Nerve Repair and Reconstruction*. Philadelphia, JB Lippincott, 1991, p 1525.

130. Hutchinson MR, Bederka B, Kopplin M: Anatomic structures at risk during minimal incision endoscopically assisted fascial compartment releases in the leg. *Am J Sports Med* 31:764-769, 2003.

131. Kenzora JE: Symptomatic incisional neuromas on the dorsum of the foot. *Foot Ankle* 5:2-15, 1984.

132. Lidor C, Hall RL, Nunley JA: Centrocentral anastomosis with autologous nerve graft treatment of foot and ankle neuromas. *Foot Ankle Int* 17:85-88, 1996.

133. Mass DP, Ciano MC, Tortosa R: Treatment of painful hand neuromas by their transfer into bone. *Plast Reconstr Surg* 74:182-185, 1984.

134. Miller SD: Dorsomedial cutaneous nerve syndrome: Treatment with nerve transection and burial into bone. *Foot Ankle Int* 22:198-202, 2001.

135. Nunley JA, Gabel GT: Tibial nerve grafting for restoration of plantar sensation. *Foot Ankle Int* 14:489-492, 1993.

136. Petropoulos PC, Stefanko S: Experimental observations on the prevention of neuroma formation. Preliminary report. *J Surg Res* 1:241-248, 1961.

137. Redfern DJ, Sauve PS, Sakellariou A: Investigation of incidence of superficial peroneal nerve injury following ankle fracture. *Foot Ankle Int* 24:771-774, 2003

138. Robbins TH: Nerve capping in the treatment of troublesome terminal neuroma. *Br J Plast Surg* 39:239-240, 1986.

139. Solomon LB, Ferris L, Tedman R, Henneberg M: Surgical anatomy of the sural and superficial fibular nerves with an emphasis on the approach to the lateral malleolus. *J Anat* 199(Pt 6):717-723, 2001

140. Sunderland S: *Nerves and Nerve Injuries*, ed 2. New York, Churchill Livingstone, 1978.

141. Tupper JW, Booth DM: Treatment of painful neuromas of sensory nerves in the hand: A comparison of traditional and newer methods. *J Hand Surg Am* 1:144-151, 1976.

142. Whipple RR, Unsell RS: Treatment of painful neuromas. *Orthop Clin North Am* 19:175-185, 1988.

143. White JC, Hamlin H: New uses of tantalum in nerve suture, control of neuroma formation and prevention of regeneration after thoracic sympathectomy, illustration of technical procedures. *J Neurosurg* 2:402, 1945.

Lateral Plantar Nerve Entrapment

144. Baxter DE, Pfeffer GB: Treatment of chronic heel pain by surgical release of the first branch of the lateral plantar nerve. *Clin Orthop Relat Res* 279:229-236, 1992.

145. Gould JS: Treatment of the painful injured nerve incontinuity. In Gelberman GH (ed): *Operative Nerve Repair and Reconstruction*. Philadelphia, JB Lippincott, 1991, pp 1541-1550.

146. Henricson AS, Westlin NE: Chronic calcaneal pain in athletes: Entrapment of the calcaneal nerve? *Am J Sports Med* 12:152-154, 1987.

147. Schon LC: Nerve entrapment, neuropathy, and nerve dysfunction in athletes. *Orthop Clin North Am* 25:47-59, 1994.

148. Schon LC: Plantar fascia and Baxter's nerve release. In Myerson M (ed): *Current Therapy in Foot and Ankle Surgery*. St. Louis, Mosby–Year Book, 1993, pp 177-182..

149. Schon LC, Anderson CD, Easley ME, et al: Surgical treatment of chronic lower extremity neuropathic pain. *Clin Orthop Relat Res* 389:156-164, 2001.

150. Schon LC, Baxter DE: Heel pain syndrome and entrapment neuropathies about the foot and ankle. In Gould JS (ed): *Operative Foot Surgery*. Philadelphia, WB Saunders, 1994, pp 192-208.

151. Schon LC, Baxter DE: Neuropathies of the foot and ankle in athletes. *Clin Sports Med* 9:489-509, 1990.

152. Schon LC, Glennon TP, Baxter DE: Heel pain syndrome: Electrodiagnostic support for nerve entrapment. *Foot Ankle* 14:129-135, 1993.

153. Watson TS, Anderson RB, Davis WH, Kiebzak GM: Distal tarsal tunnel release with partial plantar fasciotomy for chronic heel pain: An outcome analysis. *Foot Ankle Int* 23:530-537, 2002.

Medial Plantar Nerve Entrapment

154. Kopell HP, Thompson WAL: *Peripheral Entrapment Neuropathies*, ed 2. Huntington, NY, Robert E Kreiger Publications, 1976.

155. Marinacci AA: Neurological syndrome of the tarsal tunnels. *Bull L A Neurol Soc* 33:90-100, 1968.

156. Murphy PC, Baxter DE: Nerve entrapment of the foot and ankle in runners. *Clin Sports Med* 4:753-763, 1985.

157. Rask MR: Medial plantar neuropraxia (jogger's foot): Report of three cases. *Clin Orthop Relat Res* 134:193-195, 1978.

Superficial Peroneal Nerve Entrapment

158. Banerjee T, Koons DD: Superficial peroneal nerve entrapment: Report of two cases. *J Neurosurg* 55:991-992, 1981.

159. Cozen L: Bursitis of the heel. *Am J Orthop* 3:372-374, 1961.

160. Heimkes B, Posel P, Stotz S, et al: The proximal and distal tarsal tunnel syndromes: An anatomic study. *Int Orthop* 11:193-196, 1987.

161. Husson JL, Blouet JM, Massé A: Le syndrome du défilé de l'aponévrose superficielle postérieure surale. *Int Orthop* 11:245-248, 1987.

162. Kernohan J, Levack B, Wilson JN: Entrapment of the superficial peroneal nerve. Three case reports. *J Bone Joint Surg Br* 67:60-61, 1985.

163. Lowdon IM: Superficial peroneal nerve entrapment. A case report. *J Bone Joint Surg Br* 67:58-59, 1985.

164. Mackey D, Colbert DS, Chater EH: Musculocutaneous nerve entrapment. *Ir J Med Sci* 146:100-102, 1977.

165. McAuliffe TB, Fiddian NJ, Browett JP: Entrapment neuropathy of the superficial peroneal nerve. A bilateral case. J Bone Joint Surg Br 67:62-63, 1985.

166. Quirk R: Ballet injuries: The Australian experience. *Clin Sports Med* 2:507-514, 1983.

167. Radin EL: Tarsal tunnel syndrome. *Clin Orthop Relat Res* 181:167-170, 1983.

168. Rondhuis JJ, Huson A: The first branch of the lateral plantar nerve and heel pain. *Acta Morphol Neerl Scand* 24:269-279, 1986.

169. Rosson GD, Dellon AL: Superficial peroneal nerve anatomic variability changes: surgical technique. *Clin Orthop Relat Res* 438:248-252, 2005.

170. Schepsis AA, Fitzgerald M, Nicoletta R: Revision surgery for exertional anterior compartment syndrome of the lower leg: Technique, findings, and results. *Am J Sports Med* 33:1040-1047, 2005.

171. Sarrafian SK: *Anatomy of the Foot and Ankle: Descriptive, Topographic, Functional*. Philadelphia, JB Lippincott, 1983.

172. Sridhara CR, Izzo KL: Terminal sensory branches of the superficial peroneal nerve: An entrapment syndrome. *Arch Phys Med Rehabil* 66:789-891, 1985.

173. Styf J: Entrapment of the superficial peroneal nerve. Diagnosis and results of decompression. *J Bone Joint Surg Br* 71:131-135, 1989.

174. Styf JR, Korner LM: Chronic anterior-compartment syndrome of the leg. Results of treatment by fasciotomy. *J Bone Joint Surg Am* 68:1338-1347, 1986.

175. Tanz SS: Heel pain. *Clin Orthop Relat Res* 288:169-178, 1963.

Deep Peroneal Nerve Entrapment

176. Akyuz G, Us O, Turan B, et al: Anterior tarsal tunnel syndrome. *Electromyogr Clin Neurophysiol* 40:123-128, 2000.

177. Borges LF, Hallett M, Selkoe DJ, Welch K: The anterior tarsal tunnel syndrome: Report of two cases. *J Neurosurg* 54:89-92, 1981.

178. Gessini L, Jandolo B, Pietrangeli A: The anterior tarsal tunnel syndrome: Report of four cases. *J Bone Joint Surg Am* 66:786-787, 1984.

179. Gutmann L: Atypical deep peroneal neuropathy in presence of accessory deep peroneal nerve. *J Neurol Neurosurg Psychiatry* 33:453-456, 1970.

180. Krause KH, Witt T, Ross A: The anterior tarsal tunnel syndrome. *J Neurol* 217:67-74, 1977.

181. Lambert EH: The accessory deep peroneal nerve. A common variation in innervation of extensor digitorum brevis. Neurology 19:1169-1176, 1969.

182. Lindenbaum BL: Ski boot compression syndrome, Clin Orthop Relat Res 140:109-110, 1979.

Sural Nerve Entrapment

183. Aktan Ikiz ZA, Ucerler H, Bilge O: The anatomic features of the sural nerve with an emphasis on its clinical importance. *Foot Ankle Int* 26:560-567, 2005.

184. Fabre T, Montero C, Gaujard E, et al. Chronic calf pain in athletes due to sural nerve entrapment. A report of 18 cases. *Am J Sports Med* 28:679-682, 2000.

185. Gould N, Trevino S: Sural nerve entrapment by avulsion fracture of the base of the fifth metatarsal bone. *Foot Ankle* 2:153-155, 1981.

186. Pringle RM, Protheroe K, Mukherjee SK: Entrapment neuropathy of the sural nerve. *J Bone Joint Surg Br* 56:465-468, 1974.

187. Solomon LB, Ferris L, Tedman R, Henneberg M: Surgical anatomy of the sural and superficial fibular nerves with an emphasis on the approach to the lateral malleolus. *J Anat* 199(Pt 6):717-723, 2001.

188. Webb J, Moorjani N, Radford M: Anatomy of the sural nerve and its relation to the Achilles tendon. *Foot Ankle Int* 21:475-477, 2000.

Saphenous Nerve Entrapment

189. Dumitru D, Windsor RE: Subsartorial entrapment of the saphenous nerve of a competitive female bodybuilder. *Phys Sports Med* 17:116-125, 1989.

190. Garland R, Frizelle FA, Dobbs BR, Singh H: A retrospective audit of long-term lower limb complications following leg vein harvesting for coronary artery bypass grafting. *Eur J Cardiothorac Surg* 23:950-955, 2003.

191. Hutchinson MR, Bederka B, Kopplin M: Anatomic structures at risk during minimal-incision endoscopically assisted fascial compartment releases in the leg. *Am J Sports Med* 31:764-769, 2003.

192. Morrison C, Dalsing MC: Signs and symptoms of saphenous nerve injury after greater saphenous vein stripping: Prevalence, severity, and relevance for modern practice. *J Vasc Surg* 38:886-890, 2003.

193. Mozes M, Ouaknine G, Nathan H: Saphenous nerve entrapment simulating vascular disorder. *Surgery* 77:299-303, 1975.

194. Romanoff ME, Cory PC Jr., Kalenak A, et al: Saphenous nerve entrapment at the adductor canal. *Am J Sports Med* 17:478-481, 1989.

195. Tranier S, Durey A, Chevallier B, Liot F: Value of somatosensory evoked potentials in saphenous entrapment neuropathy. *J Neurol Neurosurg Psychiatry* 55:461-465, 1992.

196. Upton RM, McComas AJ: The double crush syndrome in nerve entrapment syndromes. *Lancet* 2:359-362, 1973.

MISCELLANEOUS

Plantar Heel Pain

Thomas H. Lee • Peter B. Maurus

HISTORY

Plantar heel pain is a common disease process that continues to challenge orthopedic surgeons. Because of the complex anatomy around the heel and the plantar surface of the foot, the function and etiology of pain have been difficult to understand. Researchers continue to debate whether the source of pain is trauma around the plantar calcaneal tuberosity from traction and shear forces from the plantar fascia or whether it is from a compressive neuropathy.

DEMOGRAPHICS

Wood originally described plantar fasciitis in 1812 and believed it was infectious in origin.[64] With fewer than 20 articles published concerning plantar fasciitis prior to 1960, surgical researchers obviously had little interest in this subject. However, an increase in the reported incidence of heel pain over the last 20 years has led researchers to publish more than 300 independent articles addressing this disorder since the last edition of this text.

Demographic studies estimate that more than two million patients receive treatment for plantar fasciitis each year in the United States.[78] An estimated one in 10 people will develop heel pain during their lifetime,[24] and 1% of all visits to orthopedic surgeons are thought to be for heel pain.[85]

EPIDEMIOLOGY

With the advent of x-ray technology, early diagnoses of heel pain commonly involved the heel spur. Steindler and Smith (1938) performed rotational osteotomies to move the spur from the weight-bearing surface.[101] In 1957, DuVries promoted the concept of physical impingement onto the plantar fat pad and believed that even some large spurs were asymptomatic because the angle of growth did not cause plantar impingement.[30] DuVries believed some spurs were delivered into the plantar soft-tissue structures as a result of a depression of the longitudinal arch and that some small jagged spurs indicated a subacute inflammatory process.

After a review of 323 patients, Lapidus and Guidotti suggested a mechanical cause for heel pain but did not believe it was caused by physical plantar impingement from the heel spur.[62] They thought the foot functioned as a truss (a triangular structure with two beams connecting the base with a rod) (Fig. 12–1). When a load is applied to the truss, the struts are under compression and the tie rod is under tension.[52,63,91] Patients might better understand the analogy of a bow and arrow; pressure placed on the apex of the bow causes

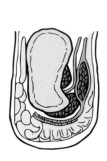
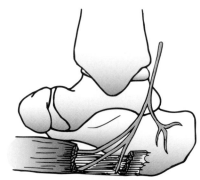

Figure 12–2 The concept of nerve entrapment was initially put forward by Tanz.

the bowstring to become tense and pull tension at the insertion points. Because so many patients recovered despite the presence of the heel spur, Lapidus and Guidotti concluded that the mechanism of pain might result from the "concentrated tension" of the plantar fascia.[62]

After performing a cadaveric dissection study, Tanz proposed nerve entrapment as a cause of pain (Fig. 12–2).[102] He found that a branch of the lateral plantar nerve, which innervates the abductor digiti quinti muscle, passes around the plantar medial border of the heel. These early concepts laid the foundation of our current understanding of the anatomy, mechanism, and cause of plantar heel pain.

ANATOMY

Plantar Fascia

The plantar fascia is a broad-band, multilayered, fibrous aponeurosis. Fibrofatty subcutaneous tissue along the plantar surface of the foot cushions its surface, and the fascia itself covers the intrinsic musculature and neurovascular structures.

The plantar fascia originates from the anterior and medial aspect of the calcaneus. The fibers of the fascia spread into a broad sheet as they course distally and divide into five digital bands at the metatarsophalangeal (MTP) joints. Strong vertical septa divide the medial, central, and lateral portions of the plantar fascia and create three distinct compartments of intrinsic plantar muscles. Each digital band divides to pass on either side of the flexor tendons and inserts into the periosteum of the base of the proximal phalanges. Fibers of the fascia also blend with the dermis, transverse metatarsal ligament, and flexor tendon sheath.[116]

The plantar fascia is relatively inelastic. Postmortem studies found a maximum elongation of 4%, with failures occurring at 90 kg at the clamp margins.[120] The

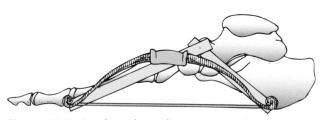

Figure 12–1 Load on the arch compresses the struts and therefore places tension on the plantar fascia.

fascia itself requires more than 1000 N to fail.[61] Because of these inelastic properties, high tensile forces concentrate on the heel tuberosity during the push-off phase of gait due to the dorsiflexion of the MTP joints. In addition, the gastrocnemius–soleus complex pulls simultaneously and concentrates additional body weight onto the forefoot.[77] Further, the downward acceleration of the body concentrates ground reaction forces by an additional 20%. Activities such as running and prolonged weight bearing, which concentrate forces to the plantar fascia during stance and push off, can increase the risk of injury by increasing the forces exerted on the MTP joint and, subsequently, on the plantar fascia origin.

Heel Fat Pad

The fat pad on the calcaneus functions as an important cushion to the hindfoot. A typical healthy man has a gait velocity of approximately 82 m/min and a cadence of 116 gait cycles/min.[92] Each heel strike generates 110% of body weight but can concentrate up to 250% of body weight with running. With walking, the impact load over the calcaneal tuberosity is about 5 kg/cm², with more than 1160 impacts per mile.[77] The unique design of the human heel fat pad can accommodate these impact forces.

The anatomy was first described by Teitze in 1921.[79] The structure is a honeycombed pattern of fibroelastic septa, which completely enclose fat globules (Fig. 12–3). The closed-cell structure of the fat pad provides the mechanical integrity for its shock-absorbing func-

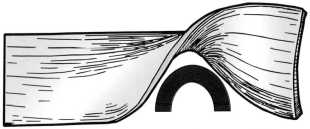

Figure 12–4 The foot functions like a twisted plate.

tion. The tissue septa are U-shaped around the tuberosity and anchored to the calcaneus and skin. Elastic transverse and diagonal fibers that separate the fat into compartments reinforce the chambers internally. After approximately age 40 years, the fat pad begins to deteriorate; with the loss of collagen, elastic tissue, and water, the overall thickness and height of the fat pad decrease. These changes result in softening and thinning of the heel fat pad, decreased shock absorbency, and reduced protection of the heel tuberosity.[56]

Mechanics

Sarrafian described the structural mechanism of the foot.[91] The foot functions like a twisted plate (Fig. 12–4). The posterior segment of the plate is compressed side to side, and the anterior segment is compressed in a dorsal–plantar direction. The twisting of the plate determines a longitudinal and midsegment transverse arch. At rest, continued twisting of the footplate creates a high-arched, shorter plate.

The forefoot pronates relative to the supinated hindfoot. Untwisting of the footplate creates a low-arched plate (Fig. 12–5). Conversely, the forefoot supinates relative to the pronated hindfoot. The foot has the structural and functional characteristics of a beam and truss. The plantar fascia spans the distance from the calcaneus to the proximal phalanx to act as a truss. When under tension, the plantar fascia relieves the

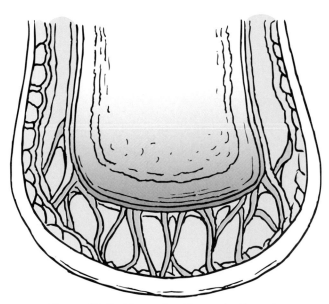

Figure 12–3 Human heel fat pad with septa.

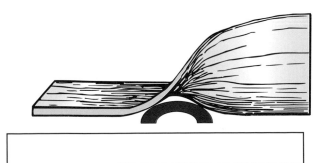

Figure 12–5 The forefoot pronates relative to the supinated hindfoot. Untwisting of the footplate creates a low-arched plate.

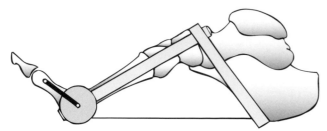

Figure 12–6 Dorsiflexion of the toes causes tension on the plantar fascia. This is the windlass effect of the plantar fascia.

tensile forces from the plantar surface of the foot, which is subjected to compressive forces. With weight bearing, the forward movement of the leg increases the tension in the plantar fascia and creates dorsiflexion forces at the MTP joints. With external rotation of the ankle, the foot twists further and reshapes into a high-arched structure; the hindfoot is supinated or is in varus, the midfoot is supinated, the forefoot is pronated, the plantar fascia is relaxed, the foot is more rigid, and it becomes a more efficient lever arm. A low-arched position results in more tension on the plantar fascia.

In the gait cycle, there is little activity of the intrinsic musculature during quiet standing.[66] The plantar intrinsic muscles do not elicit a substantial response until 30% of the gait cycle (midstance) or just prior to heel rise. Therefore, in the first half of stance phase, the passive structures (bones and ligaments) bear the entire weight of the body, and the arch descends to its lowest point.

In 1954, Hicks reported that the plantar fascia plays an important role during the second half of the stance phase.[53] Because the attachment of the plantar fascia is distal to the MTP joints, dorsiflexion of the toes causes tension on the plantar fascia. Hicks named this mechanism "the windlass effect" of the plantar fascia (Fig. 12–6). Additionally, the intrinsic muscles assume some of the load as they contract during the second half of stance. The arch is also at its highest point, held in place by the plantar fascia and intrinsic muscles, both acting as the truss of the bony arch.

At the high-arched position, the tension on the truss required to support the arch is less than during a low-arched position. A high-arched position results in less tension on the plantar fascia. Therefore, when the foot is vertically loaded with torque, the plantar fascia is under its greatest amount of tension when the leg is internally rotated onto the foot. The foot unwinds, enters a low-arched position, and puts tension on the plantar fascia. In addition, as greater pressure is placed on the MTP joint with concomitant dorsiflexion of the joint, the windlass mechanism exerts greater tension on the plantar fascia.

ETIOLOGY

Heel pain arises from three distinct sources. Mechanical derangements cause classic proximal plantar fasciitis, distal plantar fasciitis, plantar fascia ruptures, and stress fractures of the calcaneus. Rheumatologic conditions cause a wide variety of presentations of pain around the heel. Finally, neurologic conditions from impingement of critical nerves about the foot and ankle cause substantial pain in the heel.

Early investigators proposed an infectious origin for heel pain. In the 1930s, investigators implicated gonorrhea, syphilis, tuberculosis, and streptococcal infections.[21] As research discredited these theories, attention turned to the presence of the heel spur. DuVries categorized the calcaneal spurs.[30] Contrary to early thoughts, the spurs did not lie within the plantar fascia but dorsal to it. Cadaveric studies confirmed the presence of the spur within the flexor digitorum brevis, as well as within the abductor hallucis.[33] The abductor digiti minimi and quadratus plantae origins lie lateral and superior to the spur.[33]

Approximately 50% of patients with heel pain have heel spurs (Fig. 12–7).[98,100] Shmokler et al[98] found a 13.2% incidence of heel spurs in 1000 patients chosen randomly, and only 5.2% of the total patients with heel spurs reported any history of heel pain. Williams et al[118] found that 75% of patients who had heel pain also had spurs, compared with 63% of patients who had no heel pain. Although heel spurs can occur with heel pain, they are not considered the cause.

Chronic inflammation resulting from repetitive traction at the origin of the plantar fascia and flexor digitorum brevis muscle might cause heel spurs. Some investigators postulated that the fat pad loses its compressibility secondary to thinning and loss of structural integrity of the septa. Although some authors believe the thickness of the fat pad is the single most important determinant in heel pain,[56] some authors

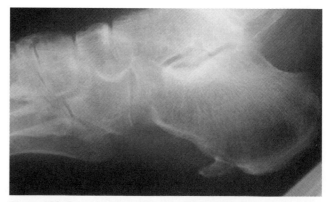

Figure 12–7 A large heel spur is seen extending from within the muscle belly of the flexor digitorum brevis.

have actually found an increased thickness of the fat pad in patients with heel pain.[5]

The elasticity of the heel fat pad may be more important than the actual thickness. Prichasuk found that heel pad elasticity is reduced in patients with heel pain and that the elasticity decreases with increasing age and body weight.[82] More fat in a closed space, combined with loss of elasticity of septa, might increase pressure on the calcaneal tuberosity.[82]

PHYSICAL EXAMINATION

As with any pathologic process, a thorough history and physical examination most often guide the clinician to the appropriate diagnosis and treatment plan. It is important to exclude other causes of plantar heel pain before making the diagnosis of plantar fasciitis, because the conservative and surgical management of the various disorders differ. The differential diagnosis includes calcaneal stress fractures, tumors, infections, disorders of the fat pad, distal plantar fasciitis, plantar fibromatosis, flexor hallucis tendinitis, and nerve entrapment of the posterior tibial nerve.

Clinicians should first review the patient's general health, including a treatment history for the heel pain (e.g., therapy, medications, injections, orthoses, or surgeries). Constitutional symptoms such as weight loss, fevers, chills, and night sweats should lead the clinician to investigate a systemic condition. Further questioning should focus on the patient's activities, both recreational and occupational. Specifically, one should inquire about a change in weight or activity coincident with the onset of symptoms.

Athletes who perform running and jumping activities are particularly prone to plantar heel pain. It is important to differentiate pain during heel strike versus pain with push off. In addition, pain at the onset of physical activity can differ from pain occurring during activity or after activity.

Obesity is a risk factor for plantar fasciitis and is associated with a worse long-term outcome in many studies.* In addition, the amount of time spent weight bearing throughout the day is a causative and provocative factor.[85] The type of shoe and its cushioned insole, as well as the surface type, can help differentiate the diagnosis.

Typically, patients describe the pain as gradual in onset. Pain with the first few steps after awakening or after a prolonged rest suggests the diagnosis of plantar fasciitis. The pain might subside with progressive activity during the day only to return at the end of the day.

Unrelenting pain at rest or night pain is a red flag that the pain may be related to a tumor or an infectious process. Bilateral heel pain suggests a systemic process, such as ankylosing spondylitis, Reiter's syndrome, or other seronegative spondyloarthropathies. A neuritic, dysesthetic type of pain is likely caused by nerve compression and irritation. Pain occurring after an acute injury is more likely a plantar fascia rupture or acute fracture within the hindfoot. Patients with ruptures of the plantar fascia often have a history of corticosteroid injection.[1,95] Paradoxically, these patients can have less pain after rupture of the plantar fascia, although there can be a subtle collapse of the longitudinal arch.

Clinicians should perform a comprehensive physical examination of the foot and ankle in search of the primary source of pain, concomitant disorder, or a locus of referred pain. A pes planus or a cavus foot deformity may be a causative or contributing factor. Assess Achilles tendon tightness. Examining the spine and extremities can help to elucidate any neurologic component to the pain; radiculopathy in an L5-S1 distribution could explain plantar heel pain.

The location of the pain is important in making the correct diagnosis. With plantar fasciitis, the pain is typically localized to the medial tubercle of the calcaneus at the origin of the central band of the plantar fascia. Distal plantar fasciitis produces pain in the distal aspect of the plantar fascia. Passive dorsiflexion of the toes with tightening of the windlass mechanism can exacerbate the pain in both proximal and distal plantar fasciitis. Plantar fibromatosis causes pain over the midportion of the fascia; the clinician can palpate nodules within the fascial substance. Flexor hallucis longus tendinitis at the level of the master knot of Henry can manifest as plantar heel pain. Tenderness with resisted flexion of the great toe can differentiate this condition from other etiologies. Calcaneal stress fractures cause more diffuse calcaneal pain and are likely to produce associated warmth and swelling. Grasping the calcaneus between the examiner's hands (the squeeze test) evokes pain with a calcaneal stress fracture.

Neurogenic pain from compression of the nerves on the medial side of the ankle or the first branch of the lateral plantar nerve is sometimes difficult to distinguish from plantar fasciitis. Pain from compression within the tarsal tunnel or at the medial calcaneal nerve usually produces diffuse pain that is typically not worsened through passive dorsiflexion of the toes. Tinel's sign may be found over these nerves. Compression of the first branch of the lateral plantar nerve (Baxter's nerve) results in more focal pain that can be easily confused with plantar fasciitis. Due to the nerve's close proximity to the medial tubercle of the calcaneus, both conditions are often present. Patients

---

*References 34, 41, 54, 62, 84, 100, 102, 113, 117, and 119.

who have undergone a previous surgical procedure might have neuromas within the operative field. Neuromas are most often seen in the medial calcaneal nerve. A ruptured plantar fascia produces a palpable gap within the substance of the fascia while stretching the plantar surface. Ecchymosis and tenderness likely occur over the proximal extent of the plantar fascia.

Disorders of the fat pad cause pain that is centered more proximally than the plantar fascia's origin. Palpation of the fat pad reveals a softened and flattened surface. Erythema and inflammation can occur over the plantar aspect of the heel, a finding unique to this condition. The fat pad may be unstable from the underlying calcaneal tuberosity, with a concomitant bursitic reaction between the bone and the pad.

DIAGNOSIS

A thorough history and physical examination leads to the diagnosis of most causes of plantar heel pain. Further investigation through imaging or laboratory studies is warranted only rarely. In some cases, however, special studies may be needed to identify or confirm the source of the disorder.

Mechanical

Plain radiographs of the foot can provide information about the bony structures and alignment. Standing anteroposterior and lateral films can be obtained easily in most office settings. Occasionally, axial and 45-degree medial oblique views are helpful. Although the soft tissues cannot be visualized adequately with radiographs, conditions such as tumors, osteomyelitis, fractures, or fat pad atrophy can be detected in some instances.

The presence of a calcaneal heel spur has been a long-standing source of controversy in the diagnosis and treatment of plantar heel pain. Tanz has shown that heel spurs exist in approximately 50% of the patients with plantar fasciitis. However, only approximately 15% of the general population have heel spurs.[102] Researchers have yet to elucidate the pathophysiology responsible for the development of heel spurs or the importance of their formation. A recent study, however, suggests that spur formation can be the end result of fasciitis.[76] A calcaneal lucency (saddle sign) is often seen just proximal to the calcaneal spur on a lateral radiograph. Amis et al[5] found this saddle sign and an increase in fat pad thickness in 60% of their patients who had unilateral heel pain. They also observed cortical abnormalities with thickened, disorganized trabeculae in 85% of these patients on 45-degree medial oblique views of the heel.

A triple-phase bone scan can be a useful diagnostic tool for calcaneal stress fractures or plantar fasciitis. Previous studies have shown predictable uptake in the heels of patients with plantar fasciitis.[43,96] Williams et al[118] reported uptake in 60% of patients with painful heels, with no false positives in painless heels. Graham[43] studied 36 patients with unilateral heel pain and found that more than 97% of the patients showed uptake in the inferomedial aspect of the heel. Sewell et al[96] reported similar uptake in patients with plantar fasciitis and that symptomatic improvement paralleled a decrease in uptake. Ozdemir et al[76] demonstrated specific osseous and fascial uptake patterns that they believed corresponded to diagnosis and prognosis, with heel spurs likely the end result of a long-standing inflammatory process within the fascia. A decrease in uptake over time correlates with symptomatic improvement.[96]

Advances in musculoskeletal imaging have led to an increased interest in magnetic resonance imaging (MRI) and ultrasound (US) imaging for evaluation of heel pain. Unlike conventional radiographs, both MRI and US provide details about the soft tissues of the foot and ankle. Many studies have evaluated the use of MRI for heel pain.* MRI is more likely useful for excluding other causes of heel pain than confirming the presence of plantar fasciitis. Proponents of MRI argue that its superior soft-tissue contrast resolution and multiplanar capability provide more information than other imaging techniques do. Typical MRI findings are fascia thickening and perifascial, calcaneal, and subcutaneous edema. Increased signal intensity is best seen on the T2 and STIR image sequences. The degree of signal intensity might correlate with symptomatic improvement. Furthermore, MRI can identify other pathologic entities, such as plantar fibromatosis, tumors, and infection.[104] MRI has even been shown to accurately identify the course of the plantar nerves and sources of entrapment.[32] The disadvantages of MRI are its high cost and low specificity.

Ultrasound of the plantar aspect of the foot can also detect plantar fascia thickening and soft tissue edema.† Ultrasound is inexpensive, fast, and painless. Successful imaging, however, is operator dependent. Recent studies suggest that ultrasound is superior to MRI, and researchers argue that ultrasound provides an earlier detection of edema and degeneration of the fat pad.[57] Ultrasound has also been shown to be equally effective to bone scan in diagnosing plantar fasciitis.[58] Typically, ultrasound shows thickened and hypoechoic plantar fascia and perifascial edema.†

---

*References 13, 32, 44, 46, 57, 70, 103, 104, and 121.
†References 2, 40, 45, 57, 58, 109, and 111.

Advances in technique, such as power Doppler ultrasound, can improve the value of ultrasound by providing additional information about local hyperemia.[111]

Rheumatologic

In most instances, laboratory studies of patients with subcalcaneal heel pain are normal. Serum hematologic and immunologic testing can detect systemic disorders that contribute to heel disorders. Patients with recalcitrant unilateral or bilateral heel pain might suffer from a seronegative spondyloarthropathy such as Reiter's syndrome, ankylosing spondylitis, or psoriatic arthritis. Inflammatory bowel arthritis and Behçet's syndrome can also manifest as heel pain. Sacroiliitis is the hallmark of these conditions, occurring in 100% of patients with ankylosing spondylitis, 54% of patients with Reiter's syndrome, and 57% of patients with psoriatic arthritis.[28] Heel pain is common in these patients, manifesting more commonly as bilateral pain than as unilateral pain.

There are few recent studies on this subject. Gerster's[37] study of 150 patients with plantar fasciitis or Achilles tendinitis showed that 22% suffered from a seronegative spondyloarthropathy and 91% tested positive for human leukocyte antigen-B27 (HLA-B27). When comparing this group to 220 patients with rheumatoid arthritis, Gerster rarely found plantar fasciitis in the rheumatoid arthritis group. Gerster and Piccinin[38] presented 18 patients with juvenile-onset seronegative spondyloarthropathy. Four patients had severe pain at the plantar fascial insertion and all were HLA-B27-positive. Four other patients had mild pain. Severe pain was associated with a poor long-term prognosis. Gerster et al[39] also studied 30 patients with seronegative spondyloarthropathy and found that 24 patients complained of severe heel pain. Four patients underwent surgical treatment with partial plantar fascia release or resection of a calcaneal heel spur, or both. They concluded that heel surgery is contraindicated during the inflammation phase, because it can cause local aggravation and risk of ankylosis of the talocalcaneal articulation.

Clinicians should consider HLA-B27 testing in patients with bilateral or recalcitrant heel pain. Other helpful studies include complete blood count, erythrocyte sedimentation rate, rheumatoid factor, antinuclear antibodies, and uric acid.

Neurologic

Electromyography (EMG) and nerve conduction velocity (NCV) studies can show signs of neuropathy in cases of nerve compression about the foot and ankle. Schon et al[93,94] found abnormal studies in 23 of 38 heels with suspected nerve entrapment. These studies are more useful for diagnosing tarsal tunnel compression than plantar entrapment. The first branch of the lateral plantar nerve, the most common offending nerve, is difficult to examine with neurodiagnostics, and nerve-conduction studies may not be reliable. EMG and NCV are effective at isolating a spinal source of radiculopathy or a double crush syndrome, with a coincident spinal and local compressive source.

CONSERVATIVE TREATMENT

Mechanical

Nonoperative treatment is the mainstay of treating subcalcaneal heel pain. Wolgin et al[119] found that the heel pain of 82 of their 100 patients improved with conservative therapy, and 15 patients continued to have mild symptoms with no limitation of work or activity. Callison[19] studied 400 patients treated with rest, casting, anti-inflammatory medications, stretching, orthoses, and steroid injections. Seventy-three percent had significant improvement within six months, 20% failed to improve, and the rest were lost to follow-up. Davis et al[27] studied 132 symptomatic heels in 105 patients. Pain resolved in 89% of the patients within 11 months with a treatment protocol of anti-inflammatory medications, rest, viscoelastic polymer heel cushions, Achilles tendon stretching, and occasional injections. They also found that obesity, sex, or heel spur morphology did not affect the outcome. The authors approached surgical treatment for the other 11% cautiously.[27] Davies et al[26] showed that less than 50% of patients who had a surgical procedure for heel pain were completely satisfied with the results. A combination of the following nonoperative treatments will likely lead to a successful result.

Stretching and Physical Therapy

A home program of stretching should be the primary treatment modality for patients with plantar fasciitis. A traditional protocol involves Achilles tendon stretching and eccentric Achilles strengthening exercises. Porter et al[81] showed these exercises to be effective in 122 painful heels, with flexibility correlating with symptomatic improvement. Tissue-specific plantar fascia stretching exercises improve outcome in these patients. Eighty-two patients were treated with prefabricated soft insoles, a cyclooxygenase-2 (COX-2) inhibitor, and either an Achilles tendon or a plantar fascia stretching program. The plantar fascia stretching group had significantly better outcomes with regard to pain, activity, and satisfaction.[29] Stretching involves sustained passive dorsiflexion of the toes before taking the first steps after awakening.

Heel Pads and Orthoses

Shoe inserts are available as an adjunct to other conservative measures. The commonly used orthoses include prefabricated silicone or rubber heel cups, prefabricated arch supports, felt pads, custom longitudinal arch supports, or a UCBL (University of California Biomechanics Laboratory) orthosis. Pfeffer et al[78] compared custom orthoses to prefabricated orthoses in 236 patients with heel pain. They found that all prefabricated inserts, especially the silicone insert (95% improvement), and stretching alone (72% improvement), performed better than a polypropylene custom orthosis (68% improvement). All patients who stood for more than 8 hours per day had a poorer outcome in all categories, thus indicating the importance of a period of relative rest.[78] The use of a more shock-absorbent material for the custom orthoses, such as medium-density polyethylene foam (Plastizote), may perform better than polypropylene. Campbell and Inman showed that a UCBL custom insert was successful in treating heel pain recalcitrant to other treatments and inserts in 31 out of 33 patients.[20] The two patients without improvement had pain associated with a seronegative spondyloarthropathy

Steroids

Clinicians often give steroid injections for heel pain. In a study of 233 orthopaedic surgeons, 170 used steroid injections for heel pain.[31] Evidence exists that steroids provide relief, but the effects are temporary in the majority of patients. Miller et al[68] reviewed the records of 24 patients (27 heels) injected with lidocaine and betamethasone and followed for 5 to 8 months. Ninety-five percent of these patients had good to excellent relief of their heel pain within the first few days after injection. At final follow-up, however, only 41% of the patients maintained this level of pain relief.

Several complications, including fascia rupture and fat pad atrophy, can occur with steroid injections for plantar fasciitis. In evaluating 51 patients with plantar fascia rupture, Acevedo et al[1] found that 44 of these patients previously had a steroid injection. Sellman[95] presented a report on 37 patients with presumed plantar fascia ruptures, all with previous steroid injections. Clinicians can reduce the incidence of complications by placing the needle superior to the fascia, typically from the medial side. This technique spreads the solution across the fascia layer and typically avoids the plantar nerves and fat pad.

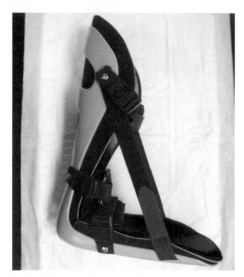

Figure 12–8   Night splints have been shown to be successful adjunctive treatment for plantar fasciitis.

Casting and Night Splints

In the small percentage of patients who have continued symptoms despite other forms of conservative treatment, night splints and casting can be beneficial (Fig. 12–8). Theoretically, night splints prevent shortening of the plantar fascia during long periods of rest, thus preventing the excessive stretch placed on the fascia during morning ambulation. Ryan[88] treated 30 recalcitrant patients successfully with night splints. Likewise, Wapner and Sharkey[113] reported success in 11 of 14 patients; they recommended 5 degrees of dorsiflexion in the splint. Mizel et al[69] reported resolution or improvement of symptoms in 77% of patients treated with night splinting and shoe modification. Berlet et al[14] cited improvement in 75% of patients with night splinting at one-month follow-up with no tendency toward deterioration of results at 6 months. Barry et al[8] had better results with night splints than with Achilles stretching alone in 160 patients. In a prospective randomized study, Batt et al[9] had only three treatment failures with night splinting in 33 patients.

Not all studies are as conclusive, however. In a large prospective randomized study of 116 patients, Probe et al[83] found no added benefit of night splinting when added to anti-inflammatory medications and stretching. A short period of casting with a below-knee walking cast can have a similar benefit to night splinting. Tisdel and Harper[107] demonstrated complete relief or improvement in 86% of patients following casting for an average of 6 weeks. Gill et al[41] found casting to be the most effective treatment among a series of other conservative modalities in 11 of their most refractory cases of plantar fasciitis. Much of the benefit from casting may be from the forced rest period inherent in cast immobilization.

Rheumatologic

Clinicians should consider systemic disease in patients with bilateral or continued recalcitrant heel pain, especially in patients who are HLA-B27 positive or have concurrent joint complaints. In these instances, consultation with a rheumatologist is recommended. Conservative treatment of heel pain associated with systemic conditions follows the same protocol as for mechanical pain. Treatment with nonsteroidal anti-inflammatory medications usually produces a dramatic response. The duration of treatment corresponds to the duration of antecedent symptoms.

Neurologic

Compression of the first branch of the lateral plantar nerve typically responds to the same conservative treatment protocol employed for plantar fasciitis. A combined approach, using anti-inflammatory medications, rest, ice, stretching, and steroid injections is usually sufficient. Prefabricated heel cups made of rubber or silicone can act as a cushion to lessen pressure over the affected area. For patients with excessive pronation, a medial longitudinal arch support can decrease compression over the area of the medial heel.

EXTRACORPOREAL SHOCK WAVE THERAPY

Extracorporeal shock wave therapy (ESWT) is the newest technology used to treat chronic plantar fasciitis (Fig. 12–9). Based on lithotripsy technology, ESWT uses powerful shock waves to break up scar tissue and allow healing of the inflamed fascia. International studies using low-energy ESWT for chronic heel pain have reported 57% to 80% good or excellent results.[51,87,88] Studies using high-energy shock wave therapy, as used in the United States, have reported success rates ranging from 56% to 94%.* Hammer et al[49] demonstrated that up to 80% of their 49 painful heels had complete or near complete relief with three weekly sessions of ESWT. At 2-year follow-up, all patients noted a greater than 90% decrease in pain during activities of daily living.[47]

Current indications for ESWT include proximal plantar heel pain that has lasted longer than 6 months and has been recalcitrant to at least three conservative

_____
*References 3, 22, 72, 90, 99, 112, and 122.

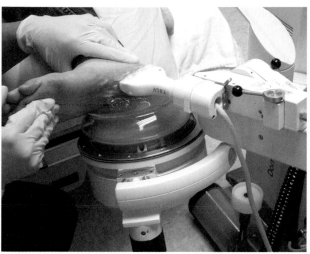

Figure 12–9 Extracorporeal shock wave allows for a noninvasive intervention for plantar fasciitis.

therapies, such as cortisone injections, strapping, custom orthotics, stretching, NSAIDS, and physical therapy.

Various modalities are used to generate the shockwave including electrohydraulic (OssaTron, SanuWave, Marietta, Ga),[90] electromagnetic (Dornier Epos Ultra, Dornier MedTech America, Kennesaw, Ga), and piezoelectric generators. Regardless of the generator, all create shockwaves by converting electrical energy into mechanical energy.[74] The resultant shockwave is an acoustic impulse created in a water medium, which spreads through tissue without losing substantial energy due to similar acoustic impedance of anatomic tissue.[80]

The shock wave is defined by the focus geometry (length and diameter), focus pressure maximum, and focus energy density (mJ/mm^2).[48] For shockwaves to be effective in a clinical situation, the maximally beneficial pulse energy must be concentrated at the point of treatment.[74] Today, ESWT is classified based on the energy level as either low level (0.04-0.12 mJ/mm^2) or high level (>0.12 mJ/mm^2).[48]

Currently, ESWT can treat various musculoskeletal pathologies. Researchers believe the shock waves stimulate a reactivate healing process in tendons and bones through microdisruption of avascular or minimally vascular tissues to encourage revascularization, release of local growth factors, and recruitment of appropriate stem cells conducive to more normal tissue healing.[105] The onset and immediate disappearance of cavitation bubbles exert a deep tissue effect that causes the rupture of microcapillaries and, thus, leakage of chemical mediators, stimulating neoangiogenesis and improving the resolution of the chronic process.[80] Contraindications for ESWT use include any type of hemophilia or coagulopathy, malignancy, or open growth plates.[74]

Currently, two devices are Food and Drug Administration (FDA) approved for ESWT for chronic plantar fasciitis: the Dornier Epos Ultra and the OssaTron. Published studies using the OssaTron machine report varied success. Pilot studies for FDA approval of the OssaTron reported that 56% of the patients had a successful result at 3-month follow-up.[72,73] One year after treatment, a study involving 20 patients treated with the OssaTron reported that 90% had good or excellent results, and another study with 79 patients reported that 94.1% were complaint free or significantly better.[3,112] Studies in Taiwan using the OssaTron found that 73.5% of patients reported no complaint or significant improvement at the 3-month follow-up and 87% at the 6-month follow-up.[22] Interestingly, Helbig et al[51] showed a possible correlation between duration of plantar fascia pain and the success rate of treatment. In their study, patients with symptoms for more than 35 months achieved good or very good results, whereas those with symptoms for only 3 to 12 months had poorer results.

Predicting which patients will have successful results versus unsuccessful or less-than-desirable results is difficult. One potential predictor, however, is the presence of calcaneal bone marrow edema and not the thickness of the plantar fascia on pretherapeutic MRI.[65] In a meta-analysis encompassing 840 total patients, Ogden et al[71] found that high-energy shockwave impulses appear to provide more relief and more quickly, and with fewer treatments. They recommend ESWT as a safe and effective nonoperative treatment for plantar fasciitis.

SURGICAL TREATMENT

Mechanical

Open Plantar Fascia Release

In some difficult cases, symptoms persist despite all efforts at nonoperative intervention; thus, surgery may be indicated. Attempt conservative treatment for at least 6 months to a year prior to resorting to surgery. The procedure of choice is an open partial plantar fascia release with decompression of the first branch of the lateral plantar nerve. Surgical results have been good, with up to 95% of patients having satisfactory results in multiple studies.[12,25,42,107,115] Much of the benefit from surgical treatment might be due to the enforced period of rest dictated by the postoperative protocol.

DuVries[30] postulated that the subcalcaneal heel spur was the source of heel pain and found that 100% of patients had relief of symptoms with resection of the spur at early follow-up. Manoli et al[67] reported calcaneal fractures after spur removal due to extensive bone resection. Snook and Chrisman[100] believed that removing only a portion of the medial calcaneal tuberosity, rather than the entire heel spur, eliminated the offending structure and maintained a broad weight-bearing surface.

Ward and Clippinger[114] reported excellent results in seven of eight patients with a medial plantar fasciectomy. Gormley and Kuwada[42] reported 95% complete pain relief in 94 patients with partial medial plantar fasciectomy and heel spur excision. Daly et al[25] studied the surgical results in 14 patients with plantar fasciitis and found that 71% of their patients had good or excellent results. Force-plate analysis showed subtle biomechanical changes, however, despite satisfactory clinical results. Baxter and Thigpen[12] reported good results in 32 of 34 heels treated by partial medial plantar fasciectomy, nerve decompression, and heel spur removal. They stressed the importance of decompressing the first branch of the lateral plantar nerve as it passes over the abductor hallucis and under the calcaneus. Watson et al[115] studied 75 patients (80 heels) and reported that 93% of their patients had a satisfactory outcome with the same procedure. They did not remove the heel spur in any of their patients.

Endoscopic Plantar Fascia Release

Many researchers advocate endoscopic plantar fascia release as a safe and effective alternative to open release (Fig. 12–10). Proponents argue that it offers a safer approach with a more rapid return to activity.[6,17,50,89,108] Although a great deal of the early literature on this procedure touted excellent results, however, a more critical review of the findings leaves many questions unanswered.

Barrett et al's[7] study of 652 cases of endoscopic plantar fascia release by 25 surgeons is the largest study to date on this topic. The results are difficult to interpret, however, due to the variation in patient selection, follow-up, and subjective outcome measurements. Despite these shortcomings, the authors continue to report that 97% of their patients believed the procedure was successful. There were 62 complications in 53 of the patients. These complications included midfoot pain, heel pain, and wound infections.

A recent study by O'Malley et al[75] demonstrated promising results in 20 patients with heel pain; 90% reported improvement or complete relief and 10% had no relief. Patients with bilateral symptoms had worse results and none of them had complete relief. They recommend this procedure for recalcitrant heel pain.

Hogan et al[55] recently published their results on endoscopic plantar fascia release in 22 consecutive

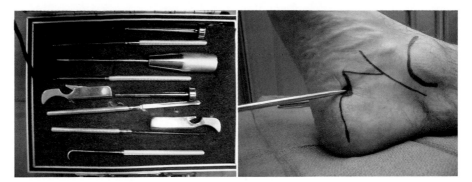

Figure 12–10 Endoscopic plantar fascia release allows for the percutaneous release of the medial two thirds of the plantar fascia. The technique is limited by the lack of thorough visualization of the neurovascular bundle and the risk of destabilizing the lateral column.

patients with plantar fasciitis that had failed an average of at least seven months of conservative treatment. At an average of 8.48 months of follow-up they found a 97.7% satisfaction rate, and all patients reported at least 50% improvement in their heel pain. Bilateral symptoms and previous ankle trauma or surgery (or both) were significantly correlated with inferior results.

Concerns with endoscopic release are poor visualization and the possibility of unintended complete release. Complete release of the plantar fascia has been associated with instability of the lateral column and calcaneal cuboid joint pain. Furthermore, heel spurs and compression of the nerve to the adductor digiti minimi cannot be addressed endoscopically.

Endoscopic plantar fascia release remains a controversial procedure. Recognizing this fact, the American Orthopaedic Foot and Ankle Society (AOFAS) has released a position statement reinforcing correct diagnosis, conservative treatment, operative indications, and surgical planning.[4]

Neurologic

Compression of the first branch of the lateral plantar nerve remains a common cause of recalcitrant heel pain. Neurolysis or neurectomy of the nerve often affords relief to patients with this condition. Kenzora[59] reported 100% satisfactory results in six patients after release of the nerve through a midline plantar incision. Baxter et al[10,11] reported up to 89% good or excellent results in two studies after release of the first branch of the lateral plantar nerve.

Complications

As with any surgical procedure, open and endoscopic plantar fascia releases have known complications. Persistent and recurrent pain are the most common complications, most often due to failure to correctly diagnose the source of the pain or the failure to treat the condition appropriately. A careful reexamination

of the patient can provide clues about why the intervention failed.

If a neural decompression has not been performed or was performed inadequately, pain could result from compression in the tarsal tunnel or over the first branch of the lateral plantar nerve. Endoscopic releases cannot address the nerve and thus should not be performed in patients with expected nerve compression symptoms. Patients with systemic disorders, such as seronegative spondyloarthropathies, do not respond well to surgery. Failure to make the diagnosis of a systemic cause of heel pain can lead to a poor surgical outcome. Postoperative complications with plantar fascia release, whether open or endoscopic, are rare. Complications include neuritis, superficial or deep infections, incision pain, adhesions, deep venous thrombosis, and transfer pain associated with biomechanical abnormalities.

Open Release

Many studies have reported complications associated with open plantar fascia release.* Sammarco et al[89] found four complications in 35 patients after open release. These complications included two superficial wound infections, one deep venous thrombosis, and one superficial phlebitis. All responded to conservative treatments. Baxter and Thigpen[12] reported only one complication, a superficial infection, in a group of 26 patients. Watson et al[115] reported one deep venous thrombosis and one wound dehiscence in 80 heels. Manoli et al[67] presented four cases of calcaneus fracture after heel spur removal.

Endoscopic Release

Endoscopic plantar fascia release has a similar mix of related complications.[7,15,16,60,75] Kinley et al[60] reported a 41% complication rate with this procedure, although this high number includes mostly minor complications. Gentile et al[36] reported a case of traumatic

---

*References 12, 18, 23, 25, 26, 35, 89, 110, and 115.

pseudoaneurysm of the lateral plantar artery after endoscopy of the plantar heel. They attributed this complication to the poor exposure inherent in this procedure The most concerning problems with endoscopic procedures are the inability to address nerve compression and the possibility of inadequate or overaggressive release due to poor visualization.

Most of these complications are minor and respond well to conservative measures. A major complication of plantar fascia release, however, is development of biomechanical changes and resultant transfer pain. Transfer pain occurs commonly along the dorsal midfoot and lateral column and is sometimes referred to as "lateral column syndrome."

The plantar fascia assists in maintaining the natural arch of the foot. Sarrafian found that both partial and complete release of the plantar fascia transmit compressive forces to the dorsal and lateral midfoot.[91] Brugh et al[18] evaluated lateral column symptomatology after plantar fascia release. They found that regardless of surgical technique (endoscopic or open release), lateral column symptoms were more likely to result when more than 50% of the plantar fascia was released. These changes can lead to pain with weight bearing. Thorardson et al[106] studied the effect of release of the plantar fascia and found that sequential release reduces the arch-supporting function of the fascia.

Daly et al[25] evaluated the results of plantar fasciotomy in 16 feet. They found a decrease in the arch height and the ratio of arch height to arch length and a decreased angle of the first talotarsal joint (talotarsal-1). Gait analysis using force plates determined that their patients spent less time on their heels after release.

Using a finite element model for analysis, Gefen[35] showed that with total plantar fascia release, tension stresses caused by the long plantar ligaments increased significantly and might exceed the normal average stress by more than 200%. Sharkey et al[97] performed stress analysis on eight cadaver feet. They showed that complete fasciotomy increased the magnitude of strain in the dorsal aspect of the second metatarsal by more than 80%, suggesting that plantar fascia release or rupture accelerates the accumulation of fatigue damage in these bones. Careful patient selection and surgical technique will help the surgeon avoid these complications.

AUTHORS' PREFERRED METHOD OF TREATMENT

Initial Visit

We first obtain a thorough history and perform a comprehensive physical examination to identify the cause of the patient's complaints. We carefully describe the diagnosis and disease process to the patient, because understanding the mechanism of subcalcaneal heel pain leads to better patient acceptance of the treatment and compliance with the postoperative protocol. If the diagnosis of plantar fasciitis is in question, further testing with advanced imaging, such as MRI, bone scan, or serum studies, may be indicated to guide the treatment plan. However, advanced imaging techniques are infrequently ordered.

The initial treatment consists of conservative management, with antiinflammatories to control pain, modification of activity, and passive stretching. For patients with a mechanical need for an orthosis, we use a prefabricated heel cushion in conjunction with the conservative therapy. In the case of foot-based neurogenic symptoms, a relief area should be placed below the course of the medial and lateral plantar nerves. A custom orthosis may be beneficial if a traction neurogenic cause is suspected. Stretching of the heel cord and plantar fascia is demonstrated to the patient, stressing plantar fascia–specific stretching, as described by DiGiovani et al.[29] Formal physical therapy with modalities and teaching of a home program may be necessary.

First Follow-up Visit

We reexamine the patient and review the treatment history between 3 and 6 months postoperatively. We perform a repeat physical examination and, possibly, diagnostic and confirmatory testing. If the patient is having difficulty following the prescribed treatment regimen, the initial treatment plan should be reinforced and repeated. A dorsiflexion night splint can help prevent contracture of the plantar fascia and lead to resolution of some recalcitrant cases. If pain continues, we recommend complete rest in a short-leg walking cast for 6 to 8 weeks. If symptoms persist despite these interventions, ESWT should be considered. We prefer a single session using a high-energy generator under regional ankle block anesthesia.

Second Follow-up Visit

At the second follow-up visit, we again assess the effectiveness of the treatment regimen. If the patient had ESWT, the effects are evaluated. If the patient is improving clinically or tolerating the current symptoms, we maintain the program of conservative management. If the patient has unacceptable continued pain or worsening symptoms, an open plantar fasciotomy with release of the first branch of the lateral plantar nerve should be considered.

The indications for operative intervention are continued unremitting pain for more than 1 year, failure of all nonoperative modalities, and failure of one ESWT session. Relative contraindications include inadequate conservative management or inadequate compliance and unrealistic expectations. Specific medical contraindications, such as vascular insufficiency, diabetes, and infection, are also considered.

Before performing any surgical procedure, the patient must understand the disorder completely, and all other causes of heel pain must be excluded. In cases of recurrent pain after a previous procedure, evaluate the foot for the presence of neuromas within the plantar and calcaneal nerves.

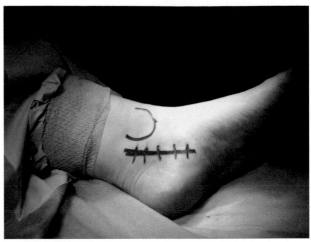

Figure 12–11 The skin incision follows the path of the posterior tibial nerve as it courses toward the plantar aspect of the foot.

OPEN PLANTAR FASCIOTOMY WITH RELEASE OF THE FIRST BRANCH OF THE LATERAL PLANTAR NERVE

Surgical Technique

1. Position the patient supine on the operating table.
2. Apply a tourniquet to the affected extremity and inflate to 300 mm Hg.
3. Make a 5-cm curvilinear incision along the posteromedial neurovascular bundle starting proximally from midway between the medial malleolus and the medial border of the Achilles tendon to the inferior border of the abductor hallucis muscle distally. Typically, the incision ends at the junction of the medial and plantar skin surfaces. For greater exposure, extend the incision distally approximately one-quarter across the plantar aspect of the heel just anterior to the heel fat pad (Fig. 12–11).
4. The abductor hallucis brevis muscle and flexor retinaculum (laciniate ligament) will be visible. Release the superficial fascia and the flexor retinaculum over the posterior tibial nerve. Retract the abductor hallucis muscle first dorsally, then plantarly, to fully visualize the deep fascia. Release the deep fascia of the abductor hallucis to fully decompress the bifurcation of the posterior tibial nerve (Fig. 12–12).
5. At this level, identify the lateral plantar nerve and its first branch to the abductor digiti minimi. Free these nerves from the surrounding tissues, and follow with blunt dissection to verify that there is no proximal or distal impingement. Often the fascia of the quadratus plantae will be released (Fig. 12–13).
6. Release one half to two thirds of the plantar fascia.
7. Reflect a portion of the flexor digitorum brevis to access the plantar heel spur. Palpate and assess the spur. If the spur is large and requires resection, remove the spur in line with the plantar cortex using an osteotome, taking care to maintain the contour of the plantar cortical profile. Smooth the edges with a power rasp.

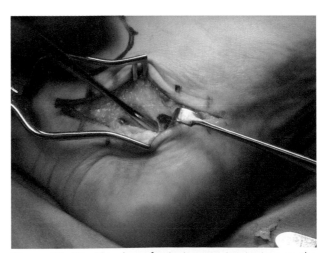

Figure 12–12 The deep fascia is seen impinging on the medial and lateral plantar nerve. Release of the deep fascia is an important component to the plantar fascia release.

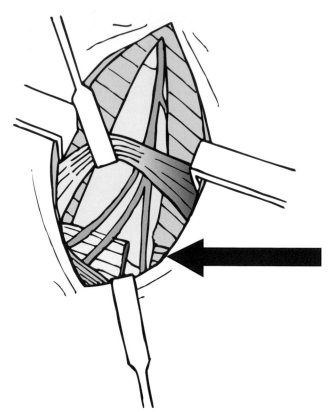

Figure 12–13 After the release of the deep fascia of the abductor hallucis muscle, the muscle is reflected dorsally to expose and transect the plantar fascia.

8. Irrigate the wound and close the skin with nonabsorbent sutures.
9. Apply a bulky dressing and a short-leg cast.

Postoperative Protocol

1. The patient maintains non–weight-bearing status with the limb in a bulky Jones dressing for 10 to 14 days. Immobilization protects the heel from scar formation and calcaneus fracture due to spur removal.
2. At the first postoperative visit, the bulky Jones dressing and sutures are removed, and the limb is placed in a short-leg, full weight-bearing cast for 3 weeks.
3. At the next visit, the cast is changed to a weight-bearing walking boot for 3 weeks.
4. The patient may return to regular daily activities with a shoe insert that supports the heel and arch. Patients should continue daily use of these inserts for 6 months postoperatively.
5. Heel cord and plantar fascia–specific stretching exercises should continue indefinitely.

ACKNOWLEDGMENT

The authors acknowledge editorial assistance and review provided by Janet L. Tremaine, ELS, Tremaine Medical Communications, Dublin, Ohio.

REFERENCES

1. Acevedo JI, Beskin JL: Complications of plantar fascia rupture associated with corticosteroid injection. *Foot Ankle Int* 19(2): 91-97, 1998.
2. Akfirat M, Sen C, Gunes T: Ultrasonographic appearance of the plantar fasciitis. *Clin Imaging* 27(5):353-357, 2003.
3. Alvarez R: Preliminary results on the safety and efficacy of the Ossatron for treatment of plantar fasciitis. *Foot Ankle* 23:197-203, 2002.
4. American Orthopaedic Foot and Ankle Society: AOFAS Position Statement: Endoscopic and open heel surgery. Available at http://www.aofas.org/displaycommon.cfm?an=1&subarticlenbr=31 (accessed March 10, 2006).
5. Amis J, Jennings L, Graham D, Graham CE: Painful heel syndrome: Radiographic and treatment assessment. *Foot Ankle* 9:91-99, 1988.
6. Barrett SL, Day SV: Endoscopic plantar fasciotomy for chronic plantar fasciitis/heel spur syndrome. Surgical technique—early clinical results. *J Foot Surg* 30:568-570, 1991.
7. Barrett SL, Day SV, Pignetti TT, Robinson LB: Endoscopic plantar fasciotomy: A multi-surgeon prospective analysis of 652 cases. *J Foot Ankle Surg* 34(4):400-406, 1995.
8. Barry LD, Barry AN, Chen Y: A retrospective study of standing gastrocnemius–soleus stretching versus night splinting in the treatment of plantar fasciitis. *J Foot Ankle Surg* 41(4):221-227, 2002.
9. Batt ME, Tanji JL, Skattum N: Plantar fasciitis: A prospective randomized clinical trial of the tension night splint. *Clin J Sport Med* 6(3):158-162, 1996.
10. Baxter DE, Pfeffer GB, Thigpen M: Chronic heel pain. Treatment rationale. *Orthop Clin North Am* 20(4):563-569, 1989.
11. Baxter DE, Pfeffer GB: Treatment of chronic heel pain by surgical release of the first branch of the lateral plantar nerve. *Clin Orthop* 279:229-236, 1992.
12. Baxter DE, Thigpen CM: Heel pain—operative results. *Foot Ankle* 5(1):16-25, 1984.
13. Berkowitz JF, Kier R, Rudicel S: Plantar fasciitis: MR imaging. *Radiology* 179(3):665-667, 1991.
14. Berlet GC, Anderson RB, Davis H, et al: A prospective trial of night splinting in the treatment of recalcitrant plantar fasciitis: The Ankle Dorsiflexion Dynasplint. *Orthopedics* 25(11):1273-1275, 2002.
15. Blanco CE, Leon HO, Guthrie TB: Endoscopic treatment of calcaneal spur syndrome: A comprehensive technique. *Arthroscopy* 17(5):517-522, 2001.
16. Boyle RA, Slater GL: Endoscopic plantar fascia release: A case series. *Foot Ankle Int* 24(2):176-179, 2003.
17. Brekke MK, Green DR: Retrospective analysis of minimal-incision, endoscopic, and open procedures for heel spur syndrome. *J Am Podiatr Med Assoc* 1998 88(2):64-72, 1998.
18. Brugh AM, Fallat, LM, Savoy-Moore RT: Lateral column symptomatology following plantar fascial release: A prospective study. *J Foot Ankle Surg* 41(6):365-371, 2002.
19. Callison WI: Heel pain in private practice [abstract]. Presented at the Orthopaedic Foot Club, Dallas, Texas, April, 1989.

20. Campbell JW, Inman VT: Treatment of plantar fasciitis and calcaneal spurs with the UC-BL shoe insert. *Clin Orthop Relat Res* 103:57-62, 1974.

21. Chang CC, Miltner LJ: Periostitis of the os calcis. *J Bone Joint Surg* 16:355-64, 1934.

22. Chen H, Chen L, Huang T: Treatment of painful heel syndrome with shock waves. *Clin Orthop Relat Res* 387:41-46, 2001.

23. Conflitti JM, Tarquinio TA: Operative outcome of partial plantar fasciectomy and neurolysis to the nerve of the abductor digiti minimi muscle for recalcitrant plantar fasciitis. *Foot Ankle Int* 25(7):482-487, 2004.

24. Crawford F, Thomson C: Interventions for treating plantar heel pain. *Cochrane Database Syst Rev* 3:CD000416, 2003.

25. Daly PJ, Kitaoka HB, Chao EY: Plantar fasciotomy for intractable plantar fasciitis: Clinical results and biomechanical evaluation. *Foot Ankle* 13(4):188-195, 1992.

26. Davies MS, Weiss GA, Saxby TS: Plantar fasciitis: How successful is surgical intervention? *Foot Ankle Int* 20(12):803-807, 1999.

27. Davis PF, Severud E, Baxter DE: Painful heel syndrome: Results of nonoperative treatment. *Foot Ankle Int* 15(10):531-535, 1995.

28. Deesomchok U, Tumrasvin T: Clinical comparison of patients with ankylosing spondylitis, Reiter's syndrome and psoriatic arthritis. *Med Assoc Thai* 76(2):61-70, 1993.

29. DiGiovanni BF, Nawocznski DA, Lintal ME, et al: Tissue-specific plantar fascia-stretching exercises enhances outcomes in patients with chronic heel pain. A prospective, randomized study. *J Bone Joint Surg Am* 85:1270-1277, 2003.

30. DuVries HL: Heel spur (calcaneal spur). *Arch Surg* 74:536-542, 1957.

31. Fadale PD, Wiggins ME: Corticosteroid injections: Their use and abuse. *J Am Acad Orthop Surg* 2(3):133-140, 1994.

32. Farooki S, Theodorou DJ, Sokoloff RM, et al: MRI of the medial and lateral plantar nerves. *J Comput Assist Tomogr* 25(3):412-416, 2001.

33. Forman WM, Green MA: The role of intrinsic musculature in the formation of inferior calcaneal exostoses. *Clin Podiatr Med Surg* 7(2):217-223, 1990.

34. Furey JG: Plantar fasciitis: The painful heel syndrome. *J Bone Joint Surg Am* 57:672-673, 1975.

35. Gefen A: Stress analysis of the standing foot following surgical plantar fascia release. *J Biomech* 35(5):629-637, 2002.

36. Gentile AT, Zizzo CJ, Dahukey A, et al: Traumatic pseudoaneurysm of the lateral plantar artery after endoscopic plantar fasciotomy. *Foot Ankle Int* 18(12):821-822, 1997.

37. Gerster JC: Plantar fasciitis and Achilles tendinitis among 150 cases of seronegative spondarthritis. *Rheumatol Rehabil* 19:218-222, 1980.

38. Gerster JC, Piccinin P: Enthesopathy of the heels in juvenile onset seronegative B-27 positive spondyloarthropathy. *J Rheumatol* 12(2):310-314, 1985.

39. Gerster JC, Saudan Y, Fallet GH: Talalgia. A review of 30 severe cases. *J Rheumatol* 5(2):210-216, 1978.

40. Gibbon WW, Long G: Ultrasound of the plantar aponeurosis (fascia). *Skeletal Radiol* 28(1):21-26, 1999.

41. Gill LH, Kiebzak GM: Outcome of nonsurgical treatment for plantar fasciitis. *Foot Ankle Int* 17(9):527-532, 1996.

42. Gormley J, Kuwada GT: Retrospective analysis of calcaneal spur removal and complete fascial release for the treatment of chronic heel pain. *J Foot Surg* 31(2):166-169, 1992.

43. Graham CE: Painful heel syndrome: Rationale of diagnosis and treatment. *Foot Ankle* 3(5):261-267, 1983.

44. Grasel RP, Schweitzer ME, Kovalovich AM, et al: MR imaging of plantar fasciitis: Edema, tears, and occult marrow abnormalities correlated with outcome. *AJR Am J Roentgenol* 173(3):699-701, 1999.

45. Griffith JF, Wong TY, Wong SM, et al: Sonography of plantar fibromatosis. *AJR Am J Roentgenol* 179(5):1167-1172, 2002.

46. Hall RL, Erickson SJ, Shereff MJ, et al: Magnetic resonance imaging in the evaluation of heel pain. *Orthopedics* 19(3):225-229, 1996.

47. Hammer DS, Adam F, Kreutz A, et al: Extracorporeal shock wave therapy (ESWT) in patients with chronic proximal plantar fasciitis: A 2-year follow-up. *Foot Ankle Int* 24(11):823-828, 2003.

48. Hammer DS, Rupp S, Ensslin S, et al: Extracorporeal shock wave therapy in patients with tennis elbow and painful heel. *Arch Orthop Trauma Surg* 120:304-307, 2000.

49. Hammer DS, Rupp S, Kreutz A, et al: Extracorporeal shockwave therapy (ESWT) in patients with chronic proximal plantar fasciitis. *Foot Ankle Int* 23(4):309-313, 2002.

50. Hawkins BJ, Langermen RJ Jr, Gibbons T, et al: An anatomic analysis of endoscopic plantar fascia release. *Foot Ankle Int* 16(9):552-558, 1995.

51. Helbig K, Herbert C, Schostok T, et al: Correlations between the duration of pain and the success of shock wave therapy. *Clin Orthop* 387:68-71, 2001.

52. Hicks JH: The foot as a support. *Acta Anat* (Basel) 25:34-45, 1955.

53. Hicks JH: The mechanics of the foot. II. The plantar aponeurosis and the arch. *J Anat* 88:25-30, 1954.

54. Hill JJ Jr, Cutting PJ: Heel pain and body weight. *Foot Ankle* 9:254-255, 1989.

55. Hogan KA, Webb D, Shereff M: Endoscopic plantar fascia release. *Foot Ankle Int* 25(12):875-881, 2004.

56. Jahss MH, Kummer F, Michelson JD: Investigations into the fat pads of the sole of the foot: Heel pressure studies. *Foot Ankle* 13; 227-232, 1992.

57. Kamel M, Eid H, Mansour R: Ultrasound detection of heel enthesitis: A comparison with magnetic resonance imaging. *J Rheumatol* 30(4):774-778, 2003.

58. Kane D, Greaney T, Shanahan M, et al: The role of ultrasonography in the diagnosis and management of idiopathic plantar fasciitis. *Rheumatology* 40(9):1002-1008, 2001.

59. Kenzora JE: The painful heel syndrome: An entrapment neuropathy. *Bull Hosp J Dis Orthop Inst* 47:178-189, 1987.

60. Kinley S, Frascone S, Calderone D, et al: Endoscopic plantar fasciotomy versus traditional heel spur surgery: A prospective study. *J Foot Ankle Surg* 32(6):595-603, 1993.

61. Kitaoka HB, Luo ZP, Growney ES, et al: Material properties of the plantar aponeurosis. *Foot Ankle Int* 15(10):557-560, 1994.

62. Lapidus PW Guidotti FP: Painful heel: Report of 323 patients with 364 painful heels. *Clin Orthop* 39:178-186, 1965.

63. Lapidus PW: Kinesiology and mechanical anatomy of the tarsal joints. *Clin Orthop* 30:20-35, 1963.

64. Leach RE, Seavey MS, Salter DK: Results of surgery in athletes with plantar fasciitis. *Foot Ankle* 7(3):156-161, 1986.

65. Maier M, Steinborn M, Schmitz C, et al: Extracorporeal shock wave application for chronic plantar fasciitis associated with heel spurs: Prediction of outcome by magnetic resonance imaging. *J Rheumatol* 27:2455-2462, 2000.

66. Mann R, Inman VT: Phasic activity of intrinsic muscles of the foot. *J Bone Joint Surg Am* 46:469-481, 1964.

67. Manoli A 2nd, Harper MC, Fitzgibbons TC, et al: Calcaneal fracture after cortical bone removal. *Foot Ankle* 13(9):523-525, 1992.

68. Miller RA, Torres J, McGuire M: Efficacy of first-time steroid injection for painful heel syndrome. *Foot Ankle Int* 16(10):610-612, 1995.

69. Mizel MS, Marymont JV, Trepman E: Treatment of plantar fasciitis with a night splint and shoe modification consisting of a steel shank and anterior rocker bottom. *Foot Ankle Int* 17(12):732-735, 1996.

70. Narvaez JA, Narvaez J, Ortega R, et al: Painful heel: MR imaging findings. *Radiographics* 20(2):333-352, 2000.

71. Ogden JA, Alvarez RG, Marlow M: Shockwave therapy for chronic proximal plantar fasciitis: A meta-analysis. *Foot Ankle Int* 23(4):301-308, 2002.

72. Ogden JA, Alvarez R, Levitt R, et al: Shock wave therapy for chronic proximal plantar fasciitis. *Clin Orthop* 387:47-59, 2001.

73. Ogden JA, Alvarez RG, Levitt R, et al: Shock wave therapy (orthotripsy) in musculoskeletal disorders. *Clin Orthop* 387:22-40, 2001.

74. Ogden JA, Toth-Kischkat A, Schultheiss R, et al: Principle of shock wave therapy. *Clin Orthop* 387:8-7, 2001.

75. O'Malley MJ, Page A, Cook R: Endoscopic plantar fasciotomy for chronic heel pain. *Foot Ankle Int* 21(6):505-510, 2000.

76. Ozdemir H, Ozdemir A, Soyucu Y, et al: The role of bone scintigraphy in determining the etiology of heel pain. *Ann Nucl Med* 16(6):395-401, 2002.

77. Perry J: Anatomy and biomechanics of the hindfoot. *Clin Orthop* 177:9-15, 1983.

78. Pfeffer G, Bacchetti P, Deland J, et al: Comparison of custom and prefabricated orthoses in the initial treatment of proximal plantar fasciitis. *Foot Ankle Int* 20(4):214-221, 1999.

79. Pfeffer GB: Plantar heel pain. In Myerson MS (ed): *Foot and Ankle Disorders.* Philadelphia, WB Saunders, 2000, pp 834-850.

80. Pigozzi F, Giombini A, Parisi A, et al: The application of shock waves therapy in the treatment of resistant chronic painful shoulder. *J Sports Med Phys Fitness* 49:356-361, 2000.

81. Porter D, Barrill E, Oneacre K, et al: The effects of duration and frequency of Achilles tendon stretching on dorsiflexion and outcome in painful heel syndrome: A randomized, blinded, control study. *Foot Ankle Int* 23(7):619-624, 2002.

82. Prichasuk S: The heel pad in plantar heel pain. *J Bone Joint Surg Br* 76:140-142, 1994.

83. Probe RA, Baca M, Adams R, et al: Night splint treatment for plantar fasciitis. A prospective randomized study. *Clin Orthop* (368):190-195, 1999.

84. Riddle DL, Pulisic M, Pidcoe P, et al: Risk factors for plantar fasciitis: A matched case-control study. *J Bone Joint Surg Am* 85(5):872-877, 2003.

85. Riddle DL, Schappert SM: Volume of ambulatory care visits and patterns of care for patients diagnosed with plantar fasciitis: A national study of medical doctors. *Foot Ankle Int* 25(5):303-310, 2004.

86. Rompe JD, Hopf C, Nafe B, Burger R: Low-energy extracorporeal shock wave therapy for painful heel: A prospective controlled single-blind study. *Arch Orthop Trauma Surg* 115:75-79, 1996.

87. Rompe JD, Schoellner C, Nafe B: Evaluation of low-energy extracorporeal shock wave application for treatment of chronic plantar fasciitis. *J Bone Joint Surg Am* 84:335-341, 2002.

88. Ryan J: Use of posterior night splints in the treatment of plantar fasciitis. *Am Fam Physician* 52:891-898, 1995.

89. Sammarco GJ, Helfrey RB: Surgical treatment of recalcitrant plantar fasciitis. *Foot Ankle Int* 17(9):520-526, 1996.

90. SanuWave: Plantar fasciitis. Available at http://www.ossatron.com/pf_procedure.asp (accessed March 10, 2006).

91. Sarrafian SK: Functional characteristics of the foot and plantar aponeurosis under tibiotalar loading. *Foot Ankle* 8(1):4-18, 1987.

92. Sarrafian SK: *Anatomy of the Foot and Ankle,* ed 2. Philadelphia, JB Lippincott, 1993.

93. Schon LC: Plantar fascia and Baxter's nerve release. In: Myerson MS (ed): *Current Therapy in Foot and Ankle Surgery.* St Louis, Mosby, 1993, pp 177-182.

94. Schon LC, Glennon TP, Baxter DE: Heel pain syndrome: Electrodiagnostic support for nerve entrapment. *Foot Ankle* 14(3):129-135, 1993.

95. Sellman JR: Plantar fascia rupture associated with corticosteroid injection. *Foot Ankle Int* 15(7):376-381, 1994.

96. Sewell JR, Black CM, Chapman AH, et al: Quantitative scintigraphy in diagnosis and management of plantar fasciitis (calcaneal periostitis): Concise communication. *J Nucl Med* 21(7):633-636, 1980.

97. Sharkey NA, Donahue SW, Ferris L: Biomechanical consequences of plantar fascial release or rupture during gait. Part II. Alterations in forefoot loading. *Foot Ankle Int* 29(2):86-96, 1999.

98. Shmokler RL, Bravo AA, Lynch FR, et al: A new use of instrumentation in fluoroscopy controlled heel spur surgery. *J Am Podiatr Med Assoc* 78:194-197, 1988.

99. Smith S: Inside insights on shockwave therapy. *Podiatr Today* 8:38-42, 2001.

100. Snook GA, Chrisman OD: The management of subcalcaneal pain. *Clin Orthop* 82:163-168, 1972.

101. Steindler A, Smith AR: Spurs of the os salcis. *Surg Gynecol* 66:663, 1938.

102. Tanz SS: Heel pain. *Clin Orthop* 28:169-178, 1963.

103. Theodorou DJ, Theodorou SJ, Kakitsubata Y, et al: Plantar fasciitis and fascial rupture: MR imaging findings in 26 patients supplemented with anatomic data in cadavers. *Radiographics* 20 Spec No:S181-S197, 2000.

104. Theodorou DJ, Theodorou SJ, Resnick D: MR imaging of abnormalities of the plantar fascia. *Semin Musculoskelet Radiol* 6(2):105-118, 2002.

105. Thiel M: Application of shock waves in medicine. *Clin Orthop* 387:18-21, 2001.

106. Thorardson DB, Kumar PJ, Hedman TP, et al: Effect of partial versus complete fasciotomy on the windlass mechanism. *Foot Ankle Int* 18(1):16-20, 1997.

107. Tisdel CL, Harper MC: Chronic plantar heel pain: Treatment with a short leg walking cast. *Foot Ankle Int* 17(1):41-42, 1996.

108. Tomczak RL, Haverstock BD: A retrospective comparison of endoscopic plantar fasciotomy to open plantar fasciotomy with heel spur resection for chronic plantar fasciitis/heel spur syndrome. *J Foot Ankle Surg* 34(3):305-311, 1995.

109. Tsai WC, Chiu MF, Wang CL, et al Ultrasound evaluation of plantar fasciitis. *Scand J Rheumatol* 29(4):255-259, 2000.

110. Vohra PK, Giorgini RJ, Sobel E, et al: Long-term follow-up of heel spur surgery. A 10-year retrospective study. *J Am Podiatr Med Assoc* 89(2):81-88, 1999.

111. Walther M, Radke S, Kirschner S, et al: Power Doppler findings in plantar fasciitis. *Ultrasound Med Biol* 30(4):435-440, 2004.

112. Wang C, Chen H, Huang T: Shockwave therapy for patients with plantar fasciitis: A one-year follow-up study. *Foot Ankle* 23:204-207, 2002.

113. Wapner KL, Sharkey PF: The use of night splints for treatment of recalcitrant plantar fasciitis. *Foot Ankle* 12(3):135-137, 1991.

114. Ward WG, Clippinger FW: Proximal medial longitudinal arch incision for plantar fascia release. *Foot Ankle* 8(3):152-155, 1987.

115. Watson TS, Anderson RB, Davis WH, et al: Distal tarsal tunnel release with partial plantar fasciotomy for chronic heel pain: An outcome analysis. *Foot Ankle Int* 23(6):530-537, 2002.

116. Williams PL, Warwick R, Dyson M, et al, (eds): *Gray's Anatomy,* ed 37. London, Churchill Livingstone, 1989, p 652.

117. Williams PL: The painful heel. *Br J Hosp Med* 38:562-563, 1987.

118. Williams PL, Smibert JG, Cox R, et al: Imaging study of the painful heel syndrome. *Foot Ankle* 7:345-349, 1987.

119. Wolgin M, Cook C, Graham C, et al: Conservative treatment of plantar heel pain: Long-term follow-up. *Foot Ankle Int* 15(3):97-102, 1994.

120. Wright DG, Rennels DC: A study of the elastic properties of plantar fascia. *J Bone Joint Surg Am* 46:482-492, 1964.

121. Yu JS: Pathologic and post-operative conditions of the plantar fascia: Review of MR imaging appearances. *Skeletal Radiol* 29(9):491-501, 2000.

122. Zingas CN, Collon D, Anderson K: Shock wave therapy for plantar fasciitis [abstract]. Presented at the AOFAS Annual Summer Meeting, Traverse City, Mich, 2002.

Soft Tissue and Bone Tumors

Arthur K. Walling

Primary malignant tumors of the soft tissues or bones of the foot and ankle develop infrequently.* Similarly, metastatic and marrow cell lesions are exceedingly rare.[22,43] Soft tissue lesions are considerably more common than their skeletal counterparts, and fortunately, most of these lesions are benign. Although the rarity of malignant disease is encouraging, unfortunately it carries the potential for misdiagnosis and increased morbidity in patients who do have a malignancy.

Because malignant bone and soft tissue tumors are uncommon, many foot and ankle surgeons are unfamiliar with their presentation, imaging features, biopsy techniques, and treatment. Improper treatment can result in not only loss of limb but even loss of life. The onus thus falls on the treating physician to maintain respect for all foot and ankle lesions. It is better to regard a lesion of uncertain origin as potentially malignant and to treat it with this possibility in mind.

This chapter outlines the proper steps in staging lesions and the appropriate techniques for biopsy. This helps the physician avoid undertreating a malignant lesion or overtreating a benign one.

CLINICAL EVALUATION

The evaluation of a foot and ankle tumor includes a thorough patient history, careful physical examination, and appropriate radiographic studies. Lesions of the foot and ankle manifest early in their course partly because of the thin soft tissues covering these areas. Even small masses are usually easily palpable. Dorsal lesions produce symptoms because of pressure against the thin dorsal skin from shoes, and plantar lesions are aggravated by weight bearing. Pain and discomfort can also be produced, even by small lesions, secondary to mechanical impediment of the tightly bound gliding mechanisms of muscles and tendons. However, not all lesions are painful or small. The statement that benign lesions are painless and malignant lesions are painful is inaccurate. Likewise, size is not a predictor of malignancy; all large lesions start out small. An unfortunate example is synovial sarcoma, which can occur as a small painless lesion that has been present for months to years.[12,13]

During the physical examination the physician should note whether the lesion is fixed to the skin, tendons, or bone. However, diagnosis based on palpation alone is notoriously unreliable. The consistency of tumors often depends on the tension that they exert on the surrounding tissue. Even a ganglion may be

soft, firm, or hard. Transillumination and auscultation provide additional information in the evaluation of fluid-containing and vascular lesions. Careful aspiration of suspected ganglia is an easy and acceptable method of verifying their suspected diagnosis, but if typical ganglion fluid is not obtained, the clinician should not assume that the fluid was too thick to aspirate. Serious consideration should be given to the possibility of the lesion's being a solid tumor and of greater consequence.

RADIOGRAPHIC EVALUATION

The goal of imaging is to form a differential diagnosis, to assign a probable Musculoskeletal Tumor Society stage, and to plan biopsy and subsequent treatment. Plain anteroposterior (AP) and lateral radiographs remain the most informative imaging tests for osseous lesions.[47] Special views to place lesions in their optimal position may be necessary.

It is sometimes possible to characterize osseous lesions as geographic or permeative by their appearance. A *geographic pattern* is a concentric loss of bone with a well-delineated margin between normal and abnormal bone, as is seen in giant cell tumors of bone. A *permeative pattern* is harder to identify because there is only a subtle difference between the involved and uninvolved bone and usually accompanying periosteal elevation, such as is seen with marrow cell lesions. The type of matrix produced by the tumor also offers clues to the diagnosis. Cartilage mineralization forms stipples and rings, whereas osteoid is more cloudlike.

Imaging Modalities

Standard radiographs can offer important information, even in soft tissue tumors. Fat density may be appreciated, and the presence of soft-tissue calcification is an important diagnostic consideration. Computed tomography (CT) occasionally provides additional information regarding penetration of lesions beyond the subchondral plate.

Radionuclide bone scans are used to rule out additional skeletal lesions, to identify lesions that might not have been apparent on conventional radiographs, and to provide information regarding the intensity of uptake in a specific lesion. The examiner must be careful not to overinterpret areas of increased uptake if no confirmatory plain films are available; the bone scan is sensitive to inflammatory conditions, synovitis, and unrecalled trauma that can produce osteoporosis. The bone scan also provides some information regarding soft tissue lesions. Soft tissue lesions that show increased uptake could be benign or malignant;

---

*References 10, 12, 13, 20, 22, 35, and 41.

however, lesions that show no uptake on scanning are invariably benign.

Angiography can provide information regarding proximity of lesions to neurovascular bundles; however, its role has been limited by the advent of CT and magnetic resonance imaging (MRI). CT scanning is superior for cross-sectional bone detail and, with the use of vascular contrast, provides good evaluation of soft tissue detail. MRI provides superior soft tissue detail in multiple planes and defines marrow involvement in osseous lesions. These sophisticated scanning tests are primarily used for anatomic localization in preoperative surgical planning. These studies do not distinguish between benign and malignant disease, and much more diagnostic information is gained from the routine radiographs of bone lesions. The overuse of MRI to rule out occult pathologic processes about the foot and ankle has become unconscionable.

Radiographic Features and Locations

Some tumors share certain radiographic features and locations. In formulating a differential diagnosis, the physician should keep these similarities in mind. The following situations, however, are by no means all inclusive or infallible.

Lesions can cross the epiphysis or epiphyseal scar. The epiphysis represents a relative barrier to lesions; however, these tumors and conditions can appear as epiphyseal and metaphyseal lesions. Giant cell tumors and chondroblastomas begin as epiphyseal lesions but can extend into the metaphysis. Infection and eosinophilic granuloma can also manifest in this manner.

Lesions can occur around joints. With lesions around joints, the physician should consider which lesions could arise from the bone and which from the joint. The latter conditions include chondroblastoma, giant cell tumor, intraosseous ganglion, infection, and pigmented villonodular synovitis, which can occur on both sides of the joint. Less common conditions that can occur around joints include amyloidosis and gout.

Calcification within the soft tissue has a variety of causes; the differential should include collagen vascular disease, especially scleroderma; postpyogenic myositis, which forms bone but can appear as calcification; calcinosis universalis or tumor calcinosis; ochronosis; hemangioma, which forms phleboliths in the vascular spaces; and synovial sarcoma.

Lesions can occur in the diaphysis of bone. Diaphyseal tumor involvement is uncommon. These lesions, which do *not* usually occur in the diaphysis, include Ewing's sarcoma, eosinophilic granuloma, fibrous dysplasia, adamantinoma, and ossifying fibroma.

STAGING

Preoperative staging of lesions provides a rationale for definitive surgical treatment and long-term prognosis. The staging incorporates radiographic, histologic, and clinical data to categorize tumors. Enneking[12] has devised staging systems for benign and malignant tumors. The staging applies to both bone and soft tissue lesions.

Benign Lesions

Benign tumors can be classified as follows:

- Stage 1: Lesions are static or tend to heal spontaneously.
- Stage 2: Lesions have a more aggressive radiographic appearance, are less mature histologically, and show evidence of continued growth.
- Stage 3: Lesions are locally aggressive and histologically immature and show progressive growth that is not limited by natural barriers.

Malignant Lesions (Sarcomas)

Sarcomas are designated *low-grade* (stage 1) or *high-grade* (stage 2) lesions based on histologic appearance, and their radiographic aggressiveness is also taken into consideration (Table 13–1). They are then termed *intracompartmental* (A) or *extracompartmental* (B) based on anatomic location. Sarcomas with distant metastasis are stage 3 lesions.

Low-grade and intracompartmental lesions are more amenable to limb salvage surgery because there is less chance of metastasis or primary recurrence. High-grade and extracompartmental lesions carry a more guarded prognosis and require more extensive surgery. There are fewer true compartments because of the longitudinal course of tendons and nerves in the foot and ankle. The proximity of neurovascular bundles and the sparseness of soft tissue coverage around the foot and ankle can make adequate

TABLE 13–1

Classification of Malignant Tumors

Stage	Grade	Site	Metastasis
IA	Low	Intracompartmental	None
IB	Low	Extracompartmental	None
IIA	High	Intracompartmental	None
IIB	High	Extracompartmental	None
III	Any	Either	Present

surgical treatment of benign aggressive and malignant tumors incompatible with preservation of a functional foot.[12,49] The most functional reconstructions and the ways a preferred surgical margin can be obtained through amputation are discussed later in this chapter.

ANATOMIC FACTORS

Certain anatomic structures help to form compartments that serve as relative barriers to tumor growth. The distal tibia and fibula with their attached interosseous membrane separate the distal leg into anterior and posterior soft tissue compartments. The articular cartilage surfaces of the malleoli are good barriers to tumor growth, but the thin cortices of the epiphyseal regions have multiple vascular perforations that allow easy extension into the soft tissues. The bones of the hindfoot, as well as the individual tarsal bones, are separate compartments and have multiple articular surfaces that provide good containment of lesions; however, their other surfaces are quite thin and possess multiple vascular perforations that allow easy ingress or egress of lesions. The rays of the foot form individual compartments, but no effective fascial barriers separate the soft tissues and prevent extracompartmental extension. Because of these anatomic considerations and the paucity of soft tissues covering the osseous components of the foot and ankle, soft tissue extensions of bone lesions and bone invasion by soft tissue lesions occur early in the development of benign aggressive and malignant lesions.

BIOPSY

Although the biopsy is part of the staging sequence, its importance cannot be underestimated, and it should be considered a major surgical procedure. Tumor implantation or extension, primarily by dissection of hematoma, can result from the biopsy. Depending on the malignant potential or implantability of the tumor, extension of the tumor's influence can result, converting an intracompartmental lesion into an extracompartmental one. This in turn can require a more extensive procedure to remove this extension or convert a lesion amenable to limb salvage to one requiring amputation.[12] It also is imperative to consider the surgical margins that may be needed for definitive treatment before the biopsy so that the incision can be placed in a position to be completely excised as part of the specimen at final resection.

An *excisional biopsy* should be performed for lesions that are presumptively benign or small enough that they can be removed with a surrounding cuff of normal tissue. This removes the entire lesion, avoids potential seeding, and serves as adequate treatment for benign or low-grade malignant lesions. An *incisional biopsy* is preferred for larger lesions or presumptive malignant lesions that would require undue sacrifice of normal tissue to achieve a wide margin with the biopsy.

Frozen-section histologic confirmation should be obtained from all lesions at their biopsy. In lesions amenable to excisional biopsy, no further treatment is necessary if the diagnosis is compatible with the surgical margin. With an incisional biopsy or in lesions that were not removed with a satisfactory margin, the incision is closed meticulously and the extremity prepared again and draped. The closed incision is then covered with a protective barrier (Ioban), and operating room personnel are regowned and regloved. With fresh instruments, the lesion is completely excised with the appropriate surgical margin (see Fig. 13–7D).

If the frozen-section histology is inconclusive or if the lesion is one for which adjunctive therapy (chemotherapy or radiation therapy) is appropriate before definitive surgical excision, the biopsy site should be closed in layers over a small drain brought out in line with the biopsy incision. Meticulous hemostasis should be obtained before closure. These steps are taken to decrease the formation of hematoma and potential spread of the tumor. The drain site is positioned so that it can be excised at definitive surgical resection. The biopsy should be performed under tourniquet control but without exsanguination. Biopsy incisions should be longitudinal, and unnecessary dissection and spreading must be avoided (Fig. 13–1).

Major vascular bundles and tendon sheaths should be excluded from biopsy sites because of the potential for spread. Lesions in the talus can require medial malleolar osteotomy (see Fig. 13–23D) for adequate visualization or may be approached through a posterolateral approach just lateral to the edge of the Achilles tendon if the lesion is posterior. Calcaneal lesions may be reached either medially or laterally, with incisions paralleled to the border of the transition from weight-bearing to non–weight-bearing skin. In the midfoot, incisions should be made medial or lateral to the anterior tibial tendon and common toe extensors. In the forefoot, direct incision over the metatarsal allows for future ray resection.

Needle biopsy should be reserved for lesions whose diagnosis is obvious from the staging studies. The quantity of specimens obtained might not be sufficient for adequate diagnosis. Also, because of the paucity of soft tissues, the depth of needle penetration or subse-

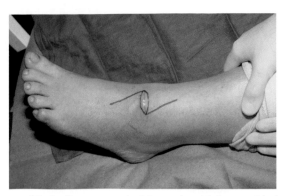

Figure 13–1 Transverse incisions should be avoided on extremities. Longitudinal incisions are more amenable to reexcisions, either for definitive treatment or for treatment of recurrences. As illustrated here, a transverse incision was initially used to remove this soft tissue lesion around the ankle. When the lesion recurred, large flaps were needed to excise all the tumor and previous surgical site.

quent hematoma formation can cause inadvertent extension of the lesion.

Not all lesions need to be biopsied. For instance, enchondromas of the metatarsals or phalanges are often found incidentally on x-ray. If these lesions are asymptomatic and their radiographic features are benign, serial radiographic evaluation for a reasonable length of time may be all that is necessary.

TREATMENT OF SOFT TISSUE LESIONS

The primary treatment for benign and malignant soft tissue tumors is surgical resection, and results are directly related to the adequacy of the surgical margins.[12] The *surgical margins* are defined as follows:

Intralesional: The lesion is removed from within the reactive pseudocapsule.

Marginal: The lesion is removed by dissection around the outside of the pseudocapsule (may leave microscopic disease).

Wide: The lesion (and biopsy tract) is removed with a cuff of normal tissue so that the reactive pseudocapsule is not exposed.

Radical: The entire anatomic compartment containing the lesion is removed.

The choice of surgical margin is determined by the stage of the lesion. The choice of reconstruction after the resection is determined by the anatomic site of the lesion and the anticipated disability from the resec-

tion. It is unwise to think of amputation as a definitive procedure. An amputation, depending on its proximity to the reactive pseudocapsule, could represent any of the four surgical margins. It is more appropriate to consider amputation a method of *reconstruction.* If the surgical resection required to achieve the appropriate margin will result in a significant disability, an amputation may not only achieve the desired surgical margin but also afford the best means for reconstruction and rehabilitation.

Benign stages 1 and 2 lesions of the soft tissue are appropriately treated by marginal excision or wide excision if this can be achieved without sacrificing functional structures. Benign stage 3 and malignant stage 1A (low-grade) soft tissue lesions require wide margins for treatment. Because of involvement of adjacent tendons, neurovascular structures, and bone, wide excision might sacrifice too much tissue to leave a functional foot. Wide excision may only be obtainable when the lesion is small, confined to a toe or metatarsal ray, or situated in the subcutaneous tissues. Malignant stage 2 lesions and some stage 1B lesions require margins that usually necessitate amputation. Lesions of the toe may be treated with disarticulation at the metatarsophalangeal level. Lesions around the metatarsal need a ray resection, midfoot lesions require a Syme amputation, and lesions around the hindfoot or periarticular soft tissues of the ankle require below-knee amputations above the musculotendinous junction.

Alternatives of more conservative marginal or wide resection plus adjuvant radiation therapy may occasionally be used, but the tolerance of the foot and ankle to this regimen is less satisfactory than in other anatomic sites.[12] The resulting function and disability may be worse than that achieved with more radical surgery (e.g., amputation and satisfactory prosthesis). Chemotherapy is used primarily to control possible micrometastasis rather than to create the potential for a lesser surgical procedure.[8,35] A lesser surgical margin that increases the risk of local recurrence has a direct bearing on the possibility of developing distant metastasis.

As stated earlier, soft tissue lesions are more common than their osseous counterparts and are much more often benign than malignant. Around 5% of sarcomas are thought to occur about the foot and ankle; of these, synovial sarcoma and epithelioid sarcoma have a relatively higher incidence. Lesions can arise from any of the mesenchymal tissues, including fibrous, vascular, perineural, lipomatous, synovial, and muscular.[13] Table 13–2 lists some of the lesions encountered around the foot and ankle, and several of these are examined in detail.

TABLE 13-2

Types of Soft Tissue Tumors

Benign	Malignant
Fibrous	
Plantar fibroma (fibromatosis)	Fibrosarcoma
Pseudosarcomatous fasciitis	Malignant fibrous histiocytoma
Vascular	
Glomus tumor	Angiosarcoma
Hemangioma	Hemangioendothelioma
	Hemangiopericytoma
Neural	
Neurilemoma	Neurosarcoma
Neurofibroma	
Fat	
Angiolipoma	Liposarcoma
Lipoma	
Synovial	
Ganglion	Synovial sarcoma
Giant cell tumor of tendon sheath	
Pigmented villonodular synovitis	
Synovial chondromatosis	
Muscle	
Leiomyoma	Leiomyosarcoma
	Rhabdomyosarcoma
Miscellaneous	
Xanthoma of tendon	Kaposi's sarcoma
	Malignant melanoma
	Soft tissue sarcoma

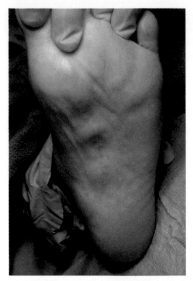

Figure 13–2 Typical size and appearance of plantar fibroma along the medial border of the plantar fascia.

Fibrous Tumors

Fibroma, Plantar Fibroma, and Fibromatosis

Fibroma is a soft tissue lesion composed of dense, mature fibrocytes. It usually occurs around fibrous structures and fascial planes, may be noticed at any age, and is usually asymptomatic. If it is symptomatic, marginal extracapsular excision is easily accomplished and has a negligible recurrence rate. This entity has a much different prognosis and should be distinguished from plantar fibroma and fibromatosis.

Plantar fibroma usually manifests as a solitary lesion or multiple nodules, occurring most often along the medial border of the plantar fascia (Fig.13–2). It occurs more often in adolescents and young adults. Lesions are firm and fixed to the plantar fascia and produce discomfort on weight bearing because of the irregular contour of the plantar surface in the arch of the foot. Growth is usually slow, stops once the lesion

reaches a size of approximately 2 cm, and then remains unchanged indefinitely. Older patients may have associated Dupuytren's contracture of the hands or Peyronie's disease. Although no specific staging study helps to separate this benign disease from its malignant counterparts, the location along the medial border of the plantar fascia makes the diagnosis clinically quite evident.

Asymptomatic patients require no treatment. Symptomatic patients should be given a persistent trial of nonsurgical therapy, including shoe modification and nonsteroidal anti-inflammatory drugs (NSAIDs). Attempted surgical resection is best avoided. If these lesions are left undisturbed and are treated symptomatically, their presence rarely cannot be tolerated; it is with surgical manipulation that they become a problem. Because the lesion extends into dermis and skin as well as the underlying fascia, it is difficult to obtain satisfactory surgical margins. Accordingly the recurrence rate after marginal excision is not only high but often astonishingly rapid. It is these inadequately excised lesions that take on a more aggressive and debilitating course. If excision is to be undertaken, the resection must remove the adherent overlying dermis, skin, and a significant amount of normal-appearing plantar fascia. The remaining defect often requires skin grafting and, because of the proximity of the plantar nerves, may leave a hypersensitive plantar arch. Even this approach can result in additional recurrence if employed in treatment of recurrent lesions. Seldom is more than one attempt at excision prudent. Despite this aggressive behavior, malignant degeneration of these lesions is virtually unknown.

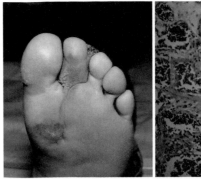
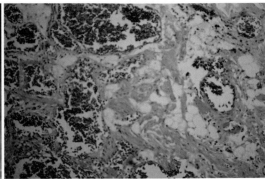

Figure 13–3 A, Skin and soft tissue changes in a patient with hemangioma. **B,** Histologic section demonstrating multiple vascular channels with thin endothelial lining and a benign fibrous supporting stroma.

A   B

Everything known about these lesions seems to indicate an extremely cautious approach to their treatment, but the literature is full of reports of attempted surgical treatment and results.* None of these articles has shown a success rate that would justify the morbidity encountered in the unsuccessfully treated patient.

Fibromatosis (desmoid) is distinguished from plantar fibroma by its different anatomic site, more aggressive clinical course, more aggressive pathologic characteristics, and different response to treatment.[3,12,13] It is more often encountered in and around the large muscles of the proximal portions of the extremities and the trunk. It manifests in the foot as a soft tissue mass deep in the plantar arch and not superficial, as is a plantar fibroma. Fibromatosis grows actively and occasionally rapidly, producing a mass of considerable size.

Imaging studies depict a soft tissue mass without particular distinguishing characteristics. Clinically the differential diagnosis includes possible soft tissue sarcoma. These lesions are usually large enough to be amenable to Tru-Cut needle biopsy, which confirms their diagnosis. Again, because of their size and location, marginal excision is usually the best margin that can usually be obtained. Multiple recurrence can require amputation for effective rehabilitation.

Pseudosarcomatous Fasciitis

Pseudosarcomatous fasciitis straddles the transition between fibromatosis and fibrosarcoma. It is more common in young adults and in the deep subcutaneous tissue. It may be quite tender and can exhibit a local inflammatory response. Staging studies are nonspecific. On biopsy the histology shows mitotic structures but without evidence of necrosis or vascular invasion.

Because of the difficulty in distinguishing between pseudosarcomatous fasciitis and fibrosarcoma, treatment decisions based on frozen sections are inappropriate. A skilled pathologist is required for accurate diagnosis. Although histologically it resembles a stage 3 lesion, its response to treatment may be better.

Vascular Tumors

Glomus Tumor

Glomus tumors are benign vascular tumors that have their peak incidence in the 20- to 40-years age range. Subungual glomus tumors are associated with a female predominance of 3:1.[44] These tumors typically manifest with a bright-red to bluish discoloration beneath the nail bed and are associated with lancinating pain that worsens with cold exposure or direct pressure. They are usually less than 1 cm in diameter. Radiographs may show a well-marginated bony erosion over the dorsal surface of the distal phalanx.

Treatment involves marginal excision for this stage 1 or 2 benign lesion. Pain relief is prompt, and recurrence is unusual. In any lesion found under the nail, the possibility of malignant melanoma should always be considered in the preoperative differential diagnosis.

Hemangioma

Hemangiomas are benign vascular tumors believed to represent hamartomatous malformations of normal vascular tissues or benign neoplasms.[12,32] These tumors can be of the cavernous, capillary, or mixed type; the port-wine capillary hemangiomas are most common in the foot. Hemangiomas arise in childhood and adolescence. When these tumors are superficial, a noticeable bluish discoloration is observed, associated with a soft, doughy mass (Fig. 13–3). More extensive lesions can have associated localized gigantism of adjacent bone and soft tissue. Plain radiographs can

*References 2, 3, 12, 41, 49, and 51.

show multiple small calcified phleboliths. Other imaging studies (MRI, CT, and angiography or venography) can further identify the hemangioma's anatomic extent.

Hemangiomas are best treated symptomatically. NSAIDs have been found useful, as have compression stockings, which in some early presentations have led to partial involution. Because these lesions are infiltrative and lack a pseudocapsule, marginal excision is associated with a high local recurrence rate. Surgical resection should be reserved for cases that cause significant disability. Preoperative embolization, when possible, has facilitated their removal.

Neural Tumors

Neurilemoma

Neurilemoma (neurilemmoma, neurolemmoma) is a benign tumor of nerve sheath (Schwann cell) origin with a peak incidence in the fourth and fifth decades of life. No predilection toward either gender is shown. The tumor is usually solitary, well encapsulated, and on the surface of a peripheral nerve. Patients present with a painful nodule associated with a positive Tinel sign in the distribution of the affected nerve. These are usually stage 2 benign lesions, and marginal excision is curative. The tumor can be shelled out of the nerve sheath without damage to the nerve fibers themselves (Fig. 13–4). Recurrence is rare, and these tumors have little malignant potential.

Neurofibroma

Neurofibromas are spindle cell tumors of peripheral nerves that may be solitary or multiple. Ninety percent are solitary and usually located in the dermis or subcutaneous tissue. Ten percent of cases are associated with von Recklinghausen's disease and manifest with multiple lesions that may be associated with scoliosis, localized gigantism, or tibial pseudoarthroses. Neurofibromas are the most common neurogenic tumor. They are stage 2 benign lesions and diffusely invasive, permeating between nerve fibers with no clear plane of dissection. Resection usually requires removal of the affected portion of the nerve as well. Because of this, the surgeon must often choose between the disability caused by the lesion and the disability resulting from resection. The tumor can recur, and 10% of patients with Recklinghausen's disease (neurofibromatosis) develop neurosarcomas.[12,13]

Fat Tumors

Lipoma

Lipomas are the most common benign soft tissue tumors. Lipomas can occur in the soft tissue, muscle, or bone. Most lipomas of the foot are located in the subcutaneous tissue. The mass is soft, nontender, mobile, and usually asymptomatic unless it compresses local tissue. Radiographs reveal a well-marginated, fatlike density with rare calcification

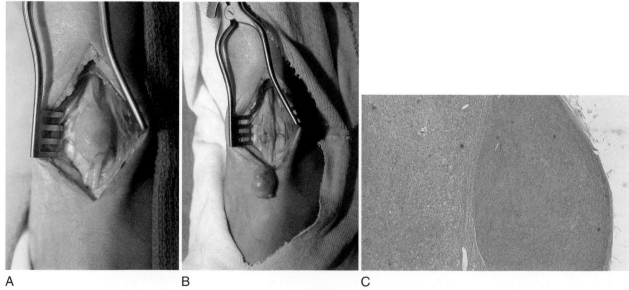

A   B   C

Figure 13–4   A, Neurilemoma on the dorsal surface of the ankle. **B,** Lesion removed, leaving nerve fibers intact. **C,** Low-power photomicrograph showing admixture of spindle and round cells with palisading of the spindle cell nuclei.

secondary to fat necrosis. CT is diagnostic and shows a well-defined lesion with the same density (−90 to −120 Hounsfield units) as normal fat.[30,47] MRI is likewise diagnostic. Treatment consists of marginal excision, with little chance for local recurrence.

Angiolipoma

Angiolipomas are tumors composed of mature fat with multiple vascular channels. They are usually subcutaneous, less than 2 cm in diameter, and exquisitely tender to palpation.[48] An angiogram or MR image may show the tortuous blood vessels seen in hemangiomas. Because of angiolipomas' infiltrative nature, marginal excision is more difficult and is associated with a higher recurrence rate than with simple lipomas.

Synovial Tumors

Ganglion

The lowly ganglion occurs so frequently about the dorsum of the foot and ankle that it has all too often led to the casual assumption that every asymptomatic, soft, movable mass is benign.[4,12] Occasionally this unwarranted optimism can lead to misdiagnosis and disaster. If the physician suspects a solid, potentially malignant lesion instead of a benign, fluid-filled, cystic ganglion, attempted aspiration for confirmation is recommended. This requires a large-bore needle, and lesions that do not yield fluid should be treated as potentially malignant. The aspiration causes no morbidity if the lesion proves to be a ganglion, and if the lesion is found to be solid, the site is treated as a biopsy tract.

The ganglion is the product of mucoid degeneration in an area of the joint capsule or tendon sheath. Ganglia can remain stationary, increase in size, or spontaneously rupture and disappear. Plain films are usually of little help unless underlying arthritic changes are seen in the joint adjacent to the lesion. CT and MRI can identify the well-defined reactive pseudocapsule with decreased density within.

Treatment is usually reserved for cases that produce mechanical pain. Although aspiration is excellent for verification, a 70% rate of recurrence is a common result.[20] Marginal excision is curative if the entire cyst wall with surrounding degenerative capsular or tendon sheath is removed (Fig. 13–5).

Giant Cell Tumor of Tendon Sheath

As its name implies, the giant cell tumor of tendon sheath often arises from the synovial lining of tendon sheaths but also can occur distant to synovial tissue. It also is referred to as *benign fibrous histiocytoma* and *fibroxanthoma*.[25,26] This lesion typically is found in both the hand and the foot. Most lesions manifest initially as small, painless masses that slowly enlarge (Fig. 13–6). The lesions can invade adjacent structures (Fig. 13–7) and produce mechanical pain as they enlarge. Imaging studies define their anatomic extent.

These lesions are usually well circumscribed, and a wide excision is preferred and curative. Histologically they are composed of fibrous stroma with giant cells and cholesterol-laden histiocytes. Intralesional or piecemeal excision can lead to implantation and recurrence.

Pigmented Villonodular Synovitis

Pigmented villonodular synovitis most often occurs around joints but can also occur around tendon sheaths and bursae linings.[17,31] It manifests as an intermittent swelling, with minimal discomfort, and without a history of antecedent trauma. Joint aspiration reveals bloody or brownish fluid and does not appreciably reduce the swelling because of the resid-

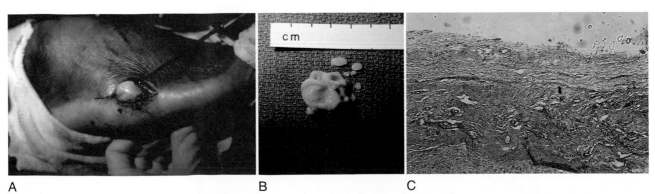

Figure 13–5 **A,** Ganglion arising from the fifth metatarsocuboid joint. **B,** Gross specimen consisting of a fibrous capsule and several "rice" bodies that were contained within the capsule. **C,** Representative section demonstrating a fibrous capsule with collagenous matrix and vascular tissue, all with benign features.

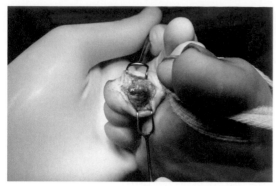

Figure 13–6 This lesion manifested as a small, painful mass on the flexor side of the third toe. Giant cell tumors of the tendon sheath have a characteristic dark-red to brown color.

ual thickening of the capsule. Radiographic findings are variable, and long-standing involvement can show bone erosion or degenerative changes within the affected joint. Imaging studies are usually not needed for diagnosis but can show a more extensive process than was suspected on clinical examination alone (Fig. 13–8). The course of the disease and risk of recurrence vary with the lesion's stage.

When the lesion is symptomatic or has radiographic evidence of progressive joint destruction, synovectomy is the treatment of choice. Synovectomy can be performed arthroscopically or open, depending on the location and extent of involvement. More extensive lesions require extracapsular synovectomy, which

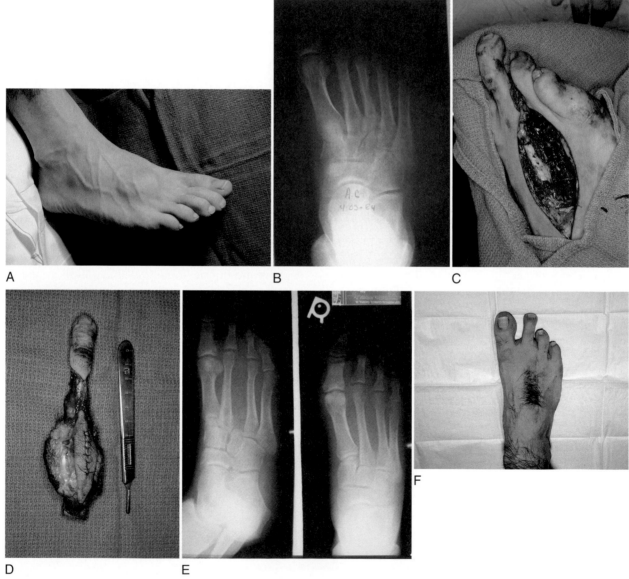

Figure 13–7 A, Painful mass of 2.5 years' duration overlying and fixed to the third metatarsal. **B,** Plain radiograph shows erosion of the lateral border of the third metatarsal. **C,** Biopsy confirmed giant cell tumor of tendon. Because of extension into the metatarsal, the lesion was treated with a wide margin that included third ray resection. **D,** Specimen with incisional biopsy tract completely excised. **E,** Postresection radiograph. **F,** Clinical appearance of the foot after resection. Patient has no functional limitations and has returned to all activities, including vigorous sports.

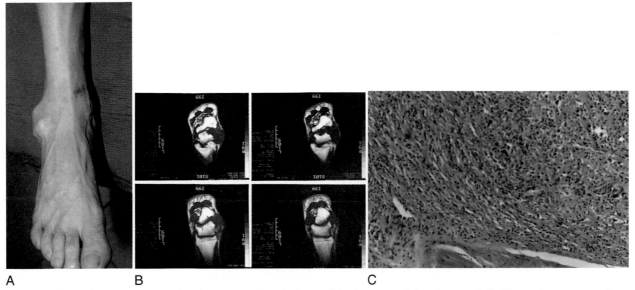

A   B   C

Figure 13–8 **A,** Patient presented with a mass primarily located in the area of the sinus tarsi. **B,** Magnetic resonance image demonstrates extension of the lesion into the ankle joint as well as unrecognized medial subtalar involvement. Surgery confirms the presence of PVS. **C,** Medium-power view demonstrating a dense collagenous stroma, with deeper cells containing brown pigment characteristic of hemosiderin.

might not be possible technically because of the risk of serious disability to the patient. Recurrence is common and often disabling. Radiation therapy has been used as an adjuvant therapy for recurrences; unfortunately, it also is less effective with the most aggressive lesions and when the surgeon needs the most help. Restraint may be the best treatment for recurrence.[31]

Synovial Chondromatosis

Synovial chondromatosis is a tumor that results from chondral metaplasia within the synovial tissue. This tumor has a peak incidence in early adult life and a male-to-female ratio of 2:1. Greater than 50% of cases occur around the knee, but synovial chondromatosis can also occur in and around the ankle. This tumor can cause numerous cartilaginous bodies within a joint, bursa, or tendon sheath, or it may be solitary.

On gross examination, multiple cartilaginous and osteocartilaginous nodules are embedded in the synovium, often with additional free loose bodies in the joint. Microscopically these nodules are composed of cartilage with varying degrees of calcification or ossification and can have atypical cytology that should not be misinterpreted as low-grade chondrosarcoma. If the pathologist gives a diagnosis of low-grade chondrosarcoma for a particular lesion, the surgeon should specifically question the possibility of synovial chondromatosis before proceeding with a definitive procedure.

Radiographs can show variable amounts of speckled calcifications depending on the maturity of the lesions,

and often more disease is present than radiographs indicate because of numerous uncalcified nodules (Fig. 13–9). Treatment consists of synovectomy and removal of the extruded, loose cartilaginous bodies from the joint. This amounts to a marginal excision; recurrence after synovectomy is not unusual. Persistent, long-standing synovial chondromatosis leads to severe degenerative arthritis. Isolated case reports of sarcomatous transformation exist.[33]

Miscellaneous Lesions

Xanthoma of Tendon

Xanthomatous deposits can develop in tendons as an expression of essential familial hypercholesterolemia.

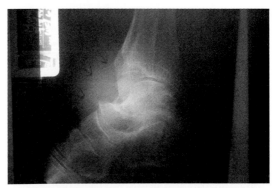

Figure 13–9 Patient with a mass over the anterior ankle. Plain radiograph demonstrates a soft tissue mass and erosion of the talus. At surgery, the ankle was filled with uncalcified nodules of synovial chondromatosis that were not apparent on radiographic examination.

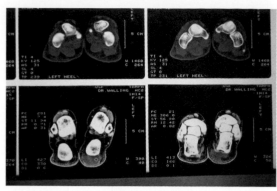

Figure 13–10 Computed tomography scan identifies soft tissue tumor of the left heel in a patient initially thought to have plantar fasciitis. Biopsy revealed myxoid chondrosarcoma, which was treated with amputation. Imaging tests provide mostly anatomic information and only rarely distinguish benign from malignant disease.

A common site is the Achilles tendon. Clinically it manifests as a painful fusiform swelling, which can suggest an inflammatory synovitis. The swelling is firm and moves with the tendon. Various imaging tests demonstrate a mass within the substance of the tendon. Treatment should be symptomatic. Debulking of the lesion has been reported to reduce pain but is technically difficult because of the infiltrative nature of the process, which involves the full complement of the tendon.[20] Postoperative protection to avoid rupture is recommended.

Soft Tissue Sarcoma

As mentioned previously, although soft tissue sarcomas of the foot and ankle are rare, they do exist. Although all the histologic varieties listed in Table 13–2 can occur, it is appropriate to discuss them as a group. Very little distinguishes one tumor from another with respect to their clinical appearance, staging, and recommendations for treatment.*

Clinically it can be difficult to distinguish benign from malignant disease. Even sarcomas may be small and slow growing (synovial sarcomas can follow an indolent course for several years), and solid lesions that do not yield fluid on aspiration should be regarded with suspicion. Radiographs are usually unrevealing unless the tumor invades the bone, but occasionally calcification within the lesion alerts the astute observer to the possibility of a synovial sarcoma. A plain chest radiograph is important to rule out distant metastasis when a primary sarcoma is suspected.[47] Additional staging studies (CT, MRI) primarily provide anatomic information (Fig. 13–10).

Treatment of soft tissue sarcomas is surgical and based on the tumor grade. Stage 1 lesions require at least a wide margin, whereas stage 2 lesions require more. The primary surgical limitation with foot and ankle lesions involves the tumor's anatomic location. Amputation often offers the best method of obtaining adequate surgical margins and functional reconstruction.

With foot and ankle sarcomas, the ability to obtain local control has always been good, even if it requires amputation. Unfortunately, the risk of distant metastasis remains significant. Most of the soft tissue sarcomas spread hematogenously and most often to the lungs. The role of adjuvant chemotherapy in suppressing or preventing metastasis and its effect on long-term survival continue to be evaluated. Lymphatic spread is much less common and most often associated with synovial sarcoma. Lymphatic mapping to guide node dissection holds significant promise.

Malignant Melanoma

The incidence of malignant melanoma is increasing at the highest rate of any malignancy. Unlike many other forms of cancer that primarily affect older people, melanoma often occurs in younger people.[14,16] The median age for patients with melanoma is in the low 40s.[14,46]

The poorer survival rates reported for patients with foot and ankle melanomas reflect the advanced stage and depth of these lesions at presentation and underscore the problem of early recognition compared with melanomas at other sites. The plantar surface of the foot and the subungual areas are relatively inconspicuous to the patient. The ABCDs of asymmetry, border irregularity, color variegation, and diameter greater than 6 mm are suspicious for melanoma when associated with a precursor lesion, but an even higher index of suspicion is needed for plantar and subungual lesions.[14]

Subungual lesions are notoriously difficult to diagnose. Ominous features that should raise the suspicion of melanoma include spontaneous nail liftoff or nail loss attributed to trauma that fails to regenerate a new nail, nail bed pigmentation that spills into the nail fold (Hutchinson's sign), and de novo nail bed pigmentation that fails to migrate distally with time, as occurs with subungual hematoma (Fig. 13–11). In addition, any nonhealing plantar ulceration in a patient without a predisposing condition (e.g., neuropathy) should be approached with a high index of suspicion, and biopsy should be the rule rather than the exception.

Surgical treatment is determined by site, depth, and stage of the lesions.[14] This can vary from wide local excision with skin grafting to amputation. Recent

---

*References 1, 8, 12, 13, 20, 41, and 49.

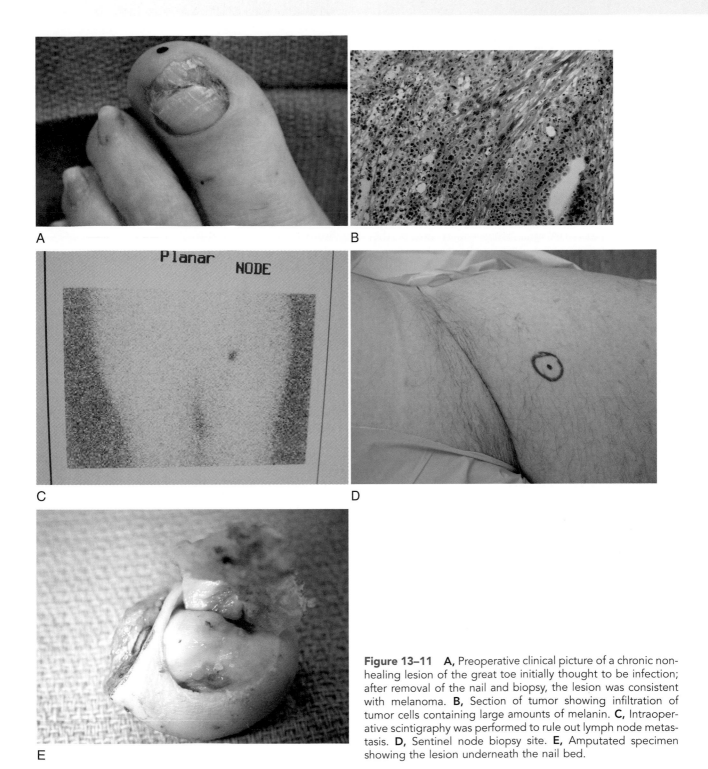

Figure 13–11 **A,** Preoperative clinical picture of a chronic non-healing lesion of the great toe initially thought to be infection; after removal of the nail and biopsy, the lesion was consistent with melanoma. **B,** Section of tumor showing infiltration of tumor cells containing large amounts of melanin. **C,** Intraoperative scintigraphy was performed to rule out lymph node metastasis. **D,** Sentinel node biopsy site. **E,** Amputated specimen showing the lesion underneath the nail bed.

protocols have used isotope-directed lymphatic mapping to assess the need for lymphatic node dissection. Adjuvant chemotherapy, limb perfusion, and specific immunotherapy are also being studied for their long-term effects on survival and local recurrence. The 5-year survival for melanoma at all sites is approx-imately 80%. Fortin et al[14] identified a 60% 5-year sur-vival for site-specific foot and ankle melanomas and concluded that these patients present with advanced tumor stage and depth. The foot and ankle surgeon must be familiar with the features of melanoma and its treatment.

Kaposi's Sarcoma

In 1872 Kaposi described five cases of an unusual tumor that principally affected the skin of the lower extremities in a multifocal and often symmetric fashion.[13] Interest in Kaposi's sarcoma in the United States has been renewed because of its increased incidence in renal transplant patients and in acquired immunodeficiency syndrome (AIDS).[9] Approximately 0.4% of patients with renal transplants develop Kaposi's sarcoma, which represents a 150- to 200-fold increase in incidence compared with the general population.[21] Approximately 30% of AIDS patients develop Kaposi's sarcoma. However, it affects the known risk groups unequally. It rarely occurs in transfusion recipients but affects about 40% of homosexual patients with AIDS.[9,18]

Current evidence suggests that Kaposi's sarcoma is a viral-associated, if not viral-induced, tumor.[13] It has a predilection for the skin of the hands and feet, particularly the great toe.[28] The lesions appear as flat, pink patches that slowly enlarge, becoming blue-violet and papular in appearance (Fig. 13–12). They are often associated with edema secondary to lymphatic obstruction.

The microscopic findings are variable. Early lesions can show a proliferation of miniature vessels that are so bland that they resemble normal capillary or lymphatic endothelium. The more advanced stages demonstrate a characteristic spindle cell component but are typically devoid of pleomorphism and significant meiotic activity. Histologically aggressive forms of Kaposi's sarcoma can also be seen.

Recognition of the early changes of Kaposi's sarcoma, especially in AIDS patients, remains a difficult diagnostic problem.[18] The overall prognosis varies considerably and depends on a number of interrelated factors, such as the immunologic competence of the host, the stage of the disease, and the presence or absence of opportunistic infections. As for treatment, surgery is no longer indicated except for tissue diagnosis. Radiation and chemotherapy are the preferred therapies. Staging of Kaposi's sarcoma provides a means of comparing treatment protocols.

Stage I: Cutaneous, locally indolent

Stage II: Cutaneous, locally aggressive, with or without regional lymph node involvement

Stage III: Generalized mucocutaneous with or without lymph node involvement

Stage IV: Visceral

Subtype A: No systemic signs or symptoms

Subtype B: Systemic signs including 10% weight loss or fever higher than 38° C (100° F) (orally) unrelated to an identifiable source of infection and lasting more than 2 weeks

TREATMENT OF OSSEOUS LESIONS

Various skeletal lesions have a special affinity for specific anatomic regions around the foot and ankle (Table 13–3). For example, intraosseous ganglion is the most common lesion of the medial malleolus. Aneurysmal bone cyst, chondroblastoma, and giant cell tumor are seen much more often in the distal tibia and the talus than in the distal fibula. Surface osteosarcomas can occur around the distal tibia and fibula and be mistaken for osteochondromas. Unicameral bone cyst and aneurysmal bone cyst have a peculiar affinity for the area just below the angle of Gisane in the calcaneus. Chondrosarcoma is the most common

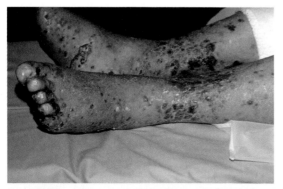

Figure 13–12 Late-stage Kaposi's sarcoma with violet papular appearance. (Courtesy of Wayne Cruse, MD, H. Lee Moffitt Cancer Center, Tampa, Fla.)

TABLE 13–3

Types of Bone Tumors

Benign	Malignant
Osseous	
Osteochondroma	Osteosarcoma (variants)
Osteoid osteoma	
Osteoblastoma	
Cartilaginous	
Enchondroma	Chondrosarcoma
Chondroblastoma	
Periosteal chondroma	
Fibrous	
Fibrous cortical defect	Fibrosarcoma
	Malignant fibrous histiocytoma
Miscellaneous	
Infection	
Fracture	

sarcoma about the foot and occurs more often in the calcaneus, as does osteosarcoma, its less common counterpart.

Surgical margins for skeletal lesions follow the same guidelines as those for soft tissues. Benign stage 1 and stage 2 lesions may be treated with extended intralesional curettage. Defects from curettage or marginal excision may be reconstructed by cancellous bone grafting or methacrylate augmentation. The exothermic reaction from the methacrylate serves to extend the curettage and also provides immediate structural support to lesions requiring removal of subchondral bone. In some stage 2 lesions and in stage 3 lesions where a local recurrence would be difficult to manage, it may be better to overtreat with a marginal excision that removes the intraarticular surface. This sacrifices a portion of the articular cartilage with the subsequent necessity for fusion across the area of sacrifice. The disability from the arthrodesis is usually less than that of a recurrence, which would require a wide margin that might not be obtainable without amputation.[6] As discussed with soft tissue lesions, malignant stage 1 osseous lesions require a wide margin, which usually necessitates partial or complete amputations at appropriate levels. Malignant stage 1B and stage 2 lesions usually require reconstruction by amputation.

Osseous Tumors

Osteochondroma

Osteochondromas are aberrant developmental anomalies that arise from the periphery of the cartilaginous growth plates. They occur most often around the rapidly growing, long tubular bones and rarely in the small bones of the hand or foot. They are composed of bone and cartilage, and their cartilage cap has all the features of a physeal growth plate. Because of this, osteochondromas continue to enlarge throughout growth. The lesion increases in size and moves away from the physeal plate with age. Enlargement stops with the cessation of growth and closure of the physeal plates, and the lesion remains inactive. Rarely, sarcomatous transformation can occur in the cartilage cap, giving rise to a secondary chondrosarcoma. Malignant transformation is much more common in conjunction with multiple hereditary osteochondromas than with the solitary form.

Symptoms are usually caused by mechanical factors. Clinically, osteochondromas manifest as a hard, fixed mass. Their radiographic picture is characteristic enough to preclude biopsy, unless the lesion is symptomatic, and it should reveal a confluence of the cancellous bone into the stalk of the osteochondroma (Fig. 13–13). Radiographically, osteochondromas may

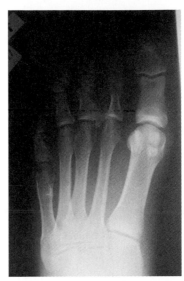

Figure 13–13 Osteochondroma of the proximal phalanx of the third toe in a patient with multiple hereditary osteochondroma. Contrast the location adjacent to the old epiphysis to the location and appearance of the subungual exostosis seen in Figure 13-19.

be confused with subungual exostosis, from which they are distinctly different and which occur primarily on the distal phalanges.[50]

Osteochondromas can be distinguished from surface osteosarcomas, which do not have a cancellous bridge, and radiographically can demonstrate a string sign. Treatment of osteochondromas consists of simple excision.

Osteoid Osteoma and Osteoblastoma

Osteoid osteoma can occur in any bone of the foot but is more common in the tarsal bones.[42,45,52] It most often occurs before the third decade of life. Although classically associated with a history of localized nocturnal pain relieved by aspirin, this presentation only occurs in about one third of patients. With plain radiographs, the examiner may have difficulty identifying the small nidus (less than 1 cm) with its characteristic surrounding halo of reactive bone. With a compatible patient history but negative radiographs, bone scanning usually confirms its presence. Further localization can be achieved with CT or MRI (Fig. 13–14).

Although these lesions have been known to resolve spontaneously over time, most often the patient's discomfort dictates surgical intervention. The critical step in treatment is accurate identification and removal of the nidus. To aid in this, some authors recommend intraoperative bone scanning. The isotope is administered before surgery, and a sterile Neoprobe is used intraoperatively to help localize the lesion. I have not found this to be necessary with good imaging studies.

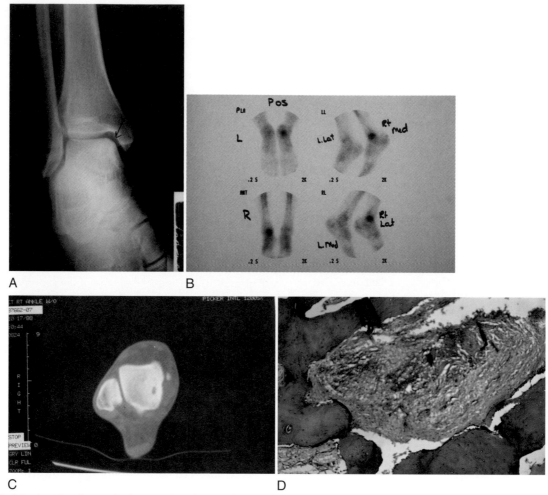

Figure 13–14   A, AP radiograph shows only a faint nidus in the medial talus of an osteoid osteoma. **B,** Bone scan confirms suspicion. **C,** CT scan demonstrates nidus and adjacent halo of reactive bone. **D,** Representative histologic section showing a thickened rim of reactive bone surrounding a well-vascularized central nidus of mesenchymal tissue.

En bloc excision is curative, but the majority of lesions are successfully treated with intralesional curettage. The overlying reactive bone is carefully shaved away until the nidus is visually identified. It is then entirely removed with additional deep shaving or a high-speed burr. Local recurrence is rare and most often can still be treated with re-excision.

Osteoblastoma is arbitrarily designated by its larger size (greater than 1 cm) compared with osteoid osteoma. However, the histologic picture truly distinguishes one from the other. Radiographically, osteoblastoma is more of a radiolucent lesion without the characteristic reactive bone seen with osteoid osteoma. Typical locations are the same, with the talus being most common. Osteoblastoma has a peculiar affinity for the subperiosteal region of the dorsal head–neck junction of the talus.[52] Whereas osteoid osteoma is nonprogressive and might heal spontaneously, osteoblastoma is progressive and can exhibit both local aggressiveness and malignant transformation. Treatment consists of extended intralesional curettage and grafting. Recurrences require more aggressive treatment and are at higher risk for more malignant behavior.

Cartilaginous Tumors

Enchondroma

Enchondroma (true chondroma, enchondrosis) is a common benign tumor of cartilage seen slightly less frequently in the foot than in the hand. It often is asymptomatic unless associated with a pathologic fracture (Fig. 13–15). Plain radiographs show a typical punched-out appearance dominated within by stippled calcification. Asymptomatic lesions may be followed clinically. Symptomatic lesions are treated by curettage and bone grafting. Malignant degeneration

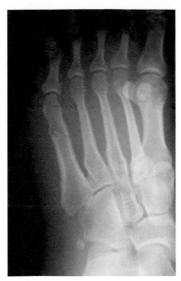

Figure 13–15 Pathologic fracture through a previously asymptomatic enchondroma of fifth metatarsal.

is observed less often in the small bones of the hand and foot than in long bones, and the key to this malignant degeneration is endosteal scalloping seen radiographically.

Chondroblastoma

Chondroblastoma typically occurs in the epiphysis before closure of the growth plate (Fig. 13–16). When seen in the foot, the talus and calcaneus are the most common locations. Presentation usually consists of pain, with associated joint discomfort and swelling secondary to the tumor's subchondral location. Radiographs show a radiolucent lesion with a slight reactive rim, and calcification is evident in approximately 25% of cases. CT scanning provides anatomic detail, especially when penetration through the subchondral

bone and into the adjacent joint is suspected. Because of its usual proximity to the joint, initial treatment most often requires intralesional curettage and grafting. Occasional recurrence results from this treatment. Because stage III lesions and recurrence require wide surgical margins, the surgeon should consider removing the articular cartilage and primary arthrodesis rather than accept the risk of added disability from additional recurrences.

Chondromyxoid Fibroma

Chondromyxoid fibroma is rarely seen in my practice, but Wold et al[52] found the hindfoot to be the third most common site of occurrence. Radiographs identify a radiolucent lesion without calcification (Fig. 13–17). Histologically the lesion demonstrates chondroid, myxoid, and fibrous areas. Treatment consists of intralesional curettage and bone grafting or marginal excision if possible.

Periosteal Chondroma

Periosteal chondroma is a cartilaginous lesion that is often an incidental finding. Clinically it can manifest as a painless mass on the surface of a metatarsal. Periosteal chondroma shows a typical saucerization of the underlying bone along its long axis, with a thin rim of reactive bone. Radiographic differential diagnosis should include both periosteal osteosarcoma and periosteal chondrosarcoma. Treatment is by intralesional curettage.

Miscellaneous Lesions

Infection

Acute osteomyelitis can be confused with an osseous tumor. In this age of overuse of antibiotics the typical findings of erythema, swelling, increased temperature,

Figure 13–16 A, Tomogram of ankle demonstrates typical epiphyseal location of a chondroblastoma of the fibula in a patient with open growth plates. **B,** Biopsy specimen showing a cartilaginous matrix surrounded by a fibrous stroma and interspersed giant cells.

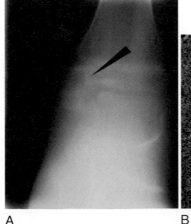

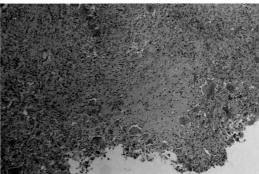

A   B

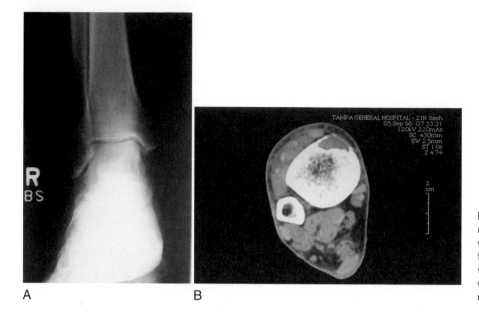

A   B

Figure 13-17 A, Metaphyseal radiolucency of the tibia in a patient with biopsy-proven chondromyxoid fibroma. **B,** Computed tomography scan further characterizes the lesion, which shows no evidence of cartilaginous calcification.

and elevated white blood cell count may be lacking. Because the incidence of infection is much higher than with either benign or malignant tumors, a high index of suspicion remains important, especially when coupled with a compatible clinical history of penetrating injury to the foot or previous infectious episode associated with high fever.

Radiographic changes in acute osteomyelitis may be subtle. Metaphyseal radiolucency with early periosteal elevation and a permeative radiographic appearance are diagnostic clues (Fig. 13-18). Differential diagno-

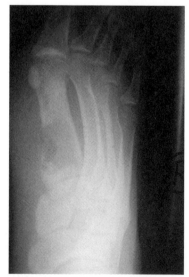

Figure 13-18 Radiograph demonstrates painful mass overlying dorsum of first metatarsal. Needle aspiration yielded gross pus, and cultures revealed *Staphylococcus aureus* infection.

sis includes eosinophilic granuloma and Ewing's sarcoma. Focal infection (Brodie's abscess) might resemble osteoid osteoma both clinically and radiographically.[24]

Subungual Exostosis

Subungual exostosis is a benign osteochondral lesion that causes pain and nail deformity.[11,34,50] This lesion arises from the tip of the distal phalanx and manifests as a periungual or subungual nodule. The characteristic radiographic appearance is diagnostic (Fig. 13-19). Ossification varies with the maturity of the lesion. This lesion is distinctly different from an osteochondroma that arises from the physeal growth plate. Complete surgical excision is the treatment of choice, and if the entire cartilaginous portion is excised, the recurrence rate is low.

Unicameral Cyst and Intraosseous Lipoma

In the foot, *unicameral cysts* occur most often in the calcaneus.[12] In children and teenagers these lesions are usually discovered incidentally and require no treatment when asymptomatic. In contrast to unicameral cysts in long bones, which often undergo spontaneous involution with skeletal maturity, unicameral cysts of the calcaneus persist through adulthood usually without consequence (Fig. 13-20). If there is pain or evidence of continued growth, with a concern of impending pathologic fracture, treatment may be considered. Treatment options include aspiration and injection of methylprednisolone, injection of allograft demineralized bone matrix, bone graft substitutes, and open curettage and bone grafting.[49] The patient's age

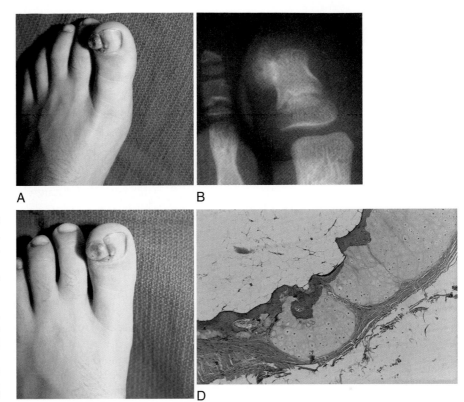

Figure 13–19   A, This patient had an 8-month history of pain and deformity of the lateral border of great toe. **B,** Anteroposterior radiograph demonstrates a mature osteochondral lesion (subungual exostosis) arising from the metaphysis area of the distal phalanx. Contrast this with the radiograph of the osteochondroma in Figure 13–13. **C,** Appearance of toe after complete excision of the lesion and a portion of the overlying nail bed. **D,** Typical histopathology showing a stalk of trabecular bone with a fibrocartilaginous cap and islands of cartilage.

and lesion's maturity affect the success of all methods; the older the patient, the lower the recurrence rate, regardless of the treatment used.

Unicameral cysts of the calcaneus must be distinguished from a radiolucency in the angle of Gisane, which is also usually an incidental finding in adults. In this case the radiolucency is filled with fat and represents an *intraosseous lipoma* or *pseudocyst* (Fig. 13–21). CT and MRI confirm the presence of fat within the lesion.[12,19] These lesions are asymptomatic and require no treatment.

Aneurysmal Bone Cyst

Aneurysmal bone cysts (ABCs) develop in the first two decades of life and have eccentric metaphyseal locations.[7,15] The radiographic picture is of a radiolucent, expansive lesion with a thin shell of reactive periosteal bone (Fig. 13–22). At biopsy the lesion consists of clotted and unclotted blood in a friable network of mesenchymal tissue. Histologically it consists of blood-filled cavities surrounded by spindle-shaped fibroblastic cells and multinucleate giant cells. Treatment consists of curettage and bone grafting. All tissue should be submitted for histologic examination because ABCs may be a secondary feature of a more aggressive tumor. Recurrence is a possibility. ABCs of

the talus might require malleolar osteotomy for adequate exposure and treatment (Fig. 13–23).

Epidermoid Inclusion Cyst

The epidermoid inclusion cyst typically occurs beneath the nail bed of the distal phalanx of the toe. It results from trauma that causes displacement of nail matrix into or adjacent to the phalanx. As these ectopic cells grow, they form a keratin-lined cyst. Clinically this cyst causes enlargement of the digit and is painful. Radiographically, it produces a radiolucency in the subungual area of the distal phalanx (Fig. 13–24). Treatment consists of confirmatory biopsy followed by curettage and grafting if necessary.

Giant Cell Tumor

Giant cell tumors usually occur in the epiphysis of long bones or in equivalent apophyseal areas after closure of the growth plates.[5,36] Although these tumors are most common in the third decade, they have been reported in all age groups. Giant cell tumors can occur in the distal tibial epiphysis or the hindfoot. Localized pain and swelling are common.

Plain radiographs show a geographically identifiable, radiolucent lesion with a small rim of reactive bone. Staging studies provide further anatomic local-

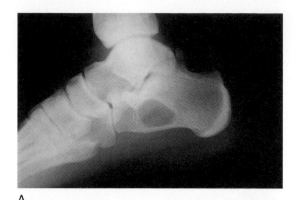

A

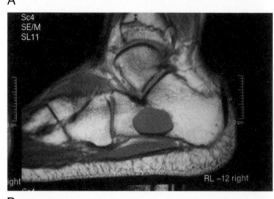

B

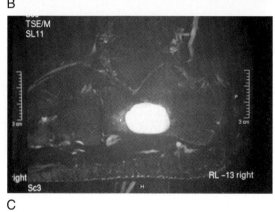

C

Figure 13–20 A, Unicameral cyst of the calcaneus persisting into adulthood and discovered incidentally. **B,** T1-weighted magnetic resonance image distinguishes cyst from fat. **C,** T2-weighted image demonstrates a bright signal, confirming fluid content.

ization (Fig. 13–25). These lesions are stage 2 or 3. Stage 2 lesions are best treated with extended curettage because of their proximity to subchondral bone and adjacent cartilage. If pathologic fracture has occurred, treatment is delayed until early healing of the fracture has taken place (approximately 3 to 4 weeks). This allows for margination and containment of the tumor.

Adjuvant agents (cryotherapy, cauterization, phenol, methacrylate) all have their advocates.[29,38] I prefer to use phenol and methacrylate because of its thermal extension of the curettage and its instantaneous mechanical support. Recurrence rates with these techniques are 10% to 30%. Marginal excision results in fewer recurrences than intralesional curettage but is usually impractical because of the giant cell tumor's subchondral location. Stage 3 or recurrent lesions require a wide resection, and reconstruction usually requires arthrodesis or even amputation.[6] So-called benign metastasis occurs in about 5% of cases.[39]

Intraosseous Ganglion and Degenerative Bone Cyst

The most common site for an *intraosseous ganglion* is the medial malleolus.[12] These lesions are usually asymptomatic and incidentally noted on radiographs, appearing as a rounded, circumscribed radiolucency with a distinct margin (Fig. 13–26).[37] When biopsied, usually to rule out other possible diagnoses, the intraosseous ganglion appears as a dense fibrous wall filled with a clear or yellow amorphous material. Treatment consists of curettage and bone grafting.

Degenerative bone cysts are also called *synovial, subchondral,* or *subarticular cysts.* Degenerative cysts may be related to intraosseous ganglia, but their clinical presentations are distinctly different. Intraosseous ganglia are usually asymptomatic or minimally symptomatic and are often discovered incidentally. They are not associated with arthritis and do not have a communication with the joint. They are usually biopsied for diagnostic and not necessarily therapeutic reasons. Histologically they have a thin- or thick-walled lining containing a viscous fluid. Degenerative bone cysts are usually symptomatic, are associated with articular cartilage changes (chondromalacia or arthritis), communicate with the joint, are treated because of symptoms or increasing size, and histologically have little associated lining, with the cavity basically just fluid (Fig. 13–27).

Treatment of degenerative cysts also consists of curettage and bone grafting. However, patients with degenerative cysts often remain symptomatic because of the overlying cartilaginous abnormality.

Malignant Bone Tumors

Chondrosarcoma

Chondrosarcoma is rarely observed in the foot but is still the foot's most common malignant bone tumor.[23,35,52] This tumor most often arises in the hind-

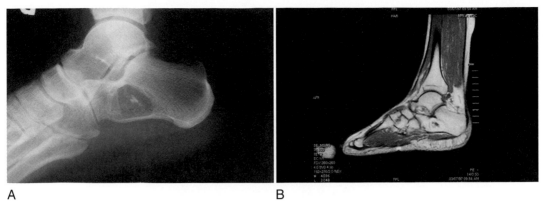

Figure 13–21 A, Intraosseous lipoma with central calcification. **B,** Magnetic resonance (MR) image confirms the presence of fat within the lesion. Compare this to the MR characteristics of the unicameral cyst in Figure 13-20.

foot and may be primary or secondary (arising in a preexisting benign cartilage tumor). The most common symptomatic complaint is pain. Radiographs reveal a destructive lesion with areas of calcification (Fig. 13–28).

Primary chondrosarcomas usually display less calcification than lesions that have undergone malignant transformation to secondary chondrosarcomas. *Sec-*

ondary chondrosarcomas are usually lower grade (1A or 1B) and, if present in the toes or metatarsals, may be treated by amputation of only the toe or by resection of the ray. Primary chondrosarcomas are high grade (2A or 2B) and require removal of the affected bone with at least a wide margin. Because of their typical location in the hindfoot, this usually results in amputation.[8]

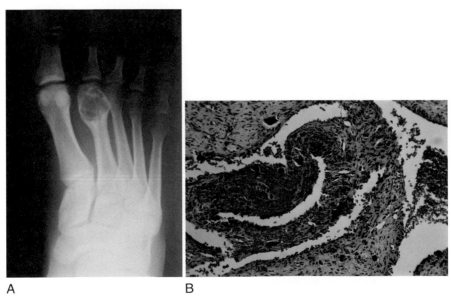

Figure 13–22 A, Aneurysmal bone cyst (ABC) derives its name from its characteristic radiographic appearance. This ABC of the second metatarsal demonstrates expansile radiolucency and shell of reactive periosteal bone typically associated with its presence. **B,** Medium-power view demonstrating vascular channels with numerous red blood cells surrounded by fibrous stroma and occasional giant cells.

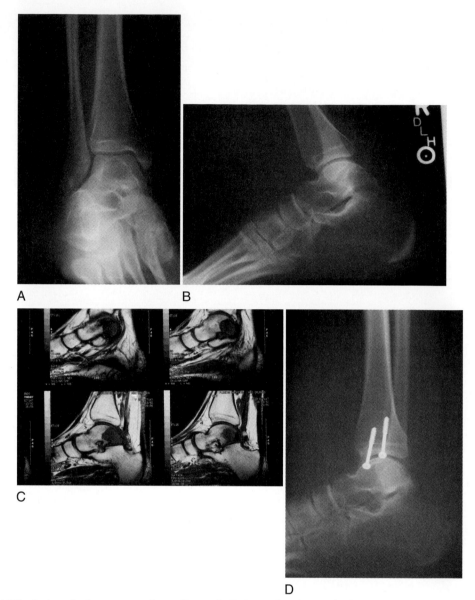

Figure 13–23 ABC of talus. **A,** Anteroposterior radiograph. **B,** Lateral radiograph. **C,** Magnetic resonance image. **D,** Postoperative lateral radiograph demonstrates stabilization of malleolar osteotomy and appearance of the lesion after extended curettage and bone grafting.

Distant metastasis, usually to the lung, occurs more often in primary chondrosarcomas. As with all suspected malignant tumors, preoperative work-up should include CT of the lungs. Radiation therapy plays no role in the treatment of chondrosarcomas. Likewise, chemotherapy is only occasionally considered as adjunctive treatment in high-grade tumors or with metastasis.

Osteosarcoma

Osteosarcoma is seen less often than chondrosarcoma but also usually occurs in the hindfoot.[12,24,52] The most common presenting symptom is pain. Plain radiographs show a lesion both destroying and making bone (Fig. 13–29). Staging should include CT of the lungs to rule out distant metastasis before treatment.

Osteosarcomas are high-grade lesions (2A or 2B). Treatment consists of confirmatory biopsy and then usually a course of induction systemic chemotherapy. Definitive surgery usually requires amputation and is followed by additional chemotherapy. This sequence of treatment allows assessment of the effectiveness of the chemotherapy by calculating the amount of

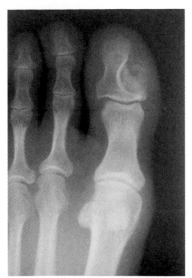

Figure 13–24 Radiograph demonstrates extrinsic erosion of the distal phalanx from an epidermoid inclusion cyst.

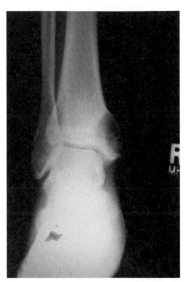

Figure 13–26 Typical location and appearance of intraosseous ganglion. In this location, giant cell tumor should be considered part of the differential diagnosis.

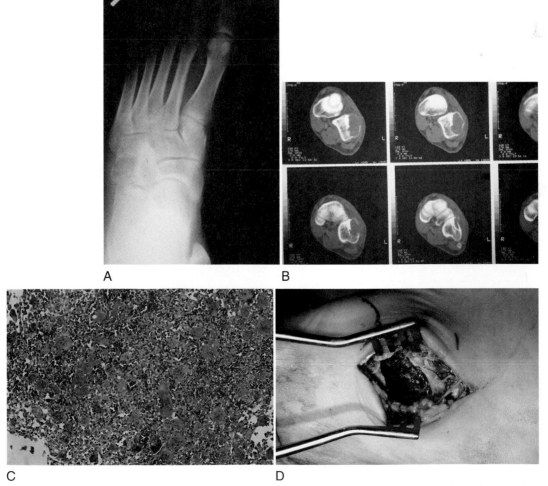

A

B

C

D

Figure 13–25 **A,** Radiolucent lesion of cuboid demonstrates a geographic pattern of bone loss and mild rim of reactive bone attempting to contain the lesion. This is typical of giant cell tumors. Additional differential diagnoses include aneurysmal bone cyst and cartilage lesions. **B,** CT confirms the geographic nature of the lesion and indicates loss of cortex, which should raise concern of soft tissue extension of the tumor. **C,** Low-power view of curetting showing giant cells, mononuclear stromal cells, and areas of hemorrhage. **D,** Cavity remaining after extended curettage can be treated by various methods in an attempt to decrease local recurrence (see text).

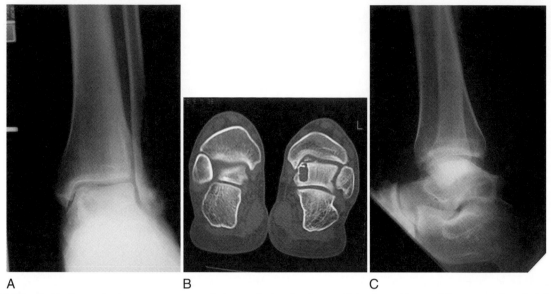

A   B   C

Figure 13–27 **A,** Radiograph demonstrates a radiolucent lesion in the medial talus with overlying osteochondral fracture. **B,** CT confirms subchondral communication with the joint and likelihood of this being a degenerative cyst. **C,** Lateral radiograph reveals the posterior extent of the lesion in the talus. This location is more difficult to access and treat arthroscopically and might require malleolar osteotomy for adequate exposure.

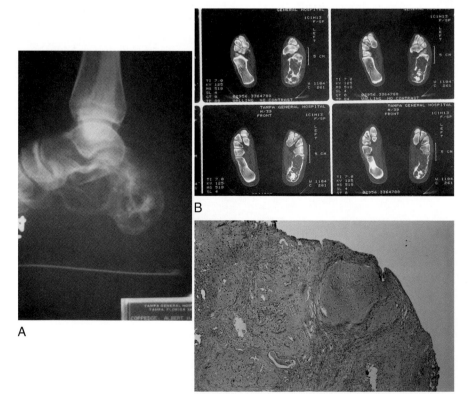

A

B

C

Figure 13–28 **A,** Lateral view of calcaneus demonstrates a destructive lesion with central calcification. **B,** CT confirms the destructive nature of the tumor and demonstrates both cortical breakthrough and soft tissue extension. **C,** Low-power micrograph of the biopsy specimen shows nodular cartilaginous tissue surrounded by vascular fibrous tissue consistent with chondrosarcoma.

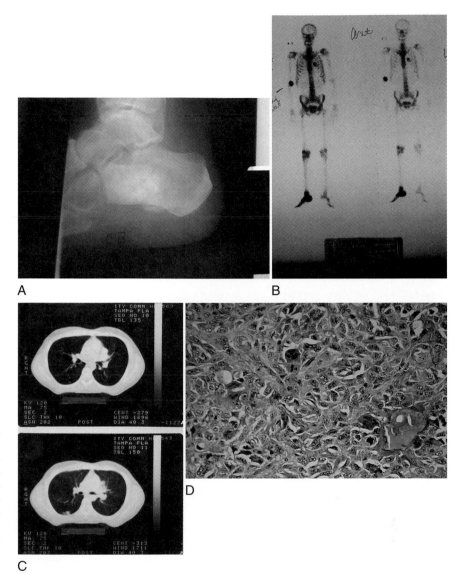

Figure 13–29 A, Lateral radiograph of the hindfoot typifies the abnormal production and destruction of bone seen in osteosarcoma. **B,** Bone scan demonstrates intense uptake in the calcaneus as well as a region of uptake in chest. **C,** CT of lung confirms the presence of lung metastasis at presentation. **D,** High power photomicrograph of the biopsy demonstrating bizarre cellular forms, mitoses, and pink matrix consistent with osteoid production.

necrosis found within the tumor at surgery (90% is considered a good response). Pulmonary metastasis does occur; however, surgical resection of these lesions has shown encouraging 5-year survival results.

Figure 13–30 is a radiograph of a typical metatarsal stress fracture. Because of the associated pain and swelling, these may initially be mistaken for osteosarcoma. A thorough history should clarify the diagnosis and prevent unwarranted biopsy.

Ewing's Sarcoma

Ewing's sarcoma is a round cell malignancy believed to arise from the nonmesenchymal elements of the bone marrow. It occurs most often in children and young adults. It has a peculiar affinity for the diaphysis of the fibula and is one of the few childhood malignancies that affects the small bones of either the hand or the foot.[27] The Mayo Clinic has reported a 5% incidence of Ewing's tumors in the foot.[52]

The typical radiographic appearance is one of subtle radiolucency with a permeative pattern and periosteal elevation, and thus the differential diagnosis includes osteomyelitis and eosinophilic granuloma.[26] The soft tissue component of the lesion may be quite extensive compared with the bone involvement. As with other sarcomas, work-up should always include CT evaluation of the lungs. Current treatment of Ewing's sarcoma employs systemic chemotherapy and surgery (Fig. 13–31).

Metastatic Carcinoma

Although metastatic carcinoma is the most common malignant tumor of bone, it is seldom found distal to the knee.[22] Of the five carcinomas most likely to metas-

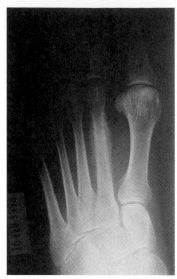

Figure 13–30 Second metatarsal stress fracture in postal carrier. Although new periosteal bone formation is present, no associated destruction is seen, as in osteosarcoma.

tasize to bone (lung, breast, prostate, kidney, thyroid), bronchogenic carcinoma of the lung is most common to occur below the knee. If another primary lesion is found in a metastatic location distal to the knee, the primary carcinoma often has already metastasized to the lung. Treatment to prevent pathologic fracture or for palliation is indicated to maintain quality of life.

METABOLIC CONDITIONS SIMULATING TUMORS

Fibrous Dysplasia

Fibrous dysplasia is a developmental skeletal disease consisting of immature fibrous connective tissue and poorly formed immature trabecular bone. Fibrous dysplasia ranges from small, single monostotic lesions to widespread, disseminated polyostotic lesions involving large areas in more than one bone. The

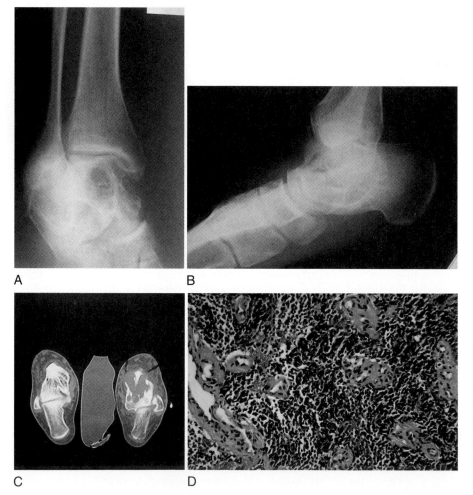

A

B

C

D

Figure 13–31 **A,** Anteroposterior x-ray of the ankle showing a lesion of the medial talus with preservation of the cortex. **B,** Lateral x-ray of the same patient. **C,** CT scan showing significantly more soft-tissue extension than would have been expected based on the plain x-rays. **D,** Biopsy material demonstrating a darkly staining "blue cell" lesion showing the poorly differentiated small round cells of Ewing's sarcoma.

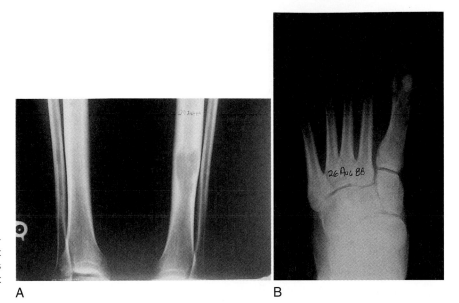

Figure 13–32 A, Patient with polyostotic fibrous dysplasia and involvement of the tibia. **B,** Typical ground glass appearance in the ipsilateral first metatarsal.

A   B

polyostotic variety is often confined to one extremity or one side of the skeleton (Fig. 13–32A). The lesions appear during childhood, remain active during growth, and become latent during adulthood. Malignant degeneration is rare, occurring in the adult polyostotic form.[24]

Clinical presentation may be incidental or secondary to pathologic fracture. It can occur as one aspect of Albright's syndrome, a combination of skeletal lesions, cutaneous lesions (café au lait spots), and precocious puberty. The characteristic radiographic picture is one of loss of trabecular detail and a homogeneous ground glass appearance. The lesions occur most often in the metaphysis, but it is one of the few lesions that develop in the diaphysis of the bones (Fig. 13–32B).

Treatment may be necessary for repetitive stress fractures or deformity. Because healing of dysplastic bone is with the same type of defective tissue, internal fixation and grafting are necessary for support. Cortical allograft is clinically superior because it has less tendency to be completely remodeled.

Gout

The term *gout* denotes a heterogenous group of diseases in which tissue deposition of monosodium urate (MSU) or uric acid crystals from supersaturated extracellular fluids results in expression of one or more clinical events.[40] Manifestations of the syndrome include acute gouty arthritis, with recurrent attacks of a specific type of severe articular and periarticular inflammation; tophi, with accumulation of articular, osseous, soft tissue, and crystalline deposits; gouty

nephropathy with renal impairment; and uric acid urinary calculi.

Gouty arthritis is seen primarily in middle-aged men and postmenopausal women and represents the most common form of inflammatory disease in men older than 30 years. The metatarsophalangeal joint of the great toe is involved most often and is involved at some time in 75% of patients (Fig. 13–33). Subcutaneous MSU-containing tophi occur only with fairly advanced gout (Fig. 13–34). Tophi can also form in the synovium and subchondral bone.

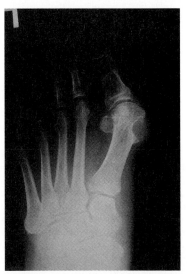

Figure 13–33 Erosion of the first metatarsal at the capsular insertion secondary to repeated gouty attacks.

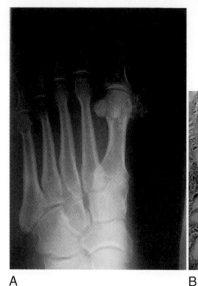

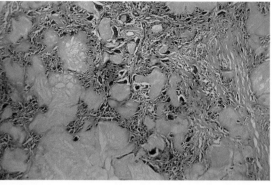

Figure 13–34 A, Subcutaneous gouty tophi. **B,** Sectioned tophus showing the urate crystals, which are lightly stained, surrounded by inflammatory cells and large macrophages, which are the most deeply stained.

A   B

Treatment of gout is determined by each patient's clinical manifestations. Therapy is designed to halt acute attacks, prevent recurrence, and reverse or prevent complications secondary to the deposition of MSU crystals. The surgical treatment is limited to correction of the arthritic effects of the disease and occasionally involves debridement of unresponsive soft tissue tophi once the overall disease is controlled.

REFERENCES

1. Allard MM, Thomas RL, Nicholas RW: Myositis ossificans: an unusual presentation in the foot. *Foot Ankle Int* 18:39-42, 1997.

2. Aluisio FV, Mair SD, Hall RL: Plantar fibromatosis: Treatment of primary and recurrent lesions and factors associated with recurrence. *Foot Ankle Int* 17:672-678, 1996.

3. Barbella R, Fox IM: Recurring desmoid tumor of the foot: A case study. *Foot Ankle Int* 17:221-225, 1996.

4. Begin LR, Guy P, Mitmaker B: Intramural leiomyosarcoma of the dorsal pedal vein: A clinical mimicry of ganglion. *Foot Ankle* 15:48-51, 1994.

5. Burns TP, Weiss M, Snyder M, Hopson CN: Giant cell tumor of the metatarsal. *Foot Ankle* 8:223-226, 1988.

6. Casadei R, Ruggieri P, Guiseppe, et al: Ankle resection arthrodesis in patients with bone tumors. *Foot Ankle Int* 15:242-249, 1996.

7. Casadei R, Ruggieri P, Moscato M, et al: Aneurysmal bone cyst and giant cell tumor of the foot. *Foot Ankle Int* 17:487-495, 1996.

8. Chou LB, Malawer MM: Analysis of surgical treatment of 33 foot and ankle tumors. *Foot Ankle Int* 15:175-181, 1994.

9. Cohn DL, Judson FN: Absence of Kaposi's sarcoma in hemophiliacs with the acquired immunodeficiency syndrome. *Ann Intern Med* 101:401, 1984.

10. Dahlin DC, Unni KK (eds): *Bone Tumors,* ed 4. Springfield, Ill, Charles C Thomas, 1986.

11. dePalma L, Gigante A, Specchia N: Subungual exostosis of the foot. *Foot Ankle Int* 17:758-763, 1996.

12. Enneking WF: *Musculoskeletal Tumor Surgery.* New York, Churchill Livingstone, 1983.

13. Enzinger FM, Weiss SW (eds): *Soft Tissue Tumors,* ed 2. St Louis, Mosby, 1988.

14. Fortin PT, Freiberg AA, Rees R, et al: Malignant melanoma of the foot and ankle. *J Bone Joint Surg Am* 77:1396-1403, 1995.

15. Fraipont MJ, Thordarson DB: Aneurysmal bone cyst of the navicular: A case report and review of the literature. *Foot Ankle Int* 17:709-711, 1996.

16. Friedman RJ, Rigel DS, Silverman MK, et al: Malignant melanoma in the 1990s: The continued importance of early detection and the role of physician examination and self-examination of the skin. *CA Cancer J Clin* 41(4):201-226, 1991.

17. Friscia DA: Pigmented villonodular synovitis of the ankle: A case report and review of the literature. *Foot Ankle Int* 15:674-678, 1994.

18. Giraldo G, Beth E, Buonaguro FM: Kaposi's sarcoma: A natural model of interrelationship between viruses, immunologic responses, genetics, and oncogenesis. *Antibiot Chemother* 32:1-11, 1984.

19. Greenspan A, Raiszadeh K, Riley GM, Matthews D: Intraosseous lipoma of the calcaneus. *Foot Ankle Int* 18:53-56, 1997.

20. Harrelson JM: Tumors of the foot. In Jahss MH (ed): *Disorders of the Foot and Ankle,* ed 2. Philadelphia, WB Saunders, 1991.

21. Harwood A: Kaposi's sarcoma in renal transplant patients. In Friedman-Kien AE, Laubenstein LJ (eds): *AIDS: The Epidemic of Kaposi's Sarcoma and Opportunistic Infections.* New York, Masson, 1984, pp 41-44.

22. Hattrup SJ, Amadio PC, Sim PH, Lombardi RM: Metastatic tumors of the foot and ankle. *Foot Ankle* 8:243-247, 1988.

23. Huvos AG: *Bone Tumors: Diagnosis, Treatment and Prognosis.* Philadelphia, WB Saunders, 1979.

24. Johnston JO: Tumors and metabolic disease of the foot. In Mann RA, Coughlin MJ (ed): *Surgery of the Foot and Ankle,* ed 6. St Louis, Mosby, 1992.

25. Jones FR, Soule EH, Coventry MD: Fibrous xanthoma of synovium. *J Bone Joint Surg Am* 51:76-86, 1969.

26. Kauffman SL, Stout AP: Histocytic tumors (fibrous xanthoma and histiocytoma) in children. *Cancer* 14:469-482, 1961.

27. Leeson MCF, Smith MJ: Ewing's sarcoma of the foot. *Foot Ankle* 10:14151, 1989.

28. Lewis GM: *Practical Dermatology,* ed 3. Philadelphia, WB Saunders, 1967.

29. Marcove RC, Weis LD, Vaghaiwalla MR, et al: Cryosurgery in the treatment of giant cell tumors of bone: A report of 52 consecutive cases. *Cancer* 41:957-969, 1978.

30. Math KR, Pavlov H, DiCarlo E, Bohne WH: Spindle cell lipoma of the foot: A case report and literature review. *Foot Ankle Int* 16:220-226, 1995.

31. Matthews RS, Hart JA: Benign synovioma (pigmented villonodular synovitis). *Surg Forum* 26:513–515, 1975.

32. McNeill TW, Ray RD: Hemangioma of the extremities. *Clin Orthop Relat Res* 101:154-166, 1974.

33. Mullins F, Berard CW, Eisenberg SH: Chondrosarcoma following synovial chondromatosis. A case study. *Cancer* 18:1180-1188, 1965.

34. Multhopp-Stephens H, Walling AK: Subungual exostosis: A simple technique of excision. *Foot Ankle Int* 16:88-91, 1995.

35. Murari TM, Callaghan JJ, Berrey BH Jr, Sweet DE: Primary benign and malignant osseous neoplasms of the foot. *Foot Ankle* 10:68-80, 1989.

36. O'Keefe RJ, O'Donnell RJ, Temple HT, et al: Giant cell tumor of bone in the foot and ankle. *Foot Ankle Int* 16:617-623, 1995.

37. Patterson RH, Jones M, Tuten R: Intraosseous ganglion cyst of the talus: A case report. *Foot Ankle* 14:538-539, 1993.

38. Persson BM, Wouters HW: Curettage and acrylic cementation in surgery of giant cell tumors of bone. *Clin Orthop Relat Res* 120:125-133, 1976.

39. Rock MG, Pritchard DJ, Unni KK: Metastases from histologically benign giant cell tumor of bone. *J Bone Joint Surg Am* 66:269-274, 1984.

40. Schumacher HR: *Primer on the Rheumatic Diseases,* ed 9. Atlanta, Arthritis Foundation, 1988.

41. Seale KS, Lange TA, Monson D, Hackbarth DA: Soft tissue tumors of the foot and ankle. *Foot Ankle* 9:19-27, 1988.

42. Shereff MJ, Cullivan WT, Johnson KA: Osteoid osteoma of the foot. *J Bone Joint Surg Am* 65:638-641, 1983.

43. Singh DP, Dhillon MS, Sur RK, et al: Primary lymphoma of the bones of the foot: Management of two cases. *Foot Ankle* 11:314-316, 1991.

44. Smyth M: Glomus-cell tumor in the lower extremity. Report of two cases. *J Bone Joint Surg Am* 53:157-159, 1971.

45. Snow SE, Sobel M, DiCarlo EF, et al: Chronic ankle pain caused by osteoid osteoma of the neck of the talus. *Foot Ankle Int* 18:98-101, 1997.

46. Sober AJ: Cutaneous melanoma: Opportunity for cure. *CA Cancer J Clin* 41(4):197-199, 1991.

47. Walling AK: The orthopaedic perspective. In Greenfield G, Arrington J (eds): *Imaging of Bone Tumors.* Philadelphia, JB Lippincott, 1994.

48. Walling AK, Companioni GR, Belsole RJ: Infiltrating angiolipoma of the hand and wrist. *J Hand Surg [Am]* 10:288-291, 1985.

49. Walling AK, Gasser SI: Soft-tissue and bone tumors about the foot and ankle. *Clin Sports Med* 13:909-938, 1994.

50. Walling AK, Multhopp-Stephens H: Subungual (Dupuytren's) exostosis. *J Pediatr Orthop* 15:582-584, 1995.

51. Wapner KL, Ver, vereli PA, Moore JH Jr, et al: Fibromatosis: A review of primary and recurrent surgical treatment. *Foot Ankle Int* 16:548-551, 1995.

52. Wold LE, et al: *Atlas of Orthopaedic Pathology.* Philadelphia, WB Saunders, 1979.

Toenail Abnormalities

James K. DeOrio • Michael J. Coughlin

The nails are special cutaneous appendages that have the primary function of protecting the distal phalanx. Only primates have toenails, and whether the first primates with flat nails had an advantage over their peers by being able to remove parasites better from their bodies (thus promoting their evolutionary superiority) is a matter of fascinating speculation.[177]

In humans, diseases and deformities of the toenails are among the most common and disabling of foot problems. They can result from local or systemic disorders or from congenital malformations. Only a small percentage of toenail abnormalities result from systemic diseases, such as psoriasis and endocrine disorders. The majority are caused by intrinsic factors and are directly or indirectly related to tinea infections. The other deformities stem from mechanical problems and constitute some of the most common yet difficult foot problems for the treating physician.

Although few studies of physicians' reports have documented the frequency of nail disorders, Krausz[96] did examine the incidence of nail disorders (Table 14–1). During 41 years of practice, Krausz reported on 7670 patients displaying one or more nail disorders.[119]

The nail has only a few pathologic responses to disease and can demonstrate abnormalities as a manifestation of either systemic or dermatologic diseases. Before examining specific examples of nail disorders, this chapter reviews the anatomy and physiology of the toenail and supporting structures to facilitate an understanding of the pathologic conditions.

ANATOMY

The toenail or *nail plate* is composed of several layers of dense, overlapping keratinized cells. There are three layers, each originating from a different area of the nail unit. The relatively thin dorsal layer is stiff and brittle and covers the relatively thick middle layer. The deep layer is thought to be derived in part from the nail bed itself.[74,90,91] The nail plate differs from hair or skin in that it does not desquamate skin cells. The hardness of the nail plate can be attributed to its high sulfur content[47] and to the paucity of water within the plate. Although the nail plate is ten times more permeable to water than the skin, the nail plate, unlike the skin, has a low fat content and thus cannot retain water.[12]

The normal nail plate grows distally approximately 0.03 to 0.05 mm/day, and it has a thickness of 0.5 to 1 mm.[85] The nail plate is supported by the nail unit,[52] or *perionychium*,[177] an area of epithelial tissue that is divided into four components (Fig. 14–1)[173]: nail bed, hyponychium, proximal nail fold, and nail matrix. Synonyms are common for various anatomic units (Box 24–1).

The nail plate lies on the *nail bed*, a roughened epithelial surface consisting of longitudinal grooves

Table 14–1

Incidence of Pathologic Nail Conditions	
Condition	**Incidence (%)**
Onychocryptosis	26
Onychogryphosis or onychauxis	23
Onychophosis	19
Onychomycosis	8
Onychotrophia	4

Data from Krausz CE: Nail survey (1942-1970). *Br J Chir* 35:117, 1970; and Nzuzi SM: Common nail disorders. *Clin Podiatr Med Surg* 6:273-294, 1989.

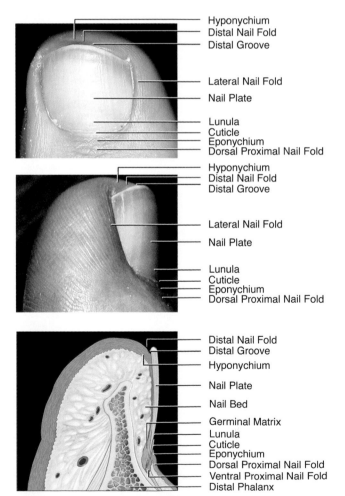

Figure 14–1 Anteroposterior *(top)* and lateral *(middle)* photographs of a toenail and a sagittal–lateral cross-sectional drawing *(bottom)* showing the various anatomic parts of the toenail unit. (By permission of Mayo Foundation for Medical Education and Research.)

that interdigitate with corresponding grooves on the undersurface of the toenail. This interdigitation firmly bonds the nail plate to the nail bed. The nail bed or sterile matrix has only one or two layers of germinal cells, which produce the nail plate.[177] At the distal end of the nail bed, where the nail bed and the nail plate separate, a smooth border of skin called the *hyponychium* forms a seal between the distal end of the toenail and the nail bed.

On the tibial and fibular borders of the toenail, the nail plate is surrounded by epidermal skin folds termed *lateral nail folds*. The base of the toenail is covered by the *proximal nail fold*, a complex structure that has germinal cells on the proximal half of the dorsal roof of the nail fold.[177] The dorsal surface of the nail fold is composed of skin on the dorsal surface of the toe. On the plantar surface of this fold, the *eponychium* forms a thin surface that attaches to the nail plate. The distal surfaces of these two components of the proximal nail fold compose the cuticle.

The *nail matrix* or *germinal matrix* is the main germinal area of the toenail. The nail matrix extends from a point just distal to the lunula and as far laterally as the entire width of the nail plate,[46] and it extends 5 to 6 mm proximally to the edge of the cuticle and closely borders the insertion of the long extensor tendon and the interphalangeal joint.[74] The nail matrix is seen beneath the nail plate as the *lunula*, the opaque, crescent-shaped area at the base of the nail. It lacks color because it is less vascular than the heavily vascularized nail bed. Distally, the nail matrix is contiguous with the nail bed. The nail matrix is covered by a small epidermal surface but does not have the epidermal ridges characteristic of the nail bed. At the distal end of the lunula, the nail matrix terminates. As noted above, at the proximal margin of the matrix, a small area on the plantar surface of the proximal nail fold appears to contribute to the growth of the nail plate.[74,106,141] This is important to remember when trying to permanently ablate the nail by removing the germinal matrix from which the nail grows.

Most matrix germination occurs between the apex of the matrix and the distal border of the lunula. The area covered by the proximal nail fold forms the thin dorsal layer of the nail plate. The area of the lunula produces the thicker, softer middle portion of the nail plate and joins with the dorsal area to form the nail plate.[74] Although the nail matrix is the major germinal area for toenail growth, microscopic areas of nail matrix may be present within the nail folds and the distal nail bed.[90,91,99] These produce a thin layer of the ventral toenail plate, a factor that occasionally accounts for postoperative regrowth.[46,74,106]

The matrix cells of the nail plate are oriented longitudinally. Because of pressure from the proximal nail fold, the nail plate grows distally rather than in an elevated direction. However, if the nail matrix is injured or altered because of trauma or surgery, the nail plate may grow in an abnormal direction. Likewise, the nail plate gives a certain rigidity to the soft tissue of the distal part of the toe. If the toenail is removed or ablated, the distal nail bed and soft tissue can grow in an elevated direction because of upward pressure on these soft tissues (Fig. 14–2). As the new nail plate begins to grow distally, it can abut these soft tissues and lead to a club nail or an ingrown toenail.

Common diseases involving the nail include infection, psoriasis, contact dermatitis and eczema, tumor, trauma, and general or systemic diseases.[163] A systematic review of nail disorders by Pardo-Castello and Pardo[128] provides a useful classification for both common and uncommon nail abnormalities and also discusses disorders caused by trauma and neoplasia. The classification includes the following:

- Dermatologic and systemic diseases
- Congenital and genetic nail disorders
- Common nail abnormalities and onycho-dystrophies

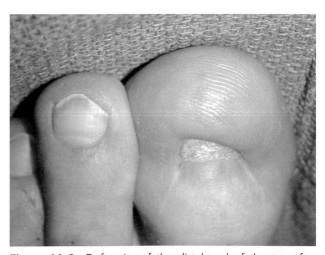

Figure 14–2 Deformity of the distal end of the toe after attempted permanent ablation of the nail. Without nail support, clubbing has resulted, with impingement of the growth of the remaining nail.

Nzuzi[120] presented the following logical classification of common nail disorders *(onychopathies)* based on the anatomic structures primarily involved:

- Nail plate disorders
- Nail bed disorders
- Nail fold disorders
- Nail matrix disorders

Use of Pardo-Castello's general classification for an overview of nail disorders and Nzuzi's classification for onychopathies provides a complete and systematic approach for a discussion of toenail disorders.

DERMATOLOGIC AND SYSTEMIC NAIL DISORDERS

Skin disorders involving the nails are usually within the province of the dermatologist, and systemic disorders involving the nails are typically within the internist's scope of practice. Few of these entities require localized or systemic treatment. Nonetheless, an awareness of the underlying pathologic processes and an understanding of the nail changes associated with specific dermatologic and systemic disorders helps to inform a consulting physician about the myriad of generalized signs and symptoms associated with toenail abnormalities and assists in making a definitive diagnosis. Pathologic conditions of the toenail are defined in Box 14-2 and terms describing infections are defined in Box 14-3.

Psoriasis

Psoriasis of the toenails often accompanies cutaneous disease, and patients often mistake it for fungal involvement of the nail (Fig. 14–3A). Involvement of the nails is seen in 80% of patients with psoriatic arthritis and in 30% of patients who have psoriasis without arthritic symptoms.[136] The most severe form of nail involvement with psoriasis, which sometimes involves shedding and loss of the nail *(onychomadesis),* is associated with psoriatic arthritis. However, many patients without arthritic changes who have psoriasis have the following abnormal findings in either their toenails or their fingernails:[170]

- *Stippling* or *geographic pitting* (tiny, often grooved depressions in the surface of the nail plate) (Fig. 24–3B and C), which is not unique to psoriasis and is seen in alopecia areata
- *Onycholysis,* especially laterally and distally, sometimes with yellowing and opacity of the nail plate, which separates and then detaches from the nail bed (Fig. 14–3D)

- Crumbling of the nail plate
- Subungual keratosis (Fig.14–3A)
- Possibly extensive skin involvement (Fig. 14–3E).

Often these changes are confused with onychomycosis. Before therapy is instituted, scrapings of the nails should be made for microscopic examination with potassium hydroxide, and fungal cultures should be started.

Treatment of psoriatic nail changes of the feet is generally unsatisfactory. Intralesional injection of corticosteroids may be effective for treating psoriasis in fingernails,[24] but similar therapy for involved toenails is administered less often.

Eczema and Contact Dermatitis

Eczema and contact dermatitis often involve not only the skin on the dorsum of the toes but also the lateral and proximal nail folds. With chronic inflammatory changes, abnormalities of the nail plate can occur. Transverse ridging and scaling as well as discoloration of the nail plate can develop. Accumulation of serous fluid can lead to onycholysis and subsequent onychomadesis. Allergic reaction to nail polish, resins, dyes, solvents, detergents, and other chemicals can cause eczema, and atopic dermatitis with no known cause can lead to the development of similar nail changes.

With the resolution of acute inflammation, the chronic changes of fissuring and dryness may be treated with topical corticosteroids. The primary objective of the treatment of eczema and contact dermatitis is the resolution of the acute inflammatory process surrounding the toenail unit.

Pyodermas

Bacterial infections occur commonly in the feet and are divided into primary and secondary pyodermas. *Impetigo* is a superficial skin infection that is often caused by *Staphylococcus* or *Streptococcus* species, or both, and usually affects younger children. The typical lesion consists of a thin-walled vesicle on an erythematous base. The vesicles form yellow crusts, and peripheral extension results in irregular serpiginous lesions. The lesions are common on the face but can occur anywhere on the body except the palms and soles. *Ecthyma* is a form of pyoderma that begins as small vesicles or pustules on an erythematous base and quickly develops a purulent, irregular ulcer. These lesions are common on the lower extremities and, as with impetigo, readily respond to systemic antibiotics. Burow's compresses are helpful in removing the crusts,

Acral: Of or belonging to the extremities of peripheral body parts.

Anonychia: Absence of nails. When anonychia is congenital, usually all the nails are absent and the condition is permanent. It can occur temporarily from trauma or systemic or local disease. Also seen in nail–patella syndrome.

Beau's lines: Transverse lines or ridges marking repeated disturbances of nail growth. May be associated with trauma or a systemic disease process.

Clubbing: Hypertrophied, curved nail with flattened angle between the nail and the cuticle. Associated with chronic pulmonary and cardiac disease.

Hapalonychia: Extremely soft nails that may be prone to splitting; associated with endocrine disturbances, malnutrition, and contact with strong alkali solutions.

Hemorrhage: Bleeding. Beneath toenail, bleeding may be associated with vitamin C deficiency, subacute bacterial endocarditis, and dermatologic disorders. *Subungual hematoma* occurs after trauma to toenail bed.

Hutchinson's sign: Hyperpigmentation spreading from nail to surrounding soft tissue. Pathognomonic for melanoma.

Hyperkeratosis: Thickening of the stratum corneum layer of the epidermis.

Hyperkeratosis subungualis: Hypertrophy of the nail bed. May be associated with onychomycosis, psoriasis, and other dermatologic disorders.

Koilonychia: Concavity of the nail plate in both longitudinal and transverse axes. Associated with nutritional disorders, iron deficiency anemia, and endocrine disorders.

Lentigo: A small melanotic spot without pigment, which is potentially malignant and is unrelated to sun exposure.

Leukonychia: White spots or striations in the nail resulting from trauma and systemic diseases, such as nutritional and endocrine deficiencies.

Melanonychia: A longitudinal streak of pigment visible in or beneath the nail.[41]

Onychauxis: Greatly thickened nail plate caused by persistent mild trauma and onychomycosis.

Onychia: Inflammation of the nail matrix, causing deformity of the nail plate and resulting from trauma, infection, and systemic diseases, such as exanthemas.

Onychitis: Inflammation of the nail.

Onychoclasis: Breakage of the nail plate.

Onychocryptosis: Ingrowing of nails or, more specifically, hypertrophy of the nail lip; also referred to as *hypertrophied ungualabia* or *unguis incarnatus*; one of the most common pathologic conditions of the toenail.

Onychogryphosis: "Claw nail" or "ram's horn nail"; extreme hypertrophy of the nail gives the appearance of a claw or horn. May be congenital or a symptom of many chronic systemic diseases, such as tinea infections. See *onychauxis*.

Onycholysis: Loosening of the nail plate beginning along the distal or free edge when trauma, injury by chemical agents, or diseases loosen the nail plate. Associated with psoriasis, onychomycosis, acute fevers, and syphilis.

Onychoma: Tumor of the nail unit.

Onychomadesis: Complete loss of the nail plate.

Onychomalacia: Softening of the nail.

Onychomycosis: Fungal infection of the nail associated with fungal disease of the foot.

Onychophosis: Accumulation of callus within the lateral groove, involving the great toe more often than the lesser toes.

Onychoptosis defluvium: Nail shedding.

Onychorrhexis: Longitudinal ridging and splitting of nails caused by dermatoses, nail infections, systemic diseases, senility, or injury by chemical agents.

Onychoschizia: Lamination and scaling away of nails in thin layers caused by dermatoses, syphilis, or chemical agents.

Onychosis: Disease or deformity of the nail plate. Also called *onychopathy*.

Onychotrophia: Atrophy or failure of development of a nail caused by trauma, infection, endocrine dysfunction, or systemic disease.

Orthonyx: Mechanical bracing of nails to correct curvature.

Pachyonychia: Extreme thickening of all the nails. Thickening is more solid and more regular than in onychogryphosis. Usually a congenital condition associated with hyperkeratosis of the palms and soles.

Paronychia: Inflammation of soft tissues around the nail margin, which can occur after trauma or infection (bacterial or fungal).

Pincer nail: Ingrown toenail with both sides of the nail turned in, nearly forming a complete circle.

Pterygium: Growth of cuticle distal to the nail plate, splitting the nail into two or more portions that gradually decrease in size as the growth widens. Can result from trauma and decreased circulation in the toes.

Stratum corneum: The most superficial layer of the epidermis.

Subungual hematoma: Blood that has collected beneath the nail plate, usually secondary to trauma. Also known as "tennis toe" or "jogger's toe."

Trachyonychia: "Rough nails." A reaction or morphologic pattern with various clinical appearances and causes.

Yellow nail syndrome: Keratohyalin granules within the nail plate seen only with electron microscopy.

Ecthyma: Ulcerative infection usually caused by group A β-hemolytic *Streptococci*. Often occurs at the site of minor trauma, frequently on the dorsal aspect of the foot.

Erythrasma: Chronic superficial bacterial infection involving the web space. The peripheral edge may be sharply demarcated and scaling.

Impetigo: Contagious skin infection caused by group A *Streptococci* or *Staphylococcus aureus* and characterized by discrete vesicles with erythematous borders. Pustules may rupture, discharging a purulent fluid that dries and forms yellowish crust.

Intertrigo: Superficial dermatitis on adjacent skin surfaces, such as between toes, caused by moisture and friction and characterized by maceration, erythema, itching, and burning.

Whitlow: Infection, often viral, occurring near the nail. Because of the similarity in appearance, subungual melanoma has been termed *melanotic whitlow.*

and topical antibiotic ointment is usually applied several times a day (Box 14–4).

Secondary pyodermas that affect the feet can be grouped into three categories: infectious eczematoid dermatitis, infected intertrigo, and miscellaneous pyogenic infections of the web space.

Infectious eczematoid dermatitis results from a discharge of wet drainage seeping over the skin from underlying cellulitis or pyodermic infection. Autoinoculation often occurs, and the infection spreads by contiguous drainage.

Infected intertrigo results from friction, moisture, and sweat retention. It is common between the toes, where it is often diagnosed as a tinea infection. Treatment consists of promoting dryness with cool, drying compresses and a bland absorbent powder. Secondary infection is treated with an appropriate topical antibiotic.

Miscellaneous pyogenic infections of the web space, which are caused by gram-negative bacteria such as *Pseudomonas* and *Proteus,* produce clinical pyodermic infections that are resistant to the usual antibacterial therapy. Identification of the organisms and appropri-

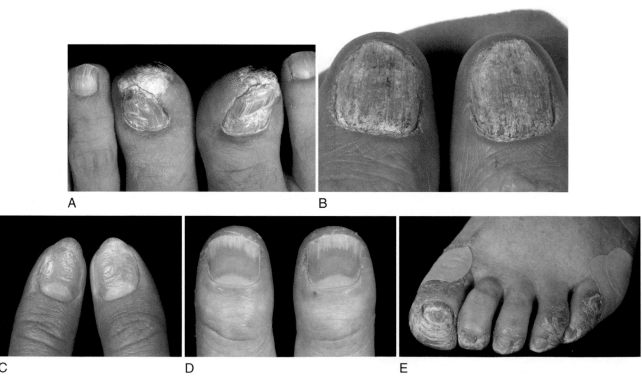

Figure 14–3 **A,** Psoriatic toenail dystrophy. The nail is thick, discolored, and distorted owing to psoriasis of the nail matrix. The symmetry is striking, and the skin is also involved. **B,** Psoriatic pits can occur in a linear fashion and produce longitudinal lines. Symmetry is a feature of psoriasis. **C,** Psoriatic parakeratotic areas are weaker than the surrounding nail and fall out, forming pits. **D,** A yellow margin between the onycholysis and the normal nail is a particular feature of psoriatic onycholysis. **E,** Psoriatic involvement of the skin is often extensive, prompting patients to protect their feet. (**A-D** from du Vivier A: *Atlas of Clinical Dermatology,* ed 3. Edinburgh, Churchill Livingstone, 2002, p 604.)

BOX 14–4 Medicinal Solutions Used in Treatment of Cutaneous Foot Disorders

Burow's solution: Aluminum sulfate in water (1:40 dilution)
Carbolic acid (phenol): 88% carbolic acid, 70% isopropyl alcohol
Castellani's paint: Mixture of phenol, alcohol, water, resorcinol, acetone, and fuchsin
Whitfield's ointment: 12% benzoic acid, 6% salicylic acid

ate antibiotic therapy should be determined by culture and sensitivity testing.

The infection should be carefully investigated to determine the presence of any underlying systemic disorders, such as diabetes, lymphoma, or an immunodeficiency syndrome that could predispose the patient to such cutaneous infections. Amonette and Rosenberg[5] found that the best treatment regimen was topical management with a combination of bed rest, exposure to air, and application of silver nitrate solution, Castellani's paint, and gentamicin sulfate cream. *Erythrasma* is often seen in intertriginous areas such as the web spaces. The causative organism is *Corynebacterium minutissimum*, which produces a well-demarcated, reddish brown, fine desquamation that fluoresces orange-red or coral-pink under a Wood lamp. Wearing loose stockings and shoes and using antibacterial soaps usually prevent this infection or eliminate it after it has been established. Treatment occasionally requires appropriate oral antibiotics.

Not every form of intertrigo of the web space is linked to infection by a fungal or bacterial organism. With psoriasis, the skin of the feet can be extensively involved, and usually the web space is involved as well. A therapeutic trial of a topical steroid cream can effectively eliminate this form of intertrigo.

Systemic Diseases

Diseases of the toenail can accompany many systemic disease processes, but the nail is underused as an aid in diagnosing systemic diseases. Often a provisional diagnosis of a fungal infection or trauma is made when, instead, a systemic disease process has caused changes in the color, shape, rate of growth, or texture of the toenail. Although many of these changes are nonspecific, they can give a diagnostician reason to suspect the presence of a systemic disease.

The consistency and color of the nail plate can change with systemic disease. Several eponyms are associated with these changes and, although

confusing, they are in general use for specific pathologic descriptions. These include Beau's lines, Mees' lines, Muehrcke's lines, half-and-half nail, blue nail, and Terry's nail.

With the sudden arrest in longitudinal nail growth, a *Beau line,* a transverse sulcus, develops that is 0.1 to 0.5 mm deep (Fig. 14–4A). With further growth of the nail plate, the Beau line progresses distally. This is associated with severe febrile episodes, peripheral vascular disease, diabetes, trauma, Hodgkin's disease, and infections such as malaria, rheumatic fever, syphilis, leprosy, typhoid fever, and various parasitic infections.

Mees's lines are also associated with growth arrest of the nail plate. Mees's lines are horizontal striations that typically involve more than one nail. They are usually 1 to 3 mm wide and are associated with Hodgkin's disease, myocardial infarction, malaria, and arsenic and thallium poisoning.[119,120]

Muehrcke's lines are white lines that occur in pairs, parallel to the lunula, and do not progress distally with nail plate growth. They occur with hypoalbuminemia and the nephrotic syndrome as well as with chronic liver disease.

Half-and-half nail is a biphasic discoloration of the nail in which the distal portion is brown, red, or pink, and the proximal portion appears normal. Half-and-half nails are associated with chronic liver disease and chronic kidney disease.

Blue nail or blue-gray nail is a bluish discoloration of the nail that is associated with subungual hematoma, melanotic whitlow, and poor oxygen perfusion in methemoglobinemia, pulmonary disease, and cyanosis.

In *Terry's nail,* characteristic changes involve opacification of the nail plate with a 1- to 3-mm pinkish band at the distal edge of the nail plate. Often this condition is connected with chronic changes associated with diabetes mellitus and liver disease (Fig. 14–4B).

Kosinski and Stewart[95] described pathologic nail conditions that are often associated with systemic disease entities. These nail changes may be manifested in cardiovascular disorders (yellow nail syndrome or splinter hemorrhages, Fig. 14–4C and D and Table 14–2), hematologic diseases (Table 14–3), endocrine disorders (Table 14–4), connective tissue diseases (Table 14–5), local and systemic infections (Table 14–6), neoplasia (Table 14–7), and renal, hepatic, pulmonary, and gastrointestinal disorders (Table 14–8).

GENETIC DISORDERS WITH NAIL CHANGES

Heritable traits can influence the appearance of toenails. Many genetic diseases with collagen

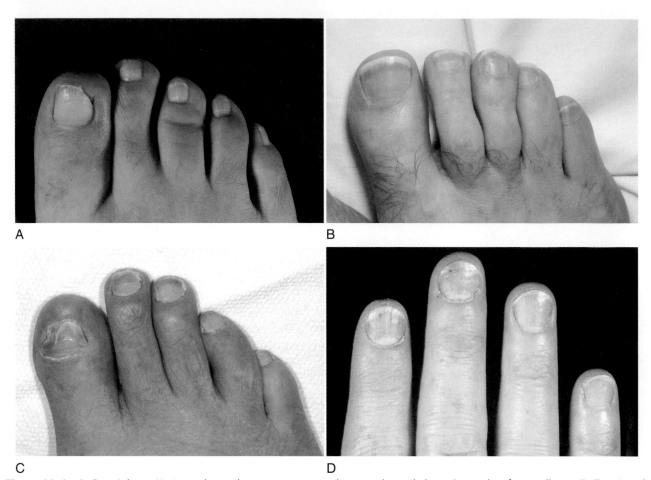

Figure 14–4   A, Beau's lines. Horizontal troughs are apparent midway up the nail about 3 months after an illness. **B,** Terry's nail. Diabetes and liver disease can produce a pinkish band located at the distal edge of the nail plate. **C,** Yellow nail syndrome. The nail is discolored yellow and is excessively curved, particularly across the horizontal axis. **D,** Splinter hemorrhages. Tiny subungual hemorrhages result in pigmented, linear splinter-like lesions. Trauma is the most common cause, but they can also be a feature of certain systemic diseases. (**D** from du Vivier A: *Atlas of Clinical Dermatology*, ed 3. Edinburgh, Churchill Livingstone, 2002, p 610.)

Table 14–2

Cardiovascular Disorders and Associated Toenail Conditions

Disease	Pathologic Changes
Arterial emboli	Splinter hemorrhages
Arteriosclerosis obliterans	Leukonychia partialis
Bacterial endocarditis	Clubbing, splinter hemorrhages
Hypertension	Splinter hemorrhages
Ischemia	Onycholysis, pterygium
Mitral stenosis	Splinter hemorrhages
Myocardial infarction	Mees' lines, yellow nail syndrome
Vasculitis	Splinter hemorrhages

Modified from Kosinski MA, Stewart D: Nail changes associated with systemic disease and vascular insufficiency. *Clin Podiatr Med Surg* 6:295-318, 1989. Used with permission.

Table 14-3

Hematologic Disorders and Associated Toenail Conditions

Disease	Pathologic Changes
Cryoglobulinemia	Splinter hemorrhages
Hemochromatosis	Brittleness, koilonychia, leukonychia, longitudinal striations, splinter hemorrhages
Hemophilia	Ingrown toenails,[77] pyogenic granulomata
Histiocytosis X	Onycholysis, pitting, splinter hemorrhages
Hodgkin's disease	Leukonychia partialis, Mees' lines, yellow nail syndrome
Hypochromic anemia	Koilonychia
Idiopathic hemochromatosis	Brittleness, koilonychia, longitudinal striations, splinter hemorrhages
Osler–Weber–Rendu disease	Splinter hemorrhages, telangiectasia
Polycythemia rubra vera	Clubbing, koilonychia
Porphyria	Onycholysis
Sickle cell anemia	Leukonychia, Mees' lines, splinter hemorrhages
Thrombocytopenia	Splinter hemorrhages

Modified from Kosinski MA, Stewart D: Nail changes associated with systemic disease and vascular insufficiency. *Clin Podiatr Med Surg* 6:295-318, 1989. Used with permission.

Table 14-4

Endocrine Disorders and Associated Toenail Conditions

Disease	Pathologic Changes
Addison's disease	Brown bands, diffuse hyperpigmentation, leukonychia, yellow nail syndrome, longitudinal pigmented deep-yellow bands
Diabetes mellitus	Beau's lines, koilonychia, leukonychia, onychauxis, onychomadesis, paronychia, pitting of nail plate, proximal nail bed telangiectasia, pterygium, splinter hemorrhages, yellow nail syndrome
Hyperthyroidism	Clubbing, increased nail growth, onycholysis, splinter hemorrhages, yellow nail syndrome
Hypothyroidism	Onycholysis, koilonychia, yellow nail syndrome
Thyroiditis	Yellow nail syndrome
Thyrotoxicosis	Koilonychia, onychomadesis, splinter hemorrhages, yellow nail syndrome

Modified from Kosinski MA, Stewart D: Nail changes associated with systemic disease and vascular insufficiency. *Clin Podiatr Med Surg* 6:295-318, 1989. Used with permission.

Table 14-5

Connective Tissue Disorders and Associated Toenail Conditions

Disease	Pathologic Changes
Alopecia areata	Leukonychia partialis, nail pitting
Atopic dermatitis/eczema	Onycholysis, onychorrhexis
Lichen planus	Atrophy of nail plate, onycholysis, onychorrhexis, pterygium
Psoriasis	Beau's lines, leukonychia, Mees' lines, nail pitting, onycholysis, splinter hemorrhages
Raynaud's syndrome	Koilonychia, yellow nail syndrome
Reiter's syndrome	Onycholysis, nail pitting
Rheumatoid arthritis	Splinter hemorrhages, yellow nail syndrome
Scleroderma (62% of patients)[142]	Absent lunula, koilonychia, leukonychia, onycholysis, onychorrhexis, pterygium
Systemic lupus erythematosus	Clubbing, hyperpigmented periungual tissue, nail pitting, onycholysis, subungual petechiae, yellow nail syndrome

Modified from Kosinski MA, Stewart D: Nail changes associated with systemic disease and vascular insufficiency. *Clin Podiatr Med Surg* 6:295-318, 1989. Used with permission.

Table 14-6

Systemic and Localized Infections and Associated Toenail Conditions

Disease	Pathologic Changes
Bacterial endocarditis	Clubbing, splinter hemorrhages
Hansen disease	Loss of lunula, nail plate dystrophy, onychogryphosis, onychauxis, onycholysis, onychodesis, onychomadesis, onychorrhexis
Malaria	Grayish nail bed, leukonychia
Measles	Onychomadesis
Recurrent cellulitis	Yellow nail syndrome
Scarlet fever	Onychomadesis
Syphilis	Koilonychia, leukonychia partialis, onychauxis, onychia, onycholysis, onychomadesis, onychorrhexis, paronychia
Trichinosis	Splinter hemorrhages, leukonychia
Tuberculosis	Leukonychia partialis, yellow nail syndrome
Typhoid fever	Leukonychia, Mees' lines
Yaws and pinta	Hypopigmentation, nail atrophy, onychia, onychauxis, paronychia, pterygium

Modified from Kosinski MA, Stewart D: Nail changes associated with systemic disease and vascular insufficiency. *Clin Podiatr Med Surg* 6:295-318, 1989. Used with permission.

Table 14-7

Tumors and Associated Toenail Conditions

Disease	Pathologic Changes
Breast carcinoma	Yellow nail syndrome
Bronchogenic carcinoma	Clubbing, Muehrcke's lines, onycholysis
Hodgkin's disease	Leukonychia partialis, Mees' lines, yellow nail syndrome
Laryngeal carcinoma	Yellow nail syndrome
Metastatic malignant melanoma	Clubbing, yellow nail syndrome
Multiple myeloma	Onycholysis

Modified from Kosinski MA, Stewart D: Nail changes associated with systemic disease and vascular insufficiency. *Clin Podiatr Med Surg* 6:295-318, 1989. Used with permission.

abnormalities are associated with dermatologic abnormalities and hair and nail disorders (Table 14–9).

Darier's disease (Darier–White disease or keratosis follicularis)[116] is an autosomal dominant disease characterized by distal subungual wedge-shaped keratoses, red-and-white longitudinal striations (Fig. 14–5A), splinter hemorrhages, notching of the distal nail plate, subungual hyperkeratosis, and thinning of the nail plate with splintering along the edge.

Pachyonychia congenita (Jadassohn–Lewandowsky syndrome),[98,118] another autosomal dominant genetic disorder,[117,118] is characterized by hypertrophy of the nail plate with severe thickening and yellowish-brown discoloration of the nail plate (Fig. 14–5B). The extreme thickening is more solid and more regular than with onychogryphosis and is accompanied by palmar and plantar keratoses. The thickening of the nail plate can lead to elevation of the distal nail plate and an incurved and elevated toenail. Tauber et al[153] reported a case of pachyonychia congenita and reviewed published reports of this disease.

Table 14-8

Hepatic, Renal, Pulmonary, and Gastrointestinal Disorders and Associated Toenail Conditions

Disease	Pathologic Changes
Hepatic	
Chronic hepatitis	Half-and-half nails, leukonychia
Cirrhosis	Clubbing, Muehrcke's lines, splinter hemorrhages, Terry nails
Renal	
Nephritis	Leukonychia
Nephrotic syndrome	Half-and-half nails, Muehrcke's lines, yellow nail syndrome
Renal failure	Brown lunula, half-and-half nails, Mees' lines
Pulmonary	
Asthma	Yellow nail syndrome
Bronchiectasis	Clubbing, inflammation of nail fold and nail bed, onychauxis, onycholysis, yellow nail syndrome
Chronic bronchitis	Clubbing, yellow nail syndrome
Interstitial pneumonia	Clubbing, yellow nail syndrome
Pleural effusion	Clubbing, onycholysis, yellow nail syndrome, leukonychia, Mees' lines
Pneumonia	Clubbing, yellow nail syndrome
Pulmonary fibrosis	Cyanosis, multiple paronychia, nail pitting
Pulmonary tuberculosis	Onychauxis
Gastrointestinal	
Peptic ulcer disease	Splinter hemorrhages
Plummer-Vinson syndrome	Koilonychia
Postgastrectomy syndrome	Koilonychia
Regional enteritis	Clubbing
Ulcerative colitis	Clubbing, leukonychia

Modified from Kosinski MA, Stewart D: Nail changes associated with systemic disease and vascular insufficiency. *Clin Podiatr Med Surg* 6:295-318, 1989. Used with permission.

Table 14-9

Genetic Disorders and Associated Nail Changes

Disease or Syndrome	Genetic Inheritance	Pathologic Nail Findings
Darier's disease	Autosomal dominant	Longitudinal red-and-white striations, atrophy or hypertrophy of nail plate, splinter hemorrhages, distal subungual wedge-shaped keratoses
Pachyonychia congenita	Autosomal dominant	Massive hypertrophy of nail plates, brown or yellow discoloration
Nail–patella syndrome	Autosomal dominant	Atrophy or hemiatrophy of nail, triangular-shaped lunula
Dyskeratosis congenita	X-linked recessive or autosomal dominant	Atrophy of nail plate, ridging, fusion of proximal nail fold
DOOR syndrome*	Autosomal recessive	Anonychia or atrophic nails

*DOOR: Deafness, onycho-osteodystrophy, and mental retardation.
Modified from Norton LA: Nail disorders: A review. *J Am Acad Dermatol* 2:451-467, 1980. Used with permission.

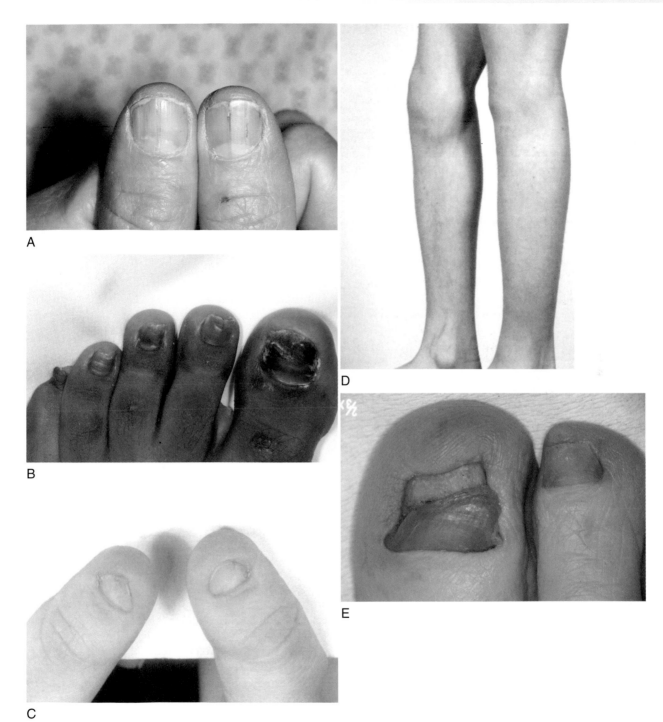

Figure 14–5 **A,** Darier's disease of the nail. There are notches in the distal margins of the nail, which is thin and friable and has alternating red-and-white lines. **B,** Pachyonychia congenita. Within the first year after disease onset, the nails become thickened, particularly at the tip, and wedge shaped. **C,** Nail–patella syndrome. The thumbnails are either absent or partially formed. Other nails may be involved to a lesser extent. **D,** Nail–patella syndrome. The patellae are either rudimentary or absent. **E,** Congenital malalignment of the big toe. (**C** and **D** from du Vivier A: *Atlas of Clinical Dermatology*, ed 3. Edinburgh, Churchill Livingstone, 2002, p 623. **E** courtesy of Dr. Robert Baran.)

The *nail–patella syndrome* (onycho-osteodysplasia)[118,149] is an autosomal dominant disease characterized by a triangular lunula and total atrophy or hemiatrophy of the nail plate (Fig. 14–5C). Other orthopaedic conditions associated with this disease include subluxation or dislocation of the radial head, presence of iliac horns, joint hypermobility, and a subluxated or dislocated hypoplastic patella (Fig. 14–5D).

Dyskeratosis congenita[118] (Zinsser–Cole–Engman syndrome) can be transmitted as an autosomal dominant or X-linked recessive trait and is characterized by ridging and thinning or atrophy of the nail plate.

DOOR syndrome[118] (*d*eafness, *o*nychodystrophy, *o*steodystrophy, and mental *r*etardation) is an autosomal recessive trait characterized by mental retardation and deafness. It may also be associated with absent or atrophic nails and curved fifth digits.

Congenital malalignment of the big toenail may be transmitted by an autosomal dominant gene of variable expression (Fig. 14–5E). It is characterized by lateral deviation of the long axis of the nail relative to the distal phalanx. Complications of this condition are local, such as perionychium onychocryptosis. In one review, 50% of cases spontaneously improved or resolved; however, the misdirected nail matrix can be rotated surgically.[15]

Congenital nail abnormalities are errors of development that can produce other anomalies, such as *anonychia* (absence of the nails) and *polyonychia* (presence of more than one nail on a digit) or *micronychia* (small nails) (Fig. 14–6).

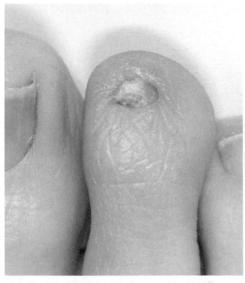

Figure 14–6 Micronychia. Nails may be totally or partially absent as the result of a congenital defect.

TRAUMA

The nail plate and nail bed can be damaged by trauma. Injury to the nail matrix can cause abnormalities such as ridging, pitting, and grooving. After an injury to the toenail, the regrowth can be a thickened, discolored nail, and after a toenail is lost, a new nail plate can grow abnormally or normally. Trauma to the distal phalanx can cause a subungual exostosis, which often causes nail plate deformity, and an osseous injury to the distal phalanx can cause callus formation that can affect the new toenail. Thickening of the distal phalanx can cause an incurved toenail that pinches the underlying soft tissue.

Trauma to the nail plate may be caused by biomechanical abnormalities as well (see later discussion on subungual hematoma). The second toe can compress the lateral nail fold adjacent to the second toe, causing an overgrowth of soft tissue with secondary infection. With more acute trauma, when the nail bed over the distal phalanx is crushed, after the nail bed is repaired, the fragmented nail can be replaced and secured with 2-octyl cyanoacrylate (Dermabond, Ethicon, Somerville, NJ).[72] This material creates a bond between the nail fragments and the skin for 7 to 14 days, when the new nail pushes it off. The material serves as a rigid splint for a fracture as well as a biologic covering to minimize desiccation and hyperkeratinization of the nail matrix. It also prevents the cuticle from adhering to the underlying germinal matrix.[147]

Similar to nail plate repairs in the hand,[30] germinal and nail bed repairs in the foot may be made under loupe magnification using 7-0 chromic suture to repair the tissue, with the intention of preventing functional or cosmetic problems. Replacing the nail prevents the eponychium from adhering to the nail bed. It may be held in place with a distal suture or two side sutures (5-0 nylon), which are removed at 7 to 10 days to prevent an epithelialized tract. If the nail is crushed too severely, similar to hand injuries, 0.020-inch silicon sheeting may be placed under the proximal nail fold to protect the nail fold.[30] If a portion of the nail bed is absent, a split-thickness graft (not a full-thickness graft) from the adjacent nail bed may be used to fill a defect to prevent later deformity of the nail.[30] One could also remove the nail longitudinally, excise the scar tissue or lesion, and undermine the nail bed all the way to the perionychial tissues to achieve a tension-free closure, as is done for split fingernail injuries.[6] A figure-of-eight suture may be used to hold the nail in place.[89]

A germinal matrix graft could also be harvested from adjacent nail tissue, and the nail narrowed as in a Winograd procedure, or harvested from another toe.

Few studies are available, however, on toenail bed reconstruction. Nonetheless, it makes sense that similar procedures could be used on the toes and the fingers.

On the medial aspect of the nail plate, with excessive pronation, hypertrophy of the ungualabia can result in an ingrown toenail. Parrinello et al[129] compared the shape of the great toenail with the base of the distal phalanx and found a significant correlation between the shape of the proximal aspect of the nail plate and the shape of the phalangeal base. However, they found no correlation between the shapes of the proximal and distal portions of the nail plate. They concluded that many other factors besides trauma influence the shape of the nail, including constricting footwear, snug-fitting stockings and hosiery, inadequate or inappropriate pedicures, and heritable traits that can lead to incurvation of the nail border with subsequent inflammation and infection.

Split-nail deformities may be treated surgically with nail removal, elliptical nail bed scar removal, and careful elevation of the matrix off the bone with extension of this dissection laterally until the nail matrix can be closed without tension.[67] Defects in the nail bed from excisional biopsy can be repaired with a free graft from the lesser toes or with split-thickness, sterile matrix grafts from the adjoining nail matrix.[43] Subungual splinters may be removed by sequential thin, sharp filings of the nail until the splinter is exposed along its entire length. This allows complete splinter removal without having to remove the entire nail.[146]

TUMORS

Tumors of the soft tissue adjacent to the toenails or involving the nail unit itself can be benign or malignant. Periungual and subungual warts *(verrucae)* are common soft tissue growths (Fig. 14–7A-C). *Fibro-*

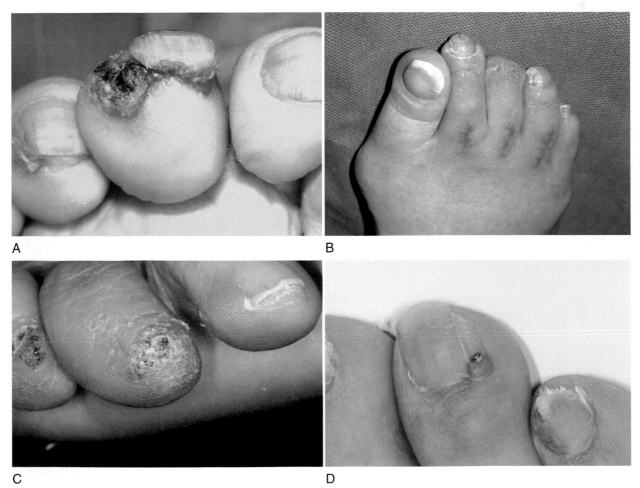

Figure 14–7 **A,** Subungual wart (verruca) on the third toe was refractory to topical treatments. **B,** Treatment of verruca on the third toe was by amputation at the distal interphalangeal joint. **C,** Verrucae on multiple toes. **D,** Angiofibroma. This may be the first evidence of tuberous sclerosis or ectodermal dysplasia.

BOX 14–5   Tumors Associated with Toenail Conditions

BENIGN NAIL TUMORS

Verruca
Fibroma
Fibrokeratoma
Neurofibroma
Myxoid cyst
Pyogenic granuloma
Glomus tumor
Pigmented nevus
Keratoacanthoma

MALIGNANT NAIL TUMORS

Squamous cell carcinoma
Malignant melanoma
Basal cell carcinoma
Metastatic carcinoma
Bowen's disease

BONE TUMORS

Bone cysts (solitary or aneurysmal)
Enchondroma
Osteochondroma
Subungual exostosis

Modified from Gunnoe RE: Diseases of the nails: How to recognize and treat them. *Postgrad Med* 74:357-362, 1983. Used with permission.

mas[140] and *fibrokeratomas* can result from trauma to the toes with consequent nodule formation impinging on the nail plate (Box 14–5). These lesions can also develop beneath the nail plate itself and cause elevation and deformity. These are benign tumors composed of connective tissue, but they can lead to thinning or destruction of the nail plate. Pressure on the nail matrix can create a longitudinal defect in the nail plate as well. A periungual fibroma or angiofibroma (Fig. 14–7D) may be the first evidence of tuberous sclerosis or ectodermal dysplasia. In general, fibromas respond readily to excision or cauterization. Glomus tumors, pyogenic granulomas, and keratoacanthomas must all be considered in the differential diagnosis.

Glomus Tumor

A glomus tumor is most commonly encountered on the acral portions of the extremities. This lesion is often in the subungual area and consists of a purplish nodule measuring only a few millimeters in diameter.

It is tender and gives rise to severe paroxysmal pain. Glomus tumors rarely ulcerate or bleed, and excision usually results in a cure, although subungual lesions are more difficult to eradicate. The differential diagnosis includes melanoblastoma, melanoma, neuroma, chronic perionychium, gout, arthritis, foreign body granuloma, and Kaposi's sarcoma.

The glomus tumor appears to be a controlled arteriovenous anastomosis or shunt between terminal vessels arising from the glomus body, a thermoregulatory structure found throughout the body; hence, it tends to give the patient cold insensitivity.[84]

The only effective treatment for glomus tumor is surgery.[30] Previously it was necessary to remove the nail, incise the nail matrix, remove the tumor, and repair the nail bed. A study of seven cases,[84] however, demonstrated that creating an L-shaped incision 5 mm distal and 5 mm medial or lateral to the nail and lifting off the entire vascular flap allowed removal of the tumor (Fig. 14–8A-C). The flap was then sutured back to its origin after hemostasis.[84] There were no recurrences or nail irregularities. T2-weighted magnetic resonance imaging (MRI) may be used to determine the precise location of the tumor (Fig. 14–8D and E). This technique might lend itself to other subungual operations as well, such as treatment of subungual exostosis. This approach has been used by others and is recommended for all noninvasive space-occupying subungual lesions regardless of type.[139]

Another type of glomus tumor, which is characterized by multiple painless hemangiomas, often has a familial pattern.[37] These multiple lesions are usually asymptomatic.

Subungual Exostosis

A subungual exostosis is a reactive bony growth typically occurring on the dorsomedial aspect of the distal phalanx of the hallux (Fig. 14–9A-D).[33,35,45,110,113] Originally described by Dupuytren in 1817, subungual exostosis has a definite predilection for the hallux, although occasionally it develops in one of the lesser toes. A subungual exostosis typically has a moderate growth rate, resulting in a unilateral growth that rarely exceeds 0.5 cm. Rarely, the exostosis develops a cartilage-capped surface, and a diagnosis of osteochondroma may be made.

Osteochondroma characteristically occurs close to the epiphyseal line (Table 14–10),[110] and it occurs more often in adolescent boys than girls (2:1 ratio). In contrast, the diagnosis of subungual exostosis is made more often in young adults aged 20 to 40 years. Ippolito et al[86] found that subungual exostoses occurred more often in the female population (2:1

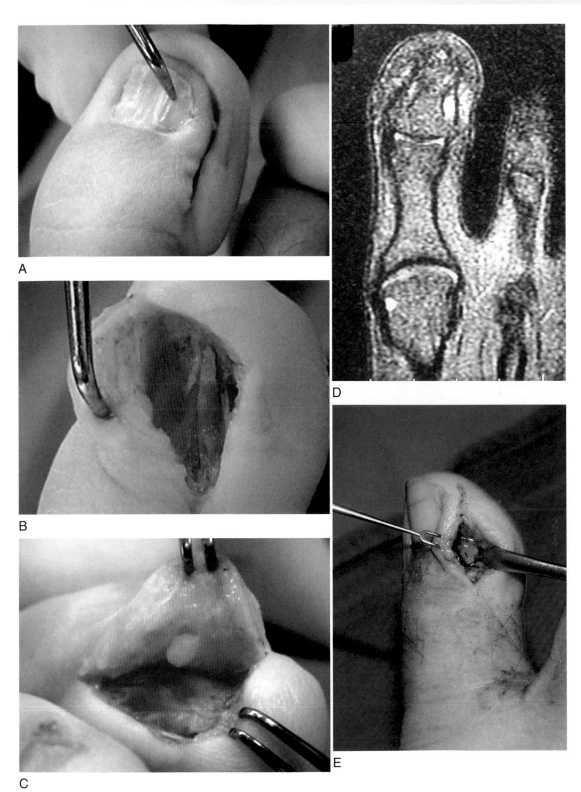

Figure 14–8 Glomus tumor. **A,** L-shaped incision to lift the entire vascular flap from the bone. **B,** The flap is lifted. **C,** The flap is elevated, showing the glomus tumor. **D,** T2-weighted magnetic resonance imaging scan with glomus tumor on the lateral side of the distal phalanx. **E,** Glomus tumor exposed surgically. (**A-C** from Horst F, Nunley JA: *Foot Ankle Int* 24:949-51, 2003; courtesy of Dr. James A. Nunley. Used with permission. **D** and **E** courtesy of Dr. Richard Marks.)

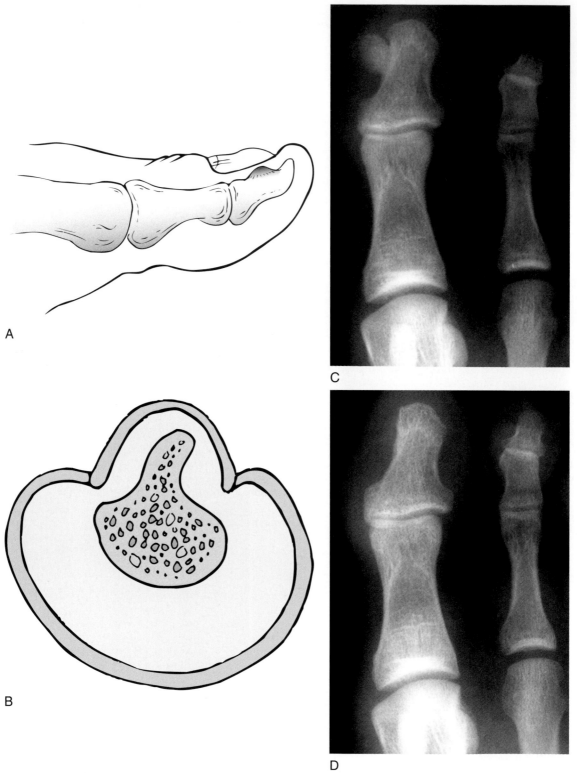

Figure 14–9 **A,** Lateral view of toe shows the effect of subungual exostosis on the configuration of the nail plate. **B,** Cross section of distal phalanx shows deformation of the nail plate by subungual exostosis. **C,** Radiograph shows subungual exostosis before excision. **D,** Radiograph after excision of exostosis.

Table 14–10

Distinguishing Features of Subungual Exostosis and Subungual Osteochondroma

Condition	Typical Age at Diagnosis (years)	Male-to-Female Ratio	Traumatic Cause	Growth Rate	Radiographic Appearance
Exostosis	20-40	1:2	Frequent[159]	Moderate	Osseous growth with expanded cap, often trabeculated (fibrocartilage cap)
Osteochondroma	10-25	2:1	Often	Slow	Sessile bone lesion, often trabeculated (hyaline cartilage cap)

Modified from Norton LA: Nail disorders: A review. *J Am Acad Dermatol* 2:457-467, 1980. Used with permission.

ratio), whereas Miller-Breslow and Dorfman[110] reported an equal distribution between male and female patients.

The cause of subungual exostosis is thought to be trauma.[57,113,121] Fikry et al[57] found a history of trauma or repetitive microtrauma in 21 of 28 cases. However, in a review of subungual osteochondroma, Vazquez-Flores et al[159] also noted that in 27 cases, trauma was recalled by 40.7% of the patients. Thus, it appears that most of these lesions are related to trauma.

In distinguishing between subungual exostosis and subungual osteochondroma, the histologic characterization of the cartilage cap is diagnostic. A subungual exostosis has a cartilaginous cap that is a reactive fibrous growth with cartilage metaplasia.[110] Jahss[87] noted that a subungual exostosis is characterized histologically as chronic fibrosis caused by irritation. A trabecular bony pattern connecting with the distal phalanx can underlie the fibrocartilaginous cap.[110] However, the distal tuft of the phalanx is usually not involved. In a subungual osteochondroma, a hyaline cartilage cap can overlie a trabeculated bony pattern.

Reporting on 21 cases of subungual exostosis, Ippolito et al[86] noted that 12 patients were athletes involved in activities such as dancing, gymnastics, or football. It is believed that increased pressure against the dorsal aspect of the nail plate from a constricting toe box can cause irritation that leads to the development of a subungual exostosis. The connection between a specific traumatic incident and the subsequent development of a subungual exostosis can also explain the increased incidence of this abnormality in athletes. Many patients describe pain that is aggravated by activities such as running or walking and is most likely from the pressure of an expanding lesion against the toe box.

A subungual exostosis can be misdiagnosed or confused with other toenail abnormalities.[86] Elevation of the nail plate (Fig. 14–10A) and discoloration can resemble chronic onychomycosis or a subungual hematoma. Chinn and Jenkin[35] reported two cases of patients with pain in the proximal nail groove who had undergone an unsuccessful surgical matrixectomy and who later received a diagnosis of subungual exostosis. The differential diagnosis includes subungual verruca, pyogenic granuloma, glomus tumor, keratoacanthoma, subungual nevus, and epidermoid inclusion cyst as well as malignant lesions, such as carcinoma of the nail bed and subungual melanoma.

The diagnosis of subungual exostosis is determined by radiographic evidence of the exostosis. A dorsoplantar radiograph might not show the exostosis, but a lateral or oblique radiograph often helps to identify the lesion (Fig. 14–10B). The exostosis typically arises from the dorsomedial aspect of the distal phalanx. It is often oval and has irregular density. Although the cartilage cap may be quite large, the radiographic appearance of the exostosis may be smaller than its actual size. The possibility that these lesions can occur on lesser toes, which are more unusual locations, needs to be kept in mind (Fig. 14–10C).

De Palma et al[45] reported on 11 cases of surgical excision of a subungual exostosis with partial onychectomy. Using histochemical and immunohistochemical methods, they concluded that most subungual bony masses exhibited the characteristics of conventional osteochondromas and that the distance of the lesion from the epiphyseal line was unrelated to its histologic features.

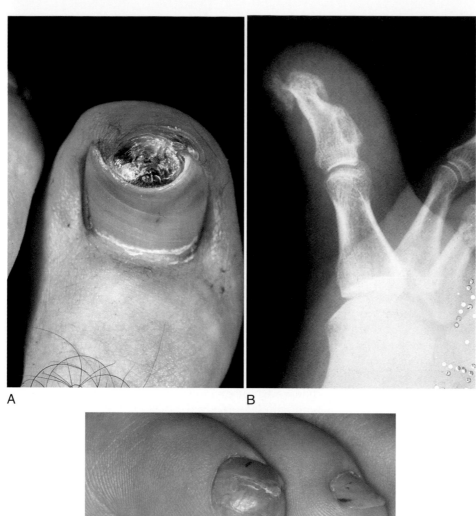

A

B

C

Figure 14–10 A, A subungual exostosis is commonly mistaken for a wart. It is a bony outgrowth that occurs beneath the big toe particularly. **B,** Calcification can be seen under the nail on a radiograph. **C,** This patient has a deformity of the fifth toenail. (**A** and **B** from du Vivier A: *Atlas of Clinical Dermatology,* ed 3. Edinburgh, Churchill Livingstone, 2002, p 618.)

RESECTION OF SUBUNGUAL EXOSTOSIS

Although a small asymptomatic lesion may be observed and treated conservatively, surgical resection of a subungual exostosis or subungual osteochondroma is the most common treatment of a symptomatic lesion. The operation involves either the above-described procedure for glomus tumor (see Fig. 14–8A-C) or the following procedure (Fig. 14–11A-D).

Surgical Technique

1. A digital anesthetic block is administered and a 0.25-inch Penrose drain or a commercially available tubular tourniquet (Mar-Med, Grand Rapids, Mich) is applied.
2. A partial or complete toenail avulsion is performed.
3. A longitudinal incision is made in the nail bed. The nail bed is reflected off the exostosis with care to avoid damage to the nail matrix.
4. The exostosis is resected with an osteotome or bone cutter. The base of the lesion is curetted.
5. The nail bed is relocated and closed with absorbable suture.
6. A compression dressing is applied and changed 24 hours postoperatively. Dressing changes are continued until drainage subsides. The nail bed is protected with a plastic bandage strip until tenderness resolves.

Recurrence

An exostosis recurs infrequently but can develop after an incomplete resection. Recurrence may be a continuing source of irritation to the toenail. Miller-Breslow and Dorfman[110] reported a 53% incidence of recurrence when a subtotal excisional biopsy was performed. After wide local excision with curettage of the base, however, a 5% to 6% rate of recurrence is expected.[121]

Melanotic Whitlow and Malignant Melanoma

Hutchinson[85] published the first significant report on subungual melanoma in 1886. Koenig and McLaughlin[94] stated that 0.025% of all reported cancer is caused by subungual melanoma. Melanomas that involve the nails are termed *melanotic whitlows*.[64] Blackish discol-

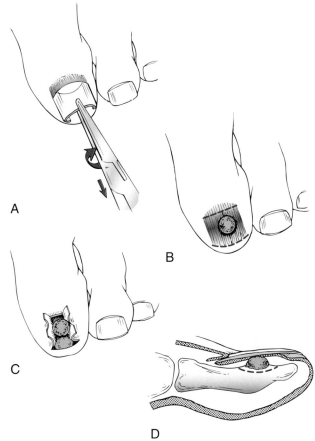

Figure 14–11 Technique for surgical excision of subungual exostosis. **A,** The toenail is completely avulsed to expose the exostosis. **B,** Longitudinal incision is made in the nail bed, avoiding injury to the nail matrix. **C,** Nail bed is reflected. **D,** Exostosis is excised with wide margins, and the nail bed is then repaired.

oration develops, especially in the nail bed (Fig. 14–12A), but minimal pigmentation (Fig. 14–12B) or the absence of pigment does not exclude the diagnosis of melanoma. The Hutchinson sign (pigment spreading beyond the nail plate into the proximal or lateral nail folds, or both) is considered pathognomonic of subungual melanoma (Fig. 14–12B).[102]

Twenty-three percent of melanomas involving the nail may be amelanotic.[14,150] Other reported colors include tan, brown, and blue.[137] A greenish tinge to the nail is most likely due to a *Pseudomonas* infection (Fig. 14–12C).

On physical examination, a melanoma may be accompanied by a splitting or loss of the nail, ulceration, and localized erythema. These malignant tumors are more common on the fingers than on the toes. Aulicino and Hunter[10] reported on 72 cases of subungual melanoma, of which two thirds were on the thumb or great toe. The most common cause of darkening of the nails is trauma, but other causes include

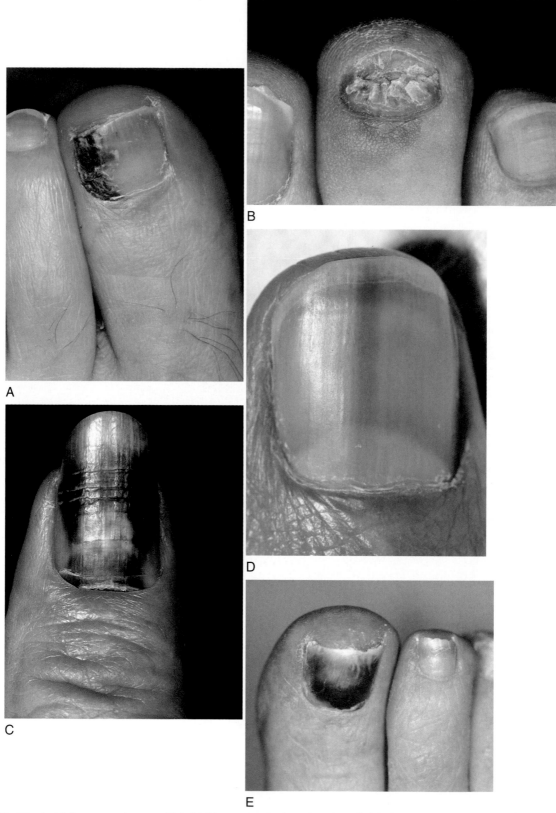

Figure 14–12 **A,** Malignant melanoma. This friable tumor, partly red and partly black, is rising up the side of the nail. There is a bluish discoloration of the nail plate and pigmentation around the base of the nail. **B,** Malignant melanoma of the nail bed. The nail is growing abnormally and has become thickened. There is pigmentation under the nail and around the posterior nail fold (Hutchinson's sign). **C,** *Pseudomonas* infection. The green discoloration from the infection is distinguishable from the black of the melanoma. **D,** Linear melanonychia. A straight black line runs longitudinally from the nail fold. It is benign. Sometimes it rises from a benign mole in the nail. **E,** Trauma. The color may be black generally, but there is usually a red-brown or russet discoloration as well as pinpoint dots of hemorrhage. The configuration may be straight as it grows out. (**B** and **C** from du Vivier A: *Atlas of Clinical Dermatology*, ed 3. Edinburgh, Churchill Livingstone, 2002, pp 620, 621.)

Addison's disease and Peutz–Jeghers syndrome. The differential diagnosis of malignant melanoma also includes glomus tumor, benign nevus, paronychia, onychomycosis, pyogenic granuloma,[94] linear melanonychia (Fig. 14–12D), and onychomycosis.

Often malignant melanoma is misdiagnosed as a benign condition, which can lead to long delays in diagnosis and appropriate treatment. With malignant melanoma, unlike a benign condition such as subungual hematoma (Fig. 14–12E), discoloration of the nail does not change as the nail grows distally and does not improve with time. A malignant melanoma might not damage the overlying nail plate, whereas a subungual hematoma can cause plate elevation. Typically, a malignant melanoma is deep black, in contrast to the less distinct color of a subungual hemorrhage.

Many patients with a subungual melanoma report the occurrence of trauma, which makes an early diagnosis difficult. Approximately 4% occur in the foot,[137] and two thirds of these appear on the hallux.[127] Melanoma occurs more often in female patients and in white patients and has an incidence of 10% to 31% among nonwhite patients.[13,92] The typical age at presentation is 50 to 60 years. A poor prognosis is associated with lymph node involvement and nail destruction or ulceration, and the long-term survival rate varies from 18% to 40%.[55,100,104,152,162] Because the lesion is often mimicked by other conditions, it is most important to do an excisional biopsy for any suspicious lesion (such as a nonhealing ulcer, subungual discoloration, or subungual hematoma) that does not advance with the nail.

Pack and Oropeza[123] and Papachristou and Fortner[127] reported that one third of patients initially present with regional lymph node involvement and that biopsy should be done for any suspicious lesion. Early amputation is the treatment of choice, usually at the metacarpophalangeal joint, because resections more than 3 cm from the lesion are not of clinical value even for the thickest melanomas.[81] However, studies of the hand suggest that a more functional, distal removal of the affected tissue can be equally effective.[111]

Other Tumorous Conditions

Bowen's disease is a relatively rare premalignant dermatologic disorder originally described by Bowen in 1912. It is typically a well-circumscribed, erythematous, papular, nodular, crusting lesion that can be mistaken for psoriasis. Bowen's disease is described as a variant of squamous cell carcinoma, an in situ carcinoma that does not usually metastasize. Patients with Bowen's disease are more likely to develop other primary malignancies,[21] and Graham and Helwig,[66]

reporting on 35 cases, noted that 80% of patients died of primary malignancies within 9 years after the appearance of Bowen's disease. Lemont and Haas[103] reported that peak occurrence is in the eighth decade, typically on the plantar aspect of the foot. Treatment is usually surgical excision or curettage, but surgical excision is the treatment of choice. If the basement membrane is disrupted, however, the potential exists for distant metastases. When maximal tissue must be preserved, Mohs surgery is 90% effective,[122] and when there is no osseous involvement, Mohs surgery is considered the treatment of choice.[170] The key is to perform a biopsy of any chronic lesion involving the nail.[122]

Basal cell carcinoma is rare in the foot,[8] and squamous cell carcinoma (Fig. 14–13A and B),[9,26,40] Kaposi's sarcoma, and other metastatic diseases are relatively rare malignant lesions. Patients with abnormal radiographic findings, chronic pain, swelling, inflammation, infection, or persistent splitting of the nail plate should be evaluated for an underlying tumor of the distal phalanx. A specific diagnosis is essential. After the diagnosis of a malignant tumor has been made by biopsy, amputation of the digit is the typical treatment.

Biopsies of suspicious lesions are always important. With the nail removed, the recommendation is to take longitudinal biopsy specimens from the nail bed and transverse biopsy specimens from the nail matrix, with subsequent repair if possible.[134]

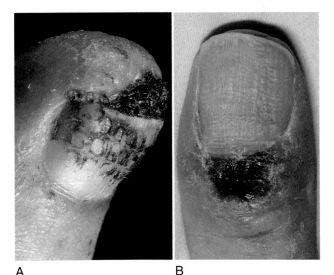

A   B

Figure 14–13 **A,** Squamous cell carcinoma under the nail. There is a thickening under the nail that has bled. Biopsy is indicated to establish the nature of the lesion which, in this case, is squamous cell carcinoma. **B,** Squamous cell carcinoma involving the proximal nail fold. (**A** from du Vivier A: *Atlas of Clinical Dermatology*, ed 3. Edinburgh, Churchill Livingstone, 2002, p 620.)

ONYCHOPATHIES AND OTHER COMMON NAIL ABNORMALITIES

Onychopathies[119,120] and other abnormalities of the toenails are most easily discussed by dividing them into abnormalities of the nail plate, nail bed, nail fold, and nail matrix (Boxes 14-6 and 14-7). Congenital and genetic nail disorders, traumatic nail disorders, tumors, and dermatologic and systemic nail disorders are discussed elsewhere in this chapter.

BOX 14-6   Onychopathies and Other Common Toenail Abnormalities

NAIL PLATE

Onychocryptosis
Onychauxis
Onychogryphosis
Onychomycosis
Onychia
Onycholysis or onychomadesis

NAIL BED

Subungual exostosis
Subungual tumor
Subungual clavus
Subungual hematoma
Subungual verruca

NAIL FOLD

Paronychia
Onychophosis
Pyogenic granuloma
Herpetic whitlow
Periungual verruca

MATRIX

Anonychia
Pterygium
Atrophy or hypertrophy (onychauxis)

KERATINIZATION DISORDERS

Psoriasis
Mycotic infections
Onychoschizia
Koilonychia
Leukonychia
Onycholysis
Onychorrhexis

Modified from Nzuzi SM: Common nail disorders. *Clin Podiatr Med Surg* 6:273-294, 1989. Used with permission.

BOX 14-7   Causes of Nail Deformities

EXTERNAL PRESSURE

Footwear

- Excessive tightness
- High heels
- Pointed toe box
- Short toe box

Stockings: excessive tightness
Casts extending beyond nail
Hallux rigidus
Hallux valgus
Hallux varus
Lesser toes

- Impingement on hallux
- Hammer toes
- Overlapping or underlapping toes
- Soft tissue neoplasm
- Pronation of feet

INTERNAL PRESSURE

Subungual exostosis or osteoma
Subungual keratosis
Subungual hematoma
Subungual neoplasm
Onychia or paronychia
Trauma

SYSTEMIC CONDITIONS

Cardiac disorders
Circulatory disorders
Endocrine disorders
Renal disorders
Metabolic disorders
Infection
Genetic disorders
Geriatric nail changes
Obesity

Modified from Johnson KA: *Surgery of the Foot and Ankle.* New York, Raven Press, 1989, p 84. Used with permission.

Common Nail Plate Disorders

Onychocryptosis, onychauxis, onychogryphosis, onychomycosis, onychia, onycholysis, and onychomadesis are the nail plate disorders seen most often.

Onychocryptosis

Onychocryptosis occurs when the border of the nail plate penetrates the adjacent soft tissue of the nail fold (Fig. 14-14). Synonyms for this condition include "ingrown toenail," "unguis incarnatus," and "ungua-labial hypertrophy."[50,51] The term "ingrown toenail" is misleading because it implies that the side of the nail

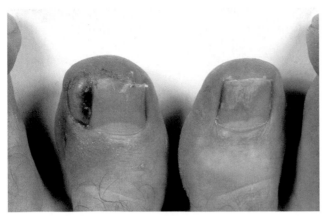

Figure 14–14 Onychocryptosis. As the skin becomes irritated it hypertrophies, exacerbating the impingement of the nail into the soft tissue. (From du Vivier A: *Atlas of Clinical Dermatology*, ed 3. Edinburgh, Churchill Livingstone, 2002, p 615.)

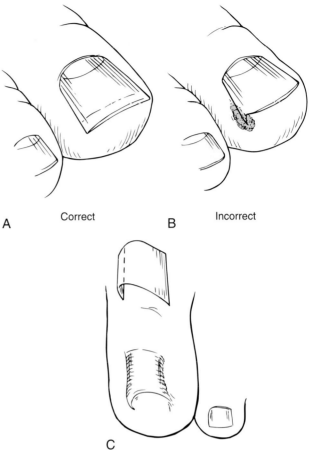

A Correct   B Incorrect

C

Figure 14–15 A, Correct nail trimming prevents ingrowth into the adjacent nail fold. **B,** Incorrect trimming can lead to a fishhook-shaped spur in the lateral nail fold, with subsequent infection. **C,** Abnormal incurving of the medial border can predispose to infection.

plate grows laterally and extends farther into the nail groove. All evidence indicates, however, that the growth of nails in vertebrates is determined by the matrix width and that the width of the nail is directly related to matrix width.[22,23,128] There is no evidence that the matrix becomes wider in a person with an ingrown toenail. The term "ingrown toenail" was chosen on the assumption that an ingrowth of the nail or its downward growth into the nail groove was caused by an increasing width in the convexity of the nail. Thus, initial attempts by surgeons at treating this disease were aimed at narrowing the nail margin. Frost[61] described three types of ingrown toenails: a normal nail plate that, with improper nail trimming, develops a fishhook-shaped spur in the lateral nail groove (Fig. 14–15A and B); an inward distortion of one or both of the lateral margins of the nail plate (incurved nail) (Fig. 14–15); and a normal nail plate with soft tissue hypertrophy of the lateral border (Fig. 14–16).

Lloyd-Davies and Brill[107] stated that complete avulsion of the nail plate, which in the past was a common treatment for an ingrown toenail, probably leads to hypertrophy of the distal lip of the nail and causes the entire nail to become embedded and clubbed. If the nail of the great toe is removed, the new toenail, unlike a fingernail, often becomes deformed as it grows distally because of upward pressure placed on it during weight bearing (see Fig. 14–2). Elliptically excising the distal soft tissue can reduce this phenomenon (Fig. 14–17A-C).

The main conditions that produce symptoms of onychocryptosis are primary hyperplasia of the nail groove in approximately 75% of cases and a deformity of the nail plate in 25% of cases. The latter is caused

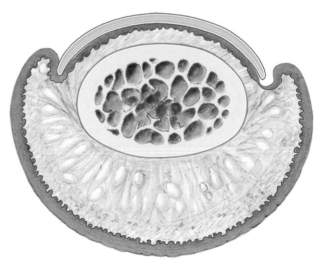

Figure 14–16 Cross-sectional view of toe through the distal phalanx. Hypertrophy of the nail leading to occlusion of the nail groove is shown on the *left.* Normal relationship between nail margin and lateral nail groove is shown on the *right.* (Courtesy of The Mayo Foundation for Medical Education and Research.)

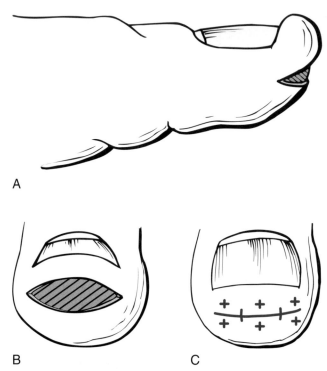

Figure 14–17 Ingrown toenail. **A** and **B,** Elliptical incision is used to resect redundant skin and soft tissue. **C,** Closure of the elliptical incision tends to reduce distal impingement against the advancing distal nail plate.

by an osseous malformation of the dorsum of the distal phalanx[105] or by hypertrophy and irregular thickening of the nail bed, often as a result of a tinea infection. The normal nail plate and its bed are 2 to 3 mm thick. The contour is largely determined by the dorsal shape of the distal phalanx. The shape and contour of the nail can vary widely because of secondary changes in the distal phalanx from irritation and pressure.[129] Such variations often produce nail deformities and accompanying symptoms that can all be classified as ingrown toenail. The most common type is incurvation of the nail margin.

Normally the space between the nail margin and the nail groove is approximately 1 mm. The groove is lined with a thin layer of epithelium that lies immediately beneath and beside the nail margins. Under normal conditions, this space sufficiently protects the groove from irritation. With a narrow toe box or tight-fitting stockings, downward pressure can develop on the nail plate, the nail lip, or the lateral nail fold. This pressure obliterates the space between the nail plate margin and the nail groove and produces constant irritation. The reactive swelling in the groove leads to gradual hyperplasia of the adjacent soft tissue and ultimately to permanent hypertrophy. As this process continues, the nail groove is finally incised by the nail margin, often with ensuing secondary infection.

To relieve the acute symptoms, after using local anesthesia or a digital block, the longitudinal border of the nail may be excised (Fig. 14–18A-G).[34] Merely excising a triangular section of the nail margin often leads to development of a thick fishhook-shaped deformity of the lateral nail plate (Fig. 14–19A and B). Hypertrophy of the adjacent soft tissue fills the space of the excised nail margin. As the nail continues to grow distally, it impinges on the elevated nail groove and gives rise to recurrent episodes of infection and formation of granulation tissue.

A congenitally thickened lateral nail margin predisposes to an ingrown toenail. This congenital factor explains why ingrown toenails sometimes occur in infants or even in neonates who have thick nail lips or no free margin between the nail groove and nail margin. In adults the condition is typically acquired. Sometimes the symptoms are so chronic and the nail changes are so severe that a terminal Syme amputation of the entire nail unit with shortening of the toe is appropriate (Fig. 14–20A and B). A subungual exostosis can cause nail deformities with subsequent incurvation, infection, and pain (Fig. 14–21A and B).

The size, shape, and contour of the nail plate and bed are usually normal. Hyperplastic changes of the nail groove and lip are accompanied by formation of granulation tissue on the lip and groove. The granulation tissue bleeds freely with slight provocation. Hypertrophied tissue can cover a large part of the nail or most of the nail. Heifetz[75] proposed a classification of ingrown toenails with the following three distinct stages:

Stage 1: Swelling and erythema are present along the lateral nail fold. The edge of the nail plate may be embedded in an irritated nail fold.

Stage 2: Increased pain accompanies acute or active infection. Drainage is present.

Stage 3: With chronic infection, granulation tissue develops in the lateral nail fold. The surrounding soft tissue is hypertrophied.

The differential diagnosis includes trauma, paronychia, subungual exostosis, onycholysis, and onychophosis.

TREATMENT

Various procedures have been reported for the cure of an ingrown toenail, but postoperative recurrence is common. Procedures generally practiced include simple avulsion of the border of the nail plate (this can temporarily resolve the infection, but a strong tendency exists for recurrent infection unless definitive treatment is performed later), reduction of the hypertrophied lip, and partial or total ablation (surgical, chemical, or laser) of the germinal matrix.

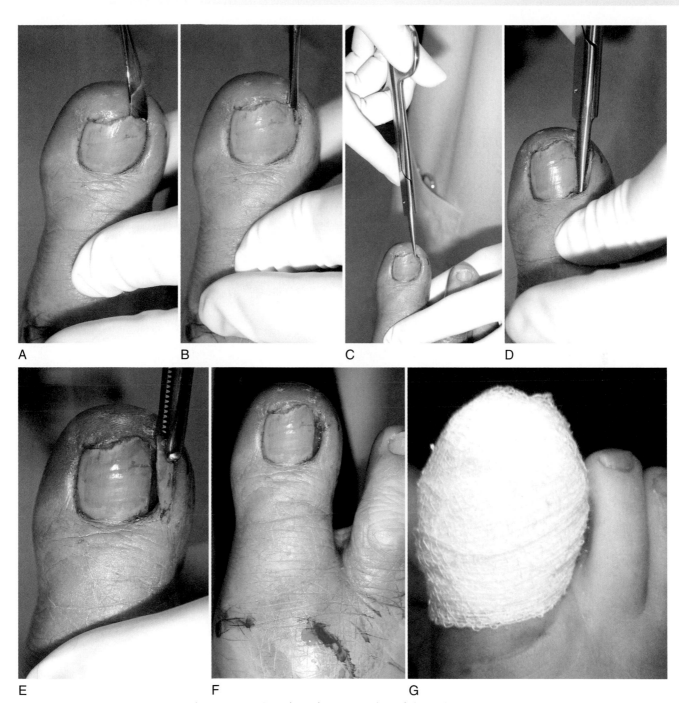

A   B   C   D

E   F   G

Figure 14–18   Treatment of onychocryptosis. **A** and **B,** The outer edge of the nail plate is elevated proximal to the cuticle. **C** and **D,** The nail border is incised longitudinally. **E** and **F,** A longitudinal portion of the nail is removed to relieve symptoms of acute infection. **G,** Gauze dressing is applied after the toenail procedure.

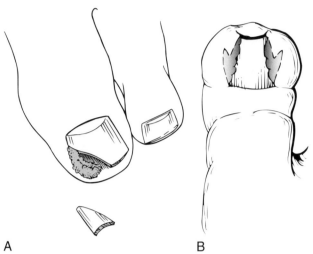

A   B

Figure 14–19 A, Symptoms of acute infection may be relieved with diagonal trimming of the nail plate. **B,** As the nail plate regrows, infection can recur.

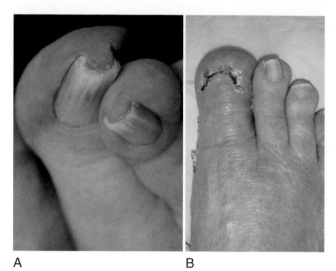

A   B

Figure 14–20 Terminal Syme's amputation. **A,** Clinical example of nail incurvature in an elderly patient. Because of the chronicity of symptoms, the patient opted for a terminal Syme's amputation. An osteotomy of the proximal phalanx was also performed to allow the toe to be straightened and to relieve impingement of the second toe. **B,** Three weeks postoperatively.

There is evidence that the second type of ingrown nail, the pincer nail, is associated with broader proximal bases of the distal phalanges, which force the nail to grow broader proximally and curve tighter distally. It is not uncommonly associated with a dorsal distal osteophyte on the phalanx. Hence, good therapeutic results have been achieved from a combination of removing the lateral matrix horns, lifting up the nail bed from the bone, removing the distal tuft of bone,[18] and suturing the lateral dermis and subcutaneous tissue beneath the nail bed. This leaves "a flat nail bed with support on each side. The nail will then grow out straight."[67]

Unquestionably, patient education is necessary in the treatment of an ingrown toenail, both to treat an acute condition and to prevent a recurrence of infec-

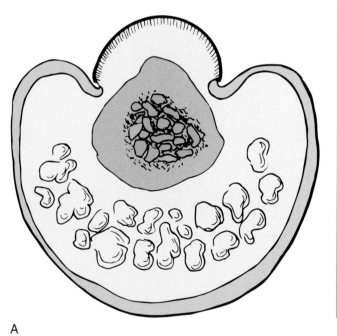

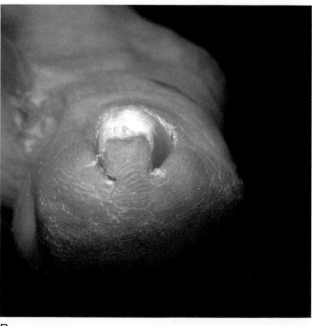

A   B

Figure 14–21 Subungual exostosis. **A,** Subungual exostosis can cause deformity of the nail plate. **B,** Clinical example of nail incurvation in an elderly patient.

tion. The patient should be instructed in proper footwear, use of loose-fitting stockings or hose, and proper nail-cutting procedures. Patients with excessive pronation may be treated with an orthotic device to decrease axial pressure on the border of the hallux. (Specific surgical procedures are discussed later in this chapter.)

Onychauxis and Onychogryphosis

Onychauxis (club nail) refers to a hypertrophied nail plate. This usually involves the great toenail, but the lesser toes may be affected as well. The deformity may be caused by systemic problems, such as nutritional deficiencies or psoriasis. The toenail may be yellow, brown, gray, or black. Most cases result from local conditions, such as trauma to the nail matrix or nail bed and tinea infection, which is the most common cause. The undersurface of the nail can become tremendously thickened from the accumulation of debris from a chronic mycotic infection.[38,172] The affected nail and its bed are thickened and deformed. When the disorder is caused by *Microsporum gypseum*, the surface of the nail might have white streaks or patches that can be excised readily. When the undersurface of the nail contains a yellowish or brown powdery substance, destruction of the nail bed has been caused by *Trichophyton purpureum*. In approximately 10% of cases of club nail, the nail bed and dorsal distal surface of the distal phalanx undergo hypertrophic changes.

Onychogryphosis refers to hypertrophy of the nail plate, especially of the hallux (Fig. 14–22A and B). The nail resembles a claw or horn, and, although uncommon, its frequency in men who have tended horses has led to the appellation "hostler's toe." It has also been referred to as "ram's horn nail." The massive growth of the nail plate overlies the dorsal surface of the toe and often terminates on the plantar surface of the toe. This condition does not appear to have any relationship to a tinea infection. In most cases, it is the result of a congenital condition or repeated trauma to the nail matrix, along with poor hygiene. In some extreme cases, the nail measures several

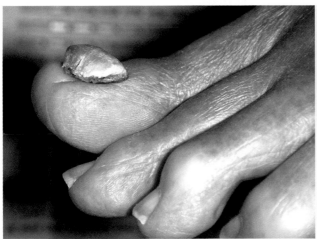

A

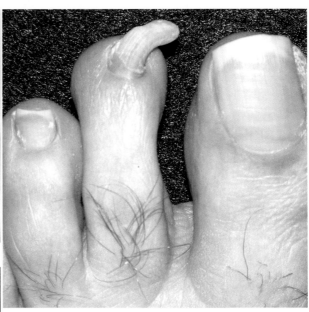

B

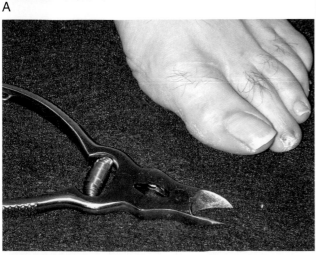

C

Figure 14–22 Onychogryphosis. **A** and **B,** With onychogryphosis, nails may become grossly thickened. **C,** With the use of a special nail cutter, these nails can be trimmed in the office.

centimeters in length and curves on itself to resemble a ram's horn.

TREATMENT

To treat onychogryphosis, a strong pair of special nail clippers is used to remove the entire nail horn up to where the nail is attached securely to the nail bed (Fig. 14–22C). Subsequent trimming and debridement help the nail become asymptomatic.

To treat onychauxis, the hypertrophied nail is gradually reduced by grinding it with a motorized tool. According to Frank and Freer,[60] *Current Procedural Terminology* code 11721 (debridement of six or more nails) was the most frequently used code (of 300 foot and ankle codes) in 1999. The cost to Medicare for this procedure was $245 million that year. Abramson and Wilton[2,3] advocated reducing hyperkeratotic nails with nail drills and burs. However, they noted that particles 0.5 to 5 μm can become airborne and be inhaled in the respiratory tract. Chronic exposure to nail dust aerosols can lead to conjunctivitis, rhinitis, asthma, coughing, impaired lung function, and hypersensitivity. Of the physicians with chronic exposure to nail dust from grinding hyperkeratotic nails, 31% had abnormally elevated immunoglobulin E levels on radioimmunoassay.

Antifungal medication may be applied either topically or beneath the nail plate. For severely deformed club nails, avulsion of the nail is advised. Later or concurrently, the nail matrix may be ablated with a surgical ablation technique, chemical nail plate destruction, or a terminal Syme amputation.

Onychomycosis

Onychomycosis is a progressive, recurring fungal infection that originates in the nail bed and accounts for 50% of all toenail abnormalities. Usually the entry is between the hyponychium and the nail plate. The infection progresses to the nail, resulting in the typical appearance of yellowing and thickening of the nail. A mycotic infection of one or more of the toenails often accompanies tinea pedis (athlete's foot).[124]

Although many people consider this primarily a cosmetic problem, a portion of the patients also experience pain (36%–48%) or limited mobility (41%) as a direct result of onychomycosis.[49,143,144] Pressure necrosis from the nail bed or severe bacterial infections can even cause limb-threatening complications in older patients.[133] The greatest predisposing factors are increasing age and male sex; men are 1.7 to 3.0 times more likely to have a fungal infection than women.[68,69] Patients with vascular disease or diabetes, as well as immunocompromised patients (e.g., patients infected with human immunodeficiency virus [HIV]), also have a higher incidence of onychomycosis than the general population (Box 14–8). With the effectiveness of the newer antifungal agents, diagnosis and treatment are more efficacious.

Zaias[172] has classified onychomycoses into four categories (Box 14–9). *Distal subungual onychomycosis* primarily involves the distal nail bed and hyponychium, with secondary involvement of the undersurface of the nail plate (Fig. 14–23A and B). *White superficial onychomycosis* is an invasion of the toenail plate on the surface of the nail by such organisms as *Trichophyton mentagrophytes* and by *Acremonium* and *Aspergillus* species (Fig. 14–23C). *Proximal subungual onychomycosis* is rare. *Candidal onychomycosis* involves the entire nail plate (Fig. 14–23D).

Onychomycosis is a common disorder of the nail, present in possibly 20% of the population. The prevalence may be much higher than this, but culture or biopsy is not usually done. In patients older than 60 years, involvement can approach 75% of the population. Infection with dermatophytes, such as *Trichophy-*

BOX 14–8   Risk Factors Associated with Onychomycosis

NEUROLOGIC DISORDERS

Hansen's disease (leprosy)
Multiple sclerosis
Peripheral neuropathy
Syphilis

VASCULAR DISORDERS

Arteriosclerotic vascular disease
Buerger's disease (thromboangiitis obliterans)
Chronic thrombophlebitis
Ischemia
Venous stasis

METABOLIC DISORDERS

Chronic alcohol abuse
Diabetes mellitus
Malabsorption syndrome
Malnutrition
Pernicious anemia
Thyroid disease

OTHER SYSTEMIC DISORDERS

Cardiac disease
Congestive heart failure
Chronic obstructive pulmonary disease
Chronic renal disease
Hypertension
Uremia

Modified from Helfand AE: Onychomycosis in the aged: An administrative perspective. *J Am Podiatr Med Assoc* 76:142-145, 1986. Used with permission.

DISTAL SUBUNGUAL ONYCHOMYCOSIS

Dermatophytes

Epidermophyton floccosum
Trichophyton rubrum
Trichophyton mentagrophytes

Yeasts and Molds

Acremonium
Aspergillus
Candida parapsilosis
Fusarium
Scopulariopsis brevicaulis

PROXIMAL SUBUNGUAL ONYCHOMYCOSIS

Dermatophytes

T. rubrum
Trichophyton megninii
Trichophyton schoenleinii
Trichophyton tonsurans

WHITE SUPERFICIAL ONYCHOMYCOSIS

Dermatophytes

T. mentagrophytes

Yeasts and Molds

Acremonium
Aspergillus
Fusarium

CANDIDAL ONYCHOMYCOSIS

Yeasts and Molds

C. parapsilosis
Candida albicans

Modified from Norton LA: *J Am Acad Dermatol* 2:451-467, 1980. Used with permission.

ton rubrum, *T. mentagrophytes*, and *Epidermophyton floccosum*, is much more common than with *Candida* species. Nondermatophytes account for less than 1% of cases of onychomycosis.[119,120] More typically, *Candida* is the cause of infection in children.

With chronic infection, the nail plate thickens and becomes discolored, brittle, and deformed. A buildup of chronic debris beneath the nail plate occurs over time. The thickened nail plate can become detached from the underlying nail bed and become painful when compressed by tight stockings or a constricting toe box.

DISTAL SUBUNGUAL ONYCHOMYCOSIS

Distal subungual onychomycosis is the most common of the four types of mycotic infections (Fig. 14–23A

and B). This deeply seated form of onychomycosis results in yellowish longitudinal streaks within the nail plate. Although the incubation period is unknown, the mode of transmission is thought to be through direct contact of a traumatized nail predisposed to mycotic infection.[78] Serologic and genetic analysis of HLA class I in a homogeneous population showed that persons lacking the HLA-DR53 phenotype were at increased risk for developing *Trichophyton rubrum* onychomycosis.[175] Therefore, HLA-DR53 might provide the immune response necessary to prevent a fungal infection.[145]

The disease often occurs before the sixth decade of life. The infectious organism invades insidiously from the free edge of the nail plate toward the base, resulting in a thickened, discolored, and deformed nail plate. The initial infection occurs in the stratum corneum, the superficial layer of the epidermis. As the inflammation continues, the response of the nail bed is cellular accumulation, nail elevation, and discoloration. With the accumulation of debris beneath the nail, further fungal and microorganism growth occurs. After invading the nail bed, the fungus penetrates the nail plate and causes delamination of the toenail.

Several dermatophytes are associated with subungual onychomycosis. *Trichophyton*, *Epidermophyton*, and *Microsporum* are the usual dermatophytes, and *T. rubrum* is the most common. *Trichophyton interdigitale* and *T. mentagrophytes* can also be present, and *E. floccosum* and nondermatophytes (*Scopulariopsis*, *Aspergillus*, *Fusarium*, and *Candida* species) have been reported.[108] This disease entity is not believed to be contagious.

Endonyx onychomycosis is a variant of distal subungual onychomycosis in which the fungi reach the nail via the skin but invade the nail plate directly instead of infecting the nail bed.[131] Endonyx onychomycosis does not cause hyperkeratosis. Despite the milky-white discoloration of the nail, the nail plate itself is of normal thickness and smooth.[19]

WHITE SUPERFICIAL ONYCHOMYCOSIS

White superficial onychomycosis appears as opaque, white, well-demarcated islands on the surface of the nail plate (Fig. 14–23C). In this infection, the pathogen invades the superficial dorsal aspect of the nail plate, which results in the development of white plaques. This is the rarest form of onychomycosis and is seldom seen except in immunologically compromised patients.[27] The infection typically starts in the periuticle nail plate and then grows distally, involving and destroying the entire nail plate. These plaques of localized fungal growth can progress to more diffuse involvement, invading the entire surface of the nail plate. The toenail can turn brownish and become

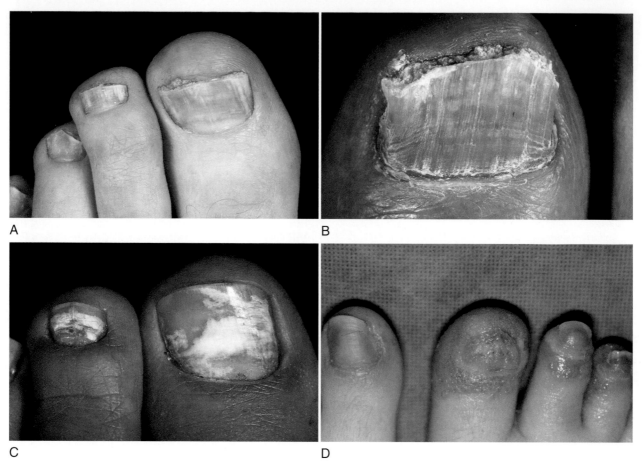

A   B

C   D

Figure 14–23   A, Distal subungual onychomycosis. This is the most common of the four types of mycotic infection. The nails are yellow and thickened, with hyperkeratotic material underneath. **B,** In this advanced case of distal subungual onychomycosis, the involved nail is thickened and opaque, with crumbly material distally. **C,** White superficial onychomycosis. *Trichophyton mentagrophytes* produces a superficial white discoloration of the nail. **D,** In this untreated case, *Candida* infection of the nail plate, with brown discoloration and onycholysis, is present in addition to swelling of the nail fold. (**A-C** from du Vivier A: *Atlas of Clinical Dermatology*, ed 3. Edinburgh, Churchill Livingstone, 2002, p 601.)

roughened and pitted from chronic infection. The most common infectious organism is *T. mentagrophytes* (Table 14–11).[108] Topical antiseptics may be an effective early treatment for this type of onychomycosis.

PROXIMAL SUBUNGUAL ONYCHOMYCOSIS

Proximal subungual onychomycosis occurs infrequently and is typified by whitish discoloration extending distally from underneath the proximal nail fold. *T. rubrum* is the most usual infectious organism. This entity is more common in people infected with HIV.[48,139]

CANDIDAL ONYCHOMYCOSIS

Candidal onychomycosis, characterized by generalized thickening of the nail plate, results from *Candida albicans* or *Candida parapsilosis* infection (Fig. 24–23D). Initially, longitudinal white striations appear within the nail plate. The nail bed thickens, and the distal end

Table 14–11	
Prevalence of Infectious Organisms in White Superficial Onychomycosis	
Organism	**Prevalence (%)**
Trichophyton mentagrophytes	68
Trichophyton rubrum	8
Candida albicans	4
Miscellaneous	8
No growth	12

Modified from Bodman MA, Brlan MR: Superficial white onychomycosis. *J Am Podiatr Med Assoc* 85:205-208, 1995. Used with permission.

of the digit appears bulbous and clubbed. The nail plate can become opaque as well.

DIAGNOSIS

An early sign of mycotic infection is thickening of the distal and lateral borders of the nail plate. The nails can become opaque, and discoloration can occur with chronic infection. The edges of the nail plate can erode and partial or complete loss of the nail plate can occur. As time passes with advanced onychomycosis, it is difficult for the clinician to distinguish among the patterns of mycotic penetration of the nail plate. Although total dystrophic onychomycosis may be considered a separate class of onychomycosis, it is actually a progression of any of the above types, with involvement of the entire nail unit leading to possible permanent scarring of the nail matrix.[131]

When a fungal infection is suspected, diagnosis is attempted by examining a specimen under a light microscope. Vigorous scraping of the nail produces debris that can be moistened with a few drops of 10% potassium hydroxide solution. Hyphae may be seen microscopically. Samples cultured on an appropriate medium can aid in the diagnosis. Although culturing finely ground nail material or debris from beneath the nail is the optimal method of making the diagnosis of onychomycosis, 30% of the results are false negatives.[42,53] Furthermore, the sensitivity of direct microscopy with potassium hydroxide is not foolproof because the procedure is affected by many variables, including the skill of the slide preparer, the microscope used, and the sampling technique. Other methods of diagnosis include staining nail clippings with periodic acid–Schiff stain[101,132] and using in vivo confocal microscopy.[83] It is important, but not always easy, to distinguish onychomycosis from psoriasis. Beginning antifungal medication without a confirmatory diagnosis can be both futile and expensive.

In a review of 169 patients with nail disease, 32% had positive findings on both direct examination and culture, and 20% had positive findings on direct microscopy alone.[58] Only four historical and clinical diagnostic features significantly correlated with positive mycologic results: a history of tinea pedis in the past year; scaling on one or both soles; white, crumbly patches on the nail surface; and an abnormal color of the nail.

SYSTEMIC TREATMENT

In a cumulative meta-analysis that evaluated randomized, controlled trials of systemic antifungal agents for the treatment of onychomycosis, the cure rates with many antifungal drugs were similar.[70] The overall cumulative average (±SD) for mycologic cure with these drugs was as follows: terbinafine (Lamisil), 76% (±3%); pulse-dosed itraconazole (Sporanox), 63% (±7%); continuous-dosed itraconazole, 59% (±5%); fluconazole (Diflucan), 48% (±5%); and griseofulvin (Fulvicin), 60% (±6%). For open studies, the rates were somewhat higher: terbinafine, 83% (±12%); pulse-dosed itraconazole, 84% (±9%); and fluconazole, 79% (±3%).

One open study[174] evaluated the use of terbinafine for the treatment of *T. rubrum* nail bed onychomycosis. With pulse-dosed oral terbinafine (250 mg daily for 7 days every 3 months for approximately 12 months), 39 of 42 patients (93%) were cured. However, only 10 of 17 (59%) were cured when terbinafine was given every 4 months. It was thought that this regimen would not only save money but also lower drug-induced side effects. This use, however, is still off-label. The standard dosage is 250 mg by mouth every day for 90 days.

One study reported on a relatively small number of patients with onychomycosis in high-risk groups (immunocompromised patients, patients with diabetes, and patients with HIV). In these groups, terbinafine was well tolerated and equally effective in patients in all risk groups.[39]

With the use of all pharmacologic agents for treating onychomycosis, whether topical, oral, or parenteral, a frank discussion with the patient should cover side effects, including hypersensitivity, liver toxicity, gastrointestinal disorders, and cardiovascular effects. These drugs are contraindicated during pregnancy because of their teratogenic effects. Hepatotoxicity has been reported in patients, especially older ones, who have a history of liver dysfunction.[44] Other adverse effects include nausea and vomiting, pruritus, abdominal pain, and idiosyncratic liver dysfunction. Elevated liver enzyme levels are uncommon but have been reported in approximately 1 in 10,000 patients.[82]

LOCAL TREATMENT

Local therapy includes mechanical grinding and debridement of the thickened nail plate with a motorized device, curettage of the necrotic subungual tissue, and adequate trimming of the thickened nail plate. For many patients, simple debridement adequately relieves pain and discomfort without the need for surgical or pharmacologic intervention.

TOPICAL TREATMENT

The only topical brush-on treatment for onychomycosis that is approved by the U.S. Food and Drug Administration is an 8% solution of ciclopirox (Penlac) in a lacquer solution, but its effectiveness is limited. A combination of oral and topical antifungal agents has also been advocated. Use of amorolfine 5% nail lacquer (at publication, not approved for use in the

United States) resulted in improved cure rates in severe toenail onychomycosis.[16]

Ciclopirox 1% cream (Loprox), terbinafine 1% cream, and ketoconazole 2% cream (Nizoral) have also been used for topical treatment. Typically, these creams are applied twice daily to the involved toenail and surrounding soft tissue.

Some clinicians prefer avulsion of the thickened nail plate, debridement of the necrotic tissue, and treatment of the matrix and nail bed twice daily. Hettinger and Valinsky[80] advocate nail avulsion to help reduce the overall duration of treatment. After nail avulsion, the area is treated with a thin layer of cream. Therapy is continued until the nail plate has regrown. The authors reported that all nails that grew back were free of mycotic infection. They reported a 96% success rate at an average of 11 months of follow-up. After removal of the infected nail plate, patient compliance was critically important to the overall success rate. Chemical nail plate destruction, surgical ablation, or a terminal Syme amputation may be considered as well. These techniques are discussed elsewhere.

Onychia

Onychia, also known as *onychitis*, occurs with inflammation of the nail matrix and accumulation of granulation tissue around the toenail. It may be associated with poorly fitting footwear or tight stockings, or it can occur after trauma to the distal phalanx, such as stubbing the toe or dropping an object onto the toe. On occasion, osteomyelitis or osteitis occurs and causes painful symptoms.

Initial treatment requires removal of the causative agent. Minimizing trauma or pressure over the toenail can alleviate symptoms. In the presence of an acute bacterial or fungal infection, culture and sensitivity testing should be performed. Appropriate antibiotic therapy may be instituted.[176] Radiography is used to identify any osseous involvement. If acute infection is present, local surgical care includes incision and drainage. Toenail avulsion and, on occasion, surgical ablation of the toenail may be necessary. Localized treatment with topical antifungal agents such as clotrimazole (Lotrimin) or nystatin cream may be helpful. The simultaneous use of roomy footwear or sandals might help to remove pressure from the painful toenail. Often, symptoms subside with time and aggressive conservative treatment.

Onycholysis and Onychomadesis

Onycholysis is separation of the nail plate from the nail bed along the lateral and distal borders. *Onychomadesis* is separation of the entire nail plate, beginning proximally and ending distally. Onychomadesis may be associated with drug reaction, eczema, scarlet fever,

leprosy, lead poisoning, or trauma.[120] Nail ablation may be necessary to treat a chronic condition.

Onycholysis, which occurs more frequently in female patients than in male patients, seems to be associated with local trauma as well as with drug and allergic reactions, eczema, hypothyroidism, hyperthyroidism, lichen planus, bacterial and fungal infections, and vascular insufficiency. *C. albicans* and *Pseudomonas* species are the most common infectious organisms. Trimming of the separated nail plate and application of topical antifungal medication may be helpful in treating this condition. For more severe symptoms, toenail ablation may be necessary.

Nail Bed Disorders

The structure and function of the nail bed may be altered by subungual exostosis, subungual tumors, subungual clavus, subungual hematoma, or subungual verruca.

Subungual Exostosis

Abnormalities of the underlying bone can be diagnosed with the aid of a radiograph. Typically, these involve the distal phalanx. A subungual exostosis must be distinguished from an osteochondroma (see previous section on tumors). Likewise, usually when a lytic lesion is present in the distal phalanx, a benign tumor such as an enchondroma or solitary bone cyst should be considered.

In a patient with chronic complaints of pain, swelling, inflammation, and chronic paronychia, the physician should consider radiography to evaluate the patient for an underlying bone tumor. The development of chronic subungual ulceration should alert the clinician to the possibility of squamous cell carcinoma, probably the most common malignant tumor of the toe.

Subungual Tumors

Subungual and periungual fibromas, exostoses, mucous cysts (Fig. 14–24), glomus tumors, enchondromas, keratoacanthomas, pyogenic granulomas, and other benign lesions occur in the area of the distal phalanx. Malignant tumors, such as squamous cell carcinoma, basal cell carcinoma, and malignant melanoma, can develop in this area as well (see previous section on tumors).

Subungual Clavus

A hyperkeratotic lesion in the subungual region is characterized by the accumulation of debris beneath the nail plate. A callus can develop in this area because of pressure from a confining toe box or long-term use of tight stockings. Vascular insufficiency, psoriasis, dia-

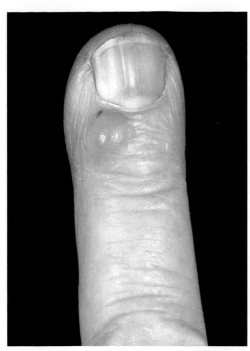

Figure 14–24 Mucous cyst. A smooth, well-circumscribed, firm, flesh-colored nodule overlies the distal interphalangeal joint, causing a deformity in the nail. This lesion is best treated by excision of the osteophytes at the distal interphalangeal joint or fusion of the joint. (From du Vivier A: *Atlas of Clinical Dermatology*, ed 3. Edinburgh, Churchill Livingstone, 2002, p 619.)

betes, localized fungal infection, and various systemic diseases also can cause subungual clavus. As the amount of debris accumulates, a yellowish-gray cast develops in the toenail. Typically, a patient complains of pain caused by external pressure from a closed-toe shoe. The differential diagnosis includes subungual exostosis, subungual osteochondroma, trauma, subungual verruca, and glomus tumor.

Debridement of the hyperkeratotic clavus is the treatment of choice. Trimming of the detached nail plate facilitates debridement of the necrotic tissue.

Subungual Hematoma

Hemorrhagic accumulation between the nail bed and the nail plate is a *subungual hematoma*. Typically, this occurs with trauma to the nail bed and rupture of small capillaries in this region. Crushing or shearing trauma to the nail produces painful subungual hemorrhage manifested by a dusky swelling of the nail plate. The differential diagnosis of a discolored nail includes subungual exostosis, malignant melanoma, Kaposi's sarcoma, nevus, glomus tumor, and trauma. Within hours after injury, pressure builds up because of bleeding beneath the nail plate. Edema, pain with movement of the digit, and blue or black discoloration

under the nail can prompt the patient to seek evaluation and treatment. Fracture of the distal phalanx occurs in 25% of patients.

A syringe needle, nail drill, trephine, dental bur, fine-point scalpel blade (no. 11), heated paper clip, or carbon dioxide laser[79] may be used to penetrate the nail bed and evacuate a trapped hematoma (Fig. 14–25A and B). Palamarchuk and Kerzner[125] describe using a handheld cautery unit to decompress a subungual hematoma. With minimal pressure on the nail, the cautery unit creates a small hole in the nail, and the hematoma is easily evacuated. Radiographs may be necessary to rule out a fracture. Further therapy may include oral antibiotics.

Tucker et al[157] studied crush injuries of the distal phalanx with concomitant nail bed injuries. In general, if the hematoma was less than 20% of the area of the nail plate, patients were not treated. A larger area of hematoma suggests the possibility of a nail bed injury and possible fracture of the distal phalanx. With an open injury, inspection of the nail bed and repair of a lacerated nail bed or matrix may be necessary. An open fracture should be treated routinely like any open fracture. Fox[59] reported a case of osteomyelitis after an open nail bed injury and recommended aggressive irrigation and debridement and parenteral antibiotics to minimize the risk of subsequent infection.

Subungual Verruca

A subungual or periungual verruca can occur beneath the nail plate or in the nail groove (see Fig.14–7). The appearance of a verruca is similar to that of a wart on any other part of the foot. When a verruca involves the subungual tissue, care must be taken in the treatment plan to avoid damage to the nail matrix. Usually the wart can be ablated with chemical treatment, excision, or electrocautery or with a combination of these treatments.

Nail Fold Disorders

Nail fold disorders include paronychia, onychophosis, pyogenic granuloma, herpetic whitlow, and periungual verruca.

Paronychia

Paronychia is an inflammation of the nail groove that usually affects the hallux but can affect the lesser toes as well (Fig. 14–26A). It either is accompanied by an ingrown toenail or is a forerunner of an ingrown toenail. Paronychia varies in severity and can occur as a mild cellulitis. More severe cellulitis of the nail fold is characterized by swelling, erythema, pain, tenderness, and often a purulent discharge from beneath the nail fold. Secondary dystrophic changes of the nail are

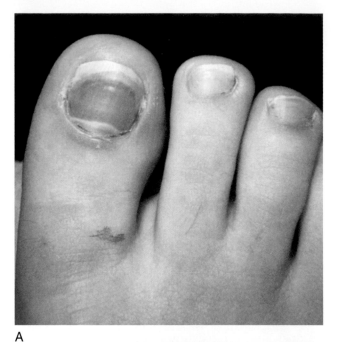

A

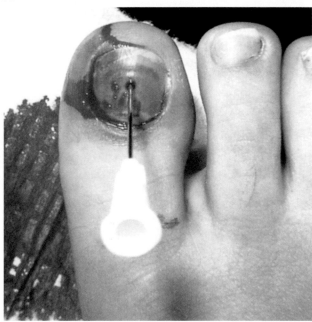

B

Figure 14–25 Subungual hematoma. **A,** When there is considerable pain or swelling under the nail after hematoma formation, the hematoma may be released. **B,** A small hole created in the nail allows blood to drain, but the procedure must be done soon after injury because coagulated blood cannot be drained. (From Dockery GL, Crawford ME: *Color Atlas of Foot and Ankle Dermatology.* Philadelphia, Lippincott-Raven, 1999, p 344.)

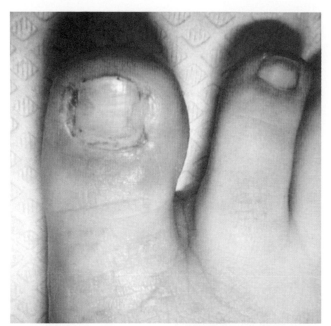

A

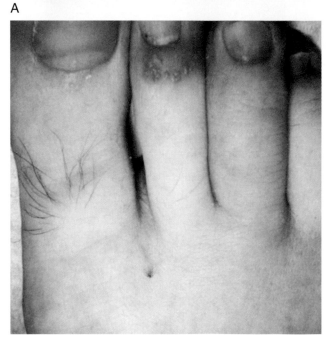

B

Figure 14–26 **A,** Paronychia. Typical appearance of *Staphylococcus* infection with localized swelling, erythema, and draining at the toenail border. Paronychia either is accompanied by an ingrown toenail or is a forerunner of an ingrown toenail. **B,** Herpes simplex. The characteristic foot lesion is a cluster of minute painful red lesions on the second toe, proximal to the nail bed. This condition rarely results in herpetic whitlow or paronychia. (**A** from Dockery GL: *Cutaneous Disorders of the Lower Extremity.* Philadelphia, WB Saunders, 1997, p 41. Used with permission. **B** from Dockery GL, Crawford ME: *Color Atlas of Foot and Ankle Dermatology.* Philadelphia, Lippincott-Raven, 1999, p 158.)

commonly seen, and chronic paronychia involvement with *Candida* infection can occur. At times the infection extends to the nail matrix, in which case it is termed *onychia*. Unlike onychia, paronychia by itself is rarely caused by skin disorders such as herpes simplex (Fig. 14–26B). When extrinsic pressure from a confining toe box crowds the tissue on the medial aspect of the nail, a severe infection can result. Granulation tissue and extensive ulceration in the nail groove are characteristic of chronic changes.

TREATMENT

Treatment of paronychia consists of the following steps:

1. Relieve extrinsic pressure from footwear.
2. Excise a 2-mm linear portion of the nail margin to relieve the cutting effect of the edematous nail groove.
3. Paint the granulation tissue with a silver nitrate stick.
4. Apply a fungicidal ointment and cover with a sterile dressing.

Onychophosis

Onychophosis occurs with an accumulation of callus within the lateral nail groove and involves the great toe more often than the lesser toes. This can occur with extrinsic pressure from a tight-fitting toe box, with pronation of the foot and abduction of the hallux, or with an incurved nail plate. Erythema and swelling typically occur in the nail groove, and this can develop into an ingrown toenail. Pain is often associated with this condition. The differential diagnosis includes subungual clavus, onychia, paronychia, and onychocryptosis.

The initial treatment involves shaving or debridement of the callus. With a purulent infection, partial avulsion of the nail and eventual ablation of the nail matrix may be necessary. Radiographs may be helpful in ruling out a subungual exostosis, which can occur with similar symptomatic findings.

Pyogenic Granuloma

Pyogenic granuloma, first described by Hartzell[73] in 1904, is a vascular lesion that develops from connective tissue.[25,54] The cause is unknown, but trauma is often suspected. It can occur at any age, range from red to dark blue or black, and grow to be 2 to 10 mm. It grows rapidly and tends to bleed and ulcerate. It can develop secondary to trauma along the lateral nail fold (Fig. 14–27A). The differential diagnosis includes onychia, Kaposi's sarcoma, glomus tumor, periungual verruca, melanoma, fibroma, hemangioma, angiosarcoma, and basal cell carcinoma. It may be pedunculated or sessile and is often complicated by a staphylococcal infection (Fig. 14–27B).

Typical treatment involves surgical excision, cauterization with silver nitrate, electrocautery, or laser. After treatment, moist dressings and antibiotics may be indicated. If the bone becomes infected, the lesion must be curetted and left to drain, or it can be filled with a bone graft substitute mixed with the appropriate antibiotic (Fig. 14–27C-E).

Herpetic Whitlow

Herpetic whitlow[88] is a primary infection with a herpesvirus. It often occurs symptomatically as a painful group of vesicles on one or more swollen toes (see Fig. 14–26B). The vesicles are often surrounded by an erythematous base. Regional lymphangitis may be associated with this condition, and the infection may be confused with bacterial infection or impetigo.

Herpetic whitlow should be distinguished from a bacterial infection, which can require systemic antibiotics and incision and drainage. A typical antibiotic regimen is not effective with a viral infection. Oral antiviral medication, such as acyclovir (Zovirax), may be successful in decreasing symptoms.

Periungual Verruca

A periungual wart is located on the margin of the nail plate and resembles warts found elsewhere on the foot (see Fig. 14–7). Of viral origin, verrucae require careful treatment to prevent trauma to the nail matrix, which can cause a permanent nail deformity. Treatment varies from chemical ablation of the wart to electrocautery or cryotherapy. Surgical excision may also be considered. If a lesion persists despite treatment, or if there is recurrence or atypia, a biopsy should be done to rule out verrucous carcinoma, the treatment of which is wide and deep surgical excision. Amputation is reserved for advanced lesions not amenable to excision.[158]

Nail Matrix Disorders

Disorders of the nail matrix can result in an abnormality of the nail plate. Ridging, atrophy, partial or complete anonychia, and pterygium formation can occur after trauma.

Anonychia

Anonychia, or the absence of toenails, may be an inherited condition[161,176] or it can occur after surgical destruction of a nail matrix (Fig. 14–28). It can also occur with systemic illnesses, vascular insufficiency, Raynaud's disease, and frostbite. Often the destruction of the nail matrix that leads to anonychia is surgically induced as a treatment of chronic nail conditions. No

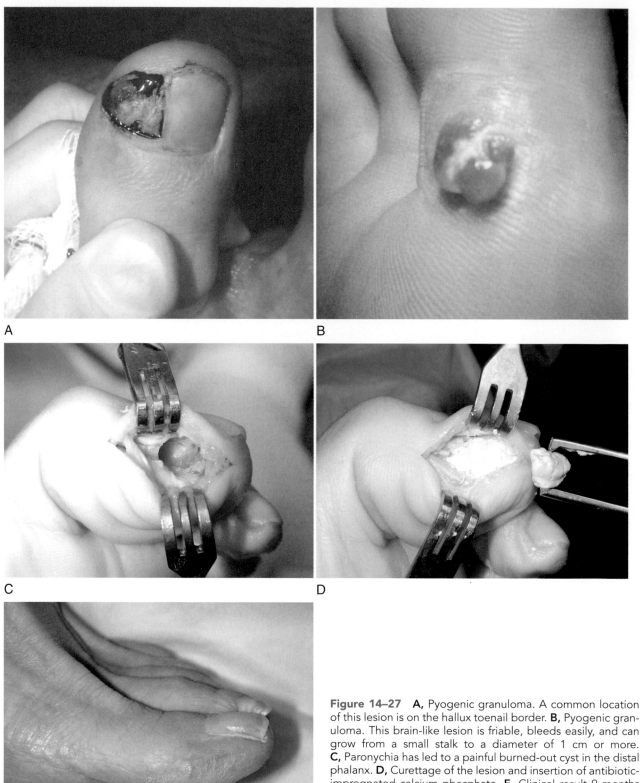

Figure 14–27   A, Pyogenic granuloma. A common location of this lesion is on the hallux toenail border. **B,** Pyogenic granuloma. This brain-like lesion is friable, bleeds easily, and can grow from a small stalk to a diameter of 1 cm or more. **C,** Paronychia has led to a painful burned-out cyst in the distal phalanx. **D,** Curettage of the lesion and insertion of antibiotic-impregnated calcium phosphate. **E,** Clinical result 9 months postoperatively. (**A** from Mann RA, Coughlin MJ: *The Video Textbook of Foot and Ankle Surgery.* St. Louis, Medical Video Productions, 1990. Used with permission. **B** from Dockery GL: *Cutaneous Disorders of the Lower Extremity.* Philadelphia, WB Saunders, 1997, p 42.)

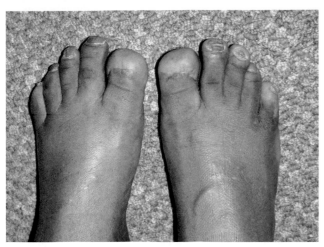

Figure 14–28 Anonychia. Anonychia may be an inherited condition, but in this patient it resulted from a bilateral terminal Syme's amputation for onychogryphosis.

treatment is usually warranted for acquired or congenital anonychia.

Pterygium

With pterygium, the cuticle grows forward on the nail plate and splits it into two or more portions. Zaias[173] noted that it occurs more often in the fourth and fifth digits. Pardo-Castello and Pardo[128] reported that it occurs more commonly in association with leprosy and peripheral neuritis. Other disease entities that can occur with pterygium include vascular insufficiency, Raynaud's disease, scleroderma, and lichen planus.

Atrophy and Hypertrophy

Hypertrophy of the nail matrix results in increased thickness of the nail plate and nail bed. The nail plate can become grooved, abnormally raised, and elongated. With hypertrophy, onychogryphosis or onychauxis develops.[176] At the other end of the spectrum, atrophy of the matrix can develop temporarily, with resultant transverse ridges or lines in the nail plate, which are called *Beau's lines*. These occur when the growth of the nail matrix is suddenly arrested. As regrowth occurs, a normal nail plate develops and leaves a transverse line. This appears to be associated with increased fever, infection, and arthritis. Thinning of the nail plate can occur with anemia and lichen planus.

Pathologic Keratinization

The cells of the nail matrix can differentiate abnormally in association with a systemic disease, such as psoriasis, when keratin formation is increased in the nail bed. An abnormal rate of keratinization can occur

with a fungal infection and may be associated with onychoschizia, koilonychia, and leukonychia.

Onychoschizia is a distal fissuring or splitting of the nail plate (Fig. 14–29A). Delamination can occur, with longitudinal separation of the layers of the nail plate. Hematologic disorders, trauma, infection, hypovitaminosis, and dermatologic disorders can lead to onychoschizia.

Koilonychia is a concavity of the nail plate or a spoon-shaped nail (Fig. 14–29B). Genetic factors, endocrine disorders, thyroid disease, infection, hematologic abnormalities, Raynaud's disease, and nail bed tumors are all causes of koilonychia. The thickness of the nail plate varies, but it remains smooth and commonly opacifies.

Leukonychia is a whitish discoloration or spot on the nail plate (Fig. 14–29C). Several nails may be involved. Variations of leukonychia include punctate discoloration or transverse striations 1 to 2 mm in width that resemble Mees's lines. Opacification may be partial (as in Hodgkin's disease), complete (as in Hansen's disease), or longitudinal (as in Darier's disease).

Conservative and Surgical Treatment

Conservative treatment is often used with stage I infections of the toenail and with a prominent and painful toenail edge. Typical conservative treatment involves elevation of the lateral toenail plate from an inflamed or impinged nail fold. A wisp of cotton is carefully inserted beneath the edge of the nail plate (Fig. 14–30A and B).[34,75,114] With elevation of the nail plate, care must be taken not to fracture the toenail when the cotton is inserted. A digital anesthetic block may be used to decrease pain when the nail plate is elevated. Collodion may be added to the cotton wisp for longevity.

The patient is encouraged to soak the toe twice daily in a tepid salt solution. The toenail region is then dried and the inflamed area coated with a desiccating solution, such as gentian violet or alcohol. Usually the patient returns for a follow-up visit when the cotton wisp is to be removed. As the erythema diminishes, the patient is instructed to replace the cotton wisp. Desiccating agents are used until inflammation has subsided. The cotton packing must be replaced until the nail plate has grown beyond the distal extent of the nail fold. Usually nail growth is approximately 2 mm per month, so the estimated duration of treatment can be calculated for the patient.

After the length of the nail plate is adequate, the patient is instructed in proper transverse trimming of the nail plate. Care is taken not to pick or tear the nail plate because this can cause recurrent infection.

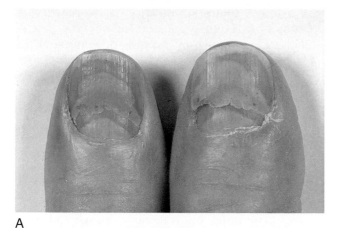

A

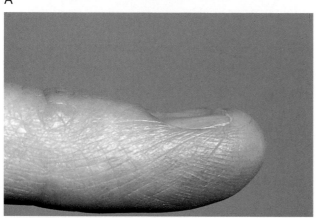

B

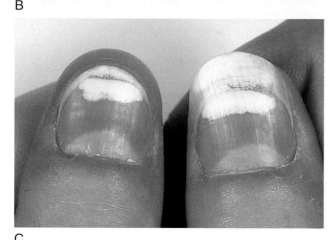

C

Figure 14–29 **A,** Onychoschizia. Shedding of the nails. This results from a severe illness when nail growth slows or ceases temporarily. **B,** Koilonychia. The nail is concave rather than convex and is thus spoon shaped. **C,** Leukonychia. White spots in the nails are common. Gross lesions can occur. The cause is unknown, but trauma may be relevant. (**A-C** from du Vivier A: *Atlas of Clinical Dermatology,* ed 3. Edinburgh, Churchill Livingstone, 2002, pp 611, 613.)

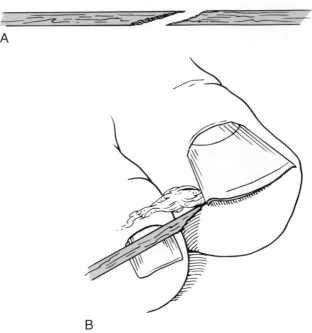

A

B

Figure 14–30 Method of elevating the lateral margin of the nail plate. **A,** A cotton-tipped applicator is broken to create a sharp point. **B,** A wisp of cotton is placed under the impinging edge of the nail plate.

Diagonal trimming of the nail can initially decrease the inflammation associated with acute infection, but it tends to postpone definitive treatment. Dixon[46] noted that "the nail fold tissue will quickly exploit the absence of the nail and can result in recurrence" (see Fig. 14–19).

Treatment of ingrown toenails is individualized for each patient. Heifetz[75] observed that only during stage I can conservative methods be adequately used. When conservative care has been unsuccessful or when acute (stage II) or chronic (stage III) infection has occurred, aggressive nail care is necessary. Alternatives include partial nail plate avulsion; complete toenail avulsion; plastic reduction of the nail lip; partial onychectomy; nail splinting with a hemicylindrical, longitudinal plastic tube cut from thin plastic tubing[1,71]; packing the lateral nail fold with a rolled, alcohol-soaked strip of cotton; complete onychectomy; Syme's amputation of the toe; and carbon-dioxide laser matrixectomy (83% effective in one study[168]).

Digital Anesthetic Block

A digital anesthetic block is usually sufficient anesthesia for any of the toenail procedures.[109] A toe is usually anesthetized within 10 minutes after injection of 1% lidocaine (4 mL in each side of the toe and 1 mL as a dorsal subcutaneous block, using a 1.5-inch 25-gauge needle and a 10-mL syringe).

Buffering 1% lidocaine with a small amount of sodium bicarbonate (in a 9:1 ratio with sodium bicarbonate, 44 mEq/50 mL) decreases the pain of the injection by increasing the pH of normally acidic anesthetic solutions.[20] It can also increase the effectiveness of the lidocaine and prolong its duration of action. Lidocaine (1% and 2%), 0.5% bupivacaine, and 0.5% ropivacaine have all been effective as local anesthetic agents. However, sodium bicarbonate precipitates in bupivacaine and ropivacaine, so it is best used with lidocaine.

The technique involves using the anesthetic solution to raise a small skin wheal on the dorsomedial aspect of the hallux. The needle is directed in a dorsoplantar direction to anesthetize the dorsal and plantar digital sensory nerves. After this is completed, the needle is turned horizontally and the dorsal aspect of the great toe infiltrated. The needle is then withdrawn and inserted at the lateral base of the great toe, and the dorsolateral and plantar lateral digital nerves are anesthetized (Figs. 14–31A-C and 14–32A-C).

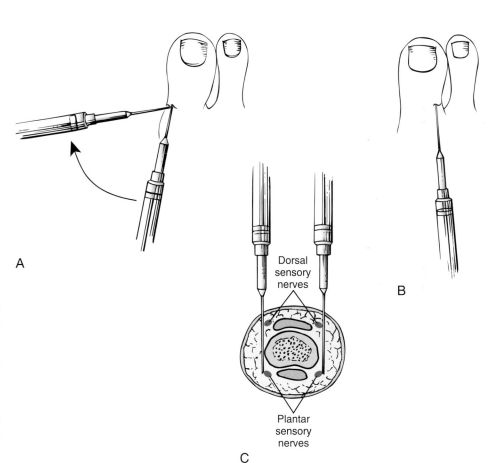

A

B

C

Dorsal sensory nerves

Plantar sensory nerves

Figure 14–31 Technique of digital anesthetic block with 1% lidocaine. **A,** Initially, a medial wheal is raised, and the needle is advanced in a dorsoplantar direction. The needle is then turned horizontally, and the dorsum of the toe is blocked. **B,** A second injection is done to anesthetize the lateral aspect of the toe. **C,** A cross section shows the path of the needles.

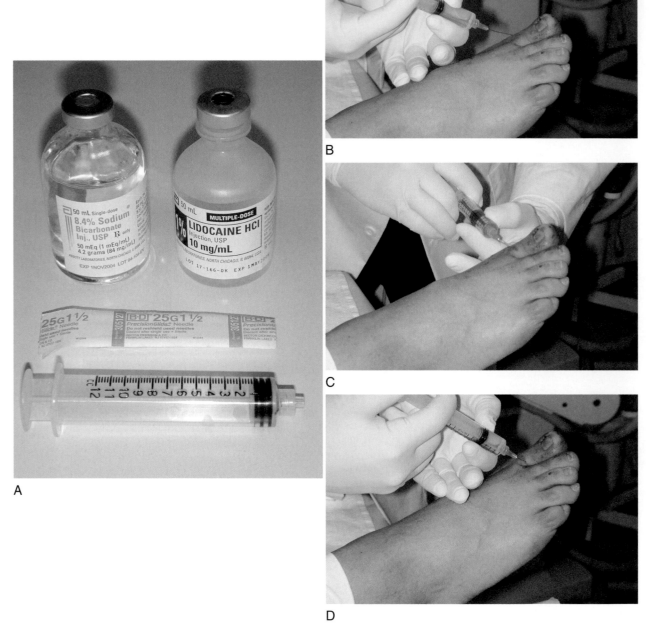

Figure 14–32   Technique of digital anesthetic block with 1% lidocaine. **A,** A 25-gauge needle, 1% lidocaine anesthetic solution without epinephrine, and sodium bicarbonate (44 mEq/50 mL) are used in the digital block. **B,** Initially a medial wheal is raised, and the needle is advanced in a dorsoplantar direction. **C,** The needle is then turned horizontally, and the dorsum of the toe is blocked. **D,** The needle is then inserted in a dorsoplantar direction on the lateral side of the toe to anesthetize the lateral digital nerve.

PARTIAL NAIL PLATE AVULSION

Surgical Technique

1. A digital anesthetic block is established and the toe is cleansed in a routine manner.
2. A 0.25-inch Penrose drain or commercially available doughnut tubing is used as a tourniquet.
3. The outer edge of the toenail plate is elevated proximally to the cuticle (see Fig. 14–18A and B and video clip 55).
4. Scissors or small bone cutters are used to section the nail longitudinally (see Fig. 24–18C and D).
5. Care is taken to remove only as much nail as necessary. The nail is then grasped with a hemostat and avulsed (see Fig. 14–18E and F). The nail bed is examined to ensure that no spike of nail tissue remains.
6. A gauze compression dressing is applied and changed as needed until drainage subsides, usually within a few days (see Fig. 14–18G).

Postoperative Care

After removal of the edge of the nail plate, acute or chronic infection usually subsides. Antibiotics may be used, depending on the severity of the infection.

Aftercare is important for a successful outcome following partial toenail avulsion. With distal growth of the nail plate, the advancing edge is at risk for recurrent infection. A cotton wisp is placed beneath the advancing edge to elevate the nail plate. A digital block may be necessary to replace subsequent packs. The patient is instructed in the technique of packing the toenail plate edge with a cotton wisp, and packing is continued until the nail edge has advanced past the distal extent of the nail groove.

Lloyd-Davies and Brill[107] reported a 47% recurrence rate of infection after partial nail plate avulsion. Another 33% of patients reported residual symptoms. Keyes[93] reported a 77% incidence of recurrence.

COMPLETE TOENAIL AVULSION

With a more extensive infection, complete toenail avulsion may be performed.

Surgical Technique

1. A digital anesthetic block is used and the toe cleansed as usual.
2. A 0.25-inch Penrose drain or a commercially available tubular tourniquet may be applied.
3. The nail plate is elevated from the nail bed and matrix (Fig. 14–33A).
4. The cuticle is incised and elevated from the nail plate.
5. The toenail is avulsed by grasping it with a hemostat (Fig. 14–33B). Usually this is associated with immediate bleeding, and a compression dressing is applied. Hemostasis is usually prompt.
6. After 24 hours, daily soaking is begun in a tepid salt solution.
7. The bandage is replaced and changed daily until drainage has subsided.

Antibiotics may be prescribed, depending on the severity of the infection. Reepithelialization of the nail bed occurs over 2 to 3 weeks. As the nail grows, the advancing edges should be elevated with a cotton wisp to prevent recurrence of a toenail infection.

Murray and Bedi[115] reviewed a series of 200 patients who underwent various toenail procedures. Of the 145 patients who underwent a simple toenail avulsion, 64% experienced recurrent symptoms after the initial procedure, 86% experienced recurrence after a second procedure, and 80% had recurrence after more than two avulsions.

Although toenail avulsion can give dramatic relief of not only infection but also symptoms, the rate of cure after toenail avulsion is quite low. Typically a second procedure must be performed. Dixon[46] noted a much higher recurrence rate of infection when multiple avulsions of a single toenail were performed. Lloyd-Davies and Brill[107] reported that within 6 months, 31% of patients required further treatment after total nail plate avulsion. Palmer and Jones[126] reported a 70% recurrence of symptoms.

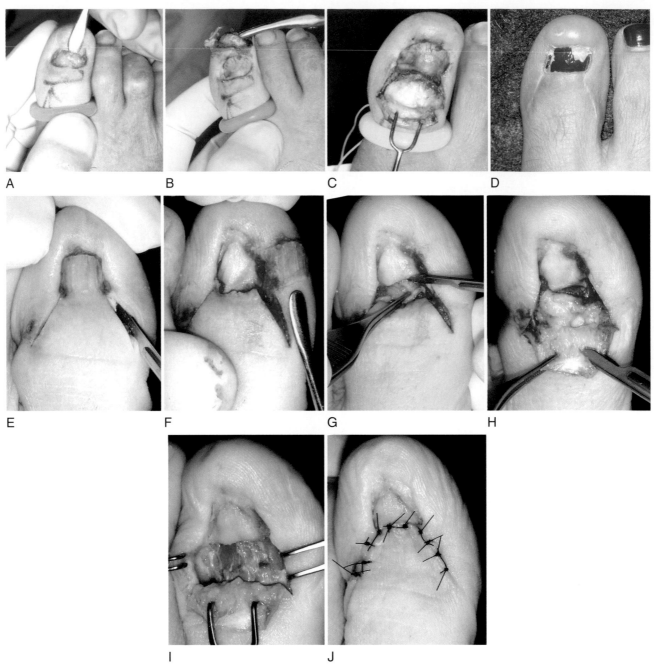

Figure 14–33 Technique of complete toenail avulsion with the Zadik procedure. **A,** Nail is freed from the nail bed. **B,** Nail is removed. **C,** Oblique cuts in soft tissue at the base of the nail allow the germinal matrix to be removed. Afterward, the proximal nail fold is repaired to the nail bed. Care is taken so that the extensor tendon is not excised from the distal phalanx. **D,** Clinical results 8 months later. **E,** Oblique cuts are made at the base of the nail plate. **F,** The nail plate is released with an elevator and removed. **G,** The germinal matrix is sharply excised from the nail bed and removed. **H,** The ventral nail fold is retracted. **I,** Complete removal of the germinal matrix. **J,** Closure of the ventral nail fold to the nail bed.

PLASTIC REDUCTION OF THE NAIL LIP

A plastic nail lip reduction may be used for a younger patient who has mild to moderate disease. With an acute infection, a partial toenail avulsion is performed initially. After the acute infection resolves, a plastic nail lip reduction is performed.

Surgical Technique

1. A digital anesthetic block is used and the toe is cleansed in the usual manner.
2. A 0.25-inch Penrose drain or a commercially available tubular tourniquet is used for hemostasis.
3. A spindle-shaped section, approximately 3 mm × 1 cm and triangular in cross section, is excised from the site of the nail lip.
4. The incision extends from the distal portion of the toe to approximately 5 mm proximal to the nail fold and is located about 2 mm from the lateral nail groove (Fig. 14–34A and B).
5. Excess subdermal fat is excised.
6. The skin margins are coapted with interrupted 3-0 nylon sutures. The closure draws the nail groove laterally and downward (Fig. 14–34C and D).
7. A sterile dressing is applied and changed as needed until drainage has subsided.
8. Sutures are removed 3 weeks after the procedure.

Alternative Procedure

Bouche[29] has described distal dermatoplasty of the hallux to treat clubbing of the tip of the great toe after total nail plate loss (see Figs. 14–2 and 14–17). In a small series of four patients, Keyes[93] reported a 25% recurrence rate with this procedure.

PARTIAL ONYCHECTOMY (WINOGRAD'S OR HEIFETZ'S PROCEDURE)

Partial onychectomy is performed only after an acute infection has resolved, usually after a partial nail plate avulsion.[75,76,164,165] Cadaveric studies have shown that a straight needle passed proximally along the floor of the lateral

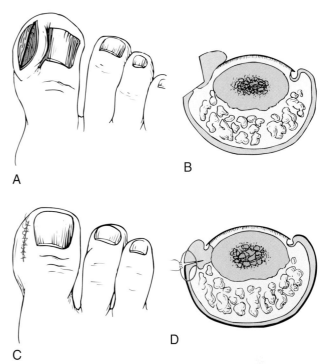

Figure 14–34 Soft tissue wedge resection for ingrown toenail. **A,** A triangular section is removed from the lateral aspect of the nail groove. **B,** Cross section after excision. **C,** The nail lip and groove are pulled down after the nail margins are sutured. **D,** Cross section after suturing.

nail groove defines the lateral extent of the nail matrix.[11] This helps the operator identify the lateral extent of the germinal matrix.

Surgical Technique

1. A digital anesthetic block is used, and the toe is cleansed as usual.
2. A 0.25-inch Penrose drain or a commercially available tubular tourniquet is used for hemostasis.
3. The border of the nail is freed up from surrounding tissue, as previously described, and the border of the nail is cut using heavy, strong scissors or wire cutters. The nail is then removed (Fig. 14–35A-G).
4. With the Heifetz procedure (video clip 56), the resection is carried just distal to the terminal extent of the lunula (Fig. 14–36A). With the Winograd procedure (video clip 57), not only is the nail matrix excised, but the nail bed is resected as well (Fig. 14–36B).

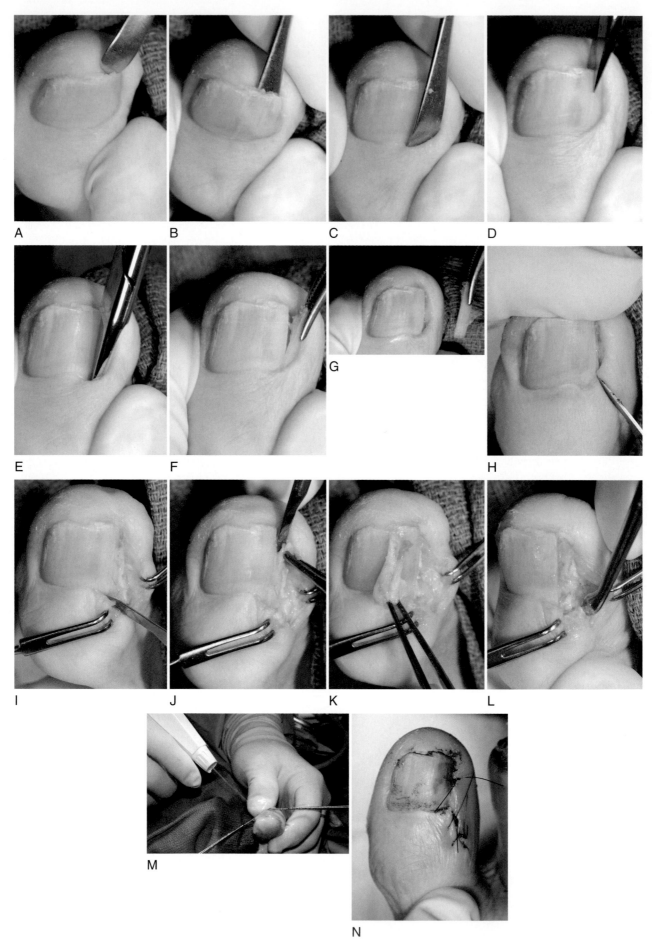

Figure 14–35 Winograd's procedure for partial onychectomy. This patient had a history of repeated lateral ingrown toenail of the right great toe. Onychocryptosis is not present in these photos. **A,** A Freer elevator is used to release the lateral nail from the nail bed. **B,** A Freer elevator is pushed past the germinal matrix. **C,** The eponychium is released from the nail. **D,** The nail is cut along the lateral border using sharp, strong scissors or a wire cutter. **E,** Scissors are pushed proximally to cut the entire nail. **F,** The nail is grasped with a hemostat. **G,** The nail is pulled free from the nail bed. **H,** An oblique 6-mm incision is made from the corner of the eponychium. **I,** The germinal matrix is excised in line with the nail cut. **J,** The nail bed is excised from the proximal phalanx. **K,** The nail bed and germinal matrix are removed. **L,** Remaining remnants of the germinal matrix and nail bed are curetted. **M,** The wound is irrigated thoroughly. **N,** At 2 weeks, the 4-0 nylon sutures may be removed.

5. An oblique incision is made at the apex of the nail bed (Fig. 14–35H). The proximal nail matrix and edge of the cuticle are excised. Care is taken to avoid injury to the extensor tendon insertion and to avoid penetration of the interphalangeal joint.

6. The germinal matrix has a pearly white color and a leathery texture. It extends into the nail fold laterally, and for the Winograd procedure it must be completely excised along with the nail bed (Fig. 14–35 I-K). Applying methylene blue to stain the nail matrix can help the surgeon identify the lateral extent of the germinal matrix.

7. In the Winograd procedure, the remaining nail bed and matrix are curetted from the cortex of the distal phalanx (Fig. 14–35L).

8. The wound is thoroughly irrigated and the skin edges are coapted with interrupted nylon suture (Fig. 14–35M and N).

9. A compression dressing is applied and changed at 24 hours (see Fig. 14–18G). Sub-sequent dressings are changed weekly until drainage resolves. Prophylactic antibiotics may be prescribed, depending on the surgeon's preference or the patient's risk of infection. Sutures are removed 2 weeks postoperatively.

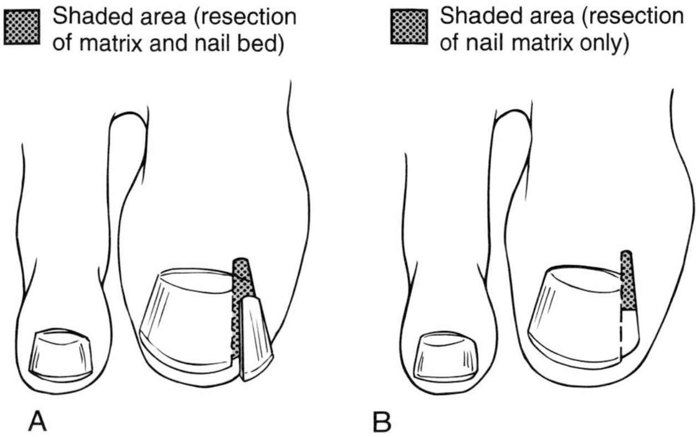

Results and Complications

Murray and Bedi,[115] in a review of 200 patients, reported a 27% recurrence rate after a Winograd procedure and a 50% recurrence rate after a double Winograd procedure. Clarke and Dillinger[36] reported their experience with the Winograd procedure: Of 29 procedures evaluated, one third had unsatisfactory results, including nine recurrences and two patients who reported continued discomfort at follow-up (range, 8 to 18 months). Palmer and Jones[126] reported a 29% recurrence rate after a Winograd resection. In a series of 528 patients who had an ablation of the lateral matrix, Gabriel et al[62] reported a 1.7% recurrence rate and a 79% satisfaction rate. Winograd[165] reported a 15% recurrence rate among 20 patients. Pettine et al[130] reported that with the Heifetz procedure, the satisfaction rate was 90% and the recurrence rate was 6%. Keyes[93] reported a 12% recurrence rate with the Heifetz procedure.

Wadhams et al[160] reported the development of 10 epidermal inclusion cysts after 147 partial matrixectomies (6.8%), typically a Winograd procedure. The average time from treatment to development of the inclusion cyst was 5.5 months. Excision of the inclusion cyst was recommended. A well-encapsulated, white, glistening mass was noted at surgery.

Alternative Procedure

Electrocautery ablation has been recommended as yet another procedure. A single-sided Teflon-coated spatula (to protect the dorsal tissues) is used to perform a lateral matrixectomy after lateral nail plate removal.[178]

▨ Shaded area (resection of matrix and nail bed)

▨ Shaded area (resection of nail matrix only)

A   B

Figure 14–36 Proposed soft tissue excision for partial onychectomy (shaded area is excised). **A,** Heifetz's procedure. **B,** Winograd's procedure. (**B** from Mann RA, Coughlin MJ: *The Video Textbook of Foot and Ankle Surgery.* St. Louis, Medical Video Productions, 1990.)

COMPLETE ONYCHECTOMY (ZADIK'S PROCEDURE)

On occasion, a patient requires complete and permanent removal of the toenail.[169] This procedure is not performed in the presence of acute infection but usually after an initial toenail avulsion. Surgery should be delayed until infection and inflammation have subsided.

Surgical Technique

1. A digital anesthetic block is performed and the toe is cleansed in the usual manner.
2. A 0.25-inch Penrose drain is used for hemostasis. Alternatively, commercial tourniquets are easy to use; exsanguination is accomplished as they are applied.
3. An oblique incision is made at the medial and lateral apex of the nail folds, and the toenail, if present, is avulsed (see Fig. 14–33B, E, and F and video clip 58). Alternatively, the proximal portion of the nail is removed to explore the nail matrix.
4. The cuticle, eponychium, and proximal nail bed are completely excised.
5. The matrix is excised proximally to the cuticle, laterally into the nail folds, and distally as far as the distal extent of the lunula (see Fig. 14–33G). To assist the surgeon in identifying the lateral extent of the nail matrix, the nail matrix may be stained with methylene blue and dried.[17]
6. The nail matrix is curetted and the remaining tissue excised. Care must be taken to avoid the extensor tendon (see Fig. 14–33C, H, and I). In the fingers, the distance between the nail matrix and the extensor tendon averages 1.2 mm (range, 0.9-1.8 mm).[148]
7. The skin edges are approximated with interrupted 3-0 nylon sutures (Fig. 24–33J). Excess tension should be avoided along the suture line because it can lead to sloughing of the skin.
8. A compression dressing is applied and changed 24 hours postoperatively. Further dressing changes are performed as needed, depending on the amount of drainage.

Postoperative Care

Sutures are removed 2 to 3 weeks postoperatively. The patient should be informed about possible partial regrowth of the toenail. Cosmetic results are usually better than with a Syme amputation, and the remaining nail bed accepts nail polish (see Fig. 14–33D).

Results and Complications

Murray and Bedi[115] reported a 16% recurrence rate with the Zadik procedure. Palmer and Jones[126] reported a 28% failure rate and Townsend and Scott[155] a 50% failure rate with complete onychectomy. Eighty-nine percent of patients reported acceptable results despite the small regrowth, typically in the central region.

Alternative Procedure

The use of a carbon dioxide laser for matrixectomy has had variable success. Apfelberg et al[7] reported a 22% recurrence rate. Wright[167] reported a recurrence rate of 50% after laser toenail ablation and recommended that it not be used for either partial or complete toenail ablation.

TERMINAL SYME'S AMPUTATION (THOMPSON–TERWILLIGER PROCEDURE)

For symptomatic regrowth of toenail tissue or when a patient requires a more reliable excision, a terminal Syme amputation of the distal phalanx may be considered (Figs. 14–37A-C and 14–38 A-D and video clip 59).[154] Nonetheless, a proximal matrixectomy is almost always preferable cosmetically to the bulbous amputation stump that is left with Syme's amputation.

Surgical Technique

1. A digital anesthetic block is used and the toe cleansed in the usual manner.
2. A 0.25-inch Penrose drain or a commercially available tubular tourniquet is used.
3. An elliptical incision is used to resect the nail bed, matrix, and proximal and lateral nail folds. The cuticle and proximal border of skin are excised as well.
4. Any remaining toenail matrix and toenail bed are curetted from the dorsal surface of the distal phalanx.
5. Approximately half the distal phalanx is removed, and the remaining edges of bone are beveled with a rongeur (Fig. 14–38B and C).

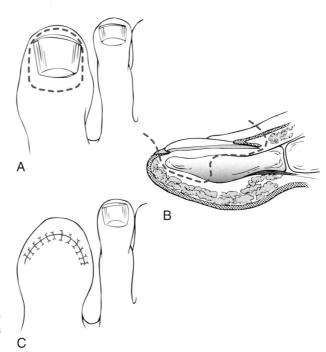

Figure 14–37 Terminal Syme's amputation. **A,** An elliptical incision is used to excise all adjacent soft tissue as well as the toenail bed and matrix. **B,** Distal phalanx is excised. **C,** Excess skin is excised, and the skin edges are approximated.

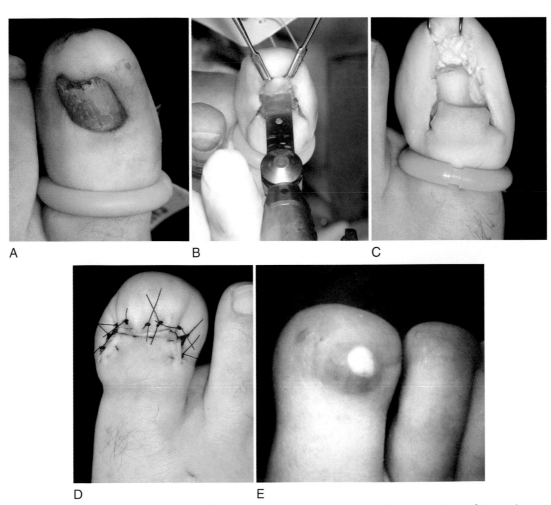

Figure 14–38 Terminal Syme's amputation. **A,** Chronic onychomycosis is present with surrounding soft tissue hypertrophy that is painful. **B,** The entire nail complex has been removed. A saw is used to remove enough of the distal phalanx to close the wound without tension. **C,** A rasp has been used to round off the distal phalanx. There is ample tissue for closure of the hyponychium to the proximal nail fold. **D,** Wound closure. **E,** Regrowth of the nail after incomplete removal of the germinal matrix can produce a cyst. (**E** from Mann RA, Coughlin MJ: *The Video Textbook of Foot and Ankle Surgery.* St. Louis, Medical Video Productions, 1990.)

6. Excess skin is removed, and the skin edges are approximated with nylon suture (Fig. 24–38D).

7. A compression dressing is applied and changed 24 hours postoperatively.

Postoperative Care

Dressing changes are performed as needed until drainage has subsided. Prophylactic antibiotics may be used, depending on the surgeon's preference. Sutures are removed 3 weeks postoperatively.

Results and Complications

Murray and Bedi[115] concluded that the terminal Syme amputation is the definitive technique for recurrent nail plate growth after repeated ablation procedures. Thompson and Terwilliger,[154] in a series of 70 terminal Syme's amputations, reported excellent results with a 4% recurrence rate (Fig. 14–38E). Pettine et al[130] reported a 12% recurrence rate.

Because the cosmetic result is unsightly, some authors suggest that this procedure is appropriate only for malignant tumors invading the distal portion of the terminal phalanx.[17] Otherwise, a proximal matrixectomy (Zadik's procedure) may be performed.

PHENOL-AND-ALCOHOL MATRIXECTOMY

A phenol-and-alcohol matrixectomy may be done instead of a surgical resection (Fig. 14–39A-C). Burzotta et al[31] advised that this procedure could be performed in the presence of concurrent infection. Various techniques for application of phenol, with various success rates, have been reported.

Surgical Technique

1. A digital anesthetic block is used and the toe cleansed as usual.

2. A 0.25-inch Penrose drain or a commercial tourniquet is applied for hemostasis.

3. The nail plate edge is avulsed (Fig. 14–40A) as previously described (see Fig. 14–18A-G).

4. The skin around the matrixectomy site may be coated with petroleum jelly to prevent injury.

5. A cotton-tipped applicator from which most of the cotton has been removed is used to apply the phenol solution. Fresh 88% carbolic acid (phenol) is used.

6. After the cotton-tipped applicator is moistened with phenol, the excess phenol is blotted on a gauze pad. The applicator is inserted into the nail groove and matrix area for 30 seconds to 1 minute (Fig. 14–40B).[4,32,38,135,166] Bostanci et al[28] recommend rubbing the phenol into the tissue for 3 minutes.

7. After the applicator is removed, the area is flushed with alcohol to dilute the phenol

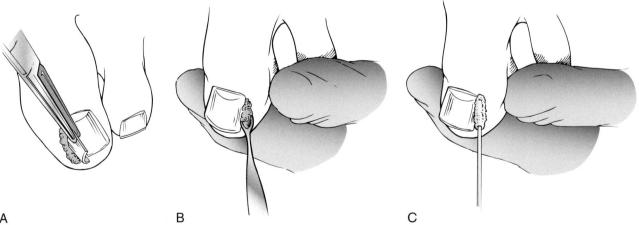

A   B   C

Figure 14–39   Phenol matrixectomy. **A,** The edge of the nail plate is cut with scissors and then avulsed. **B,** The lateral toenail groove and matrix are curetted. **C,** Phenol is applied to cauterize the nail matrix.

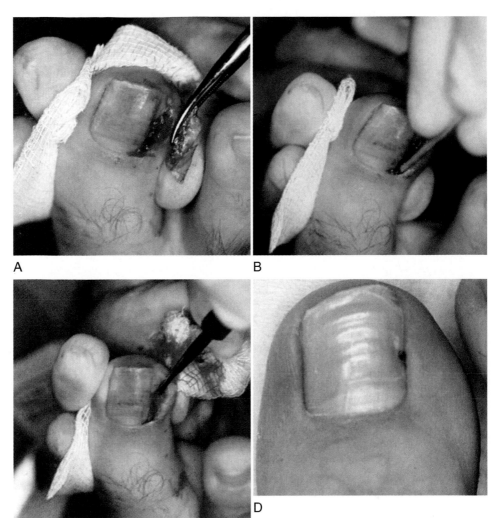

Figure 14–40 Phenol matrixectomy. **A,** The lateral edge of the nail has been removed. **B,** A sterile applicator with the cotton partially removed is used to place 88% carbolic acid on top of the germinal matrix and nail bed. **C,** The granulation tissue may be curetted. **D,** Results 6 months later. (From Salasche SJ. In Sher RK, Daniel CR III [eds]: *Nails: Therapy, Diagnosis, Surgery,* ed 2. Philadelphia, WB Saunders, 1997, p 346.)

and clear it from the wound. The alcohol probably acts less as a neutralizer and more as a diluter, but because the phenol is more soluble in the alcohol, its use is appropriate.

8. Two subsequent 1-minute phenol applications are performed. A tourniquet must be used to keep the wound free of blood because blood dilutes the phenol and reduces its effectiveness.

9. After each phenol application, alcohol is used to flush the nail groove and matrix region.

10. The granulation tissue may be curetted (Fig. 14–40C).

Postoperative Care

A sterile dressing is applied and changed daily until drainage has subsided. The patient is allowed to soak the foot in a tepid salt solution. Although moderate inflammation can occur initially, good results are usually achieved (Fig. 14–40D).

Results and Complications

Regrowth of part or all of the nail plate is the most frequent complication after phenol ablation of the toenail. Chemical matrixectomies have an 80% to 95% satisfaction rate, with recurrence rates of 1% to 40%.

In his long-term analysis of 733 cases, Kuwada[97] reported a recurrence rate of 4.3% after partial matrixectomy and 4.7% after complete matrixectomy. The overall reported complication rate with partial phenol matrixectomies was 9.6% and with total matrixectomies 10.9%. Mori et al,[112] in a review of 75 patients, reported a recurrence rate of 3.9% for the matrix phenolization method and 4.1% for the nail bed periosteal flap procedures. Postoperative pain was less in the matrix phenolization group, but that group had a longer duration of healing than the periosteal flap group.

However, Bostanci et al[28] concluded that phenolization was the treatment of choice for 172 patients who had 350 phenol ablations, with a recurrence rate of 0.57% (nail spikes). This procedure has been reported to be as effective in diabetic patients as in nondiabetic patients.[56,63] Complications can occur from its use, however, including extensive burns resulting in distal toe amputation.[151] In another study, when simple nail avulsion was performed, the addition of phenol dramatically decreased recurrences, but there was increased postoperative inflammation.[138] Finally, in another study, the in vitro maximal effective duration of use of 88% phenol was 1 minute, with little increase in damage with applications between 1 and 2 minutes. Thus, the placement of the phenol is probably more important than the duration of contact between the phenol and tissues.

In their evaluation of phenol matrixectomies, Gilles et al[65] noted that periostitis and mixed bacterial infections developed postoperatively. Rinaldi et al[135] reported a high rate of wound cultures positive for bacteria (87.5%). Altman et al[4] found a decreased incidence of inflammation after using silver sulfadiazine and 1% hydrocortisone cream postoperatively. Although minimal postoperative pain is associated with phenol matrixectomies, prolonged healing is common because of the chemical burn induced.

Alternative Procedure

Sodium hydroxide (10% solution) has been used in a manner similar to phenol. In those cases, however, neutralization of the strong base with 5% acetic acid is important.[156]

REFERENCES

1. Abby NS, Roni P, Amnon B, et al: Modified sleeve method treatment of ingrown toenail. *Dermatol Surg* 28:852-855, 2002.
2. Abramson C, Wilton J: Inhalation of nail dust from onychomycotic toenails: Part I, characterization of particles. *J Am Podiatr Med Assoc* 75:563-567, 1985.
3. Abramson C, Wilton J: Nail dust aerosols from onychomycotic toenails: Part II, clinical and serologic aspects. *J Am Podiatr Med Assoc* 75:631-638, 1985.
4. Altman MI, Suleskey C, Delisle R, et al: Silver sulfadiazine and hydrocortisone cream 1% in the management of phenol matricectomy. *J Am Podiatr Med Assoc* 80:545-547, 1990.
5. Amonette RA, Rosenberg EW: Infection of toe webs by gram-negative bacteria. *Arch Dermatol* 107:71-73, 1973.
6. Antony AK, Anagnos DP: Matrix-periosteal flaps for reconstruction of nail deformity. *Plast Reconstr Surg* 109:1663-1666, 2002.
7. Apfelberg DB, Rothermel E, Widtfeldt A, et al: Progress report on use of carbon dioxide laser for nail disorders. *Curr Podiatr* 32:29-31, 1983.
8. Ashby BS: Primary carcinoma of the nail-bed. *Br J Surg* 44:216-217, 1956.
9. Attiyeh FF, Shah J, Booher RJ, et al: Subungual squamous cell carcinoma. *JAMA* 241:262-263, 1979.
10. Aulicino PL, Hunter JM: Subungual melanoma: Case report and literature review. *J Hand Surg [Am]* 7:167-169, 1982.
11. Austin RT: A method of excision of the germinal matrix. *Proc R Soc Med* 63:757-758, 1970.
12. Baden HP: The physical properties of nail. *J Invest Dermatol* 55:115-122, 1970.
13. Banfield CC, Dawber RP: Nail melanoma: A review of the literature with recommendations to improve patient management. *Br J Dermatol* 141:628-632, 1999.
14. Banfield CC, Redburn JC, Dawber RP: The incidence and prognosis of nail apparatus melanoma: A retrospective study of 105 patients in four English regions. *Br J Dermatol* 139:276-279, 1998.
15. Baran R: Significance and management of congenital malalignment of the big toenail. *Cutis* 58:181-184, 1996.
16. Baran R, Feuilhade M, Combernale P, et al: A randomized trial of amorolfine 5% solution nail lacquer combined with oral terbinafine compared with terbinafine alone in the treatment of dermatophytic toenail onychomycoses affecting the matrix region. *Br J Dermatol* 142:1177-1183, 2000. Erratum in: *Br J Dermatol* 144:448, 2001.
17. Baran R, Haneke E: Matricectomy and nail ablation. *Hand Clin* 18:693-696, 2002.
18. Baran R, Haneke E, Richert B: Pincer nails: Definition and surgical treatment. *Dermatol Surg* 27:261-266, 2001.
19. Baran R, Hay RJ, Tosti A, et al: A new classification of onychomycosis. *Br J Dermatol* 139:567-571, 1998.
20. Bartfield JM, Ford DT, Homer PJ: Buffered versus plain lidocaine for digital nerve blocks. *Ann Emerg Med* 22:216-219, 1993.
21. Bartolomei FJ, Brandwene SM, McCarthy DJ: Bowen's disease. *J Am Podiatr Med Assoc* 76:153-156, 1986.
22. Bean WB: Nail growth: A twenty-year study. *Arch Intern Med* 111:476-482, 1963.
23. Bean WB: Nail growth: 30 years of observation. *Arch Intern Med* 134:497-502, 1974.
24. Bedi TR: Intradermal triamcinolone treatment of psoriatic onychodystrophy. *Dermatologica* 155:24-27, 1977.
25. Berlin SJ, Block LD, Donick II: Pyogenic granuloma of the foot: A review of the English literature and report of four cases. *J Am Podiatry Assoc* 62:94-99, 1972.
26. Berlin SJ, Stewart RC, Margolies MC, et al: Squamous cell carcinoma of the foot with particular reference to nail bed involvement: A report of three cases. *J Am Podiatry Assoc* 65:134-141, 1975.
27. Bodman MA, Brlan MR: Superficial white onychomycosis. *J Am Podiatr Med Assoc* 85:205-208, 1995.
28. Bostanci S, Ekmekci P, Gurgey E: Chemical matrixectomy with phenol for the treatment of ingrowing toenail: A review of the literature and follow-up of 172 treated patients. *Acta Derm Venereol* 81:181-183, 2001.

29. Bouche RT: Distal skin plasty of the hallux for clubbing deformity after total nail loss. *J Am Podiatr Med Assoc* 85:11-14, 1995. Erratum in: *J Am Podiatr Med Assoc* 85:176, 1995.

30. Brown RE: Acute nail bed injuries. *Hand Clin* 18:561-575, 2002.

31. Burzotta JL, Turri RM, Tsouris J: Phenol and alcohol chemical matrixectomy. *Clin Podiatr Med Surg* 6:453-467, 1989.

32. Cangialosi CP, Schnall SJ: A comparison of the phenol–alcohol and Suppan nail techniques (onychectomy/matrixectomy). *Curr Podiatr* 30:25-26, 1981.

33. Cavolo DJ, D'Amelio JP, Hirsch AL, et al: Juvenile subungual osteochondroma: Case presentation. *J Am Podiatry Assoc* 71:81-83, 1981.

34. Ceh SE, Pettine KA: Treatment of ingrown toenail. *J Musculoskel Med* 7:62-82, 1990.

35. Chinn S, Jenkin W: Proximal nail groove pain associated with an exostosis. *J Am Podiatr Med Assoc* 76:506-508, 1986.

36. Clarke BG, Dillinger KA: Surgical treatment of ingrown toenail. *Surgery* 21:919-924, 1946.

37. Conant MA, Wiesenfeld SL: Multiple glomus tumors of the skin. *Arch Dermatol* 103:481-485, 1971.

38. Coughlin M: Ingrown toenails: Procedures to relieve pain and forestall recurrence. *Consultant* 35:965-975, 1995.

39. Cribier BJ, Bakshi R: Terbinafine in the treatment of onychomycosis: A review of its efficacy in high-risk populations and in patients with nondermatophyte infections. *Br J Dermatol* 150:414-420, 2004.

40. Dale SJ, Simons J: Subungual squamous cell carcinoma. *J Am Podiatry Assoc* 70:421-425, 1980.

41. Daniel CR: Longitudinal melanonychia and melanoma: An unusual case presentation. *Dermatol Surg* 27:294-295, 2001.

42. Daniel CR III, Elewski BE: The diagnosis of nail fungus infection revisited. *Arch Dermatol* 136:1162-1164, 2000.

43. Das SK: Nail unit matrix transplantation: A plastic surgeon's approach. *Dermatol Surg* 27:242-245, 2001.

44. DeBenedette V: The safe and effective uses of four oral antifungal agents. *Cosm Dermatol* 7:44-46, 1994.

45. de Palma L, Gigante A, Specchia N: Subungual exostosis of the foot. *Cosm Dermatol* 17:758-763, 1996.

46. Dixon GL Jr: Treatment of ingrown toenail. *Foot Ankle* 3:254-260, 1983.

47. Dockery GL: Nails: Fundamental conditions and procedures. In McGlamry ED (ed): *Comprehensive Textbook of Foot Surgery.* Baltimore, Williams & Wilkins, 1987, pp 3-37.

48. Dompmartin D, Dompmartin A, Deluol AM, et al: Onychomycosis and AIDS: Clinical and laboratory findings in 62 patients. *Int J Dermatol* 29:337-339, 1990.

49. Drake LA, Scher RK, Smith EB, et al: Effect of onychomycosis on quality of life. *J Am Acad Dermatol* 38:702-704, 1998.

50. DuVries HL: Hypertrophy of ungual labia. *Chirop Rec* 16:11, 1933.

51. DuVries HL: Ingrown toenail. *Chirop Rec* 27:155-164, 1944.

52. Dykyj D: Anatomy of the nail. *Clin Podiatr Med Surg* 6:215-228, 1989.

53. Ellis DH: Diagnosis of onychomycosis made simple. *J Am Acad Dermatol* 40:S3-S8, 1999.

54. Estersohn HS, Stanoch JF: Pyogenic granuloma: A literature review and two case reports. *J Am Podiatry Assoc* 73:297-301, 1983.

55. Feibleman CE, Stoll H, Maize JC: Melanomas of the palm, sole, and nailbed: A clinicopathologic study. *Cancer* 46:2492-2504, 1980.

56. Felton PM, Weaver TD: Phenol and alcohol chemical matrixectomy in diabetic versus nondiabetic patients: A retrospective study. *J Am Podiatr Med Assoc* 89:410-412, 1999.

57. Fikry T, Dkhissi M, Harfaoui A, et al: Subungual exostoses: A retrospective study of a series of 28 cases [French]. *Acta Orthop Belg* 64:35-40, 1998.

58. Fletcher CL, Hay RJ, Smeeton NC: Onychomycosis: The development of a clinical diagnostic aid for toenail disease: Part I, establishing discriminating historical and clinical features. *Br J Dermatol* 150:701-705, 2004.

59. Fox IM: Osteomyelitis of the distal phalanx following trauma to the nail: A case report. *J Am Podiatr Med Assoc* 82:542-544, 1992.

60. Frank SC, Freer HL: Onychauxic dystrophic toenails requiring debridement in Medicare patients: Prevalence and anatomical distribution. *J Am Podiatr Med Assoc* 93:388-391, 2003.

61. Frost L: Root resection for incurvated nail. *J Am Podiatr Med Assoc* 40:19, 1950.

62. Gabriel SS, Dallos V, Stevenson DL: The ingrowing toenail: A modified segmental matrix excision operation. *Br J Surg* 66:285-286, 1979.

63. Giacalone VF: Phenol matricectomy in patients with diabetes. *J Foot Ankle Surg* 36:264-267, 1997.

64. Gibson SH, Montgomery H, Woolner LB, et al: Melanotic whitlow (subungual melanoma). *J Invest Dermatol* 29:119-129, 1957.

65. Gilles GA, Dennis KJ, Harkless LB: Periostitis associated with phenol matrixectomies. *J Am Podiatr Med Assoc* 76:469-472, 1986.

66. Graham JH, Helwig EB: Bowen's disease and its relationship to systemic cancer. *Arch Dermatol* 80:133-159, 1959.

67. Gruver DI: Treatment of tubular toenail. *Plast Reconstr Surg* 112:934, 2003.

68. Gupta AK, Jain HC, Lynde CW, et al: Prevalence and epidemiology of onychomycosis in patients visiting physicians' offices: A multicenter Canadian survey of 15,000 patients. *J Am Acad Dermatol* 43:244-248, 2000.

69. Gupta AK, Konnikov N, MacDonald P, et al: Prevalence and epidemiology of toenail onychomycosis in diabetic subjects: A multicentre survey. *Br J Dermatol* 139:665-671, 1998.

70. Gupta AK, Ryder JE, Johnson AM: Cumulative meta-analysis of systemic antifungal agents for the treatment of onychomycosis. *Br J Dermatol* 150:537-544, 2004.

71. Gupta S, Sahoo B, Kumar B: Treating ingrown toenails by nail splinting with a flexible tube: An Indian experience. *J Dermatol* 28:485-489, 2001.

72. Hallock GG, Lutz DA: Octyl-2-cyanoacrylate adhesive for rapid nail plate restoration. *J Hand Surg [Am]* 25:979-981, 2000.

73. Hartzell M: Granuloma pyogenicum (botryomycosis of French authors). *J Cutan Dis* 22:520-525, 1904.

74. Hashimoto K: Ultrastructure of the human toenail: Cell migration, keratinization, and formation of the intercellular cement. *Arch Dermatol Res* 240:1-22, 1970.

75. Heifetz CJ: Ingrown toe-nail: A clinical study. *Am J Surg* 38:298-315, 1937.

76. Heifetz CJ: Operative management of ingrown toenail. *J Mo Med Assoc* 42:213-216, 1945.

77. Heim M, Schapiro J, Wershavski M, et al: Drug-induced and traumatic nail problems in the haemophilias. *Haemophilia* 6:191-194, 2000.

78. Helfand AE: Onychomycosis in the aged: An administrative perspective. *J Am Podiatr Med Assoc* 76:142-145, 1986.

79. Helms A, Brodell RT: Surgical pearl: Prompt treatment of subungual hematoma by decompression. *J Am Acad Dermatol* 42:508-509, 2000.

80. Hettinger DF, Valinsky MS: Treatment of onychomycosis with nail avulsion and topical ketoconazole. *J Am Podiatr Med Assoc* 81:28-32, 1991.

81. Ho VC, Sober AJ: Therapy for cutaneous melanoma: An update. *J Am Acad Dermatol* 22:159-176, 1990.

82. Holub PG, Hubbard ER: Ketoconazole in the treatment of onychomycosis. *J Am Podiatr Med Assoc* 77:338-339, 1987.

83. Hongcharu W, Dwyer P, Gonzalez S, et al: Confirmation of onychomycosis by in vivo confocal microscopy. *J Am Acad Dermatol* 42:214-216, 2000.

84. Horst F, Nunley JA: Glomus tumors in the foot: A new surgical technique for removal. *Cosm Dermatol* 24:949-951, 2003.

85. Hutchinson J: Melanosis often not black: Melanotic whitlow. *BMJ* 1:491-493, 1886.

86. Ippolito E, Falez F, Tudisco C, et al: Subungual exostosis: Histological and clinical considerations on 30 cases. *Ital J Orthop Traumatol* 13:81-87, 1987.

87. Jahss MH: Disorders of the Foot and Ankle: Medical and Surgical Management, ed 2. Philadelphia, WB Saunders, 1991, pp 937, 1548-1572.

88. Jarratt M: Herpes simplex infection. *Arch Dermatol* 119:99-103, 1983.

89. Jeys LM, Khafagy R: A useful technique for securing nails: The figure-of-eight suture [letter]. *Br J Plast Surg* 54:651, 2001.

90. Johnson M: The human nail and its disorders. In Lorimer DL, Neale D (eds): *Neale's Common Foot Disorders: Diagnosis and Management: A General Clinical Guide*, ed 4. Edinburgh, Churchill Livingstone, 1993, pp 123-139.

91. Johnson M, Comaish JS, Shuster S: Nail is produced by the normal nail bed: A controversy resolved. *Br J Dermatol* 125:27-29, 1991.

92. Kato T, Suetake T, Sugiyama Y, et al: Epidemiology and prognosis of subungual melanoma in 34 Japanese patients. *Br J Dermatol* 134:383-387, 1996.

93. Keyes EL: The surgical treatment of ingrown toenails. *JAMA* 102:1458-1460, 1934.

94. Koenig RD, McLaughlin KS: Subungual melanoma. *J Am Podiatr Med Assoc* 84:95-96, 1994.

95. Kosinski MA, Stewart D: Nail changes associated with systemic disease and vascular insufficiency. *Clin Podiatr Med Surg* 6:295-318, 1989.

96. Krausz CE: Nail survey (1942-1970): *Br J Chir* 35:117, 1970.

97. Kuwada GT: Long-term evaluation of partial and total surgical and phenol matrixectomies. *J Am Podiatr Med Assoc* 81:33-36, 1991.

98. Langford JH: Pachyonychia congenita. *J Am Podiatry Assoc* 68:587-591, 1978.

99. Lapidus P: The ingrown toenail. *Bull Hosp Joint Dis* 33:181-192, 1972.

100. Lawrence W Jr: Management of malignant melanoma. *Am Surg* 38:93-106, 1972.

101. Lawry MA, Haneke E, Strobeck K, et al: Methods for diagnosing onychomycosis: A comparative study and review of the literature. *Arch Dermatol* 136:1112-1116, 2000.

102. Lemon B, Burns R: Malignant melanoma: A literature review and case presentation. *J Foot Ankle Surg* 37:48-54, 1998.

103. Lemont H, Haas R: Subungual pigmented Bowen's disease in a nineteen-year-old black female. *J Am Podiatr Med Assoc* 84:39-40, 1994.

104. Leppard B, Sanderson KV, Behan F: Subungual malignant melanoma: Difficulty in diagnosis. *BMJ* 1:310-312, 1974.

105. Lerner LH: Incurvated nail margin with associated osseous pathology. *Curr Podiatr* 11:26-28, 1962.

106. Lewis BL: Microscopic studies of fetal and mature nail and surrounding soft tissue. *Arch Dermatol Syphilol* 70:732-747, 1954.

107. Lloyd-Davies RW, Brill GC: The aetiology and out-patient management of ingrowing toe-nails. *Br J Surg* 50:592-597, 1963.

108. Lundeen GW, Lundeen RO: Onychomycosis: its classification, pathophysiology and etiology. *J Am Podiatry Assoc* 68:395-401, 1978.

109. Mann RA, Coughlin MJ: Toenail abnormalities. In Mann RA, Coughlin MJ (eds): *The Video Textbook of Foot and Ankle Surgery*. St. Louis, Medical Video Productions, 1990, pp 56-66.

110. Miller-Breslow A, Dorfman HD: Dupuytren's (subungual) exostosis. *Am J Surg Pathol* 12:368-378, 1988.

111. Moehrle M, Metzger S, Schippert W, et al: "Functional" surgery in subungual melanoma. *Dermatol Surg* 29:366-374, 2003.

112. Mori H, Umeda T, Nishioka K, et al: Ingrown nails: A comparison of the nail matrix phenolization method with the elevation of the nail bed-periosteal flap procedure. *J Dermatol* 25:1-4, 1998.

113. Multhopp-Stephens H, Walling AK: Subungual exostosis: A simple technique of excision. *Cosm Dermatol* 16:88-91, 1995.

114. Murray WR: Onychocryptosis: Principles of non-operative and operative care. *Clin Orthop Relat Res* 142:96-102, 1979.

115. Murray WR, Bedi BS: The surgical management of ingrowing toenail. *Br J Surg* 62:409-412, 1975.

116. Nagata F, Chu C, Phipps R: Nail involvement in Darier's disease: A case report. *J Am Podiatry Assoc* 70:635-636, 1980.

117. Norton LA: Disorders of the nails. In Moschella SL, Pillsbury DM, Hurley HJ (eds): *Dermatology*. Philadelphia, WB Saunders, 1975, pp 1222-1236.

118. Norton LA: Nail disorders: A review. *J Am Acad Dermatol* 2:451-467, 1980.

119. Nzuzi SM: Common nail disorders. *Clin Podiatr Med Surg* 6:273-94, 1989.

120. Nzuzi SM: Nail entities. *Clin Podiatr Med Surg* 6:253-271, 1989.

121. Oliveira Ada S, Picoto Ada S, Verde SF, et al: Subungual exostosis: Treatment as an office procedure. *J Dermatol Surg Oncol* 6:555-558, 1980.

122. Ongenae K, Van De Kerckhove M, Naeyaert JM: Bowen's disease of the nail. *Dermatology* 204:348-350, 2002.

123. Pack GT, Oropeza R: Subungual melanoma. *Surg Gynecol Obstet* 124:571-582, 1967.

124. Page JC, Abramson C, Lee WL, et al: Diagnosis and treatment of tinea pedis: A review and update. *J Am Podiatr Med Assoc* 81:304-316, 1991.

125. Palamarchuk HJ, Kerzner M: An improved approach to evacuation of subungual hematoma. *J Am Podiatr Med Assoc* 79:566-568, 1989.

126. Palmer BV, Jones A: Ingrowing toenails: The results of treatment. *Br J Surg* 66:575-576, 1979.

127. Papachristou DN, Fortner JG: Melanoma arising under the nail. *J Surg Oncol* 21:219-222, 1982.

128. Pardo-Castello V, Pardo OA: *Diseases of the Nails*, ed 3. Springfield , Ill, Charles C Thomas, 1960, pp 19-20.

129. Parrinello JF, Japour CJ, Dykyj D: Incurvated nail: Does the phalanx determine nail plate shape? *J Am Podiatr Med Assoc* 85:696-698, 1995.

130. Pettine KA, Cofield RH, Johnson KA, et al: Ingrown toenail: Results of surgical treatment. *Foot Ankle* 9:130-134, 1988.

131. Ratz J, Blumberg M: Onychomycosis. Available at http://www.emedicine.com/derm/topic300.htm (accessed March 20, 2006).

132. Reisberger EM, Abels C, Landthaler M, et al: Histopathological diagnosis of onychomycosis by periodic acid–Schiff-stained nail clippings. *Br J Dermatol* 148:749-754, 2003.

133. Rich P: Special patient populations: Onychomycosis in the diabetic patient. *J Am Acad Dermatol* 35:S10-S12, 1996.

134. Rich P: Nail biopsy: Indications and methods. *Dermatol Surg* 27:229-234, 2001.

135. Rinaldi R, Sabia M, Gross J: The treatment and prevention of infection in phenol alcohol matricectomies. *J Am Podiatry Assoc* 72:453-457, 1982.

136. Rodnan GP: Psoriasis. In Rodnan GP, Schumacher HR (eds): *Primer on the Rheumatic Diseases,* ed 8. Atlanta, Arthritis Foundation, 1983, pp 151-152.

137. Rose J, Cohen RS, Mauro G: Subungual malignant melanoma. *J Foot Surg* 25:154-159, 1986.

138. Rounding C, Hulm S: Surgical treatments for ingrowing toenails. *Cochrane Database Syst Rev* 2:CD001541, 2000.

139. Rozmaryn LM, Schwartz AM: Treatment of subungual myxoma preserving the nail matrix: A case report. *J Hand Surg [Am]* 23:178-180, 1998.

140. Saltzman BS: Periungual fibroma: A case report. *J Am Podiatry Assoc* 68:696, 1978.

141. Samman PD: The human toe nail: Its genesis and blood supply. *Br J Dermatol* 71:296-302, 1959.

142. Sari-Kouzel H, Hutchinson CE, Middleton A, et al: Foot problems in patients with systemic sclerosis. *Rheumatology (Oxford)* 40:410-413, 2001.

143. Schein JR, Gause D, Stier DM, et al: Onychomycosis: Baseline results of an observational study. *J Am Podiatr Med Assoc* 87:512-519, 1997.

144. Scher RK: Onychomycosis is more than a cosmetic problem. *Br J Dermatol* 130 Suppl 43:15, 1994.

145. Scher RK, Joseph W, Robbins J: Progression and recurrence of onychomycosis. Available at http://www.medscape.com/viewprogram/2334_pnt (accessed March 20, 2006).

146. Schwartz GR, Schwen SA: Subungual splinter removal. *Am J Emerg Med* 15:330-331, 1997.

147. Shepard GH: Management of acute nail bed avulsions. *Hand Clin* 6:39-56, 1990.

148. Shum C, Bruno RJ, Ristic S, et al: Examination of the anatomic relationship of the proximal germinal nail matrix to the extensor tendon insertion. *J Hand Surg [Am]* 25:1114-1117, 2000.

149. Silverman ME, Goodman RM, Cuppage FE: The nail–patella syndrome: Clinical findings and ultrastructural observations in the kidney. *Arch Intern Med* 120:68-74, 1967.

150. Spencer JM: Nail-apparatus melanoma. *Lancet* 353:84-85, 1999.

151. Sugden P, Levy M, Rao GS: Onychocryptosis–phenol burn fiasco. *Burns* 27:289-292, 2001.

152. Takematsu H, Obata M, Tomita Y, et al: Subungual melanoma: A clinicopathologic study of 16 Japanese cases. *Cancer* 55:2725-2731, 1985.

153. Tauber EB, Goldman L, Claassen H: Pachyonichia congenita. *JAMA* 107:29-30, 1936.

154. Thompson TC, Terwilliger C: The terminal Syme operation for ingrown toenail. *Surg Clin North Am* 31:575-584, 1950.

155. Townsend AC, Scott PJ: Ingrowing toenail and onychogryposis. *J Bone Joint Surg Br* 48:354-358, 1966.

156. Travers GR, Ammon RG: The sodium hydroxide chemical matricectomy procedure. *J Am Podiatry Assoc* 70:476-478, 1980.

157. Tucker DJ, Jules KT, Raymond F: Nailbed injuries with hallucal phalangeal fractures: Evaluation and treatment. *J Am Podiatr Med Assoc* 86:170-173, 1996.

158. Van Geertruyden JP, Olemans C, Laporte M, et al: Verrucous carcinoma of the nail bed. *Cosm Dermatol* 19:327-328, 1998.

159. Vazquez-Flores H, Dominguez-Cherit J, Vega-Memije ME, et al: Subungual osteochondroma: Clinical and radiologic features and treatment. *Dermatol Surg* 30:1031-1034, 2004.

160. Wadhams PS, McDonald JF, Jenkin WM: Epidermal inclusion cysts as a complication of nail surgery. *J Am Podiatr Med Assoc* 80:610-612, 1990.

161. Weiner AL: Alopecia areata with nail changes. *Arch Dermatol* 72:469, 1955.

162. Welvaart K, Schraffordt Koops H: Subungual malignant melanoma: A nail in the coffin. *Clin Oncol* 4:309-315, 1978.

163. White CJ, Laipply TC: Diseases of the nails: 792 cases: Clinical and microscopial findings with resume of newer therapeutic methods. *Ind Med Surg* 27:325-327, 1958.

164. Winograd AM: Modification in technique of operation for ingrown toe-nail. *JAMA* 92:229-230, 1929.

165. Winograd AM: Results in operation for ingrown toe-nail. *Illinois Med J* 70:197-198, 1936.

166. Witt CS, Zielsdorf LM, Wysong DK: A modified partial chemical matricectomy. *J Am Podiatr Med Assoc* 76:684-685, 1986.

167. Wright G: Laser matricectomy in the toes. *Foot Ankle* 9:246-247, 1989.

168. Yang KC, Li YT: Treatment of recurrent ingrown great toenail associated with granulation tissue by partial nail avulsion followed by matricectomy with Sharpulse carbon dioxide laser. *Dermatol Surg* 28:419-421, 2002.

169. Zadik FR: Obliteration of the nail bed of the great toe without shortening of the terminal phalanx. *J Bone Joint Surg Br* 32:66-67, 1950.

170. Zaiac MN, Weiss E: Mohs micrographic surgery of the nail unit and squamous cell carcinoma. *Dermatol Surg* 27:246-251, 2001.

171. Zaias N: Psoriasis of the nail. A clinical-pathologic study. *Arch Dermatol* 99:567-579, 1969.

172. Zaias N. Onychomycosis. *Arch Dermatol* 105:263-274, 1972.

173. Zaias N: *The Nail in Health and Disease,* ed 1. New York, SP Medical, 1980, pp 1-43.

174. Zaias N, Rebell G. The successful treatment of *Trichophyton rubrum* nail bed (distal subungual) onychomycosis with intermittent pulse-dosed terbinafine. *Arch Dermatol* 140:691-695, 2004.

175. Zaitz C, Campbell I, Moraes JR, et al: HLA-associated susceptibility to chronic onychomycosis in Brazilian Ashkenazic Jews. *Int J Dermatol* 35:681-682, 1996.

176. Zimmerman P, Prior J, McGuire J, et al: Onychia of a macronychia in congenital aphalangia. *J Am Podiatr Med Assoc* 82:380-381, 1992.

177. Zook EG: Understanding the perionychium. *J Hand Ther* 13:269-275, 2000.

178. Zuber TJ: Ingrown toenail removal. *Am Fam Physician* 65:2547-2552, 2554, 2002.

Workers' Compensation and Liability Issues

Gregory P. Guyton

A BRIEF HISTORY

Every industrialized nation now employs some form of workers' compensation system to manage the substantial costs associated with workers' injuries. Although the bureaucracies that manage these systems are of legendary complexity, the alternative of unrestricted tort litigation is clearly worse. From the perspective of the employer as well as the worker, the relative predictability of workers' compensation insurance premiums and the emphasis on worker rehabilitation are indispensable features of a modern business environment. A historical perspective can provide some insight into how and why the modern systems exist.[6]

Workers' compensation has been considered so essential that it is as old as recorded law. The first codes

relied upon "schedules" that equated specific injuries, usually amputations, with specific awards. Evidence of such a schedule has been uncovered in the codes of Ur-Nammu, an early ruler of the city-state of Ur in ancient Sumeria, the original cradle of civilization. Similar schedules were present in other cultures, including ancient Egypt and Rome.[11]

The industrial revolution rapidly created conditions for the average worker that were socially unsustainable over the long term. During the early part of the 19th century, three features of common law throughout Europe and America substantially tipped the scales against the worker[9]: contributory negligence, the fellow servant rule, and the doctrine of assumption of risk.

Contributory negligence implied that if the worker was in any way responsible for his or her injury, the employer held no liability. For instance, one celebrated

791

American case of the era involved a railroad worker severely injured due to a loose handrail on a railcar. Because the worker's job description included inspecting the railcar, he was denied any compensation.

The fellow servant rule implied that if any fellow employee was responsible for a worker's injury, the employer was not held liable.

The doctrine of assumption of risk essentially amounted to an implicit liability release. It held that employees essentially know the hazards of their employment when they sign on and the employers were expected only to meet the general safety standards of the industry as a whole. In the case of the 19th century coal industry, to take one example, those standards could be remarkably low. The assumption of risk was often codified explicitly in employment papers, which became known as "right to die" contracts.[5]

Access to the courts was generally poor, and workers at the time had few options. As a response, private organizations such as the English "Friendly Societies" and the German "Krankenkassen" were formed to provide at least more affluent workers with some rudimentary disability insurance.[4]

Workers' conditions played a central role in the political pressures upon European governments by the latter half of the 19th century. This proved most acute in Prussia, where Karl Marx and other social activists were successfully agitating for reform. As the socialist movement gained strength, an unlikely champion of workers' rights emerged in the form of Chancellor Otto von Bismarck. Faced with the necessity of concentrating on his foreign-policy adventures, the resourceful practitioner of realpolitik sought to co-opt the agenda of his political opponents to keep the home front quiet. He was directly responsible for a variety of social reforms including the first elements of a modern social security system, public aid, and no-fault disability insurance. Also among these was the landmark Workers' Accident Insurance enacted in 1884 as the first modern widespread system of workers' compensation.[5,8,9] While co-opting their agenda, Bismarck also ruthlessly suppressed his political opposition. The Social Democratic Party was outlawed outright in 1875.

Workers' compensation reforms came to the United States in the early 20th century. As in Prussia before, a socialist movement was beginning to agitate for the working class. Substantial socialist political activity occurred, accompanied by a literary movement of muckrakers who sought to expose a variety of social ills. Most famous among these was Upton Sinclair, the author of the popular and lurid short novel *The Jungle,* which exposed the abysmal conditions in the meat-processing industry of Chicago.

At the same time, the business community came to realize the benefits of workers' compensation. Access to tort litigation was growing, and the German experience was proving successful in controlling costs. As early as 1893, the U.S. Department of Labor commissioned a report outlining the beneficial aspects of the German experience entitled *Compulsory Insurance in Germany.*[2]

Growing public sentiment for and diminishing capitalist fear of workers' compensation led to the gradual adoption of a modern system in the United States. The federal government led the way within its own jurisdiction. In 1908, President Taft pushed through legislation creating a compensation system for workers involved in interstate trade.[9] There followed a vigorous debate on adopting some form of a national standard for compensation, as companies argued that a competitor in an unregulated state would have an unfair advantage. To address the problem, a national conference was convened in Chicago in 1910 by representatives of all the major industrial states to outline a uniform set of guidelines for workers' compensation law.[6]

Between 1911 (Wisconsin) and 1948 (Mississippi), every state in the nation developed broadly similar workers' compensation systems. The critical features of the modern American systems are as follows:

- With few exceptions, most cases are administered by special workers' compensation boards rather than through the courts.
- Considerable emphasis is placed upon rehabilitation, including returning the worker at least to limited duty as soon as practicable.
- Cases are administered on a no-fault basis. The concepts of contributory negligence, the fellow-servant rule, and a worker's acceptance of the intrinsic risk of the profession no longer play a role.
- Employers are provided with a substantial measure of tort immunity for work-related injuries.

An additional feature was added after the fact in most states. In Oklahoma in 1920, a one-eyed man lost sight in his remaining eye in an industrial accident. Under the existing system, the employer was held responsible for the workers' total disability even though the first eye was lost because of unrelated circumstances. The effect was predictable; a vast number of one-eyed, one-armed, or one-legged workers were fired in the state over the next year. The legislative solution was the creation of second-injury funds. These serve as reinsurance plans that are usually state-administered. Insurance carriers or self-insured employers pay into the fund, which then covers the unique circumstances of second injuries. Although these funds represent a small percentage of the total financial burden of workers' compensation, they are critical in encouraging the rehabilitation and ultimate reemployment of a worker with a prior history of injury.[6]

The medical community initially responded with equanimity to the spread of workers' compensation systems in the United States. By the 1950s, however, demand by physicians to participate in independent medical examinations led to the publication in the *Journal of the American Medical Association* of a series of guides to perform impairment ratings. These were later compiled into a separate text, the *Guides to the Evaluation of Permanent Impairment.*[1] Now in its fifth edition, this collection of rating scales, known as the AMA *Guides,* serves as a common framework across multiple workers' compensation schemes to simplify the physician's task of rating impairment.[3]

THE UNIQUELY RESILIENT FOOT

The majority of issues involved in the care of the injured worker are simply those encountered in the routine practice of foot and ankle surgery. The most difficult decision making comes when the legal questions of causation are raised. This is particularly the case when cumulative trauma is purported to be the cause of disease.

Unlike the situation in the upper extremity, it is rare that the lower-extremity stresses seen on the job differ substantially from those encountered in everyday living. Additionally, the time away from work is quantitatively more important; a 40-hour workweek implies that the worker is on the job roughly 25% of the time. There is no substantial epidemiologic evidence that cumulative trauma from the exposures of an industrial occupation can be linked to any common foot and ankle disorder.[7]

It is true that almost no careful studies have been done in the area, but it is also true that the human foot is perhaps the most resilient part of the body to repetitive mechanical stress. During normal gait, the peak forces seen by the foot are approximately 110% of body weight, and the stance phase accounts for 62% of the gait cycle.[13] When jogging, an activity that numerous cultures such as the Masai in East Africa spend their lifetimes doing, the peak forces are 240% of body weight spread over just 38% of the gait cycle. This simple act therefore quadruples the impulses applied to the foot with each step. Any additional forces applied from ordinary ambulation in an industrial setting pale by comparison.

In the medical–legal setting of workers' compensation, it is absolutely critical to keep any judgments of causation on a firm scientific footing. The concept of cumulative industrial trauma as a cause of the common disorders of the foot and ankle cannot currently be supported.[7]

MEDICAL–LEGAL REPORTS IN THE FOOT AND ANKLE

The Independent Medical Examination

In addition to the routine medical notes, some unique reports are commonly required in workers' compensation and other medical–legal work. The first of these, the independent medical examination (IME), is an interaction in which the physician provides a summary of the patient's history and current status and answers any specific questions posed by the sponsor of the examination. IMEs might be requested (and paid for) by workers' compensation carriers, employers themselves, disability boards, or attorneys for either side.

Regardless of the sponsor, the independent medical report requires an objective evaluation. These reports are always rendered as a second opinion, not as the opinion of the treating physician. In fact, some attorneys recommend avoiding the use of the word "patient" at all. Although some IME subjects ultimately seek treatment with their examiner, the IME is not the appropriate forum for soliciting clinical business. It is important that the subject also understand that the examiner is not his or her physician.

By definition, an IME does not establish a physician–patient relationship and therefore should not be subject to malpractice or state regulation. The legal issues surrounding this issue remain murky, however. It is imperative to clarify the requirements of any state medical board before performing an IME in a jurisdiction for which the physician is not licensed. Some states require that temporary medical privileges be obtained.

There are many acceptable forms of an IME report, but several critical issues must always be addressed. First, the questions posed by the requesting sponsor must always be answered explicitly. IME reports are typically lengthy; conclusions should be made easy for the reader by simply cutting to the chase. Second, an IME should always contain sufficient information to be able to generate a permanent impairment rating later if necessary. Third, superfluous commentary should be avoided. Although the IME is impartial, it is also a sponsored exam in which only certain items of information are requested. Items that would be routinely included in a medical report should be mentioned, but it is careful practice to exclude opinions that are only of legal importance, regardless of which party might benefit, unless they are specifically sought. These might include, for instance, speculation on the cause of a disease or apportionment of a subjects' impairment among multiple injury episodes.

Inevitably, patients with vague complaints that cannot be clearly substantiated by the physical findings eventually are encountered in any medical–legal practice. In these cases, it is best to objectively state the presence or absence of physical findings and include statements about the reliability of the examination. The presence of breakaway weakness, tenderness that disappears with patient distraction or change in position, dramatic hyperesthesia, and nonanatomic distributions of nerve complaints should all be appropriately documented. A simple, objective summation statement that avoids accusation is appropriate for the assessment in these cases. It is more professional to state "the examination reveals no objective evidence of organic disease" than to use the more pejorative "the patient is malingering."

An example construct for an IME report for the foot and ankle is provided with annotations.

An Example Independent Medical Examination

The Request Letter

Dear Dr. Guyton,

We have scheduled an independent medical examination for Mr. William Jones on July 1, 2005. Mr. Jones was injured in a fall while working for AAA Roofing on August 15, 2003. He subsequently underwent open reduction and internal fixation by Dr. Shannon Apple. He underwent extensive physical therapy and work-hardening courses but has continued to complain of limited motion and burning pain in the foot. He returned to work in a sedentary capacity on May 5, 2004. The diagnosis of tarsal tunnel syndrome has recently been suggested. We are asking you to address the following questions:

1. What is Mr. Jones's current diagnosis?

2. Is Mr. Jones at maximal medical improvement? If not, when would you estimate this to be?

3. Is further diagnostic testing recommended?

4. Is surgery recommended? Are further nonoperative measures required? What degree of recovery can be expected?

5. Please provide a rating of permanent impairment if appropriate. Restrict your analysis to the right foot and ankle.

6. What are his appropriate work restrictions?

Your report is due by July 21, 2005. Please fill out the attached work status worksheet and fax it to us upon completion of the examination.
Sincerely,
Tracy Bird, IME Scheduler
AAA Medical Evaluations

The IME Report

Independent Medical Examination
Mr. William Jones
Medical Record Number WC-22222
Social Security Number 111-11-1111
Case Number 333333

Mr. William Jones was evaluated in my office on July 1, 2005, for the purpose of an independent medical examination. He arrived promptly and was appropriate during the interview. He was accompanied by Nurse Case Manager Kelly Jenkins of American Case Management.

> A short preamble should identify the examination as an IME. A comment on the subject's level of cooperation is usually appropriate, as is mention of any person(s) present during the exam.

History of Present Illness

Mr. Jones is a 42-year-old white male roofer who was injured in a 15-foot fall from a commercial property roof on August 15, 2003. He suffered a comminuted right intraarticular calcaneus fracture and was evaluated by Dr. Shannon Apple. Open reduction and internal fixation was performed on August 26, 2003. Postoperatively he began early motion and was transferred to a removable splint by the end of the first week. His wound healed uneventfully, and physical therapy was begun initially for motion only within the first week. Weight bearing was begun at 8 weeks postoperatively.

> A routine history of present illness is provided. Special attention should be paid to postoperative management, immobilization history, and physical therapy.

Following the institution of weight bearing, Mr. Jones began to complain of increasing burning and pain and numbness on the plantar aspect of the foot. His pain included the dorsal and plantar aspects of the forefoot at that time. He was fitted with a pair of orthotics when he was weaned from his CAM walker boot at 3 months postoperatively. The orthotics were subsequently revised on two occasions.

An orthotic and bracing history is also important. Modification of these devices is often the most time-consuming portion of a postinjury rehabilitation course. If no orthotics or braces have been used, this should be stated.

An electromyography/nerve conduction velocity (EMG/NCV) study was performed on March 22, 2004, by Dr. Dale Atkins, a neurologist. These studies were interpreted as demonstrating mild tarsal tunnel syndrome. Reports reviewed today indicated the NCV showed a motor latency of the medial plantar nerve across the ankle of 5.2 ms and a motor latency of the lateral plantar nerve across the ankle of 4.7 ms. No EMG abnormalities were noted. A tarsal tunnel release was discussed, but the patient declined consideration of further surgery at that time. Dr. Apple performed a single injection into the tarsal tunnel on April 2, 2004, but Mr. Jones states this did not improve his pain.

Nerves play a prominent role in workers' compensation cases. The interpretation of EMG/NCV can be surprisingly subjective, and these data should be recorded as accurately as possible. This includes the name of the examiner, his or her specialty, date, numerical motor latencies, and EMG findings. Comparing subsequent EMG/NCV examinations on the basis of the electromyographer's general impression alone is not reliable.

There are absolutely no data to suggest how EMG/NCV results should be interpreted after a prior tarsal tunnel release; whether or not these values can be expected to normalize is not known. Serial electrical studies are common in workers' compensation cases, and overinterpretation of the studies should be avoided if a nerve has already been released.

Shortly following the EMG/NCV, Mr. Jones states that his symptoms became more focal on the lateral aspect of the foot. He describes shooting pains along the fifth ray into the fourth and fifth digit that are inconstant in character. His cold tolerance is poor, and he occasionally notes color changes in the toes. He does not believe the orthotics have improved the situation.

A brief summary of the subject's current complaints should be included at the end of the history.

Mr. Jones was released to work on May 1, 2004, on restricted duty. He was released to a medium level of activity including maximum lifting of 50 pounds but restricted from climbing ladders. He relates that his company did not have a position available that matched those conditions, and he remained off work until July 15, 2004. At that time, a sedentary clerical position opened up and he has worked in the company office since.

The subject's work release history, along with any physician-provided restrictions, is critical. Whether or not the subject actually returned to work should also be stated.

Past Medical History
Significant for exercise-induced asthma and a meniscal injury to the right knee (remote).
Surgical History
Significant for a right knee arthroscopy in 1987 and the calcaneal open reduction and internal fixation (ORIF).
Social History
Mr. Jones is married with one child. He does not smoke and drinks approximately one drink per week. In the 3 years prior to his injury he had become an avid marathon runner. He has not returned to running since.

The subject's habits are important, including smoking history, alcohol use, and any unusual avocations.

Family History
Noncontributory.
Work History
The subject has worked as a roofer for approximately 10 years and has worked in general construction since the age of 18. He began working for AAA Roofing in 1999 and has no history of prior work-related injury.

Work history should be a separate section that includes the length of time with the current employer, the subject's previous type of employment, and any prior work-related injuries.

Review of Systems

Negative for any neurologic, cardiac, pulmonary, infectious, or other musculoskeletal symptoms. He has no history of psychiatric illness.

Physical Examination

Demonstrates a muscular white male who appears his stated age of 42. He is 5 feet 11 inches tall and weighs 170 pounds. He ambulates with a mildly antalgic gait on the right side and does not use supports or braces. He does have 3/4-length semirigid arch supports that are well-fitted.

> The physical and radiographic examinations should be able to provide the basis for an impairment rating independent of any other information. A few special items are included to cover all the requisite information.
>
> The subject's height and weight should be recorded. Gait pattern and the use of any walking supports or braces are potentially important for determining an impairment rating.

Examination of the right lower extremity demonstrates 4 cm of calf circumference atrophy measured at its maximum extent compared to the left. He has a strip of anhidrosis in the forefoot consistent with the distribution of the sural nerve. No other skin changes are noted. He has diminished sensation and dysesthesia objectively in a sural distribution. A Tinel sign is present over the lateral aspect of the calcaneus. He has no Tinel's sign over the tarsal tunnel and no plantar paresthesias. There is no allodynia. No evidence of vascular instability is present. He has mild chronic edema about the hindfoot and a well-healed lateral approach incision to the calcaneus.

> Atrophy of the calf is also a potential factor in the calculation of an impairment rating.
>
> Any objective signs of nerve dysfunction are very useful (anhidrosis, dependent rubor, temperature, etc.). When present, these provide more concrete bases for evaluating nerve disease than the subjective findings of patient-reported dysesthesia.

He has normal ankle range of motion of 35 degrees of dorsiflexion and 50 degrees of plantarflexion, which is symmetric with the uninjured left side. Subtalar motion is restricted to 50% of that on the contralateral side, with 7 degrees of eversion and 15 degrees of inversion. It is associated with moderate pain. The remainder of the foot has a normal conformation and motion.

He is able to fire all motor groups with 5/5 strength to manual testing including the peroneals, anterior tibialis, gastroc–soleus, posterior tibialis, and extensor hallucis longus.

Radiographs

Weight-bearing radiographs of the right foot taken today demonstrate significant subtalar arthritis involving the posterior facet. There is less than 1 mm of joint space remaining. The changes are progressive compared to films dated September 12, 2004, from Dr. Apple's office and include further loss of joint space and osteophyte formation. The calcaneal height has been appropriately restored and a Brodén view does not demonstrate any evident malreduction of the posterior facet of the subtalar joint. There are no hardware complications.

> Radiographically based impairment ratings can use a system that grades the remaining joint space in millimeters according to the AMA *Guides*. Although this is often not as useful to the orthopaedist as other radiographic features of arthritis, it should be commented upon, when possible, to conform to this admittedly awkward standard.

Assessment

Mr. Jones has progressive post-traumatic subtalar arthritis following a calcaneus fracture treated with open reduction and internal fixation. He also has objective evidence of sural nerve dysfunction related to the injury. The diagnosis of tarsal tunnel syndrome is not supported by today's examination. His previous NCV findings included only mildly prolonged latencies and no EMG abnormalities.

> The assessment should be as concise as possible, enumerating the diagnoses and addressing any previous controversies in the record. A specific treatment plan is not required unless it is solicited by the report sponsor. The independent medical examiner is not the treating physician, and the purpose of the IME might not be to recommend further medical care.

In response to the specific questions posed in the request letter from Tracy Bird:

> The report should be made as easy to understand by the sponsor as possible. When an enumerated list of questions is provided, answer them in a separate section one by one. Not everyone who reads the report will be familiar with the format of medical records, and this simple list makes the conclusions immediately obvious.

1. Mr. Jones's diagnosis is outlined above.

2. Mr. Jones is not at maximal medical improvement. He has progressive subtalar arthritis and should benefit from surgical intervention. Should surgery be undertaken, MMI would occur roughly 6 months postoperatively.

3. No further diagnostic tests are required at this time.

4. Mr. Jones has progressive symptomatic subtalar arthritis and would be expected to benefit from a subtalar fusion. In addition, exploration and neurolysis of the sural nerve is recommended. He is appropriately motivated and his ultimate return to work as a manual laborer is likely, but following a subtalar fusion he would be permanently restricted from working on sloping roof surfaces.

5. A permanent impairment rating is not appropriate at this time because further surgery is recommended.

> Permanent impairment ratings should be provided only when the patient is at maximal medical improvement. If this is not the case or if further recommended medical interventions would push the timing of MMI further into the future, this should be stated.

6. His current work restrictions as outlined by Dr. Apple are appropriate. These include an 8-hour day at a medium physical demand level, a 50-pound intermittent weight-lifting restriction, and no crawling or ladder climbing.

Thank you for allowing me to participate in the evaluation of Mr. Jones. Please contact my office if I can be of further assistance.

The Impairment Rating

The second common medical–legal report is the impairment rating. It is generated upon request by either an independent medical examiner or, in more straightforward cases, the treating physician. Impairment is usually assessed when the medical situation is not expected to change in the near future. This point in time is usually referred to as "maximal medical improvement" or "MMI." Impairment is usually considered permanent for purposes of reaching a financial settlement between the parties involved.

Impairment and *disability* are distinct concepts, and the terms should not be used interchangeably.

Impairment means simply what is physically wrong with a subject, whereas *disability* encompasses how that impairment affects how that subject can make a living. Impairment is determined by a physician, and disability is determined through a legal proceeding based in part upon that impairment. For instance, the impairment rating following a traumatic amputation of the hallux would be the same for an office worker and a professional soccer player, but their disability would obviously be dramatically different.

The formal definitions according to the AMA *Guides* are as follows.[3] Impairment is "a loss, loss of use, or derangement of any body part, organ system, or organ function." A disability is "an alteration of an individual capacity to meet personal, social, or occupational demands or statutory or regulatory requirements because of an impairment."

As in the case of the IME, there are many acceptable forms of documenting impairment ratings. Because they usually involve a substantial amount of additional administrative work, it is common to bill and document them separately from either an IME or a routine follow-up note.

In general, the AMA *Guides to the Evaluation of Permanent Impairment* provide the basis for generating impairment ratings. Some jurisdictions require the use of the AMA *Guides* by statute, others by common practice. A few jurisdictions, such as Florida, North Carolina, and Oregon, have their own published methodologies, but these are based largely upon the AMA *Guides* as well.[10] Calculating the rating can be quite complex, and the AMA *Guides* include a tutorial in the methods required. It is critical to read the "Lower Extremity" chapter carefully when rating the foot and ankle.

Ratings are expressed in terms of the "whole person," "lower extremity," or "foot." In the tables in the AMA *Guides,* specific impairments are listed with values for each of these categories. The final rating can be converted between the different expressions if necessary.

Reviewing the physical examination section of the sample IME indicates an inordinate amount of attention to several usually unimportant features. Although they may or may not be important in determining a treatment course, factors such as the degree of atrophy, the gait pattern, and the use of supports or braces are important to document for a possible impairment rating. Nerve dysfunction also plays a more prominent role in medical–legal work than in routine surgical practice. Sensory deficits and autonomic nerve dysfunction are usually added to the rating. The skin examination is extremely important; anhidrosis or other autonomic change may be visible in a specific nerve distribution.

Importantly, the "Lower Extremity" chapter is used to evaluate problems in *specific peripheral nerves*. If a subject's pain cannot be localized to specific nerve distributions and is characterized by a global pattern of hyperesthesia, dysesthesia, or allodynia, the physician must determine whether or not there is a diffuse metabolic cause for the pain, a causalgic pain syndrome is present, or the subject is malingering. Diffuse pain from peripheral neuropathy or complex regional pain syndrome is usually evaluated according to the very loose guidelines in the "Central and Peripheral Nervous System" chapter of the AMA *Guides*. In more complex cases with causalgic pain as the central feature, it is entirely appropriate for an orthopaedic surgeon to state that the evaluation is beyond his or her scope of practice and to recommend that the determination of maximal medical improvement and the impairment rating be calculated by a pain management specialist.

The impairment rating is generated for use in a specific workers' compensation settlement proceeding within a specific state or federal jurisdiction. The AMA *Guides* provide a common framework across the country, but additional factors may be considered by state or federal statute. Some state laws still perversely stipulate the use of the fourth edition of the AMA *Guides*, a book now long out of print. The request letter usually states under what jurisdiction the rating is required, and it is good practice to state the jurisdiction and any specific additional factors that might be considered as a result in the opening of the report.

Calculating the Rating

Calculating impairment ratings is, at best, an imprecise science. Although often vague and incomplete, the AMA *Guides* at least provide a systematic approach to organizing the process.[10] There are many different pathways to determine impairment, and it is up to the physician to determine which calculation is most appropriate, relevant, and focused in any given clinical situation. In general, the AMA *Guides* list 13 separate categories that can be considered, including nine based upon anatomic criteria, three based upon functional criteria, and a separate category when the diagnosis itself is most appropriate.

To guide the process, a clinical worksheet is provided in the AMA *Guides* (5th edition) to record the various components of lower extremity impairment. Its use is optional, but it helps document the steps in the process. To calculate an impairment rating for the foot and ankle, the following steps are recommended.

CONSIDER CATEGORIES

Consider all of the thirteen categories separately and record the possible impairments for each subcategory.

Use the bracketed [foot] values in the tables to make the initial calculations if a foot rating is requested, or the (lower extremity) values if a lower extremity rating is requested.

Anatomic

1. *Limb length discrepancy* should be measured by radiography if possible.

2. *Muscle atrophy* should be measured by comparing maximum girth of the calf or thigh, or both.

3. *Ankylosis* helps to differentiate the impairment when the joint is stiffened in an optimal or nonoptimal position.

4. *Arthritis* requires a radiographic, not physical exam, measurement. It is based upon the cartilage intervals (in millimeters) measured on a preferably weight-bearing radiograph.

5. *Amputation* impairments are based upon the level of amputation

6. *Skin loss* is determined from specific situations of full-thickness skin loss, which are listed in the chapter and essentially cover full-thickness loss on the weight-bearing areas.

7. *Vascular disorders* are rare, but specific conditions are outlined.

8. *Peripheral nerve injuries* require nerve deficit ratings, which are based upon loss of motor and sensory function for a series of listed peripheral nerves. In the foot, not all cutaneous nerves are listed, and the physician has to use his or her judgment. For instance, a saphenous nerve neuroma might be considered in similar fashion as a sural nerve injury. Nerve injuries represent a common source of additional impairment in foot and ankle ratings and should be carefully considered.

Functional

9. *Gait derangement*, which includes limps and the use of supportive devices, is used as a rating tool alone in the presence of arthritis. This is the most nonspecific rating category, and a more specific means of generating the rating is almost always appropriate. Nevertheless, gait derangement can provide a useful overall check for the rating generated by other means. For instance, a patient with a 50% impairment of the foot and ankle would be expected to have a substantial gait derangement, and gait derangement can be mentioned—even if it is not used to calculate the rating—to demonstrate the internal consistency of the other method(s) used.

10. *Causalgia* is rated when causalgic pain is present, indicated by a regional pain disturbance beyond

the distribution of discrete nerves. In this case, the peripheral nerve ratings should not be used. These are among the most difficult ratings to address, and the "Lower Extremity" chapter should be abandoned in favor of the "Central and Peripheral Nervous System" chapter, section 13.8, entitled "Criteria for Rating Impairments Related to Chronic Pain."

11. *Manual muscle testing* is used for muscle weakness from direct injury. The section on peripheral nerve injury is used if the weakness comes from that source.

12. *Range-of-motion* rating is subdivided by joint.

Diagnosis-based

13. *Diagnosis-based estimates* are the preferred method when a diagnosis-based impairment is given that closely matches the clinical situation, such as the case for most fractures. It includes muscle weakness and atrophy in the estimate. Additional impairment can be given for other factors such as an associated nerve palsy.

USE THE CROSS-USAGE CHART

Use the cross-usage chart at the beginning of the chapter to determine what combinations of impairment values can be used. Not all elements of potential impairment can be combined. For instance, the diagnosis-based estimates already include the muscle atrophy and weakness expected with the given fracture or ligamentous injury they describe, whereas additional nerve palsies represent something out of the ordinary that can then be factored in. A standard methodology is outlined in the AMA *Guides* in the form of the "cross-usage chart" at the beginning of each chapter. This matrix determines what can and what cannot be combined to determine the final impairment.

DETERMINE THE APPROPRIATE CATEGORY

Of all the different combinations of impairment values, determine which is most appropriate for the clinical situation. The physician is expected to choose which method most accurately reflects the clinical circumstance. There is considerable latitude in determining whether a combination of anatomic factors, a diagnosis-based estimate, or the very general gait assessment is most appropriate. The goal, when possible, is to use the pathway that is most direct and focused.

In general, a diagnosis-based estimate or simple anatomic feature such as an amputation that closely matches the clinical situation is preferred, and it can be modified by the presence of other factors such as a nerve impairment. A general assessment, such as that afforded by gait or the very nebulous assessment of causalgic pain, provides for the most variable rating determinations and should be used only when other options are not available. If two rating methods are roughly similar in their suitability, the higher rating is used by convention.

COMBINE RATINGS

Combine the rating, if necessary, with other ratings from the same lower extremity. If two parts of one extremity are concurrently evaluated, the ratings generated for each part have to be combined to generate a lower-extremity rating. The Combined Values Chart in the AMA *Guides* is used to make this determination. If no additional parts of the lower extremity are being rated, the foot rating can be converted to a lower-extremity rating by multiplying by 0.7.

HIGHLIGHT PERTINENT PARTS OF THE RATING

Pull out those parts of the rating due to the current injury, if asked. Commonly a preexisting injury or disease is present. The request usually asks to have a full rating calculated and then asks that you state what portions are due to the injury or incident in question.

RATE THE BODY PART

Put the rating in terms of the body part required by the requesting entity. Most requests for foot ratings ask that the report be restricted to the foot and ankle or the lower extremity. This request should be respected. It only creates confusion if the rating is expressed as a "whole person" value and must then be recalculated. For uncomplicated ratings in which no other parts of the lower extremity or whole person are also impaired, the following conversion is used:

Whole Person Rating = Lower Extremity Rating × 0.4
Lower Extremity Rating = Foot Rating × 0.7

IDENTIFY ALTERNATIVE RATING PATHWAYS

Consider mentioning the alternative rating pathways to corroborate the final result. The most defensible impairment ratings are those that clearly use a primary method to calculate the number but can also be substantiated by demonstrating that other methods would yield a broadly similar figure. Although this corroboration is not mandatory, it at least serves as an internal check to ensure that the final calculated result is not completely out of bounds. The physician should consider how well his or her impairment rating would hold up against another; that is, after all, what often happens in the legal proceeding.

An Example Impairment Rating Report

The Request Letter

Dear Dr. Guyton,

You evaluated Mr. William Jones for the purpose of an independent medical evaluation on July 1, 2005. A subtalar fusion was recommended both by you and Mr. Jones's treating physician, Dr. Apple. Mr. Jones has elected not to undergo surgery at this time. As we discussed on the phone, he would be considered at maximal medical improvement at this time unless surgery were performed. Please provide a rating of permanent impairment for Mr. Jones. Restrict your rating to the right lower extremity. Include consideration of the factors required by the State of Maryland in your report.

Sincerely,

Tracy Bird, IME Scheduler

AAA Medical Evaluations

Permanency ratings are appropriately performed when the subject is at maximal medical improvement. Sometimes, as in this case, the timing of MMI depends on what treatment options the patient chooses to pursue.

Many ratings in foot and ankle orthopaedic practice are restricted to the lower extremity of the foot and ankle.

Commonly, the letter mentions the jurisdiction under which the case is being handled. The jurisdiction should be mentioned in the report along with any special considerations that are required.

Impairment Rating Report
Evaluation of Permanent Impairment

Mr. William Jones

Medical Record Number WC-22222

Social Security Number 111-11-1111

Case Number 333333

The following impairment rating is based upon my evaluation of Mr. William Jones on July 1, 2005. It is calculated according to the methodology of the State of Maryland and includes consideration of the factors of atrophy, pain, weakness, and loss of endurance, function, and range of motion as required by section 9-721 of the Annotated Code of Maryland.

The jurisdiction under which the case is being handled, any special considerations that are required by law in that jurisdiction, and the date of the examination upon which the rating is based should be included in the lead paragraph. The state codes governing workers' compensation ratings are commonly available online through state government websites.

Mr. Jones has post-traumatic subtalar arthritis with limited motion and 0 mm of radiographic joint space. Table 17-3 of the AMA *Guides* specifies a 25% impairment of the foot and ankle as a result of the radiographic evaluation. He also has anatomic evidence of sural nerve dysfunction including anesthesia in a sural distribution. By Table 17-37, this accounts for 5% impairment of the lower extremity. The cross-usage chart (Table 17-2) allows these two impairments to be combined for a total of 30% impairment of the right lower extremity.

Many methods of calculating the impairment rating are possible under the AMA *Guides*, and it is at the discretion of the physician to determine the appropriate ones. The specific tables used to make the calculations should be mentioned, along with confirmation that any methods used can or cannot be combined according to the AMA *Guides*.

The above method is generally concordant with impairment calculated by alteration of gait. Mr. Jones has a mildy antalgic gait that does not require the use of supports. This corresponds to a range of whole body impairment of less than 15% according to Table 17-5, which translates to a range of less than 38% impairment of the lower extremity. The calculation by means of the direct assessment of his arthritis and nerve dysfunction is more focused and accurate.

If possible, the calculation can be further supported by demonstrating that one or more alternate methods would yield broadly similar results. A rationale for choosing the primary method can also be stated.

My final rating for Mr. Jones is a 30% impairment of the right lower extremity.

Leave no doubt as to the final rating and the body part it refers to (e.g., whole person, lower extremity, or foot).

INTERACTING WITH OTHER WORKERS' COMPENSATION PROFESSIONALS

The Case Manager

The case manager is a position unique to workers' compensation systems. He or she is usually, but not always, a nurse who works for a case management company that is contracted by the workers' compensation insurance carrier. In the ideal setting, their role is not to advocate either for the employer or for the worker but to ensure that the patient receives high-quality, efficient care and that the case progresses efficiently. This task can entail simple items such as making certain that return-to-work forms are filled out at the time of a patient visit, or it can require seeking a second opinion when a patient's progress is slow.

It is important to recognize that case managers and the insurance company adjusters with whom they correspond have independent sources of information about the progress a patient should make following specific injuries.[12] It is their role to make inquiries if the patient does not meet these benchmarks. Most use a compilation of tables called *The Medical Disability Advisor* (known as "Reed's," after its author) to project disability for various injuries as well as give them a background on the injury (Table 15–1).[14] The process of involving a case manager is expensive, but it is cost effective when viewed from a global societal perspective. The rate of ultimate return-to-work diminishes rapidly as the time off increases (Fig. 15–1). Avoiding even a few cases of complete permanent disability in an injured worker by using case managers to increase the efficiency of the system easily justifies the added expense.

The Physical or Occupational Therapist

In addition to the vital role the therapist plays in routine injury rehabilitation, there are two special

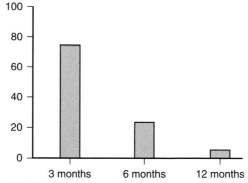

Figure 15–1 Percentage of ultimate return-to-work versus time on disability. After 1 year of disability, only 5% of workers return to employability. (Adapted from Work Loss Data Institute: *Official Disability Guidelines.* Corpus Christi, Tex: Work Loss Data Institute, 1999.)

roles that a physical therapist can play in workers' compensation settings.

Work hardening is an intensive physical therapy regimen that is done at the end of a worker's rehabilitation course. It is analogous to the beginning of sports-specific activities in the rehabilitation of an athlete. At this point, the worker will already have progressed beyond basic tasks such as weight bearing and range of motion. Work hardening is primarily used to increase endurance and maximal capability by simulating as much of the job task as possible in a protected therapeutic environment. Typically, the regimen entails at least 4 hours per day of therapy and the subject attends 5 days a week, just as on the job. The tasks involved are designed to replicate key job elements, and the session is run for 2 to 6 weeks with the express goal of returning to work at the end.

A *functional capacities evaluation* (FCE) is typically administered by a specially trained physical or occupational therapist to assist the physician in setting parameters for the patient's return to work. It involves a battery of tests designed to provide some objective basis for determining time and physical demand limitations. Not every case requires an FCE, but as the complexity of the situation increases or the length of time off stretches past several months, an FCE can be a very useful tool. Without it, the physician is essentially forced to use his or her intuition and the general impressions formed during the often very short follow-up clinic visits.

The U.S. Department of Labor publishes the *Dictionary of Occupational Titles*,[15] which defines the physical demands of specific work, the standards for intensity (Box 15–1), and the definitions of frequency (Box 15–2). The goal of the functional capacities evaluation is to determine how well the worker can meet the

TABLE 15–1

Expected Length of Disability based on Job Classification for Medial or Lateral Malleolus Fracture (Days)*

USDOL Job Classification	Minimum	Optimum	Maximum
Sedentary	7	14	42
Light	14	28	56
Medium	28	56	84
Heavy	42	84	112
Very heavy	42	112	168

*An example optimal disability table from *The Medical Disability Advisor* used by case managers and insurance adjusters to predict the length of disability.
USDOL, United States Department of Labor.
From Reed P (ed): *The Medical Disability Advisor: Workplace Guidelines for Disability Duration*, ed 3. Boulder, Colo, Reed Group, 1997.

BOX 15–1   U.S. Department of Labor Definitions of Work Intensity[15]

Sedentary: Exerting up to 10 pounds of force occasionally and/or a negligible amount of force frequently to lift, carry, push, pull, or otherwise move objects, including the human body. Involves sitting most of the time but may involve walking or standing for brief periods of time.

Light: Exerting up to 20 pounds of force occasionally and/or up to 10 pounds of force frequently and/or a negligible amount of force constantly. Even when weight is negligible, a job is rated light when it involves walking or standing to a significant degree; it requires sitting most of the time but involves pushing and/or pulling of arm or leg controls; it involves working at a production rate that requires constant pushing or pulling of materials.

Medium: Exerting 20 to 50 pounds of force occasionally and/or 10 to 25 pounds of force frequently and/or up to 10 pounds of force constantly. Physical demand requirements are greater than that required for light work.

Heavy: Exerting 50 to 100 pounds of force occasionally and/or 25 to 50 pounds of force constantly. Physical demand requirements are greater than that required for medium work.

Very Heavy: Exerting greater than 100 pounds of force occasionally and/or greater than 50 pounds of force frequently and/or greater than 20 pounds of force constantly. Physical demand requirements are greater than that required for heavy work.

---

physical demands of the job at the required intensity and frequency.

A typical FCE report includes a description of the items that were tested, the patient's projected endurance, and, in summary, the patient's overall level of function, which is typically stated as a combination of overall strength and frequency. If a specific occupation is a goal (called an "own job" FCE), the FCE also states the requirements of that position. Others state the requirements of a general occupation (an "own

---

BOX 15–2   U.S. Department of Labor Definitions of Work Frequency[15]

Never: Activity or condition does not exist.
Occasionally: Activity or condition exists up to one third of the time.
Frequently: Activity or condition exists from one third to two thirds of the time.
Constantly: Activity or condition exists two thirds or more of the time.

---

occupation" FCE), and some have no comparative standard if the patient is currently unemployed (an "any occupation" FCE). The patient's perceived effort is also indicated.

An FCE does not rigidly set return-to-work parameters but instead comes back to the involved parties for the physician to make a final determination. There is usually little reason to doubt the objective strength capacities contained in an FCE. The most subjective part of the report is endurance. Regardless of how thorough the examiner is, no FCE fully replicates an 8-hour day. The endurance capability is *projected*, and some leeway in interpretation may be used by the physician.

As a general rule, FCEs are underused in more complex compensation settings. They provide a very useful tool to the physician near the end of a long rehabilitation course when some objective return-to-work limitations are required, and there should be no hesitation in asking the case manager or adjuster to obtain one in these situations.

REFERENCES

1. American Medical Association Staff: *Guides to the Evaluation of Permanent Impairment*, ed 1. Chicago, American Medical Association, 1971.
2. Brooks JG: *Compulsory Insurance in Germany*. Washington, DC, United States Department of Labor, 1893.
3. Cocchiarella L, Andersson GBJ (eds): *Guides to the Evaluation of Permanent Impairment*, ed 5. Chicago, American Medical Association, 2000.
4. Geerts A, Kornblith B, Urmson J: *Compensation for Bodily Harm*. Brussels, Fernand Nathan, 1977, p 211.
5. Gerdes DA: Worker's compensation, an overview for physicians. *S D J Med* 43(7):17-23, 1990.
6. Guyton GP: A brief history of workers' compensation. *Iowa Orthop J* 19:106-110, 1999.
7. Guyton GP, Mann RA, Krieger LE, et al: Cumulative industrial trauma as an etiology of seven common disorders in the foot and ankle: What is the evidence? *Foot Ankle Int* 5(2):317-326, 2000.
8. Hadler NM: The disabling backache. An international perspective. *Spine* 20:640-649, 1995.
9. Haller JS Jr: Industrial accidents—worker compensation laws and the medical response. *West J Med* 148(3):341-348, 1988.
10. Harper JD: Determining foot and ankle impairments by the AMA fifth edition guides. *Foot Ankle Clin N Am* 7:291-303, 2002.
11. Kramer SN: *History Begins at Sumer*. London, Thames and Hudson, 1958, p 93.
12. Kunkel M, Miller SD: Return to work after foot and ankle injury. *Foot Ankle Clin N Am* 7:421-428, 2002.
13. Mann RA, Coughlin MJ (eds): *Surgery of the Foot and Ankle*, ed 7. St. Louis, Mosby, 1999, chapter 1.
14. Reed P (ed): *The Medical Disability Advisor: Workplace Guidelines for Disability Duration*, ed 3. Boulder, Colo, Reed Group, 1997.
15. United States Department of Labor: *Dictionary of Occupational Titles*, ed 4, revised. Washington, DC, US Government Printing Office, 1991. Available at http://www.oalj.dol.gov/libdot.htm (accessed February 20, 2006).
16. Work Loss Data Institute: *Official Disability Guidelines*. Corpus Christi, Tex: Work Loss Data Institute, 1999.

Arthritis, Postural Disorders, and Tendon Disorders

Arthritic Conditions of the Foot

Paul S. Shurnas • Michael J. Coughlin

The foot and ankle are subject to disabling arthritides at many sites and from various causes. Nontraumatic isolated degenerative arthritis can be a disabling cause of foot dysfunction, but early radiographic changes facilitate the diagnosis and treatment. Inflammatory arthritis, on the other hand, may be difficult to diagnose because of the age of the patient, magnitude and location of specific joint involvement, and progression of the arthritic process, which vary significantly depending on the individual inflammatory disease process. Basic science research has implicated an imbalance between the class I and II subgroups of the major histocompatibility complex (MHC) in diseases like psoriatic arthritis,[10] and further research might identify a specific genetic locus for other inflammatory diseases. Treatment with natural medications like glucosamine has been shown to reduce swelling in an animal model of collagen-induced arthritis.[341]

The foot pain, disability, and activity restrictions associated with rheumatoid arthritis can be reliably measured, as demonstrated by a validated instrument called the foot function index (FFI), and in the future this will help to standardize comparisons of many of the different types of surgical procedures used in treating rheumatoid arthritis.[294] Inflammatory arthropathy can be categorized depending upon the underlying pathophysiology into synovial inflammatory diseases, including seropositive disorders (rheumatoid arthritis) and seronegative disorders (Reiter's syndrome, psoriatic arthritis, ankylosing spondylitis); crystal deposition disease, including gout and pseudogout; and connective tissue disorders (systemic lupus erythematosus and mixed connective tissue diseases).[319]

INFLAMMATORY ARTHROPATHIES

Rheumatoid Arthritis

Rheumatoid arthritis is a systemic disease that affects 1% to 2% of the general population.[288] Rana[275] has estimated that five million people in the United States suffer from rheumatoid arthritis. Women are affected much more often than men. Although onset can occur

at any age, often the peak incidence is during the third to fifth decades. This symmetric polyarthropathy affects both small and large joints in both the upper and lower extremities.[288]

The diagnosis of rheumatoid arthritis is based on clinical evaluation, radiographic examination, and laboratory testing. The histopathology of bone lesions in rheumatoid arthritis is characterized by fibroblast proliferation; infiltration of macrophages, lymphocytes, and plasma cells; collagen deposition; and new bone formation. The hyaline cartilage surface is usually necrotic, and pannus is absent except at the margins of the capsular attachments. The process appears reparative in nature, but the inflammatory cell infiltrate or aggregate around small blood vessels in deeper bone marrow regions helps to confirm the diagnosis.[369] Furthermore, in a study of 223 patients with seropositive rheumatoid arthritis, rheumatoid nodules or areas of soft tissue necrosis have been characterized histologically into three classical zones: a necrotic central area, a surrounding wall of cells, and a marginal zone associated with the subcutaneous tissue or joint capsule. Such nodules appeared to develop after 4 or more years of disease duration and were associated with pain and deformity in nearly 70% of patients studied. Such necrosis or nodule formation may be an important factor that worsens the clinical prognosis in seropositive patients.[21]

Although rheumatoid arthritis typically has an insidious onset, acute presentation is by no means rare. Much attention has been centered on rheumatoid deformities of the hand in terms of initial involvement of individual joints; with acute onset, however, the feet are involved slightly more often than the hand (15.7% vs. 14.7%) (Short et al cited by Calabro[34]). Moreover, persons affected with mild to moderate rheumatoid arthritis with concomitant foot involvement have marked reduction in mobility and functional capacity.[357] An increased incidence of foot problems occurs with duration of the disease process,[235] and in chronic rheumatoid arthritis, Vainio[345] has reported that the incidence of foot deformities approaches 90%. Michelson[235] reported that ankle and hindfoot symptoms were much more common (42%) than forefoot symptoms (28%) in a series of 99 patients followed in an outpatient setting. In chronic rheumatoid arthritis, symmetric involvement is common; early on, asymmetric involvement may be observed.

History and Physical Examination

Early complaints of patients with rheumatoid arthritis involve poorly defined forefoot pain and metatarsalgia. Typically these complaints result from synovitis and an intra-articular effusion, which lead to painful ambulation. Poorly defined metatarsalgia can indicate an interdigital neuroma; in time, however, synovitis and deformity can make the diagnosis more straightforward. Zielaskowski[374] has reported an association of rheumatoid synovitis, nodule formation, and interdigital neuroma.

A variable course of presentation occurs in the symptomatic rheumatoid foot. Nonspecific forefoot swelling is characterized by tenderness to palpation and pain on ambulation. The most common forefoot deformities are hallux valgus, subluxation or dislocation of the lesser metatarsophalangeal (MTP) joints, and fixed hammer toe or claw toe deformities of the lesser toes (Fig. 16–1). In patients with nonspecific pain or diffuse foot pain, or both, with no visible radiographic findings and subtle or minimal clinical findings, a ^{99}Tc bone scan can help to localize disease.[260] The bone scan, together with hematologic laboratory work—erythrocyte sedimentation rate (ESR), C-reactive protein (CRP), rheumatoid factor (RF), antinuclear antibodies (ANAs), and serum uric acid—can help confirm an inflammatory cause. Magnetic resonance imaging (MRI) is increasingly used to evaluate forefoot symptoms and may be helpful in diagnosing joint erosion, chondrolysis, and other specific features of various inflammatory diseases that have characteristic MRI findings.[8]

Preoperative assessment, including attention to the vascular supply of the foot, is important. Although rheumatoid vasculitis is uncommon, it can present an increased risk to wound healing with surgery. The diagnosis of vasculitis is difficult, but nail splinter hemorrhages, neuritis or paresthesias in peripheral nerves (necrotizing vasculitis of nerve sheath vessels), skin ulcerations, poor capillary refill, and laboratory tests (antiphospholipid antibodies, RF level, CRP, ESR) can help facilitate the diagnosis. Anticoagulation, antiplatelet, and immunosuppressive treatment may be necessary in the treatment of this condition.[251,258,286]

Radiographic Examination

The classic radiographic signs of rheumatoid arthritis are that of a synovial inflammatory disease. The hyperemia involved with acute synovitis leads to periarticular osteoporosis,[126] and early radiographic examination might reveal only soft tissue swelling and diffuse juxtaarticular osteoporosis. Normal bone mineralization is usual in psoriasis, Reiter's syndrome, ankylosing spondylitis, and crystalline arthropathies.[207] Synovial inflammation eventually leads to marginal cortical erosions[116] at the reflection of synovium and capsule attachment (Fig. 16–2). These peripheral erosions eventually progress to central erosions with resultant joint space narrowing, subluxation, and dislocation. Eventual destruction of the articular cartilage occurs as the rheumatoid pannus spreads around the cartilaginous surface. The articular cartilage is thought to be destroyed by proteolytic enzymes, resulting in joint space narrowing.[33]

Gold and Bassett[116] have noted that rheumatoid arthritis tends to strike earliest at the first, fourth, and fifth MTP joints. They reported that the medial aspect of the first, second, third, and fourth metatarsals and

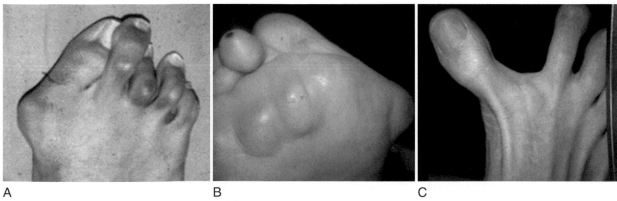

Figure 16–1 A, Clinical photo of hallux valgus deformity with subluxation of the lesser metatarsophalangeal (MTP) joints. **B,** Progression of the arthritis leads to dislocation of lesser MTP joints and the development of intractable plantar keratoses. The plantar fat pad is drawn distally so that it is no longer in a functional position. **C,** A severe hallux varus deformity in rheumatoid arthritis after rupture of the lateral capsule and adductor tendon.

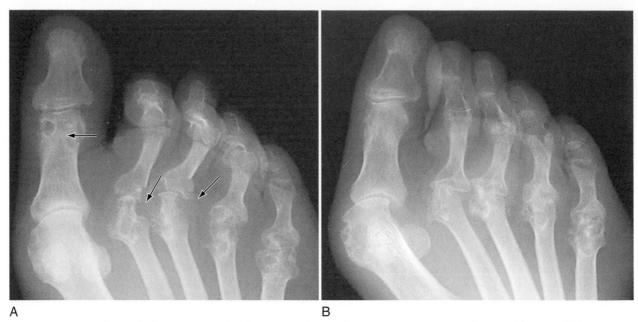

A   B

Figure 16–2 A, Radiograph demonstrates articular marginal cortical erosions and juxtaarticular osteoporosis of lesser metatarsophalangeal (MTP) joints. **B,** Severe hallux valgus. Subluxation and dislocation of lesser MTP joints with central erosion and joint space narrowing.

the lateral aspect of the fifth metatarsal were involved initially. The earliest visible erosions probably occur on the lateral aspect of the fifth metatarsal.[207] The interphalangeal joints are typically spared except for the hallux.[325] Midfoot and hindfoot changes include midfoot collapse, pes planus, and subtalar sclerosis. Localized inflammation in the areas of the retrocalcaneal bursa and at the attachment of the Achilles tendon and plantar aponeurosis are common with long-standing disease.

Rheumatoid arthritis can be divided into the following four stages:

- *Stage I:* No bone deformity; discomfort and synovitis without significant joint space narrowing.
- *Stage II:* Early involvement without fixed deformity; minimal erosive changes.
- *Stage III:* Soft tissue deformity; significant joint erosive changes.
- *Stage IV:* Articular destruction; severe hallux valgus, dislocation of the lesser MTP joints with fixed hammer toe or claw toe deformities, pes planovalgus (flatfoot), and hindfoot arthroses.

Radiographic progression of rheumatoid arthritis can be evaluated by various methods, but commonly used methods are those described by Larsen,[197] Rau,[276] and Steinbrocker.[323] Rau's and Larsen's methods were found to be equivalent, as reported by Tanaka et al[331] in assessing progression of early rheumatoid arthritis, which indeed affects pharmacologic treatment. More-

over, the magnitude of 5-year disability as measured by the Health Assessment Questionnaire Disability Index (HAQ-DI) was associated with joint space narrowing scores in the first year rather than periarticular erosion.[211] Another report suggested that 59% of 190 patients with early rheumatoid arthritis could be classified as nonprogressive based on radiographic joint changes[265] and that radiographic progression may be slowed by treatment with disease-modifying antirheumatic drugs (DMARDs) and other pharmacologic agents, including antibiotics (sulfonamides, doxycycline), salicylates, cytotoxic drugs (methotrexate, leuprolide acetate, cyclophosphamide), nonsteroidal antiinflammatory drugs (NSAIDs), corticosteroids, and cytokine inhibitors (etanercept, infliximab).

These findings could change the use of newer disease-modifying agents and create a larger pool of patients with secondary osteoarthritis. In turn, this could lead to a change in the use of specific orthopaedic procedures from those that are typically joint destructive to those that are joint sparing[339] for many patients with rheumatoid arthritis who have nonprogressive disease.

Pathophysiology

When considering treatment of forefoot and midfoot problems, the hindfoot must be assessed as well. Hindfoot and midfoot deformity must be addressed or forefoot reconstruction efforts can fail.[326] Limited midfoot arthrodesis can be performed concomitantly if indicated but surgery is often staged, with the midfoot given surgical priority.

Forefoot Arthritis

In the early stages of rheumatoid arthritis, specific changes in the foot include inflammation of the synovium with distention of the MTP joint capsule. Synovial proliferation leads to chronic capsule distention, resulting in loss of integrity of both the MTP joint supporting capsular structures and the collateral ligaments. With continued ambulation in the presence of soft tissue instability and with constant dorsiflexion stress on the MTP joints, subluxation and eventual dislocation occur.[235,318] As the MTP joints of the lesser toes dislocate, the base of the proximal phalanx eventually comes to rest on the dorsal metatarsal metaphysis (Fig. 16–3). Progressive contracture of the long flexor tendons and the plantar intrinsic muscles lock the base of the proximal phalanx on the dorsometatarsal neck. The proximal phalanx becomes fixed in a dorsiflexed position, creating a plantar-directed force on the metatarsal head.[70] Simultaneously, the plantar fat pad is drawn distally over the metatarsal heads, leaving only an extremely thin soft-tissue covering on the plantar aspect of the metatarsal heads. The loss of the protective plantar fat pad cushion coupled with increased stress on the underlying skin can lead to the development of intractable plantar keratotic lesions and, in time, ulceration of the plantar skin.

Subluxation and dislocation of the lesser toes create an imbalance between the intrinsic and extrinsic muscles and give rise to progressive hammering of the lesser toes. Occasionally, a swan-neck deformity of a lesser toe develops, but more often a hyperextension deformity of the MTP joint occurs in combination with a flexion deformity of the proximal interphalangeal (PIP) and distal interphalangeal (DIP) joints (claw toe deformity). Because of severe contracture of the lesser toes, significant shoe-fitting problems result. Callosities can develop over the dorsal aspect of the PIP joint, causing areas of pressure. Large synovial cysts or rheumatoid nodules can develop in the forefoot and, when located on weight-bearing surfaces, lead to significant difficulty with ambulation. Although typically the lesser toes deviate in a lateral direction, medial deviation occasionally occurs. The resultant direction depends, to a great extent, on the direction in which the hallux deviates (varus or valgus).

Michelson et al[235] reported that within the first 1 to 3 years of rheumatoid arthritis, 65% of patients are noted to have MTP synovitis. With chronic rheumatoid arthritis, Vidigal et al[351] and others[229,318] have reported that approximately two thirds of patients develop subluxation and dislocation of the lesser MTP joints (Fig. 16–4). Michelson et al[235] and others[229,345,351] have

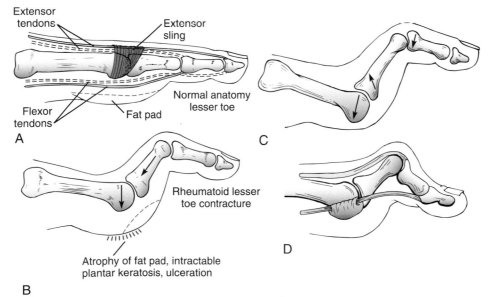

Figure 16–3 Pathophysiology of the rheumatoid forefoot. **A,** Normal alignment and balance of metatarsophalangeal (MTP) joints and toes. Fat pad is centered beneath metatarsal heads. **B,** As rheumatoid deformity progresses, an imbalance occurs with progressive dorsal subluxation of the MTP joints and deformities of the lesser toes. The fat pad is drawn distally by the contracting lesser toes. **C,** End-stage deformity. Dislocation of MTP joint with proximal phalanx ankylosed to the dorsal aspect of the metatarsal head. This forces the metatarsal head into the plantar aspect of the foot and results in severe callus formation. Lesser toes develop hammer toe deformities that often become severely contracted, and the fat pad is drawn distally and is no longer in a functional position. **D,** With chronic dorsiflexion deformity of the proximal phalanx at the MTP joint, flexor tendons subluxate dorsally, becoming functional extensors of the MTP joint.

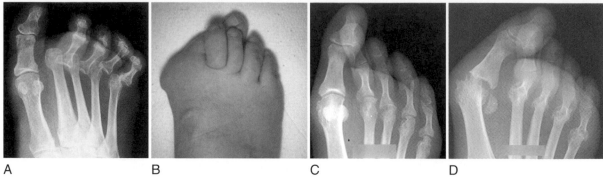

A   B   C   D

Figure 16–4   A, Preoperative radiograph demonstrates lesser metatarsophalangeal (MTP) joint dislocations, marginal erosions with chondrolysis, and relative sparing of the 1st MTP joint. **B,** Clinical photograph at presurgical follow-up demonstrates hallux valgus deformity with dislocation of lesser MTP joints. **C.** Thirty-year-old woman demonstrating marginal erosions of the third, fourth, and fifth MTP joints with chondrolysis. **D.** Eight years later, radiographs demonstrate severe hallux valgus, chondrolysis, and dislocation of lesser MTP joints.

reported that the incidence of hammer toe or claw toe deformity of the lesser toes varies from 40% to 80%.

Hallux valgus increases in incidence and severity in the chronic stages of rheumatoid arthritis.[34] Michelson et al[235] and others[318,345,351] have reported a high incidence of hallux valgus in patients with chronic rheumatoid arthritis (59% to 90%). With progressive clawing of the lesser toes, little lateral stability is afforded to the great toe, and the hallux migrates laterally to a fixed position either under or over the second and third toes. Progression of the rheumatoid process includes destruction of articular cartilage and resorption of subchondral bone, which tends to destabilize the hallux. As the hallux valgus deformity worsens, the weight-bearing function of the first ray lessens, and a greater proportion of weight is borne on

the lesser metatarsal heads. Craxford et al[72] reported increased pressure beneath the second and third metatarsal heads with chronic rheumatoid arthritis (Fig. 16–5).

Midfoot Arthritis

Vidigal et al[351] reported midtarsal joint involvement in approximately two thirds of patients with chronic rheumatoid arthritis. Associated with this, flattening of the longitudinal arch occurs in approximately 50% of patients.[318] Often a valgus deformity of the hindfoot occurs. The resultant ambulatory pattern is a shuffling, flat-footed steppage gait. Fu and Scranton[108] noted that with progressive rheumatoid arthritis the foot changes to a passive weight-bearing platform for ambulation. Chronic synovitis and eventual chondrolysis of the tarsometatarsal joints often occur with chronic disease.

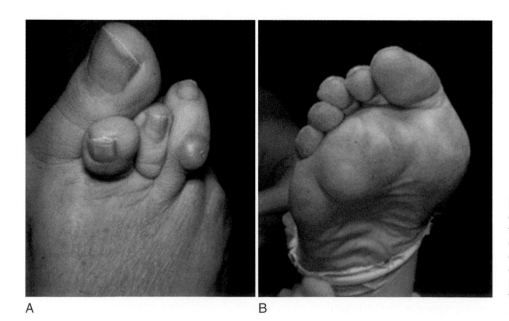

A   B

Figure 16–5   A, Hallux valgus deformity with dislocation of the lesser metatarsophalangeal (MTP) joints and hammer toe deformity. **B,** Plantar view demonstrates severe intractable plantar keratoses associated with dislocation of the lesser MTP joints.

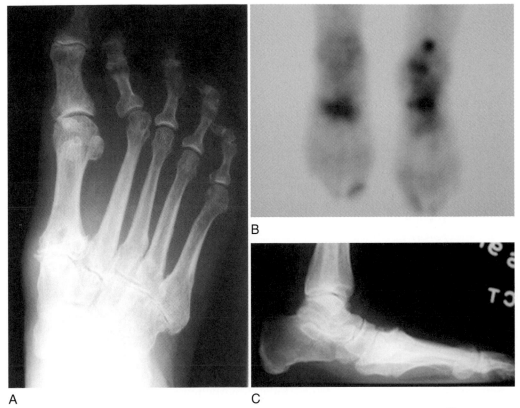

A   C

Figure 16-6 A, Anteroposterior (AP) radiograph demonstrates severe arthritis of Lisfranc's joint. **B,** ^{99}Tc bone scan shows bilateral midfoot uptake as well as uptake in the left ankle and hindfoot. **C,** Lateral radiograph demonstrates midfoot arthritis with pes planus and rocker-sole deformity.

Usually, because of the limitation of motion at midfoot joints, a fibrous or bony ankylosis develops, but reduced motion is rarely restrictive.

Occasionally the first metatarsocuneiform (MTC) joint becomes extremely hypermobile, with subsequent loss of normal weight-bearing function. Resultant transfer metatarsalgia can occur from this hypermobility. Loss of the longitudinal arch on weight-bearing lateral radiographs is demonstrated by sagging at either the MTC or the naviculocuneiform articulation. Severe deformity can occur over time and make weight bearing almost impossible (Fig. 16-6A and B).

Hindfoot Arthritis

Vainio[345] reported that 72% of women and 59% of men with chronic rheumatoid arthritis had involvement of either the midtarsal or the subtalar joint but that surgical intervention was relatively infrequent. Clayton[47] reported that the forefoot was involved 10 times more often than the hindfoot.

Changes in the hindfoot occur much later with longer duration of rheumatoid arthritis. Spiegel and Spiegel[318] observed that in patients with rheumatoid arthritis of less than 5 years' duration, only 8% demon-strated hindfoot arthrosis, whereas in those who had had rheumatoid arthritis longer than 5 years, 25% were symptomatic. They concluded that hindfoot arthrosis was an acquired deformity that developed from the mechanical stress of weight bearing. In a series of patients with rheumatoid arthritis who were evaluated with computed tomography (CT) scans, Seltzer et al[301] noted talonavicular joint involvement in 39% (Fig. 16-7), calcaneocuboid involvement in 25%, and subtalar involvement in 29%. Gold and Bassett[116] reported the talonavicular joint is typically the first tarsal joint to be involved. Vidigal et al[351] and Michelson et al[235] reported the incidence of subtalar joint involvement varied from 32% to 42%.

The underlying pathophysiology with hindfoot involvement relates to progressive destruction of the capsular and ligamentous supporting structures of the subtalar joint. Because subtalar joint function is intimately associated with transverse tarsal joint function, instability of these joints can result in altered function and gait. Often the end result is a progressive pes planovalgus deformity of the hindfoot (Fig. 16-8). Posterior tibial tendon dysfunction with rheumatoid arthritis can lead to a unilateral progressive flatfoot deformity as well.[79,222]

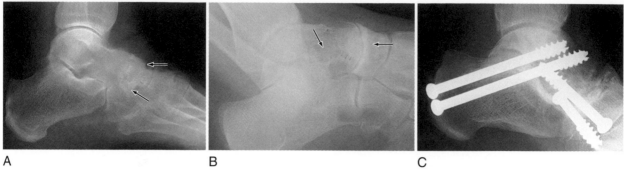

Figure 16–7 A, Fifty-year-old woman with isolated talonavicular arthritis. **B,** Talonavicular arthritis with cyst formation at the subtalar joint. **C,** After triple arthrodesis.

Keenan et al[178] reported that pes planovalgus deformities in patients with rheumatoid arthritis resulted from exaggerated pronation forces on the weakened and inflamed subtalar joint. They demonstrated that with electromyographic studies, an increased period of activity of the tibialis posterior muscle occurred, which they interpreted as an "attempt to stabilize" an unstable foot. Flattening of the longitudinal arch also can develop secondary to naviculocuneiform joint deterioration or first metatarsocuneiform joint collapse. In some patients, severe valgus of the hindfoot may be associated with a concomitant valgus deformity of the ankle joint as well (Fig. 16–9). This creates a difficult management situation, with both ankle and hindfoot involvement. Bracing is difficult, and a pantalar fusion may be necessary to realign the foot but presents the patient with a difficult surgical recovery.

With severe, long-standing hindfoot deformity, an Achilles tendon contracture can develop. Although not a primary deformity, it occurs secondarily in relation to a chronic valgus deformity of the hindfoot. At the time of a triple arthrodesis, Achilles tendon lengthening may be necessary.

Conservative care for midfoot and hindfoot degeneration includes rest to relieve swollen and inflamed joints, minimizing weight bearing during acute flare-ups, casting, padding, roomy footwear, and custom-made longitudinal arch supports. With instability, a polypropylene ankle–foot orthosis (AFO) can provide some relief. NSAIDs and occasional judicious use of an isolated corticosteroid injection can give symptomatic relief. When progressive deformity occurs or unrelenting pain is refractory to conservative treatment, surgical intervention for midfoot or hindfoot dysfunction may be necessary.

The objective in all surgeries of the midfoot and hindfoot is to obtain a plantigrade foot. The goal is to obtain heel valgus of approximately 5 degrees after arthrodesis or reconstruction. An autogenous iliac crest graft at the time of arthrodesis depends on the magnitude of the deformity and the specific fusion that is desired. If substantial realignment is part of the surgical plan, then an iliac crest autograft or a structural allograft may be necessary. Distraction or lengthening of the medial or lateral column may be needed to reestablish alignment. Failure to perform a bone graft in the presence of a severe pes planovalgus deformity can result in undercorrection or recurrent deformity (see Chapter 19).

With hindfoot involvement, a patient might misconstrue subtalar or transverse tarsal joint pain as "ankle" pain. Careful physical examination may be necessary to differentiate these symptomatic areas. Selective injections or imaging studies such as CT scan or MRI (or both) can provide conclusive information.

Ankle Joint Arthritis

Ankle joint involvement in the patient with chronic rheumatoid arthritis is manifested mainly as synovitis. Spiegel[318] reported that 63% of patients who had had rheumatoid arthritis less than 10 years were affected with ankle synovitis. Rana[274] and others[20,345,351] have reported ankle joint involvement varying from 4% to 16% (Figs. 16–9 and 16–10). This is in contradistinction to subtalar, talonavicular, and calcaneocuboid joint involvement, which is much more frequent. Often, pain and tenosynovitis around the ankle are mistaken for ankle joint pain. As a rule, significant deformity of the ankle joint does not occur. Although Wagner[353] found that severe involvement of the ankle joint that required surgical intervention was rare, Michelson[235] reported a slightly higher incidence of ankle and hindfoot involvement (42%) than forefoot involvement (28%), although these patients were not necessarily candidates for surgery.

Ankle arthrodesis or arthroplasty may be indicated with end-stage ankle arthritis refractory to conservative care (Fig. 16–11). Rarely, with arthrosis of both the subtalar and the ankle joint, a pantalar arthrodesis is performed. More reliable results are reported

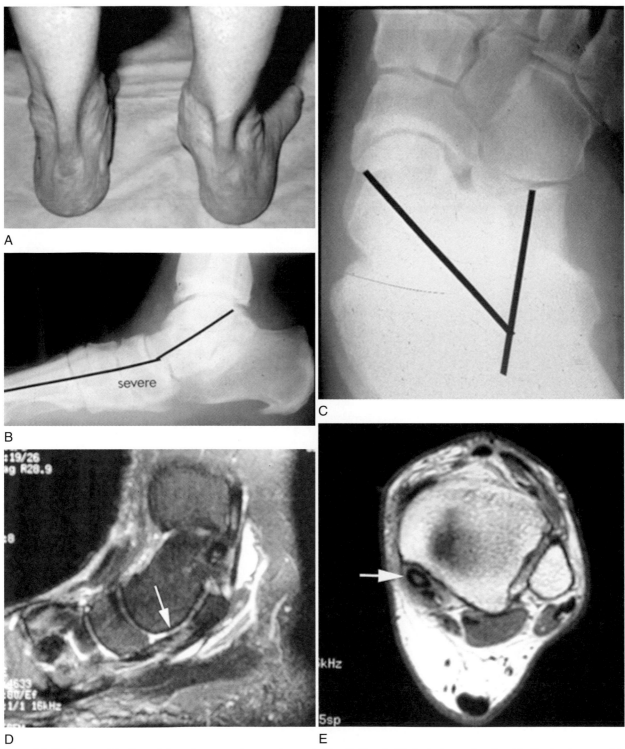

Figure 16–8 Severe hindfoot deformity secondary to rheumatoid arthritis. **A,** Clinical photo showing hindfoot valgus position. **B,** Because of inadequate support to the talus, the talus has assumed an extremely plantar-flexed position with resultant pes planus as shown on the lateral radiograph. **C,** Peritalar subluxation is notable on the anteroposterior (AP) radiograph. **D** and **E,** MRI shows posterior tibial tendon tendinosis and high-grade signal change within the tendon.

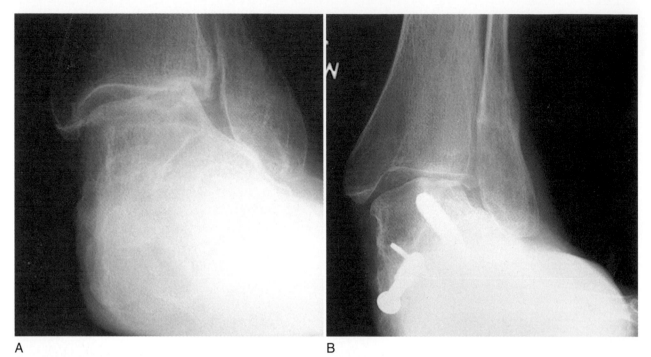

A   B

Figure 16–9   From 10% to 30% of patients with rheumatoid arthritis have severe valgus of the foot. **A,** Anteroposterior (AP) weight-bearing radiograph of the ankle joint demonstrates a valgus tilt to the mortise. **B,** Postoperative AP weight-bearing radiograph demonstrates marked valgus tilting of talus and mortise. Whether this change resulted from severe hindfoot deformity or from progressive rheumatoid involvement of the ankle joint after hindfoot arthrodesis remains unknown.

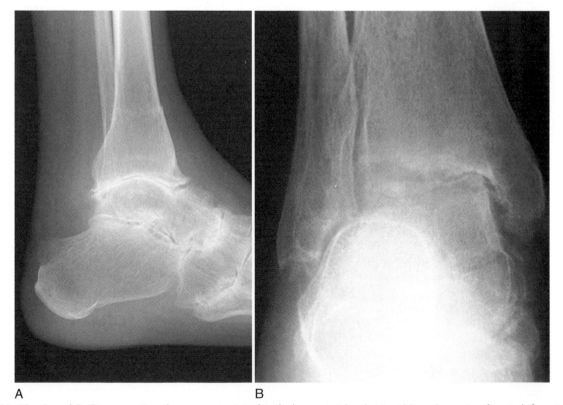

A   B

Figure 16–10   **A** and **B,** Degenerative changes associated with rheumatoid arthritis. Although no significant deformity occurs, severe chondrolysis is associated with pain and difficult ambulation.

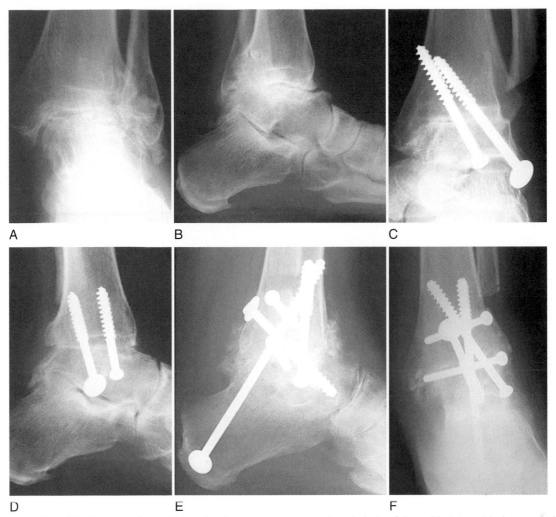

Figure 16–11 **A** and **B,** Preoperative radiographs demonstrate severe chondrolysis of the ankle joint with rheumatoid arthritis. **C** and **D,** After arthrodesis of the ankle joint with compression screw technique. **E** and **F,** With arthritis of the subtalar and ankle joint, pantalar arthrodesis is performed.

following ankle arthroplasty or hindfoot realignment using limited joint arthrodeses combined with soft tissue reconstructive procedures, so treatment with either concomitant or staged ankle arthroplasty might become more common (see Chapter 17).

A stress fracture of the distal tibia can occur in patients with long-standing rheumatoid arthritis. A stress fracture can develop from an abnormal hindfoot posture associated with marked osteopenia. A varus deformity of the ankle joint can occur (Fig. 16–12A and B), or a valgus deformity can develop with subsequent fracture of the fibula (Fig. 16–12C). Moreover, stress fracture in the lower extremity (including the metatarsals) is common in the patient with rheumatoid arthritis, and a high index of suspicion is needed for this diagnosis with complaints of pain in areas away from joints.[91,210]

Treatment

An appreciation of the clinical course of rheumatoid arthritis is essential in the decision-making process of developing a treatment program (Fig. 16–13A). Gait analysis of patients with chronic rheumatoid arthritis when compared to those of nonarthritic subjects demonstrates delayed and reduced forefoot loading, resulting in a shorter stride length.[259] This effect may be related to forefoot pain's reducing the functional lever arm of the foot during push off.

Platto et al[269] reported an association between impaired ambulation and foot deformity. They observed a greater association between hindfoot disease and gait impairment as compared with forefoot disease.[269] On the other hand, Shi et al[306] studied 100 feet with rheumatoid arthritis and reported no correla-

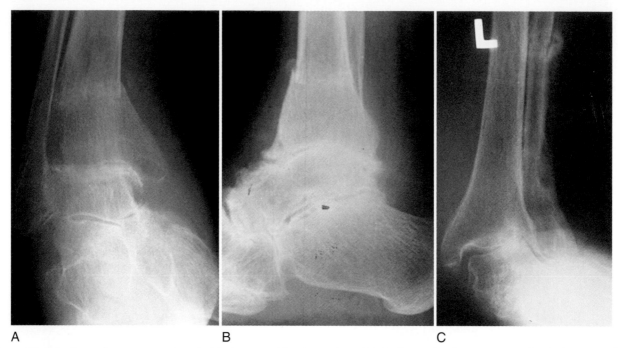

A   B   C

Figure 16–12   Stress fractures associated with rheumatoid arthritis. **A** and **B,** Radiographs demonstrate a distal tibia stress fracture that has migrated into a varus deformity. **C,** Ankle arthritis associated with a fibular stress fracture with subsequent valgus deformity.

tion between a loss of arch height and hallux valgus or forefoot splaying. Nonetheless, initial orthopaedic treatment is directed toward pain relief, prevention of deformity, correction of deformity, preservation of function, and restoration of function. Medical management throughout the entire disease process includes pharmacologic treatment as well, and this has been shown to improve ambulatory capacity.[131]

Conservative Treatment

The most important aspect of early nonsurgical care is wearing proper footwear. Likewise, modification of a patient's footwear may be beneficial. A carefully placed metatarsal pad just proximal to an intractable plantar keratotic lesion or an area of MTP joint tenderness can relieve discomfort associated with increased pressure. Excavating the insole beneath a pressure area can also decrease symptoms. Many patients with mild to moderate rheumatoid involvement of the foot can be fitted with a broad-toed, soft-soled shoe.[334] An extra-depth shoe with a Plastizote or compressible insole can help to accommodate more severe deformities. A Plastizote liner or viscoelastic insole can relieve plantar pain in a patient with an atrophied plantar fat pad. With significant lesser-toe contractures, extra-depth shoes fitted with a customized orthosis can accommodate painful plantar lesions such as intractable plantar keratoses. Although a Plastizote liner can accommodate significant forefoot deformities, it commonly needs to be

replaced every few months as the insert bottoms out. Orthotic devices and footwear that redistribute weight-bearing forces tend to decrease pressure areas, diffuse weight-bearing, decrease shearing forces, support unstable joints, and restrict motion are helpful.[69,315] Custom orthotics that incorporate a metatarsal dome pad may be more effective in reducing metatarsalgia and pressure beneath the first and second metatarsal heads.[150]

Involvement of a pedorthist and the use of orthopaedic appliances can help to prevent deformities and maintain function. There have been several studies that evaluated the use of specific custom orthotics or shoes for the treatment of rheumatoid foot deformities.[40,51,158,364] Conrad et al[51] found no benefit from posted foot orthoses compared to placebos in regard to pain relief or reduction in disability. In contrast, Woodburn et al[364] found a 19% reduction in pain, 31% reduction in disability, and 14% reduction in functional limitation with the use of custom rigid orthotics. Chalmers et al[40] reported that semirigid orthoses had a significant effect on pain reduction, and soft orthoses and supportive shoes had little or no effect. None of these orthoses had any effect on reduction of joint synovitis.

Jannink et al[158] evaluated the methodology of 11 randomized, controlled clinical trials that had studied the effect of orthopaedic shoes and orthoses. The authors reported that although all 11 studies demon-

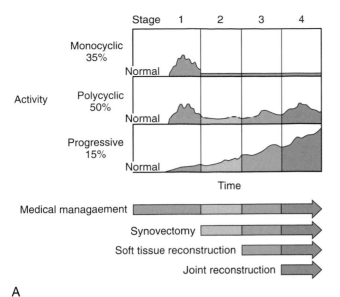

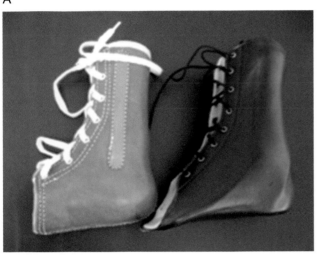

Figure 16–13 A, Clinical course of rheumatoid arthritis. **B,** Braces used to alleviate pain in ankle and hindfoot arthritis.

strated the effectiveness of their product, the studies evaluated did a relatively poor job of examining usability, efficiency, satisfaction, and reliability of patient use. It appears that orthoses designed to support rheumatoid arthritic foot deformities and to provide pain relief might yield some benefit, but patient satisfaction, usability, and the specific indications for a specified device remain vague, and specific indications are yet to be determined.

Metatarsalgia in the early stages of rheumatoid arthritis may be alleviated by a metatarsal arch support, over the-counter soft insoles, metatarsal pads, or custom-made orthotic devices. Shoes with a low heel, soft leather upper, and increased depth tend to accommodate claw toes and hammer toes. Soft-soled, rocker-bottom shoes decrease stress on the metatarsal

and the hindfoot region. An over-the-counter padded insole such as a Spenco liner or a molded insole can relieve pressure areas. Nonrigid longitudinal custom-made arch supports tend to shift pressure areas more proximally.

Patients should be instructed in foot care and careful observation of skin for potential breakdown. Patients with midfoot and hindfoot pain with no fixed deformity often can be treated with a customized arch support or a polypropylene AFO. Bracing may be necessary when foot and ankle pain becomes refractory to other methods of treatment. A molded leather ankle brace or an Arizona brace with steel stays can be worn inside a shoe and can provide significant ankle and hindfoot support (Fig. 16–13B).

During acute arthritis exacerbations, diminished activity level, rest, and cast immobilization help to reduce symptoms.

Physical therapy can be helpful in treating patients with foot problems associated with rheumatoid arthritis. Contrast baths may be used to decrease swelling and inflammation, although in the presence of Raynaud's phenomenon, they may be contraindicated. Stretching exercises for a contracted Achilles tendon and passive manipulation of the ankle and hindfoot can help to restore or maintain motion. Maintaining range of motion at the MTP joint and interphalangeal joints in the presence of acute rheumatoid arthritis may be aided by active or passive manipulation. Muscle strengthening and conditioning may be helpful in maintaining ambulatory capacity. Additionally, exercise in early rheumatoid arthritis has been shown to enhance neuromuscular performance without an obvious negative effect on disease activity or joint disease.[129] Limitation of ambulation during acute episodes, exercises, and stretching of involved joints are all important physical therapy modalities in maintaining function in the patient with chronic rheumatoid arthritis.

With the increasing involvement of numerous lower extremity joints, gait training is occasionally necessary to maintain ambulatory independence. The use of ambulatory aids such as canes and crutches can reduce weight-bearing stress, but this may be done at the expense of the upper extremities. With significant upper extremity involvement, platform crutches or canes with special handgrips may be necessary.

Pharmacologic agents that reduce inflammation and relieve pain facilitate the treatment of rheumatoid arthritis. Salicylates are often the first line of defense, although nonsteroidal antiinflammatory drugs (NSAIDs) are often used as well. The occasional judicious use of a intra-articular corticosteroid injection may be beneficial, but systemic oral steroid therapy is used less commonly because of the well-known deleterious side effects of chronic corticosteroid use.[59] Cutaneous ulcers that were likely related to methotrexate toxicity have been reported to develop spontaneously in a patient with rheumatoid arthritis.[244]

At surgery, patients who are taking or have recently been taking corticosteroids should be treated with corticosteroids during the perioperative period. Patients who have recently undergone total joint replacement should be covered with perioperative antibiotics at the time of foot and ankle surgery.[59] Some discontinue the use of methotrexate one week before and one week after surgery because of their belief that there is diminished wound-healing capacity with concomitant methotrexate therapy. Recent data suggest that discontinuing disease-modifying agents such as tumor necrosis factor inhibition agents (etanercept, infliximab) might not be necessary.[25]

Bibbo et al[25] reported no adverse affects on complication rates in 31 patients followed prospectively for 12 months after elective foot and ankle surgery. However, surgical wounds in patients with rheumatoid arthritis do not heal as rapidly when compared to patients without rheumatoid arthritis and should be monitored closely for infection, vasculitis, and other causes of delayed wound healing.[253]

The reported effect of in-office plantar callosity shaving or debridement is temporary and appears to decrease substantially within a week following debridement.[365] At best, plantar callosity shaving offers temporary relief prior to definitive surgical treatment.

Surgical Treatment

Medical management should continue throughout the progression of the rheumatoid disease process. Surgical procedures may be indicated depending on the severity and progression of the inflammatory process. A monocyclic disease process infrequently requires extensive surgery, whereas a polycyclic or progressive process increases the risk of later surgical treatment (Fig. 16–13A).

The precise timing of surgical intervention for the patient with rheumatoid foot and ankle deformities varies significantly and must be individualized for each patient. During the proliferative phase of synovitis, a synovectomy of an involved joint may slow the progression of the rheumatoid inflammatory process. At other times, conservative management provides adequate relief for a patient, and no surgical intervention is warranted. With progressive collapse of the longitudinal arch, early surgical intervention can prevent significant hindfoot deformity. Furthermore, an attempt should be made to prevent loss of ambulatory capacity with progression of the disease over a long period. Surgical reconstruction to maintain ambulation is important. Surgical intervention may be inter-spersed with periods of conservative care so that numerous surgical procedures are not clustered during a short time.

Many patients require lower extremity total joint replacement. In general, proximal joint surgery should precede distal joint surgery. For example, a total hip or total knee replacement usually should precede hindfoot surgery. Hindfoot surgery typically should precede forefoot surgery,[57] the rationale being that with a valgus or pronation deformity, a recurrent forefoot deformity may develop. Moreover, patients with valgus hindfoot deformities have been shown to have higher forefoot pressures compared to patients with a normal hindfoot based on pedobarograph studies.[326] Extensive bilateral forefoot surgery should be discouraged because of the magnitude of surgery as well as the decreased ambulatory capacity after surgery. In patients who are considered for total ankle arthroplasty, we believe that the hindfoot should be realigned prior to the implantation of the total ankle.

LESSER METATARSOPHALANGEAL JOINT SYNOVECTOMY

Synovectomy of the lesser MTP joints is indicated for painful, symptomatic MTP joints early in the disease process. Subluxation or dislocation of the lesser MTP joints with formation of intractable plantar keratoses is a contraindication to simple synovectomy because surgery will achieve limited gains. Debridement of hypertrophic synovial tissue can arrest the degenerative process, reduce MTP joint distention, and decrease soft tissue deformation, which can eventually lead to subluxation and dislocation if untreated.

The duration of remission achieved with synovectomy varies from patient to patient. A patient should be informed that a synovectomy may be a temporizing procedure and that eventually with progressive deformity, a forefoot arthroplasty may be necessary. Preoperatively, patients considered for synovectomy alone should have swollen and tender MTP joints with minimal deformity. Flexible or mild fixed hammering may be treated concomitantly. When planning the surgical synovectomy, dorsal interspace incisions are used so that they can be reused if later forefoot reconstruction is necessary.

Synovectomy has been recommended for the lesser MTP joints by Vainio[344] and others.[3,5,37,69,70,277]

Surgical Technique

1. The patient is placed supine on the operating table with a well-padded bump under the hip. Either an Esmarch bandage or a well-padded thigh tourniquet is used to maintain a bloodless field for surgery.
2. The involved MTP joint is approached through a dorsal longitudinal incision made in the second web space to approach the second or third MTP joint. The incision is made in the fourth web space to approach either the fourth or fifth MTP joints.
3. Using the extensor tendon as a guide, the dissection is carried down through the extensor hood, exposing the MTP joint.
4. The proliferative synovial tissue is excised on the dorsomedial and dorsolateral aspect through sharp dissection. Care is taken to remove hypertrophic synovium beneath the collateral ligaments.
5. With longitudinal tension placed on the toe, the resection is carried as plantarward as possible. A small rongeur is used to debride any hypertrophic synovium.
6. The joint capsule is approximated with interrupted 4-0 absorbable suture. The skin is closed in an interrupted manner.
7. For a synovectomy of the first MTP joint, a dorsal longitudinal incision is centered over the first MTP joint and the dissection carried down on either side of the extensor hallucis longus tendon. The technique otherwise is the same as described for the lesser MTP joints.

Postoperative Care

A gauze-and-tape compression dressing is applied at surgery and changed every 10 to 14 days for 6 weeks. The patient is permitted to ambulate in a postoperative shoe with weight bearing as tolerated. Active and passive joint range-of-motion exercises are initiated 3 weeks after surgery.

Results and Complications

Raunio and Laine[277] reported on 33 feet (28 patients) that underwent MTP joint synovectomy. With short-term follow-up, they found 80% of patients satisfied and noted diminished progression of rheumatoid arthritis on both clinical and radiographic examination. Cracchiolo[70]

observed that synovectomy of one or two isolated MTP joints may give temporary relief.

Vainio[344] stated that synovectomy decreased symptoms of metatarsalgia and noted reduced symptoms of interdigital neuroma in patients with synovial inflammatory disease. Higgins et al[149] reported the occurrence of interdigital neuroma associated with seronegative rheumatoid arthritis. Aho[3] reported good relief with synovectomy in 16 patients (21 feet). He noted that they were symptom free and pain free "months to years" after synovectomy.

Belt et al[17] reported the results of synovectomy on 83 patients at 15 years and 68 patients at 20 years postoperatively. They concluded that synovectomy was insufficient treatment without concomitant use of immunosuppressive drugs and that 75% of joints that had undergone synovectomy alone in their series later went on to excisional arthroplasty. The long-term effects of newer disease-modifying agents that block the inflammatory cascade and immune signaling may either be integral in the long-term success of synovectomy or eventually obviate the need for synovectomy by disease suppression.

Care must be taken in exposing the lesser MTP joints through an intermetatarsal dissection to avoid injury to an adjacent sensory nerve. A major complication after synovectomy is damage to a dorsal cutaneous nerve to a lesser toe or damage to a branch of the digital nerve. Either can result in postoperative numbness in a fairly confined area. Recurrence of synovial hypertrophy can develop in time, and the patient should be informed of this preoperatively. It is hoped with synovectomy that progression of the disease process will be significantly delayed.

RHEUMATOID HAMMER TOE DEFORMITY

Hammer toe and claw toe involvement of the lesser toes is common with chronic rheumatoid arthritis. Typically the hammer toe deformity occurs in conjunction with MTP joint subluxation and dislocation. In early stages, padding of contracted lesser toes and roomy footwear can accommodate the deformed lesser toe. Surgical correction is typically deferred until a forefoot reconstruction is performed.

The surgical treatment of a hammer toe deformity depends on the severity of the deformity. A mild deformity may be treated with passive manipulation and intramedullary Kirschner wire fixation. Closed osteoclasis in combination with forefoot arthroplasty has been advocated for a mild and moderate hammer toe deformity.[46,69,189,221,267] For more severe deformities, a proximal phalangeal condylectomy achieves realignment by bony decompression. PIP arthrodesis has been advocated by Coughlin[57] and others.[69,167,189,355]

Surgical Technique

1. An elliptical or longitudinal incision is centered over the dorsal aspect of the PIP joint, excising the callus, extensor tendon, and joint capsule, thereby exposing the PIP joint (Fig. 16–14A and B) (see Chapter 7).

2. The collateral ligaments on the medial and lateral aspect of the PIP joint are severed, allowing the condyles of the proximal phalanx to be delivered into the wound. Care is taken to protect the adjacent neurovascular bundles.

3. A portion of the proximal phalanx is resected just proximal to the flare of the condyles, and any prominent remaining edges are smoothed with a rongeur (Fig. 16–14C).

4. At this point, the toe is brought into correct alignment. If tension appears to be present at the PIP joint and correcting the deformity is difficult, more bone should be resected.

5. The articular surface of the base of the middle phalanx is resected with a rongeur (this is optional).

6. A 0.045 Kirschner wire is introduced at the PIP joint and driven distally, exiting the tip of the toe. With the toe held in proper align-

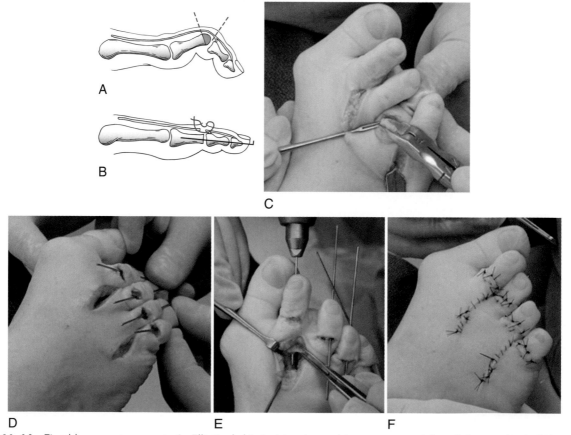

Figure 16–14 Fixed hammer toe repair. **A,** Elliptical skin incision is used to expose condyles of the proximal phalanx, which are then resected. **B,** Kirschner wire is used to stabilize the arthroplasty site. **C,** Clinical photo of proximal phalanx condyle resection. **D,** Placement of intramedullary Kirschner wires in middle and distal phalanges. **E,** Kirschner wires are advanced through the proximal phalanx into the metatarsals. **F,** Multiple hammer toe repairs are shown in conjunction with a rheumatoid forefoot reconstruction.

ment, the pin is then driven in a retrograde fashion to stabilize and align the proximal phalanx (Fig. 14D and E). Later, after the MTP joint arthroplasty, the pin is advanced into the metatarsal diaphysis and proximal metaphysis, stabilizing the arthroplasty site. The placement of intramedullary Kirschner wires to stabilize the surgical site depends on the surgeon's choice. Kirschner wires have been advocated for treatment of hammer toes and lesser MTP joint excisional arthroplasty with rheumatoid foot deformities.[58,220] Internal fixation not only helps simplify dressing changes but also seems to produce a cosmetically superior result by achieving acceptable position of the toes as well as maintaining this alignment.

Postoperative Care

Dressings are changed every 10 days, when the rest of rheumatoid foot repair is inspected and redressed. The Kirschner wire and sutures are removed 3 weeks after surgery.

Alternative Method: Closed Osteoclasis

An alternative to an open hammer toe repair is a closed osteoclasis. After the MTP joint forefoot arthroplasty, passive pressure is placed on the PIP joint, and the middle and distal phalanges are brought into hyperextension (Fig. 16–15). With significant ankylosis or deformity, it may become apparent that the magnitude of pressure needed to straighten the toe

can place the neurovascular status of the toe at risk. In this situation, a surgical decompression with a proximal phalangeal condylectomy is indicated.

An open arthroplasty technique of the PIP joint does enable easier placement of the intramedullary Kirschner wire. With a closed osteoclasis, the Kirschner wire is introduced at the base of the proximal phalanx and is driven distally out the tip of the toe. It is then retrograded in a proximal direction across the MTP joint arthroplasty site into the metatarsal diaphysis and metaphysis to stabilize the site. The skin can be protected from the Kirschner wire by using an angiocatheter sheath during retrograde placement through the base of the proximal phalanx.

Results and Complications

Coughlin[58] has reported the long-term results (mean follow-up of 74 months) of open hammer toe repair in combination with forefoot arthroplasty and first MTP joint arthrodesis (rheumatoid forefoot reconstruction) for rheumatoid arthritis. Of 188 toes, 142 had an open hammer toe repair, and in 76 (53%) of these the pulp of the toe touched the ground at final follow-up. None of the lesser toes at final follow-up were reported to be a source of pain or to limit shoe choice. Successful arthrodesis of the PIP joint did not affect pain scores.

Recurrence of a hammer toe deformity places the MTP joint at risk for recurrent deformity as

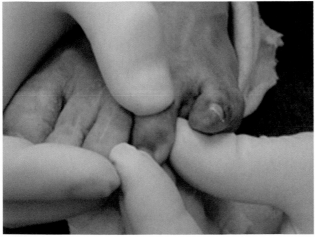
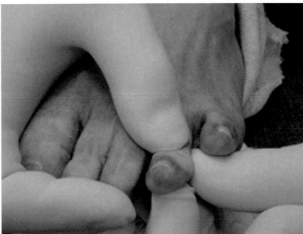

A   B

Figure 16–15 Before **(A)** and after **(B)** closed osteoclasis of the fourth toe. Fixed hammer toe deformity is manipulated into extension and can be stabilized with an intramedullary Kirschner wire.

well. Coughlin[58] reported six postoperative mallet toe deformities (4%) (five had had a hammer toe repair) and three (2%) recurrent hammer toe deformities in 142 open hammer toe repairs associated with a complete rheumatoid forefoot reconstruction in 58 feet with a mean follow-up of 74 months.

Recurrent clawing of a lesser toe leads to hyperextension of the MTP joint with eventual subluxation, dislocation, and re-deformation of the lesser toe. Recurrence of a hammer toe or claw toe deformity is to be avoided. Re-deformation can result from failed initial correction or actual recurrence. Thus a closed osteoclasis should be reserved for only mild deformities, whereas a DuVries phalangeal arthroplasty is preferred for more significant deformities (see Chapter 7). Furthermore, increased bony decompression when needed is achieved by resection arthroplasty of the lesser MTP joint.

The results after a hammer toe repair in the rheumatoid foot are consistently good. However, complications may occur, including persistent swelling, recurrent deformity, and skin or nail loss. Swelling of the toe can persist for 1 to 6 months postoperatively. It invariably subsides.

Occasionally, a mild deformity can recur, or a toe can deviate in either a medial or a lateral direction. This is rarely a significant problem. After stabilization of the first ray, adjacent pressure from the hallux is uncommon. Fusion of the first MTP joint stabilizes the first ray and helps to prevent lateral pressure on the lesser toes. This has now been verified radiographically, biomechanically, and clinically in several studies* Radiographically, arthrodesis of the first MTP joint improves the first metatarsal declination and the talometatarsal and talocalcaneal angles, suggesting it achieves stabilization of the longitudinal arch.[206]

Biomechanically, arthrodesis of the first MTP joint has been associated with a decrease in measured first ray mobility in clinical studies on patients with hallux valgus and hallux rigidus.[61,62,66] Instron testing of fixation for arthrodesis has demonstrated that the most stable construct for first MTP arthrodesis is a dorsal plate with an oblique lag screw.[270] Gait and pressure analysis before and after arthrodesis verified restoration of the weight-bearing function of the first ray. However, there was a significant change in the postoperative gait pattern, characterized by a shorter step length and a slight loss of ankle plantar flexion at toe-off, although hip and knee mechanics were not affected.[76] Clinically, Coughlin[58] has demonstrated 96% (45 of 47 feet) good or excellent results following a rheumatoid forefoot reconstruction consisting of arthrodesis of the first MTP joint, resection of the lesser metatarsal heads with preservation of the phalangeal base and extensors, and fixed hammer toe repair at a mean of 6 years of follow-up.

The toe might mold to the shape of the adjacent toes. This is uncommon after a rheumatoid foot repair. On occasion a patient has some discomfort at the hammer toe arthroplasty site, and a painful pseudarthrosis may develop. When necessary, a corticosteroid injection provides lasting relief.

---

*References 58, 61, 66, 76, 206, and 270.

Surgical Reconstruction

The treatment of choice for advanced rheumatoid arthritis complicated by hallux valgus, metatarsalgia, subluxation and dislocation of the lesser MTP joints, and fixed hammer toe deformities involves an arthrodesis of the MTP joint, multiple hammer toe repairs, and excisional arthroplasty of the lesser MTP joints (metatarsal head excision). Many procedures have been used to resect the lesser MTP joints (video clip 51). These include metatarsal head excision (*Hoffman procedure*) (Fig. 16–16A and B), resection of the base of the proximal phalanx, resection of the base of the proximal phalanx with beveling of the plantar metatarsal surface (*Fowler procedure*)[105] (Fig. 16–16C), and partial proximal phalangectomy combined with metatarsal head resection (*Clayton procedure*) (Fig. 16–16D and E). Although the use of eponyms is discouraged and these authors might not have recorded the initial description of their technique, their names have become associated with the individual procedure.

The choice of a particular surgical incision varies depending on the surgeon's preference. A transverse plantar incision[338] (Fig. 16–17A1), elliptical plantar incision[105,174] (Fig. 16–17A2 and A3), transverse dorsal incision (Fig. 16–17B1 and B2), and multiple dorsal longitudinal incisions (Fig. 16–17C1 and C2) have all been advocated. Our preference is for three dorsal longitudinal incisions, with the medial incision centered

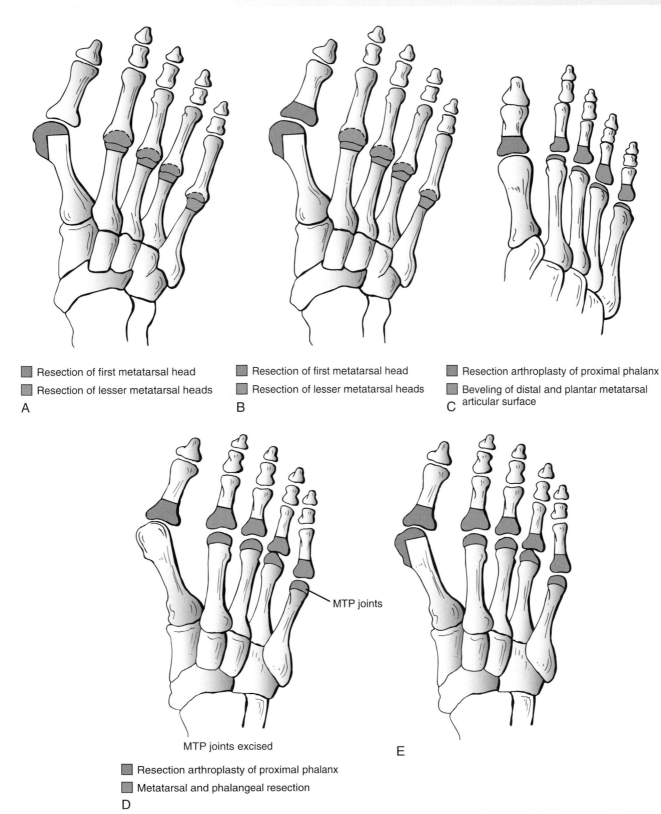

■ Resection of first metatarsal head

■ Resection of lesser metatarsal heads

A

■ Resection of first metatarsal head

■ Resection of lesser metatarsal heads

B

■ Resection arthroplasty of proximal phalanx

■ Beveling of distal and plantar metatarsal articular surface

C

MTP joints

MTP joints excised

■ Resection arthroplasty of proximal phalanx

■ Metatarsal and phalangeal resection

D

E

Figure 16–16   Treatment for dislocation of lesser metatarsophalangeal (MTP) joints with rheumatoid arthritis. **A,** Hoffman procedure (metatarsal head resection). **B,** Modified Hoffman procedure with the first MTP surfaces shaped for MTP arthrodesis rather than excisional arthroplasty. **C,** Fowler procedure (partial proximal phalangectomy and beveling of distal and plantar metatarsal articular surface). **D,** Clayton procedure (partial proximal phalangectomy with metatarsal head resection). **E,** Modified Clayton procedure with the first MTP surfaces shaped for arthrodesis rather than excisional arthroplasty.

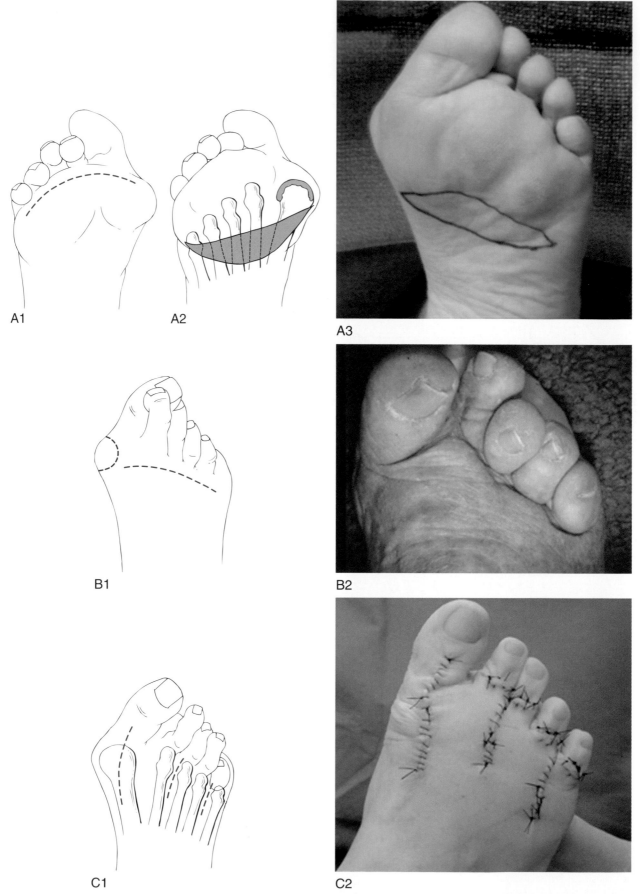

Figure 16–17 Incisions for rheumatoid forefoot reconstruction. **A1,** Transverse plantar incision. **A2** and **A3,** Elliptical plantar incision with resection of ellipse of skin. **B1,** Transverse dorsal incision. **B2,** Long-term follow-up demonstrates contractures following transverse dorsal incision. **C1** and **C2,** Multiple dorsal longitudinal incisions.

over the first MTP joint and the two lateral incisions centered in the second and fourth intermetatarsal spaces.[57]

If only one or two MTP joints are affected, deciding whether an entire forefoot arthroplasty should be performed is difficult. Without first MTP joint arthrosis, an arthroplasty on the lesser MTP joints may be performed (Fig. 16–18A and B). If one or two lesser MTP joints are involved, an arthroplasty may be performed on these joints; however, a frank discussion with the patient must detail the likely progression of the disease process, with eventual involvement of the other MTP joints. Rarely is the first MTP joint spared when all the lesser MTP joints are afflicted. And vice versa, when only the first MTP joint is involved, a fusion may be carried out and a lesser MTP resection arthroplasty is deferred (Fig. 16–19A to C). When the entire forefoot is involved except for the fifth MTP joint, an arthroplasty of the fifth MTP joint is recommended because in time the fifth toe will drift medially with resultant loss of stability of the adjacent MTP joints.

Thomas[334] recommended resection of a single symptomatic metatarsal head. If more than three joints were involved, he recommended an entire forefoot arthroplasty, and for one or two involved lesser MTP joints, a limited resection. Morrison,[245] on the other hand, reported on limited resection in two cases and stated that such a modification was not justified. Marmor[224] reported that resection of one or two metatarsal heads "has always ended in failure." We support the notion of Clayton[46,47] and others[32,205,275,346] that if two metatarsals require resection, an entire forefoot arthroplasty is the treatment of choice. Moreover, complication rates increase with revision procedures,[58] and delaying limited procedures in favor of complete reconstruction is usually preferable.

LESSER METATARSOPHALANGEAL JOINT ARTHROPLASTY

Surgical Technique

1. The lesser MTP joints are approached through two dorsal longitudinal incisions 3 cm long. The first incision is placed between the second and third metatarsals, starting at the web space and proceeding proximally. A similar incision is placed in the fourth web space and extends proximally (Fig. 16–20A and B).
2. The skin flaps are slightly undermined, and an oblique dissection is carried out medially and laterally to identify the adjacent MTP joints. The extensor tendons are identified but are usually left intact unless a significant contracture is present. The base of the proximal phalanx can be identified by tracing the distal portion of the extensor tendon. By starting the dissection in the interspace and carrying it out obliquely, the adjacent neurovascular bundles are protected.
3. With sharp dissection, the metatarsal neck is exposed. The periosteum is stripped along the metaphysis of the metatarsal in a circumferential manner. Plantar flexion of the involved toe can often deliver the metatarsal head dorsally. A synovectomy is performed as needed. A McGlamry elevator can be useful if the deformity is not severe. However, at times a significant MTP joint dislocation is present, and careful use of a small Hoke osteotome to strip the capsular tissue can help to expose the metatarsal head without sacrificing the extensor tendons. Once the base of the proximal phalanx is freed of its soft tissue attachments, the phalanx can be pulled somewhat distally, increasing the exposure of the metatarsal head.
4. A bone-cutting rongeur or microtooth saw is used to transect the metatarsal in the proximal metaphyseal region (Fig. 16–20C1 and C2). The amount of bone removed depends on the magnitude of the overlap of the proximal phalanx on the metatarsal head. An osteotome or Freer elevator can be used to release the remaining adhesions, allowing delivery of the metatarsal head. The metatarsal head is then grasped with a rongeur and pulled from the wound. Ideally, the metatarsal head is removed in one piece to avoid leaving remnants of bone, which can cause recurrence of plantar callosities (Fig. 16–20D1 and D2). Enough head is resected so that the resection arthroplasty accommodates the tip of the surgeon's index finger with gentle longitudinal traction of the digit, or about 1 cm (Fig. 16–20F).
5. After the metatarsal head has been removed, the plantar aspect of the remaining metatarsal shaft is beveled with a rongeur to minimize the risk of recurrent callosities.
6. Once the metatarsal head has been excised, any significant synovial cysts or

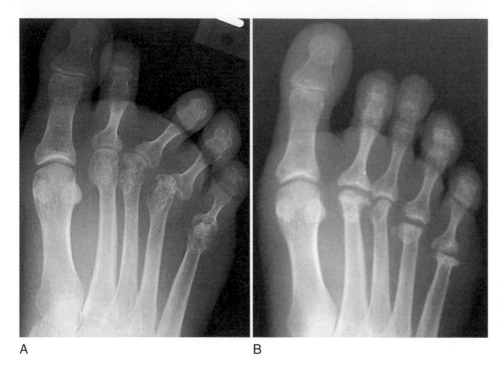

A   B

Figure 16–18 Rheumatoid involvement of lesser metatarsophalangeal (MTP) joints with sparing of first MTP joint. Preoperative **(A)** and postoperative **(B)** radiographs demonstrate resection arthroplasties of lesser MTP joints.

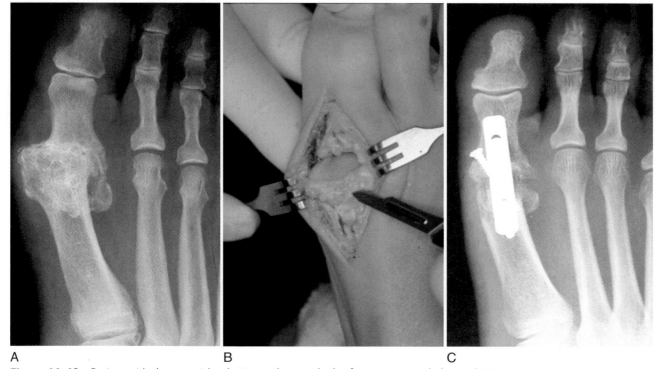

A   B   C

Figure 16–19   Patient with rheumatoid arthritis involving only the first metatarsophalangeal (MTP) joint. **A,** Preoperative radiograph demonstrates hallux valgus and destructive joint changes. **B,** Clinical picture verifies destructive erosion of the MTP joint. **C,** Postoperative radiograph demonstrates correction of hallux valgus with MTP arthrodesis.

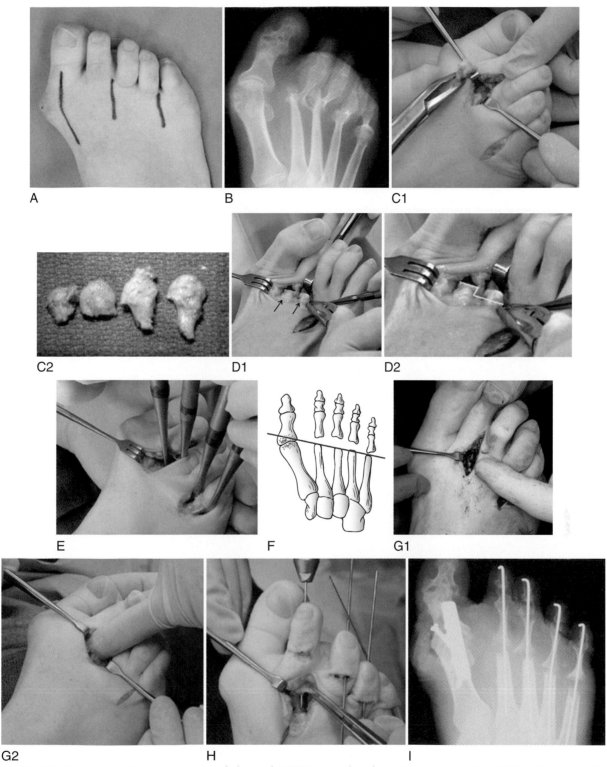

Figure 16–20 Technique of lesser metatarsophalangeal (MTP) joint arthroplasty. Preoperative clinical **(A)** and radiographic **(B)** appearance of severe rheumatoid forefoot deformity. **C1,** A bone-cutting rongeur is used to transect the metatarsal in the metaphyseal–diaphyseal region. It is grasped with a rongeur and removed. **C2,** Multiple metatarsal heads are removed. **D1,** After each metatarsal shaft is transected, the distal portion is removed. **D2,** Inset shows that the shaft of the third metatarsal is too long and needs to be shortened. **E,** Technique of using vertical osteotomes to gauge the cascade of metatarsal lengths when dorsal longitudinal incisions are used and direct comparison of the individual lengths is difficult. **F,** A diagram demonstrates the desirable anatomic cascade that is the goal with the resection arthroplasty so that each successive resection is a few millimeters shorter than the previous one. **G1** and **G2,** Tip of index finger (approximately 1 cm in diameter) is used to gauge the magnitude of resection. **H,** Kirschner wires are used to stabilize hammer toe repair and lesser MTP resection arthroplasties. **I,** Radiograph demonstrates first MTP joint arthrodesis with 1 cm resection arthroplasty at each of the lesser MTP joints.

plantar subcutaneous bursae are resected in the depths of the wound. Care must be taken on the plantar aspect to remove only the dorsal half of a synovial cyst in order to avoid excessive resection of soft tissue.

7. The procedure is repeated for the remaining metatarsal heads. Care is taken to assure that the anatomic cascade of metatarsal length is recreated with the resections (Fig. 16–20D to F). Again, a rongeur is used to bevel the plantar aspect of the remaining metatarsal surfaces to remove any prominent plantar spikes.

8. The base of the proximal phalanx is preserved because it forms a wide concave surface that affords stability to the pseudoarticulation that has been created. (Removal of the base of the proximal phalanx leaves a greatly narrowed diaphyseal region that articulates with the remaining metatarsal diaphysis.) By removing the contracture at the MTP joint, the fat pad will realign without resection of plantar skin.[57]

9. The most important aspect of the excisional arthroplasty is achieving adequate decompression at the MTP joint. Usually a 1-cm space between the base of the proximal phalanx and the prepared metatarsal surface is sufficient (Fig. 16–20E1 and E2). The tip of the index finger is used as a gauge to measure an adequate amount of resection. With minimal longitudinal tension on the toe, there should be a minimal amount of pressure on the tip of the index finger that has been placed in this interval.

10. With a symmetric resection of the metatarsal heads, an even distribution of pressure beneath the metatarsals should be achieved. Usually the first and second metatarsals are of equal length, whereas the third, fourth, and fifth are progressively shorter from the medial to the lateral aspect of the forefoot. Avoiding a prominent metatarsal prevents new pressure points from developing. At this point, attention is directed toward the hammer toe deformities of the lesser toes. With a significant deformity, it is preferable to resect the condyles of the proximal phalanx in order to decompress the joint. This also aids in placement of the intramedullary Kirschner wires. On occasion, a closed osteoclasis or manipulation of the interphalangeal joint is performed to reduce the hammer toe deformity.

11. To align the lesser toes, a 0.045-inch Kirschner wire is introduced at the PIP joint and driven distally through the middle and distal phalanges (Fig. 16–20H and I). A Kirschner wire of adequate length is used so that the proximal tip of the wire is eventually embedded in the proximal metatarsal base across the resection arthroplasty, giving stability to the arthroplasty site. The pin is advanced through the proximal phalanx into the metatarsal diaphysis and proximal metaphysis. The pin is bent at the tip of the toe to prevent proximal migration. A similar technique of pin placement is carried out for all the lesser MTP joint arthroplasties (Fig. 16–21A and B).

12. The MTP joint arthroplasty sites are irrigated with antibiotic solution, and the skin is approximated with 3-0 or 4-0 nylon sutures. The incisions for the hammer toe repairs are approximated as well.

13. Attention is then directed to the first MTP joint (discussed later). Once the lesser toes have been realigned and the MTP joint space is reduced, the surgeon has an idea of the amount the first ray needs to be shortened. Often at least 1 cm of shortening is achieved laterally, and extra bone must be removed from the first ray to achieve its appropriate length (Fig. 16–22A to C).

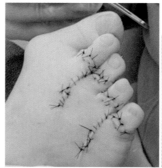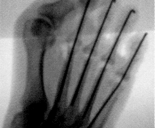

A   B

Figure 16–21 **A,** Clinical photo shows completion of forefoot arthroplasty before the first metatarsophalangeal joint arthrodesis. **B,** Intraoperative fluoroscopy demonstrates resection of the lesser metatarsals and relative excess length of the first metatarsal, which can now be corrected during arthrodesis.

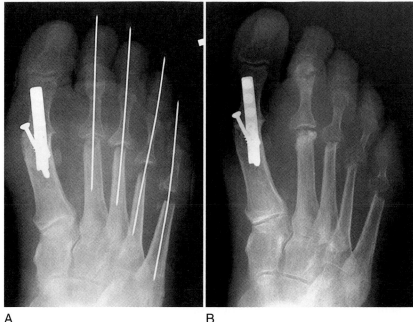

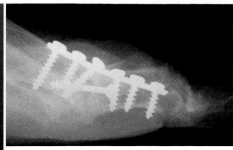

Figure 16–22 A, Radiograph demonstrates metatarsophalangeal (MTP) arthrodesis and multiple Kirschner wire fixation of lesser MTP joints. **B,** After Kirschner wire removal. **C,** Lateral radiograph after forefoot arthroplasty.

Postoperative Care

A gauze-and-tape compression dressing is applied at surgery and changed 2 to 3 days later. The patient is permitted to ambulate in a postoperative shoe or short walking boot with weight bearing on the heel. Compression dressings are changed every 7 to 10 days for approximately 6 weeks after surgery. Typically the Kirschner wires are removed 3 to 5 weeks after surgery. Postoperative radiographs are obtained as necessary.

In the immediate postoperative period, circulatory status of the toes must be monitored. With severe deformities, vascular compromise can develop. Removal of intramedullary Kirschner wires can allow revascularization of a compromised toe. If a toe remains blue or white 15 minutes after surgery, loosening the compression dressing or removing the Kirschner wire is often necessary. Application of nitro paste to the distal aspects of the digits will improve blood flow and can allow fixation to remain in place.

Results and Complications

The results after a rheumatoid forefoot repair in general are gratifying. Coughlin[58] reported 96%

good or excellent results of rheumatoid forefoot reconstruction in 47 feet using Hoffman's technique of metatarsal head resection, fixed hammer toe repair, and great toe MTP joint arthrodesis. There was a 2% to 3% recurrence rate of hammer toe and mallet toe deformities, no reported first MTP joint nonunions, and 7% re-dislocation of the lesser MTP joints (70% were dislocated preoperatively). Pain was absent or mild in 91% (43 of 47 feet) and moderate in four feet at a mean follow-up of 6 years. There were no special shoe requirements, 15 feet had no functional limitation, 28 feet had some limit of recreational activity, and four had limitation of daily activity. Based on the most recent biomechanical, radiographic, and clinical data, Coughlin's rheumatoid forefoot reconstruction is the procedure of choice for chronic rheumatoid forefoot deformity.

Using first MTP arthrodesis and lesser MTP joint arthroplasty techniques, Mann and Thompson[221] reported 89% (18 cases) good and excellent results at final follow-up. Mann and Schakel[220] reported 90% good or excellent results using a similar technique (two threaded Steinman pins for first MTP joint arthrodesis) in 28 feet with minimal recurrence of deformity at 3.7 years of follow-up.

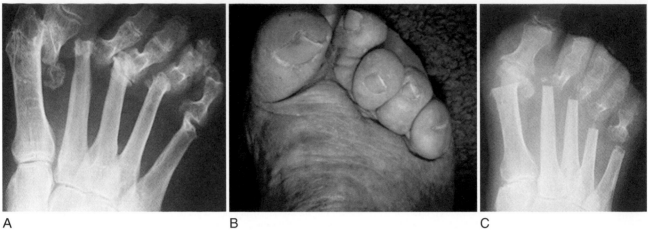

A   B   C

Figure 16–23 Keller resection arthroplasty. **A** and **B,** Clinical appearance with recurrent hallux valgus and subluxation of the lesser metatarsophalangeal (MTP) joints. **C,** Radiographs demonstrate recurrence of the lateral forefoot deformity after the first MTP silicone implant and Hoffman procedure (resection of first through fifth metatarsal heads).

A major reason for dissatisfaction with many forefoot arthroplasties reported in the literature is that they were combined with first MTP joint resection arthroplasty. Watson[355] concluded that a Keller arthroplasty did not receive support from the lateral toes. Craxford et al[72] reported recurrent deformation and dissatisfaction after forefoot arthroplasty associated with resection of the first MTP joint. Indeed, progression of hallux valgus leads to re-deformation of the lesser MTP joints and recurrent lesser toe deformity (Fig. 16–23A to C). Maintenance of first MTP joint alignment with an arthrodesis protects not only the hallux but also the lesser MTP joints from recurrent deformity and subsequent metatarsalgia. The relocated fat pad is maintained in a normal position after MTP arthroplasty. The lesser MTP joints do not have much motion, but this does not appear to be a problem for patients. Typically, patients no longer walk with a heel-to-toe gait but rather by placing the foot flat on the ground.

Of 1874 cases reported in several series describing various surgical techniques of lesser MTP joint arthroplasty, an overall 81% satisfactory rate has been reported. Partial proximal phalangectomy as a treatment for claw toe deformities and subluxated MTP joints achieved a satisfaction rate of 65% (180 of 278 cases).[50,83,255,294] Partial proximal phalangectomy with beveling of the metatarsal condyle, as described initially by Fowler,[105] has a lower reported success rate of 43% (116 of 177 cases). Partial proximal phalangectomy combined with metatarsal head resection, as described by Clayton[47] and others,[130] has a higher reported success rate, with 80% good and excellent results (507 of 636 cases).

Saltzman[294] reported on the results of partial phalangectomy and syndactylization for mild rheumatoid

forefoot deformities. Postoperatively, 64% of patients reported limitation in activity due to metatarsalgia, and 36% of patients considered the result cosmetically unsatisfactory. Some authors have used a combination of partial proximal phalangectomy with beveling of the metatarsal condyles for more moderate deformities and resorted to metatarsal head resection for more severe deformities. A metatarsal head excision, as described by Hoffman[151] and others, has the highest published success rate of 89% good and excellent results (748 of 843 cases).

Barton,[11] who compared different forefoot arthroplasty procedures, concluded that individual surgical techniques did not make a difference. However, he combined a first MTP joint excisional arthroplasty with lesser MTP arthroplasties, which likely influenced the end results. Mulcahy et al[247] reported the surgical results of two groups of patients whose treatment differed based on arthrodesis or resection of the first MTP joint and concluded that a stable first MTP joint (with an arthrodesis) and resection of the lesser metatarsal heads with Kirschner wire fixation led to a more cosmetic forefoot and a more even distribution of forefoot pressures postoperatively.

In another study, radiographic follow-up following Keller's resection in 23 feet demonstrated first MTP joint erosive changes that continued even after the resection in more than 50% of cases.[17] Furthermore, the same authors noted that the need for revision surgery was much higher in those who underwent a Keller procedure. Raunio[277] reported a similar increase in the need for second surgery following a Keller procedure and recommended arthrodesis of the first MTP joint.

Comparing panmetatarsal forefoot resection arthroplasty techniques, Fuhrmann[109] reported better success with the Hueter–Mayo resection in 188 patients who had undergone either a Keller or a Hueter–Mayo resection arthroplasty of the first metatarsophalangeal joint but 30% of the Hueter–Mayo group still experienced persistent metatarsalgia. Thomas et al[333] reported satisfactory results at an average follow-up of 65 months. Of the 20 patients (39 feet), 60% reported problems with balance, and only 12% of the feet could be fitted with footwear of choice following surgery. Mild to severe recurrent hallux valgus was noted in 51% of cases. Thomas et al[333] reported good or excellent results in only 30% of cases.

Hasselo et al[142] reported short-term results with forefoot arthroplasty from eight surgeons using several different reconstruction techniques for the first MTP joint, including simple bunionectomy, silicone first MTP implant, excisional arthroplasty, and arthrodesis. Little can be concluded from the long-term results because of the numerous procedures and numerous surgeons involved. Craxford et al[72] reported an initial 80% satisfaction rate after forefoot arthroplasty but noted that it diminished to 55% at 4.5 to 8.5 years of follow-up. No first MTP arthrodeses were used in this study.

Postoperative complications of resection arthroplasty techniques without first MTP arthrodesis, including claw toes, intractable plantar keratoses, metatarsalgia, and recurrent pain, have been reported in many series. Petrov et al[268] found that 28% of 15 patients who underwent panmetatarsal head resection for rheumatoid forefoot arthritis developed recurrent plantar ulceration as early as 6 months postoperatively. The most common apparent cause of reulceration was recurrent bone growth, most commonly under the second metatarsal head.

However, the major reason for dissatisfaction postoperatively in most series is the progressive hallux valgus deformity. Notably, Pastalis et al[264] found restriction of walking ability due to forefoot pain (56%), recurrent great toe deformity (72%), and recurrent painful callosities (61%) at a mean follow-up of 10.5 years. These complications can often be prevented with first MTP arthrodesis.

Vandeputte et al[347] reported the results of two separate groups of patients compared to evaluate the results of resection compared to arthrodesis of the first MTP joint and lesser MTP resection arthroplasty. The authors concluded that when a fusion was achieved, it protected and unweighted the lesser metatarsals more effectively than resection or pseudarthrosis. Hasselo et al[142] recommended that fusion and stability of the first ray should be the primary goal for surgical intervention of the rheumatoid forefoot.

Flint and Sweetnam[101] and Nissen[257] recommended amputation of the lesser toes as the treatment of choice for severe rheumatoid forefoot deformity. However, it appears that forefoot reconstruction offers better cosmetic results and improved ease in fitting footwear than amputation procedures do (Fig. 16–24A to E).

The most common complication after forefoot arthroplasty is recurrence of intractable plantar keratoses or recurrent pain from inadequate bone resection.[253] Clayton[46,47] noted a 10% repeat surgery rate following inadequate resection of the lesser metatarsal heads. Adequate decompression of the MTP joints at surgery is extremely important. If a metatarsal is significantly longer than an adjacent metatarsal, a high risk exists for the development of postoperative recurrent intractable plantar keratoses. Chronic swelling in the forefoot is a common postoperative complaint, but the swelling usually subsides with time. Isolated excision of one or two metatarsal heads is, in general, to be avoided, because an intractable plantar keratotic lesion often develops beneath remaining metatarsal heads.

Repeat surgery for the rheumatoid forefoot is necessary for the following reasons:

* Bone regrowth in the area of lesser metatarsal head resections
* Irregular lesser metatarsal head resections
* Limited surgery with only one or two metatarsal heads resected
* Re-deformity caused by hindfoot or ankle joint disease.

A meticulous technique with attention to a regular resection of the metatarsal heads in a line in which the first and second metatarsals are of equal length and the third, fourth, and fifth metatarsals are progressively shorter helps to prevent recurrent intractable plantar keratoses (Fig. 16–20D and F). Meticulous care in debridement of the area of the metatarsal head resection is necessary so that all bone fragments are removed, because this minimizes bone regrowth. In general, all four lesser metatarsal heads should be removed. Limited surgery in which only one or two metatarsal heads are removed should be avoided.

In a long-term report on his practice experience, Graham[124] recommended that even with minimal involvement of the first MTP joint, an arthrodesis is warranted in combination with a forefoot arthroplasty (Fig. 16–25). He suggested that deterioration of the first MTP joint with time would likely lead to recurrent lateral forefoot deformities. Thordarson et al[337] reported similar findings in seven patients (13 feet) with initially well preserved first MTP joints and reported that 11 of 13 feet developed recurrent hallux valgus following an attempt at joint preservation at a mean follow-up of only 24 months.

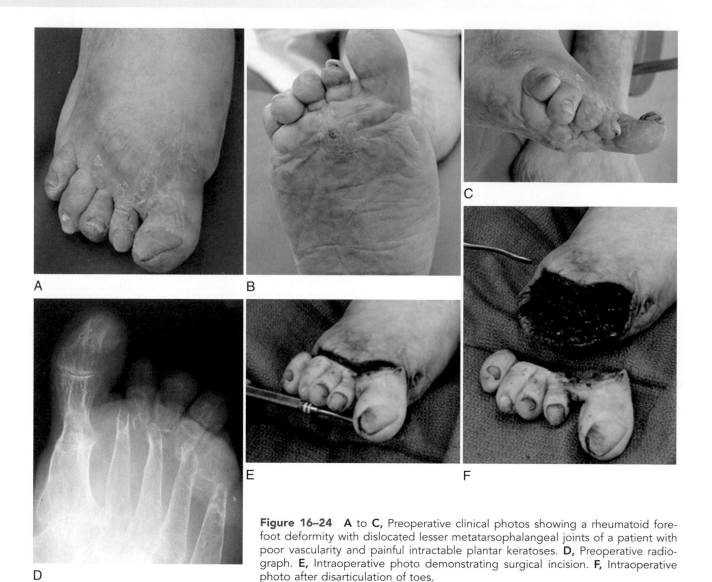

Figure 16–24   A to **C,** Preoperative clinical photos showing a rheumatoid forefoot deformity with dislocated lesser metatarsophalangeal joints of a patient with poor vascularity and painful intractable plantar keratoses. **D,** Preoperative radiograph. **E,** Intraoperative photo demonstrating surgical incision. **F,** Intraoperative photo after disarticulation of toes.

Others maintain that joint-sparing procedures should be considered. Hanyu et al[137] reported 83% satisfactory results in 75 feet (47 patients) with a mean of 6 years of follow-up using either Mitchell's osteotomy (23 feet) or first MTP joint Silastic arthroplasty (52 feet) combined with lesser metatarsal shortening oblique osteotomies. Although the authors reported that more than half of the feet appeared to look normal postoperatively, recurrent hallux valgus was observed in 15% of cases, lesser MTP joint subluxation was noted in 21%, recurrent hammer toes in 13%, and recurrent callosities in 12%. Shi et al[305] found that 17 of 21 feet with rheumatoid arthritis had great or moderate pain relief after a Lapidus procedure but found statistically significant recurrent hallux

valgus (mean of 20 degrees) at a follow-up of almost 4 years. The most reliable results for reconstructive rheumatoid forefoot surgery were reported by Coughlin[58] in terms of pain relief, use of regular footwear, subjective patient satisfaction, and minimal complications.

If hindfoot or ankle disease is present, it is preferable to treat these areas before a forefoot arthroplasty. Furthermore, surgery should be reserved for patients with severe pain and disability, because the procedure is considered a salvage procedure and the resultant lesser toes will have little active function. Surgery does not restore functional capacity to the foot but does improve ambulatory capacity and achieves pain relief, improves cosmesis, and in general gives gratifying results.

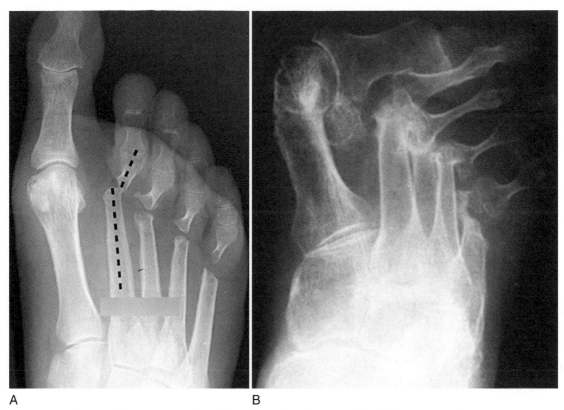

A   B

Figure 16–25 A, Radiograph demonstrates lateral forefoot arthroplasty (modified Clayton procedure). First ray was uninvolved. Note excess length of first ray. **B,** Long-term follow-up after simple bunionectomy and lesser forefoot arthroplasty (Hoffmann procedure) is complicated by severe valgus deformity of the hallux and recurrent deformity of the lesser MTP joints.

FIRST METATARSOPHALANGEAL JOINT ARTHROPLASTY

Resection arthroplasty of the first MTP joint has been recommended in the past for reconstructing the severely deformed rheumatoid forefoot.[109] McGarvey and Johnson[229] and others[147,246] have stated that the Keller procedure in combination with forefoot arthroplasty is often unsuccessful.

McGarvey and Johnson[229] reported a 33% satisfaction rate when excisional arthroplasty was combined with lesser MTP resection arthroplasty (see Fig. 16–23). In reporting their experience with excisional arthroplasty in patients with rheumatoid arthritis, they noted recurrence of hallux valgus in 53%, recurrent metatarsalgia in 20%, and foot instability in 27%. Only one third of patients were satisfied with their postoperative result. They concluded that a first MTP arthrodesis was the treatment of choice in combination with forefoot resection arthroplasty. van der Heijden et al[346] reported that 29 of 41 (71%)

of the resection arthroplasties of the first MTP joint were unsatisfactory (video clip 28).

Initially a resection arthroplasty may give significant relief of symptoms in the treatment of a hallux valgus deformity in the rheumatoid patient. Hasselo et al[142] reported that initial acceptable results with excisional arthroplasty deteriorated rapidly, resulting in poor push off of the first ray, recurrent deformity, unacceptable cosmetic results, and recurrent pain. Craxford et al[72] found little difference between patients who had resection arthroplasty and patients treated conservatively with special shoes to manage their rheumatoid forefoot deformity. (For the surgical technique of excisional arthroplasty, see the later discussion under hallux rigidus.) Furthermore, more recent reports suggest long-term function of the foot is compromised with an unstable first ray created by the resection arthroplasty.[333] There may be a difference in extent of compromised gait postoperatively depending on the resection technique used (Keller or Mayo).[110]

Silicone elastic (Silastic) implant arthroplasty of the first MTP joint has been recommended as an alternative to resection arthroplasty (Fig. 16–26). Cracchiolo[69] and Jenkin and Oloff[160] recommended Silastic implant replacement of the great toe and lesser MTP joints. The reported results by Hanyu et al[136] found 74% good or excellent results in 60 feet at 12 years of follow-up. However, nine implants were noted to have fractured, four were removed because of infection or recurrent deformity, and 59% had sinking of the implant with findings of silicone synovitis in 12 joints (21%).

Silastic implants have been fraught with short-term and long-term complications (see later discussion of first MTP implant arthroplasty under hallux rigidus). Although satisfactory results have been reported in some cases, many long-term complications have been noted, including fracture, silicone synovitis, osteolysis, and recurrent pain. Moreover, salvage of a failed implant arthroplasty is technically demanding and usually requires an interposition graft from the iliac crest or proximal tibia[145] or simultaneous arthrodesis of both the interphalangeal and MTP joint.[97] In general, silicone prosthetic replacement of the first MTP joint is rarely indicated in treatment of the rheumatoid forefoot with hallux valgus. For lesser MTP joint replacement, there appears to be little difference between resection arthroplasty and silicone implant replacement.[160] Thus, the added expense and risk of implant arthroplasty in most situations are unwarranted.

Stabilization of the first ray with a first MTP arthrodesis has been recommended by DuVries[83] and others on the premise that an arthrodesed first MTP joint stabilizes the first ray. This has been verified by Coughlin et al[61,65-67] in clinical studies on hallux rigidus and hallux valgus.

A forefoot arthroplasty itself weakens support for the great toe. Consequently, during gait the hallux and lateral toes displace dorsally and lat-

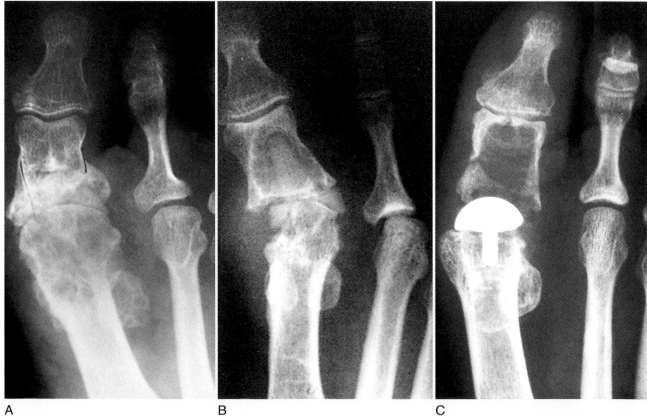

A   B   C

Figure 16–26 Complications following silicone implant arthroplasty. **A,** Severe osteolysis of proximal phalanx. **B,** Fragmentation, synovitis, and osteolysis after single-stem implant placement. **C,** Severe collapse, bone overgrowth, synovitis, and osteolysis after metal and silicone implant arthroplasty.

erally. As the toes migrate dorsolaterally, weight bearing is increased on the previously resected lesser metatarsal shafts and there is an increased incidence of metatarsalgia. After an arthrodesis, lateral translation of pressure beneath the lesser metatarsals is uncommon. Following arthrodesis, in the latter half of stance phase, the foot lifts off the ground slightly earlier,[218] decreasing stress on the lesser MTP joints, decreasing metatarsalgia, and protecting the lesser toes from recurrent deformity.

Preoperative foot imprints have been compared with postoperative pressure studies. Minns and Craxford[239] reported two to three times increased pressure developing beneath the metatarsal heads before surgical resection. Also, repositioning of the plantar fat pad has been speculated to improve tolerance of pressure. Fu and Scranton[108] found significant increase of pressure developing beneath symptomatic metatarsal heads after irregular resection arthroplasty. Henry and Waugh[147] reported improved weight-bearing function of the hallux after arthrodesis and hypothesized that this accounted for the improved function.

In a long-term follow-up study after forefoot arthroplasty, Watson[355] stated that the major effect of surgical intervention was pain relief and concluded that arthrodesis was the treatment of choice for a rheumatoid forefoot deformity. After resection arthroplasty, he noted that the valgus position of the hallux was not supported by the lesser toes. He concluded that first MTP resection arthroplasty gave mediocre results in comparison with first MTP arthrodesis.

Direct comparisons between excisional arthroplasty and arthrodesis of the first MTP joint have demonstrated that arthrodesis is superior as noted previously. Beauchamp et al[14] concluded that arthrodesis resulted in better forefoot balance, cosmesis, and shoe fitting.

Occasionally a patient has an uninvolved first ray and significant forefoot deformity with lateral metatarsalgia. Cracchiolo[70] recommended that if the hallux was neither malaligned nor involved with MTP synovitis, it should "be left alone." With significant hallux valgus deformity without chondrolysis (Fig. 16–27), he recommended a routine hallux valgus repair, and with significant dysfunction, he recommended an arthrodesis or implant. Graham,[124] however, in a long-term report on his practice experience, recommended that with even minimal involvement of the first MTP joint, an arthrodesis was warranted in combination with a forefoot arthroplasty. He suggested that valgus angulation of the first MTP joint in time would likely necessitate forefoot realignment. Thordarson[337] reported a high failure rate following first MTP joint preservation techniques in patients with rheumatoid arthritis and concluded an arthrodesis was preferable, even with minor deformity.

FIRST METATARSOPHALANGEAL ARTHRODESIS

Arthrodesis of the first MTP joint provides stability to the joint and achieves permanent correction of a hallux valgus deformity. It often permits the use of ordinary footwear and, in combination with excisional arthroplasty of the lesser MTP joints, helps to achieve lasting relief of disabling pain. Arthrodesis of the first MTP joint in rheumatoid arthritis provides stability to the first ray, and the rigidity minimizes stress to the lesser MTP joints. It protects the position of the repositioned plantar fat pad beneath the lesser metatarsals and often results in a painless foot with little likelihood that further surgical intervention will be necessary. For these reasons and those mentioned previously, arthrodesis of the first MTP joint in rheumatoid arthritis is the treatment of choice for the first ray in reconstructing the rheumatoid forefoot.

Arthrodesis of the first MTP joint was first described by Clutton[49] in 1892. Numerous surgical techniques have been proposed describing various approaches, techniques of joint preparation, and methods of internal fixation to improve alignment capability and the success rate of fusion. First MTP arthrodesis has been recommended as a means to salvage various great toe deformities, including hallux valgus associated with rheumatoid arthritis, hallux rigidus, and severe hallux valgus, as well as recurrent hallux valgus,[114,217,342] neuromuscular instability,[114,217,218,335,342] and traumatic arthritis.[161]

The alignment of the hallux postoperatively plays a significant role in patient satisfaction. Reporting on his long-term experience with MTP arthrodesis and the relationship of first ray

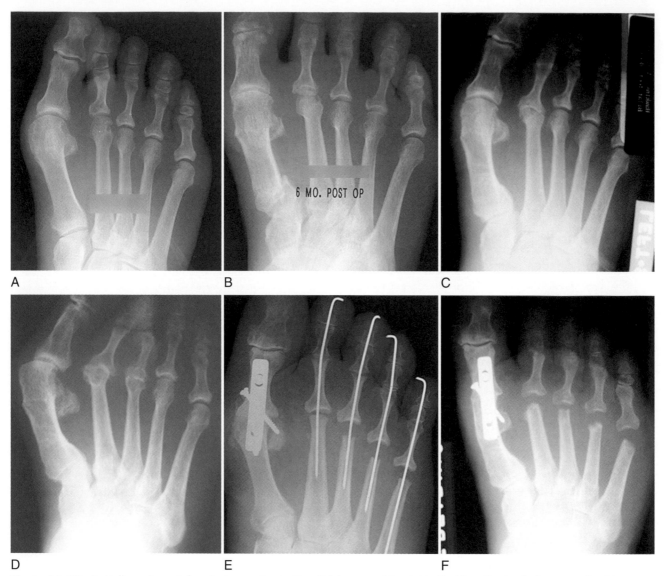

Figure 16–27 **A,** Hallux valgus deformity in a patient with mild rheumatoid arthritis. **B,** After distal soft tissue repair with a proximal first metatarsal osteotomy, realignment is achieved. **C,** Three years following surgery, mild subluxation of the first MTP joint has developed. **D,** Nine years postoperatively there is a severe recurrence of the hallux valgus deformity with dislocation of the second and third MTP joints. **E,** After MTP fusion and forefoot arthroplasty. **F,** One year postoperatively, adequate realignment is maintained.

alignment to later interphalangeal arthritis, Fitzgerald[98] noted a correlation between degenerative interphalangeal joint arthritis and the magnitude of MTP valgus. He suggested that arthrodesis in less than 20 degrees of valgus (Fig. 16–28) tripled the incidence of interphalangeal joint arthritis. Thus the magnitude of varus/valgus alignment of the arthrodesis site has been a subject of controversy. Recommendations for valgus alignment vary from 15 to 30 degrees, with 15 degrees most commonly recommended (Fig. 16–29A). If the MTP joint is

fixed in a straight position (minimal valgus or a slight varus), the medial border of the hallux can impact against the medial border of the toe box, causing discomfort. In time, degenerative arthritis of the interphalangeal joint can develop.

Although Coughlin[58] could not substantiate Fitzgerald's finding of an increased incidence of IP joint arthritis with decreased valgus angulation, he did observe that MTP joint dorsiflexion of less than 20 degrees was associated with IP joint degeneration in patients with rheumatoid arthritis. He recommended an MTP fusion angle

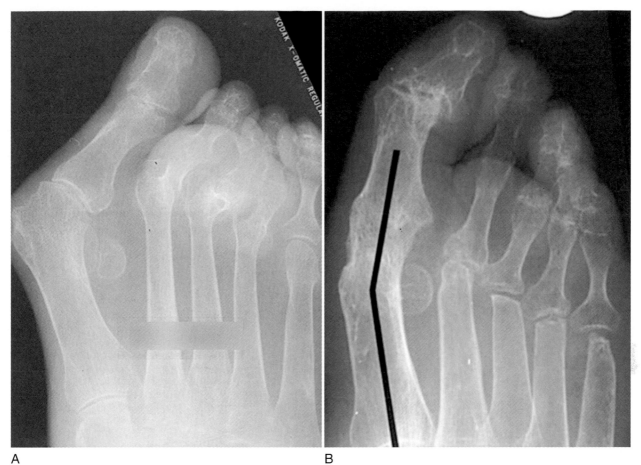

A   B

Figure 16–28 **A,** Severe hallux valgus deformity with subluxation of second, third, and fourth metatarsophalangeal joints. **B,** After arthrodesis in a relatively straight position, there is marked interphalangeal joint arthritis of the hallux 2 years following surgery.

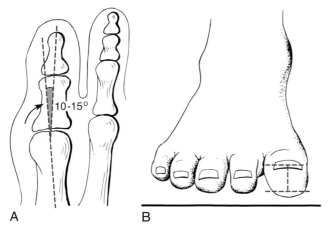

A   B

Figure 16–29 **A,** Metatarsophalangeal fusion in 15 degrees achieves acceptable alignment of the first ray. **B,** Excessive pronation or medial rotation of the hallux can lead to pressure along the medial border. Rotational malalignment should be avoided.

between 21 and 25 degrees with respect to the metatarsal shaft.[58] Although increased valgus and dorsiflexion angles may decrease the incidence of postoperative interphalangeal joint arthritis,[58,98] first MTP arthrodesis itself increases stress at the interphalangeal joint. Progressive IP joint arthritis can develop over time after MTP fusion, even with significant valgus at the MTP joint, although it is rarely symptomatic.[58,221] Thus, the authors recommend arthrodesis in 10 to 15 degrees of valgus (Fig. 16–30A) because it achieves a more acceptable alignment of the first ray in relationship to the lesser metatarsals. Excessive valgus at the fusion site leaves a widened forefoot and a less desirable cosmetic appearance (Fig. 16–30B).

Recommendations for dorsiflexion (in relationship with the ground) vary from 10 to 30 degrees, with an average recommendation of

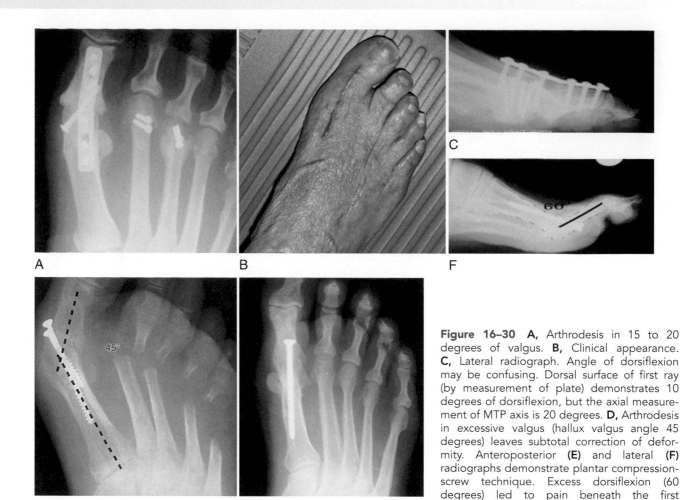

Figure 16–30 **A,** Arthrodesis in 15 to 20 degrees of valgus. **B,** Clinical appearance. **C,** Lateral radiograph. Angle of dorsiflexion may be confusing. Dorsal surface of first ray (by measurement of plate) demonstrates 10 degrees of dorsiflexion, but the axial measurement of MTP axis is 20 degrees. **D,** Arthrodesis in excessive valgus (hallux valgus angle 45 degrees) leaves subtotal correction of deformity. Anteroposterior **(E)** and lateral **(F)** radiographs demonstrate plantar compression-screw technique. Excess dorsiflexion (60 degrees) led to pain beneath the first metatarsal head.

slightly more than 20 degrees with respect to the metatarsal shaft (Fig. 16–30C). For women preferring high-heeled shoes, increased dorsiflexion at the fusion site may be desirable. Dorsiflexion of less than 10 degrees can cause a complaint of pressure at the tip of the toe,[58,246] whereas dorsiflexion greater than 40 degrees can lead to increased pressure beneath the first metatarsal head[14] (Fig. 16–30D to F).

Recommendations in the literature vary depending on the reference of measurement of dorsiflexion (first metatarsal axis, proximal phalangeal axis, plantar aspect of the foot). The plantar inclination of the first metatarsal averages 15 degrees, and with dorsiflexion of the phalanx 5 to 15 degrees, which translates into 20 to 30 degrees of angulation at the arthrodesis site.

Rotation of the hallux is important, and the toe should be placed in a neutral position.[140,204] Excessive pronation or medial rotation can lead to pressure on the medial border of the toenail, causing infection[246] (see Fig. 16–29B).

McKeever[230] and others[61,278,281] have reported that an increased angle between the first and second metatarsals (1-2 intermetatarsal angle) is not a contraindication for MTP fusion. Harrison and Harvey[140] and others[55,60,61] have reported a significant reduction in the 1-2 intermetatarsal angle after arthrodesis. Mann and Katcherian[217] and Humbert et al[155] reported an average decrease of approximately 6 degrees in the 1-2 intermetatarsal angle after arthrodesis. Coughlin[58] found a mean reduction of 3 degrees after first MTP joint arthrodesis in patients with rheumatoid arthritis. Thus a first metatarsal osteotomy is rarely, if ever, indicated in combination with first MTP arthrodesis (Fig. 16–31A to C).

Many patients express concern about their gait following MTP arthrodesis. Mann and Oates,[218] Fitzgerald,[98] and Coughlin and

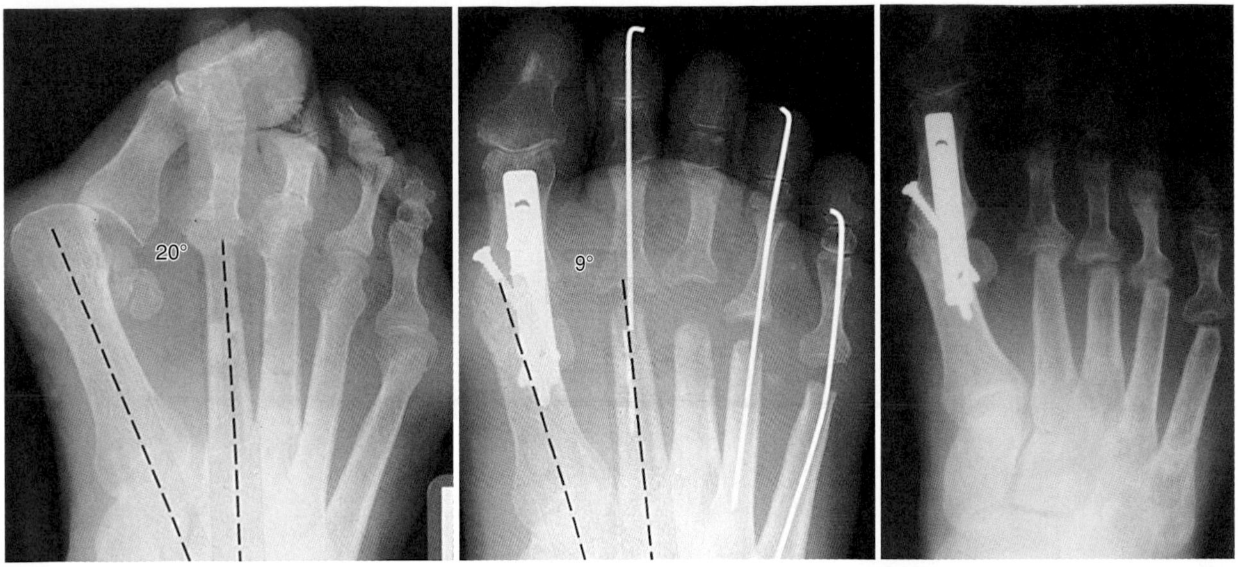

Figure 16–31 A, Preoperative radiograph demonstrates severe hallux valgus with dislocation of metatarsophalangeal (MTP) joint and angle of 20 degrees between first and second metatarsals. **B,** After arthrodesis and forefoot arthroplasty, angle between first and second metatarsals is reduced to 9 degrees. **C,** Final radiographs at 1 year after surgery.

Grebing[61] have reported an excellent gait pattern postoperatively. Mann and Oates[218] concluded that the "foot lifts off slightly early" after an arthrodesis because dorsiflexion of the MTP joint is limited. If a first MTP arthrodesis is fixed in a proper position, Turan and Lindgren[343] stated that a patient has a "nearly normal gait." Gait analysis before and after first MTP joint arthrodesis has demonstrated restoration of the weight-bearing function of the first ray.[76] DeFrino et al,[76] however, have demonstrated a significantly shorter step length and slight loss of ankle plantar flexion at toe-off following MTP joint fusion.

The success rate of MTP arthrodesis varies significantly depending on the preoperative diagnosis, the surgical technique, and the method of internal fixation used.

The use of flat surfaces for MTP arthrodesis has been popularized because of the simplicity of creating horizontal osteotomies of the proximal phalanx and metatarsal articular surfaces (Fig. 16–32). The technique, however, requires exact precision to obtain the desired alignment. If further correction of any one of these alignment variables is necessary, the first ray must be shortened to realign the prepared surfaces. Further attempts to alter any one of these variables may have a simultaneous, undesirable affect on other alignment variables. Curved sur-

faces enable adjustment of one variable without necessarily altering other alignment variables (Fig. 16–33).

Preparation of first MTP joint surfaces with conical reamers was first proposed by G.K. Rose in 1950.[360] Later, Bingold,[26] Moynihan,[246] and others advocated conical reamers to fashion the first MTP joint in preparation for fusion. Wilson[360] reported the use of a "hole-saw" to shape the metatarsal head to a cylindrical shape and then used convex and concave power reamers to prepare the MTP surfaces. Marin[223] developed a hand-held convex and concave reamer system. Coughlin[54,55,60] and Jeffery and Freedman[159] also have advocated power reamers.

Depending on the sclerosis of the subchondral bone, shaping of the arthrodesis site by hand-held reamers can be relatively difficult.[218,223,360] Complications of the conical arthrodesis technique include loss of fixation,[281] malposition,[41,246,343,359] first ray shortening,[246,360] nonunion,[14,41,223,246,343] and excess shortening at the fusion site.[59]

In an attempt to simplify the surgical technique of first MTP arthrodesis, congruous cup-shaped power reamers were designed[54,55] (Fig. 16–34). Power driven to increase torque strength in comparison to hand-held reamers, all reamers were cannulated to accept a 0.062-

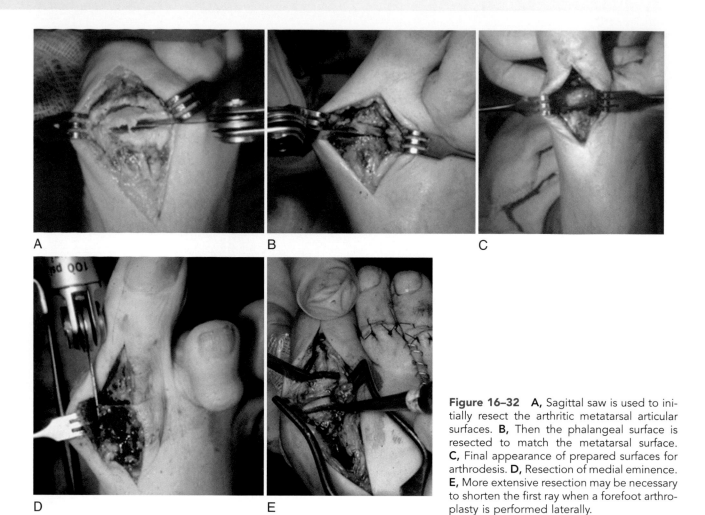

Figure 16–32 **A,** Sagittal saw is used to initially resect the arthritic metatarsal articular surfaces. **B,** Then the phalangeal surface is resected to match the metatarsal surface. **C,** Final appearance of prepared surfaces for arthrodesis. **D,** Resection of medial eminence. **E,** More extensive resection may be necessary to shorten the first ray when a forefoot arthroplasty is performed laterally.

inch Kirschner wire to ensure precise orientation of each instrument. The concave female portion of the reamer shapes the metatarsal surface to a uniform curved hemisphere, and the convex male reamer excavates the proximal phalanx to a concave, congruous surface. The cup-shaped surfaces resect less bone, reducing ultimate first ray shortening. The cup-shaped surface allows preparation without predetermination of the varus/valgus, rotation, and plantar flexion/dorsiflexion alignment. After joint preparation, the surgeon can then select the appropriate alignment for arthrodesis.

Various methods of internal fixation have been advocated, including screw fixation (see Fig. 16–33A to C), dorsal plate (see Fig. 16–33F and G),[55,58,60,61] wire loop,[98,99,358,360] Kirschner wire[98,113,114,310,373] (see Fig. 16–33C and D), cat gut suture,[343] Steinmann pin fixation* (see Figs.

*References 54, 63, 214, 215, 217, 218, 220, and 221.

16–36E and 16–37H), staples,[215] and an external fixator.[35,140] A stable construct for internal fixation is necessary. Rongstad et al[290] found that a dorsal mini-plate technique required two and a half times greater force to failure and had three times greater initial stiffness than an oblique cancellous screw. Instron testing of fixation for arthrodesis showed that the most stable construct involved machined conical reaming and a dorsal Vitallium (cobalt, chromium, and molybdenum alloy) mini-plate with an oblique lag screw,[270] which was twice as strong as an oblique lag screw alone.[270]

Curtis et al[73] evaluated crossed Kirschner wires and flat fusion surfaces, flat surfaces with a dorsal plate and screws, flat surfaces with interfragmentary screws, and curved surfaces with lag screw fixation. They showed that the stability achieved with conical reaming "is significantly greater than that with planar joint excision." Although this study demonstrated that a

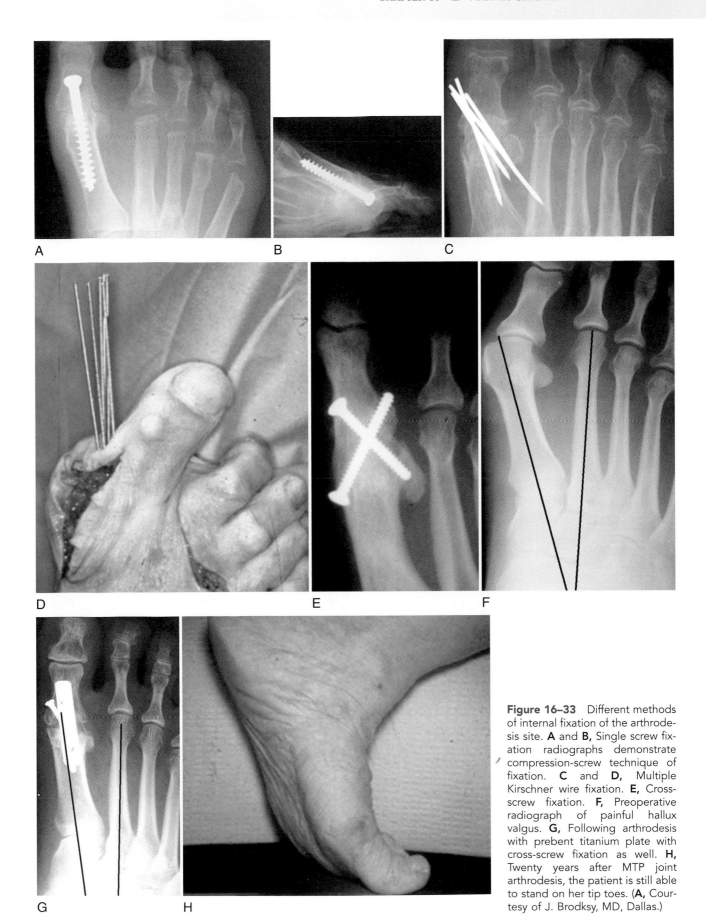

Figure 16–33 Different methods of internal fixation of the arthrodesis site. **A** and **B,** Single screw fixation radiographs demonstrate compression-screw technique of fixation. **C** and **D,** Multiple Kirschner wire fixation. **E,** Cross-screw fixation. **F,** Preoperative radiograph of painful hallux valgus. **G,** Following arthrodesis with prebent titanium plate with cross-screw fixation as well. **H,** Twenty years after MTP joint arthrodesis, the patient is still able to stand on her tip toes. (**A,** Courtesy of J. Brodksy, MD, Dallas.)

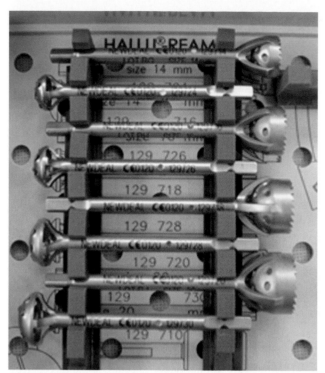

A

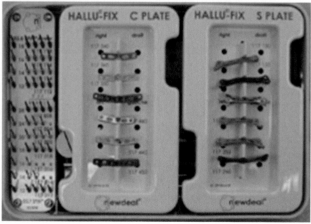

B

Figure 16–34 A, Power reamers are used to shape corresponding phalangeal and metatarsal articular surfaces for fusion. **B,** The complete set includes the reamers, plates (primary and revision), and screws.

single interfragmentary screw produced more stability than a plate, adding a screw to a dorsal plate further increases stability. The authors concluded that a dorsal Vitallium plate provided significantly greater bending and torsional strength than a stainless steel plate and that a power conical reaming system provided a significant advantage in obtaining fusion of the first MTP joint.[73]

Active infection is an absolute contraindication to MTP joint arthrodesis. Degenerative arthritis of the interphalangeal joint is a relative contraindication to first MTP fusion.* Marin[223] stated that at least 45 degrees of interphalangeal joint motion should be present if an MTP fusion is performed. Severe osteoporosis can make it difficult to stabilize a fusion site with routine methods of internal fixation.[54,55]

Surgical Technique

1. A dorsal longitudinal incision is centered over the first MTP joint, extending from just proximal to the interphalangeal joint to a point 3 cm proximal to the MTP joint (Fig. 16–35A and video clip 29).
2. The dissection is deepened to the joint capsule along the medial aspect of the extensor hallucis longus tendon. The extensor tendon may be incised to obtain adequate exposure if necessary and is repaired at the conclusion of the procedure.
3. A sagittal saw is used to remove the medial eminence. A thin wafer of bone is removed from the metatarsal and phalangeal articular surfaces. (When further shortening is desired, more bone may be removed from the metatarsal head.) By decompressing the MTP joint, exposure is increased for preparation of the MTP joint surfaces.
4. A 0.062-inch Kirschner wire is centered on the distal metatarsal head surface and driven in a proximal direction. A power-driven small joint reamer is then used to prepare the surfaces for arthrodesis (Fig. 16–35B and C).
5. A cannulated metatarsal barrel reamer is used to reduce the metaphysis to a cylinder of constant dimension and to create a convex cup-shaped surface. Alternatively, an osteotome can be used to shave any prominence and a combination metatarsal barrel and head reamer can be used. Any debris or excess bone along the periphery is removed with a rongeur (Fig. 16–35D to F).
6. A Kirschner wire is centered on the base of the proximal phalanx and driven distally.
7. A cannulated (convex) fluted phalangeal male reamer is used to prepare a concave

*References 14, 20, 26, 161, 223, and 352.

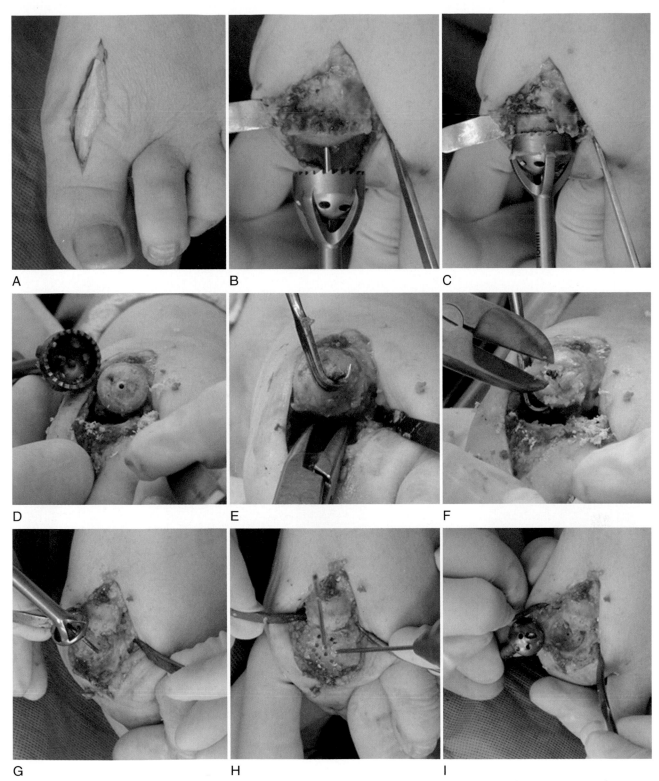

Figure 16–35 Technique of metatarsophalangeal (MTP) joint preparation. **A,** Dorsal longitudinal incision. **B,** Kirschner wire placed in the center of the metatarsal head for control of the power reamer. **C** and **D,** Over the 0.062-inch Kirschner wire, a cannulated reamer is used to shape the metatarsal head to a convex surface at the end of a cylinder of constant dimension. **E,** Remaining debris on the plantar aspect of the first metatarsal head is removed. **F,** When the prepared surface is sclerotic, it may be perforated with multiple drill holes or fish scaled with a bone-cutting forceps. **G,** Placement of the Kirschner wire into the center of the phalangeal articular surface. **H,** Reaming of the phalangeal surface with a cannulated phalangeal reamer is used to create corresponding cup-shaped concave surface. **I,** If the reamed surface is sclerotic, it is perforated with several drill holes.

Continued

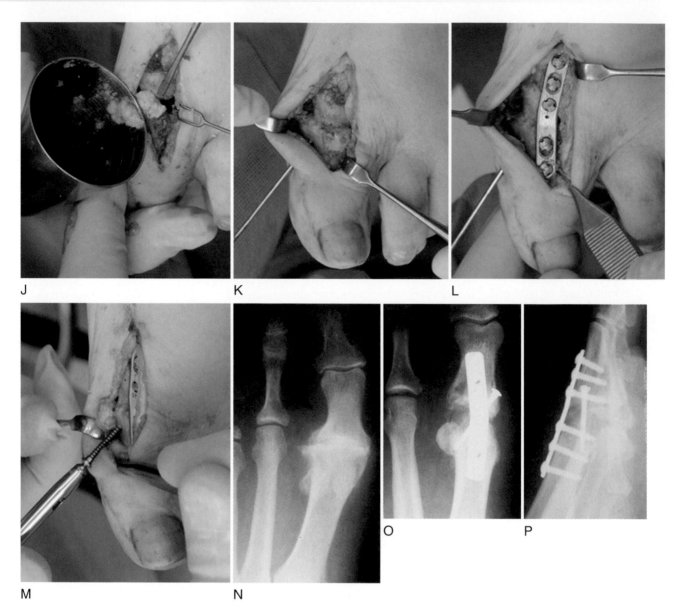

Figure 16–35—cont'd **J,** Rinsed reamings may be used as an autologous bone graft. **K,** The phalanx is temporarily stabilized with a crossed Kirschner wire. **L,** A prebent low-profile compression plate is placed on the dorsal aspect of the MTP joint to stabilize the fusion site. **M,** A cross screw is added for further internal fixation. **N,** Preoperative radiograph demonstrates end-stage MTP joint arthritis. **O** and **P,** Postoperative radiographs demonstrate correct alignment with 15 degrees of valgus and 20 degrees of dorsiflexion.

cup-shaped surface in the proximal phalanx (Fig. 16–35G to I).

8. The Kirschner wire is removed, and the rongeur is used to remove any remaining joint debris. Washed metatarsal reamings of cancellous bone may be used for autograft (Fig. 16–35E).

9. The congruous cancellous joint surfaces are then coapted in the desired dorsiflexion/plantar flexion, varus/valgus, and rotation. The desired position is 20 to 25 degrees of dorsiflexion (first metatarsal–phalangeal axis), 10 to 15 degrees of valgus, and neutral rotation. All angular measurements relate to the axis of the first metatarsal shaft and proximal phalanx. With the cup-shaped surfaces, rotation or any other dimension may be altered without disturbing other alignment variables.

10. After obtaining proper alignment, the fusion site is temporarily stabilized with one or two crossed 0.062-inch Kirschner wires (Fig. 16–35J and K).

11. The fusion site is rigidly fixed with a mini-fragment six-hole plate that is prebent in both dorsiflexion and valgus (Fig. 16–35L). A primary or revision plate with more variable fixation holes can be used depending on the bone quality. The plates come prebent to set both the dorsiflexion and valgus angles and are best placed over the dorsal aspect of the prepared MTP joint surfaces. Fixation with bicortical self-tapping twist-off screws is used.

12. The Kirschner wires are removed, and a cross-compression screw is placed to augment fixation when a primary plate is used (Fig. 16–35M).

13. If incised, the extensor hallucis longus tendon is repaired. The capsule and skin are closed in a routine manner (Fig. 16–35N to P).

Postoperative Care

A gauze-and-tape compression dressing is applied at surgery and changed weekly. The patient is allowed to ambulate in a wooden-soled postoperative shoe or short walking boot, with weight initially borne on the heel and lateral aspect of the foot. If the patient is considered unreliable, a below-knee cast is applied. Dressings and casting are discontinued 8 to 12 weeks after surgery with radiographic evidence of a successful arthrodesis.

Alternative Method of Fixation

On occasion, after failure of a resection arthroplasty or with significant osteoporosis, intramedullary fixation might be needed to stabilize an arthrodesis site. Infrequently, an interposition iliac crest graft may be needed to restore length to the first ray, especially for the salvage of a failed excisional or silicone arthroplasty.

1. After the MTP joint surfaces have been prepared, a 1/8-inch, double-pointed threaded Steinmann pin is centered on the base of the proximal phalanx and is driven distally across the interphalangeal joint, through the distal phalanx, and out through the tip of the toe.

2. Once the pin has been advanced out through the tip of the toe, the drill is attached to the distal end of the pin, and the pin is pulled, under power, farther distally until its tip is flush with the prepared surface of the base of the proximal phalanx. A pin cutter is used to remove 10 cm (4 inches) of the pin's distal aspect so that it will not interfere when the second pin is attached to the drill and pulled distally (video clip 30).

3. A second 1/8-inch, double-pointed threaded Steinmann pin is then centered just to the medial aspect of the first pin and driven in a similar manner across the interphalangeal joint and out the tip of the toe. The drill is then attached to the distal end of the second pin, and this pin is pulled farther distally until its proximal point is flush with the prepared surface of the proximal phalanx (Fig. 16–36A to C).

4. The toe is now positioned in the desired amount of rotation, valgus, and dorsiflexion.

5. With the prepared surface of the phalanx compressed on the prepared metatarsal surface, the longest pin is driven in a retrograde manner across the MTP joint into the metatarsal shaft. After the pin penetrates the proximal cortex of the first metatarsal, further advancement is not necessary. A pin cutter is then used to sever this pin, leaving approximately 1/8 inch extending beyond the tip of the toe.

6. The power drill is attached to the distal aspect of the remaining pin. This pin is driven

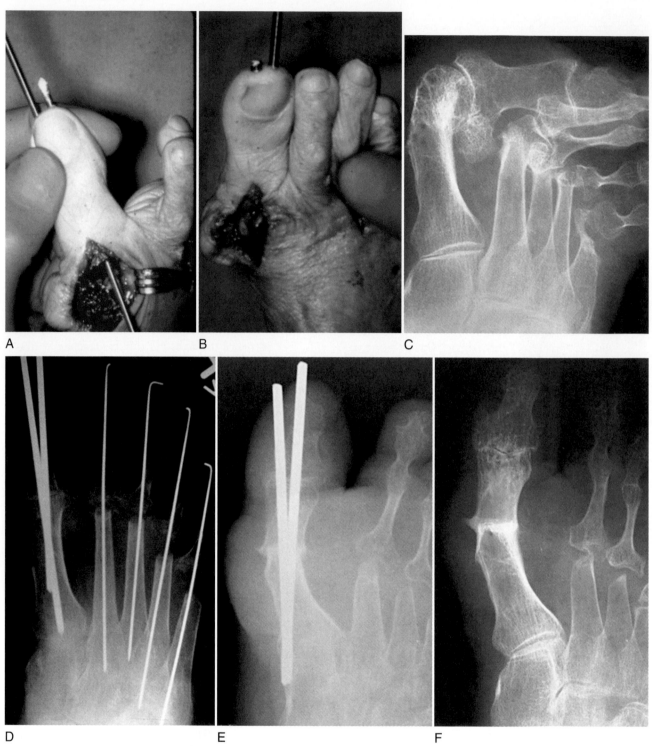

A

B

C

D

E

F

Figure 16–36 **A** and **B,** Stabilization of arthrodesis site with 1/8-inch double-pointed threaded Steinmann pins. Pins are first drilled out through the tip of the toe and then are drilled back in a retrograde manner proximally across the metatarsophalangeal joint to secure the fixation. Preoperative **(C),** intraoperative **(D),** and postoperative **(E** and **F)** radiographs demonstrate repair of a recurrent rheumatoid foot deformity with severe osteoporosis. Intramedullary Steinmann pins were used for fixation.

in a retrograde manner and advanced until it penetrates the metatarsal cortex. The remaining pin extending beyond the toe tip is cut, leaving 1/8 inch protruding for ease in later pin removal (Fig. 16–36D to F).

7. Routine closure of the joint capsule and skin is performed. Pins are often removed from the patient using local anesthesia in an office setting once radiographic union has been demonstrated, usually at 12 to 16 weeks after surgery.

Alternative Technique with Interpositional Graft

1. A bicortical or tricortical graft is obtained from the iliac crest graft (Fig. 16–37A). The graft is shaped to fit the desired gap (defect) at the MTP joint (Fig. 16–37B and C). After debridement of the MTP joint, the interposition graft is shaped and placed in the interval between the prepared surfaces of the proximal phalanx and first metatarsal. Cancellous bone is packed into any bone defects. The bicortical or tricortical graft is trapezoidal (wider plantarward and medially, narrower on the dorsolateral aspect) to allow slight valgus and dorsiflexion alignment of the arthrodesis site (Fig. 16–37D).

2. Three doubled-pointed, 5/64-inch threaded Steinmann pins are individually introduced at the MTP joint, centered on the prepared phalangeal articular surface, and driven distally, crossing the interphalangeal joint and exiting at the tip of the toe using the technique previously described. They are then pulled distally until they are flush with the prepared surface.

3. Using a lamina spreader to distract the prepared surface, the interposition bone graft is keyed into place (Fig. 16–37E and F).

4. After placement of the intercalary graft, the threaded Steinmann pins are individually driven across the interposed bone graft and into the metatarsal metaphysis. They are advanced in a retrograde manner until they penetrate the proximal metatarsal cortex (Fig. 16–37G and H).

5. Each pin is then severed at the tip of the toe, leaving 1/8 inch extending to aid in later pin removal. The subcutaneous tissue and skin are closed in a routine fashion.

Postoperative Care

A gauze-and-tape compression dressing is applied at surgery and changed weekly. Ambulation is allowed on the heel and lateral aspect of the foot in a wooden-soled postoperative shoe or short walking boot. The pins are left in place until radiographic evidence of successful arthrodesis is demonstrated, usually at a minimum of 16 weeks.

Results and Complications

In series where patients were evaluated for rate of successful postoperative arthrodesis, 1394 of 1536 arthrodeses successfully united for a 91% fusion rate (range, 77% to 100%).

Coughlin[58] reported a fusion rate of 100% using machined conical reamers and a mini-fragment plate in a series of 32 patients (47 feet) with rheumatoid arthritis who underwent arthrodesis as part of a rheumatoid forefoot reconstruction with mean follow-up of 74 months. The hallux valgus deformity was corrected to a mean of 20 degrees. Subsequent IP joint arthritis correlated with an MTP dorsiflexion angle of 20 degrees or less.

Mann and Thompson[221] reported on MTP arthrodesis in 18 feet (average follow-up, 4 years). In 12 feet a total forefoot reconstruction was performed, and in 6 feet a subtotal forefoot reconstruction was performed. Results were classified as excellent or good in 16 feet; 17 of 18 first MTP joints went on to successful fusion, and the one fibrous ankylosis was not painful. Interphalangeal degenerative arthrosis was noted radiographically but was not found to be clinically significant.

A 92% fusion rate (1074 of 1164 feet) has been reported using conical reamers.*

Coughlin and Abdo[60] reported on 47 patients (58 feet) who underwent first MTP arthrodesis. The diagnosis in 28 cases was rheumatoid arthritis and in 16 was hallux rigidus. A 98% fusion rate was achieved. The average preoperative 1-2 intermetatarsal angle was reduced from 11.9 to 9.5 degrees and the average hallux valgus angle from 35.5 to 17.1 degrees. The average dorsiflexion was 22.6 degrees (measured on a lateral radiograph of the angle subtended by the axis of the first metatarsal and proximal phalanx). Average shortening was 4 mm. Ten

*References 54, 55, 58, 60, 61, 64, 66, 212, and 223.

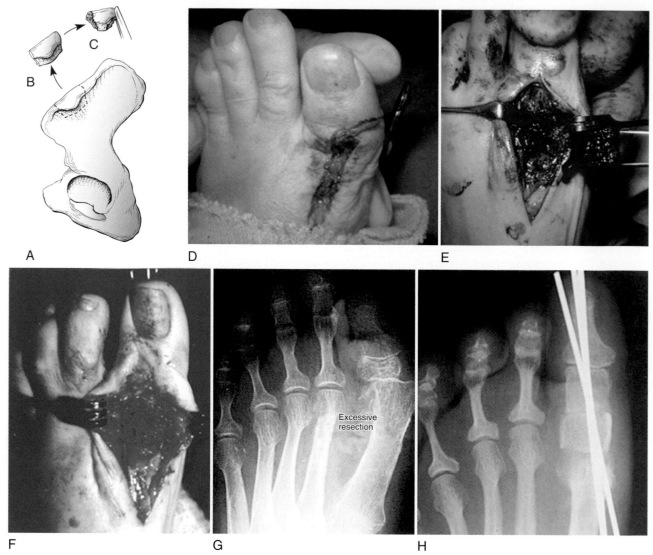

Figure 16–37   A, Diagram demonstrates removal of bicortical iliac crest graft. **B** and **C,** Either trapezoidal graft or football-shaped graft is used to span the defect at the metatarsophalangeal (MTP) joint. **D,** Photo demonstrates marked shortening after debridement of the arthroplasty site. **E,** Intraoperative photo demonstrates interposition graft before insertion. **F,** Interposition graft after insertion. It has been stabilized with three axial Steinmann pins. **G,** Radiograph demonstrates marked shortening after excisional arthroplasty. **H,** Radiograph of a different patient's foot demonstrates intercalary graft stabilized with threaded Steinmann pins.

patients were noted to have slight progression of interphalangeal joint arthritis, but only one was symptomatic.

Coughlin and Grebing[61] reported a similar high percentage of good and excellent clinical and radiographic results when arthrodesis was used for severe hallux valgus deformity. von Salis-Soglio and Thomas[352] reported on 48 cases with a successful fusion rate of 92%, and Mankey and Mann[212] reported on 51 cases with a similar 92% success rate. Coughlin,[55] using a relatively bulky yet flexible mini-fragment plate, reported on 35 cases with 100% fusion rate.

Chana et al[41] suggested that "subsequent procedures to remove hardware should not be necessary." Indeed, removal of hardware adds a further postoperative expense. Coughlin and Abdo[60] removed only 4 of 58 plates (6%), but Coughlin[55] removed 12 of 35 larger dorsal stainless steel plates (34%). Mankey and Mann[212] reported removal of 8 of 56 dorsal plates (14%).

When MTP fusion is combined with a lateral MTP resection arthroplasty, the first ray is often shortened to achieve an acceptable cosmetic appearance as well as to avoid an excessively long first ray, which can impact against the toe box. The comparative length of the first and second ray rarely has been analyzed after MTP arthrodesis. Mann and Oates[218] reported that three of 41 patients thought their hallux was "too short" after MTP fusion. Coughlin reported 3-mm average shortening in one series[55] and 4 mm in another series.[60]

Complications after arthrodesis are uncommon and include nonunion[155,343] and malunion.[98,99,155,343,373] Nonunion[343] can occur because of the small contact area at the fusion site (Fig. 16–38). Unsuccessful arthrodesis does not necessarily lead to painful pseudoarthrosis,[14] and McKeever[230] and others[14,41,114,155,223] have stated that a nonunion can still lead to an acceptable result. If a nonunion occurs, significant shortening can lead to metatarsalgia.[246] Results tend to vary depending on the selected method of internal fixation and the specific technique. However, an average 10% failure rate has been noted in the literature.[55] The highest rate of nonunion (23%) was reported by Gimple et al,[113] who used crossed Kirschner wires for internal fixation. Marin[223] and Turan and Lindgren[343] observed that inadequate internal fixation was the most common cause of nonunion (Fig. 16–39).

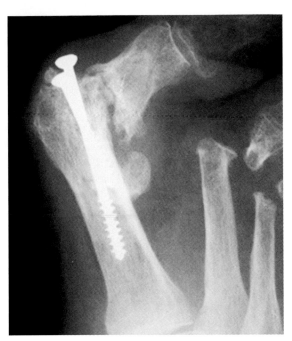

Figure 16–38 Radiograph demonstrates nonunion after compression screw fixation of arthrodesis site.

Failure of internal fixation has been reported as well. Mankey and Mann[212] reported an 8% failure rate (4 of 51 cases) with a stainless steel plate. With a Vitallium plate and an absence of screw holes at the fusion site, Coughlin and Abdo[60] reported a 2% failure rate (1 of 58).

Malunion in any plane is poorly tolerated and underscores the need for meticulous attention to the final position of arthrodesis. Malunion can occur in any of three planes: varus/valgus, dorsiflexion/plantar flexion, or rotation.

Interphalangeal joint arthritis after first MTP fusion has been reported to vary from 6% to 60% (Fig. 16–40). Coughlin and Abdo[60] reported a 10% incidence of progressive arthritis, but only 2% of cases were symptomatic. Chana et al[41] reported a 21% incidence of interphalangeal arthritis at 10-year follow-up in all joints fused in less than 20 degrees of valgus. Mann and Thompson[221] reported a 65% incidence of arthritis but did not believe this was clinically significant. Mann and Schakel[220] noted a 60% incidence, but only one third of cases were symptomatic. In both series, internal fixation (threaded Steinmann pins) crossed the interphalangeal joint, which might have been a factor in the high rates of arthritis.[220,221] Interphalangeal joint hypermobility[343] can develop

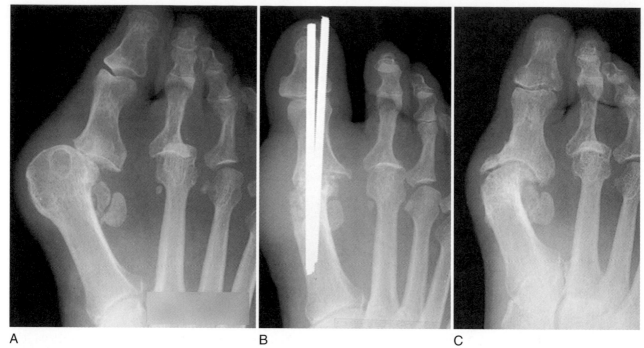

A   B   C

Figure 16–39 A, Radiograph demonstrates severe subluxation of the first metatarsophalangeal (MTP) joint in a steroid-dependent patient with rheumatoid arthritis. **B,** After arthrodesis with intramedullary Steinmann pin fixation. **C,** Seven years after surgery, nonunion has developed. Despite this, the patient was pleased with correction of her deformity and reported no pain.

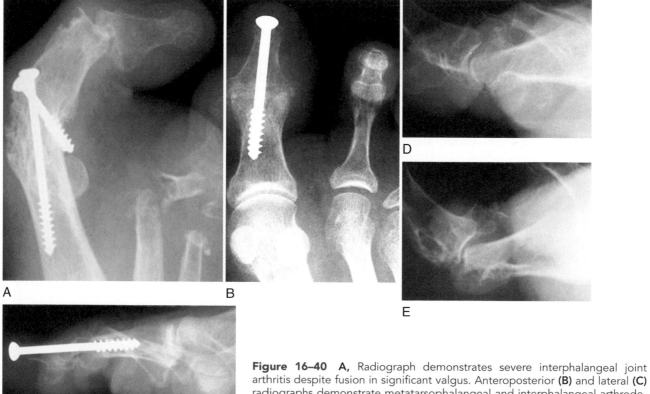

Figure 16–40 A, Radiograph demonstrates severe interphalangeal joint arthritis despite fusion in significant valgus. Anteroposterior **(B)** and lateral **(C)** radiographs demonstrate metatarsophalangeal and interphalangeal arthrodeses for arthritis. **D** and **E,** Hyperextension deformity of interphalangeal joint in time develops owing to arthrodesis in less-than-adequate dorsiflexion.

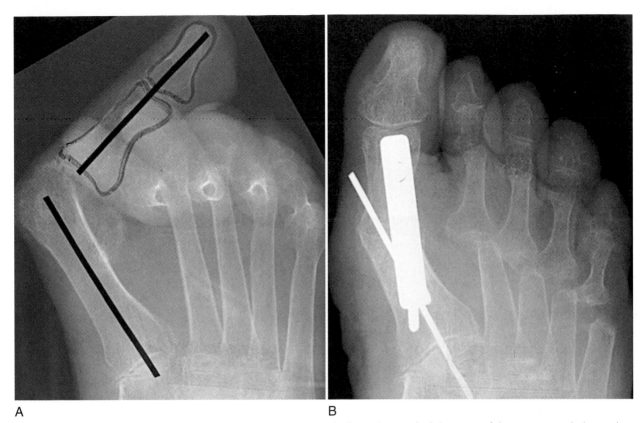

A   B

Figure 16–41   A, Preoperative radiograph demonstrates severe hallux valgus with dislocation of the metatarsophalangeal joint and angle of 20 degrees between the first and second metatarsals. **B,** After arthrodesis and forefoot arthroplasty, angle between the first and second metatarsals is reduced to 9 degrees.

after fusion with inadequate dorsiflexion at the MTP joint.

Arthrodesis of the first MTP joint creates a stable medial buttress that protects the lesser toes from further deformity (Fig. 16–41A to C). Fusion tends to provide first ray stability, preserve first ray length, and maintain strength of the hallux. Often after a fusion, increased weight bearing on the inner aspect of the foot leads to a reduction in lateral metatarsalgia. This is in contradistinction to excisional arthroplasty, where weight bearing of the first ray is decreased and lateral metatarsalgia increased.

Reviewing their experience with the Keller procedure, Rogers and Joplin[289] noted a 63% incidence of metatarsalgia after excisional arthroplasty but only a 9% incidence after first MTP arthrodesis. Henry and Waugh[147] reported significant weight bearing on the first ray in only 40% of cases after excisional arthroplasty but in approximately 80% after MTP arthrodesis.

Marin[223] and others[98,155] reported minimal metatarsalgia after first MTP arthrodesis. Often a patient is able to wear ordinary footwear after arthrodesis.

The technique of first MTP joint arthrodesis should be simple to perform and should achieve predictable postoperative results. The ideal method of arthrodesis should allow easy adjustment of joint surfaces during surgery to vary the final arthrodesis alignment. The shaping of congruous cancellous bone surfaces that can easily be adjusted to the desired position of fusion is important in maintaining position and achieving a high rate of bony union. As McKeever[230] noted, "It is the arthrodesis and its position that [are] important and not the method by which it is produced." The ultimate goal of MTP arthrodesis is correction of a permanent deformity and creation of a stable, comfortable gait pattern that allows the patient to wear ordinary footwear.

UNCOMMON PROBLEMS ASSOCIATED WITH RHEUMATOID ARTHRITIS

Subluxation or Dislocation of a Single Metatarsophalangeal Joint

An isolated dislocation of a lesser MTP joint occurs infrequently with rheumatoid arthritis. If it develops, it typically occurs at the second or third MTP joint. When the condition is present and symptomatic, pain usually develops beneath the metatarsal head where dislocation has occurred. Pain also can occur in the area of a contracted lesser toe with hammer toe or claw toe formation. Initial treatment centers on conservative management including an extra-depth shoe, soft insole, and metatarsal arch support.

When conservative care is unsuccessful, surgical intervention can require a hammer toe repair, synovectomy, and flexor tendon transfer (see earlier discussion) and occasionally a metatarsal head excision. Isolated metatarsal head excision has been discouraged by Rana[275] and others[46,47,245,346] but recommended by Thomas.[334] A physician must explain to the patient that limited forefoot surgery can alleviate symptoms and provide short-term relief of pain, but with time and progression of the rheumatoid arthritis, the other lesser MTP joints can become malaligned. On the other hand, it is difficult for a physician to recommend a complete forefoot reconstruction based on the presence of pain and deformity at a single lesser MTP joint.

Interphalangeal Joint Arthritis of the Hallux

Occasionally, after an arthrodesis of the first MTP joint, degenerative arthritis develops at the interphalangeal joint of the hallux, possibly because of progression of the inflammatory arthritic process. Other causes of interphalangeal joint arthritis include fusion of the first ray in a relatively straight position or lack of dorsiflexion and crossing of the interphalangeal joint with internal fixation (see Fig. 16–40D and E). Valgus deviation at the interphalangeal joint can develop with a rather grotesque appearance of the tip of the toe. Occasionally, ulceration can occur on the plantar–medial aspect of the interphalangeal joint. Hyperextension of the distal phalanx can occur as well, and in these isolated cases an arthrodesis of the first interphalangeal joint is indicated (video clip 32).[307] The great toe is shortened slightly to decompress the joint. Neutral rotation with minimal varus or valgus is achieved when the arthrodesis is performed. Although there

may be some concern about the postoperative gait pattern, the patient with long-standing rheumatoid arthritis usually tolerates simultaneous MTP and interphalangeal joint fusion surprisingly well.

Rheumatoid Nodule or Cyst

On occasion, rheumatoid nodules or cysts form on the plantar aspect of the foot, in a weight-bearing area, or over a bony prominence. This makes wearing shoes difficult. A rheumatoid cyst or nodule should be excised, often under local anesthesia. Care should be taken to avoid superficial sensory nerves in the area of the resection.

When a cyst develops in the heel pad region, the heel pad can become unstable. This presents a difficult situation to treat because with aggressive resection there is often inadequate padding between the calcaneus and the plantar skin. Conversely, with an inadequate resection, a patient can continue to have symptoms. Thus the dorsal aspect of the cyst should be excised, leaving a portion of the plantar cyst near or in contact with the plantar skin. The area should be drained to prevent hematoma formation. It is hoped that adhesions will form between the plantar skin and the undersurface of the calcaneus to achieve a stable plantar fat pad.[165]

Splaying of the Rheumatoid Foot

At times, significant 1-2 and 4-5 intermetatarsal angles develop with a rheumatoid forefoot deformity. The question can arise whether an osteotomy of either the first or the fifth metatarsal should be performed at the time of first MTP joint arthrodesis and lesser metatarsal head resection arthroplasty. In general, the 1-2 intermetatarsal space significantly reduces after a first MTP arthrodesis (see Fig. 16–41A and B). Likewise, the 4-5 intermetatarsal angle often reduces after resection arthroplasty. Thus it is rarely necessary to perform a first or fifth metatarsal osteotomy.

CRYSTAL-INDUCED ARTHROPATHIES

The pathogenesis of *crystal deposition disease* occurs with the inclusion of crystalline material within the synovium, capsule, ligaments, and osseous tissue, where an inflammatory response occurs. The common causes of crystalline deposition disease in foot and ankle disease are *monosodium urate deposition disease* (gout) and *calcium pyrophosphate dihydrate deposition disease* (pseudogout).

Gouty Arthropathy

History and Incidence

Gout has been known since early recorded medical history.[196] Rana[275] noted that Hippocrates described gout in the foot as "podagra" (*pous* meaning "foot," *agra* meaning "attack"), and this term is used in much of the early medical literature. Hyperuricemia occurs from an inborn error of metabolism and is the cause of *primary gout*, whereas *secondary gout* occurs as an acquired disorder or after the use of certain pharmacologic agents. A gouty attack is characterized by the precipitation of monosodium urate crystals in the synovial tissue, leading to an acute inflammatory response. It is estimated that the incidence of gout in the United States is 1.3% of the general population.[371] The mean age of onset is 40 years, and gout is familial in 75% of patients.[282,284] Gout typically occurs in men, although women develop gout after menopause.

Pathophysiology

Gout develops as a monoarticular arthritis, with the first MTP joint involved in most cases. Sixty percent of patients have a second attack within a year. The first MTP joint is affected in greater than 50% of patients in initial attacks of gout,[194,226] and on a long-term basis, involvement of the great toe can approach 90%.[31,194]

The acute phase of gout is characterized by the rapid onset of exquisite pain and tenderness, periarticular swelling and erythema, and increased tissue temperature that mimics cellulitis. Dactylitis, or a sausage-shaped digit, has been reported to occur in patients with gout, psoriatic arthritis, Reiter's syndrome, and undifferentiated spondyloarthropathy but rarely in rheumatoid or osteoarthritic patients unless flexor tendon sheath infection is present.[292] However, cases of concomitant gout and rheumatoid arthritis have been reported,[317] and psoriasis can also be a cause of hyperuricemia.[138] A gout attack represents a complication of prolonged hyperuricemia, which can be influenced pharmacologically by decreased renal excretion or increased production of uric acid.

In the acute phases of gout, urate crystals can deposit not only in the synovium and capsular tissues but over time also in the articular cartilage and subchondral bone. After an acute flare-up, an interval phase can occur with few or no symptoms. This interval phase can develop 72 to 96 hours after an acute attack and can last for weeks or years. In the chronic phase of gout, urate deposits or gouty tophi develop as a chalky precipitate in the soft tissue[201] (Fig. 16–42). These tophi can produce ulceration and secondary infection and are typically seen only after several attacks.[196] Control of hyperuricemia through strict diet or medications such as allopurinol can prevent formation of

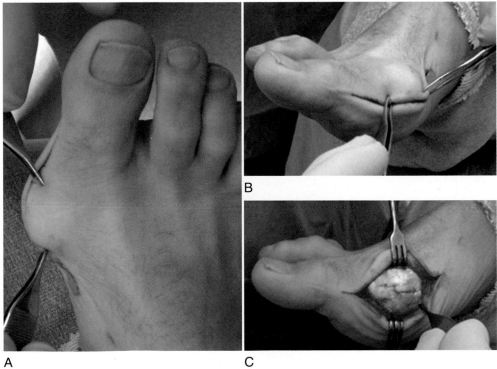

A   C   B

Figure 16–42 Gouty arthritis. **A** and **B,** Marked swelling and enlargement of the first metatarsophalangeal joint. **C,** Surgical debridement of white, chalky gouty deposits.

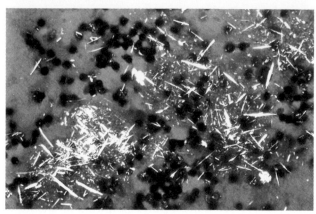

Figure 16–43 Pathologic specimen from biopsy of patient with gout. Birefringence seen under polarized light in a specimen from a patient with gouty tophi. (Courtesy of D. Claassen, MD, Boise, Idaho.)

tophi. A diagnosis is made by microscopic evaluation of the crystals after an arthrocentesis or debridement of the joint. Sodium urate crystals are typically needle shaped in appearance and range from 2 to 10 μm in length but can be significantly longer. Under polarized light the crystals display negative elongation (*birefringence*), a characteristic finding with sodium urate crystals (Fig. 16–43).

The risk of an attack of gouty arthritis increases with higher serum levels of uric acid (greater than 7.0 mg/dL in men and greater than 6.0 mg/dL in

women).[126,284] In a supersaturated state, monosodium urate crystals can precipitate. Serum uric acid levels do not always correlate with an acute attack of gout, although persons with uric acid levels greater than 6 mg/dL are at increased risk for gouty attacks. Silent hyperuricemia is present in 25% to 33% of patients.[282] The predilection of gouty attacks for the lower extremity and specifically the MTP joint of the hallux has been explained as being caused by the decreased pH in the foot, increased urate solubility with the lower temperatures exhibited in the foot, and the first MTP joint's being subject to significant stress during normal gait. Landry[194] also noted that at 37° C the solubility of uric acid is 6.8 mg/mL and at 30° C, 4.5 mg/mL. With decreased temperatures in peripheral tissues, decreased solubility of uric acid may be characterized by increased precipitation of monosodium urate crystals. Boss[31] noted that the intraarticular temperature of the normal knee joint is 33° C and the intra-articular temperature of the normal ankle joint is 29° C. The temperature of a peripheral joint such as the MTP joint of the hallux is thus well below 37° C.

On radiographic examination the initial finding merely may be soft tissue swelling. With time, crystalline deposition can cause the development of well-marginated erosions bordered by sclerotic margins at a distance from the joint (Fig. 16–44). As eventual reparative attempts are made by the adjacent bone, an elevated bony margin develops that appears to over-

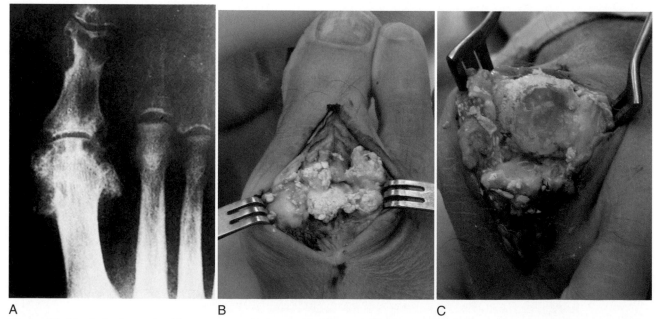

A   B   C

Figure 16–44   **A,** Radiograph of first metatarsophalangeal joint demonstrates periarticular erosion characteristic of gouty arthritis. **B,** Accumulation of crystalline deposits in capsular tissue. **C,** Clinical photo shows the associated destructive joint changes of gouty arthropathy.

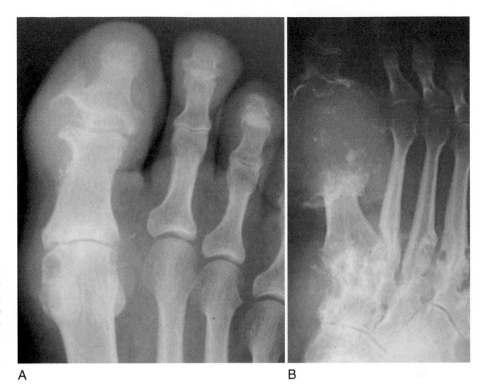

Figure 16–45 A, Radiograph demonstrates arthritis of the interphalangeal joint with overhanging bone sign. **B,** Typical osseous erosion of the first metatarsophalangeal joint associated with chronic gout. (**B,** Courtesy of A. Smith, MD, Prince Rupert, Canada.)

A   B

hang the tophaceous deposit as though it were displaced by it, forming a characteristic radiographic finding (overhanging edge sign)[86,225,325] (Fig. 16–45). The articular space is often well maintained. In the subcortical bone, a lacy pattern of bone erosion is pathognomonic of this disease process. Punched-out areas of bony lysis can grow to greater than 5 mm in diameter.[194,226] A distinguishable feature of gouty arthropathy is the presence of erosive lesions somewhat remote from the articular surface. Periarticular erosion just proximal to the MTP joint can occur on both the medial and the lateral aspect of the metatarsal head. Arthritic involvement of the interphalangeal joint of the great toe occurs not only in gouty arthropathy but also with psoriasis and Reiter's syndrome. Radiographic findings can vary from no detectable abnormality to severe destruction of foot joints. Miskew and Goldflies[240] have described avascular necrosis of the talus as a complication of gouty arthropathy.

Treatment

Pharmacologic treatment focuses on increasing uric acid excretion, decreasing uric acid formation, and decreasing acute inflammation. In acute phases of gout, indomethacin is an effective agent because it inhibits prostaglandin synthesis. Boss[31] has recommended 25 to 100 mg orally every 4 hours until symptomatic relief is obtained; however, 50 mg every 6 hours with gradual tapering after reduction in inflam-

mation is a reasonable regimen.[287] Colchicine may be given orally or intravenously. The recommended oral dosage is 0.6 mg every hour until the patient experiences relief of pain or develops gastrointestinal side effects such as nausea or diarrhea.[31,273,287] Side effects from large doses of colchicine have included alopecia, aplastic anemia, and respiratory depression,[31] and long-term effects include peripheral neuropathy. Approximately 25% of the population does not respond to colchicine.[103] Uricosuric agents (probenecid) increase renal excretion of uric acid by approximately 50%.[287] In the acute phases of gout, symptomatic treatment also includes foot elevation and bed rest.

With resolution of the acute phase of gout, allopurinol may be used to prevent further attacks. Allopurinol inhibits the enzyme xanthine oxidase and effectively decreases uric acid production. A daily oral dose of 300 to 800 mg is well tolerated by most patients.[287] Gastrointestinal discomfort occasionally is present, although serious side effects such as hepatitis, agranulocytosis, and hypersensitivity reactions are rare.[31] The patient should be under the continued supervision of a rheumatologist. Approximately 10% of patients with untreated gout will develop chronic tophaceous deposits with eventual destruction of bone and joints. Patients with a serum urate level of 9 mg/dL or less typically do not develop tophi even if they are not treated. Once the serum urate level exceeds 11 mg/dL, tophaceous deposits are more common, and if preventive measures are not taken, recurrent attacks can occur.

Surgery for gouty arthropathy depends on the specific deformity. In the presence of gouty tophi an ulceration or sinus tract may be debrided. After debridement, application of moist dressings and administration of parenteral antibiotics often result in the rapid resolution of lesions with minimal scarring. Debulking of the tophaceous material by curettage usually decreases symptoms.[196,367]

The medical and surgical treatment of chronic tophaceous gout, however, can result in not only the rapid dissolution of tophi but also the destruction of bone, because much of the bone matrix is replaced by sodium urate crystals (Fig 16–45). Significant shortening of the phalanges and metatarsals can occur, but Larmon and Kurtz[196] emphasized that amputation is rarely indicated.

The frequency of surgery for the treatment of chronic tophaceous gout has decreased in recent years because of improved diagnosis and medical management. Occasionally, however, an untreated patient who has had numerous attacks of chronic gout can develop tophaceous gout that requires surgical intervention. Kurtz[192] and Larmon and Kurtz[196] have described in detail the surgical debridement of tophaceous lesions. Kumar et al[190] reported on their experience of 45 patients who underwent surgery for tophaceous gout. The main indication for surgery was sepsis control or prevention of ulcerated tophaceous gout. Eighty-nine percent of patients were male. Renal impairment was the most common medical problem in 38%, hypertension in 27%, heart disease in 20%, and diabetes in 18%. In their study, 53% of patients experienced delayed wound healing and 7% required digital amputation.

Articular degenerative changes that lead to pain, deformity, and decreased function may be treated with either excisional arthroplasty or arthrodesis. The arthrodesis and forefoot reconstructive techniques used are similar to those used for rheumatoid forefoot disease (see earlier discussion).

Calcium Pyrophosphate Dihydrate Deposition Disease (Pseudogout)

Incidence

Calcium pyrophosphate dihydrate (CPPD) deposition disease is also known as *chondrocalcinosis* or *pseudogout*. The incidence of pseudogout is about half the incidence of gout in the United States.[23] It occurs most often between the sixth and eighth decades of life. A familial form of pseudogout manifests at a slightly younger age.[23] No conclusion has been made regarding the mode of genetic transmission.[371] The male-to-female ratio is 1.5 : 1 for pseudogout.[4,23] It can have a polyarticular presentation.

Pathophysiology

CPPD crystals might be deposited in synovial and capsular tissues as well as within tendons and ligaments. The development of acute synovitis appears to develop with crystal shedding, in which crystals deposited in articular cartilage are shed into the joint. After phagocytosis of the crystals, enzymatic and lysozymal release by leukocytes leads to an intense inflammatory response. The most common areas of involvement are the MTP joints in the foot, where periarticular calcification can develop. Crystals are radiopaque and are demonstrated as linear calcifications within joint hyaline cartilage or as diffuse opacifications within soft tissues. Joint destruction, although uncommon, resembles the typical changes of osteoarthritis, including chondrolysis, subchondral sclerosis, and cyst formation. Pseudogout can be precipitated by trauma.

Chondrocalcinosis often affects the upper extremity joints and the knees, as opposed to gout, which more often involves lower extremity joints. The joints of the hindfoot are occasionally involved. Often the knee is affected, with a linear calcification within the menisci (Fig. 16–46A).

Joint aspiration and microscopic identification of crystals are necessary to establish a diagnosis. No underlying enzymatic defect or metabolic abnormality leads to CPPD arthropathy. The disorder is typically diagnosed by the microscopic demonstration of weakly (positive) birefringent crystals of varying shapes under polarized light (1 to 20 μm in length) (Fig. 16–46B).

Treatment

Pharmacologic treatment with NSAIDs and the occasional judicious use of an intraarticular steroid injection may be warranted.[2] Colchicine is relatively inconsistent in relieving symptoms, but NSAIDs may be more helpful. Recurrent attacks separated by asymptomatic periods and eventual chronic degenerative arthropathy can develop. Surgery, when necessary, uses techniques of arthrodesis and joint debridement typically used for osteoarthritis.

SERONEGATIVE ARTHROPATHIES

Enthesopathy is a characteristic finding of seronegative arthropathies. The site of insertion of a ligament, tendon, joint capsule, or fascia is called the *enthesis*, and inflammation of this site is called *enthesopathy*.

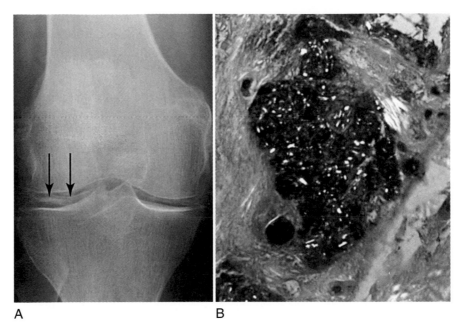

Figure 16–46   A, Chondrocalcinosis often affects the knee joint with calcification of menisci. **B,** With chondrocalcinosis, microscopic evaluation demonstrates crystals characterized by positive birefringence under polarized light. The soft tissue is infiltrated with crystals in the central area of the specimen. (**B,** Courtesy of D. Claasen, Boise, Idaho.)

A   B

Inflammation can lead to osteolysis, new bone formation, and capsular fibrosis. The large number of tendinous insertions and joints in the foot increases the vulnerability of this region for inflammation. Seronegative arthropathies are characterized by the absence of a positive rheumatoid factor. The arthritic process often involves the axial skeleton. Because musculoskeletal pathologic findings are often indistinguishable from rheumatoid arthritis, the presence of other findings (gastrointestinal or genitourinary disorders, dermatologic abnormalities, nail changes) may be necessary to make a conclusive diagnosis.

The three common seronegative arthropathies (psoriatic arthritis, Reiter's syndrome, ankylosing spondylitis) involving the lower extremity are characterized by radiographic features that differentiate them from rheumatoid arthritis. Key radiologic features include absence of generalized osteoporosis because of a less profound synovitis, presence of whiskering or adventitious calcification around the involved joints with erosive bony changes, and intraarticular ankylosis. The seronegative arthropathies are often associated with heel pain syndrome (20% incidence).[127,287] Rheumatoid arthritis rarely manifests with initial symptoms of heel pain (see Fig. 16–51).

Psoriatic Arthritis

Definition and Incidence

Psoriatic arthritis is an asymmetric polyarthritis often, but not always, associated with skin and nail disorders. The association of arthropathy and psoriasis was initially described by Alibert[5] in 1818, but Bazin[13] coined the term *psoriatic arthropathy* in 1860. The prevalence of psoriasis in the general population is less than 3%.[93,249,324] Onset of arthritis is typically insidious, but it can have an acute onset mimicking gout. Typically the onset occurs in the third or fourth decade, but any age group can be affected. Unlike rheumatoid arthritis, the male-to-female ratio is 1:1.[43,93,100] A heritable tendency, probably polygenic in nature, has been reported.[249] Farber and Nall[93] have noted a 36% familial onset in affected subjects.

Two different patterns of dermatologic presentation occur with psoriasis. *Psoriasis vulgaris* (Fig. 16–47A) is characterized by silvery papules and white scaly plaques. *Psoriasis pustulosis* (Fig. 16–47B) is characterized by pustules and vesicles on the thenar eminence and along the longitudinal arch of the foot.[43] Nail involvement is characterized by onycholysis, pitting subungual hyperkeratosis, and splinter hemorrhages. Disease with obvious nail and dermatologic disease (74%) tend to be easier to diagnose than disease with limited skin involvement.[133]

Fitzpatrick et al[100] noted arthritis associated with psoriasis in 3% to 4% of the population. Hammerschlag et al[133] reported that 14% of patients with psoriatic arthritis had skin lesions in hidden areas (gluteal fold, axilla, beneath hairlines). In 12% to 16% the arthropathy precedes the onset of skin abnormalities.[133,285] In one series the average onset of psoriasis was 32 years of age and the average onset of arthritis was 36 years.[133] Although Moll and Wright[243] reported arthritic involvement of the hands as a characteristic finding, Hammerschlag et al[133] reported that the foot and ankle were involved as the initial area of disease

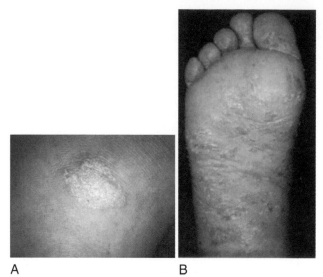

A   **B**

Figure 16–47   A, Psoriasis vulgaris is characterized by silvery papules and white scaly plaques. **B,** Psoriasis pustulosis is characterized by vesicles on the plantar aspect of the foot. (From Dockery G: *Cutaneous Disorders of the Lower Extremity.* Philadelphia, WB Saunders, 1997.)

presentation three times more often than the hand (foot and ankle 55%, hand and wrist 20%).

Psoriatic arthritis should be suspected with a familial history of psoriasis, skin and nail lesions, multiple joint arthropathy, and a sausage digit.[104] Involvement of the nails is seen in 63% of patients with psoriatic arthritis, compared with 37% of those with psoriasis without arthritic symptoms.[298] Although psoriatic arthritis characteristically has been reported to affect the DIP joints, Rodnan and Schumaker[287,288] noted that only 5% to 10% of patients exhibit classic DIP joint arthropathy (Fig. 16–48A).

Patients with asymmetric arthropathy involving only two or three joints and those with a pattern of symmetric polyarthritis are clinically indistinguishable from those with rheumatoid arthritis. Evaluating patients with psoriatic arthritis, Roberts et al[285] noted arthritis indistinguishable from rheumatoid arthritis in 78%, distal joint arthritis in 17%, and arthritis mutilans in 5%.

Psoriatic arthritis appears to be progressive. It progresses in almost 50% of patients despite disease-modifying pharmacologic treatment.[115,173] Moreover, foot and ankle involvement was reported to be the most common site of involvement in 86% of patients in one study.[133] Psoriatic arthritis differs from rheumatoid arthritis mainly in the pattern of arthritic involvement. Typically in this seronegative arthropathy the rheumatoid factor is negative. Human leukocyte antigen

(HLA)-B27 testing is positive less often than with ankylosing spondylitis or Reiter's syndrome.[175]

Examination

Physical examination is characterized by the presentation of arthritis, with swelling, joint tenderness, and pain with erythema. The MTP joints are involved slightly more often than the ankle or interphalangeal joints. Nail dystrophy is common. Gold and Bassett[116] and others[100,133] have noted involvement of the interphalangeal joint of the hallux. Although these patients are not seriously ill, they can exhibit chronic fatigue, lymphadenopathy, fever, weight loss, and splenomegaly. Ultrasonographic evaluation of psoriatic dactylitis has demonstrated that the digital swelling is due to flexor tenosynovitis (96%) as well as articular synovitis (52%).[171]

The radiographic appearance of psoriatic arthritis is similar to that of rheumatoid arthritis.[116,126] The os calcis typically develops spurring or sclerosis on the posterior plantar surface. Erosion of the distal tuft of the terminal phalanx (*acro-osteolysis*) can occur,[243] along with whittling of the phalanges and metatarsals and cupping of the proximal aspect of the phalanges and metatarsals. Whittling and cupping occurring simultaneously is termed *pencil-in-cup deformity.* Ankylosing of the digits can occur.

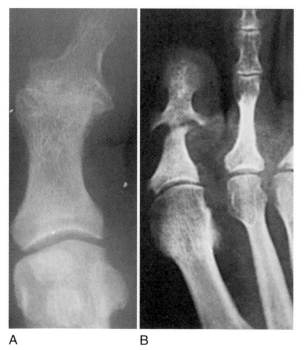

A   **B**

Figure 16–48   A, Classic distal interphalangeal joint (DIP) arthropathy characteristic of psoriatic arthritis. **B,** Psoriatic arthritis with extensive destruction of the interphalangeal joint of the hallux. (Courtesy of A. Smith, MD, Prince Rupert, Canada.)

Characteristically a predilection exists for the PIP and DIP joints with relative sparing of the MTP joint,[236] but separation of patients with DIP involvement into a distinct subclass is not warranted because clinical and radiographic outcome appears to be affected by the number of joints involved (oligoarticular versus polyarticular).[172] In 5% of patients with distal arthritis, one or more joints progress to severe osteolysis of the phalanx, with severe deformities often described as *arthritis mutilans* (complete resorption of bone), and an opera-glass or telescoping deformity of the digit can occur (Fig. 16–48B). All these findings have been well described, but Moll and Wright[243] have noted that they are relatively uncommon. Erosions in the periarticular region and poorly defined periostitis can occur along the short diaphyseal regions of the phalanges.[126]

Treatment

Heel pain symptoms are indistinguishable from Reiter's syndrome (see Fig. 16–51). The pathogenesis is similar to, although less marked than, that of rheumatoid arthritis with inflammatory cellular infiltrates. The treatment of heel pain is usually nonsurgical, with immobilization, rest, padding, stretching, and use of pharmacologic agents. In general, much of the medical treatment is pharmacologic, with administration of NSAIDs and occasional use of intraarticular corticosteroid injections for symptomatic MTP and DIP joints. The treatment of skin lesions can involve methotrexate and corticosteroids.

Surgical treatment of forefoot deformities associated with psoriasis is uncommon but, when necessary, follows the surgical principles of rheumatoid arthritis, with MTP or interphalangeal joint fusions of the hallux, lesser MTP joint excisional arthroplasty, and hammer toe or mallet toe repairs. Kitaoka[183] has reported a high level of good and excellent results (89%) with arthrodesis procedures, forefoot arthroplasty, and rheumatoid-type surgical procedures in psoriatic arthritis patients followed over a 15-year period. However, Stern et al[324] reported an increased infection rate in patients with psoriatic arthritis who had undergone total joint arthroplasty and suggested preventive preoperative prophylactic measures, including perioperative antibiotics and localized skin care. It is preferable to have clear skin to operate through, and aggressive dermatologic efforts can reduce skin-related complications.

The priority is the identification of the disease process. Poorly defined metatarsalgia may be the first sign of psoriasis. The presentation of seronegative arthritis with poorly defined forefoot pain can initially be misdiagnosed as an interdigital neuroma, and the patient could undergo unnecessary surgery.[133]

Reiter's Syndrome

Presentation and Etiology

Reactive arthritis was initially described by several authors in the eighteenth century, but a report by Hans Reiter[280] in 1916 of a triad of conjunctivitis, urethritis, and asymmetric arthritis has become associated with this disease entity.[42] More recently, this syndrome has been expanded to include the symptoms of mucosal ulceration, balanitis circinata, and keratoderma blennorrhagicum. *Keratoderma blennorrhagicum* describes a pustular lesion on the sole of the foot that is seen in approximately 10% of those with Reiter's syndrome. It may be confused with psoriasis and in time can form a hyperkeratotic lesion. Keat[176] has reported that these other symptoms can differ in frequency depending on the underlying infectious organism.

Although the cause of Reiter's syndrome is unknown, 60% to 80% of patients have a positive HLA-B27 test, suggesting an immunologic predisposition.[102,176] Most investigators suspect an infectious cause, although no single organism has been isolated. The disease is often reported to follow gastrointestinal or genitourinary tract infection.[126] It is associated with gonococcal infections, gastrointestinal disorders, and diarrhea. *Salmonella*, *Shigella*, *Yersinia*, and *Campylobacter* organisms have all been implicated. *Balanitis circinata* is associated with either *Shigella* dysentery or sexually acquired Reiter's syndrome, but it is infrequently associated with *Salmonella*, *Campylobacter*, or *Yersinia* infections.

The association between a bacterial infection and an elevated HLA-B27 led Fan and Yu[92] to propose a genetic predisposition, with arthropathy being secondarily induced by the infection.

Chand and Johnson[42] reported on 120 patients with Reiter's syndrome at the Mayo Clinic over a 10-year period. The median age of onset was 26 years, and 50% of these patients had foot and ankle symptoms. A definite predilection for the lower extremity has been observed,[29,42,116,126,325] and the most frequently affected locations are the interphalangeal joints, MTP joints, ankle, and calcaneus. The knee was involved in two thirds of patients. Physical findings are similar to those of other seronegative spondyloarthropathies.[237]

Symptoms and physical findings include pain, swelling, tenderness, mild stiffness, and erythema of the involved joints. Often a patient describing the onset of ambiguous foot pain has undiagnosed Reiter's syndrome. The onset is typically insidious and occurs in young men (10:1 ratio)[176] with asymmetric involvement of the lower extremity. Symptoms often occur less than 30 days after an infection[176] (more than 80% of patients). Because arthritis can appear following an infectious process, Reiter's syndrome should be suspected in a patient with any asymmetric polyarticular symptoms of the lower extremity, especially if one of the areas of involvement is the calcaneus.

Significant swelling of a digit can cause a sausage toe[104,236] (Fig. 16–49). Because it is not seen exclusively in Reiter's syndrome, other diagnoses to be considered with a sausage toe are cellulitis, trauma, osteomyelitis, and psoriasis. Chand and Johnson[42] noted a sausage toe in 26% of patients with Reiter's syndrome, and Gold and Bassett[116] reported frequent involvement of the interphalangeal joint.

Although radiographic findings are not present in up to one third of patients, soft tissue swelling is often demonstrated early in the disease process, similar to rheumatoid arthritis, psoriasis, and ankylosing spondylitis. The radiographic pattern can demonstrate concomitant joint involvement of the heels, sacroiliac joints, ankle, and tarsus.[308] In the presence of calcaneal pain, fluffy periostitis, or exuberant new periosteal bone formation can occur at the insertion of the plantar fascia or Achilles tendon. Intraarticular and extraarticular joint erosion also may be noted, especially in the area of the interphalangeal and MTP joints. Guerra and Resnick[126] reported large, painful calcaneal spurs occurring with Reiter's syndrome.

Bony ankylosis and severe joint destruction are uncommon, but over time, radiographic findings can mimic psoriasis, rheumatoid arthritis, and ankylosing spondylitis.

Treatment

Treatment may be unnecessary because in many cases the disease is self-limited. Spontaneous resolution can occur, although symptoms in some patients can linger chronically.[102] Nonsurgical treatment includes the occasional judicious use of an intraarticular corticosteroid injection and short periods of NSAID administration. Fan and Yu[92] have suggested a 3-month course of tetracycline to reduce the chronicity and severity of the arthritis. Calcaneal pain may be treated with immobilization, viscoelastic heel pads or heel lifts, and dorsiflexion night splints (see Chapter 12).

HIV, AIDS, Reiter's Syndrome, and Inflammatory Arthropathy

Seronegative arthritides (Reiter's syndrome, psoriatic arthritis, unclassified arthritic disorders with enthesopathy) may be associated with human immunodeficiency virus (HIV) infection and acquired immunodeficiency syndrome (AIDS).[177,315,361] The foot and ankle are often involved, and occasionally the enthesopathy has a fulminant course with severe limitation of ambulatory capacity. Foot and ankle involvement is reported to involve one to four sites, including the Achilles tendon (85%), MTP joint (54%), subtalar joint (23%), and the phalanges (dactylitis) (13%).[361] Radiographic changes are identical to those seen in psoriatic arthritis, with osteolysis and pencil-in-cup deformities. Inflammation, joint ankylosis, osteolysis, and periarticular erosive changes can result from severity, persistence, and recurrence of the enthesopathy.

According to Espinoza et al,[87] some patients with subclinical HIV infection and concomitant Reiter's syndrome are treated with an immunosuppressive agent (e.g., methotrexate) and then develop Kaposi's sarcoma, fulminant AIDS, or an opportunistic infection (e.g., *Pneumocystis jiroveci* pneumonia). In some patients, depletion of circulating CD4+ lymphocytes is noted at initial presentation of arthritis. Often the response to NSAIDs is impressive, although a small percentage of patients remain refractory to pharmacologic treatment.

Systemic Lupus Erythematosus

Presentation, Etiology, and Incidence

Systemic lupus erythematosus (SLE) is an autoimmune disease in which autoantibodies are directed

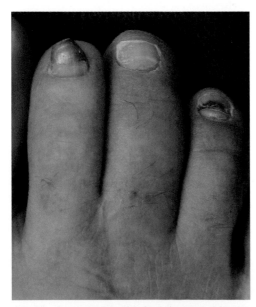

Figure 16–49 Sausage toe (third toe here) occurs in approximately one fourth of patients with psoriatic arthritis.

against components of the cell nucleus. Its onset typically is in the second or third decade of life, and it is more common in blacks and women than men (8:1). The estimated incidence is 1 in 2000 in the general population.[287] Although the cause is not known, an immune complex deposition (immunoglobulins M, G, and A) occurs in the small arteries and arterioles. Osteonecrosis can occur in 5% to 8% of patients when disease duration is 5 years or longer. SLE can also be induced by pharmacologic agents such as antibiotics, antiarrhythmics, antihypertensives, anticonvulsants, and antithyroid medications. The deposition of immune complexes in vessel walls can result not only in vasculitis but also in osteonecrosis and arthritis. Vasculitis can lead to periungual hemorrhages and punched-out cutaneous lesions forming leg ulcers. SLE is a classic autoimmune disease with multisystem involvement.

The clinical course is variable and may be insidious or fulminant in onset. The patient can also experience repeated episodes of febrile illness, weight loss, severe fatigue, joint pain, and swelling, which can occur for months before other symptoms develop. Arthralgia and joint deformity occur because of soft tissue laxity, but rarely does bone deformity result. Arthritis and arthralgia are seen in 95% of SLE patients.[287] Involvement of the hands and feet is common. The foot may be the initial site of onset and the only site of symptoms.

Raynaud's disease is noted in 15% of SLE patients.[15] Dermatologic changes include hyperkeratosis and atrophy of the epidermis. Peripheral neuropathy might also be noted. Musculoskeletal symptoms include myalgia secondary to myositis.

Any four of the following 11 criteria can indicate a diagnosis of SLE: macular rash, discoid rash, photosensitivity, oral ulcers, arthritis, serositis, renal disorders, neurologic disorders, hematologic disorders, immunologic disorders, and positive test for antinuclear antibody (ANA).[287]

Laboratory abnormalities associated with SLE include anemia and thrombocytopenia. A positive lupus erythematosus cell test occurs in 60% to 80% of patients,[15] and a positive test for ANAs is present in 99%. One fifth of patients with SLE have a positive rheumatoid factor.[287]

On radiographic evaluation the characteristic difference between SLE and rheumatoid arthritis is that although both patients experience joint pain, no erosive arthropathy is associated with SLE. However, SLE is noted as a deforming arthropathy and is a multisystem disease that can lead to myositis, polyarthritis, spontaneous tendon rupture, osteonecrosis, septic arthritis, soft-tissue calcification, and osteomyelitis.[203] Osteoporosis[325] may be present without articular erosion. Joint space narrowing can occur, as well as soft tissue calcifications. (Soft tissue calcifications can also be seen with hyperthyroidism, scleroderma, and dermatomyositis.) Periarticular cystic changes occur in 50% of patients, as does resorption of the distal tufts of the distal phalanges.[15] With repeated synovitis, subluxation, eventual dislocation, and deviation can occur in joints of the forefoot, but this joint laxity typically is painless without swelling, synovitis, or restricted motion.

Treatment

Pharmacologic therapy is the mainstay of SLE treatment. Salicylates, NSAIDs, corticosteroids, cytotoxic drugs, and antimalarial medications may be used. Rest during the active phases of the disease can decrease symptoms. Immobilization or support with orthoses and casting may be necessary. Although surgery is performed infrequently for SLE, with progressive subluxation and dislocation, arthroplasty and fusion techniques similar to those used in the treatment of rheumatoid forefoot and hindfoot deformities may be necessary. Beilstein and Hawkins[15] recommend avoiding penicillin analogues at surgery because of possible drug-induced lupus syndrome.

Ankylosing Spondylitis
Presentation and Etiology

Ankylosing spondylitis is an inflammatory arthropathy affecting the axial skeleton and peripheral joints. The sacroiliac joints are often involved. Ankylosing spondylitis is characterized by onset in the second and third decades of life, typically in the male population (male-to-female ratio, 4:1). There appears to be a strong familial tendency.[363]

Foot and ankle symptoms are uncommon,[116,325] and lower extremity symptoms infrequently lead to an initial diagnosis of ankylosing spondylitis, because spine and sacroiliac symptoms are more common and more severe. Sacroiliitis and asymmetric involvement of the heel and foot, however, can herald the onset of ankylosing spondylitis. The forefoot is eventually involved in 60% of patients with chronic ankylosing spondylitis.[116] The MTP joints are affected in a way similar to that of rheumatoid arthritis, but because of less significant synovitis, less periarticular osteoporosis is present, which can help to differentiate spondylitis from rheumatoid arthritis. The overwhelming involvement of the axial skeleton with ankylosing spondylitis can make foot and ankle symptoms seem relatively insignificant. Enthesopathy is a characteristic feature of seronegative spondyloarthropathies such as ankylosing spondylitis, and radiographic changes in the calcaneus are indistinguishable from those of Reiter's syndrome.[202]

Ankylosing spondylitis may be confused with *diffuse idiopathic skeletal hyperostosis* (DISH) syndrome. DISH syndrome occurs in older and middle-aged men and is characterized by stiffness of the spine and peripheral hyperostosis. It is not associated with sacroiliitis or a positive HLA-B27. The foot is often a site of ossification in DISH syndrome because of the multiple sites of ligament, tendon, and fascial attachments. More than 70% of DISH patients have radiologic abnormalities of the foot.[111] Posterior calcaneal spurring is common. Spurs are often large, vary in shape, may be multiple and bilateral, and are not associated with underlying bone erosion or sclerosis. The sesamoid bones are often involved. Treatment of DISH parallels that of degenerative arthritis, with frequent use of NSAIDs. Surgery is rarely necessary but may be done for significant bone enlargements or excision of prominent exostoses (Fig. 16–50). Radiographs of the spine can show a characteristic flowing hyperostosis or candle wax calcification adjacent to several vertebral segments.[111] In the juvenile patient, Levi et al[202] reported frequent hindfoot involvement and spontaneous arthrodesis of the tarsometatarsal joints.

Calcaneal pain at the plantar aponeurosis or the Achilles tendon insertion sites (Fig. 16–51) is often indistinguishable from Reiter's syndrome.

A strong association exists between HLA-B27 and ankylosing spondylitis.[299] Bluestone[29] reported a positive HLA-B27 in 75% to 100% of patients, although this test can be positive with Reiter's syndrome and psoriatic arthritis as well.[279] Wollheim[363] reported that 90% of patients with ankylosing spondylitis test positive for HLA-B27. Positive tests are noted more often in white and Asian populations, and the incidence is lower in the black population.

Back pain and spine stiffness might not occur until 4 to 6 months after onset of other symptoms. MTP joint involvement is similar to that of rheumatoid arthritis, but the synovitis is often less intense. Sub-

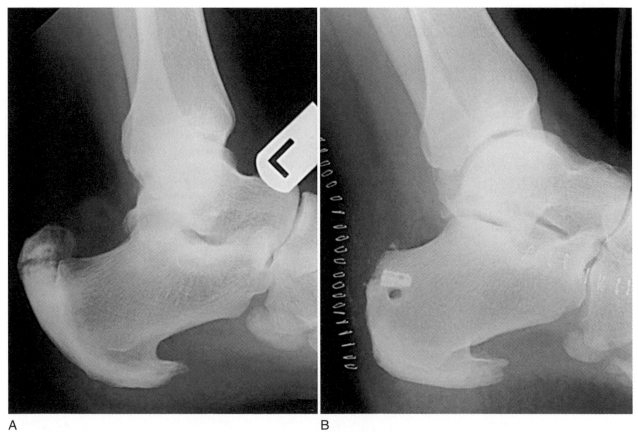

A   B

Figure 16–50   A, Large bone spurs occurring at the plantar fascia insertion and the Achilles tendon insertion associated with diffuse idiopathic skeletal hyperostosis (DISH) syndrome. Note fracture of the dorsal spur. **B,** After resection of a painful fractured spur and reinsertion of the Achilles tendon with a flexor hallucis longus tendon augmentation transfer.

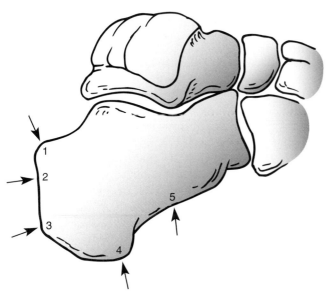

Figure 16–51 Common areas of enthesopathy associated with inflammatory arthritis. *1*, Superior aspect of calcaneus. *2* and *3*, Achilles tendon insertion. *4*, Plantar fascia insertion. *5*, Plantar aspect of calcaneus.

chondral sclerosis is more evident than osteoporosis, which can help to differentiate ankylosing spondylitis from rheumatoid arthritis. A more chronic inflammatory process can lead to lesser MTP joint deformities resembling rheumatoid arthritis.

Radiographic findings include periostitis and new bone formation, which can result in joint capsule ossification or bone ankylosis. A radiographic index to assess tarsal involvement in patients with possible spondyloarthropathy has shown that oblique and lateral radiographic views of the foot provide the most useful information in determining the diagnosis.[262] Bony proliferation or "whiskering" often occurs adjacent to areas of osseous erosion and is pathognomonic of ankylosing spondylitis.[126,325] Periostitis and erosions in the calcaneus along the plantar surface and in the area of Achilles tendon insertion are virtually indistinguishable from psoriasis and Reiter's syndrome (Fig. 16–51).

Treatment

Pharmacologic treatment of ankylosing spondylitis involves NSAIDs and corticosteroids. Surgery is uncommon, but when it is necessary, forefoot reconstruction techniques are similar to those used for rheumatoid arthritis.

MISCELLANEOUS ARTHROPATHIES OF THE FOOT AND ANKLE

Lyme Disease

Presentation and Etiology

First described in 1977 after the investigation of symptoms of arthropathy in young children living near Lyme, Connecticut, this disease is now recognized in endemic areas in the Northeastern, Northern Midwest, and Pacific Northwest United States. Lyme disease is the most common arthropod-borne infectious disease diagnosed in the United States.[77,90] Although Lyme disease has been diagnosed in almost every state, almost 50% of the cases have been reported in New York (state) alone.[356] Eighteen states with endemic populations of the vectors *Ixodes dammini* and *Ixodes pacificus* have contributed greater than 90% of the reported cases.[77] In 1996 more than 16,000 cases of Lyme disease were reported in the lower 48 states, representing a 41% increase from 1995.[6]

Lyme disease is caused by a tick bite from the *Ixodes* species that is infected by a spirochete, *Borrelia burgdorferi*. Deer support the adult population of the *Ixodes* ticks that transmit the disease. Mice serve as the host of immature stages of the tick and as the primary reservoir of the spirochete. Infected deer transmit the tick to humans, who then contract Lyme disease from the spirochete. The tick is small, and often the infectious bite is not appreciated. The spirochete infection manifests in stages similar to syphilis, with multisystem involvement.

A skin rash, fever, and general malaise may be subclinical, and the disease can progress quietly to a tertiary phase with neurologic, cardiac, and musculoskeletal involvement. Erythema chronicum migrans (ECM), the characteristic rash, is an erythematous macular skin lesion that appears anywhere from 3 days to a month after the tick bite[321,322] (Fig. 16–52). The rash is noted to have expanding edges that are characterized by a central clearing over time. It can grow to as large as 30 cm or more. An ECM rash is not recognized in approximately one third of patients with Lyme disease.[287]

Although many patients do not recall a tick bite because of the tick's small size,[90] a rash or flulike illness during the summer months[199] can indicate Lyme disease. Joint involvement may be the initial symptom and is noted by approximately one third of those infected. Lyme arthritis usually occurs 3 to 4 weeks after the onset of the skin lesion.

In *stage I* a rash occurs, and symptoms are characterized by a nonspecific flulike condition.[320] *Stage II* occurs days to weeks later. The neurologic and cardiac

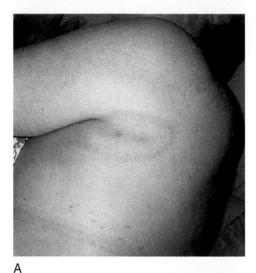

A

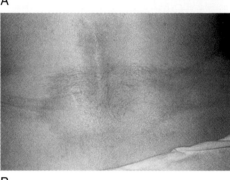

B

Figure 16–52 Characteristic erythema chronicum migrans (ECM) rash associated with Lyme disease. **A,** Axilla. **B,** Lumbar region.

manifestations include atrioventricular block, pericarditis, congestive heart failure, neuritis, peripheral neuropathy, and aseptic meningitis.[198] Sixty percent of patients develop asymptomatic involvement of large joints,[169] with the knee being most often involved. Joint effusions are typically large and out of proportion to a patient's complaints.[198]

Stage III (tertiary presentation) of Lyme disease with musculoskeletal involvement is characterized by arthropathy and tendinitis. Faller et al[90] reported on 10 patients with subtalar and first MTP joint pain, tendinitis, heel pain syndrome, and dysesthesias on the plantar aspect of the foot. Symptoms were present for 6 weeks to 6 years after the alleged infections, and symptoms in many patients had been misdiagnosed and treated with other modalities. Lyme disease in its tertiary stage can be confused with many other problems, including metatarsalgia and interdigital neuroma. Dennis[77] and Lawrence[198] note that there are many similarities between Lyme disease and syphilis. Lyme disease has been called "the great imitator" because it is difficult to diagnose clinically and is often

confused with other diagnoses, including septic arthritis, juvenile arthritis in younger patients, or inflammatory arthritis in older patients. A high level of suspicion is necessary to make the correct diagnosis, which is confirmed by laboratory tests.

Lawson and Steere[199] reported stage III developing within an average of 5 months after a tick bite (range, 1 to 32 months). If untreated initially, more than half the patients develop musculoskeletal symptoms within 2 years. Stage III is characterized by transient joint symptoms, although they are usually recurrent. Over time, recurrences tend to occur less often and attacks tend to be shorter.[198] Chronic arthritis develops in 10% of patients with Lyme disease,[198] and approximately 60% of untreated patients develop an intermittent arthritis.[170] Findings consistent with inflammatory arthritis are typical of the chronic stages of Lyme disease. Prolonged joint synovitis can lead to juxtaarticular osteoporosis, chondrolysis, and cortical or marginal erosions. With chronic arthritis, chondrolysis, subchondral sclerosis, juxtaarticular osteoporosis, bone erosion, and osteophyte formation can occur.[189]

Lyme disease is diagnosed by serologic confirmation on indirect fluorescent antibody tests or enzyme-linked immunosorbent assay (ELISA).[198,356] However, wide variation exists in test results, and sensitivity can vary from laboratory to laboratory. The erythrocyte sedimentation rate is often elevated with the disease process.

Treatment

Antibiotic treatment is preferred regardless of the stage of infection. Conventional antibiotic treatment for 4 to 6 weeks is associated with clinical improvement of symptoms in most patients and with a decrease in antibody titers.[90] Early diagnosis and treatment can limit symptoms. A high index of suspicion for patients in endemic areas or who have traveled in endemic areas aids in the early diagnosis and the institution of antibiotic treatment.

For stage I disease, typical treatment is doxycycline (100 mg three times a day) or amoxicillin (500 to 1000 mg four times a day) for 2 to 3 weeks[7,198] (Table 16–1). NSAIDs may be of some benefit in treating joint symptoms.[320]

Fibromyalgia

The term *fibromyalgia* was coined by Hench[146] in 1976 to describe generalized musculoskeletal pain associated with a large number of localized areas that were tender to palpation. Fatigue and sleep disorders were associated with the condition as well.[141] Localized areas of tenderness (tender points) are reproducible

TABLE 16-1

Treatment of Lyme Disease

Stage	Serology	Laboratory Data	Antibiotic Regimen*
I	Usually negative	Sedimentation rate 40-60 mL/h	Doxycycline 100 mg bid or tid × 2-3 wk Amoxicillin 500-1000 mg qid × 2-3 wk
II	Usually positive		Ceftriaxone 2 g/day × 2 wk Penicillin G 20 million U qd/6 doses × 3 wk
III	Usually positive		Ceftriaxone 2 g qd × 2 wk Penicillin G 20 million U qd/6 doses × 3 wk

*Erythromycin, 250-500 mg qid for 2 to 3 weeks, may be given to patients with allergies to penicillin or cephalosporins; however, this treatment might not be as effective.
Modified from Lawrence S: *Orthopaedics* 15:1331-1335, 1992.

on repeated examination[362] (Table 16-2), and 11 of 18 positive points must be elicited to diagnose fibromyalgia.

Sleep disorders include insomnia, difficulty remaining asleep, or wakening unrefreshed after sleeping.[238] Laboratory tests and radiographic evaluation do not play a role in the diagnosis of fibromyalgia but are important in ruling out other disorders, such as hypothyroidism, polymyalgia rheumatica, rheumatoid arthritis, polymyositis, SLE, metabolic myopathy, metastatic cancer, neurosis, and chronic fatigue syndrome.[18,146] Goldenberg[117] has estimated that 3 to 6 million Americans carry the diagnosis of fibromyalgia, a majority being women. The diagnosis is one of exclusion.

Fibromyalgia is unresponsive to steroids and NSAIDs alike.[18] Bennett[19] has recommended aerobic exercise as therapeutic, although fatigue and pain tend to restrict activity. Tricyclic antidepressants may be

helpful, as is the supportive concern of the treating physician. Many patients are relieved to receive a "diagnosis," but this obviously does not treat the symptoms. Fibromyalgia is described as a *pain syndrome* and *is not* an arthritic condition. The treating physician must differentiate it from the pain of an underlying arthritic condition.

Other symptoms often associated with fibromyalgia include Raynaud's phenomenon, headache, morning stiffness, paresthesias, depression, and anxiety.

Recognition of fibromyalgia as an entity is important because the treating physician should include it in the differential diagnosis of metatarsalgia and other areas of pain and discomfort in the foot. Although the presence of this chronic pain syndrome in other areas does not preclude surgical intervention in the area of the foot and ankle, it is unlikely that generalized foot and ankle discomfort will be relieved by surgical intervention. A frank preoperative discussion with the patient with fibromyalgia in whom foot and ankle surgery is contemplated is important regarding patient expectations and the possibility of continued pain after surgery.

Juvenile Arthritis

Foot and ankle problems are common in patients with juvenile rheumatoid arthritis (JRA) and psoriatic arthritis (JPA). Most of the problems encountered with these patients can be treated nonoperatively. In a descriptive study by Spraul and Koenning[319] that evaluated JRA patients, the authors found all but 9 of 144 children had foot problems. The deformities included pronated hindfoot (73%), midfoot deformity (72%), and splayfoot (36%); 35% had ankle limitation in motion. Subjects with polyarticular disease had a higher incidence of hallux valgus and lesser toe deformity, and pauciarticular subjects had more pronation deformity of the forefoot. Ankle joint stiffness was related to the duration of disease but not the

TABLE 16-2

Tender Points Associated with Fibromyalgia

Location*	Tender Points
Knee	Medial fat pad proximal to joint line
Greater trochanter	Lateral hip region
Gluteal region	Upper outer aspect of buttocks
Lateral epicondyle	Slightly distal to epicondyle
Costochondral junction	Second costochondral junction
Supraspinatus muscle	Proximal medial border of scapular spine
Trapezius muscle	Upper border of trapezius
Lower cervical region	C5-C7 region
Occiput	Suboccipital muscle insertion

*Each location can have bilateral involvement, for a total of 18 specific areas.
Adapted from Wolfe F, Smythe H, Yunus M, et al: *Arthritis Rheum* 33:160, 1990. Copyright American College of Rheumatology.

subtype of arthritis. The pattern of joint involvement at disease onset can distinguish juvenile psoriatic and rheumatoid arthritis. Small joint disease (MTP, IP, and wrist or MCP joints) was more common with oligoarticular juvenile psoriatic arthritis compared with pauciarticular juvenile rheumatoid arthritis.[154] Furthermore, nearly 50% of patients with juvenile psoriatic arthritis progress over time from oligoarticular to polyarticular arthritis and commonly present with MTP, DIP joint, second toe dactylitis, and chronic anterior uveitis.[283]

Degenerative Joint Disease

Degenerative arthritis of the joints of the foot and ankle typically occurs in middle-aged and older patients, but it can occur in younger persons after osteochondral injuries or trauma. Factors that can affect the onset and progression of arthritis include physical activity, occupation, and obesity, although many cases of degenerative arthritis, such as in the first metatarsophalangeal (MTP) joint and first metatarsocuneiform (MTC) joint, are not associated with any specific known injury.

Although the cause of degenerative joint disease is unknown, biochemical and histologic changes from both an intraarticular and an extraarticular standpoint can lead to distortion of the joint surface. As the degenerative process progresses, changes in the anatomic structure of the joint result in restricted range of motion and loss of function. This in turn can place abnormal stresses on adjacent joints, which can lead to an abnormal gait and discomfort.

The history elicited from a patient with degenerative arthritis varies depending on the number and location of joints involved. Typically, symptoms are aggravated by walking, standing, or physical activity and decrease with rest. As the day progresses, symptoms either appear or become progressively more severe.

Physical examination often demonstrates a tender, swollen joint with restricted motion. Crepitation may be present, and with forced motion, pain may be elicited. Bone proliferation around the margin of the affected joint may be obvious to palpation and can cause a superficial bursitis or skin ulceration.

Radiographic evaluation often demonstrates a decreased joint space or chondrolysis, sclerosis in the periarticular region, subchondral cyst formation, and proliferative bone formation at the periphery of the joint. Evidence of joint inflammation is uncommon with osteoarthritis, and thus periarticular osteoporosis rarely occurs. Chondrolysis of articular cartilage may be evidenced by asymmetric joint space narrowing. Intraarticular loose bodies may be present as well.

Conservative treatment methods often can significantly reduce symptoms. NSAIDs may be efficacious, and the occasional judicious use of an intraarticular steroid injection can relieve symptoms. Pharmacologic agents can often reduce symptoms of inflammation and synovitis.

Weight reduction, decreased activity, and occasional joint immobilization can reduce symptoms. Reduced athletic activity or cross-training may be of benefit (e.g., joggers may bike or swim; standing jobs may be supplemented by more sedentary occupations).

Over-the-counter footwear or prescription footwear can reduce symptoms over bony prominences.[70] Orthoses can support unstable areas and areas with rigid deformities. Semiflexible orthoses appear to be better tolerated than rigid orthoses in treating degenerative joint disease of the hindfoot and midfoot. Orthoses that may be considered include ankle–foot orthoses (AFOs) for ankle, hindfoot, and midtarsal deformities; rocker-bottom shoe modifications for decreased ankle and hindfoot motion; molded-leather ankle braces for hindfoot arthritis; and custom-made and prefabricated orthoses for midfoot and forefoot problems.

The primary indication for surgery for degenerative arthritis of the foot and ankle is intractable pain or deformity that is not relieved with local or systemic pharmacologic treatment or biomechanical aids such as immobilization or bracing. Surgical techniques vary from arthrodesis to excisional arthroplasty to osteotomy. Joint implants in general have been disappointing in the forefoot, hindfoot, and ankle (see later discussion of first MTP implants).

DEGENERATIVE ARTHRITIS OF THE INTERPHALANGEAL JOINT

Degenerative arthritis of the interphalangeal joint of the hallux can result from trauma, after arthrodesis of the MTP joint,[99] or from inflammatory arthritis (rheumatoid arthritis, psoriatic arthritis, Reiter's syndrome, gout). Clawing of the toe can occur as a result of contracture of the flexor hallucis longus tendon and can lead to a fixed plantar flexion deformity.

Conservative treatment options include an extradepth shoe, a foam sleeve that pads both the tip of the toe and the dorsal interphalangeal (DIP) joint region, or an excavated insole to decrease pressure at the tip of the hallux. With a fixed contracture or intractable interphalangeal joint pain, arthrodesis of the interphalangeal joint of the hallux is indicated.

The arthrodesis is performed through a dorsal L-shaped or elliptical incision. The joint surface is excised and the arthrodesis fixed with a small-fragment cancellous screw inserted at the tip of the hallux (Fig.

16–53A to C). One or two Kirschner wires or Stein-mann pins may be added to control rotation.[306] Shives and Johnson[307] reported an overall pseudarthrosis rate of 44% with the use of only crossed Kirschner wires for interphalangeal joint fusion. With a compression arthrodesis technique, the pseudarthrosis rate was reduced to 10% (Fig. 16–53D to F; video clip 32).

Degenerative arthritis of the interphalangeal joints of the lesser toes can occur after trauma but also may be associated with Freiberg's infraction (Fig. 16–54). Degenerative arthritis of the interphalangeal joints of the lesser toes may be treated with arthrodesis or exci-sional arthroplasty (see Chapter 7 for treatment of hammer toe deformities).

HALLUX RIGIDUS

Definition

The term *hallux rigidus* describes a painful condition of the MTP joint of the great toe characterized by restricted motion (mainly dorsiflexion) and prolifera-tive periarticular bone formation. It was initially reported in 1887 by Davies-Colley,[75] who described a plantar-flexed position of the proximal phalanx in relationship to the first metatarsal head and proposed the name "hallux flexus." A few months later, Cotter-ill[53] reported on the same condition but coined the term "hallux rigidus." Other terms, such as hallux limitus, dorsal bunion, hallux dolorosus, hallux malleus, and metatarsus primus elevatus, have been advocated.[180] The terms *hallux rigidus* and *hallux limitus* are used interchangeably, although, to some, *hallux limitus* is distinguished by a decrease in dorsiflexion, whereas hallux rigidus describes an absence of motion.[112] DuVries[84] in 1959 and Moberg[241] observed that other than hallux valgus, hallux rigidus is the most common condition to affect the first MTP joint and may be even more disabling than hallux valgus because of the limitations on ambulation that occur in more severe cases. Gould et al[121] stated that 1 in 40 patients older than 50 years develop hallux rigidus.

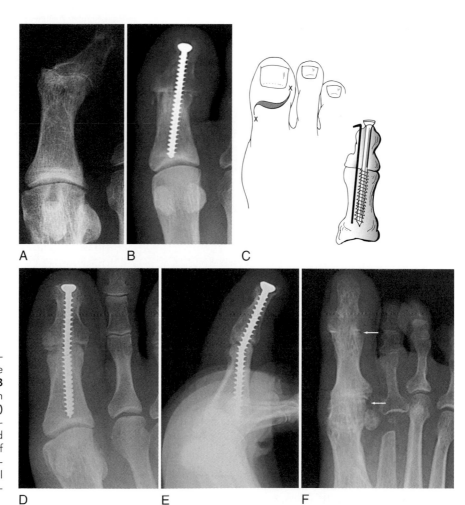

Figure 16–53   A, Preoperative radio-graph demonstrates degenerative arthritis of interphalangeal joint. **B** and **C,** Arthrodesis after compression screw fixation. Anteroposterior **(D)** and lateral **(E)** radiographs demon-strate failure of fixation and pseudoarthrosis after arthrodesis of the interphalangeal joint. **F,** Success-ful fusion of metatarsophalangeal and interphalangeal joint for degen-erative arthritis.

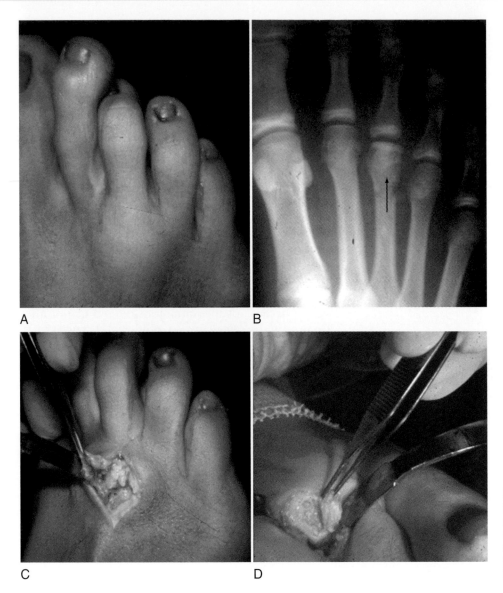

A   B   C   D

Figure 16–54 Freiberg's infraction. Clinical photo **(A)** and radiograph **(B)** showing huge osteophyte formation *(arrow)* at the third metatarsophalangeal joint. **C,** Operative exposure. **D,** Removal of distal free fragment.

Incidence

Hallux rigidus has been described in two distinct age groups by Nilsonne[256] and others: the adolescent and the adult. Nilsonne[256] hypothesized that hallux rigidus in the adolescent was a primary deformity, whereas in the adult, hallux rigidus was a secondary deformity resulting from the development of degenerative arthritis. Bingold and Collins[27] suggested that the two entities were merely a continuum of the same degenerative process. Goodfellow[118] reported on three patients who demonstrated classic findings of osteochondritis dissecans of the metatarsal articular surface, and McMaster[231] described seven patients with similar findings. Coughlin and Shurnas[65] found no evidence to support a requirement for a distinction based on age.

Although Gould[120] and Nilsonne[256] suggested that hallux rigidus typically is characterized by bilateral involvement, studies reporting results of surgery have emphasized mainly unilateral involvement. However, if follow-up is continued for a long enough period, 80% or more of patients can be expected to have bilateral symptoms.[65]

Gould[120] reported a higher male involvement in those over age 30 with complaints of hallux rigidus, but in those undergoing surgical repair, most studies have reported an overwhelmingly higher incidence of female involvement.*

Bonney and MacNab[30] also noted that in those with onset in teenage years, there was a 50% incidence of a family history. Coughlin and Shurnas[65] found in their series of patients with hallux rigidus that nearly 95%

---

*References 30, 63, 65, 80, 213, and 256.

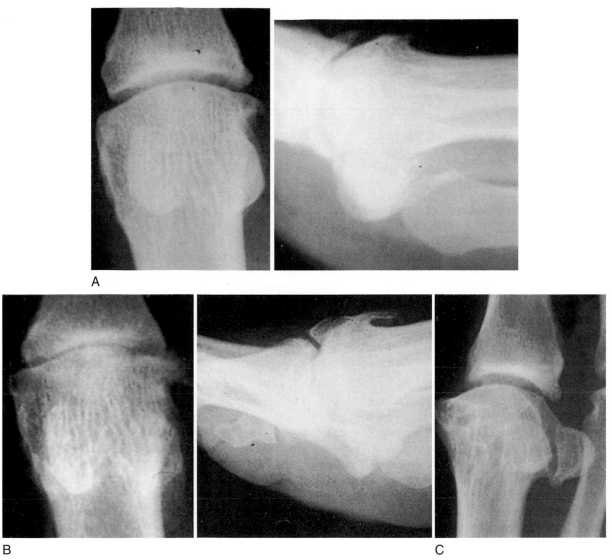

Figure 16–55 **A,** Anteroposterior (AP) and lateral radiographs demonstrate grade 1 hallux rigidus deformity. **B,** Over 10 years, significant progression of disease occurred to a grade 2 hallux rigidus deformity. **C,** Oblique radiograph demonstrates adequate joint space present although the AP radiograph did not show an adequate joint space because of overhanging.

of patients with a positive family history of great toe problems had bilateral hallux rigidus and that nearly 80% of all patients with hallux rigidus had a positive family history.

Signs and Symptoms

Although initially hallux rigidus is characterized by pain, swelling, and MTP synovitis, restricted dorsiflexion is a classic finding. As the degenerative process proceeds, proliferation of bony osteophytes on the dorsal and dorsolateral aspect of the first metatarsal head develop, creating a prominent bony ledge against which the proximal phalanx abuts (Fig. 16–55A). A significant amount of new bone rarely forms along the medial border of the first

MTP joint. Hallux valgus is uncommon with hallux rigidus.

With time and further osteophyte formation, increased bulk around the MTP joint can lead to significant discomfort with constricting footwear (Fig. 16–55B). However, the joint space often remains reasonably preserved despite the narrowed appearance on the anteroposterior (AP) view as verified on the oblique radiograph (Fig. 16–55C). With enlargement of the dorsal exostosis, the proximal phalanx can become positioned in plantar flexion with limitation of dorsiflexion, the condition for which the term *hallux flexus* was coined. With severe deformity, almost complete bony ankylosis can occur.

In adults with hallux rigidus the basic pathologic entity is that of degenerative arthritis.[30] Mann and

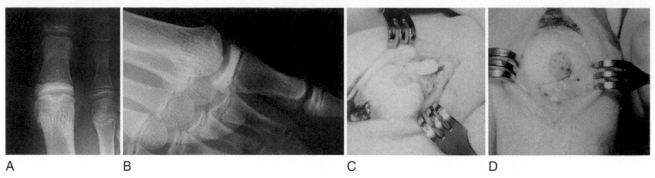

A   B   C   D

Figure 16–56 **A** and **B,** Radiographs demonstrate juvenile hallux rigidus secondary to osteochondral defect of the metatarsal head. **C** and **D,** Intraoperative photos demonstrate osteochondral lesion. Loose fragment has been removed. The lesion was debrided and its base was drilled.

Clanton[213] noted that with increasing age, increasing degenerative arthritis occurs. The classic location of the cartilage loss is on the dorsal half to two thirds of the metatarsal head,[143,241] often at a site between the apex of the articular surface and the dorsal margin of the proximal phalanx.

Etiology

The cause of hallux rigidus or hallux limitus has not been determined, although several predisposing factors have been cited. The most common cause cited is trauma, which can occur as a single episode such as an intraarticular fracture or crush injury, but hallux rigidus can occur with repetitive microtrauma as well. In a patient who sustains an acute injury to the MTP joint, forced hyperextension[56] or forced plantar flexion[48] can create compressive forces through jamming of the toe, with development of an acute chondral or osteochondral injury. What may begin as an acute sprain or turf toe can evolve into chronic discomfort.

An osseous injury can be diagnosed with radiographs, but with a cartilaginous injury, a diagnosis can only be made by physical examination (possibly with newer MRI techniques) and a high clinical index of suspicion of an intraarticular injury (Fig. 16–56A-D). A clear traumatic episode is most likely the cause of unilateral hallux rigidus based on long-term follow-up.[65] In the adolescent patient with hallux rigidus, an osteochondral defect is often identified on radiographic examination or can be verified by MRI.[118,134,182,231,300]

Other suggested causes of hallux rigidus include a congenital flattened or squared metatarsal head,[84] a long first metatarsal, a short first metatarsal,[80,156,216] tight intrinsic muscles,[82] pes planus or hindfoot pronation, and a congruent MTP joint[84,112] (Fig. 16–57).

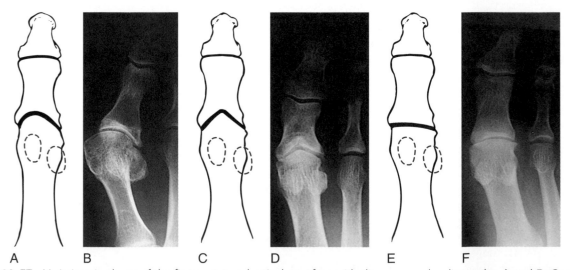

A   B   C   D   E   F

Figure 16–57 Variations in shape of the first metatarsal articular surface with diagrams and radiographs. **A** and **B,** Oval shape can allow valgus position to occur. Chevron surface (**C** and **D**) and flat surface (**E** and **F**) resist lateral pressure on the hallux. Although hallux valgus is uncommon, traumatic osteoarthritis can develop, resulting in hallux rigidus.

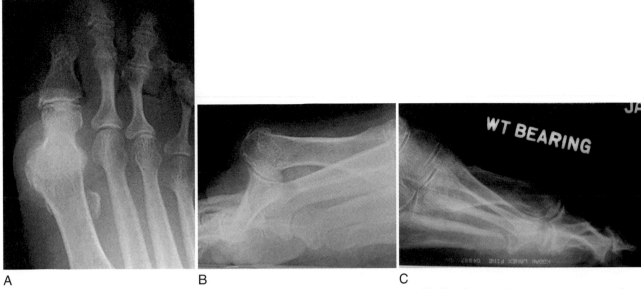

Figure 16–58 Anteroposterior **(A)** and lateral **(B)** radiographs of a severe case of hallux flexus with metatarsus primus elevatus. **C,** Severe postsurgical elevatus.

Although investigators have hypothesized that these factors play a major role in the development of hallux rigidus, other than for osteochondritis, the only documented factors associated with the cause of hallux rigidus are a flat or chevron shaped joint, hallux valgus interphalangeus, metatarsus adductus, bilaterality in those with a positive family history, trauma in unilateral cases, and female gender.[65,66] There have been no proven associations with first ray mobility, metatarsal length, Achilles or gastrocnemius contracture, any type of abnormal foot posture, hallux valgus, adolescent onset, footwear, occupation, or metatarsus primus elevatus.[65,66]

One of the more controversial areas regarding etiology is the condition known as *metatarsus primus elevatus* (Fig. 16–58), which describes a dorsal elevation of the first metatarsal in relationship to the lesser metatarsals. Although Lambrinudi[193] in 1938 and Jack[156] in 1940 initially called attention to hyperextension of the first ray, Root et al[291] advanced a popularly accepted concept that hypermobility of the first ray "is the most frequent cause of hallux limitus." Numerous other authors have supported the notion that an elevated first metatarsal is causally related to hallux rigidus or hallux limitus, but others[153,233] dispute the relevance of this claim.

Bingold and Collins[27] and others[80,291] have distinguished between a structural (fixed) and a functional (flexible) elevation of the first metatarsal. Both conditions are believed to lead to restricted dorsiflexion of the first MTP joint, but with a flexible deformity, range of motion is decreased only with weight bearing. A fixed elevation of the first metatarsal is present whether the foot is weight bearing or not. (Examples of a fixed metatarsus primus elevatus deformity are a dorsiflexed malunion of a first metatarsal osteotomy or fracture; a flexible elevation might occur with posterior tibial tendon insufficiency, muscle weakness, spasticity, or paralysis.)

Elevation can occur anywhere along the axis of the first ray (MTC, cuneiform–navicular, or talonavicular joint). As the first metatarsal elevates, the hallux impacts or jams into the dorsal metatarsal articular surface, leading initially to limited or restricted dorsiflexion and eventually to injury to the metatarsal articular surface.[80,291]

Smith[312] and others[39,94,95,291] have implicated subtalar joint pronation as the cause of first ray hypermobility. Some investigators[153,233] have questioned the frequency and significance of metatarsus primus elevatus in relationship to hallux rigidus, and we believe it occurs less than 5% of the time in association with hallux rigidus.

Recent studies[68] have evaluated the notion of an elevated first ray in patients with hallux rigidus and demonstrated when elevation was present, it was a secondary phenomenon most likely due to a malfunctioning first MTP joint. Elevatus was reduced substantially following cheilectomy or interposition arthroplasty and could be corrected preoperatively or postoperatively to neutral with a dorsiflexion stress test on the first MTP joint. If the first MTP joint was arthrodesed, then postoperative elevation was corrected to almost neutral. This reduction in elevatus was associated with a decrease in first ray mobility.[65,66] Elevatus is most commonly a secondary change with hallux rigidus, and not a primary cause. It is directly related to the severity of the disease and the restriction of MTP joint motion.

Reporting on nine patients, Kessel and Bonney[182] noted two adults with acquired metatarsus primus elevatus after surgery and one patient who developed an elevated first metatarsal after developing MTP joint synovitis. Whether the primary cause was hallux rigidus or metatarsus primus elevatus was not clear.

From an anatomic standpoint, Meyer et al[233] have stressed that the abnormal measurements associated with metatarsus primus elevatus can result from a combination of the increased dorsoplantar diameter of the first metatarsal, the sesamoid mechanism, and the plantar soft tissue structures, which all tend either to elevate the first metatarsal or to influence the measurement of first metatarsal elevation. Coughlin and Jones[62] found that selected release of the plantar soft tissue attachments of the first MTP joint significantly increased measured first ray mobility. Bonney and MacNab[30] and Jack[156] reported that many of their patients had an elevated first ray, but no control groups were included in these studies to suggest a relationship between hallux rigidus and metatarsus primus elevatus.[233] Moberg[241] stated, "I have not seen many adult patients in which metatarsus primus elevatus has been part of the problem." Nonetheless, once metatarsus primus elevatus was implicated as a cause of hallux rigidus, several authors devised or advocated procedures to decrease first ray elevation.[182,193,231,241]

Meyer et al[233] reported that no statistical correlation existed between hallux rigidus and an elevated first metatarsal. In analyzing lateral weight-bearing radiographs in both normal subjects and patients with hallux rigidus, they reported that two thirds of the subjects had evidence of an elevated first metatarsal greater than 5 mm. Based on this observation, the authors concluded that an elevated first ray may be "perfectly normal during midstance" and that the presence of a radiographically elevated first metatarsal

"should no longer be considered a pathologic entity." They further concluded that in a large majority of patients an elevated first metatarsal did not correlate with first MTP joint disease.

Horton and Myerson[153] confirmed Meyer et al's study, showing no difference in average elevation of the first metatarsal between a control group and those with demonstrated hallux rigidus. Coughlin and Shurnas[65,66] confirmed these findings and, as noted, the authors concluded that elevatus is most likely a secondary finding that follows first MTP joint motion restriction. We suggest that procedures are designed to correct elevatus were treating a secondary anatomical finding and not a primary cause of hallux rigidus.

History and Physical Examination

A patient with hallux rigidus typically complains of stiffness with ambulation and pain localized to the first MTP joint that is aggravated by walking and standing and relieved by rest. Pain typically is insidious in onset.

Physical examination can reveal a variety of findings, varying from mild synovial thickening early in the disease process to significant bone hypertrophy and osteophyte formation with long-term disease. The classic finding is limitation or absence of passive MTP joint dorsiflexion,[74] often in the presence of normal or adequate plantar flexion. Interphalangeal joint hyperextension can develop to compensate for restricted MTP joint dorsiflexion.[95,120] A prominent ridge of bone on the dorsal first metatarsal head and the dorsal base of the proximal phalanx is easily palpable (Fig. 16–59). Skin irritation can develop with pressure from footwear over the dorsal exostosis.

On forced dorsiflexion, pain often is elicited with bone impingement between the base of the proximal phalanx and dorsal metatarsal osteophytes. On forced plantar flexion, pain may be elicited from stretching of the extensor hallucis longus, MTP joint capsule, and

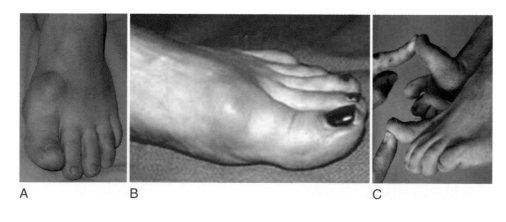

A   B   C

Figure 16–59 First metatarsophalangeal joint of a patient with hallux rigidus. Note increased bulk dorsally **(A)** and medially **(B)**. **C,** There is restricted dorsiflexion compared with the contralateral side.

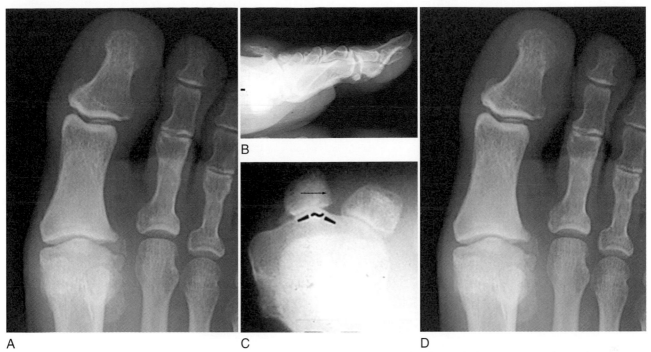

Figure 16–60   Grade II hallux rigidus. **A,** Anteroposterior radiograph. **B,** Lateral radiograph demonstrates a large dorsal osteophyte resembling dripping candle wax. **C,** Axial view demonstrates unusual occurrence of osteoarthritis of the medial sesamoid *(arrow)* associated with hallux valgus. **D,** Nonuniform narrowing of the articular surface of metatarsophalangeal joint. More chondrolysis occurs medially.

inflamed synovium over the dorsal osteophyte. With ambulation, the patient often directs weight bearing to the outer aspect of the foot to minimize dorsiflexion of the first MTP joint. Tingling, hyperesthesia, or a positive Tinel sign over the dorsal digital nerve in the first web space can occur from compression against the dorsolateral osteophyte.

Radiographic Evaluation

Standing AP, lateral, and sesamoid radiographs are obtained to evaluate the foot with hallux rigidus (Fig. 16–60A to C). The AP radiograph often demonstrates nonuniform joint space narrowing with widening and flattening of the first metatarsal head (Fig. 16–60D). An oblique radiograph can demonstrate an adequate joint space, which is obscured on the AP radiograph by overlying osteophytes. Subchondral cysts and sclerosis in the first metatarsal head, widening of the base of the proximal phalanx, and hypertrophy of the sesamoids can develop in more advanced stages.

Osteophyte formation on the AP radiographs occurs more often on the lateral than the medial aspect of the metatarsal head. An osteochondral defect may be visualized in the central metatarsal articular surface area

(Fig. 16–61). On the lateral radiograph, in advanced cases, the dorsal metatarsal osteophyte can resemble dripping candle wax as the osteophyte courses proximally along the dorsal first metatarsal metaphyseal shaft. Dorsophalangeal osteophytes and loose bodies may be present, and on a dorsiflexion stress view dorsal impingement may be observed and confirms that extension is blocked.

Lateral weight-bearing radiographs are also used to evaluate the presence of an elevated first metatarsal in relationship to the lesser metatarsals. With a true lateral radiograph, the central diaphyseal axes of the first and second metatarsals are marked. Meyer et al[233] noted that in normal feet, up to 5 mm of elevation is normal (Fig. 16–62).

Evaluation of the metatarsal–sesamoid articulation with axial radiographs is important, although involvement of the sesamoid complex occurs infrequently except with severe arthroses (Fig. 16–63).

Several different attempts have been made to classify hallux rigidus. A classification scheme is helpful in standardizing terminology both for describing the magnitude of the arthritic process and for recommending treatment. Table 16–3 outlines the recommended clinical and radiographic classification of hallux rigidus based on long-term evaluation and follow-up.

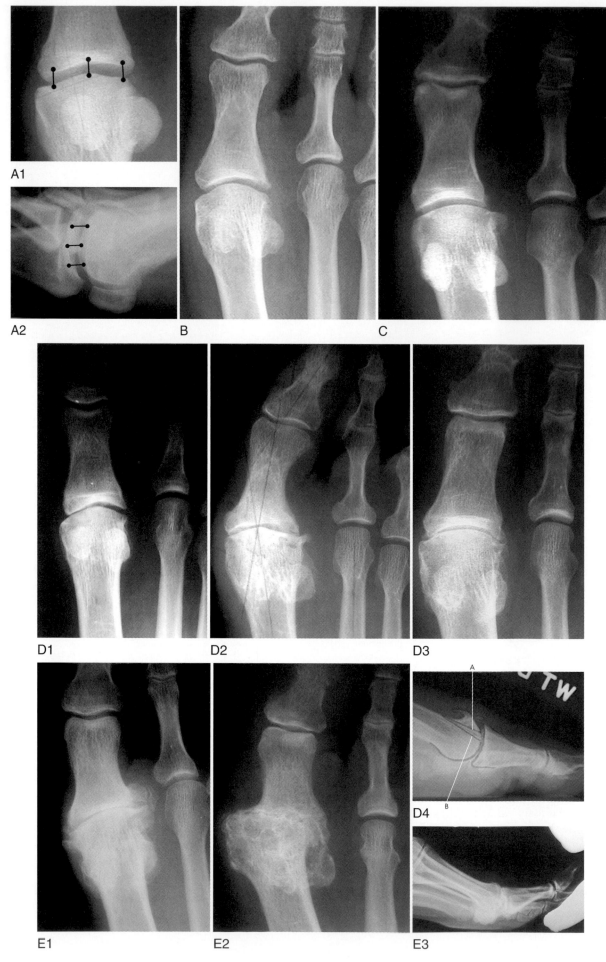

A1

A2

B

C

D1

D2

D3

D4

E1

E2

E3

Figure 16–61 Anteroposterior (AP) **(A1)** and lateral **(A2)** radiographs demonstrating our technique of measuring the width of the metatarsophalangeal (MTP) joint space. Marks are made medially, centrally, and laterally along the joint surface on both the AP and lateral radiographs. The distance between the marks is measured with a goniometer corrected for magnification. The measurements are averaged and compared to the contralateral side or a normal articular length if there is bilateral disease. In this example, this is grade 0 hallux rigidus; the radiograph demonstrates essentially a normal joint on both AP and lateral views. **B,** Grade 1 hallux rigidus. The radiograph shows mild periarticular osteophyte formation, but notable loss of passive motion is detected clinically. **C,** Grade 2 hallux rigidus with notable increase in periarticular osteophytes. **D1** to **D3,** Grade 3 hallux rigidus with progressive chondrolysis and osteophyte formation. **D4,** Lateral radiograph shows substantial cartilage space remaining in the joint. Line *A* is a flat cut of the osteophyte, and line *B* demonstrates a more aggressive cheilectomy, which typically results in greater postoperative range of motion. **E1** and **E2,** Grade 4 hallux rigidus with pain in the mid range of motion and substantial or complete chondrolysis of the MTP joint. **E3,** Grade 3 is distinguished clinically from grade 4 by the absence of pain at the mid range of motion, but the two can be identical radiographically.

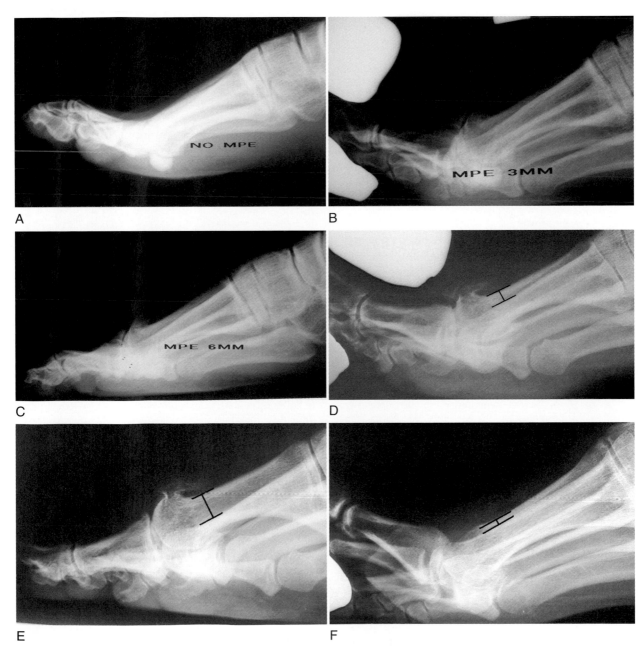

Figure 16–62 The effect of dorsiflexion stress on the first metatarsophalangeal (MTP) joint with hallux rigidus. Metatarsus primus elevatus (MPE) correlates with MTP joint arthrosis noted in sequential radiographs taken over an 11-year period. **A,** Early grade 1 hallux rigidus with no metatarsus elevatus. **B,** Six years later, elevatus is 3 mm with or without stress test. **C,** Eleven years later, elevatus is 6 mm. **D,** Dorsiflexion stress reduces elevatus to 3 mm. **E,** Elevatus does increase with increasing grade of hallux rigidus. **F,** It is often reduced following either a cheilectomy or MTP arthrodesis.

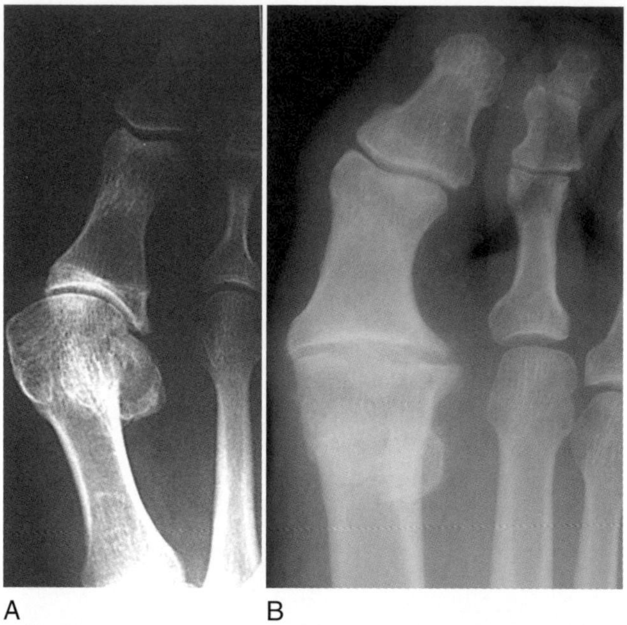

A   B

Figure 16–63 **A,** Hallux valgus is rarely seen in association with hallux rigidus. **B,** Hallux valgus interphalangeus is commonly seen. An average HVI angle of 17 degrees is reported.[65] (From Coughlin MJ, Shurnas PS: *J Bone Joint Surg Am* 85[11]:2072-2088, 2003.)

Conservative Treatment

Conservative management of symptomatic hallux rigidus depends on a patient's symptoms and the magnitude of the degenerative process. Early disease (characterized by synovial irritation) is treated with NSAIDs and a stiff insole to reduce excursion of the MTP joint. Several commercially available orthoses provide rigidity to the forepart of the shoe. Orthoses have been shown to provide greater and longer-term pain relief than NSAIDS alone.[336]

An insole with a Morton's extension can also reduce MTP range of motion and can be moved from shoe to shoe. The addition of an extended steel or fiberglass shank between the inner and outer sole may be effective in reducing MTP motion. Prefabricated and custom-made orthoses can reduce midfoot pronation, which can reduce symptoms. Unfortunately, many orthoses decrease available room in the toe box, which can increase pressure on the dorsal exostosis. A shoe with a low heel and roomy upper can accommodate the enlarged MTP joint associated with a more advanced hallux rigidus deformity. Taping of the

TABLE 16–3

Clinical and Radiographic Classification of Hallux Rigidus

Grade	Range of Motion	Radiograph	Clinical
0	Dorsiflexion 40-60 degrees and/or 10%-20% loss compared to normal side	Normal or minimal findings	No subjective pain, only stiffness; loss of passive motion on examination
1	Dorsiflexion 30-40 degrees and/or 20%-50% loss compared to normal side	Dorsal spur is main finding, minimal joint narrowing, minimal periarticular sclerosis, minimal flattening of metatarsal head	Mild or occasional subjective pain and stiffness; pain at extremes of dorsiflexion and/or plantarflexion on exam
2	Dorsiflexion 10-30 degrees and/or 50%-75% loss compared to normal side	Dorsal, lateral, and possibly medial osteophytes give flattened appearance to metatarsal head, no more than 25% dorsal joint space involvement on lateral radiograph, mild to moderate joint narrowing and sclerosis, sesamoids not usually involved but may be irregular in appearance	Moderate to severe subjective pain and stiffness that may be constant; pain just before maximal dorsiflexion and/or plantar flexion on exam
3	Dorsiflexion of 10 degrees or less and/or 75%-100% loss compared to normal side and notable loss of plantar flexion (often 10 degrees or less plantar flexion)	As in grade 2 but with substantial narrowing, possibly periarticular cystic changes, more than 25% dorsal joint may be involved on lateral side, sesamoids are enlarged and/or cystic and/or irregular	Nearly constant subjective pain and substantial stiffness; pain throughout range of motion on exam (but not at mid range)
4	Dorsiflexion of 10 degrees or less and/or 75%-100% loss compared to normal side and notable loss of plantar flexion (often 10° or less plantar flexion)	As in grade 2 but with substantial narrowing, possibly periarticular cystic changes, more than 25% dorsal joint may be involved on lateral, sesamoids are enlarged and/or cystic and/or irregular	Nearly constant subjective pain and substantial stiffness; pain throughout range of motion on exam plus definite pain at mid range of motion

From Coughlin MJ, Shurnas PS: *J Bone Joint Surg Am* 85(11):2072-2088, 2003.

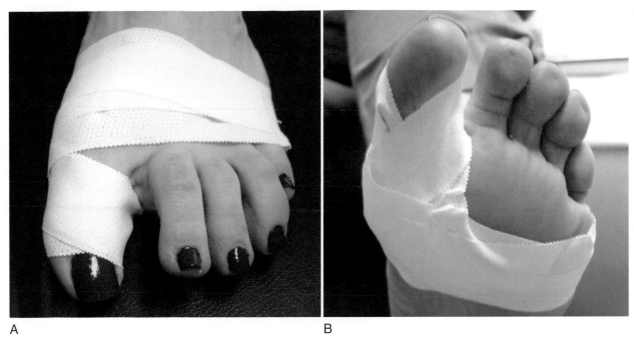

A   B

Figure 16–64   Taping of the hallux to decrease dorsiflexion excursion may reduce pain. **A,** Dorsal view. **B,** Plantar view.

hallux (Fig. 16–64) to decrease dorsiflexion excursion may be effective as well. Symptoms often subside if the first MTP joint is protected.

On occasion the judicious use of an intra-articular steroid injection provides temporary relief. Repeated injections can accelerate the degenerative process and are discouraged. When continued symptoms restrict activity, surgical intervention may be considered.

The results of nonoperative treatment have been evaluated. Solan et al[314] noted approximately 6 months of benefit using intraarticular steroid injection and joint manipulation for mild to moderate hallux rigidus but found limited benefit for its use in more

advanced grades of disease.[314] Smith et al[311] reported the long-term results of 22 patients (24 feet), with a mean follow-up of 14 years, who were treated nonoperatively for hallux rigidus. They found that 75% of patients still chose not to have surgery. The intensity of pain remained similar in 22 feet, improved with time in one, and worsened in one. Most patients were able to minimize pain by wearing a roomy, stiff-soled shoe. Others[123] have reported successful treatment in nearly 60% of patients treated nonoperatively with footwear modifications, orthoses, injections, and taping. Follow-up ranged from 1 to 7 years (Fig. 16–65).

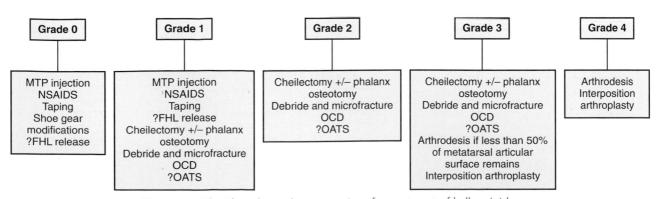

Grade 0	Grade 1	Grade 2	Grade 3	Grade 4
MTP injection NSAIDS Taping Shoe gear modifications ?FHL release	MTP injection NSAIDS Taping ?FHL release Cheilectomy +/– phalanx osteotomy Debride and microfracture OCD ?OATS	Cheilectomy +/– phalanx osteotomy Debride and microfracture OCD ?OATS	Cheilectomy +/– phalanx osteotomy Debride and microfracture OCD ?OATS Arthrodesis if less than 50% of metatarsal articular surface remains Interposition arthroplasty	Arthrodesis Interposition arthroplasty

Figure 16–65   Algorithm indicating options for treatment of hallux rigidus.

The geriatric patient deserves special consideration because the mortality rate in patients older than 90 years who undergo elective surgery has been reported to be 2.3%.[1] Age alone is not the sole determinant of whether elective procedures should be considered,[38] but the severity of diseases and comorbidities are good predictors of surgical outcome.[81] Cardiovascular complications account for nearly 50% of mortality.[128] With the increase in the aging population, many geriatric patients benefit from elective operative management when indicated, but they should be counseled about the increased risks.[1,31,38]

Surgical Treatment

Decision making in the surgical treatment of hallux rigidus is based on the degree of arthrosis present clinically and radiographically (Fig. 16–66). In the presence of synovial thickening without radiographic demonstration of degenerative arthritis, an MTP joint synovectomy is the treatment of choice. Moreover, synovitis and limited MTP joint motion without radiographic changes should be evaluated by ruling out an inflammatory or potentially erosive joint process (serum complete blood count [CBC], ESR, CRP, ANA, RF, HLA-B27, and uric acid) or considering the possibility of other causes of joint restriction. Michelson and Dunn[234] reported flexor hallucis stenosing tenosynovitis indicated by retromalleolar or arch tenderness over the FHL and increased signal on MRI as a cause of hallux limitus in patients without radiographic changes in the first MTP joint but with restricted passive joint motion.

With an osteochondral defect, removal of cartilaginous loose fragments and drilling of the osseous base can aid in the regeneration of a fibrocartilaginous surface. In a younger patient, an osteochondral autogenous transfer system (OATS) procedure can be considered. In a juvenile or adult patient with restricted passive dorsiflexion but no significant dorsal exostosis (without clinical findings of flexor hallucis stenosis), a dorsal closing wedge phalangeal osteotomy can improve joint function.[182,241,312,332]

In an adult patient with impingement of the proximal phalanx against a dorsal osteophyte on the metatarsal head, a cheilectomy is the preferred treatment. If an unsatisfactory result occurs, other opportunities for salvage remain. Cheilectomy is the mainstay of surgical treatment for hallux rigidus and can be combined with other procedures tailored to a specific problem such as an OATS procedure for a large central defect or microfracture for smaller defects, phalangeal osteotomy for severe interphalangeus or to enhance dorsiflexion, or soft tissue interposition for end-stage hallux rigidus in a patient who is opposed to an arthrodesis.

Typically with grade 0 or 1 hallux rigidus, careful examination for FHL stenosing tenosynovitis is performed. If FHL stenosing tenosynovitis is diagnosed, then an FHL release is performed and MTP joint synovectomy or phalangeal osteotomy may be added depending on the individual case. In grade 2 or 3 hallux rigidus, a cheilectomy, or occasionally a cheilectomy combined with a phalangeal osteotomy,[335] may be considered. With grade 4 hallux rigidus (severe degenerative arthritis), salvage procedures include arthrodesis, excisional arthroplasty, soft tissue interpositional arthroplasty, or prosthetic replacement.

Preoperative planning includes careful inspection of the preoperative AP and especially the lateral radiograph for loss of joint space. A careful physical examination is performed to assess pain with gentle loading of the hallux in a neutral position with respect to dorsiflexion and plantar flexion.[85] If this maneuver elicits pain at the mid range of motion, the remaining cartilage surface is inadequate and portends a poor prognosis for the success of cheilectomy.[66]

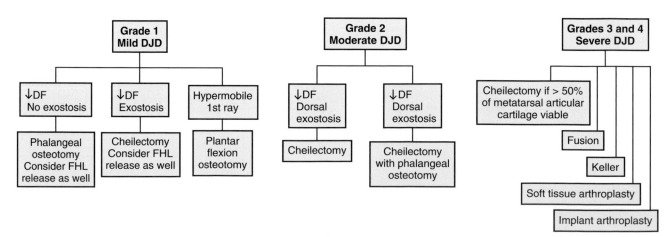

Figure 16–66 Treatment considerations of hallux rigidus. ↓, decreased; DF, dorsiflexion; DJD, degenerative joint disease; FHL, flexor hallucis longus; Keller, Keller arthroplasty.

To establish a pain-free MTP joint, an arthrodesis, interposition arthroplasty, or joint resection arthroplasty may be necessary. We do not advocate a Keller or Mayo resection arthroplasty; rather, we recommend soft tissue interposition arthroplasty as described by Coughlin[68] or Hamilton.[132]

Although many activities are possible after an arthrodesis, many younger patients often prefer to preserve motion. Procedures to reestablish motion at the MTP joint often do so at the expense of stability. Resection arthroplasty has been favored for hallux rigidus,[75,168,256,309,368] but not in the younger patient. Often with an excisional arthroplasty, weakness of plantar flexion at the MTP joint occurs and can lead to transfer metatarsalgia.[63] In an older, less-active patient, a resection arthroplasty or resection arthroplasty with interposition of soft tissue may be considered.

For patients who want moderate physical activity, resection arthroplasty should be discouraged. However, less-destructive resection arthroplasties such as the Valenti procedure (resection of the dorsal proximal phalanx and metatarsal head in a V shaped cut) have reported a high proportion of good and excellent results (33 of 36 procedures) in younger patients (mean age, 50.6 years) with a mean follow-up of 4.2 years.[191] Implant arthroplasty has been advocated for treatment of hallux rigidus,[327,329,330] but reported complications and severe difficulty with revision procedures have made this procedure less popular (see later discussion of implants for the first MTP joint).

PROXIMAL PHALANGEAL OSTEOTOMY

A dorsal closing wedge proximal phalangeal osteotomy was initially proposed by Bonney and MacNab[30] for the treatment of adolescents with hallux rigidus. Kessel and Bonney[182] reported on the results of this technique. Heaney,[144] Harrison,[139] and later Moberg[237] recommended phalangeal osteotomy to use available plantar flexion and create a "functional transfer of plantar flexion to dorsiflexion" with this osteotomy.[271]

The indications for a dorsal closing wedge proximal phalangeal osteotomy for hallux rigidus are in the adolescent patient with no significant osteophyte formation. This may be used in combination with an FHL release when indicated and less often in combination with cheilectomy in the older patient.[332]

Surgical Technique

1. A medial longitudinal incision extending from the interphalangeal joint to a point 1 cm proximal to the first MTP joint exposes the proximal phalanx.[182,241]
2. The MTP joint is identified. A dorsal closing wedge osteotomy is performed just distal to the MTP joint space. In the adolescent patient, care must be taken to avoid injury to an open proximal phalangeal epiphysis. The size of the resected wedge is determined by the degree of plantar flexion at the MTP joint. This osteotomy should permit the toe to be dorsiflexed to 35 degrees in relationship to the metatarsal shaft (15 degrees in relationship to the plantar surface of the foot) (Fig. 16–67A).
3. The osteotomy is firmly secured with crossed or parallel Kirschner wires, with compression staples, or with sutures placed through drill holes at the osteotomy site (Fig. 16–67B). If a phalangeal osteotomy is combined with a cheilectomy, stable internal fixation is mandatory because early motion is necessary for a successful cheilectomy. The wound is closed in a routine manner.

Postoperative Care

A gauze-and-tape compression dressing is applied at surgery and changed weekly. The patient is allowed to ambulate in a postoperative shoe. Dressing changes and guarded ambulation are necessary until the osteotomy site is healed 4 to 6 weeks after surgery. Internal fixation is removed when necessary after successful healing is demonstrated.

Results and Complications

Kessell and Bonney[182] reported on nine adolescents with short-term follow-up (average 14 months), noting pain relief in more than 90% and an average increase in dorsiflexion of 39 degrees. Although this procedure was originally recommended for adolescent patients, Moberg[241] extended the indications to the adult population. Unfortunately, he reported no follow-up of results. In a long-term follow-up of phalangeal osteotomies (average follow-up 11 years), Citron[45] reported that 50% of patients had complete relief of pain, although further degenerative arthrosis was noted. Thomas and Smith[332] reported on 17 patients who underwent a combination cheilectomy and phalangeal osteotomy for grades 1 and 2 hallux rigidus. All osteotomies healed. Although the average increase in dorsiflexion was only 7 degrees, 96%

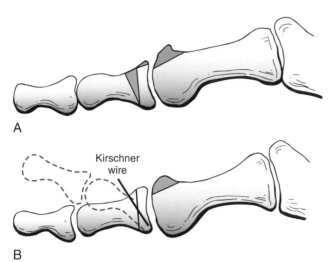

Figure 16–67 Moberg procedure. Dorsal and closing wedge osteotomy of proximal phalanx is used to correct hallux rigidus. This exchanges plantar flexion for dorsiflexion. **A,** Proposed osteotomy and cheilectomy. **B,** After closing wedge osteotomy.

of patients were satisfied with their surgical result. Southgate et al[316] reported similarly good results following proximal phalangeal osteotomy and found comparable results to arthrodesis in terms of pain relief in 10 patients with osteotomies compared to 20 patients with arthrodeses with a mean of 12 years of follow-up.[316]

The indications for phalangeal osteotomy in relationship to hallux rigidus remain to be clearly delineated. For an adolescent with hallux rigidus, a phalangeal osteotomy appears to be advantageous, but the osteotomy must avoid an open phalangeal physis when present. In an adolescent a cheilectomy might not be necessary because there is rarely significant arthrosis or osteophyte formation; however, inspection of the metatarsal articular surface is important because an osteochondral defect should be treated. For an adult with grade 1 hallux rigidus, a phalangeal osteotomy may be sufficient. With significant MTP arthrosis, an isolated phalangeal osteotomy might not be sufficient treatment and occasionally may be combined with a cheilectomy for grades 2 and 3 disease. Whether Thomas and Smith's [332] or Southgate's studies[316] will be confirmed with greater numbers of longer-term positive results remains to be determined.

CHEILECTOMY

Cheilectomy, or excision of the dorsal exostosis of the metatarsal head, was first proposed by Nilsonne,[256] who attempted the procedure in two cases but thought it offered only temporary relief. Bonney and Macnab[30] later used this technique for cases of "polyarthritis" and noted poor results. In 1959 DuVries[84] advocated removal of the proliferative bone at the MTP joint to enable dorsiflexion. Although he noted 90% satisfactory results, no long-term follow-up was reported. In 1979 Mann, Coughlin, and DuVries[216] described their technique of cheilectomy and reported successful results at long-term follow-up. Most recently, Coughlin and Shurnas[66] reported 92% successful results using Mann's technique of cheilectomy in 80 patients with 9.6 years of follow-up. This study clearly defined the role of cheilectomy in treating all grades of hallux rigidus and proposed a clinical and radiographic classification to help select appropriate surgical treatment (see Table 16–3).

Although some have stressed the temporary nature of the procedure[28,82] or limited indications,[312] we perform cheilectomy for grades 1 and 2 hallux rigidus, in younger athletic patients, and in patients with more advanced degenerative arthrosis (grade 3 hallux rigidus with more than 50% of the metatarsal articular surface remaining) who wish to avoid the risk and morbidity of a more extensive procedure. Geldwert et al[112] have demonstrated that for grades 1 and 2 hallux rigidus (using a different classification scheme), a cheilectomy relieved pain significantly in 93% of patients, but for grade 3 hallux rigidus the success rate fell to 29%. A cheilectomy is a simple procedure that leaves a stable joint, has low morbidity,[112] and preserves strength and joint motion.[95,112,143]

Surgical Technique

1. A dorsal longitudinal incision extends from the middle of the proximal phalanx to 3 cm proximal to the MTP joint. The extensor hood and joint capsule are incised, and the dissection is deepened on the medial or lateral aspect of the extensor hallucis longus tendon (Fig. 16–68A and video clip 33).
2. A thorough synovectomy is carried out, and the MTP joint is inspected to locate osteophytes or loose bodies and to assess the

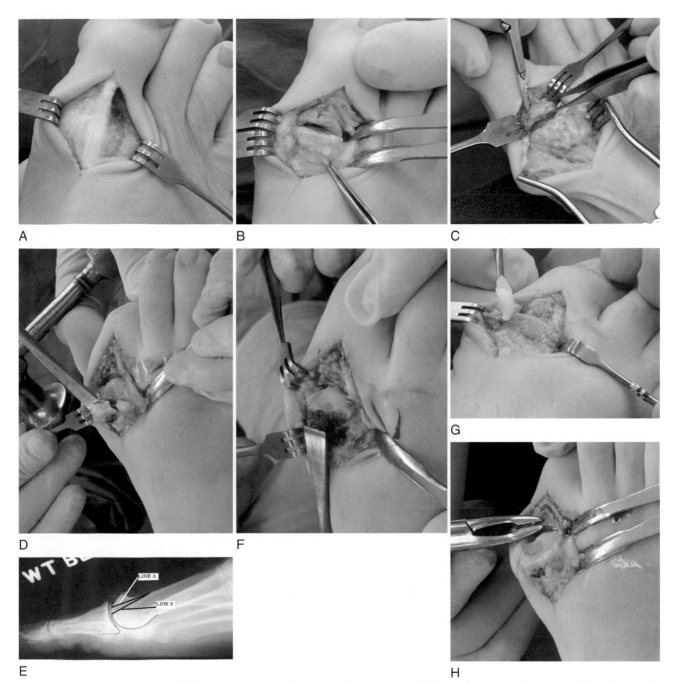

Figure 16–68 **A,** A dorsomedial skin incision is used to expose the metatarsophalangeal joint. **B,** The extensor hood is incised, the extensor tendon is retracted laterally (or medially), and the joint space is exposed. **C,** A synovectomy is performed, the joint is inspected, and any loose bodies are removed. **D,** A cheilectomy is performed to include any cartilage defect if possible. **E,** About 25% to 30% of the dorsal metatarsal head is resected. **F,** The osteotome denotes the dorsal axis of the first metatarsal; thus, actually more bone is removed below this level. **G,** Bone wax is used to decrease postoperative bleeding. **H,** Any osteophytes on the dorsal base of the proximal phalanx are removed with a rongeur.

extent of the articular cartilage damage (Fig. 16–68B). The proximal phalanx is plantar flexed to aid in exposure, and any dorsal phalangeal osteophyte is resected (Fig. 16–68C and H).

3. The joint is inspected to determine the amount and location of cartilage loss (Fig. 16–68D). If a cheilectomy is indicated (more than 50% of metatarsal articular cartilage is viable), then the metatarsal osteophyte is generously resected on the dorsal, dorsomedial, and dorsolateral aspects using a 6-mm osteotome (Fig. 16–68E). It is critical that at least 20% to 30% of the dorsal metatarsal head is removed with this oblique osteotomy. The decision regarding the extent of bone resection depends on the size of the dorsal exostosis, the amount of articular cartilage destruction, and the need to establish adequate dorsiflexion at the conclusion of the procedure.

4. The resection is initiated just dorsal to the edge of the remaining viable metatarsal articular cartilage. (Thus, with more severe arthrosis, more metatarsal head is resected.) However, more extensive resection can increase the risk of MTP subluxation, and greater than 30% to 40% resection is discouraged. Any remaining eburnated bone or defects can be microfractured or drilled, and if less than 50% of the metatarsal articular surface is viable, an arthrodesis is recommended (Fig. 16–68F).

5. Any articular cartilage irregularities are removed, including loose cartilaginous fragments. Dorsiflexion of approximately 60 degrees is desirable after an extensive cheilectomy. Any dorsal or medial osteophytes are removed from the base of the proximal phalanx and along the upper border of the metatarsal head.

6. The raw bone surfaces are smoothed with a rasp or rongeur and may be coated with a thin layer of bone wax to impede further bleeding. The joint capsule is closed in a routine manner. A gauze-and-tape compression dressing is applied and changed weekly (Fig. 16–68E).

Postoperative Care

At 7 to 10 days after surgery, aggressive active and passive range-of-motion exercises are initiated. The patient is allowed to ambulate in a postoperative shoe with weight bearing on the heel and along the outer border of the foot. Patients are encouraged to mobilize the MTP joint 5 minutes of every hour. Weekly office visits are scheduled to monitor the patient's progress with range of motion. At 2 to 3 months after surgery, most swelling and thickening of the periarticular tissue subside. Maximal improvement in motion is usually achieved at this point.

Physical therapy can be scheduled depending on a patient's compliance and success with joint mobilization. On occasion, chronic thickening and swelling can take several months to subside and the use of a short course of oral steroid may be useful in resolving this problem.

Results and Complications

Mann, Coughlin, and DuVries[216] reported on their experience with 20 patients and noted 85% pain relief with cheilectomy. The remaining patients had only mild discomfort. Postoperative dorsiflexion averaged 30 degrees, with minimal progression of arthrosis.

Mann and Clanton[213] later reported an average increase in postoperative range of motion of 19 degrees (average dorsiflexion, 48 degrees) after cheilectomy; 74% of patients had improvement in joint motion, and 25% had no change or lost motion. Complete or considerable relief of pain was noted by 90% of patients. Only one patient noted recurrence of a dorsal osteophyte. The authors stressed that a patient must be counseled that after surgery, some will continue to have pain, some do not gain MTP joint motion, and some actually lose MTP motion.

This concept was well demonstrated by Mulier et al[248] in 20 athletes (22 feet) at a mean age of 31 years who underwent Mann's cheilectomy for all grades of hallux rigidus with a mean follow-up of 5.1 years. Subjectively, 14 feet were rated excellent, 7 good, and 1 fair, but only 13 athletes were able to play at the same or higher level, and seven played at a lower level. Two patients had symptoms clearly related to persistent symptoms of hallux rigidus.

A cheilectomy resects bone and removes bony impingement but does not repair the intraarticular damage. Thus some pain or aching might remain after surgery. Over time the results of cheilectomy can deteriorate, depending on the severity of the degenerative process.[332]

Ultimately, even with failure, a cheilectomy does not "burn bridges" and leaves options for other salvage techniques available. Likewise, it does not trade one problem for another.[85]

Feltham[96] reported on cheilectomy results using Mann's technique on 67 patients with a mean of 65 months of follow-up and noted a 91% satisfaction rate with four failures. Better results were observed in patients older than 60 years; the technique was used for all grades of hallux rigidus. Coughlin and Shurnas[66] recommended cheilectomy for grades 1, 2, and 3 hallux rigidus (with more than 50% metatarsal articular cartilage remaining at the time of surgery). They reported 97% good and excellent subjective results (mean follow-up, 9.6 years) and 92% long-term successful results for pain relief and function following cheilectomy,

It is critical that patients with more advanced clinical and radiographic disease (grades 3 [less than 50% metatarsal cartilage surface remaining at surgery] and 4 [end-stage disease]) understand that a cheilectomy is very likely to fail based on the results of the study. Such patients would be better served with an arthrodesis or interposition arthroplasty depending on the individual patient's needs (see Fig. 16–73). Moreover, the effect of microfracture performed on any remaining small (<5 mm) defect after the cheilectomy has been completed can extend the indications for a cheilectomy, but the results of this additional technique are not completely known (Fig. 16–69). Coughlin and Shurnas[66] reported no adverse effect on the long-term results of a small number of patients who underwent microfracture with cheilectomy, but any patient with less than 50% of the metatarsal articular surface remaining had a significantly increased risk of failure of the cheilectomy (Fig. 16–70).

Probably the main reason for failure of cheilectomy as reported in the literature (in appropriately selected patients) centers on inadequate bone resection (Figs. 16–71 to 16–75). Feldman et al[95] and others[80,143,209] have advocated excision of osteophytes flush with the metatarsal shaft. This might explain Hattrup and Johnson's[143] high failure rate of greater than 30%. Only 53% of their patients were satisfied after their surgery. A cheilectomy should not remove bone "in line" with the dorsal metatarsal cortex, but it should remove up to 30% to 40% of the metatarsal head in an oblique fashion. Using Mann's technique as elaborated by Coughlin,[64] predictable and reliable long-term results can be expected. Unfortunately, with inadequate resection, MTP joint motion is not restored, and if impingement persists, ultimately the procedure can fail (Figs. 16–71 and 16–72).

A more extensive bone resection has been advocated by Saxena[297] and Grady and Axe[122] using the Valenti procedure (Fig. 16–76), which resects a sizable portion of the articular surface of the proximal phalanx and metatarsal head while retaining first ray length and the plantar intrinsic muscle insertions. Saxena[297] reported an average increase in dorsiflexion of 28 degrees, and Grady and Axe[122] reported an average 12-degree improvement in dorsiflexion. Excessive resection of bone, however, can lead to an unstable MTP joint with subluxation of the proximal phalanx.[143]

Although we do not have experience with the Valenti procedure and do not necessarily advocate this procedure, this technique supports the premise that a more extensive resection with cheilectomy improves postoperative range of motion and relieves impingement. With more advanced arthrosis, the normal gliding MTP joint motion is replaced by a rocking or hinged motion. Shereff and Baumhauer[303] noted that motion analysis of the MTP joint in hallux rigidus has demonstrated a greatly displaced center of rotation as more advanced arthritis ensues.

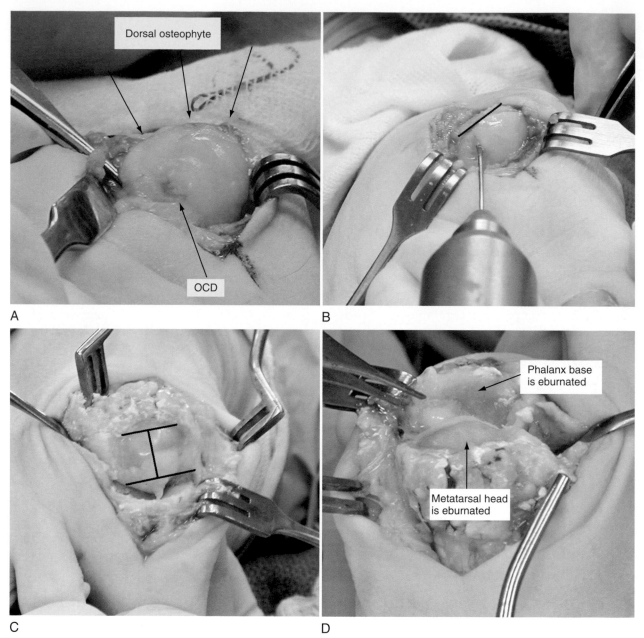

Figure 16–69 Treatment of osteochondral defect (OCD). **A** and **B,** If an area of full-thickness cartilage loss remains after a cheilectomy of up to 33% of the metatarsal head, the area may be drilled or perforated with a small Kirschner wire after a cheilectomy (indicated by the black line) of up to 33% to 40% of the metatarsal head. **C,** Dorsal/plantar extent of the metatarsal head articular surface is indicated by the black lines prior to excision. Cartilaginous loss extends well into the remaining metatarsal and phalangeal articular surface. Greater than 50% loss of the cartilaginous surface portends a poorer prognosis for success following a cheilectomy. In this case, the patient was treated with a metatarsophalangeal joint arthrodesis. **D,** Substantial loss of cartilage on the phalangeal articular surface.

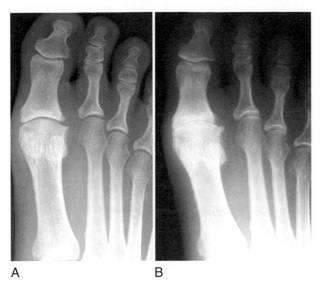

A   **B**

Figure 16–70 **A,** Preoperative radiograph with grade 2 hallux rigidus. **B,** Following cheilectomy, complete chondrolysis has occurred. This is very unusual and can necessitate metatarsophalangeal joint arthrodesis.

EXCISIONAL ARTHROPLASTY

Excisional arthroplasty was first described by Davies-Colley[75] in 1887 and was popularized by Keller[181] in 1904. The MTP joint is decompressed by resecting the base of the proximal phalanx, thereby relaxing contracted soft tissue structures. Excisional arthroplasty can relieve pain and has traditionally been accepted as treatment for more advanced degenerative arthritis of the first MTP joint. Gould[120] reported good relief of pain but observed that a hallux extensus deformity can occur after excisional arthroplasty. Bonney and MacNab[30] concluded that excisional arthroplasty had no place in the treatment of patients with generalized arthritis or metatarsus primus elevatus.

The Keller procedure is indicated in the older, more sedentary patient or household ambulator with grade 3 or 4 hallux rigidus in whom extensive surgery is contraindicated. It is not advocated for younger, more active patients with extensive hallux rigidus,[30,312] because a flaccid, nonfunctional hallux can be a worse problem than the original hallux rigidus deformity.

Surgical Technique

1. A medial longitudinal incision is used to approach the first MTP joint. The incision extends from just proximal to the interphalangeal joint to 1 cm proximal to the medial eminence (video clip 28).
2. A proximally based medial capsular flap is developed, exposing the MTP joint.
3. A cheilectomy is performed, and if a prominent medial eminence is present, it is resected (see previous discussion). A sagittal saw is used to remove the proximal one third of the proximal phalanx (Fig. 16–77A and B).
4. To reestablish flexor power, the plantar aponeurosis and capsule are reattached to the plantar base of the proximal phalanx through several drill holes in its base. This can also prevent a cock-up deformity at the MTP joint (Fig. 16–77C).
5. A 0.062-inch Kirschner wire is introduced at the MTP joint and driven in a distal direction, exiting the tip of the toe. It is then retrograded proximally into the metatarsal head

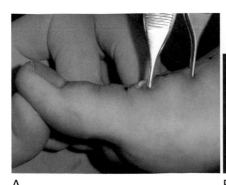
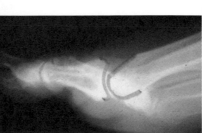
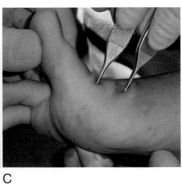

A   **B**   **C**

Figure 16–71 **A,** Preoperative motion. Following the dorsal incision, the forceps hold the skin apposed, but marked restriction of dorsiflexion is noted. **B,** Lateral radiograph following cheilectomy. **C,** Dorsiflexion immediately following cheilectomy.

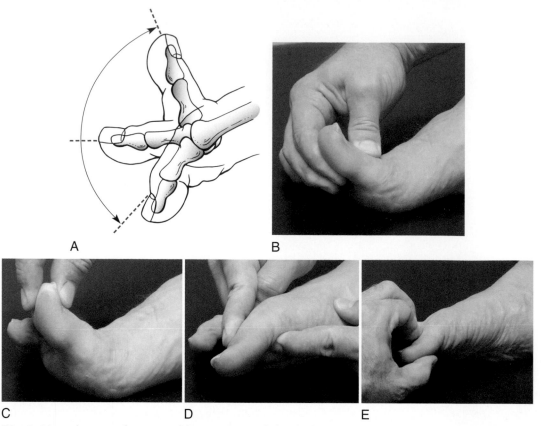

Figure 16–72 **A,** Normal range of motion of first metatarsophalangeal (MTP) joint. **B,** Technique of dorsiflexion mobilization (with plantar pressure on the proximal phalanx). **C,** Incorrect technique that places pressure on the distal interphalangeal joint. **D,** Technique of plantar flexion mobilization. **E,** Although one can grasp the distal phalanx, better pressure can be applied to the MTP joint by grasping the proximal phalanx and pushing downward.

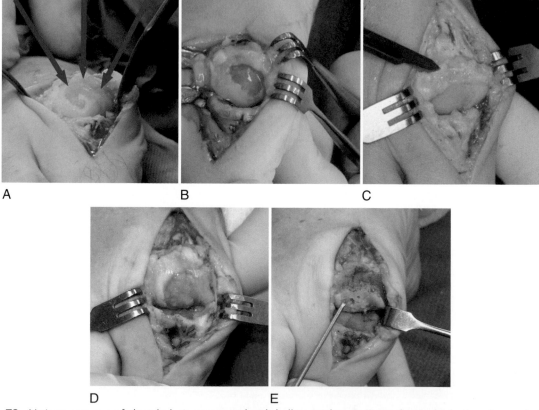

Figure 16–73 Various patterns of chondrolysis associated with hallux rigidus. **A,** Central articular lesion. Arrows indicate complete loss of cartilage. **B,** A dorsocentral articular lesion can often be resected with the cheilectomy; in this case some full loss area remains and can lead to postoperative pain. **C,** Complete lateral articular chondrolysis of this magnitude is best treated by arthrodesis. **D,** V-shaped central articular chondrolysis that extends plantarward for 50% of the height of the metatarsal head. **F,** It may be resected with cheilectomy and drilling of remain articular defect.

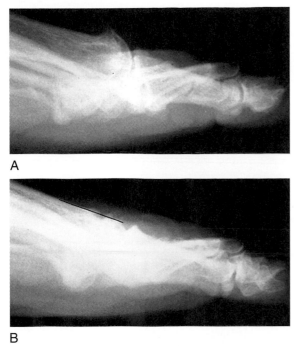

A

B

Figure 16–74 Preoperative **(A)** and postoperative **(B)** radiographs demonstrate inadequate resection of bone from metatarsal head. For a successful cheilectomy, at least 20% to 30% of dorsal metatarsal head should be excised.

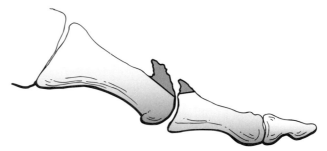

Figure 16–75 Proposed "correct" resection of the osteophyte from the base of the proximal phalanx and metatarsal head.

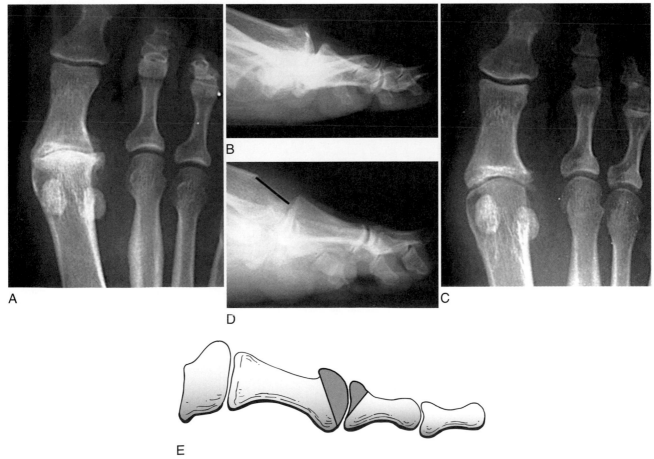

A

B

D

C

E

Figure 16–76 Cheilectomy. Preoperative anteroposterior (AP) **(A)** and lateral **(B)** radiographs demonstrate significant osteophyte formation. Postoperative AP **(C)** and lateral **(D)** radiographs demonstrate removal of approximately one third of the dorsal metatarsal head. **E,** Diagram of the Valenti procedure. Bone has been extensively resected from the base of the proximal phalanx and the metatarsal head.

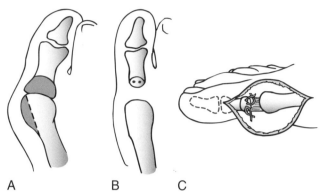

A   B   C

Figure 16–77   Diagram of excisional arthroplasty. **A,** Shaded area shows resected area of bone. **B,** After partial proximal phalangectomy. **C,** Reattachment of intrinsics to the base of the proximal phalanx. (With interpositional arthroplasty, intrinsics are not reattached to the base of the proximal phalanx.)

to stabilize the MTP joint. The pin is bent at the tip of the toe to prevent proximal migration.

6. The medial capsular flap is sutured to the periosteum of the proximal phalanx with interrupted sutures.

7. The skin is closed in a routine manner (Fig. 16–78).

Postoperative Care

A compression dressing is applied and changed weekly. The patient is allowed to ambulate in a wooden-soled shoe. The Kirschner wire is removed 3 weeks after surgery, and gentle passive and active range-of-motion exercises are then commenced.

SOFT TISSUE INTERPOSITIONAL ARTHROPLASTY

A modified resection arthroplasty has been advocated by Ganley et al,[110] Hamilton et al,[132] and Barca[9] for hallux rigidus associated with more severe degenerative arthroses. An excisional arthroplasty is combined with a capsular interpositional arthroplasty technique, with this tissue serving as a biologic spacer. Indications include grade 3 and 4 hallux rigidus and situations when an arthrodesis, excisional arthroplasty, or implant might be considered. According to Hamilton et al,[132] the relative length of the first and second metatarsals should be equal. A short first metatarsal is a con-

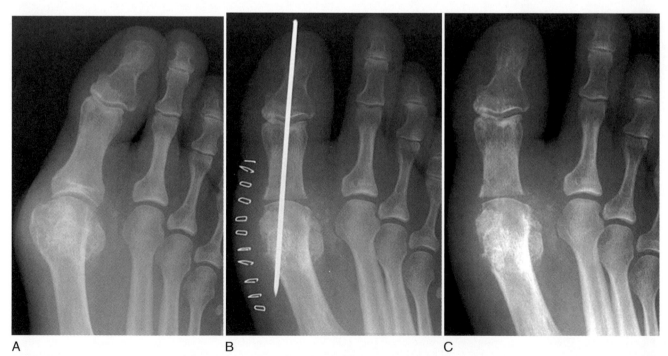

A   B   C

Figure 16–78   Excisional arthroplasty. **A,** Preoperative radiograph demonstrates combined hallux valgus and hallux rigidus. **B,** After excision arthroplasty with Kirschner wire stabilization. **C,** After excisional arthroplasty.

traindication to this procedure because of the increased risk of a transfer lesion or lateral metatarsalgia. Coughlin and Shurnas[68] reported similar indications using an autologous gracilis tendon biologic spacer with conical bone resection of the base of the proximal phalanx and metatarsal head using power reamers to create an effective joint space for placement of the tendon interposition graft. Disruption of the plantar intrinsics is avoided.

Hamilton's Surgical Technique

1. A medial longitudinal incision is centered over the first MTP joint. The MTP capsule is incised longitudinally. A periosteal elevator is used to reflect the dorsal, medial, and lateral capsule.
2. A cheilectomy is performed, and 25% or less of the proximal phalanx is resected with a transverse phalangeal osteotomy. The flexor hallucis brevis tendon is detached with this procedure and is not reattached (Fig. 16–79A).
3. The extensor hallucis brevis tendon and capsule are transversely incised approximately 3 cm proximal to the MTP joint line.

The tendon and capsule are mobilized and rotated distally and plantarward and sutured to the tendon of the flexor hallucis brevis with 2-0 nonabsorbable sutures (Fig. 16–79B and C).
4. A 0.062-inch Kirschner wire is driven distally through the proximal and distal phalanx and then advanced in a retrograde manner to stabilize the MTP joint. The pin is bent at the tip of the toe to prevent proximal migration (Fig. 16–79D).
5. The medial capsule is imbricated with interrupted absorbable sutures. The skin is approximated with a routine closure (Fig. 16–80).

Coughlin's Surgical Technique (Fig. 16–81)

1. A dorsomedial approach to the MTP join is made and centered over the joint. The capsule is opened longitudinally and reflected in a subperiosteal fashion to expose the metatarsal head and phalanx as described for an MTP joint arthrodesis (Fig. 16–81A to D).
2. The osteophytes are debrided off the phalanx and metatarsal head, and concave

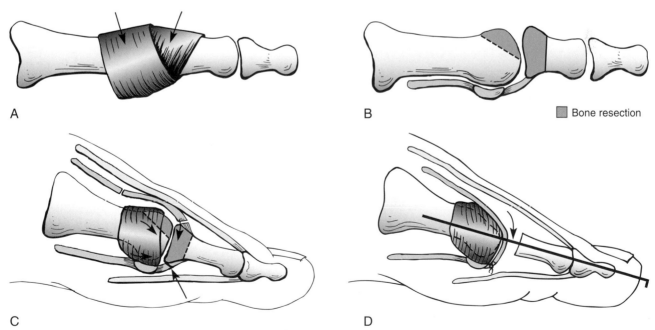

A

B   ■ Bone resection

C

D

Figure 16–79 Capsular interpositional arthroplasty.[132] **A,** Anatomy of extensor expansion. **B,** Shaded area of bone marks the resection (25% of the length of the proximal phalanx is removed). Dorsal cheilectomy is performed. **C,** The extensor hallucis brevis tendon and dorsal capsule are released proximally and transposed as an interpositional arthroplasty. **D,** The tendon and capsule are sutured to the plantar plate. The flexor hallucis brevis is not reattached to the base of the proximal phalanx. A Kirschner wire is used to stabilize the repair.

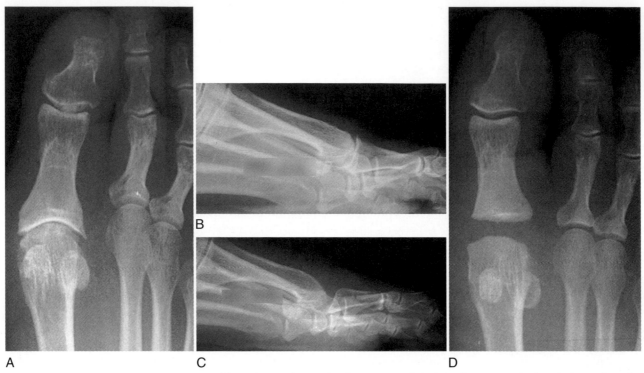

A   C   D

Figure 16–80   Anteroposterior (AP) **(A)** and lateral **(B)** radiographs demonstrate failed cheilectomy with chondrolysis of the first metatarsophalangeal joint. Postoperative lateral **(C)** and AP **(D)** radiographs after Hamilton's interpositional arthroplasty.

reaming is performed on both the phalanx base and metatarsal head based on the size of the proximal phalanx base. The plantar tissues are not disturbed (Fig. 16–81E and F).

3. A gracilis free graft is then harvested via a longitudinal incision centered over the hamstrings group insertion on the proximal medial tibia. The sartorius fascia is incised, and the gracilis tendon is identified and detached from its distal insertion. The distal end is secured with a Krakow suture and then harvested with a tendon stripper. Alternatively, an allograft tendon may be used.

4. The graft is prepared on the back table, cleaned of muscle tissue with an elevator, and rolled into a ball and sutured to maintain the oval shape (Fig. 16–81G).

5. The graft is placed into the prepared joint surface, and the capsule closed over the graft and sutured into it during the closure (Fig. 16–81H).

6. A Kirschner wire may be used if needed for stability and is placed the same as in the resection arthroplasty, but it is usually not

required. It is removed 3 weeks postoperatively (Fig. 16–81I).

Postoperative Care

Postoperative care is the same for both techniques. The foot is placed in a gauze-and-tape compression dressing at surgery and changed weekly for 6 weeks. The Kirschner wire is removed 3 weeks after surgery. Passive range of motion in the dressing is initiated at 2 to 3 weeks after surgery when skin healing is complete. The patient is permitted to ambulate in a wooden-soled postoperative shoe, initially with weight bearing on the heel and on the outer aspect of the foot. Plantigrade ambulation is permitted 3 weeks after surgery following removal of the Kirschner wire.

Results and Complications

Reported rates of subjective satisfaction with excisional arthroplasty vary from 76% to 96%.[48,368] Bonney and MacNab[30] observed that functional results can deteriorate over time. Rogers and Joplin[289] reported generally poor

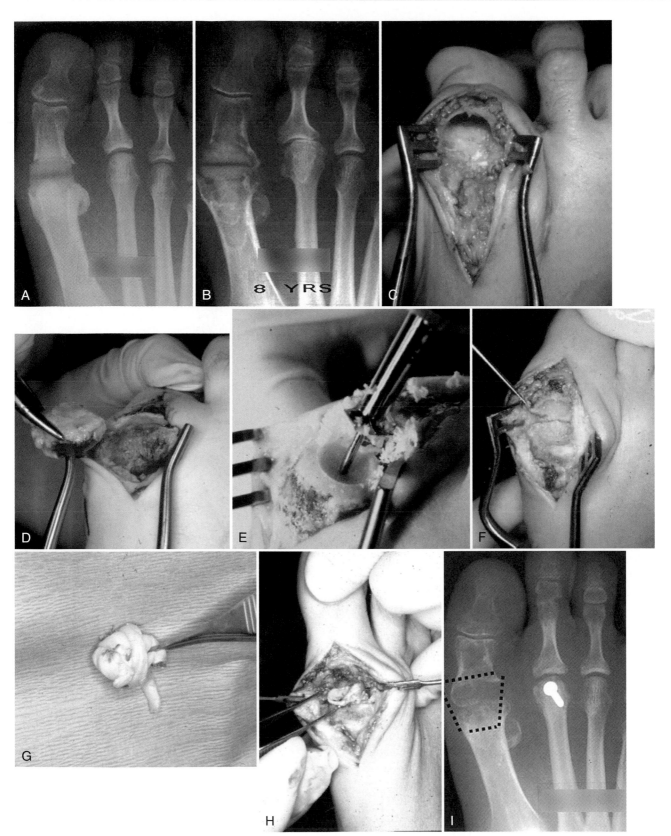

Figure 16–81 Technique of Coughlin's soft tissue interposition arthroplasty. **A,** Following removal of silicone double stemmed implant for hallux rigidus **B,** Eight years later, severe erosion has occurred around the implant. **C,** Intraoperative photo after implant removal. **D,** Following dorsal cheilectomy, which may be necessary. **E,** Preparation of metatarsal head by reaming with power cup-shaped reamer to create a convex surface (a cannulated phalangeal reamer was used). **F,** Following preparation of the phalangeal surface with a phalangeal reamer. **G,** Preparation of the tendon bundle harvested from the gracilis muscle. **H,** Placement of the tendon anchovy. **I,** Radiograph one year after soft tissue arthroplasty.

results with excisional arthroplasty and noted marked objective improvement in only 9%, no change in 71%, and postoperative deterioration in 20% of patients after surgery. Henry and Waugh[147] noted an association between increased phalangeal resection and lateral metatarsalgia. Weight bearing on the great toe was noted in 73% of the feet from which one third or less of the proximal phalanx was resected but in only 19% of the feet from which more than one third was resected.

An excisional arthroplasty appears to have fewer postoperative complications and improved patient satisfaction when performed for hallux rigidus in comparison to a hallux valgus deformity. Coughlin and Mann[63] reported significant postoperative metatarsalgia after excisional arthroplasty. Other complications include cock-up deformity of the great toe,[63,208] stiffness of the interphalangeal joint, marked shortening, impaired control and function, and decreased flexor strength of the great toe. Because of the high frequency of complications, excisional arthroplasty is recommended for elderly, low-demand patients who have no lateral metatarsalgia. It is best reserved for household ambulators who are poor candidates for any other procedure.

Hamilton[132] reported results on 30 patients (34 feet), all of whom had advanced degenerative arthrosis of the first MTP joint (less than 1 mm of joint space). A soft tissue arthroplasty was performed in these patients (see Figs. 16–79 and 16–80). Dorsiflexion increased an average of 40 degrees, and 93% of patients were satisfied with the procedure. No lateral metatarsalgia was noted. Careful selection of patients was recommended regarding first metatarsal length. Wrighton[368] reported only 59% satisfactory results with interpositional arthroplasty versus 76% satisfactory results with a standard Keller procedure. Ganley et al[110] reported on 50 patients with similar follow-up (average 2 years) and noted 92% satisfaction. A 2% transfer lesion rate was noted. Barca[9] used a slightly different arthroplastic interpositional technique in which a rolled-up plantaris tendon was positioned at the base of the proximal phalanx. He reported an average increase in dorsiflexion of 42 degrees (Fig. 16–82A and B).

Although Hamilton et al[132] reported generally encouraging results with interpositional arthroplasty, further follow-up is needed to document

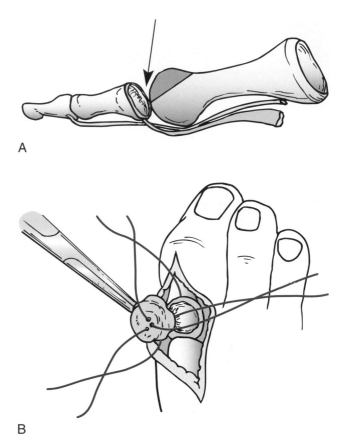

A

B

Figure 16–82 A, Cheilectomy and excavation of base of proximal phalanx as described by Barca.[9] **B,** Preparation of the anchovy for placement in the base of the proximal phalanx.

the long-term reliability of this procedure. Coughlin and Shurnas[68] reported the results of interposition arthroplasty on eight active younger patients (mean age of 40 years) with a minimum of four years of follow-up. They reported that all patients were satisfied with the procedure, although there was slight weakness in toe flexion power in most patients. No clear transfer lesions were noted, but two patients had mild pain in the second MTP joint and increased pressure beneath the second metatarsal as demonstrated by Harris mat studies. It was not clear if these two patients had subtle second MTP joint capsular instability prior to the index procedure or if this problem developed subsequent to their surgery. In any case, none of the patients had limits in activity and no further surgeries have been performed.

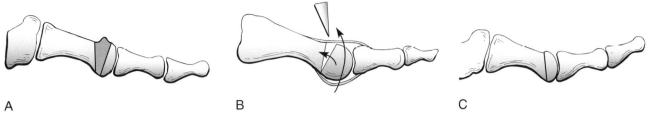

A

B

C

Figure 16–83 Diagram of Watermann osteotomy. **A,** Proposed closing wedge dorsal osteotomy. **B,** Rotation of the articular surface in the dorsal direction. **C,** Modified Watermann procedure with the osteotomy located more proximally.

FIRST METATARSAL OSTEOTOMY

Many osteotomy techniques have been described and recommended, but there are no long-term studies to substantiate their claims of successful treatment of hallux rigidus. However, there are studies that describe complications of these procedures; salvage options are difficult at best. Osteotomies of the first metatarsal have been advocated in the treatment of hallux rigidus.[39,74,80,180,354]

Eponyms have become commonplace in describing different osteotomy techniques. The *Watermann osteotomy* uses functional articular cartilage on the plantar first metatarsal head by rotating the metatarsal articular surface dorsally[39] by means of a dorsal closing wedge distal metatarsal osteotomy (Fig. 16–83). The *Green–Watermann osteotomy* (Fig. 16–84) plantar flexes the first metatarsal by means of a modified chevron osteotomy that can present a degenerated metatarsal cartilaginous surface to the articular base of the proximal phalanx. It can also lead to development of an intractable plantar keratosis beneath the first metatarsal head. Feldman[94] recommended the Green–Watermann osteotomy as the procedure of choice for hallux limitus, noting that it achieves success by means of a dorsal cheilectomy, plantar transposition of the

first metatarsal, and shortening of the first metatarsal.

A shortening osteotomy is said to relax periarticular structures[39] (Fig. 16–85). In theory, these osteotomies appear to offer realignment for hallux rigidus associated with an elevated first metatarsal. However, Jahss[157] stated that limited application exists for these osteotomies. No long-term studies substantiate claims that these procedures are efficacious.[312] Cavalo et al[39] reported on two cases and Youngswick[372] on 10 cases but with no long-term follow-up. Feldman[94] described the surgical procedure but presented no series. The original Watermann osteotomy[354] rotates the metatarsal articular surface dorsally. If metatarsus primus elevatus is present, further dorsiflexion is contraindicated. Complications from osteotomies have been reported and will be discussed later.

A plantar flexion osteotomy can depress an elevated first metatarsal, and Davies[74] and Bonney and MacNab[30] have recommended this type of procedure (Fig. 16–86). Davies[72] noted "very positive results" and stated this osteotomy can "re-establish normal function and preserve the first metatarsophalangeal joint cartilage." Again, no series has been presented on this technique. Shereff and Baumhauer[303] stated, "The lack of statistical methods in small retrospective case series make the confirmation

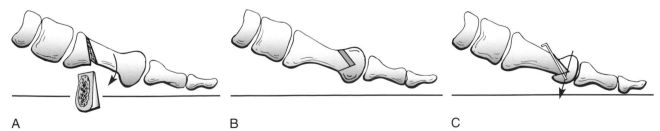

A

B

C

Figure 16–84 **A,** Plantar flexion closing wedge osteotomy presses first metatarsal. **B** and **C,** Green–Watermann osteotomy plantar flexes the first metatarsal by means of a modified chevron osteotomy.

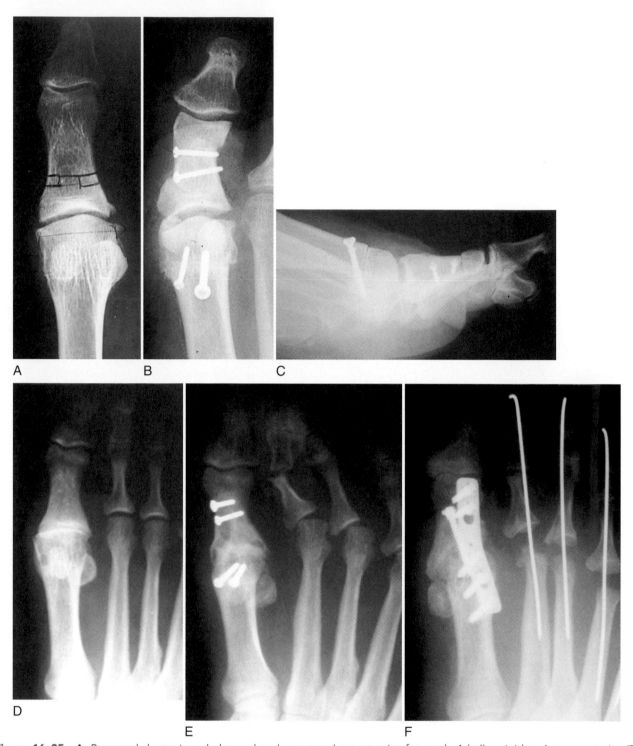

Figure 16–85   **A,** Proposed shortening phalangeal and metatarsal osteotomies for grade 1 hallux rigidus. Anteroposterior **(B)** and lateral **(C)** radiographs after shortening phalangeal and metatarsal osteotomies. **D,** Grade 4 hallux rigidus treated with attempted periarticular osteotomies. **E,** Complete chondrolysis, severe pain, and subluxation of lesser metatarsophalangeal (MTP) joints. **F,** Salvaged with MTP arthrodesis and forefoot arthroplasty.

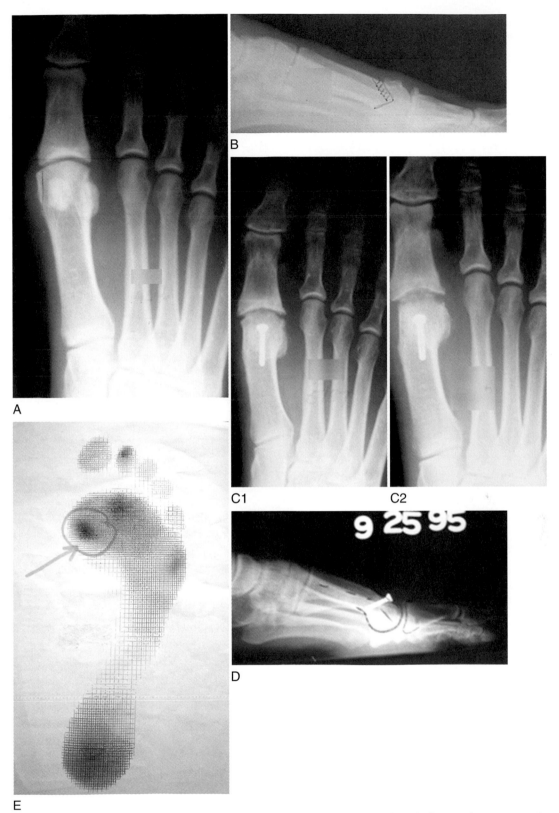

Figure 16–86 **A,** Preoperative anteroposterior (AP) radiograph demonstrates grade 1 hallux rigidus. **B,** Lateral radiograph demonstrates proposed plantar flexion osteotomy (modified Green–Watermann procedure). Note dorsal osteophytes on phalanx and metatarsal. There is no evidence of hallux metatarsus primus elevatus. Postoperative AP radiograph immediately after **(C1)** and 2 years after **(C2)** osteotomy. **D,** Lateral radiographs 3 years after plantar flexion osteotomy. **E,** Note the area of increased pressure beneath the first metatarsal head.

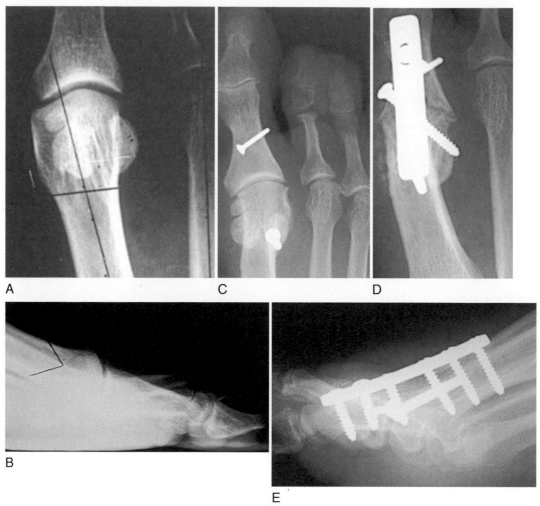

Figure 16–87 Anteroposterior (AP) **(A)** and lateral **(B)** radiographs demonstrate grade 1 hallux rigidus. **C,** After decompression shortening osteotomy of the proximal phalanx and first metatarsal. Postoperative AP **(D)** and lateral **(E)** radiographs after fusion for a painful first metatarsophalangeal joint.

of reported good results impossible" with osteotomy techniques. Horton et al[153] concluded that a plantar flexion osteotomy of the first metatarsal cannot be recommended based solely on the radiographic appearance of metatarsus primus elevatus.

Coughlin and Shurnas[66] found that any apparent elevation of the first metatarsal correlated with the grade of hallux rigidus and that it corrected to almost neutral on follow-up radiographs after either cheilectomy or arthrodesis. Therefore, we believe it is undesirable, in general, to perform a surgical procedure for the treatment of a secondary problem. Osteotomies designed to rotate good plantar cartilage into the joint space are done by employing a cheilectomy of the damaged cartilage surface, and thus the results of such

procedures must be compared to Mann's cheilectomy alone. As previously noted, the results reported by Coughlin and Shurnas[66] with Mann's cheilectomy alone in properly selected patients yielded a high percentage of good and excellent results (97%) at long-term follow-up (9.6 years). That leaves little room for improvement but rather bases the selection of an osteotomy procedure on a surgeon's anecdotal experience, with potentially substantial inherent complications that leave difficult salvage options.

Thus the results obtained with these procedures are difficult to interpret and compare because the authors have not documented results in detail. More research is needed to establish the indications, if any, and document results (Fig. 16–87).

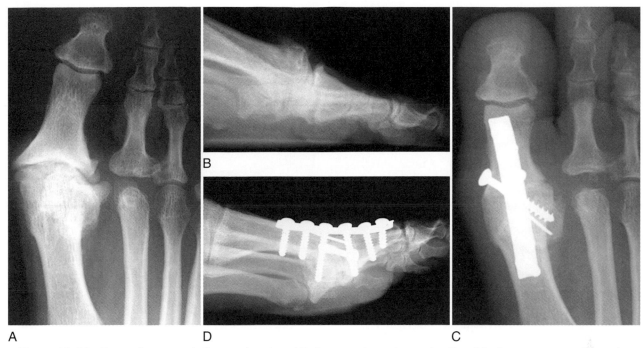

Figure 16–88 Fusion for severe hallux rigidus. **A** and **B,** Preoperative radiographs. **C** and **D,** Postoperative radiographs.

METATARSOPHALANGEAL JOINT ARTHRODESIS

Arthrodesis of the MTP joint for hallux rigidus has been advocated in several reports. This is a salvage procedure that may be used for grade 3 or 4 severe hallux rigidus. With this procedure the length and stability of the first metatarsal are preserved. The indications, besides hallux rigidus, are a failed implant, failed excisional arthroplasty, or failed osteotomy. Relatively few contraindications exist for arthrodesis, although careful counseling is necessary so patients can appreciate the restricted MTP motion that arthrodesis achieves.

Surgical Technique

1. The MTP joint is approached through a dorsal longitudinal incision.
2. Joint surfaces are prepared for arthrodesis by resection of the remaining cartilage and subchondral bone (video clip 29).
3. Various methods of internal fixation may be used depending on the surgeon's preference (Fig. 16–88; see also Fig. 16–35 and video clip 30).

Results and Complications

The success rate for MTP arthrodesis varies significantly depending on the preoperative diag-nosis, surgical technique, and method of internal fixation. Reported success rates vary from less than 77% to 100%.[30,55,56,60,61,89,113,212,352]

With cup-shaped surfaces, a high rate of fusion has been achieved. Coughlin and Abdo[60] reported subjective good or excellent results in 93% of patients; 98% of cases went on to fusion. Other authors have reported on a dorsal compression plate for MTP arthrodesis. von Salis-Soglio and Thomas[352] reported on 48 cases with a successful fusion rate of 92%, and Mankey and Mann[212] reported on 51 cases, also with a 92% fusion rate. Coughlin[55] reported on the use of a stainless steel small-fragment plate in 35 cases with a 100% fusion rate. The main advantage of rigid internal fixation is that it allows early ambulation in a postoperative shoe. Coughlin and Abdo[60] noted that hardware removal occurred infrequently (less than 7%) and that patient acceptance of an arthrodesis was quite high.

Coughlin and Shurnas[66] reported 32 successful fusions of 34 (94%) and 100% good or excellent results (including the two patients with a fibrous union) and a low complication rate at a mean of 6.7 years of follow-up after arthrodesis for end-stage hallux rigidus. A low-profile Vitallium plate was used for fixation after power reaming was used to create cup-shaped arthrodesis surfaces. Only two patients required hardware removal. Moreover, measured first ray mobility was significantly reduced after arthrodesis. Lombardi et al[206] have used first MTP joint arthrodesis with good results for lower grades of hallux rigidus and reported a high proportion of good and excellent results using only screws or Steinman pins (or both). They reported reliable improvement in radiographic measures of the first ray angular deformities at a mean of 28 months. Similarly, Ettl et al[89] found a 100% union rate with screw fixation or Kirschner-wire fixation (or both) with tension-band technique alone for end-stage hallux rigidus at a mean of 54 months of follow-up. The authors reported good functional results and significant pain reduction.

The main complications of arthrodesis are malalignment, nonunion, and degenerative arthritis of the interphalangeal joint of the hallux. In a review of 1451 cases in the literature, Coughlin[55] noted a 90% success rate of fusion. With an interfragmentary screw and dorsal plate, a fusion rate of 93% to 100% has been reported.[60] When nonunion occurs, it is often painless, and a fibrous union may be an acceptable result. Alignment of the arthrodesis site, however, is quite important.

Malunion in any plane is poorly tolerated, which underscores the need for meticulous attention to the final position of the arthrodesis. Malunion can occur in any one of three planes: In the frontal plane a varus/valgus malalignment can occur; in a sagittal plane a dorsiflexion/plantar flexion malalignment can develop; and in a transverse plane a rotational deformity may be noted. With excessive dorsiflexion, pain can occur at the tip of the toe, over the interphalangeal joint, and beneath the first metatarsal head. With inadequate dorsiflexion, the patient might feel pressure at the tip of the toe. Varus/valgus alignment is critical as well (Fig. 16–89).

Fitzgerald[98] observed an increased incidence of arthrosis at the interphalangeal joint with MTP fusion in less than 20 degrees of valgus. He noted a threefold increase in the prevalence of osteoarthrosis of the interphalangeal joint with a straighter toe. Nonetheless, 10 to 20 degrees of valgus is still thought to be an acceptable position. Furthermore, Coughlin[58] found that the dorsiflexion angle was a primary determinant on the degree of IP joint arthritis and noted that 22 degrees of dorsiflexion relative to the

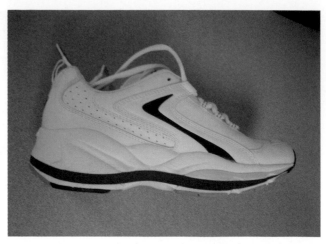

Figure 16–89   A rocker-bottom shoe can help ambulation in the patient whose first metatarsophalangeal joint was fused in inadequate dorsiflexion.

metatarsal had the lowest correlation with subsequent IP joint arthritis, whereas less dorsiflexion was associated with an increased incidence of IP joint degenerative arthritis.

METATARSOPHALANGEAL JOINT ARTHROPLASTY

First MTP joint replacement arthroplasty has been advocated for hallux rigidus, rheumatoid arthritis, and hallux valgus and as a salvage for failed first ray surgery.[327] Various implants composed of different materials have been manufactured to replace the base of the proximal phalanx, distal first metatarsal articular surface, or both. Initial attempts at proximal phalangeal articular replacement using metallic prostheses involved mainly case reports with limited follow-up[44,88,166,327] (Fig. 16–90A and B). Although Townley[340] reported a large series with long-term follow-up and generally satisfactory results, experience with metallic hemiprosthetic replacements has been limited, and this technique is not generally used at this time. Roukis and Townley[293] reported one-year follow-up on periarticular osteotomy in 16 feet compared with endoprosthetic replacement in nine feet. The authors showed minimal improvement in first MTP joint dorsiflexion with either technique, although pain relief was good.

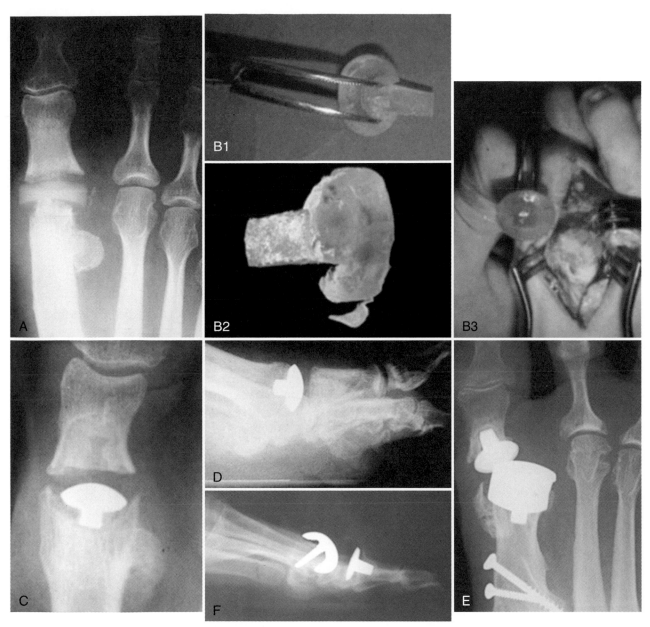

Figure 16–90 **A,** Radiograph demonstrates failed single-stem silicone arthroplasty. **B1** to **B3,** Failed silicone hemiarthroplasty implants. **C** and **D,** Failed cemented phalangeal and metatarsal implant with subsidence of the metatarsal component. **E** and **F,** Subluxation of the porous ingrowth component with loosening of the phalangeal implant 1 year after surgery. (**C** and **D** courtesy of K. Johnson, MD.)

Metal–Polyethylene Joint Replacements

Based on reported success with metal–polyethylene cemented total knee replacements, Johnson and Buck[164] designed a cemented nonconstraining first MTP total joint replacement. At greater than 3.5 years' follow-up of 21 feet, more than 50% implant loosening was noted, and the use of the implant was later discontinued[163] (Fig. 16–90C and D). Other reports have documented short-term experience.[28,185,187]

With short-term follow-up (18 months), Koenig[186] reported a 12% revision rate when repeat bony in-growth prostheses were implanted for revision of failed Silastic implants. In a larger study, Koenig and Horwitz[187] reported 61 implants that had been placed for a variety of indications. No information regarding long-term follow-up was provided (Fig. 16–90E and F). Likewise, Freed[106] reported that more than 360 implants have been placed to revise failed silicone implants, but again, no information on the subjective or objective results was reported.

Ess et al[88] reported 5 excellent, 1 good, 2 fair, and 1 poor results with 2 years of follow-up after total endoprosthetic replacement (ReFlexion). Radiographic loosening was noted on one cementless phalangeal component, one prosthetic subluxation, one superficial infection and one recurrent severe valgus deformity. Only long-term follow-up will provide further information as to whether these uncemented first MTP total joint replacements will have greater success than the cemented MTP joint replacements implanted during the 1970s and 1980s. The paucity of information available with even short-term subjective and objective results makes use of these implants questionable until investigators report further information. Metal–polyethylene total joint replacement of the first MTP joint has fallen into disfavor with the use of silicone elastomer joint replacement.

Silicone Elastomer Joint Replacement

The major experience with first MTP joint replacement was initiated with the introduction of the silicone elastomer hemiphalangeal implant by Swanson.[327] Initially described as safe and simple, it was offered as the preferred method for surgical treatment of hallux rigidus.[330] Touted as biocompatible and inert, early in vitro studies and in vivo studies by Swanson et al[330] and others[4,33] led to widespread use. Later reports of single-stem implant failure[200,350] heralded the introduction of the double-stem silicone elastomer implant,[354] which also was greeted with great enthusiasm. Freed[106] has estimated that more than 2 million first MTP joint hinged silicone implants were implanted over the following two decades. Initial in vivo studies reporting few failures gave the impression that silicone elastomer implants would perform satisfactorily over a long-term period. Later studies with longer follow-up have demonstrated higher failure rates (57% to 74%).[106,125]

Failure of an elastomer implant can occur for many reasons.[348,349] Intrinsic failure can result from the physical property of the materials, as evidenced by implant deformation, fatigue fracture, and microfragmentation. Intrinsic failure can occur with the use of a joint implant in a situation that exceeds the implant's design capability (e.g., younger patient, insufficient soft tissue, or bone realignment with hallux valgus deformity). When implant surgery is considered, the need for soft tissue[125,302,329] and bone balancing[44,170,186,250,266,302] cannot be overemphasized.

The viability of the silicone prosthesis appears to be directly related to the length of time it has been implanted. In early studies, Swanson[327] reported no fracture of hemistem and double-stem components, LaPorta et al[195] (average 1 year follow-up) noted only two fractures in 536 implants, and others[4,78,250] with relatively short-term studies found fractures to be uncommon. Implant deformation with eventual fracture has been widely reported in other series. Granberry et al[125] hypothesized that this is caused by the cumulative effect of cyclic loading of large forces (body weight) on the implant (Fig. 16–91).

Reported complications include avascular necrosis, infection, transfer metatarsalgia,[120,125,250,295] delayed wound healing,[304] recurrent deformity,[148,232] bone proliferation, bone resorption (Fig. 16–92A), subchondral cyst formation, implant displacement (Fig. 16–92B), and interphalangeal joint penetration of the silicone stem.[12]

Granberry et al[125] reported a twofold increase in lateral metatarsal weight bearing compared with the contralateral foot after first MTP joint replacement. Initial hopes that joint replace-

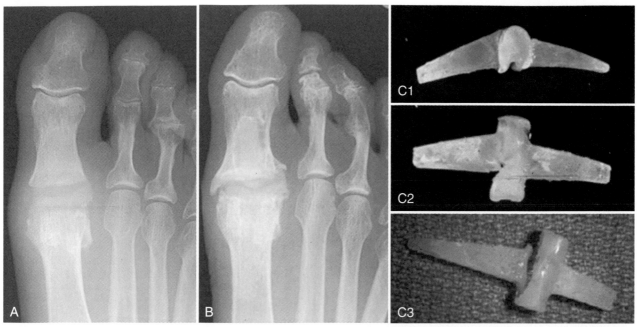

Figure 16–91 A, Radiograph demonstrates placement of double-stem silicone implant. **B,** Seven-year follow-up radiograph shows failed implant with silicone synovitis and bony resorption. **C1** to **C3,** Example of failures of double-stem implants.

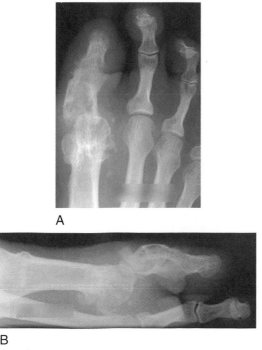

Figure 16–92 A, Anteroposterior radiograph demonstrates bone resorption. **B,** Oblique radiograph demonstrates implant displacement.

ment would facilitate a normal gait pattern[330] were high, but the authors[125] found that normal plantar weight bearing with standing was not restored and that weakened plantar-flexion power decreased toe purchase. Pain relief[330] as a primary indication for joint replacement has been reported, but with inconsistent results. Freed[106] reported moderate and severe first MTP pain in 16 of 51 joints (31%) following MTP arthroplasty. Based on survivorship analysis, Granberry et al[125] predicted a 50% failure rate with a hinged silicone implant component at 4 years.

Swanson et al[330] stated that MTP silicone replacement arthroplasty allowed good joint mobility, but limited range of motion of the hallux has been observed in several series.[78,106,125,135,254] Increased bony overgrowth in the periprosthetic region is associated with decreased range of motion.[78,125] Granberry et al[125] reported that 30% of cases in his series had less than 15 degrees of total MTP joint motion, and Freed[106] reported 33 of 51 (65%) had less than 20 degrees of motion.

The biocompatibility of silicone elastomer appears to be the greatest long-term problem. Initially thought to be inert and associated with little or no tissue reaction,[327,328,330] silicone elastomer in small particle form (1 to 100 μm) leads to a significant inflammatory response. Hemiarthroplasty articulation with a degenerated incongruent metatarsal articular surface is thought to cause abrasion and microscopic particle formation.[12,36,119,200,366] Particulate synovitis has been reported with both upper- and lower-extremity implants. Gordon and Bullough[119] observed a reactive synovitis and foreign body giant cell reaction both in soft tissue and in intramedullary bone. Freed[106] has cited 64 different reports questioning the long-term viability of first MTP joint silicone elastomer implants.

Shards of silicone generated by shear and compressive forces lead to synovitis,[232,348,349] which is followed by encapsulation of these fragments both intracellularly and extracellularly. This florid synovial and periarticular soft tissue reaction is characterized by foreign body giant cell reaction.[170,261] Medical-grade silicone has been reported to be innocuous and benign,[328] but this evaluation applies to non-fragmented implants.[52] Stress and fatigue, joint overuse, poor fit, abrasion of joint surfaces, and pistoning of the prosthesis can lead to microfragmentation. Migration of these microscopic silicone fragments can occur through the lymphatic system,[119] with secondary adenopathy as a foreign body reaction. Lymphadenopathy has been reported in association with silicone elastomer failure in a number of series.

Although joint replacement has been recommended as a means of preserving great toe length,[330] Verhaar[350] and Granberry et al[125] have reported shortening of 3 to 11 mm in follow-up studies after first MTP implant placement. Granberry et al[125] observed increased shortening with longer follow-up; the shortening resulted from resorption of bone and collapse of the prosthesis.

Many implants have functioned well with little or no reactivity on a long-term basis; however, the number of complications reported raises questions regarding the viability of long-term survival of silicone elastomer first MTP implants.[148] Papagelopoulos et al[263] reported that patient age affected survivorship of the implant in 79 patients and reported 90% implant survivorship at 10 years in patients older than 57 years at the time of surgery and 82% survivorship when patients younger than 57 years of age underwent surgery. Radiographically, 40% of

feet demonstrated bone resorption, 9% had cysts, 25% had severe implant wear, and 3% had obvious implant fracture.

Townley and Taranow[340] and others[125,227] have stated that silicone possesses neither the biologic surface characteristics nor the structural durability to withstand the tension and shear stresses at the first MTP joint (associated with normal ambulatory activity). Others have noted that the implant is not durable,[125] and McCarthy and Chapman[227] reported that with the growing body of information, silicone elastomer may be unsuitable for weight-bearing joints. There is now a shift toward implantation with titanium grommets to reduce stress on the silicone elastomer, but longer-term results are pending. Likewise, long-term results with cemented MTP replacements have not been satisfactory.[232]

Freed[106] has estimated that more than 2 million hinged silicone implants have been placed over a two-decade period, and he estimates that three quarters of the implants in his series required removal. These estimates make it evident that revision surgery will be a common occurrence in many of these patients. Needelman et al[254] stated that a considerable number of revisions of MTP joint implants are occurring each year.

Salvage of Joint Replacement

Implants have introduced a whole new series of complications and have necessitated innovative salvage techniques.

The choices regarding surgical salvage depend on the disease present. With significant synovitis and joint reaction (characterized by swelling, pain, soft tissue thickening, infection, or radiographic evidence of bony encroachment or osteolysis), implant removal, debridement, and synovectomy may be indicated. Implant removal often leads to joint fibrosis with shortening of the first ray and decreased range of motion. Nonetheless, this can lead to a relatively stable joint and, with minimal pain, can be an acceptable result. Others have advocated revision of a failed silicone elastomer implant with a total joint revision. McDonald et al[228] and Perlman et al[266] recommended revision of a hemicomponent implant to a double-stem component but reported failure of the revision second silicone component as well. Koenig[186] reported installing a metal–polyethylene component to replace a failed silicone elastomer implant but noted a 40% failure rate. Freed[106] reported 360 metal–polyethylene implants placed for failed silicone implants but provided no follow-up.

Another option after failed MTP joint implant is first MTP arthrodesis following removal of the failed components. Fusion may be difficult to achieve because of poor bone quality. The need for supplemental bone graft and prolonged immobilization may be necessary before bony union is achieved. When successful, arthrodesis can achieve a stable first ray with improved weight-bearing function. Myerson et al[252] reported their results on 24 patients (mean age of 46 years) using interposition autograft (proximal tibia or iliac crest) or allograft interposition arthrodesis with plate and screw fixation or Steinman pins (or both), Kirschner wires for failed metatarsal osteotomy, silicone arthroplasty, total joint replacement, and Keller resection. The authors reported two painless fibrous unions and three painful nonunions that were successfully revised to solid fusion. The authors underscored the technical challenge of salvaging these difficult cases. Indications for first MTP joint replacement arthroplasty with a double-stem silicone elastic implant remain severe degenerative joint disease in older, more sedentary patients or household ambulators for whom excisional arthroplasty and MTP fusion are not acceptable options.

Surgical Technique[327,329,330]

1. A dorsomedial longitudinal skin incision is centered over the MTP joint.
2. A proximally based capsular flap is developed, exposing the MTP joint.
3. An oscillating saw is used to remove 3 to 4 mm of the articular surface of the metatarsal head and 2 mm of the base of the proximal phalanx (Fig. 16–93A).
4. Any osteophytes in the area of the metatarsal metaphysis are resected.
5. With a power bur, the intramedullary canal is enlarged for placement of the phalangeal and metatarsal intramedullary silicone stems.
6. A trial reduction with various-sized MTP implants is performed to choose the appropriate size. Oversized implants should be avoided. The stem of the implant should fit well into the prepared canal, allowing the

transverse midsection of the implant to abut against the prepared phalangeal and metatarsal surfaces (Fig. 16–93B).

7. Some surgeons may select a titanium grommet to minimize adjacent wear at the silicone hinged-stem interface.
8. With an enlarged 1-2 intermetatarsal angle, a proximal first metatarsal osteotomy may be necessary. With significant valgus alignment of the first MTP joint, soft tissue balancing is mandatory because the double-stem implant does not provide sufficient stability to achieve joint alignment.
9. With placement of the appropriate-sized silicone prosthesis, the first MTP joint should be aligned properly in slight valgus, and the intramedullary stem should be well seated.
10. The joint capsule is closed with an interrupted absorbable suture. Sutures may be used to secure the phalangeal and metatarsal capsule, with drill holes placed in the metaphyseal region to anchor the capsular repair. The skin is approximated in a routine manner (Fig. 16–93C).

Postoperative Care

A gauze-and-tape compression dressing is applied at surgery and changed every 7 to 10

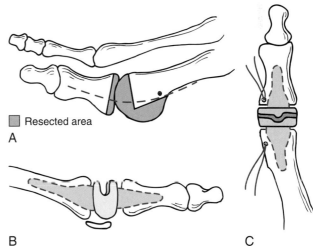

Resected area

A

B   C

Figure 16–93 **A,** Dorsomedial longitudinal skin incision is used to approach the metatarsophalangeal joint. A sagittal saw is used to remove 2 mm of bone from the base of the proximal phalanx and medial eminence and 3 to 4 mm of distal metatarsal articular surface. **B,** After broaching of the canal, the double-stem implant is placed. **C,** Capsule is repaired with interrupted closure. Drill holes in the base of the proximal phalanx and in the metatarsal metaphysis may be used to secure the capsule closure.

days. Mobilization of the MTP joint is important to achieve adequate dorsiflexion and plantar flexion after the surgical procedure. Physical or occupational therapy may be advantageous in regaining range of motion and strength at the first MTP joint.

FIRST METATARSOPHALANGEAL IMPLANT RESECTION ARTHROPLASTY

Indications for resection arthroplasty of the first MTP joint are a failed joint implant caused by infection, chronic synovitis, pain, and severe hallux rigidus in an older, sedentary patient in whom an arthrodesis is not an acceptable option.

Surgical Technique

1. A dorsal longitudinal incision is centered over the first MTP joint along the medial border of the extensor hallucis longus tendon. Z-plasty or lengthening of the tendon may be necessary to expose the MTP joint.
2. The hypertrophic synovium and pseudocapsule are excised, exposing the silicone implant.
3. After the implant is removed, a complete synovectomy excises thickened synovium in the periarticular area (Fig. 16–94A).
4. The intramedullary area is curetted to remove remaining synovial tissue.
5. If an excisional arthroplasty is desired, two 0.062-inch Kirschner wires are introduced at the MTP joint and driven distally through the tip of the toe. An alternative is crossed Kirschner wire fixation to stabilize the MTP joint (Fig. 16–94B). They are then driven in a retrograde manner into the first metatarsal head to stabilize the hallux. (In the presence of infection, internal fixation is not used.) The pins are bent at the tip of the toe to prevent proximal migration. Crossed Kirschner wires are cut off level with the surface of the skin.
6. The soft tissue and skin are approximated with an interrupted closure.

Postoperative Care

A gauze-and-tape compression dressing is applied at surgery and changed at 10-day intervals for 6 weeks. The patient is allowed to ambulate in the postoperative shoe. Intramedullary pins are removed three to four weeks after surgery.

FIRST METATARSOPHALANGEAL INTERPOSITIONAL ARTHRODESIS[145]

Surgical Technique

1. Similar incision, dissection, and debridement are performed as discussed previously for excisional arthroplasty.
2. A bicortical or tricortical graft is obtained from the iliac crest (Fig. 16–95). The graft is shaped to fit the desired gap (defect) at the MTP joint. Cancellous bone is packed into defects in the intramedullary canals. Often the bicortical or tricortical shaft is trapezoidal (wider plantarward and medially, narrower on dorsolateral aspect) to allow varus/valgus and dorsiflexion/plantar flexion at the fusion site (Fig. 16–94C to E; video clip 30).
3. Internal fixation is determined by the quality of the phalangeal metatarsal bone as well as the length of the bone graft (Fig. 16–96).
4. Axial Steinmann pins or mini-fragment plate fixation may be used for fixation depending on the surgeon's preference (Fig. 16–97).
5. With plate fixation, a low-profile revision plate (Integra) may be used and placed on the dorsomedial/dorsolateral aspect of the proximal phalanx and first metatarsal (Fig. 16–98). (See the discussion of arthrodesis in the rheumatoid arthritis section earlier in this chapter.)

Postoperative Care

A gauze-and-tape dressing is applied at surgery and changed every 10 days for 8 weeks. The patient is allowed to ambulate in a wooden-soled shoe with weight bearing on the heel and the lateral aspect of the foot. When Steinmann pins are placed, they are typically removed 16 weeks after surgery under local anesthesia after radiographic confirmation of a successful fusion. Plates may be removed if they are symptomatic, but the use of low-profile Vitallium plates often makes this unnecessary.

Results and Complications

Kitaoka et al[183] reported on excisional arthroplasty as a revision technique for silicone implant failure (average follow-up, 3.5 years). At surgery the implant was removed and a joint debridement was performed. At long-term follow-up, 80% good and excellent results were reported. No significant alignment changes

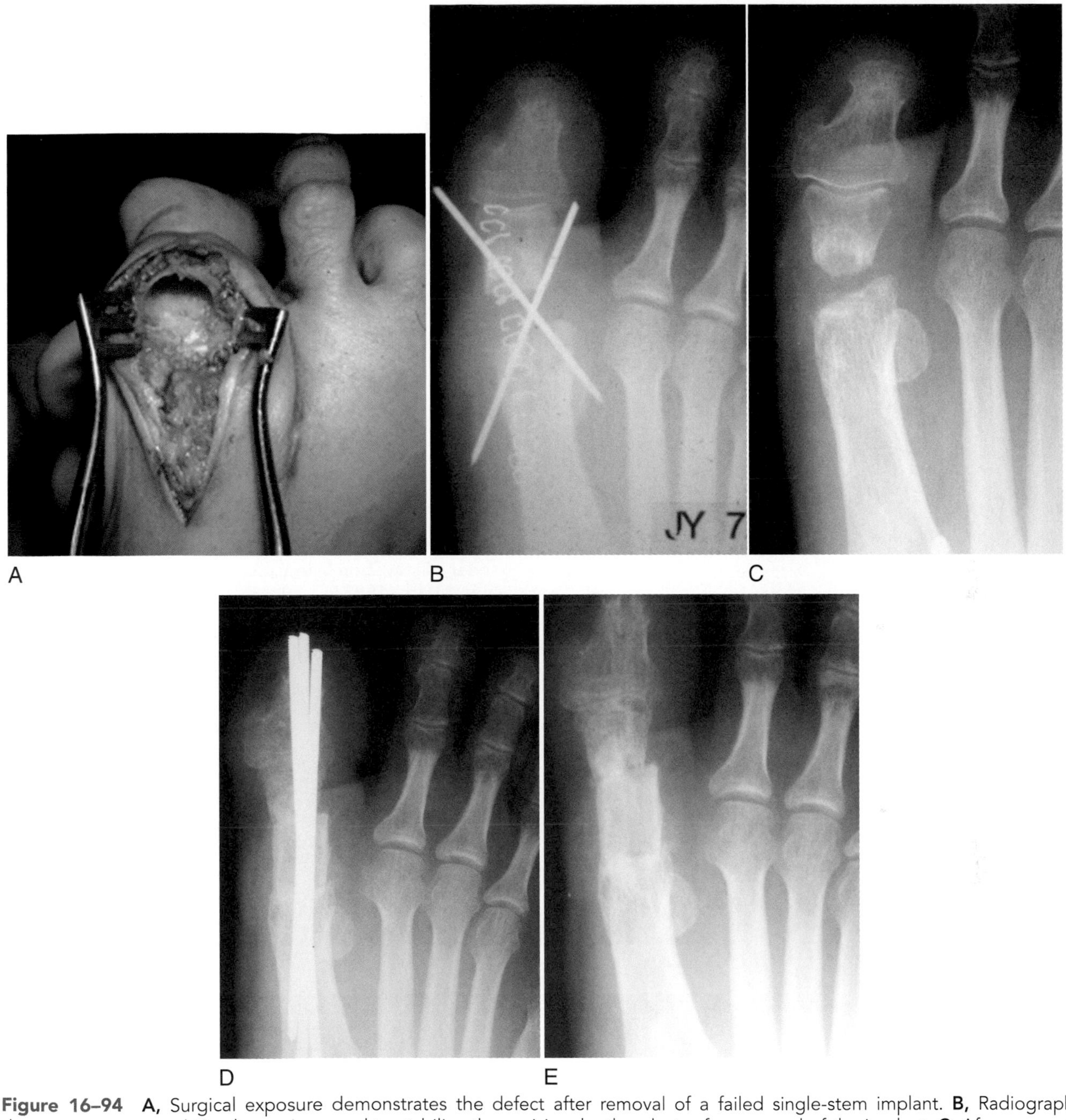

Figure 16–94 A, Surgical exposure demonstrates the defect after removal of a failed single-stem implant. **B,** Radiograph demonstrates crossed Kirschner wires used to stabilize the excisional arthroplasty after removal of the implant. **C,** After removal of Kirschner wires. **D,** Interpositional graft and arthrodesis with internal fixation. **F,** A successful fusion following removal of internal fixation.

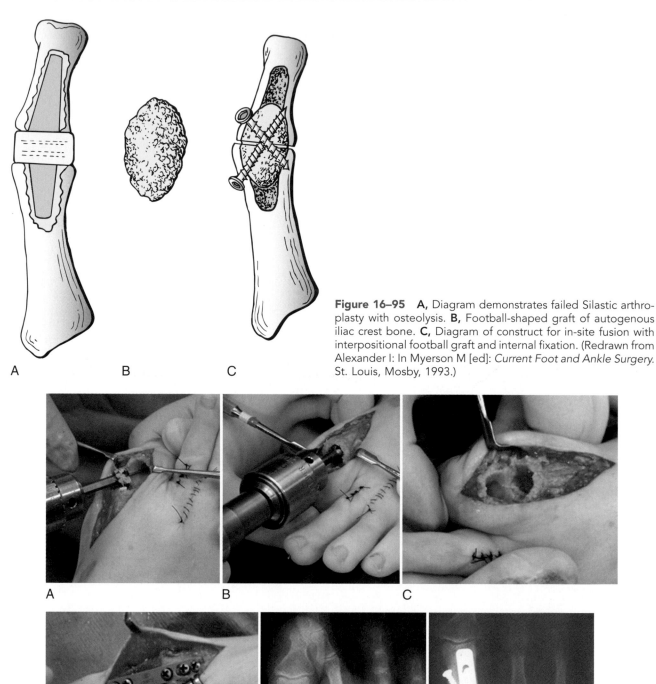

Figure 16–95   A, Diagram demonstrates failed Silastic arthroplasty with osteolysis. **B,** Football-shaped graft of autogenous iliac crest bone. **C,** Diagram of construct for in-site fusion with interpositional football graft and internal fixation. (Redrawn from Alexander I: In Myerson M [ed]: *Current Foot and Ankle Surgery.* St. Louis, Mosby, 1993.)

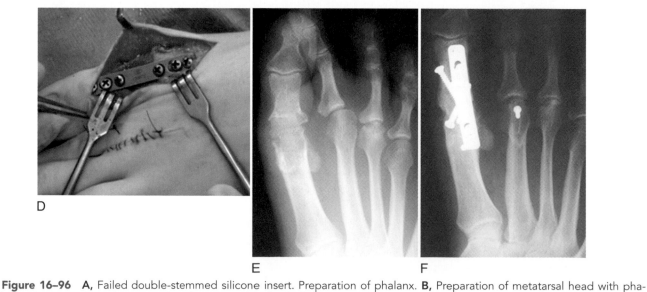

Figure 16–96   A, Failed double-stemmed silicone insert. Preparation of phalanx. **B,** Preparation of metatarsal head with phalangeal reamer. **C,** Both prepared surfaces. **D,** After football-shaped graft is inserted, a dorsal plate established adequate fixation of the arthrodesis site and graft. **E,** Preoperative radiograph. **F,** After arthrodesis with interposition graft.

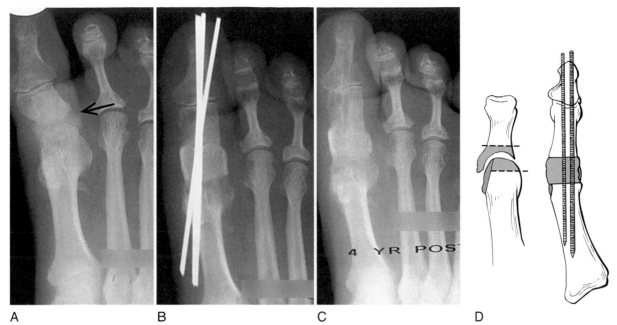

Figure 16–97 **A,** Anteroposterior radiograph demonstrates failed hemisilicone implant with shortening and extrusion of component. **B,** Radiograph after interpositional iliac crest arthrodesis. **C,** Radiograph 7 years after surgery demonstrates successful arthrodesis. **D,** Diagram of salvage arthrodesis.

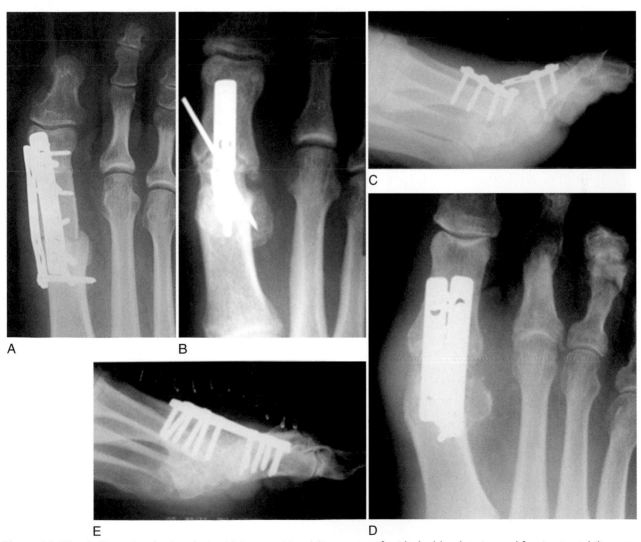

Figure 16–98 **A,** Example of arthrodesis with interpositional iliac crest graft with double-plate internal fixation to stabilize autograft. **B** and **C,** Failure of internal fixation and nonunion. **D** and **E,** Salvage with double dorsal plate technique.

907

occurred, probably because of postoperative periarticular fibrosis. The authors noted decreased pressure beneath the tip of the hallux, decreased MTP range of motion, and a tendency toward hallux extensus.

With single-plate or dual-plate fixation, a strong mechanical construct is created to protect the intercalary bone graft. With Steinmann pin fixation, two or three Steinmann pins are used to "shish-kebob" the phalanx, graft, and first metatarsal[63] (Fig. 16–99). Steinmann pins are introduced at the prepared surface of the proximal phalangeal base and driven distally across the interphalangeal joint, exiting the tip of the toe. The pins are then retrograded longitudinally through the graft and into the metatarsal head and metatarsal metaphysis. The threaded pins are cut with 1/8 inch protruding from the tip of the toe to aid in later pin removal.

Arthrodesis in the salvage of a failed Keller procedure was reported both with primary fusion and with an intercalary bone graft.[63] Five cases were reported in which an interpositional graft was used for the salvage of a failed excisional arthroplasty. All five cases went on to a successful fusion. No significant complications were noted, although this extensive type of salvage carries an increased risk of failure. Wound necrosis, infection, and delayed union or nonunion of the intercalary graft can lead to failure of the salvage technique (Fig. 16–100). A fibrous union can leave an acceptable result with some residual motion. However, infection or wound problems can eventually lead to toe amputation or ray resection as an ultimate salvage procedure. Myerson's technique,[252] as noted earlier, produced reliable results and an acceptable union rate with autograft or allograft interposition as a salvage procedure for failed implants, resection arthroplasty, or metatarsal osteotomy.

The placement of longitudinal Steinmann pins for stabilization of a first MTP fusion in which the threaded pins have crossed the interphalangeal

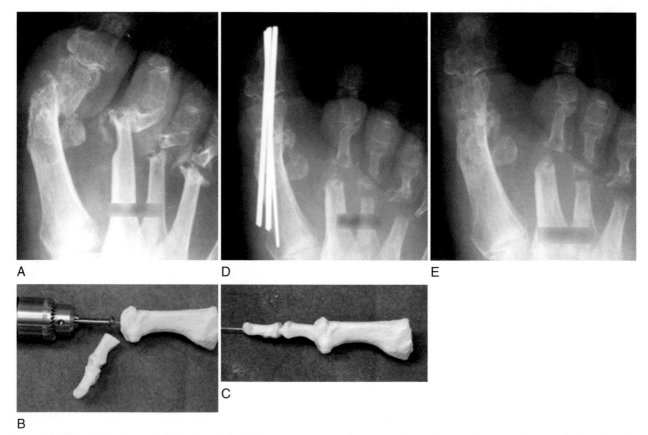

A   D   E

B   C

Figure 16–99   A, Radiograph following failed Keller resection arthroplasty. **B** and **C,** Technique of peg-in-hole arthrodesis demonstrated with sawbones model. A power phalangeal reamer is used to create a hole in the metatarsal head. **D,** Fixation with axial Steinman pins. **E,** Following successful fusion of the metatarsophalangeal joint.

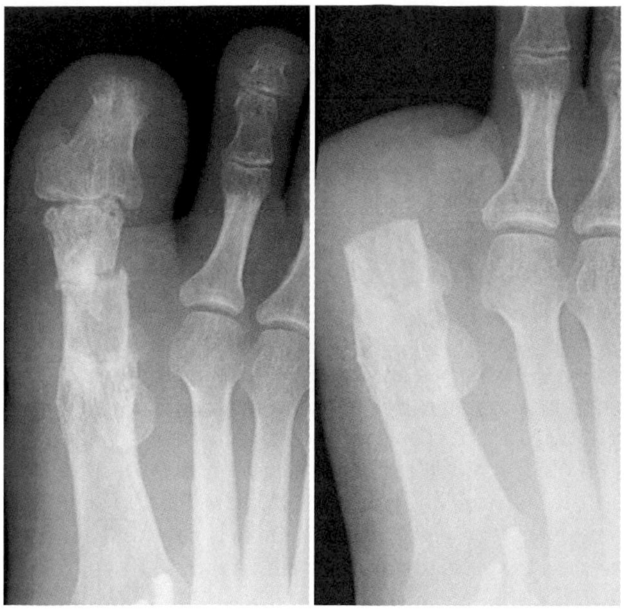

Figure 16–100 **A,** Following removal of hardware after interposition iliac crest graft and arthrodesis. **B,** Following amputation for subsequent infection following arthrodesis attempt (follow-up of case illustrated in Figure 16–90E and F). Interposition arthrodesis salvage procedures are difficult and can be fraught with significant complications.

joint has been associated with an inordinately high rate of radiographic interphalangeal joint degenerative arthritis. Nonetheless, it may be necessary to use this longitudinal pin fixation technique in the presence of significant bone loss or osteoporosis.[54] Often when this type of fixation is necessary, minimal interphalangeal joint motion is present. Mann and Thompson[221] reported a 65% incidence of interphalangeal joint arthritis with this technique, although they did not believe the observed arthrosis was clinically significant. Mann and Schakel[220] reported a 60% incidence of interphalangeal arthritis, but only one third of patients were symptomatic.

Shereff and Jahss[304] stated that because of the high biomechanical demands placed on the first MTP joint and the complex joint interactions of the first ray, routine use of joint replacement arthroplasty cannot be recommended for the first ray until consistently good or excellent results over time are obtained. It does not appear that such results are forthcoming, and the high rate of complications associated with MTP implant surgery reported in long-term follow-up has dampened the initial enthusiasm for prosthetic replacement of the first MTP joint. This enthusiasm has been supplanted by caution in the placement of implants in younger, more active patients. Implants may still be considered in older, more sedentary patients. The options of cheilectomy and excisional arthroplasty and even arthrodesis appear much less onerous than the occasional significant complications associated with various implant arthroplasties.

We strongly recommend against implant arthroplasty. We have had experiences similar to those reported by Myerson et al[252] in treating failures of implants, metatarsal osteotomies, and resection arthroplasties. We conclude that such cases present a substantial surgical challenge to achieve an acceptable salvage. Appropriate use of MTP implant arthroplasty for the correct narrow indications[135] with meticulous surgical technique will significantly reduce the frequency of this surgery as well as the morbidity and high complication rate reported in some series.[71,242]

DEGENERATIVE ARTHRITIS OF THE MIDFOOT

Anatomy and Progression

Degenerative arthritis of the first metatarsocuneiform (MTC) joint is often the result of trauma. It may be a sequela of Lisfranc's joint fracture or dislocation, but arthrosis can develop spontaneously in the midfoot as a sequela of osteoarthritis or inflammatory arthritis. In either situation, an extremely disabling condition develops because of stress placed on the longitudinal arch with weight bearing. Progressive pain and progression of a pes planus deformity can make ambulation difficult. A moderate degree of bony proliferation can cause a prominence on the dorsal aspect of the midfoot, which makes wearing shoes difficult. A progressive flatfoot deformity can also develop from instability of the MTC joint, with development of a plantar bony prominence and subsequent callus formation (Fig. 16–101). With progressive deformity, an abduction and dorsiflexion deformity of the midfoot occurs.

In evaluating a patient with arthritis of the MTC joint who cannot recall a history of trauma, the physician should be cognizant that this can represent an early Charcot's deformity (joint). Charcot's arthropa-

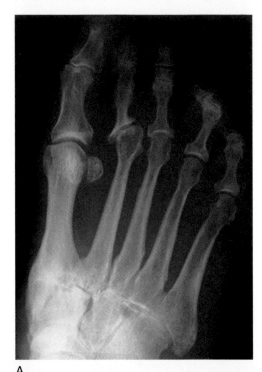

A

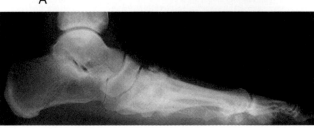

B

Figure 16–101   Anteroposterior **(A)** and lateral **(B)** radiographs demonstrate degenerative arthritis of the midfoot.

In examination of the foot, passive manipulation of the midfoot involves abduction of the forefoot and a pronation stress test to determine the location of maximal pain. The piano key test, which uses dorsal cantilever stress at each of the tarsometatarsal articulations, is a sensitive indicator of a symptomatic joint or joints.[179]

Treatment

Conservative management of midfoot degenerative arthritis includes a soft or rigid custom-molded orthosis that provides support to the longitudinal arch. This may aid in ambulation. Shoe modifications include a stiff insole and a rocker-bottom outer sole that may be added to the shoe to improve ambulation. A polypropylene AFO may be used for more advanced degenerative arthrosis. Cast immobilization and occa-

thy can develop with diabetes as well as with peripheral neuropathy and other neurologic disorders (Fig. 16–102).

Anatomically the tarsometatarsal joint is divided into three columns: the medial column (first MTC joint), the middle column (second and third MTC joints), and the lateral column (fourth and fifth metatarsocuboid joints). Radiographically the medial column is reduced when the medial border of the first metatarsal is aligned with the medial border of the medial cuneiform. The middle column is aligned when the medial border of the second metatarsal is aligned with the medial border of the intermediate cuneiform. For the lateral column, reduction is achieved when the medial border of the fourth metatarsal is aligned with the medial border of the cuboid. On the lateral radiograph, restoration of the first metatarsal declination angle and arch height are imperative.

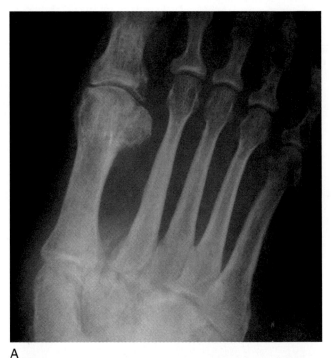

A

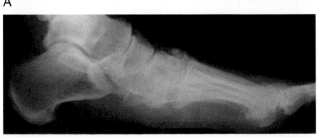

B

Figure 16–102   Anteroposterior **(A)** and lateral **(B)** radiographs demonstrate Charcot's joint in a patient with long-term diabetes. This is a painful, progressive deformity.

sionally a short-leg brace may be used to diminish pain. Unfortunately, as arthritis of the MTC joint progresses with subsequent loss of the longitudinal arch and abduction of the forefoot, the use of AFOs becomes more limited. An AFO does not reorient the foot but does add support and stability to the foot (see Chapter 4). In time and with progression of deformity, surgical intervention is indicated.

A complicating factor with midfoot arthropathy is a simultaneous hindfoot deformity. Malalignment at the transverse tarsal joint and a valgus deformity of the hindfoot often are associated with severe midfoot arthritis. A careful preoperative physical examination is necessary to determine the extent of the midfoot and hindfoot malalignment. In the subtle cavus foot with degenerative arthritis, the Coleman block test helps to determine the need for associated hindfoot procedures such as the addition of a calcaneal osteotomy or creation of plantar flexion through the first MTC joint with the arthrodesis. Correctable or supple hindfoot valgus associated with medial column arthritis should reduce with proper restoration of alignment (reduction of any varus or rotational deformity, abduction, and dorsiflexion) during the midfoot arthrodesis but any fixed or residual valgus deformity without arthritis should be addressed with a medial displacement osteotomy or lateral column lengthening. Moreover, gastrocnemius recession or Achilles lengthening may be necessary after correction is achieved and bone alignment is restored to obtain a plantigrade foot.

Surgery consists of an arthrodesis of the involved midfoot joints. Most often the second and third metatarsal middle cuneiform joints are involved. The first metatarsal–medial cuneiform articulation is involved less often and the fourth and fifth metatarsocuboid articulation least often.[188,272] The intercuneiform articulation may be involved, and if any doubt exists, Mann et al[219] suggest incorporating the intercuneiform joint within the arthrodesis.

In the patient with a pes planus deformity and abduction of the forefoot, it is important to reestablish the normal alignment of the midfoot at surgery. This is accomplished by bringing the medial Lisfranc joint into normal alignment with the hindfoot by adducting and plantar flexing the first, second, and third MTC articulations. Although a lateral column arthrodesis is much more difficult to achieve, on occasion it may be necessary to realign the entire Lisfranc's joint in the presence of severe deformity. Komenda et al[188] recommended reduction of the lateral column and temporary pin fixation until ambulation is initiated. They found a lateral column arthrodesis typically is unnecessary even in the presence of arthrosis (see Chapter 20).

Promising results have been obtained with interposition arthroplasty for lateral column arthritis,[22] and this procedure may be used as a second-stage procedure if needed for continued symptoms. Alternatively, reliable results have been reported with arthrodesis of the fourth and fifth tarsometatarsal joints as isolated procedures or in combination with medial column arthrodesis for neuropathic conditions.[272]

The potential concern with lateral midfoot arthrodesis as part of a medial column or central column procedure is that it creates an extremely rigid midfoot. In neuropathic conditions it may be necessary to achieve the additional stability afforded by inclusion of the lateral column joints, but in post-traumatic or inflammatory cases we prefer to avoid arthrodesis of the lateral column.

Whether to perform reduction of a midfoot deformity has been a controversial topic. Johnson and Johnson[162] reported on patients with mild and moderate midfoot deformities (Fig. 16–103). They performed in situ fusions using Kirschner wire internal fixation with a supplemental autogenous iliac crest graft technique. Nine of 13 patients (70%) reported good or excellent results and three nonunions. The most often fused joints were the second and third tarsometatarsal (66%) joints.

In a review of 16 patients, Sangeorzan et al[296] advocated reduction of the pes planus and abduction deformity and noted 11 of 16 cases with satisfactory results

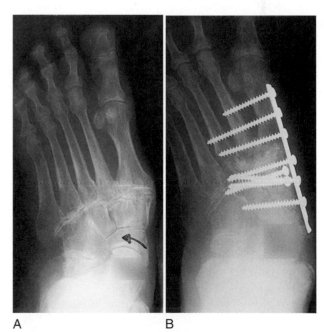

A   B

Figure 16–103 Preoperative **(A)** and postoperative **(B)** radiographs of midfoot arthrodesis for degenerative arthrosis without correction of the deformity.

(69%). Few patients had excellent results or a normal foot, but many "returned to work."

Horton and Olney[152] performed three in situ fusions and six realignment arthrodeses on eight patients (nine feet) for post-traumatic or degenerative arthrosis of Lisfranc's joint. They used a five-hole, one-third semitubular plate that spanned the tarsometatarsal joint. An iliac crest graft was packed into the intervals between the tarsometatarsal joints and between the first and second metatarsals. The authors noted a strong correlation between reduction of the deformity and the outcome and reported seven of nine good and excellent results.

Mann et al[219] reported that 38 of 41 patients with primary, traumatic, or inflammatory arthrosis of the midfoot were satisfied. They advocated reduction of the deformity. Eleven patients had an autogenous bone graft placed at the time of arthrodesis (Fig. 16–104).

Komenda et al[188] and Sangeorzan et al[296] recommend that the lateral column not be included in the arthrodesis, because this area is usually asymptomatic even with significant radiographic evidence of arthrosis. They emphasized that realignment of the midfoot contributes to a successful result. Komenda et al[188] stated that if there is 15 degrees of malalignment in the transverse or sagittal plane or greater than 2 mm of displacement, reduction of the deformity is indicated. They did use temporary internal fixation when the lateral column was realigned but did not routinely perform arthrodesis for the lateral column.

Shereff et al[303] reported 81% successful results using iliac crest bone graft and Kirschner wire fixation in 16 patients. They found that fusion of the fourth and fifth TMT joints was associated with significantly poorer functional and subjective scores.

Whether to include the intercuneiform articulations depends on inspection of these areas for arthrosis. Sangeorzan et al[296] infrequently incorporated the intercuneiform joints (one of 16), whereas Mann et al[219] and Horton and Olney[152] incorporated them in the arthrodesis technique more often. Mann et al[219] stated that if the viability of the intercuneiform articulation is in question, it is better to include it in the arthrodesis.

The use of an autogenous iliac crest graft often increases the success rate of arthrodesis. Sangeorzan et al[296] stated that an additional graft was not necessary. Komenda et al[188] used an ancillary graft in one third of cases and Mann et al[219] in one fourth of cases.

We prefer to avoid using iliac crest unless structural defects require its use. However, the use of bone healing and enhancing substrates such as Symphony (Johnson & Johnson–Depuy) or immediate postoperative application of external bone stimulators (or

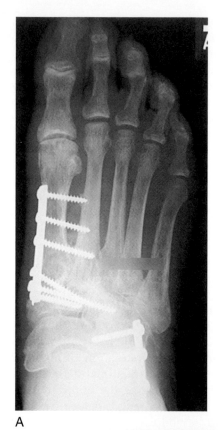

A

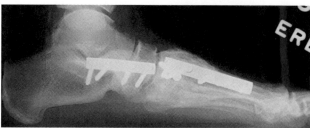

B

Figure 16–104 Anteroposterior **(A)** and lateral **(B)** postoperative radiographs demonstrate midfoot arthrodesis and lateral column lengthening to correct midfoot and hindfoot deformity.

both) is being evaluated to lower the incidence of nonunion. We believe that realignment with compression screw fixation across the respective TMT joints, and a medial column plate as a neutralization or primary construct, is needed to obtain a successful result in most cases. There is no consensus on the preferred approach for all midfoot arthritic problems, and the technique used must be tailored to the individual patient's problem and the surgeon's experience.

Our preferred approach is to incorporate the medial column joints and to leave the lateral column mobile. Generally, we use a two-incision technique for the arthrodesis, with a medial and dorsal incision spaced as far apart as possible to minimize wound-healing problems.

The magnitude of surgery requires a lengthy postoperative convalescence. After midfoot arthrodesis, most workers have difficulty returning to an occupation that requires standing for a full 8-hour day. Postoperative complications include skin slough, metatarsalgia, and incisional neuromas.[24,188,219]

Moreover, in a review of complications associated with midfoot and hindfoot arthrodesis, Bibbo, Anderson, and Davis[24] reported that wound problems can be expected in 3 to 5 percent of nondiabetic patients undergoing elective arthrodesis procedures, but that rate increased up to 53% in diabetic patients. Given the increasing numbers of diabetic patients in the United States and other countries, every effort should be made to prevent complications by evaluating and treating the vascular, neurologic, and general nutritional status of the patient prior to arthrodesis. Hindfoot alignment must be considered prior to midfoot arthrodesis as well, and concomitant osteotomies of staged hindfoot reconstruction, or both, should be considered.

REFERENCES

1. Adkins RB Jr, Scott HW Jr: Surgical procedures in patients aged 90 years and older. *South Med J* 77(11):1357-1364, 1984.
2. Agarwal AK: Gout and pseudogout. *Prim Care* 20(4):839-855, 1993.
3. Aho H: Synovectomy of MTP joints in rheumatoid arthritis. *Rheumatology* 11:126-130, 1987.
4. Albin RK, Weil LS: Flexible implant arthroplasty of the great toe: An evaluation. *J Am Podiatry Assoc* 64(12):967-975, 1974.
5. Alibert J: Précis Théorique et Pratique sur les Maladies de la Peau. Paris, Calille et Revier, 1818, p 21.
6. Anonymous: Clinical update: Lyme disease looms larger than ever. *J Musculoskel Med* 14:110-111, 1997.
7. Anonymous: Treatment of Lyme disease. *Med Lett Drugs Ther* 39(1000):47-48, 1997.
8. Ashman CJ, Klecker RJ, Yu JS: Forefoot pain involving the metatarsal region: differential diagnosis with MR imaging. *Radiographics* 21(6):1425-1440, 2001.
9. Barca F: Tendon arthroplasty of the first metatarsophalangeal joint in hallux rigidus: Preliminary communication. *Foot Ankle Int* 18(4):222-228, 1997.
10. Bardos T, Zhang J, Mikecz K, et al. Mice lacking endogenous major histocompatibility complex class II develop arthritis resembling psoriatic arthritis at an advanced age. *Arthritis Rheum* 46(9):2465-2475, 2002.
11. Barton NJ: Arthroplasty of the forefoot in rheumatoid arthritis. *J Bone Joint Surg Br* 55(1):126-133, 1973.
12. Bass SJ, Gastwirth CM, Green R, et al: Phagocytosis of Silastic material following Silastic great toe implant. *J Foot Surg* 17(2):70-72, 1978.
13. Bazin P: Leçons théoriques et cliniques sur les affections cutanées de nature arthritique et dartreux. Paris, Delahaye, 1860, pp 154-161.
14. Beauchamp CG, Kirby T, Rudge SR, et al: Fusion of the first metatarsophalangeal joint in forefoot arthroplasty. *Clin Orthop Relat Res* 190:249-253, 1984.
15. Beilstein DP, Hawkins ES: Pedal manifestations of systemic lupus erythematosus. *Clin Podiatr Med Surg* 5(1):37-56, 1988.
16. Belt EA, Kaarela K, Kauppi MJ, Lehto MU: Outcome of Keller resection arthroplasty in the rheumatoid foot. A radiographic follow-up study of 4 to 11 years. *Clin Exp Rheumatol* 17(3):387, 1999.
17. Belt EA, Kaarela K, Lehto MU: Destruction and arthroplasties of the metatarsophalangeal joints in seropositive rheumatoid arthritis. A 20-year follow-up study. *Scand J Rheumatol* 27(3):194-196, 1998.
18. Bennett RM: Confounding features of the fibromyalgia syndrome: A current perspective of differential diagnosis. *J Rheumatol Suppl* 19:58-61, 1989.
19. Bennett RM: Physical fitness and muscle metabolism in the fibromyalgia syndrome: An overview. *J Rheumatol Suppl* 19:28-29, 1989.
20. Benson GM, Johnson EW Jr: Management of the foot in rheumatoid arthritis. *Orthop Clin North Am* 2(3):733-744, 1971.
21. Berger I, Martens KD, Meyer-Scholten C: Rheumatoid necroses in the forefoot. *Foot Ankle Int* 25(5):336-339, 2004.
22. Berlet GC, Hodges Davis W, Anderson RB: Tendon arthroplasty for basal fourth and fifth metatarsal arthritis. *Foot Ankle Int* 23(5):440-446, 2002.
23. Beutler A, Schumacher HR Jr: Gout and "pseudogout." When are arthritic symptoms caused by crystal deposition? *Postgrad Med* 95(2):103-106, 109, 113-116 passim, 1994.
24. Bibbo C, Anderson RB, Davis WH: Complications of midfoot and hindfoot arthrodesis. *Clin Orthop Relat Res* (391):45-58, 2001.
25. Bibbo C, Goldberg JW: Infectious and healing complications after elective orthopaedic foot and ankle surgery during tumor necrosis factor-alpha inhibition therapy. *Foot Ankle Int* 25(5):331-335, 2004.
26. Bingold AC: Arthrodesis of the great toe. *Proc R Soc Med* 51(6):435-437, 1958.
27. Bingold AC, Collins DH: Hallux rigidus. *J Bone Joint Surg Br* 32(2):214-222, 1950.
28. Blair MP, Brown LA: Hallux limitus/rigidus deformity: A new great toe implant. *J Foot Ankle Surg* 32(3):257-262, 1993.
29. Bluestone R: Collagen diseases affecting the foot. *Foot Ankle* 2(6):311-317, 1982.
30. Bonney G, Macnab I: Hallux valgus and hallux rigidus; a critical survey of operative results. *J Bone Joint Surg Br* 34(3):366-385, 1952.
31. Boss GR, Seegmiller JE: Hyperuricemia and gout. Classification, complications and management. *N Engl J Med* 300(26):1459-1468, 1979.
32. Brattstrom H, Brattstrom M: Resection of the metatarsophalangeal joints in rheumatoid arthritis. *Acta Orthop Scand* 41(2):213-224, 1970.
33. Burra G, and Katchis SD: Rheumatoid arthritis of the forefoot. *Rheum Dis Clin North Am* 24(1):173-180, 1998.
34. Calabro JJ: A critical evaluation of the diagnostic features of the feet in rheumatoid arthritis. *Arthritis Rheum* 5:19-29, 1962.
35. Calderone DR, Wertheimer SJ: First metatarsophalangeal joint arthrodesis utilizing a mini–Hoffman External Fixator. *J Foot Ankle Surg* 32(5):517-25, 1993.
36. Caneva RG: Postoperative degenerative changes of the metatarsal head following use of the Swanson implant: Four case reports. *J Foot Surg* 16(1):34-37, 1977.
37. Caputi RA: Synovectomy. *Clin Podiatr Med Surg* 5(1):249-257, 1988.
38. Caselli MA, George DH: Foot deformities: Biomechanical and pathomechanical changes associated with aging, Part I. *Clin Podiatr Med Surg* 20(3):487-509, ix, 2003.

39. Cavolo DJ, Cavallaro DC, Arrington LE: The Watermann osteotomy for hallux limitus. *J Am Podiatry Assoc* 69(1):52-57, 1979.

40. Chalmers AC, Busby C, Goyert J, et al: Metatarsalgia and rheumatoid arthritis—a randomized, single blind, sequential trial comparing 2 types of foot orthoses and supportive shoes. *J Rheumatol* 27(7):1643-1647, 2000.

41. Chana GS, Andrew TA, Cotterill CP: A simple method of arthrodesis of the first metatarsophalangeal joint. *J Bone Joint Surg Br* 66(5):703-705, 1984.

42. Chand Y, Johnson KA: Foot and ankle manifestations of Reiter's syndrome. *Foot Ankle* 1(3):167-172, 1980.

43. Cheleuitte E, Fleischli J, Tisa L, Zombolo R: Psoriasis and elective foot surgery. *J Foot Ankle Surg* 35(4):297-302; discussion 371, 1996.

44. Chen DS, Wertheimer S: The Keller arthroplasty with use of the Dow Corning titanium hemi-implant. *J Foot Surg* 30(4):414-418, 1991.

45. Citron N, Neil M: Dorsal wedge osteotomy of the proximal phalanx for hallux rigidus. Long-term results. *J Bone Joint Surg Br* 69(5):835-837, 1987.

46. Clayton ML: Surgery of the forefoot in rheumatoid arthritis. *Clin Orthop Relat Res* 16:136-140, 1960.

47. Clayton ML: Surgery of the lower extremity in rheumatoid arthritis. *J Bone Joint Surg Am* 45:1517-1536, 1963.

48. Cleveland M, Winant EM: An end-result study of the Keller operation. *J Bone Joint Surg Am* 32(1):163-175, 1950.

49. Clutton H: The treatment of hallux valgus. *St Thomas Hosp Rep* 22:1-12, 1891-1893.

50. Conklin MJ, Smith RW: Treatment of the atypical lesser toe deformity with basal hemiphalangectomy. *Foot Ankle Int* 15(11):585-594, 1994.

51. Conrad KJ, Budiman-Mak E, Roach KE, et al: Impacts of foot orthoses on pain and disability in rheumatoid arthritics. *J Clin Epidemiol* 49(1):1-7, 1996.

52. Corrigan G, Kanat IO: Modification of the total first metatarsophalangeal joint implant arthroplasty. *J Foot Surg* 28(4):295-300, 1989.

53. Cotterill J: Stiffness of the great toe in adolescents. *BMJ* 1:1158, 1888.

54. Coughlin MJ: Arthrodesis of the first metatarsophalangeal joint. *Orthop Rev* 19(2):177-186, 1990.

55. Coughlin MJ: Arthrodesis of the first metatarsophalangeal joint with mini-fragment plate fixation. *Orthopedics* 13(9):1037-1044, 1990.

56. Coughlin MJ: Conditions of the forefoot. In DeLee J, Drez D (eds): *Orthopaedic Sports Medicine: Principles and Practice.* Philadelphia, WB Saunders, 1994, pp 221-244.

57. Coughlin MJ: The rheumatoid foot. In Chapman M (ed): *Operative Orthopaedics.* Philadelphia, JB Lippincott, 1993, pp 2311-2322.

58. Coughlin MJ: Rheumatoid forefoot reconstruction. A long-term follow-up study. *J Bone Joint Surg Am* 82(3):322-341, 2000.

59. Coughlin MJ: The Scandinavian total ankle replacement prosthesis. *Instr Course Lect* 51:135-42, 2002.

60. Coughlin MJ, Abdo RV: Arthrodesis of the first metatarsophalangeal joint with vitallium plate fixation. *Foot Ankle Int* 15(1):18-28, 1994.

61. Coughlin MJ, Grebing BR, Jones CP: Arthrodesis of the first metatarsophalangeal joint for idiopathic hallux valgus: Intermediate results. *Foot Ankle Int* 26(10):783-792, 2005.

62. Coughlin MJ, Jones CR: Unpublished data.

63. Coughlin MJ, Mann RA: Arthrodesis of the first metatarsophalangeal joint as salvage for the failed Keller procedure. *J Bone Joint Surg Am* 69(1):68-75, 1987.

64. Coughlin MJ, Shurnas PS: Hallux rigidus. *J Bone Joint Surg Am* 86 Suppl 1(Pt 2):119-130, 2004.

65. Coughlin MJ, Shurnas PS: Hallux rigidus: Demographics, etiology, and radiographic assessment. *Foot Ankle Int* 24(10):731-743, 2003.

66. Coughlin MJ, Shurnas PS: Hallux rigidus. Grading and long-term results of operative treatment. *J Bone Joint Surg Am* 85(11):2072-2088, 2003.

67. Coughlin MJ, Shurnas PS: Hallux valgus in men. Part II: First ray mobility after bunionectomy and factors associated with hallux valgus deformity. *Foot Ankle Int* 24(1):73-78, 2003.

68. Coughlin MJ, Shurnas PS: Soft-tissue arthroplasty for hallux rigidus. *Foot Ankle Int* 24(9):661-672, 2003.

69. Cracchiolo A 3rd: Management of the arthritic forefoot. *Foot Ankle* 3(1):17-23, 1982.

70. Cracchiolo A 3rd: Rheumatoid arthritis of the forefoot. In Gould J (ed): *Operative Foot Surgery.* Philadelphia, WB Saunders, 1994, pp 141-159.

71. Cracchiolo A 3rd, Weltmer JB Jr, Lian G, et al: Arthroplasty of the first metatarsophalangeal joint with a double-stem silicone implant. Results in patients who have degenerative joint disease failure of previous operations, or rheumatoid arthritis. *J Bone Joint Surg Am* 74(4):552-563, 1992.

72. Craxford AD, Stevens J, Park C: Management of the deformed rheumatoid forefoot. A comparison of conservative and surgical methods. *Clin Orthop Relat Res* 166:121-126, 1982.

73. Curtis MJ, Myerson M, Jinnah RH, et al: Arthrodesis of the first metatarsophalangeal joint: A biomechanical study of internal fixation techniques. *Foot Ankle* 14(7):395-359, 1993.

74. Davies GF: Plantarflexory base wedge osteotomy in the treatment of functional and structural metatarsus primus elevatus. *Clin Podiatr Med Surg* 6(1):93-102, 1989.

75. Davies-Colley M: Contraction of the metatarsophalangeal joint of the great toe. *BMJ* 1:728, 1887.

76. DeFrino PF, Brodsky JW, Pollo FE, et al: First metatarsophalangeal arthrodesis: A clinical, pedobarographic and gait analysis study. *Foot Ankle Int* 23(6):496-502, 2002.

77. Dennis DT: Lyme disease. Tracking an epidemic. *JAMA* 266(9):1269-1270, 1991.

78. Dobbs B: LaPorta great toe implant. Long-term study of its efficacy. Student Research Group. *J Am Podiatr Med Assoc* 80(7):370-373, 1990.

79. Downey DJ, Simkin PA, Mack LA, et al: Tibialis posterior tendon rupture: A cause of rheumatoid flat foot. *Arthritis Rheum* 31(3):441-446, 1988.

80. Drago JJ, Oloff L, Jacobs AM: A comprehensive review of hallux limitus. *J Foot Surg* 23(3):213-220, 1984.

81. Dunlop WE, Rosenblood L, Lawrason L, et al: Effects of age and severity of illness on outcome and length of stay in geriatric surgical patients. *Am J Surg* 165(5):577-580, 1993.

82. Durrant MN, Siepert KK: Role of soft tissue structures as an etiology of hallux limitus. *J Am Podiatr Med Assoc* 83(4):173-180, 1993.

83. DuVries H: Arthritides. In DuVries H (ed): *Surgery of the Foot,* ed 2. St. Louis, Mosby, 1965, pp 318-329.

84. DuVries H: Static deformities. In DuVries H (ed): *Surgery of the Foot.* St. Louis, Mosby, 1959, pp 392-398.

85. Easley ME, Davis WH, Anderson RB: Intermediate to long-term follow-up of medial-approach dorsal cheilectomy for hallux rigidus. *Foot Ankle Int* 20(3):147-152, 1999.

86. Egan R, Sartoris DJ, Resnick D: Radiographic features of gout in the foot. *J Foot Surg* 26(5):434-439, 1987.

87. Espinoza LR, Aguilar JL, Berman A, et al: Rheumatic manifestations associated with human immunodeficiency virus infection. *Arthritis Rheum* 32(12):1615-1622, 1989.

88. Ess P, Hamalainen M, Leppilahti J: Non-constrained titanium–polyethylene total endoprosthesis in the treatment of hallux rigidus. A prospective clinical 2-year follow-up study. *Scand J Surg* 91(2):202-207, 2002.

89. Ettl V, Radke S, Gaertner M, Walther M: Arthrodesis in the treatment of hallux rigidus. *Int Orthop* 27(6):382-385, 2003.

90. Faller J, Thompson F, Hamilton W: Foot and ankle disorders resulting from Lyme disease. *Foot Ankle* 11(4):236-238, 1991.

91. Fam AG, Shuckett R, McGillivray DC, Little AH: Stress fractures in rheumatoid arthritis. *J Rheumatol* 10(5):722-726, 1983.

92. Fan P, Yu D: Reiter's syndrome. In Kelley WN, Harris ED Jr, Ruddy S, Sledge CB (eds): *Textbook of Rheumatology*, ed 4. Philadelphia, WB Saunders, 1993, pp 961-973.

93. Farber EM, Nall ML: The natural history of psoriasis in 5,600 patients. *Dermatologica* 148(1):1-18, 1974.

94. Feldman KA: The Green–Watermann procedure: Geometric analysis and preoperative radiographic template technique. *J Foot Surg* 31(2):182-185, 1992.

95. Feldman RS, Hutter J, Lapow L, Pour B: Cheilectomy and hallux rigidus. *J Foot Surg* 22(2):170-174, 1983.

96. Feltham GT, Hanks SE, Marcus RE: Age-based outcomes of cheilectomy for the treatment of hallux rigidus. *Foot Ankle Int* 22(3):192-197, 2001.

97. Fink BR, Mizel MS, Temple HT: Simultaneous arthrodesis of the metatarsophalangeal and interphalangeal joints of the hallux. *Foot Ankle Int* 21(11):951-953, 2000.

98. Fitzgerald JA: A review of long-term results of arthrodesis of the first metatarso-phalangeal joint. *J Bone Joint Surg Br* 51(3):488-493, 1969.

99. Fitzgerald JA, Wilkinson JM: Arthrodesis of the metatarsophalangeal joint of the great toe. *Clin Orthop Relat Res* (157):70-77, 1981.

100. Fitzpatrick T, Johnson R, Polano M, et al: Psoriasis. In Fitzpatrick TB, Johnson RA, Polano M, et al (eds): *Color Atlas and Synopsis of Classical Dermatology* ed 2. New York, McGraw Hill, 1992, pp 40-53.

101. Flint M, Sweetnam R: Amputation of all toes. *J Bone Joint Surg Br* 42:90-96, 1960.

102. Ford DK: The clinical spectrum of Reiter's syndrome and similar postenteric arthropathies. *Clin Orthop Relat Res* (143):59-65, 1979.

103. Ford TC: Surgical management of chronic tophaceous gout. A case report. *J Am Podiatr Med Assoc* 82(10):514-519, 1992.

104. Forrester DM: Radiologic vignette. The "cocktail" digit. *Arthritis Rheum* 26(5):664-667, 1983.

105. Fowler AW: A method of forefoot reconstruction. *J Bone Joint Surg Br* 41:507-513, 1959.

106. Freed JB: The increasing recognition of medullary lysis, cortical osteophytic proliferation, and fragmentation of implanted silicone polymer implants. *J Foot Ankle Surg* 32(2):171-179, 1993.

107. Frey C, Andersen GD, Feder KS: Plantarflexion injury to the metatarsophalangeal joint ("sand toe"). *Foot Ankle Int* 17(9):576-581, 1996.

108. Fu F, Scranton P: Forefoot arthroplasty in rheumatoid arthritis: Clinical appraisal and force plate analysis. *Orthopedics* 5:163-168, 1982.

109. Fuhrmann RA, Anders JO: The long-term results of resection arthroplasties of the first metatarsophalangeal joint in rheumatoid arthritis. *Int Orthop* 25(5):312-316, 2001.

110. Ganley JV, Lynch FR, Darrigan RD: Keller bunionectomy with fascia and tendon graft. *J Am Podiatr Med Assoc* 76(11):602-610, 1986.

111. Garber EK, Silver S: Pedal manifestations of DISH. *Foot Ankle* 3(1):12-16, 1982.

112. Geldwert JJ, Rock GD, McGrath MP, Mancuso JE: Cheilectomy: Still a useful technique for grade I and grade II hallux limitus/rigidus. *J Foot Surg* 31(2):154-159, 1992.

113. Gimple K, Anspacher J, Kopta J: Metatarsophalangeal joint fusion of the great toe. *Orthopedics* 1:462-467, 1978.

114. Ginsburg AI: Arthrodesis of the first metatarsophalangeal joint: A practical procedure. *J Am Podiatry Assoc* 69(6):367-369, 1979.

115. Gladman DD, Stafford-Brady F, Chang CH, et al: Longitudinal study of clinical and radiological progression in psoriatic arthritis. *J Rheumatol* 17(6):809-812, 1990.

116. Gold RH, Bassett LW: Radiologic evaluation of the arthritic foot. *Foot Ankle* 2(6):332-341, 1982.

117. Goldenberg DL: Fibromyalgia and its relation to chronic fatigue syndrome, viral illness and immune abnormalities. *J Rheumatol Suppl* 19:91-93, 1989.

118. Goodfellow J: Aetiology of hallux rigidus. *Proc R Soc Med* 59(9):821-824, 1966.

119. Gordon M, Bullough PG: Synovial and osseous inflammation in failed silicone-rubber prostheses. *J Bone Joint Surg Am* 64(4):574-580, 1982.

120. Gould N: Hallux rigidus: Cheilotomy or implant? *Foot Ankle* 1(6):315-320, 1981.

121. Gould N, Schneider W, Ashikaga T: Epidemiological survey of foot problems in the continental United States:1978-1979. *Foot Ankle* 1(1):8-10,1980.

122. Grady JF, Axe TM: The modified Valenti procedure for the treatment of hallux limitus. *J Foot Ankle Surg* 33(4):365-367, 1994.

123. Grady JF, Axe TM, Zager EJ, Sheldon LA: A retrospective analysis of 772 patients with hallux limitus. *J Am Podiatr Med Assoc* 92(2):102-108, 2002.

124. Graham CE: Rheumatoid forefoot metatarsal head resection without first metatarsophalangeal arthrodesis. *Foot Ankle Int* 15(12):689-690, 1994.

125. Granberry WM, Noble PC, Bishop JO, Tullos HS: Use of a hinged silicone prosthesis for replacement arthroplasty of the first metatarsophalangeal joint. *J Bone Joint Surg Am* 73(10):1453-1459, 1991.

126. Guerra J, Resnick D: Arthritides affecting the foot: radiographic–pathologic correlation. *Foot Ankle* 2(6):325-331, 1982.

127. Gutierrez F, Espinoza LR: [Reactive arthritis. A review]. *Rev Med Chil* 118(7):796-804, 1990.

128. Hackford AW: Surgical principles for the aged. In Reichel W (ed): *Care of the Elderly: Clinical Aspects of Aging*, ed 4. Baltimore, Williams & Wilkins, 1995, pp 408-415.

129. Hakkinen A, Hakkinen K, Hannonen P: Effects of strength training on neuromuscular function and disease activity in patients with recent-onset inflammatory arthritis. *Scand J Rheumatol* 23(5):237-242 1994.

130. Hamalainen M, Raunio P: Long-term followup of rheumatoid forefoot surgery. *Clin Orthop Relat Res* (340):34-38, 1997.

131. Hamilton J, Brydson G, Fraser S, Grant M: Walking ability as a measure of treatment effect in early rheumatoid arthritis. *Clin Rehabil* 15(2):142-147, 2001

132. Hamilton WG, O'Malley, MJ, Thompson FM, Kovatis PE: Roger Mann Award 1995. Capsular interposition arthroplasty for severe hallux rigidus. *Foot Ankle Int* 18(2):68-70, 1997.

133. Hammerschlag WA, Rice JR, Caldwell DS, Goldner JL: Psoriatic arthritis of the foot and ankle: Analysis of joint involvement and diagnostic errors. *Foot Ankle* 12(1):35-39, 1991.

134. Hanft JR, Mason ET, Landsman AS, Kashuk KB: A new radiographic classification for hallux limitus. *J Foot Ankle Surg* 32(4):397-404, 1993.

135. Hanft JR, Merrill T, Marcinko DE, et al: Grand rounds: First metatarsophalangeal joint replacement. *J Foot Ankle Surg* 35(1):78-85, 1996.

136. Hanyu T, Yamazaki H, Ishikawa H, et al: Flexible hinge toe implant arthroplasty for rheumatoid arthritis of the first metatarsophalangeal joint: Long-term results. *J Orthop Sci* 6(2):141-47, 2001.

137. Hanyu T, Yamazaki H, Murasawa A, Tohyama C: Arthroplasty for rheumatoid forefoot deformities by a shortening oblique osteotomy. *Clin Orthop Relat Res* 338:131-138, 1997.

138. Harris MD, Siegel LB, Alloway JA: Gout and hyperuricemia. *Am Fam Physician* 59(4):925-934, 1999.

139. Harrison M: Hallux limitus. *J Bone Joint Surg Br* 53:772, 1971.

140. Harrison M, Harvey F: Arthrodesis of the first metatarsophalangeal joint for hallux valgus and rigidus. *J Bone Joint Surg Am* 45:471-480, 1963.

141. Harvey CK, Cadena R, Dunlap L: Fibromyalgia. Part I. Review of the literature. *J Am Podiatr Med Assoc* 83(7):412-415, 1993.

142. Hasselo LG, Willkens RF, Toomey HE, et al: Forefoot surgery in rheumatoid arthritis: Subjective assessment of outcome. *Foot Ankle* 8(3):148-151, 1987.

143. Hattrup SJ, Johnson KA: Subjective results of hallux rigidus following treatment with cheilectomy. *Clin Orthop Relat Res* (226):182-191, 1988.

144. Heaney S: Phalangeal osteotomy for hallux rigidus. *J Bone Joint Surg Br* 52:799, 1970.

145. Hecht PJ, Gibbons MJ, Wapner KL, et al: Arthrodesis of the first metatarsophalangeal joint to salvage failed silicone implant arthroplasty. *Foot Ankle Int* 18(7):383-390, 1997.

146. Hench PK: Evaluation and differential diagnosis of fibromyalgia. Approach to diagnosis and management. *Rheum Dis Clin North Am* 15(1):19-29, 1989.

147. Henry AP, Waugh W, Wood H: The use of footprints in assessing the results of operations for hallux valgus. A comparison of Keller's operation and arthrodesis. *J Bone Joint Surg Br* 57(4):478-481, 1975.

148. Hetherington VJ, Mercado C, Karloc L, Grillo J: Silicone implant arthroplasty: A retrospective analysis. *J Foot Ankle Surg* 32(4):430-433, 1993.

149. Higgins KR, Burnett OE, Krych SM, Harkless LB: Seronegative rheumatoid arthritis and Morton's neuroma. *J Foot Surg* 27(5):404-407, 1988.

150. Hodge MC, Bach TM, Carter GM: Novel Award First Prize Paper. Orthotic management of plantar pressure and pain in rheumatoid arthritis. *Clin Biomech (Bristol, Avon)* 14(8):567-575, 1999.

151. Hoffman P: An operation for severe grades of contracted or clawed toes. *Am J Orthop Surg* 9:441-449, 1911.

152. Horton GA, Olney BW: Triple arthrodesis with lateral column lengthening for treatment of severe planovalgus deformity. *Foot Ankle Int* 16(7):395-400, 1995.

153. Horton GA, Park YW, Myerson MS: Role of metatarsus primus elevatus in the pathogenesis of hallux rigidus. *Foot Ankle Int* 20(12):777-780, 1999.

154. Huemer C, Malleson PN, Cabral DA, et al: Patterns of joint involvement at onset differentiate oligoarticular juvenile psoriatic arthritis from pauciarticular juvenile rheumatoid arthritis. *J Rheumatol* 29(7):1531-1535, 2002.

155. Humbert JL, Bourbonniere C, Laurin CA: Metatarsophalangeal fusion for hallux valgus: Indications and effect on the first metatarsal ray. *Can Med Assoc J* 120(8):937-941, 956, 1979.

156. Jack EA: The aetiology of hallux rigidus. *Br J Surg* 27:494-497, 1940.

157. Jahss M: Personal communication, June 26, 1997.

158. Jannink MJ, van Dijk H, de Vries J, et al: A systematic review of the methodological quality and extent to which evaluation studies measure the usability of orthopaedic shoes. *Clin Rehabil* 18(1):15-26, 2004.

159. Jeffery JA, Freedman LF: Modified reamers for fusion of the first metatarsophalangeal joint. *J Bone Joint Surg Br* 77(2):328-329, 1995.

160. Jenkin WM, Oloff LM: Implant arthroplasty in the rheumatoid arthritic patient. *Clin Podiatr Med Surg* 5(1):213-226, 1988.

161. Johansson JE, Barrington TW: Cone arthrodesis of the first metatarsophalangeal joint. *Foot Ankle* 4(5):244-248, 1984.

162. Johnson JE, Johnson KA: Dowel arthrodesis for degenerative arthritis of the tarsometatarsal (Lisfranc) joints. *Foot Ankle* 6(5):243-253, 1986.

163. Johnson KA: Personal communication, 1994.

164. Johnson KA, Buck PG: Total replacement arthroplasty of the first metatarsophalangeal joint. *Foot Ankle* 1(6):307-314, 1981.

165. Jones RO, Chen JB, Pitcher D, et al: Rheumatoid nodules affecting both heels with surgical debulking: A case report. *J Am Podiatr Med Assoc* 86(4):179-182, 1996.

166. Joplin RJ: The proper digital nerve, vitallium stem arthroplasty, and some thoughts about foot surgery in general. *Clin Orthop Relat Res* 76:199-212, 1971.

167. Joplin RJ: Surgery of the forefoot in the rheumatoid arthritic patient. *Surg Clin North Am* 49(4):847-878, 1969.

168. Jordan HH, Bordsky AE: Keller operation for hallux valgus and hallux rigidus. An end result study. *AMA Arch Surg* 62(4):586-596, 1951.

169. Jouben LM, Steele RJ, Bono JV: Orthopaedic manifestations of Lyme disease. *Orthop Rev* 23(5):395-400, 1994.

170. Kampner SL: Total joint prosthetic arthroplasty of the great toe—a 12-year experience. *Foot Ankle* 4(5):249-261, 1984.

171. Kane D, Greaney T, Bresnihan B, et al: Ultrasonography in the diagnosis and management of psoriatic dactylitis. *J Rheumatol* 26(8):1746-1751, 1999.

172. Kane D, Stafford L, Bresnihan B, FitzGerald O: A classification study of clinical subsets in an inception cohort of early psoriatic peripheral arthritis—"DIP or not DIP revisited." *Rheumatology (Oxford)* 42(12):1469-1476, 2003.

173. Kane D, Stafford L, Bresnihan B, FitzGerald O: A prospective, clinical and radiological study of early psoriatic arthritis: An early synovitis clinic experience. *Rheumatology (Oxford)* 42(12):1460-1468, 2003.

174. Kates A, Kessel, L, Kay A: Arthroplasty of the forefoot. *J Bone Joint Surg Br* 49(3):552-557, 1967.

175. Katz W: Psoriatic arthritis in Reiter's disease. In Katz W (ed): *Rheumatic Diseases: Diagnosis and Management.* Philadelphia, JB Lippincott, 1977, pp 540-555.

176. Keat A: Reiter's syndrome and reactive arthritis in perspective. *N Engl J Med* 309(26):1606-1615, 1983.

177. Keat AC: Should all patients with Reiter's syndrome be tested for HIV infection? *Br J Rheumatol* 28(5):409, 1989.

178. Keenan MA, Peabody TD, Gronley JK, Perry J: Valgus deformities of the feet and characteristics of gait in patients who have rheumatoid arthritis. *J Bone Joint Surg Am* 73(2):237-247, 1991.

179. Keiserman LS, Cassandra J, Amis JA: The piano key test: A clinical sign for the identification of subtle tarsometatarsal pathology. *Foot Ankle Int* 24(5):437-438, 2003.

180. Kelikian H: Hallux Valgus Allied Deformities of the Forefoot and Metatarsalgia, Philadelphia, WB Saunders, 1997, pp 262-281.

181. Keller W: The surgical treatment of bunions and hallux valgus. *N Y Med J* 80:741-742, 1904.

182. Kessel L, Bonney G: Hallux rigidus in the adolescent. *J Bone Joint Surg Br* 40(4):669-673, 1958.

183. Kitaoka HB, Holiday AD Jr, Chao EY, Cahalan TD: Salvage of failed first metatarsophalangeal joint implant arthroplasty by

implant removal and synovectomy: Clinical and biomechanical evaluation. *Foot Ankle* 13(5):243-250, 1992.

184. Kitaoka HB, Patzer GL, Ilstrup DM, Wallrichs SL: Survivorship analysis of the Mayo total ankle arthroplasty. *J Bone Joint Surg Am* 76(7):974-979, 1994.

185. Koenig RD: Koenig total great toe implant. Preliminary report. *J Am Podiatr Med Assoc* 80(9):462-468, 1990.

186. Koenig RD: Revision arthroplasty utilizing the Biomet Total Toe System for failed silicone elastomer implants. *J Foot Ankle Surg* 33(3):222-227, 1994.

187. Koenig RD, Horwitz LR: The Biomet Total Toe System utilizing the Koenig score: A five-year review. *J Foot Ankle Surg* 35(1):23-26, 1996.

188. Komenda GA, Myerson MS, Biddinger KR: Results of arthrodesis of the tarsometatarsal joints after traumatic injury. *J Bone Joint Surg Am* 78(11):1665-1676, 1996.

189. Kuhns JG: The foot in chronic arthritis. *Clin Orthop Relat Res* 16:141-151, 1960.

190. Kumar S, Gow P: A survey of indications, results and complications of surgery for tophaceous gout. *N Z Med J* 115(1158):U109, 2002.

191. Kurtz DH, Harrill JC, Kaczander BI, Solomon MG: The Valenti procedure for hallux limitus: A long-term follow-up and analysis. *J Foot Ankle Surg* 38(2):123-130, 1999.

192. Kurtz J: Surgery of tophaceous gout in the lower extremity. *Surg Clin North Am* 45:217-228, 1965.

193. Lambrinudi P: Metatarsus primus elevatus. *Proc R Soc Med* 31:1273, 1938.

194. Landry JR, Schilero J: The medical/surgical management of gout. *J Foot Surg* 25(2):160-175, 1986.

195. LaPorta GA, Pilla P Jr, Richter KP: Keller implant procedure: A report of 536 procedures using a Silastic intramedullary stemmed implant. *J Am Podiatry Assoc* 66(3):126-147, 1976.

196. Larmon WA, Kurtz JF: The surgical management of chronic tophaceous gout. *J Bone Joint Surg Am* 40(4):743-772, 1958.

197. Larsen A, Dale K, Eek M: Radiographic evaluation of rheumatoid arthritis and related conditions by standard reference films. *Acta Radiol Diagn (Stockh)* 18(4):481-491, 1977.

198. Lawrence SJ: Lyme disease: An orthopedic perspective. *Orthopedics* 15(11):1331-1335, 1992.

199. Lawson JP, Steere AC: Lyme arthritis: Radiologic findings. *Radiology* 154(1):37-43, 1985.

200. Lemon RA, Engber WD, McBeath AA: A complication of Silastic hemiarthroplasty in bunion surgery. *Foot Ankle* 4(5):262-266, 1984.

201. Lerman RL, Danna AT, Boykoff TJ: Tophaceous deposition in the absence of known antecedent gout. *J Am Podiatr Med Assoc* 81(5):273-275, 1991.

202. Levi S, Ansell BM, Klenerman L: Tarsometatarsal involvement in juvenile spondyloarthropathy. *Foot Ankle* 11(2):90-92, 1990.

203. Lin SS, Bono CM, Treuting R, Shereff MJ: Limited intertarsal arthrodesis using bone grafting and pin fixation. *Foot Ankle Int* 21(9):742-748, 2000.

204. Lipscomb PR: Arthrodesis of the first metatarsophalangeal joint for severe bunions and hallux rigidus. *Clin Orthop Relat Res* 142:48-54, 1979.

205. Lipscomb PR: Surgery for rheumatoid arthritis—timing and techniques: Summary. *J Bone Joint Surg Am* 50(3):614-617, 1968.

206. Lombardi CM, Silhanek AD, Connolly FG, et al: First metatarsophalangeal arthrodesis for treatment of hallux rigidus: A retrospective study. *J Foot Ankle Surg* 40(3):137-143, 2001.

207. Loredo R: Radiographic manifestations of rheumatic diseases affecting the foot and ankle. *Clin Podiatr Med Surg* 16(2):215-258, v, 1999.

208. Love TR, Whynot AS, Farine I, et al: Keller arthroplasty: A prospective review. *Foot Ankle* 8(1):46-54, 1987.

209. Mackay DC, Blyth M, Rymaszewski LA: The role of cheilectomy in the treatment of hallux rigidus. *J Foot Ankle Surg* 36(5):337-340, 1997.

210. Maenpaa HM, Soini I, Lehto MU, Belt EA: Insufficiency fractures in patients with chronic inflammatory joint diseases. *Clin Exp Rheumatol* 20(1):77-79, 2002.

211. Maillefert JF, Combe B, Goupille P, et al: The 5-yr HAQ-disability is related to the first year's changes in the narrowing, rather than erosion score in patients with recent-onset rheumatoid arthritis. *Rheumatology (Oxford)* 43(1):79-84, 2004.

212. Mankey M, Mann RA: Arthrodesis of the first metatarsophalangeal utilizing a dorsal plate. Presented at the Seventh Annual Summer Meeting of the American Orthopaedic Foot and Ankle Society, Boston, Mass, July 17, 1991.

213. Mann RA, Clanton TO: Hallux rigidus: Treatment by cheilectomy. *J Bone Joint Surg Am* 70(3):400-406, 1988.

214. Mann RA, Coughlin MJ: Arthrodesis of the foot and ankle. In Mann RA, Coughlin MJ (eds): *Video Textbook of Foot and Ankle Surgery.* St Louis, Medical Video Productions, 1991, pp 105-144.

215. Mann RA, Coughlin MJ: The rheumatoid foot: Review of the literature and method of treatment. *Orthop Rev* 7:105-112, 1979.

216. Mann RA, Coughlin MJ, DuVries HL: Hallux rigidus: A review of the literature and a method of treatment. *Clin Orthop Relat Res* 142:57-63, 1979.

217. Mann RA, Katcherian DA: Relationship of metatarsophalangeal joint fusion on the intermetatarsal angle. *Foot Ankle* 10(1):8-11, 1989.

218. Mann RA, Oates JC: Arthrodesis of the first metatarsophalangeal joint. *Foot Ankle* 1(3):159-166, 1980.

219. Mann RA, Prieskorn D, Sobel M: Mid-tarsal and tarsometatarsal arthrodesis for primary degenerative osteoarthrosis or osteoarthrosis after trauma. *J Bone Joint Surg Am* 78(9):1376-1385, 1996.

220. Mann RA, Schakel ME 2nd: Surgical correction of rheumatoid forefoot deformities. *Foot Ankle Int* 16(1):1-6, 1995.

221. Mann RA, Thompson FM: Arthrodesis of the first metatarsophalangeal joint for hallux valgus in rheumatoid arthritis. *J Bone Joint Surg Am* 66(5):687-692, 1984.

222. Mann RA, Thompson FM: Rupture of the posterior tibial tendon causing flat foot. Surgical treatment. *J Bone Joint Surg Am* 67(4):556-561, 1985.

223. Marin GA: Arthrodesis of the metatarsophalangeal joint of the big toe for hallux valgus and hallux rigidus. A new method. *Int Surg* 50(2):175-180, 1968.

224. Marmor L: Resection of the forefoot in rheumatoid arthritis. *Clin Orthop Relat Res* 108:223-227, 1975.

225. Martel W: The overhanging margin of bone: A roentgenologic manifestation of gout. *Radiology* 91(4):755-756, 1968.

226. Mauro G, Rubin RP, Kanat IO: Atypical gouty arthritis. *J Foot Surg* 24(4):280-282, 1985.

227. McCarthy DJ, Chapman HL: Ultrastructure of collapsed metatarsophalangeal silicone elastomer implant. *J Foot Surg* 27(5):418-427, 1988.

228. McDonald RJ, Griffin JM, Edelman RO: Consecutive bilateral failures of first metatarsophalangeal joint prostheses. *J Foot Surg* 25(3):226-233, 1986.

229. McGarvey SR, Johnson KA: Keller arthroplasty in combination with resection arthroplasty of the lesser metatarsophalangeal joints in rheumatoid arthritis. *Foot Ankle* 9(2):75-80, 1988.

230. McKeever DC: Arthrodesis of the first metatarsophalangeal joint for hallux valgus, hallux rigidus, and metatarsus primus varus. *J Bone Joint Surg Am* 34(1):129-134, 1952.

231. McMaster MJ: The pathogenesis of hallux rigidus. *J Bone Joint Surg Br* 60(1):82-87, 1978.

232. Merkle PF, Sculco TP: Prosthetic replacement of the first metatarsophalangeal joint. *Foot Ankle* 9(6):267-271, 1989.

233. Meyer JO, Nishon LR, Weiss L, Docks G: Metatarsus primus elevatus and the etiology of hallux rigidus. *J Foot Surg* 26(3):237-241, 1987.

234. Michelson J, Dunn L: Tenosynovitis of the flexor hallucis longus: A clinical study of the spectrum of presentation and treatment. *Foot Ankle Int* 26(4):291-303, 2005.

235. Michelson J, Easley M, Wigley FM, Hellmann D: Foot and ankle problems in rheumatoid arthritis. *Foot Ankle Int* 15(11):608-613, 1994.

236. Michet CJ: Psoriatic arthritis. In Kelley WN, Harris ED Jr, Ruddy S, Sledge CB (eds): *Textbook of Rheumatology*, ed 4. Philadelphia, WB Saunders, 1993, pp 974-984.

237. Michet CJ, Machado EB, Ballard DJ, McKenna CH: Epidemiology of Reiter's syndrome in Rochester, Minnesota:1950-1980. *Arthritis Rheum* 31(3):428-431, 1988.

238. Millott M, Berlin R: Treating sleep disorders in patients with fibromyalgia. *J Musculoskel Med* 14:25-34, 1997.

239. Minns RJ, Craxford AD: Pressure under the forefoot in rheumatoid arthritis. A comparison of static and dynamic methods of assessment. *Clin Orthop Relat Res* 187:235-242, 1984.

240. Miskew DB, Goldflies ML: Atraumatic avascular necrosis of the talus associated with hyperuricemia. *Clin Orthop Relat Res* 148:156-159, 1980.

241. Moberg E: A simple operation for hallux rigidus. *Clin Orthop Relat Res* 142:55-56, 1979.

242. Moeckel BH, Sculco TP, Alexiades MM, et al: The double-stemmed silicone-rubber implant for rheumatoid arthritis of the first metatarsophalangeal joint. Long-term results. *J Bone Joint Surg Am* 74(4):564-570, 1992.

243. Moll JM, Wright V: Psoriatic arthritis. *Semin Arthritis Rheum* 3(1):55-78, 1973.

244. Montero LC, Gomez RS, de Quiros JF: Cutaneous ulcerations in a patient with rheumatoid arthritis receiving treatment with methotrexate. *J Rheumatol* 27(9):2290-2291, 2000.

245. Morrison P: Complications of forefoot operations in rheumatoid arthritis. *Proc R Soc Med* 67(2):110-111, 1974.

246. Moynihan FJ: Arthrodesis of the metatarso-phalangeal joint of the great toe. *J Bone Joint Surg Br* 49(3):544-551, 1967.

247. Mulcahy D, Daniels TR, Lau JT, et al: Rheumatoid forefoot deformity: A comparison study of 2 functional methods of reconstruction. *J Rheumatol* 30(7):1440-1450, 2003.

248. Mulier T, Steenwerckx A, Thienpont E, et al: Results after cheilectomy in athletes with hallux rigidus. *Foot Ankle Int* 20(4):232-237, 1999.

249. Murphy G, Kwan J, Mihm M: The skin. In Robbins S, Cotran R, Kumar V (eds): *Pathologic Basis of Disease*, ed 3. Philadelphia, WB Saunders, 1984, pp 1291-1293.

250. Myers SR, and Herndon JH: Silastic implant arthroplasty with proximal metatarsal osteotomy for painful hallux valgus. *Foot Ankle* 10(4):219-223, 1990.

251. Myerson MS: Adult acquired flatfoot deformity: Treatment of dysfunction of the posterior tibial tendon. *Instr Course Lect* 46:393-405, 1997.

252. Myerson MS, Schon LC, McGuigan FX, Oznur A: Result of arthrodesis of the hallux metatarsophalangeal joint using bone graft for restoration of length. *Foot Ankle Int* 21(4):297-306, 2000.

253. Nassar J, Cracchiolo A 3rd: Complications in surgery of the foot and ankle in patients with rheumatoid arthritis. *Clin Orthop Relat Res* 391:140-152 2001.

254. Needelman LM Vogler, HW Lemont H et al: A retrospective study of the Swanson great toe hemi-prosthesis. *J Foot Ankle Surg* 32(3):286-290, 1993.

255. Newman RJ, Fitton JM: Conservation of metatarsal heads in surgery of rheumatoid arthritis of the forefoot. *Acta Orthop Scand* 54(3):417-421, 1983.

256. Nilsonne H: Hallux rigidus and its treatment. *Acta Orthop Scand* 1:295-303, 1930.

257. Nissen K: The place of amputation of all toes. *J Bone Joint Surg Br* 35:488, 1953.

258. Nousari HC, Kimyai-Asadi A, Stebbing J, Stone JH: Purple toes in a patient with end-stage rheumatoid arthritis. *Arch Dermatol* 135(6):648-650, 1999.

259. O'Connell PG, Lohmann Siegel K, et al: Forefoot deformity, pain, and mobility in rheumatoid and nonarthritic subjects. *J Rheumatol* 25(9):1681-1666, 1998.

260. O'Duffy EK, Clunie GP, Gacinovic S, et al: Foot pain: Specific indications for scintigraphy. *Br J Rheumatol* 37(4):442-447, 1998.

261. Ognibene FA, Theodoulou MH: Long-standing reaction to a hemi-Silastic implant. *J Foot Surg* 30(2):156-159, 1991.

262. Pacheco-Tena C, Londono JD, Cazarin-Barrientos J, et al: Development of a radiographic index to assess the tarsal involvement in patients with spondyloarthropathies. *Ann Rheum Dis* 61(4):330-334, 2002.

263. Papagelopoulos PJ, Kitaoka HB, Ilstrup DM: Survivorship analysis of implant arthroplasty for the first metatarsophalangeal joint. *Clin Orthop Relat Res* 302:164-172, 1994.

264. Patsalis T, Georgousis H, Gopfert S: Long-term results of forefoot arthroplasty in patients with rheumatoid arthritis. *Orthopedics* 19(5):439-447, 1996.

265. Paulus HE, Oh M, Sharp JT, et al: Classifying structural joint damage in rheumatoid arthritis as progressive or nonprogressive using a composite definition of joint radiographic change: A preliminary proposal. *Arthritis Rheum* 50(4):1083-1096, 2004.

266. Perlman MD, Schor AD, Gold ML: Implant failure with particulate silicone synovitis (detritic synovitis). *J Foot Surg* 29(6):584-588, 1990.

267. Peterson LF: Surgery for rheumatoid arthritis—timing and techniques: The lower extremity. *J Bone Joint Surg Am* 50(3):587-604, 1968.

268. Petrov O, Pfeifer M, Flood M, et al: Recurrent plantar ulceration following pan metatarsal head resection. *J Foot Ankle Surg* 35(6):573-577; discussion 602, 1996.

269. Platto MJ, O'Connell PG, Hicks JE, Gerber LH: The relationship of pain and deformity of the rheumatoid foot to gait and an index of functional ambulation. *J Rheumatol* 18(1):38-43, 1991.

270. Politi J, John H, Njus G, Bennett GL, Kay DB: First metatarsalphalangeal joint arthrodesis: A biomechanical assessment of stability. *Foot Ankle Int* 24(4):332-337, 2003.

271. Purvis CG, Brown JH, Kaplan EG, Mann I: Combination Bonney-Kessel and modified Akin procedure for hallux limitus associated with hallux abductus. *J Am Podiatry Assoc* 67(4):236-240, 1977.

272. Raikin SM, Schon LC: Arthrodesis of the fourth and fifth tarsometatarsal joints of the midfoot. *Foot Ankle Int* 24(8):584-590, 2003.

273. Rana NA: Gout. In Jahss M (ed): *Disorders of the Foot and Ankle: Medical and Surgical Management*, ed 2. Philadelphia, WB Saunders, 1991, pp 1712-1718.

274. Rana NA: Juvenile rheumatoid arthritis of the foot. *Foot Ankle* 3(1):2-11, 1982.

275. Rana NA: Rheumatoid arthritis, other collagen diseases and psoriasis of the foot. In Jahss M (ed): *Disorders of the Foot and*

Ankle: Medical and Surgical Management, ed 2. Philadelphia, WB Saunders, 1991, pp 1719-1751.

276. Rau R, Wassenberg S, Herborn G, et al: A new method of scoring radiographic change in rheumatoid arthritis. *J Rheumatol* 25(11):2094-2107, 1998.

277. Raunio P, Laine H: Synovectomy of the metatarsophalangeal joints in rheumatoid arthritis. *Acta Rheumatol Scand* 16(1):12-17, 1970.

278. Raymakers R, Waugh W: The treatment of metatarsalgia with hallux valgus. *J Bone Joint Surg Br* 53(4):684-687, 1971.

279. Reinherz RP, Sheldon DP, Kwiecinski MG: Calcaneal involvement in inflammatory disease. *Clin Podiatr Med Surg* 5(1):77-88, 1988.

280. Reiter H: Über eine bisher unerkannte Spirochateninfektion. *Dtsch Med Wochenschr* 42:1535-1536, 1916.

281. Riggs SA Jr, Johnson EW Jr: McKeever arthrodesis for the painful hallux. *Foot Ankle* 3(5):248-253, 1983.

282. Robbins S: Gout. In Robbins, S, Cotran R, Kumar V (eds): *Pathologic Basis of Disease*, ed 3. Philadelphia, WB Saunders, 1984 pp 290-295.

283. Robbins S, Cotran R, Kumar V: Diseases of immunity. In Robbins S, Cotran R, Kumar V (eds): *Pathologic Basis of Disease*, ed 3. Philadelphia, WB Saunders,1984, pp 180-184.

284. Roberton DM, Cabral DA, Malleson PN, Petty RE: Juvenile psoriatic arthritis: Followup and evaluation of diagnostic criteria. *J Rheumatol* 23(1):166-170, 1996.

285. Roberts ME, Wright V, Hill AG, Mehra AC: Psoriatic arthritis. Follow-up study. *Ann Rheum Dis* 35(3):206-212, 1976.

286. Rocca PV, Siegel LB, Cupps TR: The concomitant expression of vasculitis and coagulopathy: Synergy for marked tissue ischemia. *J Rheumatol* 21(3):556-560, 1994.

287. Rodnan G, Schumacher H: Gout. In Rodnan G, Schumacher H (eds): *Primer on the Rheumatic Diseases*, ed 8. Atlanta, Arthritis Foundation, 1983, pp 120-127.

288. Rodnan G, Schumacher H: Psoriasis. In Rodnan G, Schumacher H (eds): *Primer on the Rheumatic Diseases*, ed 8. Atlanta, Arthritis Foundation, 1983, pp. 49-183.

289. Rogers W, Joplin R: Hallux valgus, weak foot and the Keller operations: An end-result study. *Surg Clin North Am* 27:1295-1302, 1947.

290. Rongstad KM, Miller GJ, Vander Griend RA, Cowin D: A biomechanical comparison of four fixation methods of first metatarsophalangeal joint arthrodesis. *Foot Ankle Int* 15(8):415-419, 1994.

291. Root M, Orien W, Weed J: *Normal and Abnormal Function of the Foot*, vol 2. Los Angeles, Clinical Biomechanics, 1977, pp 48, 266, 362, 367.

292. Rothschild BM, Pingitore C, Eaton M: Dactylitis: implications for clinical practice. *Semin Arthritis Rheum* 28(1):41-47, 1998.

293. Roukis TS, Townley CO: BIOPRO resurfacing endoprosthesis versus periarticular osteotomy for hallux rigidus: Short-term follow-up and analysis. *J Foot Ankle Surg* 42(6):350-358, 2003.

294. Saltzman CL, Johnson KA, Donnelly RE: Surgical treatment for mild deformities of the rheumatoid forefoot by partial phalangectomy and syndactylization. *Foot Ankle* 14(6):325-329, 1993.

295. Sammarco GJ, Tabatowski K: Silicone lymphadenopathy associated with failed prosthesis of the hallux: A case report and literature review. *Foot Ankle* 13(5):273-276, 1992.

296. Sangeorzan BJ, Veith RG, Hansen ST Jr: Salvage of Lisfranc's tarsometatarsal joint by arthrodesis. *Foot Ankle* 10(4):193-200, 1990.

297. Saxena A: The Valenti procedure for hallux limitus/rigidus. *J Foot Ankle Surg* 34(5):485-488; discussion 511, 1995.

298. Scarpa R, Oriente P, Pucino A, et al: Psoriatic arthritis in psoriatic patients. *Br J Rheumatol* 23(4):246-250, 1984.

299. Scherer PR, Gordon D, Kashanian A, Belvill A: Misdiagnosed recalcitrant heel pain associated with HLA-B27 antigen. *J Am Podiatr Med Assoc* 85(10):538-542, 1995.

300. Schweitzer ME, Maheshwari S, Shabshin N: Hallux valgus and hallux rigidus: MRI findings. *Clin Imaging* 23(6):397-402, 1999.

301. Seltzer SE, Weissman BN, Braunstein EM, et al: Computed tomography of the hindfoot with rheumatoid arthritis. *Arthritis Rheum* 28(11):1234-1242, 1985.

302. Sethu A, D'Netto DC, Ramakrishna B: Swanson's Silastic implants in great toes. *J Bone Joint Surg Br* 62(1):83-85, 1980.

303. Shereff MJ, Baumhauer JF: Hallux rigidus and osteoarthrosis of the first metatarsophalangeal joint. *J Bone Joint Surg Am* 80(6):898-908, 1998.

304. Shereff MJ, Jahss MH: Complications of Silastic implant arthroplasty in the hallux. *Foot Ankle* 1(2):95-101, 1980.

305. Shi K, Hayashida K, Tomita T, et al: Surgical treatment of hallux valgus deformity in rheumatoid arthritis: Clinical and radiographic evaluation of modified Lapidus technique. *J Foot Ankle Surg* 39(6):376-382, 2000.

306. Shi K, Tomita T, Hayashida K, et al: Foot deformities in rheumatoid arthritis and relevance of disease severity. *J Rheumatol* 27(1):84-89, 2000.

307. Shives TC, Johnson KA: Arthrodesis of the interphalangeal joint of the great toe—an improved technique. *Foot Ankle* 1(1):26-9, 1980.

308. Sholkoff SD, Glickman MG, Steinbach HL: The radiographic pattern of polyarthritis in Reiter's syndrome. *Arthritis Rheum* 14(4):551-555, 1971.

309. Smith NR: Hallux valgus and rigidus treated by arthrodesis of the metatarsophalangeal joint. *BMJ* 2(4799):1385-1387, 1952.

310. Smith RW, Joanis TL, Maxwell PD: Great toe metatarsophalangeal joint arthrodesis: A user-friendly technique. *Foot Ankle* 13(7):367-377, 1992.

311. Smith RW, Katchis SD, Ayson LC: Outcomes in hallux rigidus patients treated nonoperatively: A long-term follow-up study. *Foot Ankle Int* 21(11):906-913, 2000.

312. Smith T, Malay O, Ruch J: Hallux limitus and rigidus. In McGlamry E (ed): *Comprehensive Textbook of Foot Surgery*. Baltimore, Williams & Wilkins, 1987, pp 238-250.

313. Sobel E, Giorgini RJ: Surgical considerations in the geriatric patient. *Clin Podiatr Med Surg* 20(3):607-626, 2003.

314. Solan MC, Calder JD, Bendall SP: Manipulation and injection for hallux rigidus. Is it worthwhile? *J Bone Joint Surg Br* 83(5):706-708, 2001.

315. Solomon G: Inflammatory arthritis. In Jahss M (ed): *Disorders of the Foot and Ankle: Medical and Surgery Management*, ed 2. Philadelphia, WB Saunders, 1991, pp 1681-1702.

316. Southgate JJ, Urry SR: Hallux rigidus: The long-term results of dorsal wedge osteotomy and arthrodesis in adults. *J Foot Ankle Surg* 36(2):136-140; discussion 161, 1997.

317. Spector AK, Christman RA: Coexistent gout and rheumatoid arthritis. *J Am Podiatr Med Assoc* 79(11):552-558, 1989.

318. Spiegel TM, Spiegel JS: Rheumatoid arthritis in the foot and ankle—diagnosis, pathology, and treatment. The relationship between foot and ankle deformity and disease duration in 50 patients. *Foot Ankle* 2(6):318-324, 1982.

319. Spraul G, Koenning G: A descriptive study of foot problems in children with juvenile rheumatoid arthritis (JRA). *Arthritis Care Res* 7(3):144-150, 1994.

320. Steere AC: Musculoskeletal manifestations of Lyme disease. *Am J Med* 98(4A):44S-48S; discussion 48S-51S, 1995.

321. Steere AC, Malawista SE, Hardin JA, et al: Erythema chronicum migrans and Lyme arthritis. The enlarging clinical spectrum. *Ann Intern Med* 86(6):685-698, 1977.

322. Steere AC, Malawista SE, Snydman DR, et al: Lyme arthritis: An epidemic of oligoarticular arthritis in children and adults in three Connecticut communities. *Arthritis Rheum* 20(1):7-17, 1977.

323. Steinbrocker O, Traeger CJ, Batterman RC: Therapeutic criteria in rheumatoid arthritis. *J Am Med Assoc* 140:659-665, 1949.

324. Stern SH, Insall JN, Windsor RE, et al: Total knee arthroplasty in patients with psoriasis. *Clin Orthop Relat Res* (248):108-110; discussion 111, 1989.

325. Stiles RG, Resnick D, Sartoris DJ: Radiologic manifestations of arthritides involving the foot. *Clin Podiatr Med Surg* 5(1):1-16, 1988.

326. Stockley I, Betts RP, Rowley DI, et al: The importance of the valgus hindfoot in forefoot surgery in rheumatoid arthritis. *J Bone Joint Surg Br* 72(4):705-708, 1990.

327. Swanson AB: Implant arthroplasty for the great toe. *Clin Orthop Relat Res* 85:75-81, 1972.

328. Swanson AB: Letter to the editor. *J Am Med Assoc* 238:939, 1977.

329. Swanson AB, de Groot Swanson G, Maupin BK, et al: The use of a grommet bone liner for flexible hinge implant arthroplasty of the great toe. *Foot Ankle* 12(3):149-155, 1991.

330. Swanson AB, Lumsden RM, Swanson GD: Silicone implant arthroplasty of the great toe. A review of single stem and flexible hinge implants. *Clin Orthop Relat Res* (142):30-43, 1979.

331. Tanaka E, Yamanaka H, Matsuda Y, et al: Comparison of the Rau method and the Larsen method in the evaluation of radiographic progression in early rheumatoid arthritis. *J Rheumatol* 29(4):682-687, 2002.

332. Thomas PJ, Smith RW: Proximal phalanx osteotomy for the surgical treatment of hallux rigidus. *Foot Ankle Int* 20(1):3-12, 1999.

333. Thomas S, Kinninmonth AW, Kumar CS: Long-term results of the modified Hoffman procedure in the rheumatoid forefoot. *J Bone Joint Surg Am* 87(4):748-752, 2005.

334. Thomas WH: Surgery of the foot in rheumatoid arthritis. *Orthop Clin North Am* 6(3):831-835, 1975.

335. Thompson F, McElveney R: Arthrodesis of the first metatarsophalangeal joint. *J Bone Joint Surg Am* 22:555-558, 1940.

336. Thompson JA, Jennings MB, Hodge W: Orthotic therapy in the management of osteoarthritis. *J Am Podiatr Med Assoc* 82(3):136-139, 1992.

337. Thordarson DB, Aval S, Krieger L: Failure of hallux MP preservation surgery for rheumatoid arthritis. *Foot Ankle Int* 23(6):486-490, 2002.

338. Tillmann K: Surgery of the rheumatoid forefoot with special reference to the plantar approach. *Clin Orthop Relat Res* (340):39-47, 1997.

339. Toolan BC, Hansen ST Jr: Surgery of the rheumatoid foot and ankle. *Curr Opin Rheumatol* 10(2):116-119, 1998.

340. Townley CO, Taranow WS: A metallic hemiarthroplasty resurfacing prosthesis for the hallux metatarsophalangeal joint. *Foot Ankle Int* 15(11):575-580, 1994.

341. Tsi D, Khow A, Iino T, et al: Effect of Brand's glucosamine with essence of chicken on collagen-induced arthritis in rats. *Life Sci* 73(23):2953-2962, 2003.

342. Tupman S: Arthrodesis of the first metatarsophalangeal joint. *J Bone Joint Surg Br* 40:826, 1958.

343. Turan I, Lindgren U: Compression-screw arthrodesis of the first metatarsophalangeal joint of the foot. *Clin Orthop Relat Res* (221):292-295, 1987.

344. Vainio K: Morton's metatarsalgia in rheumatoid arthritis. *Clin Orthop Relat Res* (142):85-89, 1979.

345. Vainio K: The rheumatoid foot; a clinical study with pathological and roentgenological comments. *Ann Chir Gynaecol Fenn* 45(Suppl 1):1-107, 1956.

346. van der Heijden KW, Rasker JJ, Jacobs JW, Dey K: Kates forefoot arthroplasty in rheumatoid arthritis. A 5-year followup study. *J Rheumatol* 19(10):1545-1550, 1992.

347. Vandeputte G, Steenwerckx A, Mulier T, et al: Forefoot reconstruction in rheumatoid arthritis patients: Keller-Lelievre-Hoffmann versus arthrodesis MTP1-Hoffmann. *Foot Ankle Int* 20(7):438-443, 1999.

348. Vanore J, O'Keefe R, Pikscher I: Complications of silicone implants in foot surgery. *Clin Podiatry* 1(1):175-198, 1984.

349. Vanore J, O'Keefe R, Pikscher I: Silastic implant arthroplasty. Complications and their classification. *J Am Podiatry Assoc* 74(9):423-433, 1984.

350. Verhaar J, Vermeulen A, Bulstra S, Walenkamp G: Bone reaction to silicone metatarsophalangeal joint-1 hemiprosthesis. *Clin Orthop Relat Res* 245:228-232, 1989.

351. Vidigal E, Jacoby RK, Dixon AS, et al: The foot in chronic rheumatoid arthritis. *Ann Rheum Dis* 34(4):292-297, 1975.

352. von Salis-Soglio G, Thomas W: Arthrodesis of the metatarsophalangeal joint of the great toe. *Arch Orthop Trauma Surg* 95(1-2):7-12, 1979.

353. Wagner FW Jr: Ankle fusion for degenerative arthritis secondary to the collagen diseases. *Foot Ankle* 3(1):24-31, 1982.

354. Watermann H: Die Arthritis deformans des Großzehengrundgelenkes als selbständiges Krankheitsbild. *Z Orthop Chir* 48:346-355, 1927.

355. Watson MS: A long-term follow-up of forefoot arthroplasty. *J Bone Joint Surg Br* 56B(3):527-533, 1974.

356. White DJ, Chang HG, Benach JL, et al: The geographic spread and temporal increase of the Lyme disease epidemic. *Jama* 266(9):1230-1236, 1991.

357. Wickman AM, Pinzur MS, Kadanoff R, Juknelis D: Health-related quality of life for patients with rheumatoid arthritis foot involvement. *Foot Ankle Int* 25(1):19-26, 2004.

358. Wilkinson J: Cone arthrodesis of the first metatarsophalangeal joint. *Acta Orthop Scand* 49(6):627-630, 1978.

359. Wilson CL: A method of fusion of the metatarsophalangeal joint of the great toe. *J Bone Joint Surg Am* 40(2):384-385, 1958.

360. Wilson JN: Cone arthrodesis of the first metatarso-phalangeal joint. *J Bone Joint Surg Br* 49(1):98-101, 1967.

361. Winchester R, Bernstein DH, Fischer HD, et al: The co-occurrence of Reiter's syndrome and acquired immunodeficiency. *Ann Intern Med* 106(1):19-26, 1987.

362. Wolfe F, Smythe HA, Yunus, et al: The American College of Rheumatology 1990 Criteria for the Classification of Fibromyalgia. Report of the Multicenter Criteria Committee. *Arthritis Rheum* 33(2):160-172, 1990.

363. Wollheim F: Ankylosing spondylitis. In Kelley WN, Harris ED Jr, Ruddy S, Sledge CB (eds): *Textbook of Rheumatology*, ed 4. Philadelphia, WB Saunders, 1993, pp 943-960.

364. Woodburn J, Barker S, Helliwell PS: A randomized controlled trial of foot orthoses in rheumatoid arthritis. *J Rheumatol* 29(7):1377-1383, 2002.

365. Woodburn J, Stableford Z, Helliwell PS: Preliminary investigation of debridement of plantar callosities in rheumatoid arthritis. *Rheumatology (Oxford)* 39(6):652-654, 2000.

366. Worsing RA Jr, Engber WD, Lange TA: Reactive synovitis from particulate Silastic. *J Bone Joint Surg Am* 64(4):581-585, 1982.

367. Woughter HW: Surgery of tophaceous gout; a case report. *J Bone Joint Surg Am* 41(1):116-122, 1959.

368. Wrighton JD: A ten-year review of Keller's operation. Review of Keller's operation at the Princess Elizabeth Orthopaedic Hospital, Exeter. *Clin Orthop Relat Res* 89:207-214, 1972.

369. Wyllie JC: Histopathology of the subchondral bone lesion in rheumatoid arthritis. *J Rheumatol Suppl* 11:26-28, 1983.

370. Wynn AH, Wilde AH: Long-term follow-up of the Conaxial (Beck-Steffee) total ankle arthroplasty. *Foot Ankle* 13(6):303-306, 1992.

371. Wynngaarden J, Kelley W: Gout. In Stanbury, J, Wyngaarden, J, Fredrickson, D (eds): *The Metabolic Basis of Inherited Disease*, ed. 3. New York, McGraw Hill, 1972, pp 889-968.

372. Youngswick FD: Modifications of the Austin bunionectomy for treatment of metatarsus primus elevatus associated with hallux limitus. *J Foot Surg* 21(2):114-116, 1982.

373. Zadik FR: Arthrodesis of the great toe. *BMJ* 5212:1573-1574, 1960.

374. Zielaskowski LA, Kruljac SJ, DiStazio JJ, Bastacky S: Multiple neuromas coexisting with rheumatoid synovitis and a rheumatoid nodule. *J Am Podiatr Med Assoc* 90(5):252-255, 2000.

Ankle Arthritis

Charles L. Saltzman

Advances in understanding of the special features of the ankle joint and the pathogenesis of degenerative joint disease have led to new approaches in the treatment of ankle arthritis. Compared to the other major lower extremity joints, the ankle joint possesses unique epidemiologic, anatomic, biomechanical, and biological characteristics.

Unlike the hip and knee, which are prone to develop primary osteoarthritis, the ankle develops arthritis usually because of a traumatic event. Ankle articular cartilage has characteristic differences from hip or knee cartilage that might protect the ankle against developing primary osteoarthritis. Ankle articular cartilage preserves its tensile stiffness and fracture stress better than hip articular cartilage. Metabolic differences between knee and ankle articular cartilage can also help to explain the relative rarity of primary ankle osteoarthritis.

In developed nations, physicians have noted a progressive increase in the incidence of disabling ankle arthritis, which may in part be due to the combined effects of the widespread use of life-protecting thoraco-abdominal level airbag restraints and the general aging of the population.[15,16] The increased incidence of painful post-traumatic ankle osteoarthritis has spurred interest in finding therapeutic solutions to this often disabling condition.

UNIQUE CHARACTERISTICS OF THE ANKLE JOINT

The differences in anatomy and motion between the ankle joint and the other major joints of the lower limb, the hip, and the knee are readily apparent. Other differences such as the area of contact between opposing articular surfaces and articular cartilage thickness, tensile properties, and metabolism are less apparent. Taken together, the unique mechanical and biological characteristics of the ankle affect the development, clinical presentation, and course of osteoarthritis and the response to arthritis treatment in this joint.

Anatomy and Motion

The bony anatomy of the ankle joint determines the planes and ranges of joint motion and confers a high degree of stability and congruence when the joint is loaded. The three bones that form the ankle joint—the tibia, fibula, and talus—support three sets of opposing articular surfaces. The tibial medial malleolus and the medial facet of the talus form the medial articular surfaces, the fibular lateral malleolus and the talar lateral articular surface form the lateral articular surfaces, and the distal tibia and the superior dome of the talus form the central articular surfaces (Fig. 17–1).

The distal tibial articular surface has a longitudinal convexity that matches a concavity on the surface of the talus. The center of matching convexity and concavity divides the tibiotalar articulation into the medial and lateral compartments for evaluation of ankle loading and degenerative changes (Fig. 17–1). The distal tibia and the medial malleolus together with the lateral malleolus form the ankle mortise, which contains the talus. Firm anterior and posterior liga-

ments bind the distal tibia and fibula together to form the distal tibiofibular syndesmosis. Medial and lateral ligamentous complexes and the ankle joint capsule stabilize the relationship between the talus and the mortise.

The bony anatomy, ligaments, and joint capsule guide and restrain movement between the talus and the mortise so that the talus has a continuously changing axis of rotation as it moves from maximum dorsiflexion to maximum plantar flexion relative to the mortise. The talus and mortise widen slightly from posterior to anterior. Thus when the talus is plantar flexed, its narrowest portion sits in the ankle mortise and allows rotatory movement between the talus and mortise. When the talus is maximally dorsiflexed, the tibiofibular syndesmosis spreads and the wider portion of the talar articular surface locks into the ankle mortise, allowing little or no rotation between the talus and the mortise. In most normal ankles, the soft tissue structures, including joint capsule, ligaments and muscle tendon units that cross the joint, prevent significant translation of the talus relative to the mortise.

Articular Surface Contact Area

When loaded, the human ankle joint has a smaller area of contact between the opposing articular surfaces than the knee or hip. At 500 N of load, the contact area averages 350 mm[8] for the ankle joint,[8,64] compared with 1120 mm^2 for the knee[54] and 1100 mm^2 for the hip.[11] Although in vivo contact stress has not been measured in the ankle, the smaller contact area must make the normal peak contact stress higher in the ankle than in the knee or hip.

Articular Cartilage Thickness and Tensile Properties

Ankle joint articular cartilage differs from that of the knee and hip in thickness and tensile properties. The thickness of ankle articular cartilage ranges from less than a millimeter to slightly less than 2 mm.[7] In contrast, some regions of articular cartilage in the hip or knee are more than 6 mm thick and in most load-bearing areas are at least 3 mm thick.[6]

Work by Kempson[61] shows that the tensile properties of ankle and hip articular cartilage differ and that these differences increase with age (Figs 17–2 and 17–3). In particular, the tensile fracture stress and tensile stiffness of ankle articular cartilage deteriorate less rapidly with age than those of the hip.[61] The tensile fracture stress of hip femoral articular cartilage is initially greater than that of talar articular cartilage. However, with age it declines exponentially in the hip

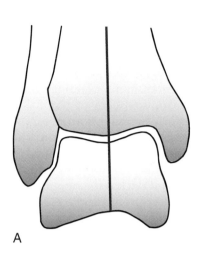

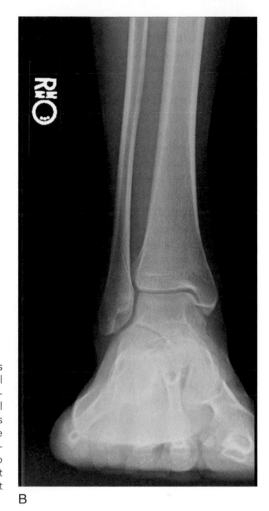

B

Figure 17–1 Ankle joint structure. **A,** The drawing shows how the talus fits in the mortise formed by the distal ends of the fibula and tibia. The medial malleolus and the medial surface of the talus form the opposing medial articular surfaces, the distal tibia and the superior talus form the opposing central articular surfaces, and the lateral malleolus and the lateral surface of the talus form the opposing lateral articular surfaces. Notice how the convexity of the distal tibial articular surface matches the concavity of the superior talar articular surface. The center of the matching convexity and concavity is used to divide the joint into medial and lateral compartments for the study of joint loading and joint degeneration. **B,** Standing radiograph of the ankle joint showing the features outlined in the drawing.

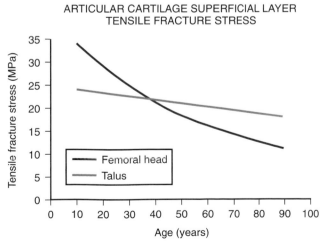

Figure 17–2 Femoral head and talus articular cartilage superficial layer tensile fracture stress versus age. Notice that the tensile fracture stress of ankle articular cartilage is greater beginning in middle age than the tensile fracture stress of femoral head articular cartilage and that the difference increases with increasing age. These illustrations were developed from data reported by Kempson.[61] (Graph courtesy of Joseph A. Buckwalter, MD.)

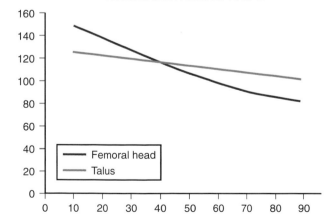

Figure 17–3 Femoral head and talus articular cartilage superficial layer tensile stiffness versus age. Notice that the tensile stiffness of ankle articular cartilage is greater beginning in middle age than the tensile fracture stress of femoral head articular cartilage and that the difference increases with increasing age. These illustrations were developed from data reported by Kempson.[61] MPa, megapascals. (Graph courtesy of Joseph A. Buckwalter, MD.)

but linearly in the ankle (Fig. 17–2). As a result of these aging differences, ankle articular cartilage can withstand greater tensile loads than hip articular cartilage beginning in middle age, and this difference increases with increasing age. Age-related changes in hip and ankle articular cartilage tensile stiffness follow a similar pattern (Fig. 17–3).

Presumably, age-related declines in articular cartilage tensile properties result from progressive weakening of the collagen fibril network in articular cartilage. The cause of the age-related weakening of the articular cartilage matrix has not been explained, but age-related changes in collagen fibril structure and collagen cross-linking have been identified that might contribute to changes in matrix tensile properties.[13,14] Kempson has suggested that these differences in tensile properties might explain the apparent vulnerability of the hip and knee to degenerative changes with increasing age and the relative resistance of the ankle to development of primary osteoarthritis.[61]

Articular Cartilage Metabolism

Ankle articular cartilage can differ from that of other joints in the expression of an enzyme that can degrade articular cartilage and in response to the catabolic cytokine interleukin-1 (IL-1). Chubinskaya and colleagues detected messenger RNA for neutrophil collagenase (MMP-8) in chondrocytes of human knee articular cartilage but not in those of ankle articular cartilage.[21] IL-1 inhibited proteoglycan synthesis by chondrocytes in knee articular cartilage more effectively than in those of ankle articular cartilage.[53] The difference in the response to IL-1 between chondrocytes in knee and ankle articular cartilage appears to be due to a greater number of IL-1 receptors in the chondrocytes of knee articular cartilage. These observations need further study, but they suggest that metabolic differences exist between knee and ankle articular cartilage, which might help to explain the relative rarity of primary ankle osteoarthritis.

PREVALENCE OF ANKLE OSTEOARTHRITIS

Determining the prevalence of ankle osteoarthritis is more difficult than it might seem at first. As in other joints, the correlation between degenerative changes in the joint and the clinical syndrome of osteoarthritis is not consistent.[32,123] In addition, it is extremely expensive and difficult to obtain and study unbiased samples of populations to determine the prevalence of osteoarthritis. For these reasons, studies of the prevalence of osteoarthritis by examination of autopsy specimens, evaluation of radiographs of populations of patients, and evaluation of patients presenting with symptomatic osteoarthritis have significant limitations.

Autopsy Studies

Despite their limitations, including relatively small numbers of joints examined and lack of random or systematic sampling of populations, autopsy studies can provide useful information concerning differences in prevalence of degeneration among joints.

Meachim et al[81-84] examined knee, shoulder and ankle joints at autopsies performed on adults. They found full-thickness chondral defects in one of 20 ankle joints from people older than 70 years.[81] Cartilage fibrillation was much more frequent than full-thickness defects in all joints.

Huch et al[53] resected 36 knees and 78 ankles from both limbs of 39 organ donors to evaluate the prevalence of ankle osteoarthritis. The joints were evaluated using a scale described by Collins.[25] Grade 0 is normal gross appearance of a joint, grade 1 is fraying or fibrillation of the articular cartilage, grade 2 is fibrillation and fissuring of the cartilage and osteophytes, grade 3 is extensive fibrillation and fissuring with frequent osteophytes and 30% or less full-thickness chondral defects, and grade 4 is frequent osteophytes and greater than 30% full-thickness chondral defects. In these studies, grades 3 and 4 were defined as osteoarthritis and grade 2 was defined as early osteoarthritis.[53] However, the authors did not have information concerning possible symptoms associated with the joints studied, so it is not certain if the degenerative changes they identified were associated with clinical osteoarthritis. Using the Collins grading scale, Huch's group found grade 3 and 4 degenerative changes in five of 78 (6%) ankle joints and in 9 of 36 (25%) knee joints (see Fig. 17–2). Degenerative changes were most commonly found on the medial aspect of the ankle.

In another series of investigations, Muehlman et al[87] examined seven joints including the knee and ankle of both lower legs in 50 cadavers. The cadavers studied ranged in age from 36 to 94 years, with a mean age of 76 years. Sixty-six percent of the knee joints had grade 3 and 4 degenerative changes compared with 18% of the ankle joints (Fig. 17–4). Ninety-five percent of the knees had grade 2, 3, or 4 degenerative changes compared with 76% of the ankles. The authors also observed that the medial compartments of both the knees and the ankles were more commonly involved than the lateral compartments. Radiographs often showed no evidence of degenerative changes, although direct examination of the joints showed regions of full-

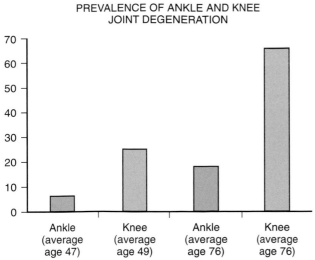

PREVALENCE OF ANKLE AND KNEE
JOINT DEGENERATION

Figure 17–4 Histograms showing the prevalence of ankle joint degeneration in autopsy studies reported by Huch and colleagues and Muehlman and colleagues.[53,87] In these studies, the criteria for joint degeneration (osteoarthritis) were extensive articular cartilage fibrillation, osteophytes, and regions of full thickness cartilage loss (Collins grades 3 and 4). Notice that joint degeneration was more than three times as common in the knee as in the ankle and that the prevalence of joint degeneration in the knee and the ankle increased with age. (Histogram courtesy of Joseph A. Buckwalter, MD.)

thickness cartilage erosion. Overall, the autopsy studies demonstrate that advanced degenerative changes are at least three times more prevalent in the knee than in the ankle and that the prevalence of degenerative changes in both joints increases with increasing age (Fig. 17–4).

Radiographic Evaluations

Although epidemiologic studies based on radiographic evaluations document a striking increase with increasing age in the prevalence of degenerative changes of all joints, including those of the foot and ankle, the reported studies have not focused on ankle osteoarthritis. Radiographic studies of ankle joint degeneration have important limitations because there is no strong correlation between formation of osteophytes and development of clinical osteoarthritis[123] and because it is difficult to evaluate the thickness of ankle articular cartilage, particularly on radiographs that were not performed in a standardized fashion. Furthermore, ankle radiographs often do not show signs of joint degeneration even when the ankle joint has regions of full-thickness erosion of articular cartilage.[87] Attempts to evaluate the prevalence of ankle degeneration and osteoarthritis by plain radiographs alone therefore have limited value.

Clinical Studies

Very few studies of the prevalence of osteoarthritis have included patients with ankle osteoarthritis. The available information suggests that knee osteoarthritis is eight to ten times more common than ankle osteoarthritis.[28,53] Yet the best currently available estimates suggest that knee replacements are performed more often than ankle replacements and ankle fusions combined. These observations, combined with the data from autopsy studies showing that advanced knee joint degeneration is about three to five times more common than advanced ankle joint degeneration, suggest that surgical procedures are performed less often for patients with advanced ankle osteoarthritis than for those with advanced osteoarthritis of the knee.

The reasons for this are unclear. It is possible that joint degeneration and osteoarthritis cause less severe pain and functional limitation in the ankle than in the knee. Lack of understanding of the evaluation and treatment of ankle osteoarthritis among physicians, the efficacy of nonsurgical treatments for ankle osteoarthritis, and the lack of effective and widely accepted surgical treatments for ankle osteoarthritis can also explain the apparent difference in the frequency of surgical treatment of ankle and knee osteoarthritis.

PATHOGENESIS OF ANKLE OSTEOARTHRITIS

Clinical experience and published reports of the treatment of ankle osteoarthritis indicate that primary ankle osteoarthritis is rare and that secondary ankle osteoarthritis, which develops after ankle fractures or ligamentous injury, is the most common cause of ankle osteoarthritis.[30,46,107,111,127] Over a 13-year period in my practice, 445 of 639 patients (70%) with Kellgren–Lawrence grade 3 and 4 ankle arthritis were post-traumatic cases, and only 46 (7.2%) had primary arthritis (Table 17–1).[107] The most common causes of post-traumatic arthritis were rotational ankle fractures (37%), and recurrent ankle instability (15%) (Table 17–2). Curiously, 61 patients in this group gave a history of a single major ankle sprain that never healed completely. This suggests an undiagnosed initial chondral injury as the causative event. Of the 46 patients who were classified as having primary ankle osteoarthritis, 23 (59%) had clinically significant hindfoot malalignment, which emphasizes the intrinsic resistance of the ankle joint to primary articular degeneration and the relative rarity of primary osteoarthritis of the ankle (Table 17–3).

TABLE 17–1

All Ankle Arthritis Patients* in the Author's Practice over a 13-Year Period

Type of Arthritis	Number of Patients	Percentage of Total	Age	
			Average	SD
Septic	10	1.6	56.7	16.94
Rheumatoid	76	11.9	58.7	12.6
Osteonecrosis	14	2.2	49.5	14.91
Neuropathic	31	4.9	53.8	13.95
Hemophiliac	12	1.9	24.3	16.86
Gouty	5	0.8	46.0	18.1
Primary	46	7.2	67.2	12.4
Post-traumatic	445	70.0	51.5	14.4

*Total of 639 patients.
SD, standard deviation.

Patients with neuropathic degenerative disease of the ankle and degenerative disease following necrosis of the talus with collapse of the articular surface make up a small portion of the patients with degenerative disease of the ankle. Primary osteoarthritis is the most common diagnosis for patients treated with hip and knee replacements. In contrast, post-traumatic osteoarthritis is the most common diagnosis in patients treated with ankle arthrodesis or replacement. This observation raises the possibility that the ankle may be at least as vulnerable as, and perhaps more vulnerable than, the hip and knee to development of severe post-traumatic osteoarthritis.

The relative rarity of primary osteoarthritis of the ankle might be the result of the congruency, stability,

TABLE 17–2

Post-traumatic Ankle Arthritis Patients in Author's Practice over a 13-Year Period

Presentation	Number	Percentage	Age (Years)	
			Average	SD
Tibial and fibular shaft	18	4.0	54.9	11.5
Tibia fracture	38	8.5	49	16.3
Plafond fracture	40	9.0	43.1	11.5
Rotational ankle fracture	164	37.0	50.8	14.2
Talar fracture	38	8.3	46.9	14.5
Osteochondritis dissecans	21	4.7	44.6	12.62
Recurrent ankle instability	65	14.6	57.7	13.29
Single sprain with continued pain	61	13.7	50	16.17
TOTAL	445			

SD, standard deviation.

TABLE 17–3

Primary Ankle Arthritis Patients in Author's Practice over a 13-Year Period

Deformity	Number	Percentage
Congenital foot deformity	7	15
Planovalgus foot	6	13
Cavovarus foot	10	22
No foot deformity	23	50
TOTAL	46	

and restrained motion of the ankle joint, tensile properties and metabolic characteristics of ankle articular cartilage, or a combination of these factors. The thinness of ankle articular cartilage and the small contact area leading to high peak contact stresses can make the joint more susceptible to post-traumatic osteoarthritis. In particular, the thinner, stiffer articular cartilage of the ankle may be less able to adapt to articular surface incongruity and increased contact stresses than the thicker articular cartilage of the hip and knee, and the contact stresses may be higher in the ankle.

Joint injuries can cause damage of articular cartilage and subchondral bone that, if not repaired, creates articular surface incongruencies and decreases joint stability. Long-term incongruence or instability can increase localized contact stress. The ankle osteoarthritis that occurs after injuries appears to follow a pattern that is consistent with the hypothesis that post-traumatic ankle osteoarthritis results from elevated contact stress that exceeds the capacity of the joint to repair itself or adapt. According to this hypothesis, the development of post-traumatic ankle osteoarthritis progresses through three overlapping stages: articular cartilage injury, chondrocyte response to tissue injury, and decline in the chondrocyte response.

Neuropathies and necrosis of the talus that cause incongruity of the articular surface also lead to secondary ankle osteoarthritis. Patients with neuropathies can develop rapidly progressive joint degeneration after minimal injury or in the absence of a history of an injury. This can occur because the loss of positional sense leads to undetected ligamentous or articular surface injuries that create localized regions of increased contact stress. Articular surface incongruence due to necrosis of the talus can have the same effect.

Consistent with the hypothesis that excessive contact stress causes degeneration of ankle articular cartilage, the significant residual joint incongruity and severe disruption of the ankle joint articular surface predictably lead to joint degeneration, commonly within 2 years of injury. Advanced joint degeneration can also develop within 2 years after injuries that cause relatively little apparent damage to the articular surface. In some of these latter cases, the joint surface might have sustained damage that is not apparent by radiographic evaluation. In others, joint instability due to alterations of the anatomy of the mortise—such as spreading of the distal tibiofibular syndesmosis, shortening and rotation of the fibula, or capsular and ligamentous laxity—can cause degeneration of the joint. However, some patients develop progressive joint degeneration following ankle injuries without apparent articular surface damage, alteration of the joint anatomy, or joint instability. On the other hand, some patients with articular surface incongruity or joint instability do not develop progressive joint degeneration. The pathogenesis of post-traumatic ankle osteoarthritis is therefore more complex than it appears and needs extensive further study.

APPROACH TO THE PATIENT WITH ANKLE ARTHRITIS

History and Physical Examination

Taking a good history and performing a careful physical examination are essential. First, determine if there is a clear history of trauma contributing to the development of ankle arthritis. Although a past fracture is the most common cause of ankle degeneration, recurrent sprains (or even one major sprain without resolution) can also be responsible. Ankle arthritis is usually not the first manifestation of generalized inflammatory arthritis, but certainly it is relatively common in patients with severe multiarticular disease. Hemophilia, gout, talar avascular necrosis (AVN), or infection can all contribute to the development of end-stage arthritis. Patients with diabetes mellitus, multiple secondary comorbidities, and low bone density are prone to major fractures and the development of Charcot's arthritis.[51]

Next, determine which activities cause ankle pain or limit function. Walking uphill causes bony impingement in the anterior ankle or the talonavicular joints. Pain caused by downhill walking suggests a problem at the back of the ankle and can include posterior soft tissue impingement, trigonal problems, or synovial chondromatosis. Pain that is primarily caused by walking on uneven ground and that is experienced in the back or lateral aspect of the ankle can indicate subtalar joint disease. Subfibular pain might not be from the ankle or subtalar joints but might be due to malalignment and secondary bony impingement of the calcaneus on the lateral process of the talus, peroneal tendons, or fibula. Posteromedial pain

typically indicates a tendon problem rather than ankle arthritis.

The examination should be done with the patient sitting and standing. In the seated position, a careful vascular and neurologic assessment can be made, joint motion estimated, and points of maximal tenderness identified. The ligaments around the ankle should be tested for stability. All major extrinsic tendons need to be palpated to determine if there are associated tendinopathies. Alignment of the foot should be evaluated. Patients with recurrent instability often have a declinated first ray, whereas patients with severe flatfeet and secondary ankle disease often have clinical instability of the medial column. In patients with rheumatoid arthritis, careful attention should be given to the skin and nails to rule out punctate infarcts suggestive of ongoing vasculitis.

The standing and walking examinations complement the seated examination. Alignment of the hindfoot is assessed from behind. Excessive varus or valgus angulation of the heel should be noted. Restriction of ankle motion can lead to early heel rise or back-knee gait. The posture of the forefoot upon striking the ground should be noted. Patients who load the lateral part of the foot might have fixed varus deformity of the ankle or transverse tarsal region.

Ankle Joint Imaging

Radiography

Plain radiographs should be taken with the patient standing whenever possible. At our center, we have a standard minimum series of radiographs taken for patients with ankle problems. These include *standing* ankle lateral, anteroposterior, mortise, and hindfoot alignment views.[104] The hindfoot alignment view is particularly important in situations where the heel is in varus or valgus and the ankle has coronal plane tilting (Fig. 17–5). If we are considering any surgery distal to the tibiotalar joint, we also obtain standing views of the entire foot.

Magnetic Resonance Imaging

Magnetic resonance imaging (MRI) is a very useful adjunct for imaging the ankle. It is excellent in delineating abnormalities of soft tissues around the ankle joint. However, in assessing ankle arthritis, the value of standard MRI is often limited. First, any hardware near the ankle joint generates major artifacts that obscure visualization of articular features. Second, the articular surfaces of the ankle are naturally close packed and congruous. Unlike the knee, where joint surfaces are not congruent, there is no clear separation of articular surfaces of the tibiotalar joint. Third, the now standard, hospital-based MRI, using a 1.5-tesla

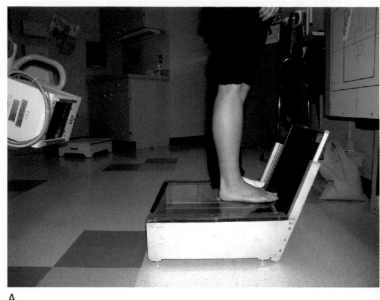

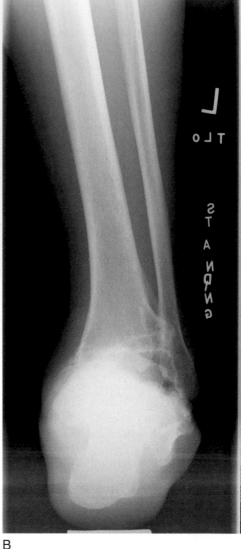

Figure 17–5   A, The hindfoot alignment view is taken with the patient standing on a platform, with the toes pointed straight ahead at the film plate. **B,** The x-ray beam directed toward the ankle in a posterior to anterior direction tilted 20 degrees caudad. The film is placed near the toes also tilted 20 degrees oriented exactly perpendicular to the beam.[104] A line passing down the central longitudinal axis of the tibia should bisect the calcaneus.

magnet, only captures three to four pixels across a healthy ankle articular surface. Instruments with smaller magnets (i.e., 0.50 or 0.75 T) cannot capture any articular features of normal ankles. In cases of degeneration, current standard MRI magnets cannot easily distinguish focal articular features, even with distraction.

Computed Tomography

Advances in computed tomography (CT) have revolutionized ankle imaging. First with the advent of four-slice CT, then 16-slice CT, and now 64-slice CT, the fidelity of CT scans has begun to eclipse MRI for imaging of the degenerated ankle. The total time for scanning has been reduced to 2 to 5 minutes compared to an average capture time of 20 minutes for MRI. As a result, CT images are much less susceptible to motion artifacts. The 4- and 16-slice helical units

now capture anisotropic, 1 mm[64] voxel-based data sets that can be postprocessed to show two- or three-dimensional renderings of any feature of interest (e.g., bone, tendons, cartilage). Noninvasive joint distraction plus air-contrast arthrography enhances the accurate visualization of ankle articular features (Fig. 17–6).[36] Computed tomography also has the large advantage over MRI of being able to work in an environment near retained hardware. CT scans to image post-traumatic ankle degeneration is now a standard adjunct to plain radiography at our center. We use double-contrast air arthrography with distraction for all imaging.

Selective Injections

I use selective injections to help identify the source of pain for patients who have clinical or radiographic

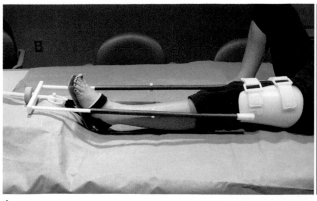

A

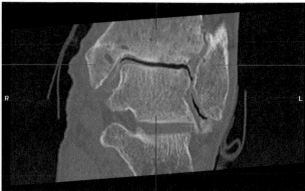

B

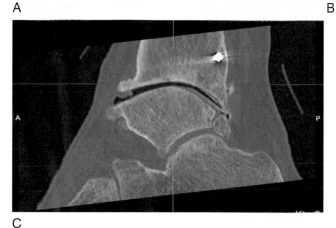

C

Figure 17–6 Noninvasive distraction facilitates imaging of ankle cartilage by separating the joint surfaces. **A,** A modified Hare splint distractor is used for this purpose. Air-contrast arthrography helps delineate the articular surfaces at the air–cartilage interface in both the coronal **(B)** and sagittal **(C)** plane projections. In this example, cartilage appears preserved primarily in the posterior third and medial and lateral gutters of the ankle joint.

findings that suggest more than one focal source of pain.[62] Before the injection, the patient is asked to perform activities that cause pain in the ankle (e.g., walk on uneven ground, walk up or down stairs, run). Diagnostic injections are done under fluoroscopic control. Contrast dye is first instilled to confirm the exact location of the injection. This is followed by injecting a local anesthetic. If the pain is not reduced by at least 75%, we look for a second source. In a study of foot and ankle fusion patients, Khoury et al[62] reported that the reduction in pain following an intra-articular injection correlated to the response from surgery.

Global Ankle Arthritis versus Focal Ankle Arthritis

When evaluating the patient with ankle pain and apparent arthritis, one of the first tasks of the clinician is to determine whether the problem is global (affects the majority of the joint), or focal (affects a specific region of the joint). Inflammatory arthritides such as rheumatoid disease and seronegative spondyloarthropathies are, by definition, global processes. Similarly, hemophiliac, gouty, crystalline deposition, and septic arthropathies are diffuse joint processes.

Intraarticular pilon fractures and neuroarthropathic fractures that cause ankle arthritis generally induce a global arthritic response, especially with multiple fracture lines involving the tibiotalar joint. Conversely, tibial shaft malunions, ankle instability, and foot malalignment problems that lead to ankle cartilage loss initially often cause well-localized focal problems.

TREATMENT OF GLOBAL ANKLE ARTHRITIS

Conservative Treatment

Little has been written about the nonoperative treatment of diffuse ankle arthritis. Indeed, no retrospective or prospective clinical trials have been reported. Nonoperative treatment is based on experience and patient preferences. In my experience, the efficacy of nonsteroidal anti-inflammatory drugs (NSAIDs) varies. Care must be exercised when prescribing these medications because of their known and sometimes substantial side effects. A judiciously timed injection of the joint with steroids can help a patient enjoy an important life event (wedding, vacation). We do not like to give repeated injections of steroids because of the catabolic risks to soft tissues.

The standard nonoperative treatment for end-stage ankle arthritis is mechanical unloading. A cane can be very helpful. If patients accept the cosmetic and functional limitations of an ankle–foot orthosis (AFO), they often obtain partial pain relief. We like to use an AFO that can be intimately molded to the contour of the posterior calf muscles. This permits some unloading of the ankle. The two designs that appear to work best are a leather ankle lacer with an imbedded polypropylene shell for structural support or a calf lacer AFO.[108] The former fits in a shoe; the latter requires metal drop locks fixed to a single shoe (Fig. 17–7). Adding a solid ankle cushion heel (SACH) and a rocker sole can help by further limiting ankle motion.

Operative Treatment

The decision to operate on ankle arthritis requires a clear assessment of the patient's functional needs and a complete understanding of the cause of the patient's problem. Isolated, primary global ankle osteoarthritis is relatively rare. More commonly, malalignment secondary to trauma, ligamentous instability, or foot deformity is present with painful and arthritic ankles. Regardless of treatment strategy, reestablishing normal foot alignment encourages improved foot function. With total ankle replacement, perfect coronal and anteroposterior alignment of the ankle holds the greatest promise of giving long-lasting function and low wear rates. With ankle fusion, correct alignment helps to maintain residual natural motion, especially in the subtalar joint, and can delay the development of secondary hindfoot arthritis. Conversely, periankle osteotomies done for focal ankle osteoarthritis can create secondary deformities, which can make the hindfoot stiff or excessively lax.

The indications for surgery continue to evolve as techniques change and evidence for effectiveness accumulates. Since the mid-1990s, we have witnessed the emergence of several alternative strategies to treat end-stage ankle arthritis. Periankle osteotomies hold promise of prolonging ankle function by redistributing forces across joints. Ankle joint distraction with tensioned wires can similarly prolong ankle function. Ankle replacement is emerging as a viable alternative

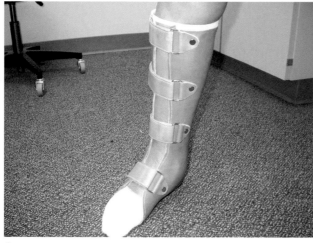

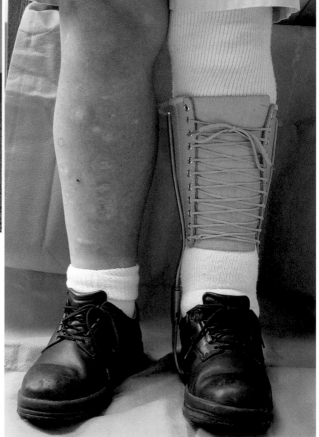

A

B

Figure 17–7 Brace treatment of ankle arthritis is directed at limiting motion and reducing axial loading. The two braces we use are a custom-made leather-lined polypropylene AFO **(A)** and a calf lacer with metal drop locks fitted to a rocker bottom shoe **(B)**. These usually are made with lace-up straps, but they can be fitted with hook-and-loop (Velcro) straps as shown in **A** for patients with profound loss of grip strength from end-stage rheumatoid disease.

for selected patients. Of all the surgical techniques, though, ankle fusion remains the workhorse of surgical reconstruction.

Primary Ankle Fusion

SURGICAL CONSIDERATIONS

In a general sense, ankle fusion has a few clear advantages over other techniques. When the pain originates within the ankle joint, a successful arthrodesis usually eliminates it. Short-term results and complication rates have been markedly improved by modern techniques of limited periosteal stripping, rigid internal fixation, and meticulous attention to alignment and position. Pain relief is more reliable with fusion than with most other techniques. Secondary operations, other than occasional hardware removals, are relatively rare.

However, ankle fusion is not entirely without problems. First, tibiotalar bone bridging after attempted fusion surgery is not completely reliable, and reported rates of initial fusion range from 60% to 100%.* Second, initial pain relief can be elusive if other causes of pain are present or revealed by ankle fusion. Third, functional limitations are common, even with clinically successful fusions (Table 17–4).[88] Fourth, shoe modifications may be needed to improve the transition from heel strike and toe-off, including use of a SACH heel or a rocker-bottom sole. Finally, accelerated degeneration of other foot joints, especially the subtalar and talonavicular joints, occur after ankle fusion after a fairly long time.[24] This, in turn, can lead to further bracing or fusion surgery and must be considered when contemplating an ankle arthrodeses for a young patient.

After an ankle fusion, approximately 50% of patients demonstrate arthroses distal or proximal to the fusion site within 7 years. Although most of these changes are seen on radiographs, their presence at 7 years does not bode well for what will develop at these joints over the next 20 to 30 years. Many factors probably affect the onset of this arthrosis besides the increased stress. One factor is probably related to the overall stiffness or laxity of the surrounding joints. The stiffer the surrounding joints, the less the patient is able to dissipate the increased stress created by the fusion compared with a patient with more joint laxity. Because an arthrodesis is often performed on a traumatized limb, the adjacent joints, although not demonstrating arthrosis, might have sustained tissue damage at the time of the initial injury that makes them more prone to develop arthrosis when subjected to increased stress. Patients with generalized flexibility and ample residual foot flexibility after the development of ankle arthritis tend to have improved outcomes after fusion than those who have intrinsic stiffness.

Once it has been decided to perform an arthrodesis, the next most critical factor is to establish the proper alignment of the fusion site. To do this, the surgeon must consider the entire lower leg and not just the foot. The position of the knee or the bow of the tibia, which can occur either naturally or because of prior trauma, must be carefully examined when planning the arthrodesis. The alignment of the extremity distal to the fusion site is also important to create a plantigrade foot. Sometimes when an ankle arthrodesis is being contemplated, an underlying postural deformity of the foot precludes placing the ankle in the optimal position. If a patient has a significant forefoot varus deformity, the ankle joint needs to be aligned in a little more valgus position to create a compromised plantigrade foot. Placing the ankle into its normal alignment of 5 degrees of valgus can keep the patient from placing the forefoot flat on the ground. Conversely, if the patient has a cavus foot with a fixed forefoot valgus, the ankle fusion might be placed into neutral or slight varus to create a foot that is as plantigrade as possible. Sometimes a selective osteotomy or arthrodesis of the forefoot is necessary to create a plantigrade foot after an ankle fusion if it cannot be created by the fusion alone.

The biomechanics of the foot dictates its optimal alignment. When the subtalar joint is placed into an *everted position*, it provides instability to the joint, creates flexibility of the transverse tarsal joint, and results in a supple forefoot. When the subtalar joint is in an *inverted position*, it provides stability to the joint,

TABLE 17–4

Functional Limitations after Ankle Fusion for 28 Highly Satisfied Patients[88]

Tasks	Number	Percentage
Walking on uneven ground	22	79
Difficulties with stair ascent or descent	21	75
Modify the way they pick objects up off the floor	20	71
Alter use of driving pedals	20	71
Aching with prolonged standing, working, or walking	18	64
Difficulty putting on boots	10	36
Difficulty getting out of a bath	6	21
Difficulty sleeping prone or supine	5	19
Swimming	3	11

*References 2, 4, 12, 23, 39, 55, 59, 73, 77, 78, 86, and 101.

locks the transverse tarsal joint, and creates a rigid fore-foot. It is therefore important to place the subtalar joint in 5 to 7 degrees of valgus when a fusion is done in order to maintain flexibility of the forefoot. A fusion in varus position creates a rigid forefoot and increased stress under the lateral aspect of the foot, which is poorly tolerated by the patient.

Soft tissue considerations are paramount to a good surgical result. Avoid making incisions through contracted, scarred skin because wound sloughs and soft tissue coverage are challenging in this anatomic region. When making an incision, the surgeon must always be cognizant of the location of the cutaneous nerves around the ankle. Although cutaneous nerves tend to lie in certain defined anatomic areas, great variation exists. It is therefore important to be always on the lookout for an aberrant cutaneous nerve as the incision is continued through the subcutaneous tissues. The most common nerves injured during ankle surgery are the medial branch of the superficial nerve encountered in anterior longitudinal approaches and the anterior branch of the sural nerve encountered beneath the lateral malleolus during transfibular approaches. The cutaneous nerves can be quite superficial and easily transected or can become adherent within scar tissue. If this occurs, a painful scar or dysesthesias distal to the injury can cause the patient to be dissatisfied with an otherwise a successful fusion.

Basic Surgical Principles

Respect the soft tissues. Retract carefully. Meticulously avoid local cutaneous nerve injury or entrapment during all stages of the procedure, including closing of the wound. Remove all cartilage, and feather and penetrate into subchondral bone. Create congruent cancellous surfaces that can be placed into apposition to permit a fusion to occur. Use bone graft or bone graft substitutes only to fill defects. Stabilize the arthrodesis site with rigid fixation, if possible. Align the hindfoot to the lower extremity and the forefoot to the hindfoot to create a plantigrade foot. For really stiff feet, slight (less than 5 degrees) dorsiflexion may be preferred. Immobilize the ankle and limit weight-bearing activity until bone bridging is certain.

Open Ankle Arthrodesis

INDICATIONS

The main indication for ankle arthrodesis is arthrosis that causes pain or deformity (or both) of the ankle joints. The arthrosis may be primary or secondary. The secondary form is caused by post-traumatic changes, postsepsis condition, avascular necrosis of the talus, failed total ankle replacement, or malalignment from a paralytic deformity. In some cases, a subtalar or transverse tarsal joint fusion (or both) is included, which results in a pantalar arthrodesis.

POSITION OF ARTHRODESIS

The desired position of the arthrodesis is as follows:

- Dorsiflexion/plantar flexion: Neutral
- Varus/valgus: 5 degrees of valgus
- Rotation: Equal or slightly more externally rotated than the opposite extremity
- Posterior displacement: Anterior aspect of the talar dome is brought to anterior aspect of tibia

Under some circumstances, such as weakness of the quadriceps muscle, the arthrodesis can be placed with the foot in 10 degrees of equinus, which will help to stabilize the knee joint. Conversely, for *really stiff feet*, slight (less than 5 degrees) *dorsiflexion* may be preferred. Generally, however, both equinus and calcaneus positioning should be minimized to prevent a back-knee thrust with the equinus and excessive weight bearing by the calcaneus. The foot is externally rotated slightly (5 degrees) compared to the other side to allow normal knee motion. This, in turn, avoids the problem of requiring the knee to externally rotate in stance phase, which can result in gradual laxity of the medial collateral knee ligament.

MANN TECHNIQUE

Preparation

1. Alignment of the normal and abnormal limb is assessed to evaluate the degree of deformity. This is done by aligning the patella parallel to the operating table and observing the degree of rotation of the foot in relation to a perpendicular line from the patella. In this way the surgeon can determine the degree of internal or external rotation of both the normal and the abnormal extremity. The advantage of this measurement approach is that it is relatively easy to check the alignment of the arthrodesis site at surgery.
2. A thigh tourniquet is applied and a sandbag is placed under the ipsilateral hip to enhance the visibility of the lateral side of the foot and ankle.

Lateral Approach

3. The skin incision begins approximately 10 cm proximal to the tip of the fibula, is

carried down over the shaft of the fibula, and then swings gently distally another 10 cm toward the base of the fourth metatarsal. Although this incision extends between nerves, with the sural nerve passing posteriorly and the superficial peroneal nerve passing anteriorly, the surgeon must be aware of an anterior branch of the sural nerve that might pass through the plane of the incision (Fig. 17–8A and video clip 10).

4. The skin flaps are developed to create a full-thickness flap along the skeletal plane. The periosteum is stripped from the fibula anteriorly and posteriorly, and the incision is carried on distally to expose the posterior facet of the subtalar joint and the sinus tarsi.
5. The dissection is carried across the anterior aspect of the tibia and ankle joint. With a periosteal elevator, the surgeon strips soft tissue from the distal end of the tibia, ankle joint, and proximal talar neck and then medially to the medial malleolus. Care is taken not to dissect distally over the neck of the talus to protect the blood supply into the talus.
6. The fibula is osteotomized approximately 2 cm proximal to the level of the ankle joint and beveled to relieve the sharp prominence (Fig. 17–8B). The distal portion of the fibula is removed by sharp and blunt dissection to expose the lateral aspect of the tibia and ankle joint as well as the posterior facet of the subtalar joint. As this is carried out, the peroneal tendons are reflected posteriorly.
7. An incision is made through the deep fascia along the posterior aspect of the distal tibia, which was exposed by the removal of the fibula. A periosteal elevator is gently moved medially across the posterior aspect of the tibia and then distally toward the calcaneus. This strips the soft tissues from the posterior aspect of the tibia and ankle joint.
8. Malleable retractors are placed anteriorly and posteriorly around the distal end of the tibia, exposing the anterolateral aspect of the ankle joint.
9. The initial cut for the arthrodesis is made in the distal part of the tibia with a sagittal saw using a short, wide blade, and the cut is completed with a deep, wide blade. This cut is made as perpendicular as possible to the long axis of the tibia, and as little bone as possible is removed from the dome of the ankle joint. This cut is brought across the ankle joint and stops just where the curve of the medial malleolus begins (Fig. 17–8C).

Medial Approach

10. A 4-cm incision is made over the anteromedial aspect of the medial malleolus over the ankle joint and swung slightly inferior around the malleolus to obtain adequate exposure of the tip of the malleolus.
11. The soft tissue is stripped anteriorly and then posteromedially around the tip of the medial malleolus, with care being taken to do as little damage to the deltoid ligament structure as possible.
12. The lateral intraarticular aspect of the medial malleolus is made visible, and the surgeon can see that the cut made in the distal tibia has not been completed. Using a 10-mm osteotome, the surgeon cuts along the lateral aspect of the medial malleolus. The articular cartilage is removed while starting to free up the initial cut that was made from the lateral side. Cutting along the lateral aspect of the medial malleolus decreases the possibility of fracturing it when mobilizing the initial cut in the distal tibia.

Lateral Approach Revisited

13. The tibial fragment is freed medially by placing a broad osteotome into the osteotomy site and gently levering it distally to break any remaining attachment to the medial malleolus, then removing it. Removal of this fragment has been facilitated by stripping the periosteum posteriorly before the cut and then making the cuts along the lateral aspect of the medial malleolus through the medial approach. Occasionally, if significant deformity exists, the entire distal end of the tibia is removed. When this is done, the tibia fragment must be split and removed in two pieces to prevent damage to the neurovascular bundle along the posteromedial corner of the joint.
14. The foot is now placed into the desired alignment in regard to dorsiflexion/plantar flexion and varus/valgus. The superior

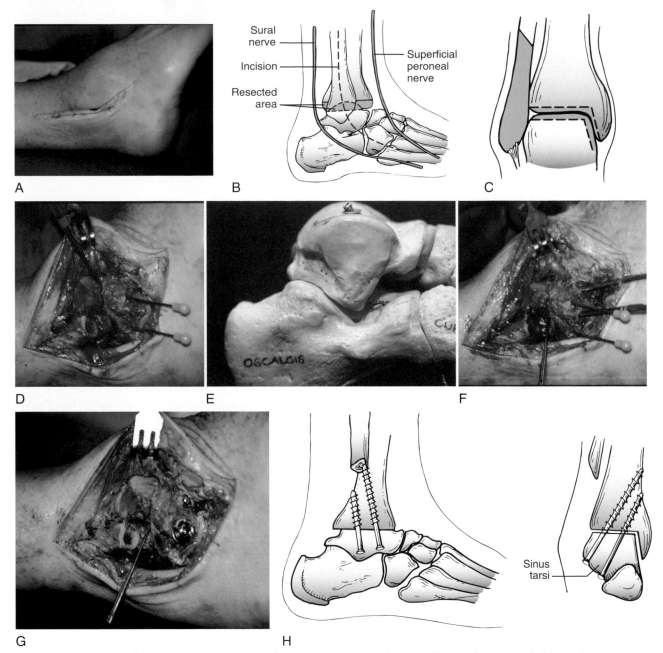

Figure 17–8   A, Line of skin incision. **B,** Diagram demonstrates cuts made in the fibula, distal end of tibia, and talus. Incision is between the superficial peroneal nerve and sural nerve. **C,** The cut in the tibia is made perpendicular to the long axis of the tibia. **D,** After the cut has been made in the talus, absolute bone apposition should exist without tension when the foot is in neutral position with regard to dorsiflexion/plantar flexion. **E,** Model demonstrates sites for placement of two screws across arthrodesis site: one on the plantar aspect at the junction between the neck of the talus and body and the other in the lateral process. **F,** The arthrodesis site is stabilized with two K-wires. Two 3.2-mm drill bits are placed from distal to proximal across the arthrodesis site, marking the site of screw placement. **G,** Following placement of 6.5-mm screws across arthrodesis site. **H,** Placement of screws in lateral and AP projections.

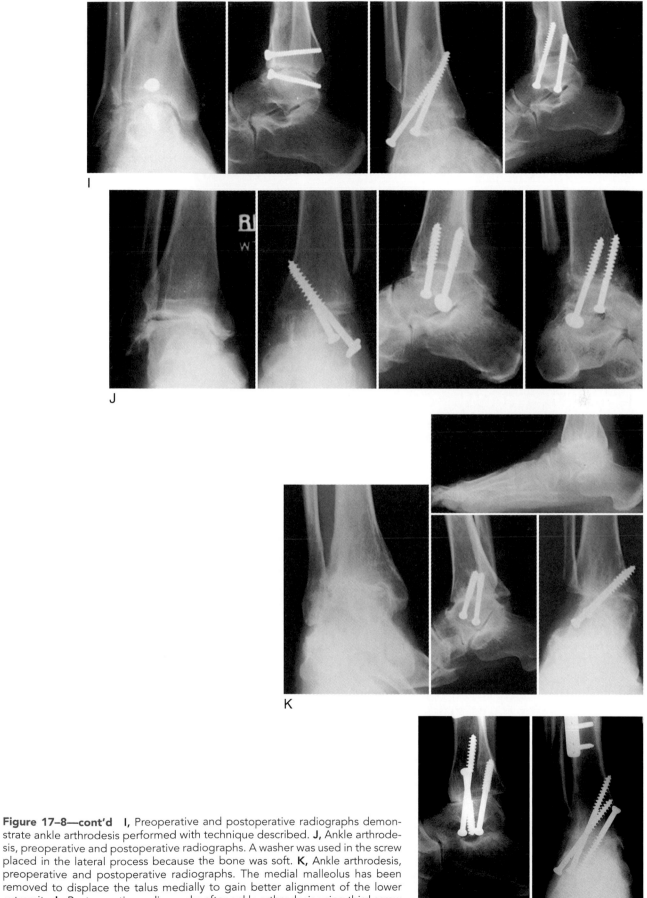

Figure 17–8—cont'd **I,** Preoperative and postoperative radiographs demonstrate ankle arthrodesis performed with technique described. **J,** Ankle arthrodesis, preoperative and postoperative radiographs. A washer was used in the screw placed in the lateral process because the bone was soft. **K,** Ankle arthrodesis, preoperative and postoperative radiographs. The medial malleolus has been removed to displace the talus medially to gain better alignment of the lower extremity. **L,** Postoperative radiographs after ankle arthrodesis using third screw from side to gain increased fixation.

L1   L2

surface of the talar dome is identified through the lateral wound, and a cut removes 3 to 4 mm from the superior aspect of the talus. The cut must be made parallel to the one that has been made in the distal end of the tibia (Fig. 8C and D).

Intraoperative Alignment

15. Once the talar cut has been made, the surfaces are brought together and the alignment is carefully checked. If any malalignment exists at this time, more bone is removed from the distal end of the tibia or occasionally from the talus to align the joint properly. As this alignment is carried out, the talus is displaced posteriorly so that the anterior aspect of the cut in the talus matches the anterior cut of the tibia. This ensures a correct amount of posterior displacement.
16. If the joint surfaces do not come together without tension, the medial malleolus is too long and needs to be shortened. Through the medial incision, sufficient bone is removed from the distal portion of the malleolus to permit the tibia and talus to come together. Usually, about 1 cm of malleolus is removed. When removing the medial malleolus, caution must be used so as not to cut the posterior tibial tendon, which can be quite adherent to the posterior aspect of the malleolus.
17. The joint surfaces can now be easily brought together and satisfactory alignment achieved (Fig. 17–8D).
18. Holding the foot in correct alignment with the two bone surfaces approximated, the surgeon inserts provisional fixation from the lateral aspect using 0.062-inch Kirschner wires. These are placed through the lateral wound and may be driven from proximal to distal, or vice versa, but they should be placed to avoid the tract used for the fixation screws.
19. With the Kirschner wires in place, alignment is again checked for the final time by palpating the patella and checking all four planes of alignment.

Internal Fixation

20. The arthrodesis site is now further stabilized by placing two 3.2-mm drill bits across the arthrodesis site. One begins within the sinus tarsi area and the other just above the lateral process (Fig. 17–8E and F). As the initial drill hole is made in the sinus tarsi, it is important to invert the calcaneus to gain access to the undersurface of the talus. The drill bit is positioned almost parallel to the floor, aimed medially and as far proximally as possible, and inserted until the bit passes through the distal medial end of the tibia. The drill bit is disconnected from the chuck and a second drill hole placed just above the lateral process and almost parallel to the first drill bit. From a technical standpoint, if the patient has stiffness of the subtalar joint that makes it difficult to angle the first drill bit proximally enough, a small trough can be cut in the lateral aspect of the calcaneus so that the drill bit can be placed at a more oblique angle.
21. One of the drill bits is removed, the depth measured, the hole tapped, and a 6.5-mm screw inserted (Fig. 17–8G). Usually a 60- to 70-mm screw with long threads is used. If the threads will not completely cross the arthrodesis site, a short-threaded screw is used. It is extremely important, however, for the threads to engage the medial cortex of the tibia to gain maximum interfragmentary compression. The screw placed into the lateral process area must be high enough so that it will not impinge against the posterior facet and oblique enough that it will not crack the bone over the lateral aspect of the talus. In patients with soft bone, it is occasionally helpful to use a washer (Fig. 17–8H and I).
22. The rigidity of the arthrodesis site is now checked by stressing it. If there is any motion, the surgeon should first check for adequate apposition of the bone along the fusion site, especially medially, and if the surfaces appear to be apposed, then check that both screws are as tight as they can be without stripping them. If worrisome motion still exists, the surgeon should consider inserting a third screw through the medial incision, bringing the screw from proximal to distal into the body of the talus. If the medial malleolus has been removed, a seam of staples can be used along the medial aspect of the joint to increase the rigidity of the construct (Fig. 17–8K to M).

Closure

23. A drain is inserted and brought out proximally along the area of the anterior compartment.
24. The deep layers are closed, followed by the subcutaneous tissue and skin.
25. Approximately 20 mL of 0.25% plain bupivacaine is instilled through the drain, which is not connected to suction until after the dressing has been applied to permit it to set.
26. A compression dressing is applied and supported with two plaster splints.
27. The tourniquet is released and the drain hooked to a suction pump.

Postoperative Care

In the recovery room, when the patient begins to experience pain, the anesthesiologist performs a popliteal block. This usually provides 18 to 36 hours of pain relief. If the block is not effective for more than 12 to 16 hours, a second block can be used. The drain is removed the following day.

The postoperative dressing is left in place for 10 to 12 days, and then it is removed along with the sutures. A short-leg, non–weight-bearing cast is applied. Removable casts are not used for an ankle fusion. They do not provide enough immobilization at the arthrodesis site because of the lever arm created by the foot and the tibia.

Six weeks after surgery the cast is removed, radiographs are taken, and if adequate healing appears to be occurring, a new short-leg fiberglass walking cast is fitted and the patient is permitted to bear weight as tolerated.

Twelve weeks after surgery the second cast is removed, radiographs are taken, and if healing is satisfactory, the patient is permitted to walk with an elastic stocking and to bear weight as tolerated. If the fusion site is not complete, the ankle is placed back into a cast for another month. Although in this series[25] the average time to fusion was 14 weeks, we did not hesitate to keep the ankle immobilized until adequate fusion occurred, which in some cases took 26 weeks. The patient must be made aware of this possibility before surgery to lessen the disappointment if the fusion is not complete at 12 weeks.

Clinical Experience

A review of Mann's[76] experience with the transfibular approach in 81 fusions in 77 patients (46 men and 31 women; average age, 56 years; range, 24 to 82 years) noted a chief complaint of pain in 67 of 81 (83%), deformity in 10 (12%), and instability in 4 (5%). The follow-up averaged 35 months (range, 12 to 74 months). Symptoms were present an average of 6.4 years (±1.9 years). Seventy-five percent of the patients used an AFO for approximately 1 year before surgery.

Mann's results demonstrated that 71 of 81 (88%) arthrodeses fused in an average of 13.8 weeks (±6 weeks) and that 10 (12%) failed to unite. In the subgroup of ankles treated for a nonunion, 9 of 12 healed after revision surgery. The time to union was 22.9 weeks compared with 13.8 weeks for the entire group. This compares favorably with other series in the literature: 21 weeks,[65] 54 weeks,[34] and 22 weeks.[74] Mann's technique of arthrodesis was the same as for the other cases, that is, creating fresh bone surfaces and using screws for interfragmentary compression without a bone graft.

Fusion occurred in 9 of 12 (75%) in our subgroup, compared with 20 out of 26 (77%) reported by Kitaoka et al,[67] who used a bone graft and external fixation with fusion; Kirkpatrick et al,[65] who used a bone graft and internal fixation with a fusion rate of 9 of 11 (81%); and Levine et al,[74] who used bone graft and internal fixation with a fusion rate of 20 of 22 (92%). Mann's series shows that bone grafting is not necessary to obtain a union in a revision operation for nonunion, especially if a defect does not exist. If necessary, however, the surgeon should not hesitate to use a bone graft.

In the seven virgin cases in which Mann obtained a nonunion, fusion was achieved in all cases with revision surgery that consisted of opening the nonunion site, unscrewing the screws, curetting the joint surfaces to obtain fresh bleeding bone, and reinserting the internal fixation. The average time to union in this group was 16 weeks. In this subgroup he could not identify the cause for nonunion, because all his patients had been treated in a similar manner.

Ninety percent of the patients believed that the surgery helped them, 70% were satisfied without reservation, 18% were satisfied with reservation, and 12% were dissatisfied. The reason for dissatisfaction was pain in four cases, nonunion in two, a limp in one, and a wound slough in one. No shoe modification was necessary in 77%. A rocker-bottom sole was used by 16%, and 7% continued to use an AFO.

The physical examination demonstrated that the calf size was reduced an average of 3.2 cm, and shortening averaged 9 mm for the entire series. In those with primary arthrosis who had no shortening preoperatively, however, it was 4 mm. No patient had problems with the peroneal tendon, and 82% demonstrated a peroneal strength of 4+ or more. The range of motion in the sagittal plane was 23 degrees (±9), subtalar joint motion was 9 degrees (±3), and transverse tarsal joint motion was 15 degrees (±5). This represented 26%, 30%, and 70%, respectively, of these motions in the uninvolved extremity. The alignment of the fusion site was determined to be excellent in 93% of cases and poor in 7%. Those in the poor category were dissatisfied with the degree of valgus of the hindfoot.

Lateral radiographs during weight bearing demonstrated that the total motion between the talus and first metatarsal in forced plantar flexion and dorsiflexion was 24 degrees (±7 degrees), at the talonavicular joint 14 degrees (±6 degrees), and at the talocalcaneal joint 8 degrees (±6 degrees). This is similar to the motion observed by Abdo and Wasilewski.[1] There was a positive correlation with patient's functioning, satisfaction, and calf size with increased motion in the foot. This correlates with the gait analysis by Mazur et al,[80] who also demonstrated that increased motion permitted better compensation for an ankle fusion.[55]

Preoperative radiographs demonstrated that 56% of the patients had degenerative changes in the hindfoot, with the subtalar joint affected twice as often as the talonavicular joint and the calcaneocuboid joint rarely involved. After surgery, 20% of Mann's patients demonstrated an increase in the arthrosis, and two required a subtalar arthrodesis.[76]

In Mann's series,[76] 10 patients had no prior history of inflammatory arthritis or trauma and were classified as having primary arthrosis. The average age of this subgroup was 69 years (range, 59 to 78) compared with 52 years for the other 71 patients. The age difference was statistically significant (P < 0.05).

When the entire medial malleolus was excised to obtain alignment or translate the talus medially, or both, 41 cases with more than a 1-cm resection had an average union time of 15.4 weeks, and there were three delayed unions and seven nonunions. The time to union in this subset was significantly longer (P < 0.05) than the 40 ankles (12.9 weeks) with less than 1 cm resected. The reason for this delay in union is not apparent, but on these ankles there had been more previous surgical procedures (1.8 versus 1.6) and greater preoperative deformity. The procedure required greater exposure and probably more periosteal stripping. The medial malleolus can also provide greater surface area at the fusion site. From an anatomic standpoint, the blood supply to the medial malleolus can be compromised, but at surgery, special care was always taken to preserve the deltoid arterial supply to the talus.

Other authors have reported successful fusion with resection of both malleoli. Scranton[113] achieved fusion in all 13 patients using fixation with a T plate, and Marcus et al[77] achieved fusion in 12 of 13 patients using a medial onlay graft in addition to lateral fixation with staples. Myerson and Quill[91] reported two delayed unions when they used a bimalleolar resection in 16 patients. In our experience, the medial malleolus should be preserved to enhance the possibility of a more rapid union, but if it must be excised to achieve better alignment, the surgeon should not hesitate to do so.

Variations on the Transfibular Ankle Arthrodesis Technique

I have used the Mann technique with several key adaptations (Fig. 17–9).

Regional anesthetics are administered preoperatively. This reduces the need for analgesics intraoperatively and appears to reduce postoperative nausea. Indwelling femoral and sciatic catheters are now available for home use and can prolong the postoperative pain-free period. Care with placing the splint is paramount when using any regional anesthetic.

The distal malleolus is rotated posteriorly on its posterior–inferior soft tissues, and its medial third is removed with a saw (Fig. 17–9D). This opens up the cancellous bone of the malleolus. All shavings from the medial third are kept for bone graft. At the end of the procedure, a small

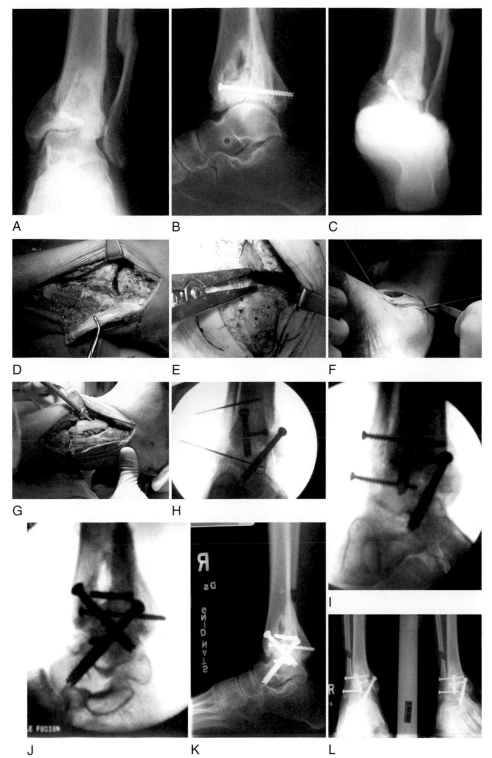

Figure 17–9 The modified lateral approach using a fibular onlay graft. These are the radiographs from a 55-year-old woman 2 years after a pilon fracture. The mortise **(A)**, lateral **(B)**, and hindfoot alignment views **(C)** show joint space narrowing, incongruity, and malalignment. She was unable to walk without pain. In this surgery, a transmalleolar approach was used. **D,** The distal fibula was posteriorly reflected on its soft tissue envelope, and the medial wall was removed to expose cancellous bone. The matching surfaces of the talus and tibia were similarly prepared to enhance healing of the fibula as part of the fusion construct. **E,** From this approach, a laminar spreader facilitates removal of residual joint contents. **F,** A separate anteromedial incision is often needed to prepare the medial gutter. **G,** The first screw is placed percutaneously from the posteromedial side of the tibia, anterior to the posterior tibial tendon, into the talus. This screw is used to compress the talus up into the medial shoulder of the ankle joint. A second derotation screw can be placed from immediately above the region of the Chaput fragment into the posterior talus. **H,** The lateral malleolus is clamped to the lateral border of the ankle and first secured with two nonparallel pins. **I** and **J,** This is fixated with either two small cancellous screws or a short one-third plate and screws, depending on the quality of host bone. **K** and **L,** The postoperative radiographs show a well-aligned and completely healed arthrodesis construct.

segment of fibula is removed above, and the lateral malleolar piece is moved superiorly 0.5 to 1.0 cm and placed as a lateral onlay buttress graft to the ankle arthrodeses construct.

When deformity is minimal or moderate, the distal tibia and proximal talar dome surfaces are removed to preserve the natural dome-shaped sagittal plane contour (Fig. 17–9E). This reduces the loss of limb length, which naturally results from joint preparation. We use 1/4-inch to 3/8-inch osteotomes and side cutting router bits to remove the joint contents. The subchondral bone is drilled with multiple small and shallow holes.

The anteromedial approach described earlier is used, and the lateral surface of the medial malleolus is denuded of cartilage and subchondral bone.

Screw placement is slightly different across the tibiotalar joint because we usually try to place two large screws out of plane from each other. The first is placed from posteromedial to anterocentral in the talus (Figure 17–9F). The leg is arranged in the figure-of-four position. A 1-cm incision is made along the posteromedial edge of the tibia 3 cm above the joint line. Skin and soft tissues need to be retracted throughout this percutaneous approach. The screw traverses the posteromedial corner of the ankle into the talus heading anteriorly. A partially threaded large cannulated screw usually compresses the construct back into the posteromedial corner.

If compression is adequate, we place one derotation screw from the anterolateral corner of the distal tibia (above the typical Chaput fragment region) into the central posterior talus (Fig. 17–9G). This is typically a 35- to 40-mm fully threaded large (6.5- to 8.0-mm) cancellous screw. If initial compression it is not adequate, we first place another large compression screw—either as described in the Mann technique or in a straight posterior-to-anterior direction starting lateral to the Achilles tendon—then place the fully threaded derotation screw.

The lateral malleolus is placed back onto the distal tibia and lateral talus as a vascularized lateral bone graft and to maintain the contour of the ankle. This is typically compressed first with a bone tenaculum, transfixed with nonparallel 0.062-inch Kirschner wires, and then held in place with two partially threaded 4.0-mm can-

cellous screws (Fig. 17–9G and H). In osteopenic bone, a three-hole semitubular plate is also used.

We deflate the tourniquet before closure, obtain hemostasis, and do not use a drain or bupivacaine in the wound.

Postoperative immobilization type and duration are the same as described with the Mann technique.

Complications

Although malalignment after an arthrodesis was not a significant problem in Mann's series (only 4 of 81 patients were not satisfied with the position of the fusion), it can be a difficult problem for the individual patient. In the patients seen after a successful arthrodesis, the most common malalignment observed is internal rotation and varus and the second most common is equinus. Malalignment after an ankle fusion can produce several gait problems.

Excessive dorsiflexion places increased stress on the heel pad, and in the patient with an insensate foot, this can cause skin breakdown. This problem can be managed with a rocker-bottom shoe.

Excessive plantar flexion can result in a back-knee thrust and a vaulting type of gait pattern. The patient often rotates the leg to be able to roll over the foot, thus placing increased stress along the medial aspect of the knee and hind-foot. The use of a SACH shoe can help to alleviate this problem.

A *varus deformity* can result in subtalar joint instability and increased stress along the lateral aspect of the foot, particularly under the base of the fifth metatarsal, and some patients develop a large callus in this area. Treatment consists of a shoe modification to redistribute pressure on the bottom of the foot.

Excessive valgus deformity produces stress along the medial aspect of the knee and hind-foot. This also results in a flatfoot posture. This deformity can be managed with an orthotic device to tilt the foot into varus.

Excessive internal or external rotation is very difficult to compensate for with any type of a shoe modification. This often results in abnormal rotation of the lower leg, sometimes giving rise to a painful hip or knee.

ARTHROSCOPIC ANKLE ARTHRODESIS

Experience with ankle arthroscopy and improved instrumentation have led to the ability to perform arthroscopically assisted surgical procedures. Schneider, Morgan, and others first developed this in the mid 1980s. Since then, several authors have reported their experience with arthroscopic ankle arthrodesis. All suggest relatively rapid healing with minimal nonunion rates.

Indications

Well-aligned or easily realignable arthritic ankles are indicated for this procedure (Fig. 17–10). Patients with global inflammatory, postseptic, or hemophilic arthritis are particularly good candidates. Patients with poor soft tissue coverage or vasculopathy at increased risk of wound problems are also given strong consideration for this procedure. Contraindications are a need for realignment of more than 5 degrees, ankles with significant focal bone loss and deformity, and very stiff immobile ankles.

Room Set-up

The anesthetic must paralyze all the musculature from the gastrocnemius–soleus complex to the ankle. A regional anesthetic can work, but it must also anesthetize the muscles under a thigh tourniquet. We typically use femoral and sciatic blocks.

The table is placed in a beach chair position and then slight Trendelenburg so that the leg is nearly parallel to the floor. The heel is positioned just off the edge of the table. The break in the table at the knee allows the surgeon to put traction on the limb without moving the patient.

We use a pump, large (4.5 mm) arthroscope, 4.5-mmm aggressive (toothed) shaver, and 4.0-mm bur and curettes. In general, we do not use a distractor because it tends to tighten the anterior capsule and make removal of the anterior talar dome cartilage more difficult. Because the goal is to remove residual cartilage and fenestrate subchondral bone, the need for noninvasive distraction is less than with other types of arthroscopy.

With a marking pen, we draw out the palpable branches of the superficial peroneal nerve the malleoli and the presumed level of the tibiotalar joint space.

Joint Preparation

1. The limb is elevated and the thigh tourniquet is inflated.
2. Instill 10 to 15 mL of saline through an anteromedial approach.
3. The medial portal is then established. A no. 15 blade is used to incise skin immediately medial to the anterior tibial tendon and 1 cm distal to the ankle. After blunt dissection is performed, the arthroscope is introduced into the anterior part of the joint.
4. The ankle is distended with the pump. We use the pump inflation as needed to distend the joint. The lateral portal is then visualized by placing the arthroscope up to the lateral margin of the peroneus tertius tendon. An incision is placed just distal to the joint, avoiding injury to any branch of the superficial peroneal nerve.
5. After blunt dissection is performed to enter the joint, the aggressive shaver is placed and a simple anterior synovectomy is performed.
6. All residual cartilage in the joint is removed with the shaver or curettes. If the lateral gutter does not show significant articular wear, we do not remove any cartilage from it. However, if it has degenerative changes, we remove all residual cartilage and incorporate the fibula into the fusion.
7. The bur is used to make multiple pockmarks through the subchondral cortex. It is critical to do this across the entire undersurface of the tibia and the anterior two thirds of the talar dome. Care is continuously taken to maintain the natural contour of the ankle joint.
8. In cases of very tight joints that are unresponsive to noninvasive distraction, we extend the incisions and place a laminar spreader in the joint to facilitate cartilage removal. (See the procedure for miniarthrotomy ankle fusion later.)
9. The tourniquet is then deflated, the pump is temporarily turned off, and the joint is inspected for adequate punctate bleeding (Fig. 17–10C).

Alignment

10. The most critical step is to position the foot correctly under the tibia. With mild or minimal deformity, the focus is on getting

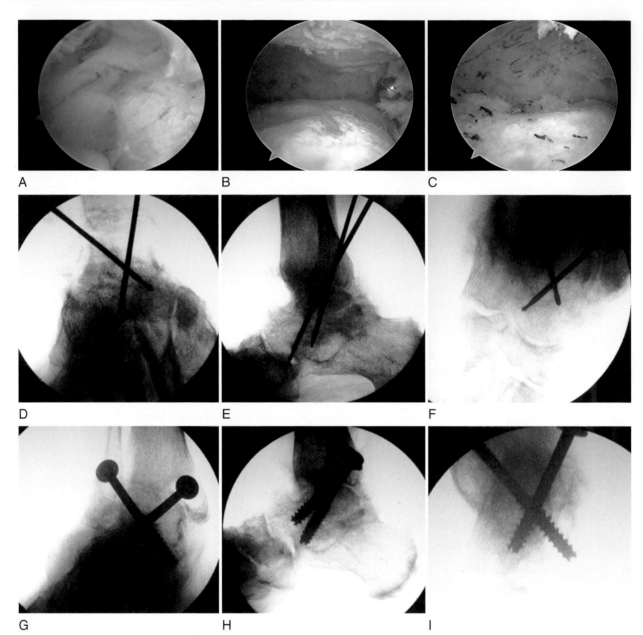

Figure 17–10 Arthroscopic ankle arthrodesis. **A,** Initial intraoperative view of anterior ankle shows bare bone, loose cartilage, and abundant soft tissue. **B,** An aggressive full-radius resector facilitates removal of the soft tissue. **C,** After the subchondral cortex is penetrated by a small bur multiple times, we reverse the tourniquet to ensure we have bleeding bone exposed for the fusion. **D** to **F,** Two guide wires are placed across the joint, into the talus without penetration of the subtalar or talonavicular joints. **G** to **I,** The position of the ankle is confirmed clinically before proceeding to screw fixation. Usually, we include the fibula with screw fixation as shown in these fluoroscopic intraoperative shots. Washers can help with compression but are not always necessary.

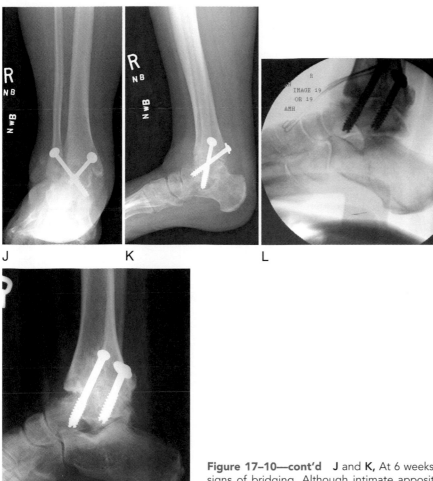

J   K   L

M

Figure 17–10—cont'd   J and **K,** At 6 weeks, the joint is already showing radiographic signs of bridging. Although intimate apposition of the tibia to the talus is a laudable goal, it might not be necessary for arthroscopic (or even mini-open; see Fig. 17–11) arthrodeses. **L,** Intraoperative radiograph shows a 1- to 2-mm gap between the tibia and talus. **M,** At 3 months this is completely filled in with bone.

the foot plantigrade and neutral in the sagittal plane. This seemingly easy task can befuddle even experienced surgeons. The reasons for this can relate to several factors. My suggestions to avoid problems are as follows:

- Place the ankle in the best position and temporarily fix it with two large Kirschner wires or cannulated pins (Fig. 17–10D to F).
- Have your assistant hold the *leg* (not the foot) and go to the side of the room to assess the sagittal position of the ankle with the foot dorsiflexed. Do not accept anything less than perfect.
- *Do not use fluoroscopy* to evaluate the position of the foot.
- Always check to ensure that the foot is in a natural or slightly increased external rotation.

- Remember the orthopaedist's "eleventh commandment": Thou shalt not varus. Varus is poorly tolerated after an ankle fusion.

Fixation

11. For a tibiotalar fusion, we use two large cannulated screws. A mini C-arm can be used to check position and length of the cannulated pins before screws are placed.
12. The first pin is placed from posteromedial to anterocentral in the talus. The leg is arranged in the figure-of-four position. A 1-cm incision is made along the posteromedial edge of the tibia 3 cm above the joint line. Skin and soft tissues need to be retracted throughout this percutaneous approach. The screw traverses the postero-

medial corner of the ankle down the center of the neck of the talus. A partially threaded large cannulated screw usually compresses the construct back into the posteromedial corner.

13. We then place a derotation screw percutaneously from the anterolateral corner of the distal tibia (above the typical Chaput's fragment region) into the central posterior talus. Care must be taken to avoid damage to local nerves with this approach.

14. When the fibulotalar joint has no apparent arthritis, it is not debrided or fixated. However if the fibulotalar joint is included in the fusion construct, a single large, partially threaded cannulated screw is used to secure the fibula to the talus. This is placed from posterolateral to inferocentral into the talar neck and body (Fig. 17–10H and I).

15. If the joint does not easily coapt, we judiciously inject a mixture of 5 to 7 mL of finely ground allograft cancellous bone and demineralized bone matrix into the regions with poor contact. This should not be done in areas of natural contact. Inclusion of the lateral malleolus increases the likelihood of grafting because the first screw tends to pull the talus over medially, leaving a small gap laterally.

Postoperative Care

The surgery can be done on an outpatient basis. This depends more on the structure of home help than medical need.

A well-padded posterior U splint is applied in the operating room. The splint and sutures are removed and a cast is applied 7 to 14 days postoperatively. The patient is allowed 5 to 10 pounds of heel weight bearing—just enough to maintain their balance.

At 6 weeks, plain radiographs are taken. These generally show a bridging cancellous ingrowth, which appears as a hazy cloud in the joint space (Fig. 17–10J to M). As long as there is good evidence of bridging bone, the leg is put in a removable boot. This is removed for sleeping, bathing, and sitting but is worn full time when standing. Progressive weight bearing is permitted as tolerated.

At ten weeks postoperatively, new radiographs are taken. If the patient has no pain with standing and the radiographs are satisfactory, the patient is weaned from the boot.

Although formal physical therapy is often unnecessary, I have found a 4- to 8-week course of balance and gait retraining after removal of the boot to speed recovery in elderly patients. For laborers or those who need to stand at work, the minimum total time off full duty is 4 months.

Clinical Experience

At least 15 case series comprising 7 to 116 patients each were reported between 1986 and 2005.* Myerson et al[91] retrospectively compared open to arthroscopic fusion in 33 patients. In patients who underwent arthroscopy, union was achieved at an average of 8.7 weeks. In patients who underwent arthrodesis by a conventional open technique using similar fixation methods, union was achieved, on average, by 14.5 weeks. Fusion rates were similar for both techniques. The two groups were not similar, because patients with more deformity or extensive osteonecrosis were selectively placed in the open group. Average hospital stay was 4 nights for the open group and 1 night for the arthroscopy group. O'Brien et al[94] reported the results of surgeries performed on 36 patients. Retrospectively, the two groups were matched for preoperative clinical deformity. A fusion rate of 82% in the open group and 84% in the arthroscopic group was achieved. Similar to Myerson's report, hospital stays averaged 3 nights for the open group and 1 night for the arthroscopic group.

Fusion rates of 90% to 100% occurred in 8 reports[†]; two reported rates of 80% to 89%,[38,95] and two listed clinical fusions of 93% and 100% but radiographic evidence of fusion in 74%[27] and 50%,[31] respectively.

Six studies had average fusion times of 7 weeks or less.[‡] An additional five studies reported up to 16 weeks' average time to fusion.[10,19,29,57,95] Another study, comprising 42 patients, had an average time for fusion based on radiographs of 5.5 months, possibly attributable to two delayed unions that required 20 months to heal. This protocol used demineralized bone matrix with autogenous bone marrow graft.[27]

---

*References 10, 19, 26, 27, 29, 31, 37, 43, 57, 91, 95, 96, 121, 125, and 128.
[†]References 10, 19, 26, 37, 43, 96, 121, and 125.
[‡]References 26, 37, 38, 43, 121, and 128.

Five studies listed good, very good, or excellent results in 80% to 100% of patients at follow-up ranging from 14 months to 8 years.[37,43,95,125,128] Crosby et al[27] reported 85% satisfied at an average of 27 months. Corso and Zimmer[26] rated 88% completely satisfied at follow-up. Paremain et al[96] noted improved American Orthopaedic Food and Ankle Society (AOFAS) scores; however, these were retrospectively assigned by the investigators. Winson et al[125] reported 80% good or excellent patient outcomes in a cohort of 104 patients at an average of 65 months of follow-up. Three further studies mentioned favorable results without using a rating scale.[19,38,121]

Complications

The most frequent complication reported has been painful hardware requiring removal.* Other major sequelae were delayed union or nonunion,[10,27,125] subtalar pain or arthritis,[19,26,27,125] subtalar joint penetration,[29] cutaneous nerve injury,[26,95] infection,[19,27,57,125] malunion,[10,38,43] dorsalis pedis pseudoaneurysm,[43] broken drill bit, deep venous thrombosis,[125] stress fracture,[125] and fracture through external fixator pin site.[27] The rates of these complications are generally not higher than those reported with open techniques.

---

*References 19, 26, 31, 43, 96, 121, 125, and 128.

MINIARTHROTOMY ANKLE FUSION

Paremain et al[96] have described a method of ankle fusion that is meant to "combine the advantages of both open and arthroscopic techniques." This approach uses enlarged arthroscopic portals for exposure and removal of cartilage.

Surgical Technique

1. Two 2- to 3-cm incisions are made anterolaterally and anteromedially (Fig. 17–11).
2. A laminar spreader is alternately placed on both sides, allowing one to see the joint directly, while avoiding the soft-tissue disruption of full open arthrotomy. Visibility can be less than that achieved with a scope

fusion. The posterior one third of the joint is often not easily seen from this approach.
3. Autogenous bone slurry or bone substitute material can be instilled to fill gaps.

Postoperative Results

Paremain et al[96] reported early radiographic evidence of healing, which occurred at an average of 6 weeks. Radiographic evidence of fusion across the anterior two thirds of the joint as well as clinical fusion was obtained in 100% of 15 cases. The authors acknowledge that the long-term sequelae of not fusing the posterior one third of the joint are unknown.

A similar mini-open technique on the lateral side only combined with an anteromedial portal was described by Hartel et al[47] They also achieved a fusion in all 8 patients reported. For the occasional ankle arthroscopist, this approach can shorten operation time compared with conventional arthroscopic approaches, which can be more technically demanding. We use this approach when the insertion of arthroscopic instruments is not easy due to large anterior joint spurs or arthrofibrosis.

Ankle Replacement

Early results with total ankle arthroplasty were disappointing. In the search for a workable ankle design, a number of different approaches were tried. Our current ability to critically analyze design strategies from the 1970s and 1980s is limited by the paucity of published data documenting the results of total ankle arthroplasties. Most clinical series from that period included 20 to 40 patients followed for an average of 5 years or less. Patient satisfaction with first-generation, cemented ankle implants varied from 19 percent to 81 percent.* The length of follow-up was a major factor affecting figures for patient satisfaction, because satisfaction generally declined with longer follow-up.

Rates of radiographic evidence for loosening with early implant designs were extremely high, ranging from 22 percent to 75 percent.† A review of the data suggests that the major factors implicated in loosening were highly constrained designs and cement fixation. We do not know whether the cement alone, or cement plus the space needed for cement fixation, was the

---

*References 18, 33, 44, 56, 66, and 68.
†References 9, 44, 50, 56, 66, and 68.

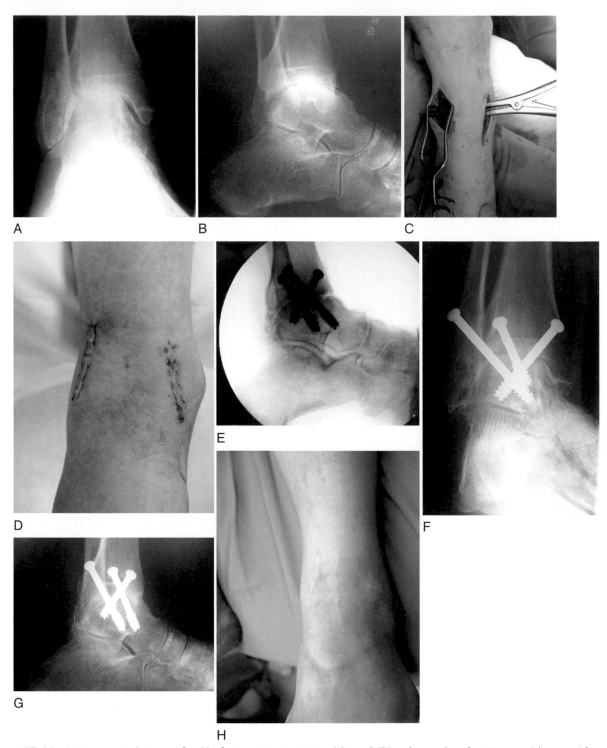

Figure 17–11   Mini-open technique of ankle fusion. Mortise **(A)** and lateral **(B)** radiographs of a 70-year-old man with painful ankle osteoarthritis. A mini-open approach was selected because his ankle moved very little and he had no deformity. The approach involves two incisions through which the joint is easily debrided of its contents. **C,** This is easily accomplished by placing a laminar spreader in one side and preparing the joint surfaces of the other side. **D,** The lateral incision can be extended to facilitate screw placement. **E,** Two or three large cannulated screws are typically used to maintain stability during the fusion process. **F** and **G,** The postoperative radiographs show a solid and well-aligned ankle, and the clinical photographs show the well-tolerated scar appearance.

chief contributing factor in these high rates of loosening.

Total ankle arthroplasty has also been associated with a relatively high incidence of wound problems. Soft tissues around the ankle, especially in elderly patients and those with rheumatoid arthritis, provide a relatively thin envelope for arthroplasty containment. Initial problems with superficial and deep infections, resection arthroplasty, attempted reimplantations or arthrodeses, and the occasional need for below-knee amputation to control infection dampened the orthopaedic surgeon's enthusiasm for total ankle replacement.

Since the 1990s, interest in total ankle arthroplasty has resurged with improved designs, better fixation approaches, and a new generation of optimistic surgeons. Whether the optimism is warranted is not yet fully known; however, intermediate-term results with the newer approaches appear to justify the optimism. Both fixed and mobile bearings are now available, but which of the two is better remains a matter of debate. The fixed bearings are less likely to break or subluxate. The mobile bearings offer the opportunity for greater congruence and theoretically less wear. Head-to-head comparison of fixed and mobile bearing-generated wear particles show no major difference at short term and similar overall characteristics as for total knee replacements.[71]

In the United States, at the time of writing, only the Agility implant (Depuy Inc, Warsaw, Ind) is approved by the U.S. Food and Drug Administration (FDA) for general use. The Scandinavian Total Ankle Replacement (STAR) (Waldemar Link, Hamburg, Germany) is on an FDA trial; the release date is unknown. All other implants used in the United States at this time must be prescribed on a case-by-case custom basis, and fall under the scrutiny of the FDA, which regulates the use of these devices in the United States.

Worldwide, many other implants are being used, most with mobile bearing designs. To my knowledge, all use an anterior approach for access to the joint. Among the currently popular designs are the Buechel Pappas (Endotec, Orange, NJ), Salto (Tornier SA, Montbonnot, France), Hintegra (Integra Life Sciences, Plainsboro, NJ), and Ankle Evolution System (Biomet, Warsaw, Ind). These vary in the area covered (some cover part of the medial or lateral recesses), contours of the articulating surfaces, materials, and fixation techniques. Limited early and intermediate results have been published for several of these implants with remarkably good results.* Most of the clinical results with these implants are from the inventors' initial series; further independent studies are clearly needed

*References 16, 17, 70, 72, 93, 114, 115, 122, and 126.

to determine true efficacy. Initial reports, though, show lower rates of early complications than previously published. Several issues are likely affecting this change, including improved surgical selection, refined indications, meticulous handling of tissues, less dissection for lower-profile implants, and better postoperative care.

Nonetheless, a learning curve affects all new procedures, and total ankle arthroplasty is not immune to this worry. To date, three studies have looked at the problems of early learners of total ankle replacement. The study by Saltzman et al[102] evaluated the records of the first 10 cases performed by nine surgeons. The number of minor and major complications was worrisome. In a further study from nine contributing surgeons who documented complications in their first 10 ankle replacements, of the total 90 ankles, these authors reported 19 intraoperative complications and 7 major revision surgeries within 2 years.

Similar initial difficulties were reported by Myerson and Mroczek.[89] In their first 25 procedures, they had 10 intraoperative complications, whereas in their next 25 procedures they reported only two. Many surgeons have commented on the need to perform enough of these procedures to get over the learning curve. This is partially borne out by the study of Haskell and Mann,[49] who looked at the initial and later cases from surgeons implanting a STAR prosthesis. Volume of surgery has an impact on the technical ease and reliability of total ankle replacement. To some extent, this is likely due to the nature of the implant because all present implants have different designs, each with its own problems to be mastered.

For all current designs, an anterior approach is used to access the ankle joint. The Agility ankle is unusual as it requires a solid distal tibiofibular synostosis for functional longevity. The tibiofibular region can be prepared for grafting either from a separate extensile lateral approach[98] or through the anterior incision.[89] If the anterior incision is used, fixation of the syndesmosis can be performed with a quasi-percutaneous technique.

TOTAL ANKLE ARTHROPLASTY BY ANTERIOR APPROACH

Surgical Technique

1. The patient is positioned supine with a bump under the ipsilateral hip.
2. A thigh tourniquet is applied. We prepare the area and then drape with a skin drape (Ioban, 3M Corporation, Minneapolis, Minn).

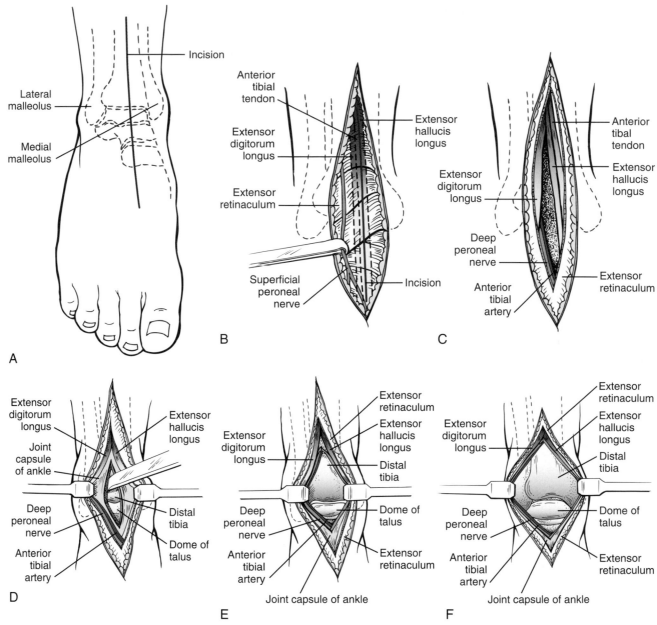

Figure 17–12   Anterior approach to the ankle. **A,** An incision is made directly anterior. **B,** The medial branch of the superficial peroneal nerve is often encountered and gently retracted laterally. **C,** The lateral bed of the extensor hallucis brevis is incised, the tendon is swept medially, and the deep neurovascular structures are retracted laterally. Often the surgeon encounters a medially directed vascular leash that requires cautery. **D,** The capsule is incised longitudinally to preserve it for later closure. **E,** Subperiosteal dissection then allows good visualization of the anterior tibiotalar joint.

3. After exsanguination by elevation, the thigh tourniquet is inflated.
4. A longitudinal incision is made in line with the extensor hallucis longus (EHL) tendon, starting 10 to 15 cm proximal to the ankle joint and just lateral to the anterior tibial crest. (Fig. 17–12).
5. The incision is brought down through the skin only. The medial fascicles of the superficial peroneal nerve's medial branch are identified and dissected free into the foot. These are usually retracted laterally. Occasionally, we intentionally transect a fine fascicle coursing medially across the neck of the talus to gain exposure. Before the operation, we tell the patient not to be surprised postoperatively by some areas of numbness along the medial aspect of the foot.
6. After the nerve has been carefully retracted, we open the extensor retinaculum in line

with EHL tendon sheath and retract the EHL medially.

7. The deep neurovascular bundle is gently teased free and retracted laterally. This preserves the lateral branch of the dorsalis pedis. This vessel supports the extensor digitorum brevis muscle, which is the best local muscle for the salvage of soft tissue coverage for anterior wound dehiscence.

8. The incision is deepened to the level of the joint. It is important to try to preserve the periosteum for later closure. In patients with rheumatoid arthritis or soft bone, the subperiosteal dissection can result in inadvertent malleolar avulsions. Care must be taken to do this gently in those at risk for bone injury. The EHL interval allows the surgeon to see into the lower lateral recess with reflection of the anterior talofibular ligament. The ligament typically heals without any instability in a well-aligned hindfoot.

9. After the joint is exposed, the first step is to remove all anterior osteophytes.

10. Implantation is performed following the guidelines of the manufacturer. Every effort must be made to avoid injury to the shoulder region of the medial malleolus because this can cause intraoperative or postoperative fracture. Because the lateral malleolus in some patients is more posterior than usual, it can be inadvertently cut with approaches from front to back.

11. We close the soft tissue in layers starting with the periosteum, then the extensor retinaculum, subcutaneous tissue, and skin. We close the skin with 4-0 nylon but usually do not use drains, although other surgeons often use them.

12. The final dressing must allow drainage and swelling. A very well padded short-leg splint seems to work best.

13. Elevation for the first 2 days is absolutely critical. Some surgeons permit early motion. Because most implants are the ingrowth type, we prefer to wait 6 weeks before initiating active motion.

14. The anterior approach can be used for ankle fusion procedures. It gives excellent visibility of the joint. An anteriorly placed plate can be used to secure fixation (Fig. 17–13). In some cases, a more limited incision than described here works very well and limits operative time and morbidity.

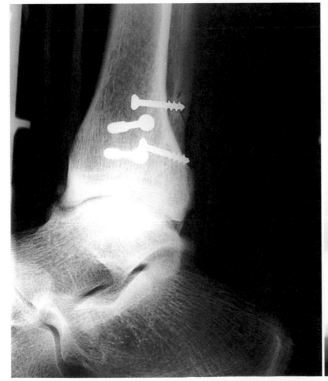
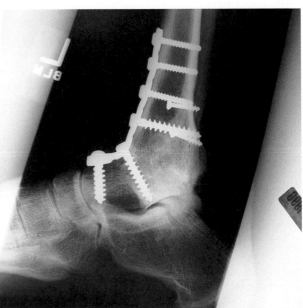

A

B

Figure 17–13 Preoperative and postoperative radiographs of an osteoarthritic ankle treated with an anterior plate via anterior approach. Unicortical screws must be used in the talus.

Osteochondral Allograft Ankle Joint Resurfacing

Limited studies suggest the potential efficacy of fresh or freshly preserved osteochondral allografts in selected patients.[45,63,120] The development of precise cutting jigs for total ankle arthroplasty has facilitated the accurate placement of allograft parts. Anatomic matching and the relatively limited supply of donor ankles remain the limiting factors. Immunologic matching or immunosuppression has not been used for these cases, but it can have a role. Further study of this issue and risk of disease transmission is necessary.

Despite widespread interest and anecdotal accounts of great success, at the time of writing, I could only find two peer-reviewed articles describing results of joint resurfacing with osteochondral allografts. Allan Gross and his colleagues in Toronto described the outcomes in nine patients treated for focal defects of the ankle articular cartilage using fresh osteochondral allografts.[45] All defects were greater than 1 cm in diameter. Three required fusion at 3, 5, and 7 years postoperatively. The remainder were intact at an average of 11 years postoperatively, most with good function, no pain, and patient satisfaction with the procedure (Fig. 17–14). Kim et al[63] reported on the experience of the UCSD (University of California at San Diego) group using shell allografts preserved at 4° C for up to 5 days. In seven patients with global arthritis, the results at an average 12 years after operation were considered poor for three, good for two, and excellent for two. Failure was primarily thought to be due to poor donor–host graft fit, and this stimulated the UCSD group to use total ankle cutting jigs in more recent cases. Their preliminary results in 12 patients (13 ankles) at an average follow-up of 21 months have been documented.[120] The group included 10 tibiotalar grafts, 1 talar graft, and 1 tibial graft. In this preliminary report, the authors revised a collapsed lateral talar dome graft to a bipolar graft and debrided two lateral gutters for impingement. Further study is clearly needed before this procedure becomes more commonly used.

SPECIAL CIRCUMSTANCES

Talar Avascular Necrosis

Avascular necrosis (AVN) of the talus is a difficult problem to treat. Fortunately, not all cases of talar AVN are clinically significant. After trauma, it is relatively common to see signs of focal talar AVN on the radiographs of asymptomatic patients. Others, though, have pain and need further evaluation.

Many treatment regimens have been devised for these patients. However, none has been subjected to rigorous testing, primarily because of the relatively low prevalence of symptomatic talar AVN. For example, in my busy tertiary clinical practice, only about 10 new patients with symptomatic talar AVN are seen each year. No one surgeon or center has had enough experience in treating these patients to provide a good scientific basis for decision making. The following describes my personal preference in handling these unusual problems.

First, I try to determine three things: Is the AVN focal or global? Is the pain coming from a joint or from the bone? Has the talus collapsed or not?

If the AVN is focal and the pain is coming from the bone, treatment can be directed at the source of pain. Fluoroscopically controlled injections of the ankle and subtalar joints with a local anesthetic should help to determine the source of pain. If these injections fail to reduce it, the pain is coming from within the talus.

Typically, surgical treatment of focal and painful talar AVN involves core decompression and grafting. Mont et al[85] reported the average of 7-year follow-up results of 11 patients (17 AVN tali without collapse) treated with core decompression and grafting. Three later required fusion, but the remaining (82%) had good results. They used autograft. Our experience mirrors theirs. Whether bone allograft is as effective as autograft has not been studied, but in our limited experience both have provided similar positive results, suggesting that the pathogenesis of pain is related to stress fracturing and bone edema rather than osteonecrosis alone.

Gilbert et al[42a] have proposed local vascularized pedicle bone grafts for treatment of these problems. In their elegant anatomic report, they show the potential for rotating a dorsal fragment of the cuboid to the ankle region while it is still fully attached to its vascular pedicle from the lateral tarsal artery. Whether this form of treatment will help to improve the relatively good results already reported for simple decompression and grafting needs further careful clinical study.

When the AVN is focal but (pain is coming from a joint, the patient is usually treated with fusion surgery. We use fluoroscopically controlled injections of the ankle and subtalar joints with a local anesthetic to determine the source of pain. These injections can also be used to help to illustrate to the patient the likely response to fusion surgery.[62] The extent and location of talar collapse should be carefully evaluated. In young patients with focal problems, osteochondral autografts or allografts may be considered for partial joint resurfacing (Fig. 17–15).

If the AVN is global or diffusely distributed throughout the talar dome and body, local measures are not generally helpful. Some of these patients present with intense pain, especially with weight bearing, and no

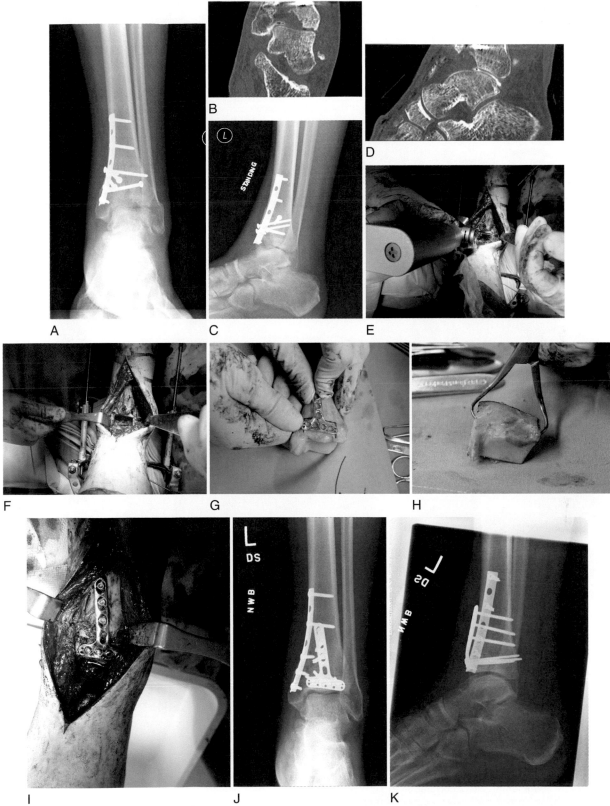

Figure 17–14 Segmental osteochondral allograft resurfacing is an option for ankles with focal post-traumatic ankle osteoarthritis and bone loss. In this case, a 24-year-old policeman sustained a pilon injury with bone loss. **A** to **D,** The central anterior segment of the distal tibia was completely absent when the patient was referred for definitive treatment. The dye-injected distraction computed tomographic (CT) images show preserved cartilage elsewhere. After an anatomically suitable fresh donor specimen was secured, an allograft replacement was performed. To facilitate the procedure, the joint was distracted with a simple tensioned wire frame **(E),** and a box defect was created **(F).** The allograft was prepared to fit the defect **(G),** adhering to the wise adage "measure twice, cut once" **(H). I,** After placement, we secured it with a wrist plate (Zimmer Holdings, Warsaw, Ind). **J** and **K,** The postoperative radiographs show excellent joint preservation and alignment.

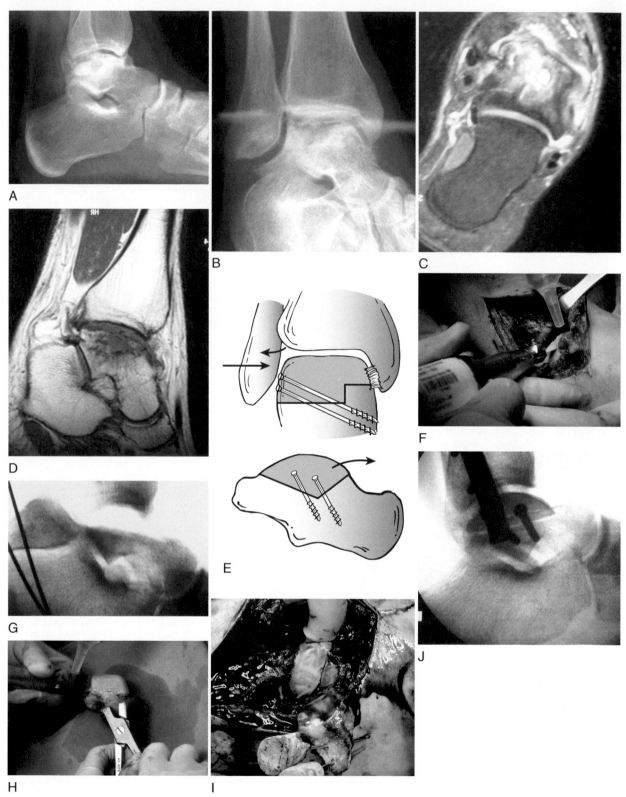

Figure 17–15   Segmental osteochondral allograft resurfacing is also an option for ankles with focal talar avascular necrosis (AVN). **A** and **B,** The preoperative radiographs of the right ankle of a 17-year-old boy with idiopathic onset of bilateral talar AVN. **C** and **D,** Magnetic resonance imaging (MRI) revealed large segmental involvement. **E,** The preoperative plan for partial joint replacement. **F** and **G,** A transmalleolar approach was used, with the lateral malleolus pinned to the calcaneus. The ankle joint was opened and the defect removed with a small saw. **H** and **I,** The allograft was prepared and placed into the defect. **J,** Two buried screws were used to secure the construct, and the distal fibula was reconstructed with standard plate and screws.

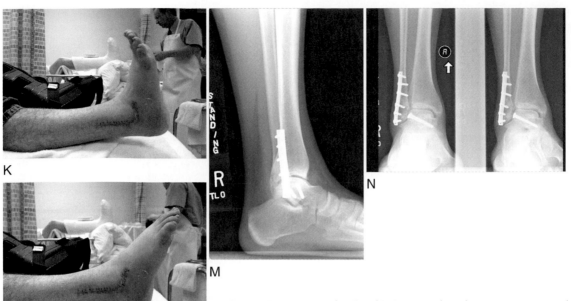

Figure 17–15—cont'd K and L, Motion when the cast was removed at 6 weeks was not painful. The patient is pain free 18 months after surgery (M and N) and is planning to have the same surgery on the opposite side. (Courtesy of Ned Amendola, MD.)

joint collapse. In the talus with MRI evidence of global or diffusely patchy AVN *and no subchondral collapse,* the AVN has the potential for resolving. In these circumstances, I simultaneously use three modalities for treatment because my experience has been positive. First, I prescribe an unloader brace, usually with a patellar tendon–bearing component or with a calf-lacer design. The ankle joint must be locked for the brace to unload. Second, I prescribe an ultrasound bone stimulator and ask that it be used in two locations, 20 minutes per day. Third, I prescribe an oral bisphosphonate for a minimum of 4 months to tip the balance of bone resorption and deposition toward deposition. In some circumstances, where pain is unbearable on the first visit, we organize a single intravenous (IV) infusion of a longer and more immediately acting bisphosphonate. With this program, we have treated eight patients (10 tali) who have experienced near complete resolution of their symptoms and no collapse over the past 8 years.

Most tali with subtotal AVN, however, develop subchondral collapse and secondary arthritis. This can occur at the ankle or subtalar joint or in both joints simultaneously. Often it involves one joint at first, and typically this is the ankle joint. Fusion of the involved joint(s) is the treatment of choice. The use of uncemented, ingrowth total ankle implants is relatively contraindicated because the potential for good ingrowth and component fixation is low.

The keys to a successful fusion in the face of talar AVN are identifying the painful joint with fluoroscopically controlled injections of a local anesthetic, resecting the entire necrotic segment, adding autogenous bone graft or a substitute as a biostimulant, and obtaining and maintaining compression with fixation.

Five current methods of fixation with their advantages and disadvantages are listed in Table 17–5. The technique for each type of fixation is different. With ankle arthritis alone, these can be used with a transfibular approach as described for an open ankle arthrodesis. The following variations must be included to make the procedure successful. For fusion of the ankle and subtalar joints, lengthen the incision distally and inferiorly and avoid injury to the sural nerve. With a blade or locking plate, extend the incision slightly anteriorly and proximally 10 to 15 cm from the ankle, and identify and retract the superficial peroneal nerve. For bone resection, leave no necrotic bone. When a plate is to be applied on the lateral side, plane the incisura fibularis so the plate adheres to the distal tibia and remove a 7- to 10-cm segment of the distal fibula to allow the plate access to the lateral side of the tibia. With significant collapse, remove the distal half of the medial malleolus to enable compression of the ankle joint. Leaving some of the medial malleolus confers better rotational control.

In certain circumstances, a posterior approach is favored over a transfibular approach. These include revision cases with a history of anterior, lateral, or medial wound problems and severe coronal plane deformity from collapse. The theoretical advantage of the posterior approach is that it does not cause disruption of the main residual blood supply to the head and neck of the talus. The technique is described next.

TABLE 17-5

Advantages and Disadvantages of Fixation Methods

Fixation	Advantages	Disadvantages	Indications
Large cannulated screws	Ease of use, familiarity	Poor axial compression, insufficient fixation of short segments	Minimal bone loss; one or both joints involved, initial cases
Blade plates	Rigid fixation, axial compression with an external compression device	Less familiar, technique dependent, no room for error, more dissection needed	One or both joints involved, significant instability from collapse, revision cases
Locking plates	Same as blade plate and easier to apply	Limited sizes, difficult to modify or bend	One or both joints involved, significant instability from collapse, revision cases
Locked intramedullary rod	Good bending fixation, relatively easy to use	Inconsistent axial compression, relatively poor distal fixation, requires removal of ~1-cm diameter dowel of bone from joints	Complete body collapse with two-joint arthritis, revision cases
Multiplane thin wire external fixator	Rigid axial compression, continuous wound evaluation, early weight bearing	Less well tolerated by patient, higher postoperative local infection rate	Infected cases, revision cases

SURGICAL TREATMENT OF TALAR AVASCULAR NECROSIS

Indications

Indications include talar AVN, complete body collapse with two-joint arthritis, and revision cases.

Contraindications

Contraindications include marginal vascular supply to the extremity, need for anterior ankle incisions, and simultaneous foot surgeries.

Preparation

1. The patient is positioned prone, with the foot dangling and the ankle supported by the end of the table.
2. A tourniquet is applied to the thigh. The limb is exsanguinated and the tourniquet is inflated.
3. The prep area includes midthigh to toes and ipsilateral posterior iliac crest if an autogenous graft is needed.

Posterior Approach and Technique of Intramedullary Nail Fixation

4. A direct longitudinal incision is made in the midline starting 10 to 15 cm above the calcaneal tuberosity. In the proximal aspect of the wound, dissection is done meticulously to avoid injury to the sural nerve and short saphenous vein (Fig. 17–16 and video clip 15).
5. The Achilles tendon can be lengthened in a Z fashion with a distal medial hemisection and a proximal lateral hemisection. The flaps can be full thickness to include tendon, subcutaneous tissue, and skin. If the tendon detaches from the skin flap, it is wrapped in a moist cloth.
6. The deep crural fascia is identified and incised laterally to the midline. Mayo scissors are used to gently spread and release any attachments anterior to the fascia. The fascia is then incised while the tibial nerve and vessels are protected.
7. The belly of the flexor hallucis longus (FHL) muscle then becomes visible. Release part of the attachment of this muscle from the fibula and interosseous ligament to bluntly sweep the muscle and tendon medially. This protects the tibial nerve and vessels during the remainder of the operation.
8. The ligaments of the posterior aspect of the ankle and subtalar joints are removed with a rongeur. When the fibula must be shortened or removed, an inside-out technique is used. The peroneal artery is tied off or electrocoagulated, the peroneal tendons are reflected, and a subperiosteal dissection

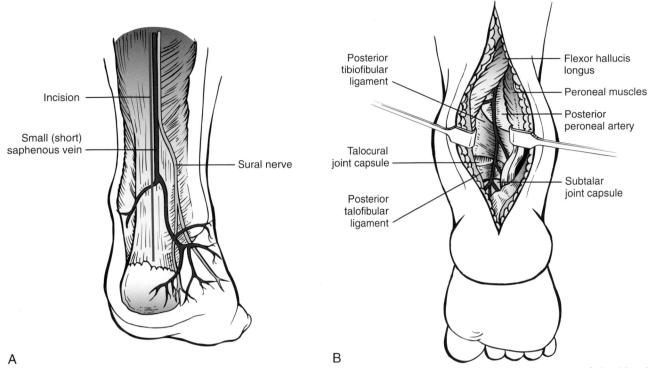

Figure 17–16 A central longitudinal approach to the posterior ankle joint respects the natural watershed area of skin blood supply. **A,** This direct central incision is well tolerated as long as the skin is not dissected free of the underlying subcutaneous tissue and is closed delicately. **B,** In the proximal part of the incision, the sural nerve is at risk for injury. The tendo Achilles is transected in a paracoronal fashion, exposing the deep crural fascia. This is incised longitudinally, exposing the belly of the flexor hallucis longus (FHL) muscle. Retracting the FHL muscle medially then exposes the investing ligaments of the posterior ankle and subtalar joints.

of the lateral malleolus is performed. Be careful not to buttonhole through the skin when dissecting anterior to the fibula. Any bone removed is used for grafting. Segments can be used for a structural graft, although this will need to be supplemented with more graft material.

9. Typically, a Gallie-type extra-articular fusion is attempted to supplement the direct tibio-calcaneal fusion. Preparation for this includes partial denudement of cortical bone from the posterior inferior tibia and superior calcaneal tuberosity.

10. The posterior talus is removed with fluoro-scopic guidance. All necrotic bone needs to be removed. Necrotic bone often has the consistency and appearance of soft chalk with fatty infiltration. With total dome involvement, the resection needs to be extensive, usually to the anterior aspect of the ankle where healthy talar neck bone remains.

11. The four sides facing the resected dome region (tibial, lateral and medial malleolar,

and calcaneal articular surfaces) are pre-pared by removing all cartilage and fenes-trating the subchondral bone.

Bone Grafting

The choice of bone graft is made individually by the surgeon and patient. Traditionally, the pos-terior iliac crest was the source of graft for this operation, and it is still an excellent choice. A large structural piece can usually be fashioned from the crest for internal support. However, other options are promising and less prone to morbidity. Case series report the successful use of allograft or bone substitutes for foot or ankle fusion procedures, suggesting potential efficacy of these approaches.[90,112,117]

At present I prefer bulk previously frozen allo-graft (usually femoral head) with some form of concurrent biological adjuvant. For young, healthy, nonsmoking patients, we add bone marrow from the posterior iliac crest admixed with demineralized bone matrix.

For older or less healthy patients we use a limited trap-door approach to the posterior iliac crest. With a pituitary rongeur we can usually harvest 10 to 15 mL of cancellous autograft through an 8 × 5-mm window. This is added around the interfaces of the bulk allograft, especially on the anterior part that is prepared on both sides of the neck to promote healing and on the extra-articular portion of the graft.

For patients with a high chance of nonunion (smokers, patients undergoing revision, the elderly) or those who object to the use of allograft, we use a structural posterior iliac crest graft. As with a bulk allograft, this must be cut to dovetail into the construct. The reconstruction can be limited by the amount of bone available, and height restoration is often less with an autograft than with an allograft.

Fixation

12. The anterior aspect of the graft is prepared and autogenous bone or aspirate with demineralized bone matrix are placed deep into the wound against the exposed talar neck.
13. The structural graft is tamped into place with fluoroscopic guidance. The graft should fill the space in all six directions. The cortical surfaces on any face requiring fusion should be resected or fenestrated to promote healing.
14. An incision is made on the plantar aspect of the heel. The position of the incision is very important both in terms of proper access to the calcaneus and avoiding potential damage to the plantar nerves. We usually draw the presumed location of the nerves with a marking pen and always stay posterior to that location. The exact location for the incision is checked fluoroscopically in the sagittal plane. Typically, it is 1.5 to 2.5 cm posterior to the calcaneocuboid joint. The transverse incision starts 0.5 cm medial to the midline and courses 1.5 to 2.0 cm lateral to the midline. Dissection to the calcaneus is performed in the transverse direction with blunt curved Mayo scissors. A nasal speculum is then placed into the wound against the calcaneus while the guide pin is placed and checked and for all aspects of the reaming.
15. Under C-arm guidance, we place a guide pin onto the inferior surface of the calca-neus approximately 2 cm proximal to the calcaneocuboid joint. The pin is then drilled inferior to superior, with its tip directed slightly posteriorly and laterally. After checking that it is centered in the tibia, it is left in place and the bone is reamed to the size of the implant.
16. Reaming usually does not have to be much wider than the implant because a scratch fit in the medullary canal is unusual with these short nails. We usually ream to the exact nail diameter and try to insert the nail. If we meet a lot of resistance, we increase reaming in 0.5-mm increments and try to insert the nail after each reaming.
17. All bone fragments from reamings are saved and placed in the medial and lateral gutters around the graft.
18. At present, the manufacturers of these nails offer two different methods for compression of the arthrodesis site. Neither is perfect. We base the decision of which nail to use on the density of the calcaneal bone. If the patient has osteopenia from rheumatoid disease or long-standing non–weight bearing, we use a rod designed to gain compression with a temporary external fixator pin in the tibia. The compression is done against locking screws placed across the calcaneal segment of the rod. In all other cases we use a rod with an inline compression device. This uses a worm screw mechanism pushed up against the inferior aspect of the calcaneus. With this approach, the first locking screws are placed across the tibial segment of the rod. Compression is then applied against that construct. When using the inline device, the surgeon must realize that the flange of the pusher is wider than the area previously reamed; the soft tissues must be retracted anteriorly so the plantar nerves are not compressed (Fig. 17–17).

Closure

19. We close in two layers. A closed suction drain may be used if bleeding is excessive. The skin is closed with interrupted 4-0 nylon sutures to avoid injury to the skin.

Postoperative Care

A very well padded posterior U splint is used. If bleeding is minimal, the splint is maintained for

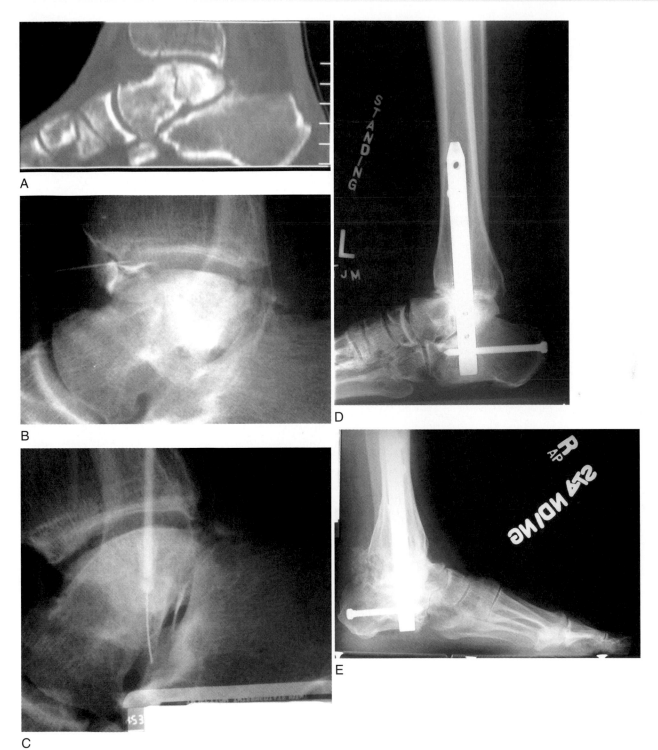

Figure 17–17 Tibiocalcaneal fusion with an intramedullary device. **A,** This patient had pain in the ankle and subtalar regions related to nonunion, avascular bone, and secondary arthritis. **C,** Selective, fluoroscopically controlled local anesthetic injections into the subtalar and ankle joints each contributed to pain relief, suggesting at least two separate sources of pain. **D** and **E,** Both joints were fused simultaneously with an intramedullary nail. Another example of the use of a nail for a tibiotalocalcaneal fusion with bone graft placed in the posterior recess of both joints.

10 to 14 days. In all other cases we change the splint on postoperative day 1 to 3 to a short-leg cast. The limb is elevated for the first 2 to 5 days.

We now frequently use long-acting peripheral nerve blocks or indwelling catheters. The rates of constipation, nausea, and other more serious complications of morphine-related analgesics have dropped significantly with this practice, and patients are more satisfied. At the first postoperative visit (10 to 14 days) it is now not uncommon for patients to tell us they had no or minimal pain with the surgery.

Weight bearing is restricted until good radiographic evidence of bridging trabeculae is obtained. Starting at 2 weeks, we allow patients to put 5 pounds of weight on the heel for balance. We generally do not allow full weight bearing or heel-to-toe transfer weight bearing until we are sure the fusion is progressing. Imaging the fusion site with a large rod present is difficult, and for this reason the average length of partial weight bearing is 3 months, average length of cast immobilization is 4 months, and average length of total immobilization is 5 to 6 months.

Rocker-bottom shoes help with initial transition to shoes. Eventually most patients do not use them.

Pitfalls

Carefully select your pin starting point. The entry point on the calcaneus is the key. The best, and sometimes only, distal fixation screw is the posterior-to-anterior screw. The entry point must be posterior enough to allow the screw to engage 1.0 to 1.5 cm of cancellous bone anterior to the rod. The entry point must be carefully selected on a case-by-case basis. Erring in the posterior direction will translate the entire foot anteriorly, which can accelerate development of midfoot or hindfoot pain and arthritis.

Keep a very careful eye on rotation when compressing the construct and placing the locking screws. Err 5 degrees toward external rotation, and if the patient has limited hip rotation, consider erring by 10 degrees. Most patients need to rotate the limb externally to vault over the foot after a tibiocalcaneal arthrodesis.

Do not remove the locking screws to dynamize the frame. If you remove the locking screws, the construct will become rotationally unstable and will fail.

Do not allow patients to lie on their backs the whole time for the first 12 to 24 hours. Encourage them to lie on their side or prone. This will reduce the incidence of posterior wound problems.

Be patient. Some of these fusions take a long time to heal, but they will heal. The patient should expect long-term immobilization of more than 6 months.

Ankle Neuroarthropathy

Ankle neuroarthropathy is a relatively uncommon disorder. In developed nations, ankle neuroarthropathy is primarily an end-stage complication of long-standing diabetes (see Chapter 23). My group reviewed our experience of treating patients with this disorder over a 20-year period at the University of Iowa.[105] Between 1983 and 2003, we treated and carefully followed a cohort of 115 patients with foot or ankle Charcot's arthropathy. Of these, 22 (19%) had ankle neuroarthropathic disease. In the past few years, the number of new patients presenting each year with Charcot's arthropathy has been increasing at our center. This is consistent with the increasing prevalence of diabetes mellitus in the United States.

Ankle Charcot problems require some unique considerations, because they pose a higher risk of limb-threatening problems and are the more common disorders of the midfoot.

Ankle fractures in diabetic patients with other major end-stage diabetic morbidities are at much higher risk for initial treatment complications or development of florid Charcot's destructive changes. Conversely, ankle fractures in diabetic patients with no other comorbidities appear to have equal risk of complications from initial treatment.[58]

Patients with Charcot's ankle generally have very low systemic bone density.[51] Surgeons have long experienced difficulty in treating Charcot's ankle problems. In retrospect, it appears that many of these problems are related to profound loss of bone density and difficulty with standard techniques of fixation, which have been developed for use in bone of normal density.

Coronal plane instability is poorly tolerated. Both varus and valgus instability patterns occur. Neither is easily braced. With fracture of the medial malleolus, the foot can invert, driving the distal tip of the fibula into the floor (or brace). Ulceration of this region usually ensues, which makes the use of casts or braces very difficult. Ulcers on the medial border of the foot often develop with uncontrolled fibular fractures.

The choice of treatment must be seen in the light of what is best for the patient, not what is best for the ankle. These patients often have multiple and serious systemic comorbidities. Some require hemodialysis or immunosuppressive agents for a renal transplant. Others have severe end-stage myocardial dysfunction or are blind. Most patients do not consider prolonged bracing a failure of treatment. The risks of surgical reconstruction and the difficulties of postoperative convalescence can be considerable and should not be underestimated. Sometimes an amputation of the leg is better than an attempt at complete reconstruction of the ankle.

Surgical Decision Making for Charcot's Ankle

The surgical treatment for an unstable or infected Charcot ankle is an arthrodesis procedure. The major decisions regarding the technique for performing this surgery revolve around the answers to three simple questions: Is the ankle joint injury open or closed? What is the exact instability pattern, varus, valgus, or both? What joints are involved: ankle, subtalar, talonavicular, or some combination?

Open Ankles

We treat open Charcot's ankles with complete debridement and a multiplane, thin-wire external fixation. We have had satisfactory results from salvage of diffuse ankle osteomyelitis by single-stage resection and circumferential frame compression arthrodesis. Whether this is done in a single stage or as multiple debridements followed by an arthrodesis depends on the surgeon's experience and individual decision making.

In my limited series of these types of cases, eight patients with diffuse ankle osteomyelitis were treated by resection of all infected tissue and hybrid-frame compression arthrodesis.[102] At presentation, five had open wounds. According to the Cierny–Mader classification, all had diffuse anatomic involvement and six of eight were compromised hosts. Seven had central distal tibial column involvement and one had primarily talar involvement. Surgery involved a two-incision approach, removal of all infected tissue, and application of a compression circumferential frame with five thin wires across the foot, two across the tibia, and two half pins in the tibia. (This technique is described in Chapter 18). Fusion of eight ankles and four subtalar joints was attempted. All patients received 6 weeks of IV antibiotics. Open wounds were treated with vacuum-assisted wound closure (wound VAC) to closure. Frames were removed at 3 months and walking casts were applied for 1 to 2 more months.

In this series, ankle sepsis was eradicated in all patients. Seven of 8 ankles fused at an average of 13.5 weeks (range, 10 to 16 weeks) (Fig. 17–18). One limb had to be amputated below the knee at 5 weeks due to untreatable vascular insufficiency. Three of four subtalar joints fused. Fixation problems included two pin tract infections that cleared with oral cephalexin and one broken half-pin. Two diabetic Charcot's patients required long-term AFO use due to subtalar instability. At an average of 3.4-years' follow-up, none of the seven fused ankles have required further surgery.

These findings are similar to those reported by others who used external fixation to treat ankle infection with ultimate arthrodesis. These series are not specifically of diabetic Charcot's patients, but together the results lend support to the efficacy of external fixation for these difficult problems. In Cierny's original series of 36 patients, he used aggressive reconstructive techniques for the time, and the limb salvage rate was 74%.[22] Patients with substantial central column involvement had staged reconstruction with antibiotic bead placement, multiple bone grafting, and liberal use of free muscle transfers. They reported that 86% of the major complications and all of the treatment failures occurred in compromised hosts. Of the 12 non-amputated ankles classified as Cierny–Mader type IVB (similar to my series above), five required re-treatment with an eventual 92% union rate and 83% infection-free rate. The average number of procedures required was 4.9.[22]

Before the Cierny–Mader classification system was developed, Lortat-Jacob et al[75] reported successful fusion with external fixation and multiple Papineau graftings in 18 of 24 (75%) ankles. Thordarson et al[116] reported their center's experience with staged reconstruction in five patients with distal tibial osteomyelitis with open wounds. The treatment protocol involved staged debridements, soft tissue transfer, unilateral external fixation, and a 6-week course of intravenous antibiotics. These authors had a high rate of salvage and infection eradication.

Richter et al[99] reported the results for 45 ankle or subtalar (or both) infections treated by a combination of debridements, a combination of internal and simultaneous large pin external fixation, and selective iliac crest grafting. Patients required an average of 2.8 surgical procedures until fusion. Solid fusion was achieved in 39 of 45 patients with this protocol. Six patients required further pin tract surgery for continuous septic drainage. This cohort of patients was different from those in my series because only five of their 45 patients had diabetes mellitus. The complications were higher in the patients with systemic comorbidities.

Kollig et al[73] presented a series most similar to my series.[102] In their series of 15 patients with septic ankles, 12 were treated with hybrid external fixation

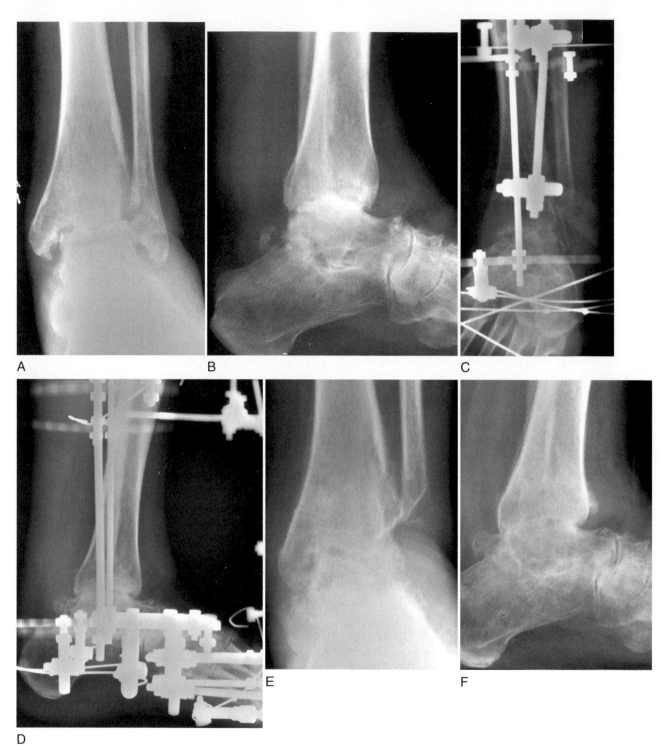

Figure 17–18   Anteroposterior **(A)** and lateral **(B)** radiographs of massively swollen (closed) ankle of a 54-year-old man with type 2 diabetes mellitus. He had received 6 weeks of intravenous nafcillin. According to the Cierny–Mader classification, he had diffuse involvement (type IV) and was a systemically compromised host (type IVB). The central and lateral columns are involved. He was treated with debridement of all infected tissue, removal of joint cartilage from the ankle and subtalar joints, and modified Ilizarov external fixation **(C** and **D)**. Anteroposterior **(E)** and lateral **(F)** radiographs at 2 years show solid fusion of both joints.

and three with a combination of external fixation and internal screw fixation. Open wounds were treated with dressing changes and skin graft as needed. Tensioned thin wires were used in the foot and distal tibia. Systemic comorbidities were present in 6 of 15 patients, and one other patient was noted to have" mental illness." One patient required revision ankle arthrodesis and two required extension of fusion to the subtalar joint. Fourteen of the 15(93%) ankles ultimately fused, but three patients had a persistently draining fistula.[73]

Unstable Ankles

The main indication for arthrodesis of Charcot's ankle is uncontrolled and unbraceable coronal plane instability. The pattern of instability determines the method of fixation. If the foot is unstable in a varus direction, we apply a plate on the medial side to buttress against further deformity. For the fibula we often simply use an intramedullary rod because the standard plate-and-screw construct has little mechanical leverage to prevent the foot from drifting into varus. Likewise, if the foot is unstable in a valgus direction we apply a plate on the lateral side of the tibiotalar joint to buttress against further deformity. If the foot is grossly unstable in all directions, either we use two plates or we sacrifice the subtalar joint and place an intramedullary rod. The rod can be placed through an extensile lateral transmalleolar approach with the patient positioned supine.

Multijoint Arthropathy

Patients can present with neuroarthropathy, which involves several joints in addition to the ankle. The goals of surgery are limited to establishing a stable, plantigrade, braceable foot. With dissolution of the talus, the objective is a stable tibiocalcaneal fusion, which can be done with an intramedullary rod, plating, or thin wire external fixation. If the fusion must extend into the foot, rod fixation is less preferable because of the difficulties with the placement of hardware around a rod.

SURGICAL TREATMENT OF ANKLE NEUROARTHROPATHY

Extensile Lateral Approach to Ankle and Subtalar Joints

1. Alignment of the normal and abnormal limb is compared to evaluate the degree of deformity. This is done by aligning the patella parallel to the operating table and observing the degree of rotation of the foot in relation to a perpendicular line from the patella. In this way, the surgeon can determine the degree of internal or external rotation of both the normal and the abnormal extremity. The advantage of this measurement is that it is relatively easy to check the alignment of the arthrodesis site at surgery. If the fusion must include both the ankle and subtalar joints, we externally rotate the foot five degrees more than the unaffected side.

2. A thigh tourniquet is applied and a sandbag is placed under the ipsilateral hip to allow the surgeon to see the lateral side of the foot and ankle.

3. The skin incision begins approximately 10 cm proximal to the tip of the fibula, is carried down over the shaft of the fibula, and swings gently distally another 10 cm toward the base of the fourth metatarsal. Although this incision extends between nerves, with the sural nerve passing posteriorly and the superficial peroneal nerve anteriorly, the surgeon must be aware of an anterior branch of the sural nerve that crosses through the plane of the incision.

4. The skin flaps are developed to create a full-thickness flap along the skeletal plane. The periosteum is stripped from the fibula anteriorly and posteriorly, and the incision is carried distally to expose the posterior facet of the subtalar joint and the sinus tarsi.

5. The dissection is continued across the anterior aspect of the tibia and ankle joint. With a periosteal elevator, the surgeon strips soft tissue from the distal end of the tibia, ankle joint, and proximal talar neck and then dissects to the medial malleolus. Care is taken not to dissect distally over the neck of the talus in order to protect the blood supply into the talus.

6. The fibula is osteotomized next at a level determined by the fixation techniques. When a rod or multiplane external fixator is used, the osteotomy is performed approximately 2 cm proximal to the level of the ankle joint and beveled to relieve the sharp prominence. If a blade or locking plate is used, the distal fibula should be transected at least 10 cm above the ankle joint. The level of resection is higher than the level of the plate to permit intraoperative compres-

sion with the distraction/compression device. The distal portion of the fibula is removed by sharp and blunt dissection to expose the lateral aspect of the tibia and ankle joint as well as the posterior facet of the subtalar joint. As this is carried out, the peroneal tendons are reflected posteriorly. The bone is cleared of soft tissue and used for grafting

7. An incision is made through the deep fascia along the posterior aspect of the distal tibia, which was exposed by the removal of the fibula. A periosteal elevator is gently moved medially across the posterior aspect of the tibia and then distally toward the calcaneus. This strips the soft tissues from the posterior aspect of the tibia and ankle joint and allows access to the posterior facet if needed.

Medial Side Decision-Making

8. The choice of a medial approach and preparation of the joint depends on the amount of ankle joint destruction and instability. With Charcot's arthropathy, the medial malleolus has almost always fragmented and the tibial plafond–talar dome structure has collapsed. However, in a few cases, the medial side remains intact or the tibial plafond–talar dome is relatively preserved, or both. Such cases are best treated by using a 4-cm anteromedial incision to the medial malleolus, with the lateral surface denuded of cartilage and subchondral bone. Otherwise, we use a 6-cm directly medial incision that starts above the medial malleolus and courses to its tip. The soft tissue is then stripped anteriorly and posteriorly around the tip of the medial malleolus in preparation for an osteotomy.

Bone Preparation

9. When deformity is minimal or moderate and the medial side remains intact, the distal tibia and proximal talar dome surfaces are removed to preserve the natural dome-shaped sagittal plane contour. This reduces the loss of limb length that naturally results from joint preparation. We use 1/4-inch to 3/8-inch osteotomes or side cutting router bits (or both) to remove the joint contents. The subchondral bone is drilled with multiple small and shallow holes.

10. When the deformity is severe, instability is gross, the tibial plafond–talar dome is collapsed, or the medial side is unstable, we use flat cuts to prepare the fusion site. From the lateral side, malleable retractors are placed anteriorly and posteriorly around the distal end of the tibia, exposing the anterolateral aspect of the ankle joint.

11. The initial cut for the arthrodesis is made in the distal part of the tibia with a sagittal saw using a short, wide blade, and the cut is completed with a deep, wide blade. This cut is made as perpendicular as possible to the long axis of the tibia, and as little bone as possible is removed from the dome of the ankle joint. This cut is brought across the ankle joint. With Charcot's arthropathy we generally bring the cut straight across to remove the medial malleolus while protecting the medial side with a Weitlaner retractor.

12. The foot is then positioned so that the plantar surface is perpendicular to the long axis of the tibia. A smooth 2- to 3-mm Steinmann pin is inserted through the heel across the subtalar joint and talar dome into the tibia. Varus/valgus and sagittal plane position are confirmed, and if they are satisfactory, a second flat cut is made across the dome of the talus perfectly parallel to the distal tibial cut. The saw cut is again started with a short, wide blade up to and around the sides of the pin and then completed with a deep, wide blade after the pin is removed.

Fixation

The choice of fixation can be difficult, and it must be tailored to the individual patient. (See the earlier discussion of surgical decision making). Internal fixation is used when there is no history of ulceration. An isolated ankle problem is treated with a blade plate or locking plate, which is often supplemented with a second short, out-of-plane plate to help control rotation. If the problem extends to the subtalar joint alone, we typically use an intramedullary rod. However, if the problem extends farther into the midfoot, a plate construct is used for the tibiocalcaneal region to allow screw fixation between the midfoot and the hindfoot.

Blade and Locking Plate Technique

Until recently, we used blade plates for a number of these reconstructions. This was initially performed as originally described by Alvarez,[3] to include either the ankle joint alone or both the ankle and subtalar joints. We changed to use cannulated plates when they were introduced for treatment of proximal humeral fractures. In particular, the 3.5-mm cannulated titanium plates with 30-mm blades were easy to shape along the side of the tibiotalar surface. The stainless steel version is a little more resistant to fatigue and a good alternative for selected patients.

Locking plates have supplanted the blade plates in our practice because of ease of use and more options for distal fixation. With a locking plate, we can usually place 3 or 4 screws into the talus at different angles, and this appears to give better fixation with less disruption of osteoporotic bone.

13. With the foot held in the optimal position for fusion, the joint is manually compressed and two smooth 2- to 3-mm Steinmann pins are placed across the ankle. If the ankle and subtalar joints are to be fused, these pins are placed from the sole across the calcaneus into the distal tibia. The pins are always placed across the most anterior and posterior regions of the ankle joint to allow placement of the plate without disruption of the initial joint position.

14. Look at the position of the foot from all perspectives. Step away from the table to view the sagittal position. From the bottom of the table, ensure that the foot is in appropriate coronal and axial alignment. The most common mistake is not enough external rotation. Replace the pins across the joint(s) until the position seems ideal.

15. The plates are often applied from the lateral side, although they can be placed from the medial side with a varus instability pattern. When the lateral side is used, the distal tibial syndesmotic incisura needs to be flattened to accept the plate. The lateral-most margin of Chaput's tubercle is similarly removed.

16. A moldable template is used to determine the shape of the plate. A large bending press may be needed to mold the plate accordingly. This step is really critical; it is worth taking extra time to ensure this is done as well as possible.

17. The choice of plate depends on the specific needs of the patient. No plate is designed for this reconstruction. At the time writing, we use either a proximal humeral or a distal tibial Synthes (Paoli, Penn) plate, because those are the most appropriate currently available. With these, the most eccentric fixation tabs often are removed.

18. The first step of plate application is to obtain a distal fixation, with the proximal section of the plate held by hand against the midline of the tibia. The first screw is usually nonlocking to get initial intimate plate-and-bone fixation. Several locking screws are then placed in the distal fragment under fluoroscopic control. The screws do not necessarily require cortical fixation.

19. Place a temporary smooth 1.5- or 2-mm pin through the second most proximal screw hole.

20. Apply the external tensioning device (AO Basic Set) with a unicortical 4.5-mm screw drilled and tapped proximal to the plate. The device is hooked to the most proximal screw hole. Remove all the smooth pins and fully compress the fusion construct into the green zone of the tensioning device.

21. Place a nonlocking screw though one of the proximal screw holes, and then place locking screws as needed though the rest.

22. We often obtain fixation across the fusion site with out-of-plane fixation. This can be done with a second short plate, a large staple, or a large screw. The use of a small plate at 90 degrees from the first seems to work well and is now our preferred approach (Fig. 17–19).

Intramedullary Rod Method of Tibiocalcaneal Fixation

23. With the foot held in the optimal position for fusion, an incision is made on the plantar aspect of the heel. The position of the incision is very important both for proper access to the calcaneus and for avoiding potential damage to the plantar nerves. We typically draw the presumed location of the nerves with a marking pen and always stay posterior to that location. The exact location for the incision is checked fluoroscopi-

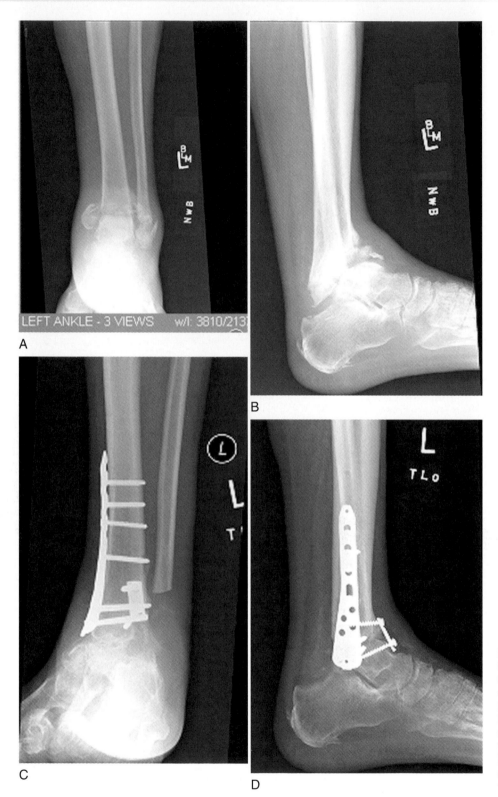

Figure 17–19 Anteroposterior **(A)** and lateral **(B)** radiographs of a Charcot ankle with good coronal plane alignment. **C** and **D,** The ankle was fused using a locking plate and a 90-degree small plate to confer out-of-plane stability. Given the excellent coronal plane alignment and strong fixation, we decided not to use a neutralization frame.

cally in the sagittal plane. Typically, it is 1.5 to 2.5 cm posterior to the calcaneocuboid joint. The transverse incision starts 0.5 cm medial to the midline and courses 1.5 to 2.0 cm lateral to the midline. Dissection to the calcaneus is performed in the transverse direction with a blunt, curved Mayo scissors. A nasal speculum is then placed into the wound against the calcaneus while the guide pin is inserted and checked and for all aspects of the reaming.

24. Under C-arm guidance, we place a guide pin onto the inferior surface of the calcaneus approximately 2 cm proximal to the calcaneal cuboid joint. The pin is then drilled inferior to superior, with its tip directed slightly posterior and lateral. After it is confirmed to be centered in the tibia, it is left in place and the bone is reamed up to the size of the implant.

25. Check alignment of the foot again. *Do not accept malalignment in the sagittal or coronal planes.* If necessary, replace the pin until the alignment is ideal.

26. Reaming usually does not have to be much wider than the implant because scratch fit in the medullary canal is unusual with these short nails. We usually ream to the exact nail diameter and try to insert the nail. If we meet a lot of resistance, we increase reaming with 0.5-mm increments and try to insert the nail after each reaming.

27. All bone shavings from reamings are saved and used for grafting.

28. At present, the manufacturers of these nails offer two different methods for compression of the arthrodesis site. Neither is perfect. We base the decision of which nail to use on the density of the calcaneal bone. Usually the patient with Charcot's arthropathy has osteoporosis. For these patients we use a rod designed to gain compression with a temporary external fixator pin in the tibia. The compression is done against locking screws placed across the calcaneal segment of the rod. In the rarer cases of normal bone density, we use a rod with an in-line compression device. This uses a worm screw mechanism that pushes up against the inferior aspect of the calcaneus. With this approach, the first locking screws are placed across the tibial segment of the rod. Compression is then applied against

that construct. When using the in-line device, the surgeon must realize that the flange of the pusher is wider than the bone previously reamed. The soft tissues must be retracted anteriorly so the plantar nerves are not compressed.

Closure

We close in two layers and rarely use a closed suction drain. The skin is closed with interrupted 3-0 nylon or 2-0 Prolene sutures.

Casting Protocol

A very well padded posterior U splint is used for the first 2 days. The patient and nursing staff must be completely aware of the importance of not bearing weight. Some patients do not have any pain and walk on the foot immediately after surgery if this restriction is not strictly enforced.

A non–weight-bearing total-contact plaster cast is applied and is changed at 1 week, 2 weeks, 5 weeks, 8 weeks, and 12 weeks after surgery, then monthly after that. X-rays are taken at 8 weeks and 12 weeks and at monthly intervals after that.

Weight bearing is restricted until good radiographic evidence of bridging trabeculae is obtained. Imaging the fusion site is difficult. With flat cuts and a locking plate placed under compression, the joint looks fused on the initial radiographs, so lack of peri-implant lucencies on later radiographs can be the best sign of satisfactory fusion. Alternatively, with an intramedullary rod, the fusion site can be obscured, and lack of implant motion may be the best guide to suggest that fusion is progressing.

With Charcot ankle reconstruction, the average time of non–weight bearing is 3 to 6 months, average time of cast immobilization is 6 to 8 months, and total immobilization time is 6 to 12 months. We typically change the patient's walking aid to either an Aircast boot (Aircast Inc, Summit, NJ) or a Charcot restraint orthotic walker. As mentioned earlier, this might be a reason to consider transtibial amputation as a serious alternative in selected patients.

Rocker-bottom shoes help with the initial transition to shoes. Loss of limb length is common, and most patients require some buildup on the bottom of the shoe.

External Fixation Protocol

Patients with severe osteopenia, proven difficulty with non–weight bearing, bilateral active Charcot's processes, or wounds that cause concern are treated with multiplane circular external fixation as a neutralization/immobilization device. Transplant patients are generally not treated with these devices because they have a higher infection risk.

We apply a static frame with 3 half pins off two separate levels into the anteromedial tibia and four or five tensioned thin wires in the foot (Fig. 17–20).[102] The frame is positioned so that the anteromedial crest of the tibia is close to the rings, because this minimizes bending of the half pins.[92] Thin wires in the foot include two or three across the calcaneus, one though the talar neck (when present), and two across the metatarsals.

Postoperative care is straightforward. Dressings on the wounds are changed at 2 days and then as needed until sutures are out. Patients are allowed to shower and are asked to pat dry the pin sites. On discharge, all patients are given a written prescription for an antibiotic that covers staphylococcus infection. If they see a pin site reddening, they are asked to fill the prescription, start antibiotic therapy, and contact the surgeon. If the symptoms worsen, they must return for a full evaluation.

Patients are allowed to put limited weight on the frames to balance, but they are asked to use two crutches or a walker until we are certain the fusion is stable.

Because these patients suffer from neuropathies, they are at high risk for injuring their healthy leg with the frame. They must sleep with a pillow wrapped to the frame to prevent undetected contralateral injury.

Frames are worn until the fusion site is healed radiographically. They are typically removed 3 to 4 months after application.

A total-contact cast is applied when the frame is removed. We generally change the cast at 1 week and then 3 weeks later. Weight bearing and cast or boot immobilization are progressed as described for the cast postoperative protocol.

Author's Experience with External Fixators in Treatment of Charcot's Arthropathy

My experience indicates that this form of treatment is associated with a high number of complications, although most are self-limited and of no major consequence. Between 1999 and 2003, I applied 40 frames as part of fusion treatment of patients with foot or ankle Charcot's arthropathy. For this cohort, the average duration of wearing a frame was 110 days. Thirty-one patients had at least one postoperative complication and several had more than one. Twenty-eight had pin-tract infections. Five of these required one 7- to 10-day course of an oral antibiotic and 21 required more than one 7- to 10-day course of antibiotic. Two patients had thin wires removed for infection. Five others broke a pin or wire, one broke the foot frame, and one had a pulmonary embolus with a negative leg venous Doppler examination.

Failed Previous Fusion Surgery

Nonunion

Reported nonunion rates vary from 0% to 40%.* They are appear to be more common in susceptible populations (smokers, elderly patients, noncompliant patients, and patients with neuroarthropathy, history of open trauma, or poor soft tissues)[23,97] and less common following minimally invasive surgeries. When to consider a nonunion a true nonunion is a controversial matter because some apparent cases of nonunion eventually unite after a year or more of immobilization.

Treatment of nonunions requires careful consideration of the patient's situation. Patients with several serious risk factors for failure or with debilitated health may be best advised not to undergo additional attempts at obtaining a solid ankle fusion. These patients should be treated with either a transtibial amputation[52] or long-term full-contact bracing.[108]

Kitaoka[67] reviewed the Mayo Clinic's experience treating ankle nonunions with external fixation. Twenty (77%) of 26 ankles successfully fused; however, at 5-year follow-up, 10 (39%) of the 26 had fair or poor results. Kirkpatrick et al[65] reported on 11 ankle nonunions primarily treated with a fibular onlay–inlay graft and internal fixation. They reported nine of 11 successful fusions, one painless nonunion, and one below-knee amputation. Similarly, Anderson et al[4] reviewed 20 patients treated for ankle nonunions or malunions with internal fixation. In their initial

---

*References 34, 40, 41, 79, 80,91, 97, 100, and 124.

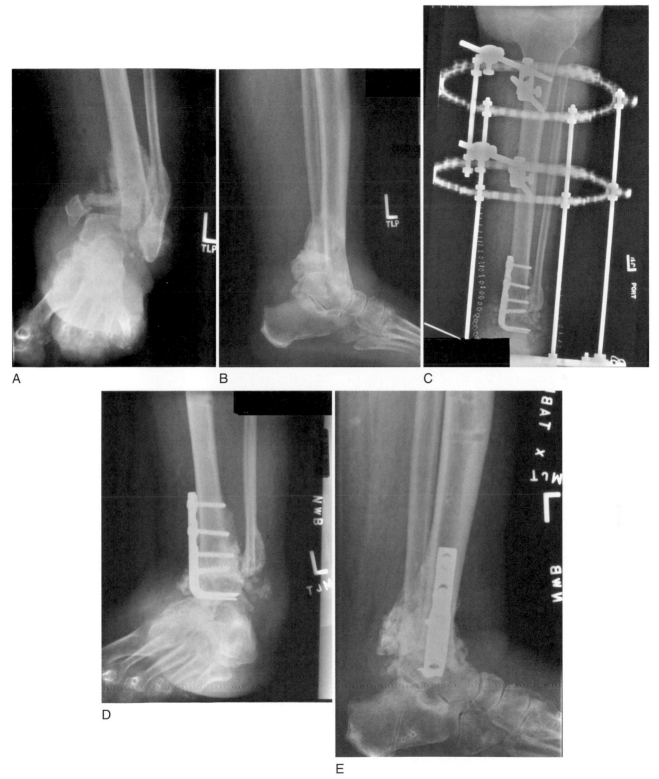

Figure 17–20 Anteroposterior (**A**) and lateral (**B**) radiographs of a Charcot ankle with unstable coronal plane alignment and severe osteoporosis. **C,** The ankle was fused using a proximal humeral blade plate, partial resection of the distal fibular, and 3-month application of a neutralization, multiplane, thin-wire fixator. **D** and **E,** Postoperatively, the ankle is well aligned and stable, and the patient is ulcer and brace free.

series they had 15 (75%) satisfactory fusions, with an additional 19 operations, 17 (85%) satisfied patients, and three (15%) below-knee amputations. Levine et al[74] described a series of 23 patients with ankle nonunions treated with either revision ankle fusions (15) or extensile fusions (9). At short follow-up, they reported fusion in 21 (91%) and satisfactory results in 19 (83%).

The basic principles of successful revision surgery are essentially the same as described for primary surgery. Some caveats do apply, though. First, patient education, expectations, and ultimately compliance with postoperative protocols are essential for obtaining a successful result. It has been my experience that patients who do not want to participate in getting well are much more likely to fail. I am reluctant to consider revision surgery unless the patient shows real interest and motivation. This somewhat intangible aspect of the evaluation does require a number of discussions with the patient to the optimal time for treatment. I have treated a number of these patients in unloading braces until they are psychologically, socially, and physically ready to take on the challenge of this operation. I discuss with all of them the reported results and the possibility that a below-knee amputation might be necessary.

The technical aspects of the surgery are straightforward. Only the minimum soft tissues are stripped to allow full access to the joint. All fibrous tissue and dead bone is removed. Infection is ruled out when indicated. Autogenous bone graft is used liberally. Fixation must be rigid. Weight bearing and smoking are restricted until full consolidation, often 4 to 5 months. CT scans can help monitor healing and give a more accurate picture of the progression of bone bridging. External electrical or ultrasound stimulation can be helpful as an adjunct to surgery,[35] but alone this is not likely to have a substantial and positive effect on the resolution of an established nonunion.[106]

Malunion

Varus or valgus malunion combined with equinus are the most common deformities that occur after ankle fusion.[60] Realignment is generally done with closing wedge procedures, although some can be treated with accurate double-plane osteotomies as described by Sangeorzan et al.[110] The advantage of closing wedges are that they do not generally stretch nerves, they are more likely to heal than opening wedges, and they offer a source of bone graft for other simultaneous foot procedures. When performing them, though, the surgeon must be aware that they often change the orientation of the foot and related joints, the two segments rarely fit and overhanging bone can irritate tendons, and they can change the length tension rela-

tionship of the musculotendinous structures that pass across the osteotomy, in effect lengthening and weakening these structures. Dome-shaped osteotomies placed around the center of rotation are less likely to have these effects, especially with single plane deformities (e.g., equinus) (Fig. 17–21).

Arguably, the best approach to realigning the leg and foot is with Ilizarov frames. The indications, techniques, and outcomes are fully discussed in Chapter 18. This approach is particularly useful in the circumstances of limb shortening, concomitant infection, or nonunion. However, the use of the frames carries its own inherent set of problems, including frequent (usually minor) adverse events, which are tolerated poorly by some patients, and techniques that are unfamiliar to most surgeons. The development of the Spatial Frame hardware and software (Richards, Inc, Memphis, Tenn) will likely ultimately make the application of corrective frames for malunions much more accessible to surgeons who do not subspecialize.

Secondary Subtalar Arthritis

The subtalar joint is the most common joint to develop arthritis after an ankle fusion. The rate of development of arthritis is unpredictable; however, after 20 years, essentially all patients develop radiographic evidence of subtalar joint degeneration.[24] This is believed to be the result of increased stresses across the subtalar joint. After ankle fusion, most patients walk with the foot externally rotated in order to vault over the planted foot in the terminal stages of the stance phase. In so doing they roll through the subtalar joint in an unnatural, medial-to-lateral direction, which presumably results in focal mal-loading of articular cartilage and, ultimately, development of osteoarthritis.

Treatment of painful subtalar arthritis is fusion surgery. Because the ankle does not move, the subtalar joint is less accessible to surgical debridement than usual. I prefer to use an internervous frown-shaped incision from the tip of the fibula anterior calcaneal process to perform this surgery. After the short extensor is reflected, the entire contents of the subtalar joint are removed. For very tight joints, a Midas Rex thin router bit helps prepare the joint. Bone graft can be harvested from the distal tibia.

The key to this procedure, though, is to use either two screws or a screw and a staple to fixate the joint. After an ankle fusion and with the foot in a short-leg cast, the rotation of the foot with respect to the leg will be transmitted directly through the subtalar joint. One single large screw is not sufficient to stop that rotation (Fig. 17–22). Two screws—somewhat spaced and out of plane—work well as a screw and a 90-degree out-of-plane staple. The first screw is generally put in

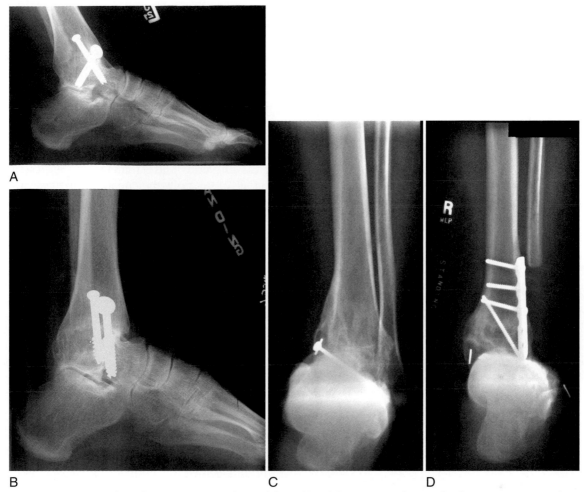

Figure 17–21 Two examples of osteotomies performed for ankle malunion. **A** and **B**, In the first, an equinus malunion after fusion involving a partial distal fibulectomy was treated by recutting the arc of the talar dome and rotating the foot into better position. Indeed, one of the original tibial screw holes was reused for fixation. **C**, In the second example, the ankle was fused in varus, as is seen on the hindfoot alignment view. **D**, The foot was reoriented under the tibia using a laterally closing wedge and blade plate fixation. Use of the plate requires partial distal fibulectomy.

compression; the second method of fixation does not need compression.

Failed Previous Replacement Surgery

Little has been written on the treatment of failed previous total ankle replacements; indeed, no series have been published specifically on total ankle replacement revision at the time of writing. Most information is anecdotal or can be gleaned from larger reports of primary surgeries.

Four major problems warrant specific discussion: infection, progressive intracomponent instability and deformity, subsidence, and polyethylene failure.

Infection

Data on wound problems and infection with ankle replacement are scarce. Accordingly, I apply basic total

joint principles derived from data on infection in the knee and hip to my treatment of wound problems and infection after total ankle replacement. The key to avoiding bad problems is prevention.

Proper patient selection is the first step. Any patient with a history of ankle infection needs a careful workup to rule out persistent sources of infection. Patients with bad skin from multiple operations, long-standing steroid dependence, dermatologic conditions, or vascular insufficiency should not have an ankle replacement. Indeed, when surgical treatment is necessary to keep these patients mobile, we try to perform arthroscopic ankle fusions.

Surgeon technique is an equally important factor. Meticulous nondestructive handling of the soft tissues should be part of every surgery. Excellent hemostasis should be followed by careful multilayered closure starting at the periosteal–capsular layer. The dressings

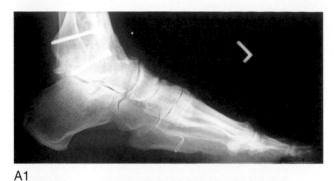

A1

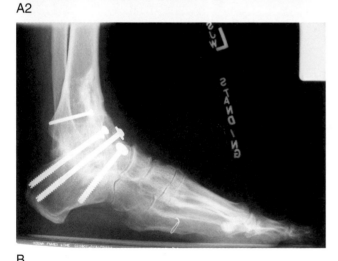

A2

B

Figure 17–22 Fusion of arthritic subtalar joint after ankle fusion. **A1** and **A2,** Nine years after ankle fusion this patient developed incapacitating subtalar arthritis and pain. **B,** An attempt to fuse the subtalar joint with one large screw failed and was successfully revised with multiple-screw fixation of the subtalar joint. After ankle fusion, the eventual development of subtalar joint arthritis and pain is common. When this is treated with a fusion surgery, the subtalar joint is best secured by using more than one screw.

need to have several soft layers encased in a harder carapace. During the first few postoperative days, the leg is elevated above the heart and the toes are monitored for swelling, which indicates that a splint needs to be changed.

Despite all these measures, wound problems and infections do occur. The treatment of superficial wound breakdown without infection is local dressing changes and prophylactic oral antibiotic coverage. Superficial wound breakdown and local infection require an aspirate of the joint through uninfected tissue to rule out deep infection. If deep infection is ruled out, the patient should be given parenteral antibiotics and started on local dressing changes. If the dehiscence reaches the joint and is recognized early, surgical incision and drainage is indicated with exchange of the polyethylene. If the wound cannot be primarily closed, a local flap using the extensor digitorum brevis (Fig. 17–23) should be swung over the wound and skin grafted. Late, deep infections generally require removal of all implants and an attempt at fusion (Fig. 17–24). A methyl methacrylate antibiotic spacer can be used to help sterilize the wound, and the fusion can be performed either in situ or with structural bone (Fig. 17–25). Carlsson et al[20] reviewed 21 cases of septic and nonseptic revision of total ankle replacements to fusions. Most were done with compressive external fixation. Thirteen fused on the first attempt, 4 fused on the second attempt, and 4 did not fuse.

Progressive Intracomponent Instability and Deformity

Recognition and correction of intracomponent instability and deformity requires *standing* radiographs. I prefer to obtain a hindfoot alignment view to help understand the force vectors across the ankle joint in quiet standing (Fig. 17–26).[104] Tilting of components can lead to instability, pain, subsidence, and progressive polyethylene wear.

Haskell and Mann[49] evaluated the influence of preoperative ankle alignment to immediate and average 2-year postoperative alignment in 35 patients with initial malalignment of at least 10 degrees who received a STAR implant. They subclassified the malalignments by preoperative varus or valgus and congruent or noncongruent. The latter is based on the fit of the articulating surfaces: When the surfaces were within 10 degrees of parallel they were considered congruent; all others were considered noncongruent. Preoperatively, 15 were varus-congruent, five were valgus-congruent, 10 were varus-incongruent, and five were valgus-incongruent. Immediately after the operation, the distribution was the same, suggesting the lack of influence of the surgery on the deformity. After an average of 2 years, eight of 34 ankles (24%) with adequate follow-up had progressive edge loading, and four required surgery for this. Of this eight, seven cases of edge loading were in ankles that were considered incongruent on preoperative radiographs. The authors

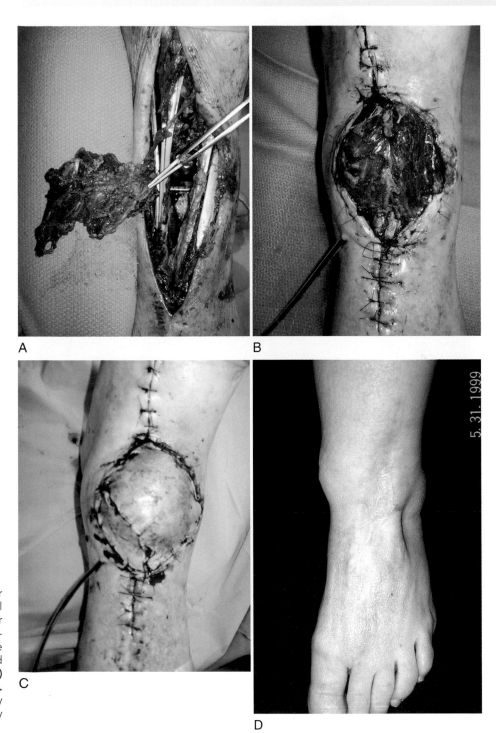

Figure 17–23 The extensor digitorum brevis is the best local muscle flap for a failed anterior ankle surgery. The deep peroneal nerve is cut to reflect the muscle on its pedicle (A) and then placed into the defect (B) and covered with skin graft (C). The muscle will eventually atrophy to form a cosmetically acceptable result (D).

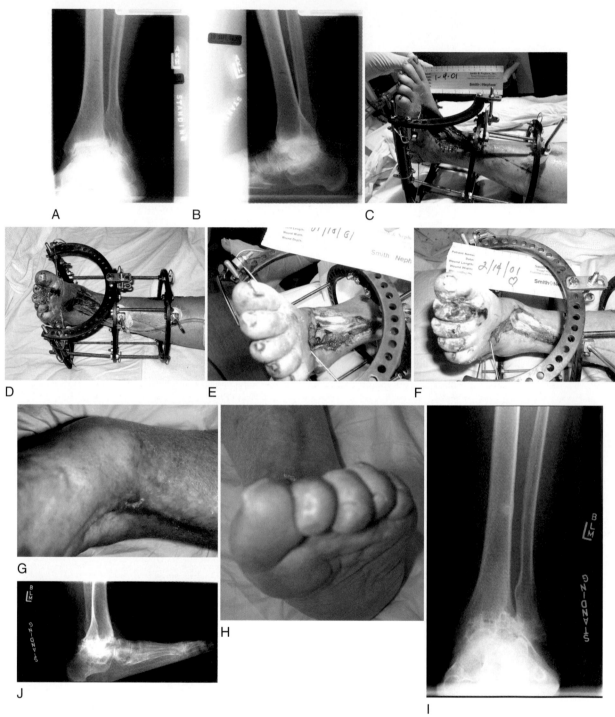

Figure 17–24   Treatment of infected ankle replacement and flap failure with fusion. This patient with end-stage rheumatoid ankle arthritis underwent a total ankle replacement that became massively infected and required extensive peri-implant debridement. **A** to **C,** We placed a multiplane, thin-wire external fixator on her to fuse the ankle and facilitate wound care **(D).** A wound vacuum-assisted closure (wound VAC) device was used for nearly 3 months, which resulted in complete re-epithelization **(E** to **G)** and preservation of blood supply to the second toe **(H). I** and **J,** During this time, the ankle fused satisfactorily, and the patient walks without use of ambulatory aids.

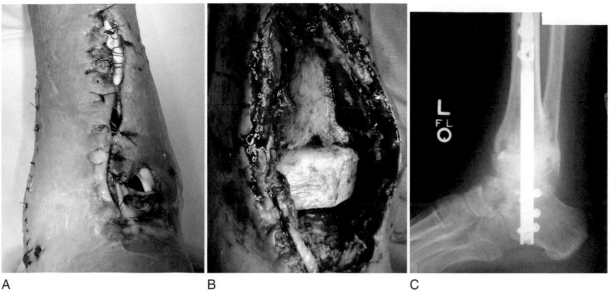

Figure 17–25 Treatment of massive ankle implant infection **(A)** with a methyl methacrylate antibiotic spacer **(B)** and staged fusion using bulk allograft **(C).** (Photographs courtesy of Chris Attinger, MD, and Paul Cooper, MD.)

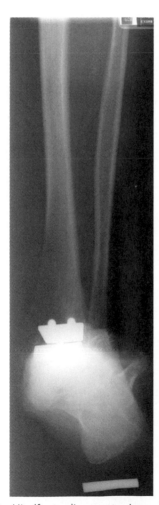

Figure 17–26 Hindfoot alignment view showing severe valgus deformity after Scandinavian Total Ankle Replacement (STAR) implant. This imbalance will lead to nonuniform mobile bearing stress and increase the risk of bearing subluxation, wear, fracture, or component subsidence.

concluded that patients with preoperative incongruent joints are 10 times more likely to develop edge loading after a STAR implant than those with a preoperative congruent joint.

Subsidence

Subsidence has been a problem with total ankle arthroplasty since it was first performed. With the use of noncemented designs, subsidence of the tibial component has become less frequent, although it can still occur. There are several causes of subsidence, including insufficient bone ingrowth; insufficient bone stock; mal-loading of the ankle replacement; overstuffing of the joint, with increased stress transmitted to the bone; and overstressing the joint with high activity or weight (Fig. 17–27). In our laboratory, we have tested native ankle ligament strain in a functional range of motion and have then done the same with both Agility and STAR ankle replacements placed in positions of perfect and abnormal alignments.[109,118,119] These studies suggest that the periankle ligaments do not strain during the normal stance phase of the gait cycle.[118] With both the Agility and STAR, however, periankle ligaments are strained in the normal range of motion, and these strains are worsened by malaligned implantations.[109,119]

Together these studies tell us that the loosening or subsidence of total ankle components might be related to abnormal strains imposed by ligaments on the bone–implant interface. The exact incidence of these problems remains a little unclear and depends on the devices. In an average 7-year radiographic follow-up of the Agility ankle, Knecht et al[70] reported 14% (16 of

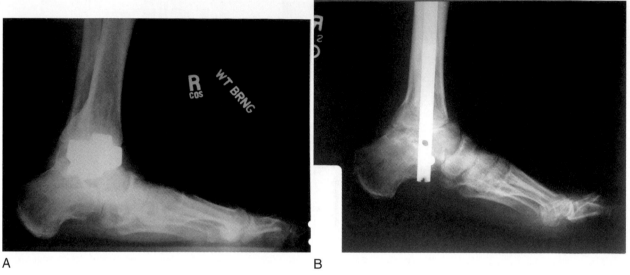

A   B

Figure 17–27   This Agility ankle was implanted in a 300-pound man who ignored his postoperative instructions and began playing golf 3 weeks after surgery. **A,** The talar component subsided deeply through the talus into the subtalar joint. **B,** This was salvaged with a tibiotalocalcaneal arthrodesis using an intramedullary rod. (Photos courtesy of Mark Scioli, MD.)

117) ankles had 5 mm or more of subsidence or 5 degrees or more of angular change, or both. Four percent (5 of 117) ankles had only tibial subsidence of 5 mm or more (average, 8 mm; range, 7 to 8 mm). Eight percent (9 of 117) ankles had only talar subsidence of 5 mm or more (average, 10 mm; range, 5 to 20 mm). The survival curve on the tibial side showed stable fixation at after 4 years but continued subsidence on the talar side up to 11 years.

My experience with 98 STAR implants over the past 6 years has been similar. Subsidence on the tibial side is almost nonexistent; however, it is an occasional problem on the talar side. In my series with an average 3.5-year follow-up, I have four patients whose talar components have subsided into the subtalar joint. Three subtalar joints have been fused, and the fourth is scheduled. Ten other patients have sustained lesser degrees of subsidence of clinical significance, usually requiring removal of impinging bone either medially or laterally. The problem, though, is if the subsidence continues, bone removal is counterproductive because the forces are retransmitted back to the ankle replacement, increasing the risk of further subsidence. In these cases, removal of the implant and replacement with a wider talar implant or conversion to an ankle fusion can be the best treatment.

A few case series have focused on conversion of a subsided or loose ankle replacement to a fusion. In the largest of these series, Kitaoka[69] reported on the experience at the Mayo clinic with 38 total ankles revised to fusion. A variety of different methods was used depending on the amount of bone loss and involvement of the subtalar joint. They reported 33 (89%) solid fusions for this often difficult mix of clinical problems. In a smaller series, Gabrion et al[42] reported successful fusion in seven of eight patients but satisfactory clinical results only in five patients.

Not all subsided ankle replacements need conversion to fusion. Indeed, some clinical situations warrant a second attempt at an ankle replacement. If the original implant was inserted incorrectly, an early revision is often the best option. Errors related to component positioning are easy to determine on early radiographs, and seeing them in an otherwise healthy and active patient should prompt a straightforward revision. If the subsidence has resulted in substantial bone loss, then a decision needs to be made about how to handle the loss.

In general there are two options, not mutually exclusive, for dealing with bone loss in total ankle revisions. One is to use a custom or revision implant that is larger than the original implant (Fig. 17–28); the other is to use bone graft. The first option works well for both tibial and talar sides; however, the bone graft option may be best for the tibial side because the initial fixation of graft to the residual, and often very deficient, talus is technically much harder. If the subtalar joint is sacrificed, then fixation is somewhat easier, because long screws can be placed through graft into the calcaneus. When allograft is used, the component should be secured to the implant with methyl methacrylate. We prefer to use anatomically matched segments of allograft for this purpose (Fig. 17–29).

Polyethylene Failure

Polyethylene can fail catastrophically with fracture or slowly with generation of bioactive submicron wear particles. Catastrophic failure is relatively rare, but

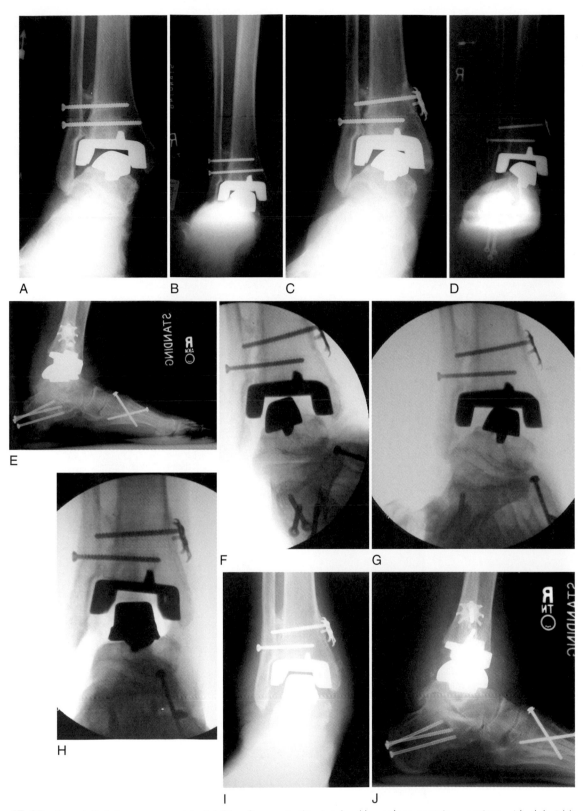

Figure 17–28 **A** and **B,** Intracomponent instability after an Agility total ankle replacement in a patient with deltoid ligament insufficiency and benign joint hypermobility syndrome. My first attempt to realign the component with extra-component surgery failed. **C** to **E,** This first revision surgery involved Achilles tendon allograft replacement of the deltoid, medialization of the cal-caneal tuberosity, and first metatarsocuneiform fusion. **F** and **G,** One year later, we performed a fluoroscopic evaluation of the joint with forced varus/valgus positioning. The talar component was found to easily displace in every direction, including straight distraction. A custom prosthesis was designed to reduce the extra volume between the components. **H,** Intraoperative imaging during the second revision showed excellent stability and alignment. **I** and **J,** Standing radiographs 2 years later show preser-vation of excellent alignment consistent with the good clinical outcome.

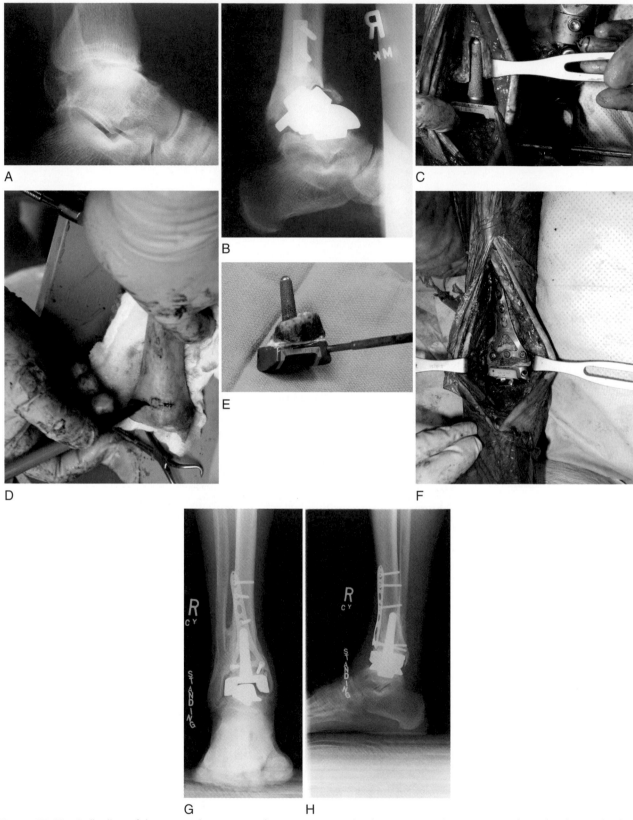

Figure 17–29 Bulk allograft bone supplementation for component subsidence. **A,** Initial preoperative lateral radiographs show anterior subluxation of the talus under the tibia. **B,** The talar implant was initially placed too anterior and never developed secure ingrowth of bone to the tibial component, ultimately resulting in anterior cortical collapse. **C,** First the implant was removed under mechanical distraction, and a trough for stem of a custom designed revision tibial component was created and trialed. An anatomically matched distal tibia **(D)** was cut to fill the bony defect and secured to the tibial component with methyl methacrylate **(E). F,** The allograft-component construct was fixated to the tibia with a low-profile plate followed by insertion of a standard revision talar component. **G** and **H,** Radiographs at 3 years show bony remodeling around the allograft and stable fixation without further subsidence.

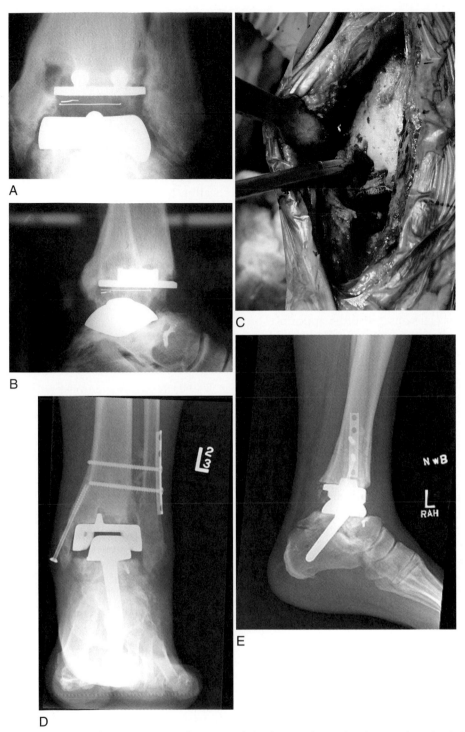

Figure 17–30 Total ankle revision for massive osteolysis. **A** and **B,** These radiographs show early polyethylene wear in a 55-year-old man 3 years after total ankle replacement. **C,** During revision surgery, large areas of osteolysis were found involving the tibial and talar sides. **D** and **E,** This was salvaged with the use of extra-thick poly and a slightly taller, stemmed talar implant for better fixation and support.

cases have been reported at scientific meetings.[5] Mobile bearings may be particularly prone to fracture because they can become extruded across the edge of the components. Fractures have generally occurred with thin bearings, because the thicker bearings are less likely to fatigue fracture. Uncorrected deformity and secondary focal elevated internal polyethylene loading are causes for catastrophic failure.

Wear of polyethylene in total ankle replacements has not yet become a major concern because long-term results are not yet available. Analyses of particles in synovial fluid from 15 of my total ankle replacement patients were compared to those from 11 patients with posterior-stabilized total knee arthroplasties.[71] Polyethylene particles were isolated and analyzed using scanning electron microscopy. Particle size (equivalent circle diameter) and concentration in ankles were the same as in knees after replacement surgery. These data suggest that the long-term result of total ankle arthroplasty should be as good as posterior-stabilized total knee arthroplasties in terms of polyethylene wear and the prevalence of osteolysis.

In a study of medium-term results with the Agility ankle (Depuy, Inc, Warsaw, Ind), Knecht et al[70] reported at an average of 7.2 years of follow-up. In this study, 15% (18 of 117) of ankles had expansile lysis. Of these, four (22%) showed definite signs of progression over time on serial x-ray evaluation, and 14 appeared relatively stable on serial radiographs. Expansile lysis was a late-onset disorder appearing, on average, 35 months after total ankle arthroplasty (range, 9 to 85 months).

Treatment of progressive and ballooning peri-implant osteolysis should be undertaken when recognized. Serial radiographs or CT scans may be needed to confirm an initial clinical suspicion. These lesions tend to enlarge, destroy bone, undermine stable fixation, and lead to more severe problems. At first patients are generally asymptomatic and not willing to undergo a large revision operation. If they insist on waiting and the problem increases, painful symptoms usually arise and the reconstruction is more difficult.

In cases where the damage is limited, the initial surgery involves exchange to a thicker polyethylene insert, complete curettage of the lesions, and bone grafting. Mobile bearings are much easier to exchange than fixed bearings. At the time of surgery, the polyethylene is inspected for signs of bearing wear, and the corresponding metal articulating surfaces are closely inspected for any surface irregularities. If irregularities are present, that surface of the implant must be replaced, or the problem will recur. If the damage to peri-implant bone is extensive and has caused subsidence of the implant, the implant might need to be replaced with a new implant. With significant bone loss, a revision implant may be necessary (Fig. 17–30).

If the wear is due to unbalanced loading of the implant, the mechanical imbalance must be corrected or the problem will recur. The surgeon must decide if this is a problem that can or will respond to revision or reconstructive surgery. In some cases—especially with severe rigid varus deformities—the surgeon might find it impossible to completely realign ankle loading to a well-balanced joint. In these circumstances it is best to perform an ankle fusion. When reconstruction

of the implant and ankle is considered feasible, the surgeon should determine if the problem has arisen from malalignment of the components or from malalignment of the ankle and foot. Treatment is then directed at the source of the problem. Revision implantations are performed to correct imbalances between components and corrective osteotomies and selective fusions are performed to balance the foot.

In my opinion, the key to reconstruction is bone alignment, not ligament or muscle support. If the bone alignment does not ensure that the weight-bearing force goes directly through the center of the implant with quiet standing, the implant will eventually tilt and expose the ankle to the risk of host reaction to accelerated polyethylene wear. Any surgeon who performs ankle replacements needs extensive experience with total joint replacement techniques and must understand how to align and balance the bony and articular architecture of the leg, ankle, and foot.

REFERENCES

1. Abdo RV, Wasilewski SA: Ankle arthrodesis: A long-term study. *Foot Ankle* 13(6):307-312, 1992.
2. Ahlberg A, Henricson AS: Late results of ankle fusion. *Acta Orthop Scand* 52(1):103-105, 1981.
3. Alvarez RG, Barbour TM, Perkins TD: Tibiocalcaneal arthrodesis for nonbraceable neuropathic ankle deformity. *Foot Ankle Int* 15(7):354-359, 1994.
4. Anderson JG, Coetzee JC, Hansen ST: Revision ankle fusion using internal compression arthrodesis with screw fixation. *Foot Ankle Int* 18(5):300-309, 1997.
5. Assal M, Greisberg J, Hansen ST Jr: Revision total ankle arthroplasty: Conversion of New Jersey Low Contact Stress to Agility: Surgical technique and case report. *Foot Ankle Int* 25(12):922-925, 2004.
6. Ateshian GA, Soslowsky LJ, Mow VC: Quantitation of articular surface topography and cartilage thickness in knee joints using stereophotogrammetry. *J Biomech* 24(8):761-776, 1991.
7. Athanasiou KA, Niederauer GG, Schenck RC Jr: Biomechanical topography of human ankle cartilage. *Ann Biomed Eng* 23(5):697-704, 1995.
8. Beaudoin AJ, Fiore SM, Krause WR, Adelaar RS: Effect of isolated talocalcaneal fusion on contact in the ankle and talonavicular joints. *Foot Ankle* 12(1):19-25, 1991.
9. Bolton-Maggs BG, Sudlow RA, Freeman MA: Total ankle arthroplasty. A long-term review of the London Hospital experience. *J Bone Joint Surg Br* 67(5):785-790, 1985.
10. Bonnin M, Carret JP: [Arthrodesis of the ankle under arthroscopy. Apropos of 10 cases reviewed after a year]. *Rev Chir Orthop Reparatrice Appar Mot* 81(2):128-135, 1995.
11. Brown TD, Shaw DT: In vitro contact stress distributions in the natural human hip. *J Biomech* 16(6):373-384, 1983.
12. Buchner M, Sabo D: Ankle fusion attributable to posttraumatic arthrosis: A long-term follow-up of 48 patients. *Clin Orthop Relat Res* 406:155-164, 2003.
13. Buckwalter JA, Woo SL, Goldberg VM, et al: Soft-tissue aging and musculoskeletal function. *J Bone Joint Surg Am* 75(10):1533-1548, 1993.

14. Buckwalter JA, Mankin HJ: Articular cartilage: Tissue design and chondrocyte–matrix interactions. *Instr Course Lect* 47:477-486, 1998.

15. Buckwalter JA, Saltzman C, Brown T: The impact of osteoarthritis: Implications for research. *Clin Orthop Relat Res* 427 Suppl:S6-S15, 2004.

16. Buechel FF Sr, Buechel FF Jr, Pappas MJ: Ten-year evaluation of cementless Buechel–Pappas meniscal bearing total ankle replacement. *Foot Ankle Int* 24(6):462-472, 2003.

17. Buechel FF Sr, Buechel FF Jr, Pappas MJ: Twenty-year evaluation of cementless mobile-bearing total ankle replacements. *Clin Orthop Relat Res* 424:19-26, 2004.

18. Buechel FF, Pappas MJ, Iorio LJ: New Jersey low contact stress total ankle replacement: Biomechanical rationale and review of 23 cementless cases. *Foot Ankle* 8(6):279-290, 1988.

19. Cameron SE, Ullrich P: Arthroscopic arthrodesis of the ankle joint. *Arthroscopy* 16(1):21-26, 2000.

20. Carlsson AS, Montgomery F, Besjakov J: Arthrodesis of the ankle secondary to replacement. *Foot Ankle Int* 19(4):240-245, 1998.

21. Chubinskaya S, Huch K, Mikecz K, et al: Chondrocyte matrix metalloproteinase-8: Up-regulation of neutrophil collagenase by interleukin-1 beta in human cartilage from knee and ankle joints. *Lab Invest* 74(1):232-240, 1996.

22. Cierny G 3rd, Cook WG, Mader JT: Ankle arthrodesis in the presence of ongoing sepsis. Indications, methods, and results. *Orthop Clin North Am* 20(4):709-721, 1989.

23. Cobb TK, Gabrielsen TA, Campbell DC 2nd, et al: Cigarette smoking and nonunion after ankle arthrodesis. *Foot Ankle Int* 15(2):64-67, 1994.

24. Coester LM, Saltzman CL, Leupold J, Pontarelli W: Long-term results following ankle arthrodesis for post-traumatic arthritis. *J Bone Joint Surg Am* 83(2):219-228, 2001.

25. Collins DH: In *The Pathology of Articular and Spinal Diseases.* London, Edward Arnold, 1949, pp 23-37.

26. Corso SJ, Zimmer TJ: Technique and clinical evaluation of arthroscopic ankle arthrodesis. *Arthroscopy* 11(5):585-590, 1995.

27. Crosby LA, Yee TC, Formanek TS, Fitzgibbons TC: Complications following arthroscopic ankle arthrodesis. *Foot Ankle Int* 17(6):340-342, 1996.

28. Cushnaghan J, Dieppe P: Study of 500 patients with limb joint osteoarthritis. I. Analysis by age, sex, and distribution of symptomatic joint sites. *Ann Rheum Dis* 50(1):8-13, 1991.

29. De Vriese L, Dereymaeker G, Fabry G: Arthroscopic ankle arthrodesis. Preliminary report. *Acta Orthop Belg* 60(4):389-392, 1994.

30. Demetriades L, Strauss E, Gallina J: Osteoarthritis of the ankle. *Clin Orthop Relat Res* 349:28-42, 1998.

31. Dent CM, Patil M, Fairclough JA: Arthroscopic ankle arthrodesis. *J Bone Joint Surg Br* 75(5):830-832, 1993.

32. Dieppe P, Cushnaghan J, Tucker M, et al: The Bristol "OA500 study": Progression and impact of the disease after 8 years. *Osteoarthritis Cartilage* 8(2):63-68, 2000.

33. Dini AA, Bassett FH 3rd: Evaluation of the early result of Smith total ankle replacement. *Clin Orthop Relat Res* 146:228-230, 1980.

34. Dohm M, Purdy BA, Benjamin J: Primary union of ankle arthrodesis: Review of a single institution/multiple surgeon experience. *Foot Ankle Int* 15(6):293-296, 1994.

35. Donley BG, Ward DM: Implantable electrical stimulation in high-risk hindfoot fusions. *Foot Ankle Int* 23(1):13-18, 2002.

36. El-Khoury GY, Alliman KJ, Lundberg HJ, et al: Cartilage thickness in cadaveric ankles: Measurement with double-contrast multi-detector row CT arthrography versus MR imaging. *Radiology* 233(3):768-773, 2004.

37. Ferkel RD, Hewitt M: Long-term results of arthroscopic ankle arthrodesis. *Foot Ankle Int* 26(4):275-280, 2005.

38. Fisher RL, Ryan WR, Dugdale TW, Zimmerman GA: Arthroscopic ankle fusion. *Conn Med* 61(10):643-646, 1997.

39. Fitzgibbons TC: Arthroscopic ankle débridement and fusion: Indications, techniques, and results. *Instr Course Lect* 48:243-248, 1999.

40. Frey C, Halikus NM, Vu-Rose T, Ebramzadeh E: A review of ankle arthrodesis: Predisposing factors to nonunion. *Foot Ankle Int* 15(11):581-584, 1994.

41. Fujimori J, Yoshino S, Koiwa M, et al: Ankle arthrodesis in rheumatoid arthritis using an intramedullary nail with fins. *Foot Ankle Int* 20(8):485-490, 1999.

42. Gabrion A, Jarde O, Havet E, et al: [Ankle arthrodesis after failure of a total ankle prosthesis. Eight cases]. *Rev Chir Orthop Reparatrice Appar Mot* 90(4):353-359, 2004.

42a. Gilbert BJ, Horst F, Nunley JA: Potential donor rotational bone grafts using vascular territories in the foot and ankle. *J Bone Joint Surg Am* 86(4):1857-1873, 2004.

43. Glick JM, Morgan CD, Myersonn MS, et al: Ankle arthrodesis using an arthroscopic method: Long-term follow-up of 34 cases. *Arthroscopy* 12(4):428-434, 1996.

44. Goldie IF, Herberts P: Prosthetic replacement of the ankle joint. *Reconstr Surg Traumatol* 18:205-210, 1981.

45. Gross AE, Agnidis Z, Hutchison CR: Osteochondral defects of the talus treated with fresh osteochondral allograft transplantation. *Foot Ankle Int* 22(5):385-391, 2001.

46. Harrington KD: Degenerative arthritis of the ankle secondary to long-standing lateral ligament instability. *J Bone Joint Surg Am* 61(3):354-361, 1979.

47. Hartel RM, Van Dijk CN, Van Kampen A, De Waal Malefijt M: Arthroscopic arthrodesis of the ankle—a new technique [abstr]. *Acta Orthop Scand* 64:10, 1993.

48. Haskell A, Mann RA: Perioperative complication rate of total ankle replacement is reduced by surgeon experience. *Foot Ankle Int* 25(5):283-289, 2004.

49. Haskell A, Mann RA: Ankle arthroplasty with preoperative coronal plane deformity: short-term results. *Clin Orthop Relat Res* 424:98-103, 2004.

50. Helm R, Stevens J: Long-term results of total ankle replacement. *J Arthroplasty* 1(4):271-277, 1986.

51. Herbst SA, Jones KB, Saltzman CL: Pattern of diabetic neuropathic arthropathy associated with the peripheral bone mineral density. *J Bone Joint Surg Br* 86(3):378-383, 2004.

52. Honkamp N, Amendola A, Hurwitz S, Saltzman CL: Retrospective review of eighteen patients who underwent transtibial amputation for intractable pain. *J Bone Joint Surg Am* 83(10):1479-1483, 2001.

53. Huch K, Kuettner KE, Dieppe P: Osteoarthritis in ankle and knee joints. *Semin Arthritis Rheum* 26(4):667-674, 1997.

54. Ihn JC, Kim SJ, Park IH: In vitro study of contact area and pressure distribution in the human knee after partial and total meniscectomy. *Int Orthop* 17(4):214-218, 1993.

55. Jackson A, Glasgow M: Tarsal hypermobility after ankle fusion—fact or fiction? *J Bone Joint Surg Br* 61(4):470-473, 1979.

56. Jensen NC, Kroner K: Total ankle joint replacement: A clinical follow up. *Orthopedics* 15(2):236-239, 1992.

57. Jerosch J, Steinbeck J, Schroder M, Reer R: Arthroscopically assisted arthrodesis of the ankle joint. *Arch Orthop Trauma Surg* 115(3-4):182-189, 1996.

58. Jones KB, Maiers-Yelden KA, Marsh JL, et al: Ankle fractures in patients with diabetes mellitus. *J Bone Joint Surg Br* 87(4):489-495, 2005.

59. Kats J, van Kampen A, de Waal-Malefijt MC: Improvement in technique for arthroscopic ankle fusion: Results in 15 patients. *Knee Surg Sports Traumatol Arthrosc* 11(1):46-49, 2003.

60. Katsenis D, Bhave A, Paley D, Herzenberg JE: Treatment of malunion and nonunion at the site of an ankle fusion with the Ilizarov apparatus. *J Bone Joint Surg Am* 87(2):302-309, 2005.

61. Kempson GE: Age-related changes in the tensile properties of human articular cartilage: A comparative study between the femoral head of the hip joint and the talus of the ankle joint. *Biochim Biophys Acta* 1075(3):223-230, 1991.

62. Khoury NJ, el-Khoury GY, Saltzman CL, Brandser EA: Intraarticular foot and ankle injections to identify source of pain before arthrodesis. *AJR Am J Roentgenol* 167(3):669-673, 1996.

63. Kim CW, Jamali A, Tontz W Jr, et al: Treatment of post-traumatic ankle arthrosis with bipolar tibiotalar osteochondral shell allografts. *Foot Ankle Int* 23(12):1091-1102, 2002.

64. Kimizuka M, Kurosawa H, Fukubayashi T: Load-bearing pattern of the ankle joint. Contact area and pressure distribution. *Arch Orthop Trauma Surg* 96(1):45-49, 1980.

65. Kirkpatrick JS, Goldner JL, Goldner RD: Revision arthrodesis for tibiotalar pseudarthrosis with fibular onlay–inlay graft and internal screw fixation. *Clin Orthop Relat Res* 268:29-36, 1991.

66. Kirkup J: Richard Smith ankle arthroplasty. *J R Soc Med* 78(4):301-304, 1985.

67. Kitaoka HB, Anderson PJ, Morrey BF: Revision of ankle arthrodesis with external fixation for non-union. *J Bone Joint Surg Am* 74(8):1191-1200, 1992.

68. Kitaoka HB, Patzer GL: Clinical results of the Mayo total ankle arthroplasty. *J Bone Joint Surg Am* 78(11):1658-1664, 1996.

69. Kitaoka HB, Romness DW: Arthrodesis for failed ankle arthroplasty. *J Arthroplasty* 7(3):277-284, 1992.

70. Knecht SI, Estin M, Callaghan JJ, et al: The Agility total ankle arthroplasty. Seven to sixteen-year follow-up. *J Bone Joint Surg Am* 86(6):1161-1171, 2004.

71. Kobayashi A, Minoda Y, Kadoya Y, et al: Ankle arthroplasties generate wear particles similar to knee arthroplasties. *Clin Orthop Relat Res* 424:69-72, 2004.

72. Kofoed H: Scandinavian Total Ankle Replacement (STAR). *Clin Orthop Relat Res* 424:73-79, 2004.

73. Kollig E, Esenwein SA, Muhr G, Kutscha-Lissberg F: Fusion of the septic ankle: Experience with 15 cases using hybrid external fixation. *J Trauma* 55(4):685-691, 2003.

74. Levine SE, Myerson MS, Lucas P, Schon LC: Salvage of pseudoarthrosis after tibiotalar arthrodesis. *Foot Ankle Int* 18(9):580-585, 1997.

75. Lortat-Jacob A, Beaufils P, Coignard S, Elahmadi J: [Tibiotarsal arthrodesis in a septic milieu]. *Rev Chir Orthop Reparatrice Appar Mot* 70(6):449-456, 1984.

76. Mann RA, Rongstad KM: Arthrodesis of the ankle: A critical analysis. *Foot Ankle Int* 19(1):3-9, 1998.

77. Marcus RE, Balourdas GM, Heiple KG: Ankle arthrodesis by chevron fusion with internal fixation and bone-grafting. *J Bone Joint Surg Am* 65(6):833-838, 1983.

78. Marsh JL, Rattay RE, Dulaney T: Results of ankle arthrodesis for treatment of supramalleolar nonunion and ankle arthrosis. *Foot Ankle Int* 18(3):138-143, 1997.

79. Maurer RC, Cimino WR, Cox CV, Satow GK: Transarticular cross-screw fixation. A technique of ankle arthrodesis. *Clin Orthop Relat Res* 268:56-64, 1991.

80. Mazur JM, Schwartz E, Simon SR: Ankle arthrodesis. Long-term follow-up with gait analysis. *J Bone Joint Surg Am* 61(7):964-975, 1979.

81. Meachim G: Cartilage fibrillation at the ankle joint in Liverpool necropsies. *J Anat* 119(3):601-610, 1975.

82. Meachim G: Cartilage fibrillation on the lateral tibial plateau in Liverpool necropsies. *J Anat* 121(1):97-106, 1976.

83. Meachim G, Emery IH: Cartilage fibrillation in shoulder and hip joints in Liverpool necropsies. *J Anat* 116(2):161-179, 1973.

84. Meachim G, Emery IH: Quantitative aspects of patello-femoral cartilage fibrillation in Liverpool necropsies. *Ann Rheum Dis* 33(1):39-47, 1974.

85. Mont MA, Schon LC, Hungerford MW, Hungerford DS: Avascular necrosis of the talus treated by core decompression. *J Bone Joint Surg Br* 78(5):827-830, 1996.

86. Moran CG, Pinder IM, Smith SR: Ankle arthrodesis in rheumatoid arthritis. 30 cases followed for 5 years. *Acta Orthop Scand* 62(6):538-543, 1991.

87. Muehleman C, Bareigher D, Huch K, et al: Prevalence of degenerative morphological changes in the joints of the lower extremity. *Osteoarthritis Cartilage* 5(1):23-37, 1997.

88. Muir DC, Amendola A, Saltzman CL: Long-term outcome of ankle arthrodesis. *Foot Ankle Clin North Am* 7(4):703-708, 2002.

89. Myerson MS, Mroczek K: Perioperative complications of total ankle arthroplasty. *Foot Ankle Int* 24(1):17-21, 2003.

90. Myerson MS, Neufeld SK, Uribe J: Fresh-frozen structural allografts in the foot and ankle. *J Bone Joint Surg Am* 87(1):113-120, 2005.

91. Myerson MS, Quill G: Ankle arthrodesis. A comparison of an arthroscopic and an open method of treatment. *Clin Orthop Relat Res* 268:84-95, 1991.

92. Nielsen JK, Saltzman CL, Brown TD: Determination of ankle external fixation stiffness by expedited interactive finite element analysis. *J Orthop Res* 23(6):1321-1328, 2005.

93. Nishikawa M, Tomita T, Fujii M, et al: Total ankle replacement in rheumatoid arthritis. *Int Orthop* 28(2):123-126, 2004.

94. O'Brien TS, Hart TS, Shereff MJ, et al: Open versus arthroscopic ankle arthrodesis: A comparative study. *Foot Ankle Int* 20(6):368-374, 1999.

95. Ogilvie-Harris DJ, Lieberman I, Fitsialos D: Arthroscopically assisted arthrodesis for osteoarthrotic ankles. *J Bone Joint Surg Am* 75(8):1167-1174, 1993.

96. Paremain GD, Miller SD, Myerson MS: Ankle arthrodesis: Results after the miniarthrotomy technique. *Foot Ankle Int* 17(5):247-252, 1996.

97. Perlman MH, Thordarson DB: Ankle fusion in a high risk population: An assessment of nonunion risk factors. *Foot Ankle Int* 20(8):491-496, 1999.

98. Pyevich MT, Saltzman CL, Callaghan JJ, Alvine FG: Total ankle arthroplasty: A unique design. Two to twelve-year follow-up. *J Bone Joint Surg Am* 80(10):1410-1420, 1998.

99. Richter D, Hahn MP, Laun RA, et al: Arthrodesis of the infected ankle and subtalar joint: Technique, indications, and results of 45 consecutive cases. *J Trauma* 47(6):1072-1078, 1999.

100. Ross SD, Matta J: Internal compression arthrodesis of the ankle. *Clin Orthop Relat Res* 199:54-60, 1985.

101. Said E, Hunka L, Siller TN: Where ankle fusion stands today. *J Bone Joint Surg Br* 60(2):211-214, 1978.

102. Saltzman CL: Salvage of diffuse ankle osteomyelitis by single-stage resection and circumferential frame compression arthrodesis. *Iowa Orthop J* 25:47-52, 2005.

103. Saltzman CL, Amendola A, Anderson R, et al: Surgeon training and complications in total ankle arthroplasty. *Foot Ankle Int* 24(6):514-518, 2003.

104. Saltzman CL, el-Khoury GY: The hindfoot alignment view. *Foot Ankle Int* 16(9):572-576, 1995.

105. Saltzman CL, Hagy ML, Zimmerman B, et al: How effective is intensive nonoperative treatment of diabetic Charcot feet? *Clin Orthop Relat Res* 435:185-190, 2005.

106. Saltzman C, Lightfoot A, Amendola A: PEMF as treatment for delayed healing of foot and ankle arthrodesis. *Foot Ankle Int* 25(11):771-773, 2004.

107. Saltzman CL, Salamon ML, Blanchard GM, et al: Epidemiology of ankle arthritis: Report of a consecutive series of 639 patients from a tertiary orthopaedic center. *Iowa Orthop J* 25:44-46, 2005.

108. Saltzman CL, Shurr D, Kamp L, Cook TA: The leather ankle lacer. *Iowa Orthop J* 15:204-208, 1995.

109. Saltzman CL, Tochigi Y, Rudert MJ, et al: The effect of agility ankle prosthesis misalignment on the peri-ankle ligaments. *Clin Orthop Relat Res* 424:137-142, 2004.

110. Sangeorzan BP, Judd RP, Sangeorzan BJ: Mathematical analysis of single-cut osteotomy for complex long bone deformity. *J Biomech* 22(11-12):1271-1278, 1989.

111. Schafer D, Hintermann B: Arthroscopic assessment of the chronic unstable ankle joint. *Knee Surg Sports Traumatol Arthrosc* 4(1):48-52, 1996.

112. Scranton PE Jr: Use of bone graft substitutes in lower extremity reconstructive surgery. *Foot Ankle Int* 23(8):689-692, 2002.

113. Scranton PE Jr: Use of internal compression in arthrodesis of the ankle. *J Bone Joint Surg Am* 67(4):550-555, 1985.

114. Su EP, Kahn B, Figgie MP: Total ankle replacement in patients with rheumatoid arthritis. *Clin Orthop Relat Res* 424:32-38, 2004.

115. Takakura Y, Tanaka Y, Kumai T, et al: Ankle arthroplasty using three generations of metal and ceramic prostheses. *Clin Orthop Relat Res* 424:130-136, 2004.

116. Thordarson DB, Patzakis MJ, Holtom P, Sherman R: Salvage of the septic ankle with concomitant tibial osteomyelitis. *Foot Ankle Int* 18(3):151-156, 1997.

117. Thordarson DB, Kuehn S: Use of demineralized bone matrix in ankle/hindfoot fusion. *Foot Ankle Int* 24(7):557-560, 2003.

118. Tochigi Y, Rudert MJ, Amendola A, et al: Tensile engagement of the peri-ankle ligaments in stance phase. *Foot Ankle Int* 26(12):1067-1073, 2005.

119. Tochigi Y, Rudert MJ, Brown TD, et al: The effect of implantation accuracy on range of movement of the Scandinavian total Ankle Replacement. *J Bone Joint Surg Br* 87:736-740, 2005.

120. Tontz WL, Jr, Bugbee WD, Brage ME: Use of allografts in the management of ankle arthritis. *Foot Ankle Clin* 8(2):361-73, xi, 2003.

121. Turan I, Wredmark T, Fellander-Tsai L: Arthroscopic ankle arthrodesis in rheumatoid arthritis. *Clin Orthop Relat Res* 320:110-114, 1995.

122. Valderrabano V, Hintermann B, Dick W: Scandinavian total ankle replacement: A 3.7-year average follow-up of 65 patients. *Clin Orthop Relat Res* 424:47-56, 2004.

123. van der Schoot DK, Den Outer AJ, Bode PJ, et al: Degenerative changes at the knee and ankle related to malunion of tibial fractures. 15-year follow-up of 88 patients. *J Bone Joint Surg Br* 78(5):722-725, 1996.

124. Wang CJ, Tambakis AP, Fielding JW: An evaluation of ankle fusion in children. *Clin Orthop Relat Res* 98:233-238, 1974.

125. Winson IG, Robinson DE, Allen PE: Arthroscopic ankle arthrodesis. *J Bone Joint Surg Br* 87(3):343-347, 2005.

126. Wood PL, Deakin S: Total ankle replacement. The results in 200 ankles. *J Bone Joint Surg Br* 85(3):334-341, 2003.

127. Wyss C, Zollinger H: The causes of subsequent arthrodesis of the ankle joint. *Acta Orthop Belg* 57 Suppl 1:22-27, 1991.

128. Zvijac JE, Lemak L, Schurhoff MR, et al: Analysis of arthroscopically assisted ankle arthrodesis. *Arthroscopy* 18(1):70-75, 2002.

Ankle Arthritis: Deformity Correction and Distraction Arthroplasty

Douglas N. Beaman • Richard E. Gellman • Elly Trepman

Symptomatic ankle arthritis is often accompanied by distal tibial or foot deformity. The goal of deformity correction in the distal tibia and foot is to improve function by creating a stable, plantigrade foot beneath a mechanically aligned lower extremity. Deformity in the ankle often is complicated by the presence of compensatory deformities in the hindfoot and forefoot. Pain symptoms can decrease despite arthritis in the foot or ankle after all primary and secondary deformities are corrected.

Ankle distraction arthroplasty is a new technique gaining interest for younger patients with ankle arthritis who seek to defer ankle arthrodesis or joint replacement. Distraction arthroplasty is based on the hypothesis that healing of arthritic cartilage can occur when the joint is unloaded and subjected to intermittent intraarticular fluid pressure changes.[13] Mechanical unloading is achieved for 3 months with an Ilizarov external fixator to distract the joint. During this period, loading and unloading of the joint during weight-bearing gait results in intermittent intraarticular fluid pressure changes because of the flexibility of the wires or joint motion through hinges in the fixator.[13,14] In vitro and animal studies have demonstrated that mechanical unloading and intermittent fluid pressure changes can reduce inflammation and normalize cartilage matrix turnover.[13] Clinical studies have demonstrated an increase in joint space and improved pain and mobility.[7,9,14] As techniques evolve and more clinical follow-up studies are done, the role of ankle distraction arthroplasty in the spectrum of treatment options for ankle arthritis should become better defined.

PRINCIPLES OF DEFORMITY EVALUATION AND CORRECTION

Normal Alignment

In all ankle arthritis patients, it is necessary to assess ankle deformities and deformities proximal and distal to the ankle that contribute to malalignment (Table 18–1). In the frontal plane, normal alignment of the lower extremity above the ankle follows a straight line (the mechanical axis) from the center of the hip through the center of the knee to the center of the ankle joint, ending at the weight-bearing point of the calcaneus (Fig. 18–1).[6] The weight-bearing point of the calcaneus is medial to the vertical anatomic axis of the calcaneus, which is parallel and 5 to 10 mm lateral to the mechanical axis (Fig. 18–2). Variations in the weight-bearing line of the tibia lie within 15 mm of the lowest calcaneal point in 95% of asymptomatic patients.[10] In the sagittal plane, the midtibial line intersects the midpoint of the talar dome and extends through or near the lateral talar process (Fig. 18–3);

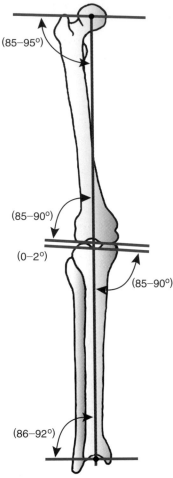

Figure 18–1 The normal mechanical axis of the lower extremity follows a straight line from the center of the hip through the center of the knee to the center of the ankle joint.

the exact location varies with the position of ankle dorsiflexion or plantarflexion or internal/external rotation.[12]

Rotation is measured using the foot–thigh angle to determine tibial external or internal torsion. Normal rotation is defined as a perpendicular line extending out from the tibial tubercle that matches the axis of the second toe. Clinically, if the uninvolved limb is asymptomatic and has no obvious deformity, it is common practice to match rotation to the symptomatic side. However, if there is major deformity in the foot or ankle joint, then measuring rotation by palpation of the malleoli may be more accurate because the normal axis of the ankle joint is described by a line between the tips of the medial and lateral malleoli, oriented from posteroinferolateral to anterosuperomedial.

Radiographic Evaluation

Deformity can be measured precisely with radiographs obtained in a typical orthopaedic office. Instruction to

---

TABLE 18–1

Considerations in Evaluating the Limb with Deformity with or without Arthritis

Primary Considerations

Deformity of the tibia and fibula: length, angulation, rotation, and translation

Primary or compensatory hindfoot, midfoot, or forefoot deformities

Secondary Considerations

Infection (previous or current)

Nonunion of fracture or arthrodesis (hypertrophic, atrophic)

Soft tissue coverage (previous wounds, free tissue transfers, skin grafts)

Musculotendinous or joint contractures

Muscle weakness

Ligamentous instability

Arthritis of the ankle, hindfoot, or midfoot

Vascular insufficiency (arterial, venous)

Neuropathy

Medical problems (diabetes, smoking, renal failure)

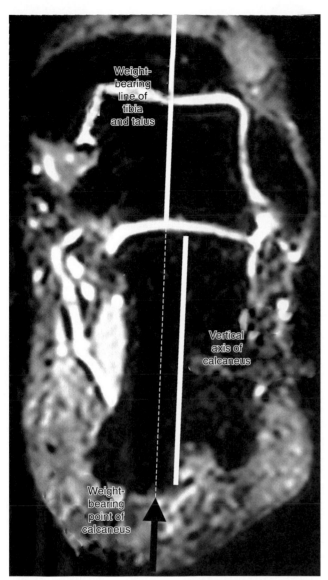

Figure 18–2 Below the ankle, the weight bearing line of the tibia and talus is parallel to and 5–10 mm medial to the vertical axis of the calcaneus. The weight-bearing point of the calcaneus (black arrow) is positioned medial to the longitudinal axis of the calcaneus and beneath the longitudinal axis of the tibia.

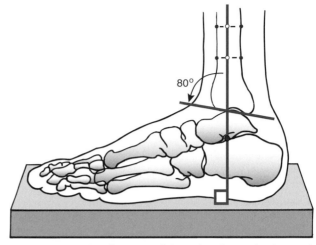

Figure 18–3 On the normal lateral radiograph, the mid-diaphyseal line of the tibia falls through the lateral talar process. The normal angle of the anterior distal tibial plafond is 80 degrees off the mid-diaphyseal tibial line.

block placed under the shorter limb to eliminate the limb length discrepancy. This allows direct measurement of the limb length discrepancy, instead of relying solely on measurements from the radiograph. The long lateral view of the limb is made with the knee in full extension to assess deformity proximal to the distal tibia and to exclude either knee flexion contracture or recurvatum from hyperlaxity that can affect limb length.

Radiographic evaluation of distal tibial and foot deformity includes weight-bearing tibial, ankle, hindfoot, and foot radiographs (Table 18–2). The radiographic angles for the ankle described below are general guidelines used in comparison with the uninvolved limb. AP tibial radiographs are made with the patella facing forward. The x-ray beam is centered on the ankle to include the tibia. If a rotational deformity of the limb is present on clinical exam, an AP ankle radiograph is made in the foot-forward position to

technicians should be simple and radiographs should be cost-efficient and time-efficient. Standard weight-bearing radiographs provide sufficient information for the majority of ankle deformities. CT scans, with or without reformations, are occasionally ordered to better evaluate complex deformity.

If clinical alignment or standing tibial radiographs demonstrate a deformity above the distal tibial region or there is a known limb-length discrepancy, then it is important to obtain standing full-length lower-extremity anteroposterior (AP) and lateral radiographs from the hip to the ankle. The pelvis is leveled with a

TABLE 18–2
Radiographic Evaluation of Deformities of the Distal Tibia and Foot
Usual Studies
Standing anteroposterior and lateral tibia
Standing anteroposterior, lateral and mortise ankle
Hindfoot alignment standing view[10] or long axial non–weight-bearing view
Standing anteroposterior and lateral foot
Special Studies
Stress radiographs of the ankle
Fluoroscopy to assess arc of ankle motion

evaluate intraarticular wear or malalignment. Lateral ankle radiographs are made in the plane of the ankle malleoli.

The hindfoot alignment view is a weight-bearing radiograph that enables observation of the tibia, ankle joint, and calcaneal tuberosity on a single view. It is the only radiograph that requires a specialized mounting box to angle the radiographic plate 20 degrees from the vertical plane. An alternative radiograph is the long axial view, which is usually done without weight bearing and visualizes the tibia, subtalar joint, and calcaneal tuberosity. A line drawn on the vertical axis of the midbody of the calcaneus should be parallel and approximately one centimeter lateral to the mid-diaphyseal line of the tibia. Valgus deformity and lateral translation indicate a pes planus deformity, and varus angulation and medial translation indicate cavovarus type deformity.

The weight-bearing AP foot radiograph is measured for the talus–first metatarsal angle, navicular coverage, and joint subluxation or arthritis. The lateral foot view is measured for the talus–first metatarsal angle, calcaneal pitch, and joint subluxation or arthritis. Other angles are used when necessary. If the opposite limb is pain free and has no obvious deformity, comparison radiographs may be made for preoperative planning.

Rotational deformity usually is not measured radiographically. If clinical examination is insufficient, computed tomography scans of the hip, distal femur, proximal tibia, and ankle malleoli accurately describe a rotational deformity.

Measurement of Deformity

In general, deformity at or near the ankle does not alter the mechanical axis of the lower extremity (see Fig. 18-1). If deformity is suspected in the mid tibia and above, the mechanical axis will deviate more than 1 cm from the center of the knee joint. Foot and ankle deformity arises from the bones, joint laxity, or intraarticular wear and malalignment. Each bone deformity is described regarding length, angulation, rotation, and translation.

In the tibia, the mechanical axis is a straight line connecting the center of the knee to the center of the ankle. The anatomic axis is a line connecting two mid-diaphyseal points of a long bone. Deformity measurements can be made from either the mechanical or anatomic axes. Terminology and values of the joint angles have been described.[8] Mid-diaphyseal tibial deformities are measured as the intersection of the anatomic axes proximal and distal to the deformity.

On an AP radiograph of the distal tibia, the frontal plane joint angle (varus, normal, or valgus) is measured between the anatomic axis of the tibia and the line parallel to the distal tibial plafond, defined as the lateral distal tibial angle (LDTA). The normal average LDTA is 89 degrees (normal range, 86 to 92 degrees). In cases of bilateral deformities, a normal LDTA of 90 degrees is assumed.

Distal tibial metaphyseal and juxta-articular ankle deformities are measured as the intersection of the proximal tibial anatomic axis and a line perpendicular to the tibial plafond. These types of deformities are common after distal tibial growth arrest or intraarticular collapse from pilon fractures.

In the sagittal plane, the anterior distal tibial angle (ADTA), defined as the angle between the mid-diaphyseal line of the tibia and the articular surface of the tibial plafond, is 80 degrees (normal range, 78 to 82 degrees). As in the evaluation of the frontal plane, comparison radiographs are useful and a standard ADTA of 80 degrees is assumed when there are bilateral deformities.

The ankle joint is different from the knee with respect to ligamentous laxity. A normal knee might have up to 3 degrees of joint convergence or laxity in the frontal plane on a weight-bearing radiograph. However, in the normal ankle, the distal tibial plafond is parallel to the talar dome, and any loss of parallel alignment is a result of ligamentous laxity or loss of articular cartilage.

Compensatory deformities in the foot and ankle are common. Varus and valgus deformities of the distal tibia usually are compensated for in the subtalar joint (Table 18-3). The degree of compensation depends on the mobility of the subtalar joint, which normally includes 15 to 30 degrees of inversion and 5 to 15 degrees of eversion (Fig. 18-4). Valgus deformities of the distal tibia usually are better compensated than

TABLE 18-3

Normal Joint Motions Compensatory to Different Distal Tibial Deformities

Distal Tibial Deformity	Compensatory Motion	Common Compensatory Range
Varus	1° subtalar eversion 2° forefoot pronation	15°
Valgus	1° subtalar inversion 2° forefoot supination	30°
Procurvatum	1° ankle dorsiflexion 2° knee hyperextension	20°
Recurvatum	1° ankle plantar flexion 2° knee flexion	50°
Internal torsion	1° hip external rotation 2° forefoot pronation	Varied
External torsion	1° hip internal rotation 2° forefoot supination	Varied

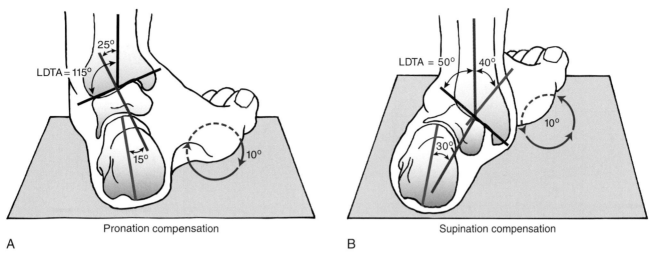

Figure 18–4 Compensation for tibial varus **(A)** or valgus **(B)** deformity with subtalar motion. LDTA, lateral distal tibial angle.

varus deformities of the distal tibia because normal subtalar inversion is greater than eversion. However, the greater translational deformity usually observed with a valgus distal tibia deformity can limit compensation imparted by subtalar joint inversion.

Farther distal in the foot, tibial varus deformity is compensated by pronation in the forefoot (see Table 18–1). When a distal tibial varus deformity is not fully compensated by subtalar joint eversion, further compensation can occur from plantar flexion of the first ray with associated rise of the arch of the foot. Similarly, compensation from first ray plantar flexion can occur when the distal tibia is normal but there is fixed subtalar joint inversion or hindfoot varus, as in a cavovarus foot.

Valgus deformity of the distal tibia that exceeds subtalar joint inversion can result in dorsiflexion of the medial column and a forefoot supination deformity. The medial dorsiflexion deformity can occur at the first ray or through the spring ligament complex and talonavicular or naviculocuneiform joints. Forefoot supination more often occurs with normal distal tibial alignment and excessive subtalar eversion, as observed with pes planus deformity or posterior tibial tendon dysfunction.

Deformity Correction

Correction of angular deformities by osteotomy involves angulating one bone segment relative to another around an imaginary axis—the angulation correction axis (ACA).[8] In common orthopaedic nomenclature, the point where the proximal and distal anatomic or mechanical axes intersect is termed the *apex* of the deformity. In most cases, the apex is the optimal location for the osteotomy and angulation,

so it also has been termed the *center of rotation of angulation* (CORA) (Fig. 18–5). Correction with osteotomy at or near the CORA avoids secondary translations.

However, if the CORA is at or near the joint, the osteotomy may be made proximal or distal to the CORA; in this case, angulation correction alone will result in a translational deformity and this translation must be corrected, either acutely at surgery or gradually in the frame. This will allow complete correction of the limb axis. For example, to correct a distal tibia varus deformity that has a CORA at the level of the ankle joint, a distal tibial osteotomy is performed proximal to the CORA in metaphyseal bone, and gradual opening distraction is performed with an external fixator to correct the angular deformity. Pure rotation at the osteotomy would result in lateral translation of the distal fragment. Therefore, the distal segment is translated medially acutely or gradually so that the mechanical axis line of the proximal tibia will intersect the center of the talus.

For a deformity in the tibial shaft, angle correction can be achieved directly at the apex of the deformity; the ACA and CORA are identical. In this case, the osteotomy is made through the CORA and ACA; the width of the bone and the type of osteotomy (e.g., opening or closing wedge) will affect the overall limb length following correction of the deformity, but no translation will occur. In certain cases, bone quality or translational deformities require the osteotomy to be made at a level other than the CORA.

To simplify the planning of hinge placement for deformity correction with external fixation, Taylor developed the hexapod spatial frame (Taylor Spatial Frame, Smith & Nephew, Memphis, Tenn). This advancement of the Ilizarov technique uses six struts

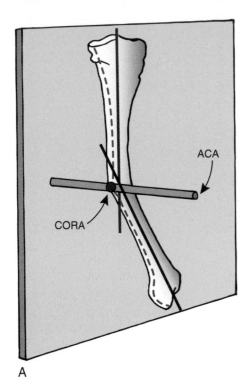

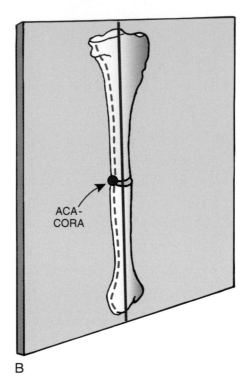

A   B

Figure 18–5   A, The center of rotation of angulation (CORA) is the intersection of the proximal and distal axis lines of the deformed bone. The axis line around which the correction is performed is the angulation correction axis (ACA). **B,** After an osteotomy that passes through the ACA-CORA, the correction produces pure angulation at the osteotomy site. In this case, an opening wedge is produced because the ACA-CORA is on the convex cortex.

connecting an upper and lower ring to correct deformities in all planes. An origin point is selected on a reference fragment and a corresponding point is selected on the other bone fragment. The relationship of these two points and their respective bone segment axis describes the deformity in terms of angulation, rotation, translation, and length. Six measurements of the deformity (angulation and translation each from the AP and lateral radiographs, plus length and axial rotation) are entered into a computer program along with information on the size and location of the external fixator to produce adjustments of the six struts to correct the deformity. This has greatly simplified deformity evaluation and correction because less time is required to calculate hinge placement and less office and operative time is expended building and modifying complex frames.

DEFORMITY CORRECTION AND FRAME APPLICATION

Patient Evaluation

Patient evaluation for ankle distraction arthroplasty includes a thorough history and physical examination. The optimal candidate is a compliant, motivated patient younger than 50 years who has post-traumatic arthritis or chronic ankle instability with arthritis, no previous history of ankle joint sepsis or ankylosis, and

an appropriate psychosocial support system to facilitate recovery and in-frame care. Specific factors important in the history include medical problems and current medications including analgesic and anti-inflammatory medication. Physically demanding occupations might not allow for optimal clinical results with ankle distraction arthroplasty. Preferred recreational activities are noted because nonimpact activities such as swimming and bicycling are advised after ankle distraction.

Physical examination includes evaluation of ankle and foot range of motion. Ankle motion (approximately 25 to 30 degrees), including dorsiflexion (5 to 10 degrees), is preferred for successful ankle distraction arthroplasty. Hindfoot motion is not required but, if present, can improve the result of distraction arthroplasty. Foot deformity such as cavovarus or flatfoot deformity is noted. Ankle joint instability is assessed clinically and may be confirmed with ankle stress radiographs in addition to the radiographic evaluation of the deformity. Fluoroscopic evaluation is used to assess the arc of ankle motion. Hinge-type motion or loss of anterior ankle articular cartilage may be associated with less successful results.

Decision Making for Immediate or Gradual Deformity Correction

Immediate correction of tibial deformity may be indicated for mild deformities without major shortening, soft tissue loss, or neurovascular compromise. However, gradual correction of deformity is preferred for severe, complex deformities, especially if the deformity is associated with major shortening of a bone segment or if immediate correction would result in minimum bone-to-bone contact. Gradual correction also may be preferred for complex deformities associated with oblique planes, rotation, translation, soft tissue compromise, or neurovascular risk.

Tibial or ankle deformities may be associated with either cavovarus or planovalgus deformity of the foot. The goal of foot deformity correction is to create a plantigrade foot with a neutral hindfoot and forefoot. Prior to application of a ring fixator in most cases, immediate correction of the foot deformity is done with soft tissue and bone procedures with or without internal fixation. However, when combined with external fixator wires, careful attention is required to avoid positioning wires and half pins near internal fixation devices (preferred minimum separation, 5 mm to 10 mm).

In patients undergoing ankle distraction, the most common tibial deformities associated with ankle arthritis are tibial valgus and distal tibial recurvatum deformities. Immediate correction is performed more commonly in patients with a supramalleolar frontal or sagittal plane deformity without shortening and with healthy bone. In these cases, a dome osteotomy may be performed with a combination of internal and external fixation. Gradual correction is preferred in oblique plane deformities or deformities associated with shortening, particularly when compensatory foot deformity is present. For example, in cases of tibial recurvatum associated with equinus deformity, the equinus can be gradually corrected with physical therapy (mild contracture) or the ring fixator (severe contracture) as the recurvatum is gradually corrected with the ring fixator.

Surgical Treatment

FOOT DEFORMITY CORRECTION AND ANKLE DEBRIDEMENT

Surgical Technique

1. The patient is positioned supine with a roll under the ipsilateral hip to position the patella forward, and a thigh tourniquet is applied. The patient position may be modified if foot deformity correction is required.

2. A C-arm fluoroscopic apparatus is placed on the contralateral side, and the instrument tables are positioned on the ipsilateral side. An additional back table is available for frame instruments and rings. The rings may be aluminum (Taylor Spatial Frame, Smith & Nephew, Memphis, Tennessee), carbon composite, or stainless steel (Ilizarov External Fixator, Smith & Nephew, Memphis, Tennessee). A large Mayo stand is used near the foot of the operative side to hold a customized sterilization tray (Quantum Medical Concepts, Hood River, Oregon) that contains the hardware required to secure half pins and wires to the rings and the threaded rods and other accessories to apply the ring external fixator.

3. Immediate correction of foot deformity and ankle debridement are performed prior to frame application. Ankle debridement is done arthroscopically or with an open approach through anteromedial and anterolateral ankle incisions. All impinging soft tissue and bone is excised from the anterior ankle and the lateral and medial gutters to facilitate ankle motion, primarily dorsiflexion.

4. Achilles tendon lengthening, gastrocnemius recession, or posterior capsulotomy is done as needed to facilitate dorsiflexion.

5. If there is hinge-type ankle motion with forced plantar flexion due to large posterior osteophytes or an os trigonum, posterior debridement is done from a posterolateral or posteromedial approach.

6. Cavovarus deformity is corrected with a varied combination of calcaneal osteotomy, plantar fascia release, first metatarsal dorsiflexion osteotomy, Jones procedure, and hallux interphalangeal arthrodesis. Depending on the specific features of the deformity, planovalgus or rocker bottom deformity correction may include hindfoot or midfoot osteotomy–arthrodesis. When reconstructing hindfoot deformities in the presence of ankle arthritis and retained hindfoot motion, it is preferable to avoid hindfoot arthrodesis because arthrodesis may be associated with increased stresses on the ankle.

OSTEOTOMY TECHNIQUES

Osteotomy techniques for deformity correction and distraction osteogenesis are designed to minimize periosteal damage and dissection.[11] The optimal osteotomy technique will preserve the periosteal blood supply and minimize thermal necrosis of bone. Although Ilizarov's early principles emphasized preservation of the intramedullary blood supply, more recent studies with the multiple drill hole or Gigli saw techniques have shown no major difference in osteotomy healing rates with preservation or disruption of intramedullary blood supply. Experimental studies have shown that corticotomy or multiple drill hole osteotomy yields more blood vessels bridging the distraction gap than an osteotomy done with an oscillating saw.[4] The Gigli saw method may be associated with faster healing than the multiple drill hole method.[3] The preferred technique varies with anatomic location.

Multiple Drill Hole Technique

The multiple drill hole technique is preferred in the diaphyseal region of the distal third of the tibia and the calcaneus (Fig. 18–6). The calcaneus can be approached either medially or laterally. Typically, a lateral approach to the calcaneal tuberosity is made just posterior to the peroneal tendons. Several drill holes are made from lateral to medial with a 3.8-mm or 4.8-mm drill, and the osteotomy is completed with an osteotome. Osteotomy completion in the calcaneus is confirmed by translating the tuberosity fragment in a dorsal-to-plantar direction.

Gigli Saw Technique

The Gigli saw technique is most useful in the proximal tibia, the metaphyseal region of the distal tibia, the supramalleolar region at the tibiofibular syndesmosis, and the midfoot (Fig. 18–7). The saw is passed around the bone with minimal soft tissue dissection, and osteotomy is performed. The Gigli saw osteotomy is also useful for open procedures with internal fixation when bone wedges are removed from the midfoot, as in correction of neuropathic deformity.

Focal Dome Osteotomy Technique

The focal dome osteotomy technique is useful for immediately correcting a deformity in the distal tibia when the CORA is at the ankle joint or within the supramalleolar metaphyseal region of the distal tibia.

1. For frontal plane deformities, a 6-mm half pin is placed in the distal tibia below the level of the osteotomy (at the CORA). Dissection is then performed proximal to the half pin.
2. Several 4.8-mm drill holes are made through a curved radiolucent jig or through connecting cubes or posts (Rancho Cube, Smith &

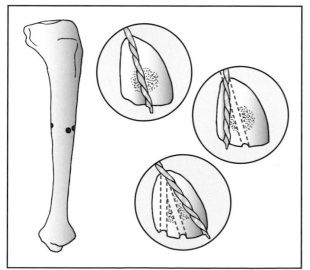
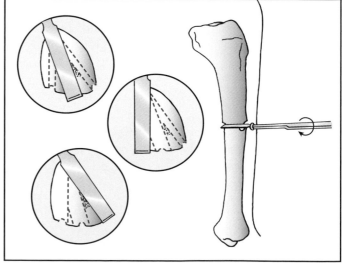

A   B

Figure 18–6 The multiple-drill-hole osteotomy technique is preferred in the diaphyseal region of the tibia. **A,** A 4.8-mm drill hole is made first from anterior to posterior, followed by two more drill holes placed posteromedial and posterolateral. **B,** The osteotomy is completed with an osteotome.

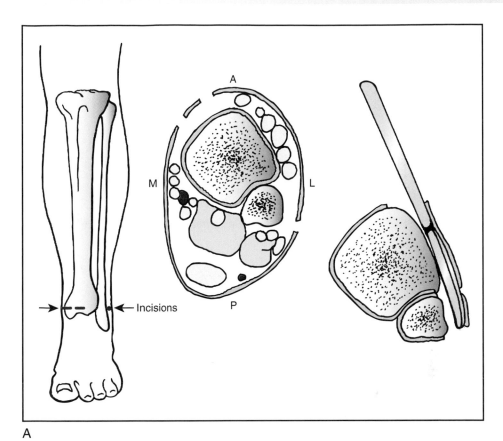

A

Figure 18–7 Percutaneous Gigli saw osteotomy in the supramalleolar region. At this level, there is no space between the tibia and fibula to pass the saw. Both tibia and fibula are cut together. **A,** Three small incisions are used. The two medial incisions are transverse, and the lateral incision is longitudinal. The periosteum is elevated anteriorly over the tibia and fibula, then the lateral incision is made over the tip of the elevator. A, anterior; L, lateral; M, medial; P, posterior. **B,** The Gigli saw is passed with a heavy suture to the posteromedial side. The medial periosteum is elevated, and the Gigli saw is used to cut the fibula and tibia from lateral to medial.

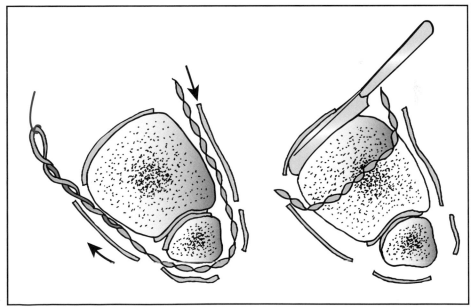

B

Nephew, Memphis, Tenn) to form the dome shape of the planned osteotomy (Fig. 18–8). The osteotomy is made as distal as possible, allowing for fixation, to take advantage of metaphyseal bone healing.

3. The remaining bone between the drilled holes is cut with a sharp osteotome. An acute correction is performed; the osteotomy can also be translated by rotation of the osteotome within the osteotomy. Some translation

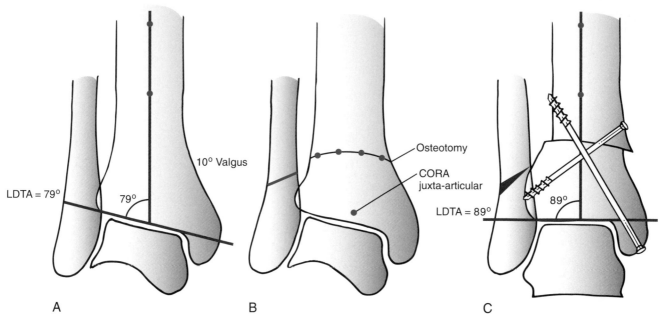

LDTA = 79°   79°   10° Valgus   A

Osteotomy   CORA juxta-articular   B

Osteotomy   CORA juxta-articular   LDTA = 89°   89°   C

Figure 18–8 Focal dome osteotomy. **A,** Preoperative measurements show a 10-degree valgus deformity of the distal tibia; LDTA = 79°. **B,** CORA is juxta-articular. Osteotomy is performed proximal to the CORA in metaphyseal bone. A radiolucent jig is available to assist in accurate placement of several 4.8-mm drill holes in the shape of a dome. Osteotomy is completed with an osteotome. Fibular osteotomy is made through a separate lateral incision. **C,** Acute correction is performed to realign proximal and distal mechanical axes. Note necessary lateral translation of the distal segment. Fixation of osteotomy is done with one or two cancellous lag screws. CORA, center of rotation of angulation; LDTA, lateral distal tibial angle.

is necessary to realign the mechanical axis because the osteotomy is not made through the CORA.

4. The osteotomy is stabilized with one or two screws. The half pin can be left in place for stabilization of the distal tibial ring if combined with Ilizarov external fixation of the foot and ankle and concurrent ankle joint distraction.

Fibular Osteotomy

Fibular osteotomy addresses fibular deformity at the time of tibial osteotomy. When the fibular deformity is similar to the tibial deformity in level and magnitude, the fibular and tibial osteotomies are made at the same level as each other. An oblique fibular osteotomy is made with a small sagittal saw or the multiple drill hole technique. If the fibula is not deformed and there is an isolated tibial deformity, the tibia may be osteotomized without a fibular osteotomy; this most commonly occurs in the posttraumatic deformity associated with a pilon fracture in which the fibula had been anatomically realigned and internally fixed and the distal tibia had healed with a malunion. Fibular osteotomy distal to the tibial osteotomy may be indicated if major translation is required for realignment.

INTERNAL FIXATION

When gradual correction of deformity is done, no internal fixation is used; the frame remains in place until the osteotomy is healed. With acute correction of deformity, osteotomies of the distal tibia and fibula usually are internally fixed.

The distal tibial osteotomy may be fixed with lag screws from the medial malleolus across the osteotomy site into the lateral cortex of the tibia. Crossed screws may be placed in the distal tibia with a separate second screw from the lateral to medial. Fixation may be augmented with a dorsally applied small fragment plate.

For calcaneal osteotomy, excessively posterior placement of the osteotomy is avoided to provide more available bone for fixation devices. The osteotomy may be fixed with one superior and one inferior calcaneal 3.5-mm or 4.5-mm screw, allowing ample room in the central part of the posterior calcaneal tuberosity for two 1.8-mm external fixation wires to further stabilize the osteotomy.

Internal fixation devices usually are avoided in the distal forefoot to allow placement of two 1.8-mm external fixation wires to engage the metatarsals. This may be achieved when the distal half to two thirds of the metatarsals are free from internal fixation devices.

APPLICATION OF THE TIBIAL BASE FRAME

Frame assembly is similar for ankle distraction arthroplasty cases with or without deformity correction (Fig. 18–9).

Surgical Technique

1. A two-ring tibial base frame is applied orthogonal to the tibia. The two rings are separated by 150-mm or 200-mm threaded rods depending on the size of the patient.
2. For the distal ring, a transverse, smooth 1.8-mm reference wire is driven through the tibia from medial to lateral, 5 cm proximal to the ankle joint.
3. The distal tibial ring is connected to this wire orthogonal to the distal tibia, with the limb centered within the ring to ensure soft tissue clearance between the limb and the rings, and the wire is tensioned.
4. The proximal ring is fixed to the tibia with two 6.0-mm half pins placed off connecting cubes or posts, one proximal and one distal to the ring in a multiplanar fashion; the most proximal half pin usually is secured to five-hole connecting cubes or posts from anterior to posterior, and the inferior half pin is secured to three-hole connecting cubes or posts placed from anteromedial to posterolateral.
5. Two additional 6.0-mm half pins are then placed and secured to the distal tibial ring, also in a multiplanar orientation, one proximal and the other distal to the distal tibial ring. Fluoroscopic imaging is helpful to ensure appropriate half pin length.

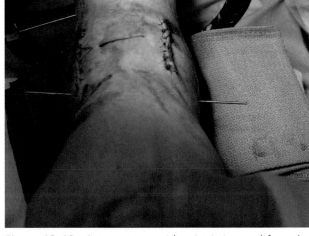

Figure 18–10 A temporary guide wire is inserted from the tip of the lateral malleolus to the tip of the medial malleolus. This wire serves as a reference for ankle hinge placement.

ANKLE HINGE PLACEMENT

Surgical Technique

1. After the tibial base frame is applied, a smooth 1.8-mm wire is placed temporarily from the tip of the lateral malleolus to the tip of the medial malleolus, and ends are cut approximately 3 cm from the skin edges (Fig. 18–10). This guide wire serves as a reference for hinge placement.
2. Ilizarov universal hinges are secured to threaded rods, which are attached to the distal tibial ring, and the hinges are aligned relative to the guide wire. The threaded rods are left 1.5 to 2.5 cm long to allow for subsequent distraction.
3. After the hinge is properly positioned, the guide wire is removed.

APPLICATION OF THE FOOT RING

Surgical Technique

1. The foot is centered in a foot ring and the hinges are attached to the ring (Fig. 18–11). In most cases the lateral hinge is placed directly on the ring, and a short threaded rod is used on the medial side (often a two-hole plate is needed off the ring to attach the medial hinge). A temporary device (Clawmaster, Quantum Medical Concepts, Hood River, Ore) can then be used to hold the foot ring in place during wire attachment.

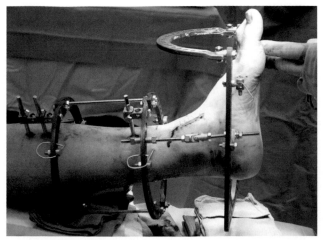

Figure 18–9 External fixator application.

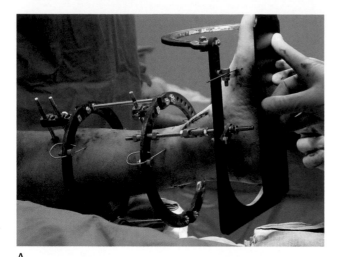

A

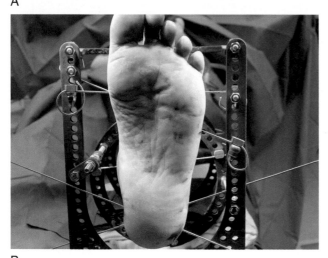

B

Figure 18–11   A, Lateral view. An assistant holds the ankle in neutral dorsiflexion with a flat plate while one calcaneal wire and one forefoot wire are inserted and tensioned to the foot plate. **B,** Plantar view. Note how foot is nicely centered in ring. Heel and forefoot wires are inserted in different planes to increase stability.

2. The foot ring is usually secured to the foot with five smooth 1.8-mm wires: one in the talar neck, two in the calcaneal tuberosity, and two in the forefoot.
3. The first calcaneal wire is placed from medial to posterolateral, avoiding the neurovascular structures on the medial aspect of the hindfoot, and the foot ring is secured to this wire parallel to the sole of the foot. Then the first forefoot wire is placed proximal to the fifth metatarsal head engaging either the fifth, fourth, and third metatarsals or the fifth and first metatarsals (plantar to the second, third, and fourth metatarsals), and care is given to

avoid distorting the normal orientation of the metatarsals relative to each other.
3. Subsequently, the second calcaneal wire is placed from distal–lateral to posteromedial. The second forefoot wire is placed medially to engage the first and second, and occasionally third, metatarsals.
4. The 1.8-mm talar neck wire is then placed to avoid subtalar joint distraction, and this wire is usually not placed under tension.
5. Tension is applied to the calcaneal wires and the forefoot wires.
6. The distal end of the foot ring can be completed with a half ring placed either in a horseshoe fashion or on the dorsal aspect of the foot ring. Ankle motion should be maintained after the foot ring has been applied.

ANKLE DISTRACTION

Surgical Technique

1. After the frame is applied, the ankle joint is acutely distracted 3 mm to 5 mm from the preoperative position using the threaded rods attached to the universal hinges (Fig. 18–12). This distraction usually is performed on the tibial ring attachment sites.
2. Fluoroscopic evaluation is done with the ankle in neutral position, and lateral radiographs are made to assess satisfactory ankle range of motion and confirm absence of ankle subluxation with motion. If the ankle distraction arthroplasty is done with either a varus-to-valgus distal tibial or immediate equinus correction, immediate ankle joint distraction is minimized to limit the risk of neurovascular compromise.
3. The ankle is held in neutral flexion by securing components (plates and threaded rods) from the distal tibial ring to the foot ring, which may be removed for range-of-motion exercises. Similarly, a frame strut (Long Fast Fix Taylor Spatial Frame Strut, Smith & Nephew, Memphis, Tenn) may be secured from the proximal tibial ring to the foot ring, released to allow range of motion, and resecured with the foot held in neutral position. A similar posterior strut can facilitate equinus correction.
4. Wounds are dressed in routine fashion, and all wires and half pins are dressed with Ilizarov sponges stacked from the skin to the

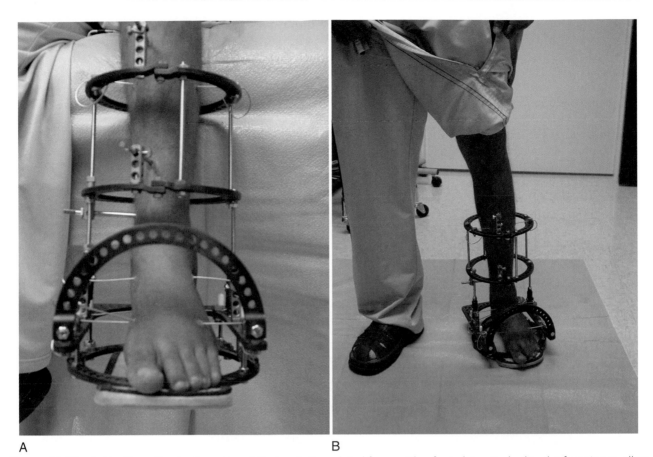

A   B

Figure 18–12 Ankle distraction by the external fixator. **A,** Completed frame with a foot plate attached to the foot ring to allow weight bearing. **B,** Patient is shown standing in frame with constrained ankle motion allowed through anatomically placed hinges. A frame strut (Fast Fix Taylor Spatial Frame Strut, Smith & Nephew, Memphis, Tenn) can be added to lock ankle in neutral or slight dorsiflexion position.

fixation attachment to provide soft tissue compression. Bulky roll (Kerlix) dressings are placed between the rings and the limb, especially about the ankle and posterior leg and heel to limit swelling. The rings are overwrapped with elastic (Ace) bandages, and an Ilizarov cover (Quantum Medical Concepts, Hood River, Oregon) is provided to optimize cleanliness.

GRADUAL CORRECTION OF TIBIAL DEFORMITIES WITH ANKLE JOINT DISTRACTION

For gradual correction of distal tibial deformities, we prefer the Taylor Spatial Frame device because of the precise ability to correct deformity with the associated Internet-based program using deformity and frame-mounting parameters. This device enables simultaneous six-axis deformity correction using the six-strut platform. With this system, a ring is placed just proximal to the ankle joint line, which can complicate hinge arrangement about the ankle joint axis and delay range of motion until there has been evidence of osteotomy healing.

Distal tibial nonunions associated with pilon fractures may be associated with ankle arthritis. However, ankle range of motion usually is avoided until the nonunion has healed. Frame extension to the foot can optimize the distal tibial osteotomy fixation, and distraction can be accomplished using threaded rods from the distal tibial ring to the foot ring. The frame is retained until the osteotomy or nonunion is healed.

GRADUAL CORRECTION OF FOOT DEFORMITIES WITH ANKLE JOINT DISTRACTION

Gradual correction of severe foot deformity is preferred when immediate correction can increase the risk of neurovascular compromise, soft tissue slough, unacceptable shortening, or osteotomy malalignment. The foot deformity may be segmental (deformities in the hindfoot and forefoot are dissimilar) or nonsegmental (deformities in the hindfoot and forefoot are similar in direction and magnitude). A segmental deformity such as a triple arthrodesis malunion can require an osteotomy with a frame configuration that maintains correct alignment of the talus to the distal tibia and allows for correction of the hindfoot malalignment separate from the forefoot.

The ankle may be difficult to distract until the foot correction has healed. Subsequently, the frame may be modified to include a foot plate, and the corrected foot is distracted as a unit from the distal tibia. A talar fixation pin is initially secured to the distal tibial ring during foot correction and is later moved to the foot ring for ankle joint distraction.

AFTERCARE

General Care

At the preoperative visit, patients are given an information packet reviewing external fixator and pin site care, and this is again reviewed with the patient after surgery. Postoperative dressings remain in place for 3 to 7 days, and pin care begins on an outpatient basis to avoid exposing pin sites in the inpatient setting. On the first postoperative day, a walking assembly, consisting of a full ring secured to a rigid rocker walking platform, is attached to the foot ring with four threaded rods to suspend the foot above the full ring by approximately 1 to 2 cm. The contralateral leg is fitted with a shoe lift to balance the pelvis for gait.

On the first postoperative day the patient is advanced from bed to chair. Physical therapy is begun on the first postoperative day, focusing on overall lower extremity function and gait. Partial weight bearing may begin on the second postoperative day and is gradually progressed during the following 1 to 2 weeks until full weight bearing is achieved. The patient is discharged from the hospital on the second or third postoperative day. Ankle range of motion generally is started on the first postoperative visit at 1 week after surgery, but this may be instituted sooner or later depending on individual circumstances.

Pin Care

At the first postoperative visit 1 week after surgery, the pin site sponges and dressings are removed and pin care is initiated with daily normal saline cleaning to remove any scabs or crusts around the pin sites. After sutures are removed at 2 weeks after surgery, the pin care is performed during a daily shower with antibacterial liquid soap and thorough water rinse to the leg

and fixator. The fixator and leg are dried with a clean towel and hair dryer at the cool setting.

Further pin care is not necessary if the pin sites remain clean and dry, but it is resumed if drainage or crust develops about the pin sites. The crusts are removed with a cotton-tipped applicator and normal saline. For draining pin sites, two adjacent pins are wrapped together with a bulky gauze roll to decrease the motion between the skin and the pin; this can limit subsequent pin site irritation that could progress to a pin site infection. Lotions, ointments, or creams generally are avoided around pin sites.

The most common problem encountered with ring fixation is a localized infection around a wire or pin. It is important to inspect all pin sites daily to assess for signs of infection or loosening, including localized redness, pain and tenderness, warmth, swelling (firm or fluctuant), and drainage from the pin or wire, which can vary in color and odor.

When early signs of pin site infection are noted, pin care is increased to twice daily, the pin site is wrapped with a gauze roll dressing, ankle range of motion is discontinued, and weight-bearing and physical therapy are limited. If signs and symptoms of a pin site infection do not rapidly improve, oral antibiotics are prescribed (cephalexin or clindamycin) for five to seven days. The pin site infection usually begins to resolve within 24 hours of starting oral antibiotic treatment. Recalcitrant pin site infection is treated with intravenous antibiotic therapy with or without pin removal. A special ring fixator cover (Quantum Medical Concepts, Hood River, Oregon) is worn when the patient is outside of the home to limit potential contamination by environmental factors.

Physical Therapy

Physical therapy is an important part of the postoperative care. This is started in the hospital and continued during the in-frame period and after frame removal. Lower extremity motion, conditioning, and gait are emphasized. Nonimpact activities including cycling, swimming, and pool therapy are encouraged, even with the fixator in place. A stationary bicycle with modified pedals is used with the ring fixator.

After adequate healing of an osteotomy, nonunion, or deformity, ankle range of motion is initiated at the first portion of each visit and continued throughout the course of the ankle distraction, with attention to optimize dorsiflexion. Ankle range of motion is initially done for 30 minutes, three to five times per day, and then progressed as tolerated by the patient and pin sites. Range of motion may be restricted with Achilles tendon lengthening or ankle ligament reconstruction and initiated 6 weeks after frame application.

Follow-up Evaluation

Weight-bearing AP, lateral, and oblique ankle radiographs are made at 1, 3, 6, and 9 weeks after frame application to confirm concentric ankle distraction and alignment. Distraction of approximately 4 mm to 5 mm greater than preoperative ankle joint space is desired, and this usually is achieved intraoperatively and maintained during the postoperative course. With associated correction of equinus or varus deformity, immediate distraction is avoided, and gradual distraction (0.5 mm per day for 10 days, starting 3 to 10 days after surgery) is performed to limit potential tibial nerve injury. Weight-bearing radiographs are necessary to confirm, add, or delete distraction.

FRAME REMOVAL

The frame typically is removed 12 weeks after application. This may be delayed until healing of a simultaneous osteotomy, nonunion correction, or malunion correction. The frame is removed under general anesthesia or in the clinic. After the frame is removed, soft dressings are applied and changed as needed for bleeding. The leg is placed in a removable fracture walker boot for ambulation. Crutches or other assistive devices are used for the first several weeks after frame removal for comfort, but weight-bearing as tolerated is allowed. Showers are resumed after the pin sites are healed, usually within 7 days after frame removal.

Care After Frame Removal

During the initial 6 to 8 weeks after frame removal, the patient gradually resumes regular foot wear and full weight bearing without assistive devices. Maintaining ankle range of motion, especially dorsiflexion, may be facilitated with nonimpact activities such as swimming, bicycling, and physical therapy. Prolonged weight bearing, as with demanding physical jobs and walking, is avoided because this can delay recovery. A removable fracture walker boot, compression stocking, or light ankle brace may be helpful to minimize discomfort and swelling. A stable level of function usually is not achieved until 6 to 12 months after frame removal.

RESULTS AND COMPLICATIONS

Ankle distraction arthroplasty is successful in 70% to 80% of patients in improving pain and function, as documented in prior studies and confirmed by our experience (Figs. 18–13 and 18–14). Patient selection is very important, and success is more likely with motivated, compliant patients who have post-traumatic or instability-related ankle arthritis and retained preoperative ankle motion (5 to 10 degrees of dorsiflexion). Patients with minimal ankle motion and marked equinus contracture are particularly susceptible to failure, and patients with previous septic ankle arthritis also have suboptimal results.

In an early study of ankle distraction for post-traumatic ankle arthritis with a hinged distraction apparatus, 13 of 16 (81%) patients had good results at 16-month follow-up.[5] A subsequent study of patients with hip arthrosis showed that articulated distraction of the hip yielded good results in 42 of 59 (71%) patients who were younger than 45 years but poor results in patients older than 45 years and in patients with inflammatory arthritis.[1]

A study of ankle distraction in 11 patients with post-traumatic arthritis showed that all patients had less pain at follow-up of 20 months.[14] Persistent ankle swelling and crepitus has been noted after removal of the external fixator, but average function improved after 1 year after surgery.[13] In a more recent prospective study of 57 patients followed for an average of 2.8 years after ankle distraction, significant clinical improvement was noted in three fourths of the patients, improvement increased over time, and joint distraction had significantly better results than ankle joint debridement alone.[7] A subsequent review by the same researchers at minimum 7 years of follow-up evaluation after ankle distraction for osteoarthritis showed that 16 of 22 (73%) patients had significant improvement of all clinical parameters and 6 (27%) patients had failed treatment.[9]

Comparable results have been achieved when ankle distraction was used for arthritis in conjunction with osteotomy for deformity correction (Figs. 18–15 and 18–16). In 11 patients with ankle arthritis associated with deformity of the distal tibia (five deformities, most commonly valgus or recurvatum and valgus) or foot (seven deformities, most commonly cavovarus), treatment consisted of ankle joint distraction with the Ilizarov device, osteotomy, and range-of-motion exercises for 3 months.[2] Tibial deformity correction was gradual in three patients and acute in two patients, and all seven foot deformity corrections were acutely performed. In 10 patients who responded to an ankle questionnaire at an average of 18 months after surgery, nine (90%) patients were very satisfied (three patients) or satisfied (six patients), one patient was not satisfied, and nine patients stated that they would undergo the procedure again.[2] The average American Academy of Orthopaedic Surgeons (AAOS) Foot and Ankle Outcome Score was 47 points (normal population average, 50 points). Dorsiflexion range directly correlated with

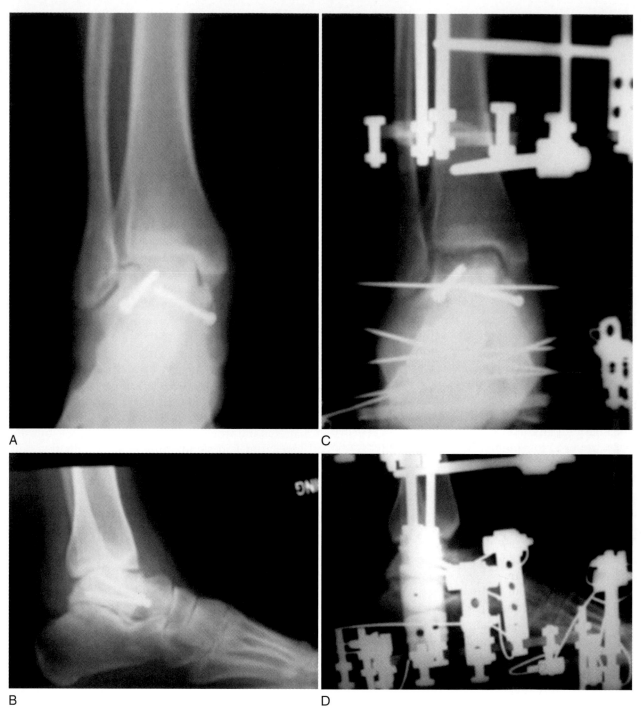

A

B

C

D

Figure 18–13   A 22-year-old woman with ankle pain was evaluated 2 years after a severe right talus fracture that had been treated acutely with open reduction and internal fixation. Anteroposterior (AP) **(A)** and lateral **(B)** radiographs show narrowing, sclerosis, and anterior osteophytes. The subtalar joint was stiff but only minimally painful. AP **(C)** and lateral **(D)** radiographs showing ankle distraction by the frame. The anterior ankle joint had been débrided with frame application.

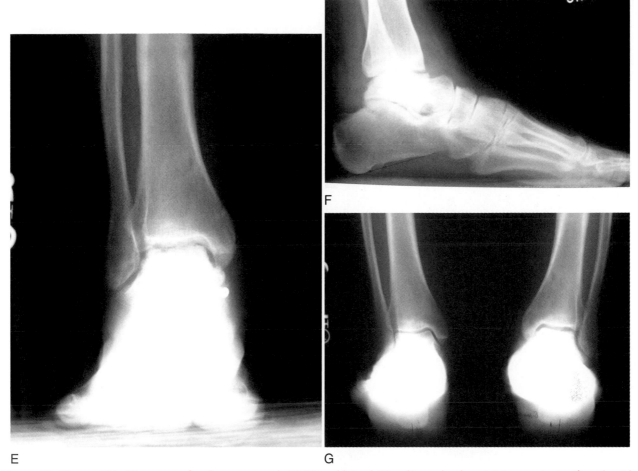

Figure 18–13—cont'd Two years after frame removal. AP **(E)** and lateral **(F)** radiographs show joint space is significantly wider than preoperatively. **G,** Hindfoot alignment view shows that the joint space is wider on the treated right ankle than the uninjured left ankle. Clinical evaluation showed improvement of symptoms.

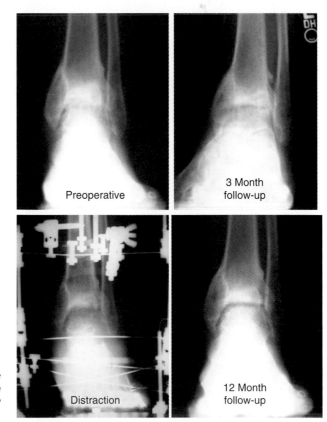

Figure 18–14 A 45-year-old-man with post-traumatic ankle arthritis treated with ankle distraction. Gradual progressive improvement in the ankle joint space correlated with gradually improved symptoms in the follow-up period.

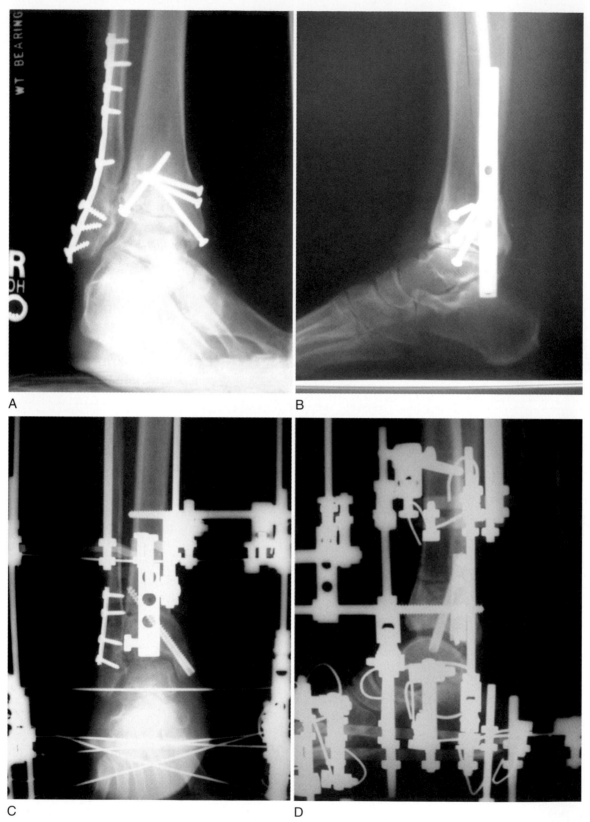

Figure 18–15 **A** and **B,** A 40-year-old woman with ankle pain was evaluated 2 years after open reduction and internal fixation of a work-related ankle fracture. Radiographs demonstrated post-traumatic arthritis and valgus deformity of the tibia and fibula. **C** and **D,** The deformity was acutely corrected with a focal dome osteotomy and internal fixation, and acute ankle distraction was applied.

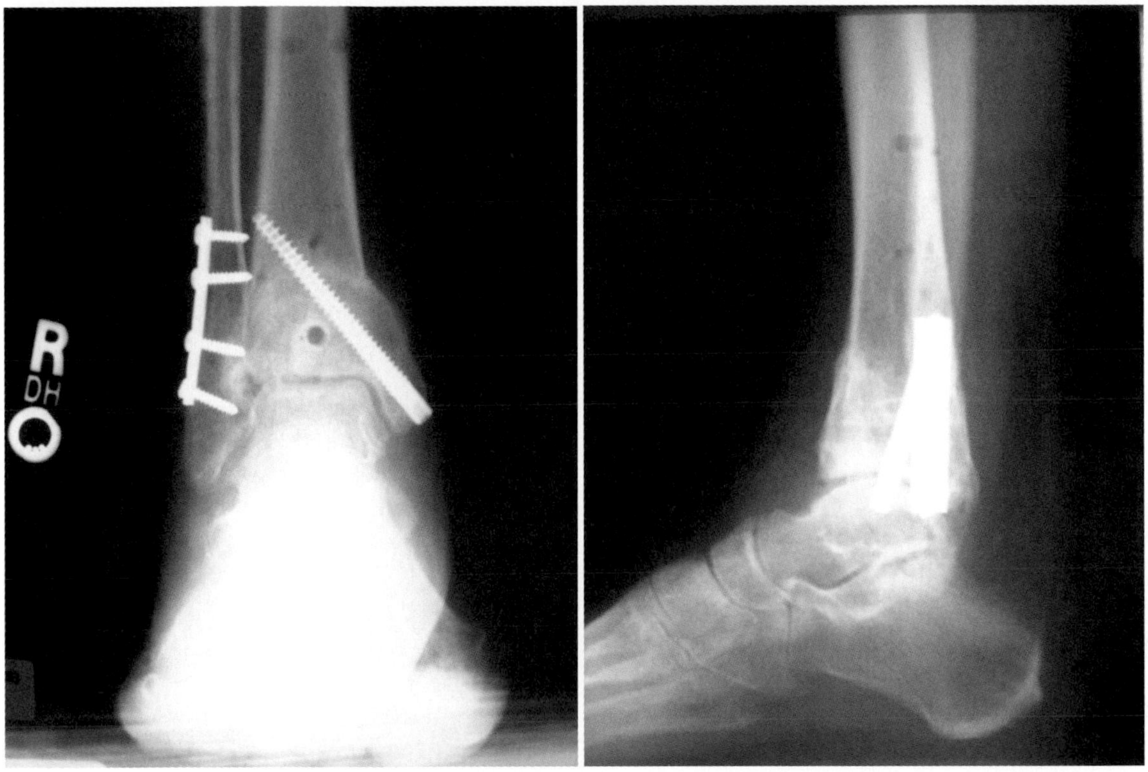

E   F

Figure 18–15—cont'd   E and **F,** Two years after the frame was removed, radiographs show maintenance of ankle joint space. The patient had improvement of preoperative pain.

AAOS score. It was concluded that deformity correction can augment the efficacy of distraction and that dorsiflexion may be an important factor in the success of an ankle distraction procedure.[2]

The most common complications of ankle distraction arthroplasty include pin site inflammation or infection, hardware failure, and failure of the procedure to relieve pain. Direct neurovascular injury resulting from pin placement can occur despite operative caution because of post-traumatic distortion of the anatomy and scarring. Other general risks include anesthetic problems, surgical wound problems and infection, and thromboembolic disease.

In patients undergoing ankle distraction with range of motion, the threaded rods attached to the universal hinges or the hinge itself can fail because of the major stresses placed on these portions of the fixator. If a half pin or wire loosens, treatment includes retensioning the wires and occasionally replacing a half pin in a new site.

Immediate correction of a deformity in the distal tibia or foot, especially with concomitant immediate ankle distraction, may be complicated by traction injury of the posterior tibial nerve and tarsal tunnel syndrome. If this occurs, the deformity may be restored and traction released to remove nerve tension, and correction and traction may be reapplied gradually. Prophylactic tarsal tunnel release can limit this complication, and careful postoperative monitoring can enable early recognition and release of traction. Gradual deformity correction and ankle distraction can limit risk of traction injury to the posterior tibial nerve. Furthermore, a postoperative anesthetic nerve block is used with caution because it can mask neuropathic symptoms, and nerve recovery may be optimized by early recognition, release of traction, and tarsal tunnel release.

For tarsal tunnel syndrome after immediate ankle distraction, the distraction is released and gradually reapplied over a 2-week period to limit further traction on the posterior tibial nerve. Tarsal tunnel release may be required in the immediate postoperative period if other measures do not restore nerve function.

Swelling and stiffness can occur after ankle distraction as a result of the underlying arthritic disorder. A period of increased pain and disability after ankle distraction can occur for 2 to 4 months after the frame is removed, occasionally persisting for up to 6 to 12 months. Nonimpact activities are emphasized during this time, including swimming and bicycling. Gradual improvement up to 9 to 12 months after fixator removal has been observed, and further procedures are

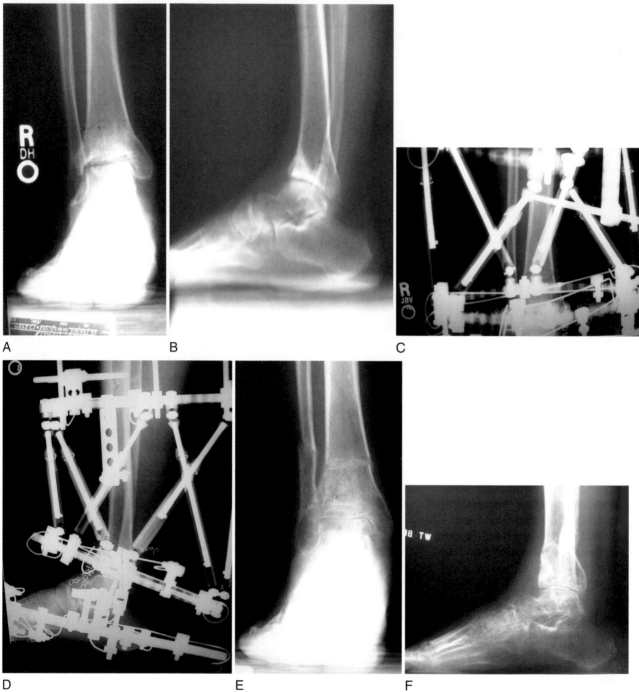

Figure 18–16   **A** and **B,** A 45-year-old man who was a former triathlete had had a distal tibia fracture 3 years earlier that healed with recurvatum and associated equinus compensation. **C** and **D,** The deformity was gradually corrected with a supramalleolar Gigli saw osteotomy. The fibular osteotomy was staged because the fibular deformity was unequal to the tibial deformity. Distraction was done acutely without range of motion until 6 weeks after surgery to allow initial healing of the osteotomy. The equinus deformity was treated with physical therapy. **E** and **F,** Radiographs at 6 months after surgery show the healed osteotomy, improved alignment, and maintenance of an ankle joint space. The patient had improvement of preoperative pain.

deferred until this time. In patients with persistent arthritic symptoms after ankle distraction, treatment options include arthrodesis and replacement arthroplasty.

REFERENCES

1. Aldegheri R, Trivella G, Saleh M: Articulated distraction of the hip. Conservative surgery for arthritis in young patients. *Clin Orthop Relat Res* 301:94-101, 1994.
2. Beaman D, Domenigoni A: Distraction and deformity correction for ankle arthritis. Paper presented at the 14th Annual Meeting of the Limb Lengthening and Reconstruction Society, Toronto, July 23-25, 2004.
3. Eralp I, Kocaoglu M, Ozkan K, Turker M: A comparison of two osteotomy techniques for tibial lengthening. *Arch Orthop Trauma Surg* 124:298-300, 2004.
4. Frierson M, Ibrahim K, Boles M, et al: Distraction osteogenesis. A comparison of corticotomy techniques. *Clin Orthop Relat Res* 301:19-24, 1994.
5. Judet R, Judet T: The use of a hinge distraction apparatus after arthrolysis and arthroplasty. Rev Chir Orthop Reparatrice Appar Mot 64:353-365, 1978.
6. Kirienko A, Villa A, Calhoun, JH: *Ilizarov Technique for Complex Foot and Ankle Deformities.* New York, Marcel Dekker, 2003.
7. Marijnissen AC, Van Roermund PM, Van Melkebeek J, et al: Clinical benefit of joint distraction in the treatment of severe osteoarthritis of the ankle: Proof of concept in an open prospective study and in a randomized controlled study. *Arthritis Rheum* 46:2893-2902, 2002.
8. Paley D, Herzenberg JE (eds): *Principles of Deformity Correction.* New York, Springer-Verlag, 2003.
9. Ploegmakers JJ, van Roermund PM, van Melkebeek J, et al: Prolonged clinical benefit from joint distraction in the treatment of ankle osteoarthritis. *Osteoarthritis Cartilage* 13:582-588, 2005.
10. Saltzman CL, El-Khoury GY: The hindfoot alignment view. *Foot Ankle Int* 16:572-576, 1995.
11. Schwartsman V, Schwartsman R: Corticotomy. *Clin Orthop Relat Res* 280:37-47, 1992.
12. Tochigi Y, Suh J-S, Amendola, A, et al: Ankle alignment determination in simple lateral radiographs. Poster presented at the 72nd Annual Meeting of the American Academy of Orthopaedic Surgeons, Washington, DC, February 23-27, 2005.
13. van Roermund PM, Lafeber FP: Joint distraction as treatment for ankle osteoarthritis. *Instr Course Lect* 48:249-254, 1999.
14. van Valburg AA, van Roermund PM, Lammens J, et al: Can Ilizarov joint distraction delay the need for an arthrodesis of the ankle? *J Bone Joint Surg Br* 77:720-725, 1995.

Flatfoot Deformity in Adults

Steven L. Haddad • *Roger Mann*

POSTERIOR TIBIAL TENDON DYSFUNCTION

Very few conditions in the realm of foot and ankle surgery incite as much controversy in management protocols as the adult acquired flatfoot. Perhaps most of this controversy extends from a lack of complete understanding of the condition, despite a time of more than 50 years since the first published reports recognizing the disorder. Like many aspects of medicine, treatment of the adult acquired flatfoot has evolved into philosophical ideas based in certain camps of academics, each camp purporting its views as reaching the ultimate solution in correcting deformity.

Wisdom gained through experience, however, leads the experienced clinician to assimilate these philoso-

phies into a spectrum of management options, incorporating components of each lesson into a unified whole. With this attitude, each patient is respected individually for the specific pathologic components in tibialis posterior tendon dysfunction that cause pain and disability. The clinician can then address these specific components from the proven methodologies created thus far. Thus, there is no one "right answer" in managing tibialis posterior tendon dysfunction, but one can gain significant insight by learning from the literature provided to date.

History

The roots of posterior tibial tendon insufficiency are found in early writings on tenosynovitis. In 1818,

Velpeau described the first case of noninfectious tenosynovitis in the hand. In 1895, De Quervain described stenosis-related tendovaginitis in the first compartment of the dorsal carpal ligament of the wrist in more than 900 patients. Kulowski in 1936[80] was the first to publish tenosynovitis of the sheath of the posterior tibial tendon, documenting one case. More than a decade later, the first large series of posterior tibial tendon tenosynovitis was published by Lipscomb at the Mayo clinic.[88] Lapidus and Seidenstein[84] commented on two cases of posterior tibial tendon tenosynovitis in 1950, stating, "nonspecific chronic tenosynovitis must be considered a rarity, particularly at the ankle." These early published reports underestimate its prevalence.

In 1955, A.W. Fowler[82] reported on seven cases of posterior tibial tendon tenosynovitis. He found "the condition was seldom diagnosed early and it was often mistaken for osteoarthritis of the ankle and treated conservatively without relief. At operation, the tendon sheath was swollen and thickened and the tendon greatly enlarged. The inflamed synovium was excised, with relief in all cases." Though anecdotal, this was the first documented series in which tenosynovectomy was used and found to be successful. This concept was reinforced by Langenskiold,[82] who in 1967 documented six cases of posterior tibial tendon tenosynovitis treated surgically after failure of conservative management. These patients experienced great pain relief after debridement of the proliferative granulation tissue.

Key,[72] in 1953, documented the first case of posterior tibial tendon rupture (partial). In his prelude, he states that the case should be of interest, showing great foresight. This worker's compensation case documented the classic signs and symptoms of the condition, including the not-so-unusual missed early diagnosis. This partial rupture was treated with excision of the torn component and debridement of the residual thickened tendon, leaving the patient with 15% disability at the ankle.

Griffiths[46] in 1965 recognized the difficulty in correcting deformity following late reconstruction of posterior tibial tendon rupture, but all of his "spontaneous" ruptures were in patients with rheumatoid arthritis. Thus, confounding factors obviate the direct correlation between posterior tibial tendon rupture and deformity correction. Sixteen years following Key's article, Kettelkamp and Alexander[71] explored spontaneous posterior tibial tendon rupture in four patients without systemic disease. Missed in this article was the prevalence of spontaneous rupture, because the authors begin by stating that it is a rarity. However, the authors pinpoint the challenge of correcting deformity created by delay in treatment. Three

of the four patients were treated operatively without correction of tendon length (the retracted tendon was bridged with extensor digitorum longus tendon graft or filled with a Z-plasty lengthening), leaving the patients with residual pain and no correction of deformity. Results at best were rated fair.

In 1974, Goldner[41] revisited the topic of progressive talipes equinovalgus in traumatic and degenerative conditions of the posterior tibial tendon. This article studied nine patients with either of these etiologies, all resulting in the common pathway of an acquired flatfoot deformity. The authors correctly recognized a disorder of the medial plantar calcaneonavicular ligament resulting in limited support through elongation due to repetitive stress. Surgical intervention was done for deformity correction as well as pain relief. Transfer of the flexor hallucis longus to substitute for the deficient or absent posterior tibial tendon was done in all cases. The tendon was sutured to the periosteum under the navicular. This tendon was chosen over the flexor digitorum longus (FDL) owing to its "more tendinous" structure, larger muscle mass, and the potential ability to elevate the sustentaculum tali to combat hindfoot valgus. In addition, the medial plantar calcaneonavicular ligament was plicated after experience in not doing so resulted in persistent or progressive deformity. The authors also found failure in simply advancing or plicating the posterior tibial tendon. They also believed that a contracted gastrocnemius–soleus complex contributes to the deformity and must be addressed at the time of surgery.

Eight years later, in 1982, the concept of spontaneous rupture of the posterior tibial tendon resurfaced with a scientific presentation by Mann and Specht.[96] The authors reviewed eight patients undergoing a variation on Goldner's flexor hallucis longus (FHL) tendon transfer by using the FDL tendon as the source replacement tendon. Rationale for avoiding the use of the FHL tendon for transfer centered on the importance of maintaining full flexion strength in the hallux in compromised patients. This paper will be reviewed more thoroughly in the surgical section of this chapter.

Following this article, the history of posterior tibial tendon dysfunction has followed the standard course of newly recognized syndromes in the history of medicine: a search for etiology, pathophysiology, and successful treatment options among multiple investigators. The ideas presented by these investigators will unfold in the following sections.

Anatomy and Function

The substance of a tendon is formed by a group of fasciculi. An epitenon surrounds the tendon and contains an outer synovial layer. Next, a paratenon, made of loose areolar tissue, surrounds the epitenon, carrying the tendinous structures. The next layer comprises the synovial sheath. The synovial sheath is usually continuous with the epitenon, forming a mesotenon that acts as a vascular channel for the tendon.[5] The mesotenon of the posterior tibial tendon sheath is not continuous. This anatomic variant will derive clinical significance as the potential for vascular insult is explored.

The posterior tibialis muscle arises from the interosseous membrane and adjacent surfaces of the tibia and fibula in the proximal one third of the leg. The myotendinous junction appears in the distal one third of the leg. The posterior tibial tendon courses directly behind the medial malleolus at a relatively acute angle. The groove is shallow, and the flexor retinaculum binds the tendon tightly into this groove. Thus, the tendon passes posterior to the axis of the tibiotalar joint and medial to the axis of the subtalar joint, plantar flexing and inverting the hindfoot.[144] In fact, the posterior tibial tendon is located farther medially from the axis of the subtalar joint than any other tendon about the ankle, and it therefore has the greatest degree of leverage to bring about inversion of the subtalar joint. It then passes beneath the calcaneonavicular ligament to insert into the tuberosity of the navicular. It is unique in that it has eleven insertion domains: the navicular, the sustentaculum tali, the medial, middle, and lateral cuneiforms, the cuboid, and the bases of the second, third and fourth metatarsals.[51,144] By its insertion into the midfoot, the tibialis posterior both adducts and supinates the forefoot.

Tendons possessing synovial sheaths have altered directional courses or are bound by tunnels or retinacula. Linear tendons (e.g., the Achilles tendon) often do not have sheaths. Tendons that contain a synovial sheath are generally located at the distal portions of the upper and lower extremities.[156] The sheath consists of three layers: a parietal layer lining the deep fibrous surface or fibroosseous canal, a visceral layer covering the tendon, and a mesotenon connecting the visceral and parietal layers serving as one source of the tendon's blood supply. The posterior tibial tendon is unique in that it does not contain a complete mesotenon and must receive its vascular supply through other channels. Synovial sheaths act to decrease the frictional forces encountered during tendon motion.[156] As gliding occurs, the visceral layer glides against the parietal layer. The mean length of the tendon sheath is 71 mm in men and 66 mm in women. The tendon sheath runs approximately 45 mm proximal to the apex of the medial malleolus and continues approximately 26 mm distal to the peak of the malleolus.[140] The excursion of the posterior tibial tendon is only 2 cm.

The posterior tibial tendon receives its blood supply from four regions: the vessels proximal to the muscle insertion, the connective tissue peritendinous arterial network, the arteries running to the tendon in the triangular vincula, and vessels from the periosteal insertion of the tendon.[140] Frey et al[35] found that the tendon receives its blood supply at the musculotendinous junction via the posterior tibial artery. They noted that a mesotenon was present in the posterior tibial tendon proximally, providing an additional network of vascular channels from the posterior tibial artery. The visceral layer also provides additional proximal blood supply, using this mesotenon as a conduit. This visceral layer remains closely adherent to the epitenon proximally. Distally, at the tendon–bone interface, the periosteal vessels provide the tendon's blood supply. These periosteal vessels are terminal segments for both the medial plantar branch of the posterior tibial artery, supplemented two thirds of the time by the medial tarsal artery, a branch of the dorsalis pedis artery.

The posterior tibial tendon functions to stabilize the hindfoot against valgus forces or eversion. The tibialis posterior is a stance phase muscle, firing from heel strike to shortly after heel lift-off.[64] It decelerates subtalar joint pronation following heel contact through eccentric contraction.[5] At midstance, it stabilizes the midtarsal joints. During the propulsive phase of stance, the tibialis posterior adducts the transverse tarsal joint, initiating inversion of the subtalar joint. This action has two beneficial effects on the gastrocnemius–soleus complex: it locks the transverse tarsal joint, allowing the gastrocnemius–soleus complex to maximize the plantar flexion force during gait, and it shifts the direction of pull of the Achilles tendon further medially, allowing the gastrocnemius–soleus complex to become the primary invertor of the subtalar joint through increased leverage. In doing so, the foot can become a rigid lever that supports the propulsive phase of gait.

Quantifying this action with respect to gait, during the normal walking cycle eversion occurs in the subtalar joint at the time of initial ground contact. The tibialis posterior becomes functional at about 7% of the cycle, the soleus muscle at about 10% of the cycle, and the lateral head of the gastrocnemius muscle at about 25% of the gait cycle. Dynamic electromyography suggests that this initial eccentric contraction of the posterior tibial muscle lasts from 7% to 30% of the gait cycle during stance. Following this, progressive inversion occurs starting at approximately 30% of the cycle through concentric contraction of the tibialis posterior.[133,145] The tibialis posterior muscle is silent during swing phase, where its antagonists enjoy maximal benefit. The primary antagonist of the posterior tibial muscle is the peroneus brevis muscle, functioning to abduct the midfoot and evert the hindfoot. Cross-sectional area studies note that the peroneus brevis muscle is 41% as strong as the posterior tibial muscle (relative strength of the posterior tibial tendon is 6.4, and of the peroneus brevis, 2.6)[137] Physiologically, this is manifested through the primary function of the peroneus brevis in unlocking the transverse tarsal joints and everting the hindfoot during the non–weight-bearing swing phase of gait.

Finally, stabilization of the longitudinal arch by the posterior tibial tendon remains a topic of debate. Most authors agree, however, that there are both static and dynamic forces at work. Static support theorists fall into two camps, those believing the foot acts as a truss, and those believing the foot acts as a beam. The truss theory is supported by Lapidus.[83] A truss works by creating two struts that meet at an apex, supported at the base by a tie rod, thus forming a triangle. As the apex is loaded, compressive forces are applied to the struts, and tensile forces are applied to the tie rod. As long as the tie rod remains intact, the struts do not collapse, and the truss holds firm. Relating this model to the anatomy of the foot, the tie rod becomes the plantar aponeurosis. Hicks[52] believes that this model becomes critical at toe-off, when the windlass mechanism has maximal effect.

The beam theory, proposed by Sarrafian,[133] supports a less rigid construct. In this model, the foot is a curved beam that sags when it is loaded. Forces generated at the midportion of the beam are compressive on the convex side of the beam and tensile on the concave side. The curved portion of the beam consists of the bones of the midtarsus. Thus, tension directly affects the structures on the concave side of these bones, namely, the plantar ligaments. Anatomically, these ligaments consist of the long and short plantar ligaments, the calcaneonavicular (spring) ligament, and the bifurcate ligament. All are attachment sites for the posterior tibial tendon.

The spring ligament consists of a stronger superior medial calcaneonavicular ligament and the inferior calcaneonavicular ligament just lateral to it.

Dynamic support of the arch revolves around the tibialis posterior muscle and the intrinsic musculature of the foot. Support of the arch by the intrinsics is discussed in the next section. With respect to the posterior tibialis muscle's contribution, Kapandji[66] suggests that contraction of the tibialis posterior adducts and plantar flexes the navicular on the talar head. In doing so, it buttresses the medial longitudinal arch against collapse. In addition, the ligamentous attachments of the posterior tibial tendon have an effect by pulling the cuboid medially along with the navicular through the bifurcate ligament. This cuboid then pulls the calcaneus medially through the strong calcaneocuboid ligament, providing additional support to the talar head through the anterior and middle facets.

Pathophysiology of Posterior Tibial Tendon Rupture

The posterior tibial tendon has a limited excursion of only 2 cm. Thus, any insult, no matter how minor, that lengthens this tendon has an adverse effect on its function. This lengthening may be gradual or acute depending on the underlying pathologic process. The inversion power provided by the posterior tibial tendon has been underestimated by some, the thought process being that all of the posterior compartment muscles act to provide this function. Jahss[62] noted that the normal inversion power of all posterior calf muscles combined is 12 to 15 pounds of torque. Patients with posterior tibial tendon rupture undergo a substantial reduction in this force, lowering the torque to 3 to 6 pounds and emphasizing the importance of this tendon.

In acute situations, the integrity of the longitudinal arch may be initially maintained through static restraints. The valgus deformity of the hindfoot created by unopposed pull of the peroneus brevis through loss of the posterior tibial tendon secondarily causes loss of this integrity. According to Duchene[29] this allows the gastrocnemius–soleus complex to act with a downward force at the talonavicular joint. Downward and medial pressure of the talar head stretches the calcaneonavicular ligaments. The plantar ligaments placed medially that unite the tarsus and metatarsus are comparatively much weaker than those on the lateral side. Eventually, the passive structures of the longitudinal arch give way under continued dynamic insult, and a flatfoot deformity results. In the beam theory, the natural curved beam of the bony architecture of the foot becomes straightened by repetitive tensile forces on its concave surface. In particular, the spring ligament is at risk of failure.

This view is supported by Niki and Sangeorzan[114] who examined the progression to flatfoot deformity in a biomechanical study. The authors evaluated the sequential cause of the acquired flatfoot by creating a custom acrylic foot-loading frame to simulate heel strike, stance, and heel rise by altering tendon tension through regulated pneumatic cylinders. Simultaneously, axial compressive loads were applied to the tibias of these cadaveric specimens. Absence of posterior tibialis function was simulated simply by not activating the pneumatic cylinder attached to this tendon, while continuing normal cylinder load on all other tendons crossing the ankle. Thus, through cyclic evaluation, the authors studied the foot architecture with all tendons loaded, in the absence of the posterior tibial tendon, and finally with activation of the posterior tibial tendon (simulating repair). Small but statistically significant changes in the angular orientation of the bone architecture of the foot were noted after release of the posterior tibial tendon. These changes were not of the magnitude seen in a true flatfoot. This led the authors to surmise that the intact osteoligamentous structure of the foot is at least initially able to maintain normal alignment following acute posterior tibial tendon dysfunction. Interestingly, when the posterior tibial tendon was restored in the flatfoot model, it did not restore the angular changes to anatomic magnitude. Again, these data support the importance of progressive longitudinal arch collapse through attenuation of the spring (and other plantar) ligaments.

The source of the attenuation may be directly related to a disorder within the gastrocnemius–soleus complex and its mechanical orientation. The valgus deformity of the hindfoot created by dysfunction of the posterior tibial tendon substantially alters the mechanical pull of the Achilles tendon. The Achilles tendon is placed lateral to the axis of the subtalar joint, allowing it to become an evertor of the hindfoot, accelerating the valgus deformity. Equally important, the moment arm of the plantar flexion force becomes the talonavicular joint rather than the metatarsal heads.[36] This proximal alteration in force concentration comes directly from the perpetual valgus hindfoot's unlocking the transverse tarsal joint, eliminating the rigid lever of the foot at toe-off. This action accelerates attrition of the spring ligament with each gait cycle.

The intrinsic musculature attempts to compensate for the deficient arch by increased work. According to Mann and Inman,[95] the intrinsics stabilize the transverse tarsal joint and thus create a more efficient lever. As expected, flatfooted persons require increased muscle action to maintain a rigid lever in light of the lack of support at other portions of the arch. Activity of the intrinsics thus begins at an earlier portion of the stance phase of gait, measured at 10% of the cycle rather than the normal 40%.

This cascade of events leads to a common pathway as the posterior tibial tendon fails and a flatfoot develops. Changes in the bone architecture are as those found by Niki,[114] involving plantar flexion of the talus, eversion together with internal rotation of the calcaneus, and eversion of the navicular and the cuboid. Clinically, the hindfoot drifts into valgus and the forefoot into abduction. The posterior tibialis muscle fires earlier and longer to stabilize the hypermobile foot and to control the increased pronation and deviation. This increased demand on the muscle leads to fatigue. The deltoid ligament becomes involved late, as the severe flatfoot deformity places increased demand on

the medial soft tissues, creating a valgus deformity and arthritic wear at the tibiotalar joint. Late term effects occur as the calcaneus falls into further valgus. Abutment against the inferior tip of the fibula creates subfibular impingement. In addition, the relative shortening of the gastrocnemius–soleus complex leads to a permanent contraction, creating a relative equinus deformity of the ankle.

Etiology

Spontaneous rupture of the posterior tibial tendon was first suggested by Kettelkamp and Alexander[71] in 1969. Prior to that time, the authors were unable to locate a case of spontaneous rupture of the posterior tibial tendon in the literature. Controversy exists as to whether spontaneous rupture is truly spontaneous. McMaster[100] noted that spontaneous rupture did not occur in rabbits. In fact, even with a 75% iatrogenic laceration of the tendon, no ruptures occurred when normal stresses were applied. He stated that some form of disease process must be present to predispose the tendon to rupture.

Trauma of the magnitude to create a complete rupture of the posterior tibial tendon is rare. Funk[36] reported that of 19 patients treated for posterior tibial tendon tenosynovitis, only 4 could recall an inciting event. The authors agreed with McMaster,[100] stating that the lack of proximity of major trauma suggests that rupture of the posterior tibial tendon is more likely related to an intrinsic abnormality or biomechanical failure rather than an extrinsic traumatic factor.

Myerson noted in a group of elderly patients with rupture of the posterior tibial tendon that only 37 (14%) recalled a specific inciting traumatic event.[113] In contrast, Funk and Johnson[36] noted antecedent trauma in one half of the younger population in their study. Thus, trauma to the tendon may be age stratified. This becomes evident from the case reports in the literature documenting acute rupture of the posterior tibial tendon resulting from ankle fractures.* The first such report, by Giblin,[39] appeared in 1980: An interposed distal stump of a ruptured posterior tibial tendon prevented reduction of an isolated medial malleolus fracture. The patient had no prior symptoms of posterior tibial tendon dysfunction. In 1983 De Zwart[25] noted that two patients sustained rupture of the posterior tibial tendon at the level of a fractured medial malleolus in bimalleolar ankle fractures. A third report[139] suggested a common theme of a small flake of bone avulsed and visualized radiographically at the medial

---

*References 1, 25, 39, 105, 116, 134, and 139.

tibial metaphysis just proximal to the medial malleolus fracture on oblique views.

A second theme[134] suggests that acute rupture of the posterior tibial tendon is more commonly seen in ankle fractures caused by pronation and external rotation. The tight binding of the posterior tibial tendon by the flexor retinaculum contributes to acute rupture through sudden trauma. Fracture of the medial malleolus is not necessary,[105] for the ruptured and interposed posterior tibial tendon may be seen with a deltoid ligament rupture associated with a pronation–external rotation fracture. This can even be seen in children,[1] raising the index of suspicion to prevent delayed flatfoot from developing following fracture of the ankle.

More likely, repetitive microtrauma can lead to the indolent progression of symptoms through an inflammatory response that ultimately leads to tendon disruption. A tendon will not tolerate more than 1500 to 2000 cycles per hour. Tendon overloading can cause microtears that trigger an inflammatory response.[5] Such microtears fail to heal, exacerbating the inflammatory response. As persons age, the tendon's elastic compliance decreases through changes in the collagen structure, predisposing the tendon to damage.[98] Myerson's[113] group of older patients reported the onset of symptoms at an average age of 60 years, seeking treatment at an average age of 64 years.

It is possible, however, that inflammation (preexisting tenosynovitis or tendinitis) has no involvement in disruption of the posterior tibial tendon. Mosier et al[107] evaluated gross and histologic specimens of 15 surgically resected posterior tibial tendons excised for rupture. Control tendons were those obtained from cadavers with no known disorder to the posterior tibial tendon, confirmed by gross inspection of the tendons at the time of harvest.

Direct inspection of the diseased tendons revealed a characteristic increased length from the malleolus to the insertion point when referenced with the cadaver tendons. Loss of normal tendon sheen and color was noted, and the tendon had a dull, white appearance. Incomplete longitudinal splitting was present without transverse rupture. Microscopic specimens stained appropriately revealed increased mucin content and myxoid degeneration. Excess mucin was found to alter the normal linear orientation of the tendon collagen bundles. Myxoid degeneration was consistent with a rupture within the substance of the tendon. At the insertion of the posterior tibial tendon, fibroblastic hypercellularity and chondroid metaplasia were present. Again, this had the effect of disrupting the linear collagen orientation. This haphazard or wavy configuration of the collagen leads to decreased tensile strength within the tendon, potentially leading to "spontaneous" rupture. This, of course, would validate McMaster's concept of predisposition. Most important, the authors found no signs of inflammatory infiltrates within either the tendon or the tenosynovium. This suggests that a degenerative condition, rather than an inflammatory one, creates disruption of the posterior tibial tendon.

Trevino in 1981[150] performed the first histopathologic examination of diseased posterior tibial tendons. The authors found a stenosing tenosynovitis characterized by a loose, wavy configuration of the collagen. Other authors[27,109] confirm this wavy configuration to the collagen, with irregular spaces between bundles. In fact, all of these investigators find little evidence of inflammation in patients with rupture of the posterior tibial tendon. Also, though no complete transverse ruptures were visualized, incompetence of the tendon in combination with elongation of the tendon was clear. Sutherland[145] suggested through electromyographic studies that the magnitude of elongation sufficient to reduce the ability of the posterior tibial tendon to act as a dynamic stabilizer of the longitudinal arch was as little as 1 cm. Clearly, degenerative changes manifested as intrasubstance collagen disruption is enough to create this length deficit.

Changes in the composition of the collagen matrix in disrupted posterior tibial tendons were explored by Goncalves-Neto et al[42] The authors confirmed the alteration in the normal linear orientation of collagen bundles in involved tendons. They noted neovascularization—an increase in size, number, and branching of blood vessels—in conjunction with an increased number of fibroblasts. These findings suggest attempts at repair. More important, they noted a shift in the type of collagen within the diseased tendon. Normal tendons are composed of type I collagen, with minor amounts of type III, IV, and V collagen. Incompetent posterior tibial tendons shifted the makeup of this collagen from 95% to approximately 56% type I. In addition, type III collagen increased 54%, and type V increased 26%. Investigators have found that as the percentages of type III and type V collagen increase within the extracellular matrix, the diameter of the collagen fibrils undergoes a marked reduction. Damaged tendon makes an attempt to heal itself, and it does so with this poorer quality collagen.

Even normal anatomic posterior tibial tendon exhibits alterations in collagen composition at specific locations. Petersen et al[117] found a change in composition of the superficial zone of the posterior tibial tendon directly adjacent to the pulley of the posterior medial malleolus. Using both light and transmission electron microscopy in combination with immunohistochemical methods, the authors noted increased type II collagen as well as acid glycosaminoglycans consistent with fibrocartilage rather than the standard composition of dense connective tissue. The authors believe the physiologic basis of this shift in composition is related to the character of the posterior tibial tendon's changing from a traction tendon to a gliding tendon (subject to intermittent compressive and shear stresses) as it courses behind the medial malleolus.

The only portion of the posterior tibial tendon that exhibited composition consistent with fibrocartilage is the portion directly adjacent to the pulley, which is consistent with the most common site of spontaneous rupture. The fibrocartilage does not penetrate the entire diameter of the tendon at this location; rather, it remains superficial. This finding is physiologic, rather than pathologic, in the posterior tibial tendon. Thus, it remains a point of weakness irrespective of the underlying disease process, but it remains vulnerable to any disease process affecting the tendon. From such an insult, a poor repair response occurs from the relatively avascular tissue. Repetitive stress or microtrauma can create such an insult owing to the suspected lower resistance to tensile forces.

Despite this information, we cannot eliminate the impact that inflammation has during the early stages of posterior tibial tendon dysfunction. Jahss first suggested a possible link between seronegative spondyloarthropathies and posterior tibial tendon tenosynovitis in 1982.[62] Seronegative disorders are inflammatory conditions occurring outside the synovium. They disproportionately involve sites of attachment of the capsule, ligament, and tendon to bone, known as the enthesis. These arthropathies are generalized and often involve multiple sites in the upper and lower extremities. Common concurrent connective tissue disorders include inflammatory bowel disease, psoriasis, urethritis, uveitis, conjunctivitis, and oral ulcers. Myerson[113] concluded that the majority of younger patients with posterior tibial tendon disorders have signs of systemic enthesopathies. This patient population was predominantly female. Symptoms of systemic disease occur at an average age of 27 years, and patients seek treatment at an average age of 39 years. Two thirds of the patients had, in addition to posterior tibial tendon tenosynovitis, other areas of inflammatory involvement. More than half had a first-degree relative with evidence of a connective tissue disorder.

Myerson[113] determined that two separate patient populations developed posterior tibial tendon tenosynovitis and subsequent dysfunction. Both populations underwent HLA typing, supporting the association between age and seronegative spondyloarthropathies. Although only two patients in the older group had positive HLA markers, a majority of the younger population had HLA markers in their blood. Of particular interest is the *Cw6* allele, the primary allele for psoriasis. Nearly half (47%) of the younger patient group had this allele compared to none in the older group. Only 12% in the institutional control group had *Cw6* in their blood. This constellation of symptoms and laboratory results strongly suggests that inflammation plays a role in the inciting event of posterior tibial tendon dysfunction, at least in persons afflicted at a younger age. The younger population had a more rapid progression toward posterior tibial tendon rupture, encouraging prompt recognition of this potential cause and allowing earlier intervention. Stratifying the condition on an age-related basis has value only in patients with associated systemic conditions, because degenerative tendinopathy has strong supportive evidence not only in Myerson's older category of patients but also in the literature just noted.

In contrast to seronegative diseases contributing to an inflammatory cause inciting posterior tibial tendon dysfunction, rheumatoid arthritis has yet to provide convincing evidence that it has a direct role in tendon destruction. Downey[28] believes that the chronic inflammatory mediators noted in rheumatoid arthritis are the predisposing factor for tenosynovitis. Michelson[102] suggested such a cause exists in as many as 64% of patients afflicted with rheumatoid disease. However, when he narrowed his criteria for diagnosis to include loss of a longitudinal arch, inability to perform a single-limb heel stance, and the inability to palpate the posterior tibial tendon, the incidence dropped to 11%.

The problem with all such studies is the concurrent destruction of the ligament complex at the subtalar and talonavicular joints known to occur in rheumatoid disease. This disorder confuses the specific cause of flatfoot. Any of the signs of posterior tibial tendon rupture noted by Michelson can be seen in patients with joint destruction from the synovitis of rheumatoid disease that creates flatfoot.

Jahss[68] examined the posterior tibial tendon in rheumatoid patients undergoing arthrodesis of the hindfoot for symptomatic flatfoot and found the tendon normal in appearance. Kirkham and Gibson[75] studied 50 patients with rheumatoid arthritis and noted no instance of posterior tibial tendon dysfunction in those with progressive longitudinal arch collapse and hindfoot valgus. Finally, Keenan[69] performed electromyography on five patients with rheumatoid arthritis and hindfoot valgus and observed that muscle activity actually increased in this patient population versus controls. These data suggest that the posterior tibial tendon is actually overpulling in an attempt to correct the hindfoot valgus, rather than undergoing destruction by the underlying disease process. Thus, attempts at linking the inflammation of rheumatoid arthritis to destruction of the posterior tibial tendon remain in question.

A vascular cause of posterior tibial tendon dysfunction has been suggested by numerous authors. Holmes and Mann[57] performed a review of 67 patients with a diagnosis of posterior tibial tendon rupture. This epidemiologic study found a statistical correlation between tendon rupture and both obesity ($P = 0.005$) and hypertension ($P = 0.025$). This patient population was older, ranging in age from 51 to 87 years, and the correlation remained strong in spite of the general population prevalence of these conditions in this age category. In addition, diabetes and steroid use (both oral and injection) were linked to posterior tibial tendon dysfunction.

All four associated conditions directly or indirectly compromise the blood supply to the posterior tibial tendon. Diabetes promotes vascular hyperplasia and sclerosis, leading to stiffness of the arterioles, luminal narrowing, and blood flow resistance. Steroids lead to local vascular attenuation, creating avascular tissue. Such ischemic insults can compromise an already tenuous blood supply to select portions of the posterior tibial tendon, leading to degenerative tendinopathy. This is supported by Kennedy and Willis,[70] who have shown through tendon-loading studies that steroid injections into the tendon sheath significantly weaken the tendon for up to 2 weeks. They found that the tendon disruption is related to collagen necrosis at the site of injection. Compromise in a tenuous blood supply can also occur in patients who have undergone previous surgery on the medial portion of the foot and ankle.

The posterior tibial tendon receives its blood supply primarily from the posterior tibial artery (although the insertion of the tendon might receive its blood supply from branches of the dorsalis pedis artery). There has been debate as to the significance of its aberrant blood supply contributing to tendon disorder. Frey and Shereff[35] used a modified Spaltholz technique to study the blood supply of the posterior tibial tendon. In doing so, they injected 28 cadaveric limbs with an India ink–gelatin suspension. This mixture was cleared via the Spaltholz technique, destroying the normal histology of the tendon while allowing visualization of the gross external and internal vasculature. To confirm isolated aberration in the posterior tibial tendon blood supply, they examined the adjacent flexor digitorum longus as a control.

Using this technique, they discovered that an important hypovascular zone (14 mm long) is present approximately 40 mm proximal to the insertion of the posterior tibial tendon.[57,144] This zone of relative avascularity generally begins at the medial malleolus as the tendon courses out of the groove. Interestingly, no mesotenon was present at this level, and the visceral layer of the synovial sheath was hypovascular. In the control flexor digitorum longus tendon, no such zone existed, and consistent vascularity was noted throughout the tendon.

This hypovascular zone has a corollary in the supraspinatus tendon, where Rathbun and Macnab[125] noted that tension in a select portion of the tendon can wring out the blood supply. Without an adequate blood supply, cells require surrounding extracellular fluid to provide nutrition through diffusion. The limits of diffusion are clear, however. Smith suggests that nutrition will not be adequate when travel distance from source to destination exceeds 1 to 2 cm. Frey and Shereff[35] thus reasoned that the hypovascular zone allows posterior tibial tendon deterioration with age. Supporting this theory are several authors documenting the common location of tendon rupture, which happens to fall directly within this zone.

There have been critics of this theory, however. In 2002, Petersen et al[118] used a different method to assess blood supply to the posterior tibial tendon. They criticize the Spaltholz technique as providing a large number of false-positive and false-negative results owing to its subjective nature. Instead, they used a combination injection of ^{99m}Tc, India ink, and gelatin, specifically studying the laminin. According to the authors, laminin is a basic component of the basement membrane, and staining with ^{99m}Tc reliably and objectively detects blood vessels in the dense connective tissues.

Macroscopic assessment of the tendon at the level of the medial malleolus revealed an avascular, rather than hypovascular, segment. The majority of the avascular tissue was concentrated directly where the tendon is in contact with the malleolus. Confirmation was achieved through the immunohistochemical findings, which revealed an absence of laminin in this same location. Laminin was noted in the posterior quarter (farthest from the contact zone against the malleolus) of the posterior tibial tendon and proximal and distal to the malleolus.

Vascular theories explaining posterior tibial tendon degeneration and rupture have been challenged by Mosier et al.[107] The disorder of the collagen was discussed earlier. In addition to the increased mucin and myxoid degeneration, the authors noted neovascularization in the degenerative zone of the posterior tibial tendon. They surmised that the tendon cannot be avascular or hypovascular in these zones, for the new blood vessels had to arise from existing circulation. In addition, they postulated that the fibroblast hypercellularity that they noted on the microscopic sections indicates increased metabolic activity within the presumed hypovascular zone, which is counterintuitive to the absence of vascular flow.

Two anatomic theories exist in the literature as to why the posterior tibial tendon is especially prone to developing long-standing inflammation and degeneration. The first potential agent is the overlying flexor retinaculum, which Jahss[62] suggests can cause compression and constriction of the tendon through synovial enlargement. This can impede circulation, fueling tendon degeneration. Secondly, the sharp turn or angle behind the malleolus creates excessive frictional forces with physical activity.[144] The excessive friction can contribute to the indolent inflammatory process.

In line with repetitive mechanical torque creating deficiency in the posterior tibial tendon are theories that congenital pes planus contributes to the disorder. Cozen[21] suggested that greater stress is placed on the posterior tibial tendon owing to both the increased subtalar motion and medial column sag seen in patients with flexible flatfoot. This is supported by Dyal et al,[32] who reviewed radiographs of patients with posterior tibial tendon insufficiency and compared them to radiographs on the contralateral (asymptomatic) side. Using angular measurements defined by Bordelon[6] and Sangeorzan,[132] the authors noted that 84% of asymptomatic feet and 86% of symptomatic feet had flatfoot deformities. These results were stratified to reveal that 23% of asymptomatic feet and 32% of symptomatic feet were moderately or severely flat. Interobserver reliability was highly correlated ($p = 0.0001$) among three surgeon observers, strengthening their results. Of course, this study does not prove that asymptomatic congenital pes planus is a potential cause of posterior tibial tendon insufficiency, but the suggestion is strong.

Indirectly, the contribution of a congenital flatfoot to posterior tibial tendon dysfunction is supported by Imhauser et al.[61] The authors created an in vitro model evaluating posterior tibial tendon function at heel rise. Unlike previous models, this construction allowed rotation of the tibia to contribute to a more physiologic gait pattern simulation. After creating a flatfoot deformity (through ligament sectioning), the authors noted a medial shift in load acting on the foot, placing undue stress on the posterior tibial tendon (and other medial structures) at heel lift. Such repetitive stress has already been discussed as a potential cause in posterior tibial tendon dysfunction.

Finally, the presence of an accessory navicular has a high correlation with developing posterior tibial tendon dysfunction.[7,67]

It is obvious that the cause of posterior tibial tendon insufficiency is most likely multifactorial and patient-specific. It is important for the clinician to assimilate the information discussed here to arrive at the correct underlying mechanism creating the disorder.

Physical Findings

Physical examination of the patient with posterior tibial tendon dysfunction begins with the patient standing barefoot, with the lower extremity exposed proximal to the knee. The examiner must ensure that the patient is standing with both knees facing forward, because the patient tends to externally rotate the involved extremity. Depending on the stage of presentation (see later), the alignment may be anatomic and symmetric, or the flatfoot deformity may be pronounced (Fig. 19–1). In this position, swelling or fullness about the medial ankle may be apparent. In advanced stages, forefoot abduction is obvious, as is impingement of the distal fibula against the calcaneus through hindfoot valgus collapse. The skin may be wrinkled laterally in this subfibular region. Direct palpation to the subfibular region with the ankle and hindfoot loaded elicits pain. In addition, in this position, with the feet symmetrically loaded, the examiner can take one finger and place it underneath the arch until striking soft tissue. By comparison with the opposite extremity in the same location, a rough estimate of arch collapse is noted.

From this position, the patient is asked to externally rotate the involved extremity 90 degrees, maintaining a fully loaded state. Collapse of the talonavicular joint may be appreciated by viewing the foot medially in this position. Calluses plantar to the talar head may be seen, and collapse at the first metatarsal–cuneiform joint may be noted. Rotating the leg 180 degrees to visualize the lateral foot and ankle, the examiner can develop a better appreciation of subfibular impingement. In this position, range of motion of the ankle may be checked and compared with the opposite extremity. It is important to examine ankle range of motion in a loaded state to avoid misrepresentation by compensation from Chopart's joint and forefoot joints. In the most advanced cases, this compensation becomes apparent as the patient passively dorsiflexes beyond neutral and the heel rises off the ground while the midfoot joints collapse.

The patient is next asked to face opposite the examiner, again with the knees symmetrically aligned forward. Hindfoot valgus should be noted and can be roughly estimated by visualizing through a goniometer to the patient's hindfoot. The proximal limb of the goniometer is positioned along the axis of the patient's leg, the hinge at the talus, and the inferior limb along the calcaneal axis. With practice, this method gives surprisingly accurate measurements of loaded valgus.

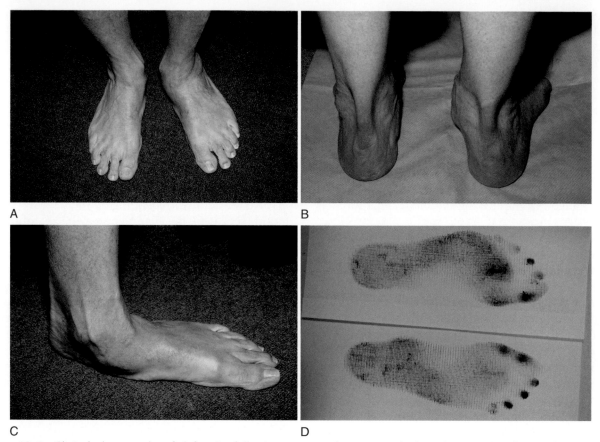

A   B

C   D

Figure 19–1   Clinical photographs of deformity following rupture of posterior tibial tendon. **A,** Dorsal view demonstrating increased abduction and a prominent talar head secondary to subluxation of the talonavicular joint. **B,** Posterior view demonstrating increased valgus of the calcaneus, increased abduction of the foot, and prominent talar head along the medial border of the foot. **C,** Medial view demonstrating collapse of the longitudinal arch and the prominence of the talar head. **D,** Harris mat demonstrating flattening of the longitudinal arch on the right in a patient with posterior tibial tendon dysfunction.

Also in this position, the examiner can note medial ankle fullness or swelling. Even in early stages, prior to valgus collapse of the hindfoot, this fullness is apparent when compared to the contralateral extremity. In addition, forefoot abduction becomes obvious when viewed from behind. The too-many-toes sign indicates more advanced disease and is sensitive in patients with congenital flatfoot as a comparative test.

One method of testing posterior tibial tendon muscle strength and integrity, the heel-rise test, is performed in this position. First, the examiner asks the patient to rise up onto both tiptoes. While doing so, the examiner looks for symmetric hindfoot inversion. Lack of symmetry indicates that the affected posterior tibial tendon is incompetent to invert the subtalar joint, lock the transverse tarsal joint, and allow heel rise through gastrocnemius–soleus complex power (Fig. 19–2). This is confirmed by asking the patient to perform a single-limb heel rise. The patient may rest a few fingers on an adjacent table or wall for balance, but the examiner ■ must be sure that the patient does

not lean forward or bend the knee while attempting to rise on one limb. Altering the body's center of gravity or recruiting adjacent muscle power by cheating in this fashion invalidates the test. In addition, the patient may be able to stand on the tiptoes of the involved

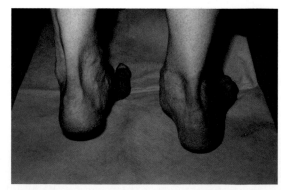

Figure 19–2   Double and single toe rise is an integral part of the physical examination. Note that on the involved *(right)* side, inversion of the subtalar does not occur.

extremity after rising up on both legs and lifting the contralateral extremity off the ground.

Returning to the truss theory, if a patient is able to remain standing on the toes without a functioning posterior tibial tendon, it is the plantar aponeurosis that brings about plantar flexion of the metatarsal heads and thus inversion of the calcaneus. In this theory, the longitudinal arch is maintained and the gastrocnemius–soleus complex maintains the ankle joint in plantar flexion. Thus, patients without a functioning posterior tibial tendon may be unable to initiate standing on tiptoes but are able to maintain the position once they have gotten on their toes, for the mechanism of action of the posterior tibial tendon is bypassed.

The examination now shifts to a seated patient. Passive range of motion of the ankle, subtalar, and the transverse tarsal joints is assessed. Excess mobility of the first metatarsocuneiform joint is assessed by firmly grasping both the first metatarsal and the midfoot and evaluating for subluxation of this joint surface in the sagittal plane. Simple dorsiflexion and plantar flexion of the first metatarsal while the midfoot is held rigid may be deceptive, and it must be compared with the opposite foot. Still, this maneuver may be useful for assessing midfoot pain and potential arthritis.

Direct palpation along the course of the posterior tibial tendon can elicit pain, although in later stage disease where tendinopathy supersedes tenosynovitis, pain might not be present. The examiner feels for increased swelling, fluid within the sheath, and increased warmth. Isolating the posterior tibial tendon for strength testing is difficult but possible. The examiner places the patient's ankle into a plantar flexed position, everting the hindfoot, to negate the effect of the anterior tibial tendon. The patient must relax the toes to prevent overpull by the flexor hallucis longus and flexor digitorum longus.[98] In this position, the patient inverts against resistance applied by the examiner's hand against the medial first metatarsal (Fig. 19-3). Strength and reproduction of pain are noted and compared with the opposite extremity. Comparison is critical, for patients can maintain some posterior tibial tendon strength with an incompetent tendon. As noted in the physiology section, the excursion of the posterior tibial tendon is only 1 to 2 cm. Thus, a length deficit of 1 cm due to rupture or tendinopathy can still provide some inversion strength while having no functional value.

The patient is then asked to lie flat, and the ankle range of motion is assessed with the knee flexed and extended. The Silversköldt test specifically measures gastrocnemius contracture by alternately relaxing and incorporating the muscle owing to its origin proximal to the knee joint. This test should be done while

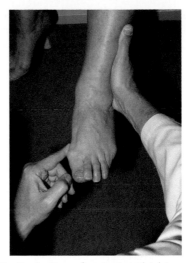

Figure 19–3 Evaluation of posterior tibial tendon function. The foot is placed into full inversion and some plantar flexion, and the patient is asked to resist pressure from the examiner's finger.

holding the subtalar joint in neutral, to avoid subtalar compensation for a tight gastrocnemius muscle. With the legs fully extended and the subtalar joint held in neutral, an assessment for fixed forefoot varus is performed. In the normal foot, a line visually drawn across the plantar metatarsal heads is perpendicular to the long axis of the tibia and calcaneus. Patients with long-standing posterior tibial tendon dysfunction can develop fixed varus (Fig. 19–4) of the forefoot as a compensation for increasing hindfoot valgus (they are attempting to maintain a plantigrade foot). The visual

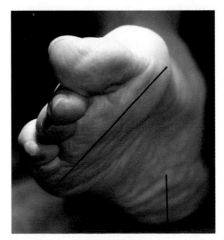

Figure 19–4 Demonstration of forefoot varus. The degree of forefoot varus is determined by placing the heel in neutral position, covering the head of the talus with the navicular, and then observing the relationship of the metatarsal heads to the neutral hindfoot. In fixed forefoot varus, the lateral border of the foot is more plantar flexed than the medial border.

metatarsal line is thus inclined medially. The rigidity of this condition may be evaluated by continuing to hold the subtalar joint in neutral while providing a manual dorsiflexion force on the lateral column of the foot through the fourth and fifth metatarsals. Normally, the lateral column of the foot is mobile, and the visual line should return to the anatomic axis. In fixed conditions, the medial inclination remains.

Finally, the patient is placed in a prone position. Here, subtalar joint motion can be measured with the knee flexed 90 degrees and the ankle plantar flexed. Relaxing the gastrocnemius–soleus complex releases outside influence on the subtalar joint and allows accurate measurements to be obtained. This may be done with a goniometer, again placing one limb of the device along the axis of the distal tibia, the hinge at the talus, and the second limb along the axis of the calcaneus. The importance of achieving accuracy in both subtalar motion assessment and fixed forefoot varus deformity will become clear as surgical procedures are discussed.

Prior to completing the examination, the patient's shoes are inspected for aberrant wear patterns. This becomes evident as medial heel wear in older shoes, because valgus hindfoot asymmetrically erodes the heel through repetitive strike.

Clinical Staging

Posterior tibial tendon dysfunction should be viewed as a syndrome in which there is a spectrum of clinical presentations. This spectrum ranges from patients with recent onset (synovitis can create pain, yet motor function is preserved) to patients with long-standing disease (marked collapse of the hindfoot and midfoot is present and motor function is absent).

The general classification system proposed by Johnson and Strom[64] enables clinicians to organize their thoughts when evaluating this condition. The authors based this classification system on disorder, clinical presentation, and radiographic findings.

Stage 1 patients present with swelling and pain along the medial aspect of the hindfoot, generally at the tip and distal to the medial malleolus along the course of the posterior tibial tendon. In this stage, tenosynovitis is the predominant source of pain. Thus, the length of the tendon is preserved and, along with it, motor strength. The patient is usually able to perform a single toe raise, with normal varus tilt to the hindfoot while on the toes. This maneuver might not cause symptoms, but repetitive toe raises reproduce the symptomatic pain. With respect to the above-mentioned parameters in physical examination, hindfoot valgus is absent, too-many-toes sign is absent, and deformity is absent.

Stage 2 patients have undergone elongation and degeneration of the posterior tibial tendon. Deformity of the foot is obvious at this stage. The hindfoot is in valgus, and the forefoot may be in abduction. Collapse at the talonavicular joint is apparent. The patient may be able to perform a single-limb heel rise early in this stage, but as the deformity progresses, the patient is unable to do so. Most important, the deformity remains flexible at this stage. Thus, the examiner can passively correct both the hindfoot valgus and forefoot abduction while the patient is seated. Recently, this stage has been subclassified into an "a" stage, where symptoms are primarily medial, the collapse is mild, and the patient can still perform a single-limb heel rise, and a "b" stage, where subfibular impingement develops along with complete incompetence of the posterior tibial tendon.

Stage 3 patients have developed a rigid deformity. Forefoot varus is fixed and usually 10 to 15 degrees at the minimum. The subtalar joint no longer reduces in a seated position, and any attempt to place the calcaneus in the anatomic axis reveals the compensatory supinated forefoot. The gastrocnemius–soleus complex is tight. Often the medial ankle pain is absent in this stage, and patients complain more of pain in the lateral ankle, which upon examination is subfibular. Pain at rest might become apparent as arthritis becomes a component of the condition. The patient is unable to perform a single-limb heel rise.

Stage 4 was added by Myerson.[110] Chronic eccentric loading of the ankle joint in valgus creates lateral compartment arthritic wear patterns. The lateral ankle pain that a patient in stage 3 presented with is now only partially subfibular impingement and more directly related to ankle arthritis. This valgus load eventually leads to a valgus deformity of the talus and attenuation of the deltoid ligament.

Imaging Evaluation

Radiography

Diagnostic modalities for evaluation of the posterior tibial tendon have evolved since Kulowski's report on tenosynovitis in 1936. However, a standard protocol for posterior tibial tendon imaging has yet to be accepted. In 1986, Funk et al[36] noted that four different types of posterior tibial tendon lesions were found during surgical exploration. The authors reported the impossibility of distinguishing the four groups by clinical or radiographic measures prior to surgery. Funk looked at 19 patients who underwent surgical exploration after failed primary conservative treatment for posterior tibial tendon dysfunction. They determined that preoperative radiographs were of little added value in diagnosis and the various lesions that might be present in the posterior tibial tendon can be suspected clinically, but a precise diagnosis cannot be made until the tendon is exposed surgically. In this study, preoperative radiographs were the only advanced imaging modality employed.

Despite this forewarning, plain radiography is a useful adjunct in evaluating posterior tibial tendon dysfunction. Weight-bearing radiographs are employed to appreciate the deformity, and they are useful in proposing management options. The standard series includes three views of the foot and, at the very least, an anteroposterior (AP) view of the ankle (Fig. 19–5). Additional radiographs can include a complete ankle series (Fig. 19–6) and a hindfoot alignment radiograph (Fig. 19–7).[130] Patients who have a congenital flatfoot undergo radiographs of the opposite foot for comparison.

Although the radiographs are normal in stage 1 disease, they are useful to rule out structural diagnoses that could be contributing to the patient's flatfoot and pain. Tarsal coalition, degenerative arthritis, accessory navicular, and old trauma such as a Lisfranc injury can be contributing to this constellation of symptoms. As the disorder progresses, characteristic changes are seen. In a general sense, lateral subluxation of the talonavicular joint is evident on the AP radiograph, and talonavicular joint sag is noted on the lateral radiograph. The lateral radiograph also provides useful information about the status of the first metatarsocuneiform joint, because subluxation or arthritis of this joint surface can contribute to the flatfoot. Subluxation also occurs at the subtalar joint, manifested as an indistinct joint surface on the lateral film. Ankle radiographs can demonstrate arthritis and subfibular impingement.

To quantify these findings, measurements have been proposed that assist in static assessment of the disorder while enabling the surgeon to follow progression. Sangeorzan et al[132] suggested that on the lateral radiograph, the important parameters are the lateral talocalcaneal angle, the lateral talometatarsal angle, and the cuneiform height. The lateral talocalcaneal angle is indicated by a line drawn midway between the superior and inferior portions of the talar body and neck and a second line drawn midway between the superior and inferior portions of both the tuberosity and the sustentaculum tali (see Chapter 3). The lateral talometatarsal angle is measured using the same line through the talus as for the lateral talocalcaneal angle and a second line drawn along a point halfway between the superior and inferior portions of the proximal and distal metaphyseal–diaphyseal junction of the metatarsal (avoiding inconsistencies with the flares distally and proximally) (see Chapter 3). Cuneiform height is measured between the medial cuneiform and

the fifth metatarsal base. Cuneiform height can also be measured between the medial cuneiform and the ground, which is less sensitive.

On the AP view, the important parameters are the talocalcaneal angle, the talometatarsal angle, and the articular congruity angle. The talocalcaneal angle uses a point midway between the medial and lateral articular surface and a second point midway between the margins of the talar neck. This line intersects with a line drawn along the lateral border of the calcaneus (see Chapter 3). The talometatarsal angle uses the talus as one axis (with the lines drawn in an identical fashion to that on the sagittal image). The second axis is drawn in the first metatarsal, midway between two points measured along the metaphyseal–diaphyseal junction (proximal and distal) (see Chapter 3).

The articular congruity angle is measured by first drawing a line connecting the articular margins of the talus and navicular. A perpendicular line is drawn at the midpoint of each line. The angle created by the intersection of these two lines represents talonavicular coverage (see Chapter 3). Normal values for these angles include an assessment by Gould,[44] who suggested that the lateral talometatarsal angle should fall between −4 degrees and +4 degrees. Saltzman[129] suggested that 95% of the population has a talocalcaneal angle of less than 12 degrees. The lateral talocalcaneal angle increases in patients with acquired flatfoot, as does the talometatarsal angle. Dyal[32] found the lowest correlation between symptomatic and asymptomatic flatfeet was at the cuneiform-to-fifth metatarsal measurement, suggesting that this might be the best measurement to determine congenital pes planus versus adult acquired flatfoot. In addition, this measurement has the best interobserver reliability, making its consistency the most accurate measurement of flatfoot.

An alternative to angular measurements as a radiographic indication to posterior tibial tendon dysfunction was proposed by Pomeroy et al.[122] Linear measurements are made to quantify uncovering of the talar head upon the navicular. A bilateral standing AP radiograph of the feet is used to evaluate this congruence by choosing an arbitrary fixed point on the medial aspect of the talar head and connecting it to an arbitrary fixed point on the medial edge of the navicular. Using identical points on the opposite foot reveals a discrepancy in length in patients with acquired flatfoot. Lateral foot radiographs of both feet undergo a similar comparison through lines drawn from the base of the fifth metatarsal to the anterior–inferior corner of the medial cuneiform. This line is drawn perpendicular to the weight-bearing axis of the floor and decreases in patients with flatfoot. The final linear measurement involves use of a bilateral AP

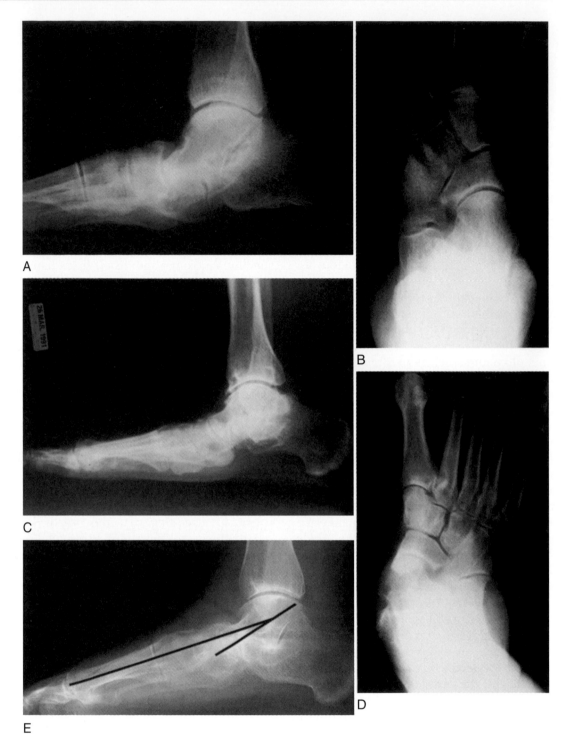

Figure 19–5   Radiographic findings associated with posterior tibial tendon dysfunction. **A** and **B,** Radiographs demonstrate significant talonavicular sag in the lateral radiograph and minimal abduction in the anteroposterior (AP) radiograph. **C** and **D,** Radiographs demonstrate minimal sag at the talonavicular joint on the lateral radiograph yet significant abduction on the AP radiograph. **E** and **F,** Moderate degree of sagging of the talonavicular joint in the lateral radiograph and abduction on the AP radiograph.

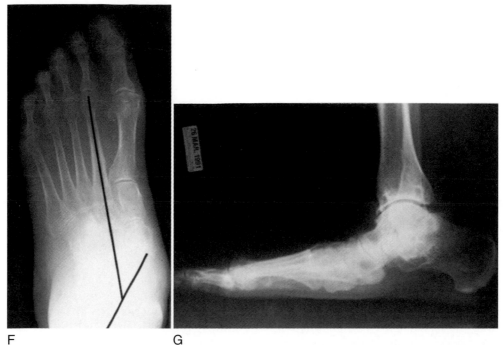

Figure 19-5—cont'd G, Minimal changes at the talonavicular joint but a moderate sag at the naviculocuneiform joint.

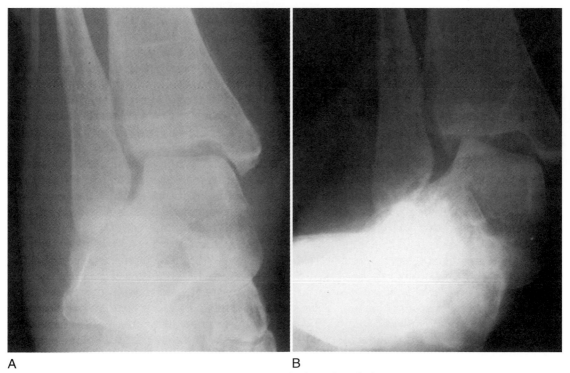

Figure 19-6 Ankle joint changes associated with posterior tibial tendon dysfunction. **A,** Anteroposterior (AP) non–weight-bearing radiograph of the ankle joint demonstrating slight talar tilt. **B,** Weight-bearing radiograph demonstrating significant valgus tilt associated with a marked valgus deformity of the calcaneus.

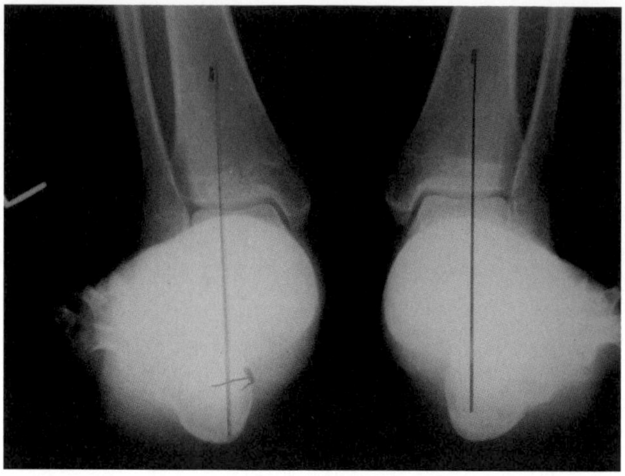

Figure 19–7 Axial radiograph of the hindfoot alignment view. This radiographic view is useful in determining the magnitude of valgus hindfoot deformity and thus planning the appropriate surgical intervention.

ankle radiograph. The total height of the ankle is measured by dropping a perpendicular line from the superior talus (in the ankle mortise) to the floor. Collapse from acquired flatfoot is evident by a decreased ankle height.

Magnetic Resonance Imaging and Computed Tomography

Advanced diagnostic modalities are also available. Before the advent of magnetic resonance imaging (MRI) and computed tomography (CT), tenography was the primary method for assessing ankle tendons.[156] Tenography is rarely used today because we have less invasive and more sensitive and specific techniques for imaging soft tissue disorders. Tenography does show the tendon structure and reveals abnormal villous thickening of the tenosynovium in tenosynovitis. It is also adequate for determining disorders within the sheath, including entrapment and sheath compression. However, it does not allow direct visualization of the posterior tibial tendon; therefore, partial ruptures or longitudinal split tears go undetected. Injections into the tendon sheath can be difficult, especially when adhesions obliterate the synovial space. Alexander et al[2] have shown that the results of tenography correlate poorly with the surgical findings. In addition, Hogan[56] explains that the flexor digitorum longus tendon, which lies directly medial to the posterior tibial tendon, can be injected inadvertently. Occasionally, the two synovial sheaths communicate, giving false negative results when true disorder exists.

CT scans show bony anatomy well, but they have limited soft tissue contrast resolution. Rosenberg et al[127] performed CT imaging on 49 patients with a suspected posterior tibial tendon rupture. By correlat-

ing surgical findings on these patients, they found CT was accurate 96% of the time in diagnosing and classifying the magnitude of tendon disruption. They were able to subclassify tendon damage into partial rupture (with tendon hypertrophy and longitudinal split tears versus tendon attenuation) and full-thickness rupture. They found periostitis of the posterior distal tibia along the course of the posterior tibial tendon in cases with rupture. This secondary phenomenon was noted in 68% of the study group, making it a useful adjunct in diagnosing posterior tibial tendon dysfunction.

Limitations, however, were noted. Longitudinal split tears were underrepresented by CT scan, with CT missing both the magnitude and volume of such tears. In addition, CT demonstrated less fraying and degeneration of the posterior tibial tendon than was seen during surgical exploration, again underestimating the magnitude of the condition. Synovial inflammation was indistinguishable from damaged tendon, underestimating tenosynovitis. In this 1988 study, the authors predicted the newly developed MRI would supplant CT as a diagnostic modality for posterior tibial tendon dysfunction. Today, CT has value only if MRI is contraindicated.

MRI is an excellent modality for detecting sheath inflammation, soft tissue resolution, and anatomic detail of the tendon.[158] It is superior to CT for tendon definition, resolution of synovial fluid, soft tissue edema, and tissue degeneration.[126] Alexander et al[2] first discussed its usefulness in a 1987 case report on a 44-year-old patient with a complete rupture of her posterior tibial tendon diagnosed by MRI and confirmed at surgery. Rosenberg et al[126] found the sensitivity of MRI versus CT is 95% versus 90%, the specificity of MRI versus CT is 100% and 100%, and the accuracy of MRI versus CT is 96% versus 91%. Elusive longitudinal split tears not visualized on CT scan were easily seen with MRI scanning. Thus, the percentage of tears that were diagnosed and classified correctly was greater with MRI (73%) than with CT (59%).

The examination should take place with the patient supine and the ankle in a neutral and slightly plantarflexed position. Axial images are most useful in assessing size, shape, and internal content of the posterior tibial tendon. However, patient position is critical to obtaining good axial images. To negate the magic angle effect of MRI, a true axial plane perpendicular to the tendon at the level of the medial malleolus is required. The magic angle effect is noted on short-TE (T1-weighted) images, where the acute 55-degree angle of the posterior tibial tendon as it exits the medial malleolus creates simulated rupture on MRI. This effect is due to the ability of the excitable protons to move in limited planes of the tightly packed collagen of the posterior tibial tendon. This effect is not visualized on long-TE (T2-weighted) images. To negate this effect, an oblique axial image may be obtained by placing the image plane approximately 45 degrees between true axial and coronal image planes.[73] Anatomically, this plane is perpendicular to the posterior facet of the subtalar joint. In addition, the tendon is occasionally lost in the homogenous signal of the medial malleolus. By plantar flexing the ankle slightly, the relaxed tendon moves away from the bone, enhancing its signal. Careful evaluation of sagittal images can reveal the location of the tendon rupture and the length of tendon involved. This ability may be enhanced by rotating the ankle slightly medially during the examination.

Normal tendon substance on MRI appears as a black and homogenous signal with an ovoid shape on all spin-echo images. This appearance is due to the dense collagen within the posterior tibial tendon. The posterior tibial tendon is normally two to three times larger than the flexor digitorum longus tendon. A small amount of fluid within the sheath is normal, though it should not be more than 1 to 2 mm wide, and it should not be circumferential. In tenosynovitis, T2-weighted images show pronounced fluid surrounding the tendon and edema within the tendon sheath. The synovial effusion appears as a bright signal and is best seen on T2 images.[65]

The hallmark of tenosynovitis is a homogenous tendon with fluid in the tendon sheath. T1 images are useful for evaluating the synovial membrane and the substance of the posterior tibial tendon (Fig. 19–8). These structures are hypertrophied, and the posterior tibial tendon occasionally reaches sizes five to ten times that of the adjacent flexor digitorum longus tendon. T1 images also evaluate intratendinous disorders by showing foci of increased signal, revealing longitudinal split tears.[65] The synovial sheath of the

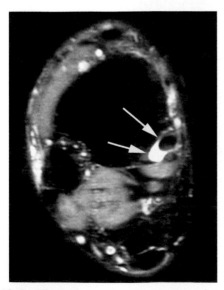

Figure 19–8 Magnetic resonance imaging demonstrates fluid (arrows) within the sheath of the posterior tibial tendon.

posterior tibial tendon ends before its insertion. Thus, there is no true tenosynovitis noted distally. Increased signal around the tendon close to its insertion is peritendinitis and is not normal.

The width of the synovial sheath is significantly increased in stage 1 posterior tibial tendon tenosynovitis.[10] In stage 2 or 3 disease it is less common to find a fluid filled synovial sheath and tendon hypertrophy. These stages are more likely to reveal tendon disorders such as split tears, ruptures, and tendon elongation.[10] Thus, MRI is especially useful for evaluation and diagnosis of stage 1 disease. MRI is more sensitive than surgical exploration in predicting disorders and successful surgical outcome.[65] MRI can detect an intrasubstance tear in the tendon that may be missed intraoperatively, leading to its predictive value.

Elongation of the tendon becomes apparent on MRI as the patient progresses to clinical stage 2 disease. The diameter of the tendon might in fact be less than the adjacent flexor digitorum longus tendon. When stage 3 deformity is reached, complete rupture is often visualized on T1 images. The inflammatory response may be absent in the tendon sheath, and mucinous degeneration may be apparent within the tendon gap. Findings in the lateral ankle may become apparent, recognized as sinus tarsi syndrome and subfibular impingement. MRI detects absence of the normal sinus tarsi fat signal with low signal on T1-weighted images. T1 images reveal fibrosis within the sinus tarsi and absence of the supporting talocalcaneal interosseous ligament and cervical ligament.[4] T2-weighted images can reveal increased signal consistent with edema in the sinus tarsi in less chronic conditions. Balen and Helms[4] found such changes in the sinus tarsi in 72% of patients who have posterior tibial tendon dysfunction (versus 36% of control patients scanned for ankle pain).

Other adjunct MRI findings in the syndrome of posterior tibial tendon dysfunction are valuable in planning surgical reconstruction. Wacker et al[152] studied the physiologic quality of both the posterior tibial and flexor digitorum longus muscle belly in patients with adult acquired flatfoot deformity. The authors found that in patients with a complete rupture of the posterior tibial tendon, the muscle belly underwent significant fatty infiltration. This nonfunctional muscle was noted within 10 months of the injury's creating complete rupture. Those with posterior tibial tendinosis without complete rupture demonstrated a mean 10.7% atrophy of the muscle belly, with compensatory hypertrophy (mean 17.2%) of the flexor digitorum longus muscle belly. The clinical implications of this study are discussed in the surgery section of this chapter.

The plantar calcaneonavicular ligament (spring ligament) has also been studied with MRI (Fig. 19–9).

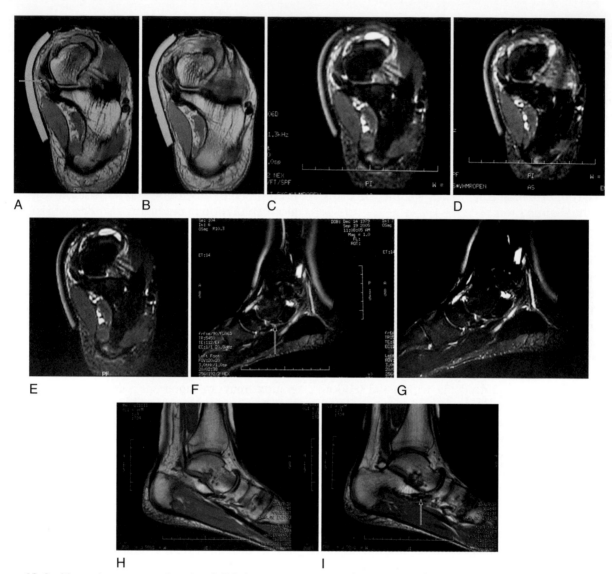

Figure 19–9 Magnetic resonance imaging (MRI) demonstrates a complete rupture of the superior calcaneal navicular portion of the spring ligament. **A** and **B,** T1 images reveal the ruptured ligament *(arrow).* **C** to **E,** T2 images reveal increased signal at the site of rupture. **F** and **G,** The sagittal T2 images emphasize the lack of support of the talar head created by the rupture of the superior calcaneonavicular ligament. **H** and **I,** The sagittal T1 images show an attenuated and ruptured ligament.

Yao[159] had independent radiologists evaluate MRI studies done *preoperatively* on patients who had intraoperative findings of spring ligament insufficiency. The MRI evaluations were done retrospectively, following definitive surgical confirmation of disorder. The control population in this series was patients without spring ligament disorder. The radiologists consistently found signal heterogeneity on axial short TE (T1-weighted) within the medial portion (superomedial calcaneonavicular) of the ligament only. Rather than finding an attenuated ligament, the medial ligament was thickened to more than 5 mm. Poor correlation between radiologists was noted with the plantar (inferior calcaneonavicular) ligament. This ligament is inherently thin, and MRI evaluation was unreliable. Biomechanical studies demonstrate that this component of the ligament plays a minor role in statically stabilizing the longitudinal arch. Overall, the sensitivity for evaluation of the medial ligament was 54% to 77%, and the specificity was 100%. Note that this evaluation was done on chronic ligament disorders, not acute ruptures. In the latter scenario, the MRI diagnosis is more reliable, because T2-weighted images demonstrate bright foci consistent with edema and hematoma.

Balen and Helms[4] found 92% of patients with advanced posterior tibial tendon dysfunction (MRI confirmed) had MRI changes consistent with superior calcaneonavicular ligament disorders. Using Yao's[159] criteria, they studied 25 patients with such disease noted in the posterior tibial tendon. Only 28% of the patients in the control group had disorders similar to the spring ligament's.

The accuracy of MRI has been supported. Khoury[73] reported that 9 of 11 preoperative MRI diagnoses of various stages of posterior tibial tendon disorder were confirmed through surgical visualization. Such pathologic states included peritendinitis, tendinosis, and partial and complete ruptures. Peritendinitis is found as fluid about the tendon sheath with a normal tendon. Tendinosis is noted with tendon thickening with or without intrasubstance degeneration or deep tears. Partial tears, normally within the portion of the tendon with tendinosis, are distinguished by reaching the surface of the tendon (whereas tears not reaching the surface are classified as tendinosis). Complete rupture reveals a gap filled with fluid or fibrous tissue, as noted above. These four entities were clearly discernible on MRI.

Ultrasound

Ultrasound is now recognized as a cost-effective and accurate modality for evaluating tendon disorders in the foot and ankle.[59] A normal tendon appears hyperechoic and a degenerated tendon hypoechoic on ultrasound (Fig. 19–10). Normal posterior tibial tendon diameter is 4 to 6 mm.[103] Tenosynovitis manifests with large amounts of fluid surrounding the tendon.[10] A hypoechoic rim visible on the longitudinal sonogram and a target sign on transverse sonogram is pathognomonic for posterior tibial tendon tenosynovitis. The term *target sign* was coined to describe a homogeneous, continuous hyperechoic tendon surrounded by a hypoechoic fluid halo. The halo represents excessive surrounding synovial fluid. Ultrasound can also reveal a swollen tendon, an irregular tendon contour, longitudinal split tears, heterogeneous echogenicity, and surrounding hypoechoic shadows in patients with tenosynovitis. In contrast, tendon rupture features an empty tibial groove at the level of the medial malleolus.[59]

Chen and Liang[10] have shown that on average the posterior tibial tendon measures 3.30 mm in diameter. A tendon afflicted with tenosynovitis averages 4.61 mm. In addition, an increased synovial sheath diameter is noted in tenosynovitis and is a reliable marker for predicting intraoperative findings. The average diameter of a normal tendon sheath is 3.64 mm. In tenosynovitis, the measurement increases to 7.24 mm ($P < 0.0001$). Therefore, ultrasound will detect both a mildly enlarged tendon and a significant increase in sheath diameter due to fluid accumulation.

Chen and Liang[10] confirmed their ultrasonographic findings through surgical exploration. All 14 patients with posterior tibial tendon tenosynovitis requiring surgical exploration had an intact posterior tibial tendon and surrounding fluid and hypertrophic tenosynovium. Though this study entertained no false-positive results, the authors caution that misdiagnosis may be common in the hands of an inexperienced examiner reviewing longitudinal scans. The authors suggest that ultrasound is superior to MRI based on speed, convenience, low cost, and its dynamic nature. This study is limited, however, by lack of double-blinding, for the surgeon was given the ultrasonic results in advance of the operation, potentially influencing intraoperative findings.

Studies have suggested that sensitivity and specificity for ultrasound is similar to those for MRI.[103] Miller et al[103] surgically explored 17 patients with posterior tibial tendon tenosynovitis who had undergone preoperative ultrasound examination. The authors found ultrasound successful in confirming intraoperative findings in all 17. They concurrently performed preoperative MRI examinations on these 17 patients. Two patients with tendon damage visible on surgical exploration had normal tendon readings on MRI.

Gerling et al[38] performed a double-blinded study on fresh cadaveric feet, creating longitudinal split tears in the posterior tibial tendon. Four separate scans were done on each cadaveric limb, the first with no tear, fol-

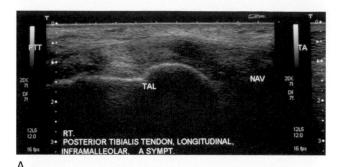

A

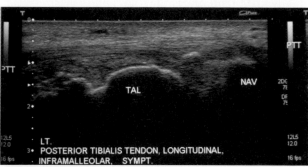

B1

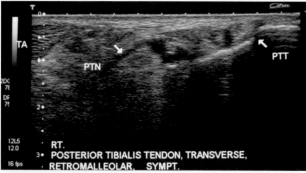

B2

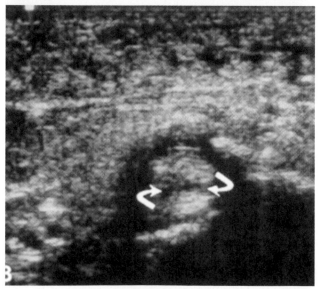

B3

Figure 19–10 Ultrasound examination of posterior tibial tendon. **A,** Normal longitudinal orientation of the posterior tibial tendon, medial to the talus (TAL) and navicular (NAV). **B,** Pathologic posterior tibial tendon. The pathologic tendon has a longitudinal split tear within it (arrows). (**B3** from Miller SD, Van Holsbeeck M, Boruta PM, et al: *Foot Ankle Int* 17[9]: 555-558, 1996.)

lowed by progressively creating a split tear of 1 cm, 2 cm, and 4 cm in length. Each limb was evaluated with ultrasound and MRI. The authors found the sensitivity of MRI versus ultrasound was 73% versus 69%; the specificity of MRI versus ultrasound was 69% versus 81%; and the accuracy of MRI versus ultrasound was 72% versus 72%. Interobserver reliability was excellent with MRI (0.86) and only fair with ultrasonography (0.37). It remains difficult to interpret the clinical value of this study, for the absence of in vivo perfusion and physiologic tendon function alters the natural environment of these radiographic modalities. The significant deviation from prior studies evaluating MRI sensitivity and specificity echo the questionable validity of this cadaveric study.

Premkumar et al[123] studied 44 tendons in patients with a clinical diagnosis of posterior tibial tendon dysfunction. The authors found the most useful criteria for diagnosing tendinosis and peritendinosis on magnetic resonance imaging was enhancement of the tendon. On color-flow Doppler sonography, increased flow was most useful in this regard. Under these criteria, the positive predictive value of MRI was 83%. The positive predictive value of ultrasound was 90%. When directly compared with MRI, the ability of ultrasound to diagnose tendinopathy was 80% sensitive and 90% specific. The ability of ultrasound to diagnose peritendinosis was 90% sensitive and 80% specific. Again, these results are difficult to interpret because no surgical exploration was performed and thus no pathologic specimens were available to confirm diagnosis.

These clinical data suggest that ultrasound is as effective a modality as MRI in the diagnostic algorithm of posterior tibial tendon dysfunction. However, careful analysis of the data finds flaws in the experimental design. Thus, readers must interpret this conclusion with caution and use the most effective modality available at their institution. These thoughts were echoed by Wertheimer, who cautions that interpretation of ultrasound requires an experienced radiologist, which is not always necessary for MRI interpretation.[156]

Magnetic Resonance Imaging Staging

Conti et al[15] have developed a classification system based on MRI observations.

Type 1, consistent with tenosynovitis, is manifested as synovial swelling, occasional fine longitudinal splits, and a homogenous black signal (tendon) on T1 images. This type is divided into two subcategories: Type 1A has one or two fine longitudinal splits, and type 1B has increased splits and mild surrounding fibrosis.

Type 2 disease consists of a narrower tendon signal, with evidence of intramural degeneration. This appears as a gray substance within the black tendon signal on T1 images. Wider longitudinal split tears are present. The tendon can taper in the diseased segment and appear bulbous at the extremes of this segment.

Type 3 is manifested as diffuse synovial swelling and prominent, uniform degeneration. This type is also divided into two subcategories: Type 3A has uniform degeneration and a few strands of intact tendon, and type 3B has complete rupture and replacement by scar tissue in the gapped segments.

This study compared the above-mentioned magnetic resonance grading with intraoperative surgical grading according to prior clinical classification schemes. The authors found that 55% of their patients had less extensive disease within the posterior tibial tendon upon direct visualization than predicted by the MRI classification. The authors found, however, that their MRI classification system did a better job of predicting successful surgical outcome than the surgical classification system. The value of this analysis, however, is clouded because the surgical techniques employed (side-to-side flexor digitorum longus tendon anastomosis to the diseased posterior tibial tendon) is no longer performed as an isolated procedure in posterior tibial tendon dysfunction of the magnitude seen in this study. Thus, it is impossible in this day to state that their MRI classification system is a better predictor of surgical outcome than surgical grading, for the techniques used at present have a far better clinical outcome. The value of MRI classification remains in question.

Treatment

Conservative Treatment

In most instances, conservative therapy should be instituted prior to contemplating surgical reconstruction for posterior tibial tendon insufficiency. Though a standard protocol has not been developed and would inherently depend on the stage of the disease when the patient presents at the office, common themes are recognized that involve rest of the tendon, medication, physical therapy, and management of orthotics and braces.

Resting or relieving the tension on the posterior tibial tendon may be done in a graduated fashion. The first level of rest involves a rigid stirrup brace or lace-up sport brace. This type of brace crosses the ankle joint and thus limits excursion of the posterior tibial tendon. However, it offloads only the inversion component to posterior tibial tendon activation, ignoring restriction on sagittal motion.[110] Thus, the posterior tibial tendon still glides within the sheath, allowing further aggravation from inflammation and repetitive stress. Still, in more mild conditions, unloading inversion is sufficient for pain relief.

If the first level of rest is ineffective, patients may wear a CAM (controlled-ankle-motion) walker boot. This device has the added benefit of eliminating motion in the sagittal plane. It retains the advantage over casting by allowing simultaneous functional rehabilitation. A below-knee cast, however, provides ultimate tendon rest and absolute compliance. Calf atrophy can compromise rehabilitation, and risk of deep venous thrombosis is present with the below-knee cast. The weight-bearing status with either device is predicated on pain relief. Patients may bear weight in a CAM boot or cast if they are completely asymptomatic. In fact, Blake and colleagues[5] emphasize that protected weight bearing encourages tendon repair by organizing new collagen along the direction of stress. Time frame of use ranges from 4 to 6 weeks.[14,90,110]

Antiinflammatory medication is used simultaneously with rest of the tendon. With controversy surrounding complications of some nonsteroidal antiinflammatory medications, the orthopedist should determine the appropriate medicine for each patient in conjunction with the patient's primary care physician. It is suggested that the patient take the medicine as prescribed for a complete 2-week course. This will allow appropriate serum concentrations to be established, and continued ingestion will maintain this therapeutic level sufficiently to eliminate the inflammatory component to posterior tibial tendon tenosynovitis.

Oral corticosteroids, and for that matter, injectable corticosteroids, are not used in our practice. As suggested in the discussion of etiology, steroids can create local microvascular attenuation, further compromising healing of the insulted posterior tibial tendon. Johnson and Strom[64] felt that steroid injections were contraindicated owing to accelerated tendon weakening. In fact, Holmes and Mann[57] reported that in an age-stratified population, 28% of the younger patients and 17% of the older patients with rupture of the posterior tibial tendon had a history of multiple steroid injections or a history of oral corticosteroid use.

Physical therapy can decrease inflammation surrounding the posterior tibial tendon in a nontoxic fashion. Iontophoresis, in which dexamethasone is repelled into the deep soft tissues with electrical current, has an antiinflammatory effect without documented risk of tendon rupture. Cryotherapy, or ice massage, can be done as part of a home program and is especially useful after exercise or activity. Extravasation of humoral mediators is highest after exercise, and icing the tendon sheath slows this release. Ultrasound is a heat-applied treatment and can exacerbate inflammatory symptoms, limiting its usefulness. Pulsed ultrasound can have a role to reduce tendinopathy pain, and it does not have the consequence of increasing inflammation through heat.

Isolated strengthening of the posterior tibial tendon should be avoided until the above-mentioned treatment protocol eliminates the patient's pain. Aggressive strengthening employed while the tendon remains painful will only exacerbate the symptoms and lengthen recovery. Selective activation of the posterior tibial tendon was explored by Kulig et al[78] The authors used MRI to evaluate changes in muscle activation during exercise. The authors found the greatest increase in posterior tibial muscle activation occurred with resisted foot adduction using resistance bands (Thera-Band) (activation increased 50%) compared to the surrounding musculature (average increase 5%). Heel rise and resisted forefoot supination produced less than half of the activation of the posterior tibial muscle when compared with foot adduction. Anatomically, the perpendicular course of the posterior tibial tendon relative to the oblique midtarsal joint axis allows contraction of the muscle belly to adduct at the oblique midtarsal axis. Therapeutic strengthening must be focused on this plane of motion to maximize effectiveness.

Orthotic and brace management has been a large focus of attention in conservative management of posterior tibial tendon dysfunction. Simply put, attempts to lessen strain across the posterior tibial tendon may be instituted by elevating the medial arch and elimi-

nating pronation. Prior to instituting orthotic management, it is important for the clinician to determine if the deformity is fixed or flexible, because the orthotist will benefit from specific instructions in fitting this device, and patient satisfaction hinges on appropriate construction.[154] When the patient has a flexible deformity, the heel must be in a subtalar neutral position when the orthotist makes the mold for the orthosis. In this case, the orthotic will have true corrective power, lessening the stress applied to the posterior tibial tendon. If the deformity is rigid, the orthotic is molded in situ, without attempts at correction. In this situation, comfort and pain relief will be enhanced by not attempting to correct an uncorrectable foot.

Patients with more mild deformities can achieve success with a semi-rigid orthosis with a medial heel wedge and a medial column post.[63] This may be particularly effective in stage 1 disease (Fig. 19–11). However, as the patient enters stage 2, with the deformity remaining flexible, a total-contact rigid orthotic or a UCBL (University of California Biomechanics Laboratory) brace may become necessary (Fig. 19–12). The UCBL brace has been shown to significantly affect the orientation and movement of the subtalar joint (and the ankle and knee joints) by reducing the degree and duration of abnormal pronation during the stance phase of gait.[87] The biomechanical principle of the UCBL is to stabilize the heel in neutral and prevent abduction of the forefoot. Abduction is blocked by building up the lateral border of the foot piece. This maneuver helps to reestablish the longitudinal arch.

Chao et al[9] used the UCBL with medial posting in patients with flexible deformities defined as less than 10 degrees of residual forefoot varus in a subtalar neutral position. Those with rigid deformities were treated with a molded solid-ankle ankle–foot orthosis (AFO). This study did not specifically look at the effectiveness of the UCBL brace; rather, its purpose was to

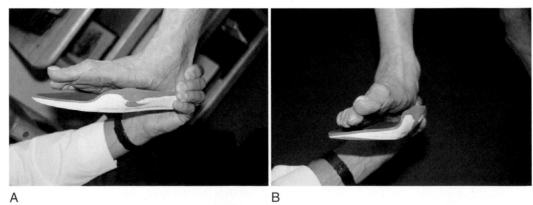

A   B

Figure 19–11   Orthotic device used for posterior tibial tendon dysfunction. **A,** Medial view demonstrates a fixed varus deformity of the forefoot, which requires medial posting to provide adequate support. **B,** Frontal view demonstrates the fixed forefoot varus in relation to the orthosis. The medial side of the foot requires adequate support for the orthotic device to be functional.

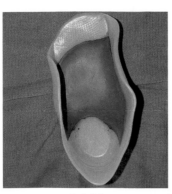

Figure 19–12 University of California Biomechanics Laboratory (UCBL) orthosis. This orthosis functions by stabilizing the heel in neutral and by building up the lateral wall of the device to prevent abduction of the forefoot, thereby helping to reestablish a longitudinal arch in the flexible foot.

assess the success of brace management for posterior tibial tendon dysfunction. The authors found that 67% of patients achieved a good to excellent result with both braces (UCBL or AFO) as a nonoperative adjunct to treating the condition.

Augustin et al[3] evaluated the use of the Arizona brace, first introduced in 1988, in nonoperative management of posterior tibial tendon dysfunction. Unlike the UCBL, this device has no significant impact on stabilizing the hindfoot, but it can restore the arch and midfoot kinematics. Augustin[3] studied 21 patients who had stage 1, 2, and 3 disease and wore the brace an average of 10 hours per day. All patients with stage 1 and 2 disease showed pain relief referable to the brace,

and 60% of patients with stage 3 disease showed similar improvement. Overall, 90% demonstrated statistically significant improvement with the Arizona brace. This thorough study evaluated patients with three separate systems, the American Orthopaedic Foot and Ankle Society (AOFAS) Hindfoot Score, the Foot Function Index, and the SF-36 Health Survey. With all three scoring systems, the Arizona brace demonstrated statistically significant improvement in patient outcome.

If patients reach stage 3 disease, where the deformity is rigid and potentially arthritic, accommodation rather than correction becomes the primary function of the brace. The orthotic or brace is not molded in subtalar neutral. A more supportive device for both the ankle and the foot, such as a thermoplastic solid-ankle AFO, may be required for pain relief (Fig. 19–13). A variety of additional braces, such as the Marzano articulated ankle brace, have been attempted with success in more advanced posterior tibial tendon dysfunction. Patients in stage 4, with arthritic ankle symptoms, require a nonarticulated brace for comfort, such as a solid-ankle AFO. Care must be taken to avoid pressure over bony prominences in patients with more severe valgus deformities. Attempting to correct such a deformity by molding the AFO to negate ankle valgus can place undue pressure across the lateral malleolus, hindfoot, or fifth metatarsal base, causing pain or ulceration.

Footwear modifications can enhance conservative treatment by stabilizing the foot, limiting pronation and strain on the posterior tibial tendon. Measuring

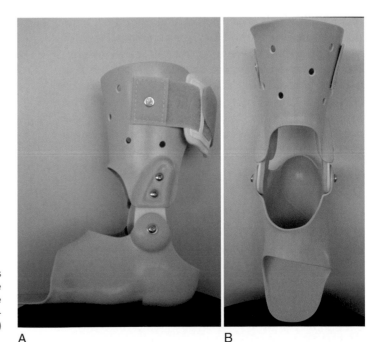

Figure 19–13 An ankle–foot orthosis (AFO). **A,** This device can be used to stabilize both the ankle and the foot in patients with stage 3 disease. **B,** The foot piece can be molded to provide support similar to a University of California Biomechanics Laboratory (UCBL) orthosis.

A   B

the offset heel area[142] can be done with the patient standing in the shoes to be modified, with equal weight on both feet. A straight ruler drops from the medial malleolus to the floor (perpendicular to the floor). This line forms a triangle with a second line drawn to the base of the shoe and a third line drawn from the base of the shoe to the malleolus. This triangle is the offset heel area, which is filled in on the shoe to establish stabilization of the longitudinal arch. According to Streb,[142] this offset should be approximately two thirds of the height of the medial shoe quarter. In addition, the offset can be made more effective by adding 1/8 inch to 1/4 inch additional medial post. Other footwear modifications include flanged heels, extended Thomas heels, and posting the medial heel and sole of the shoe from 1/4 inch to 1/2 inch to create support from heel to toe.

Often overlooked in the athlete with posterior tibial tendon dysfunction is the ability of appropriate shoe management to limit pain and lessen recurrence of tenosynovitis. According to Conti,[14] athletes should wear a running shoe with a flared heel and not run more than 400 miles on any one pair of shoes. Midfoot cushion significantly dissipates after 400 miles, resulting in less arch support, less ability to control pronation, and increased tension on the posterior tibial tendon.

Some authors[62] have suggested that conservative treatment has a limited role in posterior tibial tendon dysfunction, for it gives no relief and can allow the condition to worsen. However, most authors agree that unless a severe structural deformity is present, a 3- to 6-month trial of conservative management is indicated for posterior tibial tendon dysfunction.[5,121,128,144] The treating physician must pay careful attention to the patient, however, to look for signs of progressive deformity. The only circumstance that can cause the clinician to consider operative intervention sooner is in patients afflicted with seronegative spondyloarthropathy and posterior tibial tendon tenosynovitis. Myerson[113] suggests that failure of conservative care over a 6-week period should prompt surgical tenosynovectomy to prevent potential tendon rupture.

Surgical Treatment for Stage 1 Dysfunction

TENOSYNOVECTOMY

Indications

Though indications are defined for tenosynovectomy of the posterior tibial tendon, the procedure is often not necessary. Symptoms often resolve with conservative treatment. Still, in refractory cases, tenosynovectomy is indicated as an isolated procedure in patients with persistent inflammatory symptoms without perceptible deformity of the hindfoot. In stage 1 disease, length of the posterior tibial tendon is normal, and thus repair of the tendon is limited to small longitudinal split tears within the tendon. Timing of tenosynovectomy is influenced by the suspected cause of the condition. Patients with florid tenosynovitis due to conditions such as the seronegative spondyloarthropathies benefit from tenosynovectomy following a 6-week trial of conservative care.[113] In contrast, patients with more classic stage 1 disease, inflammation due to mechanical phenomena or more advanced age, can continue conservative care for up to 3 months before tenosynovectomy is considered.

Contraindications

The main contraindication to performing an isolated tenosynovectomy is disease within the substance of the posterior tibial tendon. Patients with degenerative changes or intrasubstance rupture of the posterior tibial tendon require more advanced procedures. Static deformity apparent through clinical and radiographic examination also warrants more advanced procedures.

Preoperative Evaluation

Direct palpation over the posterior tibial tendon medially elicits pain. The medial ankle might feel boggy or fluctuant over the posterior tibial tendon. Strength testing is normal, though repetitive single-heel rises can reproduce the patient's symptoms of pain. Clinical inspection reveals symmetric feet and ankles, without hindfoot valgus or forefoot abduction. When viewed from behind, however, there may be asymmetric posterior swelling of the medial ankle on the affected side. Radiographs are symmetric with the uninvolved side, though MRI reveals fluid within the tendon sheath on T2-weighted images and a possible longitudinal split tear within the tendon on T1-weighted images. No mucinous degeneration is visible within the substance of the tendon.

Preoperative Planning

Extensive preparation is not required for a tenosynovectomy. Review of the above-mentioned studies is appropriate, particularly the advanced diagnostic studies (MRI or ultrasound) for a potential longitudinal split tear. This is a soft tissue procedure, and thus requests for hardware or power equipment are not necessary.

Surgical Technique

1. The patient is placed in a supine position. The normal external rotation of the extremity provides adequate exposure of the medial aspect of the foot. If that is not the case, placing a rolled bump under the opposite hip provides excellent external rotation of the involved extremity.
2. A thigh tourniquet is suggested to improve visualization of the inflamed tenosynovium.
3. The incision is centered along the course of the posterior tibial tendon. The length of the incision is from the navicular insertion to approximately 4 cm proximal to the tip of the medial malleolus.
4. The tendon sheath is opened with a knife and incised with scissors. In patients with systemic conditions, there is often an effusion of fluid. Patients with degenerative disease causing posterior tibial tendon insufficiency do not have an effusion of fluid.
5. Synovitis is visible as reddish-brown friable tissue adherent to the lining of the tendon sheath as well as to the tendon itself. All such tissue must be removed (Fig. 19–14).
6. The tendon itself is carefully inspected. The surgeon evaluates the tendon for fusiform thickening and visible fissures. In particular, the surgeon must inspect the undersurface of the tendon, because friction in this loca-

tion often causes one or multiple split tears. If a fissure or split tear is noted, it should be repaired with a tubalization suture technique.
7. The surgeon must check the excursion of the tendon. As noted above, the normal excursion of the posterior tibial tendon is 1 to 2 cm. Excursion is easily detectable by marking the tendon at the apex of the medial malleolus and applying manual traction. A definitive number may be measured. If the tendon does not demonstrate this excursion, it is not a stage 1 deformity and therefore requires more aggressive intervention.
8. With respect to disorders, the posterior tibial tendon should be inspected for avulsion from its insertion on the navicular. Though it may be tempting to simply repair the tendon directly to the navicular, often this is not feasible owing to the limited excursion of the tendon and thus the higher failure rate following primary repair. In this instance, a flexor digitorum longus tendon transfer is performed (see later) followed by a side-to-side tenodesis with the nascent posterior tibial tendon. This is the only instance where the native posterior tibial tendon may be preserved, because the tendon itself has no intrasubstance disorders.
9. The sheath is then reapproximated in its entirety, preventing dislocation in the postoperative period. If a tourniquet was used, it is important to deflate it prior to closure to prevent copious scar tissue from compromising the result. The subcutaneous tissue and skin are closed, and the patient is placed in a sugar-tong plaster splint with a posterior mold or in a short-leg cast.

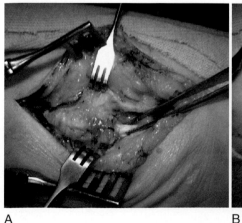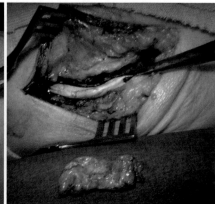

Figure 19–14 Synovitis of the posterior tibial tendon. **A,** Severe synovial proliferation about the posterior tibial tendon. Forceps are on the tendon. **B,** Appearance of the tendon following synovectomy. Synovial tissue that was encircling the tendon is below the wound.

A   B

Postoperative Care

The goal of the postoperative period is to rapidly mobilize the patient (relatively) to limit scar tissue accumulation, maximize excursion, and minimize calf atrophy. The splint or cast is removed at 10 days after surgery, and the sutures are removed. The patient is given a CAM walker boot and begins full weight bearing in this device.

The patient begins physical therapy, with attention directed toward mobilizing the tendon within the sheath. Passive and active range-of-motion therapy begins. Upon complete healing of the surgical incision, deep massage commences to prevent scar accumulation, and iontophoresis may be employed to limit inflammation around the tendon sheath. If scar tissue begins to develop, ultrasound may be used to combat it.

The CAM boot is removed by 6 weeks after surgery to limit calf atrophy and maximize the functional outcome.

Results and Complications

Funk, Cass, and Johnson[36] performed the above-mentioned procedures on 19 patients with stage 1 disease. In this 1986 paper, the authors found that 12 patients experienced complete pain relief, four had minor pain, and three had persistent moderate or severe pain. Subjectively, 11 felt significant improvement, five were somewhat better, and three were the same.

Four patients failed the surgery; three of these patients presented with a complete or partial avulsion of the posterior tibial tendon off of the navicular insertion. The authors postulate that preexisting deformity was not recognized at the time of surgery and that though the tendon proximal to the insertional rupture appeared normal, in fact it was not. Two of these patients later required triple arthrodesis to correct the deformity and eliminate the pain. This honest assessment of their data stresses that the correct surgical procedure must be chosen for this condition. The surgeon must recognize the preoperative deformity and critically assess the quality of the posterior tibial tendon intraoperatively. Failure to do so will result in less-than-adequate surgery and subsequently an unsatisfied patient.

Myerson et al[113] evaluated 76 patients with stage 1 disease caused by seronegative spondy-loarthropathies or by degenerative conditions. Fourteen of these patients underwent tenosynovectomy. All reported both subjective and objective improvement following the debridement. Just over half (57%) were afflicted by seronegative disease. It was clear to the authors that patients with seronegative disorders require earlier surgical debridement if they fail to respond to conservative measures. This type of tenosynovitis was found to be more aggressive intraoperatively and thus had a higher propensity to cause rupture of the posterior tibial tendon if left untreated.

Teasdall and Johnson[147] evaluated 19 patients undergoing tenosynovectomy for stage 1 disease. Fourteen patients experienced complete pain relief, and two complained of moderate to severe pain postoperatively. Again, this operation did not bring 100% pain relief to this population, as only 84% felt "much better" after the procedure. Two patients required subtalar arthrodesis at a later date for progressive deformity and continued pain. These results mirror Johnson's previous work on stage 1 disease and the need for a careful preoperative and intraoperative assessment of the disorder prior to performing a simple tenosynovectomy.

Crates and Richardson[22] evaluated seven patients with stage 1 dysfunction undergoing tenosynovectomy. Three patients required simultaneous repair of a split tear or fissure. None had an inflammatory arthropathy. Follow-up averaged 3.5 months, through which six out of seven patients were pain free. The seventh patient had significant intrasubstance degeneration of the posterior tibial tendon at the time of surgery. The authors still proceeded with a tenosynovectomy and repair of a degenerative split tear. This patient developed progressive deformity and pain, necessitating a lateral column lengthening procedure and flexor digitorum tendon transfer (see later for procedure description) at 1 year following the index procedure. Once again, the tendon must be accurately assessed intraoperatively, with advancement to a more aggressive procedure if indicated. Failure to do so will result in a poor outcome and necessitate additional surgery.

McCormack et al[99] reviewed eight competitive athletes with stage 1 disease undergoing tenosynovectomy at an average age of 22 years. Average time from initial evaluation by the authors to surgical intervention was 8 weeks.

One patient required repair of a longitudinal split tear in the posterior tibial tendon simultaneously. All were allowed to return to sports at 6 to 8 weeks postoperatively. No patient had tenderness or swelling about the posterior tibial tendon on follow-up examination. Telephone interviews were performed at an average of 22 months following the procedure. Seven athletes (88%) continued to participate at their sport without incident. One cited occasional pain while playing football competitively. The authors recommend early intervention in this subset of patients with stage 1 disease following an aggressive trial of conservative care.

Complications for tenosynovectomy of the posterior tibial tendon (and sheath) include infection, nerve damage causing permanent numbness, incisional wound necrosis, progression of deformity and tendon disease, and deep venous thrombosis.

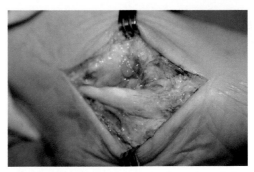

Figure 19–15 Partial avulsion at the insertion of the posterior tibial tendon into the navicular. Note the thickening of the tendon just proximal to the insertion and the way the tendon narrows more proximally.

Surgical Treatment for Stage 2 Dysfunction

The procedures for stage 2 dysfunction will be discussed in tandem. Flexor digitorum longus tendon transfer is rarely done as an isolated procedure. At the very least, it is performed in combination with a calcaneal osteotomy.

FLEXOR DIGITORUM LONGUS TENDON TRANSFER

Indications

Flexor digitorum longus (FDL) tendon transfer is indicated in stage 2 posterior tibial tendon (PTT) dysfunction (Fig. 19–15 and video clip 49). Once incompetence of the posterior tibial tendon is demonstrated, the tendon is nonviable and the diseased segment is unsalvageable. To substitute for this ineffectual tendon, a transfer is required. The FDL tendon has been chosen as the most appropriate tendon to substitute for the PTT, for several reasons. First, the origin of the FDL is the posterior tibia, directly adjacent to the origin of the PTT. These tendons are directly adjacent to each other posterior to the medial malleolus. Thus, they have the same line of pull. Second, although it has only 30% of the strength of the PTT, the FDL matches the

strength of the peroneus brevis (the PTT antagonist). Thus it is capable of balancing the valgus-deforming pull of the peroneus brevis muscle. Third, the FDL and PTT are in-phase muscles (tendons), both functioning primarily in the mid-stance phase of gait. They differ in electromyographic activity, with the PTT functioning for a longer duration than the FDL through each stance phase.[93] Finally, the FDL is expendable owing to its attachment to the flexor hallucis longus, maintaining lesser toe flexion. In addition, a majority of the push-off force during the terminal stance phase occurs through the flexor hallucis longus and the great toe, rather than through the lesser digits.

In order for the FDL tendon transfer to be functional, and thus indicated, two criteria must be met. First, there must be adequate subtalar joint motion to allow the FDL tendon to assist in overcoming the hindfoot valgus posture. Generally, 15 degrees of subtalar inversion is required. The FDL tendon cannot invert against a fixed deformity at the subtalar joint. Second, transverse tarsal motion must also be supple. In the transverse plane, the patient must demonstrate at least 10 degrees of adduction to permit motion that can lock the transverse tarsal joint, allowing heel rise during gait.

Contraindications

Contraindications for the FDL tendon transfer include rigidity to subtalar and transverse tarsal motion to the degree mentioned above. In addition, a relative contraindication is a fixed forefoot varus deformity greater than 10 to 12 degrees. In the past, this was considered an absolute contraindication, because this deformity would cause the subtalar joint to evert during midstance, negating the transfer. However, supplementary procedures, such as an opening-wedge medial cuneiform osteotomy (see later), a closing-wedge plantar flexion first metatarsocuneiform arthrodesis, or a naviculocuneiform arthrodesis to correct the fixed forefoot varus, can establish metatarsal balance and negate the impact of fixed forefoot varus. Symptomatic arthritis of the subtalar, talonavicular, or calcaneocuboid joints is a contraindication for this procedure as well. Age is *not* a contraindication in the active patient. Obesity, however, may be a contraindication owing to the limited power of the tendon transfer to correct valgus deformity. Obese patients with severe valgus deformity and dysfunction of the posterior tibial tendon might obtain better results through triple arthrodesis (see later).

Preoperative Evaluation

The clinician must carefully examine the hindfoot to ensure the supple nature of the joints mentioned above. In addition to direct manipulation, indirect estimates of a supple hindfoot may be determined through observation of a double heel rise (in patients unable to perform a single heel rise). The hindfoot should demonstrate inversion in a double heel rise. It might not be the same degree as that seen on the contralateral extremity, but it should still be visible.

Hindfoot valgus can be assessed with a goniometer while viewing the patient from behind. Holding one limb of the goniometer along the axis of the tibia, while the second limb is placed along the axis of the calcaneus, gives a relative indication of hindfoot valgus deformity. The contralateral limb must be assessed as well. More objective data can be incorporated through the hindfoot alignment view popularized by Saltzman and El-Khoury[130] (see Fig. 19–7). These authors found that 95% of asymptomatic patients have a point of heel-to-floor contact on the calcaneus within 15 mm of the long axis of the tibia. Theoretically, without increased hindfoot valgus, the FDL tendon transfer may be considered as an isolated procedure.

Fixed-forefoot varus is assessed by correcting the hindfoot to neutral with the patient in a seated position. The examiner can then assess for elevation of the first metatarsal head relative to the fifth metatarsal head, which is not passively reducible by derotation of the transverse tarsal joints (see Fig. 19–4).

Standard physical examination and radiographic examination should be performed as noted in prior sections.

Preoperative Planning

Planning for an FDL tendon transfer revolves around assessing the need for supplementary procedures. Once the surgeon has determined that the hindfoot joints are supple enough to warrant the tendon transfer, he or she needs to evaluate the foot and ankle carefully to ensure that the appropriate procedures are done in concert with the transfer. These decisions should be made *preoperatively* rather than intraoperatively, because the transfer itself will distort the architecture of the talonavicular joint, making assessment difficult. These procedures are discussed later.

Thus, in brief, if hindfoot valgus is significant, the surgeon will add a medial-slide calcaneal osteotomy to the procedure. If fixed forefoot varus is present, the surgeon can add a naviculocuneiform rotational arthrodesis to the procedure, or, if arthritis is present at the first metatarsocuneiform joint, a closing-wedge plantar flexion arthrodesis of that joint. If the surgeon corrects the hindfoot to neutral and the Silverskjöld test reveals an isolated gastrocnemius contracture, a Strayer procedure (or variation thereof) will be performed. Finally, if lateral column pain and subfibular impingement are noted, along with significant abduction of the forefoot, a lateral-column lengthening procedure may be considered. Performing any combination of these procedures should be determined *preoperatively* based on physical examination and radiographic appearance.

If an MRI is available, the surgeon should review it to determine the location of the tendinosis or rupture of the posterior tibial tendon. This will ensure that the entire compromised tendon is excised, minimizing the potential for postoperative pain medially.

Surgical Technique

1. The patient is position supine, with the leg externally rotated. A thigh tourniquet is

applied, protected with a 10 × 10-inch adhesive drape to insulate the skin underneath the tourniquet from substances involved in preparing the extremity.

2. The initial incision begins at the tip of the medial malleolus, extending toward the navicular bone. In most circumstances, this incision is extended proximally just posterior to the medial malleolus and along the posterior border of the tibia. This allows exposure of the PTT proximal to the flexor retinaculum.

3. The PTT sheath is opened with a knife. In cases with aggressive synovitis (seronegative disease), an effusion of fluid accompanies this incision. The remaining sheath is then opened with scissors.

4. The tendon is explored to determine the extent of the tendinosis. This varies from fissuring of the tendon to absence of the tendon within the sheath. In chronic situations, the diseased tendon may become adherent to the sheath, making definition of the tendon difficult. The tendon is often exposed proximal to the flexor retinaculum to allow visualization of proximal disease (Fig. 19–16A to D).

5. After confirming tendon disorder, the incision is extended along the medial aspect of the foot, along the dorsal border of the abductor hallucis to the proximal first metatarsal shaft.

6. The entire diseased segment of the posterior tibial tendon is excised. If possible, a 1-cm stump is preserved distally to facilitate attachment of the FDL tendon transfer. Proximally, the tendon is sectioned proximal to the medial malleolus.

7. The lesser toes are flexed and extended while palpating deep to the former posterior tibial tendon, distal to the medial malleolus. Flexing and extending the toes makes the FDL tendon palpable, and a knife is used to incise the sheath.

8. Scissors are used to complete the opening of the sheath proximally. This dissection is carried proximal to the medial malleolus to allow the FDL tendon to assume the position of the former PTT posterior to the medial malleolus.

9. Distally, the abductor hallucis muscle is visualized. The deep fascia is released, and the muscle belly is reflected plantarward. This brings into view the flexor hallucis brevis muscle. The muscle is traced proximally to its origin and released. This maneuver exposes the FDL and FHL tendons, which lie just laterally (Fig. 19–17A and B).

10. The FDL is now traced into the plantar surface of the foot. This is a meticulous dissection, because the plantar veins are always encountered. Bipolar cautery may be used to prevent injury to the branches of the medial plantar nerve. Plantar retraction of the abductor hallucis muscle belly assists in exposure of the FDL tendon. Emphasis is placed on achieving cauterization of all plantar veins surrounding the FDL distally, which will prevent hematoma following release of the tourniquet.

11. The fibrous connection between the FDL and flexor hallucis longus is reached and traced distally as far as possible. A side-to-side tenodesis of the two tendons is carried out.

12. A Krakow-suture weave is placed through the FDL tendon with nonabsorbable suture.

13. The dorsomedial aspect of the navicular bone is exposed by dissecting deep to the dorsal skin flap for a distance of about 2 to 3 cm. The width of the navicular bone is determined by observing the talonavicular bone and naviculocuneiform joints following this dissection. Alternatively, fluoroscopic imaging may be used to localize the most medial portion of the navicular.

14. The location of the tendon transfer is rationally determined by noting the biomechanical axis of the subtalar joint, which is the fulcrum about which the posterior tibial tendon revolves. Physics defines work as *force × distance*, so placing the lever arm of the tendon transfer as far as possible from the fulcrum of the subtalar joint will maximize force. Anatomically, the bone farthest away from this axis is the navicular bone. Therefore, the drill hole placed for the tendon transfer should be made as far medial on the navicular as possible (Fig. 19–17C and D). If a guide wire is available from screws used to secure supplementary procedures such as a calcaneal osteotomy, that guide wire may be inserted into the navicular as far medially as possible. Position is then confirmed by fluoroscopic imaging, followed by drilling with a cannu-

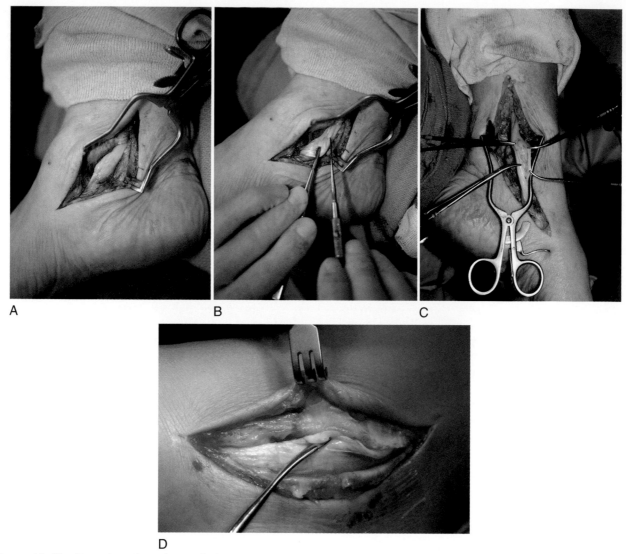

Figure 19–16 Examples of tendon pathology noted in posterior tibial tendon dysfunction. **A,** Grossly thickened tendon. **B,** Underside of tendon demonstrates fissuring. **C,** Marked cavitation of the tendon. **D,** Hypertrophy along the dorsal aspect of the tendon but otherwise minimal pathology observed.

lated drill. This method avoids inadvertent fracture of the bone bridge between the drill hole and the medial cortical wall of the navicular.

15. The inferior surface of the navicular is cleared of soft tissue attachments to facilitate the tendon transfer. Using the previously placed suture in the FDL tendon, the tendon is passed from inferior to superior through the navicular (Fig. 19–17E to F).

16. The tendon transfer is tensioned. The FDL tendon is pulled maximally while adducting the transverse tarsal joints and inverting the subtalar joint. The tendon is then marked at its position with respect to the drill hole in the dorsal navicular. All tension is released, and the tendon is marked on the dorsum of the navicular at this most relaxed state. A tendon transfer is appropriately tensioned by suturing the tendon at a point halfway between both marks. If the tendon is tensioned under maximal pull, the surgeon is functionally creating a tenodesis rather than a tendon transfer. Excursion of the FDL tendon must be maintained, while simultaneously allowing the sarcomeres to function under tension, maximizing pull. Thus, preference is given to tensioning the tendon

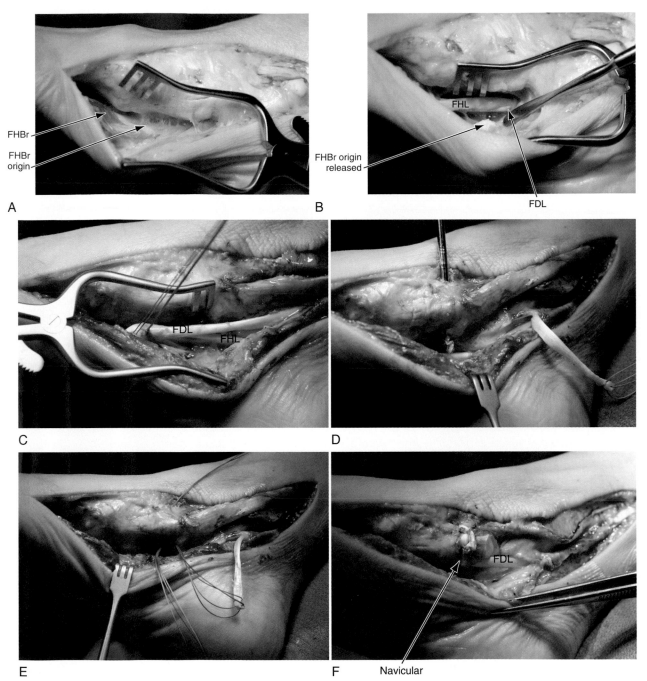

Figure 19–17 Technique of posterior tibial tendon reconstruction using the flexor digitorum longus muscle. **A,** With abductor hallucis muscle retracted plantarward, the flexor hallucis brevis (FHBr) can be visualized. Flexor hallucis brevis origin is a tendinous structure as noted in the picture. **B,** Releasing the flexor hallucis brevis origin brings the flexor hallucis longus (FHL) and the flexor digitorum longus (FDL) tendons into view. **C,** The FDL and FHL tendons are dissected distally and sutured together. The FDL tendon is then released. **D,** A vertical drill hole is made in the tarsal navicular in its medial portion. Bringing the drill through the soft tissues beneath it makes it easier to thread the tendon through the bone. **E,** The suture is passed through the hole in the navicular and the FDL tendon is pulled through the navicular, bringing the foot into some adduction and inversion. **F,** FDL tendon has been passed through the navicular and sutured to the surrounding periosteum.

halfway between maximal and minimal tension.

17. The tendon may be sutured back upon itself, if possible, under this tension. Alternatively, it is sutured to the PTT tendon stump inferiorly, and the portion placed through the drill hole is kept within the drill hole by using the previously placed Krakow suture, anchoring it to superior soft tissue (Figure 19–17F). All sutures should be nonabsorbable.

18. The proximally sectioned PTT is now evaluated. This portion is grasped firmly with a clamp, and the excursion is evaluated. If the muscle is noted to be viable proximally through adequate excursion, a side-to-side tenodesis with non-absorbable suture is performed with the FDL tendon. This is done proximal to the medial malleolus, to avoid impingement within the pulley posterior and inferior to that structure. As a general rule, younger patients with systemic or traumatic conditions causing PTT insufficiency retain viable proximal muscle, warranting tenodesis. Older patients with chronic degenerative ruptures often have poor-quality muscle proximally, which would negate the effect of the FDL tendon transfer by creating a tenodesis effect.

19. The tourniquet is now released to ensure adequate hemostasis and minimize scar tissue. The sheath is closed in its entirety with absorbable suture, the abductor hallucis fascia is reapproximated, and the subcutaneous tissue and skin are closed in a standard manner.

20. The patient is placed into a below knee cast, or sugar-tong splint with a posterior mold, in slight adduction and equinus. Immobilization does not require positioning the foot in the extremes of these planes, because the surgeon has ensured strong attachment of the tendon to the bone intraoperatively. Excessive positioning in plantar flexion and inversion can lead to rigidity not recoverable through physical therapy. It is appropriate to have some tension on the sarcomeres of the FDL muscle belly to limit atrophy during immobilization.

Postoperative Care

The patient is kept immobilized for 6 weeks of non–weight bearing on this extremity. This restriction on weight bearing is more often due to the supplementary procedures performed at the time of the FDL tendon transfer than to the transfer itself.

Following this immobilization, the patient is placed into a CAM walker boot, and physical therapy is instituted. It is important that the surgeon have a working relationship with the physical therapist so that a protocol can be followed. Overly aggressive physical therapy, such as early institution of a heel rise, can damage the tendon transfer and lead to failure of the procedure. The patient may bear full weight in the CAM boot and begins inversion strengthening with a resistance band (Thera-Band). In the first few weeks, standing balance exercises (with 25% of the weight borne on the opposite foot) may be instituted, allowing recruitment of the tendon transfer without stressing the repair. Gentle forward lunges may also be incorporated. At 9 weeks after surgery, the patient may begin leg presses on a weight machine (such as a Total Gym), with bilateral squats and double-heel rises with the plane of the bench at 30 degrees of elevation from supine. The incline is gradually increased, until 12 to 14 weeks postoperatively, the patient is standing to do these maneuvers. Activation of the tendon transfer early (without stressing the transfer) prevents the patient from delayed progression of rehabilitation upon removal from the CAM boot. Single heel rise is avoided until 3 to 4 months after surgery.

At 12 weeks after surgery, the patient may progress to a commercially available lace-up sport brace for an additional month.

Results and Complications

Studies on isolated flexor digitorum longus tendon transfer are few. Michelson et al[101] found that 50% of isolated soft-tissue reconstructions failed within one year. Other authors have not had such a dismal experience, but they admit that the indications for an isolated FDL tendon transfer are narrow.

Mann and Thompson[97] reviewed seventeen patients (14 FDL tendon transfers, 3 PTT advancements) with stage 2 posterior tibial tendon dysfunction. Twelve of their patients had an excellent result (pain free, excellent strength), one noted a good result (pain free, some loss of strength), three had a fair result (good function with persistent pain), and one had a poor result that was revised to fusion. Correction of flatfoot with an isolated transfer was not so successful, because only four achieved correction, with seven improved and four unchanged. Two patients deteriorated with respect to correction. Average follow-up for this study was 33 months. There was no difference in time of follow-up between all stratifications of results. Finally, there is no mention in the paper of a difference between the FDL tendon transfer and the PTT advancement with respect to clinical outcome.

Mann et al[92] reviewed 73 patients (75 feet) undergoing isolated FDL transfer for stage 2 disease. The average age of these patients was 54 years (range, 20 to 72 years). The mean follow-up was 73 months. The patient satisfaction demonstrated that 64 patients (88%) were satisfied and 11 (15%) were dissatisfied. Of the 11 patients who were dissatisfied, seven had either a fixed hindfoot valgus deformity or fixed forefoot varus in excess of 15 degrees. The strength of the transfer was always rated as 4 or 5 (good or normal). In the patients with no fixed deformity, the satisfaction index averaged 4.28, in which maximum satisfaction was 5, and the AOFAS score was 87. In patients who had a fixed forefoot varus deformity of greater than 15 degrees or fixed hindfoot valgus, the satisfaction index averaged 1.8 and the AOFAS score was 40.

Factors that negatively affected the results were fixed forefoot varus or fixed hindfoot valgus. Factors that were neutral (did not affect outcome) were greater than 60 months of follow-up; age greater than or equal to 60 years; spring ligament reconstruction, which was carried out in 26 or 75 feet; a proximal tenodesis of the remaining posterior tibial tendon into the tendon transfer above the malleolus; and body weight more than 40 pounds over ideal.

Mann[91] reiterated the necessity of appropriate indications of an isolated FDL tendon transfer in a more recent article in 2001. At the conclusion of this article, he agreed that flatfoot is not corrected by this procedure in isolation. He also noted that in his series of more than 100 isolated tendon transfers, less than 5% have required subsequent fusion at long-term follow-up. When he did not adhere to the indications mentioned above (i.e., supple subtalar and transverse tarsal joints without fixed forefoot supination), fully 90% of his patients required revision to a fusion at a later date. Mann also states that a medial slide calcaneal osteotomy is required with the index procedure approximately 80% of the time owing to increased hindfoot valgus.

CALCANEAL OSTEOTOMY

As noted earlier, the flexor digitorum longus transfer is rarely done as an isolated procedure. Most studies with follow-up on this procedure incorporate a medial slide calcaneal osteotomy. The idea of shifting the calcaneus or mechanically changing the axis of the calcaneus in order to restore a more neutral position of the hindfoot was first described by Gleich[40] in 1893. Dwyer[31] added interposition bone graft into the osteotomy to treat flatfoot in cerebral palsy in 1959. It was Koutsogiannis[77] who first suggested that sliding the calcaneus medially will improve outcome in flexible pes planus. This idea was resurrected in the mid-1990s and has now been supported by numerous clinical studies (see later).

Biomechanically, the purpose of the calcaneal osteotomy is twofold: First, it shifts the mechanical pull of the Achilles tendon medially, which both supports the relatively weak FDL tendon transfer and improves inversion power. Second, it shifts the weight-bearing axis of the heel closer to the long axis of the tibia. This theoretically lowers the risk of progressive valgus deformity following tendon transfer.

Cadaveric studies have explored the calcaneal osteotomy and its relationship to correcting posterior tibial tendon insufficiency and hindfoot valgus. Nyska et al[115] used ten cadaveric limbs with normal longitudinal arches to define the value of the calcaneal osteotomy with respect to the contribution of altering Achilles tendon function. The authors radiographically tested the cadavers in various stages, progressing from an unloaded foot with a normal longitudinal arch through creation of a flatfoot deformity, loading the Achilles tendon, and finally through a medial slide calcaneal osteotomy. The authors found that loading the Achilles tendon in a flatfoot model increased the flatfoot deformity. They found that the addition of a medial slide calcaneal osteotomy improved the flatfoot deformity radiographically. More important, loading the Achilles tendon following the medial slide calcaneal osteotomy did *not* increase the flatfoot deformity. From these results, the authors surmised the calcaneal osteotomy has the added effect of preventing further flatfoot deformity by eliminating the negative effect of Achilles tendon load on progressive flatfoot.

Sung et al[143] evaluated the ability of the medial slide calcaneal osteotomy to decrease the force required for the posterior tibial tendon to achieve early heel rise. The authors used 13 cadaveric limbs mounted to a loading apparatus to measure the force required by the posterior tibial tendon to achieve early heel rise (defined as 7 degrees of calcaneal plantar flexion and 5 degrees of calcaneal inversion) with and without a medial slide calcaneal osteotomy. Prior to calcaneal osteotomy, the force required for the posterior tibial tendon to achieve these parameters was 399 N. The statistically significant decrease in force required following medial slide calcaneal osteotomy was 329 N. This effect was confirmed by noting that the Achilles tendon force required to achieve heel rise decreased from 1012 N to 981 N following medial slide calcaneal osteotomy. Again, cadaveric results support the calcaneal osteotomy in improving the outcome of FDL tendon transfer.

Finally, Hadfield et al[48] evaluated pressure changes in the forefoot following medial displacement calcaneal osteotomy. Using 14 cadaveric limbs, they employed a pressure-sensitive mat to evaluate plantar foot pressures in loaded specimens both before and after medial displacement calcaneal osteotomy. The authors found a statistically significant decrease in pressure under the first and second metatarsals. The authors postulate that this alteration in load was directly due to increased pull of the Achilles tendon medially. Though not correlated clinically, this study suggests a detrimental effect of calcaneal osteotomy in patients with forefoot varus, because the lateral pressure on the metatarsal increases with the procedure.

Indications

The medial slide calcaneal osteotomy is never done as an isolated procedure in posterior tibial tendon dysfunction. It is always done in combination with the FDL tendon transfer, and thus the indications for that technique coincide with the indications for calcaneal osteotomy. However, one additional indication for the calcaneal osteotomy is a flexible hindfoot valgus deformity that is of greater magnitude when compared to the opposite extremity (Fig. 19–18A and video clip 50).

Contraindications

Again, contraindications are similar to those for the FDL tendon transfer. Risk of difficulty in healing the lateral incision should be assessed preoperatively with noninvasive arterial Doppler studies if suspicion is present.

Preoperative Evaluation

The patient is evaluated for supple hindfoot valgus by manual examination and the double heel rise. The magnitude of valgus deformity may be measured by the technique described earlier.

Preoperative Planning

The hindfoot alignment view can assist in determining the magnitude of correction required by shift of the posterior tuberosity.

Surgical Technique

1. The patient is placed into a lateral decubitus position. It is helpful to place the patient on a bean bag so the patient can be easily rolled into a supine position intraoperatively. This will facilitate the FDL tendon transfer and any additional medial procedures following the calcaneal osteotomy. A thigh tourniquet is applied, protected with a 10- × 10-inch adhesive drape to insulate the skin underneath the tourniquet from substances involved in preparing the extremity.
2. The incision begins proximally at the superior aspect of the posterior tuberosity of the calcaneus, anterior to the Achilles tendon insertion, and posterior to the peroneal tendons (Fig. 19–18B). Practically, this is approximately 1 cm posterior to the fibula and 2 cm proximal to the superior aspect of the calcaneus. This incision extends distally at a 45-degree angle with the plantar surface of the foot. Alternatively, the small fluoroscopy unit that will be used to assess

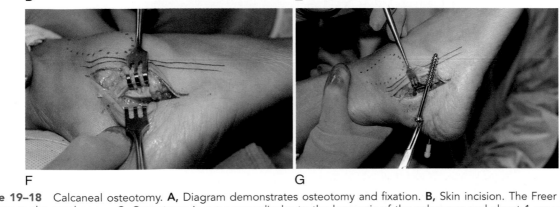

Figure 19–18 Calcaneal osteotomy. **A,** Diagram demonstrates osteotomy and fixation. **B,** Skin incision. The Freer elevator is pointing to the sural nerve. **C,** Osteotomy is cut perpendicular to the long axis of the calcaneus and about 1 cm posterior to the posterior facet of the calcaneus. **D,** Upon completion of the osteotomy, a wide osteotome is used to open the osteotomy site. **E,** A lamina spreader is used to open the osteotomy site so that the periosteum on the medial side can be gently teased off the bone. **F,** Medial displacement of the osteotomy site of about 1 cm. **G,** The partially threaded screw is used to fix the osteotomy site. Preferably the threads will all be on the distal part of the osteotomy.

the cut line and position of the calcaneal tuberosity may also be used to confirm the location of the incision.

3. The sural nerve will invariably be encountered, normally anterior to the surgical approach. Thus, initial dissection is done with scissors dissection until the nerve is mobilized anteriorly. Following retraction of the nerve safely out of the surgical field, dissection may proceed with a scalpel directly to the bone of the calcaneus. While stripping the periosteum off of the lateral wall, care is taken to avoid detachment of the insertion of the calcaneofibular ligament.

4. Again, using a mini-fluoroscopy unit is helpful to confirm location of the osteotomy in order to ensure that the osteotomy will be anterior enough to create a significant shift of the posterior tuberosity while allowing adequate bone distally (anteriorly) for screw fixation. Generally, the plane of the osteotomy is slightly posterior to the peroneal tendon sheath. The plane is perpendicular to the longitudinal axis of the calcaneus, or at an approximate 45-degree angle from the plantar surface of the foot.

5. Prior to the cut, small Hohman retractors are placed at the superior location of the osteotomy to protect the Achilles tendon, and at the inferior aspect of the osteotomy to protect the plantar fascia and lateral plantar nerve branches.

6. The cut is made with a wide and long blade from a macro-sagittal oscillating saw. This allows a smooth cut to be made through the soft cancellous bone of the calcaneus. The lateral wall is scored first, followed by penetration to the medial cortex. Upon reaching the medial cortex, the saw blade is gently bounced off the medial wall until it penetrates. Caution while penetrating the medial cortex is critical. The palm of the surgeon's opposite hand may be placed on the medial hindfoot to assist in determining penetration of the saw blade. Greene et al[45] studied the medial neurovascular anatomy in relation to the calcaneal osteotomy. The authors found, on average, that four neurovascular structures crossed the osteotomy site. Most were branches of the lateral plantar nerve and posterior tibial artery. The most common branches of the lateral

plantar nerve at risk were the calcaneal sensory branch and the second branch. The medial plantar nerve was not at risk.

7. Following completion of the osteotomy, a 25-mm straight osteotome is inserted into the plane of the cut, gently distracting the surfaces (Fig. 19–18C and D). A smooth lamina spreader is also inserted to distract the osteotomy site (Fig. 19–18E). Care must be taken to avoid crushing the soft bone of the calcaneus with this device. The medial periosteum is then freed with the use of a Freer elevator.

8. With the posterior tuberosity now mobile, the ankle is placed on an elevated bump, and the knee is flexed to release gastrocnemius tension. This allows medial translation of the posterior tuberosity without superior migration from Achilles tendon pull. Generally, the magnitude of the shift is 1 cm (Fig. 19–18F and G).

9. Provisional fixation of the osteotomy is done with an 0.062-inch Kirschner wire followed by placement of the guide wire from the cannulated screw system. The wire is placed laterally in the posterior tuberosity in order to accommodate the medial shift and stay within the anterior calcaneus (Fig. 19–18G). The mini-fluoroscopy unit can be used to ensure the appropriate placement of this guide wire on the sagittal and axial planes. The axial image can be used to determine the appropriate magnitude of tuberosity shift. The lateral image can be used to ensure that the posterior tuberosity is not superiorly or inferiorly translated. One large cannulated screw is acceptable. The contact surface of the osteotomy is large and the bone is cancellous. Thus the union rate is high.

10. The overhanging edge is beveled with a chisel and rasped smooth. Bone wax may be applied to this exposed surface to minimize adherent scar.

11. The tourniquet is released, and hemostasis is achieved to minimize hematoma formation. During closure, it is important to avoid entrapment of the sural nerve. This will create a painful neuroma or sensory deficit (or both) in the lateral foot.

12. The bean bag is released, allowing the patient to assume a supine position for the additional medial procedures.

Postoperative Care

No additional treatment besides that mentioned for the FDL tendon transfer is required for the calcaneal osteotomy. The postoperative protocol is not altered by addition of this technique.

Results and Complications

Results of the medial slide calcaneal osteotomy are based on its use in conjunction with the flexor digitorum longus tendon transfer (Fig. 19-19).

Myerson and Corrigan[112] reviewed 32 patients treated with a medial slide calcaneal osteotomy and FDL tendon transfer. Mean follow-up was 20 months. Thirty (94%) were satisfied with the outcome of the procedure, exhibiting pain relief, arch improvement, and return to normal footwear without orthotic support. Of this group, 28 (88%) experienced no pain, 3 (9%) had mild pain, and 1 had persistent pain. The last patient eventually underwent triple arthrodesis for progressive deformity and pain. By 6 months, 78% were able to perform a single heel rise, and by 12 months 88% were able to do so. Radiographic improvements were noted, with the AP talometatarsal angle improving from 26 degrees to 6 degrees and the complementary lateral angle improving from 28 degrees to 13 degrees. The talonavicular coverage angle improved from 37 degrees to 15 degrees.

Guyton et al[47] evaluated 26 patients undergoing a medial slide calcaneal osteotomy in combination with an FDL tendon transfer at an average of 36 months after surgery. Pain relief was rated excellent by 75% and good by 16%. Twenty-three (88%) could perform a single heel rise at the time of follow-up. Of the three who could not perform this maneuver, two had failures of fixation of the FDL tendon transfer, necessitating late subtalar arthrodesis. The third patient failed the procedure late, following pregnancy nearly 6 years after the index procedure. Eliminating those requiring subtalar fusion, subtalar motion averaged 81% of the contralateral (normal) extremity. Radiographic assessment showed an improvement in the AP talometatarsal angle from 21 degrees to 7 degrees and the lateral talometatarsal angle from 20 degrees to 13 degrees. Talonavicular coverage improved from 22 degrees to 10 degrees. Similar to Myerson's results, radio-

graphic improvement was present, but complete correction was not provided by these procedures. Only 50% of patients felt the conformation of their foot had noticeably changed, and only one (4%) found the improvement significant. Finally, the median length of time to the patient's rating of maximal improvement was 10 months.

Fayazi et al[34] reviewed 23 patients undergoing both calcaneal osteotomy and FDL tendon transfer at an average of 35 months. Twenty-two patients (96%) were subjectively better, one (4%) was the same. Objectively, AOFAS scores on 21 patients evaluated in person (the rest were by telephone) improved from 50 to 89. Two (9%) were able to perform a single heel rise prior to surgery, 18 (78%) were able to perform this postoperatively. Twenty-one (91%) stated they would have the procedure again (one unsatisfied patient was under workers' compensation, the second sustained a deep venous thrombosis postoperatively).

Wacker et al[153] reviewed 48 patients undergoing the procedures. Twenty-five (52%) were completely satisfied, 19 (40%) were satisfied with minor reservations, two (4%) were satisfied with reservations, and two (4%) were dissatisfied. The latter two had revision to calcaneocuboid arthrodesis. Visual analogue scores for pain noted an improvement from 7.3 to 1.7. Although improvement in visible alignment was noted in 92%, only 25% had fair clinical alignment. Sixteen required orthoses following the operation.

Myerson et al[111] reviewed 129 patients undergoing the procedure at an average of 5.2 years postoperatively. An assessment of strength with a dynamometer designed for torque measurements of concentric and eccentric muscle action revealed 95 patients (74%) experienced inversion and plantar flexion strength symmetric with the contralateral (normal) extremity. Eighteen patients (14%) were mildly weak (<25% of normal), and four (3%) were moderately weak (>50% loss of strength). With respect to the opposite extremity, subtalar motion was normal in 56 (44%), slightly decreased in 66 (51%), and moderately decreased in 7 (5%) patients. Most patients (108, 84%) were able to wear normal shoes without orthotic support. Radiographic assessment noted an improvement in the AP talometatarsal angle from 25 degrees to 6 degrees and the lateral talometatarsal angle

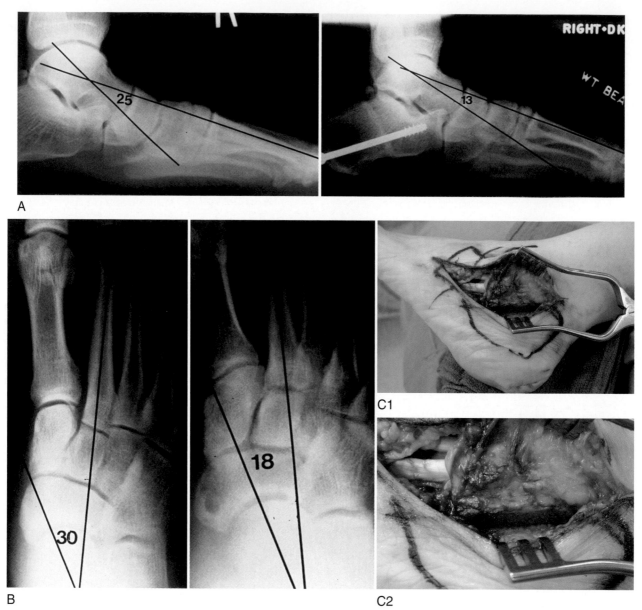

Figure 19–19   A, Preoperative and postoperative lateral radiographs demonstrating correction obtained following a medial displacement calcaneal osteotomy. **B,** Preoperative and postoperative anteroposterior (AP) radiographs demonstrate correction of the flatfoot deformity following a calcaneal osteotomy. **C,** Intraoperative photographs demonstrate the 1-cm medial shift normally performed for the procedure.

from 27 degrees to 12 degrees. Talonavicular coverage improved from 37 degrees to 16 degrees. A positive subjective outcome was directly related to radiographic improvement. The mean time to self-rated maximal improvement was 14 months.

Complications include sural nerve neuritis or neuroma, infection, incisional wound necrosis, overcorrection (varus hindfoot), nonunion and malunion (rare), injury to medial neurovascular structures (see earlier), peroneal tendon adhesions, hardware irritation, and deep venous thrombosis.

SPRING LIGAMENT REPAIR AND RECONSTRUCTION

Spring ligament insufficiency or disruption has been implicated in progressive deformity following posterior tibial tendon rupture. The spring ligament is made up of two distinct structures: the larger superomedial calcaneonavicular ligament and the inferior calcaneonavicular portion. The inferior ligament plays a minor role in arch stabilization. In advanced posterior tibial tendon dysfunction, abnormalities within the spring ligament may be seen in 92% of MRI examinations of the ankle.[4] Thus, recognition and repair of this structure is considered in conjunction with the procedures discussed earlier (not as an isolated procedure).

Indications

Spring ligament repair is indicated if rupture is visible or laxity is noted upon direct inspection intraoperatively. Indications for reconstruction of the ligament with allograft or autograft tendon weave procedures include chronic, degenerative tissue in the residual spring ligament that would preclude healing with primary repair.

Contraindications

The only relative contraindication to primary spring ligament repair is a long-standing rupture composed of degenerated ligament tissue. In that instance, ligament reconstruction with allograft or autograft may be considered.

Preoperative Evaluation

If available, the MRI is a useful adjunct to planning spring ligament repair, due to both its sen-

sitivity and specificity. The location and the poor quality of the tissue can be mapped out, assisting the surgeon in ensuring that healing will depend only on good-quality tissue following removal of this poor-quality ligament. In patients with severe abduction of the forefoot or plantar flexion of the talus, strong suspicion for ligament injury is present. This is visible both on radiographs of the foot and ankle and on clinical examination with a lax talonavicular joint.

Preoperative Planning

Major planning is not required for spring ligament repair unless the surgeon believes that the ligament has insufficiency that would warrant a tendon weave procedure (see later). In that instance, it is critical to plan incisions in locations where the proposed autograft tendon may be harvested. In addition, patient positioning becomes important. If one is going to harvest the peroneus longus tendon for a graft, this should be done while the patient is in the lateral position undergoing the medial slide calcaneal osteotomy.

Surgical Technique for Spring Ligament Repair

1. The medial incision used for FDL tendon transfer is used for plication of the ligament.
2. The easiest and strongest method to repair the spring ligament is through a transverse incision, without excising redundant tissue
3. Closure is done through a pants-over-vest suture. The foot is held in position with the talonavicular joint reduced, and markings are made on the ligament, outlining the overlap of the redundant ligament.
4. Nonabsorbable suture is then placed from the distal segment to the proximal mark. A second set of nonabsorbable sutures is placed from the proximal segment to the distal mark.
5. These sutures are not tied until the flexor digitorum longus tendon is brought through the hole drilled into the navicular. This prevents undue tension on the spring ligament repair. In fact, the appropriate tension to be applied to the FDL tendon transfer (see above) should be done before tying the spring ligament sutures (i.e., the FDL tendon must be marked at the appropriate tension as well). Once the FDL tendon is brought through the

drill hole, the ligament sutures are tied. The FDL tendon is then secured to the stump of the posterior tibial tendon, during which time the assistant continues to hold the talonavicular joint in reduction.

6. This method has value in that it is a reinforced approach to repairing the ligament. Simply excising the redundant segment and repairing the ligament end to end has a potentially higher rate of failure owing to the compromised tissue.

Surgical Technique for Spring Ligament Reconstruction

Before contemplating this method of reconstructing the spring ligament, the surgeon must realize that all studies concerning tendon weave procedures are purely cadaveric. No clinical studies have been presented to date. The most recent study[11] on tendon reconstruction for this disorder uses a peroneus longus tendon graft.

1. A curved incision is made along the posterior border of the fibula and carried toward the inferior portion of the cuboid bone.
2. The peroneus longus is freed from any soft tissue attachments, from the posterior fibula to the inferior surface of the cuboid. The tendon is then sectioned as far proximal as possible to maximize graft length.
3. The medial incision is a distal extension of the incision made for the flexor digitorum longus tendon transfer. This incision is extended to the middle of the first metatarsal.
4. The base of the first metatarsal is exposed from medial to lateral, exposing (but not detaching) the insertion of the peroneus longus tendon.
5. The peroneus longus is pulled from lateral to medial, through the plantar surface of the foot. It remains attached to its insertion.
6. The sustentaculum tali is identified in the medial calcaneus. The flexor hallucis longus tendon is retracted inferiorly, and a drill hole is made from the inferior surface of the sustentaculum tali directed transversely and slightly posteriorly, such that it exits just inferior and posterior to the lateral malleolus.
7. The tendon is passed through this drill hole from medial to lateral.

8. The assistant places tension on this tendon while restoring the alignment of the talonavicular joint. The tendon is then secured on the lateral surface of the calcaneus with a screw and spiked ligament washer.
9. A second drill hole is made 1 cm posterior and parallel to the prior drill hole, this time from lateral to medial.
10. The peroneus longus tendon graft is passed from lateral to medial.
11. A drill hole (separate from the drill hole for the FDL reconstruction) is made within the navicular, and the peroneus longus tendon graft is passed from superior to inferior and sutured back upon itself.

This method reconstructs both the superomedial and plantar (inferior) components of the spring ligament.

Results and Complications

Goldner[41] presented the first concept of the medial ligaments as a factor in acquired flatfoot deformity. His surgical technique involved creating a tongue of tissue out of the plantar calcaneonavicular ligament, advancing it proximally, and plicating it with nonabsorbable sutures. The ligament repair was then reinforced with the tendon graft used to reconstruct the insufficient posterior tibial tendon. Six patients were included in this review, all with acquired flatfoot from either traumatic disruption of the posterior tibial tendon or degenerative rupture. Goldner states that this procedure provided satisfactory function and avoidance of a triple arthrodesis. No further objective data were provided in this review.

Gazdag et al[37] evaluated 18 patients with evidence of spring ligament injury noted during reconstruction for posterior tibial tendon insufficiency. The authors found that seven patients had a longitudinal tear within the ligament complex, seven had laxity without obvious tear, and four demonstrated complete rupture. They created a grading system with grades 1, 2, and 3 corresponding to these three clinical observations (respectively). Grade 1 tears were repaired with a few nonabsorbable sutures. Of patients with grade 2 and grade 3 tears, six underwent reconstruction with the use of half of the anterior tibial tendon.

The anterior tibial tendon was detached proximally and passed through a drill hole in the navicular from superior to inferior and anchored to the sustentaculum tali with a bone anchor. Four additional patients had the interrupted nonabsorbable sutures supplemented with the stump of the resected posterior tibial tendon. Use of fibers from the superficial deltoid ligament to supplement grade 2 and grade 3 tears was discontinued owing to lack of strength. Fourteen (78%) had an excellent result, with dramatic pain relief and restoration of function. Two (11%) had a fair result, with mild pain medially and limitations in walking beyond six blocks. Two (11%) had a poor result. One of these patients developed reflex sympathetic dystrophy and arthritic changes in the talonavicular joint. The second patient had osteoarthritis of both the talonavicular and subtalar joints. The results were not consistent with the grade; the four patients with a grade 3 tear all had an excellent result. Grade 1 and grade 2 patients both demonstrated five excellent, one fair, and one poor result. The authors emphasize the importance of evaluating for and repairing the deficiency in this ligament during reconstruction for posterior tibial tendon insufficiency.

Mann[92] found no difference between repairing and not repairing the spring ligament in 75 patients, of whom 26 underwent spring ligament repair. The repair technique employed was not discussed in this presentation.

Choi et al[11] found in a biomechanical study that the peroneus longus tendon graft functioned best when the entire reconstruction was performed (i.e., both the superomedial and inferior portions). The authors tested cadavers with three circumstances: superomedial reconstruction only, inferior reconstruction only, and both superomedial and inferior reconstruction. Reconstruction was performed after creating a flatfoot model by sectioning the superomedial and inferior portions of the spring ligament, the interosseous ligament, and the medial talonavicular joint capsule. The authors admit the concern that detachment of the peroneus longus tendon might allow dorsiflexion of the first ray, accentuating flatfoot deformity. Thus, they reiterate the importance of fixing the tendon graft under tension to maintain the declination of the first metatarsal in a static fashion.

PLANTAR FLEXION OPENING WEDGE OSTEOTOMY OF THE MEDIAL CUNEIFORM

This procedure, first mentioned by Cotton[18] was created to "restore the triangle of support of the static foot." Its applicability in patients with adult acquired flatfoot deformity lies in its use as an adjunct procedure, assisting in correcting forefoot varus and improving declination of the first ray to restore a normal talar–first metatarsal angle.

Indications

This osteotomy is indicated in patients with fixed forefoot varus. In particular, following reconstruction with a lateral column lengthening procedure (see later), if the patient has elevation of the first ray with respect to the adjacent metatarsals, this procedure creates metatarsal balance. In addition, in patients with severe midfoot sag at the level of the naviculo-cuneiform joints, in which fusion has a high rate of nonunion, this procedure more predictably creates elevation of the arch and restoration of a clinically plantigrade foot.

Contraindications

This procedure is contraindicated in patients with osteoarthritis of the first metatarsocuneiform joint. These patients are better served with an arthrodesis of this joint through a closing wedge osteotomy. Patients with gapping at the plantar surface of the first metatarsocuneiform joint from hypermobility are better served with an arthrodesis of this joint.

Preoperative Evaluation

Patients are examined in both a seated and standing position for fixed forefoot varus. Correction of the subtalar joint to neutral reveals a rigid elevation of the first ray. Palpation of the plantar metatarsal heads while correcting the hindfoot to neutral reveals the magnitude of this elevation. Adequate vascularity must be present in the distal foot to support healing of the bone graft. Thus, noninvasive Doppler studies with toe pressures are helpful in this evaluation.

Preoperative Planning

Once again, thought should be given to incision placement. The incision for this osteotomy is dorsally based. One should not carry the medial incision for the FDL transfer too distal in order to avoid an insufficient skin bridge and encourage necrosis. Alternatively, if the medial incision must be carried distally, the incision should curve plantarward near the medial cuneiform to maximize this skin bridge. Planning for bone graft comes in the form of autograft, where the appropriate amount of iliac crest must be excised, or allograft, where a bone block is both structural and useful.

Surgical Technique

1. The patient is in a supine position, with the foot vertical (not internally or externally rotated).
2. A dorsal incision is made overlying the medial cuneiform (Fig. 19–20C).
3. The extensor hallucis longus is retracted medially, and dissection proceeds to the medial cuneiform. Care is taken to avoid the deep peroneal nerve and the dorsalis pedis artery.
4. Fluoroscopic imaging is used to locate the middle of the medial cuneiform, the location of the osteotomy.
5. A transverse osteotomy is made with a micro-sagittal saw from dorsal to plantar. The osteotomy should violate the deep plantar cortex.
6. A straight osteotome placed dorsal to plantar is used to lever the medial cuneiform open at the osteotomy site.
7. The width of the dorsal base of the graft can be determined by either or both of two methods. The assistant wedges the dorsal cuneiform open with an osteotome until the surgeon feels a precise balance to the metatarsal heads, and the dorsal gap is measured. It is important to measure the depth of the graft as well, to create an interference fit. The second method involves wedging the medial cuneiform open under a lateral fluoroscopic image and looking for appropriate declination of the first metatarsal. Once this is achieved, the dorsal gap is measured.
8. The bone graft is harvested in a standard fashion, or the allograft is soaked in antibiotic solution and used.
9. After interposition of the appropriate graft size, lateral fluoroscopic radiographs may be used to ensure excellent fit and appro-

priate talus–first metatarsal angle. If the fit is not precise, the surgeon can improve the fit by inserting the saw blade from the micro-sagittal saw into the osteotomy site (proximally and distally) with the graft in place and create a perfect fit by dorsal-to-plantar cutting with the blade. This technique is very helpful, but it must be done carefully to prevent shortening the graft or altering the shape of the wedge.
10. This graft is stable and thus does not require fixation. However, the surgeon can use a cannulated screw from dorsal–distal to plantar–proximal or a compression staple.
11. The wound is closed in layers.

Postoperative Care

The patient wears a short-leg cast for 6 weeks. Weight bearing is restricted until both surfaces of the wedge have incorporated (fused) with the surfaces of the medial cuneiform. If necessary, a CT scan may be used for confirmation.

Results and Complications

The only study in the literature looking specifically at this osteotomy used in conjunction with an adult-acquired flatfoot deformity and pediatric congenital flatfoot comes from Hirose and Johnson.[54] Using the above-mentioned technique, the authors reviewed 16 feet undergoing the procedure. Two separate populations were studied, adult and pediatric. The average time to union was 7 weeks in the pediatric population and 12 weeks in the adult population. The authors noted a statistically significant improvement in the lateral talus–first metatarsal angle, the calcaneal pitch, and the medial cuneiform-to-floor height. They also noted the power of this procedure to correct a wide range of forefoot varus through adjustment in wedge width and taper.

Complications include painful hardware due to the lack of fat providing cushioning between the skin and hardware in this portion of the foot; neuroma of the superficial peroneal nerve, deep peroneal nerve, and saphenous nerve; and nonunion. The Cotton osteotomy is useful in both primary reconstruction and revision surgery, where failure of the index procedure can achieve success through its powerful ability to correct the medial longitudinal arch (Fig. 19–21).

Text continued on p. 1059

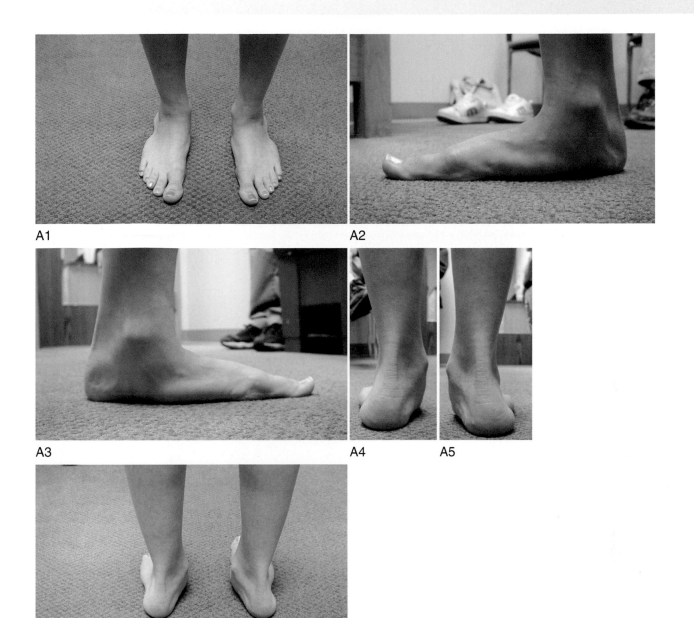

A1

A2

A3

A4   A5

A6

Figure 19–20 Cotton osteotomy used in primary reconstruction. **A,** Preoperative clinical photographs of a severe flatfoot deformity **(A2** and **A3),** with hindfoot valgus **(A4** and **A5)** and subfibular impingement **(A1** and **A6).** This deformity is flexible and remained painful with orthotic management.

Continued

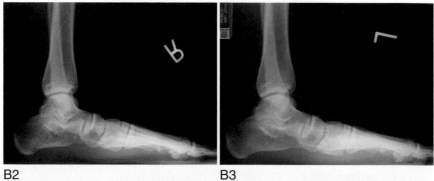

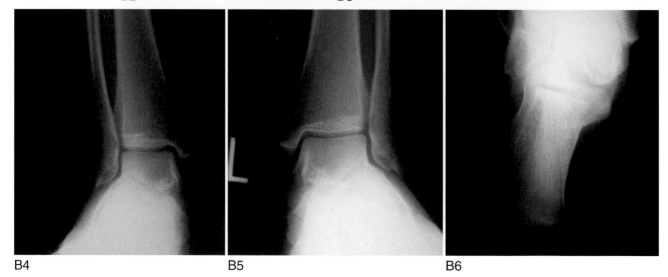

Figure 19–20—cont'd   B, Preoperative radiographic series. Note increased talus–first metatarsal angle on both the antero-posterior (AP) **(B1)** and lateral **(B2** and **B3)** foot radiographs. Note lack of adequate visualization of the subtalar joint on the lateral foot radiographs **(B2** and **B3)** due to hindfoot valgus **(B6)** and talar collapse. Subfibular impingement is evident on the AP ankle radiographs **(B5).**

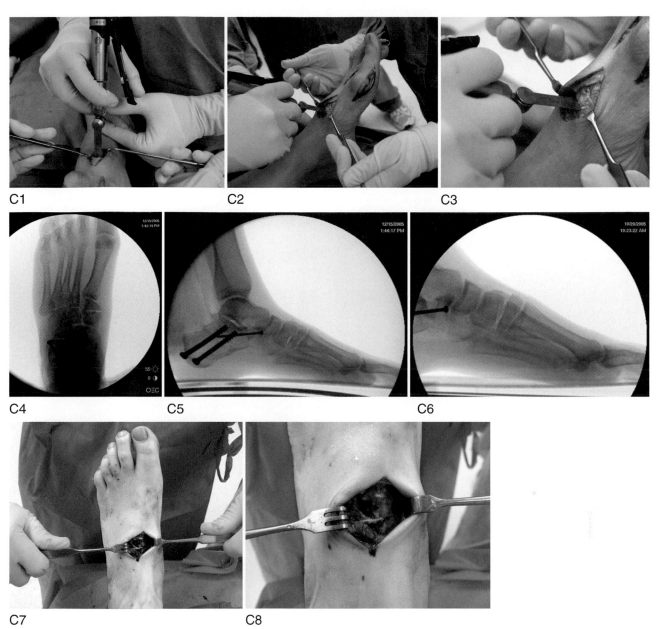

Figure 19-20—cont'd   C, Intraoperative photographs and fluoroscopy. **C1** to **C3,** Note angle of saw cut, using microsagittal saw. Visualization of the first metatarsocuneiform joint (seen distally through the open wound) is not necessary. **C4** to **C6,** Intraoperative fluoroscopy demonstrates complex correction through medial slide calcaneal osteotomy, Evans procedure, and Cotton osteotomy. **C7** and **C8,** Final photographs of graft interposition demonstrate excellent graft apposition, under compression, that does not require fixation to achieve union.   *Continued*

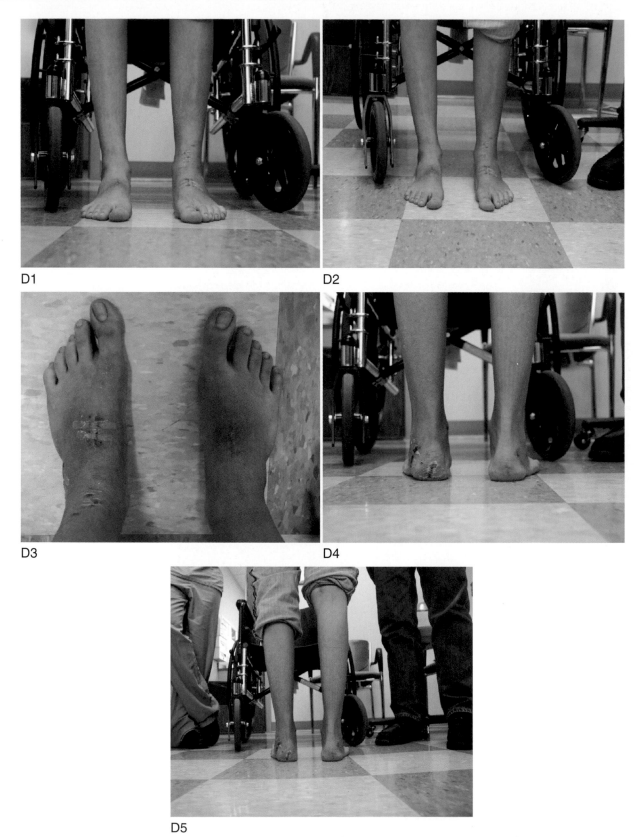

D1

D2

D3

D4

D5

Figure 19–20—cont'd   D1 through **D5,** Postoperative clinical photographs. Note correction of deformity in all planes, with restoration of the physiologic arch through the Cotton osteotomy and lack of forefoot supination following the Evans procedure (balance achieved through the Cotton osteotomy).

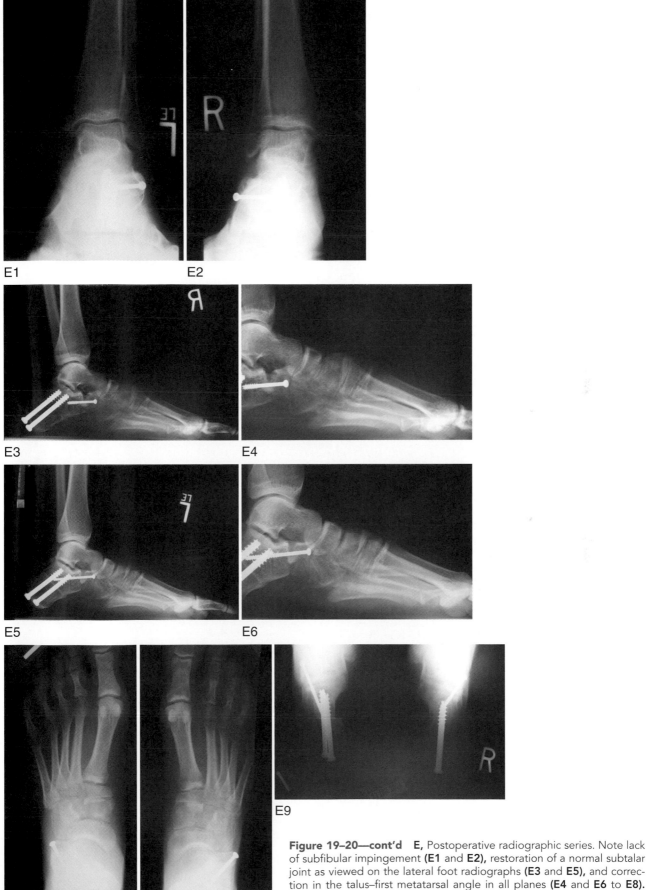

E1   E2

E3   E4

E5   E6

E7   E8   E9

Figure 19–20—cont'd **E,** Postoperative radiographic series. Note lack of subfibular impingement (**E1** and **E2**), restoration of a normal subtalar joint as viewed on the lateral foot radiographs (**E3** and **E5**), and correction in the talus–first metatarsal angle in all planes (**E4** and **E6** to **E8**). **E4** and **E6,** Note interposed wedge graft into the medial cuneiform particularly evident on the lateral radiographs. **E9,** Prior hindfoot valgus deformity has been corrected to neutral.

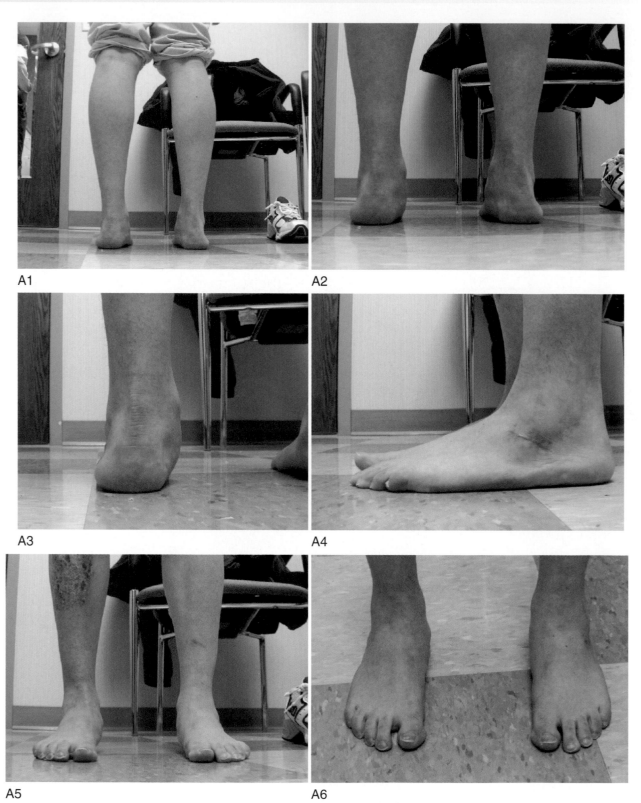

Figure 19–21   Cotton osteotomy used in revision surgery. This patient had a prior Evans procedure with excision of an accessory navicular and advancement of the posterior tibial tendon (note suture anchor). She had persistent subfibular impingement pain and lateral overload of her forefoot (fixed supination) with weight bearing. **A,** Preoperative clinical photographs. Note hindfoot valgus **(A1** to **A3),** surgical scar for lateral column lengthening **(A4),** and fixed supination of forefoot **(A5** and **A6)** with subsequent subfibular impingement.

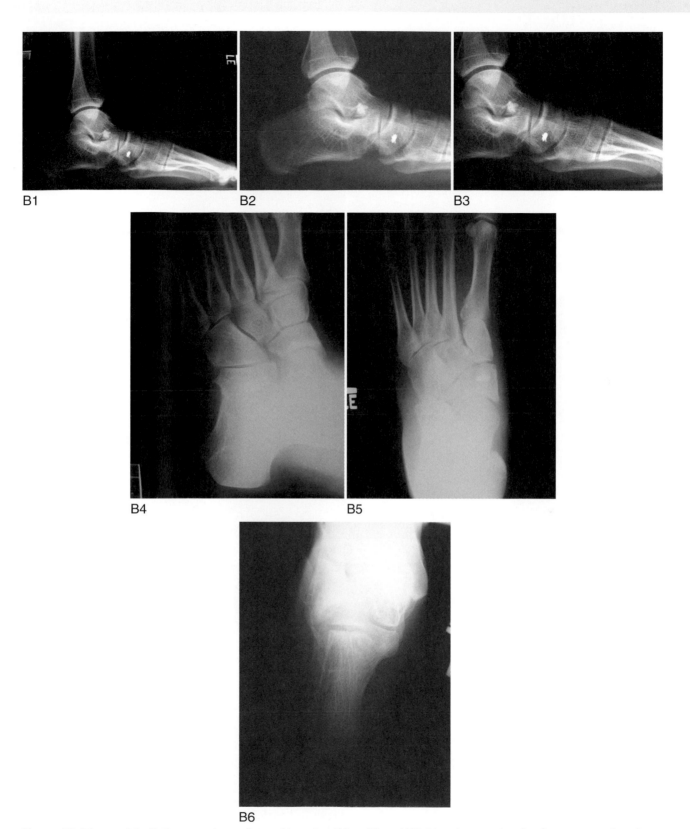

Figure 19–21—cont'd **B,** Preoperative radiographic series. **B1** to **B3** and **B5,** Note increase in talus–first metatarsal angle on both the anteroposterior (AP) and lateral foot radiographs. **B4,** Note healed Evans calcaneal osteotomy. **B5,** Note resection for accessory navicular (including ostectomy of navicular) on AP foot radiograph. **B6,** Valgus deformity of the calcaneus is evident.

Continued

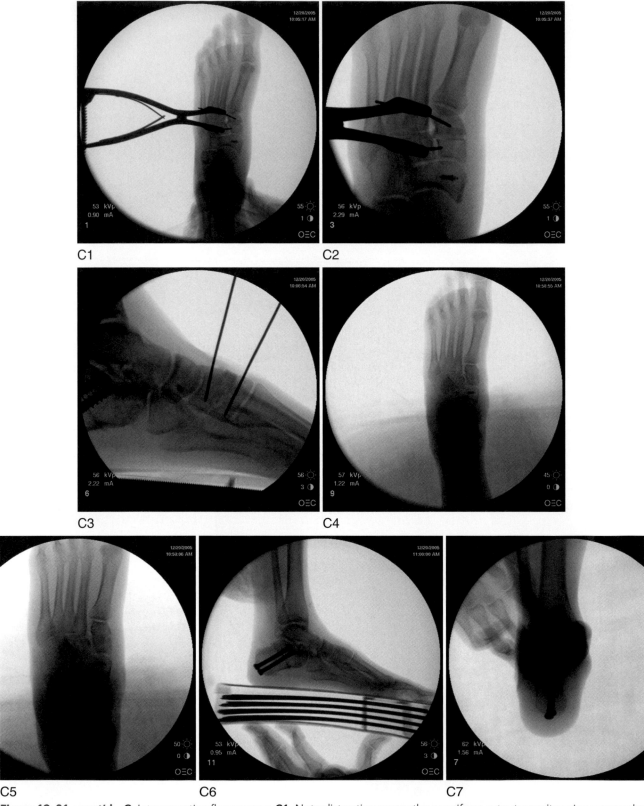

Figure 19–21—cont'd **C,** Intraoperative fluoroscopy. **C1,** Note distraction across the cuneiform osteotomy site using a spreader that is not interposed within the osteotomy site. Graft interposition is visible on the AP **(C2)** and lateral **(C3)** planes. **C4** to **C6,** Final fluoroscopic views include simulated weight-bearing radiographs, which ensure a plantigrade foot by assessing the fore-foot weight-bearing axis. **C7,** Note the medial slide calcaneal osteotomy under the intraoperative axial view demonstrating restoration of the posterior tuberosity of the calcaneus beneath the tibial weight-bearing axis.

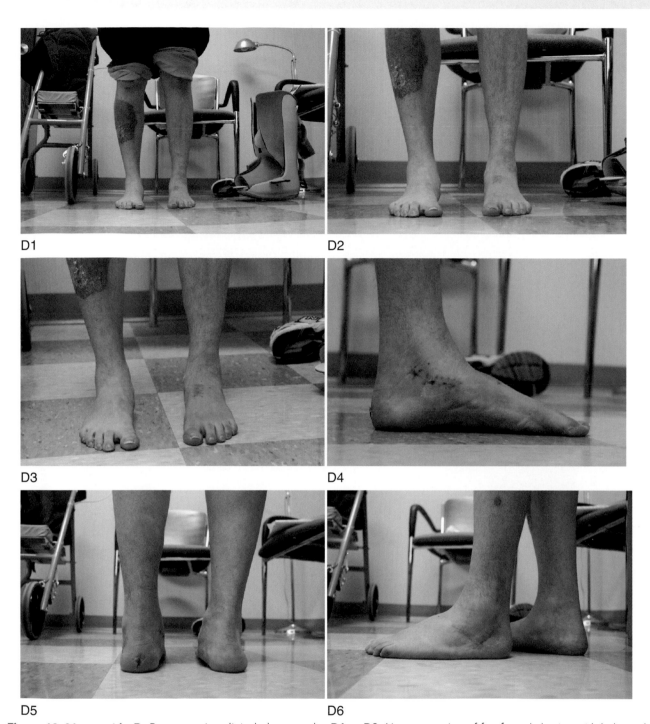

D1

D2

D3

D4

D5

D6

Figure 19–21—cont'd **D,** Postoperative clinical photographs. **D1** to **D3,** Note correction of forefoot abduction with balanced forefoot and lack of forefoot supination. **D4,** Note restoration of physiologic arch through Cotton osteotomy. **D5,** The hindfoot has been corrected to neutral. **D6,** Note healed lateral surgical incisions without necrosis despite multiple lateral incisions.

Continued

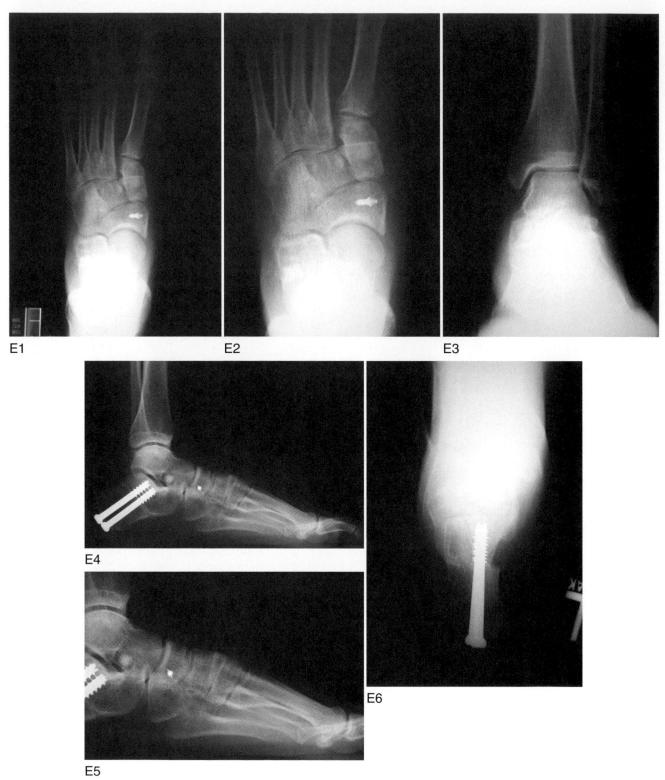

E1

E2

E3

E4

E6

E5

Figure 19–21—cont'd E, Postoperative radiographic series. **E1, E2,** and **E4,** Note the corrected talus–first metatarsal angle on both AP and lateral planes. **E4** and **E5,** In particular, note the ability of the Cotton osteotomy to correct the lateral talus–first metatarsal angle. Note the correction of the subfibular impingement **(E3)** and hindfoot valgus **(E6).**

LATERAL COLUMN LENGTHENING THROUGH EVANS PROCEDURE AND CALCANEOCUBOID JOINT ARTHRODESIS

Lengthening of the lateral column of the foot is indicated in late stage 2 disease, or what is now commonly called stage 2B posterior tibial tendon insufficiency. Progression of the disorder has led to forefoot abduction, pronation of the forefoot, and subfibular impingement. This progression suggests irreversible ligament destruction that a calcaneal osteotomy, flexor digitorum longus tendon transfer, and spring ligament repair will not be sufficient to correct.

Rather than automatically turning to the triple arthrodesis with advanced flatfoot deformity, the Evans procedure (commonly done in children for congenital flatfoot) was applied to the adult population in 1993[132] through a cadaveric study to understand its corrective value on radiographic measurements in improving flatfoot deformity. Significant improvements in the talonavicular coverage, talometatarsal angle, and calcaneal pitch angle were noted. By providing a rigid block to prevent progressive medial ligament failure to allow recurrence of flatfoot, the lateral column lengthening procedure began to be used to combat lateral impingement.

Late-term impingement has been quantified by Malicky et al[89] through the use of a device to simulate weight bearing while a CT scan is performed on the hindfoot. The authors evaluated the scans for narrowing of the sinus tarsi (sinus tarsi impingement) or osseous contact between the fibula and the calcaneus (calcaneofibular impingement). The authors found that sinus tarsi impingement was responsible for lateral impingement in flatfeet 92% of the time, and calcaneofibular impingement was responsible 66% of the time (versus 0% and 5%, respectively, in control plantigrade feet). The authors speculate that the sinus tarsi impingement occurs first, followed by calcaneofibular impingement as the disorder progresses.

The mechanism of correction is not defined. Initially, it was thought that lengthening the lateral column created tension on the plantar fascia, tightening the windlass mechanism and restoring arch height.[106] However, this theory was investigated by Horton et al,[58] who performed a cadaveric study using a liquid-metal strain gauge sutured within the medial band of the plantar fascia. The authors created a flatfoot model and then loaded the feet to 400 N both before and after a lateral column lengthening procedure. They found that lateral column lengthening actually loosens the plantar fascia by an average of 2.7 mm, refuting the windlass theory. The authors did not investigate the long plantar ligament.

More recently, Dumontier et al[30] performed a cadaveric study investigating the relationships of the various joints about the hindfoot both before and after an Evans procedure. Following creation of a flatfoot model, the authors loaded the feet to 250 N and performed three-dimensional CT scans. The navicular was found to rotate about the talus in 19 degrees of abduction, 3 degrees of pronation, and 3 degrees of plantar flexion. The cuboid rotated in 24 degrees of adduction, 14 degrees of pronation, and 2 degrees of plantar flexion. Both bones underwent translation as well: The navicular translated 5.6 mm medially and 1.8 mm plantarward, and the cuboid translated 3 mm medially. The data suggest that the correction is achieved through alteration in congruence about the various bone and joint surfaces, though the authors admit that the long plantar ligament and other soft tissue structures might have a role. With respect to bony changes, it appears that the navicular rotates about the talar head, which is not a perfect sphere. By rotating the navicular plantarward upon the talar head, the navicular moves to that portion of the head with a smaller radius of curvature, plantar flexing the forefoot upon the talus and increasing arch height. Of course, these concepts remain theories, but they begin to take the difficulty in understanding the mechanism of lateral column lengthening to a more accurate level.

Finally, the motion preserved with calcaneocuboid distraction arthrodesis has been studied by Deland et al[26] in a cadaveric study incorporating a magnetic space tracker system for accuracy. Range of motion about the measured joint surfaces was created by tendon pulls. The authors found that lengthening the lateral column by 1 cm resulted in a 52% reduction in talonavicular joint motion and a 30% reduction in subtalar joint motion. The authors found that eversion was limited more than inversion. Inversion motion in the talonavicular joint was 66% of normal following the lateral column lengthening, whereas the subtalar joint retained 88% of inversion motion. Though reduction in motion might seem dramatic, when compared to the alternative triple arthrodesis in this patient population, the lateral column lengthening becomes a useful alternative in treating progressive flatfoot.

Indications

Lateral column lengthening is indicated in patients with late stage 2 deformity with symptomatic subfibular or sinus tarsi impingement. This procedure is done in combination with any or all of the procedures described earlier.

Contraindications

Patients with stage 3 disease should not undergo this largely joint-sparing procedure. A rigid or fixed deformity precludes a lateral column lengthening. Osteoarthritis of the subtalar joint is a contraindication. Within the operative options of lateral column lengthening, an Evans procedure (see later) is contraindicated in the face of known calcaneocuboid joint arthritis.

Preoperative Evaluation

Clinically, observation of the foot and ankle, and comparison with the opposite extremity, is critical to determine the necessity of adding this procedure to others done simultaneously in flatfoot reconstruction. Standing, patients demonstrate significant hindfoot collapse into valgus, depressed or absent medial longitudinal arch, and increased abduction of the forefoot (the latter two have the talonavicular joint acting as a fulcrum in collapse). Patients demonstrate tenderness to direct palpation in the subfibular region due to sinus tarsi or calcaneofibular impingement. Forefoot varus should be noted, but it is not a contraindication if it is supple or if it is treatable with a medial cuneiform opening wedge osteotomy or a first tarsometatarsal arthrodesis.

Radiographically, evaluation for arthritis of the hindfoot joints is critical, because hindfoot arthritis can change the indicated procedure to a triple arthrodesis. If there is any question, a CT scan of the hindfoot is appropriate. Angular measurements as discussed earlier are performed and compared to the opposite foot and ankle, paying particular attention to the talo-

navicular coverage and talometatarsal angles. It is important to recognize that the source of the flatfoot is not an old or missed Lisfranc injury, which would require an entirely different treatment algorithm.

Preoperative Planning

Using radiographic parameters, estimation of the appropriate interposition graft dimensions may be made. However, confirmation of appropriate graft size is made intraoperatively. Preoperative discussion with the patient should include the merits and detractions of allograft and autograft in selecting the appropriate source for the interposition graft.

Surgical Technique for Evans Procedure

This procedure is more easily performed in the lateral decubitus position. This position allows easy access to the calcaneus for the medial slide calcaneal osteotomy and the lateral column lengthening, and the patient can be rolled supine for subsequent medially based procedures. In the lateral position, the leg can be externally rotated to achieve fluoroscopic views of the entire foot in the AP plane. This imaging should be done with a standard fluoroscopic unit with a large field of view (or, alternatively, hard-copy radiographs should be obtained intraoperatively). The purpose of the larger machine (or radiographs) is to allow visualization of the talometatarsal angle to ensure adequacy of correction before selecting graft size.

1. A thigh tourniquet is used for this procedure, but it should be deflated before closure to ensure adequate hemostasis and thus lessen the risk of incisional wound necrosis through hematoma and edema.
2. If allograft is to be used, popliteal fossa block anesthetic works well and gives longer postoperative pain relief. If iliac crest autograft is to be used, regional or general anesthetic is required (though a popliteal block assists with postoperative pain control).
3. A 5-cm lateral incision is made along the length of the anterior neck of the anterior calcaneal tuberosity, extending to the calcaneocuboid joint (Fig. 19–22).
4. The sural nerve and peroneal tendons are retracted inferiorly, and the extensor brevis musculature is retracted superiorly.

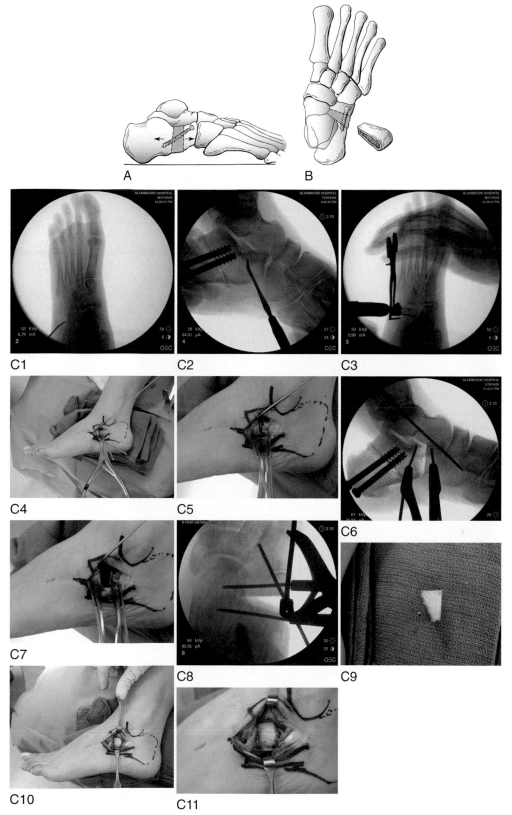

Figure 19–22 Evans calcaneal osteotomy. **A,** Anteroposterior (AP) view of completed Evans procedure with bone graft and internal fixation in place. Osteotomy is performed approximately 1 cm proximal and parallel to the distal surface of the calcaneus. Note that the osteotomy exits the medial side of the calcaneus between the anterior and middle facets. **B,** Lateral view demonstrates bone graft placed in the calcaneus. **C,** Intraoperative photographs and fluoroscopy. Note location of the osteotomy site **(C1** and **C2)** followed by completion of the osteotomy under fluoroscopic imaging **(C3),** with the location of osteotomy approximately 1 cm proximal to calcaneocuboid joint. Note distraction done with extraosteotomy spreader (pins outside the osteotomy site to facilitate graft interposition) **(C4** to **C7),** with restoration of the AP talonavicular coverage **(C8).** Note that the calcaneocuboid joint is pinned prior to distraction with a large-diameter smooth pin to prevent subluxation of this joint with distraction **(C4** to **C8). C9** to **C11,** Wedge allograft is interposed into the osteotomy site.

5. Sharp dissection exposes the neck of the calcaneus proximal to the calcaneocuboid joint.

6. Location of the osteotomy may be based on prior studies reviewing the anatomy of the middle and anterior facets of the calcaneus. Raines and Brage[124] determined the optimal osteotomy site to be 10 mm proximal to the calcaneocuboid joint by a cadaveric study evaluating the exact location of the separation between the anterior and middle facets. However, 60% of their specimens had contiguous facets, which were always violated regardless of the osteotomy position. Hyer et al[60] performed a far more extensive evaluation of 768 cadaveric calcanei, confirming that only 41% had discrete anterior and middle facets. In those with discrete facets, osteotomy placement between 11.5 mm and 15 mm proximal to the calcaneocuboid joint will avoid facet violation.

7. The calcaneocuboid joint should be located and marked, and the osteotomy site should be marked using the above-mentioned criteria.

8. A prophylactic smooth wire may be placed across the calcaneocuboid joint to prevent subluxation of this joint with distraction.

9. The osteotomy is made with an oscillating saw under iced irrigation to prevent heat necrosis of bone.

10. Distraction may be done with a variety of devices. A lamina spreader inserted directly into the osteotomy site can crush the bone on either side of the osteotomy, and it should be used with caution. Our current preference is to use a large Hinterman (Integra, New Deal, NJ) distractor, which requires pin placement on either side of the osteotomy. This allows controlled distraction without shift of the osteotomized fragments, and it allows unobstructed access to the site for graft interposition. Alternative methods include a small external fixation device or a cervical spine distractor.

11. With the leg externally rotated into a supine position (the body remains lateral), distraction of approximately 8 to 12 mm is performed. Under direct visualization with the fluoroscopic device (or hard-copy radiographs), accurate assessment of both talonavicular coverage and the talometatarsal angle is possible. Once anatomic correction is achieved, distraction stops.

12. The graft width is measured, and the graft is either harvested from the iliac crest (tricortical) or fashioned from allograft.

13. The graft is inserted and the tension on the distractor is lessened. Congruence about the graft–osteotomy interface is assessed. To achieve the best congruence, a thin saw blade may be inserted on either side of the osteotomy site (between the graft and the osteotomy), and feathered to create flat, opposing surfaces. Care must be taken to not recut the osteotomy (i.e., shorten the lateral column), because the magnitude of correction will be compromised. Alternatively, the surgeon can fashion a graft 1 mm larger than the proposed graft size, allowing for bone removal during this method of achieving congruence.

14. Fixation may be achieved with one screw (4.0-mm cancellous cannulated, 3.5-mm cortical, and 4.0-mm solid cancellous have been described) directed from the distal calcaneus, across the graft, and into the proximal calcaneus. Lag technique is employed. Multiple screws are not necessary and can compromise graft strength. The screw should be proximal to the calcaneocuboid joint, and a countersink device is helpful to prevent screw head irritation. A compression staple has also been described to achieve fixation. In all cases, fixation is performed with the assistant placing plantar-to-dorsal pressure upon the cuboid bone (i.e., pushing upward with the thumb on the plantar surface of the foot underlying the cuboid) to minimize the risk of forefoot supination's compromising the outcome.

15. The provisional wire is removed from the calcaneocuboid joint, and congruence of that joint is checked with fluoroscopy. The correction is checked simultaneously.

16. Additional cancellous bone graft may be packed around the graft site to assist with union.

17. The tourniquet is let down at this time.

18. The extensor brevis muscle is sewn back over the graft site. This is an important step, and every effort should be made to cover the graft to enhance vascularity to the fusion site and to minimize the depth of any wound complication that can occur. If a

wound complication does occur, this will minimize any additional surgery required for coverage.

19. Subcutaneous and skin closure is performed, taking tension off of the skin through dermal closure.
20. Additional procedures are performed. Specifically, the surgeon should assess the forefoot for supination following lateral column lengthening and add a medial cuneiform opening wedge osteotomy or first tarsometatarsal arthrodesis if appropriate.
21. A short-leg cast or splint is applied in the operating room.

Surgical Technique for Calcaneocuboid Distraction Arthrodesis

This technique is performed almost identically to the Evans procedure, with the following modifications:

1. The incision continues distally along the lateral wall of the cuboid for the extent of this bone.
2. Preparation of the fusion may be done with the oscillating saw under iced irrigation, though in this case the facets are not a

concern, and the entire joint is removed with flat cuts. A flat chisel or osteotome may also be used, but the surgeon must create flat cuts with these tools (Fig. 19–23).
3. A higher rate of nonunion (see later) can require more rigid internal fixation. If the one-screw method is chosen, the surgeon may direct this screw from the anterior neck of the calcaneus distally into the cuboid. This provides compression across the graft, and a countersink is used to prevent screw head irritation. Often, a large diameter (4.5-mm) screw is appropriate. The screw may be supplemented by plate fixation. An AO Cervical H-Plate (Synthes, Paoli, Penn) is often used, and it is fixed with 3.5-mm cortical screws rather than the provided screws for increased rigidity of the construct.

Postoperative Care

The patient wears a short-leg cast for 6 weeks and is strictly non–weight bearing. Careful evaluation of radiographs is necessary at 6 weeks to ensure adequacy of union. If there is concern, a CT scan can provide useful additional information. Physical therapy may be instituted at 6

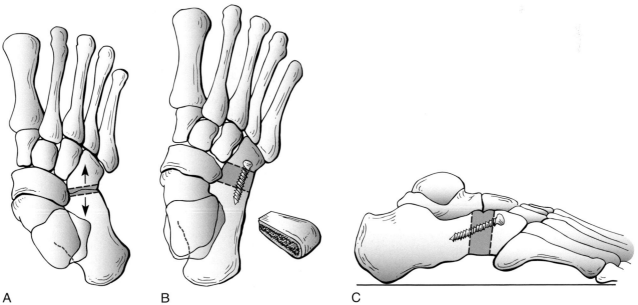

A   B   C

Figure 19–23 Calcaneocuboid distraction arthrodesis. **A,** Anteroposterior (AP) view shows severe valgus of the hindfoot and abduction deformity through the transverse tarsal joint. The area of planned arthrotomy and fusion is indicated. **B,** Articular surfaces of the calcaneus and cuboid are removed with a sharp curette, and subchondral bone is drilled. Distraction is provided between the calcaneus and cuboid, taking care to position the cuboid slightly plantarly and medially in relation to the calcaneus. This helps to correct the medial column of the forefoot's tendency to dorsiflex slightly. **C,** Postoperative lateral view with bone graft in place. Rigid internal fixation provides needed compression and torsional rigidity. Cervical H-plate is one alternative for fixation. *Continued*

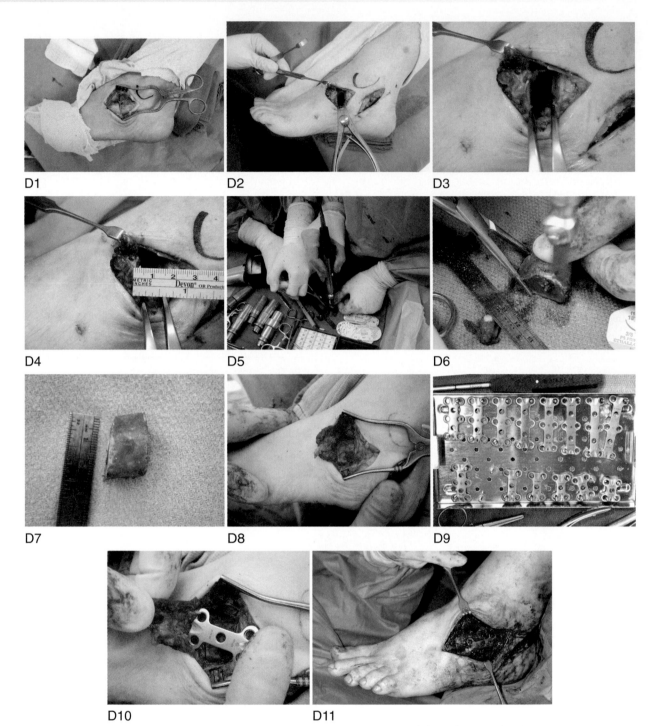

D1

D2

D3

D4

D5

D6

D7

D8

D9

D10

D11

Figure 19–23—cont'd D, Intraoperative photographs. **D1,** Lateral exposure of the calcaneocuboid joint prior to osteotomy. **D2** and **D3,** Distraction done with an intraosteotomy lamina spreader is more difficult owing to its occupied space. A smooth lamina spreader facilitates this exposure. **D4,** After fluoroscopic visualization of the restored talonavicular joint, graft size is measured. **D5** to **D7,** Autograft is prepared and measured. **D8,** Graft is interposed. **D9** to **D11,** Multiple choices for fixation include a cervical H-plate, which provides rigidity and helps to protect the graft from collapse while revascularization proceeds.

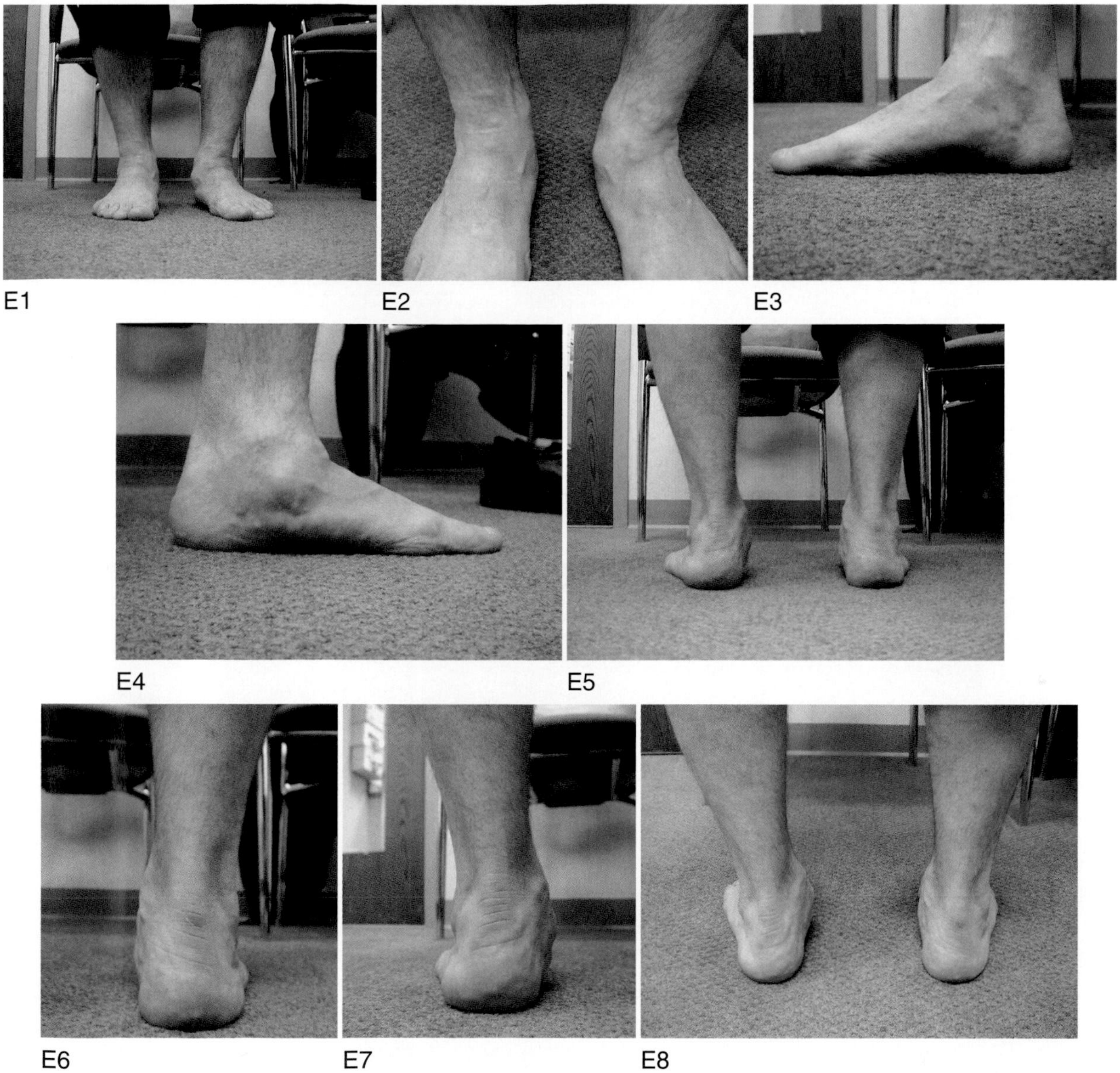

Figure 19–23—cont'd **E,** Clinical example. This patient presented with a unilateral acquired flatfoot deformity *(left)* following complete rupture of the posterior tibial tendon. He has subfibular pain in addition to medial ankle pain. Note the collapse of his arch **(E1, E2,** and **E4)** with hindfoot valgus deformity **(E5** to **E7)** and sag with bulging of the medial ankle **(E8).**

Continued

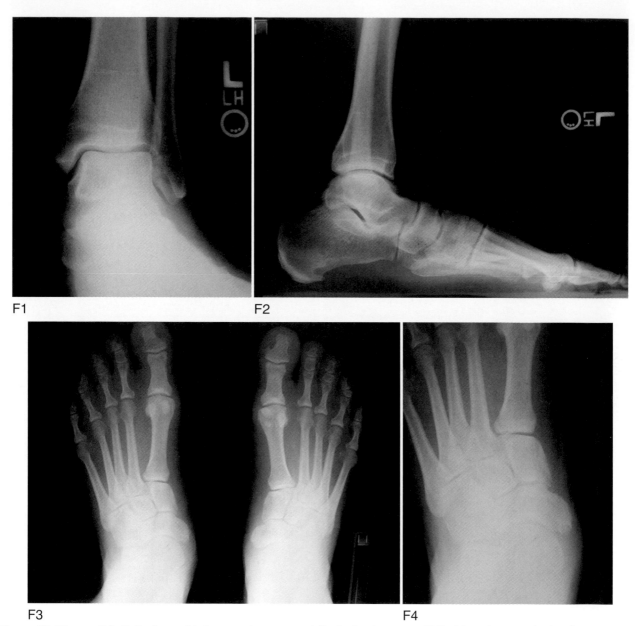

F1

F2

F3

F4

Figure 19–23—cont'd   **F,** Radiographic images document subfibular impingement **(F1)** with an increased talus–first metatarsal angle on both the lateral **(F2)** and AP **(F3 and F4)** planes. **F4,** Note peritalar subluxation.

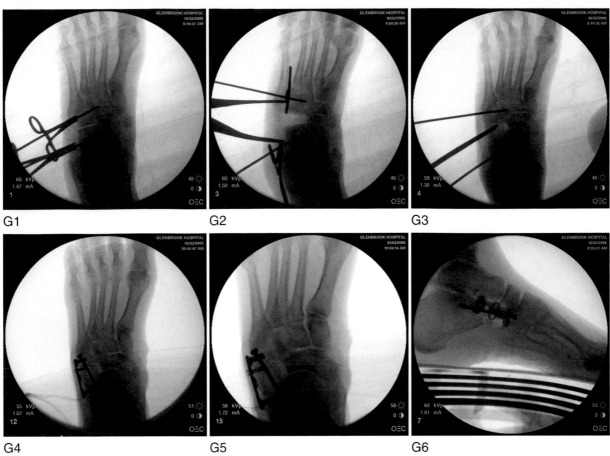

G1   G2   G3

G4   G5   G6

Figure 19–23—cont'd   G1 and **G2,** Intraoperative fluoroscopy begins with extra-articular joint distraction until talonavicular coverage is achieved. This is followed by graft interposition **(G3)** and both lag screw and plate supplementation **(G4** to **G6).**

Continued

weeks postoperatively, though weight-bearing restrictions remain.

It is difficult to provide a specific time interval when institution of weight bearing becomes safe in this patient population. Late collapse of the interposed graft has been noted (see later) and might compromise a correction that initially seems perfect. In general, I begin weight-bearing slowly over the subsequent 6 weeks if my 6-week evaluation demonstrates adequate union. I have the patient begin with standing in a CAM walking boot and advance to short distance walking by 3 months postoperatively. I reassess with radiographs, studying for any potential graft collapse or hardware failure. If this is not present, I then allow unrestricted, full weight bearing in the CAM boot for an additional month and review the radiographs again. If at 4 months postoperatively there is no loss of correction and no perceived nonunion or late graft collapse, I allow the patient to wear ath-

letic shoes, advancing to regular footwear as swelling dissipates and flexibility improves. Caution should still be used, however, because late graft collapse can still occur.

Results and Complications

The primary criticism of this procedure remains the complications associated with it. They are nonunion, late graft collapse, soft tissue complications, forefoot supination, poor fusion position, and osteoarthritis at the calcaneocuboid joint following Evans procedure

It has been suggested that the Evans procedure has a higher rate of union than the calcaneocuboid distraction arthrodesis. Danko et al[24] reviewed 130 feet undergoing lateral column lengthening, 69 with an Evans procedure and 61 with a calcaneocuboid arthrodesis. Collapse, defined as loss of correction with lucency or fragmentation and loss of graft length, was noted

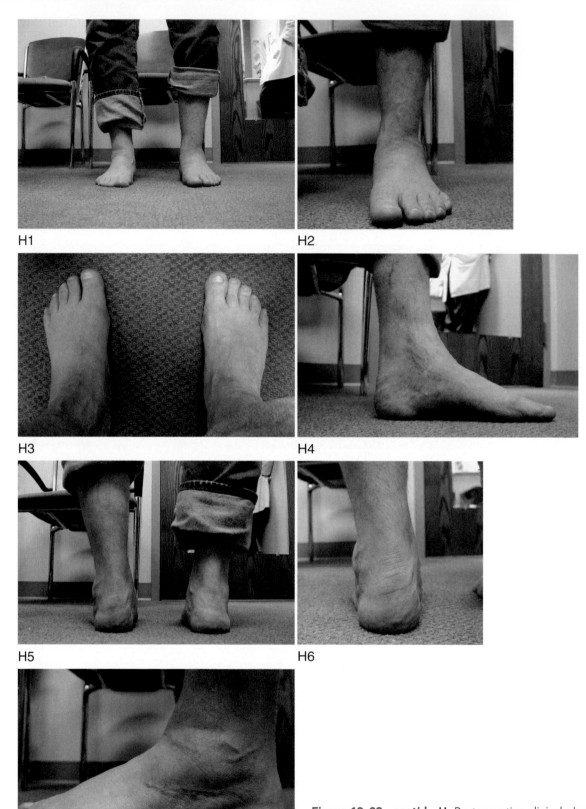

H1

H2

H3

H4

H5

H6

H7

Figure 19–23—cont'd   H, Postoperative clinical photographs. Photographs demonstrate anatomic and symmetrical correction **(H1)** without forefoot supination **(H2)** or forefoot abduction **(H3). H4,** The longitudinal arch has been restored. **H5** and **H6,** Hindfoot valgus is corrected to neutral (without a supplemental medial slide calcaneal osteotomy) through distraction arthrodesis. **H7,** The surgical incision healed without incident.

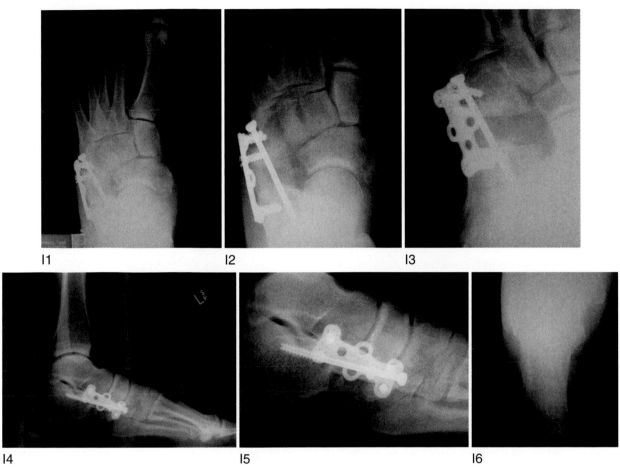

Figure 19–23—cont'd I, Postoperative radiographs demonstrate correction of the talus–first metatarsal angle **(I1),** with corrected peritalar subluxation **(I2)** and a complete union of the interposed graft **(I3).** The lateral radiograph confirms restoration of the talus–first metatarsal angle **(I4)** and graft union **(I5). I6,** Hindfoot valgus is restored to neutral without calcaneal osteotomy.

between 0.3 and 1.3 years following surgery. Twenty-nine percent of those undergoing calcaneocuboid distraction arthrodesis demonstrated collapse, but none of the feet undergoing Evans procedures demonstrated collapse.

Conti and Wong[16] evaluated 32 patients undergoing calcaneocuboid distraction arthrodesis with iliac crest autograft. The authors noted that 15 patients (47%) demonstrated inadequate incorporation of the bone graft at an average of 5 months following the index procedure. Of feet developing complete graft collapse (16%), only one was fixed with a cervical H-plate (the rest were fixed with crossed Kirschner wires). Still, the same percentage of patients with crossed Kirschner wires and cervical H-plate fixation developed inadequate incorporation in some form. In this category, some

developed union failure at the graft–host bone interface (36% of the 15 patients demonstrating failure). Commonly, this complication occurred late; the patient was initially doing well and then presented with increasing pain after minor trauma. The authors suggest that the bone graft probably united appropriately at first and collapsed later owing to failure of complete graft incorporation through creeping substitution.

Toolan et al[149] evaluated 41 feet undergoing calcaneocuboid distraction arthrodesis. They noted a 20% nonunion rate at that site, without qualifying between lack of union at the host–graft interface and late graft collapse. They found that all sites fixed with a cervical H-plate united.

Kimball et al[74] compared fixation of the lateral column lengthening with crossed 3.5-mm screws and a cervical H-plate in a biomechanical study. Following fixation, they loaded the specimens to failure and found that the average applied load necessary to create a 1-mm joint separation at the graft–host interface was 30.5 N for crossed screws and 78 N for the H-plate. They advocate the more rigid fixation device to minimize the risk of nonunion. They postulate that the rate of nonunion may be elevated in the calcaneocuboid arthrodesis population over the Evans procedure population owing to increased difficulty in healing subchondral bone over cancellous bone and the increased torque that occurs across the graft at the site of a normal joint surface.

Toolan et al[149] found 32% of their patients had anesthesia or paresthesias of the sural nerve.

Moseir-LaClair et al[108] noted 11% superficial wound complications in 28 feet undergoing an Evans procedure. Sixty-seven percent of these patients required irrigation and debridement intraoperatively, but all healed without any additional supplementary procedures. With appropriate coverage of the graft site with the extensor digitorum brevis, plastic surgical skin grafting or muscle flap procedures are avoidable and local wound care is generally sufficient.

This can be combated by supplementary procedures as noted in the surgical technique. Leaving the forefoot in fixed supination can lead to uncomfortable alterations in plantar foot pressures. Tien et al[148] studied both pre- and postoperative medial and lateral forefoot pressures in cadavers undergoing an Evans procedure and a calcaneocuboid distraction arthrodesis. Immediate stability was achieved with cervical H-plate fixation in both populations. Both procedures created statistically significant increases in lateral forefoot loading while causing decreased medial forefoot loading. Increase in pressure during the flatfoot phase of gait averaged 46% with the Evans procedure and 104% with calcaneocuboid distraction arthrodesis. Though both procedures elevated load laterally, the calcaneocuboid arthrodesis created twice as much overload. This is concerning and would argue for the surgeon ensuring plantar-applied superior pressure to the cuboid during fixation to minimize the controllable technical component to this overload.

Poor fusion position was emphasized by Sands et al,[131] who studied alteration in hindfoot kinematics by increasing length on the lateral column during fusion of the calcaneocuboid joint. In addition, they evaluated fusing the lateral column with a standard 10-mm graft in altered positions (plantar flexion and eversion, and dorsiflexion and inversion). If the calcaneocuboid joint was fused in a neutral position, no change in hindfoot motion and kinematics was noted at any lateral column length: 0 mm, 5 mm, or 10 mm. Altering the position of the foot at fusion, however, created a significant reduction in motion at both the talonavicular and subtalar joints. Again, the surgeon must pay careful attention to the position of the foot at the time of fixation during fusion for a lateral column lengthening procedure.

The potential for the Evans procedure to create osteoarthritis in the calcaneocuboid joint remains controversial. Initially, it was thought that the Evans procedure created undue stress across the calcaneocuboid joint through static increased load, leading to accelerated arthritic wear. Cooper et al[17] measured real-time calcaneocuboid joint pressure with a sensor pad at increasing lengths following an Evans calcaneal osteotomy. The authors recorded peak pressures across the calcaneocuboid joint of 2.3 megapascals (MPa) after lengthening the lateral column 10 mm. Baseline value for the unloaded calcaneocuboid joint was 0.0 MPa. The difference was statistically significant. Expected peak pressures in the 1-cm lengthening loaded calcaneocuboid joint were surmised to be even higher in vivo owing to ground reaction forces and peroneal tendon pull. The authors validated their results by testing the accuracy of the TekScan (TekScan, Boston, Mass) with known compressive forces in the laboratory.

In contrast to these findings, Momberger et al[104] performed a cadaveric study using a more recent model TekScan sensor placed within the calcaneocuboid joint after creation of a flatfoot model. Peak pressures increased significantly across the calcaneocuboid joint after creating the flatfoot model, from 8.9 kg/cm^2 to 18.5 kg/cm^2. Following Evans lateral column lengthening with a 10mm graft, peak pressures actually decreased to 15.0 kg/cm^2. The study by Cooper et al[17] did not create a flatfoot model as a component of their investigation. Thus, while these studies cannot undergo direct comparison owing to their differing design protocols, it appears that the Evans procedure does not increase the contact pressures across the calcaneocuboid joint beyond what is seen in an acquired flatfoot deformity. Theoretically, however, correcting the flatfoot deformity without a lateral column lengthening should restore the calcaneocuboid joint pressures to baseline. Thus, in both studies, it appears that the peak pressure remains elevated after an Evans procedure, though the clinical implications of this elevated pressure remain in question. There are no studies documenting the pressure value necessary to create an osteoarthritic joint.

Clinical studies support the development of osteoarthritis following an Evans procedure. In addition to the outcome studies mentioned below, Phillips[119] found 26% of his patients developed osteoarthritis at the calcaneocuboid joint at 7 to 20 years following the procedure.

Patient Outcome Studies

Toolan et al[149] reviewed 41 feet undergoing calcaneocuboid joint distraction arthrodesis at an average of 34 months postoperatively. Eighty-eight percent of feet were less painful compared to their preoperative status or were pain-free. Seventy-eight percent of patients felt an improvement in their activities of daily living. Ninety-two percent of patients felt they would have the procedure again under similar preoperative circumstances, and 85% were satisfied with the procedural outcome. Radiographically, the talus–first metatarsal angle corrected from 26 degrees to 10 degrees on the AP plane and 23 degrees to 8 degrees on the lateral plane. The talonavicular coverage improved from 36 degrees to 12 degrees on the AP plane. In addition to the above-mentioned complications noted in this study, nearly 50% of the patients required a separate procedure for removal of symptomatic hardware.

Hinterman et al[53] reviewed 19 patients undergoing an Evans procedure in combination with medial procedures. He achieved a 95% satisfaction rate with the surgery, with 32% rated clinically excellent and 58% rated good. He altered the standard surgical technique by creating his osteotomy proximal to the middle facet, between that structure and the posterior facet. On average, this site is located 12 mm to 20 mm proximal to the calcaneocuboid joint. This stable osteotomy required no internal fixation in all but three of their patients, and all but one patient achieved union. Seventy-nine percent reported complete pain relief, 16% reported minor pain. The mean functional score improved from 48.6 preoperatively to 91.1 postoperatively, and the AOFAS Hindfoot Score improved from 51.4 preoperatively to 82.8 postoperatively. Radiographically, an improvement of the AP talus–first metatarsal angle of 20 degrees was measured, and an equal improvement of 20 degrees was found in the lateral talus–first metatarsal angle. Over the course of follow-up (average, 2 years), there was not a statistically significant change in this angular measurement. Two patients demonstrated degenerative changes at the calcaneocuboid joint at the time of most recent follow-up. One required fusion of that joint.

Mosier-LaClair et al[108] reviewed 28 patients undergoing lateral column lengthening through the Evans procedure in combination with a medial slide calcaneal osteotomy and associated medial procedures. Follow-up averaged 5 years. Though no preoperative AOFAS Hindfoot Score was determined for this patient population, the authors tested the patients at final follow-up and found the average score was 90. Eighty-one percent were satisfied with the operation, and 19% were dissatisfied owing to persistent pain. Fourteen percent of their patients demonstrated radiographic signs of calcaneocuboid joint arthritis postoperatively, of which 1 patient was symptomatic.

SUBTALAR ARTHRODESIS TO TREAT POSTERIOR TIBIAL TENDON DYSFUNCTION

An isolated subtalar fusion is used when there is a fixed deformity or restricted inversion of the subtalar joint but a stable, easily correctable transverse tarsal joint and fixed forefoot varus of less than 10 degrees. The subtalar joint should be positioned in approximately 5 degrees of valgus. If the subtalar joint is placed into too much valgus, the patient may continue to have a lateral impingement type of problem, resulting in persistent hindfoot pain. See Chapter 20 for indications and the surgical technique. The main advantage of the isolated subtalar joint arthrodesis is that it maintains transverse tarsal joint motion, leaving the patient a more flexible foot (Fig. 19–24).[94]

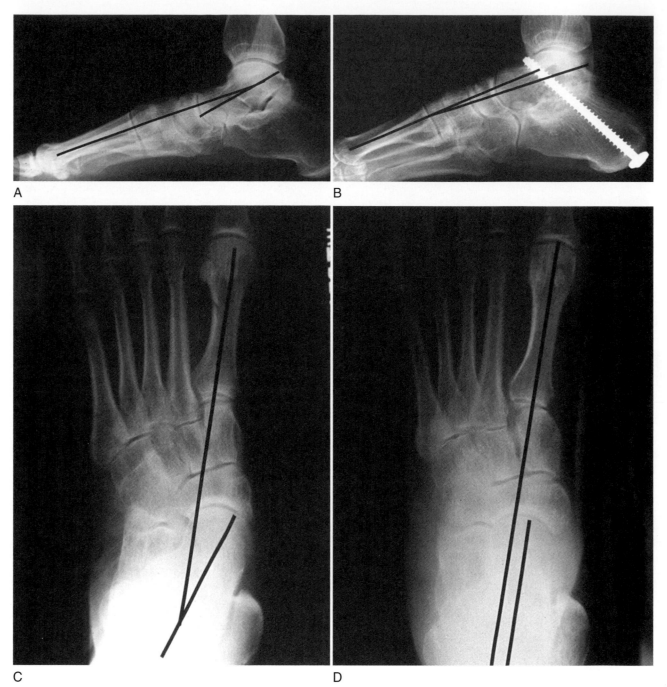

Figure 19–24   Preoperative **(A, C)** and postoperative **(B, D)** radiographs show a subtalar fusion to correct posterior tibial tendon dysfunction. Note the degree of correction that is obtained in the anteroposterior and lateral radiographs following this procedure.

TRIPLE ARTHRODESIS TO TREAT POSTERIOR TENDON DYSFUNCTION

A triple arthrodesis is indicated when there is a fixed valgus deformity or arthrosis or both of the subtalar joint, fixed abduction of the transverse tarsal joint, or a fixed varus deformity of the forefoot. Under these circumstances, in order to create a plantigrade foot the subtalar joint is corrected into 5 degrees of valgus, the transverse tarsal joint is repositioned into neutral abduction/adduction, and the forefoot varus is corrected to neutral position.

This procedure from a technical standpoint can be very challenging. An arthrodesis in situ for a severely deformed foot is not adequate to realign the foot, and the patient will have persistent symptoms due to lateral impingement and a nonplantigrade foot if correction of the deformity is not achieved (Fig. 19–25). See Chapter 20 for indications and the surgical technique.

RIGID FLATFOOT ASSOCIATED WITH ADULT TARSAL COALITION

Incidence

The majority of the world's literature pertaining to tarsal coalition involves the adolescent patient. Tarsal coalition results from failure of differentiation of the primitive mesenchyme with the resultant lack of joint formation. This concept was first proposed by Leboucq in 1890.[85] The overall incidence is less than 1%.[79] However, a number of studies debate this point, stating that tarsal coalition goes unrecognized in asymptomatic persons and in nonosseous variants. Solomon et al[138] suggest that the incidence of talocalcaneal coalition may be as high as 12.7%. The incidence of bilaterality varies in the literature, ranging from 20% to 60% in talocalcaneal coalitions and 40% to 68% in calcaneonavicular coalitions. A review of the literature by Stormont and Peterson[141] noted that the incidence of talocalcaneal coalitions was 48.1%, calcaneonavicular was 43.6%, talonavicular was 1.3%, and other coalitions were 5.7%.

While most patients with this entity present between the ages of 8 and 16 years,[49] symptomatic coalitions do occur in the adult population. Presentation is most often associated with a traumatic event, such as a severe ankle sprain sustained through sports activity or an incidental injury during activities of daily living. It is rare for such a patient to have prior problems with

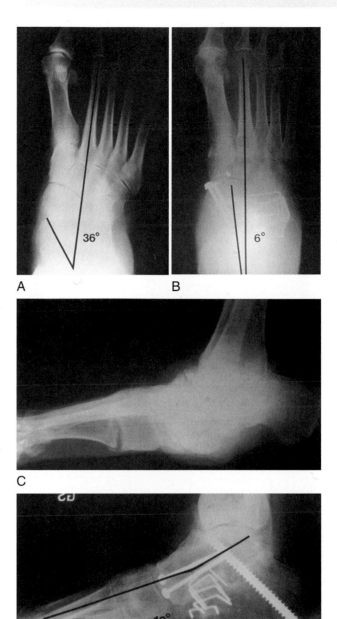

Figure 19–25 The triple arthrodesis is used to correct severe stage 3 deformity as a result of posterior tibial tendon dysfunction. Preoperative **(A)** and postoperative **(B)** anteroposterior (AP) radiographs demonstrate correction of abduction. Preoperative **(C)** and postoperative **(D)** radiographs demonstrate correction of the longitudinal arch.

the involved foot. According to Varner and Michelson,[151] the lack of prior symptoms may be due to the neutral alignment of most adults with tarsal coalition and lack of spasm about the peroneal tendons. Only 7 of 32 adults (22%) presenting with tarsal coalition had a valgus deformity of their hindfeet. In fact, their cohort included 11 asymptomatic tarsal coalitions, and only one of these patients had a valgus hindfoot.

Physical Examination

Physical examination often reveals a flatfoot deformity of variable rigidity. Patients with a talocalcaneal coalition demonstrate no inversion of the calcaneus upon single-limb heel rise, and those with a calcaneonavicular coalition might demonstrate a percentage of inversion when compared to the unaffected side. Preservation of up to 70% of subtalar motion may be found in patients with a calcaneonavicular coalition. Transverse tarsal motion is preserved in patients with a talocalcaneal coalition, but it is severely restricted in patients with a calcaneonavicular bar.

Pain may be elicited medially directly over the anterior middle facets and inferior to the medial malleolus in patients with a talocalcaneal coalition. Often the clinical appearance of a medial bony prominence is noted in patients with a talocalcaneal bar. Pain to palpation might also be noted in the anterior portion of the sinus tarsi and around the lateral and dorsolateral portion of the talonavicular joint. Stressing the coalition by manipulating the subtalar and transverse tarsal joints can elicit pain directly at the site of the coalition. Paresthesias or frank numbness may be present in the distribution of the deep or superficial peroneal nerve in patients with significant talar beaking. Tarsal tunnel syndrome has been reported in conjunction with a talocalcaneal coalition[86] owing to impingement on the medial plantar nerve from a bony prominence at the sustentaculum tali.

Peroneal spastic flatfoot is a misnomer. Patients might demonstrate periodic spasm of the peroneal tendons due to attempted inversion against relatively shortened peroneal tendons. The shortening occurs from chronic and rigid valgus of the hindfoot. The peroneal tendons elicit a protective mechanism of contracting to minimize pain specifically at the rigid subtalar joint, and thus they might go into spasm because of the length deficit.

Radiographic Studies

Plain radiography has value in the form of weight-bearing AP, oblique, and lateral images. These routine images are inspected for distortion in the normal bone architecture suggesting union (fibrous or bony) between the involved bones. In addition, the lateral radiograph can demonstrate beaking of the talus. This traction spur at the dorsum of the talus is a secondary sign of tarsal coalition and is believed to occur through an aberrant hingelike motion of the navicular upon the talus with dorsiflexion. Subtalar joint rigidity pre-

vents the normal forward subluxation of the calcaneus upon the talus with dorsiflexion, creating a rigid hinge motion of the navicular upon the talus rather than the normal gliding motion. This hinging creates periosteal disturbance upon the head of the talus, which manifests a traction spur at that specific location.

Primary signs may be visualized on the 45-degree lateral oblique radiograph, where the calcaneonavicular coalition becomes evident as either complete osseous union or extension of the anterior neck of the calcaneus to the navicular (the anteater nose sign). The talocalcaneal coalition can also be visualized on plain radiography as narrowing of the posterior subtalar joint, failure to see the middle facet, rounding of the lateral process of the talus (on ankle radiographs), or flattening or concavity of the undersurface of the talar neck. The C sign, described by Brown et al,[8] is a bean-shaped density noted on the lateral radiograph and was initially thought to be diagnostic for talocalcaneal coalition. This sign relies on a prominent inferior outline of the sustentaculum tali to create an overlap or hyperdense region in combination with the medial outline of the talar dome and a bony bridge between the talar dome and sustentaculum tali. Brown found that although the sign is specific (not sensitive) for flatfoot in general, it is neither specific nor sensitive for talocalcaneal coalition. Clearly, the ability of the technologist to obtain a true lateral radiograph of the foot is pivotal in appropriately interpreting that radiograph for tarsal coalition. A true lateral radiograph should allow visualization of the middle and posterior facets, which are parallel. Any rotation of the hindfoot, or nonperpendicular beam positioning, will erroneously lead the interpreter to suggest tarsal coalition because the facets are not visible.

An important primary sign of talocalcaneal coalition may be detected through the Harris axial view[50] and requires the patient to stand on the radiographic cassette while dorsiflexing the ankle 10 degrees. The beam is projected downward from posterior to plantar at 45 degrees from vertical. Additional views are taken at 40 degrees and 50 degrees in order to capture the parallel nature of the posterior and middle facets. Assistance in determining the appropriate orientation of the beam comes from assessing the angle of the posterior and middle facets with reference to the vertical on the true lateral radiograph. Irregularity of the joint contour suggests a fibrous coalition, and complete obliteration of the joint is pathognomonic for bony coalition.

Despite the advanced diagnostic modalities mentioned below, unenhanced radiography has value in assessment for tarsal coalition. Crim and Kjeldsberg[23] performed a two-phase study in patients with a mean age of 29 years. The first phase involved retrospectively reviewing radiographs in patients with known tarsal coalitions (confirmed by CT, MRI, or surgery) intermixed with known controls, and assessing diagnostic accuracy. Radiographs provided to the examiners were only AP and lateral foot views, to provide consistency with routine screening radiographs obtained in an office setting. The second phase was prospective, reviewing 150 radiographs in patients with nontraumatic foot and ankle pain and following up suspected coalitions with CT. The authors found that in the first phase, talocalcaneal diagnosis through plain radiographs was sensitive 100% of the time and specific 88% of the time. Calcaneonavicular coalitions ranged from 80% to 100% sensitive and 97% to 98% specific. Observers in this study were a junior musculoskeletal radiologist, a junior radiology resident, and a junior orthopaedics resident, all provided with a 30-minute tutorial prior to reviewing radiographs. In the second phase of the study, all expected coalitions were confirmed by CT scan, with no false positives noted.

CT has superseded plain radiography in diagnostic accuracy for tarsal coalition. The coronal view may be obtained by having the patient supine with the hips and knees flexed and the feet plantar flexed 20 degrees at the ankle. The image provided is perpendicular to the posterior and middle facets and will confirm an osseous talocalcaneal coalition. In addition, the coronal view will demonstrate the nature and cross-sectional area of the coalition. CT has the added benefit of detecting early degenerative joint disease at adjacent surfaces, which can influence treatment options.

In the past, the ability of CT to evaluate calcaneonavicular coalitions was questioned. Hochman and Reed[55] investigated the ability of CT to make this diagnosis. The authors found that axial CT images provided the best assessment of calcaneonavicular coalition. They also noted, however, that coronal images provide assistance through two features: lateral bridging (an abnormal bone mass lateral to the head of the talus) and abnormal rounding of the head of the talus. In particular, lateral bridging was a definitive finding in all patients studied with a confirmed calcaneonavicular coalition. Thus, the authors suggest that while reviewing the coronal CT scan for a potential talocalcaneal coalition, the examiner must focus attention on the additional signs mentioned earlier to avoid overlooking a calcaneonavicular coalition. If coalition is suspected, the axial images should be reviewed for absence of the normal triangle of soft tissue seen anterolateral to the calcaneus. If a coalition is present, this triangle is replaced by bony protrusions from the calcaneus and the navicular.

The limitations of CT stem from fibrous coalitions, where its accuracy may be compromised.[120,155] Fibrous or cartilaginous coalition is suggested indirectly by an abnormal angulation of the facet, joint space irregularity, subchondral sclerosis, or articular narrowing. However, the actual fibrous tissue is not well visualized. MRI becomes the better modality to assess this particular component. In particular, the T1-weighted images reveal intermediate-to-low signal bridging the gap in the suspected fibrous coalitions. In addition, osseous coalitions are confirmed by continuity of the bone marrow across the proposed site. More recently, an ill-defined hyperintense pattern was detected on STIR (short T1 inversion recovery) or T2 images in the subchondral bone adjacent to the coalition.[136] It is suspected that this pattern is due to abnormal stresses across the rigid coalition, creating microfractures and edema within the bone.

The value of MRI over CT in fibrous tarsal coalitions remains in question. Emery et al[33] reviewed 40 MRI and CT scans taken on 20 patients with symptoms suggesting tarsal coalition. The authors found 15 feet in 9 patients demonstrated tarsal coalition by both MRI and CT scans. Ten coalitions were confirmed through surgical exploration. In this study, 71% of the subjects were patients with a fibrous coalition. Sensitivity and specificity were compared, revealing that CT scanning was 94% sensitive and 100% specific, whereas MRI was 88% sensitive and 100% specific. The authors found a 97.5% agreement between CT and MRI in rendering diagnosis of tarsal coalition, despite the large percentage of fibrous coalitions. Thus, the choice of study depends on the physician's expected findings in a particular case; cost-effectiveness currently favors a CT scan in patients with isolated tarsal coalitions, but if additional soft tissue disorder (posterior tibial tendon disorder) is sought, MRI is the better diagnostic modality.

Treatment

Most tarsal coalitions are asymptomatic. If a coalition is detected radiographically when evaluating for a separate problem, the patient should be informed about the condition, but no treatment beyond simple observation is necessary.

Pain in conjunction with the adult tarsal coalition is often in associated with a traumatic event, most often an ankle sprain. Thus, it is important to maintain clinical suspicion when examining a patient with an ankle sprain, evaluating for rigidity in subtalar motion. Patients who present late after sustaining an ankle sprain must be carefully evaluated for tarsal coalition.

Conservative Treatment

Conservative management for tarsal coalition begins with antiinflammatory medication, icing, and modifying activity. Persistent pain mandates cast immobilization. The clinician must decide the weight-bearing status in the cast based on consultation with the patient. One may certainly use a short-leg walking cast for 6 weeks, but if the patient remains symptomatic following cast removal, a second casting (with a non–weight-bearing cast) will be required. Thus, this protocol might extend the casting for a second interval, which can be avoided by making the first cast non–weight bearing. Regardless, it is my experience that 60% to 70% of patients respond to immobilization if they have had no prior symptoms from the coalition. This experience is not supported in the literature, where only one third of patients were found to respond to conservative measures.[19,81] If the patient fails two attempts at casting, surgical intervention is appropriate.

Longer-term conservative management can incorporate a medial heel wedge, Thomas heel, or medial longitudinal arch support.[19] Generally, in rigid flatfoot, use of a rigid device that attempts to correct the collapsed arch actually increases the patient's symptoms and limits compliance with the device. Thus, accommodative orthotics made of Plastizote, or semi-rigid devices that accommodate rather than correct the arch, have higher satisfaction. A UCBL orthosis or a lace-up ankle brace may be required for continued sports participation by minimizing stress across the coalition. In patients who do not participate in sports, a polypropylene AFO may be required. Cowell and Elener[20] found that patients with a fixed hindfoot valgus deformity and a talocalcaneal coalition fared poorly with conservative care when compared with a hindfoot in neutral.

Surgical Treatment

CALCANEONAVICULAR COALITION

Surgical treatment of the calcaneonavicular coalition in an adult with minimal or no secondary changes (arthrosis) consists of resection of the coalition (Fig. 19–26). The goal is to eliminate painful motion at the coalition site while potentially increasing hindfoot motion. The suspected location of pain arising from the coalition appears to be the site around the coalition rather than the actual coalition itself. In particular, the hyperintense ill-defined areas noted on MRI of tarsal coalition[136] can represent bone contusion or edema that create coalition pain. It is clear that the hyperintensity is present in the subchondral bone, and not within the coalition itself. Thus, a generous resection of the coalition invariably removes the diseased segment of bone, providing pain relief for the patient.

Indications

Indications for resection of a calcaneonavicular coalition are pain refractory to conservative care, and limited function from extreme rigidity.

Contraindications

Improvement with conservative care is a contraindication to surgery. If the patient is asymptomatic, resection of the coalition is not indicated. In addition, if the adjacent joints are arthritic, resection of the coalition is not sufficient, and a double or triple arthrodesis becomes the best alternative.

Preoperative Evaluation

Patients are evaluated radiographically for coalition. Plain radiographs include the 45-degree oblique view, which demonstrates the coalition. CT scanning reveals the extent of the coalition and whether it is osseous or fibrous. More important, the CT scan assists in evaluating adjacent joint surfaces for arthritic wear. For example, post-traumatic arthritis of the cuboid or subtalar joint can mimic symptoms of a tarsal coalition. Such arthritis warrants fusion rather than resection.

Severity of the planovalgus foot deformity is assessed clinically. The literature does not address correction of the flatfoot deformity in conjunction with coalition resection. However, it must remain a consideration, especially in patients with subfibular impingement (separate from pain at the site of the coalition) or pain medially underlying the talar head. Such patients become candidates for simultaneous medial slide calcaneal osteotomies, lateral column lengthenings, or medial cuneiform opening wedge osteotomies.

Preoperative Planning

Radiographs are reviewed to determine the extent and location of the coalition. In certain circumstances, a polymerase chain reaction (PCR) nasal screen is appropriate to evaluate for staphylococcus species, and noninvasive blood flow studies assist in wound healing assessment.

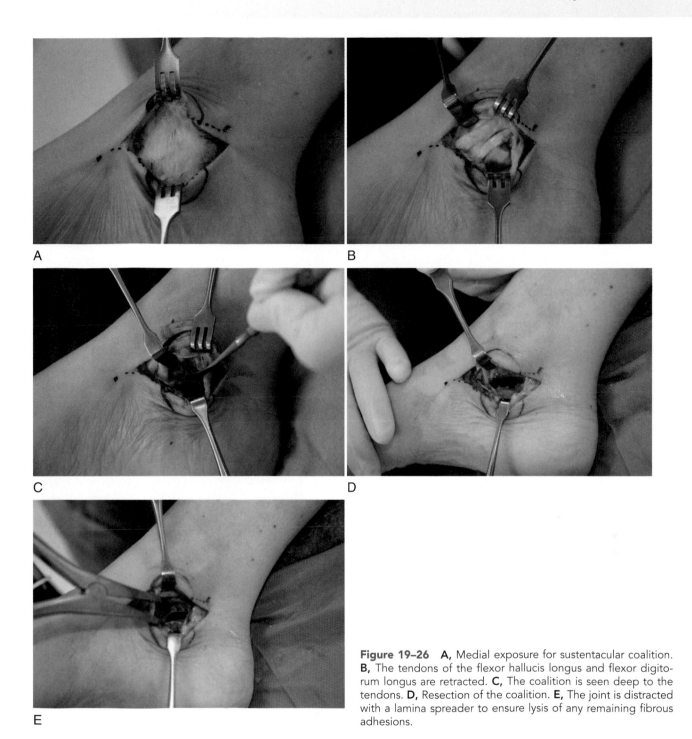

Figure 19-26 **A,** Medial exposure for sustentacular coalition. **B,** The tendons of the flexor hallucis longus and flexor digitorum longus are retracted. **C,** The coalition is seen deep to the tendons. **D,** Resection of the coalition. **E,** The joint is distracted with a lamina spreader to ensure lysis of any remaining fibrous adhesions.

Surgical Technique

1. Equipment required includes a sharp beveled chisel or a set of sharp straight osteotomes, a rongeur or large pituitary rongeur, and bone wax to cover the exposed bone surfaces (video clip 52).

2. The patient is positioned supine with adequate support placed under the ipsilateral hip. Elevation of the lateral hip allows internal rotation of the extremity, facilitating exposure of the coalition.

3. It is helpful to incorporate a popliteal block when considering anesthetic, and if an

indwelling popliteal catheter may be used, the patient will experience outstanding pain relief for at least 3 days following the procedure. In fact, the entire procedure can be performed with this block, with the use of a calf tourniquet. If a general anesthetic or spinal anesthetic is chosen, a thigh tourniquet may be used to facilitate hemostasis.

4. The incision begins 1 cm distal to the tip of the fibula and is carried obliquely to the base of the third metatarsal.

5. Two nerves that are subcutaneous at the portion of the foot are at risk. The intermediate dorsal cutaneous branch of the superficial peroneal nerve crosses the surgical path and should be identified and protected with a vessel loop. The anterior branch of the sural nerve can also be found at the proximal portion of the incision.

6. The origin of the extensor digitorum brevis muscle is detached from the lateral surface of the talus and reflected distally.

7. The anterior process of the calcaneus is identified and traced toward the navicular. The coalition is identified as a broad surface of bone (or a surface interrupted by fibrous tissue) connecting the anteromedial aspect of the calcaneus to the plantar–lateral portion of the navicular.

8. The parameters of the coalition are carefully identified. This is critical to avoid violation of the articular surface of the navicular or the calcaneocuboid joint. For confirmation, the surgeon can use intraoperative fluoroscopy.

9. The ligaments between the talus and navicular and the calcaneus and cuboid are preserved. Damage to the talonavicular ligaments will allow the navicular to sublux upon the talus. Similarly, damage to the calcaneocuboid ligament will allow the cuboid to shift upon the calcaneus.

10. With a straight osteotome or sharp chisel, the navicular portion of the coalition is resected with an oblique angle, ensuring that the plantar–lateral portion is resected. The calcaneal portion is resected with a parallel cut beginning at the superior–medial articular surface of the calcaneo-cuboid joint.

11. The block of bone and fibrous tissue removed may be as large as 2 cm using these resection margins. After removing the coalition, the surgeon looks for additional bone fragments impinging upon the talo-navicular or calcaneocuboid joint. All such fragments are removed at this time.

12. Manipulation of the transverse tarsal joint assists in evaluating for impingement along the lateral aspect of the calcaneocuboid joint. Occasionally, an abnormally shaped calcaneocuboid joint is detected that can block abduction of the foot. This abnormally shaped bone arises from the calcaneus and must be removed to facilitate abduction of the cuboid. Under normal circumstances, the amount of bone removed at this location is small.

13. Bone wax is applied to all cut bone surfaces.

14. The origin of the extensor digitorum brevis may now be interposed into the defect. Keith needles threaded with absorbable suture are placed into the tendinous origin of the muscle. These needles are passed plantarward and may be tied on either side of the plantar fascia through a small separate incision. With this technique, a button may be avoided.

15. The tourniquet is deflated prior to closure to minimize the risk of hematoma and subsequent scar formation. Hemostasis is very important at this stage, and if drainage is persistent, a suction drain is placed deep in the area of the coalition.

16. The extensor fascia is approximated, as is the subcutaneous tissue and skin.

17. A plaster splint limiting inversion and eversion, or a short-leg fiberglass cast, is applied intraoperatively.

Postoperative Care

If it was not done prior to the procedure, the popliteal block with an indwelling catheter can be performed in the recovery room to facilitate pain control.

Sutures are removed at 10 days after surgery, unless significant swelling suggests an incisional wound complication. In this instance, sutures are left in place for 3 weeks. The patient is given a CAM walker boot, and ambulation is encouraged. Physical therapy may be instituted simultaneously to encourage aggressive passive range of motion of the transverse tarsal and subtalar joints. Gains achieved intraoperatively will be maintained or enhanced through this activity. A compression stocking, or a more formal lymphedema clinic, should be used to minimize soft tissue edema. Swelling compromises motion at this critical juncture.

The CAM walker boot should be discontinued by 4 weeks postoperatively, which will further encourage range of motion of the hindfoot.

TALOCALCANEAL COALITION RESECTION

Similar to the calcaneonavicular coalition, surgical treatment of the talocalcaneal coalition in an adult with minimal or no secondary changes (arthrosis) consists of resection of the coalition. Again, the goal is to eliminate painful motion at the coalition site while potentially increasing hindfoot motion.

Indications

Surgical resection of a talocalcaneal coalition is indicated after failure of two trials of conservative care (casting). Pain is the primary indication, because recovery of subtalar motion might not be significant enough as an isolated indication.

Contraindications

Previously it was thought that a coalition that occupied more than 50% of the total articular surface of the subtalar would have a poor result.[135] Scranton[135] chose this value based on CT data, and using this arbitrary figure he evaluated his own results, finding good results in 13 of 14 patients. He has been misquoted in many orthopaedic texts over the years, leading to the misconception that he found poor results in patients with coalitions occupying greater than 50% of the *middle* facet as an isolated entity.

It has been shown by Comfort and Johnson[13] that 77% of patients undergoing resection of a talocalcaneal coalition involving less than one third of the *total* joint surface (anterior, middle, and posterior facets) experience good or excellent results. This study evaluated 20 patients using CT to map out the surface area of the posterior, anterior, and middle facets. They used these data to determine the location and extent of the talocalcaneal coalition as a percentage of the surface area of the entire joint construct. All

patients in the study group had the coalition resected for symptoms. On average, these coalitions involved 66.5% of the anterior and middle facets (these facets are contiguous 67% of the time[133]) and 29.8% of the total joint surface area. With outcome based on level of activity, pain, and subtalar motion, 60% of the results were rated good or excellent. A strong correlation was found between the size of the coalition and the clinical outcome, noting that fair or poor results were found in 75% of the patients sustaining coalitions occupying more than one third of the total joint surface. Age was not correlated with surgical outcome. It has been suggested that increased age correlates with more poor results owing to resection allowing increased motion across degenerative joint surfaces. This study places that contraindication in question.

Finally, the authors compared their results to Scranton's guidelines and found that if they had followed his initial guidelines for resection, their entire group would be candidates for resection, because no coalition involved more than 50% of the total joint surface. In that case, they would have had a much greater percentage of fair or poor results than those illustrated by Scranton. Thus, this study based on Wilde's criteria for measuring surface area of the subtalar joint[157] suggests that surgery is contraindicated in talocalcaneal coalitions occupying greater than one third of the total articular surface of all three facets of the subtalar joint.

Preoperative Evaluation

Patients are evaluated for coalition radiographically. Plain radiographs include the Harris axial view, which demonstrates the coalition. CT scanning reveals the extent of the coalition and whether it is osseous or fibrous. More important, the CT scan assists in evaluating adjacent joint surfaces for arthritic wear. For example, post-traumatic arthritis of the subtalar joint can mimic symptoms of a tarsal coalition, and if arthritis is present, it warrants fusion over resection.

Clinically, severity of the planovalgus foot deformity is assessed. The literature does not address correction of the flatfoot deformity in conjunction with coalition resection. However, it must remain a consideration, especially in patients with subfibular impingement (separate from pain at the site of the coalition) or pain medially underlying the talar head. Such patients become candidates for simultaneous medial slide calcaneal osteotomies, lateral column lengthenings, and/or medial cuneiform opening wedge osteotomies.

Preoperative Planning

Radiographs are reviewed to determine the extent and location of the coalition. In certain circumstances, a PCR nasal screen is appropriate to evaluate for staphylococcus species, and noninvasive blood flow studies assist in wound healing assessment.

Whereas the resection of a calcaneonavicular coalition is relatively simple, the resection of a talocalcaneal coalition is technically demanding and requires adequate exposure, careful orientation, and cautious dissection.

Surgical Technique

1. Equipment required includes a sharp beveled chisel or a set of sharp straight osteotomes, a rongeur or large pituitary rongeur, and bone wax to cover the exposed bone surfaces (video clip 53).
2. It is helpful to incorporate a popliteal block when considering anesthetic, and if an indwelling popliteal catheter can be used, the patient will experience outstanding pain relief for at least 3 days following the procedure. In fact, the entire procedure can be performed with this block, with the use of a calf tourniquet. If a general anesthetic or spinal anesthetic is chosen, a thigh tourniquet may be used to facilitate hemostasis.
3. The patient is positioned supine, with adequate support placed under the contralateral hip to facilitate external rotation of the operative extremity.
4. The incision is made along the inferior aspect of the posterior tibial tendon sheath, beginning 1 cm distal to the tip of the medial malleolus and extending distal to the talonavicular joint.
5. The incision is deepened through the subcutaneous tissue and fat to expose the posterior tibial tendon sheath. The inferior aspect of the sheath is opened and the tendon is retracted superiorly.
6. Deep to this, the sheath for the flexor digitorum longus is encountered. This sheath passes along the medial surface of the talus,

superior to the sustentaculum tali and thus the location of the coalition.
7. The flexor digitorum longus is retracted superiorly to expose the inferior edge of its tendon sheath. This inferior edge should be exposed from the medial malleolus to the talonavicular joint. Plantar to the flexor digitorum longus tendon is the neurovascular bundle, which should be identified and protected.
8. The area of the coalition can be identified by locating the posterior facet of the subtalar joint proximally and the tarsal canal distally. The coalition lies between these two landmarks.
9. Using an osteotome or a chisel, a wedge of bone is removed to excise the coalition. The apex of the wedge is lateral. It may be easiest to start at the proximal point of the coalition, at the medial aspect of the posterior facet, and proceed distally. The surgeon must excise sufficient bone to visualize the joint surfaces. Once a sufficient amount of bone has been removed from the middle facet, the tarsal canal is visualized. The sustentaculum tali is not removed in its entirety. In addition, though sufficient bone must be resected to regain a portion of subtalar motion, the surgeon must take care to avoid removing excessive bone, because the subtalar joint will become destabilized, accelerating arthritic wear.
10. Subtalar motion is checked and is often less than 50% of that detected on the opposite, normal side.
11. Bone wax is placed over the exposed bone surfaces.
12. The tourniquet is deflated and meticulous hemostasis is performed. Limiting hematoma will limit subsequent scar tissue and enhance motion.
13. The tendon sheaths are approximated, restoring the tendons to their normal anatomic position.
14. The subcutaneous tissue and skin are sutured.
15. A plaster splint limiting subtalar motion, or a short-leg fiberglass cast, is applied.

Postoperative Care

If not done prior to the procedure, the popliteal block with an indwelling catheter can be performed in the recovery room to facilitate pain control.

Sutures are removed 10 days postoperatively, unless significant swelling suggests an incisional wound complication. In this instance, sutures are left in place for 3 weeks. The patient is then placed into a CAM walker boot, and ambulation is encouraged. Physical therapy may be instituted simultaneously to encourage aggressive and passive range of motion of the transverse tarsal and subtalar joints. Gains achieved intraoperatively will be maintained or enhanced through this activity. A compressive stocking, or a more formal lymphedema clinic, should be used to minimize soft tissue edema. Swelling compromises motion at this critical juncture.

The CAM walker boot should be discontinued by 4 weeks postoperatively, which will further encourage range of motion of the hindfoot.

Results and Complications

Results of both talocalcaneal and calcaneonavicular coalitions are reviewed.

Swiontkowski et al[146] performed a follow-up study of 40 patients who underwent 57 procedures for tarsal coalition. In total, 44 calcaneonavicular coalitions and 13 talocalcaneal coalitions were reviewed. Thirty-nine of the 44 calcaneonavicular coalitions underwent resection, whereas 5 underwent triple arthrodesis. At an average follow-up of 4.6 years, 29 (66%) were asymptomatic and 7 (16%) had symptoms with strenuous activity. In all, 90% improved considerably through surgical intervention. In the talocalcaneal group, five patients underwent resection and nine had an arthrodesis (both triple and subtalar). At a mean follow-up of 3.1 years, 4 of 5 resections were asymptomatic. Of those undergoing arthrodesis, 78% were symptom-free. In both series, talar beaking had no influence on outcome and is not a contraindication. The authors experienced no complications in any of their procedures other than some coalition resections requiring arthrodesis for persistent pain.

Mann et al[94] evaluated 10 patients with a talocalcaneal coalition undergoing subtalar arthrodesis. This adult population (average age 26 years) was followed for an average 7.5 years. None were candidates for resection of the coalition. Preoperative pain index improved from 3.5

(out of 4) to 1, and postoperative function improved from 3.2 (out of 4) to 0.7. The final modified American Orthopaedic Foot and Ankle Society (AOFAS) score was 93. Sixty percent (6 out of 10) demonstrated radiographic evidence of mild talonavicular arthrosis, which was not present preoperatively, but none were symptomatic. The authors prefer subtalar arthrodesis for severe flatfoot associated with talocalcaneal coalition over triple arthrodesis, in order to preserve some of the motion at Chopart's joint. Such limitations clinically amounted to a 40% decrease in transverse tarsal motion, dorsiflexion decrease by 30%, and plantar flexion decrease of 9%.

Gonzalez and Kumar[43] evaluated 48 patients who underwent resection of a calcaneonavicular coalition in 75 feet. They divided their population into two groups. Group A (32 feet) patients were directly evaluated by the authors in follow-up. Group B (43 feet) patients were evaluated retrospectively. The authors found that 84% of the patients in group A achieved a good or excellent result. Those with a fair result did not warrant conversion to arthrodesis. Group B patients demonstrated 72% good or excellent results, with 7% overall requiring revision to a triple arthrodesis. Combining both groups yielded 77% good or excellent results from resection of a calcaneonavicular coalition. Again, talar beaking did not preclude a good outcome clinically. The result did not deteriorate over time, and some patients followed for more than 20 years maintained a good or excellent result.

Cohen et al[12] evaluated 13 feet undergoing resection for calcaneonavicular coalition. This cohort consisted of adult patients (average age 33 years) with 77% demonstrating preexisting degenerative arthritis radiographically. With an average 3-year follow-up, 85% (11 of 13) had subjective relief of preoperative symptoms, and 2 of 13 underwent secondary arthrodesis (one subtalar, one triple). Subtalar motion improved an average of 10 degrees. Preoperative degenerative arthritic changes were noted in the naviculocuneiform joint (23%), the subtalar joint (23%), and the talonavicular joint (46%). Preexisting arthritis was mild or minimal in 12 of 13 patients, and the one patient with moderate osteoarthritis (multiple peripheral osteophytes in the absence of significant joint space narrowing) later required a subtalar arthrodesis.

Complications stemmed from the initial use of the extensor digitorum brevis muscle as an interposition graft with a pull-out suture placed medially. This technique resulted in a 50% lateral wound-dehiscence rate. Using bone wax prior to restoring the extensor digitorum brevis to its anatomic position eliminated this complication.

REFERENCES

1. Abosala A, Tumia N, Anderson D: Tibialis posterior tendon rupture in children. *Injury* 34(11):866-867, 2003.
2. Alexander IJ, Johnson KA, Berquist TH: Magnetic resonance imaging in the diagnosis of disruption of the posterior tibial tendon. *Foot Ankle* 8(3):144-147, 1987.
3. Augustin JF, Lin SS, Berberian WS, Johnson JE: Nonoperative treatment of adult acquired flat foot with the Arizona brace. *Foot Ankle Clin* 8(3):491-502, 2003.
4. Balen PF, Helms CA: Association of posterior tibial tendon injury with spring ligament injury, sinus tarsi abnormality, and plantar fasciitis on MR imaging. *AJR Am J Roentgenol* 176(5):1137-1143, 2001.
5. Blake RL, Anderson K, Ferguson H: Posterior tibial tendinitis. A literature review with case reports. *J Am Podiatr Med Assoc* 84(3):141-149, 1994.
6. Bordelon RL: Correction of hypermobile flatfoot in children by molded insert. *Foot Ankle* 1(3):143-150, 1980.
7. Brahms MA: The posterior tibial tendon. *J Am Podiatry Assoc* 56(11):502-503, 1966.
8. Brown RR, Rosenberg ZS, Thornhill BA: The C sign: More specific for flatfoot deformity than subtalar coalition. *Skeletal Radiol* 30(2):84-87, 2001.
9. Chao W, Wapner KL, Lee TH, et al: Nonoperative management of posterior tibial tendon dysfunction. *Foot Ankle Int* 17(12):736-741, 1996.
10. Chen YJ, Liang SC: Diagnostic efficacy of ultrasonography in stage I posterior tibial tendon dysfunction: Sonographic–surgical correlation. *J Ultrasound Med* 16(6):417-423, 1997.
11. Choi K, Lee S, Otis JC, Deland JT: Anatomical reconstruction of the spring ligament using peroneus longus tendon graft. *Foot Ankle Int* 24(5):430-436, 2003.
12. Cohen BE, Davis WH, Anderson RB: Success of calcaneonavicular coalition resection in the adult population. *Foot Ankle Int* 17(9):569-572, 1996.
13. Comfort TK, Johnson LO: Resection for symptomatic talocalcaneal coalition. *J Pediatr Orthop* 18(3):283-288, 1998.
14. Conti SF: Posterior tibial tendon problems in athletes. *Orthop Clin North Am* 25(1):109-121, 1994.
15. Conti S, Michelson J, Jahss M: Clinical significance of magnetic resonance imaging in preoperative planning for reconstruction of posterior tibial tendon ruptures. *Foot Ankle* 13(4):208-214, 1992.
16. Conti SF, Wong YS: Osteolysis of structural autograft after calcaneocuboid distraction arthrodesis for stage II posterior tibial tendon dysfunction. *Foot Ankle Int* 23(6):521-529, 2002.
17. Cooper PS, Nowak MD, Shaer J: Calcaneocuboid joint pressures with lateral column lengthening (Evans) procedure. *Foot Ankle Int* 18(4):199-205, 1997.
18. Cotton FJ: Foot statics and surgery. *N Engl J Med* 214:353-362, 1936.
19. Cowell HR: Talocalcaneal coalition and new causes of peroneal spastic flatfoot. *Clin Orthop Relat Res* 85:16-22, 1972.
20. Cowell HR, Elener V: Rigid painful flatfoot secondary to tarsal coalition. *Clin Orthop Relat Res* 177:54-60, 1983.
21. Cozen L: Posterior tibial tenosynovitis secondary to foot strain. *Clin Orthop Relat Res* 42:101-102, 1965.
22. Crates JM, and Richardson EG: Treatment of stage I posterior tibial tendon dysfunction with medial soft tissue procedures. *Clin Orthop Relat Res* 365:46-49, 1999.
23. Crim JR, Kjeldsberg KM: Radiographic diagnosis of tarsal coalition. *AJR Am J Roentgenol* 182(2):323-328, 2004.
24. Danko AM, Allen B Jr, Pugh L, Stasikelis P: Early graft failure in lateral column lengthening. *J Pediatr Orthop* 24(6):716-720, 2004.
25. De Zwart DF, Davidson JS: Rupture of the posterior tibial tendon associated with fractures of the ankle. A report of two cases. *J Bone Joint Surg Am* 65(2):260-262, 1983.
26. Deland JT, Otis JC, Lee KT, Kenneally SM: Lateral column lengthening with calcaneocuboid fusion: Range of motion in the triple joint complex. *Foot Ankle Int* 16(11):729-733, 1995.
27. Delmi M, Kurt AM, Meyer JM, Hoffmeyer P: Calcification of the tibialis posterior tendon: A case report and literature review. *Foot Ankle Int* 16(12):792-795, 1995.
28. Downey DJ, Simkin PA, Mack LA, et al: Tibialis posterior tendon rupture: A cause of rheumatoid flat foot. *Arthritis Rheum* 31(3):441-446, 1988.
29. Duchene GG: *Physiology of Motion*. Philadelphia, JB Lippincott, 1949, pp 303-369.
30. Dumontier TA, Falicov A, Mosca V, Sangeorzan B: Calcaneal lengthening: Investigation of deformity correction in a cadaver flatfoot model. *Foot Ankle Int* 26(2):166-170, 2005.
31. Dwyer FC: Osteotomy of the calcaneum for pes cavus. *J Bone Joint Surg Br* 41(1):80-86, 1959.
32. Dyal CM, Feder J, Deland JT, Thompson FM: Pes planus in patients with posterior tibial tendon insufficiency: Asymptomatic versus symptomatic foot. *Foot Ankle Int* 18(2):85-88, 1997.
33. Emery KH, Bisset GS 3rd; Johnson ND, Nunan PJ: Tarsal coalition: A blinded comparison of MRI and CT. *Pediatr Radiol* 28(8):612-616, 1998.
34. Fayazi AH, Nguyen HV, Juliano PJ: Intermediate term follow-up of calcaneal osteotomy and flexor digitorum longus transfer for treatment of posterior tibial tendon dysfunction. *Foot Ankle Int* 23(12):1107-1111, 2002.
35. Frey C, Shereff M, Greenidge N: Vascularity of the posterior tibial tendon. *J Bone Joint Surg Am* 72(6):884-888, 1990.
36. Funk DA, Cass JR, Johnson KA: Acquired adult flat foot secondary to posterior tibial-tendon pathology. *J Bone Joint Surg Am* 68(1):95-102, 1986.
37. Gazdag AR, Cracchiolo A 3rd: Rupture of the posterior tibial tendon. Evaluation of injury of the spring ligament and clinical assessment of tendon transfer and ligament repair. *J Bone Joint Surg Am* 79(5):675-681, 1997.
38. Gerling MC, Pfirrmann CW, Farooki S, et al: Posterior tibialis tendon tears: comparison of the diagnostic efficacy of magnetic resonance imaging and ultrasonography for the detection of surgically created longitudinal tears in cadavers. *Invest Radiol* 38(1):51-56, 2003.
39. Giblin MM: Ruptured tibialis posterior tendon associated with a closed medial malleolar fracture. *Aust N Z J Surg* 50(1):59-60, 1980.
40. Gleich A: Beitrag zur operativen Plattfussbehandlung. *Arch Klin Chir* 46:358-362, 1893.
41. Goldner JL, Keats PK, Bassett FH 3rd, Clippinger FW: Progressive talipes equinovalgus due to trauma or degeneration of the

posterior tibial tendon and medial plantar ligaments. *Orthop Clin North Am* 5(1):39-51, 1974.

42. Goncalves-Neto J, Witzel SS, Teodoro WR, et al: Changes in collagen matrix composition in human posterior tibial tendon dysfunction. *Joint Bone Spine* 69(2):189-194, 2002.
43. Gonzalez P, Kumar SJ: Calcaneonavicular coalition treated by resection and interposition of the extensor digitorum brevis muscle. *J Bone Joint Surg Am* 72(1):71-77, 1990.
44. Gould N: Graphing the adult foot and ankle. *Foot Ankle* 2(4):213-219, 1982.
45. Greene DL, Thompson MC, Gesink DS, Graves SC: Anatomic study of the medial neurovascular structures in relation to calcaneal osteotomy. *Foot Ankle Int* 22(7):569-571, 2001.
46. Griffiths JC: Tendon injuries around the ankle. *J Bone Joint Surg Br* 47(4):686-689, 1965.
47. Guyton GP, Jeng C, Krieger LE, Mann RA: Flexor digitorum longus transfer and medial displacement calcaneal osteotomy for posterior tibial tendon dysfunction: A middle-term clinical follow-up. *Foot Ankle Int* 22(8):627-632, 2001.
48. Hadfield M, Snyder J, Liacouras P, et al: The effects of a medializing calcaneal osteotomy with and without superior translation on Achilles tendon elongation and plantar foot pressures. *Foot Ankle Int* 26(5):365-370, 2005.
49. Harris RI: Rigid valgus foot due to talocalcaneal bridge. *J Bone Joint Surg Am* 37(1):169-183, 1955.
50. Harris RJ, Beath T: Etiology of peroneal spastic flatfoot. *J Bone Joint Surg Br* 30:624-634, 1948.
51. Helal B: Tibialis posterior tendon synovitis and rupture. *Acta Orthop Belg* 55(3):457-460, 1989.
52. Hicks JH: The mechanics of the foot. II. The plantar aponeurosis and the arch. *J Anat* 88(1):25-30, 1954.
53. Hintermann B, Valderrabano V, Kundert HP: Lengthening of the lateral column and reconstruction of the medial soft tissue for treatment of acquired flatfoot deformity associated with insufficiency of the posterior tibial tendon. *Foot Ankle Int* 20(10):622-629, 1999.
54. Hirose CB, Johnson JE: Plantar flexion opening wedge medial cuneiform osteotomy for correction of fixed forefoot varus associated with flatfoot deformity. *Foot Ankle Int* 25(8):568-574, 2004.
55. Hochman M, Reed MH: Features of calcaneonavicular coalition on coronal computed tomography. *Skeletal Radiol* 29(7):409-412, 2000.
56. Hogan JF: Posterior tibial tendon dysfunction and MRI. *J Foot Ankle Surg* 32(5):467-472, 1993.
57. Holmes GB Jr, Mann RA: Possible epidemiological factors associated with rupture of the posterior tibial tendon. *Foot Ankle* 13(2):70-79, 1992.
58. Horton GA, Myerson MS, Parks BG, Park YW: Effect of calcaneal osteotomy and lateral column lengthening on the plantar fascia: A biomechanical investigation. *Foot Ankle Int* 19(6):370-373, 1998.
59. Hsu TC, Wang CL, Wang TG, et al: Ultrasonographic examination of the posterior tibial tendon. *Foot Ankle Int* 18(1):34-38, 1997.
60. Hyer CF, Lee T, Block AJ, VanCourt R: Evaluation of the anterior and middle talocalcaneal articular facets and the Evans osteotomy. *J Foot Ankle Surg* 41(6):389-393, 2002.
61. Imhauser CW, Siegler S, Abidi NA, Frankel DZ: The effect of posterior tibialis tendon dysfunction on the plantar pressure characteristics and the kinematics of the arch and the hindfoot. *Clin Biomech (Bristol, Avon)* 19(2):161-169, 2004.
62. Jahss MH: Spontaneous rupture of the tibialis posterior tendon: Clinical findings, tenographic studies, and a new technique of repair. *Foot Ankle* 3(3):158-166, 1982.

63. Janisse DJ, Wertsch JD, Del Toro DR: Foot orthoses and prescription shoes. In Redford JB, Basmajian JV, Trautman P (eds): *Orthotics, Clinical Practice and Rehabilitation Technology*, New York, Churchill Livingstone, 1995, pp 64-65.
64. Johnson KA, Strom DE: Tibialis posterior tendon dysfunction. *Clin Orthop Relat Res* (239):196-206, 1989.
65. Kadakia AR., and Haddad SL: Hindfoot arthrodesis for the adult acquired flat foot. *Foot Ankle Clin* 8(3):569-594, x, 2003.
66. Kapandji I: *The Physiology of the Joints.* New York, Churchill Livingston, 1970, pp 170-194.
67. Karasick D, Schweitzer ME: Tear of the posterior tibial tendon causing asymmetric flatfoot: Radiologic findings. *AJR Am J Roentgenol* 161(6):1237-1240, 1993.
68. Kaye RA, Jahss MH: Tibialis posterior: A review of anatomy and biomechanics in relation to support of the medial longitudinal arch. *Foot Ankle* 11(4):244-247, 1991.
69. Keenan MA, Peabody TD, Gronley JK, Perry J: Valgus deformities of the feet and characteristics of gait in patients who have rheumatoid arthritis. *J Bone Joint Surg Am* 73(2):237-247, 1991.
70. Kennedy JC, Willis RB: The effects of local steroid injections on tendons: A biomechanical and microscopic correlative study. *Am J Sports Med* 4(1):11-21, 1976.
71. Kettelkamp DB, Alexander HH: Spontaneous rupture of the posterior tibial tendon. *J Bone Joint Surg Am* 51(4):759-764, 1969.
72. Key JA: Partial rupture of the tendon of the posterior tibial muscle. *J Bone Joint Surg Am* 35(4):1006-1008, 1953.
73. Khoury NJ, el-Khoury GY, Saltzman CL, Brandser EA: MR imaging of posterior tibial tendon dysfunction. *AJR Am J Roentgenol* 167(3):675-682, 1996.
74. Kimball HL, Aronow MS, Sullivan RJ, et al: Biomechanical evaluation of calcaneocuboid distraction arthrodesis: A cadaver study of two different fixation methods. *Foot Ankle Int* 21(10):845-848, 2000.
75. Kirkham BW, Gibson T: Comment on the article by Downey et al. *Arthritis Rheum* 32(3):359, 1989.
76. Korvin H: Coalitio talocalcaneal. *Z Orthop Chir* 60:105, 1934.
77. Koutsogiannis E: Treatment of mobile flat foot by displacement osteotomy of the calcaneus. *J Bone Joint Surg Br* 53(1):96-100, 1971.
78. Kulig K, Burnfield J. M, Requejo SM, et al: Selective activation of tibialis posterior: Evaluation by magnetic resonance imaging. *Med Sci Sports Exerc* 36(5):862-867, 2004.
79. Kulik SA Jr, Clanton TO: Tarsal coalition. *Foot Ankle Int* 17(5):286-296, 1996.
80. Kulowski J: Tendovaginitis (tenosynovitis), general discussion and report of one case involving the posterior tibial tendon. *J Missouri State Med Assoc* 33:135-137, 1936.
81. Kumar SJ, Guille JT, Lee MS, Couto JC: Osseous and non-osseous coalition of the middle facet of the talocalcaneal joint. *J Bone Joint Surg Am* 74(4):529-535, 1992.
82. Langenskiöld A: Chronic non-specific tenosynovitis of the tibialis posterior tendon. *Acta Orthop Scand* 38(3):301-305, 1967.
83. Lapidus PW: Kinesiology and mechanical anatomy of the tarsal joints. *Clin Orthop Relat Res* 30:20-36, 1963.
84. Lapidus PW, Seidenstein H: Chronic non-specific tenosynovitis with effusion about the ankle; report of three cases. *J Bone Joint Surg Am* 32(1):175-179, 1950.
85. Leboucq H: De la soudure congenitale de certains os du tarse. *Bulletin de l'Academie Royale de Medecine de Belgique* 4:103-112, 1890.
86. Lee MF, Chan PT, Chau LF, Yu KS: Tarsal tunnel syndrome caused by talocalcaneal coalition. *Clin Imaging* 26(2):140-143, 2002.

87. Leung AK, Mak AF, Evans JH: Biomedical gait evaluation of the immediate effect of orthotic treatment for flexible flat foot. Prosthet Orthot Int 22(1):25-34, 1998.

88. Lipscomb P: Non-suppurative tenosynovitis and paratendinitis. Instr Course Lect 7:254, 1950.

89. Malicky ES, Crary JL, Houghton MJ, et al: Talocalcaneal and subfibular impingement in symptomatic flatfoot in adults. J Bone Joint Surg Am 84(11):2005-2009, 2002.

90. Mann RA: Acquired flatfoot in adults. Clin Orthop Relat Res 181:46-51, 1983.

91. Mann RA: Posterior tibial tendon dysfunction. Treatment by flexor digitorum longus transfer. Foot Ankle Clin 6(1):77-87, vi, 2001.

92. Mann RA: Flatfoot in adults. In Coughlin MJ, Mann RA (eds): Surgery of the Foot and Ankle. St Louis, Mosby, 1999, pp 733-767.

93. Mann RA: Tendon transfers and electromyography. Clin Orthop Relat Res 85:64-66, 1972.

94. Mann RA, Beaman DN, Horton GA: Isolated subtalar arthrodesis. Foot Ankle Int 19(8):511-519, 1998.

95. Mann R, Inman VT: Phasic activity of intrinsic muscles of the foot. J Bone Joint Surg Am 46:469-481, 1964.

96. Mann R, Specht T: Posterior tibial tendon rupture. Presented at the Annual Winter Meeting of the American Orthopedic Foot and Ankle Society, Las Vegas, Nevada, 1982.

97. Mann RA, Thompson FM: Rupture of the posterior tibial tendon causing flat foot. Surgical treatment. J Bone Joint Surg Am 67(4):556-561, 1985.

98. Marcus RE, Pfister ME: The enigmatic diagnosis of posterior tibialis tendon rupture. Iowa Orthop J 13:171-177, 1993.

99. McCormack AP, Varner KE, Marymont JV: Surgical treatment for posterior tibial tendonitis in young competitive athletes. Foot Ankle Int 24(7):535-538, 2003.

100. McMaster PE: Tendon and muscle ruptures. Clinical and experimental studies on the causes and location of subcutaneous ruptures. J Bone Joint Surg 15:705, 1933.

101. Michelson J, Conti S, Jahss MH: Survivorship analysis of tendon transfer surgery for posterior tibial tendon rupture. Orthop Trans 16:30-31, 1992.

102. Michelson J, Easley M, Wigley FM, Hellmann D: Posterior tibial tendon dysfunction in rheumatoid arthritis. Foot Ankle Int 16(3):156-161, 1995.

103. Miller SD, Van Holsbeeck M, Boruta PM, et al: Ultrasound in the diagnosis of posterior tibial tendon pathology. Foot Ankle Int 17(9):555-558, 1996.

104. Momberger N, Morgan JM, Bachus KN, West JR: Calcaneocuboid joint pressure after lateral column lengthening in a cadaveric planovalgus deformity model. Foot Ankle Int 21(9):730-735, 2000.

105. Monto RR, Moorman CT 3rd, Mallon WJ, Nunley JA 3rd: Rupture of the posterior tibial tendon associated with closed ankle fracture. Foot Ankle 11(6):400-403, 1991.

106. Mosca VS: Calcaneal lengthening for valgus deformity of the hindfoot. Results in children who had severe, symptomatic flatfoot and skewfoot. J Bone Joint Surg Am 77(4):500-512, 1995.

107. Mosier SM, Lucas DR, Pomeroy G, Manoli A 2nd: Pathology of the posterior tibial tendon in posterior tibial tendon insufficiency. Foot Ankle Int 19(8):520-524, 1998.

108. Mosier-LaClair S, Pomeroy G, Manoli A 2nd: Operative treatment of the difficult stage 2 adult acquired flatfoot deformity. Foot Ankle Clin 6(1):95-119, 2001.

109. Mueller TJ: Acquired flatfoot secondary to tibialis posterior dysfunction: Biomechanical aspects. J Foot Surg 30(1):2-11, 1991.

110. Myerson MS: Adult acquired flatfoot deformity: Treatment of dysfunction of the posterior tibial tendon. J Bone Joint Surg Am 78:780-792, 1996.

111. Myerson MS, Badekas A, Schon LC: Treatment of stage II posterior tibial tendon deficiency with flexor digitorum longus tendon transfer and calcaneal osteotomy. Foot Ankle Int 25(7):445-450, 2004.

112. Myerson MS., and Corrigan J: Treatment of posterior tibial tendon dysfunction with flexor digitorum longus tendon transfer and calcaneal osteotomy. Orthopedics 19(5):383-388, 1996.

113. Myerson M, Solomon G, Shereff M: Posterior tibial tendon dysfunction: Its association with seronegative inflammatory disease. Foot Ankle 9(5):219-225, 1989.

114. Niki H, Ching RP, Kiser P, Sangeorzan BJ: The effect of posterior tibial tendon dysfunction on hindfoot kinematics. Foot Ankle Int 22(4):292-300, 2001.

115. Nyska M, Parks BG, Chu IT, Myerson MS: The contribution of the medial calcaneal osteotomy to the correction of flatfoot deformities. Foot Ankle Int 22(4):278-282, 2001.

116. Penney KE, Wiener BD, Magill RM: Traumatic rupture of the tibialis posterior tendon after ankle fracture: A case report. Am J Orthop 29(1):41-43, 2000.

117. Petersen W, Hohmann G, Pufe T, et al: Structure of the human tibialis posterior tendon. Arch Orthop Trauma Surg 124(4):237-242, 2004.

118. Petersen W, Hohmann G, Stein V, Tillmann B: The blood supply of the posterior tibial tendon. J Bone Joint Surg Br 84(1):141-144, 2002.

119. Phillips GE: A review of elongation of os calcis for flat feet. J Bone Joint Surg Br 65(1):15-18, 1983.

120. Pineda C, Resnick D, Greenway G: Diagnosis of tarsal coalition with computed tomography. Clin Orthop Relat Res 208:282-288, 1986.

121. Plattner PF: Tendon problems of the foot and ankle. The spectrum from peritendinitis to rupture. Postgrad Med 86(3):155-162, 167-170, 1989.

122. Pomeroy GC, Pike RH, Beals TC, Manoli A. 2nd: Acquired flatfoot in adults due to dysfunction of the posterior tibial tendon. J Bone Joint Surg Am 81(8):1173-1182, 1999.

123. Premkumar A, Perry MB, Dwyer AJ, et al: Sonography and MR imaging of posterior tibial tendinopathy. AJR Am J Roentgenol 178(1):223-232, 2002.

124. Raines RA Jr, Brage ME: Evans osteotomy in the adult foot: An anatomic study of structures at risk. Foot Ankle Int 19(11):743-747, 1998.

125. Rathbun JB, Macnab I: The microvascular pattern of the rotator cuff. J Bone Joint Surg Br 52(3):540-553, 1970.

126. Rosenberg ZS: Chronic rupture of the posterior tibial tendon. Magn Reson Imaging Clin N Am 2(1):79-87, 1994.

127. Rosenberg ZS, Jahss MH, Noto AM, et al: Rupture of the posterior tibial tendon: CT and surgical findings. Radiology 167(2):489-493, 1988.

128. Ross JA: Posterior tibial tendon dysfunction in the athlete. Clin Podiatr Med Surg 14(3):479-488, 1997.

129. Saltzman CL, Brandser EA, Berbaum KS, et al: Reliability of standard foot radiographic measurements. Foot Ankle Int 15(12):661-665, 1994.

130. Saltzman CL, el-Khoury GY: The hindfoot alignment view. Foot Ankle Int 16(9):572-576, 1995.

131. Sands A, Early J, Harrington RM, et al: Effect of variations in calcaneocuboid fusion technique on kinematics of the normal hindfoot. Foot Ankle Int 19(1):19-25, 1998.

132. Sangeorzan BJ, Mosca V, Hansen ST Jr: Effect of calcaneal lengthening on relationships among the hindfoot, midfoot, and forefoot. Foot Ankle 14(3):136-141, 1993.

133. Sarrafian SK: *Anatomy of the Foot and Ankle.* Philadelphia, JB Lippincott, 1983, pp. 43-61; 216-219; 375-425.

134. Schaffer JJ, Lock TR, Salciccioli GG: Posterior tibial tendon rupture in pronation–external rotation ankle fractures. *J Trauma* 27(7):795-796, 1987.

135. Scranton PE Jr: Treatment of symptomatic talocalcaneal coalition. *J Bone Joint Surg Am* 69(4):533-539, 1987.

136. Sijbrandij ES, van Gils AP, de Lange EE, Sijbrandij S: Bone marrow ill-defined hyperintensities with tarsal coalition: MR imaging findings. *Eur J Radiol* 43(1):61-65, 2002.

137. Silver RL, de la Garza J, Rang M: The myth of muscle balance. A study of relative strengths and excursions of normal muscles about the foot and ankle. *J Bone Joint Surg Br* 67(3):432-437, 1985.

138. Solomon LB, Ruhli FJ, Taylor J, et al: A dissection and computer tomograph study of tarsal coalitions in 100 cadaver feet. *J Orthop Res* 21(2):352-358, 2003.

139. Stein RE: Rupture of the posterior tibial tendon in closed ankle fractures. Possible prognostic value of a medial bone flake: report of two cases. *J Bone Joint Surg Am* 67(3):493-494, 1985.

140. Stephien M: The sheath and arterial supply of the tendon of the posterior tibialis muscle in man. *Folia Morph (Warsz)* 32:51-61, 1973.

141. Stormont DM, Peterson HA: The relative incidence of tarsal coalition. *Clin Orthop Relat Res* 181:28-36, 1983.

142. Streb HS, Marzano R: Conservative management of posterior tibial tendon dysfunction, subtalar joint complex, and pes planus deformity. *Clin Podiatr Med Surg* 16(3):439-451, 1999.

143. Sung IH, Lee S, Otis JC, Deland JT: Posterior tibial tendon force requirement in early heel rise after calcaneal osteotomies. *Foot Ankle Int* 23(9):842-849, 2002.

144. Supple KM, Hanft JR, Murphy BJ, et al: Posterior tibial tendon dysfunction. *Semin Arthritis Rheum* 22(2):106-113, 1992.

145. Sutherland DH: An electromyographic study of the plantar flexors of the ankle in normal walking on the level. *J Bone Joint Surg Am* 48(1):66-71, 1966.

146. Swiontkowski MF, Scranton PE, Hansen S: Tarsal coalitions: Long-term results of surgical treatment. *J Pediatr Orthop* 3(3):287-292, 1983.

147. Teasdall RD, Johnson KA: Surgical treatment of stage I posterior tibial tendon dysfunction. *Foot Ankle Int* 15(12):646-648, 1994.

148. Tien TR, Parks BG, Guyton GP: Plantar pressures in the forefoot after lateral column lengthening: A cadaver study comparing the Evans osteotomy and calcaneocuboid fusion. *Foot Ankle Int* 26(7):520-525, 2005.

149. Toolan BC, Sangeorzan BJ, Hansen ST Jr: Complex reconstruction for the treatment of dorsolateral peritalar subluxation of the foot. Early results after distraction arthrodesis of the calcaneocuboid joint in conjunction with stabilization of, and transfer of the flexor digitorum longus tendon to, the midfoot to treat acquired pes planovalgus in adults. *J Bone Joint Surg Am* 81(11):1545-1560, 1999.

150. Trevino S, Gould N, Korson R: Surgical treatment of stenosing tenosynovitis at the ankle. *Foot Ankle* 2(1):37-45, 1981.

151. Varner KE, Michelson JD: Tarsal coalition in adults. *Foot Ankle Int* 21(8):669-672, 2000.

152. Wacker JT, Calder JD, Engstrom CM, Saxby TS: MR morphometry of posterior tibialis muscle in adult acquired flat foot. *Foot Ankle Int* 24(4):354-357, 2003.

153. Wacker JT, Hennessy MS, Saxby TS: Calcaneal osteotomy and transfer of the tendon of flexor digitorum longus for stage-II dysfunction of tibialis posterior. Three- to five-year results. *J Bone Joint Surg Br* 84(1):54-58, 2002.

154. Wapner KL, Chao W: Nonoperative treatment of posterior tibial tendon dysfunction. *Clin Orthop Relat Res* 365:39-45, 1999.

155. Wechsler RJ, Schweitzer ME, Deely DM, et al: Tarsal coalition: Depiction and characterization with CT and MR imaging. *Radiology* 193(2):447-452, 1994.

156. Wertheimer SJ, Weber CA, Loder BG, et al: The role of endoscopy in treatment of stenosing posterior tibial tenosynovitis. *J Foot Ankle Surg* 34(1):15-22, 1995.

157. Wilde PH, Torode IP, Dickens DR, Cole WG: Resection for symptomatic talocalcaneal coalition. *J Bone Joint Surg Br* 76(5):797-801, 1994.

158. Woll TS: Posterior tibial tendon dysfunction. *West J Med* 159(4):485-486, 1993.

159. Yao L, Gentili A, Cracchiolo A: MR imaging findings in spring ligament insufficiency. *Skeletal Radiol* 28(5):245-250, 1990.

Arthrodesis of the Foot and Ankle

Roger A. Mann

TECHNICAL CONSIDERATIONS
SOFT TISSUE CONSIDERATIONS
SURGICAL PRINCIPLES

COMPLICATIONS
SPECIFIC ARTHRODESES (video clips 11-14)

Arthrodesis plays an important role in reconstructive surgery of the foot and ankle, enabling the surgeon to create a painless, stable, plantigrade foot. It is used most often to correct a painful joint secondary to arthrosis, chronic instability of the foot and ankle from muscle dysfunction (e.g., posterior tibial tendon, poliomyelitis), or a deformity that has resulted in a nonplantigrade foot.

Arthrodesis can greatly enhance a patient's functional capacity, but it places increased stress on the joints proximal and distal to the fusion site. After an ankle or triple arthrodesis, approximately 30% of patients demonstrate arthroses distal or proximal to the fusion site within 5 years. Although most of these findings are radiographic, their presence at 5 years does not bode well for what will occur at these joints 20 to 30 years in the future.

Many factors probably affect the onset of this arthrosis besides the increased stress. One factor is probably related to the overall stiffness or laxity of the surrounding joints. The stiffer the surrounding joints, the less the patient is able to dissipate the increased stress created by the fusion compared with a patient who has more joint laxity. Because an arthrodesis is often per-formed on a traumatized extremity, the adjacent joints, although not demonstrating arthrosis, might have sustained tissue damage at the time of the initial injury that makes them more vulnerable to develop arthrosis when subjected to increased stress.

Although this chapter discusses arthrodesis of the joints of the foot and ankle, the clinician should always remember that, if possible, arthrodesis should be avoided, particularly in patients younger than 50 years. Often an osteotomy or a tendon transfer can be used to create a plantigrade foot without resorting to an arthrodesis. It is often more challenging to the surgeon's creativity to avoid an arthrodesis. If the surgeon can offer the patient 5 to 10 years of improved quality of life from a reconstructive procedure without using an arthrodesis, this is the desired approach.

TECHNICAL CONSIDERATIONS

The two basic types of arthrodeses are an in situ fusion and one that corrects a deformity. In an *in situ fusion,* positioning the foot or ankle is usually not difficult because no deformity is present. In a *deformity-*

correcting fusion, however, the surgeon must decide the precise alignment that must be obtained to produce a plantigrade foot. To determine the alignment, the surgeon first must evaluate the normal extremity. With the patient in a supine position, the patella is aligned to the ceiling, giving the surgeon a reference point from which all measurements are made. The degree of internal or external rotation, varus or valgus, and abduction or adduction is carefully noted. A particular arthrodesis is not always placed into a standard alignment; rather, it must be individualized for each patient. Using the patella as a reference point makes alignment at surgery much easier and more precise.

When evaluating the patient for an arthrodesis, the surgeon must also carefully examine the adjacent joints for range of motion and overall alignment. Because an arthrodesis places more stress on the surrounding joints, if one of these joints has mild arthrosis, the prognosis for success is diminished. As an example, when a double or triple arthrodesis needs to be performed and there is mild arthrosis of the ankle or valgus or varus tilt of the talus in the ankle mortise, following a double or triple arthrodesis the ankle joint can deteriorate more rapidly or become more symptomatic as a result of the increased stress. Therefore it is important to inform the patient who is about to undergo a triple or double arthrodesis in the presence of early arthrosis of the ankle joint that although the fusion will create a painless hindfoot, it might also result in rapid deterioration of the ankle. Similarly, if the patient has concomitant arthrosis of the tarsometatarsal joints that is not symptomatic, it can become symptomatic after a triple or double arthrodesis because of the added stress from the proximal fusion. In some cases when multiple joints are involved, it may be more desirable to treat the patient conservatively with an orthotic device such as an ankle–foot orthosis (AFO) rather than carry out an arthrodesis.

Once a decision has been made to perform an arthrodesis, the next most critical factor is to establish the proper alignment of the fusion site. To do this, the surgeon must consider the entire lower extremity and not just the foot. The position of the knee or the bow of the tibia, which can occur either naturally or as a result of prior trauma, must be carefully examined when planning the arthrodesis. The alignment of the extremity distal to the fusion site is also important to be sure a plantigrade foot is created.

The biomechanics of the foot dictates its optimal alignment. When the subtalar joint is placed into an *everted (valgus) position*, it creates flexibility of the transverse tarsal joint and results in a supple forefoot. When the subtalar joint is in an *inverted (varus) position*, it locks the transverse tarsal joint. This creates a rigid forefoot and increased stress under the lateral aspect of the foot. It is therefore important to align the subtalar joint in 5 to 7 degrees of valgus when a fusion is carried out in order to maintain flexibility of the forefoot. When a talonavicular arthrodesis is performed, the surgeon must remember that motion in the subtalar joint will no longer occur. Therefore the subtalar joint must be aligned into 5 degrees of valgus, after which the talonavicular joint is aligned while taking into account abduction or adduction of the transverse tarsal joint as well as correcting any forefoot varus that might be present. This complex alignment creates a technically challenging situation for the surgeon. If the joints surrounding the talonavicular joint are not properly aligned, a plantigrade foot will not be created.

When arthrodesing the tarsometatarsal joints, the surgeon should always try to match the abnormal foot to the normal foot by carefully evaluating the weight-bearing posture of both feet preoperatively. The most common deformity is abduction and varying degrees of dorsiflexion. Any malalignment needs to be corrected. Once the first metatarsocuneiform joint is stabilized, the other joints need to be aligned, both in the transverse and in the dorsoplantar direction. This will align the metatarsal heads and prevent one from being too prominent, which can result in an intractable plantar keratosis.

SOFT TISSUE CONSIDERATIONS

The soft tissue envelope of the foot and ankle often contains little or no fatty tissue. At times this lack of soft tissue padding has been further compromised by previous surgery or trauma to the soft tissues, resulting in adherence of the soft tissue to the underlying bone. The surgical approach should be as precise as possible to avoid placing undue tension on the skin edges. If significant realignment is to be achieved, it must not be at the expense of proper wound approximation. This occasionally occurs when attempting to correct a valgus deformity of the heel in which an opening lateral wedge osteotomy results in increased tension on the lateral skin edges, which makes closure difficult. Skin flaps should be made as full thickness as possible to diminish the possibility of a skin slough. Creating an incision down to the bone, then retracting on the deep structures and not the skin edge, is probably the best way to avoid a skin problem.

When making an incision, the surgeon must always be cognizant of the location of the cutaneous nerves about the foot and ankle. Although cutaneous nerves tend to lie in certain anatomic areas, great variation exists. Therefore, as the incision is carried down through the subcutaneous tissues, it is important to always look for an aberrant cutaneous nerve. The cutaneous nerves can be quite superficial and easily transected but sometimes become adherent within scar tissue. If this occurs, a painful scar or dysesthesias distal to the injury can result in a dissatisfied patient despite a satisfactory fusion.

Another unique problem after foot surgery is the impact of footwear, which can rub against a subcutaneous neuroma, further aggravating the problem.

If a nerve is inadvertently transected during a surgical approach, it should be carefully dissected to a more proximal level and the cut end buried beneath some fatty tissue or muscle so that it will not become symptomatic. Sometimes, although a nerve is not cut, it can be stretched as a result of retraction, which can result in a transient loss of function. Patients must be made aware of the potential for nerve injury and the area where they can experience numbness.

SURGICAL PRINCIPLES

When carrying out an arthrodesis of the foot and ankle, the following surgical principles should be carefully observed:

- A well-planned incision of adequate length to avoid undue tension on the skin edges.
- An attempt should be made to create broad, congruent cancellous surfaces that can be placed into apposition to permit an arthrodesis to occur.
- The arthrodesis site should be stabilized with rigid internal fixation. This sometimes depends on the surgeon's ingenuity in creating a rigid construct, particularly if poor bone stock is present.
- When performing a fusion, the hindfoot must be aligned to the lower extremity and the forefoot to the hindfoot to create a plantigrade foot.

After exposure of the fusion site, the soft tissues surrounding the joints are removed. This mobilizes the joints, allowing the surgeon to realign the foot. At times, because of previous trauma or severe malalignment, mobilization of the joints is not possible and bone resection needs to be carried out. In my experience, however, the majority of cases can be aligned, even when a significant deformity is present, by complete mobilization of the involved joints followed by manipulation to create a plantigrade foot.

Once the joints have been mobilized and it is determined that bone does not need to be removed, the articular surfaces are meticulously debrided of their articular cartilage and any fibrous tissue to subchondral bone. This is achieved with a curet or a small, sharp osteotome. A lamina spreader or a towel clip can facilitate distraction of the articular surfaces, making the debridement easier, but this can damage the bone if it is soft.

Once the subchondral bone is exposed, the foot is once again manipulated, placing it into the desired alignment. If this is achievable, internal fixation can be inserted. If large amounts of bone need to be removed to create a plantigrade foot, this should be done *before* removing the articular cartilage. The subchondral surfaces are heavily feathered or scaled with a 4- or 6-mm osteotome, which creates a broader, bleeding cancellous surface required for successful fusion. The articular surfaces to be arthrodesed are brought together and stabilized with provisional fixation. Then interfragmentary compression is achieved using appropriate definitive fixation.

By carrying out a fusion in this manner, broad bleeding surfaces of cancellous bone are brought together, which provides the best possible chance for a successful arthrodesis. In my experience, bone graft from the iliac crest is rarely necessary when carrying out an arthrodesis. Sometimes bone has been lost, making a bone graft necessary, but in an in situ fusion, grafting is not usually required. If a small amount of bone is needed, it can be harvested from the calcaneus, medial malleolus, or proximal medial tibia without violating the iliac crest and causing its attendant morbidity. Likewise, bone substitutes or other materials are rarely required if the bone preparation is carried out correctly.

For internal fixation, I prefer an interfragmentary screw that compresses the joint surfaces. At times a power staple, a plain staple, or a plate may be used. Although an external fixator can provide excellent fixation, if possible a closed system without an external fixator is safer due to possible pin tract problems with prolonged immobilization. Because of soft bone or soft tissue problems, however, it may become necessary to use an external fixator. Under these circumstances this device provides excellent rigid fixation.

The skin closure after a fusion is very critical. The surgeon should always attempt, if possible, to obtain a soft tissue cover underneath the skin flaps, such as fat or muscle. This is important because if a superficial wound slough occurs, it will be over an underlying bed of soft tissue rather than bone. This is not always possible, particularly on the dorsum of the foot, where bone lies directly beneath the skin. If any tension is noticeable on the skin edge, some type of a relaxing skin suture should be used. A drain is always useful if profuse bleeding is anticipated.

The initial postoperative dressing is very important and should support the soft tissues as well as the arthrodesis site. A heavy cotton gauze roll provides uniform compression about the extremity, supported by plaster splints. A circumferential cast should be avoided during the immediate postoperative period because it can result in undue pressure against the expanding extremity, increasing pain and possibly jeopardizing healing of the wound edges. The postoperative dressing is used for approximately 10 to 14 days before removing the sutures.

After most fusions, bupivacaine hydrochloride (bupivacaine) is instilled into the wounds to diminish the initial postoperative pain. A popliteal block is used, which generally provides 18 to 36 hours of pain relief. The popliteal block may be repeated after 18 to 24 hours if the patient has too much breakthrough pain. It is much easier to prevent postoperative pain than play catch-up after the pain cycle has been established.

COMPLICATIONS

The main complications after an attempted arthrodesis include infection, skin slough, nerve disruption or entrapment, nonunion, and malalignment.

The possibility of *infection* is always a postsurgical concern. During surgery, antibiotic irrigation as well as parenteral antibiotics can help minimize this complication. Good surgical technique with careful handling of the tissues, removal of devitalized tissue, and prevention of hematoma formation also play an important role in minimizing the possibility of infection. If an infection occurs, it is important to recognize and treat it promptly with appropriate antibiotics.

A *skin slough* around the foot and ankle can present a difficult management problem because of the lack of adequate subcutaneous tissue. The potential for a skin slough can be minimized by creating full-thickness skin flaps, making incisions of adequate length to minimize tension on the skin edges, using postoperative drainage when appropriate, and applying a firm compression dressing postoperatively. Placing a patient into a cast without adequate padding is not advisable. When a skin slough occurs, it is important to treat it vigorously with local debridement and application of wet-to-dry dressings to promote granulation tissue, followed by coverage with a split-thickness skin graft. Vacuum-assisted closure (wound-VAC) can be extremely useful to manage a wound slough. If the slough is too large, a plastic surgeon should be consulted.

Nerve disruption or entrapment around the foot and ankle not only creates numbness but also can cause chronic pain from footwear rubbing against the neuroma. A carefully planned surgical approach is the best treatment, but if a symptomatic neuroma occurs,

it should be identified and resected into an area not subject to pressure and then buried either beneath muscle or into bone.

A *nonunion* of an attempted fusion site is always an unfortunate event. As a general rule, of the joints around the foot and ankle, the talonavicular probably has the highest incidence of nonunion. Its curved surfaces make adequate exposure difficult, and preparation of the joint surfaces may be inadequate. Even when the bone surfaces have been adequately prepared, nonunion can occur if internal fixation is inadequate.

The vascularity of the bone plays an important role in the development of a nonunion. Avascular necrosis of the talus from any cause creates a situation that is very difficult to manage. When avascular bone is present, it is often not possible to obtain a fusion to the dysvascular bone, and an attempt must be made either to bypass the avascular area or to determine the portions of the talus that still have adequate vascularity and attempt a fusion using these areas. The navicular can develop evidence of avascular changes either spontaneously or secondary to previous injury. When this problem is encountered, the involved area needs to be resected and bone grafted. When dealing with dysvascular bone preoperatively, it is important to identify the areas of potential problems and create a surgical plan that will help solve the problem. Recognizing a dysvascular problem also helps to predict the outcome for the patient.

Occasionally an asymptomatic nonunion occurs and can be treated with observation. After a triple arthrodesis the talonavicular joint occasionally does not fuse, but because of a successful fusion of the subtalar and calcaneocuboid joints, it may not be a source of pain. If a nonunion is symptomatic, a revision of the fusion site needs to be considered. If the overall alignment of the nonunion is satisfactory, bone grafting by inlaying bone across the nonunion site often results in a fusion if internal fixation is adequate. At other times, if the nonunion site has resulted in loss of alignment, the area needs to be revised. This is done by removing the internal fixation and the fibrous tissue between the bone ends, realigning the surfaces, performing a bone graft if necessary, and inserting rigid fixation.

Malalignment after a fusion is a problem that usually can be avoided by meticulous bone preparation and rigid internal fixation. Malalignment after a triple arthrodesis is seen most often. The usual malalignment following a triple arthrodesis is varus of the heel and adduction or supination (or both) of the forefoot. This requires the patient to walk on the lateral aspect of the foot, causing patient dissatisfaction. When a fusion of the hindfoot is performed, it is important to evaluate the entire lower extremity preoperatively and intraoperatively to reduce the risk of malalignment. After carefully observing the normal extremity, the surgeon should always relate the foot alignment to the patella. Once the joint surfaces have been prepared and provisionally stabilized, the alignment should again be checked to be sure it is correct. Malalignment can only be prevented by careful observation of the extremity at surgery.

SPECIFIC ARTHRODESES

Much has been written about arthrodesis of the foot and ankle. Many surgical approaches, site preparations, and types of internal and external fixation have been proposed. This section presents the techniques I have evolved over time and that result in a satisfactory outcome with careful adherence to technique. Other techniques may be equally effective, but reproducibly good results have been achieved with subtalar arthrodesis, talonavicular arthrodesis, double arthrodesis, triple arthrodesis, naviculocuneiform arthrodesis, and tarsometatarsal arthrodesis.

SUBTALAR ARTHRODESIS

An isolated subtalar joint arthrodesis results in satisfactory correction of deformity and relief of pain that enables the patient to regain the ability to perform most activities. Of the hindfoot fusions, the patient's ability to achieve a high level of function is greatest after a subtalar arthrodesis. Biomechanically, the position of the subtalar joint determines the flexibility of the transverse tarsal (talonavicular–calcaneocuboid) joint, and therefore it is imperative that a subtalar arthrodesis be positioned in about 5 degrees of valgus to permit mobility of the transverse tarsal joint. If it is placed in varus, the transverse tarsal joint is locked, and the patient tends to walk on the lateral side of the foot. The posture of the forefoot also needs to be considered because if there is more than 10 to 12 degrees of fixed forefoot varus, after a subtalar arthrodesis the patient cannot compensate for this deformity and walks on the lateral side of the foot, resulting in discomfort beneath the fifth metatarsal head or base, or both, and in severe stress on the lateral ankle ligaments. Occasionally the fixed forefoot varus can be corrected by carrying out a simultaneous naviculocuneiform fusion.

It was previously believed that an isolated subtalar arthrodesis should not be carried out, and that a triple arthrodesis would be the procedure of choice when a hindfoot fusion was indicated. The literature has demonstrated, however, that an isolated subtalar arthrodesis produces a superior result with less stress on the ankle joint than a triple arthrodesis.*

Indications

The most common indication for a subtalar arthrodesis is arthrosis secondary to trauma, usually a calcaneal fracture, rheumatoid arthritis, primary arthrosis, or talocalcaneal coalition that cannot be resected. It is also indicated for a muscle imbalance (e.g., loss of peroneal muscle function) or posterior tibial tendon dysfunction with an unstable subtalar joint but normal transverse tarsal joint motion and a fixed forefoot varus deformity of less than 12 degrees. A subtalar arthrodesis is indicated in patients with a neuromuscular disorder such as Charcot–Marie–Tooth disease, poliomyelitis, or nerve injury with instability of the subtalar joint.

Although a subtalar fusion can have an excellent result, if the deformity can be corrected with a calcaneal osteotomy instead of a fusion, this should be strongly considered.

Position of Arthrodesis

The subtalar arthrodesis should be placed in approximately 5 degrees of valgus. Varus should be avoided because it results in increased stability of the transverse tarsal joint. Conversely, too much valgus results in an impingement against the fibula and increased stress along the medial aspect of the ankle joint.

Surgical Technique

1. The patient is placed in a supine position with a support under the ipsilateral hip to facilitate exposure of the subtalar joint (video clip 11).
2. A thigh tourniquet is applied.
3. The skin incision begins at the tip of the fibula and is carried distally toward the base of the fourth metatarsal. When an isolated subtalar arthrodesis is carried out, the incision usually stops at about the level of the calcaneocuboid joint (Fig. 20–1A).

*References 1-4, 7, 8, 10, 11, and 14-16.

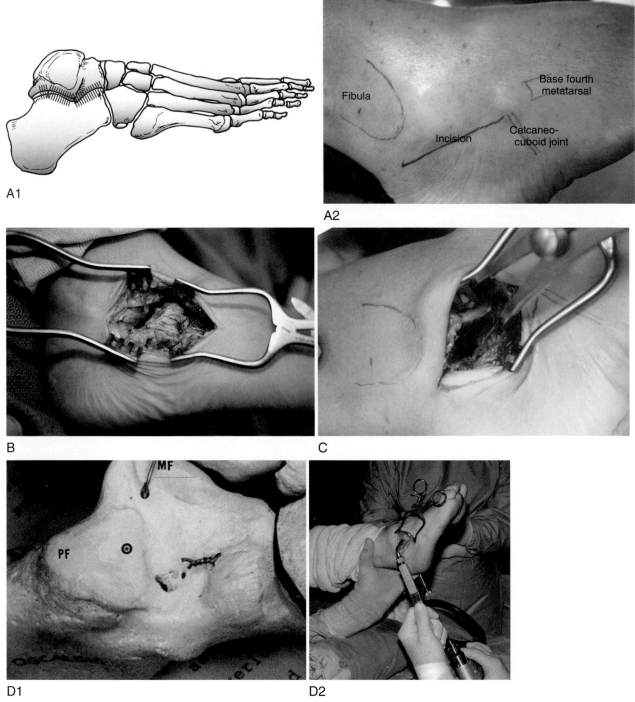

Figure 20–1 Subtalar joint fusion. **A,** Site of fusion. Incision is made from the tip of the fibula and extends toward the base of the fourth metatarsal so as to place it in the interval between a branch of the superficial peroneal nerve dorsally and the sural nerve plantarly. **B,** Exposure of subtalar joint with Weitlaner retractor. **C,** A lamina spreader placed within the sinus tarsi area exposes the posterior and middle facets. **D,** When a screw is used for fixation of the subtalar joint, it is placed through the posterior facet into the neck of the talus. *Circle* in the posterior facet *(PF)* demonstrates where the tine of the guide is placed in order to accurately place the screw. *MF* identifies the middle facet. The anterior cruciate guide is placed into the subtalar joint with the tine in posterior facet, as marked on the model. The guide is then set on the heel, after which a guide pin is placed across the subtalar joint. **E,** Preoperative and postoperative radiographs demonstrate subtalar fusion using a 7.0-mm screw. The screw begins off the weight-bearing area of the heel. **F,** Preoperative and postoperative radiographs demonstrate subtalar arthrodesis after calcaneal fracture. Interpositional bone graft is used to reestablish the talocalcaneal relationship. Interpositional bone graft is rarely required to obtain a satisfactory result. **G,** When lateral subluxation of the subtalar joint is present, the joint must be reduced and not fused in situ. The lateral aspect of the calcaneus should line up with the lateral aspect of the talus. **H,** Example of in situ fusion with persistent lateral subluxation of the subtalar joint, resulting in subfibular impingement and persistent pain. **I,** Preoperative and postoperative radiographs demonstrating subtalar fusion in a patient with prior ankle fusion who developed arthrosis of the subtalar joint.

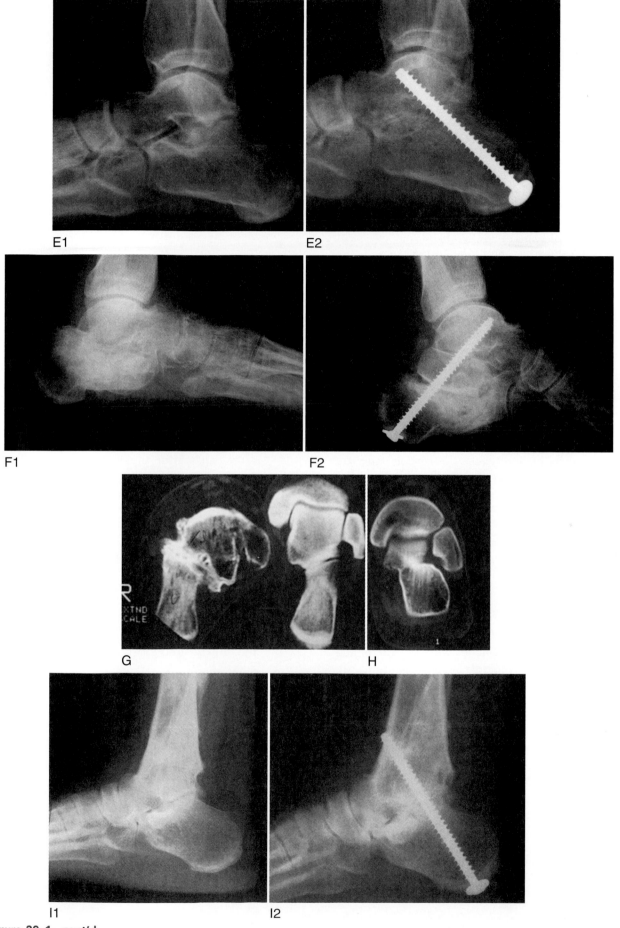

E1   E2

F1   F2

G   H

I1   I2

Figure 20-1—cont'd

4. While deepening the incision, the surgeon should be cautious, because the anterior branch of the sural nerve may be crossing the operative site.

5. The incision passes along the dorsal aspect of the peroneal tendon sheath and distally along the floor of the sinus tarsi.

6. The extensor digitorum brevis muscle origin is detached and the muscle belly reflected distally, exposing the underlying sinus tarsi, subtalar joint, and calcaneocuboid joint (Fig. 20–1B). The fat pad is dissected out of the sinus tarsi and reflected dorsally.

7. A small elevator is passed along the lateral side of the posterior facet of the subtalar joint. It is not necessary to strip the peroneal tendons off the lateral side of the calcaneus unless a lateral impingement from a previous calcaneal fracture requires decompressing.

8. With a curet, the contents of the sinus tarsi and tarsal canal are removed.

9. A lamina spreader is inserted into the sinus tarsi to visualize the posterior facet of the subtalar joint (Fig. 20–1C). When looking across the sinus tarsi, the surgeon can see the middle facet of the subtalar joint. If the surgery is being carried out for severe arthrosis or a talocalcaneal coalition, it is often not possible to open the subtalar joint very far. Under these circumstances, a small curet is used to remove the cartilage from the posterior facet. A thin wide elevator then can be inserted into the joint to pry it open, after which a lamina spreader is inserted.

10. With a curet of appropriate size, all the articular cartilage is removed from the posterior and middle facets. Using a curet, a fairly safe instrument, reduces the possibility of damaging the flexor hallucis longus tendon in the posterior aspect of the joint or the neurovascular bundle along the posteromedial aspect of the joint. When removing the articular cartilage from the middle facet, it is important not to inadvertently go too far distally and damage the cartilage on the plantar aspect of the head of the talus, which lies just in front of it.

11. Once all the articular cartilage has been removed, the lamina spreader is removed and the alignment of the subtalar joint observed. If no deformity is present, the surgeon may proceed with feathering or scaling the articular surfaces. If a varus deformity needs to be corrected, bone is removed from the lateral aspect of the posterior facet to correct the deformity. It is unusual to remove more than 3 to 5 mm of bone when correcting a deformity, although occasionally more bone needs to be removed.

12. If a previous calcaneal fracture is present in which the lateral wall needs to be decompressed, the peroneal tendons are elevated from the lateral aspect of the calcaneus as far posteriorly and plantarward as possible. The impinging lateral wall is removed so that it is approximately in line with the lateral aspect of the talus. Sometimes, up to 7 to 10 mm of bone needs to be resected in severe cases.

13. The posterior and middle facets, along with the bone in the base of the sinus tarsi, are heavily scaled. The dense bone in the floor of the sinus tarsi is deeply scaled and is mobilized so that it can be packed into the tarsal canal after the internal fixation has been inserted. The bone along the lateral aspect of the calcaneus that forms the anterior process may be mobilized to within about 0.5 cm of the calcaneocuboid joint and used for bone graft. When a lateral decompression has been carried out, even more bone is available to the surgeon. Rarely is bone harvested from the iliac crest.

14. After the bone surfaces have been scaled, the subtalar joint is manipulated and placed into the desired position of 5 degrees of valgus.

Internal Fixation

Internal fixation is carried out with a fully threaded 7.0-mm cannulated screw to obtain maximum interfragmentary compression. A washer is always used.

Screw patterns used for fixation of the subtalar joint include placing the screw from the neck of the talus into the calcaneus, placing a screw from the calcaneus into the talus, and placing two screws between the calcaneus and the talus. In most cases a single fully threaded screw inserted through a glide hole in the calcaneus, starting the screw off the weight-bearing surface, results in a rigid internal fixation with maximum purchase in the neck of the talus, which facilitates interfragmentary compression of the subtalar joint. A washer is always used because the grip of the screw in the neck of the talus is so strong it can suck the screw into the calcaneus without the washer.

15. The preferred method for stabilization, particularly with a valgus deformity, is to place the 7.0-mm cannulated screw from the heel across the subtalar joint and into the neck of the talus. Screw placement is carried out by placing an AO (Arbeitsgemeinschaft für Osteosynthese) anterior cruciate guide with the sharp tine in the anterior aspect of the posterior facet of the subtalar joint (Fig. 20–1D). The other end of the guide is placed on the heel pad just above the weight-bearing area. This alignment permits the screw to pass through the anterior aspect of the posterior facet and into the neck of the talus, but the screw does not penetrate the sinus tarsi area. This placement provides maximum purchase in the talar neck from the fully threaded 7.0-mm screw. A guide pin is drilled into the calcaneus until it is visible in the posterior facet of the subtalar joint. If placement is satisfactory, the anterior cruciate guide is removed; if not, another attempt is made to place the guide pin correctly.
16. The subtalar joint is placed into 5 degrees of valgus, and the guide pin is drilled into the talus until it just penetrates the dorsal aspect of the neck of the talus. The pin placement is confirmed by fluoroscopy.
17. With the pin properly placed, a 2-cm transverse incision is made over the entrance of the guide pin into the heel pad. This incision must be made wide enough to accommodate the screw and washer to prevent compressing the skin and fat of the heel pad. The incision is carried directly to bone, and slight stripping is done on each side of the pin to accommodate the washer. A depth gauge is used to determine the length of the screw.
18. The guide pin is advanced through the talar neck, appears on the dorsal aspect of the ankle, and is secured with a clamp. This is important so that when the holes are drilled,

the guide pin cannot come out, which can result in loss of alignment. The initial hole is drilled with a 4.5-mm bit, just penetrating the neck of the talus. A 7.0-mm drill bit is used to overdrill only the calcaneus, creating the glide hole. The hole in the talar neck is tapped, and a fully threaded, 7.0-mm cannulated screw of appropriate length is inserted. By overdrilling the calcaneus, intrafragmentary compression at the arthrodesis site is achieved. With a fully threaded screw, the maximum number of threads are placed in the neck of the talus, maximizing the compression. In placing the screw, the surgeon should not have more than 2 to 3 mm of screw exposed on the neck of the talus. The position of the screw is verified with fluoroscopy (Fig. 20–1E).
19. The guide pin is removed, and the small bone fragments that have been mobilized are packed into the tarsal canal and the sinus tarsi area. It is not necessary to fill up the sinus tarsi completely when carrying out an isolated subtalar joint fusion. If more bone is needed, it can be obtained from the calcaneus or medial malleolus, using a trephine.

Closure

20. The fat pad previously dissected from the sinus tarsi and retracted dorsally is placed back into the sinus tarsi area. The extensor digitorum brevis muscle is closed over the area, creating a cover for the arthrodesis site.
21. The subcutaneous tissue and skin are closed in a routine manner, and bupivacaine is instilled into and around the arthrodesis site.
22. The patient is placed into a compression dressing incorporating two plaster splints.

Postoperative Care

In the recovery room a popliteal block is used to control postoperative pain. The patient's dressing is changed approximately 10 days after surgery, and the sutures are removed. The patient is placed into a removable cast with an elastic bandage to control swelling but is kept non–weight bearing for 6 weeks. At 6 weeks, if the radiographs demonstrate that early union is occurring, the patient is permitted to bear weight as tolerated in a removable cast. Approximately 12 weeks after surgery, radiographs are obtained, and if satisfactory union has occurred, the patient is permitted to ambulate with an elastic stocking.

Complications

Nonunion of the subtalar joint occurs infrequently. The few nonunions that we have encountered are usually in young patients after a severe intraarticular calcaneal fracture in which the bone in the midportion of the calcaneus appears to be sclerotic and may be dysvascular. A nonunion should be repaired with bone grafting and further internal fixation.

Malalignment of the subtalar joint in too much varus results in locking of the transverse tarsal joint and increased weight bearing on the lateral side of the foot. To accommodate this, the patient often walks with the extremity in external rotation.

If the subtalar joint is placed into excessive valgus, it can impinge against the fibula, causing pain over the peroneal tendons. It can also place increased stress along the medial aspect of the ankle joint and pronation of the foot.

Sural nerve entrapment or laceration can occur and may be bothersome to the patient. Unfortunately, the anterior branch of the sural nerve can pass next to the incision, making this complication almost unavoidable, but an attempt should be made to identify it and retract it if possible. If the neuroma is too bothersome it requires resection to a more proximal level.

Author's Experience

We reviewed 101 of our subtalar arthrodeses using the single lag screw method of fixation. The average time for arthrodesis was 12.3±3.4 weeks. In the series, 99 of 101 fused (98%).[6] The presence of a prior ankle fusion significantly prolonged the time to arthrodesis to 14.9±7 weeks. Other factors including smoking, revision surgery, patient age, or sex did not affect time to arthrodesis. The fixation screw was removed in 13 (13%) of 101, at an average of 8.8 months.

We reviewed another series of 48 subtalar fusions in 44 patients (26 women and 18 men; average age, 41.3 years; range, 13 to 75 years)

at an average of 60 months (range, 24 to 177 months) after surgery.[8] The preoperative diagnosis was calcaneal fracture in 12 cases, talocalcaneal coalition in 11, subtalar joint arthrosis without calcaneal fracture in 12 (5 primary, 7 post-traumatic), posterior tibial tendon dysfunction in 11, subtalar joint instability in one, and psoriatic arthritis in one case.

Fusion occurred in 47 of 48 arthrodeses, with the one nonunion in a young patient after a calcaneal fracture. This was successfully revised using iliac crest bone graft. Sixteen (33%) of the 48 fusions underwent screw removal.

Forty-one patients (93%) were satisfied. The three dissatisfied patients (7%) had persistent pain; one foot was fused in 12 degrees of valgus and another in 7 degrees of varus. The patients observed a decrease in their pain from 3.7 out of 4.0 to 0.8 and a functional increase from 3.4 out of 4.0 to 0.9. Using the American Orthopaedic Foot and Ankle Society (AOFAS) scoring system,[5] the patients averaged 89.3, which translated to 86% good and excellent results, 7% fair, and 7% poor.

Functionally the patients did well, although half observed problems walking on uneven ground and climbing steps and inclines. Seventy percent participated in recreational sports (e.g., walking for pleasure, biking, skiing, swimming), and 14% were able to play sports that required running and pivoting (e.g., basketball, racquet sports). This is a much higher level of activity compared with patients who have undergone a triple arthrodesis.[3]

Nine patients had work-related injuries; five of these had a fracture of the calcaneus with resultant arthrosis. The two patients with bilateral fractures did not return to work, two were retrained for a sedentary job, and one retrained for a construction job. Of the four other patients, three returned to work and one retired.

All patients wore normal shoes, and six used an orthotic device.

The physical examination demonstrated that the alignment averaged 5.7 degrees of valgus, and the one patient with fusion in varus was dissatisfied. The range of motion demonstrated an average of 9.8 degrees of dorsiflexion compared with 14.2 degrees on the uninvolved side, for a 30% loss of motion, and plantar flexion averaged 47.2 degrees compared with 52.4 degrees, for a 9.2% loss of motion. This resulted in a 14% loss of sagittal plane motion. The transverse tarsal joint motion demonstrated 60% loss of abduction and adduction compared with the uninvolved side. Five feet had flexible forefoot varus with an average of 7 degrees, and six had fixed forefoot varus with an average of 4.7 degrees.

Final follow-up radiographs demonstrated an increase in arthrosis of the ankle joint in 12 of 33 patients; 11 of these had slight arthrosis (two had mild symptoms), and one had moderate changes and was symptomatic. Arthrosis increased at the transverse tarsal joint in 13 of 33 patients, 12 had slight arthrosis, and only one had mild symptoms. New osteophyte formation along the anterior aspect of the ankle was noted in 12 patients; five were slight (two symptomatic), five moderate (all were symptomatic), and two severe (both symptomatic).

Evaluation of the subgroups demonstrated that the 11 patients with a calcaneal fracture had an AOFAS score of 83. Ten of the 11 underwent an in situ fusion with lateral wall decompression. One patient with severe collapse had a bone block added to restore the height of the calcaneus. Based on our experience and that of others,[9,12] it is not necessary to add a bone block when carrying out an isolated subtalar fusion after a calcaneal fracture unless severe impaction exists with greater than 1.5 cm loss of height (Fig. 20–1F).

The 10 patients who underwent a subtalar arthrodesis for talocalcaneal coalition had an average AOFAS score of 93. Six of these patients had evidence of mild arthrosis of the talonavicular joint at follow-up, but none were symptomatic. Our study and another[13] demonstrate that isolated subtalar fusion is the treatment of choice for a nonessential talocalcaneal coalition. A triple arthrodesis is not necessary to obtain a satisfactory result, even in the presence of beaking of the talonavicular joint.

The eight patients with posterior tibial tendon dysfunction had an AOFAS score of 88. This procedure was used when the primary deformity was in the hindfoot with hindfoot valgus and calcaneal impingement against the fibula or when subtalar joint inversion was absent, precluding the use of a tendon transfer. These patients all had less than 12 degrees of fixed forefoot varus and no transverse tarsal joint hypermobility. A subtalar fusion is the procedure of choice for these patients, because a tendon transfer will fail owing to lack of subtalar inversion. A triple arthrodesis is not necessary and creates a more rigid foot.

The five patients with primary arthrosis of the subtalar joint that had not been previously described in the literature had an AOFAS score of 100. These patients did extremely well and had essentially no limitations after their procedure. The other seven patients who had arthrosis of the subtalar joint not associated with a calcaneal fracture but rather a talar fracture had an AOFAS score of 86. This again demonstrates that for an isolated subtalar joint problem, an isolated subtalar joint arthrodesis results in satisfactory correction, and that a more extensive fusion, with its increased long-term morbidity, is not necessary.

Special Considerations

Occasionally in the patient with rheumatoid arthritis, severe subluxation occurs at the subtalar joint (Fig. 20–1G and H). It is imperative that the clinician recognize this problem so that when a subtalar arthrodesis is carried out, the calcaneus is repositioned under the talus, restoring the normal weight-bearing alignment. If the surgeon fails to recognize this malalignment and places a bone block into the lateral side of the subtalar joint, wedging it open will not reposition the calcaneus into correct anatomic alignment.

Sometimes following an ankle arthrodesis patients develop arthrosis of the subtalar joint. In this situation we carry out our standard type of fusion. The screw placement is a little simpler because there is no concern about penetrating the ankle joint with the screw (Fig. 20–1I). Postoperatively these patients are placed into a short-leg cast rather than a removable cast because I believe better immobilization can be achieved. We have not had problems achieving an arthrodesis in this patient cohort, although it does take longer to occur.

TALONAVICULAR ARTHRODESIS

Although arthrodesis of the talonavicular joint involves only a single joint, biomechanically it results in almost complete loss of motion in the subtalar and transverse tarsal joints. This motion is lost because for the subtalar joint to invert and evert, the navicular must rotate over the talar head. Thus, if talonavicular movement is restricted, subtalar motion does not occur.[19,22]

An isolated talonavicular arthrodesis results in a satisfactory outcome, particularly in patients who do not place a high demand on their foot, such as rheumatoid patients.[18,20] In the high-demand patient or one working at a strenuous occupation, it is probably advisable to add a calcaneocuboid joint arthrodesis. This creates a double arthrodesis, resulting in increased stability of the transverse tarsal joint.[17] The addition of the calcaneocuboid joint to the talonavicular fusion does not result in any further loss of hindfoot motion. Therefore, I usually carry out a double arthrodesis instead of the isolated talonavicular arthrodesis, except in the low-activity patient.

Indications

The most common indication for an isolated talonavicular arthrodesis is primary arthrosis, arthrosis secondary to trauma,[20] or rheumatoid arthritis.[18] With instability of the talonavicular joint secondary to dysfunction of the posterior tibial tendon or collapse of the talonavicular joint from rupture of the spring ligament, an isolated talonavicular arthrodesis can be considered. In these circumstances, however, I usually carry out a double or triple arthrodesis.

Alignment of the Fusion

The alignment of the normal foot is observed to determine the alignment of the affected side. The positioning of an isolated talonavicular arthrodesis is very important, because the subtalar and calcaneocuboid joint motion is greatly restricted after this arthrodesis. Therefore the hindfoot and forefoot must be aligned into a plantigrade position; if not, a nonplantigrade foot will be created and may be symptomatic. The subtalar joint should be placed into 5 degrees of valgus, the talonavicular joint into neutral, and the forefoot into 0 to 5 degrees of forefoot varus (Fig. 20–2A).

Surgical Technique

1. The patient is placed in the supine position, and a thigh tourniquet is applied. Because the extremity naturally falls into external rotation, the patient does not require turning.
2. The talonavicular joint is usually approached through a longitudinal incision starting just distal to the medial malleolus and carried distally 1 cm beyond the naviculocuneiform joint (Fig. 20–2B). The incision can be curved slightly dorsally, particularly if a large dorsal osteophyte requires removal.
3. Using a periosteal elevator or a sharp, curved osteotome, the joint capsule is stripped from the dorsal, medial, and plantar aspects of the joint.
4. If dorsal osteophytes are present, they are removed at this time, using an osteotome or a rongeur.
5. Exposure of the talonavicular joint is facilitated by placing a towel clip into the proximal medial portion of the navicular and applying a distracting force in a medial direction (Fig. 20–2C).
6. The articular surfaces of the talus and navicular are identified, and the articular cartilage is removed with an osteotome or curet.
7. If the bone is hard enough, a small lamina spreader sometimes can be placed into the medial side of the joint to gain better visualization. This being a curved joint, visualization of the lateral aspect is difficult but essential if satisfactory debridement is to be achieved.
8. The joint surfaces are heavily feathered, and the foot is manipulated into anatomic alignment.
9. The calcaneus is held in one hand, placing the subtalar joint in approximately 5 degrees of valgus. The talonavicular joint is manipulated, bringing the transverse tarsal joint into a few degrees of abduction and the forefoot into a plantigrade position that is perpendicular to the long axis of the tibia. If possible, the forefoot should not have a residual of more than 5 to 7 degrees of fixed forefoot varus or valgus.
10. The type of internal fixation selected depends in part on the quality of the bone. Using two 4.0- or 4.5-mm cannulated screws

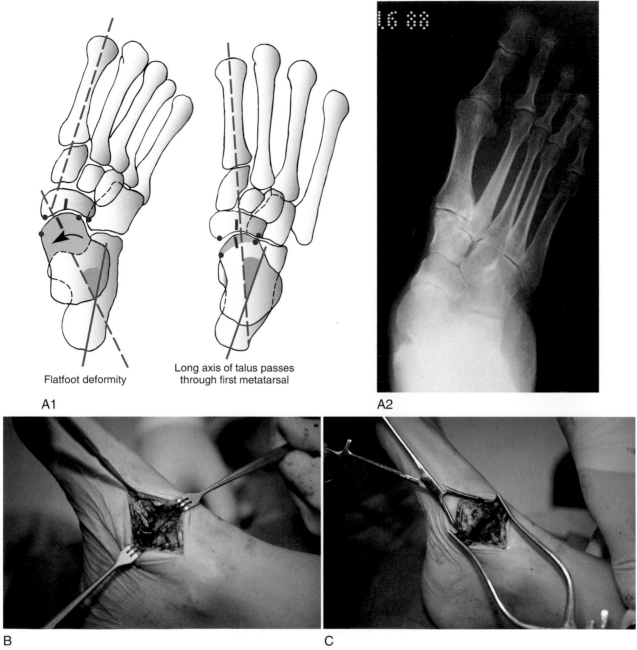

Flatfoot deformity

Long axis of talus passes
through first metatarsal

A1

A2

B

C

Figure 20–2   Talonavicular arthrodesis. **A,** Radiograph and diagram demonstrate changes that occur in the talonavicular joint with flatfoot deformity. The head of the talus deviates medially as the forefoot deviates laterally into abduction. The diagram demonstrates abnormal alignment brought about by flatfoot deformity and its subsequent correction. The navicular is once again centered over the head of the talus. **B,** Exposure of the talonavicular joint through a medial incision. The Freer elevator points to the naviculocuneiform joint. **C,** Access is gained to the talonavicular joint by distracting the joint with a towel clip.

gives excellent fixation, and the profile of the screw head is low enough that fracturing the medial aspect of the navicular need not be a concern. In a large person a 7.0-mm cannulated screw can be used. If the bone is very soft, multiple staples are useful.

11. With the surgeon holding the foot in correct alignment, a guide pin is placed starting along the medial side of the navicular at the naviculocuneiform joint and drilled obliquely across the navicular into the head and neck of the talus.

12. The alignment of the foot is then once again carefully verified, and if it is satisfactory, the pin placement is checked with fluoroscopy. A second parallel pin is inserted.

13. The navicular is overdrilled and a 40- to 50-mm, long-threaded cancellous screw is inserted. The smooth shank of the screw must completely pass across the intended fusion site. If the bone is soft, a washer is used.

14. After both screws have been inserted, the stability of the arthrodesis site is checked. If any significant motion is present, staples can be used to increase stability. This is sometimes necessary in the rheumatoid patient or the elderly patient with porotic bone.

15. If the bone is too soft, four or five staples are used for fixation. This is also useful if the navicular fractures while inserting a screw (Fig. 20–3).

16. The wound is closed in layers, with the deep fascia being approximated over the arthrodesis site. The subcutaneous tissue and skin are closed in a routine manner. The wound over the talonavicular joint rarely breaks down.

17. Bupivacaine is injected into the wound to provide postoperative analgesia.

18. The patient is placed into a compression dressing incorporating two plaster splints.

Postoperative Care

In the recovery room a popliteal block is administered to control postoperative pain. The postoperative dressing is changed in 10 to 14 days, sutures are removed, and the patient is placed into a short-leg, removable cast with an elastic bandage to control swelling. Weight bearing is not permitted. Six weeks after surgery, radiographs are obtained, and if satisfactory union is occurring, the patient is permitted to ambulate with weight bearing as tolerated in a short-leg cast. Three months after surgery, if radiographic healing is evident, the patient is

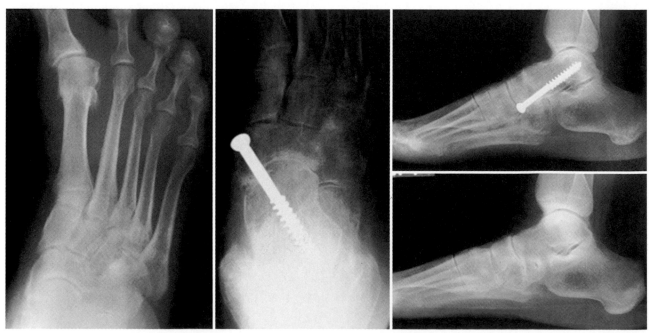

Figure 20–3 Preoperative and postoperative radiographs demonstrate talonavicular arthrodesis using a 7.0-mm cannulated screw. Note the congenital hallux varus.

permitted to ambulate without support as tolerated.

Complications

The nonunion rate of the talonavicular joint is much higher than that of the calcaneocuboid or subtalar joint, partly because of the surgeon's inability to gain adequate exposure of the entire joint in preparation for the arthrodesis. The high nonunion rate can also result from the relative avascularity of the navicular, particularly in post-traumatic cases. If a nonunion occurs and the alignment is satisfactory, carrying out a slot type of bone graft into several areas around the talonavicular joint usually results in satisfactory union.

Malalignment of the joint results in malposition of the hindfoot and forefoot. The most common malposition is a flatfoot deformity, which results from leaving the forefoot in too much abduction and the subtalar joint in valgus. This can only be corrected by revision to a triple arthrodesis.

DOUBLE ARTHRODESIS

The double arthrodesis as described by DuVries[23] consists of a fusion of the talonavicular and calcaneocuboid joints.[17,24] It is based on the biomechanical principle that if the motion in the talonavicular and calcaneocuboid joints is eliminated, no motion occurs in the subtalar joint. This results in the same degree of immobilization as a triple arthrodesis, but without the necessity of completing the subtalar portion. A double arthrodesis takes less time and probably has less patient morbidity because the subtalar joint is not included in the fusion mass.

Indications

The double arthrodesis is indicated when the malalignment involves the transverse tarsal joint or forefoot, or both. It is most often carried out for patients with posterior tibial tendon dysfunction who are not candidates for a tendon reconstruction or subtalar fusion. In these patients, the subtalar joint is flexible and no subtalar disorder is present. There is also a fixed forefoot varus, greater than 15 degrees, and abduction of the transverse tarsal joint is increased. A fusion of the talonavicular and calcaneocuboid joints is sufficient to create a plantigrade foot without including the subtalar joint. If any arthrosis is present within the subtalar joint, a triple arthrodesis is indicated.

The double arthrodesis is also indicated in patients with isolated arthrosis involving the talonavicular joint who, because of their young age or high level of activity, would be placing great stress on the foot. Although an isolated talonavicular arthrodesis is excellent for the less active patient (e.g., with rheumatoid arthritis), a more active person often has some pain in the foot if the calcaneocuboid joint is not added to the talonavicular fusion. Based on my experience in large patients, rather than do a double arthrodesis, a triple arthrodesis is a better procedure, because when a double arthrodesis is carried out, great stress is placed on the talonavicular fusion site, which can result in fixation failure and loss of alignment. When the subtalar joint is added, creating a triple arthrodesis, it stabilizes the subtalar joint, relieving stress on the talonavicular joint.

Position of Arthrodesis

The positioning of the foot for a double arthrodesis is extremely critical. The subtalar joint must be placed into 5 degrees of valgus and maintained there while the transverse tarsal joint is positioned into the same degree of abduction or adduction as the normal foot. The forefoot is placed into a plantigrade position with little or no residual fixed forefoot varus. In many patients with dysfunction of the posterior tibial tendon, one of the main components being corrected is the fixed forefoot varus of greater than 15 degrees, which precludes performing an isolated subtalar fusion.

Surgical Technique

1. The patient is placed in a supine position with a support under the ipsilateral hip to allow easy access to the medial and lateral aspects of the foot (video clip 12).
2. A thigh tourniquet is applied.
3. The skin incision is made along the lateral aspect of the foot, starting at the base of

the fourth metatarsal, and extends proximally toward the tip of the fibula, stopping about 1 cm short of the tip.

4. The incision is deepened to the extensor digitorum brevis muscle. Care is taken to identify any anterior branch of the sural nerve that might be crossing the surgical field.

5. The capsule of the extensor digitorum brevis is opened, its origin is released, and the muscle is reflected distally about 1 cm distal to the calcaneocuboid joint.

6. The calcaneocuboid joint is identified and the soft tissue stripped plantarward and dorsally using a periosteal elevator.

7. The articular cartilage is removed from the calcaneocuboid joint as thoroughly as possible using a small, sharp osteotome or curet.

8. Placing a deep retractor into the wound along the dorsal aspect, the surgeon identifies the lateral aspect of the talonavicular joint opposite the calcaneocuboid joint and removes articular cartilage if possible. Usually, cartilage can be removed from the lateral third of the talar head and occasionally from the navicular, depending on how tight the foot is.

9. The medial approach is through a longitudinal incision, starting at the tip of the medial malleolus and carried distally 1 cm past the naviculocuneiform joint (see Fig. 20–2B).

10. The incision is deepened through the capsular tissues, after which the capsule and spring ligament are stripped from the navicular. An elevator is passed over the dorsal aspect of the talonavicular joint, completely freeing the joint.

11. Using a towel clip embedded into the proximal portion of the navicular, the surgeon distracts the talonavicular joint by pulling the foot in an adducted position and longitudinally (see Fig. 20–2C). If the quality of the bone is adequate, a small lamina spreader is useful to gain exposure.

12. The articular cartilage is removed from the talonavicular joint with an osteotome or curet. Sometimes removing the cartilage is difficult, and it is important to be sure that the joint capsule has been completely stripped from the talonavicular joint to facilitate exposure.

13. The foot is manipulated into proper alignment to determine whether any bone needs to be removed from the attempted fusion site, which generally is not necessary. However, it is important to be sure no gap is created at the calcaneocuboid joint when the foot is brought into a plantigrade position.

14. To correct a severe forefoot varus deformity, the navicular must be plantar flexed on the head of the talus. This is carried out by holding the hindfoot in one hand and rotating the forefoot in such a way as to plantar flex the navicular on the head of the talus while simultaneously adducting the foot. This maneuver corrects the deformity and creates a plantigrade foot.

15. With the foot held in a plantigrade position, the calcaneocuboid joint is observed because if it is distracted, some bone needs to be removed from the talar head. This does not occur often, but again, it is important that a gap is not created between the calcaneus and cuboid.

16. Before placing the internal fixation, the bone ends are heavily scaled using a 4-mm osteotome. The talonavicular joint must be well feathered from both medial and lateral sides to ensure that the greatest amount of bone surface has been destroyed to help prevent a nonunion.

17. Many ways are available to carry out internal fixation for a double arthrodesis. If adequate bone stock exists, two 4.0-mm cannulated screws across the talonavicular joint provides excellent internal fixation. A single 7.0-mm screw can be used in a large patient, but in a smaller person or a person with soft bone, it can result in a fracture of the medial side of the navicular (Fig. 20–4A to C).

18. The foot is then manipulated into proper alignment as described earlier; and the guide pin for the 4.0-mm cannulated screw is placed across the talonavicular joint.

19. The guide pin is started at the distal end of the navicular at the naviculocuneiform joint. If one starts at the midportion of the navicular, insufficient bone may be present along the medial side of the navicular, and a fracture of the medial aspect of the navicular can occur. The surgeon should attempt to incorporate as much of the medial aspect of the navicular as possible with the screw. The placement is usually checked with

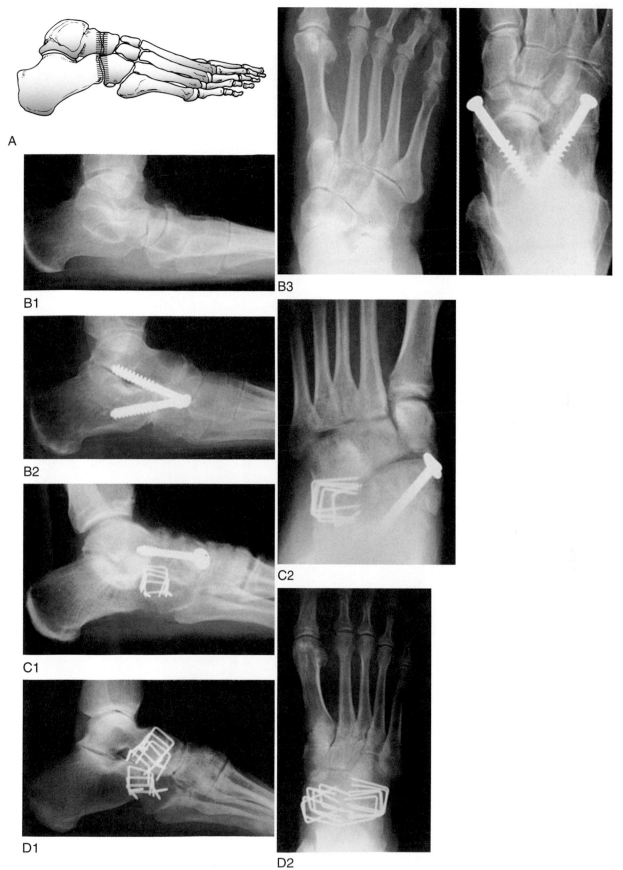

Figure 20–4 **A,** Diagram of double arthrodesis. **B,** Preoperative and postoperative radiographs demonstrating arthrodesis using 7-0 mm cannulated screws. **C,** Double arthrodesis using a cannulated screw for the talonavicular joint and power staples for the calcaneocuboid joint. **D,** Double arthrodesis using power staples in both the talonavicular and calcaneocuboid joints. This is done when the bone is soft, particularly in a patient with rheumatoid arthritis. Note the arrangement of staples around the joint to gain maximum stabilization. *Continued*

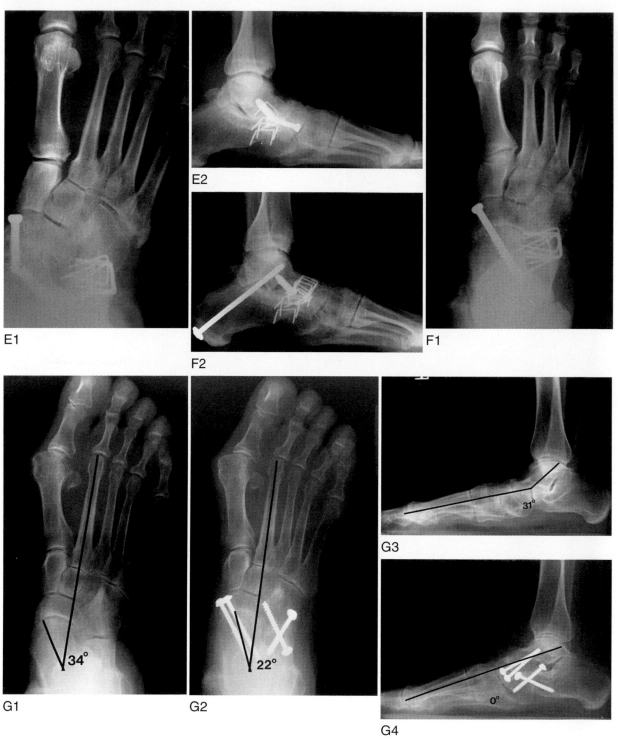

Figure 20–4—cont'd   E, Radiographs demonstrate failed double arthrodesis secondary to fracture of the talonavicular screw. **F,** Revision of double arthrodesis to a triple arthrodesis. **G,** Preoperative and postoperative radiographs demonstrate the correction that can be obtained with double arthrodesis in a patient with an acquired flatfoot secondary to posterior tibial tendon dysfunction.

fluoroscopy, and if placement is satisfactory, a parallel pin is inserted. The navicular is overdrilled with a 4.0-mm drill bit, after which 4.0-mm long threaded screws are inserted. It is important that the threads cross the joint surface. If the quality of bone is not good, washers should be employed.

20. The fixation of the calcaneocuboid joint is usually carried out using two 4.0-mm cannulated screws. As a general rule, the screws can be brought from proximal to distal, starting in the anterior process area and brought obliquely across into the cuboid. At times, however, the bone alignment is such that this is not possible, and the screws are brought from the cuboid into the calcaneus. Sometimes the bone is too soft, and a seam of staples is used (Fig. 20–4D).

21. The deep layers are closed, followed by the subcutaneous tissues and skin.

22. The wounds are instilled with 0.25% bupivacaine, after which a compression dressing incorporating plaster splints is applied.

Postoperative Care

In the recovery room a popliteal block is administered to control postoperative pain. The postoperative dressing is removed in approximately 10 days, after which the patient is placed into a removable cast with an elastic bandage to control swelling. The patient is kept non–weight bearing for 6 weeks from the time of surgery. At 6 weeks, radiographs are obtained. If satisfactory union is occurring, the patient is permitted to bear weight in a cast. Approximately 12 weeks after surgery, radiographs again are obtained. If satisfactory union has occurred, the patient is permitted to ambulate with an elastic stocking .

Author's Experience

We reviewed our experience with 32 patients (19 women, 13 men) who had undergone a double arthrodesis.[25] The average age was 62 years (range, 38 to 81 years), and average follow-up was 56 months (range, 24 to 162 months). The diagnosis was posterior tibial tendon dysfunction in 20 patients, isolated talonavicular arthrosis in five, rheumatoid arthritis in five, talar neck nonunion in one, and an acquired flatfoot deformity after a spinal cord injury in one.

The patients' satisfaction rate was 92%, and 8% were dissatisfied. Pain relief was the main benefit. The preoperative pain, assessed as 4.3 of a possible 5, diminished postoperatively to 1.4 (zero equals no pain). Functional capacity increased from 3.6 of 4 preoperatively to 1.3 postoperatively.

The fusion rate was 87.5% (28 of 32 cases). Four nonunions of the talonavicular joint occurred, all of which had staple fixation. Three of the four required a revision to a triple arthrodesis (Fig. 20–4E and F).

As a group, they noted maximum recovery at about 8 months after surgery.

The patients' level of activities demonstrated that most could walk for pleasure, and five were able to run short distances; 60% played golf, biked, hiked, and swam. Seventy-five percent of the patients noted some difficulty when walking on uneven ground or inclines or when going up and down steps.

The physical examination demonstrated that the average hindfoot position was 5.8 degrees of valgus, the transverse tarsal joint had 4.4 degrees of abduction, and the forefoot varus was 9 degrees. The range of motion of the ankle joint decreased 11 degrees compared with the uninvolved side.

The radiographic evaluation demonstrated that the anteroposterior (AP) talar–second metatarsal angle improved from 30 degrees (abduction) to 14 degrees, and the lateral talar–first metatarsal angle improved from –16 degrees (indicating dorsiflexion) to –7 degrees postoperatively (Fig. 20–4G).

The follow-up radiographs demonstrated a slight degree of ankle arthrosis in 53% of patients that was not present preoperatively, and 30% noted mild symptoms. Twenty percent demonstrated evidence of arthrosis in the subtalar joint, but none were symptomatic. The naviculocuneiform joint demonstrated an increase in arthrosis in 37% of patients, all of whom had slight symptoms, except for one patient, whose symptoms were severe. The tarsometatarsal joints demonstrated a 22% increased incidence, but none were symptomatic.

Special Considerations

Complex problems involving the talonavicular joint include its possible collapse secondary to fracture, avascular necrosis, or both. At other times, involvement of the forefoot distal to the talonavicular joint occurs, with extension into the naviculocuneiform and sometimes the tarsometatarsal joints. In these situations a modified double arthrodesis has been used to provide stability.

In many of these cases the overall alignment of the foot is satisfactory or at least adequate for a plantigrade foot. Rather than take down the involved areas and place a large bone graft, a rectangular slot is cut from the talus to the cuneiforms or into the metatarsal bases, as indicated by the clinical circumstances (Fig. 20–5). The slot is cut all the way across the foot from medial to lateral, after which a piece of iliac crest bone graft is inlaid into the slot. Fixation of the bone graft and surrounding bone is done with screws or multiple staples. At the same time the calcaneocuboid joint is arthrodesed to provide stability to the lateral column. This is obviously an extensive procedure and is only done under certain circumstances when significant deformity within the midportion of the foot is present but no significant anatomic correction needs to be carried out. In a situation with marked destruction of the midfoot and malalignment, this procedure cannot be used. Then one would need to take down the involved area and either bone graft it or possibly collapse the lateral column to realign the midfoot.

After the inlay bone graft procedure, the patient is immobilized for a prolonged period. As a general rule, weight bearing is not permitted for 3 months, after which the patient is gradually started on progressive weight bearing over the next 3 months. It is sometimes difficult to state when union has occurred, and therefore the surgeon should be very cautious in allowing patients to bear weight.

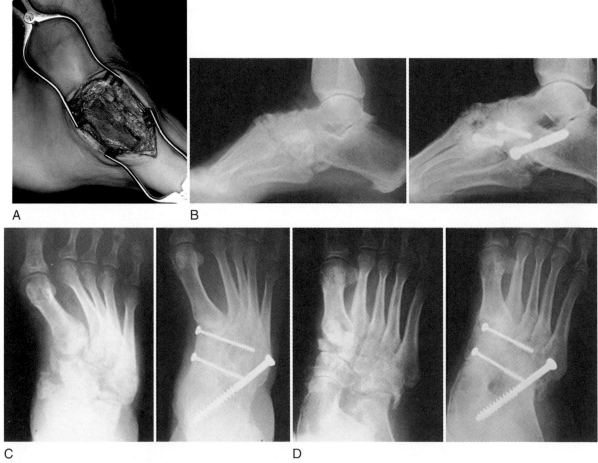

Figure 20–5 Technique for slot graft to correct disruption of tarsal joints. **A,** Outline of slot graft extending from the talus into the metatarsal bones. **B,** Preoperative and postoperative radiographs demonstrate placement of the bone block, which is held in place with two 4.0-mm screws, and fusion of the calcaneocuboid joint to help reinforce the fusion site. Preoperative and postoperative anteroposterior **(C)** and oblique **(D)** radiographs demonstrate placement and incorporation of the bone block.

TRIPLE ARTHRODESIS

The triple arthrodesis consists of fusion of the talonavicular, calcaneocuboid, and subtalar joints (Fig. 20–6A). Initially the triple arthrodesis was used to treat deformities of the foot secondary to paralysis, mainly poliomyelitis, in which severe anatomic distortion was present.[33,35,38] To correct this abnormality, large bone wedges were resected to place the foot into a plantigrade position. Little or no internal fixation was used, and at times the patient was returned to surgery in the immediate postoper-ative period to remanipulate the foot into better alignment.

As the number of patients with deformed feet secondary to paralysis declined, the triple arthrodesis was performed less often. It is now most often carried out for residuals of trauma, rheumatoid arthritis, and long-standing poste-rior tibial tendon dysfunction in which the basic bone anatomy is present. Although distorted, significant bone resection is usually not neces-sary. This allows the procedure to be done by releasing the contracted joint capsules, remov-ing the articular cartilage, scaling the exposed

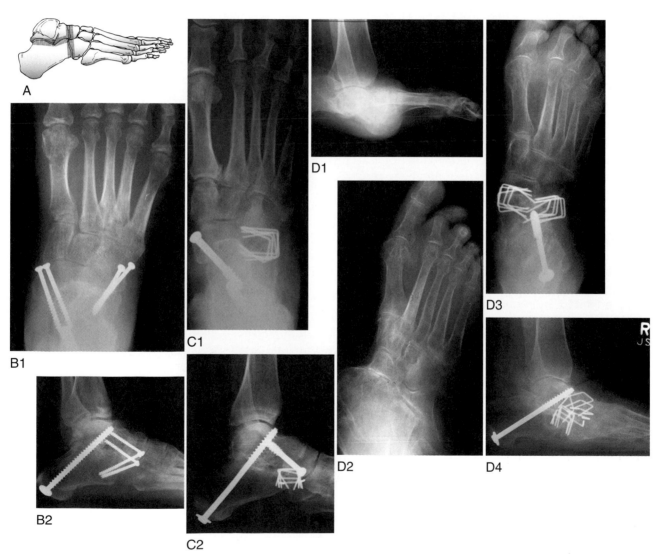

Figure 20–6   Triple arthrodesis, methods of internal fixation. **A,** Diagram of triple arthrodesis. **B,** Postoperative radiograph demonstrating triple arthrodesis with anatomic restoration of foot posture. **C,** Triple arthrodesis using 7.0-mm cannulated screws for the subtalar and talonavicular joints and multiple power staples for the calcaneocuboid joint. **D,** Correction of severe hind-foot deformity secondary to long-standing posterior tibial tendon dysfunction with restoration of the longitudinal arch using a 7.0-mm cannulated screw for the subtalar joint and power staples for the talonavicular and calcaneocuboid joints. Note that the height of the longitudinal arch has been restored and severe abduction of the foot is corrected.

bony surfaces, and using manipulation to create a plantigrade foot. It is not unusual to carry out a triple arthrodesis when no distortion of the anatomy exists, and an in situ fusion is achieved.[32]

The best way to carry out a triple arthrodesis is by meticulously releasing the joint capsules to mobilize the joint; removing the articular cartilage; scaling or feathering the bone surfaces; aligning the foot into a plantigrade position; and securing the joints with rigid internal fixation. By using these principles, a high fusion rate and a plantigrade foot can be achieved. In our experience, bone grafting from the iliac crest is rarely necessary, but if bone graft is needed, it can usually be obtained from the calcaneus, medial malleolus, or proximal tibia without violating the iliac crest and risking added morbidity.

Although the triple arthrodesis is a valuable tool for the orthopaedic surgeon, it is not without postoperative complications. The literature points out that because of the added stress across the ankle joint as a result of a triple arthrodesis, approximately 30% of patients demonstrate ankle degeneration at 5 years.[26-31,36-38] This reinforces the biomechanics of the foot and ankle complex, demonstrating that the ankle, subtalar, and transverse tarsal joints are functioning together. When a triple arthrodesis is carried out, increased stress is placed proximally on the ankle joint and distally on the midfoot. Therefore it is imperative that a more limited arthrodesis always be considered when feasible. Because of the possible ankle joint deterioration, when evaluating the patient preoperatively for a triple arthrodesis, a weight-bearing AP radiograph of the ankle must be included to ascertain if preexisting arthrosis can preclude the triple arthrodesis or at least to predict the future for the patient.

Indications

Arthrosis involving the subtalar joint and either the talonavicular or the calcaneocuboid joint, or both, is an indication for triple arthrodesis. Arthrosis of only the subtalar joint can usually be treated by an isolated subtalar joint fusion.

Triple arthrodesis can be used for the unstable hindfoot secondary to neuromuscular disorders such as poliomyelitis, nerve injury, posterior tibial tendon dysfunction, or rheumatoid arthritis in which the subtalar and transverse tarsal joints are involved. Malalignment of the foot secondary to arthrofibrosis resulting from a compartment syndrome, crush injury, or severe trauma is an indication for a triple arthrodesis. In the patient with a symptomatic, unresectable, or previously resected calcaneonavicular coalition, a triple arthrodesis is indicated. It is important to appreciate, however, that the patient with a talocalcaneal (subtalar) coalition can be treated with an isolated subtalar fusion even if there is osteophyte formation on the dorsal aspect of the talar head. The patient with a severe symptomatic pes planus deformity that is not amenable to other procedures, such as lateral column lengthening, calcaneal osteotomy, or subtalar fusion, can also be considered a candidate for a triple arthrodesis.

Whenever considering a triple arthrodesis, however, the surgeon must be mindful of the consequences of the potential degeneration at the ankle joint. If a younger person can be treated with an AFO or a more limited fusion, this may be a better method of treatment.

Position of Arthrodesis

The position of a triple arthrodesis is critical because once an arthrodesis has been achieved, the foot is in a fixed position and cannot accommodate to the ground. It is therefore essential that the hindfoot be placed in about 5 degrees of valgus, the transverse tarsal joint in 0 to 5 degrees of abduction, and the forefoot in less than 10 degrees of varus. If accurate alignment is not achieved, the patient will have a nonplantigrade foot, which can cause chronic pain that requires a revision.

Surgical Technique

1. The normal foot is examined and its alignment noted. Patients have a varying degree of forefoot adduction or abduction, and the surgeon should attempt to match this with the affected extremity (video clip 14).
2. The patient is placed in a supine position with a support under the ipsilateral hip to improve visualization of the lateral aspect of the hindfoot. (A detailed discussion of this approach is presented in the sections on subtalar and double arthrodeses.)

3. The skin incision starts at the tip of the fibula and is carried to the base of the fourth metatarsal. Caution should be used when deepening this incision, looking for the sural nerve and possibly an anterior branch (see Fig. 20–1A).

4. The extensor digitorum muscle is removed from its origin on the lateral side of the talus and calcaneus and retracted distally.

5. The subtalar and calcaneocuboid joints are visualized, and the articular cartilage is removed.

6. Through the lateral incision, the lateral aspect of the talonavicular joint is identified and as much articular cartilage is removed as possible. (A detailed discussion of this approach is presented in the section on talonavicular arthrodesis.)

7. The skin incision begins 2 cm distal to the tip of the medial malleolus in the midline and is carried 1 cm distal to the naviculo-cuneiform joint (see Fig. 20–2B).

8. The incision is deepened to expose the joint capsule, which is stripped from the talonavicular joint.

9. Using a towel clip in the navicular, the surgeon distracts the joint by pulling the foot into an adducted position to enhance visualization of the articular surfaces (see Fig. 20–2C). If the bone stock is adequate, a small lamina spreader is useful.

10. The articular cartilage is removed from the talonavicular joint.

11. At times, some articular cartilage is also removed through the lateral incision. This depends on the flexibility of the foot.

12. The foot is manipulated, first by bringing the subtalar joint into 5 degrees of valgus, then manipulating the transverse tarsal joint to eliminate the fixed forefoot varus. This is done by rotating the navicular in a plantar direction on the head of the talus and simultaneously bringing the transverse tarsal joint into about 0 to 5 degrees of abduction. This maneuver usually creates a plantigrade foot. The foot cannot be manipulated if the joints have not been completely mobilized.

13. After the manipulation, it is important to inspect the articular surfaces to be sure there is good bone apposition. If the bones are not properly apposed, it may be necessary to remove some bone, usually from the head of the talus, to shorten the medial column and close the calcaneocuboid joint.

14. Once alignment has been achieved, the joint surfaces are heavily scaled or feathered in preparation for internal fixation.

15. The internal fixation is initially achieved in the subtalar joint (see the section on subtalar arthrodesis and Fig. 20–1D).

16. The anterior cruciate guide is placed into the posterior facet of the subtalar joint and then the back of the heel. A guide pin is inserted into the posterior facet and the AO guide is removed.

17. The calcaneus is manipulated into 5 degrees of valgus, and the pin is advanced into the neck of the talus. Its position is verified by fluoroscopy.

18. The length of the screw is determined and the guide pin is drilled through to present on the dorsal aspect of the ankle joint.

19. A 4.5-mm cannulated drill is used to make the initial hole, which must pass through the anterior cortex of the talus, after which the calcaneus is overdrilled with a 7.0-mm bit. The talar neck is tapped and a 7.0-mm fully threaded cannulated screw with a washer is inserted. This fixes the subtalar component of the triple arthrodesis in correct alignment. In our experience, a single screw is adequate to stabilize the subtalar joint.

20. The transverse tarsal joint is manipulated to correct the forefoot malalignment. Once the appropriate alignment has been achieved, the talonavicular joint is fixed.

21. The fixation of the talonavicular joint is usually achieved with two 4.0-mm cannulated screws. The guide pin is inserted across the talonavicular joint, starting at the naviculocuneiform joint, and is driven obliquely into the neck of the talus. Two guide pins are inserted and their position is verified radiographically.

22. The navicular is overdrilled with a 4.0-mm drill bit, and a partially threaded cannulated screw of appropriate length is inserted; a washer may be used depending upon bone quality. The screws generally are about 45 to 60 mm in length, but this varies from patient to patient.

23. The calcaneocuboid joint is visualized and fixed with two 4.0-mm cannulated screws. The guide pin is placed from the calcaneus

into the cuboid, and two partially threaded screws of appropriate length are used. If the bone is too soft, staples are used.

24. If the surgeon is not satisfied with the coaptation of the bony surfaces, a bone graft can be used if necessary.

25. The extensor digitorum brevis muscle is closed over the lateral side of the wound, after which the subcutaneous tissue and skin are closed. On the medial side, the capsular tissue is closed over the talonavicular joint, if possible, after which the subcutaneous tissue and skin are closed.

26. Bupivacaine (0.25%) is instilled into the wound to provide initial postoperative analgesia.

27. A compression dressing incorporating two plaster splints is applied.

Postoperative Care

In the recovery room, a popliteal block is administered to control the immediate postoperative pain. The patient's initial surgical cast is changed 10 to 14 days after surgery, and the sutures are removed if appropriate. The patient is placed into a short-leg removable cast with an elastic bandage to control edema and is kept non–weight bearing for 6 weeks. Then radiographs are obtained, and if satisfactory union is occurring, the patient is permitted to bear weight as tolerated in the removable cast.

Twelve weeks after surgery, radiographs are again obtained, and if a fusion has occurred, the patient wears an elastic stocking and is permitted to bear weight as tolerated. If the fusion is somewhat tenuous, the patient is asked to walk around the house without the cast and use it outside for another month (Fig. 20–6B to D).

Complications

The most frequent complication after a triple arthrodesis is a *nonunion* of one of the fusion sites, most often the talonavicular joint, probably because its exposure is more difficult and the bone may be sclerotic. If a nonunion occurs and is not symptomatic, no treatment is indicated. Occasionally after a triple arthrodesis, if two of the three joints have fused, the joint with a nonunion is asymptomatic. If a painful nonunion is present but the alignment of the extremity is satisfactory, some type of an inlay bone block

across the area of the nonunion, possibly along with reinforcement of the internal fixation, usually results in a satisfactory fusion. If the area of the nonunion is symptomatic and the alignment is unsatisfactory, revision of the arthrodesis may be necessary.

The next most common complication is *malalignment*. In my experience the most frequent malalignment is residual varus of the calcaneus, followed by a fixed forefoot varus and then adduction of the forefoot. A valgus deformity of the hindfoot, although not as common as a varus deformity, is distressing for most patients and can result in an unsatisfactory outcome.[31,35] In this situation the surgeon might consider a medial displacement calcaneal osteotomy to correct the excessive valgus if the remainder of the forefoot alignment is satisfactory.

Entrapment of the sural nerve, particularly an anterior branch, giving rise to dysesthesias on the lateral side of the foot, can annoy the patient. This might need to be corrected by a neurolysis or resection of the nerve, then burying the stump under soft tissues or into bone.

Occasionally after a triple arthrodesis in a patient with long-standing severe valgus deformity, although a plantigrade position of the foot can be achieved, the ankle cannot be brought back to neutral position because of an Achilles tendon contracture. When the triple arthrodesis is carried out, if the ankle cannot be brought into about 5 degrees of dorsiflexion, an Achilles tendon lengthening or gastrocnemius slide should be strongly considered. One must be cautious, however, not to overlengthen the tendon, but the foot should not be left in an equinus posture. Adults recover their strength very slowly, if at all, after Achilles tendon lengthening.

Revision for Malalignment

A plantigrade foot might not be achieved after a triple arthrodesis. If the patient is symptomatic, a revision of the triple arthrodesis may be indicated. Technically these are very difficult cases and need to be carefully planned preoperatively to identify the precise nature and degree of the malalignment and which components of the triple arthrodesis need to be revised.

If the hindfoot is malaligned and the forefoot is in a plantigrade position, the hindfoot can be corrected without revising the forefoot. If a varus deformity is present, a lateral closing wedge Dwyer procedure can be used. Occasionally a lateral displacement osteotomy with some rotation of the fragment from varus into valgus can produce better alignment.

When the calcaneus is in too much valgus and there is an impingement against the fibula, a calcaneal osteotomy displacing it in a medial direction can be used to correct the deformity. However, rather than create a long oblique osteotomy, as one would for a Dwyer procedure, the cut is made more perpendicular, just posterior to the posterior facet of the subtalar joint. The osteotomy is then displaced medially about 1 cm, and occasionally the posterior fragment can be rotated slightly on its long axis if the degree of valgus has a rotational component. Fixation of the osteotomy is usually done with a cannulated 7.0-mm screw placed just lateral to the Achilles tendon and driven distally across the osteotomy site into the calcaneus. If one screw is not adequate for fixation, a Steinmann pin is used for 4 weeks until the bones have become sticky.

If the hindfoot is properly aligned and the main deformity is malalignment of the forefoot, usually from residual forefoot varus, the front portion of the triple arthrodesis can be revised and the hindfoot left intact. Besides the varus deformity, an adduction deformity is also often present. This type of revision is carried out through a medial and lateral approach through the previous incisions. The soft tissues are stripped off the fusion mass around the transverse tarsal joint, which is osteotomized, and the foot is realigned. The realignment is usually carried out by rotating the forefoot block of bone into a more pronated position. If there is residual adduction or possibly abduction in the forefoot, a lateral or medial closing wedge is removed at the same time to achieve satisfactory alignment. Fixation after a revision can usually be achieved by using large screws, but if the bone is too soft, multiple staples can be useful.

The postoperative regimen after revision of a triple arthrodesis is the same as for a triple arthrodesis, that is, non–weight bearing for 6 weeks and then weight bearing for 6 weeks.

Author's Experience

We have reviewed two groups of patients after triple arthrodesis.[30,34] The first group involved 29 fusions in 27 patients (23 women, 4 men) for treatment of posterior tibial tendon dysfunction. The average age was 62 years (range, 44 to 78 years), and average follow-up was 55 months (range, 24 to 122 months). The preoperative AOFAS score was 30, which improved postoperatively to 80. One nonunion of the talonavicular joint occurred and was asymptomatic.

The AP radiographs demonstrated that the talar–first metatarsal angle improved from 24 to 10 degrees postoperatively and the talar–second metatarsal angle from 35 to 19 degrees. In the lateral radiograph the talar–first metatarsal angle improved from 18 to 9 degrees. In all cases the final correction was greater than the contralateral foot if it was not pathologic. The radiographs further demonstrated an increase in the arthrosis in the ankle joint in 10 of 29 cases (33%), in the naviculocuneiform joint in five (17%), and at the tarsometatarsal joint in four (14%) (Fig. 20–7A and B).

A second group consisted of 17 patients (12 women, 5 men) and 18 feet, with an average age of 66 years (range, 52 to 80 years). They were evaluated to determine the effect of a triple arthrodesis in the older age group, because no paper had previously addressed this in the literature.[30] The etiology was posterior tibial tendon dysfunction in 10 patients, rheumatoid arthritis in three (four feet), diabetes mellitus in one, poliomyelitis in one, trauma in one, and poststroke effects in one. The follow-up was 42 months (range, 27 to 156 months). The procedure was carried out because of pain, deformity, or both. The pain level preoperatively was 4 on a scale of 5 and postoperatively was 1.

Fourteen patients (15 feet) were satisfied because of the improved position and diminished pain. Interestingly, however, 11 patients still thought they had some pain in the foot, but it was not sufficiently symptomatic for them to be dissatisfied with the procedure. Of the three patients who were dissatisfied, two had a valgus alignment of the heel that resulted in pain. The patients observed that the time from surgery to maximum relief was about 10 months.

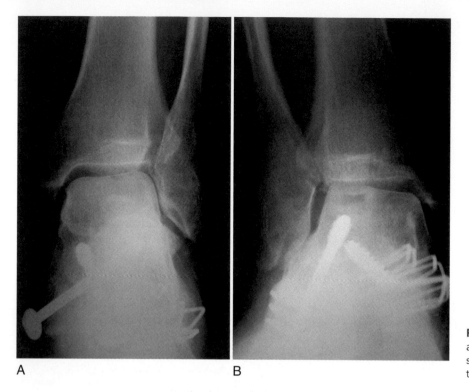

A   B

Figure 20–7   A, Mild valgus tilt of the ankle joint 2 years after triple arthrodesis. **B,** Moderate valgus tilt 3 years after triple arthrodesis.

The level of activities improved for nine patients (10 feet). Seven reported no change in their ambulatory capacity, and one believed that her ambulatory capacity was decreased. The appearance of the foot improved for 13 of 17 patients, and two were dissatisfied because of the valgus alignment of their heel. Twelve patients (13 feet) could wear any shoe they wanted, but five had some problems with footwear.

The range of motion demonstrated that dorsiflexion was equal on both feet, and plantar flexion on the affected side was 30 degrees compared to 44 degrees on the normal side, for a 32% loss.

Radiographs demonstrated that the AP talar–second metatarsal angle improved from 36 to 16 degrees and the lateral talar–first metatarsal angle from 22 to 9 degrees, which indicates plantar flexion of the first metatarsal.

Some evidence of arthrosis of the ankle joint was seen preoperatively in 14 of the 18 ankles and progressed in seven (one grade in three ankles and greater than one grade in four). Seven patients demonstrated changes at the naviculocuneiform and tarsometatarsal joints.

Three nonunions occurred, one at the talonavicular joint, which was revised successfully, and two at the calcaneocuboid joint, one requiring revision and one being asymptomatic.

In summary, the triple arthrodesis is an excellent procedure for correcting a fixed deformity of the foot, but it should be used judiciously, particularly in the younger patient, and only when a lesser procedure cannot be used.

NAVICULOCUNEIFORM ARTHRODESIS

A naviculocuneiform arthrodesis is usually carried out for arthrosis of one or more of the articulations as a result of primary arthrosis or secondary to trauma. The other reason to carry out this arthrodesis is in the patient with posterior tibial tendon dysfunction and a fixed forefoot varus deformity so that a more extensive hindfoot fusion can be avoided.

In the patient with a fixed uncorrectable forefoot varus deformity, a double or triple arthrodesis is indicated because an isolated subtalar arthrodesis would cause the patient to walk on the lateral border of the foot. If the fixed forefoot varus can be corrected, however, patients with this deformity can be treated with a subtalar arthrodesis and a naviculocuneiform arthrodesis. This spares the transverse tarsal joint, which leaves the forefoot more flexible. Approximately 15 to 20 degrees of fixed forefoot varus can be corrected through the naviculocuneiform joint, depending upon how rigid the deformity is.

Indications

The most common indication is isolated naviculocuneiform arthrosis secondary to trauma. The next most common indication is a fixed forefoot varus deformity secondary to posterior tibial tendon dysfunction.

Position of Arthrodesis

With arthrosis of the joint secondary to trauma there usually is little or no deformity of the forefoot, and an in situ fusion can be carried out. Because this is a difficult articulation to obtain an isolated arthrodesis, the fusion mass should include the first and second and, if possible, the third naviculocuneiform joints. When there is a fixed forefoot varus, the position of the arthrodesis depends upon the degree of deformity. Arthrodesis is usually carried out along with either a subtalar arthrodesis or a reconstruction of the posterior tibial tendon with an FDL transfer.

Surgical Technique

1. The patient is placed in the supine position, and a thigh tourniquet is applied. Because the extremity naturally falls into external rotation, the patient does not require turning.
2. The naviculocuneiform joint is approached through a longitudinal incision starting just distal to the medial malleolus and carried distally just dorsal to the posterior tibial tendon, distal enough to expose the first metatarsocuneiform joint.
3. The dissection is carried down to bone, using caution not to injure the posterior tibial tendon as it passes on the plantar aspect of the wound. As one proceeds distally, the tibialis anterior tendon is obliquely crossing the field and needs to be mobilized so that it can be pulled somewhat distally out of harm's way.
4. By sharp and blunt dissection the joint capsule is stripped from the medial, dorsal, and plantar aspects of the joint.
5. Using a small osteotome, the articular cartilage is removed from the first, second, and third cuneiform, as well as the corresponding surface of the navicular. Usually it is difficult to completely denude the third naviculocuneiform joint. A small lamina spreader does help facilitate exposure of these joints.
6. The articular surfaces are then feathered with a 4-mm osteotome or perforated with multiple drill holes.
7. The foot is corrected by rotating the distal portion of the foot into pronation or plantar flexion at the fusion site while holding the hindfoot in neutral position. Sometimes it takes several manipulations in this manner to gain the necessary correction. It is important, however, that as this is carried out the hindfoot is held in neutral position, otherwise inadequate correction will be obtained. If correction of the deformity seems overly difficult, it is probably due to lack of adequate capsular stripping.
8. Once the foot is manipulated into satisfactory alignment, a 0.062-inch Kirschner wire is placed across the dorsal aspect of the joint to stabilize it so that internal fixation can be inserted.
9. Rigid fixation can be achieved by placing the screws from the tubercle of the navicular and proceeding distally into the first and second cuneiforms. A third screw passing from the first cuneiform back into the navicular can also be used with caution. The problem with the screw passing in this direction is that all the threads have to pass across the fusion site and cannot enter the talonavicular joint.
10. Usually one screw is passed from the navicular into the first cuneiform and the second from the navicular into the second cuneiform. As a rule, it is not possible to get a screw from the navicular into the third cuneiform.
11. The wound is closed in layers, with the deep fascia being approximated over the fusion site. The subcutaneous tissue and skin are closed in a routine manner. Wounds along the medial border of the foot usually heal well.

Postoperative Care

A popliteal block is administered by anesthesia to control postoperative pain. The postoperative dressing is changed in 10 to 14 days, sutures are removed, and the patient is placed into a short-leg removable cast with an elastic bandage to control swelling. Weight bearing is not permitted until 6 weeks after surgery. At 6 weeks following surgery, if x-rays demonstrate early union, the patient is permitted to bear weight as tolerated in a short-leg removable cast. As a general rule, the arthrodesis occurs after about 3 months.

Complications

Nonunion of the naviculocuneiform joints does occur, but by including at least the first and second joints along with the internal fixation passing from the tubercle of the navicular into the cuneiforms, satisfactory union seems to occur in most cases (Fig. 20–8).

The other complication is incomplete correction of the fixed forefoot varus in the patient with posterior tibial tendon dysfunction. If malalignment is still present and results in a nonplantigrade foot, a double or triple arthrodesis might be necessary to create a plantigrade foot.

TARSOMETATARSAL ARTHRODESIS

Arthrodesis of the tarsometatarsal joints can involve an isolated joint, usually the second or third, or it can involve multiple joints, depending on the etiology of the arthrosis. As a general rule, patients with primary arthroses usually have fewer joints that require fusing than those with post-traumatic arthrosis. In our study of 41 feet, we observed that the patient with post-traumatic arthrosis had an average of six joints fused per foot, compared with four joints per foot in the primary arthrosis group.[41]

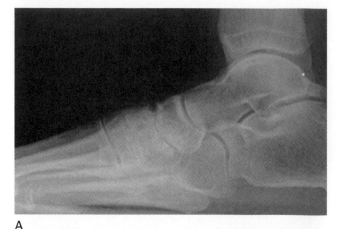

A

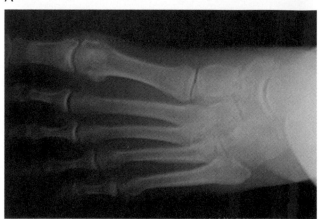

B

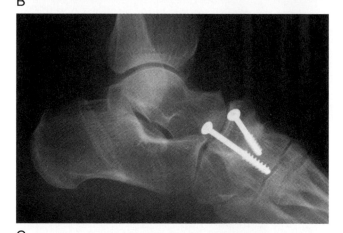

C

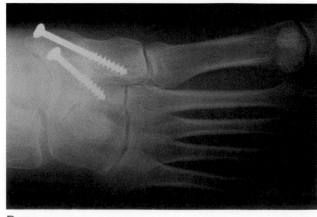

D

Figure 20–8 Preoperative (**A** and **B**) and postoperative (**C** and **D**) radiographs of a naviculocuneiform arthrodesis to correct a forefoot varus deformity. Note the placement of screws from the navicular into the cuneiforms. The fusion mass should include the navicular and at least cuneiforms 1, 2, and 3, if possible.

The extent of the deformity is also variable. This depends on the number of joints involved and whether the deformity results from primary or traumatic arthrosis. The patient with primary arthrosis tends to have more pronation and a greater degree of deformity. Usually, if a single joint is involved, particularly the second or third, little or no deformity is present and therefore only an in situ fusion is necessary. If a deformity is present, however, realignment of the foot is essential to obtain a satisfactory result.

Determining the extent of the fusion site is sometimes difficult, particularly if it appears as though only one joint is involved. Besides a careful physical examination and radiographic studies consisting of weight-bearing radiographs, a computed tomography (CT) scan and bone scan may be useful in determining the extent of the arthrosis and which joints should be included in the fusion mass. Even after careful physical and radiographic evaluation, if any doubt exists regarding the presence of arthrosis, the joint should be examined at surgery to be sure that arthritis is not being overlooked. Arthrosis may be seen at surgery when, even in retrospect, the radiograph appears to be normal. This is particularly true for the medial naviculocuneiform joint and the third metatarsocuneiform (MTC) joint. Although the most obvious arthrosis usually is present at the tarsometatarsal or intertarsal joints, the naviculocuneiform joints must always be carefully evaluated, particularly in the patient after trauma. If the naviculocuneiform joint does appear to be involved, at least the two medial joints should always be included in the fusion mass and, if necessary, the third. It is difficult to obtain an isolated fusion between the medial cuneiform and the navicular.

The question is often raised about whether the fourth and fifth metatarsocuboid articulations should be included in the fusion site or if they should undergo isolated fusion. As a general rule, the fourth and fifth metatarsocuboid articulations seem to be somewhat more forgiving and tend to be less symptomatic than the medial three MTC joints, despite the arthrosis. The reason may be that more flexibility exists in the two lateral rays than in the medial three rays, which are more rigid. Motion also occurs between the third cuneiform and cuboid, which results in more motion of the two lateral rays of the foot. If clinical examination and radiographs show arthrosis at the fourth and fifth metatarsocuboid joints and a fusion is indicated, however, the cuboid should *not* be fused to the lateral cuneiform so that some mobility can be maintained between the medial and lateral aspects of the longitudinal arch. Not fusing the cuboid to the lateral cuneiform appears to give the foot a little more flexibility to adapt to the ground.

Indications

The main indication for arthrodesis of the tarsometatarsal joints is arthrosis resulting in pain, deformity, or both. The arthrodesis can include a single joint or multiple joints.

Position of Arthrodesis

The arthrodesis site is positioned to correct any forefoot abduction or adduction or dorsiflexion. At times a complex deformity from trauma, particularly a crush injury, results in a deformity involving multiple planes, and it can be difficult to achieve a plantigrade foot. However, the surgeon should attempt to obtain a foot as close to plantigrade as possible.

Surgical Technique

1. The patient is placed in a supine position, and a tourniquet is used about the thigh (video clip 13).
2. The surgical approach varies, depending on which joints are being arthrodesed. For an isolated first tarsometatarsal arthrodesis, a dorsomedial incision is used, centered over the joint. This allows satisfactory visualization of the joint as well as access to the dorsum of the foot to insert screws for internal fixation.
3. For an isolated second MTC arthrodesis, the incision is made just lateral to the midportion of the joint. By placing the incision here, the neurovascular bundle is located medial to the incision. Subperiosteal dissection can safely mobilize and retract the neurovascular bundle medially.
4. The approach to the first, second, and third tarsometatarsal joints is carried out through two longitudinal incisions. The first is centered over the dorsomedial aspect of the first tarsometatarsal joint or possibly slightly toward the midline, compared with the isolated fusion. The second incision is made

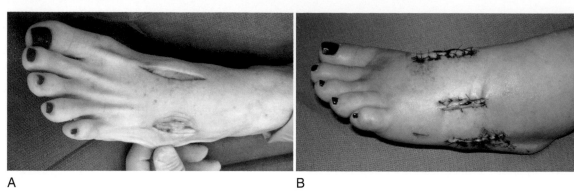

A   **B**

Figure 20–9   A, Lateral incision used to expose lateral Lisfranc's joint. **B,** Postoperative photograph demonstrating dorsal and dorsal-medial incision.

just to the lateral side of the second MTC joint. If the dorsal incision is not made lateral enough, it is very difficult to visualize the third MTC joint. It is important to make long incisions to minimize traction on the skin edges (Fig. 20–9).

5. The approach to the fourth and fifth metatarsocuboid articulations is through a dorsal incision centered between them, which provides adequate exposure.

6. When carrying out the surgical approach to the tarsometatarsal joints, the surgeon must be extremely cautious, looking for the superficial branches of the peroneal nerve that pass along the dorsum of the foot. Along the medial aspect of the foot, the surgeon is usually working in an internervous interval, although occasionally the internal division of the superficial peroneal nerve may be encountered.

7. The approach to the second MTC joint is the most hazardous, because the internal and external divisions of the superficial peroneal nerve lie in the subcutaneous tissue in a somewhat irregular pattern. As one proceeds deeper, the neurovascular bundle containing the superficial branch of the deep peroneal nerve and dorsalis pedis artery are encountered as they pass distally.

8. The incision over the fourth and fifth metatarsocuboid articulations tends to be in an internervous interval between the external division of the superficial peroneal nerve medially and the sural nerve laterally. Again, however, the nerve pattern varies greatly in this area, and nerve branches should be carefully identified and retracted.

9. When approaching tarsometatarsal joints one, two, and three, it is easier to start the subperiosteal dissection through the medial incision. From this incision the surgeon identifies the skeletal plane and, with a sharp elevator, moves along this plane, stripping the soft tissues from the bone as far as the third MTC joint. This usually allows the surgeon to pass underneath the neurovascular bundle without causing damage to it. If the foot is severely distorted, however, this might not be safe, and the neurovascular bundle should be identified through the incision over the second MTC and carefully dissected off of the bone.

10. Once exposed, the involved joints are meticulously debrided with a curet, small osteotome, or rongeur. All the soft tissue and articular cartilage around the joints are removed, including the plantar aspects.

11. Once the joints are totally mobilized, it is always impressive how readily a deformity can be reduced. Occasionally, usually in the patient after trauma, some bone needs to be removed to create congruent surfaces for the fusion to occur.

12. After the joint surfaces have been debrided, the foot is realigned by first placing the first MTC joint into a plantigrade position. To help assess alignment (in particular abduction/adduction), the surgeon should always observe the normal foot before the procedure and relate it either to the alignment of the patella or to the medial side of the talus and hindfoot. As a general rule, when a deformity is present at the first MTC joint, it is usually abduction and dorsiflexion. Therefore, the first metatarsal is usually manipulated into some adduction and plantar flexion. If the alignment appears correct and good bone apposition is present, the bone

ends are feathered and the anticipated fusion site stabilized with the guide pin from the 4.0-mm cannulated screw set. If the apposition is not satisfactory, some bone is removed, feathered, and pinned.

13. The alignment is carefully checked again, and if it is satisfactory, internal fixation can be inserted.

14. Once the first MTC joint is aligned and stabilized, the other metatarsal bases are brought over to it, which effectively realigns the deformity. The second metatarsal is adducted so that it comes to lie next to the first and then is slightly plantar flexed. As the metatarsal is plantar flexed, the surgeon palpates the first metatarsal head to be sure that the degree of plantar flexion of the second metatarsal head is not excessive. The cuneiforms usually are not very deformed and tend to fall into place as the metatarsals are manipulated into a plantigrade position.

15. If the third MTC joint is to be arthrodesed, it is aligned next in relation to the second, and in this way the deformity is corrected.

16. When the fourth and fifth MTC joints are involved, as mentioned previously, an attempt is made to carry out the fusion only to the cuboid. The surgeon must be careful not to fuse the third cuneiform–cuboid articulation.

17. The internal fixation can be carried out in many ways, but we prefer to use the 4.0-mm cannulated screw with a small head. Because the skin is thin in this area, the low-profile heads can usually be buried, so they do not require removal.

18. The first MTC joint is fixed by inserting one screw from the dorsal aspect of the first metatarsal into the medial cuneiform, after which a second screw is placed from the dorsal aspect of the medial cuneiform into the base of the first metatarsal. This gives rather rigid internal fixation to the joint. As the screws are inserted, the joint surfaces are compressed with a towel clip (Fig. 20–10).

19. The second MTC joint is fixed by placing a long oblique screw, starting in the metatarsal and passing it proximally across the joint into the cuneiform. The angle that this pin makes with the second metatarsal is extremely acute and at times is difficult to start because the guide pin tends to slide

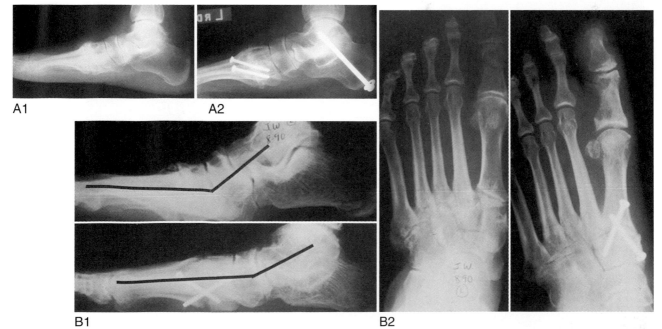

A1   A2   B1   B2

Figure 20–10 Tarsometatarsal arthrodesis. **A,** Preoperative and postoperative radiographs demonstrate arthrodesis of the first metatarsocuneiform (MTC) joint using two 4.0-mm cannulated screws. This method gives excellent internal fixation. Note the subtalar fusion as well. **B,** Preoperative and postoperative radiographs demonstrate arthrodesis at the first MTC joint with two crossed screws. Note that the deformity has been significantly improved, although not totally corrected, by the arthrodesis.

along the metatarsal proximally. This can sometimes be overcome by making a small vertical drill hole to identify where to start the guide pin, which is usually about 2 cm distal to the joint. The guide pin usually catches on this edge of bone and does not tend to slide up the metatarsal. If this screw is not placed obliquely enough, it will not engage the cuneiform adequately, and rigid fixation will not be achieved (Fig. 20–11).

20. Once the guide pin is in satisfactory position, the metatarsal is drilled with the 4.0-mm bit. The hole is countersunk to lower the profile of the head and prevent the screw head from impinging against the metatarsal when it is seated, which can fracture the dorsal portion of the metatarsal.

21. The third MTC joint is fixed in a manner similar to the second. Occasionally the screw is placed from the lateral aspect of the base of the metatarsal obliquely into the third or occasionally the second cuneiform.

22. Once the tarsometatarsal joints have been fixed, a screw is placed across the cuneiforms, depending on the extent of the fusion site. If only a single articulation is

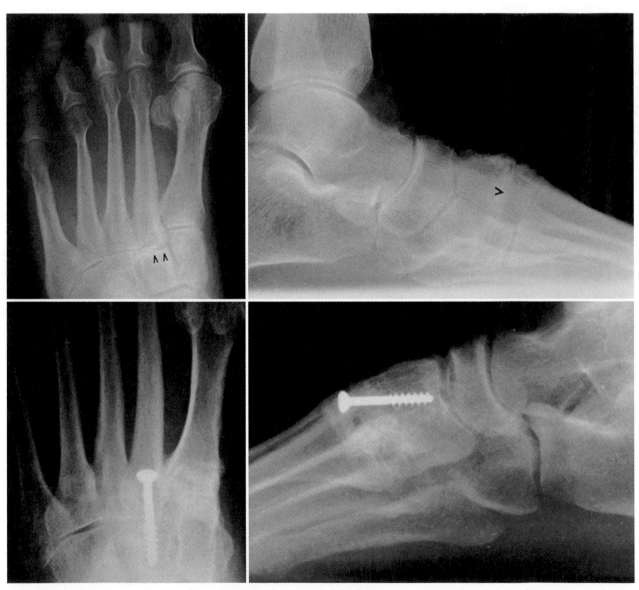

Figure 20–11 Preoperative *(top)* and postoperative *(bottom)* radiographs demonstrate isolated arthrodesis *(arrows)* of second metatarsocuneiform joint. (From Mann RA, Coughlin MJ: *The Video Textbook of Foot and Ankle Surgery.* St. Louis, Medical Video Productions, 1991.)

being fused, it is not necessary to fuse the cuneiforms to one another. If the first, second, and third MTC joints are being fused, however, a screw is placed mediolaterally across the cuneiforms to stabilize them. Another screw is then placed from the medial aspect of the first metatarsal base obliquely into the cuneiforms. This screw may also cross the second MTC joint. This screw helps to reinforce the fusion mass and ensure that rigid fixation is achieved.

23. When the naviculocuneiform joints are included in the fusion mass, a screw can be passed from the tip of the navicular into the cuneiforms, which usually provides excellent internal fixation. If the naviculocuneiform joints are to be included in the fusion site, it is imperative that at least the first and second cuneiforms be involved because an isolated fusion of the medial cuneiform and the navicular is difficult to achieve. Screws can also be placed from the cuneiforms into the navicular (Fig. 20–12).

24. Fixation of the metatarsocuboid joint is usually achieved by placing a screw from the dorsal aspect of the fourth metatarsal into the cuboid. The fixation of the fifth metatarsocuboid joint is more difficult because the actual articulating surface is quite small. An oblique guide pin may be placed percutaneously from the lateral aspect of the metatarsal base into the cuboid and a screw inserted over it.

25. Proliferative bone over the dorsal aspect of the MTC joints is removed, morselized, and packed into any existing spaces in the

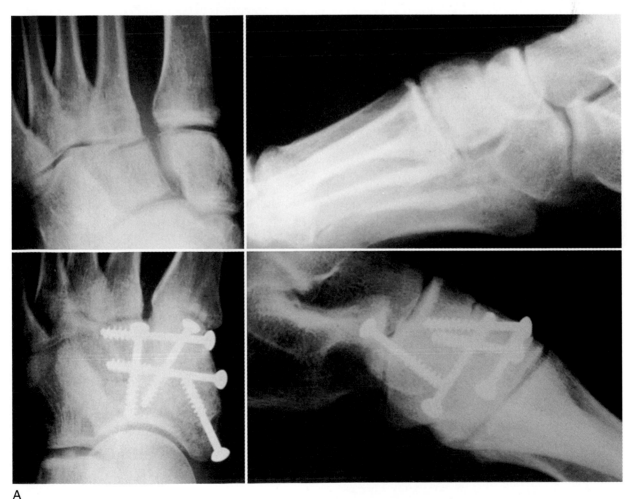

A

Figure 20–12 Midfoot arthrodesis of multiple joints. **A,** Preoperative and postoperative radiographs of intertarsal arthrodesis for degenerative arthrosis. Note that the screw pattern locks navicular to the cuneiforms; also note the intercuneiform screws. If the tarsometatarsal joints are not involved, the arthrodesis does not need to include them.   *Continued*

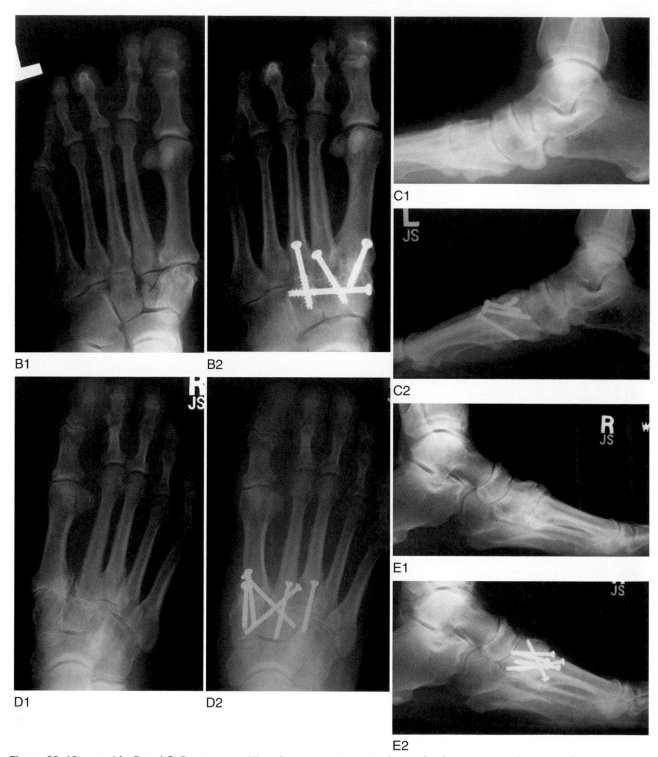

Figure 20–12—cont'd **B** and **C,** Preoperative **(1)** and postoperative **(2)** radiographs demonstrate arthrodesis of tarsometatarsal joints 1, 2, and 3, along with cuneiforms using a four-screw pattern. Note the correction of deformity in both the anteroposterior and lateral planes. **D** and **E,** Preoperative **(1)** and postoperative **(2)** radiographs demonstrate arthrodesis of tarsometatarsal joints 1, 2, and 3, along with intercuneiform joints using a six-screw pattern. The number of screws used depends on the stability of fixation needed to obtain rigid fixation. Note the correction of deformity in both the anteroposterior and lateral planes.

fusion site. If the surgeon is not satisfied with the apposition of the bone surfaces, a bone graft, generally from the calcaneus or medial malleolus, can be used.

26. The skin closure is very important in these cases. The skin is very fragile, and when multiple joints are arthrodesed, moderate swelling can occur.

27. The subcutaneous tissue is closed with 3-0 plain sutures and the skin with a running longitudinal near-far/far-near suture, which keeps tension off the skin edges.

Postoperative Care

At the conclusion of the procedure, 0.25% bupivacaine is placed into the surgical field to provide initial postoperative pain relief. A compression dressing consisting of fluffs and a heavy cotton bandage incorporating two plaster splints is applied. In the recovery room, a popliteal block is placed to control the initial postoperative pain.

The patient is kept non–weight bearing in the postoperative cast for approximately 12 to 14 days, after which the cast is removed and the patient placed into a short-leg removable cast with an elastic bandage to control swelling. The patient is keep non–weight bearing for 6 weeks. At 6 weeks radiographs are obtained, and if early union is occurring, weight bearing is permitted in the cast for another 6 weeks. Twelve weeks after surgery, radiographs are again obtained, and if satisfactory union has occurred, the patient is gradually permitted to work out of the removable cast and into a shoe. An elastic stocking is used to control swelling.

Complications

The three main complications that can occur after a tarsometatarsal arthrodesis are skin slough, nonunion, and failure to correct a malalignment.

The skin on the dorsum of the foot often has little subcutaneous fat. Combined with postoperative swelling and multiple incisions, this can lead to a *skin slough*. Therefore, meticulous care must be taken at surgery to obtain a good subcutaneous closure followed by a skin closure, with a minimum amount of tension along the skin edge. I prefer a running, horizontal mattress suture that keeps the tension off the skin edges as much as possible. If a slough occurs, local

wound care usually is adequate to resolve the problem, but sometimes a skin graft or even a flap is necessary. If the slough is not too large, vacuum-assisted wound closure (wound-VAC) maybe useful.

A *nonunion* of an attempted fusion site can occur, although infrequently. With meticulous preparation of the bone surfaces and rigid internal fixation, the tarsometatarsal joints have a high fusion rate. We were able to obtain a fusion in 176 of 179 joints for a 98% fusion rate.[41] If a nonunion occurs and is symptomatic, the fibrous tissue around the involved joint needs to be excised, the bone surfaces once again scaled, the joint bone grafted if necessary, and internal fixation reapplied.

Malalignment of the foot can be a problem. The deformity usually present preoperatively is abduction and dorsiflexion, which results in a large prominence on the plantar–medial aspect of the foot in the area of the first tarsometatarsal joint. If the forefoot is not reduced by bringing the first metatarsal into adduction and plantar flexion, this prominence remains and might continue to be a source of pain for the patient. With adequate reduction, this prominence does not strike the ground, which usually provides relief for the patient. Occasionally, malalignment of a metatarsal occurs by placing it into too much dorsiflexion or plantar flexion, which can be corrected with an osteotomy and internal fixation if necessary.

A *neuroma*, particularly on the dorsum of the foot, can also occur from entrapment or laceration of one of the sensory nerves on the dorsum. Usually a small branch is involved, and although annoying to the patient, it usually is not a major problem. Occasionally, if one of the larger branches of a superficial peroneal nerve is cut, a large, painful neuroma develops and is aggravated by footwear. If this occurs and is symptomatic, the neuroma should be identified and buried either underneath the extensor digitorum brevis muscle or into a hole in the bone. The dorsum of the foot being so devoid of fatty tissue in some patients sometimes makes it difficult to bury the nerve's cut end adequately.

Author's Experience

We reviewed a series of 40 patients (41 feet) who underwent surgery, with a follow-up of 6 years (range, 2 to 17).[41] The diagnoses were primary arthrosis in 21 patients (18 women, 3 men) and 22 feet, post-trauma effects in 17 (9 women, 8 men), and inflammatory arthritis in two (one man, one woman). The age for the primary arthrosis group was 60 years (range, 27 to 75), for post-trauma group 40 years (range, 30 to 67), and for arthritis group 44 and 70 years. The patients noted symptoms for an average 2.8 years for the post-trauma group, 10.9 years for the primary arthrosis group, and 14 years for the arthritis group.

Preoperatively, all the patients complained of pain, and 78% had a foot deformity that made wearing shoes difficult. The group with primary arthrosis had a greater degree of deformity than the patients with traumatic arthrosis.

Using the technique described previously, we were able to obtain union in 176 of 179 joints for a 98% union rate. Of the three nonunions that occurred, one required surgical repair. Patient satisfaction was 93% (38 of 41 feet). Postoperatively, five patients had a prominent metatarsal head, although none developed a callus that required trimming. The prominent head involved the second metatarsal twice, second and third metatarsals twice, and first and second metatarsals once. Three patients developed a stress fracture of the second metatarsal, and all of them healed spontaneously. Three feet demonstrated minimal neuritic symptoms along one of the dorsal scars, but none required further treatment.

The preoperative radiographic findings demonstrated that the patients with primary arthrosis had more pronation than those with traumatic arthrosis. The deformity observed in the AP radiograph was usually two times greater than that noted on the lateral radiograph. The average correction obtained in the AP plane (i.e., abduction or adduction) was 9 degrees, which compares favorably to that of Horton and Olney,[39] who obtained a 10-degree correction. In the lateral radiograph we obtained an average correction of 8 degrees, which was approximately half that reported by Horton and Olney. At follow-up, arthrosis not present preoperatively was observed in adjacent joints in three patients (five joints) in the post-trauma group and eight patients (12 joints) in the primary arthrosis group. None of these were symptomatic.

Our failure rate of the procedure was 3 (7%) of 41, which was lower than that reported by Sangeorzan et al,[42] whose failure rate was 5

(31%) of 16, and Johnson et al,[40] whose rate was 2 (15%) of 13.

The primary differences between patients with primary arthrosis and post-trauma arthrosis were age (60 versus 41 years, respectively) and the extent of the deformity, which was greater in the primary arthrosis patients. These patients had an average of six joints fused per foot, whereas the post-trauma patients had four joints per foot.

After surgery, one patient continued to use an AFO, and 11 used some type of an orthotic device (e.g., Hapad, Spenco liner) in their shoe. No patient required custom-made footwear.

REFERENCES

Subtalar Arthrodesis

1. Angus PD, Cowell HR: Triple arthrodesis: A long-term review. *J Bone Joint Surg Br* 68:260-265, 1986.
2. Bennett GL, Graham CE, Mauldin DM: Triple arthrodesis in adults. *Foot Ankle* 12(3):138-143, 1991.
3. Graves SC, Mann RA, Graves KO: Triple arthrodesis in older adults. *J Bone Joint Surg Am* 75:355-362, 1993.
4. Haritidis JH, Kirkos JM, Provellegios SM, Zachos AD: Long-term results of triple arthrodesis: 42 cases followed for 25 years. *Foot Ankle* 15(10):548-551, 1994.
5. Kitaoka HB, Alexander IJ, Adelaar RS, et al: Clinical rating systems for the ankle–hindfoot, midfoot, hallux and lesser toes. *Foot Ankle* 15(7):349-353, 1994.
6. Haskell A, Pfeiff C, Mann R: Subtalar joint arthrodesis using a single lag screw. *Foot Ankle Int* 25:774-777, 2004.
7. Mann RA, Baumgarten M: Subtalar fusion for isolated subtalar disorders: Preliminary report. *Clin Orthop Relat Res* 226:260-265, 1988.
8. Mann RA, Beaman DN, Horton G: Isolated subtalar arthrodesis. *Foot Ankle Int* 19(8):511-519, 1998.
9. Russotti GM, Cass JR, Johnson KA: Isolated talocalcaneal arthrodesis: A technique using moldable bone graft. *J Bone Joint Surg Am* 70:1472-1478, 1988.
10. Sangeorzan BJ, Smith D, Veith R, Hansen ST: Triple arthrodesis using internal fixation in treatment of adult foot disorders. *Clin Orthop Relat Res* 294:299-307, 1993.
11. Southwell RB, Sherman FC: Triple arthrodesis: A long-term study with force plate analysis. *Foot Ankle* 2(1):15-24, 1981.
12. Stephens HM, Sanders R: Calcaneal malunions: Results of a prognostic computed tomography classification system. *Foot Ankle Int* 7(7):395-401, 1996.
13. Swiontkowski MF, Scranton PE, Hansen S: Tarsal coalitions: Long-term results of surgical treatment. *J Pediatr Orthop* 3:287-292, 1983.
14. Tenuta J, Shelton YA, Miller F: Longer-term follow-up of triple arthrodesis in patients with cerebral palsy. *J Pediatr Orthop* 13:713-716, 1993.
15. Wetmore RS, Drennan JC: Long-term results of triple arthrodesis in Charcot–Marie–Tooth disease. *J Bone Joint Surg Am* 71:417-422, 1989.

16. Wukich OK, Bowen RJ: A long-term study of triple arthrodesis for correction of pes cavovarus in Charcot–Marie–Tooth disease. *J Pediatr Orthop* 9:433-437, 1989.

Talonavicular Arthrodesis

17. Clain MR, Baxter DE: Simultaneous calcaneal–cuboid and talonavicular fusion: Long-term follow-up study. *J Bone Joint Surg Br* 76:133-136, 1994.
18. Elbaor JE, Thomas WH, Weinfeld NS, Potter TA: Talonavicular arthrodesis for rheumatoid arthritis of the hindfoot. *Orthop Clin North Am* 7:821-826, 1976.
19. Elftman H: The transverse tarsal joint and its control. *Clin Orthop Relat Res* 16:41, 1960.
20. Fogel GR, Kato HY, Rand JA, Chao EY: Talonavicular arthrodesis for isolated arthrosis: 9.5 year results and gait analysis. *Foot Ankle* 3(2):105-113, 1982.
21. Harper MC, Tisdel CL: Talonavicular arthrodesis for the painful acquired flatfoot. *Foot Ankle Int* 17(11):658-661, 1996.
22. O'Malley MJ, Deland JT, Lee K: Selective hindfoot arthrodesis for the treatment of adult acquired flatfoot deformity: An in vitro study. *Foot Ankle Int* 16(7):411-417, 1995.

Double Arthrodesis

23. DuVries HL: *Surgery of the Foot.* St Louis, Mosby, 1959, p 300.
24. Inman VT (ed): *DuVries' Surgery of the Foot,* ed 3. St Louis, Mosby, 1973, pp 491-494.
25. Mann RA, Beaman DN: Double arthrodesis for posterior tibial tendon dysfunction. *Clin Orthop Relat Res* 365:74-80, 1999.

Triple Arthrodesis

26. Adelaar RS, Dannelly EA, Meunier PA, et al: A long-term study in triple arthrodesis in children. *Orthop Clin North Am* 7:895-908, 1976.
27. Angus PD, Cowell HR: Triple arthrodesis: A critical long-term review. *J Bone Joint Surg Br* 62:260-265, 1986.
28. Bennett GL, Graham CE, Mauldin DM: Triple arthrodesis in adults. *Foot Ankle* 12(3):138-143, 1991.
29. Drew AJ: The late results of arthrodesis of the foot. *J Bone Joint Surg Br* 33:496-502, 1951.

30. Graves SC, Mann RA, Graves KO: Triple arthrodesis in older adults: Results after long-term follow-up. *J Bone Joint Surg Am* 75:355-362, 1993.
31. Haritdis JH, Kirkos JM, Provellegios SM, Zachos AD: Long-term result of triple arthrodesis: Forty-two cases followed for twenty-five years. *Foot Ankle Int* 15(10):548-551, 1994.
32. Jahss MH, Godsick PA, Levin H: Quadruple arthrodesis with iliac bone graft. In Bateman JE, Trott AW (eds): *The Foot and Ankle,* New York, Thieme-Stratton, 1980, pp 93-102.
33. Lambrinudi C: New operation on drop-foot. *Br J Surg* 15:193-200, 1927.
34. Mann RA, Mann JA, Prieskorn D, Sobel M: Posterior tibial tendon dysfunction treated by fusion. Paper presented at the 18th Annual Verne T. Inman Lectureship, University of California, San Francisco, May, 1997.
35. Ryerson EW: Arthrodesing operations on the feet. *J Bone Joint Surg* 5:453-471, 1923.
36. Smith RW, Shen W, DeWitt S, Reischl SF: Triple arthrodesis in adults with non-paralytic disease. *J Bone Joint Surg Am* 86:2707-2713, 2004.
37. Southwell RB, Sherman FC: Triple arthrodesis; a long-term study with force plate analysis. *Foot Ankle* 2(1):15-24, 1981.
37. Wetmore RS, Drennan JC: Long-term results of triple arthrodesis in Charcot–Marie–Tooth disease. *J Bone Joint Surg Am* 71:417-422, 1989.

Tarsometatarsal Arthrodesis

39. Horton GA, Olney BW: Deformity correction and arthrodesis of the midfoot with a medial plate. *Foot Ankle* 14:493-499, 1993.
40. Johnson JE, Johnson KA: Dowel arthrodesis for degenerative arthritis of the tarsometatarsal (Lisfranc) joints. *Foot Ankle* 6(5):243-253, 1986.
41. Mann RA, Prieskorn D, Sobel M: Mid-tarsal and tarsometatarsal arthrodeses for primary degenerative osteoarthrosis or osteoarthrosis after trauma. *J Bone Joint Surg Am* 78:1376-1385, 1996.
42. Sangeorzan BJ, Veith RG, Hansen ST Jr: Salvage of Lisfranc's tarsometatarsal joint by arthrodesis. *Foot Ankle* 10(3):193-200, 1990.

Pes Cavus

Gregory P. Guyton • Roger A. Mann

Pes cavus describes a foot with a high arch that maintains it shape and fails to flatten out with weight bearing. A precise radiographic definition of pes cavus is difficult because the deformity is made up of various components in the forefoot and hindfoot. The predominant deformity in pes cavus may be in the hindfoot, the forefoot, or a combination of both.

BIOMECHANICAL CONSEQUENCES OF PES CAVUS

Regardless of the cause of the deformity, the consequences for the mechanics of the foot are similar. The weight-bearing area beneath the metatarsal heads and heel pad is decreased, leading to substantially higher plantar pressures in both locations. The subtalar joint axis is more vertical and the talar head tends to remain over the anterior process of the calcaneus. The result is that there is less subtalar motion during gait; both the subtalar and transverse tarsal joints are more rigid. The ability of the foot to absorb the impact of walking by pronating during the early part of stance phase is diminished. A *cavus* foot is always stiffer than one of normal conformation.

Additionally, because of the clawing and hyperextension of the metatarsophalangeal (MTP) joints, the toes do not participate in weight bearing during toe-off, and power is diminished. The plantar aponeurosis normally functions as a passive windlass mechanism to elevate the longitudinal arch, plantar flex the metatarsals, and invert the calcaneus. In the cavus foot, all three of these conditions are present permanently, and the plantar aponeurosis becomes contracted.

The muscle weakness patterns seen around the foot vary with the cause of the condition, but adduction of the forefoot is commonly seen when the posterior tibialis is active in the presence of a weak peroneus brevis. Metatarsus adductus exacerbates the already considerable tendency for excessive pressure in the lateral column of the foot, and stress reactions of the fifth metatarsal can result.

TYPES OF DEFORMITY

The most confusing aspect of pes cavus is that the condition manifests so many anatomic variations. Pes cavus must be viewed as a spectrum of deformities in which the underlying abnormality is that of an elevated longitudinal arch, but after that an almost infinite variety of bony and soft tissue deformities can be present. The spectrum can range from a mild cavus foot, with flexible claw toes as the only significant clinical problem, to a severe rigid deformity with altered weight bearing, callosities, lateral ankle laxity, stress reactions, and pain. The cavus foot is best understood by systematically analyzing the bone deformities, the soft tissue deformities, and the specific muscle functions that are imbalanced.

The Hindfoot

The bony deformity may be predominantly in the hindfoot, the forefoot, or a combination of both. A *hindfoot cavus* describes an elevated pitch of the long axis of the calcaneus, which is usually greater than 30 degrees in a cavus foot (Fig. 21–1). Hindfoot cavus was a very common deformity in the era of widespread poliomyelitis; the focal nature of the disease in the anterior horn cells of the spinal cord often led to gastrocnemius weakness but sparing of the tibialis anterior and often the foot intrinsics. The resultant imbalance of forces then often led to dramatic calcaneal pitch angles and subsequent soft tissue contractures. Pure hindfoot cavus is now less common. Elevated calcaneal pitch is usually encountered as a component of a combined deformity in the idiopathic cavus foot with no clear neurologic cause.

The Forefoot

A *forefoot cavus* describes plantar flexion of the metatarsals and is usually more pronounced along the

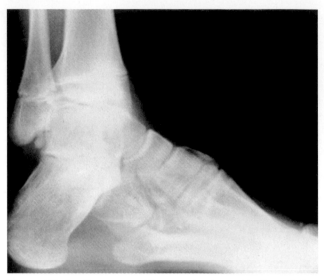

Figure 21–1   Pes cavus with a predominant hindfoot deformity. Note the dramatically high pitch angle of the calcaneus.

medial column (Fig. 21–2). Additionally, the forefoot may be adducted as well. The critical issue in a forefoot cavus is that the deformity of the forefoot *causes* the varus deformity of the hindfoot, which is secondary. For instance, the most common cause of pure forefoot cavus is Charcot–Marie–Tooth disease, in which the peroneus longus muscle function is preserved while the anterior tibialis function is lost. The unopposed plantar flexion force of the peroneus longus forces the first metatarsal head down, leaving the lateral side of the forefoot relatively unaffected. Conceptually, the foot can be thought of as a simple tripod with contact points at the heel, first metatarsal, and fifth metatarsal. If the first metatarsal is depressed and the fifth metatarsal is unaffected, a supination deformity develops that forces the hindfoot into varus.

Radiographically, forefoot cavus can be determined by drawing lines down the long axes of the first metatarsal and the talus on the lateral standing x-ray. This *talo–first metatarsal angle* should ordinarily be 0; the axes should be collinear. A drop in the first ray relative to the axis of the talus indicates an element of forefoot cavus.

Early in the development of many cases of forefoot cavus the deformities remain relatively flexible. The arch might not flatten while standing, but muscle forces are holding it in position rather than bone and joint contractures. This is typical, for instance, of a very young patient with Charcot–Marie–Tooth disease. The subtalar joint compensates for the forefoot deformity by falling into a varus alignment (Fig. 21–3). As the disease progresses, the capsule and interosseous ligament of the subtalar joint become contracted and the once-flexible hindfoot deformity becomes rigid.

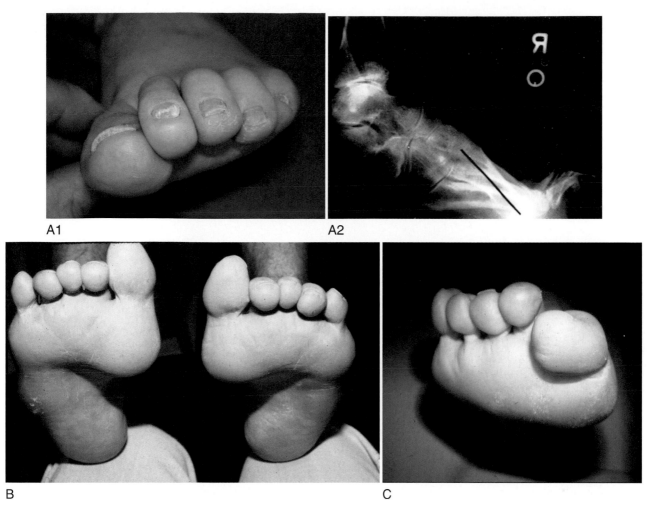

A1 A2

B C

Figure 21–2 Pes cavus with a predominant forefoot deformity. **A,** The driving force is forefoot valgus, clinically seen as depression of the first metatarsal head. The radiograph demonstrates plantar flexion of the first metatarsal relative to the axis of the talus. **B,** Bilateral plantar flexion of the first metatarsal accompanied by a varus heel deformity. **C,** Some cases demonstrate a more generalized forefoot deformity with generalized forefoot equinus.

In some early cases of forefoot cavus, surgery to correct the forefoot alone results in a balanced foot. To determine whether or not the hindfoot is still flexible in such a case, the *Coleman block test* can be applied clinically. With the patient standing, wooden blocks of whatever thickness is required are placed under the lateral column of the forefoot, leaving the medial column unsupported. The first metatarsal head is then free to drop off the side of the block. The patient is then viewed from behind. If the subtalar joint is flexible, it will follow and the heel will align into neutral or slight valgus. If the hindfoot is rigid, however, it will remain fixed in varus.

The Metatarsophalangeal Joint

The deformities of the MTP joints are variable. They might be as mild as flexible clawing of the MTP joints in association with mild flexion of the interphalangeal joints, or they can manifest as rigid claw toe deformities. Once severe rigid claw toe deformities are present, the forces from the extrinsic toe extensors serve to hold the metatarsal heads in a plantar flexed position (Fig. 21–4). Importantly, the plantar fat pad is displaced distally in severe cases as the toes pull up into extension. Not only are the metatarsal heads driven plantarward by the deformity, but they are also deprived of their normal cushioning layer of fat.

Soft Tissues

The plantar aponeurosis commonly develops a contracture with time in all forms of cavus foot. It is important to remember that anatomically the plantar aponeurosis is much more stout on the medial aspect of the foot. As the contracture develops it not only

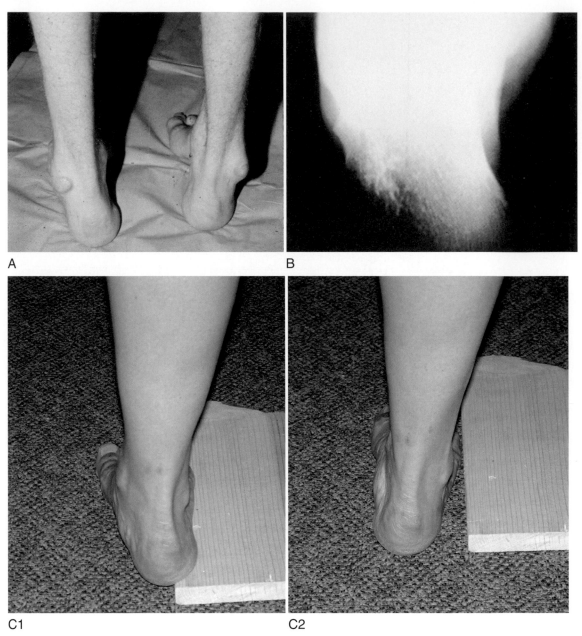

A   B

C1   C2

Figure 21–3   Varus heel deformity. **A,** In cases of forefoot-driven cavus, the varus heel is initially present as the natural standing posture of the heel when the first ray is plantar flexed and adducted. With time, the hindfoot deformity can become fixed. The presence of the deformity can be best assessed from behind. **B,** An axial view of the calcaneus demonstrates marked varus deformity. **C,** The Coleman block test can be used to demonstrate persistent flexibility of the hindfoot. If the heel can be forced into valgus by weight bearing on a block supporting only the lateral column of the foot, the subtalar joint remains flexible. In this case, the cavus can be corrected by addressing the forefoot deformity alone.

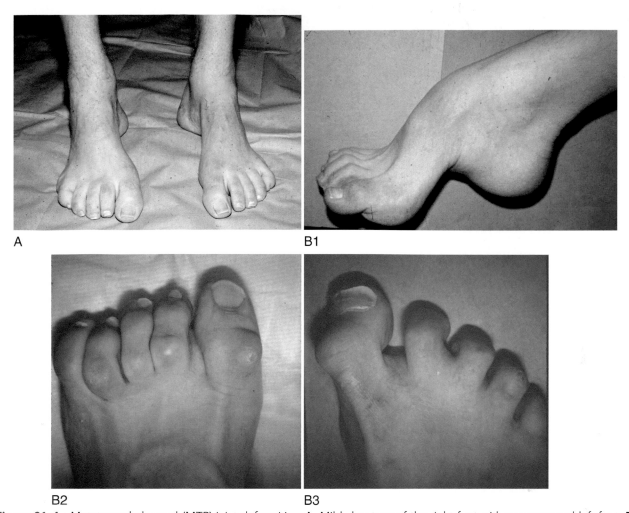

Figure 21–4 Metatarsophalangeal (MTP) joint deformities. **A,** Mild claw toes of the right foot with a near-normal left foot. **B,** Examples of severe clawing of the MTP joints, including clawing of the hallux from the use of the extensor hallucis longus (EHL) as an accessory dorsiflexor.

holds the longitudinal arch in an elevated position but also holds the forefoot adducted and keeps the calcaneus inverted (Fig. 21–5). Although some bone-surgery procedures can secondarily relax the plantar fascia by altering the shape of the arch, they are rarely adequate by themselves. The importance of the plantar fascia in maintaining deformity should always be considered.

ETIOLOGY

The pathomechanics that produce a cavus foot vary with the disease process. The common thread in all forms of cavus foot, though, is muscle *imbalance*. Historically, the attempt to attribute all forms of cavus foot to a single neurologic lesion has led to inaccuracy and immense confusion in the literature. Bentzon[2] and Hallgrimsson[14] in 1939 believed that the imbalance was always found in the extrinsic muscles. Duchenne,[8] writing in 1959, proposed that the deformity results from an imbalance between the extrinsics and the intrinsics. The simple truth is that a cavus foot is best thought of as an end result that a variety of subtle neurologic lesions can produce, and each must be evaluated on its own terms.

Brewerton et al[4] specifically looked at the cause of pes cavus in a series of 77 patients, and found subtle neurologic effects in 66% of them. That still left 26 patients with no clear diagnosis, and this "idiopathic" group still constitutes the largest subset of patients seen in clinical practice. In the idiopathic group, 11 of the 26 patients had a family history of pes cavus, and 7 of the 26 had nonspecific abnormalities upon electromyographic and nerve conduction velocity examination. Most cases of idiopathic pes cavus likely represent a very subtle neurologic lesion that is below clinical detection.

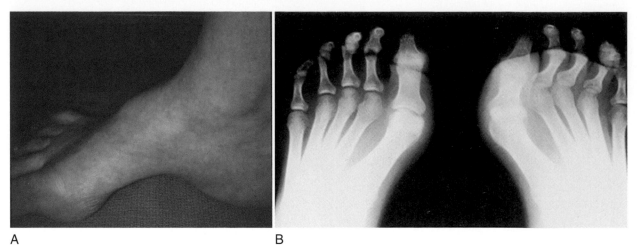

A   B

Figure 21–5   Contracture of the plantar aponeurosis contributes to and fixes the deformity. The tight medial band of the plantar fascia holds the forefoot in adduction and the hindfoot in varus. **A,** Cavus foot demonstrates adduction of the forefoot, an elevated longitudinal arch, and varus of the calcaneus. **B,** Radiograph demonstrating severe adduction of the forefoot.

Nevertheless, the majority of pes cavus patients do indeed have a neurologic diagnosis, and a thorough neurologic exam is critical. By far the most common diagnosis producing pes cavus in the Western world today is Charcot–Marie–Tooth disease, but a host of other less common conditions can also be discovered (Table 21–1).[17] An aggressive work-up including a neurology referral and central nervous system imaging is mandatory in some situations that might point toward a correctable lesion of the spinal cord, such as a syrinx or spinal cord tumor. These include rapid progression, hyperreflexia, clonus, or significant asymmetry between sides in motor pattern or deformity. For the inescapable reason that the motor pathways to the foot are the longest (and therefore most vulnerable) in the body, an alert foot and ankle surgeon will almost certainly have the opportunity to make more than a few new diagnoses of neurologic lesions over the course of his or her career.

CHARCOT–MARIE–TOOTH DISEASE

Charcot–Marie–Tooth disease (CMT) is the single most common diagnosis associated with pes cavus and should at least be considered in every patient who presents with pes cavus. Because of its special status, a deeper discussion is warranted.

CMT disease is not, in fact, a single disease but rather a heterogeneous group of disorders caused by inheritable defects in any of several constituent proteins of the myelin sheath of a peripheral nerve. The disorder was described in general terms by the great French neurologist Jean Martin Charcot and his pupil

TABLE 21–1

Etiology of Pes Cavus

Classification	Specific Etiology
I. Neuromuscular	
A. Muscle disease	Muscular dystrophy
B. Afflictions of peripheral nerves and lumbosacral spinal nerve roots	Charcot–Marie–Tooth disease
	Spinal dysraphism
	Polyneuritis
	Intraspinal tumor
C. Anterior horn cell disease of spinal cord	Poliomyelitis
	Spinal dysraphism
	Diastematomyelia
	Syringomyelia
	Spinal cord tumors
	Spinal musculature atrophy
D. Long tract and central disease	Friedreich's ataxia
	Roussy–Lévy syndrome
	Primary cerebellar disease
	Cerebral palsy
II. Congenital	Idiopathic cavus foot
	Residual of clubfoot
	Arthrogryposis
III. Traumatic	Residuals of compartment syndrome
	Crush injury to lower extremity
	Severe burn
	Malunion of fractured foot

Modified from Ibrahim K: In Evarts CM (ed): *Surgery of the Musculoskeletal System.* New York, Churchill Livingstone, 1990, pp 4015-4034.

Marie in 1886 and independently by Tooth in England later that year.[5,35] Originally Charcot attributed the disorder to a spinal defect, and it was Tooth's subsequent work that correctly classified it as a peripheral nerve disorder. The disease is the most common inheritable defect of peripheral nerve, but approximately half of the time it represents a sporadic genetic event. CMT patients usually enjoy a normal lifespan and are often normally active early in the disease, but the foot deformities and motor weakness associated with it represent a major source of pain and morbidity.

The nomenclature associated with CMT is confusing because of the historical lack of understanding of its cause. Degenerative peripheral neuromuscular diseases were once commonly referred to as *progressive muscular atrophy* (PMA). This was subsequently modified to more accurately describe CMT in the form *peroneal muscular atrophy* (also PMA) and even today this term occasionally appears in the literature. Dyck and Lambert developed an extensive classification of inheritable motor neuropathies based upon their electrodiagnostic patterns in the 1960s and 1970s.[11] Their scheme refers to a series of seven *hereditary motor sensory neuropathies* (HMSN-I through HMSN-VII). These electrically based diagnoses still appear occasionally in the literature.

Fortunately, since 1990 there has been an explosion of understanding of the specific genetic defects underlying the CMT disorders.[3] This has instigated a new and hopefully definitive round of reclassifications of the disease. The four most common types are described here, but the list is hardly definitive because research in the field is very active.

CMT-1 is the most common form and accounts for more than 50% of all cases. It is autosomal dominant and demonstrates slow nerve conduction velocities (NCVs) in the range of 10 to 30 m/sec as a result of demyelination. CMT-1 can be further subdivided.

CMT-1A accounts for 80% of CMT-1 cases and is the single most common form of the disease in general. Curiously, it is usually caused by a segmental trisomy along chromosome 17. The area contains the gene for peripheral myelin protein-22 *(PMP-22)*, whose function remains unknown. Although some cases have been linked to alternative point mutations in *PMP-22*, the segmental trisomy responsible for most cases indicates CMT can be produced from a *gene dosage effect.* This chromosomal aberration is inheritable in an autosomal dominant fashion, but many cases seem to represent sporadic chromosomal recombination events.

CMT-1B accounts for 5% to 10% of CMT-1 patients and is associated with a point mutation in the myelin P_0 gene. The phenotype is associated with a particularly aggressive form of the disease.

CMT-1C represents the small remainder of CMT-1 patients in whom the genetic defect is still unknown.

CMT-2 is the second most common general form of the disease and represents 20% of patients. It is autosomal dominant like CMT-1 but has dramatically different electrical findings: NCVs are near normal and there is no evidence of demyelination. Four separate chromosomal loci have been identified, but the product proteins involved remain unknown. In general, the course of CMT-2 is more indolent than that of CMT-1.

CMT-X shows an X-linked inheritance pattern; male patients are affected and female patients are either unaffected or mildly affected carriers. It is found in 10% to 20% of all CMT cases and is associated with defects in yet another myelin constituent protein, connexin 32.

CMT-4 is an autosomal recessive form of the disease and is quite rare. It in fact encompasses a large number of described genetic defects on different chromosomal loci; no product proteins have yet been described.

The foot deformities in CMT do not result from absolute weakness of the motor units powering the foot but of their relative *imbalance.** A specific pattern of motor weakness is common in CMT in which the anterior and lateral compartment musculature is selectively affected, with certain curious exceptions. For instance, the disease almost always affects the peroneus brevis but spares the peroneus longus. This was first observed clinically by Mann[22] and subsequently confirmed by Tynan,[36] who demonstrated that the cross-sectional area of the peroneus longus was preserved on MRI imaging of patients with the disease. An additional oddity can be observed in the anterior compartment musculature; the extensor hallucis muscle can be spared while the anterior tibialis is affected; this occurs despite the more distal location of the extensor hallucis longus (EHL) and their shared peroneal innervation.

The reasons for the unusual patterns of motor weakness in CMT remain poorly understood. The selective denervation affects certain muscles in the anterior and lateral compartments and only very late posterior compartment involvement is seen. Denervation in CMT progresses very differently from a classic symmetric polyneuropathy such as that encountered in diabetes. At least some speculation has been centered upon the possibility that some element of nerve compression can play a role.[12] An additional inheritable disorder that renders nerves susceptible to compression, hereditary neuropathy with liability to pressure palsies (HNPP), involves a gene *deletion* for PMP-22, the same

---

*References 1, 13, 15, 22, 24, and 28.

protein involved in the gene dosage effect that appears to cause CMT-1A. Anatomic dissections have indicated that the peroneal nerve in fact divides into multiple distinct pathways even before it passes around the neck of the fibula, and these separate pathways may be more or less vulnerable to compression than others. To date, however, no studies of nerve decompression in CMT patients or animal models have been performed.

Regardless of the cause of the patterns of weakness, each of the deformities of the disease can be explained in the form of a weak agonist muscle and a *more normally functioning* antagonist (Table 21–2). There is *no* evidence of spasticity in the motor units that remain innervated.

The functional peroneus longus serves to plantar flex the first ray while the denervated anterior tibialis fails to provide any counterbalancing dorsiflexion. The first metatarsal head is depressed and a forefoot cavus results. An equinus contracture develops as the gastrocnemius is unopposed by the anterior tibialis. Additionally, the toe extrinsics force the toes into a clawed position that is not counterbalanced by the denervated foot intrinsics. This also serves secondarily to depress the metatarsal heads and raise the arch. The supination and adduction of the foot is worsened because the posterior tibialis is unopposed by the weakened peroneus brevis. In cases with sparing of the EHL, the claw toe deformity of the hallux is worsened even more dramatically because the patient uses the EHL to dorsiflex the foot and compensate for the weak anterior tibialis.

As long as the functional motor units are understood, surgery to correct the foot deformities of CMT is no different from that used in other forms of cavus feet. What should be appreciated, however, is the inexorably progressive nature of the disease. It is rare in

clinical practice to encounter a patient at such an early stage of disease that the foot is entirely supple with no hindfoot or forefoot contractures. However, rebalancing the foot through tendon transfers can help prevent the development of further deformity if it is done early enough.[27] For instance, the overpull of the peroneus longus that forces the forefoot into cavus can be eliminated by transferring the tendon to the peroneus brevis. This also serves to help oppose the tibialis posterior and prevent adduction. The emphasis in early-stage surgery on CMT should be on tendon transfers rather than lengthening motor units. Strayer procedures, fractional lengthening of the posterior tibialis, and lengthening of the Achilles have their role when contractures are encountered, but they should be used with caution because of the residual weakness they produce. Because the long-term outcome of CMT is one of progressive, inexorable weakness, strength should be preserved whenever possible.

POLIOMYELITIS

The last great epidemic of polio in the United States occurred in New England in 1955. Although the residual effects of the disease are now encountered with increasing rarity, it still serves as a useful model of a process that can produce either a forefoot cavus or a hindfoot cavus.[7]

Paralytic polio is the result of an RNA virus that primarily affects the thalamus, hypothalamus, motor centers of the brain stem and cerebellum, and the anterior tracts of the spinal cord. There is a wide variety of clinical presentations depending upon what portions of the CNS are affected, but as a practical matter the

TABLE 21–2

Foot Deformities in Charcot–Marie–Tooth Disease

Deformity	Weak Agonist Muscle(s)	Intact Antagonist Muscle(s)	Action
Equinus	Tibialis anterior	Gastrocnemius–soleus	Plantar flexion
Adduction and hindfoot varus	Peroneus brevis	Tibialis posterior	Adducts the foot, inverts the subtalar joint
Plantar flexion of the first ray	Tibialis anterior	Peroneus longus	Plantar flexes the first ray, creates a secondary forefoot cavus
Toe deformities	Foot intrinsics	Long toe flexors	Clawing occurs as the extrinsic forces are unmodified by the intrinsics; also depresses the metatarsal heads and accentuates cavus
Hallux claw toe	Foot intrinsics	EHL and FHL	Severe hallucal clawing occurs when a spared EHL is used to assist a weak tibialis anterior dorsiflex the foot

EHL, extensor hallucis longus; FHL, flexor hallucis longus.
After Guyton GP, Mann RA: *Foot Ankle Clin* 5:317-326, 2000.

lower extremity weakness patterns of polio come from a strikingly selective destruction of the anterior motor neurons in the spinal cord itself.

Following an initial incubation period of 6 to 20 days, the acute phase of the disease is associated with the most dramatic paralysis and lasts approximately 7 to 10 days. Clinically detectable weakness usually occurs when more than 60% of the motor neurons to a muscle group are affected. Muscle function can recover gradually thereafter; the most substantial gains occur in the first 4 months, and some return of function is usually seen up to 2 years after the illness.

Patterns of Foot Deformity in Polio

Hindfoot Cavus

The gastrocnemius–soleus complex is the critical variable in determining what variety of foot deformity will develop. The classic cavus foot deformity resulting from polio is that of a hindfoot cavus associated with a dramatically high calcaneal pitch angle. This is the result of the paralysis of the gastroc–soleus complex with preservation of the remainder of the posterior compartment, the intrinsic foot musculature, and the anterior tibialis. When appropriate tension is missing from the Achilles tendon, the long toe flexors still function to depress the metatarsal heads, raising the arch. The intrinsics foreshorten the distance between the metatarsals and the calcaneus, functioning much like a bowstring to raise the calcaneal pitch. The result is a vertical posture of the calcaneus.

Forefoot Cavus

A lesion slightly higher in the spinal cord can spare the gastroc–soleus complex but affect the tibialis anterior selectively. This situation results in two particular imbalances that drive depression of the first ray and a forefoot cavus. First, just as in CMT, the peroneus longus is unopposed and directly plantar flexes the first ray. Second, the extensor hallucis longus is still functional and serves as an accessory dorsiflexor of the foot. This creates a claw toe as the foot is pulled up through the toe rather than the usual midfoot insertion of the tibialis anterior. The claw toe deformity itself also serves to depress the metatarsal head.

Other Deformities

Because the motor neuron destruction in poliomyelitis is often patchy and recovery is sometimes incomplete, the patterns of motor weakness cannot always be so neatly categorized. When the tibialis posterior is affected, either alone or in combination with the tibialis anterior, the result is a progressive planovalgus foot rather than a cavus foot. Rarer still is isolated involvement of the peroneals, which usually results in

a very mild cavus foot dominated more by varus of the hindfoot with attendant instability of the ankle. The critical lesson is that, like all peripheral neural lesions, the motor weakness patterns in polio all must be evaluated and treated individually.

OTHER NEUROLOGIC LESIONS

Although CMT and polio represent the most historically prominent etiologies of the cavus foot, a wide variety of other lesions can lead to the deformity.

Friedreich's ataxia is a familial progressive ataxia in which posterior column function is steadily lost.[25] It occurs in an autosomal recessive form with an earlier age of onset (11.75 years) and in a dominant form with a later age of onset (20.4 years). No cases of onset after the age of 25 have been reported. The disease is usually associated with pronounced and progressive symmetric cavus foot deformities with severe claw toe formation. In numerous instances the foot deformities have been the presenting complaint.

A heterogeneous group of *hereditary cerebellar ataxias* are also associated with cavus foot, but they are less easy to categorize than the Friedrich's ataxia, which primarily shows spinal cord involvement.

Roussy-Lévy syndrome is a rare syndrome of cavus foot, sensory ataxia without obvious long-tract signs, peripheral motor atrophy, and kyphoscoliosis. Because it shares characteristics of both diseases, it was poorly differentiated from Friedreich's ataxia and CMT for many years.[26] The onset occurs very early in childhood and runs a relatively benign course.

Spinal muscular atrophy is a heterogeneous group of disorders that are usually present from birth but have some late-onset forms.[30] They are characterized by an inexorably progressive loss of anterior motor neuron cells. The disorders are characterized by hypotonia and can be associated with the cavus foot deformity, although it is rarely the presenting feature.

Structural spinal cord disease often manifests with cavus foot deformity and requires a high degree of suspicion to detect. In particular, the unexplained onset of a progressive bilateral cavus deformity or essentially any unilateral deformity should warrant an imaging work-up. *Spinal cord tumors* are notorious for their early absence of symptoms, and foot deformity might be the initial complaint. *Syringomyelia* is a cavitation in the center of the spinal cord that usually occurs in the cervical cord but can also interrupt the neural pathways to the lower extremities and result in spasticity or deformity. *Diastematomyelia* is a rare disorder in which a spicule of bone or fibrous band sagittally divides the spinal canal in the thoracic or high lumbar regions and separates the spinal cord into two pieces, each surrounded by dura. Because the cord and axial skeleton grow at different rates, a traction myelopathy very slowly develops as the child matures. The findings can be subtle, but making the diagnosis is critical.

Spinal dysraphism in all its forms (spina bifida, myelocele, myelomeningocele) is certainly more common and can manifest with a variety of postural foot disorders depending upon the particular patterns of involvement. Fortunately, the diagnosis is almost always well established early in life.

Cerebral palsy is, by definition, a static encephalopathy and can result in a variety of foot deformities, including pes cavus. Although the neurologic lesion is not progressive, the flexibility of the postural disorders deteriorates with time.

POST-TRAUMATIC CAVOVARUS FOOT DEFORMITIES

Any traumatic condition that leads to an imbalance of the intrinsic and extrinsic foot musculature can lead to a cavus deformity. The deep posterior compartment of the leg is most commonly involved in traumatic compartment syndromes, and a Volkmann's contracture in that location will lead to a cavus foot with a prominent claw toe component. Crush injuries of the leg and severe burns or soft tissue loss can also have the same result, both from direct injuries to the musculature and indirectly through tibial nerve injury. Compartment syndromes confined to the foot most commonly occur with calcaneus fractures or with crush injuries to the forefoot; they have been associated with the late development of claw toes but not with cavus deformity.

Several forms of fracture malunion can also result in a rigid cavovarus foot. Most commonly, a talar neck fracture with substantial medial comminution can fall into a varus malunion. This substantially limits subtalar joint eversion and leads secondarily to the calcaneus assuming a varus malalignment. Alternatively, a varus hindfoot can result from residual deformity from an intraarticular calcaneus fracture or even medial impaction of the tibial plafond.

CONGENITAL PES CAVUS

Clubfoot Residuals

The cavus foot deformity is one of four components of the congenital clubfoot, easily remembered by the mnemonic CAVE (cavus, adductus, varus, equinus). Adult clubfoot residuals encountered after childhood casting usually result from a failure of early casting to

adequately elevate the first ray prior to abducting the foot about the fulcrum of the talar head as described by Ponseti.[23] The most severe deformities that result from improper casting technique are usually not those of residual cavus but of a rocker-bottom foot that results when the equinus is inappropriately corrected while the calcaneus remains locked under the talus; the foot then dorsiflexes through the midfoot rather than through the ankle.

A wave of enthusiasm for surgical clubfoot correction in the 1970s and 1980s is also now yielding residual effects in the adult foot and ankle population. The results of clubfoot correction surgery have proved to be substantially less reliable than once believed.[20,31] A patient presenting with problems with a postsurgical clubfoot is just as likely to have overcorrection into planovalgus as residual undercorrection in cavovarus. The one constant in the surgically corrected clubfoot is a remarkable amount of stiffness in adults. In a dynamic gait analysis study, Huber and Dutoit[16] specifically identified late subtalar stiffness as the primary feature associated with a poor result following childhood clubfoot surgery. It is rare that anything short of triple arthrodesis can be entertained to address the residual complaints.

The Idiopathic Cavus Foot

Despite the litany of potential known causes of the cavus deformity, the largest single group of cases encountered is symmetric and has no known cause. They can manifest because of stiffness in the hindfoot, stress fractures along the lateral column, recurrent ankle instability, or, commonly, for symptoms totally unrelated to the conformation of the arch.

Physical Examination

The patient encounter begins with a careful history of the condition and a detailed family history. The patient's gait is carefully observed for the nature of ground contact, the position of the heel, and the position of the toes during stance. Any fall of the heel toward further varus as weight transfers onto the limb should be noted by observing the patient walk from behind. During swing phase, the examiner should check for the possibility of a footdrop and cock-up deformity of the first MTP joint.

With the patient seated, the examiner observes active and passive range of motion of the ankle, subtalar, transverse tarsal, and MTP joints. Muscle function is very carefully assessed. Special attention should be paid to the ability of the peroneus longus to selectively plantar flex the first ray, because this can point to the potential for a tendon transfer to effectively assist in treatment. A patient who does not carry a known neurologic diagnosis should also undergo a neurologic screening, including testing for long tract signs, reflexes, hamstring tightness, and any asymmetry. Intrinsic wasting is usually easier to pick up in the upper extremity, and in suspected cases of CMT or other systemic peripheral neuropathies, an examination of the intrinsic musculature of the hands is in order. Subtle disease can usually be discerned in the loss of muscle mass and strength of the first dorsal interosseous along the radial border of the second metacarpal. The patient exhibits weakness in abducting the index digit away from the midline with the rest of the hand held in a neutral position to isolate the intrinsics.

The relative position of the hindfoot to the forefoot must be noted along with the rigidity of that relationship. The Coleman block test can be used to determine the ability of the hindfoot to fall back into an appropriate valgus posture. The lateral side of the foot is supported on a small flat wooden block and the medial column is allowed to fall off the side. If the hindfoot is not rigid and the deformity is being driven by a first ray fixed in plantar flexion, the calcaneus will noticeably tilt into valgus when viewed from behind. In theory, a foot that exhibits flexibility on the Coleman block test can be corrected by working on the forefoot deformity alone.

Standing radiographs of the foot are critical. A line drawn down the axis of the talus should pass through the axis of the first metatarsal on both anteroposterior (AP) and lateral weight-bearing images in the normal situation. This talus–first metatarsal angle can be used to assess the severity of a forefoot cavus because the first ray is dropped. The calcaneal pitch angle is elevated in cases of hindfoot cavus. On the AP radiograph, the presence of any associated metatarsus adductus should be noted because this can require some degree of additional surgical attention or limit the degree of correction that can be achieved.

Because of the very subtle findings associated with structural disease of the spinal cord, substantial unexplained asymmetry or rapid progression of the deformity warrants a neurologic referral and imaging.

Conservative Treatment

Many cases of cavus deformity represent stable or slowly progressive deformities that are appropriately managed, at least initially, by conservative means. In the case of an adolescent with progressive deformity and a still-supple foot, however, there may be much to be lost by inappropriate delay. Soft tissue surgery alone might manage the deformity early in the course of the disease and prevent the necessity of osteotomies or fusions.

A stretching program to maintain motion is an important component of conservative management, particularly in cases of neurologic origin. Eversion and dorsiflexion should be emphasized. Metatarsalgia might be an early presenting complaint from uncovering of the metatarsal heads as claw toes develop. A semirigid foot orthosis with a metatarsal pad can be used to address these complaints. In more severe cases, either an articulated or solid-ankle molded ankle–foot orthosis (AFO) might be necessary to control the hindfoot.

The goal of conservative management is to produce a plantigrade foot with even distribution of pressure. Once this has been achieved, periodic observation of the patient is necessary to determine whether progression of the deformity necessitates changes in the alignment of the orthosis or consideration of surgical intervention.

Surgical Treatment

Decision Making

The goal of surgical management is to produce a plantigrade, stable foot. If the foot is fairly supple, a soft tissue procedure such as a plantar fascia release with or without tendon transfer might suffice. At times in a younger patient, several procedures may be necessary during growth to maintain adequate balance of the foot and help prevent bone deformities. In some situations, such as arthrogryposis, this might not be feasible despite sound surgical management.

If a specific bone deformity coexists in a supple foot and prevents the foot from being plantigrade, such as a plantar-flexed first ray, excessive dorsiflexion, or varus of the calcaneus, an osteotomy to correct the bone deformity along with a soft tissue procedure may be beneficial. It is much better to maintain a flexible foot than to carry out a fusion, if feasible. If the foot is rigid, however, an arthrodesis might be necessary to produce a plantigrade foot.

There is no simple boilerplate approach applicable to all cavus feet. The key to surgical decision making is to adopt procedures that are necessary to match each specific deformity. It is not uncommon to have a foot with a combination of fixed and supple deformities; a particular case might require a combination of bone and soft tissue procedures. The list of procedures described here are by no means exhaustive, but they represent the mainstays of surgical treatment of the most common components of the cavus foot.

Soft Tissue Procedures

PLANTAR FASCIA RELEASE (STEINDLER STRIPPING)

The contracted plantar fascia plays a major role in maintaining height of the longitudinal arch and varus positioning of the calcaneus in the patient with pes cavus. Release and stripping of the plantar fascia often help to reduce the height of the longitudinal arch in patients who retain some degree of flexibility (video clip 16).[34] At times, the procedure may be carried out in conjunction with a Dwyer calcaneal osteotomy, a triple arthrodesis, or a first metatarsal osteotomy.

Surgical Technique

1. The patient is placed in a supine position. The normal external rotation of the lower extremity provides adequate visualization of the foot. A tourniquet is used around the thigh.
2. An oblique skin incision is made, starting distal to the weight-bearing area of the calcaneal fat pad and passing over the contracted plantar fascia. This incision does not put the medial calcaneal branches to the heel pad at risk of being cut.
3. The incision is deepened through the fat, exposing the plantar fascia on the plantar aspect of the foot as well as medially over the fascia of the abductor hallucis muscle.
4. The origin of the plantar fascia is transected while tension is being applied to it by dorsiflexing the MTP joints. In this way the plantar fascia will separate as it is cut. Often some deeper septa must be carefully transected. The lateral plantar nerve passes just distal to the cut, so the surgeon must be cautious when transecting the septa.
5. After releasing the plantar fascia, the surgeon palpates along the medial aspect of the foot, particularly in a severely deformed case, to release the superficial and deep fascia surrounding the abductor hallucis muscle. This is a very important part of the release, particularly in cases involving significant adduction of the forefoot.
6. Once the cuts have been made by blunt dissection and stretching the fascia, the wound is carefully inspected to ensure that no tight bands of fascia remain, either on the plantar aspect of the foot or along the abductor muscle.
7. The wound is closed with interrupted sutures and infiltrated with 0.25% bupivacaine hydrochloride (Marcaine).

Postoperative Care

The patient is placed into a short-leg compression dressing incorporating plaster splints. The sutures are removed in 12 to 14 days, after which the patient is placed in a short-leg cast. Weight bearing is begun as tolerated if this is the only procedure performed. Four weeks of immobilization is usually adequate if plantar fascia release is carried out as an isolated procedure.

FIRST TOE JONES PROCEDURE

The procedure is used to correct a hyperextension deformity of the first MTP joint caused by weakness of the tibialis anterior. Although the EHL is also located in the anterior compartment and is innervated more distally than the tibialis anterior, its function can be spared in a surprising number of conditions. In modern practice, this is usually seen in CMT or variants of cerebral palsy, but it was historically common in polio.[19] In these cases, the EHL is functioning as an accessory dorsiflexor of the ankle joint, which results in hyperextension of the MTP joint and secondary flexion of the interphalangeal joint (Fig. 21–6). Moving the insertion of the EHL tendon into the base of the first metatarsal facilitates dorsiflexion of the ankle and also relieves the cock-up deformity of the MTP. To prevent a floppy first toe, a fusion of the interphalangeal joint is usually performed.

Surgical Technique

1. The procedure is carried out with the patient supine under general anesthesia. A tourniquet is used around the thigh (Fig. 21–7 and video clip 20).

Interphalangeal Joint Arthrodesis

2. An elliptical skin incision is centered over the dorsal aspect of the interphalangeal joint of the hallux. The collateral ligaments are cut to expose the articular surfaces.

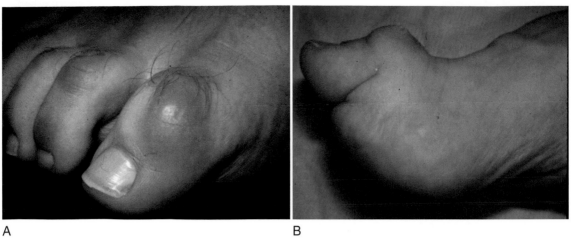

A   B

Figure 21–6 Cock-up deformity of the first metatarsophalangeal joint from the use of the extensor hallucis longus as an accessory dorsiflexor with a weak anterior tibialis. **A,** Resting. **B,** With active attempted dorsiflexion of the ankle.

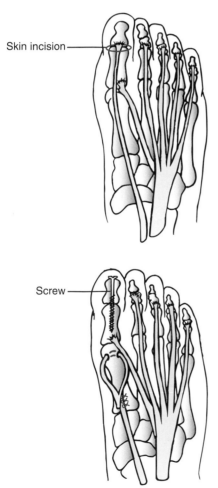

Skin incision

Screw

Figure 21–7 The first toe Jones procedure moves the pull of the extensor hallucis longus (EHL) tendon from the great toe to the neck of the first metatarsal. Interphalangeal joint arthrodesis of the hallux is then performed to prevent a floppy toe. The procedure aids the ability of the EHL to serve as an accessory dorsiflexor and helps eliminate depression of the first metatarsal head. (From Mann RA, Coughlin MJ: *The Video Textbook of Foot and Ankle Surgery.* St. Louis, Medical Video Productions, 1991.)

3. The extensor hallucis longus tendon is freed from its retinacular attachments along its mediolateral aspect.
4. The surfaces of the interphalangeal joint are removed with a power saw to create two flat surfaces. The interphalangeal joint is placed in a few degrees of plantar flexion and neutral varus/valgus alignment.
5. A 2.5-mm hole is drilled in an antegrade manner from proximal to distal through the midportion of the distal phalanx. Where the drill bit begins to pressure the skin on the tip of the toe, a generous transverse incision is made to prevent maceration of the tissue.
6. The drill bit is removed and brought back through the hole from distal to proximal. Holding the interphalangeal joint in a reduced position, the surgeon extends the drill hole into the proximal phalanx.
7. The hole is measured. A 4.0-mm solid shaft cancellous lag screw is inserted, providing compression to the arthrodesis site.
8. A Kirschner wire may be placed obliquely across the interphalangeal joint to control any rotational forces. This is removed after approximately 4 weeks.

Extensor Hallucis Longus Tendon Transfer

9. A longitudinal incision is made over the dorsal aspect of the first metatarsal.
10. The extensor tendon, which was previously freed distally, is now freed proximally and delivered into the wound.

11. A transverse drill hole is made and cleaned in the distal portion of the first metatarsal. The size is selected to snugly fit the tendon.
12. The extensor hallucis longus tendon is passed through the drill hole and sutured onto itself, holding the ankle in 10 degrees of dorsiflexion and placing a moderate amount of tension on the tendon transfer.
13. The wounds are closed in a routine manner and infiltrated with 0.25% bupivacaine.

Postoperative Care

The patient is placed into a short-leg compression dressing incorporating plaster splints. A popliteal block can be useful to control postoperative pain. The sutures are removed at 10 to 12 days and the patient is placed in a short-leg walking cast for 4 weeks. At 6 weeks postoperatively ambulation as tolerated is allowed. If the interphalangeal joint fusion is not complete at that time, an additional period of ambulation in a postoperative shoe may be necessary.

PERONEUS LONGUS TO BREVIS TRANSFER

Many cases of cavus foot, particularly in CMT, are associated with preserved function of the peroneus longus muscle in the presence of a failing tibialis anterior.[13] This pulls the first ray plantarward and leads to a forefoot cavus deformity as well as a secondary hindfoot varus. If the deformity is addressed early enough while it remains supple, a transfer of the peroneus longus to the peroneus brevis can dramatically improve the situation by both weakening the plantar pull on the first metatarsal and augmenting the function of the usually failing peroneus brevis.

Surgical Technique

1. The surgery is carried out with the patient supine. A small bump under the ipsilateral hip can facilitate access to the lateral aspect of the foot. A thigh tourniquet is used (video clip 18).
2. A 4-cm incision is made over the anterior margin of the peroneus longus on the lateral aspect of the foot as it courses toward the cuboid to turn underneath the foot. This inci-

sion is then deepened through the subcutaneous fat to access the peroneus brevis. Care should be taken to avoid injury to the sural nerve, which usually passes through the proximal aspect of the incision.
3. The peroneus longus and peroneus brevis each lie in separate sheaths in this area, and they must be released to access the tendons.
4. The peroneus longus is then cut as far distally as possible as it makes the turn around the cuboid to pass underneath the midfoot. If an os peroneum is present in the tendon, it is excised and the cut is made through this area.
5. The foot is held in maximum eversion and the peroneus longus is woven two or three times in Pulvertaft fashion through the distal aspect of the peroneus brevis. A 2-0 coated polyester suture (Ethibond) is used to join the tendons. If other procedures are to be carried out on the foot, the final tensioning and suture of the tendon is saved until the end of the case.
6. The wound is closed with interrupted sutures and infiltrated with 0.25% bupivacaine.

Postoperative Care

The foot is placed in a short-leg compression dressing reinforced with plaster splints. After 10 to 12 days, the sutures are removed and a short-leg weight-bearing cast is applied. If no other procedures are being performed, a transition to regular footwear is usually made after a total of 4 to 6 weeks of immobilization.

CLAW TOE CORRECTIONS

Treatment of the claw toe deformity depends upon whether a fixed or flexible deformity is present. With fixed deformity at the MTP joints, release of the extensor tendons and joint capsules is required. To hold the toes in the neutral position, usually a flexor tendon transfer needs to be done. With fixed deformity of the proximal interphalangeal joint (hammer toe), a DuVries phalangeal arthroplasty with removal of the distal portion of the proximal phalanx or an interphalangeal joint arthrodesis is indicated. If the claw toe deformity is passively correctible, a flexor tendon transfer alone usually suffices.

The surgical techniques for flexor tendon transfer (Girdlestone procedure), DuVries phalangeal arthroplasty to correct a hammer toe, and release of the MTP joints in a fixed contracture are described in Chapter 8.

Osteotomies

At times a specific bony deformity is present in pes cavus that significantly impairs the patient's ability to maintain a plantigrade foot, but the remainder of the foot remains relatively supple. This usually takes the form of a fixed varus deformity of the hindfoot or a fixed plantar flexion of the first ray. If the fixed deformity can be corrected, a plantigrade foot can be achieved without an arthrodesis. In general, an osteotomy that includes the first metatarsal or calcaneus or both is carried out in conjunction with a plantar fascia release and peroneus longus to brevis tendon transfer.

DORSIFLEXION OSTEOTOMY OF THE FIRST METATARSAL

Particularly in cases of CMT, plantar flexion of the first metatarsal can become fixed, with a resultant rigid forefoot valgus deformity. This forefoot equinus deformity can also involve the second and, rarely, the third metatarsal. As a result of this deformity, as the head of the first metatarsal contacts the ground, the forefoot is twisted into an inverted position. If this is associated with a varus deformity of the calcaneus, a weak peroneus brevis muscle, or a contracted plantar fascia, dramatic increases in stress on the lateral ankle ligaments can result. This stress can lead to chronic lateral ankle ligament instability over time.

In general, a first metatarsal osteotomy is not carried out as an isolated procedure but as part of a more comprehensive cavus foot correction. In the patient with very mild deformity, sometimes only a plantar fascia release and dorsiflexion osteotomy of the first are required. More often, however, a calcaneal osteotomy, plantar fascia release, and first metatarsal osteotomy are done together. The first-toe Jones procedure can also be added without complication.

Surgical Technique

1. The patient is placed in a supine position. If this is an isolated procedure, the first metatarsal osteotomy can be carried out under an ankle block only. If it is part of a more comprehensive cavus foot correction, general anesthesia is used (video clip 19).
2. An incision is made over the dorsal aspect of the first metatarsal, starting over the medial cuneiform and ending over the distal third of the metatarsal.
3. The incision is deepened to the extensor tendon, which is immobilized and retracted medially or laterally.
4. The metatarsocuneiform (MTC) joint is identified, and the proposed osteotomy site is marked on the bone starting about 1.5 cm distal to the joint (Fig. 21–8A and B).
5. A 2.7-mm or 3.5-mm screw is centered in the proximal portion of the metatarsal above the proposed osteotomy.
6. A .062-inch Kirschner wire is used to make a transverse drill hole in the dorsal part of the metatarsal 1 cm distal to the osteotomy.
7. The osteotomy is a dorsal closing wedge that usually removes 5 to 10 mm of bone, depending upon the degree of plantar flexion of the first metatarsal that must be corrected.
8. The first cut is made parallel to the MTC joint. A convergent cut is then made distally, aiming for the plantar cortex. Care is taken to leave the plantar cortex intact. A greenstick fracture is made as the osteotomy is closed, resulting in a more stable construct than if the cuts were fully completed. It is better to undercut the osteotomy than to remove too large a segment.
9. After the osteotomy has been created, the plantar cortex is loosened by rocking the bone back and forth until the dorsal gap can be closed (Fig. 21–8C).
10. To determine whether enough bone has been removed, the ankle is brought up into dorsiflexion and the forefoot is carefully evaluated, comparing the level of the first and fifth metatarsals in relation to the long axis of the leg. The surgeon must imagine that the foot is in a plantigrade position and that the first and fifth metatarsals are on the same plane.

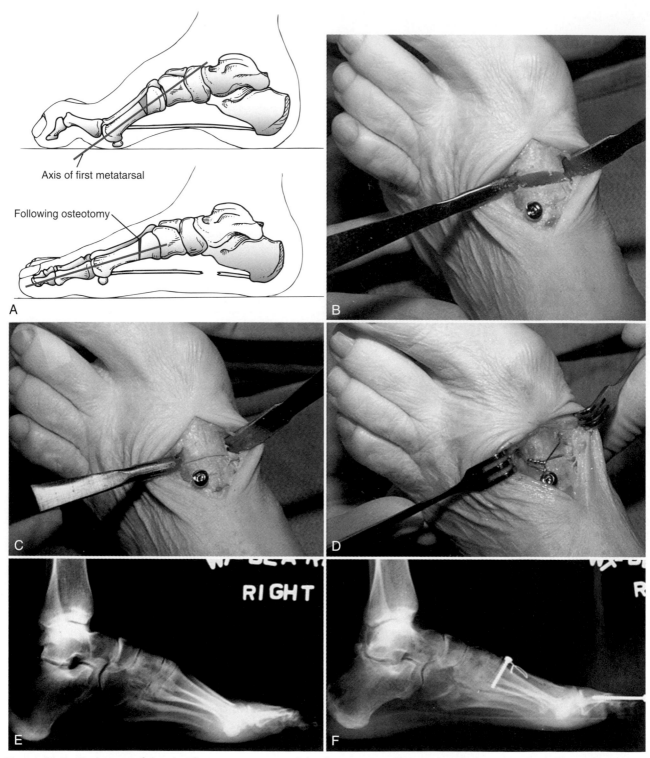

Figure 21–8   Technique of the dorsiflexion osteotomy of the first metatarsal. **A,** A dorsally based wedge of bone is removed approximately 1 cm distal to the first metatarsocuneiform joint. The plantar fascia is often released when carrying out this procedure for a cavus foot. **B,** A 3.5-mm screw has been placed in the proximal fragment to serve as a post. **C,** The osteotomy site is closed down and the plantar aspect of the foot carefully palpated. If the first metatarsal is still too plantar flexed, a larger wedge is removed. **D,** The osteotomy site is fixed by placing a length of 22-gauge wire through a transverse drill hole in the distal fragment and then fixing it to the screw. **E,** Preoperative and postoperative radiographs demonstrate dorsiflexion of the first metatarsal after proximal osteotomy. (From Mann RA, Coughlin MJ: *The Video Textbook of Foot and Ankle Surgery.* St. Louis, Medical Video Productions, 1991.)

11. If the size of the osteotomy cut is correct, internal fixation is inserted.
12. A piece of 22-gauge wire is passed through the transverse drill hole that was made distal to the osteotomy site in step 6.
13. The wire is then brought up around the screw head in the proximal portion of the metatarsal and tightened with a wire tightener while the osteotomy is held closed (Fig. 21–8D).
14. Once the osteotomy site has been completely closed, the bottom of the forefoot is again carefully examined. If the degree of dorsiflexion is adequate, the surgeon may proceed with closure of the wound. If it is not adequate, the wire is removed and more bone is removed from the osteotomy site (Fig. 21–8E).
15. Occasionally the second metatarsal needs to be dorsiflexed, which is done using the same procedure.
16. The wounds are closed in a routine manner and are infiltrated with 0.25% bupivacaine.
17. The foot is placed in a compression dressing. If this is the only procedure being carried out, splints are not required.

Postoperative Care

A popliteal block can be useful to control postoperative pain. If this is the only procedure being carried out, the patient is permitted to ambulate as tolerated in a postoperative shoe. If it is done in conjunction with other procedures, the patient is placed in a short-leg non–weight-bearing cast. Generally the osteotomy heals in approximately 6 weeks, after which ambulation is permitted as tolerated.

DWYER CALCANEAL OSTEOTOMY

Patients with a moderate-to-severe cavus deformity usually have a varus deformity of the calcaneus. When arthrodesis can be avoided, a fixed varus deformity is treated with the lateral closing wedge calcaneal osteotomy described by Dwyer.[9,10] If the patient lacks adequate dorsiflexion and has a high calcaneal pitch angle (a hindfoot cavus), a Samilson[29] osteotomy is carried out to allow the calcaneal tuberosity and the attached Achilles tendon to slide vertically, thereby effectively lengthening the gastroc-

soleus complex and correcting the effective pitch angle of the calcaneus. These procedures are usually carried out with a plantar fascia release and a first metatarsal osteotomy.

Surgical Technique

1. The patient is placed in a supine position with a bolster beneath the ipsilateral hip for adequate exposure of the lateral aspect of the calcaneus. A tourniquet is used on the thigh.
2. The skin incision begins about 2 cm posterior to the tip of the fibula and is carried obliquely past the tip of the fibula toward the plantar aspect of the calcaneocuboid joint (Fig. 21–9A and video clip 17).
3. The sural nerve is identified and retracted dorsally away from the surgical field.

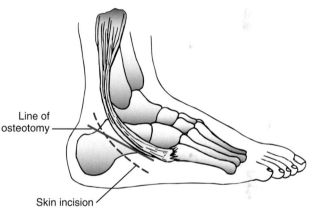

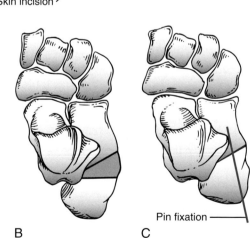

Figure 21–9 The Dwyer calcaneal osteotomy. A, Skin incision is made along the inferior margin of the peroneal tendons, with caution taken to avoid injury to the sural nerve. B, A lateral closing wedge of bone is taken of sufficient size to correct the deformity. C, Fixation is achieved with a longitudinal pin, a longitudinal screw, or a lateral staple. (From Mann RA, Coughlin MJ: *The Video Textbook of Foot and Ankle Surgery.* St. Louis, Medical Video Productions, 1991.)

4. The incision is carried just below the peroneal tendon sheath, which is stripped dorsally off of the lateral aspect of the calcaneus and left intact. The exposure of the calcaneus should extend from its dorsal aspect behind the fibula to just proximal to the calcaneocuboid joint. Dorsally, the soft tissue is stripped off the superior aspect of the calcaneus behind the ankle and subtalar joints.

5. A long oblique osteotomy is made in the calcaneus starting about 1 cm posterior to the posterior facet of the subtalar joint and ending distally about 1 cm proximal to the calcaneocuboid joint. The cut is started with a short, wide saw blade. As the line of the cut is established, the saw blade must be kept as perpendicular as possible to the long axis of the calcaneus. Once the short saw blade has reached its limit, a longer blade is used to complete the cut. If possible, the medial cortex of the calcaneus is left intact.

6. A second cut is now created, removing a pie-shaped wedge of bone from the lateral aspect of the calcaneus. The size of the wedge depends upon the severity of the varus deformity. Usually 5 to 7 mm of calcaneus is removed with the second cut (Fig. 21–9B).

7. Once the second cut is completed, a greenstick fracture is made on the medial side of the calcaneus by manipulating the fragments back and forth. The osteotomy is then closed. Sometimes, temporary insertion of a stout pin into the posterior tuberosity can serve as a joystick to facilitate closing the osteotomy. The position of the bone is carefully evaluated. If an inadequate degree of correction has been obtained, more bone needs to be removed.

8. The osteotomy site can be fixed with multiple laterally based bone staples or by a 5.0-mm to 7.3-mm screw placed down the long axis of the calcaneus through a separate stab incision (Fig. 21–9C). If a screw is used, it should be placed lateral to the midline and the patient should be warned that it can require later removal if it irritates the back of the foot against the heel counter of a shoe.

9. The wound is closed in a routine manner and infiltrated with 0.25% bupivacaine.

Postoperative Care

The patient is placed into a short-leg compression dressing incorporating plaster splints. A popliteal block can be useful in controlling postoperative pain. The sutures are removed 10 to 12 days after the procedure, and a short-leg non–weight-bearing cast is applied. Ambulation is permitted in the cast 4 weeks after the procedure, and casting is discontinued 8 weeks postoperatively if radiographs demonstrate union.

Results and Complications

The postoperative results after a Dwyer calcaneal osteotomy are usually most satisfactory (Fig. 21–10). Some minor shortening of the height of the calcaneus occurs, but this is usually not significant. Occasionally the sural nerve becomes entrapped in scar tissue or disrupted, which can create a problem for the patient.

The only significant error that can be made when performing this procedure is to fail to remove sufficient bone, leaving the hindfoot in varus. Sometimes it is difficult to judge whether adequate bone has been removed. The surgeon must attempt to line up the calcaneus with the long axis of the leg when trying to decide if a sufficient degree of correction has been achieved.

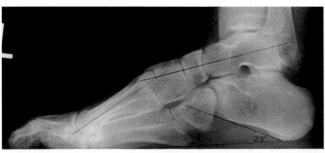 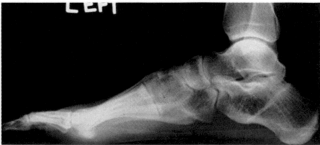

A   B

Figure 21–10 Preoperative **(A)** and postoperative **(B)** radiographs demonstrate the results of the Dwyer calcaneal osteotomy. The tarsal canal is visible on end preoperatively, indicating a varus deformity of the heel, whereas the position of the subtalar joint changes once the heel is brought into valgus.

SAMILSON CRESCENTIC OSTEOTOMY OR SLIDING CALCANEAL OSTEOTOMY

Some patients with a predominantly hindfoot cavus have remarkably high calcaneal pitch in excess of 30 degrees, either with or without a concomitant varus deformity. The Samilson osteotomy was described in the polio population to address this problem.[29] As described originally, the osteotomy was performed along a curved crescentic cut that allowed the posterior section of the calcaneus to pivot superiorly, reducing the pitch angle of the calcaneus. With more rigid internal fixation devices easily available today, a flat cut osteotomy is usually used. The flat cuts also facilitate removal of a lateral wedge of bone in addition to the sliding displacement if a varus component must also be corrected. The procedure is always carried out in association with a plantar fascia stripping, which is completed before the osteotomy.

Surgical Technique (Modified Samilson Osteotomy with a Flat Cut)

1. The patient is placed in a supine position with a bolster under the ipsilateral hip to facilitate exposure of the lateral side of the calcaneus. A thigh tourniquet is used.
2. The skin incision begins 1.5 cm above the superior aspect of the calcaneus posterior to the fibula and is carried distally in a straight line posterior to the peroneal tendon sheath, ending at the plantar aspect of the calcaneus.
3. The sural nerve is identified and retracted anteriorly.

4. An incision is made down to the calcaneus just posterior to the peroneal tendons. The exposure is developed over the superior aspect of the calcaneus behind the ankle and subtalar joints and distally onto the plantar aspect of the foot.
5. A vertical cut is made using a wide, short blade, starting about 1 cm posterior to the posterior facet. It extends distally and angulates very slightly anteriorly with the ankle held at a right angle (Fig. 21–11A). The cut is substantially more vertical than that used for a Dwyer osteotomy. When the short blade is no longer effective, a wide, longer blade is used. This cut is continued completely through the medial cortex, taking care to avoid injury to the medial structures.
6. Once the cut is completed, a broad osteotome is placed into the osteotomy site and the bone is pried apart. A smooth lamina spreader is placed into the osteotomy site to free it further. With the lamina spreader in place, a periosteal elevator is used to tease the soft tissues carefully off the medial aspect of the osteotomy cut.
7. Once the osteotomy site is freed, it is displaced dorsally approximately 1.5 to 2 cm, and the alignment of the foot is carefully observed. If a varus deformity is also present, a lateral closing wedge osteotomy is created, removing 5 to 10 mm of bone from the lateral aspect of the posterior fragment (Fig. 21–11B).
8. After correction, the alignment of the osteotomy site is carefully observed by allowing it to slide dorsally and close laterally.

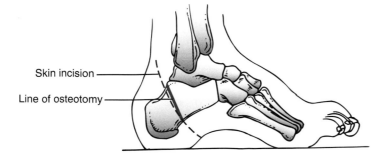 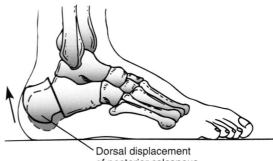

Skin incision

Line of osteotomy

Dorsal displacement of posterior calcaneus

A

B

Figure 21–11 Modified Samilson calcaneal osteotomy for hindfoot cavus. **A,** The skin incision is somewhat vertical in relation to the course of the peroneal tendons. **B,** After release of the plantar aponeurosis, the proximal fragment is displaced dorsally, lowering the longitudinal arch. If a varus deformity is present, a lateral wedge of bone can also be removed to combine the Dwyer and Samilson techniques. (From Mann RA, Coughlin MJ: *The Video Textbook of Foot and Ankle Surgery.* St. Louis, Medical Video Productions, 1991.)

9. The osteotomy can be fixed using multiple staples or one or more 5.0- to 7.3-mm screws placed down the long axis of the calcaneus.
10. The wounds are closed in a routine manner and infiltrated with 0.25% bupivacaine.

Postoperative Care

The patient is placed into a well-padded short-leg compression dressing incorporating plaster splints. A popliteal block can be useful to control

postoperative pain. The sutures are removed approximately 10 to 12 days after surgery, and the patient is placed in a short-leg, non–weight-bearing cast. Weight-bearing in a cast or boot brace is initiated after 6 weeks, and all immobilization is discontinued at 10 weeks after surgery if the radiographs demonstrate union.

Results and Complications

The results after the Samilson-type calcaneal osteotomy are usually satisfactory (Fig. 21–12).

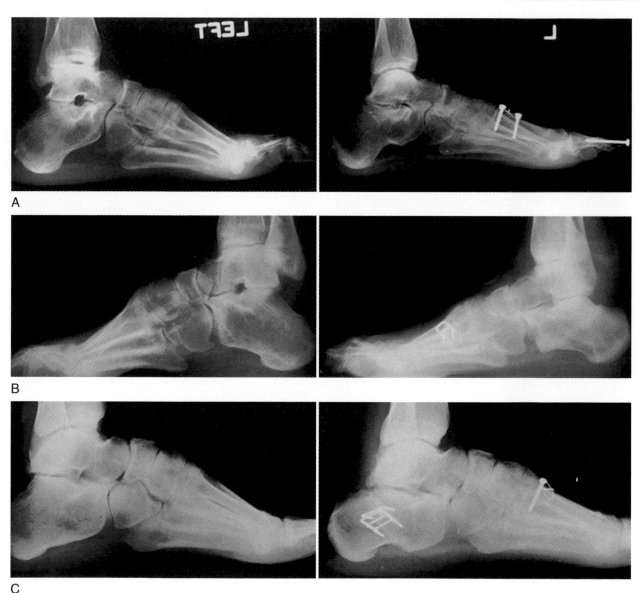

Figure 21–12 Three sets of radiographs demonstrate the results of the modified Samilson calcaneal osteotomy for a cavus deformity. Additional procedures were carried out in each case as required. Note the decreased height of the longitudinal arch and the increased length of the foot. **A,** Samilson calcaneal osteotomy, first metatarsal osteotomy, and first toe Jones procedure. **B,** Samilson calcaneal osteotomy, first metatarsal osteotomy, and plantar fascia release. **C,** Samilson calcaneal osteotomy fixed with staples, first metatarsal osteotomy, and plantar fascia release. **(A** from Mann RA, Coughlin MJ: *The Video Textbook of Foot and Ankle Surgery.* St. Louis, Medical Video Productions, 1991.)

The primary technical error is an osteotomy that is not displaced dorsally or a varus correction that is inadequate. The sural nerve is also at risk and represents a potential source of postoperative discomfort.

Midtarsal Osteotomies

Various type of midfoot osteotomies have been proposed for the patient with a forefoot equinus or anterior cavus deformity with the apex located at Chopart's joint. These include the Cole osteotomy, which consists of removing a dorsal wedge of bone from the navicular, cuneiforms, and cuboid.[6] A similar, more distal osteotomy has been proposed by Japas, in which a V-shaped osteotomy is made within the tarsal bones.[18] The distal portion is then depressed to allow the forefoot to be brought out of its equinus position.

Although, in theory, midfoot osteotomies are preferred because they correct a typical deformity closer to its apex than a basilar osteotomy of the first metatarsal, in practice this is not the case. Inevitably all variations of the midfoot osteotomies result in multiple intraarticular cuts that can lead to early arthrosis. The residual deformity from the much safer extra-articular osteotomy through the first metatarsal is well tolerated, and this approach should be universally preferred. Midfoot procedures should be reserved for patients who already have arthrosis, and the joints should then be arthrodesed in conjunction with the cavus correction.

Arthrodesis Procedures

The triple arthrodesis is the requisite operation for more severe, rigid postural deformities of the hindfoot of any kind. In the cavus foot, it is important to remember that other procedures such as a first metatarsal osteotomy or Jones procedure can be carried out in addition to a triple arthrodesis if the conditions warrant. Routine joint preparation and cartilage removal often proves adequate for milder degrees of deformity. Because the posterior facet of the subtalar joint is approached from the lateral side, there is a natural tendency to remove more bone laterally and position the calcaneus toward valgus using standard techniques, just as one would perform a triple arthrodesis for hindfoot arthritis. When this proves inadequate for more severe deformities, a variety of additional cuts can be made to facilitate a plantigrade foot.

SIFFERT TRIPLE ARTHRODESIS

The variation of the triple arthrodesis described by Siffert involves a step cut made in the talar head to facilitate reduction of the cavus deformity. It is used in more severe, rigid deformities.[32,33] The navicular is mortised underneath the head of the talus. In this way the forefoot is rotated, thereby correcting the forefoot equinus (Fig. 21–13A). This is a technically demanding procedure that should not be undertaken lightly. The patient's radiographs should be carefully studied and an outline of the procedure made before attempting it.

Lateral Approach

1. The patient is placed in a supine position with a lift under the ipsilateral hip to facilitate exposure of the lateral aspect of the foot. A tourniquet is used around the thigh.
2. The skin incision starts at the tip of the fibula and is carried toward the base of the fourth metatarsal.
3. The incision is deepened through the subcutaneous tissue and fat. Caution must be taken to look out for an anterior branch of the sural nerve.
4. The extensor digitorum brevis muscle is removed from its origin along the lateral aspect of the sinus tarsi and is reflected distally beyond the calcaneocuboid joint.
5. The joint capsule around the lateral aspect of the subtalar joint and calcaneocuboid joint are opened and the joint surfaces exposed.
6. Because the foot is often in an adducted position, the lateral aspect of the talonavicular joint can usually be easily visualized from the lateral wound. If so, the joint capsule is stripped off the joint as much as possible.

Medial Approach

7. The medial approach starts at the tip of the medial malleolus and is carried distally to the naviculocuneiform joint. It is deepened through the subcutaneous tissue and fat to expose the joint capsule.
8. The joint capsule of the talonavicular joint is widely opened and stripped off the dorsal aspect of the navicular but not off the dorsal

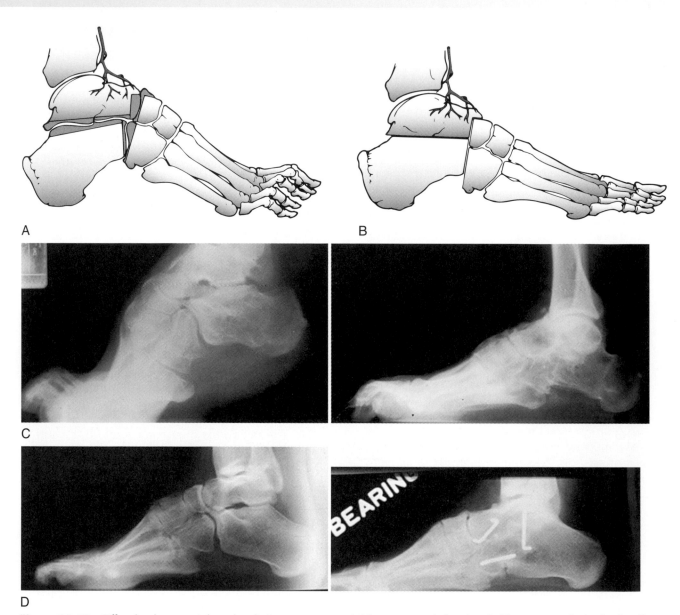

A

B

C

D

Figure 21–13 Siffert beak-type triple arthrodesis to correct a rigid cavovarus deformity. **A,** The cuts made in the hindfoot. Usually a lateral closing wedge osteotomy is made in the subtalar joint. The navicular is mortised beneath the head of the talus to reduce the height of the longitudinal arch. A lateral wedge is removed from the calcaneocuboid joint to correct the residual forefoot adduction and adjust the shortening of the medial column. **B,** Position of the foot postoperatively. **C,** Severe cavus foot correction for a case of Charcot–Marie–Tooth disease with a severe forefoot equinus. **D,** Preoperative and postoperative weight-bearing radiographs from another case demonstrate the lowering of the longitudinal arch.

neck of the talus in order to protect its blood supply.

Preparation of Joint Surfaces

9. The first bone cuts involve the posterior facet of the subtalar joint to correct the varus deformity of the heel. Usually, 3 to 5 mm of bone needs to be resected from the lateral aspect of the posterior facet to bring the calcaneus into 5 degrees of valgus.
10. The head of the talus is now visualized through the medial incision. A segment is removed from the plantar two thirds of the talar head extending about 1 cm in depth into the head (Fig. 21–13A and B). Note that the dorsal one third of the talar head is left intact, and the piece of bone removed from the head is approximately 1 cm in depth.
11. A thin slice of bone is removed from the dorsal aspect of the navicular while holding the forefoot in neutral rotation to create a flat dorsal surface that can be placed beneath the cut in the head of the talus.
12. Because the medial column has been significantly shortened, the lateral column is also shortened through the calcaneocuboid joint. This is done by first removing the end of the calcaneus with a saw, then removing a segment of bone from the cuboid to correct the abduction–adduction alignment of the foot.
13. At this point, the alignment of the foot should be satisfactory, and the osteotomy sites are inspected (Fig. 21–13B). At times, pieces of bone must be removed to be sure the fit is adequate.
14. The joints are now fixed, beginning with the subtalar joint. The talonavicular joint is secured next, followed by the calcaneocuboid joint. Staples, screws, or a combination are all acceptable.
15. The Achilles tendon should be lengthened if the foot cannot be brought up to 10 degrees of dorsiflexion.
16. Occasionally, a first and possibly second metatarsal osteotomy must also be carried out if the forefoot equinus deformity is too severe. Usually the rotation of the forefoot block of bone adequately corrects the forefoot equinus deformity in all but the most severe cases.

Wound Closure

17. The wounds are closed in layers. As the foot is being abducted in most cases, special attention should be paid to soft tissue tension on the medial side, which is being stretched. The deep layers are closed with 2-0 Vicryl or chromic sutures. The subcutaneous layers are closed with 3-0 absorbable suture, and the skin is closed with interrupted nylon sutures or staples. The wounds are infiltrated with 0.25% bupivacaine.

Postoperative Care

A short-leg compression dressing incorporating plaster splints is applied. A popliteal block can be useful in controlling postoperative pain. The cast is changed at about 2 weeks, and the patient is placed into a short-leg, non–weight-bearing cast. Six weeks after surgery, weight bearing is begun in a cast. Immobilization is weaned away after 10 weeks if radiographs are satisfactory.

Results and Complications

The Siffert beak-type triple arthrodesis can correct even the most severe forefoot cavus deformity (Fig. 21–13C and D). A routine triple arthrodesis does not address the forefoot equinus directly and is more limited in its corrective power. Large case series are not available, but the complications and risks of nonunion would be expected to be comparable to those of a standard triple arthrodesis.[21,37]

REFERENCES

1. Alexander IJ, Johnson KA: Assessment and management of pes cavus in Charcot–Marie–Tooth disease. *Clin Orthop Relat Res* 246:273-281, 1989.
2. Bentzon PGK: Pes cavus and the m. peroneus longus. *Acta Orthop Scand* 4:50, 1933.
3. Bertorini T, Narayanaswami P, Rashed H. Charcot–Marie–Tooth disease (hereditary motor sensory neuropathies) and hereditary sensory and autonomic neuropathies. *Neurologist* 10(6):327-337, 2004.
4. Brewerton DA, Sandifer PH, Sweetnam DR: Idiopathic pes cavus: An investigation into its aetiology. *BMJ* 2:659-661, 1963.
5. Charcot J-M, Marie P: Sur une forme particulaire d'atrophy musculaire progressive souvent familiale debutant par les pieds et les jambes et atteignant plus tard les mains. *Rev Med* 6:97-138, 1886.
6. Cole WH: The treatment of claw-foot. *J Bone Joint Surg Am* 22:895-908, 1940.

7. Dhillon MS, Sandhu HS: Surgical options in the management of residual foot problems in poliomyelitis. *Foot Ankle Clin* 5(2):327-347, 2000.

8. Duchenne GB: *The Physiology of Motion.* Trans EB Kaplan. Philadelphia, WB Saunders, 1959.

9. Dwyer FC: The present status of the problem of pes cavus. *Clin Orthop Relat Res* 106:254-275, 1975.

10. Dwyer FC: Osteotomy of the calcaneum for pes cavus, *J Bone Joint Surg Br* 41:80-86, 1959.

11. Dyck PJ, Lambert EH: Lower motor and primary sensory neuron diseases with peroneal muscular dystrophy. I. Neurologic, genetic, and electrophysiologic findings in hereditary polyneuropathies. *Arch Neurol* 18:603-618, 1968.

12. Guyton GP: Differential anatomy of the peroneal nerve at the fibular head: Implications for the pathogenesis of foot deformity in Charcot–Marie–Tooth disease. Presented at the American Orthopaedic Foot and Ankle Society Annual Meeting, Hilton Head, SC, June 26-29, 2003.

13. Guyton GP, Mann RA: The pathogenesis and surgical management of foot deformity in Charcot–Marie–Tooth disease. *Foot Ankle Clin* 5(2):317-326, 2000.

14. Halgrimsson S: Pes cavus, seine Behandlung und einige Bemerkungen über seine Aetiologie. *Acta Orthop Scand* 10:73, 1939.

15. Holmes JR, Hansen ST Jr: Foot and ankle manifestations of Charcot–Marie–Tooth disease. *Foot Ankle* 14(8):476-486, 1993.

16. Huber H, Dutoit M: Dynamic foot-pressure measurement in the assessment of operatively treated clubfeet. *J Bone Joint Surg Am* 86(6):1203-1210, 2004.

17. Ibrahim K: Pes cavus. In Evarts CM (ed): *Surgery of the Musculoskeletal System.* New York, Churchill Livingstone, 1990, pp 4015-4034.

18. Japas LM: Surgical treatment of pes cavus by tarsal V-osteotomy. *J Bone Joint Surg Am* 50:927-944, 1968.

19. Jones R: An operation for paralytic calcaneocavus. *Am J Orthop Surg* 5:371 1908.

20. Kremli MK: Fixed forefoot adduction after clubfoot surgery. *Saudi Med J* 24(7):742-744, 2003.

21. Mann DC, Hsu JD: Triple arthrodesis in the treatment of fixed cavovarus deformity in adolescent patients with Charcot–Marie–Tooth disease. *Foot Ankle* 13(1):1-6, 1992.

22. Mann RA, Missirian J: Pathophysiology of Charcot–Marie–Tooth disease. *Clin Orthop Relat Res* 234:221-228, 1988.

23. Morcuende JA, Dolan LA, Dietz FR, Ponseti IV: Radical reduction in the rate of extensive corrective surgery for clubfoot using the Ponseti method. *Pediatrics* 113(2):376-380, 2004.

24. Olney B: Treatment of the cavus foot. Deformity in the pediatric patient with Charcot–Marie–Tooth. *Foot Ankle Clin* 5(2):305-315, 2000.

25. Pandolfo M: Friedreich ataxia. *Semin Pediatr Neurol* 10(3):163-172, 2003.

26. Pareyson D: Differential diagnosis of Charcot–Marie–Tooth disease and related neuropathies. *Neurol Sci* 25(2):72-82, 2004.

27. Roper BA, Tibrewal SB: Soft tissue surgery in Charcot–Marie–Tooth disease. *J Bone Joint Surg Br* 71(1):17-20, 1989.

28. Sabir M, Lyttle D: Pathogenesis of pes cavus in Charcot–Marie–Tooth disease. *Clin Orthop Relat Res* 175:173-178, 1983.

29. Samilson RL: Crescentic osteotomy of the os calcis for calcaneocavus feet. In Bateman JE, (ed): *Foot Science.* Philadelphia WB Saunders, 1976, p 18.

30. Schmalbruch H, Haase G: Spinal muscular atrophy: Present state. *Brain Pathol* 11(2):231-247, 2001.

31. Simbak N, Razak M: Residual deformity following surgical treatment of congenital talipes equinovarus. *Med J Malaysia* 53 Suppl A:115-120, 1998.

32. Siffert RS, del Torto U: "Beak" triple arthrodesis for severe cavus deformity. *Clin Orthop Rel Res* 181:65-67, 1983.

33. Siffert RS, Forester RI, Nachamle B: "Beak" triple arthrodesis for correction of severe cavus deformity. *Clin Orthop Rel Res* 45:101, 1966.

34. Steindler A: Operative treatment of pes cavus: Stripping of the os calcis. Surg Gynecol Obstet 24:612, 1917.

35. Tooth HH: *The Peroneal Type of Progressive Muscular Atrophy.* London, HK Lewis, 1886.

36. Tynan MC, Klenerman L, Helliwell TR, et al: Investigation of muscle imbalance in the leg in symptomatic forefoot pes cavus: A multidisciplinary study. *Foot Ankle* 13(9):489-501, 1992.

37. Wukich DK, Bowen JR: A long-term study of triple arthrodesis for correction of pes cavovarus in Charcot–Marie–Tooth disease. *J Pediatr Orthop* 9(4):433-437, 1989.

Disorders of Tendons

Michael J. Coughlin • Lew C. Schon

EXTENSOR TENDONS

Extensor Tendon Injuries

The treatment of disruption of extensor tendons varies depending on whether a laceration or rupture has occurred. The first step in the treatment is an accurate diagnosis based on a careful physical examination. With an isolated rupture, typically only one tendon is involved. On the other hand, with a penetrating wound or laceration, several structures may be damaged. It is important to routinely assess the function of individual tendons and to evaluate the neurovascular status of the anterior ankle and dorsal foot. Knowledge of tendon anatomy, particularly the courses and insertions, is useful in determining the nature and extent of the pathologic process.

Anzel et al[2] evaluated 1014 cases of tendon injuries at the Mayo Clinic and noted that 21 injuries were to the extensors to the toes, a 2% incidence. They did not differentiate between injuries to the extensor hallucis longus (EHL) and extensor digitorum longus (EDL).

Extensor Digitorum Longus

Bell and Schon[3] have noted that the EDL proper can only be lacerated between the ankle and the midfoot because individual tendons are found below this level. The EDL is relatively superficial and easily lacerated with trauma (Fig. 22–1). Because the main function of the EDL is extension of the metatarsophalangeal (MTP) joint and the proximal and distal interphalangeal (PIP and DIP) joints of the lesser toes, when it is transected and not repaired, a claw toe deformity can develop. Patients with chronic extensor tendon lacerations report difficulty controlling the toes when attempting to put on socks or slide into shoes. During these activities the toe tends to catch on the fabric or insole and passively flex underneath the foot. Often, because of the proximity of the anterior tibial tendon to the extensor hallucis longus and the neurovascular bundle, injury to these structures can occur simultaneously.

Anatomy

The EDL originates on the lateral tibial condyle, the anterior crest of the fibula, and the interosseous membrane, and it inserts on the base of the terminal phalanges of the four lesser toes. Innervated by the deep peroneal nerve, the EDL functions to extend the toes at the DIP joint and to dorsiflex and evert the foot.

The EDL divides into two separate tendons beneath the superior retinaculum and then further divides into two lateral tendons to the fourth and fifth toes and two medial tendons to the second and third toes (Fig. 22–2). The individual tendon of the EDL to each toe is joined on the lateral aspect by the tendon of the extensor digitorum brevis. These individual tendons are anchored at the level of the MTP joint by a fibroaponeurotic dorsal digital expansion.[19]

Physical Examination

On physical examination, an absence of extension of the lesser toes at the MTP joint is demonstrated after disruption of the EDL. Weakness of extension of the toes can also be appreciated at the PIP and DIP joints. Furthermore, because the EDL affects eversion and dorsiflexion of the foot, significant weakness of this function can be noted after tendon disruption. On palpation, a gap may be noted at the area of tendon injury. An interruption of the EDL may be diagnosed by an inability to palpate this tendon in the forefoot or ankle region as well as by weakness of lesser toe extension. The status of the superficial peroneal and deep peroneal nerves should be evaluated as well as the function of the extensor digitorum brevis.

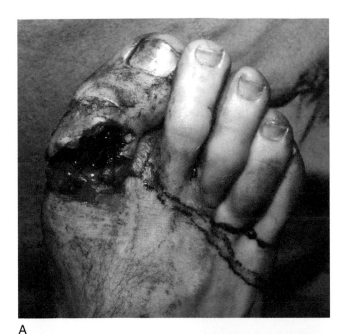

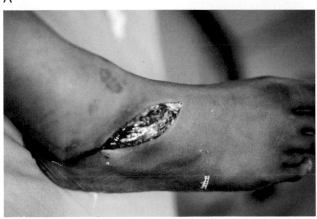

A

B

Figure 22–1 **A,** Dorsal toe laceration with distal disruption of extensor hallucis longus. After resection of the margins of the wounds, the tendon was repaired. **B,** Dorsal lateral foot laceration with disruption of the extensor tendons and preservation of the extensor hallucis longus tendon. Following wound debridement, longitudinal proximal and distal extensions of the wounds permitted repair of the tendons.

On physical examination, difficulty can surround the diagnosis because of the ability of one tendon to substitute function for another. For example, the extensor digitorum brevis (EDB) can substitute for the EDL. On the plantar aspect of the foot, the flexor digitorum longus (FDL) can substitute for the flexor hallucis longus (FHL) because of a crossover connection between the two flexor tendons. Comparison to unaffected contralateral toes can be useful. Careful assessment is important to delineate a specific tendon injury.

Surgical Treatment

Bell and Schon[3] recommend that the EDL be primarily repaired using a modified Kessler suture technique. Alternatives include a modified Bunnell or Krackow technique (Fig. 22–3). Postoperatively the foot is protected for 3 to 4 weeks with the foot and ankle in neutral position, with subsequent gradual initiation of passive range-of-motion exercises. The authors suggest night splinting after cast immobilization is discontinued.

At surgical exploration after a laceration, careful and comprehensive management is important with an open wound. All wounds should be thoroughly explored, debrided, and copiously irrigated. Any foreign bodies or materials should be removed. Inspection of adjacent neurovascular structures is important, and they should be repaired or ligated as appropriate. Parenteral antibiotics, tetanus prophylaxis, and immobilization should be used depending on the specific tissue injury. A second look operation 24 to 72 hours later should be considered for wounds with greater contamination.

Rooks[18] reviewed reports of EDL injuries[6,7,12,22,24] and noted 26 cases of EDL disruption. A preponderance of satisfactory results occurred after surgical repair. Lipscomb and Kelly[12] reported on six lacerations of the EDL in combination with other tendon injuries and reported 50% good results. Floyd et al[6] reported on

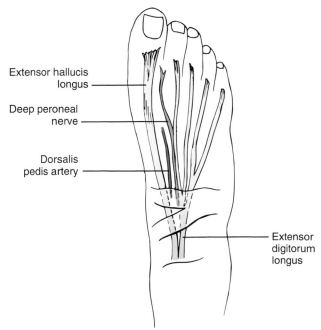

Figure 22–2 The extensor digitorum longus tendon divides into two separate tendons beneath the extensor retinaculum and then further divides into separate tendons to the four lesser toes.

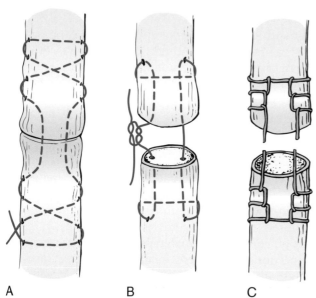

Figure 22–3 Technique of tendon repair. **A,** Modified Bunnell technique. **B,** Kessler technique. **C,** Krackow technique.

eight EDL disruptions, seven of which were primarily repaired. The one tendon that was not repaired had a poor result. Other reports note generally good results with surgical intervention.[7,22,24] Wicks et al[24] reported on four lacerations of the EDL and concluded that those not repaired did not have a significant problem. Floyd et al[6] reported a high incidence of painful dorsal scars after laceration of the dorsum of the foot. Rooks[18] advised surgical repair of a disrupted EDL if it could be accomplished with minimal extension of the wound. He advised careful attention to associated nerve injuries as well.

Akhtar and Levine[1] reported a case of spontaneous dislocation of the EDL after a rupture of the inferior extensor retinaculum. They repaired the retinaculum and relocated the tendon successfully.

In general, injuries to the EDL tendon occur with lacerations to the dorsum of the foot or anterior ankle. In the course of surgical exploration, appropriate treatment of nerve and vessel injuries should be carried out, and repair of the disrupted EDL tendons should be done when feasible.

Extensor Digitorum Brevis

The EDB tendon originates on the distal lateral and superior surface of the calcaneus and inserts on the lateral aspect of the extensor digitorum longus tendon and also on the base of the proximal phalanx of the first through fourth toes. It is innervated by the deep peroneal nerve and provides extension at the MTP joint. The muscle is the only intrinsic muscle on the

dorsum of the foot. There is no EDB tendon to the fifth toe.

The EDB is located on the lateral aspect of the forefoot and covers the lateral aspect of the subtalar joint. The tendons are quite small and are often injured following a laceration on the dorsolateral aspect of the foot. Bell and Schon[3] suggest that if the tendons are easily identified at the time of an EDL repair, an EDB repair should be performed as well. If the EDB is not repairable, EDL repair alone is adequate. No series have been reported on repairs of the EDB.

Kriza and Mushlin[10] reported an avulsion fracture of the EDB from its origin on the calcaneus. It was treated nonsurgically with a successful result. An avulsion fracture of the EDB should be distinguished from an os peroneum, a fracture of the anterior process of the calcaneus, the peroneal trochlea, a fracture of the cuboid, or a rupture of the calcaneofibular ligament.

Extensor Hallucis Longus

Anatomy

The EHL originates on the midportion of the anterior fibula and the interosseous membrane and inserts onto the base of the distal phalanx of the hallux. Innervated by the deep peroneal nerve, it extends the hallux and everts the foot. The EHL receives its motor supply much farther distally than the anterior tibial muscle and the EDL. The motor branch to the EHL travels in close proximity to the fibula for about 10 cm before penetrating the muscle belly.[20] The EHL is connected to the base of the proximal phalanx by the extensor aponeurosis, which receives contributions from the abductor and adductor hallucis. At the level of the ankle joint, the EHL becomes tendinous as it enters three successive soft tissue tunnels beneath the superior extensor retinaculum and inferior extensor retinaculum and within the extensor hood of the hallux (Fig. 22–4). These three areas play a role in a tendon entrapment or in preventing proximal retraction of the EHL tendon after injury.[9]

Lipscomb and Kelly[12] noted that as the EHL passes beneath the extensor retinacular ligaments, it is enveloped in a separate sheath, providing a gliding mechanism on the anterior aspect of the tibia and ankle.

History and Physical Examination

Attritional ruptures can occur at or around the level of the ankle joint.[15] Spontaneous ruptures of the EHL tendon occur, but lacerations are more common.

The patient might note a sudden pop with subcutaneous rupture of the EHL. Development of ecchymosis in the area of the tendon and tenderness to

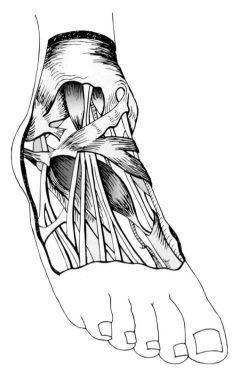

Figure 22–4 At the level of the ankle joint, the extensor hallucis longus becomes tendinous as it courses between superior and inferior extensor retinaculum.

palpation are coupled with an inability to dorsiflex the great toe (Fig. 22–5). The tendon typically is not painful after rupture. An obvious defect may be present in the region of the anterior ankle with disruption of the EHL, and a gap may be noted. The tendon might not be palpable. EHB substitution can allow weak extension of the interphalangeal joint of the hallux.[22] Depending on the location of the disruption, some function might remain. Lacerations over the dorsum of the foot and the anterior ankle may be accompanied by injury to the anterior tibial or dorsalis pedis artery, deep and superficial peroneal nerve, and anterior tibial tendon (Fig. 22–6).

Surgical Treatment

Extension of any laceration should be performed in a longitudinal direction to assess an injury to the EHL. Evaluation of the anterior tibial tendon, deep peroneal nerve, or other elements of the neurovascular bundle is important. The tendon is approximated and repaired with a 2-0 nonabsorbable suture with a modified Kessler or Krackow technique (see Fig. 22–3).

If the tendon is retracted, a more proximal incision or an extension of the exposure may be necessary in the area of the anterior ankle. The tendon might be caught beneath the more proximal extensor retinaculum. It is also very helpful to dorsiflex the ankle and

the toes to passively deliver the tendon ends into the wound. Once the ends are found, insert a long 25-gauge needle perpendicularly to skewer the tendon and keep it from retracting. This is a relatively atraumatic way to hold the tendon during repair.

After primary repair, a posterior splint or cast is used for 4 weeks. After removal of the splint, early passive range-of-motion exercises are initiated. Poggi and Hall[17] recommend a below-knee cast with the ankle positioned at a 90-degree angle and further plantar flexion blocked. A removable boot brace is best in compliant patients because it permits controlled passive but not active dorsiflexion of the toe and ankle to minimize adhesions. Avoid passive or active plantar flexion or active dorsiflexion until 4 to 8 weeks after repair.

Results and Complications

With an EHL injury, the foot often is in a dorsiflexed position with the EHL under tension. Significant retraction can develop depending on the level of the laceration. Laceration of the digit distal to the extensor expansion may be evidenced by no significant tendon retraction because the extensor expansion prevents proximal migration.[5,16] Duke and Greenberg[5] recommend nonsurgical treatment following a distal injury. Noonan et al[16] reported on three patients who sustained lacerations of the base of the nail with Salter

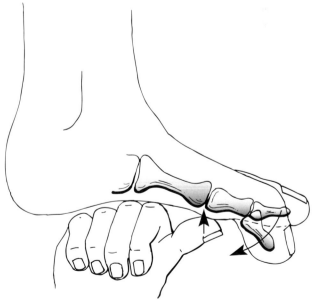

Figure 22–5 Technique of push-up test to examine function of the extensor hallucis longus (EHL). A thumb or finger is pressed on the plantar aspect of the first metatarsophalangeal joint. With unopposed function of the flexor hallucis longus, the interphalangeal joint flexes, demonstrating discontinuity or dysfunction of the EHL.

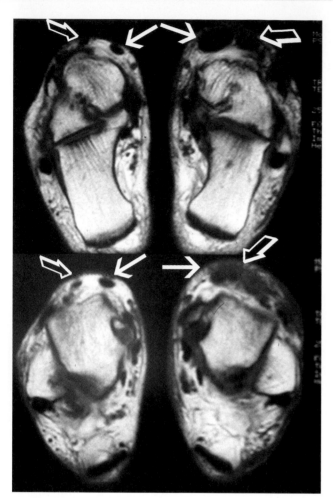

Figure 22–6 Magnetic resonance images demonstrating normal tendons on the left and injured extensor hallucis longus and anterior tibial tendon on the right following an anterior ankle deep laceration. The *solid arrows* indicate the anterior tibial tendon and the *open arrows* indicate the flexor hallucis longus.

fractures and concluded that these could be treated conservatively.

More-proximal EHL injuries have been reported by a number of authors.[6,7,12,21-24] Floyd et al[6] reported on 13 EHL lacerations, of which 11 underwent a primary repair. One was not repaired, and one had a second-ary repair. Using a modified Kessler suture technique or a modified Bunnell technique, they reported seven good and six fair results. They concluded that a primary repair of the disrupted EHL is indicated. Wicks et al[24] reported on 11 lacerations of the EHL, with seven of nine showing good results. They suggested that patients with a late, unrepaired tendon disruption may be better cared for by conservative treatment. Simonet and Sim[22] reported on five lacerations of the anterior ankle treated with a primary repair with sat-isfactory results.

Griffiths[7] reported on six cases of EHL disruption in younger patients (ages 4, 19, 21, 22, 23, and 25), five of which were repaired acutely. Based on the one patient who did not have a surgical repair, the authors concluded that "formal repair of the extensor hallucis longus seems unnecessary. Its natural tendency for spontaneous repair after tenotomy is well known." Although this suggests that the EHL does not need to be repaired, Floyd et al[6] noted that the sole justifi-cation for not repairing this tendon appears to be Griffiths' one patient, who recovered spontaneously. Indeed, Griffiths did not even note the actual location of the injury.

Kass et al[9] observed that after an isolated tenotomy with the foot in a plantar-flexed position, minimal retraction can occur. On the other hand, with the EHL under tension, significant retraction can occur, and a significant gap can develop that precludes later tendon healing. Floyd et al[6] did note significant proximal retraction of the EHL in two cases. Kass et al[9] and Floyd et al[6] concluded that tenotomies are quite different from lacerations of the EHL.

Duke and Greenberg[5] reported on 75 distal teno-tomies of the EHL and found no evidence of weakness of the great toe in 16 seen in follow-up. Bell and Schon[3] noted that the EHL, if left unrepaired, suffers no sequelae. They concluded, however, that these notions are based on the experience of Griffiths and thought it was imprudent to extrapolate that spontaneous recovery of EHL function routinely occurs and that EHL repair is not warranted. Since the time of that article, we have seen several minor chronic sequelae from a neglected laceration. The primary problems observed are clumsiness donning shoes or boots and plantar flexion deformity of the hallux. In general, based on our clinical observations, efforts to repair the tendon should be undertaken when possible.

Isolated rupture of the EHL occurs infrequently. Menz and Nettle[14] described a case with rupture at the musculotendinous junction. Poggi and Hall[17] reported on a closed rupture of the EHL at the level of the MTP joint that occurred several years after a cheilectomy. Sim and Deweerd[21] reported on a spontaneous rupture of the EHL on the anterior aspect of the ankle in a skier.

McMaster[13] stated that spontaneous rupture of a tendon rarely occurs without predisposing factors such as chronic disease. Successful surgical treatment centers around early diagnosis and prompt surgical intervention. Sim and Deweerd[21] and Skoff[23] repaired the tendon primarily, Langenberg[11] used a free tendon graft, and Menz and Nettle[14] transferred the peroneus tertius tendon to reconstruct the EHL. All had excel-lent results.

With delayed treatment of an old EHL rupture, Berens[4] noted that on initial exploration the proximal portion of the tendon could not be identified. Therefore the extensor hallucis brevis tendon was transferred into the distal stump of the flexor hallucis brevis. Menz and Nettle[14] noted that a primary repair was not possible and used the tendon of the peroneus brevis that was mobilized and sutured it directly to the EHL. Hoelzer and Kalish[8] also reported an EHL tendon disruption and noted at exploration 4 months after injury that the proximal end had retracted. The tendon of the EDL to the second toe was split and anastomosed to the distal stump of the EHL.

Postoperative scarring and adhesion formation can lead to diminished postoperative motion[23] and may be a source of pain, but this is uncommon. Floyd et al[6] reported that 38% of those injured had a painful scar.

Conclusion

With only one reported exception, the results of surgical repair of acute disruption of the EHL tendons have been good.

The actual site of injury is an important factor in developing a plan for treatment of a disruption of the EHL. If the injury is distal to the extensor expansion, nonsurgical treatment is warranted. An injury proximal to the extensor expansion may be treated with a primary repair. Treatment of EHL injuries 6 weeks or later after injury is often associated with an inability to reapproximate the tendon ends. A tendon transfer or tendon graft may be necessary to bridge the interval gap. In these cases one should assess the amount of tendon loss by placing moderate tension on the tendon ends and placing the ankle and hallux in neutral position. When the tendon ends cannot be opposed without excessive tension, a tendon slide using healthy proximal EHL tendon for defects up to 4 to 5 cm may be attempted. For anything greater than a 5-cm gap, a tendon transfer may be performed. The most common reported transfer is the peroneus tertius,[14] but a split of the extensor to the second toe for use in lacerations distal to the ankle joint[8] is a good alternative.

Aggressive surgical treatment of open lacerations about the foot is most important. Adequate exploration and debridement and anatomic restoration of tendons are usually appropriate. Although Griffiths[7] noted that the EHL tendon might heal spontaneously and that formal repair is not indicated, review of the literature does not support the notion that conservative management is warranted. Surgical repair of the EHL is important when feasible. On the other hand, with significant soft tissue loss, EHL repair might not be feasible, but secondary tendon grafting can be considered if the soft tissues are adequate and free of infection.

ANTERIOR TIBIAL TENDON RUPTURE

Subcutaneous rupture of the anterior tibial tendon has received little attention in the literature, and relatively few ruptures have been reported. Forst et al[33] reviewed the literature and noted 63 cases of anterior tibial tendon disruption: 13 were lacerations and 50 were spontaneous ruptures. More recently, in the largest series reported to date, Markarian et al[41] described 16 anterior tibial tendon disruptions, including 10 ruptures and six lacerations. Thus, fewer than 100 cases of anterior tibial tendon disruption (either laceration or rupture) have been reported. Most of these are either case reports or small series.

Anatomy

The anterior tibial tendon functions as the major dorsiflexor of the ankle,[32] primarily during the swing phase, heel strike, and early stance phase of the walking cycle.[28,52] It originates from the proximal half of the anterior tibia, the lower lateral tibial condyle, lateral tibia, and the interosseous membrane and inserts on the plantar medial aspect of the first cuneiform and the plantar base of the first metatarsal (Fig. 22–7). At the level of the lower and middle thirds

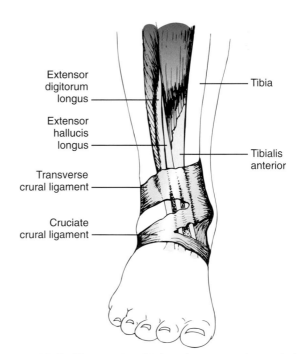

Extensor digitorum longus

Extensor hallucis longus

Transverse crural ligament

Cruciate crural ligament

Tibia

Tibialis anterior

Figure 22–7 The anterior tibial tendon courses beneath the transverse crural ligament and cruciate crural ligament before inserting on the plantar medial aspect of the first cuneiform and plantar base of the first metatarsal.

of the tibia, it becomes tendinous and is surrounded by a synovial sheath.

Innervated by the deep peroneal nerve, the anterior tibial tendon functions to dorsiflex and invert the foot and provides controlled plantar flexion at heel strike. The tendon is active in heel strike phase in an *eccentric* mode as it allows the ankle to slowly plantar flex until foot flat. It is active again in the swing phase in a *concentric* mode, dorsiflexing the ankle and keeping the forefoot from dragging.

The tendon passes beneath the superior extensor retinaculum and the upper and lower limbs of the inferior extensor retinaculum. Petersen et al[49] investigated the structure and vascular pattern of the tibialis anterior tendon using injection techniques, light and transmission electron microscopy, and immunohistochemistry. They found a well-vascularized peritenon, with blood vessels penetrating the tendon and anastomosing with a longitudinally oriented intratendinous network. Despite a well-vascularized posterior surface of the tendon, they found an avascular zone where the tendon runs under the superior and inferior retinacula.

Not only is the tendon vulnerable to spontaneous rupture here but, as the tendon passes beneath these retinacular structures, it also lies on the distal surface of the tibia and is at risk for injury with fracture of the tibia or a laceration. Lipscomb and Kelly[12] stated that the tendon had 6 to 7 cm of excursion at this level.

An acute disruption of the anterior tibial tendon can occur with trauma at any age from fracture of the tibia or laceration.[29,41] Three quarters of these disruptions occur in male patients. A spontaneous rupture can occur from an underlying degenerative process. Inflammatory arthritis,[33,37] gout, rheumatoid arthritis,[41,48] impingement from an underlying exostosis, a local steroid injection,[33,51] and diabetes[25,33,37,39,48] have all been cited as contributing factors in anterior tibial tendon rupture (Fig. 22–8).

Ruptures occur near the anterior tibial tendon's insertion, most often close to or within 2 to 3 cm of the insertion (Fig. 22–9). They can be caused by chronic wear from an exostosis at the first metatarsocuneiform (MTC) joint or by attrition from rubbing against the edge of the inferior extensor retinaculum. McMaster[13] noted that ruptures occur in the presence of an abnormal tendon structure. This correlates well with the deficiency in the tendon's vascular supply.

Markarian et al[41] have described "acute on chronic" tears manifesting as a degenerative tear in the anterior tibial tendon. These ruptures usually occur in men between the fifth and seventh decades of life and most often are reported in the seventh decade.[25,30] They appear to develop as an age-related phenomenon.

Anterior tibial tendon ruptures occur with forced or excessive plantar flexion[25,39,43,52] against a contracted anterior tibial muscle. An acute rupture is usually one of two different clinical presentations. With acute trauma in a younger patient who is involved with a higher functional level of activity, the rupture is associated with acute onset of pain but infrequently with severe trauma. Decreased dorsiflexion strength is noted at the time of injury, which usually prompts the patient to seek medical evaluation and treatment soon after injury. On the other hand, an older patient typically has no history of antecedent trauma and presents several months after the incident with a complaint of a painless drop foot.[50] Often a patient does not remember a precipitating event,[52] and the older patient often is unaware of the condition.[30] Markarian et al[41] reported an average 10-week delay in diagnosis in their series of 16 anterior tibial tendon disruptions. Late diagnosis is common, and permanent disability is rare.

The patient often experiences a snapping sensation that is associated with a brief episode of sharp pain over the anterior aspect of the ankle and is accompanied by swelling. Ambulation may be difficult in the initial few hours after rupture, but the pain subsides rapidly. A patient might note lack of coordination, a slapping gait, or an inability to clear the toes with ambulation. In time, the anterior tibial muscle atrophies.

The anterior tibial tendon is rarely involved with tendinitis, although Burman[26] and Goldman[34] have described such cases.

History and Physical Examination

A patient with anterior tibial tendon rupture often complains of swelling of the anterior ankle and foot, has weak dorsiflexion, and reports catching the foot on irregular or uneven ground.[50] Foot drop may be significant or minimal. The mild pain associated with a tendon rupture usually subsides quickly.[39,41] Swelling of the anterior ankle can disguise the rupture, although with time a palpable defect becomes apparent.[37,39,43] A fixed lump or mass on the anterior ankle can develop from the bulbous end of the proximal tendon segment (Fig. 22–10). The proximal tendon often retracts to the level of the ankle joint, and the mass is found deep to the extensor retinaculum and is often adherent to the synovial sheath.[25,39] Typically the area of the anterior tibial tendon lacks normal contour as it crosses the ankle.

A lack of dorsiflexion power might not be appreciated by the examiner unless muscle strength is compared with the contralateral side. However, weakness in dorsiflexion against resistance can make the diagnosis more apparent.[12,29,37,39] The patient is typically

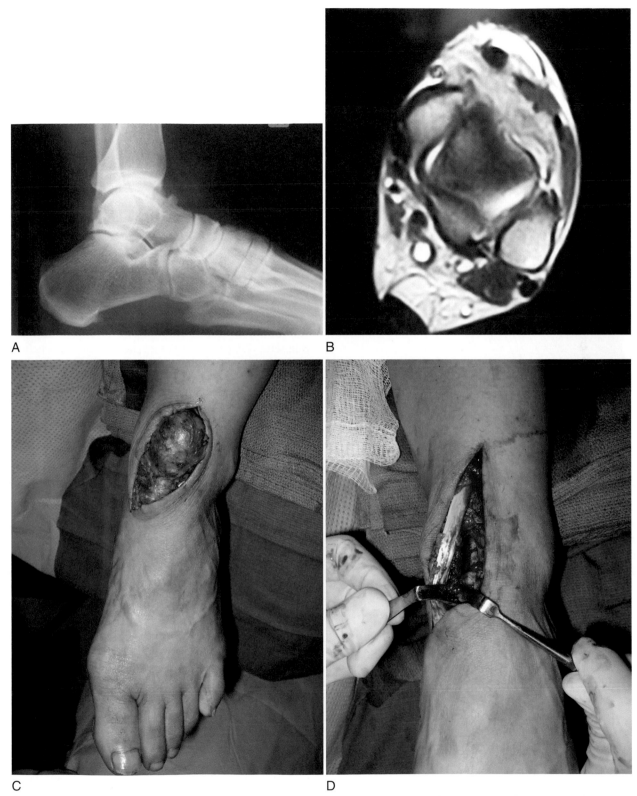

Figure 22–8 Ganglion of the anterior ankle region eroding the anterior tibial tendon, masquerading as a tendon rupture. **A,** Lateral radiograph with dorsal talar spur. **B,** Magnetic resonance image demonstrating a mass anterior to the anterior tibial tendon. **C,** Mass at surgery. **D,** Following resection, the anterior tibial tendon is intact. The joint is exposed to remove the osteophytes.

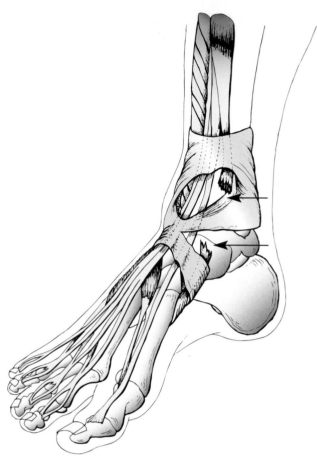

Figure 22–9 Spontaneous rupture of anterior tibial tendon (*arrows*) typically occurs in distal 3 cm of tendon.

unable to walk on the heel. Many patients are able to dorsiflex the ankle using the remaining dorsiflexors (EHL, EDL),[12] and Moberg[44] has reported that anterior tibial tendon function can be replaced to a large extent by the toe extensors. Patients often do not recognize anterior tibial dysfunction because of the remaining dorsiflexion power of the EHL and EDL and do not seek treatment until many months after injury (Fig. 22–11).

Without anterior tibial tendon function, a gait disturbance typically occurs.[25,41,52] With a drop foot, slap foot, or steppage gait, typically after heel strike, the patient is unable to plantar flex the foot slowly in a controlled manner.[12,25,42,43] The abnormal gait occurs as the patient attempts to clear the toes from catching on the ground with ambulation.

Mensor and Ordway[42] reported a slight loss (10 to 15 degrees) of dorsiflexion after anterior tibial tendon rupture. Burman[27] and Moberg[44] reported development of a spontaneous flatfoot deformity following anterior tibial tendon rupture.

This condition can be misdiagnosed as a peroneal palsy or confused with an L4-5 radiculopathy.[43,46] Per-

oneal nerve palsy and lumbar disk syndrome can easily be ruled out on neurologic examination with normal sensation on the dorsum of the foot, normal sensation in the first web space, and normal function of the other extensor tendons with active dorsiflexion of the toes.[37] Heel varus and eversion weakness in conjunction with the loss of dorsiflexion suggests a common peroneal nerve palsy or radiculopathy and makes the diagnosis of tibialis anterior rupture unlikely. In patients with acute anterior tibial disruption, the injury is often associated with laceration or a distal tibial fracture. Open injuries after a fracture or laceration can occur but require assessment of motion and strength of the anterior tibial tendon so that a tendon disruption is not overlooked. Surgical exploration of traumatic wounds should be considered if there is any notion of weakness, a gap, or deformation of the anterior ankle.

Imaging

Magnetic resonance imaging (MRI) can be helpful in defining an anterior tibial rupture.[35,36,39,47,48] Normal tendons have a low signal intensity contrast well with surrounding fat, which has a high signal intensity. Both sagittal and axial images are helpful. In patients presenting late who do not recall a precipitating accident or event, MRI can be helpful in making a diagnosis of rupture (Fig. 22–12).[52]

Treatment

Ruptures of the anterior tibial tendon are uncommon. No consensus appears to exist regarding recommendations of surgical versus nonsurgical treatment; however, the ultimate goal remains improved function. When an anterior tibial tendon rupture is diagnosed early in a younger active patient, surgical repair is likely to improve ambulation and decrease morbidity. Treatment of an old rupture is more controversial and appears to lead to unpredictable results.[52] Unfortunately, ruptures in older patients are often initially unnoticed.

For the older patient, bracing or a polypropylene ankle–foot orthosis (AFO) or a double upright brace may be prescribed. Ouzounian and Anderson[48] noted that of five patients treated conservatively, three refused a brace or found it too restrictive. Two patients who used a brace found it improved their level of activity. Compliance in the older patient can be difficult. With nonsurgical treatment the proximal tendon segment usually becomes adherent in the area of the anterior ankle. Some loss of ankle dorsiflexion strength and motion develops. In elderly, sedentary patients with a low level of activity, a normal gait

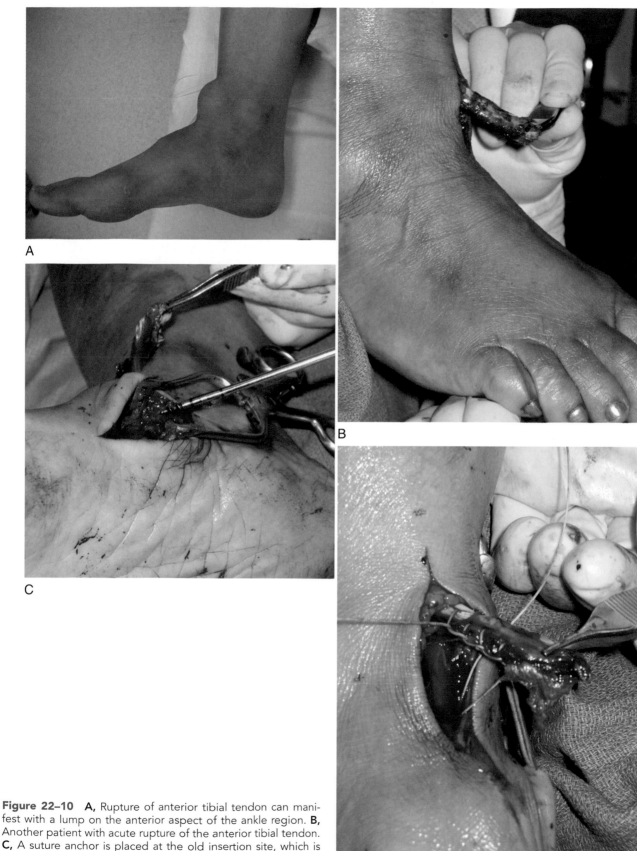

Figure 22–10 **A,** Rupture of anterior tibial tendon can manifest with a lump on the anterior aspect of the ankle region. **B,** Another patient with acute rupture of the anterior tibial tendon. **C,** A suture anchor is placed at the old insertion site, which is prepared by lifting off local periosteum. **D,** Krackow suture placed in the distal tendon stump. *Continued* D

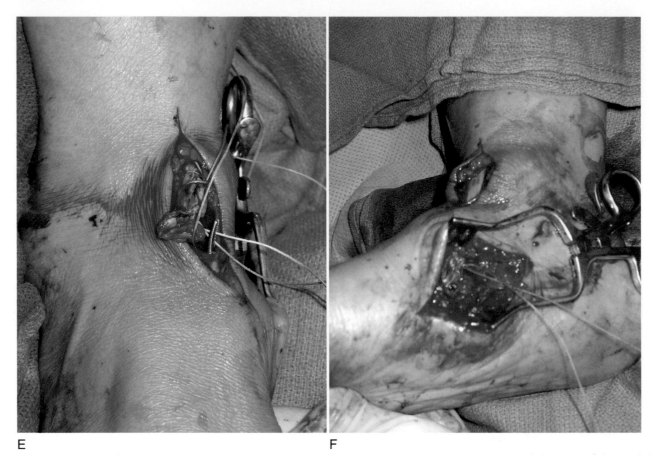

E   F

Figure 22–10—cont'd   E, Distal tendon is passed through a tunnel into its position at the plantar medial aspect of the medial cuneiform. **F,** Following repair of the anterior tibial tendon to suture anchor.

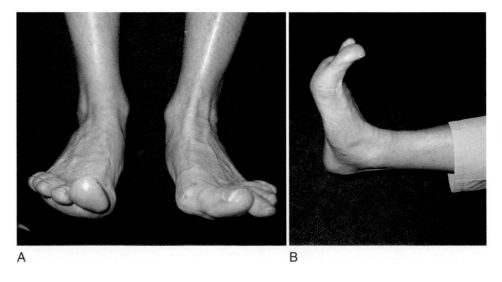

A   B

Figure 22–11   A, Intact anterior tibial tendon on the left foot, rupture on the right. **B,** The extensor digitorum longus and extensor hallucis longus are recruited to dorsiflex the ankle. Note extension of toes with ankle dorsiflexion. The injured ankle dorsiflexes less and everts more due to the tendon imbalance. The medial ray is still relatively plantar flexed.

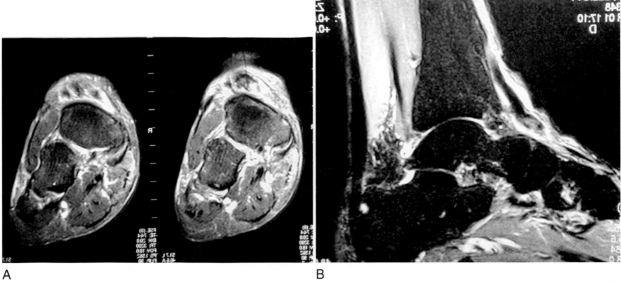

A   B

Figure 22–12 Magnetic resonance image demonstrates rupture of the left anterior tibial tendon off its insertion. **A,** At the level of the naviculum, the anterior tibial tendon is indistinct dorsomedially. **B,** Sagittal view demonstrates the anterior tibial tendon, which appears wavy due to loss of tension. It is surrounded by synovial fluid, and distally the tendon cannot be traced, ending abruptly in a widened fibrotic mass just dorsal to the naviculum.

pattern actually may be achieved, justifying conservative treatment.[30,43]

Markarian et al[41] found no significant difference in the conservative and surgical treatment in elderly patients and suggested that nonsurgical treatment was a viable option and "should not adversely affect overall foot and ankle function."

Decreased dorsiflexion strength,[33,43] incoordination or a slapping gait,[42] and progressive flatfoot deformity[33] may be associated with nonsurgical treatment. Although full functional recovery might not be obtained, function and gait in the older, less active patient may be acceptable.[30,41,43,44,46]

For patients who want a higher level of function, surgical repair is indicated. Surgical intervention can entail direct repair for the acute rupture or reconstruction of the anterior tibial tendon with either a tendon transfer or an interposition tendon graft for delayed treatment.

Both surgical and conservative treatments have been advocated for anterior tibial tendon ruptures, and treatment should be tailored to the individual patient depending on age, level of activity, time elapsed since the rupture occurred, current level of disability, and local and systemic contraindications to surgery. Nonsurgical treatment is preferred in the older patient with fewer demands, and surgical repair is typically indicated in the younger and middle-aged active athlete. Markarian et al[41] concluded that although primary repair is the optimal treatment for a ruptured anterior tibial tendon, when diagnosis is delayed longer than 4 weeks, the treating physician should "consider the physical demands and goals of the patient" before automatically recommending surgery.

Acute Surgical Treatment

With a laceration of the anterior tibial tendon, the proximal segment may be found anywhere along the course of the tendon. Often it retracts to the level of the ankle joint. With a rupture, the proximal stump is often found deep to the extensor retinaculum and is often adherent to the synovial sheath. The site of rupture is typically just proximal to the site of the tendon insertion and just distal to the inferior border of the superior extensor retinaculum.

Lipscomb and Kelly[12] and others recommend direct repair of the anterior tibial tendon. Its reinsertion into the navicular is an alternative with an avulsion fracture or distal rupture. The technique of repair and reconstruction depends on the pathologic process present and the time delay in diagnosis. Ouzounian and Anderson[48] prefer a direct repair with reinsertion of the anterior tibial tendon into bone.

With delay in diagnosis and retraction of the proximal tendon stump or with injury to a large segment of tendon, direct repair might be impossible. Tendon reconstruction is then an option. An extensor tendon graft, tendon transfer,[48] or partial tendon advancement[40] are surgical options for reconstruction. Although the tendon may be advanced through a drill hole, it may be reinforced with bone anchors or a pull-out wire as well.[31]

PRIMARY REPAIR OF RUPTURED TIBIAL TENDON

Surgical Technique

1. The patient is placed in a supine position with a thigh tourniquet for hemostasis. An anterior curvilinear incision is made on the inferomedial aspect of the anterior tibial tendon and extended from the level of the first cuneiform proximally to the level of the superior extensor retinaculum.
2. The anteroinferior extensor retinaculum is divided, and the anterior tibial tendon is identified and traced to its insertion in the first cuneiform.
3. The dorsalis pedis artery and deep peroneal nerve lie on the lateral aspect of the EHL, and the dissection is deepened on the medial aspect of the EHL to protect the neurovascular bundle.
4. Because the proximal stump of the tendon often retracts to the level of the ankle joint after rupture, exploration should proceed proximally to identify the end of the tendon. The tendon sheath is incised longitudinally and the hematoma debrided (Fig. 22–13A and B). After debridement of the tendon ends, a no. 1 nonabsorbable suture is used to approximate the tendons with a Bunnell, Krackow, or modified Kessler technique (Fig 22–13C; see also Fig. 22–3A-C). The tendon edges are then oversewn with an interrupted absorbable suture. If the tendon has avulsed or is lacerated from its distal attachment, a suture anchor can be inserted into the cuneiform and the tendon secured to the periosteum. Fig. 22–13D-F
5. The synovial sheath is repaired, but the inferior extensor retinaculum is not repaired to prevent formation of adhesions (Fig. 22–13G).
6. The skin is approximated in a routine manner.

Postoperative Care

A below-knee cast is applied with the foot in maximum dorsiflexion. Weight bearing is permitted 2 to 3 weeks after surgery. Immobilization is continued for 12 weeks during the day and at night as well. Range-of-motion exercises are initiated 6 to 8 weeks after surgery. Progressive resumption of walking then begins, followed by jogging, jumping, running, or aggressive athletic activities.

Alternate Techniques

The anterior tibial tendon also may be lengthened using a sliding anterior tibial tendon graft that spans the rupture site, anastomosing the proximal and distal segments of the tendon.[37,40] Several different tendon transfers have been described to bridge a gap in the anterior tibial tendon. Forst et al[33] accomplished a delayed repair bridging an extensive defect with a peroneus brevis tendon graft. Moberg[44] recommended an EHL tendon transfer to the distal stump of the anterior tibial tendon. The more proximal EHL tendon is tenodesed to the distal anterior tibial tendon stump, which is secured through a drill hole into the medial cuneiform or into the distal stump of the anterior tibial tendon. Postoperative care is similar to that described for a primary repair.

Results and Complications

Mankey[40] reported that uniformly good results were achieved with reconstruction of a ruptured anterior tibial tendon. Morris et al[45] reported that patients with repaired anterior tibial tendons had weakness in dorsiflexion relative to the contralateral side. Despite finding a 75% average peak torque strength and 62% of work capacity compared to the contralateral side, there was no functional impairment.[45] Most studies recommend surgical reconstruction for a symptomatic patient with moderate or greater levels of physical activity. Other than failure of reconstruction, no significant complications have been reported in the literature. The patient should be alerted to potential complications, including adhesions, rerupture, neuroma formation, and decreased function not only at the rupture site but also at the donor site, where a tendon is harvested to aid in the anterior tibial tendon reconstruction.

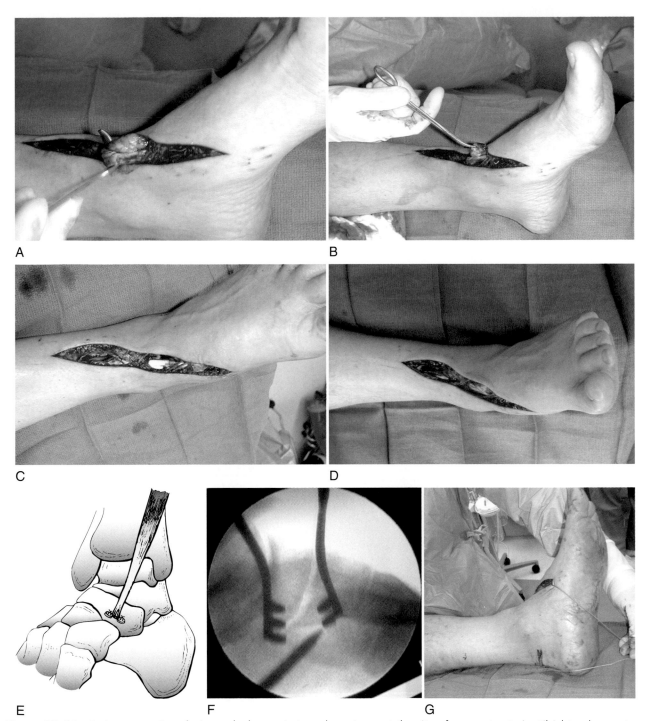

Figure 22–13 **A,** Intraoperative photograph demonstrates a hematoma at the site of a recent anterior tibial tendon rupture. **B,** Ruptured anterior tibial tendon is pulled into the wound. **C** and **D,** Intraoperative photograph demonstrates primary repair of the tendon, with adequate dorsiflexion of ankle following repair. **E** and **F,** Placement of suture anchor into the navicular. **G,** Lateral view of ankle brought into dorsiflexion with securing of the tendon to the suture anchor.

Delayed Surgical Treatment

Markarian et al[41] defined four options in the delayed treatment of an anterior tibial rupture: primary repair, reconstruction with an adjacent tendon transfer, nonanatomic repair, and conservative management. Which ever option is chosen, it is important to recognize that a secondary Achilles tendon contracture may be present. Typically if a contracture is identified, aggressive stretching pre- and postoperatively can minimize its consequences. If the Achilles is determined to be too contracted, with a 10- to 15-degree difference compared to the contralateral side, an Achilles lengthening or Strayer procedure will be beneficial.

A similar surgical approach is used for a delayed repair as for an acute repair. If an end-to-end repair is not possible after the proximal segment is mobilized, the gap may be bridged with a tendon graft. This may be a sliding tendon graft using the anterior tibial tendon, although the sliding graft can leave a scar beneath the more proximal extensor retinaculum.[38,40,41]

7. A modified Bunnell, Krackow, or Kessler suture is used to anastomose the tendon graft at the proximal and distal ends (see Fig. 22–3A-C).
8. The tendon sheath is repaired, but the inferior extensor retinaculum is not repaired in order to prevent formation of adhesions.
9. The skin is approximated in a routine manner.

Postoperative Care

A below-knee cast is applied with the foot in the maximally dorsiflexed position. Weight bearing is permitted 2 to 3 weeks after surgery using a boot brace or AFO. Immobilization is continued until 12 weeks, and range-of-motion exercises are initiated 9 to 12 weeks after surgery. The patient is cautioned to avoid jumping, running, or aggressive athletic activity for at least 12 to 16 weeks after surgery.

When the proximal stump of the anterior tibial tendon is of insufficient length for repair, the adjacent EHL or EDL tendon can be used as a graft.[30,44,47]

ANTERIOR TIBIAL TENDON SLIDING GRAFT

Surgical Technique

1. The patient is placed in a supine position with a thigh tourniquet for hemostasis.
2. An anterior curvilinear incision is made on the inferomedial aspect of the anterior tibial tendon and extended from the level of the first cuneiform proximally to the level of the superior extensor retinaculum (Fig. 22–14A).
3. The anteroinferior extensor retinaculum is divided and the anterior tibial tendon is identified. The distal stump is traced to its insertion in the first cuneiform. The proximal stump is identified. It may have retracted several centimeters proximally (Fig. 22–14B).
4. With extensive retraction, a tendon transfer may be necessary. On the other hand, to bridge a 2- to 4-cm gap, a sliding graft may be performed (Fig. 22–14C-E).
5. A sliding tendon graft may be performed if the proximal tendon is healthy or of sufficient size (Fig. 22–14F).
6. One half the width of the tendon is harvested from the proximal tendon and transferred distally. The length of tendon must be sufficient to bridge the defect.

EXTENSOR HALLUCIS LONGUS TRANSFER

1. A similar exposure is used as described for the technique of primary repair or sliding tendon graft.
2. After the fibrous tissue and hematoma are debrided at the rupture site, the EHL tendon is dissected distally at the level of the first MTP joint and detached.
3. The proximal stump of the anterior tibial tendon is sutured to the adjacent EHL tendon.
4. The EHL tendon is divided and tenodesed to the EHB (Fig. 22–15A and B).

Alternative Technique

A horizontal or vertical drill hole is made in the first cuneiform, and the tendon is passed through the bony tunnel and fixed with either a pull-out wire or a bony anchor (Fig. 22–15C). Because the EHL graft is long, it is possible to drill from the first cuneiform to the third, exiting just dorsal to the cuboid laterally. This tunnel can be drilled using the guide wire for the cannulated 6.5-, 7.0-, or 7.3-mm screw systems and then overdrilled once proper position is estab-

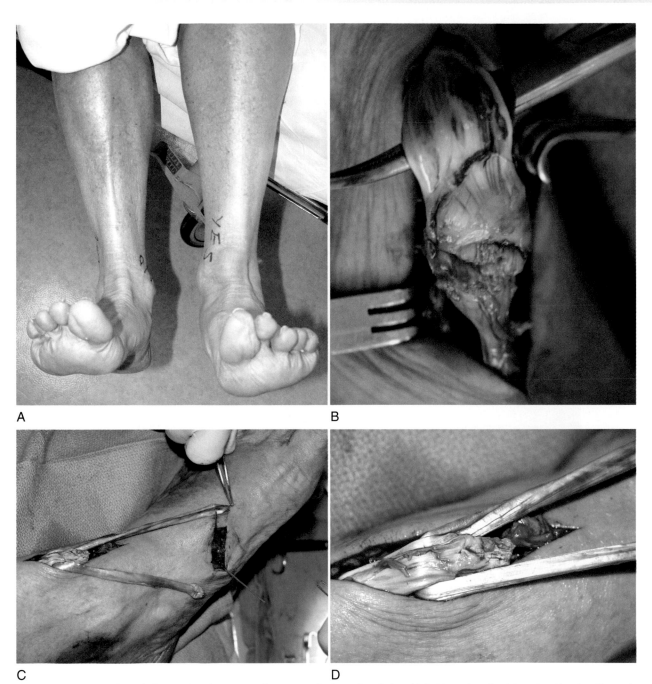

A

B

C

D

Figure 22–14   **A,** Delayed diagnosis of rupture of anterior tibial tendon (left ankle). Note that the injured ankle dorsiflexes less and everts more. The medial ray is still relatively plantar flexed. **B,** Intraoperative photo of rupture. **C,** Free tendon graft is passed through the distal end of the healthier aspect of the tendon, creating two graft ends for attachment. One limb is passed into a tunnel in the dorsal aspect of the cuneiform and the other is passed into a more plantar medial tunnel as indicated by the protruding wires. The graft is secured using 6- to 7-mm-wide soft tissue interference screws. **D,** Close-up of graft through the anterior tibial tendon.   *Continued*

lished with the set's cannulated drill bit. Using a suction tip from the lateral side, the sutures in the EHL can be passed from medial to lateral. While tension is applied on the graft with the ankle held in dorsiflexion, a soft tissue interference screw can be inserted medially and, if nec-essary, an additional one can be inserted later-ally. In the presence of a tendon avulsion from the medial cuneiform insertion or with minimal tendon retraction, the tendon can be advanced and reinserted through a drill hole in the first cuneiform (Fig. 22–16).[31]

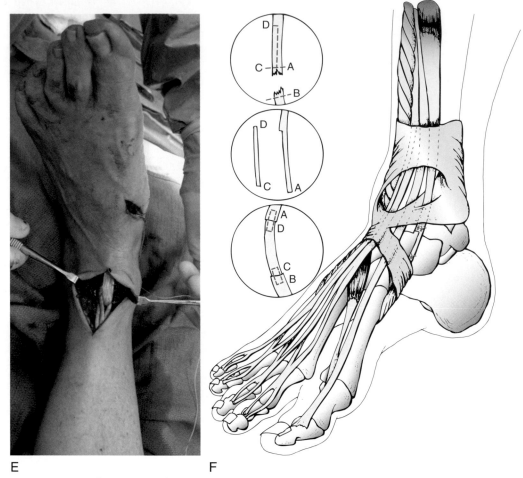

Figure 22–14—cont'd E, Following completion of repair. Tensioning the graft is critical to achieve dorsiflexion. **F,** Technique of sliding tendon graft as a delayed repair to bridge a defect in the tendon.

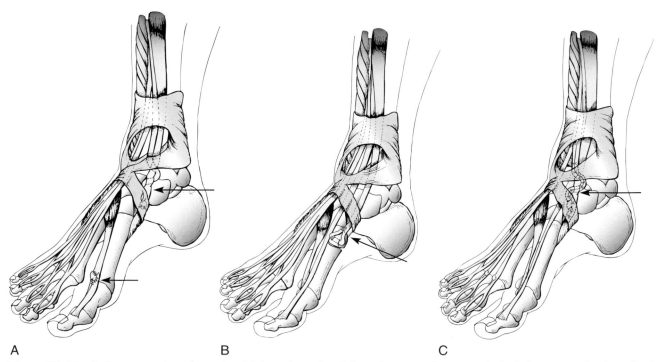

Figure 22–15 A, Reconstruction of anterior tibial tendon using Pulvertaft weave of extensor hallucis longus tendon into distal anterior tibial tendon. **B,** Reconstruction of distal rupture of anterior tibial tendon. Tendon is advanced through a horizontal drill hole in the navicular or first cuneiform and sutured to itself. **C,** Reconstruction of ruptured anterior tibial tendon using Kelikian procedure. Extensor digitorum longus (EDL) tendon to second and third toes is woven through anterior tibial tendon. EDL tendon to second and third toes is tenodesed to the extensor digitorum brevis. (**A** and **C** redrawn from Markarian G, Kelikian A, Brage M, et al: *Foot Ankle Int* 19:792-802, 1998.)

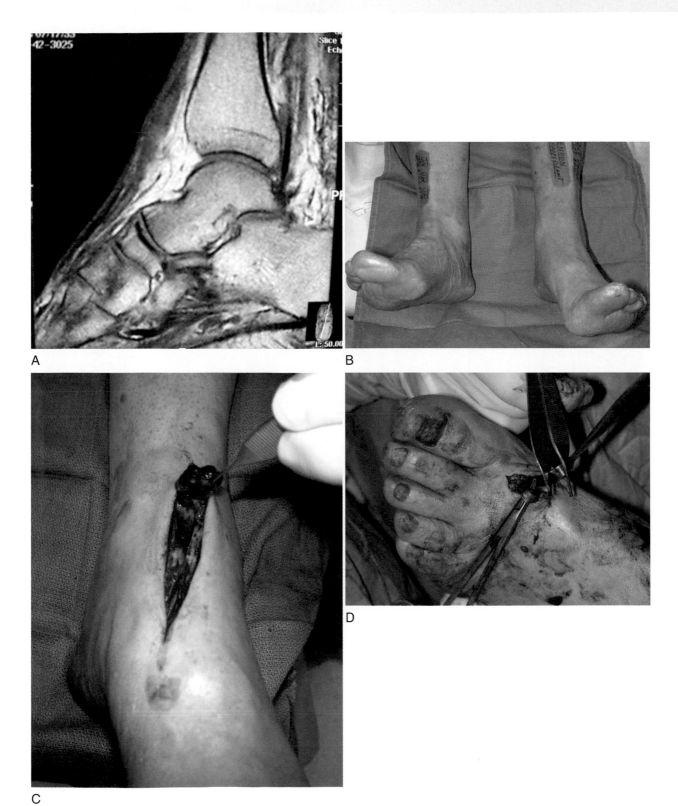

A

B

C

D

Figure 22–16 Reconstruction of chronic anterior tibial tendon with turndown and extensor hallucis longus (EHL) tendon graft. **A,** Sagittal magnetic resonance image demonstrating a long zone of fibrotic ruptured anterior tibial tendon. **B,** Clinical appearance of chronic anterior tibial tendon rupture. **C,** End of ruptured tendon. **D,** EHL tendon is identified distally and anastomosed to the extensor hallucis brevis before transection. *Continued*

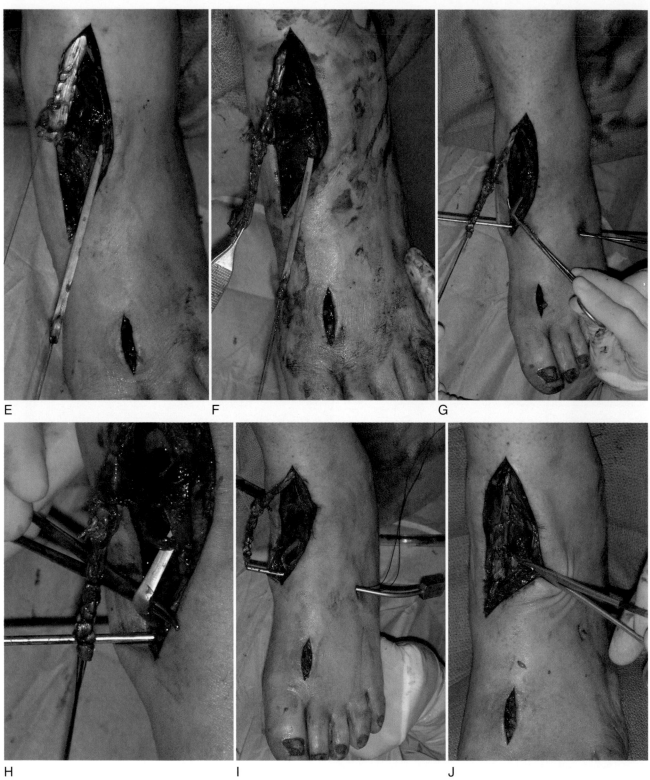

E

F

G

H

I

J

Figure 22–16—cont'd   **E,** The Krackow stitch is placed in the anterior tibial tendon and the EHL is prepared for transfer. The anterior tibial tendon is too short, so the sutures are removed and a turndown (**F**) is performed. **G,** The EHL is tunneled through a drill hole through all the cuneiforms from medial to lateral. The tunnel is wide enough to insert the anterior tibial tendon as well. The drill bit demonstrates the pathway. The clamp is under the EHL, whose suture protrudes laterally. **H,** A close-up of the transfers, **I,** A suction tip is placed from lateral to medial to help pass the anterior tibial tendon graft. **J,** The tendons are in the tunnel and fixed with suture anchors medially and laterally under proper tension.

Postoperative Care

A below-knee cast is applied with the foot in the maximally dorsiflexed position. Weight bearing is permitted 2 to 3 weeks after surgery using a boot brace or AFO. Immobilization is continued until 12 weeks, when range-of-motion exercises are initiated. The patient is cautioned to avoid jumping, running, or aggressive athletic activity for at least 12 to 16 weeks after surgery.

Other Techniques

Kelikian and Kelikian[38] suggested transferring the EDL tendon of the second and third toes to the distal stump of the anterior tibial tendon. A tenodesis of the EDB to the distal stumps of the EDL of the second and third toes is then performed (see Fig. 22–15C).

Forst et al[33] used a peroneus brevis tendon transfer, tenodesing the peroneus longus and brevis proximally. Then they resected a 9-cm segment of peroneus brevis, using this as a free graft to bridge the defect at the site of the anterior tibial tendon rupture. If the anterior tibial muscle is no longer viable as a motor, the peroneus longus can be used. It is harvested distally by the cuboid and passed from posterior behind the fibula into the anterior compartment and then inserted into the lateral cuneiform.

Conclusion

Although ruptures of the anterior tibial tendon occur infrequently, accurate early diagnosis enables a patient and physician to choose between conservative and surgical treatment. For the older patient with a lower level of activity, bracing or nonsurgical treatment may be sufficient. In those desiring a higher level of function, either acute repair or delayed reconstruction with a tendon transfer may be indicated. Although a direct primary repair is preferable, a tendon transfer or graft may be necessary to span a significant gap. The ultimate goal is improved function, and treatment should be adapted to the patient's needs. Nonsurgical treatment is probably sufficient in the older, less-active patient, and surgical repair is indicated in the more active, younger patient.

FLEXOR TENDONS

Flexor Digitorum Longus Tenosynovitis

The flexor digitorum longus (FDL) is the primary plantar flexor of the lateral four toes. Innervated by the tibial nerve, the FDL originates on the posterior tibia below the soleal line and functions to plantar flex the toes and to plantar flex and invert the foot. Lying just posterior to the posterior tibial tendon at the ankle, it courses on the plantar aspect of the tarsus in the deep midfoot before inserting on the distal phalanx of the lateral four toes. It is at risk for laceration in the toes as well as more proximally with penetrating injuries.

History and Physical Examination

Although no cases of spontaneous FDL rupture have been reported, flexor tendon ruptures following cortisone injections for interdigital neuromas have been known (Fig. 22–17). In general, FDL injury is almost

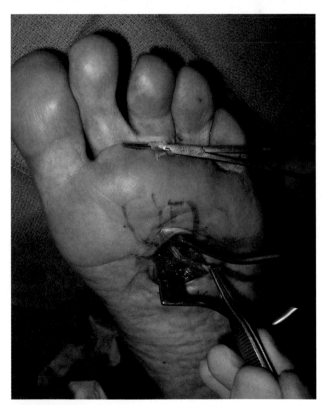

Figure 22–17 Rupture of flexor digitorum longus. The patient had received multiple cortisone injections as treatment for interdigital neuromas. He ultimately developed a bothersome dorsiflexion posture of the toe and an unstable painful metatarsophalangeal joint and an inability to flex the toe. At surgery, the flexor tendon was identified distal and proximal to the weight-bearing plantar fat pad. The tendon ends proximally and distally are sutured with a free graft of extensor digitorum brevis, which was interposed. The tendon is passed through the sheath with a clamp and secured.

always associated with a penetrating laceration. A patient often describes a history of stepping on a piece of glass or sharp object with resultant loss of plantar flexion power to one or more of the lesser toes. Concomitant sensory loss may be noted as well.

On physical examination, a laceration distal to the knot of Henry is often associated with weakness or absence of plantar flexion of the lesser toes. Most patients have poor individual control of flexion and extension of the lesser toes, but diagnosis of FDL disruption can be demonstrated by stabilizing the MTP joint and asking the patient to plantar flex the tip of the toe. Weakness or absence of plantar flexion strength to one or more of the lesser toes can demonstrate an isolated disruption of the FDL to an individual toe or a complete disruption of the FDL.[18] Because specific function of the FDL is at the DIP joint, lack of flexion power indicates a rupture (Figs. 22–18 and 22–19).

Proximal to the master knot of Henry, because of a connecting slip from the flexor hallucis longus (FHL), flexion of the DIP joint can remain despite a proximal disruption of the FHL. Often, injury to an adjacent digital sensory nerve is associated with injuries of the FHL or FDL. Chronic FDL rupture can lead to a hammer toe or swan neck deformity. Patients might complain that the toe gets caught on the inside of a shoe or sock while donning.

Surgical Treatment

While exploring a laceration, the surgeon should keep in mind the principles of trauma care, including adequate irrigation and debridement of the wound. The wound should be explored in a way that does not complicate or magnify the injury. Extension of the laceration longitudinally allows an extensile exposure. When possible, a primary repair of the injured tendons is appropriate using a Bunnell repair, modified Kessler technique, or Krackow tendon repair (see Fig. 22–3A-C).

Postoperative care necessitates immobilization in a below-knee cast for 4 to 6 weeks if the disruption is at or proximal to the master knot. Extension of the cast over the dorsal aspect of the toes prevents excessive dorsiflexion and possible disruption of the repair. If the laceration is distal to the master knot, the toe can be held flexed after repair by gluing a metal hook to the toenail and attaching it to a rubber band that is connected proximally and plantarly to a splint or dressing (Fig. 22–20).

In a review of preferences of many orthopaedic surgeons, Yancey[95] found that 80% to 93% thought repair of the FHL was important, but only 53% to 73% believed surgical repair of a lacerated FDL was indicated. One FDL laceration was not repaired and had a satisfactory result. Floyd et al[6] reported on lacerated FDL in seven patients: Five underwent a primary repair,

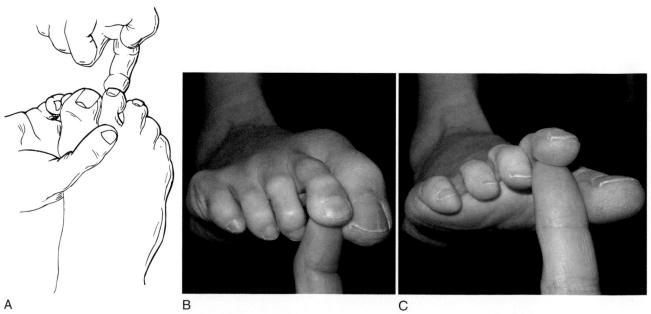

A   B   C

Figure 22–18   A, Function of the flexor digitorum longus tendon can be assessed by grasping the forefoot, stabilizing the metatarsophalangeal joint, and requesting the patient to flex the tip of the toe against resistance. **B,** Clinical photo of intact tendon. **C,** Absence of flexor strength following disruption of the flexor digitorum longus. (**A** redrawn from Rooks M: In Gould JS [ed]: *Operative Foot Surgery.* Philadelphia, WB Saunders, 1994, p 518.)

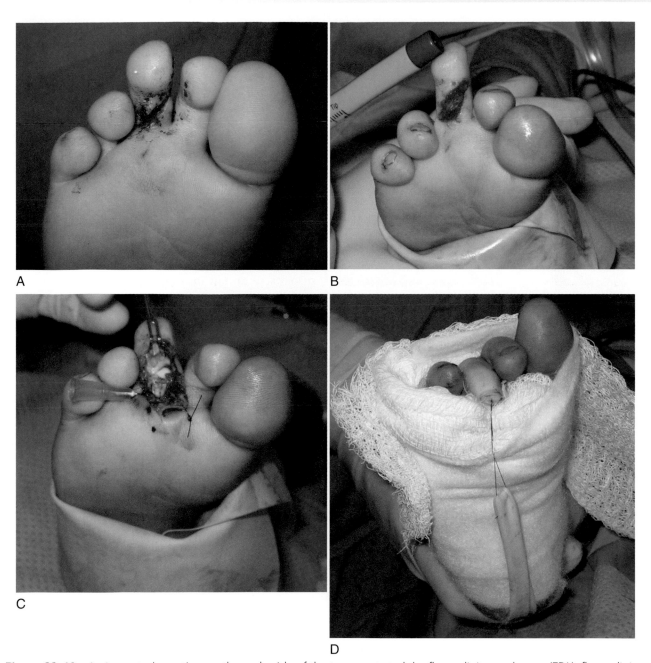

Figure 22–19 **A,** An acute laceration on the underside of the toe penetrated the flexor digitorum longus (FDL), flexor digito-rum brevis, and plantar proximal interphalangeal capsule. **B,** There is no resistance to extension of the digit. **C,** The laceration is extended, creating a Z-shaped incision. The flap of skin is sutured to the sole of the foot to permit retraction. A 25-gauge needle is passed through the proximal tendon once it is delivered into the wound to keep it in position during suturing. One limb of the FDL is repaired—not both–to avoid bulk and difficulty reestablishing tendon gliding. The flexor hallucis brevis and capsule are also repaired. The sutures were placed in all the structures and then the knots were tied with the toe in the flexed position. **D,** 3-0 nylon is placed through the tip of the nail and then looped around a Penrose drain, which is anchored into the dressing to maintain flexion.

one underwent a secondary repair, and one was left unrepaired. The six patients undergoing surgical repair did well. The patient who did not have a repair developed a claw toe deformity. Griffiths[7] reported on one patient who underwent a primary repair with an acceptable result. Wicks et al[24] reported on eight patients who underwent primary repair of a lacerated FDL, with six satisfactory results. A hyperextension deformity of the lesser MTP joint developed in the two patients with poor results.

Korovessis et al[68] reported on disruption of the FDL and posterior tibial tendon more proximally at the site

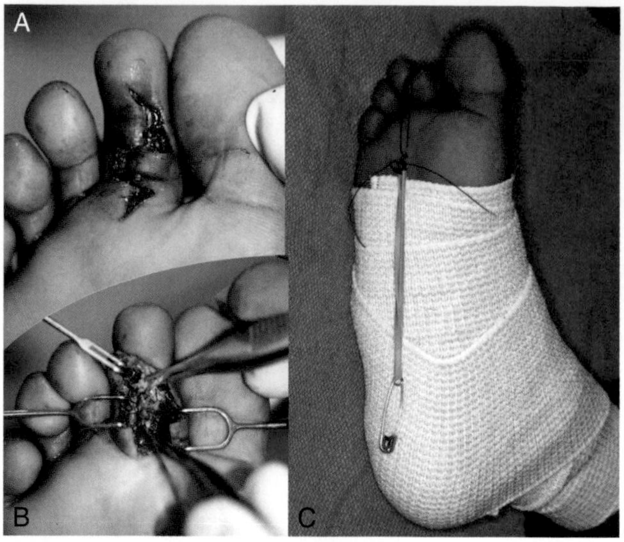

Figure 22–20 Laceration of the flexor digitorum longus in the phalangeal region. **A,** Acute injury. **B,** Following repair. **C,** Use of dynamic splint to protect repair.

of a fractured tibia that was repaired primarily with good result.

The actual site of injury is an important factor in developing a treatment plan for FDL disruption. An injury distal to the knot of Henry leaves the patient without plantar flexion power, whereas an injury proximal to the knot of Henry might leave plantar flexion power because of the crossover attachment of the FHL. Remaining function can obviate the need for a surgical repair. Treatment of an FDL injury 4 to 6 weeks or longer after injury is likely to be associated with difficulty in reapproximating the tendon.

Aggressive evaluation and repair of open lacerations around the foot are most important. The wound must be explored and debrided, and when possible, an anatomic restoration of the tendons of the FDL is warranted. With significant soft tissue loss, repair of these structures might not be possible. The overall priority is to achieve adequate wound healing and maintain a good plantar weight-bearing surface for ambulation. If a hyperextension deformity occurs postoperatively, the surgeon should consider an extensor tenotomy, extensor tendon lengthening, or MTP capsulotomy to rebalance clawed toes.

Flexor Hallucis Longus

The FHL is the major plantar flexor of the great toe. It assists with maintaining balance and generating power during walking, running, jumping, and squatting. It permits rising up onto the ball of the foot and descending downward in a controlled fashion. It

works in conjunction with the intricately structured plantar plate and the multiple short flexors to stabilize the MTP joint. Although its action occurs at the MTP, IP, and ankle joints, it assists in stabilizing the subtalar and midfoot joints as well. It is more powerful than the FDL but weaker than the posterior tibial tendons.[89] Its role is important when considering that during normal gait, twice the load of the lesser toes is supported by the great toe,[90] which during jogging and running can approach two to three times body weight. Furthermore, when a running jump is performed, these forces increase to eight times body weight.[77]

The FHL originates from the inferior two thirds of the fibula and the interosseous membrane and courses along the posterior aspect of the tibia and talus. The tendinous extension of the FHL courses inferior to the sustentaculum tali in a fibro-osseous tunnel. Distally it crosses the flexor digitorum longus at the master knot of Henry, traverses the sole of the foot, and courses between the two heads of the flexor hallucis brevis (FHB) before inserting on the plantar aspect of the distal phalanx. Innervated by the tibial nerve, the FHL flexes the distal phalanx of the hallux and plantar flexes and inverts the foot. The FHL muscle is a strong muscle because the muscle fibers run obliquely to the pull of the tendon (oblique pennation). In muscles with oblique pennation, the cross-sectional diameter of the muscle that is perpendicular to the fibers is greater than the cross-sectional diameter of muscles whose fibers are collinear with the tendon, which are typically better suited to greater excursion than to strength.[54]

Petersen et al[79] studied the blood supply of the FHL tendon using injections and immunohistochemical studies of cadaver tendons. They found that peritendinous blood vessels penetrated the tendon and anastomosed with a longitudinally oriented intratendinous network. Two avascular zones were demonstrated: one near the posterior talus and the other at the first metatarsal head. The researchers thought that these explained the most typical areas for tendon degeneration and rupture.

Flexor Hallucis Longus Tenosynovitis

Tenosynovitis of the FHL tendon has been described by Lapidus and Seidenstein[70] and others.[71-73] Approximately 50 cases have been described in the literature, mainly as case reports, although series have been reported by Hamilton[63] (17 cases) and others.[64,67,85]

Most often, tenosynovitis develops proximally at the level of the sustentaculum tali as the tendon enters the fibro-osseous tunnel. Often associated with a plantar flexion en pointe position in ballet dancers (Fig. 22–21),[58,61,63,86,94] various pathologic conditions,

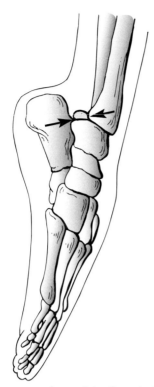

Figure 22–21 Tenosynovitis of the flexor hallucis longus may be associated with an os trigonum and may be exacerbated with forced plantar flexion typical of the en pointe position in ballet dancers.

including hypertrophy of the tendon, synovial adhesions, a more distal insertion of the FHL muscle, longitudinal degenerative tears, and nodularity in the region of the fibro-osseous tunnel, have been associated with this condition. McCarroll et al[75] and Kolettis et al[67] have implicated muscle elongation and a distal insertion of the FHL muscle as a cause of this condition.[64]

Gould[62] and Trevino et al[93] have observed that a distal stenosing tenosynovitis could occur at the level where the FHL courses between the sesamoids. Longitudinal tears of the FHL have been reported in association with tenosynovitis.[53,59,86] Hamilton[63] reported FHL tenosynovitis associated with a symptomatic os trigonum, although Kolettis et al[67] noted many cases without an os trigonum.

The spectrum of tenosynovitis, FHL triggering, nodularity, and tendon thickening in its natural course can lead to a degenerative tear of the FHL (Fig. 22–22). Frenette and Jackson[60] and others[61,63,86] have described stenosing tenosynovitis. Trepman et al[92] reported a patient who developed posteromedial ankle pain produced with active plantar flexion and passive dorsiflexion of the hallux. The patient had a tearing

sensation in the posteromedial ankle with concomitant swelling and ecchymosis. On exploration, a longitudinal tear of the FHL was identified and treated with a primary repair. Fusiform thickening, erosion of the tendon, and eventual triggering can develop from an overuse syndrome.

Another similar case is that of a professional dancer who had a history of triggering of the FHL behind the ankle and suddenly developed a more acute pain associated with a catching or locking of the hallux, which precluded dance. On exploration, a flap tear of the FHL was encountered in addition to the stenosis of the FHL sheath. Following release of the sheath and excision of the flap tear, the patient was able to return to Broadway as a principal dancer (Fig. 22–23). Thus, the mechanical irritation of the tendon not only may be a source of pain but can also be a risk factor for rupture or tear.

This has been observed by several authors including Sammarco and Miller[86] who reported fusiform thickening of the FHL tendon with rupture of the central fibers. Kolettis et al[67] reported stenosis of the tendon sheath, synovial hypertrophy, adhesions, mucoid degeneration, tendon nodularity, and several cases of partial FHL tears. Several partial ruptures have also been reported.[69,80,86] These can result from forced extension and against a contracted FHL muscle. Thickening or hypertrophy of the FHL[75] and the presence of a flexor digitorum accessorius longus[76] can lead to constriction in the fibro-osseous tunnel with subsequent tenosynovitis.

Entrapment or scarring of the FHL can also occur following distal tibial, ankle, or calcaneus fractures with a different presentation and prognosis that is important to recognize.[56,84,88] Patients complain of inability to roll through the forefoot and often a lack

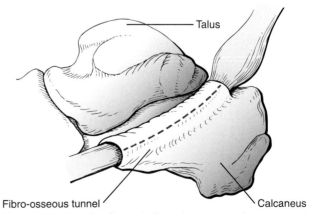

Figure 22–22 The flexor hallucis longus can be triggered from nodularity or tendon thickening with restricted motion in the fibro-osseous tunnel.

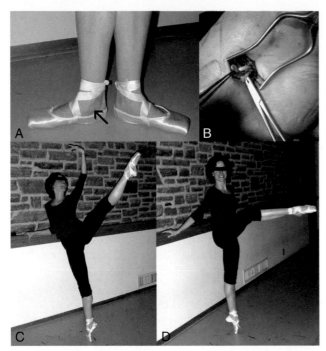

Figure 22–23 Flexor hallucis longus tenosynovitis in a professional dancer. **A,** Preoperative swelling of the tendon sheath with a painful limited range of motion of the ankle and great toe. **B,** Intraoperative photo of tendon sheath release. A flap tear of the tendon is identified and resected. Successful return to dancing with full power in the FHL to permit weight-bearing pointe work **(C)** and ability to perform flexion and extension without triggering, weakness, or pain **(D).**

of dorsiflexion flexibility at the ankle as well. In these cases, the deformity increases with dorsiflexion and decreases with plantarflexion of the ankle. This check-rein deformity has treatment implications. If the tendon is adherent to the local bone or soft tissues, it is amenable to release. If the tendon is adherent and the muscle belly is fibrosed or bound down to the posterior tibia, then release is less productive and muscle belly excision or tendon transection is necessary (Fig. 22–24).

In addition to the mechanical factors the tendon can develop pathologic processes associated with inflammatory arthropathy (rheumatoid arthritis, Reiter's syndrome, infection, gout, ulcerative colitis).[74]

History and Physical Examination

Patients often complain of a pain in the area of stenosis, a catching sensation, and some weakness during running, cutting, jumping, squatting, pushing off, or rising on the ball of the foot. Pain along the medial aspect of the ankle or subtalar joint with these mechanical stressors is often noted. Some report an audible pop or a tearing sensation in association with the onset of acute pain. In ballerinas, an en pointe

position can exacerbate symptoms. Also the dancers note that when non–weight bearing and just repetitively pointing (plantar flexing the ankle and toes) and relaxing the foot and ankle they experience pain, clicking, popping and a triggering of the hallux. Crepitus is often present on physical exam, but triggering is less common.

Kolettis et al[67] reported this condition in female ballet dancers who had chronic symptoms of FHL tenosynovitis on the medial aspect of the ankle joint. The main symptoms were pain and tenderness over the medial ankle. All patients lost the ability to stand en pointe. An os trigonum was present in only 1 of 13 cases. The differential diagnosis besides tenosynovitis includes a longitudinal tear of the FHL and systemic inflammatory arthropathy.

On examination, the FHL tendon sheath often feels thickened. Examination often reveals no active flexion of the interphalangeal joint with the hallux held in extension. There may be pain on palpation depending on the area of disease. The pain may be localized to the posteromedial ankle, in the midfoot beneath the knot of Henry, or distally in the area of the FHL insertion. Pain typically occurs with active plantar flexion of the hallux against resistance. With a partial tendon rupture, the patient can have swelling, ecchymosis, and pain with prolonged walking or running. Passive flexion and extension is typically painless. Active flexion may be absent or weak depending on the degree of stenosis or the presence of a partial rupture. The patient can develop a mild flexion tenodesis of the MTP joint with passive ankle dorsiflexion. When the condition is severe, crepitation and triggering may be noted. If a nodule becomes incarcerated in the fibro-osseous tunnel, the toe remains in extension. Passive range of motion of the hallux causes less pain than restricted active range of motion.

When flexor hallucis longus tenosynovitis manifests with pain in the posterior ankle, distinguishing between posterior ankle impingement and FHL tendinitis can be challenging. Because the two structures are close to each other, and these conditions can coexist in dancers, careful attention to diagnostic features is warranted. The trigonal or posterior ankle impingement usually occurs with passive full plantar flexion of the ankle, whereas FHL tendinitis does not. Dorsiflexion of the great toe while in the fully plantarflexed position does not usually induce symptoms in impingement conditions but can in FHL tendinitis. The point of maximum tenderness in posterior impingement is usually posterolateral, whereas it is usually posteromedial in FHL tendinitis.

Tomassen's sign is another helpful diagnostic finding for FHL stenosis. With the ankle in dorsiflexion, MTP joint dorsiflexion is lost because of the tight-

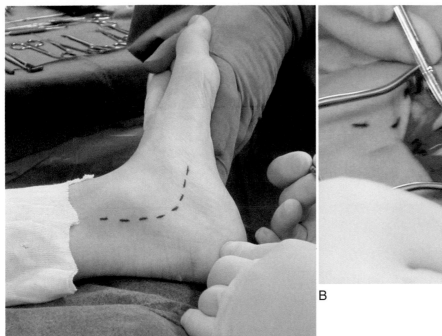

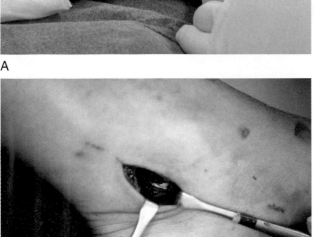

Figure 22–24 Flexor hallucis longus (FHL) tenosynovitis. **A,** Course of the tendon below the sustentaculum tali. **B,** Intraoperative photo of tendon release. Note the flexor digitorum longus tendon just superior to the FHL. **C,** Small medial incision is used to release the FHL tendon sheath. Note the distal course of the muscle belly leading to stenosis in the tunnel.

ness of the FHL tendon and low-lying muscle belly as it courses through the fibro-osseous tunnel. Further distinction is possible with lateral radiographs of the ankle taken in neutral and full plantar flexion; these views show abutment of the os trigonum between the tibia and the talus and calcaneus or subluxation of the talus and tibiocalcaneal abutment.

Radiographic Examination

Although Trepman et al[92] and others[55,83] have noted the usefulness of MRI in diagnosing FHL tenosynovitis and tears (Fig. 22–25), Boruta and Beauperthuy[53] observed that an MRI was negative in three patients with longitudinal FHL tears. In Sammarco's series[85] only eight patients had magnetic resonance imaging

(MRI) evaluations before surgery, but clinical correlation was found to be an important factor in interpreting the MRI. Oloff et al[78] reported that patients with flexor hallucis longus tendinitis also had plantar fasciitis and tarsal tunnel syndrome. In their series, they found that MRI proved valuable in establishing the correct primary diagnosis in their series.

Conservative Treatment

Nonsurgical treatment includes restricted activity, change in dancing and training technique, physical therapy, nonsteroidal anti-inflammatory drugs (NSAIDs), ice and contrast baths, whirlpool, and orthotics. Immobilization can diminish symptoms.[27] Occasionally a corticosteroid injection into the tendon

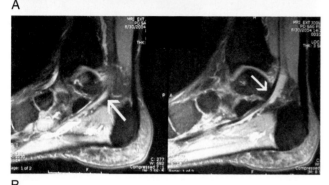

A

B

Figure 22–25 T2-weighted magnetic resonance images 5 months after an incomplete tear of the flexor hallucis longus (FHL). **A,** Coronal views demonstrate flexor tenosynovitis with increased signal intensity and abnormal but intact FHL tendon. **B,** Sagittal view demonstrates course of tendon with tenosynovitis behind the ankle and under the sustentaculum talus.

sheath is used judiciously. Kolettis et al[67] reported a risk of weakening or rupture of the FHL tendon after a steroid injection. Care must be taken to avoid an intratendinous injection, and Reinhertz[81] stressed that steroid injections are not routinely recommended because they can contribute to spontaneous rupture.

Surgical Treatment

Surgical intervention may be considered if conservative care is unsuccessful. During surgery, the sheath can be three to four times thicker than normal according to Lynch and Pupp.[74] Degenerative changes within the tendon at surgical evaluation are typically characterized by yellowing, calcification, or degenerative tears. The pathologic tendon sheath is incised in a stepwise process. If the tendon continues to catch or if the thickness is more than 1 or 2 mm wider, the thickened area of the tendon is resected. Very rarely, new pulleys in the retinacular area are needed to stabilize the tendon. If an os trigonum is present or if there is a large trigonal process, resection is considered if there were preoperative posterior impingement symptoms or if there is persistent catching after releasing. A partial FHL tear is repaired or resected or a nodular area is contoured if necessary. An alternative to open release is posterior ankle arthroscopy in the prone position.

OPEN RELEASE OF THE FLEXOR HALLUCIS LONGUS

Surgical Technique

1. With the patient in a supine position, a pneumatic tourniquet may or may not be used for hemostasis. A 3- to 5-cm curvilinear incision is made posterior to the medial malleolus and directed toward the navicular.
2. The neurovascular bundle is retracted, revealing the FHL in its fibroosseous sheath.
3. The retinaculum is released proximally to the level of the sustentaculum tali, and the tendon is inspected.
4. A tenosynovectomy is performed. Any nodules are excised. Longitudinal tears are repaired.
5. With a tear that extends into the midarch, Boruta and Beauperthuy[53] recommend releasing the knot of Henry to debride and repair a longitudinal tear. The interconnecting tendon between the FHL and FDL is excised.
6. Any prominent distal muscle fibers are excised.
7. The hypertrophic tenosynovial tissue is debrided, and if a longitudinal tear is present, it is repaired primarily. The hallux is then flexed and extended to demonstrate excursion of the tendon. The FHL is released until the retinaculum no longer prohibits its gliding motion. If the surgery is done under local anesthetic with IV sedation, it is useful to have the patient aggressively flex and extend the ankle and toes while the ankle is palpated for persistent crepitance.
8. The tendon sheath is not closed, but the distal soft tissue is approximated. The skin is closed in an interrupted fashion.

Postoperative Care

The foot and ankle are enclosed in a soft dressing and a below-knee splint or cast for 7 to 14 days, and the patient remains non–weight bearing. Then the splint or cast is removed and physical therapy is initiated, including strengthening exercises, range-of-motion activities, and full weight bearing.[74]

Results

Kolettis et al[67] reported on 13 female ballet dancers who had chronic symptoms of FHL tenosynovitis on the medial aspect of the ankle. The major symptoms were pain and tenderness over the medial aspect of the subtalar joint at an average of 6 months before surgery. All patients had lost the ability to stand en pointe. Hamilton[63] reported on 17 cases of FHL tenosynovitis and combined a soft tissue release with excision of a symptomatic os trigonum (Fig. 22–26). Routinely good and excellent results have been reported after surgical exploration, tenosynovectomy, and repair of the longitudinal degenerative tears of the FHL tendon, when present.[61,63,67,86,94]

Hamilton et al[64] reported their results of surgically treating posterior ankle pain in dancers with an average follow-up of 7 years. Thirty-seven dancers underwent 41 operations: 26 operations for tendinitis and posterior impingement, nine for isolated tendinitis, and six for isolated posterior impingement syndrome. Thirty ankles had a good or excellent result, 6 had a fair result, and 4 had a poor result. The results were good or excellent for 28 of the 34 ankles in professional dancers, compared with only two of the six ankles in amateur dancers. This discrepancy can reflect the higher expectations and a poorer ability to compensate in the amateur population.

Sammarco et al[85] reported on FHL injuries in dancers and nondancers. Thirty-one cases of flexor hallucis longus injuries in 26 patients were treated over a 16-year period. The two groups were compared with regard to age, activity, duration of symptoms, operative findings,

histopathology, and postoperative time to resumption of full activities. Twenty-seven patients required surgery for unsuccessful nonoperative treatment. In the dancers, 71% of patients had a partial longitudinal tear of the flexor hallucis longus compared with 30% in nondancers. Isolated tenosynovitis occurred in only 21% of the dancers but in 53% of the nondancers. Dancers tended to have symptoms for a longer period before seeking treatment than did nondancers. Surgical intervention for the tenosynovitis and tendon tears yielded good or excellent results in 14 of 15 dancers and 9 of 11 nondancers.

Oloff et al[78] reported on a cohort of patients with FHL tendinitis. In their retrospective series of 19 consecutive cases they reported that the condition occurred in primarily nonathletic, male, and middle-aged patients. The mean symptom duration was 20 months, with frequent previous misdiagnosis. They found overlapping signs and symptoms of flexor hallucis longus tendinitis, plantar fasciitis, and tarsal tunnel syndrome. MRI and tenography proved valuable in establishing the correct primary diagnosis in their series. Flexor hallucis longus tenolysis was successful in each case, with a mean return to regular activity at 9 weeks.

Gould,[62] who believed that trauma was a causative agent, reported three cases that responded to a lidocaine anesthetic injection that basically lysed adhesions. He also reported six other cases that required an open tenolysis. Sanhudo et al[87] described additional cases of distal stenosis at the sesamoid area.

With cases that have stenosis or synovitis at areas other than the ankle and subtalar joints, after attempted conservative treatment, consideration of a soft tissue release at the site of tendon constriction is warranted.

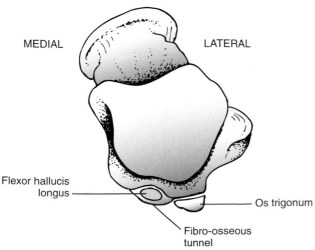

MEDIAL   LATERAL

Flexor hallucis longus

Os trigonum

Fibro-osseous tunnel

Figure 22–26 Flexor hallucis longus tenosynovitis may be exacerbated by an adjacent os trigonum.

Flexor Hallucis Longus Rupture

Although isolated spontaneous ruptures have been reported in the literature, the major reason for a loss of continuity is laceration of the tendon.[6,24,60,81,82] An injury to the FHL can occur anywhere along the course of the tendon. The site of disruption can be divided into the following zones:

- Zone 1: distal to the sesamoids in the area just proximal to the FHL insertion

- Zone 2: between the sesamoids and the knot of Henry

- Zone 3: proximal to the knot of Henry

The reason for the designation of different zones of injury is that a disruption in zone 3 leads to proximal retraction of the tendon. Injuries in zones 1 and 2 are not characterized by retraction of the proximal segment because of the fibrous slip connecting the FHL and FDL (Fig. 22–27).[57] With zone 1 injuries, a laceration leaves the tendon edges in proximity in a fairly subcutaneous region; however, the tendon is surrounded by a tendon sheath, and fibrous scarring is common. In zone 2, although the FHL is located in the deep arch of the foot, retraction is uncommon. Zone 2 injuries are characterized by a lesser degree of postoperative adhesions.

On the plantar aspect of the foot the tendons and neurovascular structures are vulnerable to penetrating injuries. Frenette and Jackson[60] reported a high incidence of nerve disruption after lacerations of the FHL. The first common digital nerve and proper digital nerve course along the medial and lateral aspect of the FHL tendon in a superficial area and are vulnerable to injury along with laceration of the FHL. The authors noted that in 75% of injuries in which a laceration was distal to the origin of the FHB, the proper or common digital nerve was lacerated as well. Wicks et al[24] reported that 60% of feet in their series demonstrated nerve injury.

Frenette and Jackson[60] reported that 80% of injuries in their series resulted from stepping on glass while barefoot. They noted 3 of 10 injuries distal to the plantar flexion crease at the MTP joint, five in the distal

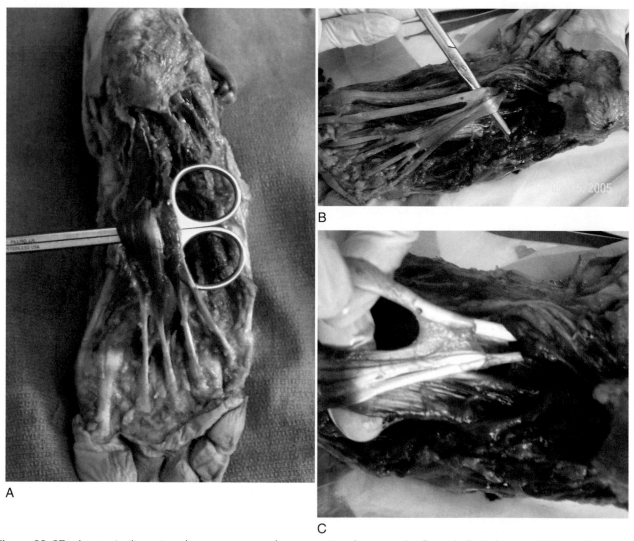

Figure 22–27 Anatomic dissection demonstrates tendon connection between the flexor hallucis longus (FHL) and flexor digitorum longus (FDL). **A,** FDL. **B,** Minor connection between FHL and FDL. **C,** Close-up. (Courtesy of Nick Goucher, MD, Ogden, Utah.)

longitudinal arch where the FHL lies between the two bellies of the FHB, and two localized to the proximal longitudinal arch.

History and Physical Examination

After injury, a patient might note subjective loss of push-off power and a feeling of giving way. A prodromal period followed by a sudden snap can herald an FHL rupture.[65,83,91] The recognition of spontaneous dorsiflexion of the toe and discomfort with pressure of the hallux against the top of the toe box may be coupled with an inability to flex the tip of the toe. A patient might give a history of forced dorsiflexion against resistance or of being involved in a repetitive activity like rising on the ball of the foot or running, cutting, and jumping. Rupture of the FHL can also be associated with systemic disease, trauma, and athletic or dance activity. In patients with a spontaneous rupture, a popping or tearing sensation may be associated with the disruption.

On physical examination, normal active extension of the hallux interphalangeal (IP) joint is present, but typically no active plantar flexion is possible. Passive flexion and extension of the hallux is typically painless. Active flexion at the MTP joint denotes function of the FHB. Occasionally, simultaneous rupture of the FHL and FHB can occur. This should be evaluated by examining for flexion of the MTP and IP joints. Further assessment of the plantar plate with attempted dorsal drawer or translation of the proximal phalanx relative to the metatarsal head should be performed. A side-by-side comparison facilitates this evaluation. After rupture, swelling and tenderness on the plantar aspect of the hallux and tenderness at the MTP joint and sesamoid region can denote a distal rupture. Pain and

swelling in the posteromedial aspect of the ankle can develop with a proximal FHL rupture. If a rupture occurs distal to the knot of Henry, active flexion of the hallux IP joint is typically absent.

The fibrous slip connecting the FHL and FDL prevents retraction of the proximal tendon into the arch or calf. When the rupture occurs proximal to this fibrous slip attachment, action of the FDL may be transmitted through the fibrous slip to the distal portion of the FHL. Thus there may be weak but apparent active flexion of the hallux. On the other hand, this allows retraction of the proximal segment.

Knowledge of position of the tendon rupture is important in planning a surgical reconstruction either in the medial plantar arch or at the level of the ankle. The location of the rupture can be at the musculo-tendinous junction, in the tendinous portion, or distally at the level of the insertion.

Radiographic Examination

Routine anteroposterior (AP) and lateral radiographs usually do not aid in the diagnosis of an FHL disruption. MRI has been advocated in the patient with weakness, pain, or dysfunction when a diagnosis is not clear or when the level of retraction of the proximal segment is unknown (Figs. 22–28 and 22–29).[83,91,92]

Surgical Treatment

Yancey,[95] in a survey of 88 foot and ankle surgeons, reported that 80% to 93% thought a primary repair of a disrupted FHL was important, whereas only half believed the other lesser toe flexor tendons were important to repair. Frenette and Jackson[60]

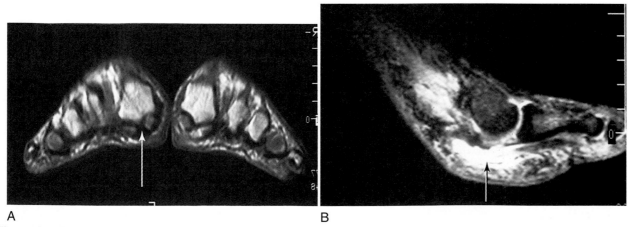

A   B

Figure 22–28 Magnetic resonance images demonstrate distal flexor hallucis longus rupture (*arrows*). **A,** Coronal view. **B,** Sagittal view. (Courtesy of M. Romash, MD, Chesapeake, Va.)

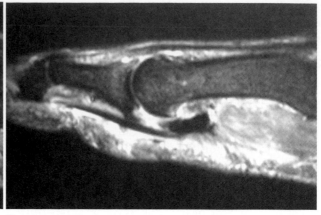

Figure 22–29   A, Sagittal view of the first metatarsophalangeal joint on magnetic resonance image showing flexor hallucis longus (FHL) tenosynovitis. The FHL can be traced from beneath the sesamoid to the base of the proximal phalanx. The sesamoidal phalangeal ligament, which is the continuation of the flexor hallucis brevis tendon, is absent, indicating rupture. **B,** The medial sesamoid shown here has retracted proximally and is no longer under the metatarsal head. The sesamoidal phalangeal ligament and plantar plate has ruptured. The FHL is visualized plantarly surrounded by edema from the ligament and plantar plate rupture. The extensor hallucis longus can be seen dorsally.

recommended repair only if the tendon ends were easily found within the depths of the laceration. They noted that the distal FHL can be tenodesed to the FHB. However, disruption of both the FHL and the FHB has a poor prognosis that can eventually lead to hyperextension of the hallux. Rasmussen and Thyssen[80] repaired the FHL after a distal rupture but observed minimal IP joint motion. They concluded that repair of the FHL tendon did not seem to be "essential in achieving good functional results in cases of rupture or laceration."

An untreated FHL laceration can lead to a cock-up deformity of the hallux. Thompson et al[91] stated that hyperextension of the great toe was an indication for surgical intervention. The options are either primary repair for a distal rupture with acute open or closed trauma or tenodesis of the FHL and FDL distal and proximal to the sustentaculum tali with a more proximal rupture. They further stated that although a tendon graft might be possible, it seemed "unnecessarily complex." When a rupture is at or adjacent to the fibro-osseous tunnel, a primary repair is often unsuccessful. In these cases, a tendon transfer using the FDL to the second toe should be considered, particularly in active or athletic patients.

Krackow[69] observed that the strength of push-off may be improved after repair, and if the patient's physical and athletic activities require high performance, repair should be considered.

PRIMARY REPAIR OF RUPTURED FHL TENDON

Surgical Technique

1. Under tourniquet control, a laceration is explored by extending the incision distally and proximally. The location of the laceration, as previously noted, determines the degree of retraction of the proximal segment. With a closed rupture the area of maximal tenderness and swelling often determines the location of surgical exploration.
2. The tendon ends are repaired with a modified Bunnell or Kessler suture technique (see Fig. 22–3A-C).

Postoperative Care

The patient is managed in a below-knee cast in plantar flexion at the ankle with an extended toe plate to prevent passive dorsiflexion at the MTP joint. At 5 to 8 weeks after surgery, active flexion is permitted and the ankle is brought to the neutral position. Depending on the tension of the reconstruction, limited dorsiflexion (usually around 20 degrees) and plantar flexion can be initiated at the MTP joint with the ankle in neutral flexion. Active inversion and eversion can be performed with some resistance to maintain muscle function. At 12 weeks, protection is discontinued.[83]

Results and Complications

Primary rupture of the FHL tendon has been described in individual case reports by eight authors (Fig. 22–30). Typically these injuries occurred in association with athletics after running, dancing, tennis, diving, and soccer, although in one case a rupture occurred after prior first ray surgery.[55] Locations include distal ruptures[55,69,80,83] and proximal ruptures at the level of the sustentaculum.[65,66,91] A rupture in the midarch just distal to the knot of Henry was reported in a marathon runner.[57]

Trepman et al[92] reported a longitudinal tear of the FHL. They performed a tenolysis, tenosynovectomy, and excision of the prominent distal muscle fibers.

The other major reports of FHL disruption are concerned with traumatic injuries. Floyd et al[6] and others[24,60] reported on a total of 35 disruptions of the FHL at varying locations along the course of the tendon.

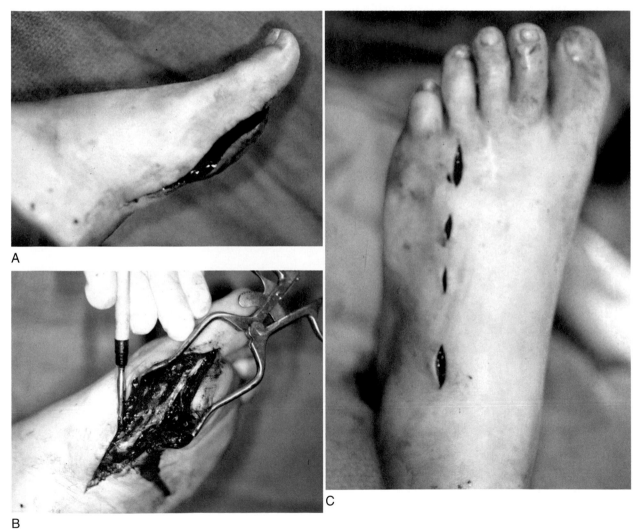

Figure 22–30 Distal rupture of the flexor hallucis longus treated with extensor digitorum brevis (EDB) free graft transfer. **A,** The patient underwent bunion surgery, which resulted in progressive weakness of the flexor hallucis longus (FHL). Once she could no longer flex her great toe, the FHL tendon was approached plantar medially. **B,** The FHL was found to be attenuated and fibrotic. **C,** The fourth toe EDB was harvested through multiple small incisions and used as a free tendon graft, successfully bridging the gap.

Primary repair of distal injuries have been reported,[69,80,83] although they are associated with minimal postoperative IP joint motion. Proximal ruptures have been treated with tenodesis of the FDL,[91] fascia lata tendon graft,[66] or primary repair.[65] Proximal repairs tend to be associated with a higher level of active IP joint motion.

Treatment of lacerations of the FHL has been reported in several series. Frenette and Jackson[60] reported on 10 lacerations, of which six underwent a primary repair and four were left unrepaired. Of those undergoing a primary repair, two thirds had no active IP joint motion. Floyd et al[6] reported on 13 lacerations, 10 of which underwent a primary repair, two underwent a delayed repair, and one was left unrepaired. Of the 12 repaired, 75% had active IP joint motion. Distal nerve lacerations were reported in 50% of cases, and 70% had acceptable results. In Floyd's series, a more proximal rupture had a greater chance of achieving postoperative IP joint motion than distal ruptures near the IP joint. With closed ruptures of the tendon at the level of the IP joint, return of IP joint motion should not be expected. A closed rupture implies a failure of the tendon under tension. On the other hand, with a laceration the tendon is cut cleanly and may be more amenable to repair, especially if this occurs in the arch. Wicks et al[24] reported 12 cases of FHL laceration that underwent a primary repair. Sensory nerve injury was noted in 60%, and 55% had acceptable results.

Primary repair has also been reported in several small series and case reports (Fig. 22–31). Boruta and Beauperthuy[53] reported three cases of longitudinal tear of the FHL at the knot of Henry primarily repaired with simultaneous resection of the interconnecting branch. Inokuchi and Usami[66] reported a proximal rupture at the level of the talus treated with a fascia lata interposition graft that achieved 50% postoperative motion of the IP joint (Figs. 22–32 and 22–33).

Thus the treatment options for disruption of the FHL include nonsurgical treatment, primary repair, tenodesis to the FDL, tenodesis of the distal FHL to the remnant of the FHB, tendon transfer using a slip of the FDL tendon to attach distally to the toe, and anastomosing the FHL to the proximal FDL and tendon graft (probably an unnecessarily complex procedure).

Significant complications after FHL repair or reconstruction include restricted IP joint motion[69,83] and contracture at the IP joint from a tight FHL tendon.[57] Coghlan and Clarke[57] reported that a Z-lengthening of the FHL was necessary to achieve an acceptable result. Romash[83] and others[69,80] did not find that a stiff IP joint led to major disability. Rasmussen and Thyssen[80] observed that FHL function does not seem to be essential in achieving a satisfactory long-term result after rupture or laceration. Floyd et al[6] stated that not repairing the FHL can result in mild deformity with essentially no functional deficit. Patients who remain untreated or who have an unsuccessful repair and develop a hyperextension deformity can ultimately be treated with an IP joint fusion and transfer of the extensor hallucis longus to the first metatarsal head (Jones transfer).

Other potential complications after surgery include postoperative scarring, pain at the surgical site, traumatic neuroma, skin slough, and infection.

Bell and Schon[3] observed that the FHL is especially vulnerable to penetrating injuries to the sole. The depth of the injury in the midfoot makes exposure of the tendon difficult and can require substantial extension of the incision. When possible, an incision should avoid the plantar aspect of the foot. A primary repair can be carried out with either a modified Kessler or Bunnell suture technique. Postoperatively the foot should be splinted in mild equinus, with weight bearing initiated 4 weeks after surgery. Cast or brace protection with limited extension of the hallux is continued for 8 to 12 weeks after repair.

Romash[83] observed that with a closed rupture, IP joint motion should not be expected postoperatively. With repair of the FHL after laceration, more than 60% of patients noted some active IP joint motion.

The surgical approach to a plantar laceration goes far beyond the question of whether the FHL should be repaired or not repaired. Adequate wound management includes irrigation, debridement, exploration to determine the magnitude of the injury and relation of injury to other structures including plantar nerves and vessels, and when possible, restoration of normal anatomy. This is best done in the operating room under adequate anesthesia where adequate exploration and wound management

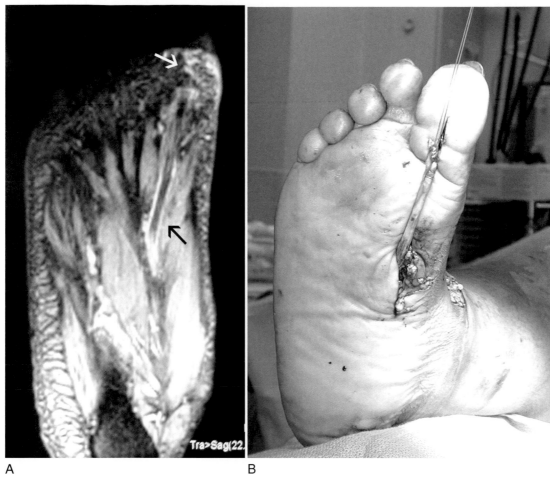

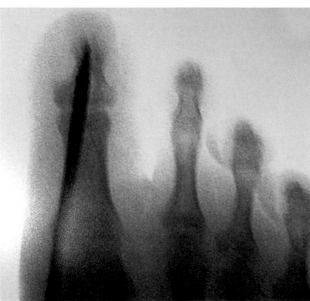

Figure 22–31 The flexor hallucis longus (FHL) tendon had spontaneously ruptured off the distal phalanx. **A,** The magnetic resonance image demonstrates the FHL is intact except for the insertion. **B,** Intraoperative photo shows ruptured FHL. **C,** The FHL is tunneled between the sesamoids and secured to the suture anchor (3.5 mm) in the distal phalanx.

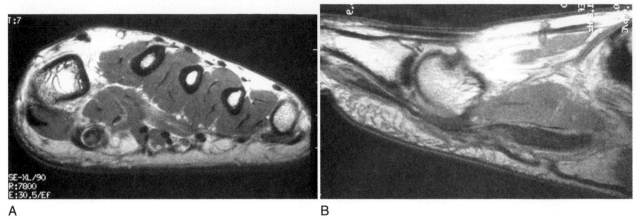

Figure 22–32 This athlete sustained an injury to the metatarsophalangeal joint, which was treated with a steroid injection. Subsequently the athlete continued to have pain and then felt a giving-way sensation and weakness in the foot. Clinically there was loss of flexion of the interphalangeal joint of the hallux. Magnetic resonance image (MRI) showed a flexor hallucis longus (FHL) rupture. **A,** Coronal MRI showing the fibrotic ruptured FHL plantar to the first metatarsal. **B,** The sagittal view demonstrates the FHL rupture proximal to the metatarsal head.

can be performed. After either a spontaneous rupture or a laceration with disruption of the FHL tendon, a repair should be performed when feasible. On the other hand, the magnitude of the exploration and the morbidity involved with such surgery should be weighed against the expected end result of surgery. If a patient develops postoperative weakness of the IP joint or a hyperextension deformity, a delayed IP joint fusion of the hallux can eliminate symptoms after nonsurgical treatment or an unsuccessful repair of an FHL injury.

Although the literature supports primary repair of an FHL laceration, a patient should be informed that after repair, active flexion of the IP joint is uncommon. Still, despite lack of IP flexion, a reasonable goal with repair may be to restore some plantarflexion power to the MTP and to the ankle joint. Perhaps there is also merit in repairing the tendon to regain some proprioceptive input from the FHL. The inconvenience or functional problems following treatment with benign neglect might not be well documented in the literature, but we recommend attempts at repair of the FHL in the case of laceration or rupture especially in young, active patients.

PERONEAL TENDONS

Peroneal Longus

Reports of dysfunction of the peroneus longus tendon are uncommon. Peroneal tendon tenosynovitis, longi-tudinal ruptures or partial tears of the peroneus longus tendon, and disruption or pathologic changes isolated to the os peroneum constitute the major pathologic conditions associated with the peroneus longus.

Anatomy

The peroneus longus muscle originates on the lateral condyle of the tibia and the head and midlateral aspect of the fibula and inserts onto the inferior aspect of the first cuneiform and the inferolateral aspect of the first metatarsal (Fig. 22–34). Innervated by the superficial peroneal nerve, the peroneus longus acts to plantar flex and evert the foot as well as to support the arch. It also plantar flexes the first metatarsal. In its muscular portion the peroneus longus lies posterior and lateral to the peroneus brevis muscle and becomes tendinous proximal to the ankle joint. It courses posterior to the peroneus brevis at the level of the distal fibula and then runs beneath the trochlear process of the calcaneus in an inferomedial direction. As the tendon crosses over the peroneal tubercle, it turns sharply and obliquely across the plantar aspect of the foot. After traversing the cuboid tunnel, it inserts on the plantar lateral aspect of the first metatarsal (Fig. 22–35).

On the lateral aspect of the calcaneus the peroneal tubercle can vary in size.[120] Along the course of the tendon from a point just proximal to the tip of the fibula and extending to the cuboid tunnel, the peroneus longus is surrounded by a synovial sheath. From a point approximately 4 cm above the lateral malleolus to the peroneal tubercle, the peroneus longus and brevis share a common sheath.[220] Distally the sheath bifurcates at the level of the peroneal tubercle (Fig. 22–36). At this point the peroneus brevis extends onward to its insertion into the base of the fifth

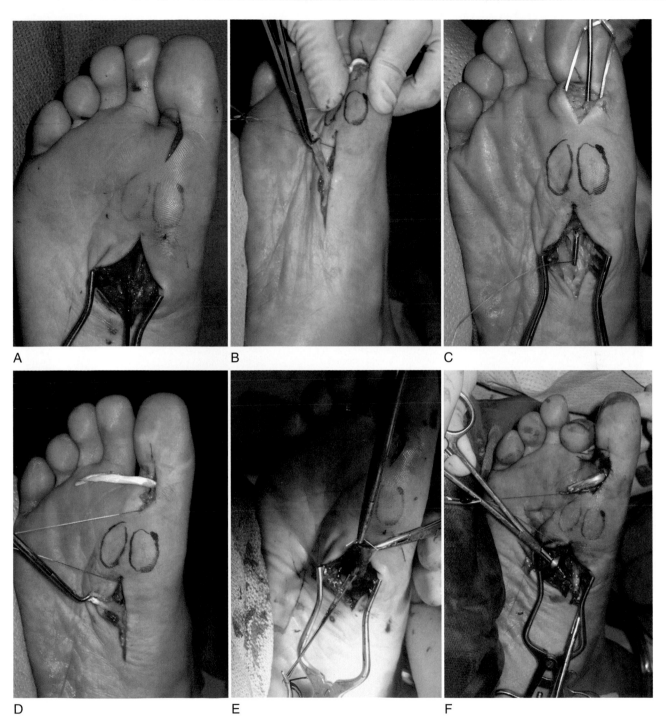

Figure 22–33 The rupture of the flexor hallucis longus (FHL) tendon occurred in the zone just proximal to the sesamoids, making an anastomosis difficult because exposure would violate the weight-bearing fat pad and be vulnerable to stenosis between the sesamoids. **A,** The tendon sheath between the sesamoids is identified and explored. **B,** The FHL is seen in the base of the proximal incision. **C,** A suture is passed through this tunnel for subsequent identification. **D,** Both tendons are brought forth from the incisions; note the length of the distal tendon stump. **E,** The proximal end is pulled distally to display where the anastomosis would have to occur if a direct repair were to be done. **F,** The flexor digitorum longus (FDL) to the second toe will be harvested to add motor strength to the weakened muscle of the FHL and to permit an anastomosis distal to the sesamoids. The FDL slip to the second toe is tensioned by the hemostat, causing flexion of the second toe. *Continued*

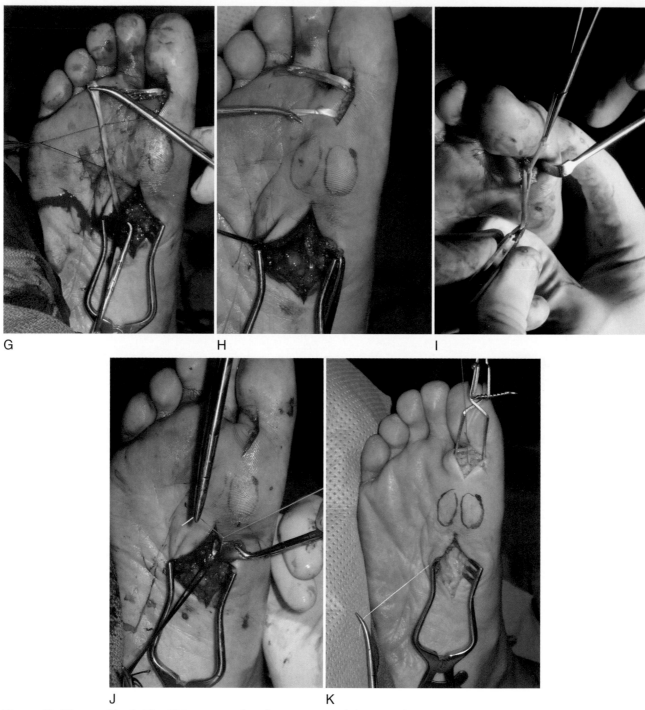

Figure 22–33—cont'd   **G,** The FDL is cut at the plantar aspect of the second toe just proximal to the distal interphalangeal crease and withdrawn from the incision. **H,** The FDL is passed with the previously placed suture through the sheath of the FHL and into the distal incision, where it lies next to the distal stump of the FHL. **I,** The FDL is secured to the FHL distally. **J,** The proximal end of the FHL is then secured to the FDL. **K,** The repaired FHL and transferred FDL from the second toe have good mechanical integrity.

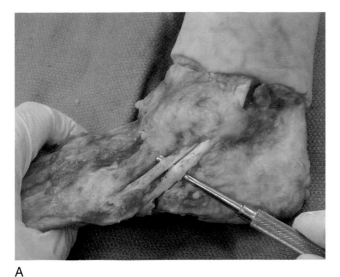

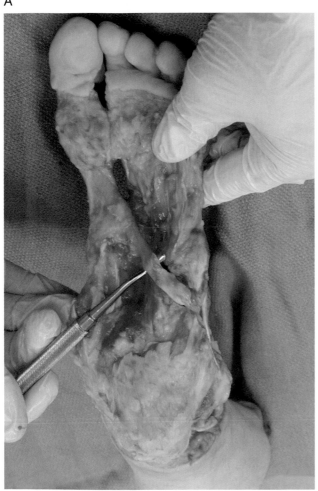

B

Figure 22–34 A, Lateral view demonstrating peroneus longus and brevis. **B,** Plantar view demonstrating the course of the peroneus longus.

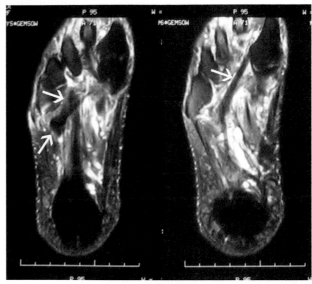

Figure 22–35 Magnetic resonance image of the course of the peroneus longus. Note the thickened tendon *(left)*, where the tendon courses around the cuboid. *Right,* The deeper slice of the same foot shows the course of the tendon proximal and plantar to the bases of the second through fourth metatarsals and onto the lateral base of the proximal first metatarsal.

metatarsal, and the peroneus longus courses toward the plantar surface of the cuboid, finally inserting on the plantar aspect of the first metatarsal.

Within the substance of the peroneus longus, the *os peroneum* may be present. Its frequency has been debated in orthothopaedic literature. Sarrafian[186] stated it is always present and may be in either a cartilaginous or a fibrocartilaginous state, whereas Pfitzner[174] noted it to be present in 8.5% of anatomic specimens. The os peroneum may be fully ossified, less than fully ossified, or multipartite. The os peroneum and tendon of the peroneus longus together are

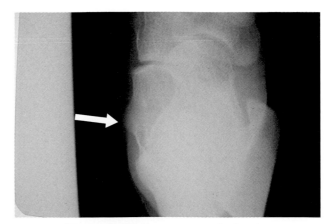

Figure 22–36 Large peroneal tubercle.

closely associated with both the lateral border of the calcaneus and the plantar lateral aspect of the cuboid (Fig. 22–37).

The blood supply of the peroneus longus has been studied by Petersen et al.[172] They found avascular regions where the peroneus longus tendon courses around the lateral malleolus and the anterior part of the tendon by the peroneal trochlea of the calcaneus. Another avascular zone exists where the tendon runs around the cuboid. These are the regions where the tendon is particularly vulnerable to tears.

Peroneal Tenosynovitis

Etiology

Tenosynovitis of the peroneal tendons was first described by Hildebrand[132] in 1907 and later by Hackenbroch.[129] Since then there have been numerous cases of peroneal tendon tenosynovitis in the literature.

Tenosynovitis can develop at different levels. It may be associated with hypertrophy of the peroneal tubercle[27,175,210,220] and can occur along the course of the peroneal tendon,[96,132] at the level of the lateral malleolus,[129] or at the ankle joint.[124,216] Burman[27] reported eight cases at the level of the peroneal tubercle. He hypothesized that this condition developed from a congenitally enlarged peroneal tubercle or following trauma to the peroneal tendons (direct blow,

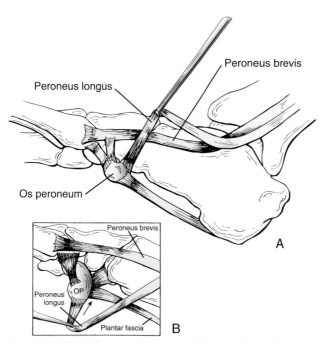

Figure 22–37 The os peroneum (OP) has four soft tissue attachments, including plantar fascial band, fifth metatarsal band, and band to peroneus brevis (A) and the fourth band to cuboid (B). (Redrawn from Sobel M, Pavlov H, Geppert M, et al: *Foot Ankle* 15:112-124, 1994.)

strain or sprain, fracture, inflammatory arthropathy, overuse, or as an injury to the os peroneum). Burman believed that Hildebrand did not describe stenosing tenosynovitis but rather subluxation of the peroneal tendons. Aberle-Horstenegg[96] described five cases of localized pain along the course of the peroneus longus as it passes beneath the cuboid that were successfully treated with conservative measures.

History and Physical Examination

With tenosynovitis of the peroneal tendons a patient typically complains of vague pain on the posterolateral aspect of the hindfoot that is increased with activity and diminished by rest. Cutting activities or running around curves can induce pain. A traumatic episode such as a lateral inversion injury to the ankle may be associated with the onset of discomfort. A patient might not recall a specific episode related to the onset of symptoms but instead might cite an increase in athletic training or physical activity associated with discomfort.

Tenosynovitis can develop following a lateral ankle sprain, direct blow to the peroneal tubercle, fracture of the calcaneus, or other episodes of direct or indirect trauma. The patient often notes pain with palpation along the course of the peroneal tendons inferior to the fibula. A palpable thickening may also be noted. Pain may be elicited with passive inversion of the foot or active eversion or pronation of the forefoot against resistance.

Radiographic Examination

Zivot et al[220] and Palmer[170] suggested that peroneal tenography may be helpful in defining the architecture of tendons and determining the presence or distortion of the peroneal tendons from tenosynovitis. MRI may be helpful in distinguishing tenosynovitis from either a complete disruption or a partial tear of the peroneus longus (Fig. 22–38).[139,193]

Conservative Treatment

Nonsurgical treatment for symptomatic peroneal tenosynovitis includes orthotic devices, physical therapy, change in training techniques, and stirrup or boot braces.[123] A below-knee walking cast may be used for 3 to 4 weeks to decrease symptoms. Because sudden changes in training patterns, alterations in surface conditions, and increases in intensity or duration of exercise (or both) can lead to symptoms, eliminating or controlling these factors can allow resolution. With continued symptoms of swelling and thickening consistent with peroneal tenosynovitis, a careful corticosteroid injection into the tendon sheath may relieve symptoms. To minimize the risk of rupture, the foot and ankle should be immobilized

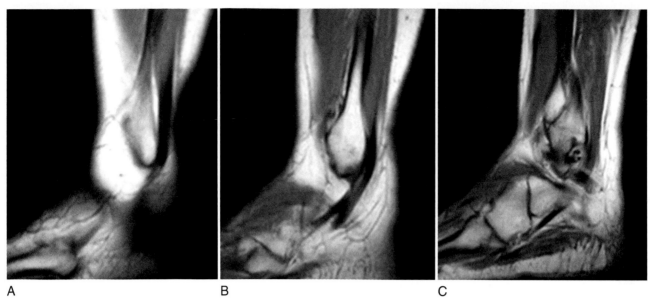

A   B   C

Figure 22–38   Magnetic resonance image of the peroneal tendons. The sequential images demonstrate the peroneal tendon anatomy. **A,** Posterior to the fibula, the peroneus longus is visualized, but on this slice the peroneus brevis is seen inserting distally onto the fifth metatarsal. **B,** The tendons are seen in the region posterior to the tip of the fibula, where peroneus brevis tears often occur. The brevis is more anterior and dorsal. **C,** This deeper slice demonstrates the peroneus longus running over the distal calcaneus toward the inferior aspect of the cuboid. This is where peroneus longus tears occur. Note in this slice posterior to the fibula the tendons are seen within the groove.

following the injection. With continued pain and swelling, surgical intervention may be indicated.

Surgical Treatment

Simple division of the tendon sheath is often effective in relieving symptoms. Anderson[100] noted that symptoms were poorly defined and that excision of the roof of the tendon sheath is usually successful. Pierson and Inglis[175] released the retinaculum and shaved a hypertrophied peroneal tubercle with good results. Interposing the retinaculum between the raw osseous surfaces of the calcaneus and the peroneus longus is recommended.

PERONEAL TENOSYNOVECTOMY

Surgical Technique

1. With the patient placed in a lateral decubitus position, a thigh tourniquet is used for hemostasis.
2. A curvilinear incision is begun at the base of the fifth metatarsal and extended to the tip of the fibula. With subcutaneous dissection, care is taken to define and protect the sural nerve.

3. The peroneal tendons are visualized through a longitudinal incision dividing the tendon sheaths (Fig. 22–39A and B).
4. With a stenotic area of the tendon sheath, a longitudinal section is removed from the sheath. Any degenerated areas of tendon or partial ruptures are resected or repaired. The peroneal tubercle is inspected and, if hypertrophied, may be resected or smoothed.
5. The peroneus longus tendon is inspected for the presence of an os peroneum. If the os peroneum is enlarged, irregular, or damaged, it may be resected and the tendon of the peroneus longus primarily repaired. With a tear of the peroneus brevis, a repair or reconstruction is performed (see discussion under "Peroneus Brevis").
6. The tendon sheaths are left unrepaired. If the superior peroneal retinaculum was incised to enable exposure, it must be repaired meticulously to prevent postoperative subluxation or dislocation.
7. The subcutaneous tissue is closed with absorbable sutures. The skin is approximated with interrupted sutures.

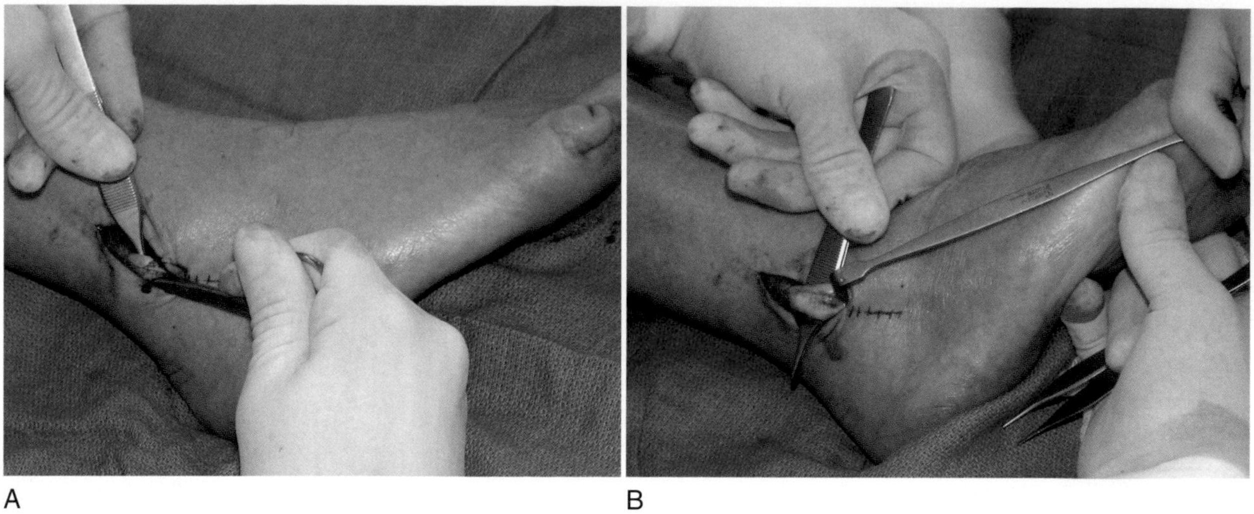

A   B

Figure 22–39 Exploration for peroneal tendon tenosynovectomy. **A,** Incision just posterior to the distal fibula. **B,** A small tear of the peroneus brevis is identified as well.

Postoperative Care

A below-knee non–weight-bearing cast or splint is placed with the foot and ankle in a neutral position. Two weeks after surgery a below-knee walking cast or brace is applied. Range-of-motion activities and physical therapy are initiated 2 to 4 weeks after surgery. Strengthening exercises are also begun.

Results

Pierson and Inglis[175] reported a case of stenosing tenosynovitis of the peroneus longus associated with hypertrophy of the peroneal tubercle and os peroneum. They released the retinaculum and excised the hypertrophied tubercle. The retinaculum was interposed between the raw osseous surface of the calcaneus and the peroneus longus.

Webster[216] reported two cases of nonspecific tenosynovitis of the peroneal tendons. At surgery, marked thickening and longitudinal fraying of the peroneus brevis tendons were noted.

Andersen[100] reported a case of tenosynovitis that developed after an inversion injury to the ankle. Surgical findings included thickening and constriction of the peroneal tendon sheath below the lateral malleolus and a bulbous enlargement of the peroneus longus. He noted that some patients complain of a "snapping ankle" with peroneal tendon tenosynovitis.

Tendon Disruption

Isolated injuries of the peroneus longus tendon are uncommon and typically limited to case reports in the literature (Fig. 22–40).[136] The os peroneum is often a useful marker in the diagnosis of the rupture. Its position is noted to be slightly proximal to the normal position, providing a clue about the rupture. Thompson and Patterson[207] thought that the presence of an os peroneum predisposed the structure to a degenerative tear in the peroneus longus tendon just distal to the sesamoid. Jahss[133] reported that spontaneous ruptures can occur in the peroneus longus secondary to rheumatoid arthritis and psoriasis. Truong et al[211] stated that concomitant diabetes, hyperparathyroidism, or local steroid injection can lead to nontraumatic rupture of either the peroneus longus or the os peroneum. Pierson and Inglis[175] found that the most common locations for irritation of the peroneus longus are at the level of the peroneal tubercle and the inferior retinaculum.

The differential diagnosis of a symptomatic peroneus longus tendon includes an acute fracture of the os peroneum or diastasis of a partite os peroneum, chronic diastasis of a previously fractured os peroneum, stenosing peroneus longus tenosynovitis (see previous discussion), a tear of the peroneus longus distal or proximal to the os peroneum, attrition or complete rupture of the peroneus longus tendon proximal or distal to the os peroneum,[136] and an enlarged peroneal tubercle (see Fig. 22–36). Sobel et al[197] suggested that painful os peroneum syndrome should be included with other diagnoses in the differential diagnosis, including lateral ankle sprain, peroneus brevis

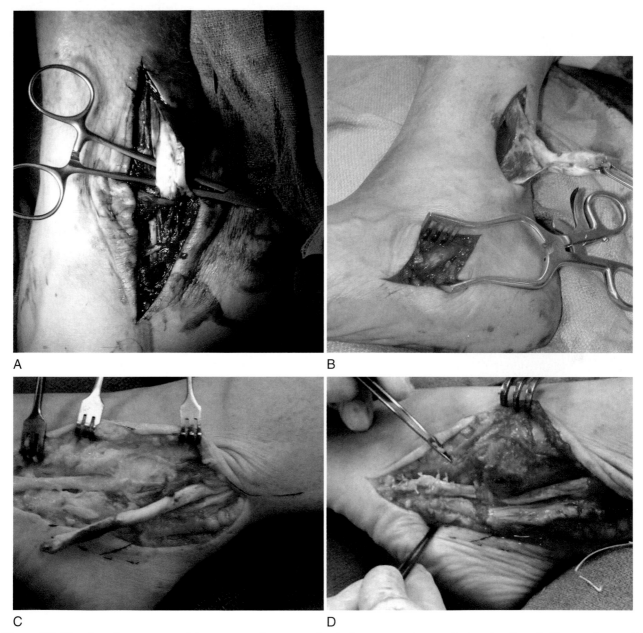

A

B

C

D

Figure 22–40 Complete rupture of the peroneus longus tendon is demonstrated at surgical exploration. **A,** Flattened tear with multiple perforations of the peroneus longus. **B,** Distal disruption with proximal migration requiring extensive exploration to retrieve the proximal portion. **C,** Rupture of the peroneus longus 10 years after a Watson–Jones repair that sacrificed the peroneus brevis. With rupture, the patient lost the ability to evert her foot. **D,** Salvage with tenodesis of the peroneus longus stump to the brevis, with takedown of the Watson–Jones repair. The patient retained good ankle stability.[136]

or extensor digitorum brevis avulsion, proximal fifth metatarsal fracture, and fracture of the anterior process of the calcaneus.

History and Physical Examination

The onset of acute plantar lateral ankle pain can occur following a traumatic episode (e.g., ankle inversion, supination injury). In chronic cases symptoms of instability and recurrent episodes of "ankle sprains" or

plantar lateral foot pain after athletic activity may be noted. The symptoms can be vague and nonspecific. MacDonald and Wertheimer[147] stressed that diagnosis may be significantly delayed with peroneus longus injuries.

Well-localized tenderness, synovitis, or thickening along the course of the distal peroneus longus tendon may be observed. Palpation may demonstrate significant tenderness over the peroneal tubercle, over the os peroneum, or where the peroneus longus enters the cuboid tunnel. Dysesthesia along the distal aspect of the sural nerve can develop. Pain may be increased with resistive plantar flexion of the first ray. Patients can also demonstrate pain or weakness with forced eversion of the foot.

Thompson and Patterson[207] did not find that a loss of function of the peroneus longus led to the formation of a dorsal bunion. They did note, however, the development of a second metatarsal stress fracture in one case.

Radiographic Examination

Initial imaging includes AP, lateral, and oblique radiographs of the foot and ankle. Thompson and Patterson[207] stated that the position of the os peroneum is a useful marker, especially with serial radiographs. Oblique radiographs can demonstrate proximal retraction of the sesamoid.[158,207] An enlarged peroneal tubercle may be observed as well (Fig. 22–41).[108,139]

Truong et al[211] encouraged the use of MRI to diagnose an os peroneum fracture, and Kilkelly and McHale[139] recommended MRI in the diagnosis of a ruptured peroneus longus tendon. A radionucleotide scan can demonstrate increased uptake in the os peroneum after a fracture or disruption (Fig. 22–42).

Ultrasound can be useful in experienced hands to diagnose peroneal tendon disease, especially in situations where a dynamic real-time evaluation is warranted.[166]

Conservative Treatment

Treatment depends on the magnitude and duration of a patient's symptoms. Nonsurgical treatment includes immobilization with a below-knee cast, air brace, or splint; taping; a compression dressing; orthotic devices; and physical therapy. Sobel et al[197] reported that in addition to their one case of successful treatment, seven other patients cited in the literature recovered successfully with nonsurgical treatment. Although acute treatment can be conservative, chronic problems are less likely to respond to these measures. Sobel et al[197] found cast immobilization was successful in 20% of patients with chronic peroneus longus symptoms but that 80% eventually required surgery. Although one cortisone injection may be considered for chronic cases, more than one corticosteroid injection should be discouraged.

The os peroneum may be excised with or without repair of the tendon. In Sobel's series the os was excised in several cases and the peroneus longus tendon repaired as well. Of nine patients with chronic symptoms, four had a complete rupture of the peroneus longus distal to the os peroneum, and five had a chronic diastasis of a multipartite os peroneum.

Surgical Treatment

With continued pain, swelling, and dysfunction, surgical intervention may be considered. The location of symptoms generally determines the surgical approach. Pain in the area of a symptomatic os peroneum combined with positive imaging studies can necessitate exploration and excision of the os peroneum. More proximal symptoms can herald a longitudinal tear or disruption of the peroneus longus tendon.

OS PERONEUM EXCISION

Surgical Technique

1. The patient is placed in a lateral decubitus position, and a thigh tourniquet is used for hemostasis.
2. A longitudinal incision is extended from the tip of the fibula approximately 4 cm distally toward the tip of the fifth metatarsal.
3. The dissection is carried down to the peroneus longus tendon, and the tendon sheath is incised. Care is taken to protect the adjacent sural nerve.
4. The os peroneum is carefully identified and, when disrupted or degenerated, is carefully shelled out of the peroneus longus tendon. If the peroneus longus is intact, it may be reinforced with interrupted no. 1 nonabsorbable suture. If the tendon is ruptured, it may be approximated with a modified Bunnell, Kessler, or Krackow suture. It can be difficult to close the void left by the os peroneum and it is often challenging to get a hold on the distal aspect of the tendon. Thus, it is useful to insert the suture distal to the os before excising it to minimize this latter problem. A strip of peroneus longus tendon may be needed to span the resultant gap to address the former situation.
5. The tendon sheath is not closed. The overlying soft tissue and skin are approximated in a routine manner.

Postoperative Care

A below-knee splint is applied with the foot in a neutral position and the ankle in slight eversion. A below-knee walking cast or boot brace is applied 2 to 4 weeks after surgery. Immobi-

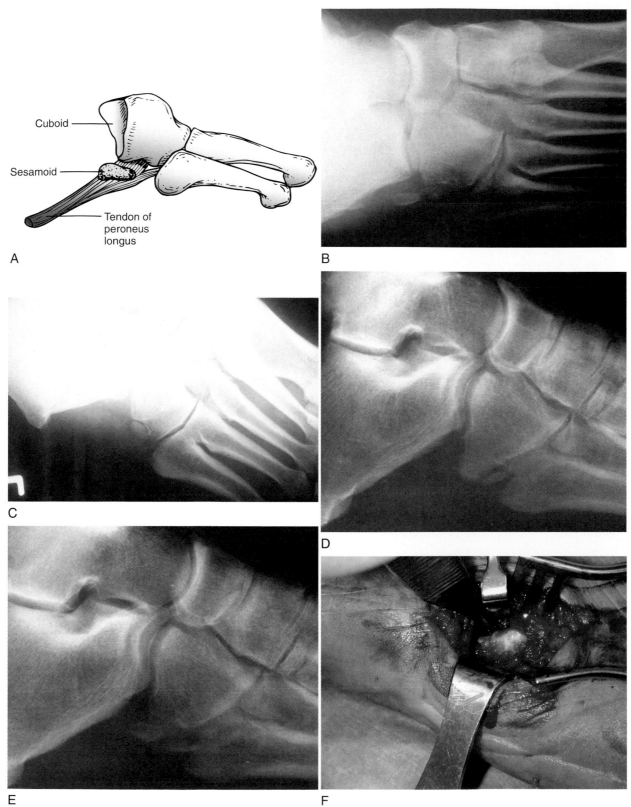

Figure 22–41 **A,** An os peroneum is contained within the tendon of the peroneus longus and articulates with the lateral border of the cuboid. **B,** More proximal location of the os peroneum can denote distal peroneus longus rupture. **C,** Normal location of os peroneum. **D,** Fragmentation of os peroneum. **E,** Proximal migration of os. Note a fragment of the os perineum is located distally, and the os has migrated proximally. **F,** Surgical excision of painful fragmented os peroneum.

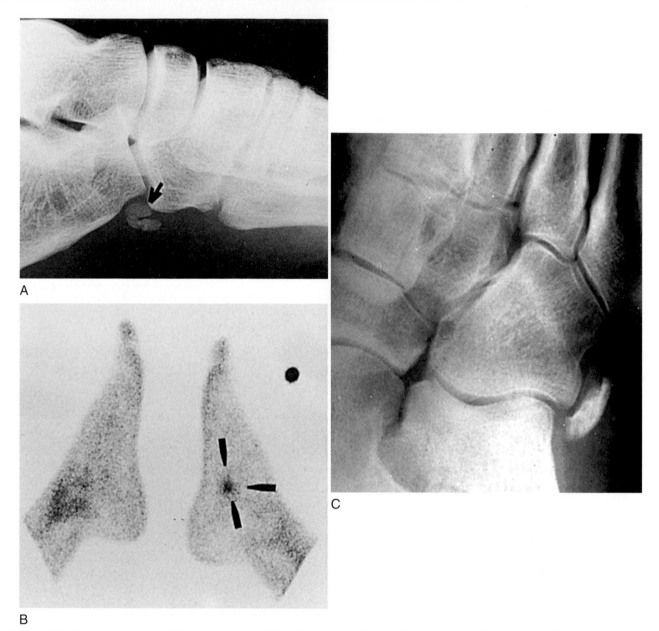

Figure 22–42   A, Osteochondritis of the sesamoid is demonstrated by its fragmentation *(arrow).* **B,** Technetium bone scan demonstrates increased uptake in os peroneum *(arrowheads).* **C,** Osteochondritis of os peroneum as demonstrated by sclerotic appearance of sesamoid. The os peroneum is at risk for rupture.

lization is continued for 6 more weeks, after which physical therapy and progressive passive and active resistive exercises are initiated. A soft brace or a stirrup brace may be helpful during the subsequent 6 to 16 weeks. Involvement in sports should be curtailed until at least 12 weeks after surgery and completion of a rigorous physical therapy regimen.

PERONEAL TENDON TENODESIS[207]

Surgical Technique

1. The patient is positioned in a lateral decubitus position with a thigh tourniquet for hemostasis.
2. A longitudinal incision is extended from the base of the fifth metatarsal to the tip of the

fibula. Care is taken to identify and protect the sural nerve.
3. The dissection is deepened to the peroneus longus and brevis tendons, and the tendon sheath is incised longitudinally.
4. The tendon of the peroneus longus is identified. With a distal rupture, the os peroneum might have migrated proximally toward the tip of the fibula, but it typically does not retract farther proximally. The proximal remnant of the peroneus longus is resected, as is the os peroneum. If it is long enough, the distal aspect of the peroneus longus is then woven through the peroneus brevis distal to the fibula and reinforced with interrupted nonabsorbable sutures. The proximal segment of the peroneus longus may be tenodesed to the peroneus brevis if sufficient tendon is present (Fig. 22–43).

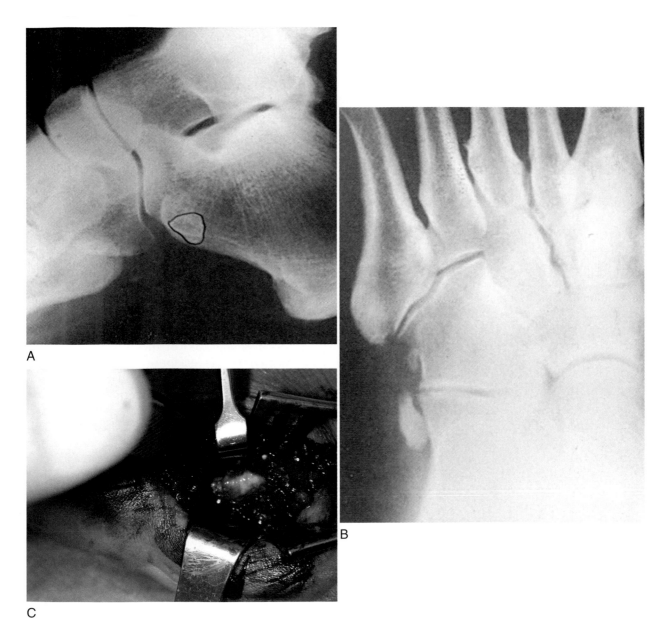

Figure 22–43 **A,** Onset of pain in a 56-year-old man on the lateral aspect of the foot and ankle with the os peroneum slightly proximal to the normal position. **B,** Oblique radiograph of a 72-year-old man 2 months after onset of lateral foot pain demonstrates proximal migration of os peroneum to the level of the calcaneocuboid joint. **C,** Intraoperative photograph demonstrates rupture of the peroneus longus at the level of the os peroneum with proximal retraction. (**A** and **B** from Thompson F, Patterson A: *J Bone Joint Surg Am* 71:293-295, 1989.)

5. The tendon sheath is not closed, but the overlying soft tissue is closed with interrupted sutures.
6. The skin is approximated in a routine manner.

Postoperative Care

A postoperative splint is applied with the foot and ankle in neutral position. Two to three weeks after surgery, sutures are removed and a below-knee walking cast or boot brace is applied. Six weeks later the full immobilization is discontinued and a stirrup or cloth brace may be used. Physical therapy commences with range-of-motion and strengthening exercises. Careful avoidance of forceful passive inversion and active eversion against resistance is recommended.

Results

Acute fractures of the os peroneum have been reported infrequently in the literature. A diagnosis may be difficult to make based on the presence of a multipartite or bipartite os peroneum. Sobel et al[197] reported on five patients with chronic diastasis of either a previous os peroneum injury or a multipartite os peroneum. They extensively reviewed the literature and identified 17 reports describing 26 patients with os peroneum and peroneus longus injuries. They concluded either that this was an overuse syndrome or that disruption of the os peroneum developed after trauma.

With an acute fracture of the os peroneum, diastasis can result with disruption of the peroneus longus tendon. Chronic diastasis with later development of stenosing peroneus longus tenosynovitis can occur as well. Likewise, attrition of the peroneus longus tendon either proximal or distal to the os peroneum, frank rupture of the peroneus longus either proximal or distal to the os peroneum, and an enlarged peroneal tubercle were all recognized by Sobel et al[197] as leading to chronic plantar lateral foot pain. With a disrupted os peroneum, thickening can develop along the course of the peroneus longus tendon inferior to the fibula or at the level of the peroneal tubercle or cuboid tunnel.

Guineys[128] and others reported on nonsurgical treatment with cast immobilization, orthoses, steroid injection, and taping and noted successful results in 12 cases.

Surgical exploration of the peroneus longus tendon with excision of the os peroneum remains a primary form of treatment. Excision of the os peroneum and tenodesis of the peroneus longus to the peroneus brevis[197] were noted to have theoretic disadvantages with the possible development of a dorsal bunion, although Thompson and Patterson[207] did not observe this in their experience. We have treated a case of peroneus longus rupture that had developed a dorsal bunion. A painful os peroneum may be surgically excised,[127,203,206] excised with primary repair of the peroneus longus tendon,[148,171,173,213] or excised with tenodesis of the peroneus longus and peroneus brevis.[197,207] In advanced cases, exploration and excision of the peroneus longus may be necessary. Grisolia[127] and others have reported 18 cases treated surgically with excision of a painful os peroneum and primary repair when necessary; 17 (94%) had acceptable results.

Longitudinal Tears

Traumatic rupture or tears of the peroneus longus tendon have been reported in the literature. Twelve tears of the peroneus longus not associated with an os peroneum disruption, one disruption of the peroneus longus at the musculotendinous junction,[113] and 32 ruptures associated with an os peroneum injury have been reported. Eighteen of these were treated surgically, and 17 had satisfactory results. Twelve ruptures that were treated conservatively had good results.

Several cases of calcific tendinitis of the peroneus longus have been reported.[110,159,183,217] Sobel et al[197] suggested that these cases actually may be a presentation of chronic degenerative changes in the peroneus longus tendon. The calcification develops in the area of the os peroneum and can follow a chronic disruption of the os peroneum. Williams[217] noted the onset of swelling, warmth, and tenderness in this region with calcification over the dorsolateral aspect of the cuboid.

Abraham and Stirnaman[97] reported simultaneous ruptures of the peroneus longus and brevis tendons in a 48-year-old diabetic woman. The tendons were repaired primarily. Evans[122] reported on a 20-year-old athlete who developed chronic lateral ankle pain. At exploration, a peroneus longus tear was noted inferior to the lateral malleolus and was treated with a tenodesis of the peroneus longus to the peroneus brevis. Burman[107] also observed a partial tear of the peroneus longus, thought to result from an enlarged peroneal tubercle. This was treated with resection of the torn portion, excision of the enlarged tubercle, and tenodesis of the peroneus longus to the peroneus brevis. Kilkelly and McHale[139] reported a traumatic rupture of the peroneus longus at the level of the peroneal tubercle successfully treated with a primary repair. Bassett and Speer[102] and others[139,189] have reported nine cases of longitudinal tears of the peroneus longus treated with primary repair with routinely good results. Thompson and Patterson[207] reported three other cases of peroneus longus disruption in older patients (average age 65 years). They were treated with tenodesis of the peroneus longus and brevis with good results.

Several studies have reported on tears of the peroneus longus and noted the presence of lateral ankle ligamentous incompetence, combined peroneal brevis and longus tears, low-lying peroneus muscle belly (see Fig. 22–43A and B), chronic peroneal tendon subluxation or dislocation, and hindfoot varus deformity. With a longitudinal tear, resection of the degenerated portion and primary repair are performed. With complete disruption and proximal migration of the proximal segment, a tenodesis of the peroneus longus and brevis is recommended. When both tendons are unhealthy or torn an FDL tendon transfer to bypass the diseased tendon is considered. Addressing the primary and associated disease is necessary for successful resolution of symptoms.[116,181,188]

Peroneus Brevis

Approximately 200 cases of longitudinal tears or ruptures of the peroneus brevis tendon have been reported in the literature. Although most references cite individual case reports. Approximately 85% of reported cases are contained in seven studies.* With the advent of accessible MRI and a growing awareness among specialists of brevis disorder, more of these acutely and chronically abnormal tendons are being identified.

Although injuries to the lateral ligamentous complex of the ankle typically involve the anterior talofibular ligament and the calcaneofibular ligament, a spectrum from various degrees of rupture, longitudinal tear, or subluxation and dislocation of the peroneal tendons can occur as well. Minor or major foot and ankle trauma could be the one event that triggers the condition, but additionally, overuse can result in tendon disorders. Furthermore, patients with idiopathic or neuromuscular cavovarus feet are vulnerable to pathologic changes in their peroneals. Whatever the cause, acute injuries or chronic insidious degenerative

tears are often associated with the signs and symptoms of synovitis of the peroneal tendon sheath.

Anatomy

The peroneus brevis muscle originates from the midportion of the lateral fibula and functions to evert and plantar flex the foot. Innervated by the superficial peroneal nerve, it becomes tendinous on the posterior aspect of the fibula. It courses on the posterior aspect of the fibula and lateral malleolus anterior to the peroneus longus. The peroneus brevis then crosses the peroneal tubercle and inserts onto the base of the fifth metatarsal. The peroneus longus, in contrast, is positioned inferior to the peroneal tubercle and runs beneath the cuboid and across the plantar aspect of the foot, inserting into the plantar base of the first metatarsal and first cuneiform. The peroneus longus is the more posterior of the two tendons and distal to the fibula. Each of the peroneal tendons is maintained within an individual tendon sheath, although they are contained within one common tendon sheath proximal to the tip of the fibula. The posterolateral aspect of the lateral malleolus forms a bony ridge that normally prevents the peroneal tendons from subluxating.

Peroneus longus and brevis injuries can be differentiated by their location. Peroneus longus injuries often are more distal and located in the region of the os peroneum, whereas peroneus brevis injuries are localized to the distal aspect of the fibula.

Etiology

Meyer[155] in 1924 initially described three anatomic specimens with attritional or longitudinal tears of the peroneus brevis localized to the area of the distal fibula. Later, Sammarco and DiRaimondo,[184] Bassett and Speer[102] and DiGiovanni et al[115] reported on several patients who underwent surgery for lateral ankle instability and were observed to have longitudinal tears of the peroneus brevis tendon.

Bassett and Speer[102] hypothesized that the cause of a longitudinal peroneus brevis tear is likely an extrinsic phenomenon, with the tendon injured by a portion of the distal fibula or the peroneus longus. In cadaver studies they observed that with plantar flexion of 15 to 25 degrees, the peroneus brevis impinged on the tip of the fibula with pressure from the peroneus longus. They found that with significant plantar flexion (greater than 25 degrees) the peroneal tendons were well seated in the fibular groove. With lesser amounts of plantar flexion (15 to 25 degrees) the tendons were "perilously draped across the distal fibula" and at risk for injury. With an inversion injury in plantar flexion, the peroneal retinaculum can be injured, with subsequent injury to the peroneus brevis tendon (Fig. 22–44).

---

*References 106, 115, 116, 145, 181, 184, and 199.

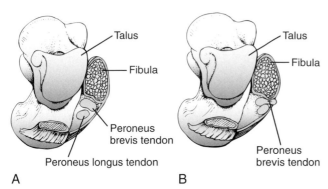

Figure 22–44 Cross section of lower leg at the ankle. **A,** Normal peroneal tendon anatomy. **B,** Compression of the peroneus brevis between the distal fibula and peroneus longus.

Longitudinal tears of the peroneus brevis probably occur from mechanical irritation or attrition within the fibular groove. Tears can occur with ankle trauma[184,195] and may be associated with lateral ankle instability or an incompetent superior peroneal retinaculum. Sobel et al,[194] in an anatomic analysis of cadaveric peroneus brevis tendons with longitudinal tears, demonstrated that the tears were centered over the posterior margin of the distal fibula. These tears demonstrated "an ample source of blood supply to the region of the tear." Vascular proliferation was noted at the site of the rupture. The authors concluded that the primary mechanism of the tendon injury was a mechanical disruption and not hypovascularity. Tears were noted to range in length from 2.5 to 5 cm (average 3.3 cm). The incidence of tears in anatomic cadaver dissections varied from 11% to 37%.[192,194] Interestingly, in these same anatomic dissections, no tears of the peroneus longus were noted. In all cases the central portion of the longitudinal tear was centered over the distal tip of the fibula in the region of the fibular groove.

Later, Sobel et al[195] inspected a large number of peroneal tendons in a laboratory setting. With tension placed on the peroneus longus and with the foot in inversion, compression was placed on the peroneus brevis at the fibular groove. The authors noted that a "flattened peroneus brevis" tendon splayed, with the anterior portion of the peroneus brevis slipping forward out of the fibular groove and over the anterior lip of the fibula. The peroneus brevis was wedged against the sharp posterior edge of the fibula, and the authors found that the peroneus brevis splits all occurred at this level. They then separated peroneus brevis splits into the following four grades:

Grade 1: splayed or flattened out (Fig. 22–45A)

Grade 2: partial-thickness split, less than 1 cm in length (Fig. 22–45B)

Grade 3: full-thickness split, 1 to 2 cm in length (Fig. 22–45C)

Grade 4: full-thickness split, greater than 2 cm in length (Fig. 22–45D and E)

Sobel et al[195] concluded that longitudinal tears or splits in the peroneus brevis were caused by acute or repetitive mechanical trauma. A sharp posterior edge of the fibula can contribute to tendon stability, but it also may be the site of peroneus brevis injury.

With redundancy or laxity of the superior peroneal retinaculum, the anterior edge of the peroneus brevis can subluxate anteriorly, resulting in attrition and longitudinal tears of the tendon. Other causes include tenosynovitis, hypertrophy of the peroneus longus, anomalous distal insertion of the peroneus brevis muscle, and presence of a peroneus quartus tendon, which can lead to overcrowding within the peroneal tendon sheath (Fig. 22–46).

Munk and Davis[164] suggested that the peroneus longus is pulled tightly against the peroneus brevis, entrapping the peroneus brevis between the peroneus longus and the fibular malleolus and peroneal tubercle. The peroneus longus thus acts as a wedge, pressing on the underlying flattened peroneus brevis and creating a longitudinal cleft in the tendon. Thus the cause of peroneus brevis tears, as Meyer[155] and Sobel et al[192,194,195] have observed, appears to emanate from compression of the peroneus brevis against the ridge on the lateral malleolus (by compression from the peroneus longus). Sobel et al[196] found the peroneus quartus present in 22% of 124 cadaver dissections. A large percentage of these cases also showed significant hypertrophy of the peroneal tubercle, which is the insertion site of the peroneus quartus. The authors concluded that the peroneus quartus may be associated with longitudinal attrition of the peroneus brevis.

In a report on 24 patients with longitudinal peroneus brevis tears, Brodsky and Krause[106] observed that all had redundancy of the superior peroneal retinaculum. The level of tears corresponded to the region of the distal 3 cm along the posterolateral edge of the fibula, where the tendon appeared to subluxate over the sharp edge of bone (Fig. 22–47). Sammarco and DiRaimondo[184] noted that all lesions occurred in a segment of tendon that "bends around the lateral malleolus during tendon excursion." They observed one case of bony impingement in the peroneal groove and suggested that compression of the peroneus brevis occurred from the peroneus longus. Of 13 patients, 12 had a history of ankle trauma.

The blood supply of the peroneus brevis has been studied by Petersen et al[172] with injection techniques and immunohistochemically by using antibodies against laminin. They found avascular regions in both

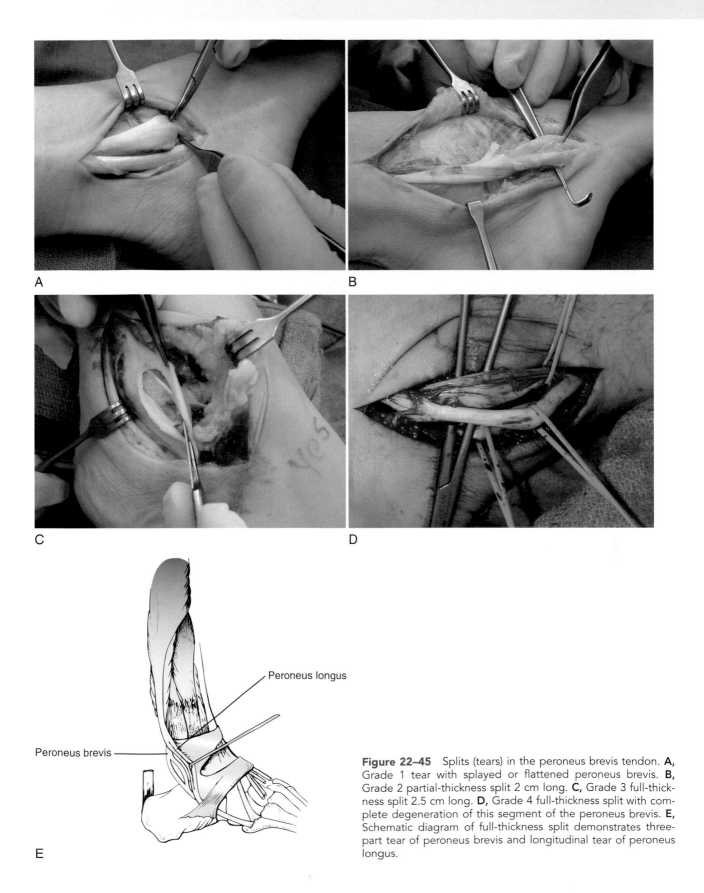

Figure 22–45 Splits (tears) in the peroneus brevis tendon. **A,** Grade 1 tear with splayed or flattened peroneus brevis. **B,** Grade 2 partial-thickness split 2 cm long. **C,** Grade 3 full-thickness split 2.5 cm long. **D,** Grade 4 full-thickness split with complete degeneration of this segment of the peroneus brevis. **E,** Schematic diagram of full-thickness split demonstrates three-part tear of peroneus brevis and longitudinal tear of peroneus longus.

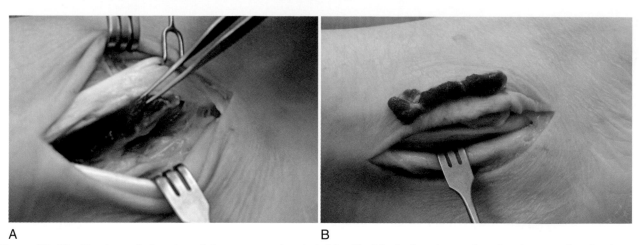

Figure 22–46 Distal muscle location of the peroneus brevis is identified (including the tendon sheath area, often leading to tendon degeneration of tears). **A,** Intraoperative photograph. **B,** Resected specimen.

the peroneus longus and brevis in the retromalleolar region. The peroneus longus had an extended zone to the peroneal trochlea and another area where the peroneus longus curves around the cuboid.[172] These are the areas where the tendon is particularly vulnerable to tears.

Geller et al[126] reported on 30 human cadaveric specimens and the location of the musculotendinous junction (MTJ) They found degenerative longitudinal tears in 4 cases. The MTJ was significantly more distal and the tendon was thicker in torn versus untorn specimens, suggesting that a lower peroneus brevis MTJ can influence the development of degenerative tears.

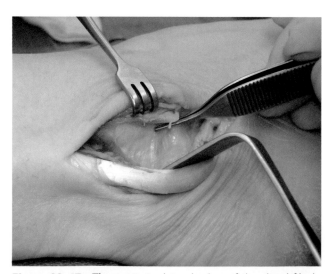

Figure 22–47 The posterior lateral edge of the distal fibula presents a sharp edge that can lead to tendon tears with subluxation.

Weber and Krause[215] reported on 30 of 70 patients who had posterolateral antiglide fibula plates who symptoms of peroneal tendinitis. In their series, of the 30 patients with symptoms, there were nine peroneus brevis lesions and three peroneus longus lesions. They recommended that a if a low placement of a plate below the distal 2 cm of the fibula (in the osteosynovial canal of the fibula) was needed for fracture fixation, avoiding screw placement in the distal hole would reduce symptoms. If a screw were needed in this distal hole then it should be fully sunk into the plate and not prominent. Thus obliquely placed distal screws in this distal hole are to be avoided.

History and Physical Examination

A patient might note a sudden pop or recall an episode of tearing in the region of the lateral ankle. Although edema may be present, ecchymosis is infrequently noted. A patient might not recall a specific traumatic episode and only seek treatment after a chronic period of discomfort or disability. Pain is typically isolated posterior to the region of the lateral malleolus and is increased with ambulation. Recalcitrant synovitis and swelling over the peroneal tendons in the region of the ankle may be presenting symptoms.

A history of ankle injury or sprain has been noted in several reports.[143,145,184,201] Sammarco and DiRaimondo,[184] reporting on 13 patients with peroneus brevis tears, noted that two tears were diagnosed preoperatively, four were suspected, and the rest were unsuspected and discovered at surgical exploration. Brodsky and Krause[106] reported that 70% of patients in their series of 24 peroneus brevis tears had a significant delay in diagnosis.

Patients with persistent lateral foot or ankle pain with a history of an ankle sprain or injury should be considered susceptible to a peroneus brevis injury. Although Sammarco and DiRaimondo[184] noted no patients with a history of inflammatory arthropathy or prior steroid injections, these conditions can predispose a patient to peroneal tendon injury.

Symptoms similar to those demonstrated with peroneal tendon tenosynovitis may be observed in a patient with a concomitant peroneus brevis tendon tear. Pain may be elicited with palpation along the course of the peroneus brevis posterior to the distal fibula. Decreased peroneal strength with eversion may be noted, and pain may be elicited with increased active eversion of the foot. Likewise, pain can occur with passive inversion of the foot. Moderate to significant soft tissue swelling may be present along the course of the peroneal tendon. Webster[216] noted a large, bulbous pseudotumor in the area of the peroneus brevis.

The magnitude of warmth and edema is often determined by the magnitude of the degenerative process. Subluxation of the peroneal tendons may be diagnosed by palpating the posterior edge of the fibula as the patient dorsiflexes and everts the foot. On examination, a painful click may be present when a longitudinal peroneus brevis split subluxates anteriorly over the anterior edge of the fibula.

Sobel et al[195] described the "peroneal compression test." With the patient sitting, the knee flexed to 90 degrees, and the foot and ankle in a relaxed plantarflexed position, the physician places a thumb over the superior retinaculum just on the posterior edge of the fibula. Slight pressure is applied to the peroneal tendons. The patient then forcibly everts and dorsiflexes the foot and ankle. Pain, crepitation, and popping with palpation over a longitudinal tear may be noted. A triggering or clicking sensation can occur with subluxation of a portion of the peroneus brevis tendon.

Mizel et al[161] used local bupivacaine injections into the peroneal tendon sheath to aid in diagnosis. They injected contrast material as well. This test might not be 100% sensitive because in approximately 15% of cases the injection communicated with the ankle or the subtalar joint, or both. They observed that the peroneus longus and brevis sheaths filled simultaneously and that the extravasation rate was 10%. Although some false-positive and false-negative results occurred, the authors believed this was a useful test in diagnosing peroneal tendon disorder.

Radiographic Examination

Although standard radiographs are obtained to evaluate the painful ankle, they usually do not demonstrate an abnormality with a peroneus brevis injury.[145] Tenography may be used[184] but largely has been replaced by MRI, which may be helpful in identifying a longitudinal tear, hypertrophy, distal insertion of the peroneal musculature, or a peroneus quartus muscle.[145,189] Sobel et al[193] suggested that MRI can aid in the diagnosis of peroneal tendon disorder and demonstrated its usefulness in evaluating a large number of cadaver specimens. Khoury et al[138] correlated the MRI findings to surgical findings and found the studies useful in establishing the diagnosis of tears. Neustadter et al[166] found sonography useful for diagnosing peroneal tendon tears. Although these studies are cost effective, results depend on technique.

Included in the differential diagnosis for chronic lateral ankle pain are lateral ankle instability, subtalar instability, peroneal tendon subluxation, tarsal coalition, lumbosacral radiculopathy, peroneal tendon rupture, longitudinal peroneal tendon tear, peroneal tendinitis, or tenosynovitis.

Conservative Treatment

Nonsurgical care for chronic lateral ankle pain includes NSAIDs, reduced activity, shoe modifications, custom insoles, and lateral heel wedges. Immobilization with a below-knee walking cast can diminish symptoms and allow the inflammatory process to subside. An ankle brace that diminishes inversion and eversion may be useful as well.

With tears of the peroneus brevis, however, symptoms typically do not subside. Brodsky and Krause[106] noted that conservative treatment failed in 20 of 24 patients (83%) with an average of 8 months of nonsurgical care. The failure of conservative care was noted in several other series as well.[116,181,188]

Surgical Treatment

Typically, two types of tears of the peroneus brevis are identified: a single longitudinal tear or multiple longitudinal tears characterized by areas of fibrillation.[145] With degenerative fibrillation the shredded fibers may be resected and the major divisions repaired primarily. An attempt should be made to tubulize the remaining tendon (Fig. 22–48).[189] Repairs are carried out with absorbable sutures on both the anterior and the posterior aspects of the tendon. With severe tendon degeneration, Brodsky and Krause[106] advocated a tenodesis proximal and distal to the peroneus longus. Tenodesis was advocated when viable tendon was less than one third the tendon diameter.

Treatment options include resection of a major tear or defect, debridement of up to one-half the tendon, or tenodesis of the peroneus brevis to the peroneus longus (video clip 54).

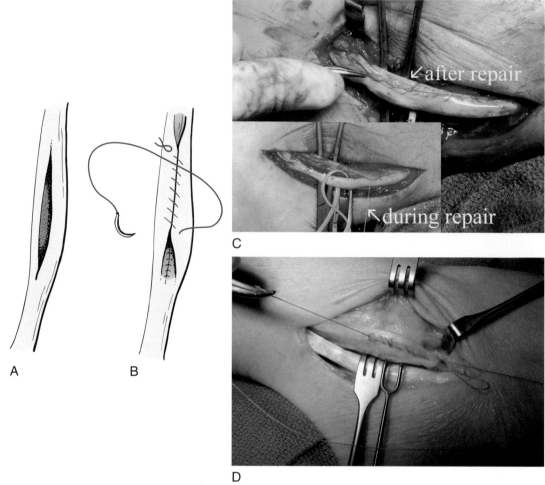

Figure 22–48   Technique of tubulization of a peroneus brevis tear. **A,** Longitudinal tear of peroneus brevis. **B,** Method used to tubulize the peroneus brevis with layered tendon repair. **C,** Tear edges are freshened and tubulization is performed on superficial and deep areas of the tear. **D,** Another example of tubulization of a peroneus brevis tear.

TENDON DEBRIDEMENT AND REPAIR

Surgical Technique

1. The patient is placed in a lateral decubitus position. A thigh tourniquet is used for hemostasis.
2. A longitudinal incision is centered over the course of the peroneal tendons beginning 1 cm posterior and proximal to the distal fibula and extended to the base of the fifth metatarsal. Care is taken to protect the sural nerve, which is posterior to the incision.
3. The superior peroneal retinaculum is identified and incised 5 mm posterior to the fibula, providing an anterior soft tissue cuff that can be repaired later.

4. Both tendons are carefully examined, especially the deep side of the peroneus brevis tendon.
5. With a low-lying peroneus muscle belly or a peroneus quartus, the muscle is excised. Proliferating synovium is debrided.
6. A peripheral tear and frayed edges should be resected (Fig. 22–49).
7. After repair or debridement, the tendons are reduced and the superior peroneal retinaculum repaired.
8. With a degenerative tear and less than one third of viable peroneus tendon available, a tenodesis is performed between the proximal peroneus brevis and longus and the distal peroneus brevis and longus. The per-

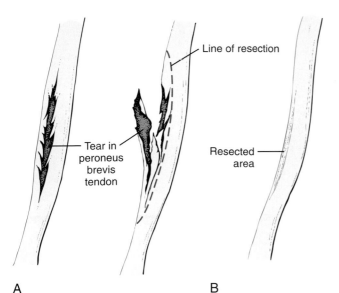

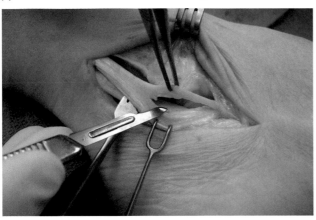

C

Figure 22–49 Technique of resection of peroneus brevis tear. **A,** Two examples of a peroneus brevis tear. **B,** After resection of the smaller portion. **C,** The smaller portion of the peroneus brevis is resected, leaving the larger segment intact.

oneus brevis tendon is woven through in a Pulvertaft repair and sutured in place with interrupted nonabsorbable sutures. It is important to appreciate where the anastomosis will move relative to the distal fibula. If at all possible, impingement and stenosis should be avoided. It may be necessary to move the connection higher or lower to avoid vulnerable locations. A direct tendon-to-tendon reconstruction with core suture technique may be useful to minimize the bulk created by the Pulvertaft weave (Fig. 22–50).

Postoperative Care

A non-weight-bearing below-knee cast is applied with the foot in neutral position. After 2 to 4 weeks of non–weight-bearing crutch ambulation, weight-bearing ambulation in a below-knee cast or fixed brace is permitted. Range of motion exercises should be initiated 2 weeks after surgery with progressive strengthening exercises initiated at 8 weeks.

Results and Complications

Brodsky and Krause[106] noted that with tenodesis, 75% of patients were satisfied postoperatively. Most patients noted gradual resolution of swelling, although a protracted postoperative course was common.

Sammarco and DiRaimondo[184] reported on a series of 14 peroneus brevis tears in 13 patients who complained of ankle instability with symptoms lasting from 8 months to 20 years. In 11 of 13 patients, lateral ankle instability was treated with a split peroneus brevis tendon graft that incorporated the peroneus brevis tear. Typically the tendon tear was present at the level of the distal fibula, with the tears 2 to 5 cm in length. Often the tendon was somewhat broader or thicker than normal in this region and was dull and yellowed with discoloration. Considerable fibrillation or fraying may be present. With passive dorsiflexion of the ankle, intraoperatively a longitudinal cleft in the peroneal brevis may be pressed forward onto the anterior aspect of the fibula.

Complications with a peroneal tendon exploration and reconstruction include sural nerve injury and injury to the superficial branch of the peroneal nerve. With an inadequate repair of the superior retinaculum, recurrent subluxation of the peroneal tendons can occur. Recurrent degenerative tears of the remaining tendon can develop, leading to recurrent pain or nonresolution of symptoms.

Saxena[188] reported on 31 peroneus brevis tears; 24 of these were isolated and 7 were combined with peroneus longus tears. The average American Orthopaedics Foot and Ankle Society (AOFAS) score was 90.8 for isolated tears, and 84.3 for combined tears. Most athletes returned to full sporting level. The average return to activity for the peroneus brevis tears group was 3.6 months, and for the group with combined lesions it was 3.7 months. Dombek[116] reported

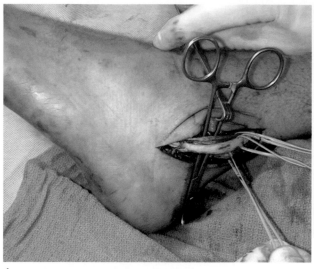

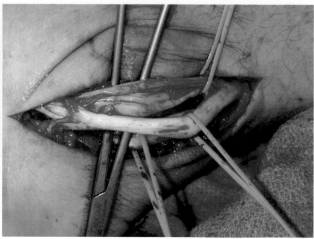

A

B

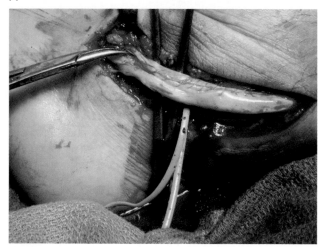

C

Figure 22–50   Tenodesis of the peroneus brevis and longus. **A,** Complex degenerative tear of the peroneus brevis, requiring tenodesis to the peroneus longus as salvage. **B,** Close-up of tear. **C,** Following Pulvertaft weave and tenodesis of two tendons.

that 98% of the patients were able to return to full activities without pain at final follow-up. The minor complication rate was 20%, but clinically significant complications (continued symptoms or revisionary surgery) occurred in an additional 10% of patients.

In Redfern and Myerson's series[181] with concomitant tears of the peroneus longus and brevis tendons, the mean postoperative AOFAS score was 82 (range, 20 to 100) points, and 91% of patients achieved normal or moderate peroneal muscle strength. Ankle instability was successfully corrected in all patients and progressive worsening of varus deformity was prevented.

Options for surgical treatment include resection of bifurcated or trifurcated fragments,[105,143,184,216] resection of degenerated tendon and primary repair,[101,102,111,145,189] reinser-

tion of the distal attachment (Figs. 22–51 and 22–52),[201] and tenodesis to the peroneus longus.[164,182,216] Mizel et al[162] and others[142,214] suggested using a Hunter tendon rod with a two-stage reconstruction technique for an absent or severely damaged peroneus brevis tendon. After trauma, tumor, or previous surgical intervention, if reconstruction cannot be accomplished with a simple tendon transfer (e.g., FHL), a staged procedure may be performed using a Hunter tendon rod to form a pseudosynovial sheath. Approximately 3 months later the Hunter tendon rod is removed, and the FHL tendon is transferred into the pseudosynovial sheath and attached to the distal tendon stump or base of the fifth metatarsal. Myerson[181] suggested considering allograft or FDL transfer, or both, when both tendons were involved.

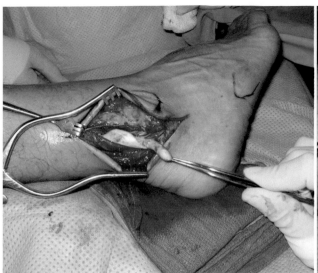

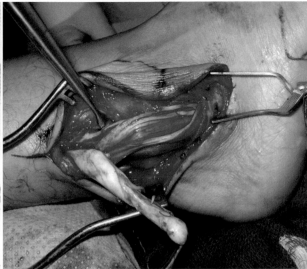

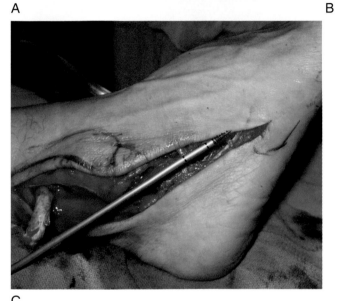

Figure 22–51 Repair of distal rupture of peroneus brevis tendon. **A,** Surgical exposure. **B,** Close-up of ruptured tendon. **C,** Placement of suture anchor for reattachment of tendon into the fifth metatarsal base.

FLEXOR DIGITORUM LONGUS TRANSFER FOR PERONEUS BREVIS LESIONS

Surgery is the procedure of choice for a more active patient who has a chronic degenerative tear of either peroneal tendon that cannot be repaired directly. A long longitudinal attritional rupture in a degenerative tendon or a chronic retracted transverse rupture is an appropriate lesion for this approach. It is an alternative to transection of the diseased tendon and tenodesis to the adjacent healthier tendon.

Because this technique adds an additional power source (the FDL muscle), it can be particularly helpful when the involved tendon's muscle is fibrotic and dysfunctional (as seen following multiple recurrent traumas or failed previous surgeries), in the face of a neurologic lesion to the peroneals (common peroneal or high superficial peroneal nerve lesion), or in cases of hereditary sensory motor nerve dysfunction (Charcot–Marie–Tooth disease). It has been successful in running athletes who require subtle proprioceptive and dynamic power needs for cutting and turning that might not be adequately restored with the tenodesis.

In our series of 17 FDL transfers for peroneal lesions, five were in athletes who had had multiple peroneal surgeries and eight were in

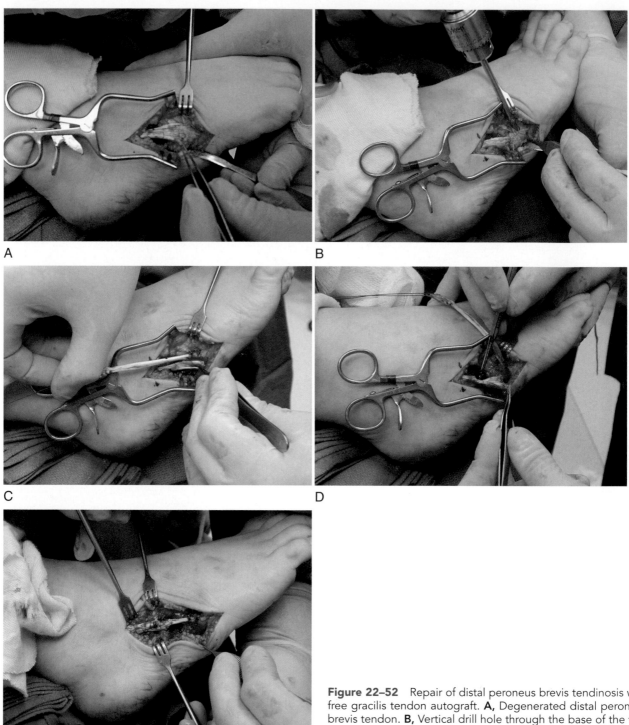

Figure 22–52 Repair of distal peroneus brevis tendinosis with free gracilis tendon autograft. **A,** Degenerated distal peroneus brevis tendon. **B,** Vertical drill hole through the base of the fifth metatarsal. **C,** Attachment of the gracilis tendon autograft through the drill hole. **D,** Resection of the degenerated distal tendon. **E,** Completion of tendon graft repair.

medium-duty or heavy-duty injured workers with prior failed surgical treatment. Six were in patients with neurologic injury or dysfunction. Eleven of the 17 patients had calcaneal varus that required a simultaneous Dwyer osteotomy.

Surgical Technique

1. The patient is positioned in the lateral decubitus position with a tilt of 45 degrees.
2. The peroneal tendons are exposed, typically using the previous incisions (Fig. 22–51A and B). Exposure should be sufficient to fully excise or debride the degenerative tendons. The muscle bellies of the involved tendons are assessed by pulling on the musculotendinous unit and feeling the springiness. When there is no springiness, the muscle is useless and should not be anastomosed to the adjacent tendon. If there is minimal muscular fibrosis, the muscle can be salvaged with a proximal tenodesis.
3. The lateral tuberosity of the calcaneus is exposed to address the varus through either prior incisions or a new one just posterior to the sural nerve (Fig. 22–53D).
4. A laterally based wedge of 5 to 10 mm of bone is removed. Laminar spreaders are placed to distract the osteotomy site by 10 mm. This permits the osteotomy to be translated laterally for additional correction.
5. The osteotomy is then secured with one or two large-fragment (typically cannulated) screws while the fragments are manually held in reduction (Fig. 22–53E).
6. More distally, the fifth metatarsal tuberosity is exposed if the brevis is the primary pathologic tendon. The zone of exposure should permit insertion of a corkscrew suture anchor deep into the metaphyseal bone. Image intensification should be used to ensure proper placement of the anchor (Fig. 22–53F and G).
7. A 5- to 10-mm zone of bone should be elevated in anticipation of attachment to the FDL. On the other hand, if the longus is to be replaced, then exposure is necessary to bypass the degenerative tendon. If there is a chronic dislocation or convex groove in the retrofibular region, a groove-deepening procedure (described later) should be considered.
8. Next, the bean bag or lateral bump is removed to initiate exposure of the FDL. When a tendon transfer is needed, the FDL

is harvested at or below the master knot of Henry. In an athlete, consideration for tenodesis of the distal FDL stump to the FHL is appropriate. When less length is needed, the tendon can be sectioned proximal to the knot (Fig. 22–53B).

9. A second incision is made 7 cm above the medial malleolus and extended for 3 cm proximally. Here the FDL is pulled proximally with preservation of the distal muscle belly (Fig. 22–53C). A Kelly clamp is passed from the medial incision along the posterior aspect of the tibia until the peroneal sheath is entered. If the tendon is not already exposed, an incision is made where the clamp penetrates. A second Kelly clamp from the lateral side is then connected to the first and the tip of the second Kelly clamp is delivered into the medial wound, where it is used to pull the tendon to the lateral side (Fig. 22–53D).
10. The FDL is then passed through the sheath and distally deep to the sural nerve to the distal anastomosis site or at the fifth metatarsal tuberosity at the corkscrew anchor site. The length of the transferred tendon is assessed with the tendon taut and the foot and ankle held in eversion. Excess tendon is resected.
11. A modified Krackow technique using one arm of the no. 0 or no. 2 suture is woven through the FDL up one side and down the other. The other suture strand is then used to advance the tendon to the tuberosity and tied securely. If the attachment is more proximal, the tuberosity site may still be preferred; otherwise an anastomosis is performed, providing the attachment site is not going to be a bulky impediment to tendon motion. For example, if the anastomosis will occur in the distal retrofibular region, a more proximal or more distal anastomosis is preferable to avoid stenosis.
12. The incisions are then closed with the foot and ankle in a relaxed plantar flexion and eversion position. A U and posterior well-padded splint is applied in this position over a sterile dressing.

Postoperative Care

Postoperatively the patient is kept non–weight bearing for 6 weeks. After the sutures are removed at 2 weeks, gentle range of motion

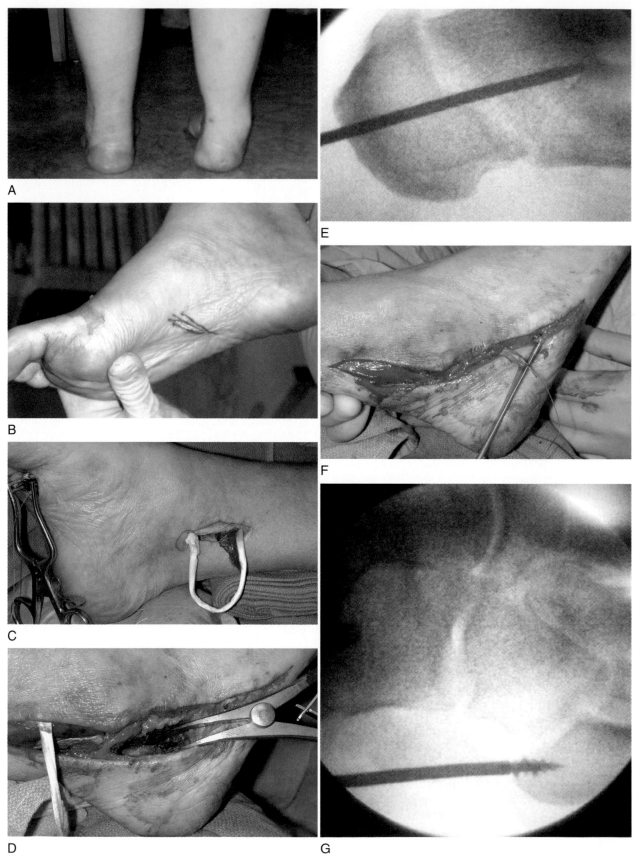

Figure 22–53 Method of reconstruction using flexor digitorum longus (FDL) tendon as free graft for absence of both peroneals. **A,** Marked varus preoperatively with peroneal brevis and longus tendon ruptures. **B,** Incision for harvest of FDL in arch. **C,** Following distal detachment of the tendon, the FDL is passed proximally into an incision above the ankle. The FDL tendon is now passed from posterior to the tibia to posterior to the fibula in the peroneal tendon sheath. **D,** A closing wedge calcaneal osteotomy to correct the varus. The osteotomy is also translated laterally. **E,** Fluoroscopy of osteotomy. **F,** Suture anchor placement into the base of the fifth metatarsal to secure the distal graft. **G,** Fluoroscopy of placement of the suture anchor.

should be performed to minimize tendon scarring. The patient should avoid dorsiflexion beyond 10 degrees of equinus and 10 degrees of inversion. Passive eversion is encouraged, but active eversion should be limited for 6 weeks. At 6 weeks the equinus splinting or bracing is discontinued and the ankle is held in neutral in a brace. Weight bearing can be initiated, followed by active eversion. At 8 to 12 weeks the boot brace can be discontinued, and a stirrup brace is worn. During the third through sixth month the stirrup is worn during walking, running, or stressful activities.

Peroneal Tendon Subluxation–Dislocation

Subluxation–dislocation of the peroneal tendons, although not rare, represent a relatively uncommon condition. Unfortunately, acute peroneal tendon dislocations are often unrecognized or misdiagnosed as "lateral ankle sprains," which often results in chronic instability that requires surgical correction.

Monteggia[163] (1803) is credited with the first description of peroneal tendon dislocation.[151] Later in the nineteenth century, Blanulet (1875) and Gutierrez (1877)[109] initially proposed surgical treatment.

Most acute peroneal tendon dislocations are associated with a traumatic episode and usually with athletic activities, often including alpine skiing. However, injuries from football, tennis, basketball, soccer, ice skating, and running have been reported as well.[101,152,185] Earle et al[118] estimated that peroneal tendon dislocation accounted for 0.5% of all skiing injuries. In a review of 265 reported cases in the literature, McGarvey and Clanton[152] observed that 71% were related to alpine skiing. Football was the second most common cause of peroneal tendon injury, cited in 7% of reports.

Several more recent reports have highlighted a slightly different perspective on peroneal dislocation and subluxation. Porter's series[178] of 14 cases of subluxation and dislocation included four from soccer, four from football, two from basketball, and one each from rugby, dancing, cycling, and baseball. Kollias and Ferkel[141] reported on 13 athletes with subluxation and dislocation. Only one was a skier; the others skated or played softball, basketball, soccer, football, or tennis.

Acute dislocations have been more frequently reported in association with fractures and dislocations of the fibula, talus, and calcaneus. These have occurred in more violent traumas such as falls, motor vehicle accidents and industrial injuries. Because more obvious bone and joint conditions are the focus of the surgeons, the tendon disorder is overlooked. Schon et al[137] reported on 23 chronic intractable peroneal subluxation–dislocations as defined by 12 months of symptoms. In this report, the average time to recognition involved several months of delay. Eight of the 23 patients were athletes, and the other 15 were workers or victims of more serious trauma. Of the seven with calcaneal fractures, six had chronic sural neuritis, one had chronic regional pain syndrome, and five had concomitant peroneal tears. In the athletic subgroup, there were four peroneal tendon tears and two patients with chronic sural neuritis.

Brodsky and Krause[106] reported on 20 patients with peroneal brevis tendon tears. Alanen et al[98] and Tan et al[205] have both reported series of peroneal tendon tears.

Anatomy

At the ankle the peroneal tendons course through a fibro-osseous tunnel at the level of the distal fibula that is bordered anteriorly by the posterior surface of the lateral malleolus; medially by the posterior talofibular ligament, posterior inferior tibiofibular ligament, and calcaneal fibular ligament[101,185]; and posterolaterally by the superior peroneal retinaculum (SPR). The peroneal tendons are enveloped by a synovial sheath that extends from the inferior border of the peroneal musculature to a point 1 cm below the fibula, where they enter separate and distinct synovial sheaths.[209] Over the course of the distal 2 cm of fibula, the synovial sheath and fascia of the lower calf condense to form the SPR, which is the main primary restraint to subluxation–dislocation of the peroneal tendons as they course around the tip of the fibula. The SPR extends from the posteroinferior edge of the fibula in an inferoposterior direction and inserts on the os calcis.

In an analysis of 30 fibular anatomic specimens, Davis et al[114] determined that the SPR originated from the posterolateral ridge of the fibula in all cases. Although averaging 10 to 20 mm in width, substantial variance was recognized in the width, thickness, and area of insertion. One or two fibrous bands course in a posteroinferior direction, inserting onto the calcaneus in 30% of cases, the Achilles tendon sheath in 60%, and the calcaneus and Achilles tendon in 10%. At least one band typically runs parallel to the calcaneofibular ligament, theoretically placing it at risk for simultaneous injury with a severe ankle sprain.

Edwards[120] examined 178 cadaver fibulas and noted a substantial recess or groove on the posterior aspect of the fibula in 82% and a plantar convex surface in

18% of the specimens. A flat or convex surface on the posterior fibula may be associated with instability of the peroneal tendons. The depth of the groove is variable (2 to 4 mm) and is accentuated by an osseous ridge that is covered by a fibrocartilaginous cap, adding another 2 to 4 mm to the overall depth of the sulcus (Fig. 22–54). Edwards[120] speculated that an insufficient lateral ridge predisposed to peroneal dislocation. The SPR has no strong attachments to the ridge itself[101] but blends with the periosteum on the lateral surface of the fibula. The inferior peroneal retinaculum attaches superiorly and inferiorly to the lateral wall of the calcaneus just below the sinus tarsi, forming a "pulley" over both peroneal tendons. The inferior peroneal retinaculum plays no role in the stability of the peroneal tendons at the level of the ankle.

Mechanism of Injury

Although a disruption or tear of the SPR has been implicated in peroneal tendon dislocation,[134,153,165,177]

rupture of the retinaculum rarely occurs.[112,118,119] Typically the retinaculum is stripped off the fibular insertion[101,112,118] or avulsed with a small fleck of fibular cortex.[180] Das De and Balasubramaniam[112] have likened this to a Bankart lesion of the shoulder, with the creation of a false pouch and laxity of the retinaculum,[202] allowing peroneal tendon dislocation anteriorly.

The mechanism of injury is typically a sudden forceful dorsiflexion and inversion injury of the ankle with a simultaneous violent contraction of the peroneal musculature, leading to a disruption of the SPR. Sobel et al[198] reported a simultaneous rupture of the calcaneofibular ligament with injury to the SPR, and in their report, this isolated case was treated with a Chrisman–Snook ankle reconstruction.

The high incidence of peroneal tendon dislocation associated with skiing injuries supports the premise of both forced dorsiflexion and acute forceful contraction of the peroneal musculature because a ski boot places

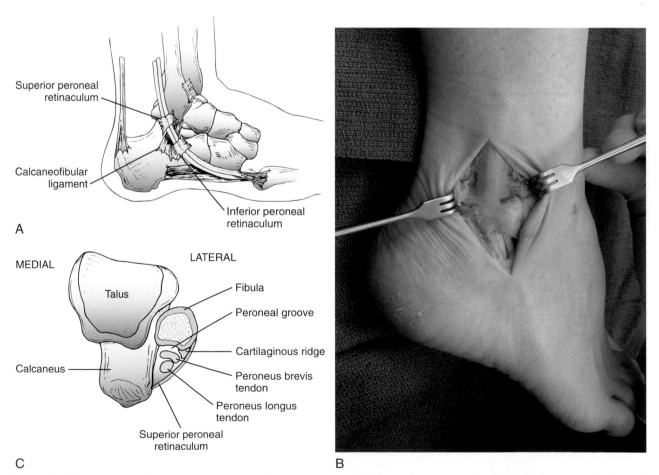

Figure 22–54 A, Lateral view of ankle demonstrates peroneal tendons beneath the superior and inferior peroneal retinacula. **B,** Clinical photo of superior peroneal retinaculum. **C,** Superior view demonstrates position of the peroneus brevis anterior to the peroneus longus tendon.

the ankle in a dorsiflexed position that limits ankle excursion, thus allowing substantial muscle contraction against a fixed ankle. The edging mechanism on the inside edge with alpine skiing places the dorsiflexed ankle in eversion as well, increasing the propensity for an injury with a caught edge.

Chronic subluxation can also occur in patients with recurrent ankle sprains. In the study of associated injuries found in chronic lateral ankle instability by DiGiovanni et al,[115] peroneal tenosynovitis was found in 47 of 61 (77%), attenuated peroneal retinaculum or retinacular avulsion was found in 33 of 61 (54%), and peroneal tendon tears were noted in 15 of 61 (25%). In these cases the chronic stretching of the SPR can allow expansion of the retrofibular ligamentous structures, thereby predisposing the tendons to roll or jump around each other more without the constraints. With time the recurrent riding of the peroneal tendons around each other and over the edge can predispose them to longitudinal splits and worsening of the subluxation.

Neuromuscular abnormalities (paralysis, polio) are also associated with peroneal tendon dislocation.[144,202] Kojima et al[140] reported congenital dislocation of the peroneal tendons in 3% of neonates, and this may be a more common entity than appreciated. When untreated, almost all cases resolve spontaneously, although one can only speculate whether these patients are at higher risk for peroneal subluxation–dislocation in later life. Some patients recall no specific history of trauma related to peroneal tendon dislocation.

Peroneal tendon subluxation–dislocation is first distinguished as either acute or chronic. Eckert and Davis[119] further differentiated different grades depending on the type of injury, and they documented the incidence of occurrence as follows:

Grade I (51%): The retinaculum is elevated from the lateral malleolus with the tendons lying between the bone and periosteum (Fig. 22–55A).

Grade II (33%): The fibrocartilaginous ridge is elevated with the retinaculum attached, and the tendons are displaced beneath the ridge (Fig. 22–55B).

Grade III (16%): A thin cortical fragment is avulsed from the fibula with the tendons displaced beneath the fibular fragment (Fig. 22–55C).

Oden[167] added also graded peroneal tendon dislocations and included a rare grade IV, with the retinaculum avulsed or ruptured from the posterior attachment (Table 22–1).

TABLE 22-1

Gradations of Peroneal Tendon Dislocations

Grade	Characteristics
I	Superior peroneal retinaculum (SPR) is still attached to the periosteum on the posterior aspect of the fibula. However, the periosteum is elevated from the underlying malleolus by the dissections that are displaced anteriorly.
II	SPR is torn free from its anterior insertion on the malleolus, and the periosteum of the tendons dissects through at this level.
III	SPR is avulsed from the insertion on the malleolus with avulsion of a small fragment of bone.
IV	SPR is torn from its posterior attachment as tendon dissects through, with the SPR lying deep to the dislocating peroneal tendon.

Modified from Oden R: *Clin Orthop Relat Res* 216:63-69, 1987.

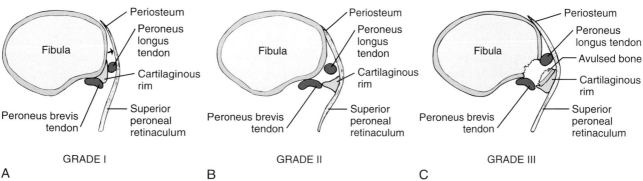

Figure 22–55 Classification of peroneal tendon subluxation–dislocation. **A,** Grade I: superior peroneal retinaculum (SPR) stripped off the fibula; peroneus longus dislocated anteriorly. **B,** Grade II injury: fibrous rim avulsed from posterolateral aspect of the fibula along with the SPR; peroneus longus dislocated anteriorly. **C,** Grade III: bony rim avulsion fracture attached to the SPR, with anterior dislocation of peroneus longus.

Grade III injuries can often be distinguished on plain radiographic examination, whereas grade I and II can only be differentiated at surgery. Eckert and Davis[119] noted that with reduction of the peroneal tendons, grade III injuries were grossly unstable after reduction. Grade II injuries were also unstable when reduced, but grade I injuries were unstable only in dorsiflexion. This can help to explain the success rate of less than 50% when nonsurgical care is elected after acute rupture. Only with a pure SPR avulsion (with disruption of either bone or fibrosseous ridge, grades II and III) can success with nonsurgical treatment be reasonably expected.

History and Physical Examination

With an *acute* dislocation the patient often recalls a significant episode of trauma. A painful snapping sensation may be associated with the actual disruption. Significant pain localized to the retromalleolar area often subsides relatively rapidly.[101] With spontaneous relocation of the peroneal tendons, a patient might relate a history of a "lateral ankle sprain." However, unlike the history of a sprain in which a patient recalls an inversion injury, with peroneal tendon dislocation the mechanism of injury is often vague. With *chronic* instability, a generalized history of "recurrent sprains" is elicited, although occasionally a patient specifically describes peroneal tendon dislocation. The patient might complain of snapping or popping or instability on uneven ground.

On physical examination, subluxation or dislocation is often missed unless it is specifically evaluated. Sarmiento and Wolf[185] and others[99,109,118,165] noted that acute dislocations are rarely diagnosed. Without early diagnosis and prompt appropriate treatment, dislocation invariably recurs.[101,121] Acutely, a variable amount of swelling and ecchymosis may be present in the retrofibular region, which can obscure the dislocated peroneal tendons. Pain is localized to the posterior aspect of the fibula more proximally and posteriorly than pain associated with an injury to the anterior talofibular ligament. It should not be difficult to differentiate peroneal tendon injury from an acute ankle sprain, but the patient should be evaluated for lateral ankle instability with a drawer and talar tilt examination as well.

With acute peroneal tendon dislocation, palpable crepitus may be noted over the posterior rim of the fibula. The ankle is passively circumducted, and with this maneuver, subluxation may be identified.[130] The patient is then asked to dorsiflex and evert the foot and ankle from a plantar-flexed, inverted position. With tensing of the peroneals, pain may be noted posterior to the fibula. Then, with resisted dorsiflexion and eversion, subluxation or dislocation of the peroneal tendons can occur. With active circumduction of the ankle and foot in clockwise and counterclockwise fashions, the peroneal tendons are palpated in the retrofibular region. Although many normal people have popping of the tendons, there are subtle side-to-side differences that are apparent in most cases. With chronic instability, swelling or ecchymosis is often minimal. An inability to dislocate the peroneal tendons does not necessarily rule out instability.[152]

On occasion a patient demonstrates anxiety when the foot and ankle are placed in a dorsiflexed and everted position. A high index of suspicion is necessary to make a diagnosis of instability of the peroneal tendons. Examination of the contralateral ankle is important in evaluating the patient for ligamentous laxity. Assessment of the patient in standing and during gait can reveal calcaneal varus. Coexisting ankle ligament instability and peroneal tendon weakness should be identified. Subtalar and ankle disorder may be found in these patients.

Radiographic Examination

Imaging of the injured ankle can occasionally be helpful in ascertaining the diagnosis of peroneal tendon instability. Routine AP, lateral, and mortise radiographs are often normal but can demonstrate a small flake of fibular cortex (0.5 to 1 cm in length), indicating a grade III injury, which is pathognomonic of a tendon dislocation. Ankle stress views for ankle instability may be performed. Computed tomography (CT) is infrequently used at present.[168,169] A CT scan may be helpful with an uncertain diagnosis to evaluate the posterior fibular groove.[101,125,204] Ultrasound evaluation is confirmatory in skilled hands.[166] MRI may be helpful in assessing a concomitant peroneal tendon injury (Fig. 22–56).[219]

Acute Dislocation

Treatment of acute peroneal tendon dislocation is controversial.[101]

Conservative Treatment

Nonsurgical treatment is always an option. McGarvey and Clanton[152] considered it a safe treatment, although they recognized the high failure rate. Sarmiento and Wolf[185] stated that an acute dislocation can be casted. Stover and Bryan[202] advocated initial conservative treatment in a well-molded below-knee cast in mild plantar flexion for 5 to 6 weeks. They reported success with casting in 57% and with taping in 40% of cases treated. The purpose of casting is to contain the peroneal tendons while the SPR heals. McLennan[153] noted that although conservative care was satisfactory "in most cases," 44% eventually required surgery. Escalas et al[121] attempted conservative

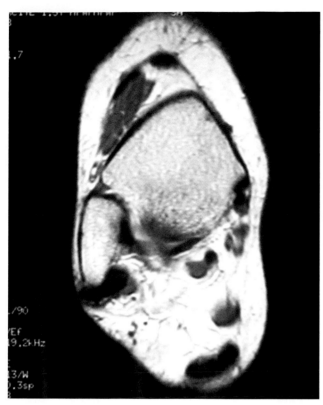

Figure 22-56 Magnetic resonance image demonstrating subluxation of peroneal tendons.

care in 38 patients, 28 of whom (74%) required eventual surgery. Earle et al[118] and others[99,119,165] noted that conservative treatment for acute peroneal tendon dislocation has a success rate of less than 50%.

These injuries tend to occur in young adults and athletes. This population generally wants a speedy return to athletic pursuits, and surgical reconstruction has a much higher rate of success compared with nonsurgical treatment.

When choosing casting, we prefer a well-molded below-knee cast in slight plantar flexion and slight inversion. A non–weight-bearing cast for 2 weeks is preferred to allow resolution of swelling.[152] This is followed by a below-knee walking cast or brace for 4 weeks, after which active range-of-motion exercises and physical therapy are initiated.

Surgical Treatment

Arrowsmith et al[101] and others advocate acute repair, citing excellent results and rapid recovery. Arrowsmith et al[101] also have called attention to peroneus brevis tears in patients with chronic peroneal instability, which significantly complicates the recovery process following delayed reconstruction and argues for early repair after peroneal tendon dislocation.

Direct reattachment of the SPR to the posterior periosteum of the fibula through multiple drill holes is the treatment of choice for repair of acute peroneal tendon dislocation.

DIRECT SUPERIOR PERONEAL RETINACULUM REPAIR

Surgical Technique

1. The patient is placed in a prone position under appropriate anesthesia and with a thigh tourniquet inflated to afford adequate hemostasis. A 6-cm longitudinal incision is centered 1 cm posterior to the fibula and extended from 5 cm proximal to 2 cm distal to the tip of the fibula. Care is taken to protect the sural nerve (Fig. 22–57A).
2. The SPR is identified and incised longitudinally 1 cm from the posterior edge of the fibula (Fig. 22–57B).
3. The fibular ridge is scarified with an osteotome, and three or four lateral-to-medial drill holes are placed vertically through the cortex and directed slightly posteriorly.
4. The sutures are passed through the drill holes and the SPR, securing the avulsed retinaculum to the fibular ridge.
5. The sutures are tied. The retinaculum is then imbricated along the incision line with absorbable sutures (Fig. 22–57C).
6. The subcutaneous tissue and skin are approximated in a routine manner (Fig. 22–58).

Postoperative Care

The foot is placed in a non–weight-bearing below-knee cast or splint with the foot in slight equinus and slight eversion. McGarvey and Clanton[152] argue that because the retinaculum has been repaired, slight eversion is acceptable, in contrast to nonsurgical treatment, where slight inversion is advocated to maintain reduction of the peroneal tendons. After 2 weeks in a non–weight-bearing cast or splint, a plantigrade below-knee cast or boot brace is applied and weight bearing is allowed for four weeks. Cast immobilization is then discontinued and may be replaced by a brace from which the patient is gradually weaned and physical therapy initiated.

Direct repair of acute peroneal tendon dislocation has been advocated by a number of authors. In 76 reported cases,[99,103,112,118,168] a 96% success rate has been reported.[152]

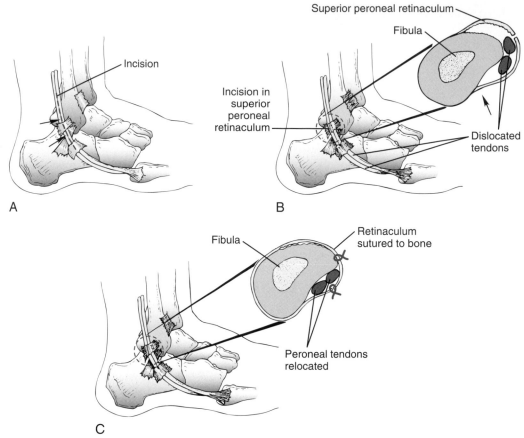

Figure 22–57 Surgical repair of acute peroneal tendon dislocation. **A,** Surgical incision. **B,** Pathologic anatomy demonstrates dislocation of peroneal tendons. **C,** Repair of superior peroneal retinaculum (SPR) with drill holes through the posterolateral portion of fibula and reefing of SPR.

CHRONIC DISLOCATION

The incidence of missed diagnosis or untreated peroneal tendon dislocation is high, leading often to recurrent dislocation. Casting and other nonsurgical methods can serve to reduce pain or diminish inflammation but have little success in permanent relocation of chronically dislocated peroneal tendons. Numerous surgical procedures have been designed to stabilize chronically dislocating peroneal tendons, attesting to no one technique's being uniformly successful in the literature (Box 22–1).

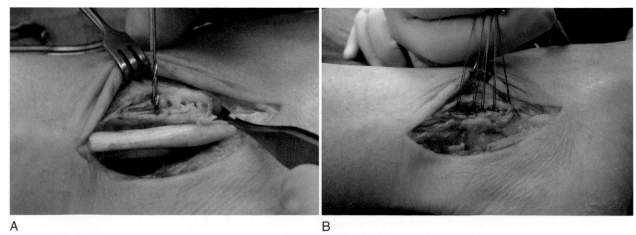

Figure 22–58 Acute repair of peroneal tendon subluxation. **A,** Following repair of small tendon tear, drill holes are placed in posterior fibular ridge. **B,** Several interrupted sutures are placed securing the superior peroneal retinaculum.

BOX 22-1 Types of Surgical Reconstruction for Peroneal Tendon Dislocation

Direct repair of peroneal retinaculum[112]
Reconstruction of peroneal retinaculum
    Achilles tendon sling[134]
    Plantaris sling[160]
    Peroneus brevis sling[101,199]
    Anomalous muscle[130]
Bone block
    Lateral malleolar osteotomy[135]
    Sliding graft (lateral malleolus)[117,156]
Groove deepening with osteoperiosteal flap[101,221]
Rerouting procedure beneath calcaneofibular ligament
    Calcaneofibular ligament mobilized with bone block from calcaneus[177]
    Calcaneofibular mobilized by osteotomizing the lateral malleolus[179]
    Peroneal tendons divided and rerouted under calcaneofibular ligament[149,185]

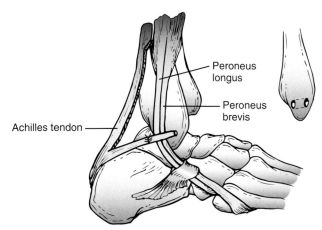

Figure 22-59 Ellis–Jones reconstruction of peroneal retinaculum employing a portion of Achilles tendon.

McGarvey and Clanton[152] have grouped the various techniques into the following areas: SPR reinforcement and repair, tissue-transfer techniques, tendon-rerouting techniques, bone-block procedures, and groove-deepening procedures.

SUPERIOR PERONEAL RETINACULUM REINFORCEMENT AND REPAIR

This technique is the same as used for an acute repair with reconstruction of the SPR. When an avulsion of the fibular ridge has occurred, it is reduced and internally fixed. Alm et al[99] and others[103,112] reported success with this procedure. Although a simple repair might not adequately stabilize peroneal tendons in the presence of a convex groove or an insufficient SPR, this technique may be combined with other techniques of reconstruction as well.

TISSUE TRANSFER TECHNIQUES

Jones[134] described the use of a distally attached slip of Achilles tendon routed through the fibula to create a reinforced retinaculum to stabilize the peroneal tendons (Fig. 22–59). Escalas et al[121] and others[119,125] also advocated this technique. The peroneus brevis[157,187,199] and the plantaris[160] have been chosen to reinforce the SPR, but no large series have been reported on these techniques. McGarvey and Clanton[152] noted a 19% complication rate with this technique.

TENDON REROUTING TECHNIQUES

Various techniques have been proposed to reroute the peroneal tendons, and most use the calcaneofibular ligament to stabilize the peroneal tendons. Platzgummer[176] and others[104,200] divided the calcaneofibular ligament near the fibular insertion (Fig. 22–60); Viernstein et al[212] and Poll and Duijfjes[177] performed a distal fibular osteotomy (Fig. 22–61); and Pozo and Jackson[179] transposed the calcaneofibular ligament

Figure 22-60 Platzgummer method for repair of dislocating peroneal tendons. Peroneal tendons are rerouted beneath the calcaneofibular ligament, which is repaired. **A,** Calcaneofibular ligament has been divided and turned down. **B,** Peroneal tendons have been relocated and calcaneofibular ligament repaired. (Modified from Platzgummer H: *Arch Orthop Unfallchir* 61:144-150, 1967.)

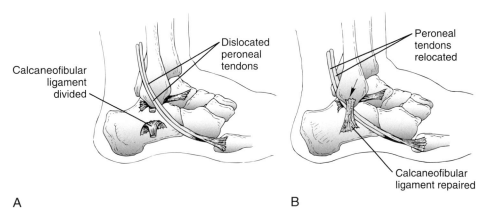

A   B

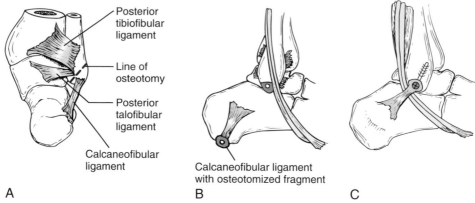

Figure 22–61 Bone block osteotomized from fibula. **A,** Line of osteotomy through fibula. **B,** Osteotomized fibular fragment is attached to the calcaneofibular ligament and turned inferiorly. The hole is predrilled in the fragment before performing the osteotomy. **C,** After peroneal tendons have been reduced, the osteotomized fragment is reattached and stabilized with internal fixation. (Redrawn from Pozo J, Jackson A: *Foot Ankle* 5:42-44, 1984.)

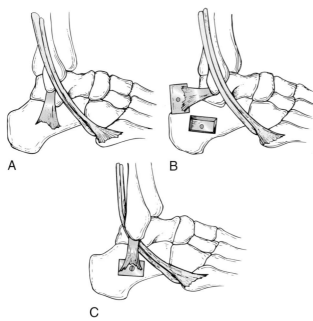

Figure 22–62 Calcaneofibular ligament transferred with bone block from calcaneus. **A,** Tendons are dislocated anteriorly. **B,** Bone block is mobilized from the calcaneus. **C,** After peroneal tendons have been relocated, bone block is internally fixed, stabilizing tendons. (Redrawn from Poll R, Duijfjes F: *J Bone Joint Surg Br* 66:98-100, 1984.)

with a calcaneal bone block (Fig. 22–62). Sarmiento and Wolf[185] and Martens et al[149] divided the peroneal tendons and repaired them after rerouting them beneath the calcaneofibular ligament. No dislocations have been reported, but a high rate of associated sural nerve injury and ankle stiffness has been noted. McGarvey and Clanton[152] note a complication rate of 61% with this technique.

One of the authors (MJC) has used the technique described by Sarmiento and Wolf[185] (Fig. 22–63) in skeletally immature patients with good success and I believe it should be included in the surgeon's armamentarium.

LeNoir[146] described a case of anterior transposition of the peroneal tendons and sheath as an alternative, routing them anterior to the distal fibula. However, no other reports are available on this procedure, and it is not recommended.

One of the authors (LCS) has also used a rerouting technique for chronic painful snapping peroneal tendons that did not respond to a groove-deepening procedure. In this procedure, the peroneus longus was placed in a channel that was created obliquely in the distal lateral aspect of the fibula, separating it from the

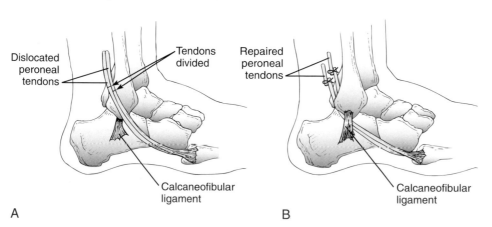

Figure 22–63 Method of rerouting peroneal tendons beneath calcaneofibular ligament by dividing tendons and repairing them. **A,** Pathologic anatomy. **B,** Peroneal tendons are relocated beneath calcaneofibular ligament after division and repair.

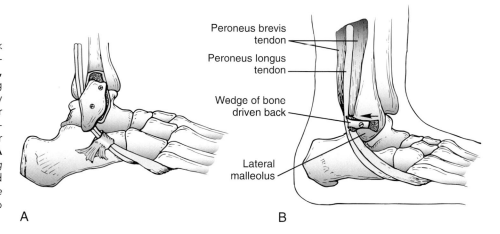

Figure 22–64 Bone block procedures for repair of subluxating peroneal tendons. **A,** Kelly technique for deepening the retromalleolar sulcus by rotating a distal fibular osteotomy. **B,** DuVries modification employing distal fibular osteotomy sliding graft. (**A** modified from Kelly R: *Br J Surg* 7:502-504, 1920; **B** modified from DuVries H: *Surgery of the Foot.* St Louis, Mosby, 1959, pp 253-255.)

brevis, which was left in the retrofibular groove. A portion of free synovial graft tacked to the bone was used to create a lining for the longus in the new fibula channel. In these two cases there was an improvement in the painful snapping, better function, and decreased swelling. Both patients continued to have some symptoms, however, despite the benefit.

BONE BLOCK PROCEDURES

Kelly[135] initially described a partial-thickness distal fibular osteotomy that was rotated posteriorly to deepen the fibular groove (Fig. 22–64A). DuVries[117] and Micheli et al[156] modified this procedure with variations of the Kelly technique (Fig. 22–64B). Wirth[218] and others[150,153,156] reported good results following distal fibular osteotomy, although a high rate of complications has been associated with internal fixation, graft fracture, tendon irritation, chronic pain, nonunion, and resubluxation.[144]

GROOVE-DEEPENING PROCEDURES

By resecting bone on the posterior aspect of the distal fibula, the peroneal groove is deepened, altering and increasing the stability of the peroneal tendon (Fig. 22–65). These procedures require some technical skill but are useful. Although McGarvey and Clanton[152] reported a 30% complication rate with groove-deepening procedures, we have used this technique with very few complications. Tracy[209] stated that peroneal groove deepening was biomechanically an unsound procedure, but Title et al[208] showed biomechanically that pressures within the middle and distal peroneal groove significantly decreased after a groove-deepening procedure when performed in the manner described next. They found it enhanced peroneal stability and decreased pressure on the peroneal tendons, and this can improve peroneal function and decrease

retrofibular pain. Zoellner and Clancy[221] and others[101,118,191] have used this technique with good success. Zoellner and Clancy[221] advocated reinforcing the SPR in combination with this procedure.

One other technique for groove deepening, which has been advocated by Mendicino et al[154] and Shawen et al,[190] deserves mention. This method involves deepening the groove by inserting progressively larger drills through the tip of the distal fibula just anterior to the calcaneofibular ligament. This weakens the posterior cancellous bone that supports the osteocartilaginous posterior aspect of the fibular groove. Next a bone tamp is inserted and the posterior fibular surface is impacted into the medullary canal. Although this procedure may be useful, further study is warranted to highlight its benefits over the flap technique as described next.

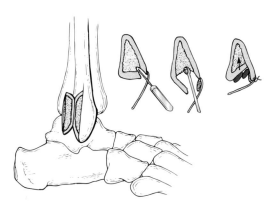

Figure 22–65 Groove deepening procedure with osteoperiosteal flaps. Decancellation of posterior surface of the lateral malleolus and recessing of cortex to deepen groove. (Modified from Arrowsmith S, Fleming L, Allman F: *Am J Sports Med* 11:142-146, 1983.)

GROOVE DEEPENING WITH A POSTERIOR OSTEOCARTILAGINOUS FLAP

Surgical Technique

1. After induction of either general anesthesia or a local ankle block with intravenous sedation anesthesia, the patient is placed in a lateral decubitus position.
2. A 4-cm incision is made over the posterior edge of the fibula, curving around the lateral malleolus anteriorly for 5 to 10 mm of the distal incision. Care is taken to avoid the branch of the sural nerve (Fig. 22–66A).
3. The subcutaneous tissues are dissected and the peroneal tendon sheaths are examined. The ankle is passively manipulated in dorsiflexion, plantar flexion, eversion, and inversion to observe subluxation of the tendons.
4. The tendon sheath is incised 1 mm posterior to the fibula. Peroneal tendons are checked for abnormal pathologic processes (tendinitis or tears), and the shape of retromalleolar groove is examined. Depending upon what is seen intraoperatively, tenosynovectomy or repair of a ruptured retinaculum or peroneal sheath is performed.
5. The anterior sheath of the retinaculum is sharply elevated off the fibula, and the fibula periosteum is raised for an area of 1 to 1.5 cm.
6. With a chisel, a 2- to 3-mm posterior osteocartilaginous flap is detached from the retromalleolar groove with subchondral bone from lateral to medial. The flap is 3 to 4 cm long and includes the distal aspect of the groove. The flap is 8 to 11 mm wide and includes the entire posterior surface of the fibula groove (Fig. 22–66B and C).
7. Two Homan retractors are placed behind the medial edge of the posterior fibula, reflecting the flap and tendons posteriorly. Using a bur, the groove is deepened by removing 4 to 7 mm of cancellous bone (Fig. 22–66D).
8. Next, 0.045-inch Kirschner wires are used to create three or four tunnels in the posterior and lateral edge of the fibula. Each wire is left in place and cut immediately before the suture is ready to be passed. The tunnels are started 4 mm anterior to the posterior edge, and they exit in the posterior cancellous bone just inside the remaining lateral wall of the fibula. These wires should not substantially block the flap from being repositioned.
9. The flap is placed onto the cancellous surface and the tendons are returned to the groove (Fig. 22–66E).
10. Using a 2-0 polyester (Ethibond) suture, a modified Kessler method is used to hold the most anterior edge (1 to 2 mm) of the posterior aspect of the sheath and retinaculum. The sutures are placed from bone to tissue and then back to bone, but they are not tied until all the throws are placed. These sutures will pull the retinaculum into the posterior lateral aspect of the groove inside the lateral wall the fibula, helping to secure the tendons and the flap and providing a cover for the raw bone surface at the fibula edge. The sutures are tied (Fig. 22–66F-H).
11. The anterior aspect of the periosteum that had been raised is advanced posteriorly and oversewn to the posterior retinaculum and sheath with 2-0 polyglactin (Vicryl) suture, taking care to avoid the tendons within. The skin is then closed with 4-0 nylon suture. The foot is placed in a bulky Jones dressing in the neutral position.

Postoperative Care

The splint is removed at 10 days and a fixed ankle boot brace applied. The patient is allowed full weight bearing and may do gentle ankle range-of-motion activities, avoiding plantar flexion of greater than 20 degrees and any inversion. At 6 weeks following surgery, a lace-up cloth or Aircast-type stirrup ankle brace is applied.

The patient may use an elliptical trainer or exercise bike with the brace and may begin jogging at 8 to 10 weeks. Cutting activities can begin after the patient has successfully progressed from large figures of eight to small figures of eight, typically at 12 weeks.

Results and Complications

This method does offer treatment to the 18% of patients who have a shallow or convex posterior fibular surface, and it can be helpful even in the presence of a normal groove. Peroneal tendon groove deepening procedures have become more widely accepted. These procedures are claimed to be less complicated than other bone procedures, while correcting the underlying

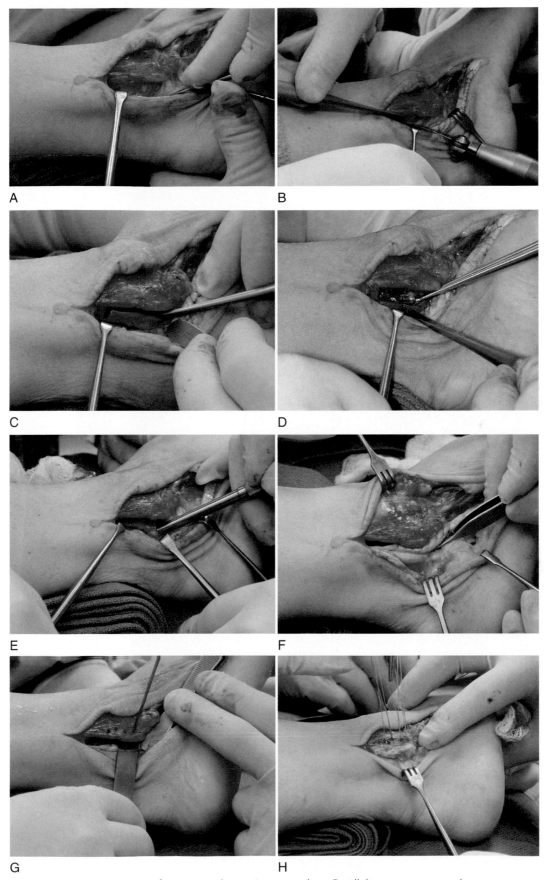

Figure 22–66 **A,** Operative exposure for groove deepening procedure. Parallel saw cuts are used to create a trap door (**B**), which is hinged (**C**) posteriorly, exposing cancellous bone. **D,** Curet or bur is used to decompress this area. **E,** Trap door is impacted into place, creating an offset and deepening the recess posterior to the fibula. **F,** Peroneal tendons are relocated. **G,** Drill holes are placed in the fibular lip. **H,** Sutures are tied securing the superior peroneal retinaculum.

anatomic deformity, preserving the gliding surface, alleviating pain and subluxation, and preserving essential tendons, ligaments, and range of motion.

Complications associated with peroneal tendon groove deepening include redislocation, decreased range of motion, sural nerve injury, and friction of the tendon after repair. In a series of 36 groove deepening procedures by one author (LCS), 23 patients had peroneal dislocations and 13 patients had chronic peroneal tendon pain. In the latter group, 10 of 13 were athletic-induced injuries and 3 of 13 were trauma-induced injuries. This group was interesting because 5 of the 13 had abnormal grooves, 3 of the 13 had revision surgery for peroneal tendon tears in the face of normal grooves, and 5 of the 13 (all athletes) had normal tendons and grooves but had chronic retromalleolar pain relieved with a local injection (I suspected excessive retrofibular pressures). Overall in the 36 patients there were no redislocations of the peroneal tendons. Two patients had snapping of the tendons, and it was necessary to reroute the tendons, creating a separate channel for the peroneus longus in the lateral aspect of the fibula, which terminated the rolling of the longus and the brevis. In this series, one patient had partial bone flap detachment and two patients had lateral distal fibula chip fractures without any consequences to the patient. Transient sural neuritis was seen in six patients, but all cases resolved spontaneously between 2 and 3 months after surgery.

Porter et al[178] used a fibular groove deepening procedure very similar to our technique, performing a complete removal of the bone flap, which allows a symmetric bone removal and deep groove. They reported no recurrences in 14 ankles, all patients returned to sports, and there were no bony complications from detachment of the bone flap.

This result might suggest that peroneal groove deepening is not only an excellent procedure to correct peroneal tendon subluxation or dislocation but also a viable option in patients with chronic retrofibular peroneal pain without obvious tendon or groove pathology, as well as in patients with peroneal tendon tears in the presence of an abnormal peroneal groove.

Although a small number of cases have been reported using this technique, a very high rate of success has been noted.[137,141,154,178,208]

The most common complication after nonsurgical or surgical treatment for peroneal dislocation is redislocation, which is decidedly higher in the nonsurgical group. Other reported complications include decreased range of motion, friction on the tendon after repair, and degenerative tendon tears. Skin sensitivity and sural nerve injury have been reported postoperatively but can be avoided with careful surgical technique.

Patients with dislocation as a result of major trauma are more likely to have sural nerve problems preoperatively.[208] Also, some patients without nerve symptoms postoperatively did have transient neuralgia that may have developed from the exposure, retraction, or the injections from the ankle block.

The reports of both peroneus longus tendon tears[149] and peroneus brevis tears[101] associated with chronic peroneal tendon dislocations make an argument for early definitive repair of peroneal tendon instability. McConkey and Favero[151] reported one case and Harper[131] two cases of subluxation of the peroneus brevis on the peroneus longus within the tendon sheath. They both report a "rising up" of the peroneus brevis tendon. A thickened peroneus brevis has been observed in two of three patients with a history of chronic ankle sprains, suggesting a concomitant peroneus brevis tendon injury. The peroneal tendons should be carefully inspected at the time of either ankle reconstruction or peroneal tendon stabilization procedures.

Conclusion

Acute subluxation and dislocation of the peroneal tendons may be misdiagnosed or not treated, leading to chronic instability. A high level of suspicion and awareness of the condition leads to early diagnosis and successful treatment. Most often these injuries occur in a young, athletically active population. Anatomically, a deficient SPR or a shallow or absent posterior fibular sulcus is often associated with instability.

Delayed conservative treatment of acute peroneal tendon dislocations is successful in approximately one half of cases. Surgical reconstruction is the treatment of choice for young, active patients and those with chronic instability. Although many surgical techniques are available, SPR reconstruction, groove deepening procedures, and occasionally tendon rerouting procedures are excellent methods with which to treat acute and chronic peroneal tendon instability successfully. Results are usually excellent after proper diagnosis and appropriate treatment of this condition.

ACHILLES TENDON

The literature concerning dysfunction of the Achilles tendon is confusing and contradictory, leaving a physician with a multitude of references that support not only varying etiologies but also treatment regimens diametrically opposed to one another. It would be impractical and impossible to cite all the major contributions from the more than 700 articles in the literature discussing methods of treatment. The purpose of this discussion is merely to present a method of clinical evaluation and treatment of various Achilles tendon disorders.

The Achilles tendon derives its name from the Greek warrior Achilles, who was dipped in the river Styx by his mother, Thetis, which rendered him invulnerable except for the unsubmerged area of his heel by which he was held. He was mortally wounded during the siege of Troy when he was struck in his heel, the only vulnerable area, by an arrow shot from the bow of the Trojan prince Paris.[282]

Anatomy

A knowledge of the anatomy of the heel region and posterior calf is essential in understanding the pathophysiology of Achilles tendon disorders. The gastrocnemius–soleus (triceps surae), the largest of the calf muscles, traverses both the ankle and the knee joint. Innervated by the tibial nerve, the triceps surae consolidates as the Achilles tendon, the largest and strongest tendon in the human body.[253,307] The gastrocnemius arises from the posterior femoral condyles and the soleus from the posterior aspect of the tibia, fibula, and interosseous membrane. The gastrocnemius is an effective plantar flexor of the ankle with the knee in extension. The soleus, which crosses only the ankle joint, is the more effective plantar flexor of the ankle with the knee in flexion.[253]

The Achilles tendon inserts over a broad area (approximately 2 × 2 cm) on the posterosuperior aspect of the calcaneal tuberosity.[244,303] Two bursae are associated with the insertional area of the Achilles tendon: the retrocalcaneal bursa, which is located between the Achilles tendon and the calcaneus, and the Achilles tendon bursa, which is located between the skin and tendon (this occurs with varying frequency) (Fig. 22–67).[263,370]

The Achilles muscle-tendon unit, during activities ranging from standing to walking to running and jumping, undergoes both eccentric lengthening and

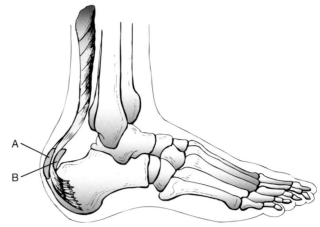

Figure 22–67 Two bursae are associated with the Achilles tendon insertion. *A*, Achilles tendon bursa superficial to tendon. *B*, Retrocalcaneal bursa located between Achilles tendon and calcaneus.

concentric contracture. Below the musculotendinous junction, the tendon is encased in a peritenon of varying thickness throughout its entire course, but no true synovial sheath exists.[247,253,356] The vascular supply to the tendon emanates from the calcaneus distally through interosseous arterioles and proximally from intramuscular arterial branches. Lagergren and Lindholm[300] described a zone of relative avascularity 2 to 6 cm proximal to the calcaneal insertion. Although the peritenon does afford a vascular supply to the area of the Achilles tendon, the paucity of circulation makes it more vulnerable to injury and degeneration. In the last 6 cm, as the Achilles tendon approaches its insertion into the calcaneus, the tendon twists 90 degrees on itself, with the fibers of the gastrocnemius oriented laterally and the fibers of the soleus medially. This anatomic characteristic, coupled with limitations of the vascular supply in the distal 6 cm, appears to predispose the Achilles tendon in this region to degenerative changes.[226,300]

Achilles Tendinitis

Pathology and Etiology

Pathologic changes occur at the tendinous insertion of the Achilles tendon into the calcaneus as well as proximal to the insertion. Besides tendinitis, others terms used include *tenosynovitis, tendinosis, peritendinitis, tendinopathy,* and *peritendinopathy,* leaving the reader with significant confusion as to what topic different authors are addressing. The term *tendinitis,* however, has commonly been used in describing Achilles tendon dysfunction. Schepsis and Leach[350] used "tendinitis" to describe any posterior heel pain, although often a dramatic lack of inflammation is noted in the tendon itself.[351] Snook[356] observed that although the term *tenosynovitis* is applicable to inflammation with most other tendons, the term is inappropriate for the Achilles tendon because it is encompassed by a peritenon and not a true synovial sheath. The paucity of vascularity within the tendon itself makes it relatively resistant to an inflammatory response; however, the peritendinous structures are at risk for inflammation. A diagnosis of pure *tendinosis* is often made after an Achilles tendon rupture on inspection of the rupture site at surgical exploration.

Achilles tendinitis is often experienced by athletes who participate in impact sports such as running and jumping. Clain and Baxter[247] observed a direct correlation between injuries and the intensity level of a training program. Clancey et al[248,249] concluded that Achilles tendinitis develops from microtears in the tendon that eventually progress to macroscopic tears without treatment. The incidence of injuries involving the Achilles tendon in athletes varies from 11% to 18%.[250,287] Clain and Baxter[247] observed that the common etiologic factor appears to be repetitive impact loading associated with running and jumping (Fig. 22–68). Forces in the area of the Achilles tendon can increase with activity and stress up to 10 times body weight, varying from 2000 to 7000 newtons (N).[247,253]

The etiology of Achilles tendon dysfunction and tendinitis can be associated with overuse syndromes, postural problems (e.g., pronation, forefoot varus, cavus deformity), surface-related injuries (e.g., training on uneven or excessively hard ground, running on a crowned road bed or slanted surface), training errors (e.g., sudden increase in duration, intensity, or distance), poor footwear (e.g., poor construction, worn-out shoes), or an underlying inflammatory arthropathy. Coupled with the aging process and other extrinsic stresses, inflammation, degeneration, and eventual rupture can occur. An overuse syndrome can develop from accumulated microtrauma with serial impact loading during sports, training, or work. An aging tendon associated with poor vascularity is also at risk for degeneration and eventual rupture.

Clancy et al[249] proposed a classification based on the duration of symptoms: *acute* with symptoms less than 2 weeks, *subacute* with symptoms for 3 to 6 weeks, and *chronic* with symptoms longer than 6 weeks.

A comprehensive classification scheme for Achilles tendinitis is helpful not only in defining the problem but also in determining a rational method of treatment. Clain and Baxter[247] separated Achilles tendon dysfunction into insertional tendinitis and noninsertional tendinitis. *Noninsertional tendinitis* occurs proximal to the tendon insertion within or on the periphery of the tendon. *Insertional tendinitis* occurs within or around the tendon at its calcaneal insertion. It may be associated with a bony prominence on the superior aspect of the calcaneus (Haglund's deformity)[275] or with the development of a calcaneal spur within or along the periphery of the Achilles insertion. Puddu et al[341] proposed three stages of inflammation. Stage 1 is peritendinitis, stage 2 is peritendinitis with tendinosis, and stage 3 is tendinosis.

Peritendinitis (stage 1) occurs with pathologic inflammatory changes localized to the peritenon (Fig. 22–69 and Box 22–2). Although the tendon is typically normal in appearance, the peritenon may be thickened, fluid can accumulate adjacent to the

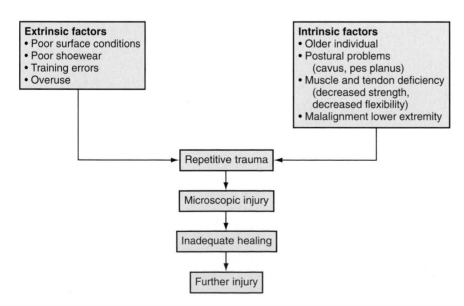

Figure 22–68 Pathophysiology of Achilles tendon dysfunction. (From DeMaio M, Paine K, Drez D: *Orthopedics* 18:195-204, 1995.)

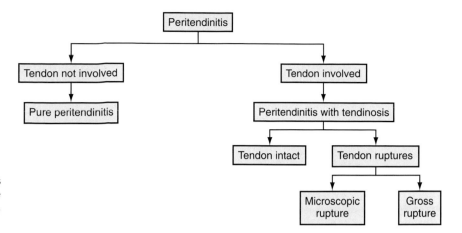

Figure 22–69 Etiology of Achilles peritendinitis. (From DeMaio M, Paine R, Drez D: *Orthopedics* 18:195-204, 1995.)

BOX 22–2 Classification of Tendon Dysfunction

Peritendinitis is an inflammation involving peritendinous structures. In the acute setting, symptoms typically last less than 2 weeks. In the subacute setting, symptoms last 2 to 6 weeks. With chronic peritendinitis, symptoms are present 6 weeks or longer. Chronic peritendinitis may be associated with tendinosis.

Peritendinitis with tendinosis is an inflammatory process involving peritendinous structures along with degeneration of tendon.

Tendinosis is typically an asymptomatic degeneration of tendon without concomitant inflammation caused by accumulated microtrauma, aging, or both. With tendinosis, an interstitial rupture, partial rupture, or acute rupture can develop.

Modified from Plattener P, Johnson K: Tendons and bursae. In Helal B, Wilson D (eds): *The Foot.* London, Churchill Livingstone, 1988; and Clancy W: *Prevention and Treatment of Running Injuries.* Thorofare, NJ, Slack, 1982.

---

tendon, and adhesions can develop. Kvist et al[299] observed peritendinous thickening and capillary and fibroblastic proliferation associated with peritendinitis.

Peritendinitis with tendinosis (stage 2) is characterized by macroscopic tendon thickening, nodularity, softening, yellowing of the tendon, decreased luster, and fibrillation. Microscopically, Puddu et al[341] observed inflammation in the peritendinous region but also focal degeneration within the tendon itself. Gould and Korson[271] reported that some tendons demonstrate extensive degeneration, whereas others have only mild changes. The earliest changes appear to be fragmentation of collagen fibers within the substance of the

tendon. At surgery, Clain and Baxter[247] observed regions of macroscopic tendon thickening and thought these were areas of focal degeneration or of partial tendon rupture and that these patients were at risk for complete tendon rupture. Burry and Pool[239] described central areas of Achilles tendon degeneration 4 to 15 mm in size and characterized by soft granulomatous and occasionally cystic changes with mucoid degeneration. These areas were associated with poor vascularity and had a striking absence of attempts at a reparative process.

Achilles tendinosis (stage 3) is characterized by degenerative lesions of the tendon without evidence of peritendinitis. Puddu et al[341] observed that a rupture of the Achilles tendon often was associated with peritendinitis with tendinosis. Microscopically with tendinosis, there is an altered tendon structure with decreased luster, yellowish discoloration, and softening of the tendon. Some patients experience a prodromal period before an Achilles tendon rupture, and others do not. Without a prodromal period, less inflammation appears to occur, and histologic changes demonstrate areas of mucoid degeneration within the tendon. Decreased cellularity and fibrillation of collagen fibers are often observed.[299] Puddu et al[341] observed that even a tendon distant from the site of the Achilles tendon rupture was abnormal. With a rupture, degenerative changes in the Achilles tendon can occur with or without peritendinitis (Table 22–2).

History and Physical Examination

Patients typically complain of pain in the area of the distal Achilles tendon, 2 to 6 cm proximal to the Achilles tendon insertion. Pain often develops with initial morning activity and can increase with exercise.[298,299] With increased tendon involvement, pain may be associated with both walking and running. Early symptoms may be characterized by

TABLE 22–2

Varieties of Peritendinitis and Tendinosis

Sign or Symptom	Peritendinitis	Peritendinitis with Tendinosis (Partial Rupture)	Tendinosis with Acute Complete Rupture
Pain	Acute	Subacute or chronic	Acute
Audible snap or pop	None	Unlikely	+
Muscle weakness	+	+	+
Antalgic gait	+	+	+
Edema	+	+	+
Pain with palpation	+	+	+
Tendon gap	−	±	+
Tendon crepitus	±	±	−
Passive dorsiflexion excursion	↓	↓	↑
Thompson test	−	−	+
Calf atrophy	−	+	±
Single-limb toe-rise test	+	±	Unable to perform
Plantar flexion strength	↓	↓	↓↓↓

sharp transient pain or recurrent episodes of sharp pain with running. Over time, less activity incites symptoms. Some patients eventually develop pain even at rest. With insertional tendinitis, pain is localized to the junction of the tendon and bone.

Clain and Baxter[247] stated that insertional Achilles tendinitis is an entirely separate entity that overlaps with the condition known as Haglund's deformity or pump bump. With this condition, discomfort is mainly noted over the posterolateral prominence of the calcaneus and is often associated with tight, constricting footwear or shoes with a closely contoured heel counter. Achilles tendinitis is infrequently associated with a pump bump.

On physical examination it is important to determine the precise area of tendon pain. The location and magnitude of soft tissue swelling should be noted. The patient should be asked to do a single-limb heel-rise test. Schepsis and Leach[350] observed that many patients demonstrated a loss of at least 5 degrees of dorsiflexion compared with the contralateral side. The calf should be examined for atrophy and a Thompson test performed to demonstrate that the Achilles tendon is intact.[362,363] The tendon should be palpated for any area of defect or nodularity. Kvist et al[299] noted the pain was localized to the lower part of the tendon in 24% of patients, the middle region in 51%, and the upper region in 10% (Fig. 22–70A-C). Diffuse tendon involvement was noted in 15% of cases and nodularity in 40%. Localized tenderness to palpation, swelling, decreased range of motion, tendon thickening, increased temperature, edema, and erythema all may be noted on physical examination. Localized crepitus is uncommon.

With peritendinitis (stage 1) the patient has notable tenderness and thickness that remains fixed with active range of motion. With a lesion of the tendon itself (tendinosis stage 3) the movement of the ankle and foot into dorsiflexion and plantar flexion is characterized by the abnormality's moving along with the tendon (painful arc sign) (Fig. 22–70D and E).

The tendon should be palpated with the joint relaxed at the level of the insertion and then palpated along its course proximally. The tendon should be examined with the ankle joint both plantar flexed and dorsiflexed. With pain localized to the insertion of the Achilles tendon, there is often increased pain with plantar flexion. With grasping of the heel and dorsiflexion of the foot, compression of the Achilles bursa can incite pain.

With insertional tendinitis, pain may be noted at the Achilles tendon insertion and may be increased with exercise. With chronic inflammation the tendon insertion can become thickened (Figs. 22–71 and 22–72).

In patients suspected of having retrocalcaneal bursitis, pain may be elicited just anterior to the Achilles tendon. Pain is elicited by squeezing in a mediolateral direction just superior and anterior to the Achilles tendon insertion (two-finger squeeze test). Pain is localized at the bone tendon interface and may be increased with eversion and dorsiflexion (Box 22–3).

Radiographic Examination

In the evaluation of Achilles tendon disorders, routine radiographs should be obtained. Radiographs can demonstrate cortical erosion associated with inflammatory arthropathy and calcification within the

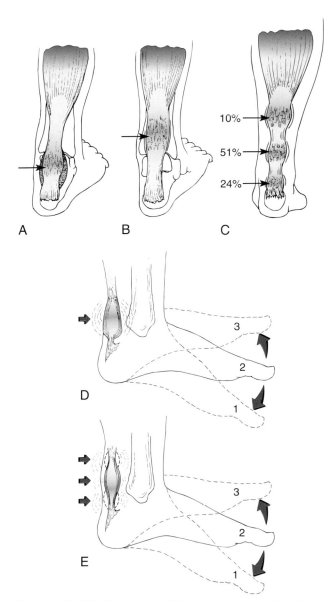

Figure 22–70 Nodularity, thickening, or tendinosis of Achilles tendon may be located in the distal region **(A),** close to insertion site, or more proximally **(B)** in the midtendon region. **C,** Frequency of occurrence by area. **D,** With peritendinitis, tenderness remains in one location despite dorsiflexion and plantar flexion of ankle. **E,** With tendinosis, the point of maximal tenderness moves proximally and distally as the ankle is dorsiflexed and plantar flexed. (Redrawn from Williams J: *Sports Med* 3:114-135, 1986.)

| BOX 22–3 | Differential Diagnosis of Achilles Tendinitis |

INCORRECT DIAGNOSES

Fracture
Other soft tissue problems
    Problems associated with gastrocnemius and soleus muscles (e.g., strain)
    Inflammation of tendons: posterior tibial, flexor hallucis longus, or flexor digitorum longus
    Inflammation of bursae: subcalcaneal, retrocalcaneal
    Inflammation of plantar fascia
    Compartment syndrome: posterior compartment, posterior tibial muscle
    Neurologic: tarsal tunnel syndrome, entrapment of medial calcaneal nerve
    Rupture: posterior tibial muscle, plantaris muscle
Bone disorders
    Calcaneal periostitis
    Sever's disease (calcaneal epiphysitis)
    Pump bumps

SYSTEMIC DISEASES

Inflammatory arthritis
Rheumatoid arthritis
Connective tissue disease
Seronegative spondyloarthropathies
    Ankylosing spondylitis
    Reiter's syndrome
Infection (e.g., tuberculosis)
Metabolic disorders
    Hyperbetalipoproteinemia
    Renal transplant

Modified from DeMaio M, Paine R, Drez D: *Orthopedics* 18:195-204, 1995.

---

tendon or at the Achilles tendon insertion. On a lateral radiograph, Haglund's deformity may be present. Schepsis and Leach[350] associated retrocalcaneal bursitis with Haglund's deformity. Pavlov et al[335] described a method of measuring the magnitude of a prominent posterosuperior calcaneal tuberosity by using parallel pitch lines (Fig. 22–73). With Haglund's deformity, the superior surface of the calcaneus projects beyond the superior calcaneal line.

Ultrasound or MRI can demonstrate a partial Achilles tendon tear, peritendinous thickening, tendinosis, nodularity, or calcification. Schepsis et al[351] found that MRI was helpful in evaluating Achilles tendon disorders (Fig. 22–74).

Conservative Treatment

Most cases of posterior heel pain are successfully managed nonsurgically.[248,350] Kvist and Kvist[298] stated that conservative management is time consuming and often unsatisfactory. Only about half of patients are successfully treated nonsurgically. One of the most significant factors influencing prognosis and recovery with conservative treatment is duration of symptoms.

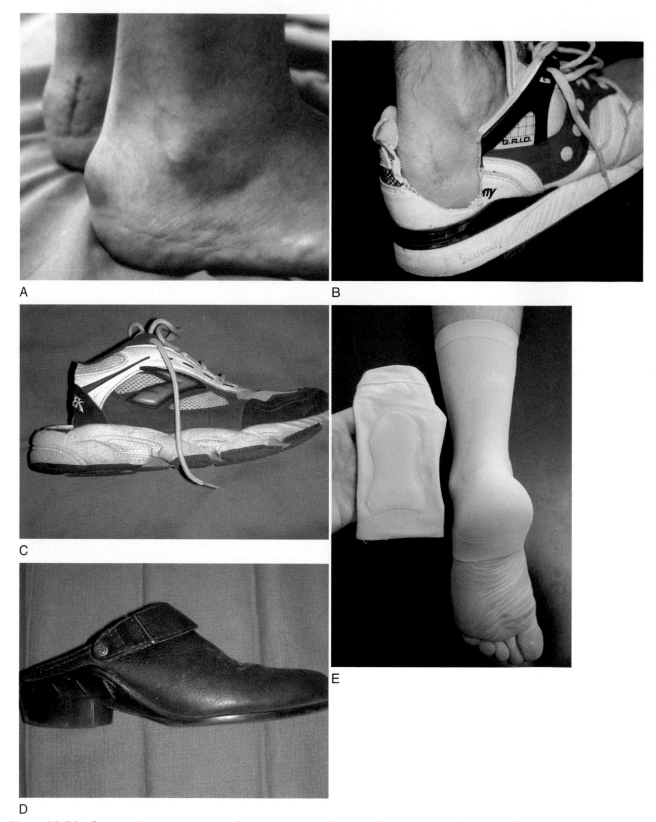

Figure 22–71 Conservative measures to reduce pressure on distal Achilles region. **A,** Obvious deformity on right heel. **B** and **C,** Cutout of shoes to reduce pressure. **D,** Backless shoe works well. **E,** Gel pad helps to reduce pressure.

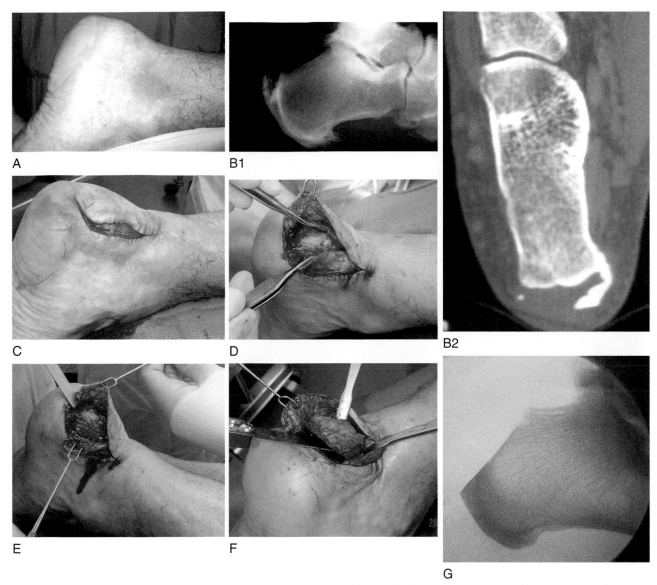

Figure 22–72   Insertional Achilles tendinitis. **A,** Enlarged area overlying Achilles insertion. **B1,** Calcification in area of insertion on lateral radiograph. **B2,** Calcification seen on magnetic resonance image. **C,** Hockey-stick incision to expose distal Achilles insertion. **D,** Tendon splitting exposure. **E** and **F,** Resection of calcific area and calcaneal tuberosity. **G,** Lateral radiograph following resection and repair.   *Continued*

If tendinosis has been present for 6 months or more, the condition is more difficult to treat nonsurgically.[351] Kvist and Kvist[298] observed that failed treatment often results from adhesions in the peritendinous region. They noted that chronic peritendinitis was much more difficult to treat successfully when it had been present 8 to 12 weeks.

Conservative treatment includes NSAIDs,[304] rest, immobilization, decreased activity, ice, contrast baths, stretching, and heel lifts (see Fig. 22–71).[281,314] A medial arch support or other orthotic devices may be used to decrease overpronation. An intratendinous injection of corticosteroid is discouraged because of the increased risk of tendon rupture.[247,307]

A peritendinous injection of local anesthetic (lidocaine or bupivacaine) can be attempted in cases of peritendinitis. This technique, called brisement, involves injecting 5 to 10 mL into the pseudosheath to break the adhesions between the mesotendon and the tendon itself. A series of 2 or 3 injections can decrease the symptoms in peritendinitis about 50% of the time.

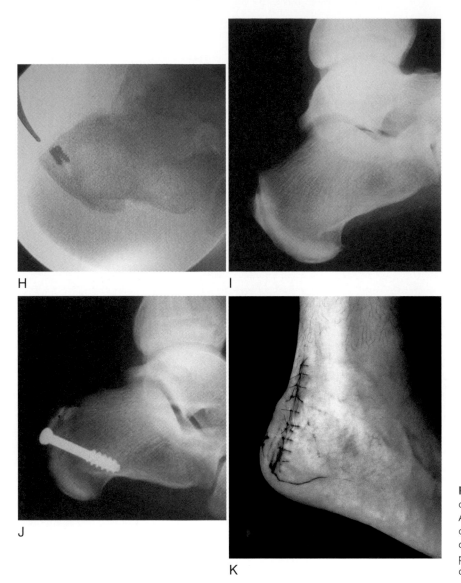

Figure 22–72—cont'd   H, Lateral radiograph with suture anchors securing the Achilles repair. **I,** Radiograph of another case with a prominent posterior tuberosity. **J,** Vertical osteotomy reduces prominence. **K,** Operative incision for osteotomy.

Activity modifications may aid in the resolution of discomfort. Occasionally, non–weight-bearing ambulation with cast immobilization is necessary.

Our preferred method of conservative treatment is a boot brace (e.g., CAM walker, Aircast walker brace, off-the-shelf AFO) either with a mild heel lift or in neutral position. The brace may be worn for 2 to 3 months for resolution of symptoms. A general rule is to use the brace until there are no symptoms for 2 weeks or until the improvement has plateaued for 2 weeks. Then the brace should be gradually discontinued, with more time spent out of the brace for progressively longer and more frequent intervals throughout the day.

With an acute episode of tendinitis, typically a patient should avoid athletic activities for 7 to 10 days. For more chronic cases, athletics might need to be avoided for 6 months. Gentle stretching exercises are initiated several times a day, with a return to athletics permitted as pain diminishes. In the patient with tendinitis, when the involved area is no longer tender to palpation, a training program may be reintroduced on a gradual basis. A decrease in running activities and intensity, initiation of stretching exercises, and a 0.25- to 0.5-inch heel lift can enable an athlete to return to sporting activities. Limiting excessive pronation can also diminish acute symptoms.

Extracorporeal shock wave therapy (ESWT) for the treatment of Achilles tendinitis is now being widely studied. Most information on ESWT comes from research on kidney stone lithotripsy, upper extremity tendinitis, and plantar fasciitis. ESWT works by creating a pressure change that propagates rapidly through a medium. When transmitted through a water medium it can either directly create high tension at a given structure or indirectly create microcavitations. Theories behind its analgesic effect in orthopaedic

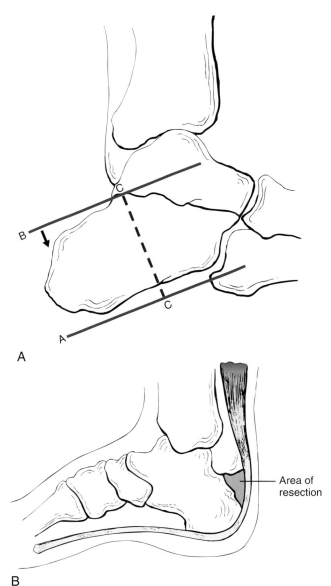

A

B

Figure 22–73 **A,** Using parallel pitch lines (lines *BC* and *AC* are parallel), magnitude of prominence of the posterosuperior calcaneal tuberosity can be assessed. **B,** When the tuberosity exceeds level of line *BC,* Haglund's deformity occurs.

Area of resection

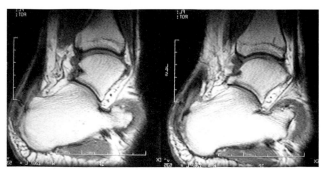

Figure 22–74 Magnetic resonance images demonstrating distal Achilles tendinoses.

applications include an alteration of the permeability of neuron cell membranes and induction of an inflammatory-mediated healing response by increasing local blood flow.[246,280]

In our practice, we have found a success rate of approximately 30%, although we have selected more severe cases to receive ESWT as a last resort before surgery. Even with this lower success rate, we offer ESWT with boot bracing for 3 months for all patients prior to surgery because this treatment has minimal side effects. Depending on the severity of the patient's condition we might allow for a more aggressive post-ESWT rehabilitation protocol. Contraindications to ESWT quoted in the literature include pregnancy, coagulopathies, bone tumors, bone infection, and skeletal immaturity.[246]

Saggini et al[346] noted successful outcomes and no complications after two treatments using ESWT on Achilles tendinitis. Several later studies reported promising results after ESWT for patients with chronic Achilles tendinitis.[255,265,330]

In general, with all forms of conservative therapy, patients with severe tendinitis should be treated until symptoms subside and rehabilitation can be initiated. A patient with only peritendinitis is at low risk for rupture. With increasing tendinosis the risk of rupture increases. A physician should have a frank discussion with an athlete regarding any predisposing factors that may have led to acute peritendinitis, including training techniques and footwear. The amount of time to recovery is variable, but subacute tendinitis (3 to 6 weeks in duration) can take a similar amount of time to resolve with a conservative program.[248] Chronic tendinitis can take much longer to resolve. Clancy[248] recommends at least 3 to 6 months of conservative treatment before surgical intervention (Box 22–4).

Surgical Treatment of Tendinitis, Tendinosis, and Haglund's Deformity

The determination of whether surgery is indicated depends on the duration and level of patient discomfort. When conservative methods are unsuccessful, Clain and Baxter[247] have used a two-incision technique on the medial and lateral aspects of the Achilles tendon (Fig. 22–75). They resected the Haglund's deformity transversely and meticulously inspected the Achilles tendon. With a prominence on the periphery of the tendon insertion, the area may be resected with a single incision and the calcific tissue excised. A suture anchor may be added to reinforce the repair (Fig. 22–76).

Excision of the retrocalcaneal bursa[371] (Fig. 22–77), excision of the prominent tuberosity,[345] and osteotomy of the calcaneus[293,375] have been advocated for treating insertional tendinitis.

BOX 22–4   Management of Peritendinitis

PATIENT ACTIVITIES

Adequate warm-up and cool-down periods
Reduced athletic activity
   Decreased duration
   Decreased training on hard surfaces
   Decreased intensity of workout
   Avoidance of hill and incline running
Stretching exercises

EQUIPMENT CHANGES

Worn-out or inadequate footwear
Worn-out or inadequate heel lifts
Worn-out or inadequate orthotic devices to reduce
   pronation

PHYSICAL THERAPY MODALITIES

Ultrasound
Heat, ice
Massage
Strengthening exercises

IMMOBILIZATION

Bracing
Casting
Decreased weight bearing

PHARMACOLOGIC TREATMENT

Nonsteroidal anti-inflammatory drugs
Corticosteroids

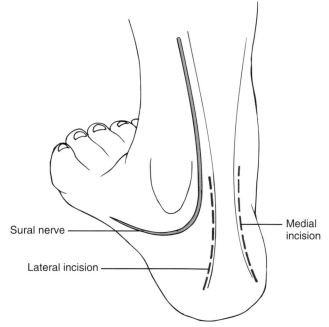

Figure 22–75 Either a two-incision technique on the medial and lateral aspects of the Achilles tendon or a single medial or lateral incision may be used to expose a prominent Haglund deformity.

EXCISION OF HAGLUND'S DEFORMITY

Surgical Technique

1. The patient is placed in a prone position under tourniquet control. A longitudinal incision is centered over the lateral margin of the os calcis, extending to a point 1 to 2 cm distal to the Achilles tendon insertion. Care must be taken to avoid injury to the sural nerve along the tendon's lateral border.
2. A retractor is used to expose the Achilles tendon, and any inflamed bursa overlying the Achilles tendon or in the retrocalcaneal area is excised.
3. The calcaneal tuberosity is inspected. If only the lateral tuberosity is enlarged, it is resected. The lateral one third of the Achilles tendon is reflected, exposing the lateral tuberosity.

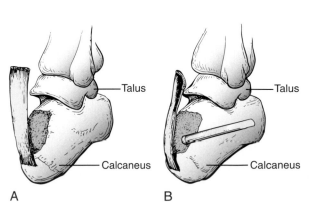

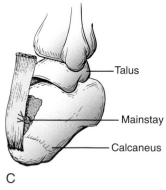

Figure 22–76 A, Prominent area of the calcaneus is resected, with care taken to protect the Achilles tendon insertion. **B** and **C,** Suture anchor may be used to reinforce the repair if the Achilles tendon insertion has been significantly weakened.

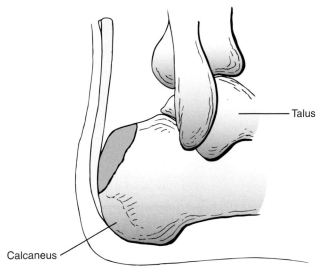

Figure 22–77 With a symptomatic Haglund deformity that extends the width of the calcaneus, the tuberosity is resected in a lateromedial direction, removing the dorsal prominence. Care is taken to protect the Achilles tendon insertion.

4. An osteotome is used to excise the lateral tuberosity, and the sharp edges are beveled with a rongeur. A power (reciprocating) rasp may also be used to effectively contour the edges.
5. If more of the tuberosity is to be removed, the foot is plantar flexed, decreasing tension on the Achilles tendon. With a retractor used to protect the Achilles tendon, an osteotomy is performed in a lateromedial direction, removing the entire Haglund's deformity (see Figs. 22–72 and 22–77 and video clip 2). After adequate bone has been removed, the tendon is secured with one or two suture anchors in the region of the lateral tuberosity.
6. Additional interrupted sutures are placed along the inferolateral margin of the Achilles tendon, securing it to the adjacent soft tissue.
7. The wound is closed in a routine manner.

Postoperative Care

A compression dressing and below-knee posterior plaster splint are applied at surgery. Two weeks after surgery the dressing is changed, sutures are removed, and a weight-bearing cast or boot brace is applied. Immobilization is dis-continued 6 weeks after surgery if the tendon attachment site was stable at the time of surgery. The patient is started on active range-of-motion exercises and physical therapy.

Results

Schepsis and Leach[350] noted a small number of patients who did not improve despite this method of treatment and who developed further tendon involvement. In these patients, a tendon transfer was necessary. In general, however, the authors noted good and excellent results with localized treatment.

Dickinson et al[256] reported on 21 patients (40 cases) in whom the superior prominence of the calcaneus was resected obliquely. Care was taken to avoid traumatizing the Achilles tendon. Immobilization was continued for 4 weeks after surgery. The authors reported a high level of good and excellent results.

Keck and Kelly[293] reported on 18 patients (26 cases). They used either an Achilles tendon-splitting incision as a direct posterior approach with resection of the calcaneal exostosis or a cuneiform osteotomy of the calcaneus, in which a dorsally based wedge of bone was removed.[375] They concluded that a prominence of the superior calcaneal tuberosity was a major factor in developing Achilles tendon bursitis and advocated excision of the Haglund deformity. Thirteen patients with 20 symptomatic heels were treated surgically. Good and excellent results were obtained in 75% of cases.

Alternative Approach: Achilles Splitting

When there is painful involvement of the Achilles insertion, the surgeon should consider a more direct approach to the pathology. This central Achilles-splitting method facilitates detachment and debridement of the tendon, resection of spurs, and contouring of the posterior superior prominence. McGarvey et al[321] reported good and excellent results with this method. Further, if needed because of poor condition of the tendon, the approach can be extended proximally to allow access to the posterior ankle for harvesting of the FHL.

Surgical Technique

1. A central incision is made directly in the midline. Alternatively, a lateral longitudinal

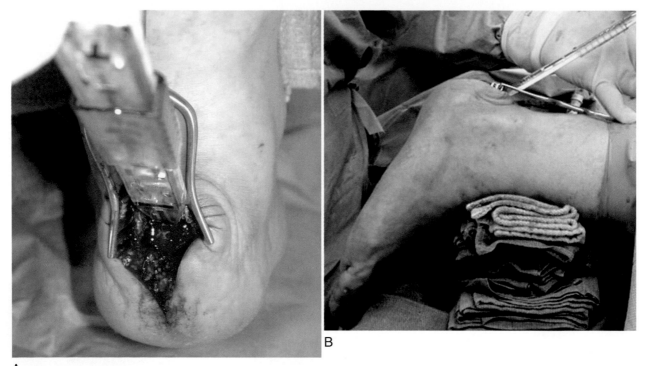

A

B

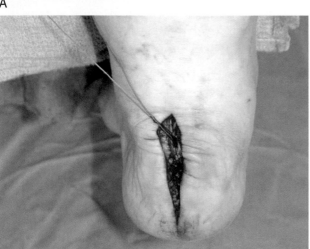

C

Figure 22–78   Resection of Haglund's deformity through a central incision. **A** and **B,** Central midline incision. Placement of suture anchor after bone resection. **C,** Tying of suture to secure the Achilles to the bone, maintaining its original tension. The knot should be buried to avoid prominence over the distal Achilles repair.

incision that traverses medially distal to the insertion also may be used.

2. The tendon is split and peeled off the posterior calcaneus.

3. With the insertional fibers detached and debrided and the posterior calcaneal tuberosity exposed, a chisel is inserted to

resect the prominent attachment site as well as the posterior superior process.

4. The edges of the bone are contoured.

5. The central Achilles is reattached to bone with a bone anchor or corkscrew suture anchor (Fig. 22–78). Care is taken to restore the proper tension to the Achilles tendon.

TENDON TRANSFERS

Three different tendon-transfer techniques have been proposed to treat insertional Achilles tendinitis. Teuffer[337] and Turco and Spinella[365] advocated transfer of the peroneus brevis. Clain and Baxter[247] observed that the peroneus brevis does not afford as much length as either the FDL or FHL, even when the peroneus brevis is released at the base of the fifth metatarsal. They advocated use of the FHL or FDL for tendon transfer. Mann et al[320] recommended use of the FDL, and Hansen[278] and Wapner et al[366,367] recommended use of the FHL. Wilcox et al[373] and others[251] noted minimal morbidity with harvesting the FHL.

Den Hartog[254] described a technique of harvesting the FHL tendon near the tip of the medial malleolus for chronic Achilles tendinosis. Good to excellent results were reported in 23 of 26 of patients without any deficit of first toe function. A recent biomechanical study showed little pressure change under the first or second MTP joint and no clinical functional deficit after FHL harvesting.[251] Prior studies also showed promising clinical results.[254,366,367,373]

In the transfer of either the FDL or the FHL, a medial arch incision is preferable for the distal release of the tendon. When length is not required for the repair, the posterior calcaneal incision can be deepened and the FHL can be harvested from behind the ankle (Fig. 22–79). The tendon is pulled cephalad into the proximal Achilles tendon incision and is either woven through the Achilles tendon and secured through a drill hole or sewed to the anterior aspect of the Achilles tendon (Fig. 22–80A-C). Schepsis et al[351] thought that a tendon transfer might be advantageous because it affords a rich vascular supply and reinforces the Achilles tendon.

Surgical Technique

See the later discussion on tendon transfer for delayed repair of Achilles tendon rupture.

1. In addition to the tendon transfer, when the segment of distal Achilles tendon is excised, a central slip from the proximal portion of the Achilles tendon may be mobilized and turned distally to bridge the distal defect (Fig. 22–80D and E).
2. A trough is created in the calcaneus just anterior to the original insertion of the Achilles tendon.

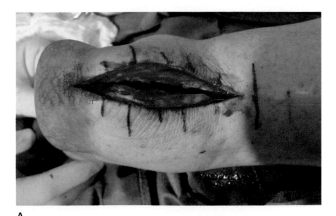

A

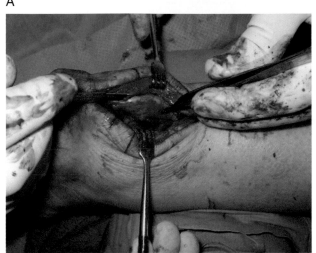

B

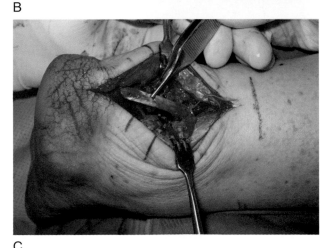

C

Figure 22–79 Resection of Achilles and flexor hallucis longus (FHL) transfer. **A,** Obvious area of distal tendinoses. **B,** Resection of diseased tendon. **C,** Transfer of FHL harvested through the same incision just above the fibro-osseous tunnel. A suture anchor or a soft tissue interference screw can be used to attach the FHL. A suture anchor is warranted to reapproximate the Achilles to the bone.

3. The central slip that is transferred distally spans the gap between the end of the Achilles tendon and the calcaneus where degenerative tendon has been resected. The slip is then cross-sutured to the FDL or FHL tendon.

4. When length allows, the proximal stump of the Achilles tendon is reattached to the calcaneus into the trough with a pull-out wire. The FHL can also be harvested at the level of the medial malleolus. (Fig. 22–81)

Postoperative Care

The foot is placed in approximately 10 degrees of equinus in a below-knee non–weight-bearing cast. The foot is brought to approximately a neutral position 4 weeks after surgery. A new cast or brace is applied for another 4 weeks. Weight-bearing ambulation is permitted 8 weeks after surgery. If a cast has been used, a removable below-knee brace is applied 3 months after surgery and used for 3 more months. Range-of-motion activities and strengthening exercises are initiated at this time. Athletic activities are restricted for 6 months after surgery.

SURGICAL TREATMENT OF PERITENDINITIS

The treatment of Achilles tendinitis and peritendinitis is the same. We differentiate between the two diagnoses because of the prognosis. Patients with peritendinitis respond more quickly than those who have peritendinitis with associated tendinosis. Peritendinitis with additional tendinosis requires not only resection of the peritenon but also debridement of the tendon and possibly augmentation with either a turn-down flap or tendon graft.

Surgical Technique

1. With the patient in a prone position under tourniquet control, a longitudinal incision is made parallel but 1 cm medial to the Achilles tendon. It extends from the musculotendinous junction inferiorly along the Achilles tendon. The incision is curved laterally at the area of the insertion.

2. The dissection is deepened to the Achilles tendon. A full-thickness flap is created between the Achilles tendon and the subcutaneous tissue to minimize the risk of a skin slough. The Achilles tendon and peritenon are inspected.

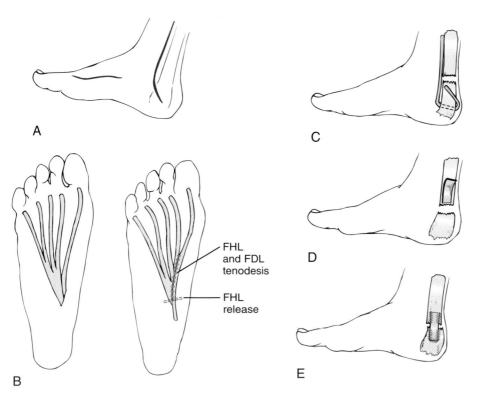

Figure 22–80 Tendon transfer technique using the flexor digitorum longus (FDL). This technique may be used after resection of Achilles tendinosis and for delayed repair of ruptured Achilles tendon. **A,** Incisions expose Achilles tendon and FDL or flexor hallucis longus (FHL). **B,** Tenodesis of FDL stump to FHL tendon. **C,** FDL (or FHL) is pulled through a transverse drill hole in the calcaneus. **D,** Augmentation of distal gap with turn-down fascial strip of the Achilles tendon. **E,** After placement of the turn-down flap within the slot in calcaneus. (Redrawn from Mann R, Holmes G, Seale K, Collins D: *J Bone Joint Surg Am* 73:214-219, 1991.)

FHL and FDL tenodesis

FHL release

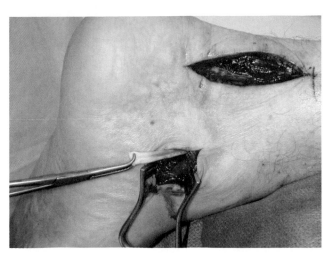

Figure 22-81 Flexor hallucis longus transfer for distal Achilles tendinosis by harvesting tendon just distal to the medial malleolus.

3. With Achilles tendinitis or peritendinitis, the peritenon is usually found to be hyperemic and thickened with adhesions. The peritenon is dissected and excised. Care is taken not to dissect the Achilles tendon circumferentially but rather to leave the anterior blood supply intact.[271]

4. The tendon is inspected and palpated for areas of thickening or degeneration. A longitudinal incision is made over the area of degeneration, when present, and this area is debrided. The tendon is then repaired.

5. The Achilles tendon insertion is inspected. With dorsiflexion of the ankle, the tendon is inspected to identify any areas of impingement on the superior surface of the calcaneus. The retrocalcaneal bursa is excised. If the bursa is prominent, the posterosuperior angle of the os calcis is removed transversely in the area just superior to the insertion of the Achilles tendon at a 45-degree angle to the long axis of the tendon. The area is then smoothed with a rasp and the ankle brought through a range of motion. Dorsiflexion should be checked to ensure impingement no longer exists.

Postoperative Care

The patient is immobilized in a below-knee cast or splint for 2 to 3 weeks. A new cast or brace is then applied, weight bearing is permitted, and active exercises are begun. Casting is discontinued 6 weeks after surgery. Jogging is permitted 8 to 12 weeks after surgery.

Results

Schepsis and Leach[350] advocated debridement and resection of the inflamed peritenon. Kvist et al[299] reported results on 182 patients (201 procedures), many of whom were high-level athletes. The crural fascia was incised, adhesions resected, and patients started on early range-of-motion activities. Of 201 cases, 36% were noted to have palpable nodules and 14% diffuse tendinosis. The disorder was localized to the upper tendon in 10%, the middle area in 51%, and the lower tendon in 24%. Nodules were thought to develop secondary to partial Achilles tendon ruptures. Results were good or excellent in 97% of cases. Twenty-six patients developed recurrent disorder, and 20 underwent second surgery and did well.

On the other hand, Puddu et al[341] stated that performing a "tenolysis" will "ensure failure" because the surgeon does nothing to revitalize circulation to the degenerated area. They recommended multiple longitudinal incisions in the peritendinous tissue to encourage ingrowth of vascularity. Tietz et al[361] recommended weaving the plantaris tendon through the degenerated area when tendinosis was present rather than excising the necrotic tissue. In advanced cases when the tendinosis involves greater than 80%, a FHL or FDL tendon can be used to augment the repair. Unlike the FHL, a potential problem when using the FDL is that its new course from its muscle belly's location to the Achilles can cross the tibial nerve, creating an inadvertent entrapment (Fig. 22-82).

A high level of good and excellent results is generally achieved in the surgical treatment of noninsertional tendinitis.[248,271,303,350,356]

Endoscopic Retrocalcaneal Decompression

Given the availability of equipment for arthroscopic procedures and surgeons familiar with these techniques, endoscopic approach to the retrocalcaneal bursa, the insertion of the Achilles, and the posterior

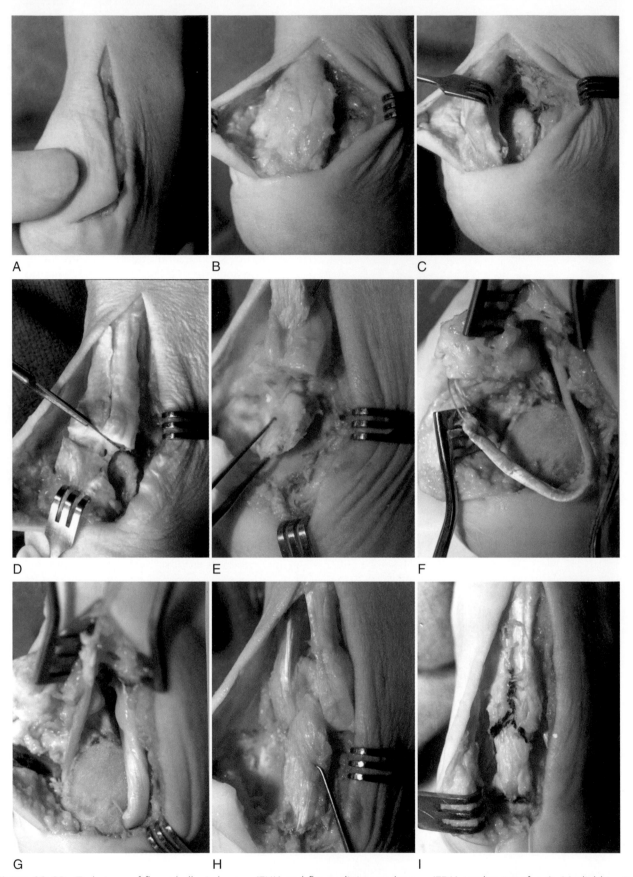

Figure 22–82 Technique of flexor hallucis longus (FHL) and flexor digitorum longus (FDL) tendon transfer. **A,** Medial longitudinal incision is curved distally over the Achilles tendon insertion. **B** and **C,** Severe tendinosis is identified with thickened distal Achilles tendon. **D,** Distal area of tendinosis is excised. **E,** Prominent Haglund's deformity is resected. **F,** After the FHL tendon is harvested, it is transferred proximally into the posterior Achilles incision. **G,** Tendon is transferred in a mediolateral direction through the drill hole in the calcaneus. **H,** Central segment of the Achilles tendon is detached proximally and turned 180 degrees. **I,** Proximal tendon is repaired side to side, and the turn-down flap is inserted into the trough in the calcaneus and secured with sutures tied through drill holes.

superior process of the calcaneus is growing in popularity. Through small portals adjacent to the Achilles tendon, the bursa is entered. Using a combination of palpation, endoscopic visualization, and image intensification, shavers and burs are inserted to address the pathology. The advantage of a smaller scar in this vulnerable area and a less traumatic debridement may prove beneficial in reducing recovery time and patient morbidity.[306]

Achilles Tendon Rupture

Ruptures of the Achilles tendon have been documented since the time of Hippocrates,[240] although Ambroise Paré[332] published the first description of this entity in 1633.

Although the true frequency of Achilles tendon ruptures in the general population is unknown, several reports suggest an incidence of less than 0.2%.[243,272,327-329] Goldman et al[270] reported only 38 cases treated at the Mayo Clinic over 20 years, and it was concluded that rupture of the Achilles tendon was an uncommon if not rare lesion.[357]

Anzel et al[2] evaluated the frequency of tendon ruptures and reported that Achilles tendon ruptures occurred less often (2%) compared with quadriceps ruptures (5%). This observation has been widely quoted, although ruptures of the Achilles tendon undoubtedly are, comparatively speaking, much more common than quadriceps ruptures. Indeed, Achilles tendon ruptures are the most common tendon rupture of the lower extremity.[272]

In recent years there has been better reporting of series of Achilles tendon ruptures. Also, however, with increased interest in physical conditioning and participation in athletic activities by middle-aged and older patients, spontaneous ruptures of the Achilles tendon are occurring with a greater frequency as well.[354]

Etiology

Achilles tendon ruptures occur in the second through eighth decades of life, although the peak incidence is during the third to fifth decades.[260,302,326-328,357] There is a marked male predominance (male-to-female ratio, 5:1).[225,230,294,301,343] A history of direct trauma is uncommon,[285] but disruption can occur anywhere along the course of the Achilles tendon. Causes include direct blows to the posterior ankle, crushing injuries, and lacerations. These injuries can cause a variable amount of adjacent soft tissue injury.

Indirect causes of rupture are the most frequently reported mechanism of injury and likely result from a combination of mechanical stress and intratendinous degeneration.[265] Arner and Lindholm[225] proposed the following three distinct mechanisms of indirect

loading or overloading resulting in tendon failure: a sharp unexpected dorsiflexion force to the ankle coupled with a strong contraction of the triceps surae (e.g., tripping on a curb, unexpectedly stepping into a hole), pushing off the weight-bearing foot with the knee in extension (e.g., lunging for a tennis shot), and a strong or violent dorsiflexion force on a plantar-flexed ankle (e.g., jumping from a height). All these mechanisms describe variations of a rapid loading process on an already-tensed tendon.

The Achilles tendon acts as a viscoelastic material with rapid loading of the muscle–tendon unit. With the modulus of elasticity increasing, the tendon becomes a stiffer structure and is more prone to rupture.[347] Ruptures are associated with strenuous activity in almost all cases.[308] Most often they are associated with athletic endeavors. Hooker[283] reported that most patients had sedentary occupations and occasionally indulged in strenuous physical activity. Fitzgibbons et al[260] observed that none of his patients had jobs that entailed manual labor. Most patients were recreational athletes. When the person is not in adequate physical condition, the onset of muscle fatigue can predispose the tendon to rupture.

Although lacerations or disruptions from external causes can occur anywhere along the length of the tendon, indirect ruptures routinely are localized to an area 2 to 6 cm proximal to the calcaneal insertion. Concomitant factors can predispose a patient to Achilles tendon rupture, including systemic inflammatory arthritis (rheumatoid arthritis, gout, systemic lupus erythematosus), endocrine dysfunction (renal failure, hyperthyroidism),[276] infection (syphilis, bacterial infection),[347] and tumor.[276] Kujala et al[297] suggested that patients with certain blood types are more at risk for Achilles tendon rupture.

The use of fluoroquinolone has been implicated in Achilles tendon rupture.[302,322,344,355] Oral corticosteroids and local injections of corticosteroids have been implicated in several reports. Ljungqvist[315] noted that 50% of patients in his series with Achilles tendon ruptures gave a history of steroid use, and Jacobs et al[286] reported five ruptures after local corticosteroid injection. Mahler and Fritschy,[318] on the other hand, reviewed 19 reports of Achilles tendon ruptures and observed that most patients receiving corticosteroids had concomitant systemic inflammatory arthritis. They questioned whether the inflammatory process or pharmacologic therapy was the causative factor in Achilles tendon rupture.

The notion that some patients are predisposed to Achilles tendon rupture is supported by familial occurrence (MJC has treated two families with father and son ruptures) and nonsimultaneous bilateral Achilles tendon ruptures. Simultaneous bilateral ruptures can occur with severe overload of the muscle–tendon unit without an underlying cause (one case during sky diving,[276] two cases during gymnastics[272]). Twenty cases of nonsimultaneous bilateral ruptures have been reported. Jessing and Hansen[288] stated that there is a 26% risk of a contralateral rupture of the Achilles tendon with return to sporting activities similar to the type that led to the initial rupture.

Intrinsic degeneration of the Achilles tendon has been proposed as a predisposing factor to rupture.[343,357] The Achilles tendon is subjected to substantial tension forces during athletic activities. In a younger patient with a normal tendon, these forces may be well tolerated. With aging, the tendon may be more vulnerable to injury.[222] Burry and Pool[239] and others[227,83] have suggested that rupture occurs only in an abnormal tendon, and the combination of intratendinous degeneration and increased mechanical stress likely results in tendon failure. The Achilles tendon 2 to 6 cm proximal to the calcaneal insertion appears to be a vulnerable region for rupture. Arner et al[227] stated that after the third decade of life the vascular supply to the Achilles tendon is diminished.

In 75 histologic examinations of Achilles tendon biopsies from the site of rupture, 74 cases demonstrated tendinous degeneration, including mucoid degeneration, tendinous calcification, or evidence of microscopic disruption of normal collagen fibers. Fox et al[261] examined histologic specimens from rupture sites of patients who had chronic symptoms and functional disability before Achilles tendon rupture and found diffuse degenerative changes in the tendon structure that they believed ultimately resulted in tendon failure. A high incidence of fibrinoid and myxomatous degeneration was observed. Jacobs et al[286] found diffuse fibrosis and degenerative changes at the tendon rupture site.

McMaster[13] concluded that a normal tendon does not rupture and that a tendon must undergo considerable damage before it will rupture. Although Schmidt-Rohlfing et al[352] stated that no relationship exists between poor blood supply and frequency of Achilles tendon rupture, vascular evaluation of cadaver and autopsy specimens by Carr[241] and others[227,300] demonstrated a decreased number and size of blood vessels in this vulnerable region. The authors concluded that diminished vascularity can predispose to tendon rupture in this region. Habusta[272] observed that circulation in this region is derived from peritendinous structures that can be interrupted or reduced by chronic tendinitis. Taylor[360] commented that "normal Achilles tendons can and do rupture," but more often predisposing factors exist.

Prodromal symptoms are reported before rupture and develop in approximately 10% of cases. Lea and Smith[302] documented the location of rupture along the course of the Achilles tendon to be 4% insertional rupture, 73% intratendinous rupture, and 24% musculotendinous junction (Fig. 22–83). Shields et al[354] reported 14% insertional rupture, 72% tendinous rupture, and 14% musculotendinous junction.

A consolidated hematoma may be present at the rupture site and, when combined with fraying of the tendon fibers and strands, resembles a mop's end or horse's mane (Fig. 22–84). The rupture occurs most often within the vulnerable area, 2 to 6 cm proximal to the Achilles tendon insertion.

History and Physical Examination

A middle-aged male patient often gives a history of prior involvement in an athletic activity. After a misstep, jump, or push off, patients report the sensation of a snap or an audible pop followed by the onset of acute pain, difficulty walking, and weakened plantar flexion power.[258] The audible pop can be likened to a rifle shot and the pain characterized as feeling as though the patient was kicked or struck in the posterior heel region. Patients might complain of lack of coordination, and many note swelling and ecchymosis in the ankle region. The left ankle is reported to be involved more often.[225,268,270,279]

A palpable gap at the rupture site and diminished plantar flexion strength are pathognomonic of an

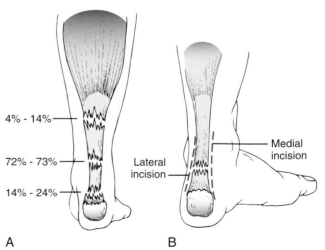

Figure 22–83 A, Achilles tendon rupture can occur anywhere along the tendon's course. Ruptures in the middle portion occur most often (72% to 73%), distal ruptures occur less often (14% to 24%), and proximal ruptures of musculotendinous junction occur least often (4% to 14%). **B,** Medial and lateral incisions.

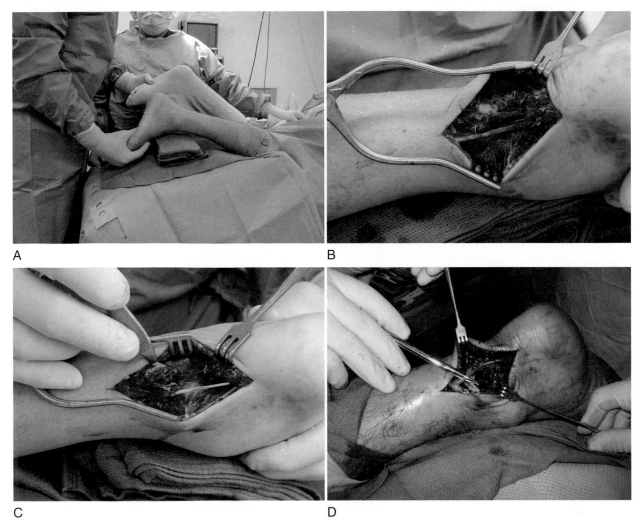

Figure 22–84 Example of an acute Achilles tendon rupture. **A,** Rupture demonstrated by excessive dorsiflexion of the right ankle. **B,** Complete rupture. **C,** Following debridement of tendon. Note intact plantaris tendon. **D,** Acute rupture with fraying of tendon.

Achilles tendon rupture.[317] Ecchymosis and swelling occur rapidly after injury and can aid in early diagnosis; within 24 hours, however, these findings can make diagnosis more difficult. The posterior indentation overlying the tendon defect may be obliterated by soft tissue swelling. Excessive dorsiflexion may be evident on the ruptured side. The acute pain initially experienced with rupture may subside and be characterized as a vague dull ache. With a more proximal rupture, diminished plantar flexion strength may be less obvious.[267] Pain on palpation is typically present, although it can subside rapidly.

Thompson and Doherty[363] described a classic clinical test used to diagnose a ruptured Achilles tendon (Fig. 22–85). With the patient kneeling on a chair with feet extended over the chair's edge or with the patient lying prone with feet extended beyond the end of the table, the examiner squeezes the calf just distal to the area of maximal calf girth on the affected and unaffected side. On the normal side the calf squeeze causes passive plantar flexion. When the same maneuver is performed on the injured side, plantar flexion of the foot is absent (a positive test), indicating a rupture of the Achilles tendon.[267,362,363] A patient with an Achilles tendon rupture is typically unable to stand on the toes on the involved side, but plantar flexion strength may be present (but decreased) because of a partial rupture, an intact plantaris muscle, or recruitment of other plantar flexors (peroneus brevis, peroneus longus, posterior tibialis, FDL).[222] Because of an absence

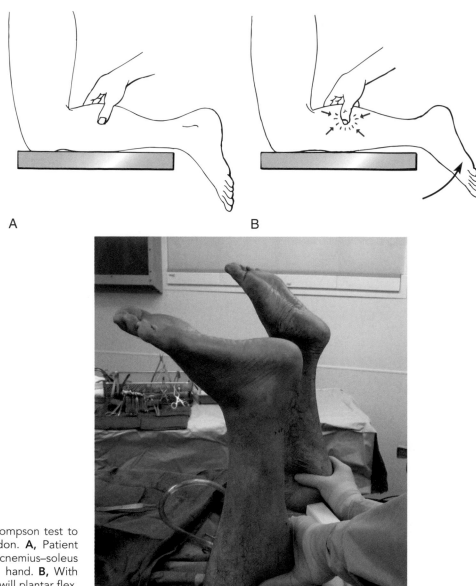

Figure 22–85 Technique of Thompson test to diagnose ruptured Achilles tendon. **A,** Patient kneels on chair, and gastrocnemius–soleus muscle complex is grasped with hand. **B,** With intact muscle–tendon unit, ankle will plantar flex. With ruptured Achilles tendon, foot typically will not plantar flex (positive Thompson sign). **C,** Clinical demonstration of Thompson test.

of pain, no palpable gap, and no obvious impairment of plantar flexion power, a diagnosis may be less than obvious.[283,343] It is estimated that in 20% to 25% of cases the diagnosis is initially missed (Fig. 22–86).[225,301,327,343]

Radiographic Examination

With a careful history and physical examination, a diagnosis is usually obvious and special diagnostic studies are rarely indicated.[279] AP and lateral radiographs on occasion can demonstrate associated tendon calcification or a tarsal fracture, although they more often show only soft tissue swelling. Arner et al[226] and others[242,301] have observed on lateral radiographs that the sharp contour of Kager's triangle (the soft tissue area bordered by the anterior aspect of the Achilles tendon, the posterior superior aspect of the calcaneus, and by the deep flexors) is disrupted after Achilles tendon rupture (Fig. 22–87A and B).[289]

Ultrasound[229,290] and MRI[229,292,368] have been suggested as diagnostic aids and may be helpful when soft tissue swelling makes physical examination more

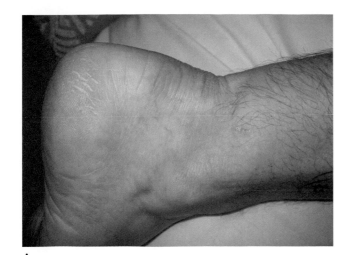

A

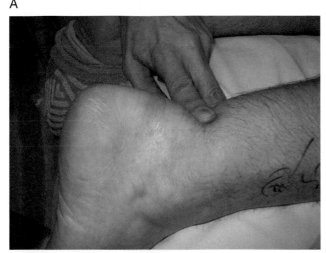

B

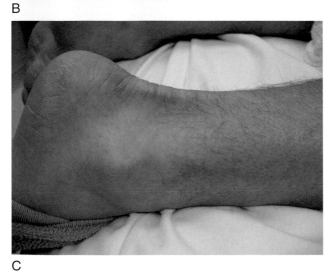

C

Figure 22–86 Clinical examination following Achilles tendon rupture. **A,** Dimple in posterior skin. **B,** Obvious defect on clinical exam. **C,** Comparison with contralateral uninjured extremity.

difficult. Astrom et al[229] stated that MRI was definitely superior to ultrasound in diagnostic specificity (Fig. 22–87C).

Conservative Treatment

Nonsurgical treatment of Achilles tendon ruptures predominated in the 1800s and 1900s. Starting in the early 1920s, surgical repair gradually increased.[258] After

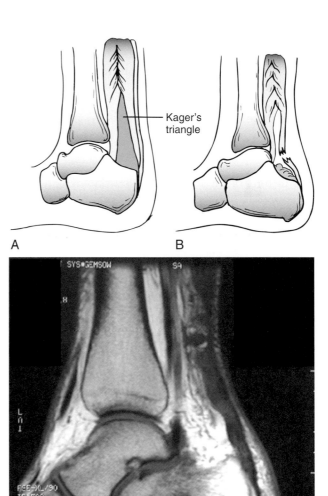

Kager's triangle

A   B

C

Figure 22–87 Kager's triangle. **A,** In normal lateral radiograph, a "crisp" Kager triangle is formed in the area posterior to the lateral malleolus. The border is formed by the anterior aspect of the Achilles tendon, posterosuperior aspect of the calcaneus, and deep flexors of the foot. **B,** After rupture, sharp definition of the triangle is obliterated. **C,** Long complex tear of the Achilles tendon. Observe the fibrotic tendon with a wavy orientation and a gap noted at 6 to 7 cm above the calcaneus.

Nistor's randomized prospective study claiming essentially no difference in the ultimate outcome of either surgical or nonsurgical treatment,[329] nonsurgical treatment has gradually become preferred for specific patients.

The basis for conservative care is that by placing the foot in an equinus position, the ends of the ruptured Achilles tendon are brought into apposition. If no attempt is made to reduce the gap with treatment, the tendon will heal in an elongated position, with resultant loss of plantar flexion power. In some cases, however, the equinus position might not produce adequate apposition, leading to residual weakness or abnormally increased length of the tendon.

Proponents of nonsurgical treatment note that cast immobilization is relatively risk free because surgical complications are avoided,[240,258,328,329,374] hospitalization is unnecessary, medical costs are minimized, time off work is less,[374] and the results are comparable to those of surgical repair.[329] The main complications of this method of treatment are increased rerupture rate and healing of the tendon with residual lengthening. In laboratory studies, Brown et al[237] and Murrell et al[325] have demonstrated that with a severed Achilles tendon in animals, those treated surgically and nonsurgically had similar strength and range of motion.

Haggmark et al[274] observed that a lengthened tendon may be characterized by increased dorsiflexion on physical examination, symptomatically can cause gastrocnemius weakness and calf fatigue, and is responsible for a high rate of posttreatment dissatisfaction.[262,274,286] One advantage of surgery is the ability to restore a proper tension length to the triceps surae unit. It is logical to assume that a functionally elongated Achilles tendon has decreased power and decreased strength. On the other hand, an Achilles tendon that has healed in a shortened position has decreased dorsiflexion, which can impair ambulation as well.

Rerupture after nonsurgical treatment is the most common complication, varying from 13% to 35% (average 18%). Nistor[329] observed that all reruptures in his series of patients treated nonsurgically occurred 1 to 7 weeks after removal of the final cast. Taylor[360] stated that most reruptures occur within the first month after 8 weeks of cast immobilization and reasoned that "the time of immobilization is inadequate." He recommended longer periods of casting or brace protection after cast removal.

Many reports favor a below-knee cast, and Blake and Ferguson[233] and others[267,283] note no recorded advantage of an above-knee cast. Freunsgaard et al[262] advocated an above-knee cast as an initial treatment and then later converted this to a below-knee cast and

reported only four reruptures in 66 patients after 12 weeks of casting. Taylor[360] advocated a regimen of 6 weeks of above-knee casting followed by 6 weeks in a below-knee cast with the ankle in neutral position. He then used a double upright brace with a neutral dorsiflexion stop for 4 to 6 weeks. He stated, "It is possible I have over-treated my patients," but he observed that normal range of motion was invariably obtained in every patient, although atrophy did not resolve.

As treatment evolves toward managing more sedentary patients nonsurgically, surgeons must not forget the lessons learned from and the treatment protocols of those who treated Achilles tendon ruptures successfully without surgery. Inadequately immobilizing an Achilles tendon rupture for an insufficient duration places a patient at risk for rerupture and increases the possibility of delayed reconstruction or a further period of immobilization (Table 22–3).

Casting Technique

Nonsurgical treatment of an Achilles tendon rupture is achieved by the application of a cast with the foot and ankle in gravity equinus. Forced plantar flexion is unnecessary and contraindicated. Although considerable controversy exists as to the length, duration, and

---

BOX 22–5   Indications for Surgery for Achilles Tendon Rupture

ABSOLUTE INDICATIONS

Acute complete rupture
Large partial rupture
Rerupture

RELATIVE INDICATIONS

Chronic tendinosis (longer than 6 months)
Chronic peritendinitis with tendinosis (longer than 6 months)
Failure of long-term conservative management (longer than 6 months)

CONTRAINDICATIONS

Older age
Inactivity
Poor health
Poor skin integrity
Systemic disease

Modified from DeMaio M, Paine R, Drez D: *Orthopedics* 18:195-204, 1995.

TABLE 22-3

Results of Treatment of Achilles Tendon Rupture

Factor	Nonsurgical Treatment	Surgical Treatment
Morbidity	↓	↑
Surgical complications	None	↑
Hospital cost	↓	↑
Physician cost	↓	↑
Strength and endurance	↓	↑
Rerupture rate	18%	2%

position of the foot and ankle within the cast, if the patient and physician are committed to nonsurgical treatment, it should be performed in a comprehensive manner (Fig. 22–88).

Taylor[360] recommended an above-knee cast applied with the knee in slight flexion (20 to 30 degrees) and the ankle in passive plantar flexion. Four weeks later the cast is changed and a below-knee cast applied with the ankle in reduced equinus or neutral plantar flexion. Weight-bearing ambulation is then initiated. Eight weeks after rupture the cast is discontinued, and a custom-molded ankle brace, a removable cast, or a stirrup brace is then used for an additional 4 weeks. A

2- to 2.5-cm heel lift may then be placed in the shoe. Range-of-motion exercises are commenced after cast removal, and active exercises are initiated 12 weeks after injury.

Surgical Treatment

Placing the ankle in equinus does not automatically approximate the two tendon ends, contrary to common assumption, as occasionally demonstrated at surgery (Box 22–5).[245] A major indication for surgery is a delay in diagnosis. Carden et al[240] found that with a delay in treatment longer than 1 week, they did not achieve results as successful as with cases treated acutely. In a long-term follow-up study (average 8 years) Boyden et al[235] demonstrated with gait analysis and Cybex testing that the functional results after delayed repair were comparable to those after an Achilles tendon rupture repaired acutely. Kellam et al[294] compared surgical and nonsurgical treatment and reported a 93% satisfaction rate after surgery and a 66% satisfaction rate after conservative treatment of Achilles tendon ruptures.

Some authors favor a medial longitudinal incision because it provides easy access to the plantaris tendon and avoids the sural nerve. Others favor a lateral incision. A midline incision has been advocated as well[258,268,283,336,343] but can result in an increased incidence of wound problems, and adhesions can develop at the surgical site. Whatever the incision, it should be deepened directly to the peritenon, and significant medial or lateral dissection should be avoided.

Reinforcement of tendon repairs has been advocated using various methods, including a pull-out wire (Fig. 22–89) to remove tension from the suture line,[286,301,342,343,363] suture anchors,[277] plantaris tendon, fascia lata,[283] and peroneus brevis.[337,363] When surgery

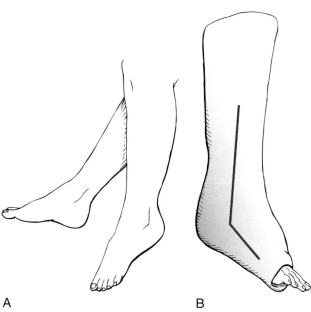

Figure 22–88 Technique of casting for nonsurgical treatment of Achilles tendon rupture. **A,** With patient sitting, foot is placed in gravity equinus. **B,** Below-knee or above-knee cast is placed with foot in gravity equinus.

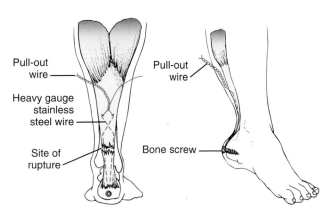

Figure 22–89 Achilles tendon repair may be reinforced with pull-out stainless steel wire or a fiber-wire type suture.

is performed, a primary repair in which the tendon ends are directly reapposed is preferable,[288] although augmentation may occasionally be used when reinforcement is necessary.

PRIMARY REPAIR OF ACHILLES TENDON RUPTURE

Surgical Technique

1. The patient is carefully positioned prone, and a thigh tourniquet is used for hemostasis. The contralateral extremity is draped and provides an intraoperative comparison, because the goal of surgery is to restore the resting length of the triceps surae.[360]
2. A 10-cm longitudinal incision is made 0.5 cm medial to the Achilles tendon and extended from the tendon insertion proximally (Fig. 22–90A; video clip 1).
3. Care is taken to avoid undermining the skin. The incision is deepened directly to the peritenon, which is incised longitudinally, exposing the rupture.
4. The ankle is plantar flexed to expose and approximate the tendon ends. The hematoma is debrided (Fig. 22–90B and C).
5. A modified Kessler, Bunnell, or Krackow[296] technique is used with a heavy nonabsorbable suture to approximate the tendon ends (Figs 22–91 and 22–92).
6. With an insecure repair, a pull-out wire is used (see Fig. 22–88).[286,301,342,343,363]
7. The repair is then reinforced with several interrupted sutures.
8. When necessary, the repair may be augmented with a turn-down fascia graft (Fig. 22–93), a plantaris tendon weave through the tendon repair,[245,283,336,342,343] or even an FHL or peroneus brevis tendon transfer.[337,365]
9. The peritenon is closed and the skin approximated with an interrupted closure.

Mini-Open Technique

To minimize the risk of wound healing complications but ensure the apposition of the tendon ends, a mini-open approach can be used for Achilles tendon repair. Instead of blindly passing the suture and risking an injury to the sural nerve, as in a percutaneous approach, a small stab incision is made and the subcutaneous soft

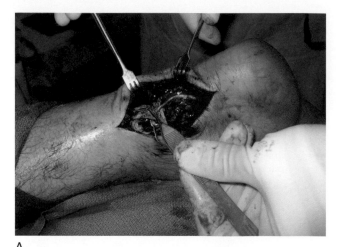

A

B

C

Figure 22–90 A, Acute rupture of the Achilles tendon. **B,** Repair with Krackow suture technique. **C,** Note tension of Achilles at conclusion of repair.

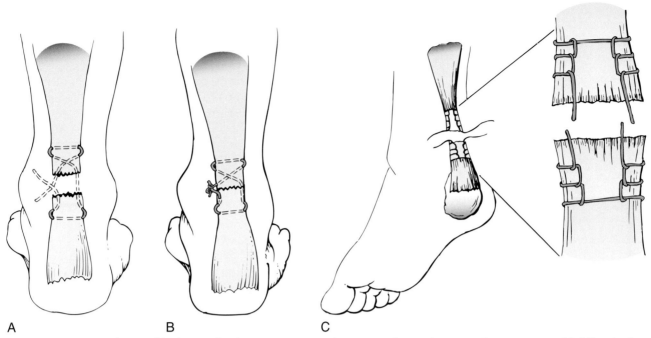

A   B   C

Figure 22–91 **A** and **B,** Modified Bunnell or box-type suture technique may be used to approximate a ruptured Achilles tendon. This technique brings the tendon into apposition, but tendon repair does not have significant strength. **C,** Krackow technique of double-lock suture to repair a ruptured Achilles tendon.

tissue is bluntly spread before passing the suture or wire.

The Achillon system (Newdeal SA, Vienne, France) facilitates this method and combines the advantage of direct visual repair with minimizing potential complications of wound and nerve problems. A small skin incision is made, and the

Achillon is introduced under the paratenon. A needle with suture is passed from the external guide through the skin into the tendon and out the opposite side. Three sutures are passed through the proximal tendon end and three are used in the distal tendon end. The device and the suture ends are pulled out from under the

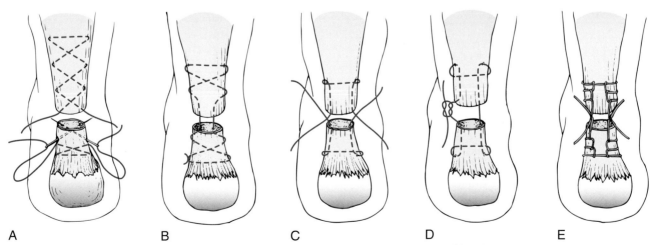

A   B   C   D   E

Figure 22–92 Various suture techniques for repair of a ruptured Achilles tendon. **A,** Double-suture Bunnell technique. **B,** Single-suture Bunnell technique. **C,** Double-suture Kessler technique. **D,** Single-suture Kessler technique. **E,** Double-suture Krackow technique.

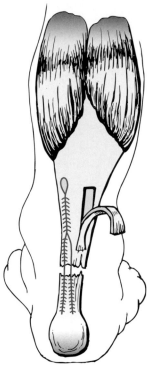

Figure 22–93   Turn-down fascial graft may be used to reinforce Achilles tendon repair.

paratenon and incision such that the end of the sutures grasping the tendon now rest entirely within the paratenon. The tendon ends are reapproximated, and the sutures are tied.

Assal et al[228] reported their experience using the Achillon device in 82 patients, noting that all patients who were elite athletes were able to return to their same level of competition.

Postoperative Care

The leg is placed in a below-knee cast or splint with the ankle dorsiflexed as much as easily possible without tension on the repair. With each cast change the ankle is gradually dorsiflexed until a neutral position is reached. At 4 weeks a walking heel is added, with the ankle in a neutral position. Six weeks after surgery the cast is removed and immobilization is discontinued. The patient may be placed in an AFO, removable cast, or a cast brace with a dorsiflexion stop if the surgeon is concerned about the security of the repair or the reliability of the patient. With a tight repair, an above-knee cast may be used.

Another method of postoperative care (LCS) implements a slightly different protocol after 2 weeks. At the time of suture removal, a boot brace dialed into 20 degrees of plantar flexion is worn. The patient is allowed to remove the brace and perform range-of-motion exercises. If the surgeon is comfortable and the patient is reliable the patient is allowed to walk somewhat like a fencer on the sole of the brace with the leg with the ruptured tendon leading and the knee held in a flexed position. The patient must not walk on the forefoot section of the brace. By 6 weeks after surgery, the patient is instructed to achieve the ankle neutral position during the range-of-motion exercises. The brace is then dialed into the neutral position and full weight bearing is permitted.

Initially, physical therapy involves gentle passive range of motion of the foot and ankle. Two weeks after cast removal, progressive resistive exercises are commenced. Four weeks after cast removal (10 weeks after surgery), aggressive walking is initiated, with a return to sports activity at 14 to 16 weeks after injury.

Early rehabilitation can minimize long-term functional deficits. Early motion after surgical treatment is recommended by some authors. Mandelbaum et al[319] initiated early motion in 29 patients after surgical repair. At 3 months a 36% functional deficit was noted, but by 6 months, 93% of patients had returned to full activity, and the functional deficit decreased to less than 3%. At long-term follow-up (3 to 5 years), Haggmark and Eriksson[273] observed that calf atrophy had largely resolved and found reproducible muscle fatigue only in those who were treated nonsurgically. Troop et al[364] advocated early protected motion using a walking boot with a dorsiflexion stop at −20 degrees. In a reliable and motivated patient this alternative can aid in a rapid return to sports activity.

Surgical Considerations

Numerous surgical procedures have been proposed to repair ruptured Achilles tendons. The basic goal of all surgical treatment is to restore the anatomic length to the triceps surae by approximating the ruptured tendon ends. In 1959 Arner and Lindholm[225] reported 77 good and excellent results after 82 surgeries and documented superior results compared with nonsurgical treatment. This led to the increased incidence of surgical repair as a treatment for Achilles tendon rupture. Indications for repair are injuries in the younger patient, active older patient, and elite athlete and patients requiring delayed treatment of an Achilles tendon rupture.[279] Contraindications to surgical repair include injury in sedentary and debilitated patients and chronically ill patients. Surgery has been advocated in several reports with routinely high levels of postoperative success.

Cetti et al[243] reported on a prospective randomized treatment of 56 patients treated surgically and 55 patients treated nonsurgically. They also reviewed 4083 Achilles tendon ruptures reported in the literature. In their review the mean time for sick leave for surgery patients averaged 10.5 weeks and for nonsurgery patients 8 weeks. The authors concluded that end-to-end repair of acute Achilles tendon ruptures resulted in a return to a higher level of sports activities. At follow-up, surgery patients had less calf atrophy, better ankle motion, and fewer post-treatment complaints. Frequency of major complications in surgery and nonsurgery patients was the same, and the authors concluded that surgery was preferable but that conservative treatment was acceptable.

In 1977 Ma and Griffith[317] described a technique of percutaneous repair of Achilles tendon ruptures under local anesthesia that appeared to minimize the risk of skin problems associated with surgery while adequately reapproximating the ruptured tendon ends (Fig. 22–94). No rerupture, infection, or nerve injury occurred in 18 cases. The initial enthusiasm with which this technique was received has been tempered by additional reports of series with higher complication rates that did not duplicate the initial success rate. Bradley and Tibone[236] reported a 12% and Aracil et al[224] a 33% rerupture rate. Sural nerve injuries have been reported.[224,260] Kakiuchi[291] reported 12 cases of percutaneous repair and stated this technique was preferable.

The ultimate assessment of treatment success is the functional result. Documentation of atrophy, muscle strength, and endurance has

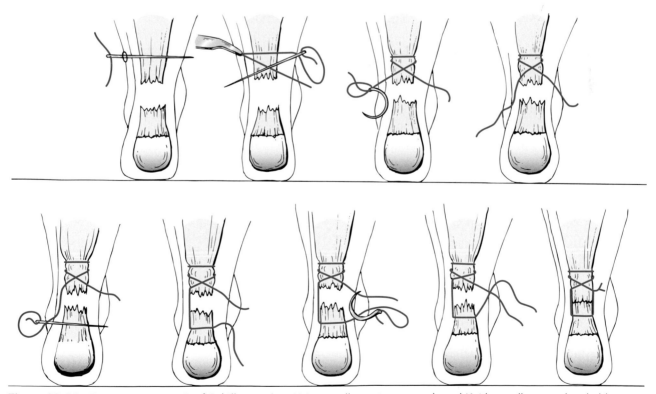

Figure 22–94 Percutaneous repair of Achilles tendon. Using small puncture wounds and Keith needles, nonabsorbable suture is woven through the proximal and distal tendons. Then, with a curved cutting needle, the suture is brought out through an enlarged medial incision. With the ankle in equinus position, the suture is tied, bringing tendon ends into apposition. (Modified from Ma G, Griffith T: *Clin Orthop Relat Res* 128:247-255, 1977.)

been quantitated with Cybex testing and other forms of muscle power evaluation, but return to prerupture activities is the standard by which all studies must be assessed. Unfortunately, a satisfactory result in one study may be at variance with the expectations of physicians and patients in other studies. Although Lea and Smith[302] reported a high level of satisfactory results with casting of Achilles tendon ruptures (48 of 52 cases), Inglis et al[285] criticized the fact that 28 different surgeons participated in this study. Post-treatment strength and endurance evaluations to some extent have standardized comparisons, but testing equipment and techniques vary in different studies. Nonetheless, these methods are much more scientific than observations of gait and manual muscle testing. However, a single-limb, multiple heel-rise test is probably the simplest and most accurate way for investigators to compare results.

The patient's age, sex, and rehabilitation effort all can affect the ultimate outcome. Leppilahti et al[310] reported significantly better recovery and strength in men than in women after repair of Achilles tendons. Parsons et al[333,334] reported that at an average 9 months after surgery, measured strength was almost equivalent to the uninjured side, confirming Taylor's notion that if one continues to rehabilitate the injured Achilles tendon, one "will continue to see improvement."[360] In an exhaustive review of the literature, Kellam et al[294] compared 608 surgery patients and 208 nonsurgery patients and found in all but one study[329] that surgical repair achieved stronger postoperative muscle power. Haggmark and Eriksson[273] noted that the recovery was best assessed by evaluating muscle fatigue or work capacity rather than strength assessment over brief intervals. They concluded that Nistor's study[329] (finding equal strength in both nonsurgical and surgical cases) did not adequately compare functional capacity. Kellam et al[294] found overall satisfaction with casting in 66% and with surgery in 93% of cases when he evaluated 13 separate studies. Wills et al[374] surveyed seven studies in which strength measurements (Cybex type) were performed after surgical and nonsurgical treatment and found superior strength after repair.

Not all patients require complete recovery of muscle strength, endurance, and functional capacity. Undoubtedly, to achieve a high functional level, a competitive athlete most often chooses surgical repair and aggressive postoperative rehabilitation. On the other hand, the sedentary patient who likely aspires to little athletic activity, when confronted with the alternatives of treatment, risks, and complications of surgery, often opts for lengthy cast immobilization. The challenging area in both patient education and physician treatment is to assist the patient who is neither sedentary nor highly competitive in choosing the best route of recovery. Some choose surgery to avoid lengthy immobilization or the risk of rerupture with further periods of immobilization. Others choose surgery because of a desire for better function. Patients must be informed of the risks of surgery because, although postsurgical complications are significantly lower than those reported in the 1970s and 1980s, a significant wound problem can require a lengthy and expensive recovery process. As Fitzgibbons et al[260] stated, "One occurrence can have catastrophic sequelae."

Complications

Lea and Smith[302] reported 17% major and 24% minor complications after surgical repair of Achilles tendon rupture. In a comprehensive review, Wills et al[374] found that 155 of 777 cases (20%) had surgical complications. Reported complications include keloid formation,[269,336] sural nerve injury,[302] adhesions,[264,302,317,336] infection, skin slough[243,269,302,317,336] (Fig. 22–95) and rerupture.[243,317]

Many of the postsurgical complications accumulated by Wills et al[374] were minor and had little effect on the functional outcome. Furthermore, postsurgical complications seen in an earlier period (30%)[227] occur with much less often with improved surgical technique and perioperative antibiotics.[285,286,312] Lieberman et al[312] more recently reported a "significant" complication rate of 0% to 3% postoperatively. However, Arner and Lindholm[225] reported 17% major complications after Achilles tendon repair. This "simple operation is associated with a curiously high incidence of complications" in an area that is quite unforgiving (Fig. 22–96).[222] A wound infection and even a small skin slough can lead to a catastrophic complication. Skin and soft tissue defects in the Achilles tendon region are difficult to treat with minor procedures.[309] Free tissue transfers have been demonstrated to be an effective method to cover

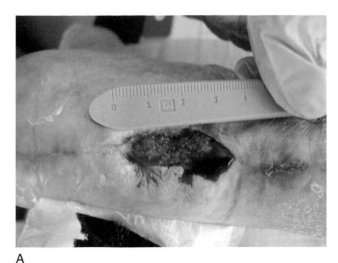

A

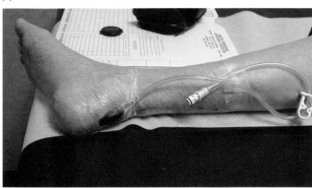

B

Figure 22–95 Skin slough following tendon repair. **A,** Full thickness skin loss. **B,** Treated with wound vacuum-assisted closure and later closure.

defects resulting from wound complications after Achilles tendon reconstruction.[309,348,358,359]

Rerupture rates after surgery are extremely low (less than 2%)[374] but vary from 13% to 35% in those treated nonsurgically.[259,338,353] Wills et al[374] reviewed 20 major studies and compiled accurate figures regarding the overall incidence of rerupture: 12 of 777 (1.5%) reruptures after surgery and 40 of 226 (18%) reruptures after nonsurgical treatment. Fruensgaard et al[262] did note a decreased rate of rerupture (7%) with 12 weeks of immobilization. This led Edna[257] to conclude that nonsurgical treatment "could not compete" with surgical repair because of the high percentage of reruptures. Nonetheless, for patients at high risk for surgical or perisurgical complications or who refuse surgery, casting is a viable alternative. Scott et al[353] noted that

most reruptures occur within 6 months of the original rupture. Patients with a second rerupture had a much lower level of satisfaction (62%) compared with those who had a primary repair (93%).

Delayed Repair

Although a delayed repair of a ruptured Achilles tendon is usually not necessary, a neglected rupture is reported to occur in up to one quarter of series. Reports in the literature use different terminology to describe this condition and treatment, including chronic rupture,[320] neglected rupture,[223,264,331,333,340] late or old repair,[367] and delayed reconstruction.[231] Dalton[252] suggested acute injuries should be defined as being diagnosed and treated at less than 48 hours after injury.

Bosworth[234] observed that contraction of the triceps surae complex can occur within 3 to 4 days after rupture and that difficulty may be experienced at surgery in "regaining coaptation" of ruptured ends. Gabel and Manoli[264] and Porter et al[340] stated that 4 weeks is the most often cited interval between rupture and repair for the condition to be considered "late." The actual definition of an old or late (or chronic) Achilles tendon rupture is debated, but the end result requires a reconstruction that most often does not permit end-to-end apposition of Achilles tendon segments with simple plantar flexion of the ankle.

The most common reason for delayed treatment occurs in association with a delay in diagnosis. However, Dalton[252] cited long-standing tendinosis with microrupture of the Achilles tendon as a secondary cause for progressive elongation of the tendon resulting in dysfunction.

Just as an acute rupture has a propensity to heal with surgical or nonsurgical treatment, a neglected or old rupture can heal without surgery, as well. The main factor in the success or failure of the healing process is the functional length of the muscle–tendon unit. An overlengthened triceps surae results in diminished strength. Although Barnes and Hardy[231] have demonstrated that abundant scar tissue forms in the rupture interval, this healing process can impair the functional end result. Inadequate plantar flexion power reduces the stability of the ankle and impairs the resultant gait pattern.

When patients are asked to recall a specific incident, they may indeed recall a traumatic episode or developing pain associated with a sporting activity. A lack of continued pain or significant swelling can lead to

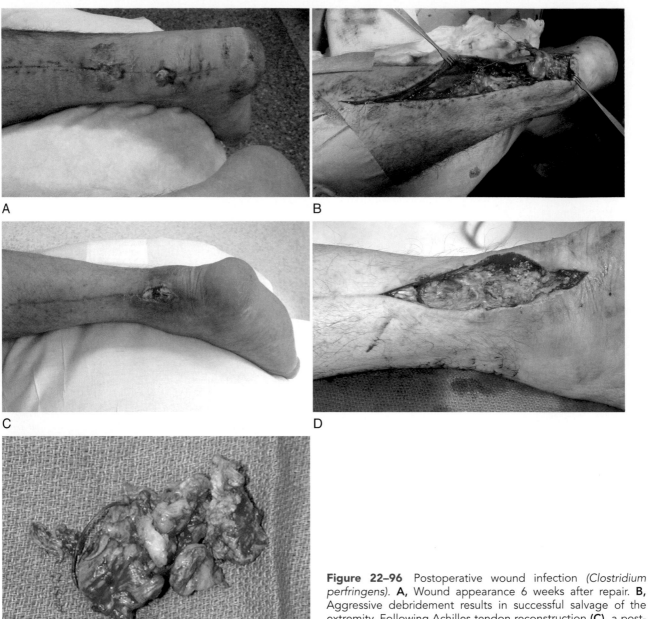

Figure 22–96 Postoperative wound infection (*Clostridium perfringens*). **A,** Wound appearance 6 weeks after repair. **B,** Aggressive debridement results in successful salvage of the extremity. Following Achilles tendon reconstruction (**C**), a postoperative infection requires aggressive debridement (**D**). **E,** Specimen following debridement. (**A** and **B** courtesy of A. Younger, MD.)

ignoring symptoms, resulting in delayed treatment. Thus at evaluation, a patient with an untreated Achilles tendon rupture may complain of an unsteady gait, difficulty ascending or descending stairs, a limp with ambulation, or difficulty in rising onto the toes. Pain is an uncommon complaint.

PHYSICAL EXAMINATION

On physical examination, a palpable gap is rarely felt at the site of the previous rupture. Increased dorsiflexion excursion of the ankle is noted compared with the

contralateral ankle, and diminished plantar-flexion strength is often observed. A patient might experience fatigue with exercise. Depending on the actual length of the Achilles tendon, the patient may be able to rise on the toes, but this ability most often is limited or absent. A repetitive toe-rise test is difficult if not impossible for the patient to perform.

CONSERVATIVE TREATMENT

Nonsurgical treatment may be necessary for reasons that include poor skin condition, diabetes mellitus, history of heavy smoking, prior surgical scarring, skin complications from prior surgery, and a patient's desire to avoid surgical intervention. Simple treatment may involve the use of high-topped boots, a laced ankle brace, or a custom-molded leather ankle lacer. With more severe dysfunction, a polypropylene AFO coupled with an aggressive calf-strengthening exercise program can enable a patient to function adequately with impaired Achilles function.

Although casting of an acute rupture is recommended by some as the primary treatment for acute rupture,[258,279,316,329] casting of the neglected or chronic rupture is more controversial. In a report on surgical and nonsurgical treatment of neglected ruptures, Cetti et al[243] found a return of some gastrocnemius-soleus function over several years. They concluded, however, that 75% of those treated with surgery had acceptable results and only 56% of those treated with casting had restoration of function. Nonetheless, gravity equinus casting remains an option for the neglected Achilles tendon rupture diagnosed within 4 weeks of rupture (see the earlier section on technique of casting) (see Fig. 22–88).

SURGICAL TREATMENT

Just as a multitude of surgical techniques have been proposed for the treatment of acute Achilles tendon ruptures, a plethora of techniques have been reported for delayed reconstruction of the neglected rupture. The purpose of any reconstruction is to restore strength and continuity to the Achilles tendon unit while minimizing the risk of surgical complications. Dalton[252] has divided the reconstruction techniques into both autologous and synthetic techniques, as shown in Box 22–6.

Ideally, a direct primary repair is preferable with any Achilles tendon rupture. Over time, contracture of the gastrocnemius-soleus complex makes this method unlikely to succeed. After excision of the interval scar tissue, the presence of a sizable gap may preclude an end-to-end repair, requiring more extensive reconstruction techniques.

Porter et al[340] reported on 11 patients who underwent proximal release of the gastrocnemius–soleus complex and imbrication of the fibrous scar tissue without excision of local tissue, thus achieving apposition of the tendon segments. Proximally the muscle complex was released by blunt dissection of any adhesions and sharp release of the posterosuperior compartment both medially and laterally. This enabled apposition of the tendon segments and closure of the rupture gap. No augmentation transfer was performed. Porter et al[340] and Carden et al[240] have reported

---

BOX 22–6 Achilles Tendon Reconstruction Techniques

I. Autologous
   A. Primary repair (uncommon)
   B. Augmentation
      1. Free fascia tendon graft
         a. Fascia lata
         b. Donor tendons (semitendinosus, peroneal, gracilis, patella tendon)
      2. Fascia advancement
         a. V-Y plasty
         b. Gastrocnemius–soleus fascia turn-down graft
      3. Local tendon transfer
         a. Flexor hallucis longus
         b. Flexor digitorum longus
         c. Peroneus brevis
         d. Peroneus longus
         e. Plantaris
         f. Posterior tibial (to be discouraged)
II. Synthetic or allograft
   A. Polyglycol threads
   B. Marlex mesh
   C. Dacron vascular graft
   D. Carbon fiber
   E. Allograft tendon substitution

Categories from Dalton G: *Foot Ankle Clin* 1: 225-236, 1996.

---

improved functional results with primary repair without augmentation in the delayed treatment of an Achilles tendon rupture. Primary repair is a very uncommon treatment for most late reconstruction techniques. As Bosworth[234] has noted, attempts at primary repair in these patients can lead to shortening of the actual length of the triceps surae if the muscle–tendon unit has significantly contracted.

Several techniques with local or distant autologous tendon tissue transfers have been proposed to reinforce or reconstruct the neglected Achilles tendon rupture. Bosworth[234] proposed a technique in which a 1.5-cm-wide longitudinal strip of tendon was dissected from the central portion of the gastrocnemius–soleus fascia. Left attached to the distal end of the proximal segment, it was then woven through the proximal and distal Achilles tendon stumps, bridging the Achilles tendon defect.

BOSWORTH REPAIR

Surgical Technique

1. A posterior longitudinal midline incision is used to expose the ruptured tendon and gastrocnemius fascia.
2. A 20-cm longitudinal strip of tendon (1.5 cm wide) is dissected free but left attached distally to the proximal stump. It is woven transversely through the proximal tendon and secured with interrupted sutures (Fig. 22–97A).
3. The fascia strip is then passed distally along the border of the Achilles tendon gap and woven transversely through the distal tendon stump (Fig. 22–97B).
4. The fascia strip is woven anteriorly and posteriorly through the proximal and distal stumps at a 90-degree angle to the initial transfer (Fig. 22–97C).
5. Each pass is secured with interrupted sutures.
6. The peritenon is approximated, if possible, and the wound is closed in layers.

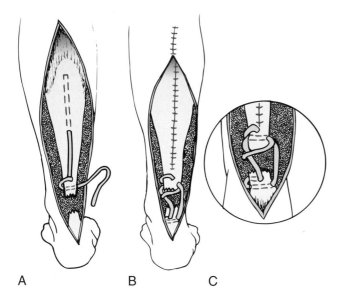

Figure 22–97 Bosworth technique. Using a fascial strip obtained from the proximal gastrocnemius–soleus complex, the Achilles tendon is reconstructed. **A,** A longitudinal strip of tendon (20 cm long, 1.5 cm wide) is left attached distally to the Achilles tendon. **B,** The strip is woven across the gap. **C,** Fascial strip is woven anteriorly and posteriorly through the proximal and distal stumps at a 90-degree angle to the initial transfer. (From Bosworth D: *J Bone Joint Surg Am* 38:111-114, 1956.)

Postoperative Care

The leg is immobilized in an above-knee cast with the knee in 45 degrees of flexion. The ankle is placed in a gravity equinus position. After subsequent cast changes, the foot is gradually brought into a neutral position. Four weeks after surgery a below-knee cast is applied and weight-bearing ambulation is commenced. Immobilization is continued for 12 weeks. An alternative approach in a reliable patient is to use a boot brace in equinus position for 6 weeks. During this time the patient may exercise the ankle to progressively obtain a neutral ankle position by the 6-week point. Then the brace is adjusted into neutral with allowance for progressive weight bearing. The brace is continued from 3 months on, and then the patient is instructed to gradually wean from the brace. Increased activity and physical therapy are begun after cast or brace removal.

Results

Barnes and Hardy[231] recommended a minimum of 8 weeks of casting and preferably 12 weeks of immobilization after reconstruction. A below-knee brace with a dorsiflexion stop at neutral or an AFO is subsequently prescribed. A 2.5-cm heel lift is used after discontinuing the brace. Bosworth[234] reported on six adult patients and noted good results with delayed reconstruction performed 1 to 14 months after the initial rupture.

Arner and Lindholm[225,313] described the use of two fascial turn-down flaps to augment an Achilles tendon repair (see Fig. 22–92). Later, Inglis et al[285] used this method for reconstructing a deficient area using slightly longer flaps (approximately 10 cm). These were woven through the distal stump and then turned back across the gap to the proximal stump, creating a total of four fascial strips bridging the defect. Others[266,270] have used modifications of a turn-down flap technique. Gerdes et al[266] used a further modification of a turn-down flap technique employing a centrally based flap in seven cases (six acute, one chronic). In cadaver studies they demonstrated that this fascial augmentation increased the strength of the repair 47% compared with a simple suture-repair technique (Figs. 22–98 and 22–101).

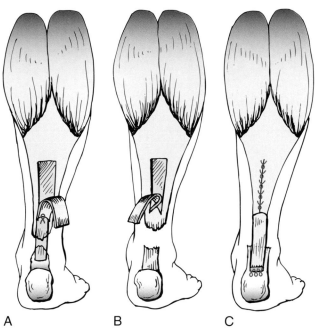

A   B   C

Figure 22–98 Technique of fascial turn-down flap. **A,** A centrally based flap is developed from the proximal segment. **B,** Flap is turned 180 degrees. **C,** Flap is sutured in place to the distal Achilles stump. (Modified from Gerdes M, Brown T, Bell A, et al: *Clin Orthop Relat Res* 280:241-246, 1992.)

ARNER AND LINDHOLM TECHNIQUE[225,313]

Surgical Technique

1. With the patient in a prone position, the extremity exsanguinated, and a thigh tourniquet inflated, a posteromedial longitudinal incision is extended from the midcalf to the Achilles tendon insertion. The deep fascia is incised in the midline, exposing the tendon rupture as well.
2. The tendon site is debrided, and the tendon ends are apposed (when possible) with an interrupted suture. A gap may be present if there is significant delay with the repair.
3. From the proximal gastrocnemius fascia, two flaps approximately 1 × 8 cm are raised. They are left attached distally at a point 3 cm proximal to the rupture site (see Fig. 22–92).
4. The flaps are twisted 180 degrees on themselves, leaving a smooth posterior surface adjacent to the subcutaneous tissue. The flaps are turned distally over the rupture site.
5. The flaps are sutured in place to the distal stump of the Achilles tendon and to each other as they cross the gap.
6. The peritenon is closed over the site of the repair. The wound is approximated with a layered closure.

ALTERNATIVE ACHILLES TURNDOWN PROCEDURE

One of us (LCS) uses this procedure. See Figures 22–98, 22–101, and 22–104.

Surgical Technique

1. After induction of anesthesia, the patient is positioned prone. Both lower extremities are prepped and draped free.
2. A medial incision is made 5 to 10 mm anterior to the medial border of the Achilles distally and more toward the midline proximally. This incision is typically long and can extend halfway up the calf.
3. Once the tendon is exposed, the chronic tendon or fibrous tissue is excised, which typically leaves a substantial gap.
4. The proximal portion of the tendon is mobilized by putting the tendon under traction (approximately 9 kg or 20 lbs).
5. Holding the foot in neutral position, the gap between the tendon edges is measured to determine the length of turndown. A 1-cm strip of tendon measuring approximately 1 cm thick is harvested centrally. The gap is measured and an additional 4 cm is then added to the length of the tendon turndown (a 2-cm distal hinge that is overlapped by the turned down flap, or 2 cm plus 2 cm). An additional 1 cm is added to account for the intended 1-cm overlap of the tendon ends distally. Thus, the total length of the needed flap equals the sum of the distance between the tendon ends as measured after the tendon debridement plus 5 cm (a 4-cm bridge plus 1 cm for overlap). For example, with an 8-cm gap, the proximal portion of the graft is 13 cm from the proximal end of the defect. There must be sufficient length to permit the tendon to be turned around on itself and enough length for distal connection to the calcaneus or the distal stump of the Achilles.
6. At 2 cm proximal to the defect, two no. 1 polyester (Ethibond) sutures anchor the corner of the turndown graft, reinforcing the high-stress junction so there is no propagation of the split between the strip and the main body of the tendon.
7. Pass the graft deep to the main tendon instead of turning down the tendon superficial to the main tendon, because there is less bulk if it is passed deep to the main tendon.

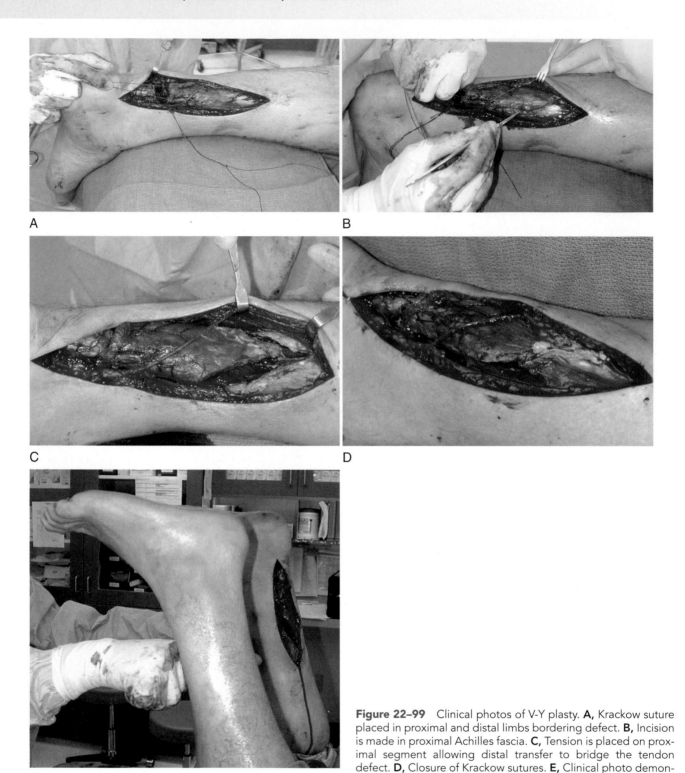

Figure 22–99   Clinical photos of V-Y plasty. **A,** Krackow suture placed in proximal and distal limbs bordering defect. **B,** Incision is made in proximal Achilles fascia. **C,** Tension is placed on proximal segment allowing distal transfer to bridge the tendon defect. **D,** Closure of Krackow sutures. **E,** Clinical photo demonstrating appropriate tension on repaired tendon.

8. Tensioning the graft requires checking the range of motion and the springiness of the operative side versus the normal side. Usually, the foot should have 15 degrees of plantar flexion in resting position and the conclusion of the reconstruction. The graft and the turndown are held in place either by hand or by suture. Once the position is established, whipstitches are used for the final anastomosis. The resting tension and

springiness are checked again at the end of the procedure.

Postoperative Care

The foot is held in 20 degrees of plantar flexion in a posterior splint. At 2 weeks, if the wound is healing well, the foot is placed in the boot brace in 20 degrees of plantar flexion, allowing weight bearing in the plantar flexed position. Range-of-motion stretching to neutral is allowed.

Six weeks following surgery, a brace is adjusted to neutral, and full weight bearing is commenced. Range-of-motion exercises are increased as well in dorsiflexion. The brace is continued for at least 12 weeks, and full recovery can take 6 months.

V-Y ADVANCEMENT

A V-Y advancement may be required if more than 80% of the tendon width is involved in a case of chronic Achilles tendinitis. It can also be performed when a zone of 1 to 3 cm of diseased tendon must be resected. It is particularly useful for treating a delayed Achilles tendon repair (4 to 12 weeks old) when there may be scar tissue that prohibits full mobilization of the tendon. In this scenario, the tendon can be primarily repaired at the rupture site and then the Achilles complex lengthened by doing the V-Y proximally to achieve the proper resting tension (see Fig. 22–100).

Surgical Technique

1. The patient is placed in the prone position. Both legs are prepped so resting tension can be checked during surgery.
2. An incision is made medial to the Achilles and extending the initial posterior incision more proximally toward the musculotendinous junction (Fig. 22–99A).
3. The diseased tendon is debrided or excised. If the technique is performed for delayed treatment of a rupture, then the tendon ends are prepared and the sutures are placed for anastomosis. The distal repair can be performed with a modified Krackow or whip stitch.
4. A V-shaped incision is made into the fascia, with the apex proximal (Fig. 22–99B and C).

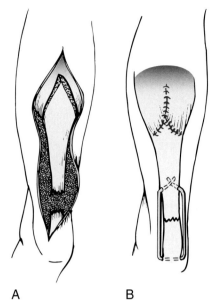

A   **B**

Figure 22–100   Reconstruction with V-Y gastroplasty. **A,** V-shaped incision is made in aponeurosis. Limbs of the V should be 1.5 times longer than the width of the gap in the Achilles tendon. **B,** Intermediate segment is advanced distally, and the gap is closed and repaired side to side. Rupture site is closed and repaired. Proximal incision is closed as a Y in lengthened position.

5. With traction on the distal tendon, an advancement of 2 to 3 cm can then be achieved without splitting the underlying muscle, which should sufficiently close the distal gap. The tendon may begin to tear and pull off the muscle base beyond an advancement of 3 to 5 cm.
6. The tendon tension is performed by checking for the resting posture of the foot and testing the springiness of the ankle as it sits in the normal slightly plantarflexed position.
7. The V-Y gap is then closed with 2-0 or 0 polyglactin (Vicryl) suture (Fig. 22–99D and E).

Postoperative Care

Postoperative care is the same as after the Bosworth repair.

Alternative Techniques

Abraham and Pankovich[223] and others[231,295,323,340] have advocated a V-Y plasty of the gastrocnemius–soleus aponeurosis to bridge the Achilles tendon defect. Using an extensive longitudinal posterior incision, the gastrocnemius–soleus

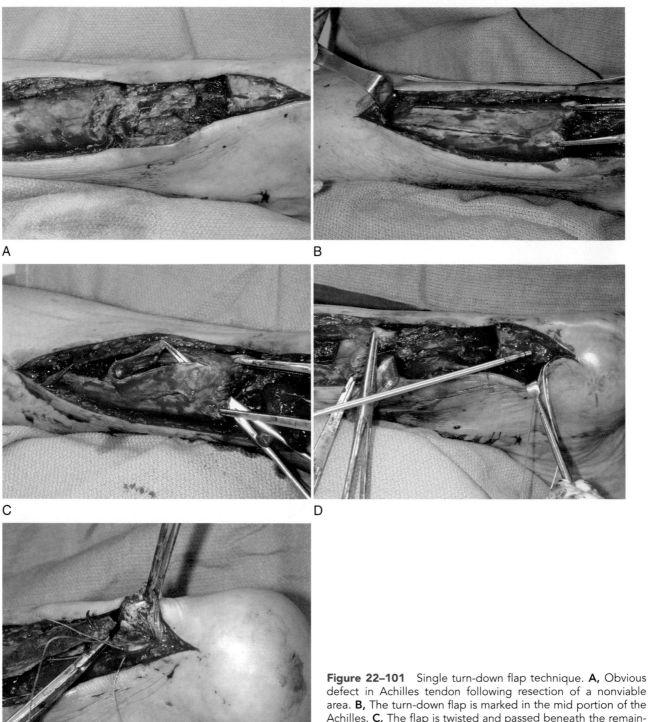

Figure 22–101   Single turn-down flap technique. **A,** Obvious defect in Achilles tendon following resection of a nonviable area. **B,** The turn-down flap is marked in the mid portion of the Achilles. **C,** The flap is twisted and passed beneath the remaining tendon bridge. This turn-down area should be reinforced with sutures to prevent propagation of the split. **D,** Sutures are placed in the distal stump of tendon. **E,** The two edges of the tendons are securely sutured together.

fascia was sectioned at the musculotendinous junction. The technique for advancement requires that the oblique limbs of the V-Y incision be 1.5 times longer than the Achilles tendon defect to allow proper apposition after the distal slide of the fascia graft (see Figs. 22–99 and 22–100). The fascia is dissected completely free from the underlying muscle, rendering the fascia a free graft, and the proximal fascial incision is repaired side to side. An end-to-end repair of the Achilles tendon is then performed. Intervening scar tissue is resected.

Bugg and Boyd[238] reported on 10 patients who underwent fascia lata grafting of an Achilles tendon defect. This requires a separate ipsilateral thigh incision to harvest a 7.5- by 15-cm fascia lata graft. This sheet is then sectioned into three separate strips (1 cm wide) and the remaining fascia sheet is left intact (Fig. 22–102). The small strips are placed obliquely across the defect and sewn to either stump. Then the remaining sheet of fascia is fashioned into a tube with the seam oriented anteriorly and the serosal surface external.

Results

Abraham and Pankovich[223] reported on four patients, three of whom regained full strength after repair. Fish[259] and Leitner et al[305] have reported similar success in relatively small series.

In the series of Bugg and Boyd,[238] follow-up results were reported for only two of the 10 patients, although the authors claimed satisfactory postoperative function for all. A pull-out wire was used to secure the proximal segment, and weight bearing was initiated 9 weeks after surgery. Cast immobilization was used for 12 weeks with this procedure (see postoperative care earlier). Others[343,376] have used fascia lata grafts in late repairs of Achilles tendon ruptures.

TENDON TRANSFERS

The use of tendon transfers to augment both acute ruptures[365] and neglected ruptures has been reported.[232,278,337,372] In 1931 Platt[339] advocated the use of the posterior tibial tendon as an augmentation transfer in the treatment of Achilles tendon rupture. Today, however, this would be considered an ill-advised treatment because several other tendon trans-

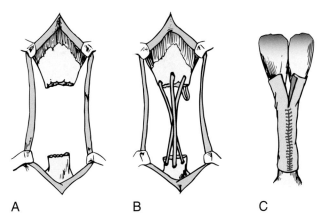

Figure 22–102 Repair using fascia lata strips. **A,** Achilles tendon rupture with gap. **B,** Three fascial strips are used to bridge the gap. **C,** Sheet of fascia lata is used to cover and reinforce the repair. (Redrawn from Bugg E, Boyd B: *Clin Orthop Relat Res* 56:73-75, 1968.)

fers are more desirable and tend to leave less deficit. Lynn[316] recommended a plantaris tendon as an augmentation to a primary repair. He chose to fan the tendon out, covering the acute Achilles repair. This technique adds little strength to the reconstruction. Others[342,343] have advocated weaving the plantaris tendon through the Achilles tendon rupture site, which does increase the overall strength of the repair. Dalton[252] proposed tendon transfer for neglected ruptures, although the plantaris is absent or is also ruptured in approximately one third of cases. In a neglected rupture the plantaris is often incorporated into scar tissue and difficult to identify. Currently the FHL, FDL, and peroneus brevis are the tendon transfers most often used either to augment primary repairs or to reconstruct a neglected rupture.

White and Kraynick[372] initially described the use of the peroneus brevis tendon in the delayed treatment of a previously ruptured Achilles tendon. Teuffer[337] and later Turco and Spinella[365] modified the technique, routing the peroneus brevis tendon through a drill hole in the calcaneus (in a lateromedial and then a proximal direction) (Fig. 22–103). Teuffer[337] reported 28 excellent and two good results but did not distinguish between early and late repairs. Turco and Spinella[365] used this technique on 40 reconstructions, eight of which were either reruptures or neglected ruptures. (In some cases the tendon was transferred through the distal Achilles stump and in other cases through a drill hole in the calcaneus.)

Although no apparent functional deficit has been reported by the authors, the importance of the per-

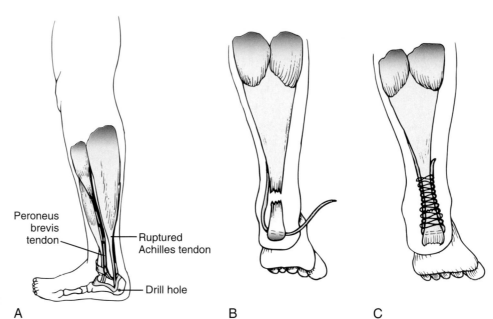

Figure 22–103 Reconstruction using peroneus brevis tendon. Peroneus brevis is isolated and detached from its insertion onto the fifth metatarsal. **A,** Transverse drill hole is placed in the calcaneus. **B,** Peroneus brevis is transferred through the drill hole. **C,** Tendon is sutured to itself and to the Achilles tendon proximally and distally. (Modified from Turco V, Spinella A: *Foot Ankle* 7:253-259, 1987.)

Peroneus brevis tendon

Ruptured Achilles tendon

Drill hole

A   B   C

oneus brevis tendon to lateral ankle stability and eversion of the foot makes this transfer less desirable than other tendon transfers.

Mann et al[320] advocated an FDL transfer for neglected Achilles tendon ruptures. They believed this transfer duplicated the medial pull of the Achilles tendon and thus was preferable to a peroneal tendon transfer. The repair was augmented with a fascial turn-down flap in seven cases. No disability of the lesser toes was reported. Routinely the FDL stump was tenodesed to the FHL at the site of the distal release.

Hansen[278] and Wapner et al[366,367] have both proposed using the FHL to reconstruct a neglected Achilles tendon rupture. The tendon was either woven through the proximal and distal Achilles tendon stumps or passed through a transverse drill hole in the calcaneus. The FHL muscle belly was approximated just anteriorly to the Achilles tendon to afford improved vascularity to this region.[264,367] Improved plantar flexion power to the foot was observed postoperatively. A tenodesis of the FHL stump to the FDL distally was rarely necessary because adequate plantar flexion strength appeared to remain in the hallux. Hansen[278] and Den Hartog[254] harvested the FHL through a direct posterior incision or a less distal incision (see Fig. 22–80), whereas Wapner et al[367] used a two-incision technique, which provides for a significantly longer tendon graft (see Fig. 22–81). This is also used for treatment of severe tendinosis with resection of a diseased distal segment and reconstruction of the Achilles tendon.

HARVEST OF LONG FLEXOR HALLUCIS LONGUS GRAFT

Surgical Technique

1. With the patient in a prone position under general or spinal anesthesia, the leg is exsanguinated and a thigh tourniquet is inflated.
2. A medial longitudinal incision beginning at the Achilles insertion is extended in a proximal direction 8 to 10 cm, with the length depending on the exposure needed (Fig. 22–104A).
3. The Achilles peritenon is opened at the site of the rupture and the rupture site is debrided. With severe tendinosis, the site of tendinosis is exposed and the tendon and bone are resected. A central turndown is shown (Fig. 22–104B-F).
4. A 7-cm longitudinal medial arch incision is made inferior and distal to the navicular and extended along the upper border of the abductor hallucis. The dissection is deepened on the dorsal aspect of the abductor hallucis, and the FDL and FHL tendons are identified.
5. The knot of Henry is released, and the FDL and FHL attachments are divided. Depending on which tendon is selected for transfer, the distal tendon is transected. The proxi-

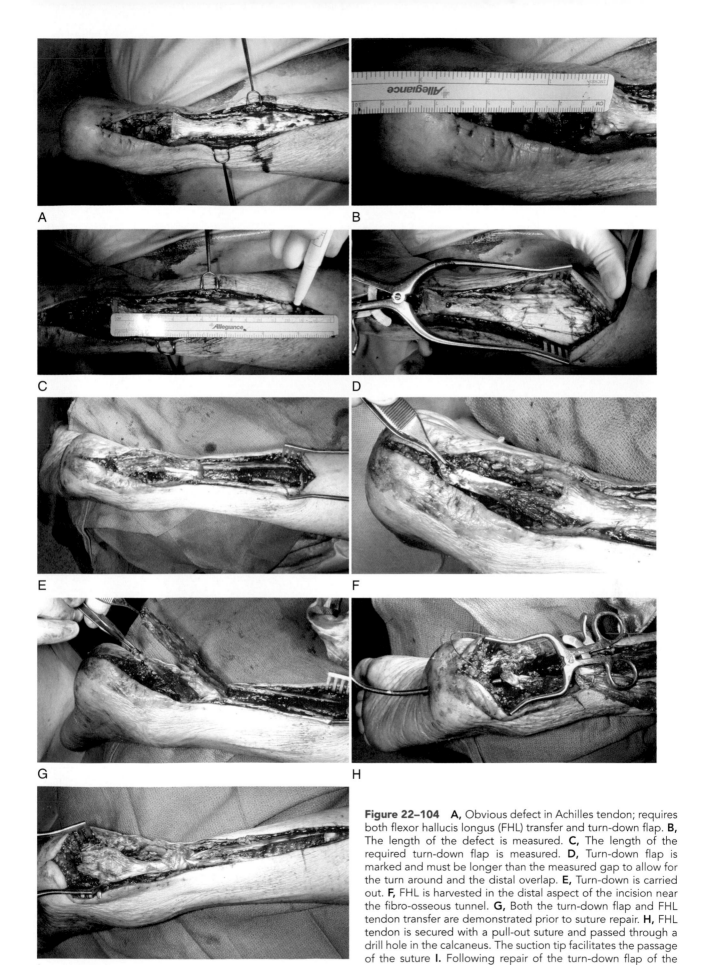

Figure 22–104 A, Obvious defect in Achilles tendon; requires both flexor hallucis longus (FHL) transfer and turn-down flap. **B,** The length of the defect is measured. **C,** The length of the required turn-down flap is measured. **D,** Turn-down flap is marked and must be longer than the measured gap to allow for the turn around and the distal overlap. **E,** Turn-down is carried out. **F,** FHL is harvested in the distal aspect of the incision near the fibro-osseous tunnel. **G,** Both the turn-down flap and FHL tendon transfer are demonstrated prior to suture repair. **H,** FHL tendon is secured with a pull-out suture and passed through a drill hole in the calcaneus. The suction tip facilitates the passage of the suture **I.** Following repair of the turn-down flap of the proximal Achilles tendon.

mal aspect of the tendon is then withdrawn into the posterior wound (Fig. 22–104G).

6. An optional procedure is available if the surgeon wishes to tenodese the distal stump of either the FDL or the FHL to the remaining adjacent tendon. Tenodesis is performed with either the lesser toes held with the interphalangeal joints in neutral extension or the hallux held in neutral position, so that tenodesis is not performed with excessive tension on either tendon.

7. A transverse drill hole is placed through the posterior aspect of the calcaneus (Fig. 22–104H).

8. With the foot held in approximately 10 to 15 degrees of plantar flexion, the transferred tendon is passed through the calcaneal drill hole in a mediolateral direction and sutured to itself with a nonabsorbable suture.

9. For a distal Achilles defect, a central slip of tendon (1 cm wide) from the proximal portion of the Achilles tendon is mobilized, turned distally, and sutured into the Achilles tendon, spanning the gap of the rupture (or area resected for chronic tendinosis) (Fig. 22–104B-F).

10. If an avulsion of the tendon or a complete degeneration of the distal insertion has occurred, a turn-down flap of the distal Achilles tendon is performed in this region. It is placed through a trough cut in the calcaneus and anchored with pull-out sutures (Fig. 22–104I).

HARVEST OF SHORT FLEXOR HALLUCIS LONGUS GRAFT

Surgical Technique

1. The patient is positioned prone.
2. Typically a medial approach to the Achilles tendon is made, staying 1 cm anterior to the medial edge of the tendon. If prior surgical scars are present it is best to use them for the approach. When the primary involvement is the Achilles insertion site, a central midline incision may be used.
3. The paratenon is opened, the degenerative tendon is excised, and the deep fascia between the superficial and deep compartments is released. Ranging the big toe while looking into the wound should allow identification of the moving FHL muscle belly.

4. The FHL tendon might have a more distal origin and might not be readily viewed in the wound. Palpation and inspection while ranging the hallux permits placement of a curved tip or right angle Kelley clamp around the tendon in the midline of the posterior ankle joint. Care should be taken while dissecting along the course of the muscle because the tibial nerve runs immediately medial to the tendon.

5. Follow and release the FHL tendon from the sheath (fibro-osseous tunnel) as it travels between the medial and lateral tubercles of the posterior talus. Continue to release the tendon for as much length as possible from the posterior approach, dissecting toward the underside of the sustentaculum tali. The tendon is cut as distal as possible, again avoiding the tibial nerve.

6. The FHL tendon is then either sewn to the Achilles repair or inserted into the calcaneus or its periosteum, depending on the tendon length and whether any calcaneus needs to be resected based on the presence of Haglund's deformity and bursitis.

7. The deep fascia between the compartments is resected, because the FHL muscle belly can provide a vascular bed for improved healing following the Achilles repair.

Postoperative Care

The foot is placed in approximately 10 degrees of equinus, and an above-knee or below-knee non–weight-bearing cast or splint is applied. Four to 6 weeks after surgery, a below-knee cast or neutral boot brace is applied with the foot and ankle in a neutral position. Eight weeks after surgery, weight bearing is allowed. Twelve weeks after surgery the patient can be gradually weaned from the brace but may still benefit from the brace or a 2.5-cm heel lift for 12 more weeks.

Results

Mann et al[320] reported five excellent and two good results with an FDL transfer. Den Hartog et al,[254] Wilcox et al,[373] and Coull et al[251] reported good and excellent results with an FHL transfer. Den Hartog[254] described a technique of harvesting the FHL tendon near the tip of the medial malleolus for chronic Achilles tendinosis. Good to excellent results were reported in 23 of 26 treated patients without any deficit in first toe function. A recent biomechanical study showed little pressure change under the first or second MTP joint and no clinical functional deficit after FHL harvesting.[251] Prior studies also showed promising clinical results.[373] Wapner et al[366] used a longer graft and reported six of seven good and excellent results with this transfer.

SYNTHETIC AND ALLOGRAFT REPAIR

Various synthetic materials have been proposed to repair neglected Achilles tendon ruptures. The major advantage of these techniques is that they avoid sacrificing other active tendon structures and avoid the more extensive dissections with other incisions and the inherent morbidity associated with them. The major drawback is that they introduce a foreign body at the rupture site, an area well known for its tenuous healing capacity. Ozaki et al[331] used a Marlex mesh graft in six patients and at 6-year follow-up noted good results. Lieberman et al[312] used a Dacron vascular graft that was woven through the tendon with a Bunnell suture technique in seven patients (all for acute repairs). No reruptures were reported. Levy et al[311] reported on five patients with recent and neglected Achilles tendon ruptures who underwent repair with this technique. They noted that immobilization could be avoided postoperatively using a Dacron vascular graft. Schedl and Fasol[349] used polyglycol threads for the repair of acute ruptures and noted two of three good and excellent subjective and functional results.

Howard et al[284] advocated carbon fiber used as synthetic lattice work for delayed repair of Achilles tendon ruptures. Weiss[369] and Parsons et al[333,334] reported its use in both acute and chronic ruptures. Nellas et al[326] used an Achilles tendon allograft to repair a neglected rupture. Mohammed et al[324] used a tissue expander in four cases to stretch and expand skin around a previous rupture site before initiating the tendon reconstruction procedure.

The use of synthetic material or the extensive dissection necessary for reconstruction for a neglected rupture can lead to wound necrosis, delayed healing, rerupture, infection, foreign body reaction, sural neuroma, and in some cases devastating tissue loss (skin, subcutaneous fat, and Achilles tendon substance), leaving a sizable soft tissue defect. A soft tissue defect can also develop following trauma (e.g., open distal tibial fracture, calcaneal fracture, crush injury, gunshot wound), lacerations, and infection. In recent years, microsurgical technical advances have enabled transfer of composite free flaps to provide a one-stage reconstruction of large defects in the Achilles tendon area. Free tissue transfers should be considered in the presence of concomitant skin and soft tissue defects with or without tendon loss.

Conclusion

Delay in diagnosis of an Achilles tendon rupture can occur because of retained ankle plantar flexion power. Plantar flexion power augmented by FHL, FDL, and posterior tibial tendon function can allow a patient to walk without obvious disability. The gap present at the rupture site can rapidly fill with hematoma, and within 48 hours[343] a defect may be difficult to palpate. The accuracy of a patient's history and the persistence of complaints may be the most helpful factors in facilitating the diagnosis at the initial evaluation. Minimal symptoms of pain can prevent a patient from even seeking medical evaluation. In time, complaints of weakness with gait, inability to ascend or descend stairs, an antalgic gait, and an inability to rise on the toes of the affected limb may necessitate a medical evaluation.

The decision to implement treatment depends on the time elapsed since the rupture, the magnitude of the disability, the desire of the patient for improved function, and risk factors associated with surgery. Bracing and nonsurgical treatment may be an acceptable alternative for a patient when weighed against the surgical risks and the necessity of a free tissue transfer should a severe wound problem develop.

Gillespie and George[268] reported on 16 patients and concluded that after delayed reconstruction of Achilles tendon ruptures, patients did not do as well as those with primary repairs. More recently, in a report of 11 patients who had undergone late reconstruction for Achilles tendon rupture, Boyden et al[235] found that those with delayed surgery had successful clinical results comparable with those after early repair. In general, patients can expect reasonably good function following late or delayed surgical reconstruction after neglected, late, or chronic rupture of the Achilles tendon.

TENDON TRANSFERS

A tendon transfer is used to help reestablish balanced muscle function around the foot and ankle to create a plantigrade foot. The plantigrade foot can also enable the patient to obtain a better gait pattern by placing the knee and hip in a more natural orientation for ambulation. Many factors need to be considered with tendon transfers.

Biomechanical Principles

The main biomechanical principle that should be considered in contemplating a tendon transfer involves the axes of the ankle and subtalar joint and the relationship of any tendon to these axes. Other factors are the specific strengths of individual muscles and their phasic activity (stance versus swing phase).

Fig. 22–105 illustrates the axes around the foot and ankle. Muscles located anterior to the ankle axis are dorsiflexors, and muscles posterior to the axis are plantar flexors. In relationship to the subtalar joint axis, muscles lying medial to this axis invert the foot, and muscles lying lateral to the axis evert the foot. Because motion can occur about both these axes simultaneously, muscles lying posterior to the ankle axis and medial to the subtalar axis plantar flex and invert the foot, whereas those posterior to the ankle axis and lateral to the subtalar joint axis plantar flex and evert the foot. Muscles lying anterior to the ankle axis and lateral to the subtalar axis dorsiflex and evert the foot. By visualizing these relationships, the surgeon can then deduce which muscles are deficient and the resultant deformity. This visualization also enables the surgeon to ascertain which muscles are still available for transfer and where they should be placed to correct the deformity.

Principles of Muscle Function

Although we tend to view muscle function around the foot and ankle as a balance of strength between dor-

siflexors and plantar flexors and invertors and evertors, Silver et al[89] have demonstrated that this balance is much more complex. In examining the relative strengths of the muscles around the ankle, they emphasized that an imbalance exists between the dorsiflexor and plantar flexor musculature. Using a numbering system based on fiber length and muscle mass, they stated that the relative strength of the dorsiflexors was 9.4 units and that of the plantar flexors 69 units. The evertors were assigned 11.9 units and the invertors 60.9 units (Table 22–4).

In view of this imbalance, control of muscle balance around the foot and ankle clearly is not based solely on one muscle group balancing another. Rather, the central nervous system (CNS) provides a modulating effect that maintains muscle balance around the foot and ankle. When the cerebral balance has been upset as a result of a CNS abnormality (e.g., cerebral palsy, cerebrovascular accident, head injury), the effects of imbalance become quite apparent. Thus after loss of

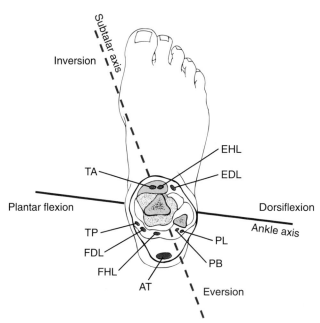

Figure 22–105 Diagram demonstrates rotation that occurs around subtalar and ankle axes. Various muscles around the subtalar and ankle axes are divided into four quadrants, using axes of the ankle and subtalar joint as reference points.

TABLE 22–4

Relative Strengths of Muscles

Tendon	Units
Plantar Flexion	
Soleus	29.9
Gastrocnemius, medial	13.7
Gastrocnemius, lateral	5.5
Flexor hallucis longus	3.6
Flexor digitorum longus	1.8
Posterior tibial	5.5
Peroneus longus	5.5
Peroneus brevis	2.6
Total Plantar Flexion	69.0
Dorsiflexion	
Anterior tibial	5.6
Extensor digitorum longus	1.7
Extensor hallucis longus	1.2
Peroneus tertius	0.9
Total Dorsiflexion	9.4
Inversion	
Posterior tibial	6.4
Flexor hallucis longus	3.6
Flexor digitorum longus	1.8
Gastrocnemius–soleus complex	49.1
Total Inversion	60.9
Eversion	
Peroneus longus	5.5
Peroneus brevis	2.6
Extensor digitorum longus	1.7
Extensor hallucis longus	1.2
Peroneus tertius	0.9
Total Eversion	11.9

this central balancing mechanism we observe in an equinovarus deformity the response to the relative strengths of the plantar flexors and invertors in relationship to the dorsiflexors and evertors.

The phasic activity of muscles must be considered as well. Muscle function around the foot and ankle is generally divided into muscles that function during swing phase and those that function during stance phase. The swing-phase muscles consist of those in the anterior compartment that bring about dorsiflexion of the ankle joint and control initial plantar flexion following heel strike. The stance-phase muscles, which include muscles from both the posterior and the lateral compartments, function during the period of midstance and control the forward movement of the tibia over the fixed foot and then initiate plantar flexion of the ankle joint.

A frequent question regarding muscle transfers is whether a stance-phase muscle can be converted to a swing-phase muscle. Most investigators agree that on a voluntary basis, a patient with a lower motor neuron (LMN) lesion can usually bring about active dorsiflexion following transfer of a stance-phase posterior tibial muscle or toe flexor muscle. When this patient walks and concentrates on using the transferred muscle, the stance-phase muscle usually functions as a swing-phase muscle. Waters,[388] however, has questioned whether over time true phase conversion persists. In general, a surgeon should attempt to transfer a swing-phase muscle to replace an absent swing-phase muscle and, conversely, transfer a stance-phase muscle to replace an absent stance-phase muscle. Occasionally this is not possible. Nonphasic transfers more likely tend to function as a tenodesis than as an active muscle transfer.

A surgeon also must be aware of the consequences of transferring a muscle from one part of the foot to another. Transferring the peroneus longus in the presence of a normal anterior tibial tendon can result in dorsiflexion of the first metatarsal and a subsequent dorsal bunion. This occurs because the normal agonist–antagonist relationship between these two muscles has been disrupted. As a result, a dorsal bunion can develop. A similar problem has been noted if the anterior tibial tendon is transferred too far laterally or if the posterior tibial tendon is transferred, particularly in a younger patient. A pronation deformity can result.

The particular type of muscle balance present plays a role in the tendon transfer selected. An LMN lesion that produces a flaccid paralysis is easier to evaluate and treat than an upper motor neuron (UMN) lesion that results in spasticity. With flaccid paralysis it is relatively simple to evaluate which muscles are functioning and the relative strength compared with a UMN lesion in which spasticity is present. When spasticity is present, it is often difficult for a patient to cooperate sufficiently to permit adequate muscle examination because of their lack of selective voluntary control. Under these circumstances a tendon release or lengthening or a tendon transfer can result in a new deformity because of a change in the balance present in the foot. For this reason, dynamic electromyographic analysis is often helpful in evaluating the patient with spasticity.[384]

The overall posture of the foot must be evaluated to ensure that the foot is plantigrade. If a deformity is present and the foot cannot be placed in a plantigrade position, other surgical procedures must be considered before a tendon transfer. A tendon transfer is unable to function if passive motion is not present in the direction that the transfer is expected to function.

Patient Evaluation

Natural History of Muscle Imbalance

A thorough understanding of the type of muscle imbalance that is present and its natural history is important in determining appropriate treatment. It is important to appreciate whether the muscle balance is progressive or nonprogressive and whether it represents a UMN or an LMN lesion. Both types of motor deficiencies can lead to a progressive deformity, but only the LMN lesion can at times result in a nonprogressive deformity. Typically the patient who has sustained an LMN lesion has a nonprogressive deformity (e.g., peroneal, sciatic nerve injury). Other types of LMN disease (e.g., peripheral neuropathies, myopathies) can demonstrate a progression of deformity. Although UMN lesions are often considered to result in spasticity (e.g., myelodysplasia), a flaccid paralysis or occasionally a mixed picture may be present.

Age of Patient

When evaluating a child with muscle imbalance, the examiner must carefully consider the effects of later growth on future deformity. In the younger child the surgeon must be concerned about what can occur after the tendon transfer (e.g., dorsal bunion, flatfoot deformity). In the older child the surgeon must be concerned that a long-standing muscle imbalance can lead to a distorted postural deformity in which the foot is no longer plantigrade. In general in the adult patient, no significant bone abnormality is present because often the muscle balance developed after skeletal maturity was reached. Fixed contractures may be present, but in general the overall bone architecture is normal.

Diagnosis

Diagnostic evaluation of a patient begins with an in-depth history of the problem, the methods of bracing used, and whether the patient's overall gait pattern is stable or deteriorating. Analysis of the range of motion of lower extremity joints and the relative muscle strengths of foot and ankle dorsiflexors and plantar flexors must be determined. When inspecting the posture of the foot, the surgeon must determine whether the foot is plantigrade. If it is not plantigrade, factors to be considered are muscle imbalance, a fixed contracture, and abnormal bone architecture. A determination must be made as to the type of gait evaluation necessary. This may be as simple as observing the patient walking or may be more sophisticated, with the use of motion analysis of the lower extremity and dynamic electromyographic data.[377,384]

Treatment

Surgical Principles

To achieve a successful tendon transfer, the surgeon should consider following basic principles.

A plantigrade foot must be present before the tendon transfer. This can be created by performing a tendon lengthening, release of a joint contracture, or, if necessary, joint arthrodesis. The tendon lengthening can involve the Achilles ir a posterior tibial or other tendon. The release of a joint contracture can consist of a posterior capsulotomy. A joint arthrodesis can vary from a subtalar or triple arthrodesis to a pantalar arthrodesis.

The muscles to be transferred should be of adequate strength and, if possible, of similar fiber length and of the same phasic activity to provide an optimal tendon transfer. A transferred muscle usually loses one grade of strength (e.g., from normal to good), and therefore, if the muscle strength is only good to fair, the transfer might not be successful.

There are several technical considerations for a tendon transfer. The tendon transfer should be performed in the presence of adequate soft tissue coverage. Dense scar tissue should be resected and if possible replaced with soft tissue coverage that provides a gliding surface for the tendon transfer. If the tendon is transferred through the interosseous membrane, a soft tissue window of adequate size should be developed. The line of tendon pull between the muscle and its insertion should be as straight a line as possible to provide maximum efficiency. The transferred tendon should preferably be implanted into bone and sutures should be placed between the periosteum and the tendon to prevent failure at the insertion site. A bone anchor may be used to reinforce the repair.

Adequate postoperative immobilization and subsequent physical therapy and retraining should be undertaken.

Tendon transfers are generally grouped into anterior, split tendon, posterior, lateral, and distal transfers. A brief discussion of each type is presented here (see Chapter 12).

ANTERIOR TENDON TRANSFER

Anterior tendon transfers are performed to reestablish dorsiflexion power. For this type of transfer to succeed, adequate passive dorsiflexion must be present before the procedure. If adequate dorsiflexion is not present, release of a posterior contracture is essential before the tendon transfer. Fig. 22–106

When the transfer is performed for flaccid paralysis, a posterior tibial transfer through the interosseous membrane is often performed.[383] At times this transfer may be reinforced by the FHL and FDL tendons. The excursion of the posterior tibial tendon is approximately 2 cm because of the shape of its muscle fibers, whereas the overall excursion of the long flexor tendons is approximately 3 cm, which enables them to move the ankle through a greater range of motion. When several tendons are transferred through the interosseous septum, an adequate soft tissue window must be created to minimize the possibility of adhesions, which can lead to restricted motion postoperatively.

With instability of the subtalar joint from loss of more than just dorsiflexor power, it may be necessary to stabilize the subtalar joint or perform a triple arthrodesis before the tendon transfer (Fig. 22–107).

Occasionally the EDL tendon may be used to provide increased dorsiflexion power at the ankle joint. This phasic transfer can provide enough extra dorsiflexion power to permit the patient to ambulate without a brace. The EDL is usually transferred into the second or third cuneiform.

After a transfer in a patient with spasticity, even with the addition of the FDL, several problems can result. The original deformity can persist or recur[386]; the original deformity can be altered, resulting in a calcaneal or calcaneovalgus deformity[386]; phase conversion can fail to occur during gait, although the patient has the ability of voluntary control.[377,386]

SPLIT TENDON TRANSFER

The split anterior tibial tendon transfer is performed to provide a yoke-type tendon configuration to the dorsum of the foot.[379] This tendon transfer is based on the principle that by tightening the lateral aspect of the yoke, a more plantigrade foot posture is achieved while using a muscle of the same phase. This transfer is most useful in a patient with spasticity with overpull

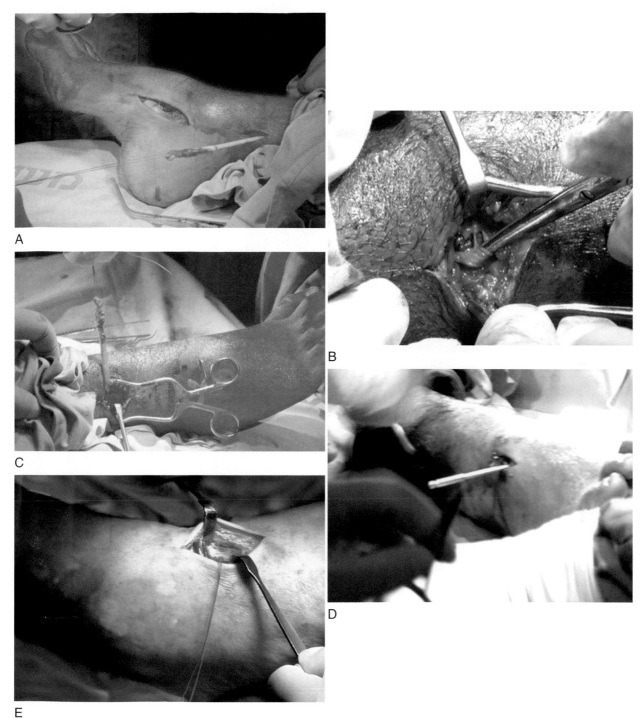

Figure 22–106 Patient with a sciatic nerve injury and foot drop. **A,** The posterior tibial tendon was harvested with additional length by distally including a strip of periosteum from the cuneiform. The hemostat was passed from posterior to anterior through the interosseous membrane. The membrane opening was widened by spreading the clamp and then pushed anteriorly through the anterior compartment. At the point where the clamp tented the skin, an incision was made. **B,** It is not uncommon to identify the superficial peroneal nerve here. **C,** With care not to damage the nerve, the tendon is passed anteriorly. **D,** The tendon is passed through a tunnel superficially over and distal to the extensor retinaculum, where another incision is placed over the lateral cuneiform. A tunnel is then created from the lateral cuneiform to the medial cuneiform. **E,** The suture will be pulled through the tunnel and the tendon secured laterally. The suture should be tied through the medial cuneiform, creating a second anchor point.

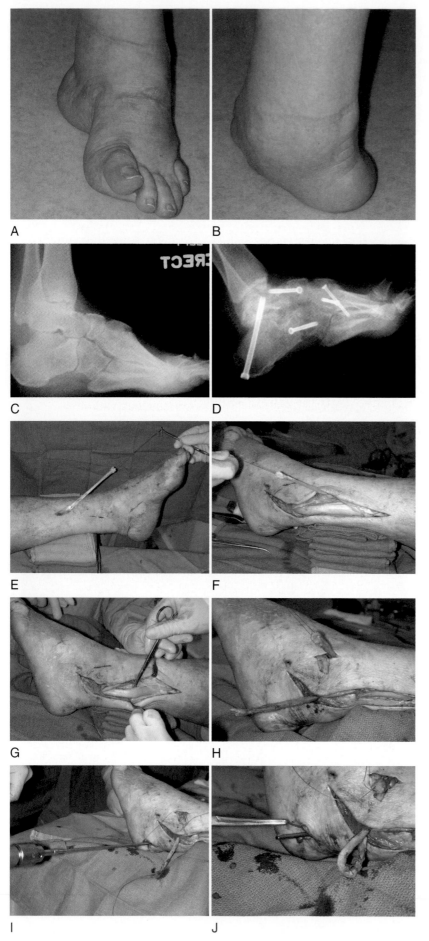

Figure 22–107 Patient had had polio. **A** and **B,** Clinical photos of severe cavo varus. **C,** Weight-bearing radiograph demonstrates the cavovarus deformity and plantar flexion of the first metatarsal. **D,** Following a triple arthrodesis to align the hind foot, a tendon transfer for a foot drop was performed because of continued dynamic varus position. The posterior tibial tendon was harvested **(E)** and transferred to the lateral side of the foot **(F)** instead of more central position. **G** and **H,** The nonfunctioning peroneal tendons were used to stabilize the lateral ankle joint through a drill hole **(I)** from lateral to medial. **J,** To pass the peroneal tendon through the calcaneus, a suction tip is used to pull the suture medialward, where it is secured.

Figure 22–108 This patient had a head injury and a mildly spastic supinated foot with severe varus and no peroneal muscular strength. Anterior clinical **(A)** and posterior clinical **(B)** views. **C,** A split anterior tibial tendon transfer (SPLATT) was performed. The incision is made over the distal aspect of the anterior tibial tendon. **D,** The tendon is split proximally above the ankle joint. **E,** The lateral half is prepared for transfer. **F,** The posterior tibial tendon was harvested from the naviculum. **G,** The posterior tibial tendon was transferred behind the tibia with assistance of Kelly clamps. **H,** The tendon is transferred into the peroneal tendon sheath to be connected to the peroneus brevis. The SPLATT is completed by attaching the lateral aspect of the tendon to the lateral cuneiform.

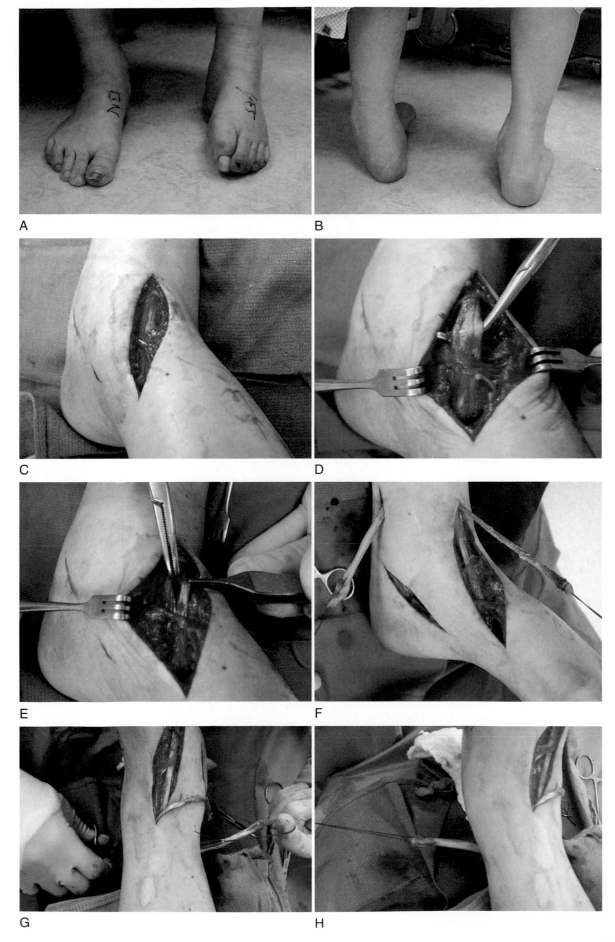

A

B

C

D

E

F

G

H

1267

of the invertors of the foot. When this procedure is performed, adequate dorsiflexion must be present. If adequate dorsiflexion is not present, Achilles tendon lengthening and possibly a posterior tibial tendon lengthening should be added to the procedure. The lateral band of the yoke must be tightened sufficiently at the tendon transfer to pull the foot into an everted position, or the procedure will fail (Fig. 22–108).

The posterior tibial split tendon transfer has been used to correct a varus hindfoot deformity. This transfer has the advantage in a younger patient of minimizing the chance of a postoperative flatfoot deformity. With this transfer, an in-phase muscle is used to provide improved muscle function.[378,381,382]

A further modification of the split tendon transfer has been used in the treatment of footdrop. Rodriguez[385] described a transfer of the posterior tibial tendon through a hole in the anterior tibial tendon. The tendon transfer was subsequently inserted into the second cuneiform. The peroneus longus tendon was then rerouted anterior to the lateral malleolus and tightened to help provide additional mediolateral balance to the foot. The advantage of this procedure is that by tightening the medial and lateral bands, a plantigrade foot is created along with simultaneous reestablishment of dorsiflexion strength.

POSTERIOR TENDON TRANSFER

Posterior tendon transfers into the Achilles tendon are typically used to prevent or retard the development of a calcaneal deformity and to restore plantar flexion power. Even if only weak plantar flexion is achieved after this type of transfer, it is better and easier to brace a foot in an equinus posture than to manage a calcaneal deformity.

Depending on the muscle function present, posterior transfer of the anterior tibial tendon through the interosseous septum or posterior transfer of the peroneus longus or posterior tibial is done. If possible, a phasic transfer is more desirable, although it appears that the anterior tibial tendon can undergo phase conversion and function as a plantar flexor during gait.[377,387]

LATERAL TENDON TRANSFER

A lateral tendon transfer is used for loss of peroneal muscle function. The peroneus brevis is a powerful evertor of the subtalar joint, whereas the peroneus longus functions mainly to plantar flex the first metatarsal and is a weak evertor. In the patient who has selectively lost peroneus brevis function (e.g., tendon laceration or rupture), the surgeon may consider using the peroneus longus as a transfer to help reestablish eversion function. A split anterior tibial transfer can likewise be used for this condition.

Because most of these muscles involve phasic transfers, uniformly good results can be expected.

DISTAL TENDON TRANSFER

The Jones tendon transfer[380] is used to correct a cock-up deformity of the first metatarsophalangeal joint that develops because of weakness of dorsiflexion by the anterior tibial muscle. Subsequently the EHL is used as a secondary dorsiflexor of the ankle joint. The EHL tendon is transferred into the first metatarsal metaphysis to provide increased dorsiflexion power of the foot. At the same time this typically corrects the chronic plantar flexion posture of the first metatarsal. A fusion of the interphalangeal joint of the hallux is necessary to offset the unopposed pull of the FHL tendon. Occasionally, an osteotomy of the base of the first metatarsal is performed to dorsiflex the first metatarsal (see Chapter 21)

An FDL tendon transfer is performed when a dynamic deformity of the lesser toes results in flexible hammering of the lesser toes. This tendon transfer involves detachment of the long flexor tendon from its insertion. The tendon is split and transferred on the medial and lateral aspect of the proximal phalanx to the extensor hood mechanism on the dorsum of the proximal phalanx. At the transfer, no fixed contracture of the proximal interphalangeal joint or spasticity must be present. Spasticity can lead to a swan-neck deformity. With a fixed contracture, the flexor tendon transfer may be unsuccessful (see Chapter 7).

REFERENCES

Extensor Tendons

1. Akhtar M, Levine J: Dislocation of extensor digitorum longus tendons after spontaneous rupture of the inferior retinaculum of the ankle. Case report. *J Bone Joint Surg Am* 62(7):1210-1211, 1980.
2. Anzel SH, Covey KW, Weiner AD, Lipscomb PR: Disruption of muscles and tendons; an analysis of 1,014 cases. *Surgery* 45(3):406-414, 1959.
3. Bell W, Schon L: Tendon lacerations of the toe and foot. *Foot Ankle Clin* 1:355-372, 1996.
4. Berens TA: Autogenous graft repair of an extensor hallucis longus laceration. *J Foot Surg* 29(2):179-182, 1990.
5. Duke HF, Greenberg PJ: Distal extensor hallucis longus tenotomy. *J Foot Surg* 30(2):133-136, 1991.
6. Floyd DW, Heckman JD, Rockwood CA Jr: Tendon lacerations in the foot. *Foot Ankle* 4(1):8-14, 1983.
7. Griffiths JC: Tendon injuries around the ankle. *J Bone Joint Surg Br* 47(4):686-689, 1965.
8. Hoelzer W, Kalish S: Traumatic severance of the anterior tibial and extensor hallucis longus tendons. *J Foot Surg* 13:96-97, 1974.
9. Kass JC, Palumbo F, Mehl S, Camarinos N: Extensor hallucis longus tendon injury: An in-depth analysis and treatment protocol. *J Foot Ankle Surg* 36(1):24-27; discussion 80, 1997.

10. Kriza CG, Mushlin TG: An avulsion fracture at the extensor digitorum brevis muscle origin. *J Foot Surg* 24(1):82-83, 1985.

11. Langenberg V: Die spontanruptur der Schne des Musculus extensor hallucis longus. *Zentbl Chir* 114:400-403, 1989.

12. Lipscomb PR, Kelly PJ: Injuries of the extensor tendons in the distal part of the leg and in the ankle. *J Bone Joint Surg Am* 37(6):1206-1213, 1955.

13. McMaster P: Tendon and muscle ruptures: Clinical and experimental studies on the causes and location of subcutaneous ruptures. *J Bone Joint Surg* 15:705-722, 1933.

14. Menz P, Nettle WJ: Closed rupture of the musculotendinous junction of extensor hallucis longus. *Injury* 20(6):378-381, 1989.

15. Mulcahy DM, Dolan AM, Stephens MM: Spontaneous rupture of extensor hallucis longus tendon. *Foot Ankle Int* 17(3):162-163, 1996.

16. Noonan KJ, Saltzman CL, Dietz FR: Open physeal fractures of the distal phalanx of the great toe. A case report. *J Bone Joint Surg Am* 76(1):122–125, 1994.

17. Poggi JJ, Hall RL: Acute rupture of the extensor hallucis longus tendon. *Foot Ankle Int* 16(1):41-43, 1995.

18. Rooks M: Tendon, vascular, nerve and skin injuries. In Gould J (ed): *Operative Foot Surgery.* Philadelphia, WB Saunders, 1994, pp 515-566.

19. Sarrafian, S: *Anatomy of the Foot and Ankle.* Philadelphia, JB Lippincott, 1983, pp 199-205.

20. Satku K, Wee JT, Kumar VP, et al: The dropped big toe. *Ann Acad Med Singapore* 21(2):222–225, 1992.

21. Sim FH, Deweerd JH Jr: Rupture of the extensor hallucis longus tendon while skiing. *Minn Med* 60(11):789-790, 1977.

22. Simonet WT, Sim L: Boot-top tendon lacerations in ice hockey. *J Trauma* 38(1):30-31, 1995.

23. Skoff H: Dynamic splinting after extensor hallucis longus tendon repair. A case report. *Phys Ther* 68(1):75-76, 1988.

24. Wicks MH, Harbison JS, Paterson DC: Tendon injuries about the foot and ankle in children. *Aust N Z J Surg* 50(2):158-161, 1980.

Anterior Tibial Rupture

25. Benzakein R, Wakim WA, DeLauro TM, Marcus R: Neglected rupture of the tibialis anterior tendon. *J Am Podiatr Med Assoc* 78(10):529-532, 1988.

26. Burman M: Stenosing tendovaginitis of the foot and ankle: Studies with special reference to the stenosing tendovaginitis of the peroneal tendons of the peroneal tubercle. *AMA Arch Surg* 67(5):686-698, 1953.

27. Burman M: Subcutaneous rupture of the tendon of the tibialis anticus. *Ann Surg* 100:368-372, 1934.

28. Cornwall M. W, McPoil T. G: The influence of tibialis anterior muscle activity on rearfoot motion during walking. *Foot Ankle Int* 15(2):75-79, 1994.

29. Crosby LA, Fitzgibbons TC: Unrecognized laceration of tibialis anterior tendon: A case report. *Foot Ankle* 9(3):143-145, 1988.

30. Dooley BJ, Kudelka P, Menelaus MB: Subcutaneous rupture of the tendon of tibialis anterior. *J Bone Joint Surg Br* 62(4):471-472, 1980.

31. Fennell CW, Ballard JM, Pflaster DS, Adkins RH: Comparative evaluation of bone suture anchor to bone tunnel fixation of tibialis anterior tendon in cadaveric cuboid bone: A biomechanical investigation. *Foot Ankle Int* 16(10):641-645, 1995.

32. Fennell CW, Phillips P 3rd: Redefining the anatomy of the anterior tibialis tendon. *Foot Ankle Int* 15(7):396-399, 1994.

33. Forst R, Forst J, Heller KD: Ipsilateral peroneus brevis tendon grafting in a complicated case of traumatic rupture of tibialis anterior tendon. *Foot Ankle Int* 16(7):440-444, 1995.

34. Goldman F: Snapping of the tibialis anterior tendon. *J Am Podiatry Assoc* 73(1):29-30, 1983.

35. Kabbani YM, Mayer DP: Magnetic resonance imaging of tendon pathology about the foot and ankle. Part I. Achilles tendon. *J Am Podiatr Med Assoc* 83(7):418-420, 1993.

36. Kabbani YM, Mayer DP: Magnetic resonance imaging of tendon pathology about the foot and ankle. Part II. Tendon ruptures. *J Am Podiatr Med Assoc* 83(8):466-468, 1993.

37. Kashyap S, Prince R: Spontaneous rupture of the tibialis anterior tendon. A case report. *Clin Orthop Relat Res* (216):159-161, 1987.

38. Kelikian A, Kelikian H: *Disorders of the Foot and Ankle.* Philadelphia, WB Saunders, 1984, pp 782-785.

39. Khoury NJ, el-Khoury GY, Saltzman CL, Brandser EA: Rupture of the anterior tibial tendon: Diagnosis by MR imaging. *AJR Am J Roentgenol* 167(2):351-354, 1996.

40. Mankey M: Anterior tibial tendon ruptures. *Foot Ankle Clin* 1:315-324, 1996.

41. Markarian GG, Kelikian AS, Brage M, et al: Anterior tibialis tendon ruptures: An outcome analysis of operative versus nonoperative treatment. *Foot Ankle Int* 19(12):792-802, 1998.

42. Mensor MC, Ordway GL: Traumatic subcutaneous rupture of the tibialis anterior tendon. *J Bone Joint Surg Am* 35(3):675-680, 1953.

43. Meyn MA Jr: Closed rupture of the anterior tibial tendon. A case report and review of the literature. *Clin Orthop Relat Res* 113:154-157, 1975.

44. Moberg E: Subcutaneous rupture of the tendon of the tibialis anterior muscle. *Acta Chir Scand* 95:455-460, 1947.

45. Morris GD, O'Malley M, Deland J, et al: Anterior tibial tendon ruptures: Results of surgical treatment. Presented at the 31st Annual Meeting of the American Orthopaedic Foot and Ankle Society, San Francisco, Calif, March 3, 2001.

46. Moskowitz, E: Rupture of the tibialis anterior tendon simulating peroneal nerve palsy. *Arch Phys Med Rehabil* 52(9):431-433, 1971.

47. Ouzounian TJ: Combined rupture of the anterior tibial and posterior tibial tendons: A new clinical entity. *Foot Ankle Int* 15(9):508-511, 1994.

48. Ouzounian TJ, Anderson R: Anterior tibial tendon rupture. *Foot Ankle Int* 16(7):406-410, 1995.

49. Petersen W, Stein V, Bobka T: Structure of the human tibialis anterior tendon. *J Anat* 197 Pt 4:617-625, 2000.

50. Prieskorn D, Plattner P: Tendons and bursae. In Helal B, Rowley D, Cracchiolo A, et al (eds): *Surgery of Disorders of the Foot and Ankle.* London, Martin Dunitz, 1996, pp 369-398.

51. Richter R, Schlitt R: [Subcutaneous rupture of the tibialis anterior tendon. (Report of 3 cases) (author's transl)]. *Z Orthop Ihre Grenzgeb* 113(2):271-273, 1975.

52. Rimoldi RL, Oberlander MA, Waldrop JI, Hunter SC: Acute rupture of the tibialis anterior tendon: A case report. *Foot Ankle* 12(3):176-177, 1991.

Flexor Tendons

53. Boruta PM, Beauperthuy GD: Partial tear of the flexor hallucis longus at the knot of Henry: Presentation of three cases. *Foot Ankle Int* 18(4):243-246, 1997.

54. Botte M: Personal communication, September 30, 2004.

55. Brand JC Jr, Smith RW: Rupture of the flexor hallucis longus after hallux valgus surgery: Case report and comments on technique for adductor release. *Foot Ankle* 11(6):407-410, 1991.

56. Carr JB: Complications of calcaneus fractures entrapment of the flexor hallucis longus: Report of two cases. *J Orthop Trauma* 4(2):166-168, 1990.

57. Coghlan BA, Clarke NM: Traumatic rupture of the flexor hallucis longus tendon in a marathon runner. *Am J Sports Med* 21(4):617-618, 1993.

58. Cowell HR, Elener V, Lawhon SM: Bilateral tendinitis of the flexor hallucis longus in a ballet dancer. *J Pediatr Orthop* 2(5):582-586, 1982.

59. Fond D: Flexor hallucis longus tendinitis—a case of mistaken identity and posterior impingement syndrome in dancers: Evaluation and management. *J Orthop Sports Phys Ther* 5:204-206, 1984.

60. Frenette JP, Jackson DW: Lacerations of the flexor hallucis longus in the young athlete. *J Bone Joint Surg Am* 59(5):673-676, 1977.

61. Garth WP Jr: Flexor hallucis tendinitis in a ballet dancer. A case report. *J Bone Joint Surg Am* 63(9):1489, 1981.

62. Gould N: Stenosing tenosynovitis of the flexor hallucis longus tendon at the great toe. *Foot Ankle* 2(1):46-48, 1981.

63. Hamilton WG: Stenosing tenosynovitis of the flexor hallucis longus tendon and posterior impingement upon the os trigonum in ballet dancers. *Foot Ankle* 3(2):74-80, 1982.

64. Hamilton WG, Geppert MJ, Thompson FM: Pain in the posterior aspect of the ankle in dancers. Differential diagnosis and operative treatment. *J Bone Joint Surg Am* 78(10):1491-500, 1996.

65. Holt KW, Cross M: Isolated rupture of the flexor hallucis longus tendon. A case report. *Am J Sports Med* 18(6):645-646, 1990.

66. Inokuchi S, Usami N: Closed complete rupture of the flexor hallucis longus tendon at the groove of the talus. *Foot Ankle Int* 18(1):47-49, 1997.

67. Kolettis GJ, Micheli LJ, Klein JD: Release of the flexor hallucis longus tendon in ballet dancers. *J Bone Joint Surg Am* 78(9):1386-1390, 1996.

68. Korovessis P, Spastris P, Katsardis T, Sidiropoulos P: Simultaneous rupture of the tibialis posterior and flexor digitorum longus tendons in a closed tibial fracture. *J Orthop Trauma* 5(1):89-92, 1991.

69. Krackow KA: Acute, traumatic rupture of a flexor hallucis longus tendon: A case report. *Clin Orthop Relat Res* 150: 261-262, 1980.

70. Lapidus PW, Seidenstein H: Chronic non-specific tenosynovitis with effusion about the ankle: Report of three cases. *J Bone Joint Surg Am* 32(1):175-179, 1950.

71. Lewin P: *The Foot and Ankle: Their Injuries, Diseases, Deformities, and Disabilities.* Philadelphia, Lea & Febiger, 1947, pp 207-208.

72. Lipscomb P: Chronic nonspecific tenosynovitis and peritendinitis. *Surg Clin North Am* 24:780-797, 1944.

73. Lipscomb P: Non-suppurative tenosynovitis and paratendinitis. *Instr Course Lect* 7:254-261, 1950.

74. Lynch T, Pupp GR: Stenosing tenosynovitis of the flexor hallucis longus at the ankle joint. *J Foot Surg* 29(4):345-348, 1990.

75. McCarroll JR, Ritter MA, Becker TE: Triggering of the great toe. A case report. *Clin Orthop Relat Res* 175:184-185, 1983.

76. Nathan H, Gloobe H, Yosipovitch Z: Flexor digitorum accessorius longus. *Clin Orthop Relat Res* 113:158-161, 1975.

77. Nigg BM: Biomechanical aspects of running. In Nigg BM (ed.): *Biomechanics of Running Shoes.* Champaign, Ill, Human Kinetics, 1986, pp 1-25.

78. Oloff LM, Schulhofer SD: Flexor hallucis longus dysfunction. *J Foot Ankle Surg* 37(2):101-109, 1998.

79. Petersen W, Pufe T, Zantop T, Paulsen F: Blood supply of the flexor hallucis longus tendon with regard to dancer's tendinitis: Injection and immunohistochemical studies of cadaver tendons. *Foot Ankle Int* 24(8):591-596, 2003.

80. Rasmussen RB, Thyssen EP: Rupture of the flexor hallucis longus tendon: Case report. *Foot Ankle* 10(5):288-289, 1990.

81. Reinherz RP: Management of flexor hallucis longus tendon injuries. *J Foot Surg* 23(5):366-369, 1984.

82. Reinherz RP, Zawada SJ, Sheldon DP: Recognizing unusual tendon pathology at the ankle. *J Foot Surg* 25(4):278-283, 1986.

83. Romash MM: Closed rupture of the flexor hallucis longus tendon in a long distance runner: Report of a case and review of the literature. *Foot Ankle Int* 15(8):433-436, 1994.

84. Rosenberg GA, Sferra JJ: Checkrein deformity—an unusual complication associated with a closed Salter–Harris type II ankle fracture: A case report. *Foot Ankle Int* 20(9):591-594, 1999.

85. Sammarco GJ, Cooper PS: Flexor hallucis longus tendon injury in dancers and nondancers. *Foot Ankle Int* 19(6):356-362, 1998.

86. Sammarco GJ, Miller EH: Partial rupture of the flexor hallucis longus tendon in classical ballet dancers: Two case reports. *J Bone Joint Surg Am* 61(1):149-150, 1979.

87. Sanhudo JA: Stenosing tenosynovitis of the flexor hallucis longus tendon at the sesamoid area. *Foot Ankle Int* 23(9):801-803, 2002.

88. Sanhudo JA, Lompa PA: Checkrein deformity—flexor hallucis tethering: Two case reports. *Foot Ankle Int* 23(9):799-800, 2002.

89. Silver RL, de la Garza J, Rang M: The myth of muscle balance. A study of relative strengths and excursions of normal muscles about the foot and ankle. *J Bone Joint Surg Br* 67(3):432-437, 1985.

90. Stokes IA, Hutton WC, Stott JR, Lowe LW: Forces under the hallux valgus foot before and after surgery. *Clin Orthop Relat Res* 142:64-72, 1979.

91. Thompson FM, Snow SW, Hershon SJ: Spontaneous atraumatic rupture of the flexor hallucis longus tendon under the sustentaculum tali: Case report, review of the literature, treatment options. *Foot Ankle* 14(7):414-417, 1993.

92. Trepman E, Mizel MS, Newberg AH: Partial rupture of the flexor hallucis longus tendon in a tennis player: A case report. *Foot Ankle Int* 16(4):227-231, 1995.

93. Trevino S, Gould N, Korson R: Surgical treatment of stenosing tenosynovitis at the ankle. *Foot Ankle* 2(1):37-45, 1981.

94. Tudisco C, Puddu G: Stenosing tenosynovitis of the flexor hallucis longus tendon in a classical ballet dancer. A case report. *Am J Sports Med* 12(5):403-404, 1984.

95. Yancey HA Jr: Lacerations of the plantar aspect of the foot. *Clin Orthop Relat Res* 122:46-52, 1977.

Peroneal Tendons

96. Aberle-Horstenegg A: Über einen eigenartigen Fußschmerz (tendovaginitis der distalen Schnenscheide des peronaeus longus). *Munchener Med Wochn* 79:946-948, 1932.

97. Abraham E, Stirnaman JE: Neglected rupture of the peroneal tendons causing recurrent sprains of the ankle. Case report. *J Bone Joint Surg Am* 61(8):1247-1248, 1979.

98. Alanen J, Orava S, Heinonen OJ, et al: Peroneal tendon injuries. Report of thirty-eight operated cases. *Ann Chir Gynaecol* 90(1):43-46, 2001.

99. Alm A, Lamke LO, Liljedahl SO: Surgical treatment of dislocation of the peroneal tendons. *Injury* 7(1):14-19, 1975.

100. Andersen E: Stenosing peroneal tenosynovitis symptomatically simulating ankle instability. *Am J Sports Med* 15(3):258-259, 1987.

101. Arrowsmith SR, Fleming LL, Allman FL: Traumatic dislocations of the peroneal tendons. *Am J Sports Med* 11(3):142-146, 1983.

102. Bassett FH 3rd, Speer KP: Longitudinal rupture of the peroneal tendons. *Am J Sports Med* 21(3):354-357, 1993.

103. Beck E: Operative treatment of recurrent dislocation of the peroneal tendons. *Arch Orthop Trauma Surg* 98(4):247-250, 1981.

104. Behfar AS: [Dislocation of the peroneal tendons]. *Sportverletz Sportschaden* 1(4):223-228, 1987.

105. Berg EE: Intraoperative peroneus brevis tendon rupture: A technique to salvage the graft during ankle ligament reconstruction. *Foot Ankle Int* 17(6):349-351, 1996.

106. Brodsky J, Krause J: Peroneus brevis tendon tears: Pathophysiology, surgical reconstruction, and clinical results. *Foot Ankle Int* 19:271-279, 1998.

107. Burman M: Subcutaneous tear of the tendon of the peroneus longus; its relation to the giant peroneal tubercle. *AMA Arch Surg* 73(2):216-219, 1956.

108. Burman M, Lapidus P: The functional disturbances caused by the inconstant bones and sesamoids of the foot. *Arch Surg* 22:936-975, 1931.

109. Cohen I, Lane S, Koning W: Peroneal tendon dislocations: A review of the literature. *J Foot Surg* 22(1):15-20, 1983.

110. Cox D, Paterson FW: Acute calcific tendinitis of peroneus longus. *J Bone Joint Surg Br* 73(2):342, 1991.

111. Cross MJ, Crichton KJ, Gordon H, Mackie IG: Peroneus brevis rupture in the absence of the peroneus longus muscle and tendon in a classical ballet dancer. A case report. *Am J Sports Med* 16(6):677-678, 1988.

112. Das De S, Balasubramaniam P: A repair operation for recurrent dislocation of peroneal tendons. *J Bone Joint Surg Br* 67(4):585-587, 1985.

113. Davies JA: Peroneal compartment syndrome secondary to rupture of the peroneus longus. A case report. *J Bone Joint Surg Am* 61(5):783-784, 1979.

114. Davis W. H, Sobel M, Deland J, et al: The superior peroneal retinaculum: An anatomic study. *Foot Ankle Int* 15(5):271-275, 1994.

115. DiGiovanni B, Fraga CJ, Cohen BE, Shereff MJ: Associated injuries found in chronic lateral ankle instability. *Foot Ankle Int* 21(10):809-815, 2000.

116. Dombek MF, Lamm BM, Saltrick K, et al: Peroneal tendon tears: A retrospective review. *J Foot Ankle Surg* 42(5):250-258, 2003.

117. DuVries H: *Surgery of the foot.* St. Louis, Mosby, 1959, pp 253-255.

118. Earle AS, Moritz JR, Tapper EM: Dislocation of the peroneal tendons at the ankle: An analysis of 25 ski injuries. *Northwest Med* 71(2):108-110, 1972.

119. Eckert WR, Davis EA Jr: Acute rupture of the peroneal retinaculum. *J Bone Joint Surg Am* 58(5):670-672, 1976.

120. Edwards M: The relations of the peroneal tendons to the fibula, calcaneus, and cuboideum. *Am J Anat* 42:213-253, 1988.

121. Escalas F, Figueras JM, Merino JA: Dislocation of the peroneal tendons. Long-term results of surgical treatment. *J Bone Joint Surg Am* 62(3):451-453, 1980.

122. Evans JD: Subcutaneous rupture of the tendon of peroneus longus. Report of a case. *J Bone Joint Surg Br* 48(3):507-509, 1966.

123. Folan JC: Peroneus longus tenosynovitis. *Br J Sports Med* 15(4):277-279, 1981.

124. Ford LT, Parvin RW: Stenosing tenosynovitis of the common peroneal tendon sheath; report of two cases. *J Bone Joint Surg Am* 38(6):1352-1357, 1956.

125. Frey CC, Shereff MJ: Tendon injuries about the ankle in athletes. *Clin Sports Med* 7(1):103-118, 1988.

126. Geller J, Lin S, Cordas D, Vieira P: Relationship of a low-lying muscle belly to tears of the peroneus brevis tendon. *Am J Orthop* 32(11):541-544, 2003.

127. Grisolia A: Fracture of the os peroneum: Review of the literature and report of one case. *Clin Orthop Relat Res* 28:213-215, 1963.

128. Guineys L: Fracture isolée d'un os sumumeriare du tarse (os peroneum) traitment par l'infiltration novocainique. *Rev Orthop* 26:943-947, 1939.

129. Hackenbroch M: Eine seltene Lokalisation der stenosierenden Tendovaginitis an der Sehnenscheide der peroneen). *Munchener Med Wochn* 74:932, 1927.

130. Hammerschlag WA, Goldner JL: Chronic peroneal tendon subluxation produced by an anomalous peroneus brevis: Case report and literature review. *Foot Ankle* 10(1):45-47, 1989.

131. Harper MC: Subluxation of the peroneal tendons within the peroneal groove: A report of two cases. *Foot Ankle Int* 18(6):369-370, 1997.

132. Hildebrand O: Tendovaginitis chronica deformans and Luxation der peronealsehnen. *Deut Z Chir* 86:526-531, 1907.

133. Jahss M: Tendon disorders of the foot and ankle. In Jahss M (ed): *Disorders of the Foot and Ankle: Medical and Surgical Management*, ed 2. Philadelphia, WB Saunders, 1991, pp 1461-1512.

134. Jones E: Operative treatment of chronic dislocation of the peroneal tendons. *J Bone Joint Surg Am* 14:574-576, 1932.

135. Kelly R: An operation for the chronic dislocation of the peroneal tendons. *Br J Surg* 7:502-504, 1920.

136. Kennedy MP, Coughlin MJ: Peroneus longus rupture following a modified Evans lateral ankle ligament reconstruction. *Orthopedics* 26(10):1059-1060, 2003.

137. Khazen GE, Adam N, Wilson MD, Schon LC: Peroneal groove deepening via a posterior osteocartilaginous flap: A retrospective analysis. Presented at the 21st Annual American Orthopaedic Foot and Ankle Society Summer Meeting, Boston, July 15-17, 2005.

138. Khoury NJ, el-Khoury GY, Saltzman CL, Kathol MH: Peroneus longus and brevis tendon tears: MR imaging evaluation. *Radiology* 200(3):833-841, 1996.

139. Kilkelly FX, McHale KA: Acute rupture of the peroneal longus tendon in a runner: A case report and review of the literature. *Foot Ankle Int* 15(10):567-569, 1994.

140. Kojima Y, Kataoka Y, Suzuki S, Akagi M: Dislocation of the peroneal tendons in neonates and infants. *Clin Orthop Relat Res* 266:180-184, 1991.

141. Kollias SL, Ferkel RD: Fibular grooving for recurrent peroneal tendon subluxation. *Am J Sports Med* 25(3):329-335, 1997.

142. LaBarbiera AP, Solitto RJ: Silastic tendon graft: Its role in neglected tendon repair. *J Foot Surg* 29(5):439-443, 1990.

143. Larsen E: Longitudinal rupture of the peroneus brevis tendon. *J Bone Joint Surg Br* 69(2):340-341, 1987.

144. Larsen E, Flink-Olsen M, Seerup K: Surgery for recurrent dislocation of the peroneal tendons. *Acta Orthop Scand* 55(5):554-555, 1984.

145. LeMelle DP, Janis LR: Longitudinal rupture of the peroneus brevis tendon: A study of eight cases. *J Foot Surg* 28(2):132-136, 1989.

146. LeNoir JL: A new surgical treatment of peroneal subluxation–dislocation. A case report with a 27-year follow up. *Orthopedics* 9(12):1689-1691, 1986.

147. MacDonald BD, Wertheimer SJ: Bilateral os peroneum fractures: Comparison of conservative and surgical treatment and outcomes. *J Foot Ankle Surg* 36(3):220-225, 1997.

148. Mains DB, Sullivan RC: Fracture of the os peroneum. A case report. *J Bone Joint Surg Am* 55(7):1529-1530, 1973.

149. Martens MA, Noyez JF, Mulier JC: Recurrent dislocation of the peroneal tendons. Results of rerouting the tendons under the calcaneofibular ligament. *Am J Sports Med* 14(2):148-150, 1986.

150. Marti R: Dislocation of the peroneal tendons. *Am J Sports Med* 5(1):19-22, 1977.

151. McConkey JP, Favero K. J: Subluxation of the peroneal tendons within the peroneal tendon sheath. A case report. *Am J Sports Med* 15(5):511-513, 1987.

152. McGarvey W, Clanton T: Peroneal tendon dislocations. *Foot Ankle Clin* 1:325-342, 1996.

153. McLennan JG: Treatment of acute and chronic luxations of the peroneal tendons. *Am J Sports Med* 8(6):432-436, 1980.

154. Mendicino RW, Orsini RC, Whitman SE, Catanzariti AR: Fibular groove deepening for recurrent peroneal subluxation. *J Foot Ankle Surg* 40(4):252-263, 2001.

155. Meyer A: Further evidences of attrition in the human body. *Am J Anat* 34:241-267, 1924.

156. Micheli LJ, Waters PM, Sanders DP: Sliding fibular graft repair for chronic dislocation of the peroneal tendons. *Am J Sports Med* 17(1):68-71, 1989.

157. Mick CA, Lynch F: Reconstruction of the peroneal retinaculum using the peroneus quartus. A case report. *J Bone Joint Surg Am* 69(2):296-297, 1987.

158. Milgram J: Muscle ruptures and avulsions with particular reference to the lower extremities. *Inst Course Lect* 10:233-243, 1953.

159. Miller C: Occupational calcaneous peritendinitis of the feet. *AJR Am J Roentgenol* 61:506-510, 1949.

160. Miller J. W: Dislocation of peroneal tendons—a new operative procedure. A case report. *Am J Orthop* 9(7):136-137, 1967.

161. Mizel MS, Michelson JD, Newberg A: Peroneal tendon bupivacaine injection: Utility of concomitant injection of contrast material. *Foot Ankle Int* 17(9):566-568, 1996.

162. Mizel M, Michelson J, Wapner K: Diagnosis and treatment of peroneus brevis injury. *Foot Ankle Clin* 1:343-354, 1996.

163. Monteggia G: *Instiuzini chirurgiche parte secondu*, Milan, Italy, 1803, pp 336-341.

164. Munk RL, Davis PH: Longitudinal rupture of the peroneus brevis tendon. *J Trauma* 16(10):803-806, 1976.

165. Murr S: Dislocation of the peroneal tendons with marginal fracture of the lateral malleolus. *J Bone Joint Surg Br* 43:563-565, 1961.

166. Neustadter J, Raikin SM, Nazarian LN: Dynamic sonographic evaluation of peroneal tendon subluxation. *AJR Am J Roentgenol* 183(4):985-988, 2004.

167. Oden R. R: Tendon injuries about the ankle resulting from skiing. *Clin Orthop Relat Res* 216:63-69, 1987.

168. Orthner E, Polcik J, Schabus R: [Dislocation of peroneal tendons]. *Unfallchirurg* 92(12):589-594, 1989.

169. Orthner E, Weinstabl R, Schabus R: [Experimental study for clarification of the pathogenic mechanism in traumatic peroneal tendon dislocation]. *Unfallchirurg* 92(11):547-553, 1989.

170. Palmer D. G: Tendon sheaths and bursae involved by rheumatoid disease at the foot and ankle. *Australas Radiol* 14(4):419-428, 1970.

171. Perlman MD: Os peroneum fracture with sural nerve entrapment neuritis. *J Foot Surg* 29(2):119-121, 1990.

172. Petersen W, Bobka T, Stein V, Tillmann B: Blood supply of the peroneal tendons: Injection and immunohistochemical studies of cadaver tendons. *Acta Orthop Scand* 71(2):168-174, 2000.

173. Peterson DA, Stinson W: Excision of the fractured os peroneum: A report on five patients and review of the literature. *Foot Ankle* 13(5):277-281, 1992.

174. Pfitzner W: Beitrage zur Kenntniss des Menschlichen extremitatenskelets: VII. Die variationen in Aufbau des Fusskelets. In Schwalbe (ed): *Morbologische Arbeiten*. Jena, Gustav Fischer, 1896, pp 245-527.

175. Pierson JL, Inglis AE: Stenosing tenosynovitis of the peroneus longus tendon associated with hypertrophy of the peroneal tubercle and an os peroneum. A case report. *J Bone Joint Surg Am* 74(3):440-442, 1992.

176. Platzgummer H: [On a simple procedure for the operative therapy of habitual peroneal tendon luxation]. *Arch Orthop Unfallchir* 61(2):144-150, 1967.

177. Poll RG, Duijfjes F: The treatment of recurrent dislocation of the peroneal tendons. *J Bone Joint Surg Br* 66(1):98-100, 1984.

178. Porter D, McCarroll J, Knapp E, Torma J: Peroneal tendon subluxation in athletes: Fibular groove deepening and retinacular reconstruction. *Foot Ankle Int* 26(6):436-441, 2005.

179. Pozo JL, Jackson AM: A rerouting operation for dislocation of peroneal tendons: Operative technique and case report. *Foot Ankle* 5(1):42-44, 1984.

180. Rask M, Steinberg L: The pathognostic sign of tendoperoneal subluxation. *Orthop Rev* 8:65-68, 1979.

181. Redfern D, Myerson M: The management of concomitant tears of the peroneus longus and brevis tendons. *Foot Ankle Int* 25(10):695-707, 2004.

182. Regan TP, Hughston JC: Chronic ankle "sprain" secondary to anomalous peroneal tendon: A case report. *Clin Orthop Relat Res* 123:52-54, 1977.

183. Roggatz J, Urban A: The calcaneous peritendinitis of the long peroneal tendon. *Arch Orthop Trauma Surg* 96(3):161-164, 1980.

184. Sammarco GJ, DiRaimondo CV: Chronic peroneus brevis tendon lesions. *Foot Ankle* 9(4):163-170, 1989.

185. Sarmiento A, Wolf M: Subluxation of peroneal tendons. Case treated by rerouting tendons under calcaneofibular ligament. *J Bone Joint Surg Am* 57(1):115-116, 1975.

186. Sarrafian SK: Osteology. In Sarrafian SK: *Anatomy of the Foot and Ankle*. Philadelphia, JB Lippincott, 1983, pp 35-106.

187. Savastano A: Recurrent dislocation of the peroneal tendons. In Bateman J, Trott A (eds): *The Foot and Ankle: A Selection of Papers from the American Orthopaedic Foot Society Meeting*. New York, Decker, 1980 pp 110-115.

188. Saxena A, Cassidy A: Peroneal tendon injuries: An evaluation of 49 tears in 41 patients. *J Foot Ankle Surg* 42(4):215-220, 2003.

189. Saxena A, Pham B: Longitudinal peroneal tendon tears. *J Foot Ankle Surg* 36(3):173-179; discussion 255, 1997.

190. Shawen SB, Anderson RB: Indirect groove deepening in the management of chronic peroneal tendon dislocation. *Tech Foot Ankle Surg* 3(2):118-125, 2004.

191. Slatis P, Santavirta S, Sandelin J: Surgical treatment of chronic dislocation of the peroneal tendons. *Br J Sports Med* 22(1):16-18, 1988.

192. Sobel M, Bohne WH, Levy ME: Longitudinal attrition of the peroneus brevis tendon in the fibular groove: An anatomic study. *Foot Ankle* 11(3):124-128, 1990.

193. Sobel M, Bohne WH, Markisz JA: Cadaver correlation of peroneal tendon changes with magnetic resonance imaging. *Foot Ankle* 11(6):384-388, 1991.

194. Sobel M, DiCarlo EF, Bohne WH, Collins L: Longitudinal splitting of the peroneus brevis tendon: An anatomic and histologic study of cadaveric material. *Foot Ankle* 12(3):165-170, 1991.

195. Sobel M, Geppert MJ, Olson EJ, et al: The dynamics of peroneus brevis tendon splits: A proposed mechanism, technique

of diagnosis, and classification of injury. *Foot Ankle* 13(7):413-422, 1992.

196. Sobel M, Levy ME, Bohne WH: Congenital variations of the peroneus quartus muscle: An anatomic study. *Foot Ankle* 11(2):81-89, 1990.

197. Sobel M, Pavlov H, Geppert MJ, et al: Painful os peroneum syndrome: A spectrum of conditions responsible for plantar lateral foot pain. *Foot Ankle Int* 15(3):112-124, 1994.

198. Sobel M, Warren RF, Brourman S: Lateral ankle instability associated with dislocation of the peroneal tendons treated by the Chrisman–Snook procedure. A case report and literature review. *Am J Sports Med* 18(5):539-543, 1990.

199. Stein RE: Reconstruction of the superior peroneal retinaculum using a portion of the peroneus brevis tendon. A case report. *J Bone Joint Surg Am* 69(2):298-299, 1987.

200. Steinbock G, Pinsger M: Treatment of peroneal tendon dislocation by transposition under the calcaneofibular ligament. *Foot Ankle Int* 15(3):107-111, 1994.

201. Stiehl JB: Concomitant rupture of the peroneus brevis tendon and bimalleolar fracture. A case report. *J Bone Joint Surg Am* 70(6):936-937, 1988.

202. Stover CN, Bryan DR: Traumatic dislocation of the peroneal tendons. *Am J Surg* 103:180-186, 1962.

203. Stropeni L: Frattura isolata di un osso soprannumerario del tarso (os peroneum externo). *Arch Ital Chir* 2:556-564, 1920.

204. Szczukowski M Jr, St Pierre RK, Fleming LL, Somogyi J: Computerized tomography in the evaluation of peroneal tendon dislocation. A report of two cases. *Am J Sports Med* 11(6):444-447, 1983.

205. Tan V, Lin SS, Okereke E: Superior peroneal retinaculoplasty: A surgical technique for peroneal subluxation. *Clin Orthop Relat Res* 410:320-325, 2003.

206. Tehranzadeh J, Stoll DA, Gabriele OM: Case report 271. Posterior migration of the os peroneum of the left foot, indicating a tear of the peroneal tendon. *Skeletal Radiol* 12(1):44-47, 1984.

207. Thompson FM, Patterson AH: Rupture of the peroneus longus tendon. Report of three cases. *J Bone Joint Surg Am* 71(2):293-295, 1989.

208. Title CI, Jung HG, Parks BG, Schon LC: The peroneal groove deepening procedure: A biomechanical study of pressure reduction. *Foot Ankle Int* 26(6):442-448, 2005.

209. Tracy E: The calcaneo-fibular ligaments and its neighborhood, based on dissections. *Bost Med Surg J* 160:369-371, 1909.

210. Trevino S, Baumhauer JF: Tendon injuries of the foot and ankle. *Clin Sports Med* 11(4):727-739, 1992.

211. Truong DT, Dussault RG, Kaplan PA: Fracture of the os peroneum and rupture of the peroneus longus tendon as a complication of diabetic neuropathy. *Skeletal Radiol* 24(8):626-628, 1995.

212. Viernstein K, Rosemeyer B: [A method of operative treatment of recurrent displacement of peroneal tendons]. *Arch Orthop Unfallchir* 74(2):175-181, 1972.

213. Wander DS, Galli K, Ludden JW, Mayer DP: Surgical management of a ruptured peroneus longus tendon with a fractured multipartite os peroneum. *J Foot Ankle Surg* 33(2):124-128, 1994.

214. Wapner K, Taras J, Lin S, et al: Peroneus brevis reconstruction with passive Hunter rods and secondary flexor hallucis longus transfer as a salvage for chronic peroneal tendon tears: A surgical demonstration. Presented at the 61st Annual Meeting of the American Academy of Orthopaedic Surgeons, New Orleans, February 24-March 1, 1994.

215. Weber M, Krause F: Peroneal tendon lesions caused by antiglide plates used for fixation of lateral malleolar fractures:

The effect of plate and screw position. *Foot Ankle Int* 26(4):281-5, 2005.

216. Webster F: Peroneal tenosynovitis with pseudotumor. *J Bone Joint Surg Am* 50:153-157, 1968.

217. Williams CR: Acute calcification of the peroneal tendons in a sheep shearer. *Foot Ankle Int* 17(1):49-50, 1996.

218. Wirth CJ: [A modified Viernstein and Kelly surgical technic for correcting chronic recurrent peroneal tendon dislocation]. *Z Orthop Ihre Grenzgeb* 128(2):170-173, 1990.

219. Zeiss J, Saddemi SR, Ebraheim NA: MR imaging of the peroneal tunnel. *J Comput Assist Tomogr* 13(5):840-844, 1989.

220. Zivot ML, Pearl SH, Pupp GR, Pupp JB: Stenosing peroneal tenosynovitis. *J Foot Surg* 28(3):220-224, 1989.

221. Zoellner G, Clancy W Jr: Recurrent dislocation of the peroneal tendon. *J Bone Joint Surg Am* 61(2):292-294, 1979.

Achilles Tendon

222. Achilles tendon rupture. *Lancet* 1(7796):189-190, 1973.

223. Abraham E, Pankovich AM: Neglected rupture of the Achilles tendon. Treatment by V-Y tendinous flap. *J Bone Joint Surg Am* 57(2):253-255, 1975.

224. Aracil J, Pina A, Lozano JA, et al: Percutaneous suture of Achilles tendon ruptures. *Foot Ankle* 13(6):350-351, 1992.

225. Arner O, Lindholm A: Subcutaneous rupture of the Achilles tendon; A study of 92 cases. *Acta Chir Scand* 116(Supp 239):1-51, 1959.

226. Arner O, Lindholm A, Lindvall N: Roentgen changes in subcutaneous rupture of the Achilles tendon. *Acta Chir Scand* 116(5-6):496-500, 1959.

227. Arner O, Lindholm A, Orell S. R: Histologic changes in subcutaneous rupture of the Achilles tendon; A study of 74 cases. *Acta Chir Scand* 116(5-6):484-490, 1959.

228. Assal M, Jung M, Stern R, et al: Limited open repair of Achilles tendon ruptures: A technique with a new instrument and findings of a prospective multicenter study. *J Bone Joint Surg Am* 84(2):161-170, 2002.

229. Astrom M, Gentz C. F, Nilsson P, et al: Imaging in chronic achilles tendinopathy: A comparison of ultrasonography, magnetic resonance imaging and surgical findings in 27 histologically verified cases. *Skeletal Radiol* 25(7):615-620, 1996.

230. Barfred T: Achilles tendon rupture. Aetiology and pathogenesis of subcutaneous rupture assessed on the basis of the literature and rupture experiments on rats. *Acta Orthop Scand Suppl* 3:1-126, 1973.

231. Barnes MJ, Hardy AE: Delayed reconstruction of the calcaneal tendon. *J Bone Joint Surg Br* 68(1):121-124, 1986.

232. Besse JL, Lerat JL, Moyen B, et al: [Distal reconstruction of the Achilles tendon with a bone–tendon graft from extensor system of the knee]. *Rev Chir Orthop Reparatrice Appar Mot* 81(5):453-457, 1995.

233. Blake RL, Ferguson HJ: Achilles tendon rupture. A protocol for conservative management. *J Am Podiatr Med Assoc* 81(9):486-489, 1991.

234. Bosworth DM: Repair of defects in the tendo achillis. *J Bone Joint Surg Am* 38(1):111-114, 1956.

235. Boyden EM, Kitaoka HB, Cahalan TD, An KN: Late versus early repair of Achilles tendon rupture. Clinical and biomechanical evaluation. *Clin Orthop Relat Res* 317:150-158, 1995.

236. Bradley JP, Tibone JE: Percutaneous and open surgical repairs of Achilles tendon ruptures. A comparative study. *Am J Sports Med* 18(2):188-195, 1990.

237. Brown TD, Fu FH, Hanley EN Jr: Comparative assessment of the early mechanical integrity of repaired tendon Achilles ruptures in the rabbit. *J Trauma* 21(11):951-957, 1981.

238. Bugg EI Jr, Boyd BM: Repair of neglected rupture or laceration of the Achilles tendon. *Clin Orthop Relat Res* 56:73-75, 1968.

239. Burry H, Pool C: Central degeneration of the Achilles tendon. *Rheum Rehabil* 12:177-181, 1973.

240. Carden DG, Noble J, Chalmers J, et al: Rupture of the calcaneal tendon. The early and late management. *J Bone Joint Surg Br* 69(3):416-420, 1987.

241. Carr AJ, Norris SH: The blood supply of the calcaneal tendon. *J Bone Joint Surg Br* 71(1):100-101, 1989.

242. Cetti R, Andersen I: Roentgenographic diagnoses of ruptured Achilles tendons. *Clin Orthop Relat Res* 286:215-221, 1993.

243. Cetti R, Christensen SE, Ejsted R, et al: Operative versus non-operative treatment of Achilles tendon rupture. A prospective randomized study and review of the literature. *Am J Sports Med* 21(6):791-799, 1993.

244. Chao W, Del JT, Bates JE, Kenneally SM: Achilles tendon insertion: An in vitro anatomic study. *Foot Ankle Int* 18(2):81-84, 1997.

245. Childress H: Spontaneous ruptures of the tendo Achilles: Etiology and treatment. *Orthop Rev* 5:13-15, 1976.

246. Chung B, Wiley JP: Extracorporeal shockwave therapy: A review. *Sports Med* 32(13):851-865, 2002.

247. Clain MR, Baxter DE: Achilles tendinitis. *Foot Ankle* 13(8):482-487, 1992.

248. Clancy W: *Prevention and Treatment of Running Injuries.* Thorofare, NJ, Stack, 1982, pp 77-83.

249. Clancy WG Jr, Neidhart D, Brand RL: Achilles tendinitis in runners: A report of five cases. *Am J Sports Med* 4(2):46-57, 1976.

250. Clement D, Taunton J, Smart G, McNicol K: A survey of overuse running injuries. *Physician Sports Med* 9:47-58, 1981.

251. Coull R, Flavin R, Stephens MM: Flexor hallucis longus tendon transfer: Evaluation of postoperative morbidity. *Foot Ankle Int* 24(12):931-934, 2003.

252. Dalton G: Achilles tendon rupture. *Foot Ankle Clin* 1:225-236, 1996.

253. DeMaio M, Paine R, Drez DJ Jr: Achilles tendinitis. *Orthopedics* 18(2):195-204, 1995.

254. Den Hartog BD: Flexor hallucis longus transfer for chronic Achilles tendinosis. *Foot Ankle Int* 24(3):233-237, 2003.

255. DePretto M, Guerra L, Pozzolini M, et al: A retrospective, multi-centre experience report of shock wave therapy on Achilles tendinitis. Presented at the Third International Congress of the International Society for Musculoskeletal Shockwave Therapy, Naples, Italy, June 1-3, 2000.

256. Dickinson PH, Coutts MB, Woodward EP, Handler D: Tendo Achillis bursitis. Report of twenty-one cases. *J Bone Joint Surg Am* 48(1):77-81, 1966.

257. Edna TH: Non-operative treatment of Achilles tendon ruptures. *Acta Orthop Scand* 51(6):991-993, 1980.

258. Fierro NL, Sallis RE: Achilles tendon rupture. Is casting enough? *Postgrad Med* 98(3):145-152, 1995.

259. Fish J: Achilles tendon: A method of repair. *Contemp Orthop* 5:21-25, 1982.

260. FitzGibbons RE, Hefferon J, Hill J: Percutaneous Achilles tendon repair. *Am J Sports Med* 21(5):724-727, 1993.

261. Fox JM, Blazina ME, Jobe FW, et al: Degeneration and rupture of the Achilles tendon. *Clin Orthop Relat Res* 107: 221-224, 1975.

262. Fruensgaard S, Helmig P, Riis J, Stovring JO: Conservative treatment for acute rupture of the Achilles tendon. *Int Orthop* 16(1):33-35, 1992.

263. Fuglsang F, Torup D: Bursitis retrocalcanearis. *Acta Orthop Scand* 30:315-323 1961.

264. Gabel S, Manoli A 2nd: Neglected rupture of the Achilles tendon. *Foot Ankle Int* 15(9):512-517, 1994.

265. Galasso O, de Durant C, Russo S, et al: Chronic achillodynia. Treatment with extracorporeal shock wave. Presented at the Third International Congress of the International Society for Musculoskeletal Shockwave Therapy, Naples, Italy, June 1-3, 2000.

266. Gerdes MH, Brown TD, Bell AL, et al: A flap augmentation technique for Achilles tendon repair. Postoperative strength and functional outcome. *Clin Orthop Relat Res* 280:241-246, 1992.

267. Giannestras N: *Foot Disorders: Medical and Surgical Management.* Philadelphia, Lea & Febiger, 1973, pp 580-583.

268. Gillespie HS, George EA: Results of surgical repair of spontaneous rupture of the Achilles tendon. *J Trauma* 9(3):247-249, 1969.

269. Gillies H, Chalmers J: The management of fresh ruptures of the tendo achillis. *J Bone Joint Surg Am* 52(2):337-343, 1970.

270. Goldman S, Linscheid RL, Bickel WH: Disruptions of the tendo Achillis: Analysis of 33 cases. *Mayo Clin Proc* 44(1):28-35, 1969.

271. Gould N, Korson R: Stenosing tenosynovitis of the pseudosheath of the tendo Achilles. *Foot Ankle* 1(3):179-187, 1980.

272. Habusta SF: Bilateral simultaneous rupture of the Achilles tendon. A rare traumatic injury. *Clin Orthop Relat Res* 320:231-234, 1995.

273. Haggmark T, Eriksson E: Hypotrophy of the soleus muscle in man after Achilles tendon rupture. Discussion of findings obtained by computed tomography and morphologic studies. *Am J Sports Med* 7(2):121-126, 1979.

274. Haggmark T, Liedberg H, Eriksson E, Wredmark T: Calf muscle atrophy and muscle function after non-operative vs operative treatment of achilles tendon ruptures. *Orthopedics* 9(2):160-164, 1986.

275. Haglund P: Contribution to the diseased conditions of tendo-Achilles. *Acta Chir Scand* 63:292-294, 1928.

276. Hanlon DP: Bilateral Achilles tendon rupture: An unusual occurrence. *J Emerg Med* 10(5):559-560, 1992.

277. Hanna JR, Russell RD, Giacopelli JA: Repair of distal tendo Achillis rupture with the use of the Mitek Anchor System. *J Am Podiatr Med Assoc* 83(12):663-668, 1993.

278. Hansen S: Trauma to the heel cord. In Jahss M (ed), *Disorders of the Foot and Ankle: Medical and Surgical Management,* ed. 2. Philadelphia, WB Saunders, 1991, pp 2355-2360.

279. Hattrup SJ, Johnson KA: A review of ruptures of the Achilles tendon. *Foot Ankle* 6(1):34-38, 1985.

280. Heller KD, Niethard FU: [Using extracorporeal shockwave therapy in orthopedics—a meta-analysis]. *Z Orthop Ihre Grenzgeb* 136(5):390-401, 1998.

281. Heneghan MA, Pavlov H: The Haglund painful heel syndrome. Experimental investigation of cause and therapeutic implications. *Clin Orthop Relat Res* 187:228-234, 1984.

282. Homer: *The Iliad.* Nagles R (trans). New York, Viking, 1996.

283. Hooker C: Rupture of the tendon calcaneus. *J Bone Joint Surg Br* 45:360-363, 1963.

284. Howard CB, Winston I, Bell W, et al: Late repair of the calcaneal tendon with carbon fibre. *J Bone Joint Surg Br* 66(2):206-208, 1984.

285. Inglis AE, Scott WN, Sculco TP, Patterson AH: Ruptures of the tendo achillis. An objective assessment of surgical and non-surgical treatment. *J Bone Joint Surg Am* 58(7):990-993, 1976.

286. Jacobs D, Martens M, Van Audekercke R, et al: Comparison of conservative and operative treatment of Achilles tendon rupture. *Am J Sports Med* 6(3):107-111, 1978.

287. James SL, Bates BT, Osternig LR: Injuries to runners. *Am J Sports Med* 6(2):40-50, 1978.

288. Jessing P, Hansen E: Surgical treatment of 102 tendo achillis ruptures—suture or tenontoplasty? *Acta Chir Scand* 141(5): 370-377, 1975.

289. Kager H: Zur klinik und diagnostik des Achillessehnenrisses. *Chirurg* 11:691-695, 1939.

290. Kainberger F. M, Engel A, Barton P, et al: Injury of the Achilles tendon: Diagnosis with sonography. *AJR Am J Roentgenol* 155(5):1031-1036, 1990.

291. Kakiuchi M: A combined open percutaneous technique for repair of tendo achillis. Comparison with open repair. *J Bone Joint Surg Br* 77(1):60-63, 1995.

292. Karjalainen PT, Ahovuo J, Pihlajamaki HK, et al: Postoperative MR imaging and ultrasonography of surgically repaired Achilles tendon ruptures. *Acta Radiol* 37(5):639-646, 1996.

293. Keck SW, Kelly PJ: Bursitis of the posterior part of the heel; an evaluation of surgical treatment of eighteen patients. *J Bone Joint Surg Am* 47:267-273, 1965.

294. Kellam JF, Hunter GA, McElwain JP: Review of the operative treatment of Achilles tendon rupture. *Clin Orthop Relat Res* (201):80-83, 1985.

295. Kissel CG, Blacklidge DK, Crowley DL: Repair of neglected Achilles tendon ruptures—procedure and functional results. *J Foot Ankle Surg* 33(1):46-52, 1994.

296. Krackow KA, Thomas SC, Jones LC: A new stitch for ligament–tendon fixation. Brief note. *J Bone Joint Surg Am* 68(5):764-766, 1986.

297. Kujala UM, Jarvinen M, Natri A, et al: ABO blood groups and musculoskeletal injuries. *Injury* 23(2):131-133, 1992.

298. Kvist H, Kvist M: The operative treatment of chronic calcaneal paratenonitis. *J Bone Joint Surg Br* 62(3):353-357, 1980.

299. Kvist M. H, Lehto M. U, Jozsa L, et al: Chronic achilles paratenonitis. An immunohistologic study of fibronectin and fibrinogen. *Am J Sports Med* 16(6):616-623, 1988.

300. Lagergren C, Lindholm A: Vascular distribution in the Achilles tendon; an angiographic and microangiographic study. *Acta Chir Scand* 116(5-6):491-495, 1959.

301. Lawrence GH, Cave EF, O'Connor H: Injury to the Achilles tendon; experience at the Massachusetts General Hospital, 1900-1954. *Am J Surg* 89(4):795-802, 1955.

302. Lea RB, Smith L: Non-surgical treatment of tendo achillis rupture. *J Bone Joint Surg Am* 54(7):1398-1407, 1972.

303. Leach RE, James S, Wasilewski S: Achilles tendinitis. *Am J Sports Med* 9(2):93-98, 1981.

304. Lehto MU, Jarvinen M, Suominen P: Chronic Achilles peritendinitis and retrocalcanear bursitis. Long-term follow-up of surgically treated cases. *Knee Surg Sports Traumatol Arthrosc* 2(3):182-185, 1994.

305. Leitner A, Voigt C, Rahmanzadeh R: Treatment of extensive aseptic defects in old Achilles tendon ruptures: Methods and case reports. *Foot Ankle* 13(4):176-180, 1992.

306. Leitze Z, Sella EJ, Aversa JM: Endoscopic decompression of the retrocalcaneal space. *J Bone Joint Surg Am* 85-A(8):1488-1496, 2003.

307. Lemm M, Blake RL, Colson JP, Ferguson H: Achilles peritendinitis. A literature review with case report. *J Am Podiatr Med Assoc* 82(9):482-490, 1992.

308. Lennox DW, Wang GJ, McCue FC, Stamp WG: The operative treatment of Achilles tendon injuries. *Clin Orthop Relat Res* (148):152-155, 1980.

309. Leppilahti J, Kaarela O, Teerikangas H, et al: Free tissue coverage of wound complications following Achilles tendon rupture surgery. *Clin Orthop Relat Res* 328:171-176, 1996.

310. Leppilahti J, Siira P, Vanharanta H, Orava S: Isokinetic evaluation of calf muscle performance after Achilles rupture repair. *Int J Sports Med* 17(8):619-623, 1996.

311. Levy M, Velkes S, Goldstein J, Rosner M: A method of repair for Achilles tendon ruptures without cast immobilization. Preliminary report. *Clin Orthop Relat Res* 187:199-204, 1984.

312. Lieberman JR, Lozman J, Czajka J, Dougherty J: Repair of Achilles tendon ruptures with Dacron vascular graft. *Clin Orthop Relat Res* 234:204-208, 1988.

313. Lindholm A: A new method of operation in subcutaneous rupture of the Achilles tendon. *Acta Chir Scand* 117:261-270, 1959.

314. Lipscomb P: Chronic nonspecific tenosynovitis and peritendinitis. *Surg Clin North Am* 24:786-796, 1944.

315. Ljungqvist R: Subcutaneous partial rupture of the Achilles tendon. *Acta Orthop Scand: Suppl* 113:1+, 1967.

316. Lynn TA: Repair of the torn Achilles tendon, using the plantaris tendon as a reinforcing membrane. *J Bone Joint Surg Am* 48(2): 268-72, 1966.

317. Ma GW, Griffith TG: Percutaneous repair of acute closed ruptured achilles tendon: A new technique. *Clin Orthop Relat Res* 128:247-255, 1977.

318. Mahler F, Fritschy D: Partial and complete ruptures of the Achilles tendon and local corticosteroid injections. *Br J Sports Med* 26(1):7-14, 1992.

319. Mandelbaum BR, Myerson MS, Forster R: Achilles tendon ruptures. A new method of repair, early range of motion, and functional rehabilitation. *Am J Sports Med* 23(4):392-395, 1995.

320. Mann RA, Holmes GB Jr, Seale KS, Collins, DN: Chronic rupture of the Achilles tendon: A new technique of repair. *J Bone Joint Surg Am* 73(2):214-219, 1991.

321. McGarvey WC, Palumbo RC, Baxter DE, Leibman BD: Insertional Achilles tendinosis: Surgical treatment through a central tendon splitting approach. *Foot Ankle Int* 23(1):19-25, 2002.

322. McGarvey WC, Singh D, Trevino SG: Partial Achilles tendon ruptures associated with fluoroquinolone antibiotics: A case report and literature review. *Foot Ankle Int* 17(8):496-498, 1996.

323. Mendicino SS, Reed TS: Repair of neglected Achilles tendon ruptures with a triceps surae muscle tendon advancement. *J Foot Ankle Surg* 35(1):13-18, 1996.

324. Mohammed A, Rahamatalla A, Wynne-Jones CH: Tissue expansion in late repair of tendo Achillis rupture. *J Bone Joint Surg Br* 77(1):64-66, 1995.

325. Murrell G. A, Lilly E. G 3rd, Collins A, et al: Achilles tendon injuries: A comparison of surgical repair versus no repair in a rat model. *Foot Ankle* 14(7):400-406, 1993.

326. Nellas ZJ, Loder BG, Wertheimer SJ: Reconstruction of an Achilles tendon defect utilizing an Achilles tendon allograft. *J Foot Ankle Surg* 35(2):144-148; discussion 190, 1996.

327. Nillius SA, Nilsson BE, Westlin NE: The incidence of Achilles tendon rupture. *Acta Orthop Scand* 47(1):118-121, 1976.

328. Nistor L: Conservative treatment of fresh subcutaneous rupture of the Achilles tendon. *Acta Orthop Scand* 47(4):459-462, 1976.

329. Nistor L: Surgical and non-surgical treatment of Achilles tendon rupture. A prospective randomized study. *J Bone Joint Surg Am* 63(3):394-399, 1981.

330. Ogden JA, Cross GL: Application of electrohydraulic orthotripsy for chronic Achilles tendinopathy. Presented at the Fifth International Congress of the International Society for Musculoskeletal Shockwave Therapy, Orlando, Florida, February 11-13, 2003.

331. Ozaki J, Fujiki J, Sugimoto K, et al: Reconstruction of neglected Achilles tendon rupture with Marlex mesh. *Clin Orthop Relat Res* (238):204-208, 1989.

332. Paré A: *Les Oeuvres d'Ambroise Paré*, ed 9. Lyon, France, C. Rigaud et C. Obert, 1633 (printed).

333. Parsons JR, Rosario A, Weiss AB, Alexander H: Achilles tendon repair with an absorbable polymer-carbon fiber composite. *Foot Ankle* 5(2):49-53, 1984.

334. Parsons JR, Weiss AB, Schenk RS, et al: Long-term follow-up of Achilles tendon repair with an absorbable polymer carbon fiber composite. *Foot Ankle* 9(4):179-184, 1989.

335. Pavlov H, Heneghan MA, Hersh A, et al: The Haglund syndrome: Initial and differential diagnosis. *Radiology* 144(1):83-88, 1982.

336. Percy EC, Conochie LB: The surgical treatment of ruptured tendo achillis. *Am J Sports Med* 6(3):132-136, 1978.

337. Perez Teuffer A: Traumatic rupture of the Achilles tendon. Reconstruction by transplant and graft using the lateral peroneus brevis. *Orthop Clin North Am* 5(1):89-93, 1974.

338. Persson A, Wredmark T: The treatment of total ruptures of the Achilles tendon by plaster immobilisation. *Int Orthop* 3(2):149-152, 1979.

339. Platt H: Observations on some tendon ruptures. *BMJ* 1:611-615, 1931.

340. Porter DA, Mannarino FP, Snead D, et al: Primary repair without augmentation for early neglected Achilles tendon ruptures in the recreational athlete. *Foot Ankle Int* 18(9):557-564, 1997.

341. Puddu G, Ippolito E, Postacchini F: A classification of Achilles tendon disease. *Am J Sports Med* 4(4):145-150, 1976.

342. Quigley TB, Scheller AD: Surgical repair of the ruptured Achilles tendon. Analysis of 40 patients treated by the same surgeon. *Am J Sports Med* 8(4):244-250, 1980.

343. Ralston EL, Schmidt ER Jr: Repair of the ruptured Achilles tendon. *J Trauma* 11(1):15-21, 1971.

344. Ribard P, Audisio F, Kahn MF, et al: Seven Achilles tendinitis including 3 complicated by rupture during fluoroquinolone therapy. *J Rheumatol* 19(9):1479-1481, 1992.

345. Ruch JA: Haglund's disease. *J Am Podiatry Assoc* 64(12):1000-1003, 1974.

346. Saggini R, Antonucci D, Bellomo RG, et al: Experimental study of shock wave therapy on Achilles tendinitis to investigate treatment parameters. Presented at the Third International Congress of the International Society for Musculoskeletal Shockwave Therapy, Naples, Italy, June 1-3, 2000.

347. Samuelson M, Hecht P: Acute Achilles tendon ruptures. *Foot Ankle Clin* 1:215-224, 1996.

348. Saunders DE, Hochberg J, Wittenborn W: Treatment of total loss of the Achilles tendon by skin flap cover without tendon repair. *Plast Reconstr Surg* 62(5):708-712, 1978.

349. Schedl R, Fasol P: Achilles tendon repair with the plantaris tendon compared with repair using polyglycol threads. *J Trauma* 19(3):189-194, 1979.

350. Schepsis AA, Leach RE: Surgical management of Achilles tendinitis. *Am J Sports Med* 15(4):308-315, 1987.

351. Schepsis AA, Wagner C, Leach RE: Surgical management of Achilles tendon overuse injuries. A long-term follow-up study. *Am J Sports Med* 22(5):611-619, 1994.

352. Schmidt-Rohlfing B, Graf J, Schneider U, Niethard FU: The blood supply of the Achilles tendon. *Int Orthop* 16(1):29-31, 1992.

353. Scott WN, Inglis AE, Sculco TP: Surgical treatment of reruptures of the tendoachilles following nonsurgical treatment. *Clin Orthop Relat Res* 140:175-177, 1979.

354. Shields CL, Jr, Kerlan RK, Jobe FW, et al: The Cybex II evaluation of surgically repaired Achilles tendon ruptures. *Am J Sports Med* 6(6):369-372, 1978.

355. Shinohara YT, Tasker SA, Wallace MR, et al: What is the risk of Achilles tendon rupture with ciprofloxacin? *J Rheumatol* 24(1):238-239, 1997.

356. Snook GA: Achilles tendon tenosynovitis in long-distance runners. *Med Sci Sports* 4(3):155-158, 1972.

357. Stein SR, Luekens CA, Jr: Closed treatment of Achilles tendon ruptures. *Orthop Clin North Am* 7(1):241-246, 1976.

358. Suominen E, Tukiainen E, Asko-Seljavaara S: Reconstruction of the Achilles tendon region by free microvascular flaps. 9 cases followed for 1-9 years. *Acta Orthop Scand* 63(5):482-486, 1992.

359. Taylor GI, Watson N: One-stage repair of compound leg defects with free, revascularized flaps of groin skin and iliac bone. *Plast Reconstr Surg* 61(4):494-506, 1978.

360. Taylor L: Achilles tendon repair: Results of surgical management. In Moore M (ed): *Symposium on Trauma to the Leg and its Sequelae*. St. Louis, Mosby, 1981, pp 371-384.

361. Teitz CC, Garrett WE, Jr, Miniaci A, et al: Tendon problems in athletic individuals. *Instr Course Lect* 46:569-582, 1997.

362. Thompson TC: A test for rupture of the tendo achillis. *Acta Orthop Scand* 32:461-465, 1962.

363. Thompson TC, Doherty JH: Spontaneous rupture of tendon of Achilles: A new clinical diagnostic test. *J Trauma* 2:126-129, 1962.

364. Troop RL, Losse GM, Lane JG, et al: Early motion after repair of Achilles tendon ruptures. *Foot Ankle Int* 16(11):705-709, 1995.

365. Turco VJ, Spinella AJ: Achilles tendon ruptures—peroneus brevis transfer. *Foot Ankle* 7(4):253-259, 1987.

366. Wapner KL, Hecht PJ, Mills RH Jr: Reconstruction of neglected Achilles tendon injury. *Orthop Clin North Am* 26(2):249-263, 1995.

367. Wapner KL, Pavlock GS, Hecht PJ, et al: Repair of chronic Achilles tendon rupture with flexor hallucis longus tendon transfer. *Foot Ankle* 14(8):443-449, 1993.

368. Weinstabl R, Stiskal M, Neuhold A, et al: Classifying calcaneal tendon injury according to MRI findings. *J Bone Joint Surg Br* 73(4):683-685, 1991.

369. Weiss A: The use of carbon fiber composites. In Jahss M (ed): *Disorders of the Foot and Ankle*, ed. 2. Philadelphia, WB Saunders, 1991, pp 2723-2727.

370. Weston WJ: The bursa deep to tendo achillis. *Australas Radiol* 14(3):327-331, 1970.

371. White C: Retrocalcaneal bursitis. *N Y Med J* 98:263-265, 1913.

372. White RK, Kraynick BM: Surgical uses of the peroneus brevis tendon. *Surg Gynecol Obstet* 108(1):117-121, 1959.

373. Wilcox DK, Bohay DR, Anderson JG: Treatment of chronic Achilles tendon disorders with flexor hallucis longus tendon transfer/augmentation. *Foot Ankle Int* 21(12):1004-1010, 2000.

374. Wills CA, Washburn S, Caiozzo V, Prietto CA: Achilles tendon rupture. A review of the literature comparing surgical versus nonsurgical treatment. *Clin Orthop Relat Res* 207:156-163, 1986.

375. Zadek I: An operation for the cure of achillobursitis. *Am J Surg* 43:542-546, 1939.

376. Zadek I: Repair of old rupture of the tendo Achilles by means of fascia lata. *J Bone Joint Surg* 22:1070-1071, 1940.

Tendon Transfers

377. Close JR, Todd FN: The phasic activity of the muscles of the lower extremity and the effect of tendon transfer. *J Bone Joint Surg Am* 41(2):189-208, 1959.

378. Green NE, Griffin PP, Shiavi R: Split posterior tibial-tendon transfer in spastic cerebral palsy. *J Bone Joint Surg Am* 65(6):748-754, 1983.

379. Hoffer MM, Reiswig JA, Garrett AM, Perry J: The split anterior tibial tendon transfer in the treatment of spastic varus hindfoot of childhood. *Orthop Clin North Am* 5(1):31-38, 1974.

380. Jones R: An operation for paralytic calcaneocavus. *Am J Orthop Surg* 5:371-383, 1908.

381. Kaufer H: Split tendon transfers. *Orthop Transplant* 1:191, 1977.

382. Kling TF Jr, Kaufer H, Hensinger R. N: Split posterior tibial-tendon transfers in children with cerebral spastic paralysis and equinovarus deformity. *J Bone Joint Surg Am* 67(2):186-194, 1985.

383. Lipscomb P, Sanchez J: Anterior transplantation of the posterior tibial tendon for persistent palsy of the common peroneal nerve. *J Bone Joint Surg Am* 43:60-66, 1961.

384. Perry J, Hoffer MM: Preoperative and postoperative dynamic electromyography as an aid in planning tendon transfers in children with cerebral palsy. *J Bone Joint Surg Am* 59(4):531-537, 1977.

385. Rodriguez RP: The Bridle procedure in the treatment of paralysis of the foot. *Foot Ankle* 13(2):63-69, 1992.

386. Schneider M, Balon K: Deformity of the foot following anterior transfer of the posterior tibial tendon and lengthening of the Achilles tendon for spastic equinovarus. *Clin Orthop Relat Res* (125):113-118, 1977.

387. Turner JW, Cooper RR: Anterior transfer of the tibialis posterior through the interosseus membrane. *Clin Orthop Relat Res* 83:241-244, 1972.

388. Waters R: Acquired neurologic disorders of the adult foot. In Mann R (ed): *Surgery of the Foot*, ed 5. St Louis, Mosby, 1986, p 339.

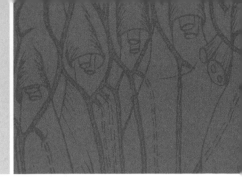

Index

Note: Page numbers followed by f indicate figures; those followed by t indicate tables; and page numbers followed by b indicate boxed material.

i